Principles and Practice of

ANESTHESIOLOGY

VOLUME ONE

Principles and Practice of
ANESTHESIOLOGY

Mark C. Rogers, M.D.
Distinguished Faculty Professor and
   Chairman
Department of Anesthesiology and Critical
   Care Medicine
Associate Dean
The Johns Hopkins Medical Institutions
Baltimore, Maryland

John H. Tinker, M.D.
Professor and Head
Department of Anesthesia
The University of Iowa College of Medicine
Iowa City, Iowa

Benjamin G. Covino, Ph.D., M.D.
Professor of Anaesthesia
Harvard Medical School
Chairman, Department of Anesthesia
Brigham and Women's Hospital
Boston, Massachusetts

David E. Longnecker, M.D.
Robert Dunning Dripps Professor of
   Anesthesia
Chairman, Department of Anesthesia
The University of Pennsylvania School of
   Medicine
Philadelphia, Pennsylvania

with 1060 illustrations

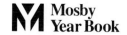
Mosby
Year Book

St. Louis Baltimore Boston Chicago London Philadelphia Sydney Toronto

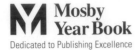

Managing Editor: Elaine Steinborn
Assistant Editor: Jo Salway
Project Manager: John A. Rogers
Senior Production Editor: Helen C. Hudlin
Manuscript Editors: Judith Ahlers, Charles Furgason, Radhika Gupta, Joseph Lawler,
Roger McWilliams, Shauna Sticht, Barbara Terrell, and Catherine Vale
Production: Jeanne Genz, Kathy Wiegand
Design: Julie Taugner
Cover Art: Christian Musselman

Printed in the United States of America

Mosby–Year Book, Inc.
11830 Westline Industrial Drive
St. Louis, Missouri 63146

Library of Congress Cataloging-in-Publication Data

Principles and practice of anesthesiology / [edited by] Mark C. Rogers
. . . [et al.].
    p.   cm.
  Includes bibliographical references and index.
  ISBN   0-8016-5818-7
  1. Anesthesiology.   I. Rogers, Mark C.
  [DNLM: 1. Anesthesiology.   WO 200 P957]
RD81.P7427   1992
617.9′6--dc20
DNLM/DLC
for Library of Congress   92-49205
                                                                            CIP

93 94 95 96 97 GW/VH 9 8 7 6 5 4 3 2 1

Contributors

Susan Albert, M.S., D.O.
Instructor
The Johns Hopkins University
Assistant Director and Clinical Coordinator
Division of Ambulatory Anesthesia
The Johns Hopkins Medical Institutions
Baltimore, Maryland

Hassan H. Ali, M.D.
Associate Professor of Anaesthesia
Harvard Medical School
Anesthesiologist
Massachusetts General Hospital
Boston, Massachusetts

James K. Alifimoff, M.D.
Anesthesia Associates of Topcka
Topeka, Kansas

Angela M. Bader, M.D.
Assistant Professor of Anaesthesia
Harvard Medical School
Staff Anesthesiologist
Brigham and Women's Hospital
Boston, Massachusetts

Mark Banoub, M.D.
Resident
Department of Anesthesia
Medical College of Ohio
Toledo, Ohio

Salvatore J. Basta, M.D.
Assistant Professor of Anaesthesia
Harvard Medical School
Assistant Anesthetist
Massachusetts General Hospital
Boston, Massachusetts

Charles Beattie, Ph.D., M.D.
Associate Professor
The Johns Hopkins University
Director of Clinical Services
Department of Anesthesiology and Critical
 Care Medicine
The Johns Hopkins Medical Institutions
Baltimore, Maryland

Robert F. Bedford, Ph.D., M.D.
Clinical Professor
Department of Anesthesiology
University of Virginia School of Medicine
Charlottesville, Virginia

Ivor D. Berkowitz, M.B., B.Ch.
Assistant Professor
Department of Anesthesiology and Critical
 Care Medicine
Associate Director, Pediatric Intensive
 Care Unit
The Johns Hopkins Medical Institutions
Baltimore, Maryland

Marina Bizzarri-Schmid, M.D.
Instructor of Anaesthesia
Harvard Medical School
Anesthesiologist
Brigham and Women's Hospital
Boston, Massachusetts

Cecil Borel, M.D.
Assistant Professor
Department of Anesthesiology and Critical
 Care Medicine
Co-Director, Neurosciences Critical
 Care Unit
The Johns Hopkins Medical Institutions
Baltimore, Maryland

Denis L. Bourke, M.D.
Associate Professor
Department of Anesthesiology and Critical
    Care Medicine
Director, Division of Regional Anesthesia
    and Pain Management
The Johns Hopkins Medical Institutions
Baltimore, Maryland

Philip G. Boysen, M.D., F.A.C.P., F.C.C.P.
Professor of Anesthesiology and Medicine
University of Florida College of Medicine
Chief, Anesthesiology Service
Co-Director, Surgical Intensive Care Unit
VHMC Gainesville
Gainesville, Florida

Michael J. Breslow, M.D., F.A.C.C.
Associate Professor
Department of Anesthesiology and Critical
    Care Medicine
Co-Director, Surgical Intensive Care Unit
Director, Combined Fellowship Program
The Johns Hopkins Medical Institutions
Baltimore, Maryland

David Bronheim, M.D.
Assistant Professor
Department of Anesthesiology
Mount Sinai School of Medicine
The Mount Sinai Medical Center
New York, New York

Daniel B. Carr, M.D.
Associate Professor
Departments of Anaesthesia and Medicine
    (Endocrinology)
Harvard Medical School
Director, Division of Pain Management
Department of Anesthesia
Massachusetts General Hospital
Boston, Massachusetts

David H. Chestnut, M.D.
Professor of Anesthesia and Obstetrics and
    Gynecology
Vice-Chairman for Administration
Department of Anesthesia
The University of Iowa College of Medicine
Iowa City, Iowa

Rose Christopherson, Ph.D., M.D.
Assistant Professor
Department of Anesthesiology and Critical
    Care Medicine
The Johns Hopkins Medical Institutions
Baltimore, Maryland

Mercedes Concepcion, M.D.
Assistant Professor of Anaesthesia
Harvard Medical School
Director of Orthopedic Anesthesia
Brigham and Women's Hospital
Boston, Massachusetts

Benjamin G. Covino, Ph.D., M.D. (Deceased)
Professor of Anaesthesia
Harvard Medical School
Chairman, Department of Anesthesia
Brigham and Women's Hospital
Boston, Massachusetts

Sanjay Datta, M.D., F.F.A.R.C.S. (ENG)
Professor of Anaesthesia
Harvard Medical School
Director of Obstetric Anesthesia
Brigham and Women's Hospital
Boston, Massachusetts

Stephen A. Derrer, M.D.
Staff Anesthesiologist
Department of Anesthesiology
Good Samaritan Hospital of Maryland
Baltimore, Maryland

Dawn P. Desiderio, M.D.
Assistant Professor
Department of Anesthesiology and Critical
    Care Medicine
Memorial Sloan-Kettering Cancer Center and
    Cornell University Medical College
New York, New York

Stanley Deutsch, Ph.D., M.D.
Professor of Anesthesiology
Department of Anesthesiology
The George Washington University Medical Center
Washington, DC

Clifford Scott Deutschman, M.S., M.D., F.C.C.M.
Assistant Professor
Surgical Intensive Care Division
Department of Anesthesiology and Critical
    Care Medicine
The Johns Hopkins Medical Institutions
Baltimore, Maryland

Michael N. Diringer, M.D.
Director, Neurology/Neurosurgery Intensive
    Care Unit
Departments of Neurology and Neurosurgery
Barnes Hospital
Washington University School of Medicine
St. Louis, Missouri

Robert T. Donham, Ph.D., M.D.
Associate Professor
Vice Chairman for Clinical Affairs
Department of Anesthesiology and Critical
  Care Medicine
The Johns Hopkins Medical Institutions
Baltimore, Maryland

David L. Dull, M.D.
Clinical Instructor
Department of Surgery
Division of Anesthesiology
Michigan State University College of Human
  Medicine
Grand Rapids Campus
Grand Rapids, Michigan

John H. Eichhorn, M.D.
Professor and Chairman
Department of Anesthesiology
School of Medicine
The University of Mississippi Medical Center
Jackson, Mississippi

James B. Eisenkraft, M.D.
Professor of Anesthesiology
Mount Sinai School of Medicine of the City
  University of New York
Attending Anesthesiologist
The Mount Sinai Medical Center
New York, New York

Marc A. Feldman, M.D.
Assistant Professor
Departments of Anesthesiology and Critical
  Care Medicine and Ophthalmology
The Johns Hopkins Medical Institutions
Division Chief of Anesthesiology
Wilmer Ophthalmologic Institute
Baltimore, Maryland

F. Michael Ferrante, M.D.
Assistant Professor of Anaesthesia
Harvard Medical School
Director, Pain Management Center
Department of Anesthesia
Brigham and Women's Hospital
Boston, Massachusetts

Hugh L. Flanagan, M.D.
Assistant Professor of Anaesthesia
Associate in Anesthesia
Brigham and Women's Hospital
Boston, Massachusetts

Robert B. Forbes, M.D., F.R.C.P.C.
Associate Professor
Chief, Division of Pediatric Anesthesiology
Department of Anesthesia
The University of Iowa College of Medicine
Iowa City, Iowa

Steven M. Frank, M.D.
Assistant Professor
Department of Anesthesiology and Critical
  Care Medicine
The Johns Hopkins Medical Institutions
Baltimore, Maryland

Kirk L. Fridrich, M.S., D.D.S.
Associate Professor
Department of Oral and Maxillofacial Surgery
The University of Iowa College of Medicine
Iowa City, Iowa

Robert P. From, D.O.
Associate Professor
Department of Anesthesia
The University of Iowa College of Medicine
Iowa City, Iowa

William R. Furman, M.D.
Associate Professor
Department of Anesthesiology and Critical
  Care Medicine
The Johns Hopkins University School of Medicine
Chairman, Department of Anesthesiology
Francis Scott Key Medical Center
Baltimore, Maryland

Joseph M. Garfield, M.D.
Associate Professor of Anaesthesia
Harvard Medical School
Anesthesiologist
Brigham and Women's Hospital
Boston, Massachusetts

Simon Gelman, Ph.D., M.D.
Professor and Chairman
Department of Anesthesia
The University of Alabama at Birmingham
Birmingham, Alabama

Lee Goldman, M.D., F.A.C.P., F.A.C.C.
Professor of Medicine
Harvard Medical School
Vice-Chairman, Department of Medicine
Brigham and Women's Hospital
Chief, Division of Clinical Epidemiology
Brigham and Women's Hospital
Beth Israel Hospital
Boston, Massachusetts

Mark N. Gomez, M.D.
Assistant Professor
Department of Anesthesia
The University of Iowa College of Medicine
Iowa City, Iowa

Jerry M. Gonzales, M.D.
Assistant Professor of Anesthesia
Department of Anesthesia
The University of Pennsylvania School of Medicine
Philadelphia, Pennsylvania

Christopher M. Grande, M.D.
Executive Director, International Trauma
    Anesthesia and Critical Care Society (ITACCS)
Special Consultant and Chief
Special Projects Branch
Department of Anesthesiology
The Shock Trauma Center
Maryland Institute for Emergency Medical
    Services Systems
University of Maryland at Baltimore
Baltimore, Maryland

Kenneth S. Haspel, M.D.
Instructor of Anaesthesia
Harvard Medical School
Assistant in Anesthesiology
Massachusetts General Hospital
Boston, Massachusetts

Mark A. Helfaer, M.D.
Assistant Professor
Departments of Anesthesiology and Critical
    Care Medicine and Pediatrics
Division of Pediatric Intensive Care and Pediatric
    Anesthesia
The Johns Hopkins Medical Institutions
Baltimore, Maryland

William W. Hesson, J.D.
Senior Assistant Director
University Hospital Administration
The University of Iowa Hospitals and Clinics
Iowa City, Iowa

Paul R. Hickey, M.D.
Associate Professor of Anaesthesia
Harvard Medical School
Anesthesiologist-in-Chief
Children's Hospital
Boston, Massachusetts

Bradley J. Hindman, M.D.
Assistant Professor of Anesthesia
Department of Anesthesia
The University of Iowa College of Medicine
Iowa City, Iowa

Carol A. Hirshman, M.D.
Professor
Departments of Anesthesiology and Critical Care
    Medicine, Environmental Health Sciences
    (Physiology), and Medicine (Pulmonary)
The Johns Hopkins Medical Institutions
Baltimore, Maryland

William D. Hoffman, M.D.
Senior Investigator
Critical Care Medicine Department
National Institutes of Health
Bethesda, Maryland
Assistant Professor
Department of Anesthesiology
University of Maryland
Baltimore, Maryland

Atul R. Hulyalkar, M.D.
Fellow, Department of Medicine
Division of Cardiology
Department of Anesthesiology and Critical
    Care Medicine
The Johns Hopkins University School of Medicine
Baltimore, Maryland

Linda S. Humphrey, M.D.
Associated Anesthesiologists
    of Reno
Reno, Nevada

Steven Karan, M.D.
Assistant Professor
Department of Anesthesiology
Uniformed Services University of the Health
    Sciences
Bethesda, Maryland

Jeffrey Katz, M.D.
Professor and Chairman
Department of Anesthesiology
University of Texas Medical School at Houston
Houston, Texas

Henrik Kehlet, Ph.D., M.D.
Professor
Surgical Gastroenterology Department
Hvidovre University Hospital
University of Copenhagen
Hvidovre, Denmark

Gerald A. Kirk, M.D.
Assistant Professor
Department of Anesthesia
The University of Iowa College of Medicine
Iowa City, Iowa

Jeffrey R. Kirsch, M.D.
Associate Professor
Department of Anesthesiology and Critical
　Care Medicine
The Johns Hopkins Medical Institutions
Baltimore, Maryland

Richard J. Kitz, M.D.
Henry Isiah Dorr Professor of Anaesthesia
Harvard Medical School
Anesthetist-in-Chief
Massachusetts General Hospital
Boston, Massachusetts

Ronald A. Kross, M.D.
Assistant Professor
Department of Anesthesiology and Critical
　Care Medicine
Memorial Sloan-Kettering Cancer Center and
　Cornell University Medical College
New York, New York

Grant D. Kruse, M.D.
Associate
Department of Anesthesia
Assistant Director, Surgical Intensive Care Unit
The University of Iowa Hospitals and Clinics
Iowa City, Iowa

Donald H. Lambert, Ph.D., M.D.
Associate Professor of Anaesthesia
Harvard Medical School
Director of Clinical Research
Department of Anesthesia
Brigham and Women's Hospital
Boston, Massachusetts

Andrea J. Layman, M.D.
Staff Anesthesiologist
St. Alexis Medical Center
Bismark, North Dakota

Thomas H. Lee, M.D., M.Sc., F.A.C.C.
Assistant Professor of Medicine
Harvard Medical School
Associate Physician
Brigham and Women's Hospital
Boston, Massachusetts

Andrzej W. Lipkowski, Ph.D., D.Sc.
Associate Professor
Medical Research Center
Polish Academy of Sciences
Warsaw, Poland

David E. Longnecker, M.D.
Robert Dunning Dripps Professor of Anesthesia
Chairman, Department of Anesthesia
The University of Pennsylvania School of Medicine
Philadelphia, Pennsylvania

Mazen A. Maktabi, M.D.
Assistant Professor
Department of Anesthesia
Neuroanesthesia Research Group
The University of Iowa College of Medicine
Iowa City, Iowa

Lynette Mark, M.D.
Assistant Professor
Department of Anesthesiology and Critical
　Care Medicine
Division of Critical Care Anesthesia and
　Cardiac Anesthesia
The Johns Hopkins Medical Institutions
Baltimore, Maryland

Lynne G. Maxwell, M.D., F.A.A.P.
Assistant Professor
Department of Anesthesiology and Critical
　Care Medicine
Clinical Director, Division of Pediatric Anesthesia
The Johns Hopkins Medical Institutions
Baltimore, Maryland

Robert W. McPherson, M.D.
Associate Professor
Department of Anesthesiology and Critical
　Care Medicine
Director, Division of Neuroanesthesia
The Johns Hopkins Medical Institutions
Baltimore, Maryland

William T. Merritt, M.D.
Head, Liver Transplantation Anesthesia
Department of Anesthesiology and Critical
　Care Medicine
The Johns Hopkins Medical Institutions
Baltimore, Maryland

Clair F. Miller, M.D.
Assistant Professor
Department of Anesthesia
Sinai Hospital of Baltimore
Baltimore, Maryland

Edward D. Miller, Jr., M.D.
E.M. Papper Professor of Anesthesiology
Chairman, Department of Anesthesiology
College of Physicians & Surgeons
Columbia University
New York, New York

Francis L. Miller, Ph.D., M.D.
Assistant Professor of Anesthesia
Hospital of the University of Pennsylvania
Philadelphia, Pennsylvania

Keith W. Miller, M.A., Ph.D.
Professor of Pharmacology
Harvard Medical School
Pharmacologist
Massachusetts General Hospital
Boston, Massachusetts

John R. Moyers, M.D.
Professor
Department of Anesthesia
The University of Iowa College of Medicine
Iowa City, Iowa

Sheila M. Muldoon, M.D.
Professor and Chairman
Department of Anesthesiology
Uniformed Services University of the Health
    Sciences
Bethesda, Maryland

Michael F. Mulroy, M.D.
Staff Anesthesiologist
Residency Program Coordinator
Department of Anesthesiology
Virgina Mason Medical Center
Seattle, Washington

David J. Murray, M.D.
Associate Professor
Department of Anesthesia
The University of Iowa College of Medicine
Iowa City, Iowa

Michael G. Muto, M.D.
Instructor, Department of Obstetrics and
    Gynecology
Harvard Medical School
Division of Gynecologic Oncology
Department of Obstetrics, Gynecology and
    Reproductive Biology
Brigham and Women's Hospital
Boston, Massachusetts

Charles Natanson, M.D.
Senior Investigator
Critical Care Medicine Department
National Institutes of Health
Bethesda, Maryland
Associate Professor of Anesthesia
Department of Anesthesia
University of Maryland
Baltimore, Maryland

Michael Nugent, M.D.
Professor and Chairman
Department of Anesthesia
Medical College of Ohio
Toledo, Ohio

Stephen D. Parker, M.D.
Assistant Professor
Department of Anesthesiology and Critical
    Care Medicine
Division of Critical Care Medicine
The Johns Hopkins Medical Institutions
Baltimore, Maryland

L. Reuven Pasternak, M.D., M.P.H.
Assistant Professor
Department of Anesthesiology and Critical Care
    Medicine
Medical Director
Ambulatory Surgery Programs
The Johns Hopkins Medical Institutions
Baltimore, Maryland

Kent S. Pearson, M.D.
Assistant Professor
Department of Anesthesia
Associate Director, Surgical Intensive Care Unit
The University of Iowa College of Medicine
Iowa City, Iowa

Beverly K. Philip, M.D.
Associate Professor of Anaesthesia
Harvard Medical School
Director, Day Surgery Unit
Brigham and Women's Hospital
Boston, Massachusetts

James H. Philip, M.E. (ENG), M.D.
Associate Professor of Anaesthesia
Harvard Medical School
Anesthesiologist and Director of Bioengineering
Brigham and Women's Hospital
Boston, Massachusetts

Daniel B. Raemer, Ph.D.
Associate Professor of Anaesthesia
Harvard Medical School
Director of Biomedical Engineering
Brigham and Women's Hospital
Boston, Massachusetts

P. Prithvi Raj, M.B.B.S., F.R.C. Anaes.
Fellow, American College of Pain Medicine
Director, Development and Research
National Pain Institute
Clinical Professor of Anesthesiology
Medical College of Georgia
Augusta, Georgia

Francis X. Riegler, M.D.
Assistant Professor of Anesthesia
The University of Pennsylvania School of Medicine
Philadelphia, Pennsylvania

James T. Roberts, M.D.
Assistant Professor of Anaesthesia
Harvard Medical School
Associate Anesthetist
Massachusetts General Hospital
Boston, Massachusetts

Peter Rock, M.D.
Associate Professor
Department of Anesthesiology and Critical
  Care Medicine
The Johns Hopkins Medical Institutions
Baltimore, Maryland

Elizabeth L. Rogers, M.D., F.A.C.P.
Professor and Associate Dean
University of Maryland School of Medicine
Chief of Staff, Veterans Affairs Medical Center
Baltimore, Maryland

Mark C. Rogers, M.D.
Distinguished Faculty Professor and Chairman
Department of Anesthesiology and Critical
  Care Medicine
Associate Dean
The Johns Hopkins Medical Institutions
Baltimore, Maryland

Brian A. Rosenfeld, M.D.
Assistant Professor
Department of Anesthesiology and Critical
  Care Medicine
The Johns Hopkins Medical Institutions
Baltimore, Maryland

Carl Rosow, Ph.D., M.D.
Associate Professor of Anaesthesia
Harvard Medical School
Associate Anesthetist
Department of Anesthesia
Massachusetts General Hospital
Boston, Massachusetts

Alan F. Ross, M.D.
Assistant Professor
Department of Anesthesia
The University of Iowa College of Medicine
Iowa City, Iowa

Neil T. Sakima, M.D.
Assistant Professor
Department of Anesthesiology and Critical
  Care Medicine
The Johns Hopkins Medical Institutions
Baltimore, Maryland

Franklin L. Scamman, M.D.
Associate Professor
Department of Anesthesia
The University of Iowa College of Medicine
Chief, Anesthesiology Service
VAMC Iowa City Hospital
Iowa City, Iowa

Charles L. Schleien, M.D., F.C.C.M.
Associate Professor
Department of Pediatrics and Anesthesiology
University of Miami School of Medicine
Director, Pediatric Critical Care Medicine
Jackson Memorial Medical Center
Miami, Florida

D. Bruce Scott, M.D., F.R.C.P.E., F.R.C. Anaes.
Consultant Anaesthetist
Royal Infirmary
University of Edinburgh
Edinburgh, Scotland

Michael J. Sendak, M.D.
Assistant Professor
Department of Anesthesiology and Critical
   Care Medicine
The Johns Hopkins Medical Institutions
Chief, Department of Anesthesiology
Maryland General Hospital
Baltimore, Maryland

Frederick E. Sieber, M.D.
Assistant Professor
Division of Neuroanesthesiology
Department of Anesthesiology and Critical
   Care Medicine
The Johns Hopkins Medical Institutions
Baltimore, Maryland

Raymond S. Sinatra, Ph.D, M.D.
Associate Professor
Department of Anesthesiology
Director, Acute Pain Management Service
Yale University School of Medicine
New Haven, Connecticut

Douglas S. Snyder, M.S., M.D.
Instructor
Department of Anesthesiology and Critical
   Care Medicine
The Johns Hopkins Medical Institutions
Baltimore, Maryland

Bruce D. Spiess, M.D.
Associate Professor
Chief of the Division of Cardiothoracic
   Anesthesiology
Department of Anesthesiology
University of Washington
Seattle, Washington

John K. Stene, Jr., Ph.D., M.D.
Director of Perioperative Anesthesia Trauma
   Services
Associate Professor
Department of Anesthesia
College of Medicine
The Pennsylvania State University
The Milton S. Hershey Medical Center
Hershey, Pennsylvania

Robert H. Stiefel
Manager, Department of Clinical Engineering
Instructor, Department of Biomedical Engineering
The Johns Hopkins Medical Institutions
Baltimore, Maryland

Judith L. Stiff, M.D., M.P.H.
Associate Professor
Department of Anesthesiology and Critical
   Care Medicine
The Johns Hopkins Medical Institutions
Attending Anesthesiologist
Francis Scott Key Medical Center
Baltimore, Maryland

Gary Strichartz, Ph.D.
Professor of Anaesthesia (Pharmacology)
Harvard Medical School
Director, Anesthesia Research Laboratory
Brigham and Women's Hospital
Boston, Massachusetts

(John) S.T. Sum Ping, M.B., Ch.B., F.F.A.R.C.S.
Assistant Professor
Department of Anesthesia
Associate Director, Surgical Intensive Care Unit
The University of Iowa College of Medicine
Iowa City, Iowa

Tommy Symreng, Ph.D., M.D.
Staff Anesthesiologist
Department of Anesthesiology
Welborn Baptist Hospital
Evansville, Indiana

Daniel M. Thys, M.D., F.A.C.C.
Director, Department of Anesthesiology
St. Luke's/Roosevelt Hospital Center
Professor, Department of Anesthesiology
College of Physicians & Surgeons
Columbia University
New York, New York

John H. Tinker, M.D.
Professor and Head
Department of Anesthesia
The University of Iowa College of Medicine
Iowa City, Iowa

Michael M. Todd, M.D.
Professor and Vice Chairman for Research
Department of Anesthesia
The University of Iowa College of Medicine
Iowa City, Iowa

Annie Umbricht-Schneiter, M.D.
Specialist in Internal Medicine and Addiction
   Medicine
The Johns Hopkins Medical Institutions
Baltimore, Maryland

Timothy R. VadeBoncouer, M.D.
Assistant Professor of Anesthesia
University of Illinois-Chicago College of Medicine
Chicago, Illinois

Leroy D. Vandam, M.D.
Professor Emeritus
Department of Anaesthesia
Harvard Medical School
Brigham and Women's Hospital
Boston, Massachusetts

Jan Van Hemelrijck, M.D.
Assistant Professor
Department of Anesthesiology
University Hospitals
Katholicke Universiteit Leuven
Leuven, Belgium

Susan Vassallo, M.D.
Instructor in Anaesthesia
Harvard Medical School
Assistant in Anesthesia
Massachusetts General Hospital
Assistant in Anesthesia
Massachusetts Eye and Ear Infirmary
Boston, Massachusetts

David S. Warner, M.D.
Associate Professor
Department of Anesthesia
The University of Iowa College of Medicine
Iowa City, Iowa

Michael E. Weiss, M.D., F.A.A.A.I.
Assistant Clinical Professor of Medicine
Division of Allergy
University of Washington School of Medicine
Seattle, Washington

Randall C. Wetzel, M.B., B.S., F.C.C.M.
Associate Professor
Departments of Anesthesiology and Critical
  Care Medicine and Pediatrics
Anesthesiologist-in-Charge
Division of Pediatric Anesthesia
The Johns Hopkins Medical Institutions
Baltimore, Maryland

Paul F. White, Ph.D., M.D., F.F.A.R.C.S.
Margaret Milam McDermott Chair in
  Anesthesiology
Department of Anesthesiology and Pain
  Management
University of Texas Southwestern Medical Center
Dallas, Texas

Alon P. Winnie, M.D.
Professor, Department of Anesthesia
University of Illinois Medical Center
Chairman, Department of Anesthesiology and
  Critical Care Medicine
Cook County Hospital
Chicago, Illinois

Myron Yaster, M.D.
Associate Professor
Departments of Anesthesiology and Critical
  Care Medicine and Pediatrics
The Johns Hopkins Medical Institutions
Baltimore, Maryland

Helen Yates, M.D.
Department of Anesthesiology and Critical
  Care Medicine
The Johns Hopkins Medical Institutions
Baltimore, Maryland

This book is dedicated to the fond memory of

Benjamin G. Covino, M.D., Ph.D.,

*whose untimely death represents a loss not only to the editors of this book,
but also to the specialty of anesthesiology.*

Ben was not only an accomplished academic anesthesiologist and an expert in regional anesthesia, he was also a friend of many of the authors and readers of this book. Those of us who were fortunate enough to have spent significant time with him will miss his warm, witty, and insightful conversation. The extended family of colleagues and students who shared time with Ben as well as his own family will always remember him fondly and with respect.

Mark C. Rogers

John H. Tinker

David E. Longnecker

Preface

Principles and Practice of Anesthesiology is the result of many hours of discussion about how the specialty should be conceptualized and practiced. We feel that anesthesiology has matured into a complete medical discipline whose focus should be on the patient. As a result, this book is clearly patient-oriented in a manner similar to that found in textbooks of medicine, surgery, and pediatrics. There are other textbooks of anesthesiology that are complete and well written, but they focus on details (e.g., administration of drugs, mechanical procedures) rather than on the complete care of the patient. The organization of this book, however, reflects what we believe is the more current and comprehensive view of the role of the anesthesiologist as the physician responsible for sound medical judgments about surgical patients, a view more in keeping with the approach of modern anesthetic practice.

One consequence of this approach is the recognition that the specialty of anesthesiology has grown increasingly complex. The sophistication needed to perform preoperative medical evaluations, to choose from a wide range of intraoperative techniques, and to manage postoperative care (especially postoperative pain management) has increased dramatically over the past decade. In fact, anesthesiology has become a discipline with many subspecialties, and of all these, traditional anesthesia practice has expanded most in the field of regional anesthesia and pain management. Compared to just a few years ago, a much greater percentage of anesthesia is being delivered by regional and combined techniques, and the anesthesiologist is being increasingly drawn into postoperative management of pain as well as a more comprehensive pain management practice that involves patients who may never have been in the operating room. Such patients include individuals with cancer-related pain,

traumatic pain, and with similar conditions for which the anesthesiologist is now considered an expert and a consultant. Therefore we have made a conscious effort in this book to emphasize this growth by discussing regional anesthesia with expanded material (including diagrams and illustrations) and by covering pain management in depth. Sections of this book have been devoted exclusively to these subspecialties in an attempt to fully integrate these areas into a major text on anesthesiology, rather than to relegate them to separate volumes.

A major investment has also been made on the part of the editors, the authors, and the publisher of this text in recognizing that a book that aspired to such goals would have to be made much more "user-friendly" than is traditionally the case. We increasingly find a computer-literate readership is accustomed to seeing displays of information in colors and in the form of icons and creative graphs. Therefore we have tried to present the information in this book in such a way that makes it easy for the reader to understand, retain, and discuss the information. In particular, innovative diagrams have been used to describe ways to administer regional anesthesia and to provide pain relief. Beyond that, the presentation of physiologic and biochemical information is offered in ways not previously tried in textbooks of anesthesiology. It is our hope that the presentation and format of this book will make it possible for the reader to use this reference not only to read but also to prepare and present slides and other illustrative media.

Finally, we made a conscious decision to acknowledge that the field of critical care medicine itself had grown to be an enormous field with many major multiple-volume texts in its own right. Attempting to cover all of critical care medicine in a few chapters seemed inconsistent with the general principles on which this book was formulated. Therefore we chose to emphasize and expand the coverage of regional anesthesia in the space traditionally reserved for a summary review of critical care medicine, which we believe will represent a better educational investment for the practicing anesthesiologist than a more superficial overview of both areas.

We clearly hope that these philosophic approaches to the understanding and presentation of the principles of anesthetic practice will provide our readership with a fresh and innovative approach to the speciality. It is our goal that the *Principles and Practice of Anesthesiology* represent a new way of looking at and of presenting the dynamic nature of modern anesthetic practice.

Mark C. Rogers
John H. Tinker
David E. Longnecker
June 1992

Contents

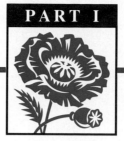

PART I

APPROACH TO THE PATIENT

CHAPTER 1

Preoperative Evaluation of the Healthy Patient

ALAN F. ROSS
JOHN H. TINKER

HOW MUCH PREOPERATIVE EVALUATION FOR THE HEALTHY PATIENT?

A healthy person, by definition, has no medical problems. Such a person scheduled for one specific surgical condition should require very little preoperative assessment. This is important because today's health care provider is increasingly challenged to trim costs.[68] Using "quality-adjusted life years," a patient's morbidity and mortality can be distilled to dollar amounts for public policy purposes.[83,177] Traditionally the clinician has used the medical history, physical examination, and laboratory tests to evaluate a patient's health. Today's anesthesiologist is discouraged from ordering tests and is advised instead to use the patient's history and physical examination as the major tool for preoperative assessment.[255] Perhaps preoperative medical evaluation is unnecessary for low-risk patients and can be eliminated to save money without affecting outcome.[113]

But how does one know that a patient is healthy? Because the surgeon says so, or because the patient has "never been sick a day," or is characterized as "spry?" This presumed healthy patient may not have seen a doctor in years. Lack of symptoms is not equivalent to good health. Significant pathology can exist without symptoms. Atherosclerosis and systemic hypertension are classic examples of silently progressive disease. The Framingham Study found that in many patients, myocardial infarction (MI) was the first sign of coronary disease.[156] Ability of patients to tolerate blood donation, kidney donation, and lung resection without symptoms attests to the tremendous reserve and compensatory capacity of the human body. Yet a compensatory response may itself become

Table 1-1	ASA physical status classification

ASA class	Description
I	No organic disease
II	Mild or moderate systemic disease without functional impairment
III	Organic disease with definite functional impairment
IV	Severe disease that is life-threatening
V	Moribund patient, not expected to survive

a problem. For example, left ventricular hypertrophy preserves normal wall stress in aortic stenosis[128] but may create severe coronary insufficiency.[198] Without symptoms, the patient may have the original and secondary pathology. **It is important to emphasize that absence of symptoms is not equivalent to American Society of Anesthesiologists (ASA) class I physical status. A true ASA I patient** *has been evaluated* **and found free of organic disease. ASA II patients who have mild-to-moderate systemic disturbances without functional limitation may also be asymptomatic (Table 1-1).** Even the truly healthy patient may present specific concerns for the anesthesiologist, such as potential airway problems, anesthetic history, volume status, gastric reflux, and so on.

This chapter will emphasize that it is invalid to assume that the asymptomatic patient is healthy. Instead, strengths and weaknesses of the history, physical examination, and laboratory testing will be explored. Our theme is that the best determination of a patient's readiness to undergo anesthesia is made by the anesthesiologist. This chapter is an assessment of the tools available for that purpose.

HISTORY AND SYMPTOM REVIEW

Patient history is of major importance in any process of diagnosis.[263] Hampton et al. considered the relative importance of history, physical examination, and laboratory testing in evaluating 80 medical outpatients.[132] In most cases the correct diagnosis was made after reading a referral letter or taking a medical history. Physical examination or laboratory findings contributed in only seven cases each. The authors concluded that time allocation for patient evaluation should concentrate on the history.

A problem with medical history is variability. Significant disagreement may occur when several physicians interview the same patient. One explanation is use of medical terminology rather than plain language to describe a patient's symptoms. Thus Koudstaal et al. found that transient cerebral ischemic attack (TIA) was overdiagnosed because of labelling symptoms as *amarosis fugax* or *dysarthria* rather than stating symptoms exactly as reported by the patient.[170] Recording symptoms in ordinary words led to greater interobserver agreement between neurologists. Variability in patient responses has also been shown. Fairbairn et al. studied the responses of 288 London postal workers to a questionnaire designed to screen for pulmonary disease.[94] Each subject was interviewed on two occasions and the responses were tape recorded. Significant discrepancies occurred when the same subject was asked the same question on a different occasion. Explanations included subject misinterpretation, ambiguous wording of the question, and occasionally, despite clear and well understood questions, the patient simply answered differently.

The issue of cost is important. The medical history requires no special equipment or technicians, but the physician's time is not free or unlimited. Roizen et al. attempted to use a six-page history questionnaire to determine which laboratory tests should be performed.[255] The system worked only when a research nurse was present to facilitate patient answers. The nurse was more expensive than the cost of the laboratory tests.

Healthy patients are often considered those who answer "no" to a list of possible symptoms and diseases. What if the patient answers "yes" when asked about shortness of breath? This may indicate a cardiopulmonary problem, lack of physical fitness, or the fact that everyone gets short of breath at *some* level of exercise! **The critical aspect of history taking is not simply asking questions, but careful listening and interpretation of the answers.**[31]

Questions to Ask Every Patient

Several items require specific inquiry because the information may not be available in the patient's chart. **Previous anesthetic history and any problems that occurred need to be known to the anesthesiologist.** For example, a previously dislodged tooth may indicate difficult laryngoscopy. A facial nerve palsy may be a clue that mask airway maintenance may be difficult. **The previous anesthetic record should be reviewed for responses to anesthetic agents, quality of airway, laryngoscopy, intubation, and all other perioperative problems.** A history of death, cardiac arrest, or high fever during an anesthetic in a family member must raise the question of malignant hyperthermia. A prolonged recovery period may indicate increased sensitivity to anesthetics, overdose, or abnormal metabolism of muscle relaxants.

History of allergy to antibiotics and contrast dyes is

often noted on the chart. Allergy to local anesthetics should be sought, and if possible the distinction made between ester vs. amide-type local anesthetics. Jaundice after general anesthesia raises concern regarding hepatic sensitivity. A patient with a long list of allergies may be sensitive to histamine-releasing drugs. Allergy to iodine soap, adhesive tape, or latex must *not* be lightly dismissed.

Although preoperative orders generally include NPO after midnight, this condition cannot be guaranteed. Outpatients may not have previously seen an anesthesiologist. Outpatient children and their parents must be thoroughly instructed that NPO includes gum, candy, and toys. Prior history of postoperative nausea and vomiting warns of possible recurrence. **The patient must always be questioned in detail about gastric reflux. Predisposing factors include pregnancy, hiatal hernia, obesity, partial bowel obstruction, and diabetes with gastroparesis.** Prolonged bowel obstruction is particularly dangerous because aspiration of feculent material is nearly always fatal. The presence of a nasogastric tube is a red flag of potential trouble ahead.

The postpubertal, premenopausal female must be informed that general anesthesia during pregnancy may be associated with miscarriage and preterm labor. Drugs such as benzodiazepines have been implicated in birth defects if given during the first trimester of pregnancy. It must be ascertained that the patient is not currently pregnant if at all possible. Home pregnancy test kit results are not reliable. A negative hospital pregnancy test is also not absolute evidence of the nongravid state because 10 days must elapse after conception for a positive reading.

Dyspnea

Dyspnea may be an indicator of pulmonary or cardiac disease. Carpenter et al. studied the relationship of episodic respiratory symptoms to long-term mortality in adults.[34] Dyspnea rather than cough, phlegm production, or wheezing was the most powerful predictor of increased mortality related to chronic obstructive lung disease. Ferris et al.[99] found dyspnea associated with increased mortality from all causes. Other studies found dyspnea associated with increased cardiovascular mortality.[51,81,140]

Patients are often asked whether shortness of breath occurs with exertion. If it occurs, the cause may not be clear because both cardiac and pulmonary conditions may contribute to this symptom[293] (Table 1-2). The infant with a rapid respiratory rate plus nasal flaring may be found to have primary cardiac disease.[8] Although wheezing is typical of asthma, it may also occur during the airway edema of congestive heart failure. Nocturnal dyspnea may be due to fluid

Table 1-2   Various causes of dyspnea

Dyspnea classification	Examples
Pulmonary	
Upper airway	Epiglottitis
	Vascular ring
Lower airway	Asthma
	Bronchitis
	Emphysema
Alveolar	Pneumonia
Interstitial	Pulmonary fibrosis
	Sarcoidosis
Vascular	Primary pulmonary hypertension
	Pulmonary embolism
Cardiac	
Valvular	Mitral stenosis
	Mitral regurgitation
Congenital heart disease	Patent ductus arteriosus
	Ventricular septal defect
Ventricular failure	Cardiomyopathy
	Congestive heart failure
	Hypertension
Atherosclerosis	Acute ischemia

shifts, leading to congestive heart failure or from accumulation of secretions in the chronic bronchitis patient. Chronic cough may be the sole presenting symptom of asthma.[56]

Some symptoms may distinguish cardiac from pulmonary dyspnea. Nocturia suggests heart failure associated with renal vasoconstriction, which occurs during daytime activity.[139] A trial of bronchodilator[235] or diuretic may be needed to aid diagnosis. Some cases of dyspnea must be distinguished with exercise testing. The cardiac patient will discontinue exercise due to muscular fatigue and lactic acidosis before reaching maximum ventilatory capacity. The pulmonary patient will stop exercise because maximum ventilatory capacity is achieved but is insufficient to provide adequate gas exchange to sustain exercise demands.[293]

Pulmonary causes

It is useful to characterize pulmonary disorders as restrictive vs. obstructive. Within the major group of obstructive diseases, the distinctions are less clear.[29] Chronic bronchitis is defined using the clinical history of cough and sputum production. Asthma is defined physiologically as reactive airway resistance. Emphysema is defined anatomically by destruction of supporting structures. **Thus the term *chronic obstructive pulmonary disease (COPD)* does not have a strict**

definition and instead is an overlap of these disorders.[289]

Progression of the different obstructive diseases may be quite different. Burrows et al. demonstrated that the yearly decline in forced expiratory volume (FEV_1) was much greater in patients with emphysema than in patients with asthma.[28] The 10-year mortality in a group with emphysematous COPD was 60%, whereas in asthmatic patients it was only 15%. The primary cause of death was respiratory in half of the patients with emphysema but in none of the patients with asthma.

Despite this favorable prognosis for patients with asthma, Sly reported that deaths from asthma have increased steadily in the United States since 1978.[288] Although most deaths have occurred in persons over age 50, mortality has also increased in children. Likely contributing factors are less than optimal treatment, poor medical follow-up, noncompliance, dysrhythmia from overuse of beta-agonist drugs and associated hypokalemia, and adrenal insufficiency from corticosteroids. In children receiving theophylline, methylprednisolone, and intravenous isoproterenol, increased cardiac-specific creatinine phosphokinase has been observed.[196] Rea et al. determined that an emergency room visit or hospitalization for asthma within the past year were factors associated with increased risk for mortality.[245]

Stein and Cassara demonstrated that preoperative optimization of pulmonary function in patients with lung disease improved outcome.[299] **Poor-risk patients treated with bronchodilator drugs, antibiotics, chest physiotherapy, and cessation of smoking had marked reductions in postoperative morbidity and mortality compared with untreated patients. Identification of the patient at-risk is thus a priority.**[319,320] Many studies have sought to correlate preoperative spirometric findings with postoperative respiratory complications.[109,216] Lawrence et al., in a literature review of spirometry before upper abdominal surgery, found that only 22 out of 135 clinical articles actually evaluated its predictive potential. Each of these had important methodologic flaws, causing Lawrence et al. to conclude that spirometry's predictive value is unproved.[180] In a series of pulmonary patients, Nunn et al. found that the two most accurate preoperative predictors of postoperative adequacy of ventilation were severe dyspnea and a low level of arterial Po_2. The FEV_1 ranged from 0.3 L to 1 L in all patients, and was not predictive of outcome.[230]

Cardiac causes

Cardiac dyspnea arises from pulmonary congestion because of excessive fluid entering the lung tissue or impaired lymphatic drainage.[179] Usually, cardiac dyspnea occurs due to poor left ventricular compliance in ischemia or ventricular hypertrophy, increased blood volume, or restricted flow as in mitral stenosis causing elevated pulmonary venous pressure. The Framingham Study determined that congestive heart failure (CHF) was usually due to coronary disease or long-standing hypertension.[208] Overt CHF carried important morbidity and mortality; namely 6-year mortality was 82% in men and 67% in women, a rate that is 4 to 8 times that of the age-adjusted general population. Risk of stroke was four times greater than in the general population, and risk of myocardial infarction was up to five times greater. Several findings are associated with the development of cardiac failure, including an enlarged heart, electrocardiogram (ECG) abnormalities such as left ventricular hypertrophy, a low or falling vital capacity reflecting engorgement of pulmonary blood, and rapid resting heart rates. Modifiable risk factors for congestive failure include hypertension, impaired glucose tolerance, cigarette smoking, obesity, elevated cholesterol level, elevated low density lipoprotein cholesterol, and both low and high levels of hematocrit.[155]

It is a widely held belief that optimizing cardiac status preoperatively will reduce perioperative morbidity. Goldman,[119] Detsky,[69] and Gerson[110] have demonstrated CHF to be a factor for increased surgical risk. Del Guerico demonstrated that preoperative optimization of cardiac function may reduce postoperative morbidity.[63]

Chest Discomfort

Cardiovascular disease has been the leading cause of death in the United States for several decades. The incidence of coronary artery disease is best illustrated by the Framingham Heart Study, which has followed 5127 persons aged 30 to 62 years who were initially free from clinical signs of coronary disease. At the 14-year follow-up, 9.6% persons had developed clinical evidence of coronary disease.[158] Recently the 30-year follow-up found 26% of the original population had developed signs of coronary disease.[157] **A disturbing finding was that approximately one of every four myocardial infarctions was discovered only by routine ECG with neither patient nor physician having previously considered the possibility of a heart attack.**[199] Unrecognized infarctions did not have a better long-term prognosis than recognized infarctions.

The patient who gives a history of chest discomfort raises important questions. Do symptoms represent angina pectoris or another thoracic condition? Does a normal ECG rule out coronary artery disease? What further workup is required? The elusiveness of the diagnosis is illustrated by the multitude of tests available to aid the clinician. Even after evaluation by experienced cardiologists, some patients will be subjected to cardiac catheterization only to find normal coronary arteries. The symptoms of angina pectoris are complicated because pain fibers traveling by sympathetic pathways interconnect in cervical and thoracic ganglia. Thus cardiac pain may be perceived throughout a band formed by the T1 to T6 thoracic dermatomes.[63] Because of shared ascending pathways, left arm pain is *not* pathognomonic of angina but may occur from any of these visceral organs. Relief of pain by nitroglycerin is also not pathognomonic for angina because esophageal spasm,[45] another T1 to T6 condition known to mimic angina pectoris, is relieved by nitrates.

Further complicating the diagnosis of angina pectoris is the variable presentation of pain. Classic angina occurs with exertion and is relieved by rest. Yet atypical angina may occur without exertion or during the early morning hours of sleep.[348] Diabetic patients may experience dyspnea instead of angina, whereas in other patients repeated episodes of clear myocardial ischemia may occur silently.[47] Despite the variable presentations of angina and its mimics, a differential diagnosis of chest pain can be organized based on its location, quality, duration, provocation, and relief of symptoms (Table 1-3).[45]

Another strategy seeks corroborative evidence in the patient's history and physical examination. Risk factors for coronary atherosclerosis have been identified[182] (Table 1-4). Although the presence of all risk factors is most predictive, individual factors are not simply additive. Some factors are positively correlated with each other. Thus, diabetes is a powerful risk factor by itself, but its predictive capacity is reduced when the hypertension and hypercholesterolemia are already present. In contrast, risk factors that are negatively correlated, such as smoking and systolic blood pressure, are stronger predictors when present together.[123] The diagnosis of angina is strengthened by a history of prior myocardial infarction. Because up to 25% of infarctions may be clinically *silent,* the ECG may provide important information. Physical examination findings may also suggest coronary artery disease (see discussion of the physical examination).

Syncope

Syncope is temporary loss of consciousness associated with inability to maintain upright posture. The

Table 1-3   Chest pain conditions resembling angina pectoris

Conditions	Duration	Quality	Provocation	Relief	Location
Mitral valve prolapse	Minutes to hours	Superficial; variable	Spontaneous	Time	Left anterior
Esophageal reflux	10 min-1 hr	Visceral; rarely radiates	Recumbency; lack of food	Food; antacid	Substernal epigastric
Esophageal spasm	5-60 min	Visceral; mimics angina	Spontaneous; cold liquids; exercise	Nitroglycerin	Substernal; radiates
Peptic ulcer	Hours	Visceral burning	Lack of food; "acid" foods	Food; antacids	Substernal; epigastric
Biliary disease	Hours	Visceral (wax and wane); colic	Spontaneous; food	Time; analgesia	Epigastric (?); radiates
Cervical disc	Variable (gradually subsides)	Superficial; not relieved by rest	Head and neck movement; palpation	Time; analgesia	Arm, neck
Hyperventilation	2-3 min	Visceral with face parathesia	Emotion; tachypnea	Stimulus removal	Substernal
Muscuolskeletal pain	Variable	Superficial tenderness	Movement; palpation	Time; analgesia	Multiple
Pulmonary disease	30 min +	Visceral (pressure) with dyspnea	Often spontaneous	Rest; time; bronchodilator	Substernal

From Christie LG, Conti CR: Systematic approach to evaluation of angina-like chest pain, *Am Heart J,* 102:897, 1981.

Table 1-4 Risk factors for coronary atherosclerosis

Status of factors	Risk factors
Fixed	Age (risk increases with age)[269]
	Sex (male > female)[269]
	Family history of coronary disease[269]
Modifiable	Elevated cholesterol[108]
	Hypertension[160]
	Smoking
	Glucose intolerance
	Body weight[238]
	Sedentary lifestyle[343]
	Personality/behavior type[249]
	Gout[100]
	Oral contraceptives

Table 1-5 One-year mortality* for patients with syncope based on causes of syncope

Author, year, patient type	Cardiac	Noncardiac	Unexplained
Day, 1982, emergency room[61]	33%	**	**
Silverstein, 1982, medical ICU[285]	19%	6%	6%
Kapoor, 1983, ER, ward, outpatient[162]	30%	12%	6.4%
Eagle, 1985, emergency room[78]	21%	0	6%

*Day study also includes major morbidity.
**Noncardiac and unexplained syncope outcomes were considered together in this study and represent 11 poor outcomes in 173 patients (~5%).

Framingham Study found that 3% of men and women experienced syncope.[265] Dermksian reported that 7% of approximately 3000 young, healthy Air Force personnel reported at least one episode of syncope.[66] Although most episodes are benign, syncope may be the presenting symptom of serious cardiovascular disease. Four studies have analyzed the diagnosis and outcome of patients evaluated for syncope.[61,78,162,285] The various causes of syncope could be categorized as cardiac, noncardiac, or unexplained. Most often the diagnosis was made by the basic workup, which included history, physical examination, basic blood tests, and ECG. Continuous ambulatory ECG monitoring or admission to an intensive care unit for monitoring also significantly contributed to the diagnosis. A cardiac cause was determined in up to 36% of cases, most frequently due to ventricular dysrhythmias, bradycardias including sick sinus syndrome and heart block, aortic stenosis, supraventricular tachycardia, and myocardial infarction. Less frequent cardiac causes were pacemaker malfunction and pulmonary embolism. In three of the four studies, the cause of syncope remained unexplained in about half the cases. As Table 1-5 shows, the 1-year follow-up outcome was much poorer for cardiac causes than other etiologies.

When a patient reports a history of syncope, a cardiac cause should first be sought. The circumstances during which syncope occurred is helpful. **A noncardiac cause is suggested when syncope occurs during hyperventilation, anxiety, coughing, urination, swallowing, or abrupt or prolonged standing.[125,143,149,347] Syncope during exercise, however, raises suspicion of a cardiac cause such as aortic stenosis,[200] hypertrophic cardiomyopathy,[89] coronary artery disease, pulmonary hypertension,[287] congenital heart dis-**

ease,[174] **or anomalous coronary anatomy.**[43] Hypertrophic cardiomyopathy was the most common cause of sudden death in a group of 29 competitive athletes reviewed by Maron et al.[201] A family history of cardiac disease or premature sudden death also raises suspicion for cardiac cause. Another major category for cardiac causes of syncope is dysrhythmia[70] (Table 1-6).

Elderly persons are more likely to acquire sick sinus syndrome. Heart block can be congenital or acquired and occurs in young and elderly patients. Symptoms such as syncope and fatigue depend on the site of the pacemaker tissue, which determines its ability to respond to autonomic innervation. **Younger patients are susceptible to tachydysrhythmias in cases of obstructive cardiomyopathy,[173,266] mitral valve prolapse, prolonged QT interval,[272] and Wolf-Parkinson-White syndrome. Medication history may provide clues about syncope because some antihypertensive regimens cause orthostatic hypotension whereas some antidysrhythmic agents may contribute to dysrhythmias.**[154]

Aspects of the physical examination useful to assessment of syncope include orthostatic changes in blood pressure, abnormalities of the pulse, the carotid upstroke, and the presence of heart murmur. The ECG is useful if it provides evidence of dysrhythmias, repolarization abnormality, conduction abnormalities, prior myocardial infarction, or ventricular hypertrophy.[306] In 134 patients with hypertrophic cardiomyopathy, normal ECGs were extremely uncommon.[267] If evidence for a cardiac cause of syncope is found, consultation should be obtained. Although unexplained syncope has a better prognosis, patients with recurrent syncope may also benefit from consultation. Dimarco et al. reported that electrophysiologic

Table 1-6	Causes of syncope
Cause	**Examples**
Central nervous system	Epilepsy
	Cerebrovascular accident
	Transient ischemic attack
Metabolic	Hyperventilation syndrome
	Hypoglycemia
	Hypoxemia
	Drug induced
Autonomic	Carotid sinus hypersensitivity
	Orthostatic hypotension
	Micturition syncope
	Deglutition syncope
	Autonomic neuropathy
Cardiac	Ventricular dysrhythmia
	Bradydysrhythmia and heart block
	Aortic stenosis
	Supraventricular tachydysrhythmia
	Myocardial infarction
	Pulmonary embolism
	Hypertrophic cardiomyopathy

Data from Day et al.,[61] Silverstein et al.,[285] Kapoor et al.,[162] and Eagle et al.[78]

techniques were able to establish a diagnosis for 17 of 25 cases of recurrent, unexplained syncope.[73] Hammill et al. have also used a tilt table to facilitate electrophysiologic diagnosis.[305]

Headache

Headache, the seventh most common cause for physician visits,[251] can be expected to be reported preoperatively with some frequency. Linet et al. surveyed over 10,000 adolescents and young adults and found that 60% to 75% had experienced at least one headache in the prior month.[188] Fortunately the incidence of serious disease is estimated to be 4 in 100,000.[71] **Adams et al. raised questions about distinguishing benign from serious headache.**[2] **Review of records of 182 patients who had documented subarachnoid hemorrhage revealed that the diagnosis was initially missed in 20% of cases.** These 41 patients were treated for 4 to 7 days with diagnoses of flu, migraine, neck trouble, sinusitis, otitis, and myocardial infarction before the correct diagnosis was made. Review of the more common headache syndromes facilitates assessment when the symptom of headache is encountered.

Headache syndromes can be organized into three groups based on their timing and etiology[146] (Box 1-1). **Recent-onset, severe headaches demand attention.** Adams et al. suggested that a *first migraine headache* may instead be due to a subarachnoid

hemorrhage.[2] "Meningism" describes headache and neck stiffness that accompanies systemic infections such as influenza and pyelonephritis. The presence of fever or infection demands investigation for meningitis. Fever is not characteristic of migraine, but may occur later in the course of subarachnoid hemorrhage. Severe headache during pregnancy may follow thrombosis of a cerebral venous sinus causing an abrupt rise in intracranial pressure.[349] Patients receiving tissue plasminogen activator for myocardial infarction have been reported to suffer intracerebral hemorrhage.[163] Suspicion is important, because headache may be otherwise attributed to nitrate therapy.

Chronic, recurrent headaches may result from systemic hypertension, in which case end organ changes, such as retinopathy, may be found.[44] In *pheochromocytoma* symptoms of paroxysmal explosive headache, palpitations, and diaphoresis may accompany a family history of pheochromocytoma, neurofibromatosis, or other endocrine tumor (multiple endocrine neoplasia).[176] Headache in a patient with a prior ventriculoperitoneal shunt raises the question of elevated *intracranial pressure* and warrants assessment of shunt function. Headache because of raised intracranial pressure is worse on awakening in the morning and is exacerbated by coughing, straining, or stooping. Accumulation of *subdural hematoma* is suspected when headache and drowsiness follow an episode of falling or head trauma, particularly in patients taking anticoagulant medication.[318] Papilledema associated with headache suggests increased intracranial pressure, but its absence does not ensure normal pressure.

Other chronic headache syndromes can be distinguished by characteristic patient history.[175] The classic *migraine* is throbbing, unilateral, and associated with visual aura of flashing lights or zigzag lines, nausea, photophobia, and focal neurologic symptoms. The patient seeks a dark, quiet room in which to lie down. In contrast, the *cluster headache* involves severe pain originating in the nostril or eye and spreading to the forehead. Tearing, nasal congestion, and Horner's syndrome occur, and the patient cannot lie still. Older patients may have headaches because of *temporal arteritis* with symptoms of unilateral blindness, scalp tenderness, transient diplopia, and masseter muscle pain termed "jaw claudication." Although elevated erythrocyte sedimentation rate is classic, it can be normal in patients with documented temporal arteritis. Persons over age 75 have a 2% to 4% incidence of *glaucoma* that causes headache beginning in the affected eye and spreading around the orbit. Associated symptoms include tunnel vision and halos around lights. Headache following a viral illness may be due to blocked drainage and bacterial overgrowth known as *sinusitis*. The headache is exacerbated by a lowered

---

BOX 1-1
GROUPS OF HEADACHE SYNDROMES

Recent onset	**Chronic recurrent**	**Referred or facial pain**
Subarachnoid hemorrhage	Tension headache	Glaucoma
Meningitis	Migraine	Otitis media
Systemic infections with "meningism"	Cluster headache	Dental causes
Venous sinus thrombosis	Hypertensive	Sinusitis
	Temporal arteritis	Trigeminal neuralgia
	Subdural hematoma	Glossopharyngeal neuralgia
	Hydrocephalus	

---

head position or externally applied pressure. The presence of fever and chills suggests systemic infection, which can lead to complications including osteomyelitis, meningitis, and cerebral abscess.

Anesthesia literature consists mostly of anecdotal reports of anesthesia in headache sufferers. McDowell et al. reported on 635 patients undergoing minor gynecologic surgery.[206] Nonopiate vs. opiate premedication did not influence the perioperative incidence of headache. The most important factor was the patient's propensity to develop headaches. Thus, while the overall incidence of headache was 42%, patients who were headache prone had an incidence of 83% whereas migraine sufferers had an incidence of 92%. Fell considered that the circumstances of preoperative fasting and anxiety may contribute to migraine headaches.[98] Strauss and Eschenroeder reported that a patient developed a hemiplegic migraine after dental extraction facilitated by local lidocaine with epinephrine, intravenous fentanyl and midazolam, and 50% nitrous oxide.[307] In contrast, Stanley reported that a dental patient suffering from a migraine had complete relief of symptoms after receiving nitrous oxide for 30 minutes.[295]

Hypertension

The Joint National Committee on Detection, Evaluation, and Treatment of High Blood Pressure (BP) has estimated that as many as 58 million people in the United States have hypertension,[228] an important risk factor in coronary artery disease, stroke, congestive heart failure, and renal failure. Patients with significant hypertension can be expected to have altered baroreflex function,[82] changes in autoregulation of the cerebral[304] and coronary[134] circulations, and altered renal function.[129] Therapy for mild, moderate, and severe hypertension has significantly reduced the possibility of stroke by 40% to 80% but has reduced the incidence of myocardial infarction by only 7%, a finding of considerable controversy.[232,334] Hypertension may be present in up to 45% of persons over age

65.[7] **Although less than 3% of United States' children have hypertension, early detection and treatment may result in substantial benefit**[316] (Table 1-7).

The finding of preoperative hypertension must take into account preoperative anxiety, appropriateness of cuff size, average of several measurements, and a quiet and comfortable sitting position with the arm at the level of the heart. Evidence of target organ involvement, such as retinal vascular changes, left ventricular hypertrophy, cardiomegaly, or renal insufficiency indicates that an elevated BP represents significant hypertension.[167,178] Special consideration should be given to the possibility of secondary causes of hypertension which, although they account for only 5% of hypertensive patients, are potentially curable. **The five major causes of secondary hypertension are renal artery stenosis,[346] primary aldosteronism,[336] Cushing's syndrome,[173] pheochromocytoma,[24] and coarctation of the aorta.[185] Clues may be present from the history and physical examination (see Table 1-10). Lesser causes of secondary hypertension include acromegaly and hyperparathyroidism. Medications can contribute to hypertension, including dermatologic steroid preparations, hormonal contraceptives, cyclosporine, and nonsteroidal antiinflammatory drugs. Ethanol and cigarette smoking have also been implicated. The Joint National Committee[228] recommends several simple laboratory tests for assessment of hypertension, including hemoglobin and hematocrit; urinalysis; serum potassium, calcium, creatinine, glucose, and uric acid; and electrocardiography.**

How should the anesthesiologist proceed if a preoperative patient is found to have hypertension? Clinical studies have addressed the risk of hypertension to the surgical patient. Bedford and Feinstein[15] demonstrated that the BP on admission to the hospital could predict a hypertensive response to endotracheal intubation. Goldman and Caldera found that surgical patients with hypertension not exceeding a diastolic pressure of 110 mg Hg did not

Table 1-7 Pediatric hypertension classification*		
Age	Diastolic	Systolic
Newborn		
7 days		≥ 96
8-30 days		≥ 104
Infant		
< 2 years	≥ 74	≥ 112
Children		
3-5 years	≥ 76	≥ 116
6-9 years	≥ 78	≥ 122
10-12 years	≥ 82	≥ 126
13-15 years	≥ 86	≥ 136
16-18 years	≥ 92	≥ 142

*Pressures listed represent significant hypertension. Values for severe hypertension are not listed.
From Report of Second Task Force on Blood Pressure Control in Children, *Pediatrics* 79(1):1, 1987.

Table 1-8 Classification of blood pressure in adults aged 18 years or older*	
BP range, mm Hg	Category
DBP	
< 85	Normal BP
85-89	High-normal BP
90-104	Mild hypertension
105-114	Moderate hypertension
≥ 115	Severe hypertension
SBP, when DBP **< 90 mm Hg**	
< 140	Normal BP
140-159	Borderline isolated systolic hypertension
≥ 160	Isolated systolic hypertension

*Classification based on the average of two or more readings on two or more occasions. *BP,* blood pressure; *DBP,* diastolic blood pressure; and *SBP,* systolic blood pressure.
From the 1988 Report of the Joint National Committee on Detection, Evaluation, and Treatment of High Blood Pressure, *Arch Intern Med* 148:1023, 1988.

have a higher incidence of perioperative myocardial infarction.[118] Unfortunately, these studies do not cover all circumstances. Medical guidelines for follow-up are determined by the severity of the hypertension. For adults, mild hypertension should be confirmed within 2 months, moderate hypertension should be evaluated or referred within 2 weeks, and severe hypertension should be referred or evaluated immediately (Table 1-8).[30] **Applying this approach to elective surgery, we recommend that mildly hypertensive patients be followed up postoperatively, whereas elective anesthesia be postponed in patients with severe hypertension. As the literature is limited, medical consultation should be obtained for the moderately hypertensive patient before anesthesia.**

Cerebrovascular Disease
Asymptomatic bruit
Stroke is the third leading cause of mortality in the United States[220] **and costs an estimated $5 billion yearly in medical care for morbidity. Despite this, the 1989 Report of the United States Preventive Services Task Force did not recommend auscultation for asymptomatic carotid bruits.**[104] The finding of a bruit is problematic for several reasons. First, a cervical bruit may be present but not indicative of carotid stenosis.[264] Hammond and Eisenger examined 1000 normal patients for the presence of bruit.[131] Patients under age 5 years had bruit in 87% of cases, and patients aged 30 to 34 had bruit in 22% of cases. Hemodialysis patients often have neck bruit presumably because of the high output circulatory state.[205] Jones reported that a cervical venous hum could be

readily perceived in 27% of subjects with an average age of 32 years.[153] The differential diagnosis also includes radiated cardiac murmurs. Chambers and Norris evaluated asymptomatic auscultated bruits in 336 patients by carotid Doppler examination. A unilateral upper neck bruit correlated to an ipsilateral stenotic lesion in 61% of cases. Bilateral upper neck bruits were the most powerful predictor of a stenotic lesion, which was found in 76% of cases. In patients with unilateral cervical bruits, a stenotic lesion was found by Doppler on the *opposite,* clinically silent side in 28% of cases.[40]

Is an asymptomatic carotid bruit a predictor of impending stroke? Population studies in Evans County, Georgia,[138] and Framingham, Massachusetts,[344] found that an asymptomatic cervical bruit, present in about 5% of patients, was associated with increased risk of stroke. However, the stroke most often was *not* related to the bruit but occurred instead because of cardiac embolism, ruptured aneurysm, or was in vascular territory different from that of the bruit. Chambers and Norris followed 500 patients with asymptomatic bruits for up to 4 years.[41] The degree of carotid stenosis on initial presentation was an important predictor of neurologic sequelae, but even in patients with severe stenosis, most experienced transient ischemic attack (TIA) rather than stroke as the initial event. **Myocardial infarctions were more frequent than strokes, and a cardiac cause of death occurred significantly more often than a**

Table 1-9 Asymptomatic carotid bruit — 1-year sequelae in 500 patients according to degree of stenosis

Sequelae	Number cases/category stenosis		
	0%-29% stenosis	30%-74% stenosis	75%-100% stenosis
TIA only	2	6	16
Stroke after TIA	1	1	2(1)*
Stroke without TIA	2(1)*	2	4(1)*
Nonfatal MI	4	8	4
Fatal MI	7	8	12

*A total of three strokes were fatal.
From Chambers BR, Norris JW: Outcome in patients with asymptomatic neck bruits, *N Engl J Med* 315:860, 1986.

neurologic cause of death[33] (Table 1-9). Another major problem with the asymptomatic bruit is that surgical therapy has been controversial.[13,332,16,204,329] Carotid endarterectomy as a procedure is currently the subject of considerable controversy and several large clinical trials.[16,204,329]

Transient ischemic attack

The presence of symptoms suggesting a first-time transient ischemic attack (TIA) is more significant than the finding of an asymptomatic bruit. Incidence of TIA in the general population is 31/100,000/year, with older age groups affected more often.[338] Outcome of patients with TIA history has been determined from population studies and from the placebo groups of multicenter studies of medical therapy for TIA.[32,101] **The highest risk of stroke is in the early months after a first time TIA.**[39] Whisnant reported that although 36% of TIA patients developed a stroke over a 5-year follow-up period, half of these strokes occurred during the first year after the original TIA, and the first month was the period of greatest risk, accounting for one fifth of all strokes.[338]

Attempts to correlate preoperative bruit or TIA to postoperative stroke have not provided clear direction.* **In summary, an asymptomatic bruit is an important marker of atherosclerosis while a *new* TIA represents an increased risk for a neurologic event. The medical history is important because *presence of symptoms* makes the distinction. Suspicion for coronary artery disease should be high in either case.**[286]

---

* References 12, 135, 136, 142, 256, 323.

Upper Respiratory Tract Infection

A frequent preoperative problem in the "healthy" patient is an upper respiratory infection (URI).[191] The Cleveland Family Study determined that the average person experienced 5.6 such episodes per year. **The highest incidence of respiratory illnesses occurred in young children, with an average of 8.3 episodes per year in the 1-year age group.**[74] Similar findings were described in separate studies in Charlottesville, Seattle,[105] and Tecumseh.[214] One large pediatric practice identified a peak in the incidence of croup in the late fall and early winter.[65] Glezen and Denny previously noted that, in general, lower respiratory tract infections had a mid-winter peak.[111]

Accurate diagnosis of the cause of URI is difficult. The symptoms of runny nose, nasal congestion, and cough may represent chronic rhinorrhea, a common cold, or the early stages of more severe lower respiratory tract illness. In fact, the "common cold" may be caused by a typical rhinovirus or more potent pathogens including influenza, varicella, rubeola, and respiratory synctial virus. Simple laboratory tests cannot distinguish viral agents, and specialized tests are too expensive and time consuming to be useful for routine preoperative evaluation.

Research has substantiated that viral respiratory illnesses may have important effects on the respiratory system. The alveolar-arterial oxygen gradient may be worsened in patients with an uncomplicated influenza infection.[152] Hyperactive bronchoconstriction can occur in nonasthmatic persons during infection with the common cold.[88] In normal adults, respiratory muscle weakness can be demonstrated during upper respiratory tract infection with normalization in 2 weeks.[212]

Clinicians have long cautioned that anesthetizing patients with URI may be accompanied by an increased incidence of bronchospasm, laryngospasm, secretions, and oxygen desaturation.[144] These concerns have recently been challenged. Tait and Knight reported that retrospective analysis of anesthetic records showed that 122 patients with symptoms of preoperative URI had no greater incidence of laryngospasm, bronchospasm, or stridor than did 3350 patients without preoperative URI,[312] although breath-holding was more frequent in the URI group. Tait and Knight also prospectively studied pediatric patients who required elective myringotomy and tympanotomy. Of the patients with URI who actually received an anesthetic, the incidence of laryngospasm was low and not different from the asymptomatic group.[311]

Criticisms of these reports are important.[124,144] Both studies failed to include those patients whose URI symptoms caused postponement of surgery. The prospective study evaluated a very short anesthetic, minimal surgical trauma, and no endotracheal intubation. Further, both studies used assessment of qualitative events such as laryngospasm for comparison of the groups.

Different conclusions were reached by Desoto et al. who studied changes in pulse oximeter saturations when pediatric patients with and without URI were anesthetized for simple otolaryngologic procedures. No intraoperative episodes of cyanosis or laryngeal spasm occurred in either group. However, in the recovery room while spontaneously breathing room air, 20% of the patients with URI had pulse oximeter saturations less than 95%. This did not occur in any patient without URI. Preoperative pulse oximeter saturations were normal in both groups.[67]

Curiously, the period following recovery from URI may be the time of heightened anesthesia risk. McGill et al. described 11 cases of unexpected intraoperative respiratory dysfunction in pediatric patients who had experienced URI in the previous 4 weeks. Despite a lack of symptoms except occasional rhinorrhea, significant atelectasis and pulmonary shunting occurred with anesthesia. This necessitated abbreviation of the surgery, additional laboratory tests such as chest radiographs and blood gases, and additional procedures such as chest percussion, postural drainage, and bronchoscopy.[209] Tait and Knight also found that the period after a URI increased the risk of laryngospasm and bronchospasm.[312] Patients who had recovered from a URI within the preceding 2 weeks had a higher incidence of respiratory complications than did patients who had ongoing URI symptoms. It is not clear why the period after a URI should pose increased risk for perioperative pulmonary dysfunction. Perhaps this represents lower respiratory tract extension of the prior upper respiratory infection. Perhaps hyperactive airway reflexes take longer to normalize than do symptoms of rhinorrhea.[88]

PHYSICAL EXAMINATION
Vital Signs

Abnormalities of the vital signs—blood pressure, heart rate, respiratory rate, and temperature—provide important clues to serious pathology. **When abnormalities are encountered, corroborating evidence must be sought in the physical examination.** Interpretation begins with an assessment of measurement accuracy. Pitfalls include incorrect BP cuff size, BP difference between arms, auscultatory gap, oral vs. rectal vs. axillary temperature, difference between apical vs. radial pulses during dysrhythmia, and estimation of respiratory rate rather than counting. **Although it is known that anxiety can alter vital signs,[195,242] a serious mistake in preoperative evaluation is to miss a serious medical condition by assuming that vital sign abnor-**

malities are due to nervousness.

Assessment of abnormality is facilitated when several vital signs are altered.[189] The combination of hypotension and tachycardia indicates significant circulatory abnormality. However, the body's compensatory mechanisms[112] may be able to maintain vital signs within the "normal" range. For example, a healthy female with ruptured ectopic pregnancy may demonstrate BP of 100/70 with a heart rate of 100, despite significant blood loss. In such cases, corroborating evidence might include signs of sympathetic activation, such as diaphoresis, tachypnea, and cool extremities; signs of hypovolemia, such as flat neck veins and diminished pulse; and provocative responses, such as orthostatic hypotension and improvement in BP with leg lift.[189] Normalcy of vital signs must consider what is "normal" for each patient.[335] A BP of 110/70 may be *abnormal* for the chronic hypertensive patient whose usual BP is 170/95.

Occasionally only a single vital sign will be perceived as abnormal. Resting tachycardia may be an important clue to hyperthyroidism,[97] diabetes,[91] cardiomyopathy, or drug effects. A chronic low BP may be due to Addison's disease.[260] Tachypnea deserves special mention because it is relatively unusual and often has an important cause. Stimuli of respiratory drive include hypoxemia, hypercarbia, metabolic acidosis, pulmonary congestion, sympathetic stimulation, anemia, fever, pregnancy, head injury, sepsis, theophylline, amphetamine, and cocaine. **Occasionally an altered vital sign is particularly related to a perioperative event, such as hypertension because of bladder distension.[93] The presence of bradycardia requires that hypoxemia be ruled out.[164]**

New evidence indicates that alterations of vital signs are sometimes complex. Whereas hypovolemia usually produces tachycardia and vasoconstriction, recent findings indicate that severe hypovolemia may instead result in abrupt inhibition of the sympathetic nervous outflow causing bradycardia and a further decrease in BP.[262] Experimental application of lower body negative pressure to simulate orthostatic hypovolemia has demonstrated this response, which is thought to explain the paradoxic bradycardia that has been observed in humans during hypotensive hemorrhage.[257]

Airway Evaluation

Airway management is a primary responsibility of the anesthesiologist, and preoperative airway assessment is essential.[261] The medical history may provide clues to potential problems such as "obstructive sleep apnea," congenital syndromes, prior neck or facial surgery, description of stridor or hoarseness,[350] pain or paresthesia during neck movement, loose or missing teeth,[342] dental work, "heartburn after eat-

---

BOX 1-2
MEDICAL CONDITIONS ASSOCIATED WITH POTENTIAL AIRWAY PROBLEMS

Soft tissue enlargement

Obstructive sleep apnea
Cushing's syndrome
Steroid therapy
Down's syndrome (tongue)
Acromegaly
Abscess: oral/pharyngeal
Tonsil enlargement
Epiglottitis
Neck hematoma (bleeding carotid
  endarterectomy)

Restrictive oral opening

Rheumatoid arthritis
Scleroderma
Facial trauma
Overbite or large teeth
Receding mandible
Radiation therapy
Treacher Collins

Cervical spine abnormality
Restricted mobility

Ankylosing spondylitis
Surgical C-spine fusion
Congenital syndrome (e.g., Klippel-
  Feil)

Excess mobility

Rheumatoid arthritis
Atlantooccipital subluxation
C-spine fracture

---

ing," and conditions prone to esophageal reflux such as hiatal hernia, diabetes, and pregnancy. The patient may volunteer that during a prior anesthetic "they had to put the tube in when I was awake." This warning must be taken seriously, but requires clarification that an endotracheal rather than nasogastric tube is described. **Previous anesthetic records should be reviewed for airway quality, laryngoscopy, and intubation.** A history of nasal polyps, fracture, deviated septum, or rhinoplasty may make the option of nasal intubation undesirable.

Physical examination of the airway assesses the individual factors of neck, mandible, and mouth structure and mobility. Medical conditions may contribute to a difficult airway because of soft tissue enlargement, restriction of oral opening, and abnormal cervical spine mobility[219] **(Box 1-2). Classical alignment of three axes (oral, pharyngeal, and tracheal) facilitates visualization of the larynx**[10] **and is accomplished by anterior flexion of the lower cervical spine plus extension of the atlanto-occipital joint.** The awake patient who can assume this position without pain or paresthesias has a favorable physical situation with respect to airway management.

Neck mobility facilitating these positions must be examined preoperatively. A short or muscular neck may impose significant limitations. Nichol and Zuck demonstrated that the atlanto-occipital distance was an important factor in neck extension.[227] Laryngoscopy and intubation is made more challenging by conditions such as a prominent maxilla, high arched palate, protruding upper teeth, limited ability to open the mouth, a small or receding mandible, and restricted mobility of the gliding temporal mandibular joint. These factors were described by Cass et al., who analyzed five cases of difficult laryngoscopy.[36] White and Kander used radiographs to evaluate 13 difficult intubation patients and found enlargement of man-

dible, reduced mobility of the temporomandibular joint, and reduction of space between the spinous processes to be factors.[339] A common guideline is that the mandibular distance between the inside of the chin and the most superiorly palpable neck structure, namely the hyoid bone, be at least two fingerbreadths. Inspection and palpation of the trachea, especially in patients who have had prior neck surgery, cancer, or radiation therapy is important. A deviated or immobile trachea warns that intubation may be difficult.

The view afforded by the open mouth has been used to predict the difficulty of laryngoscopy and intubation. Mallampati et al. used the view afforded by the open mouth to predict difficulty of laryngoscopy: faucial pillars, soft palate, and uvula (Class I), and faucial pillars and soft palate, but not uvula (Class II).[194] Cormack and Lehane described four grades of intubation difficulty depending on the view obtained by direct laryngoscopy: most of the glottis (Grade I), only posterior glottis (Grade II), only epiglottis (Grade III), and no epiglottis (Grade IV).[54] In some cases, indirect laryngoscopy may be useful to identify vocal cord motion or structural abnormalities of the larynx.

Two conditions, lower airway obstruction and atlantoaxial subluxation, pose treacherous problems even though patients may be asymptomatic. Potential lower airway obstruction must be suspected when a patient has the diagnosis of **anterior mediastinal mass.**[225,229] Several cases have been reported in which no ventilation was possible after anesthesia was induced. Despite the contention that the surgery may be minor (e.g., "just a biopsy"), anesthesia is a major concern. Preoperative evaluation should include computed tomography (CT) of the chest to determine if airway compression is present, including below the carina. **Atlantoaxial subluxation** of the cervical spine may cause symptoms of neck pain, stiffness, torticollis, and extremity paresthesia. Patients with rheumatoid arthritis,[151] infections of the posterior pharynx, neck trauma, and some congenital syndromes may be at risk.[141] Asymptomatic normal children[9] may be susceptible because of flexibility of the transverse ligament and underdeveloped odontoid process.

Respiratory Assessment

A careful physical examination may identify potential respiratory problems. Greene and Berkowitz found the quality of the preoperative cough to have a sensitivity of 81% and a specificity of 86% for prediction of postoperative pulmonary complications.[126] **Yet the physical examination may be less dependable than commonly assumed.** Schneider and Anderson reported on the examinations by 9 physicians of 13 patients with various degrees of emphysema.[270] Seventeen items, including the presence of barrel chest, lip pursing, cyanosis, coarse rales, kyphosis, use of accessory muscles, hyperresonance, diminished breath sounds, decreased chest expansion, neck vein distension, edema, and impaired cardiac dullness were assessed. There was striking disagreement as to whether a particular sign was present. Over 40% of the physicians disagreed on the presence of rales, hyperresonance, barrel chest, and use of accessory muscles in a patient with known severe emphysema. Similarly, almost 50% of the physicians disagreed on the presence or absence of hyperresonance, diminished breath sounds, and rales in a patient who was known to be without disease! Godfrey et al. also found significant observer variation in assessment of physical signs of airway obstruction.[114]

McFadden et al. found that retraction of the sternocleidomastoid muscle was the only sign that correlated with severe impairment of pulmonary function in a group of asthmatic patients during acute bronchospasm.[207] Dyspnea, wheezing, retraction, and auscultated wheezes were assumed to indicate significant disease. Resolution of dyspnea did not guarantee normal lung function; often the latter remained between 40% to 50% of predicted normal. Auscultated wheezing was the last sign to abate and remained present even when patients believed the attack had resolved. A different conclusion was reached by Shim and William, who compared the patient's rating of asthma severity with that of experienced physicians.[279] Quantitative measurement of peak expiratory flow rates revealed physicians' estimations to be quite inaccurate, and the patients' estimates closer to true values. Discrepancy in subjective vs. objective measurements was illustrated by Semmes et al., who assessed the ability of ICU personnel to estimate patients' tidal volumes.[275] The correlation to measured tidal volumes was poor.

In contrast, Stubbing et al. did find good correlation between physical signs and spirometric lung volumes in COPD patients.[308] Signs significantly related to airflow obstruction included tracheal descent, scalene muscle contraction, costal margin movement, and site of most prominent palpable cardiac contraction. Pardee et al. observed that four variables, requiring no special equipment, accurately predicted failure to wean from ventilatory support.[234] These were pulse ≥ 120 or ≤ 70, respiratory rate ≥ 30, palpable inspiratory scalene muscle recruitment, and palpable expiratory abdominal muscle tensing.

Although the *physical examination* may not be as accurate as spirometric measurement, it is useful in identifying patients with potential respiratory problems. *Inspection* may find a barrel-shaped thorax, suggestive of chronic obstructive lung disease, or kyphoscoliosis, obesity, pectus excavation, prior mastectomy, radiation therapy or burn scar suggestive of restrictive physiology. Scars from chest tube placement, tracheostomy, or thoracotomy indicate significant respiratory history. Peripheral signs of disease include cyanosis, clubbing, and nicotinc finger stains. Tachypnea is suggested when the patient must pause mid-sentence to inspire. Pursed-lip exhalation suggests obstructive disease. Accessory muscle use suggests lung disease or impaired diaphragm function. Use of extra pillows or inclined head of the bed raises the question of orthopnea. Ability to take a deep breath and cough vigorously is a basic indicator of the ability to clear atelectasis and secretions. *Palpation* identifies asymmetric chest excursion and accessory muscle use. A receding diaphragm during inspiration suggests phrenic nerve dysfunction. Abnormal tactile fremitus is present in lung disease. *Percussion* of the posterior chest measures diaphragm excursion and abnormal pleural fluid or consolidation. *Auscultation* should demonstrate clear, bilateral breath sounds. Abnormal breath sounds may occur with atelectasis, pulmonary infection, reactive airway disease, or congestive heart failure and indicate chest radiographic evaluation. Lack of auscultative abnormalities does not rule out intraoperative problems. The patient with reactive airways may be asymptomatic preoperatively, yet develop marked bronchospasm and wheezing when the trachea is intubated. Provocative preoperative maneuvers such as a forced vital capacity exhalation may elicit wheezing that is otherwise silent.

Cardiovascular System Assessment

The examination of the cardiovascular system includes the search for significant conditions including hypertension, atherosclerosis, valvular heart disease, and congestive heart failure. In addition, cardiac rhythm, rate, volume status, contractility, and reserve should be assessed.

Table 1-10 Some characteristics of secondary hypertension

Etiology	History	Physical examination	Routine laboratory tests
Renovascular	Abrupt onset or worsening of HTN; flank pain or history of abdominal trauma	Abdominal bruit; palpable kidney	May resemble aldosteronism
Primary aldosteronism	Headache; weakness; fatigue; muscle cramps; polyuria	Diastolic HTN; absent edema	Hypokalemia ECG with U waves and premature contractions; low urine specific gravity; alkalosis
Pheochromocytoma	Family history (10%); paroxysmal HTN; headaches; sweating; palpitations; weight loss; psychologic symptoms	Fever; pallor; postural hypotension; tachycardia; HTN with palpation; cutaneous lesions of neurofibromatosis	ECG with premature ventricular contractions (PVCs)
Cushing's syndrome	Weakness; fatigue; bruisability; personality changes; amenorrhea	Body habitus; truncal adipose tissue; purple striae; edema; moon facies	Glucosuria; radiographic evidence of osteoporosis
Aortic coarctation	Epistaxis; claudication	Diminished lower extremity pulses; systolic HTN	Rib notching on chest radiograph

Hypertension **must be determined with respect to patient's age, sex, and circumstance.**[228,316] A history of significant hypertension may be evident from end organ effects.[167,178] Fundoscopic examination may reveal retinal changes. Signs of secondary hypertension should be sought and may include palpable kidney, abdominal bruit, lability in BP, weight loss, pallor, enlarged thyroid gland, truncal obesity, pigmented abdominal striae, acromegalic features, absent lower extremity pulses, and differences in BP between arms and legs[24,173,185,336,346] (Table 1-10).

The physical examination may yield signs suggesting *atherosclerosis.*[283] Subcutaneous or tendinous xanthomas suggests hypercholesteremia, as does circumferential arcus senilis ring around the iris in persons under age 50.[75] An abnormal light reflex as well as an abnormal vessel caliber and tortuosity are associated with coronary artery disease.[211] A diagonal crease in the earlobe is a controversial sign.[186] Trophic changes of the skin of lower extremities may be due to impaired arterial perfusion. Hypertension, gouty changes of the great toes, and obesity also indicate risk factors. Direct evidence for atherosclerosis is present when a carotid or femoral bruit is auscultated. The examination of the heart may strengthen the diagnosis. A soft systolic murmur at the apex, radiating to the axilla and heard only during chest pain, is suggestive of ischemic papillary muscle dysfunction.[202] Accentuation of the fourth heart sound by hand grip exercise has been noted but recently debated.[292]

Auscultation of a diastolic bruit created by turbulent blood flow in a stenotic coronary artery has been reported but is likely to be a subtle finding.[62]

The physical examination may help rule out atherosclerosis.[282] Pain reproduced by palpation of a costochondral junction or ribs, or by motion of the neck or shoulder, suggests an inflammatory or traumatic cause. A pericardial friction rub suggests pericarditis,[76] whereas a midsystolic click and late systolic murmur suggest mitral prolapse. A narrowed pulse pressure and systolic murmur suggest aortic stenosis whose compensatory left ventricular hypertrophy is a recognized cause of ischemic chest pain. A difference in BP between the arms may indicate a dissecting aortic aneurysm.[254]

The discovery of a *heart murmur* **during preoperative evaluation has several implications.** The risk of surgery may be increased, as in valvular aortic stenosis. The type of murmur and compensatory changes may have implications for choice of anesthetic and monitoring. Antibiotics for endocarditis prophylaxis may be indicated. History suggesting a heart murmur may include exertional dyspnea, palpitations, fatigue, chest pain, a family history of heart disease or early death, or an episode of rheumatic fever.[19,331] Syncope may occur from aortic stenosis.[190,273] The patient's awareness of an exaggerated, bounding pulse suggests aortic insufficiency.[291] A history of hemoptysis or systemic emboli is characteristic of mitral stenosis[274] although mitral regurgitation

Table 1-11   Change in murmur intensity with diagnostic maneuver

Maneuver	Right sided	Aortic stenosis	Idiopathic hypertrophic subaortic stenosis	Mitral regurgitation	Ventricular septal defect
Inspiration	↑	↓	↓	↓	↓
Exhalation	↓	↑	↑	↑	↑
Valsalva	↓	↓	↑	↓	↓
Leg elevation	—	—	↓	—	—
Handgrip	—	—	↓	↑	↑
Arterial occlusion	—	—	—	↑	↑

Type of murmur*

*Arrows indicate the intensity of change in most patients studied. Dashes indicate that either the intensity was unchanged or that neither an increase nor decrease characterized a majority of patients.
From Lembo NJ et al: Bedside diagnosis of systolic murmurs, *N Engl J Med* 318:1572, 1988.

also causes pulmonary congestion.[23] Sharp chest pains have been associated with mitral valve prolapse.

Auscultation identifies the location, intensity, timing (systolic or diastolic), radiation pattern, pitch, and shape (crescendo, decrescendo) of the heart murmur. Whereas auscultation is a skill that grows with experience, even experienced physicians may interpret various murmurs differently. Raftery and Holland reported that when five experienced physicians examined 32 patients, significant differences of opinion occurred. Two normal patients were diagnosed to have mitral stenosis although a phonocardiogram did not detect the murmur![243] Accepting some uncertainty in the auscultatory evaluation, the physician should seek corroborating evidence. Differentiation of systolic murmurs can be facilitated by maneuvers including inspiration and exhalation, Valsalva and Mueller maneuvers, squatting vs. standing, leg elevation, handgrip, transient arterial occlusion, and amyl nitrate inhalation (Table 1-11). These techniques have enabled physicians to differentiate among hypertrophic cardiomyopathy, ventricular septal defect, mitral regurgitation, and aortic stenosis.[181] Assessment of pulse and BP is helpful.[38,239] A wide pulse pressure suggests aortic insufficiency, although patent ductus arteriosus and arteriovenous fistula may also demonstrate this sign. The large forward stroke volume of aortic insufficiency contributes to the "water hammer pulse." Aortic stenosis exhibits a diminished and delayed stroke volume giving rise to a narrow pulse pressure described as "parvus et tardus." The chest radiograph and ECG provide important information. Although heart disease can exist without cardiac enlargement, the finding of cardiomegaly on a chest radiograph is real evidence of pathology. Other findings may include increased pulmonary artery size, pulmonary vascular congestion, enlargement of left atrium, abnormal calcium

deposits, and abnormal shape of the heart. The ECG can strengthen the diagnosis of valvular heart disease by the findings of atrial and ventricular hypertrophy as well as the "strain" pattern of aortic stenosis.

Signs of *congestive heart failure* **such as third heart sound, cardiomegaly, pulmonary rales, jugular venous distension, and peripheral edema have been correlated with reduced ejection fractions.**[38,79,239] Recently, questions have been raised regarding the reliability of these signs for estimating hemodynamics in chronic heart failure.[197] Stevenson and Perloff found 18 of 43 patients lacked rales, edema, or elevated jugular pressure, yet had a pulmonary capillary wedge pressure ≥22 mm Hg.[197] They concluded that the patient's pulse pressure correlated better to the cardiac index. Another problem is that reduction in normal activity level may give a false impression of adequate compensation.[120,301]

Failure of the left ventricle is expected to produce pulmonary congestion and signs of reduced forward flow, such as fatigue.[281] Pallor, oliguria, and postprandial abdominal discomfort may occur because of vasoconstriction.[351] Failure of the right ventricle may be evidenced by jugular venous distension and pulsations, liver enlargement, peripheral edema, and abnormal neck vein distension when pressure is applied to the periumbilical region[161] (Box 1-3). Other causes of elevated venous pressure include cor pulmonale, tricuspid stenosis or insufficiency, constrictive pericarditis, pericardial effusion, and pulmonary hypertension. In congestive failure, the Valsalva maneuver causes a square wave change in pressure, whereas in normal patients, characteristic decreases and overshoot in the BP and heart rate occur.

Other characteristics of the cardiac examination include assessment of rate and rhythm. Goldman et al.[120] have identified the presence of non-sinus rhythm or premature ventricular contractions as predictive of

BOX 1-3
FRAMINGHAM CRITERIA FOR CONGESTIVE HEART FAILURE

Major criteria	Minor criteria
Orthopnea	Ankle edema
Paroxysmal nocturnal dyspnea	Night cough
	Dyspnea on exertion
Neck vein distension	Hepatomegaly
Rales	Pleural effusion
Cardiomegaly	Decreased vital
Acute pulmonary edema	capacity
S₃ gallop	Tachycardia (> 120)
Increased venous pressure (16 cm H₂O)	
Circulation time > 25 sec	
Hepatojugular reflux	

From McGee PA, Castelli WP, McNamara PM et al: The natural history of congestive heart failure: The Framingham Study, *N Engl J Med* 26:1441, 1971.

cardiac complications.[119] A regular pulse does not guarantee sinus rhythm since a junctional rhythm is quite regular. Cannon "A" waves in the jugular venous pulse may be seen in a junctional rhythm, in various degrees of heart block, or in premature beats. "A" waves will be absent in atrial fibrillation which is also suggested by an irregularly irregular pulse. A patient's volume status is influenced by intravenous fluids, diuretic use, bleeding, and other factors. Physical signs suggesting hypovolemia include tachycardia, dry mouth, absence of moisture on axillary skin, decreased skin turgor, and absence of jugular venous distension in the supine position. Changes in BP, pulse, or sensorium in the sitting vs. the supine position suggest decreased volume. A paradoxic pulse is nonspecific and may be seen in hypovolemia, as well as in conditions of cardiac tamponade, mediastinal mass, and acute asthma.[278] Adequacy of cardiac output can be estimated by urine output, warm extremities, and normal mentation. **The ability to identify the patient whose cardiovascular system is reliant upon an activated sympathetic nervous system greatly aids in planning an anesthetic.**

Abdominal Examination

Examination of the abdomen can yield useful findings to the anesthesiologist.[62,122] Each scar may prompt the patient's memory of prior anesthetics and surgery. A midepigastric scar may indicate procedures such as a vagotomy or antrectomy, which may enhance the potential for gastroesophageal reflux. Prior laparotomy predicts adhesions that may increase the length

and blood loss of abdominal surgery. Portal hypertension or vena caval obstruction may cause prominent superficial abdominal veins. Abdominal striae due to previous pregnancy are white. Striae that are red or purple suggest excess levels of cortisol. **Abdominal distension is an important finding because it represents a risk for gastroesophageal reflux.**[250] Abdominal distension may occur from swallowed air; delayed gastric emptying from anxiety, pain, or narcotics; bowel obstruction; or ascites. Hyperactive vs. absent bowel sounds facilitates diagnosis. Lower abdominal distension in a female also raises the possibility of pregnancy. Obesity may predispose to increased surgical risk.[236]

Palpation of the abdomen should include assessment for prominence or tenderness of the liver. Castell et al. have suggested that estimation of liver size by dullness to percussion technique is more accurate than the distance of the liver below the rib margin.[37] Pain on palpation may be due to congestion from ventricular failure,[46] inflammation from infectious hepatitis, or gallbladder disease.[106] Positive findings should prompt an evaluation of liver function tests. Suspicion of infectious hepatitis represents a risk to both patient and health care team.[72,107] **Tenderness of the flank or suprapubic region may occur in the presence of a urinary tract infection.** Bladder distension may be secondary to prostatic disease, neurogenic dysfunction, or polyuria of diabetes. Such findings decrease the usefulness of urine output as a monitor and may predict bladder distension in the perioperative period, a potent stimulus to hypertension.[93] Auscultation for abdominal bruits may discover findings of abdominal aortic aneurysm or renal artery stenosis.

Neurologic, Muscular, and Skeletal Examination

Assessment of neurologic function begins with an appraisal of mental alertness. Pupil size will be useful to assess anesthetic depth and narcotic effect. Preoperative anisocoria should also be noted. Cranial and facial nerve functions may be altered by surgery, positioning problems, or pressure from the face mask, hence baseline information is useful. Ability to discriminate pinprick or temperature sensation will be necessary for assessment of a spinal or epidural anesthetic. Lower extremity weakness or sensory deficit may make spinal or epidural technique undesirable. **Assessment of preoperative neurologic function is important before procedures that may affect neurologic function such as carotid artery surgery,[80] aortic cross-clamping, or cardiopulmonary bypass.**[226]

Examination of the musculoskeletal system may provide clues to important systemic disease[210] and neuromuscular diseases that increase risk of anesthesia.[52,86,127] **Patients with neuromuscular, connective**

Table 1-12 Symptoms and signs of neuromuscular disease	
Symptoms	**Signs**
Weakness	Flaccid weakness, hyporeflexia
Wasting	Atrophy
Twitching	Fasciculation
Pain	Tenderness
Swelling	Mass, enlargement, induration
Spasms	Spasms, delayed relaxation
Stiffness	Persistent contraction at rest

From Layzer RL: *Neuromuscular manifestations of systemic disease*, Philadelphia, 1985, FA Davis.

tissue, and various endocrine disorders may describe muscle weakness. Examples include myasthenia gravis, muscular dystrophy, polymyositis, dermatomyositis, hyperthyroidism, hypothyroidism, glucocorticoid excess, adrenal insufficiency, hyperaldosteronism, and hyperparathyroidism. Mineral, electrolyte, and vitamin abnormalities such as hypokalemia, hyperkalemia, hypermagnesemia, hypercalcemia, hypophosphatemia, and barium poisoning may present as weakness, whereas hypocalcemia and hypomagnesemia produce hyperreflexia. Muscular symptoms and related physical findings are illustrated in Table 1-12. Some signs of neuromuscular disease are distinctive,[240,241] such as arched foot known as *pes cavus* or inward rotation of the ankles known as *talipes equinovarus*. To the experienced eye, the patient with myotonic dystrophy has a characteristic face that includes thinned frontal hair, wasting of the temporalis muscle, and expressionless features.

Some simple muscle tests may help to clarify symptoms of weakness. Proximal muscle strength is illustrated by ability to abduct arms (deltoids) or by supine leg raising (iliopsoas). Distal muscle strength is illustrated by spreading of the fingers (intrinsic hand muscles) or dorsiflexion of the foot (tibialis anterior). The patient who fails to release a firm handshake should be suspected of having a myotonic disorder. Muscle reflexes may be diminished in muscular disease or delayed in hypothyroidism. Reflexes are more brisk in hyperthyroidism or upper motor neuron diseases. Skeletal abnormalities also provide clues important to anesthetic planning. Distinctive stature may be noted in patients with acromegaly and Marfan's syndrome.[224] Joint deformities indicating rheumatoid arthritis raise concerns for atlantooccipital instability.[55] Ankylosing spondylitis may have associated aortic insufficiency.[324] Patients with pectus excavatum may harbor other congenital cardiac abnormalities.

PREOPERATIVE LABORATORY TESTS
Controversial Issues

The American Cancer Society advocates six screening tests for malignancy.[252] The rationale is that the tests can detect *asymptomatic* disease. **Preoperative screening tests have been used to try to detect asymptomatic disease before anesthesia and surgery.** Such preoperative laboratory testing has been extensively criticized[20,252] for lack of impact on patient care, unnecessary high costs, potential for increased physician liability, and the difficulties that arise when an isolated unexplained abnormal test is found. These criticisms will be evaluated with reference to the data from which they were raised.

A major argument against routine preoperative screening tests in asymptomatic patients is that they have little impact on outcome. How was this concluded? Many studies were based on retrospective chart review. The authors determined what constituted "impact," such as cancellation or delay of surgery, and then evidence for impact was sought in the record. Unless the record specifically indicated that the test had impact, it was not considered to have been important, either way. Korvin et al., for instance, analyzed preoperative laboratory results for 1001 patients and concluded that in *only one instance* did a test contribute to patient care.[169] A postoperative elevation of liver enzymes occurred in a patient who had received halothane and the test prevented reexposure. Yet in the other 1000 cases, 87 new diagnoses were suggested by the screening tests, including 7 cases of uremia and 30 cases of hepatobiliary disease, 3 of which were viral hepatitis. Evidence was found for diabetes or hypercholesterolemia in 19 cases. Considering that these are modifiable risk factors for coronary disease, the leading cause of death in the United States, a number of patients may have benefited despite the fact that surgery was not postponed. Although retrospective chart review has obvious limitations, Kaplan et al. suggest that such review is too expensive and time consuming. They recommend that retrospective analysis of computer demographic data and discharge diagnoses could judge the appropriateness of preoperative tests. Thus, their conclusion that 60% of preoperative laboratory tests were performed on patients who lacked a recognized medical indication was based on information already processed several times. Pertinent is the finding of Kempczinski that in some cases as many as 60% of clinical events may not be recorded in discharge diagnoses.[165]

Another question is whether appropriate tests were used for assessment. Delahunt and Turnbull reported that 803 patients underwent 1792 routine preoperative tests, namely, blood chemistries and chest radiographs, before varicose vein stripping or inguinal hernia repair.[64] The authors concluded that none of the laboratory tests altered patient management. However, the one complication noted was a death that occurred in a 57-year-old hypertensive male following an intraoperative cardiac arrest. We wonder if a preoperative ECG would have led to a different conclusion.

A frequent explanation for lack of impact is that abnormal laboratory results are often ignored by physicians. Consider the work of O'Conner and Drasner who examined impact of preoperative hematocrit and urinalysis in pediatric patients. Laboratory tests suggested previously unknown anemia or microcytosis in 73 children. Appropriate follow-up testing or treatment could be documented in only seven cases, six of which received a new diagnosis or new therapy. Unfortunately, 66 of the children with anemia or microcytosis had no documented follow-up observation. Bates and Yellin used physician questionnaires to assess the impact of abnormalities found on multiphasic screening tests. The primary impediment between the reported abnormalities and new management was physician failure to confirm findings.[14] Turnball and Buck determined by chart review of 1010 cholecystectomy patients that only 4 patients could have received a conceivable benefit from a preoperative screening test.[325] Part of the reason may have been that "action was taken" in only 17 of 104 potentially significant abnormalities.[11] Of the cases where "no action was taken," five patients had postoperative urinary tract infections, five had postoperative pulmonary complications, and four had postoperative cardiac complications. **The deficiency in these examples is not in the laboratory test but in the physician responsible for patient care. If the decision is made to order *any* laboratory test, there is a valid obligation to follow up its results, whether or not that follow-up delays surgery.**

The major argument against screening tests is that most of the significant abnormal results are already suggested by the history and physical examination. Unfortunately this literature assessment has been based on retrospective review and may not have been applicable during prospective preoperative evaluation. For example, risk factors such as age, sex, hypertension, and smoking should perhaps have predicted the presence of atherosclerosis in a patient who suffered a postoperative MI. However, a routine ECG demonstrating an old silent myocardial infarction might have triggered considerably more extensive evaluation.

Cost of preoperative laboratory testing is another major issue.[25,44] Before 1986, virtually all third party payors paid hospitals for such testing. Further, the "cost/charge ratio" (e.g., the ratio of the actual cost of the test to the amount billed to the carrier) was, of course, a major source of profit for hospitals. Most hospitals are "not for profit" organizations, and these profits were used to offset losses from other unprofitable areas. This is one of many ways hospitals utilize "cost-shifting." With Medicare's adoption of the Diagnosis Related Group (DRG) system, hospitals receive a lump sum payment based on diagnosis, not treatment. Suddenly, the more preoperative testing in Medicare patients, the *less* profit! Is it entirely coincidental, therefore, that so many recent studies are now attacking the performance of routine screening tests in asymptomatic patients?

Often, the best way a physician can resist these pressures is to perform a more careful history and physical examination. If a laboratory test can be rationally *indicated*, after the history and examination, then good medical care is given, assuming that the positive test results are properly followed up.

The contention that preoperative laboratory testing may increase medicolegal liability is discussed by Kaplan et al.[159]: "A complication traceable to an overlooked result more readily suggests legal liability than does a complication possibly related to the absence of a test that neither hospital policy nor medical literature considers appropriate." Although this posture may protect physicians who ignore abnormal findings, is this a valid perspective? Are a patient's chances for good outcome improved by obtaining the test with the hope that the physician will investigate any abnormality, or by not obtaining the test at all? **The anesthesiologist is either simply a "preoperative evaluator," whose only job is to safely get the patient through tomorrow's surgery, or he/she is a physician who needs to act like a doctor preoperatively.** We most strongly disagree with this kind of negative real or imagined liability-driven reasoning.

Electrocardiogram

The electrocardiogram (ECG) has often been used to screen for evidence of cardiac disease.[48,248,290] Numerous studies used findings on the preoperative ECG as an independent predictors of perioperative cardiac complications.[69,110,119,150] **Goldman et al. established that either the presence of a non-sinus rhythm or the documentation of more than five premature ventricular contractions was an independent indicator of increased risk.**[119] These two alone accounted for one fourth of the potential risk and were as important as the risk factors determined by history, namely age > 70 years, myocardial infarction in the previous 6 months; or those determined by physical examination, namely S_3 gallop, jugular vein distension, or important valvular aortic stenosis. Detsky et al. modified the Goldman cardiac risk index significantly and expanded use of the preoperative ECG to include: prior infarction on ECG, left ventricular hypertrophy on ECG, non-sinus rhythm or premature atrial beats, and more than 5 premature ventricular beats.[69] Cooperman et al. studied peripheral vascular surgery patients and also found that dysrhythmia on the preoperative ECG was a risk factor for cardiac complication.[53] Each study probably underestimated the significance of the preoperative ECG because patients whose surgery was delayed or cancelled because of ECG abnormalities were excluded.

Numerous studies have determined that a myocardial infarction occurring within 6 months before surgery carries a significantly increased risk for reinfarction.[296,315] Because these reinfarctions have approximately 50% mortality, an important function of the preoperative evaluation is to rule out a recent infarction. If one out of every four myocardial infarctions are clinically unrecognized (e.g., the patient is asymptomatic) the preoperative ECG might be useful to detect high-risk patients. Goldberger and O'Konski point out that because the incidence of unrecognized infarctions increases markedly with age, such an unrecognized infarction occurring within the prior 6 months is unlikely in a young person[116] (Table 1-13). Yet consider that such an infarction may occur in a 35-year-old man with an incidence of 3.2 per 10,000 persons. If anesthesia and surgery within 6 months of that event precipitate a reinfarction in 30% of cases and if half these reinfarctions are fatal, the incidence of mortality would be 0.5/10,000 persons, a number similar to several recent published statistics for overall anesthetic risk of death.

An objection to the routine preoperative ECG is that important information can be acquired by patient history and physical examination. However, in the Goldman et al. analysis of over 50 preoperative history and physical findings, most were not found to be predictive of outcome. Moorman et al. evaluated this question for a routine admission ECG in 1410 general medical patients. Patients were divided into two groups on the basis of whether a cardiac problem was suggested by history or physical examination. In patients with suspected cardiac problems, the admission ECG provided new information in 6.9% of the cases, a number the authors believed justified these routine ECGs. In patients where no cardiac problem was suspected, the admission ECG provided "new information" in 1.0% of cases. Although the yield was low, the authors concluded that the cost effectiveness of these ECGs was in the same range as other accepted medical practices.[215] However, Moorman et al.'s "new information" criteria are not equivalent to abnormality. In fact, of the 1410 admission ECGs, 75% were actually abnormal (Table 1-14). Why this apparent discrepancy? If an abnormality was present on a prior ECG, it was not counted as *new information.* Therefore the Moorman study did not evaluate the usefulness of a single ECG but rather the usefulness of two ECGs. In fact, it is remarkable that for patients with already suspected cardiac problems by history, physical examination, or a prior ECG, the routine ECG *still* provided *new* information in almost 7% of the cases.

Another argument against ECG evaluation has been that many abnormalities are nonspecific changes that do not affect patient management. Recent evidence suggests that nonspecific changes may be meaningful indicators of coronary disease. Harlan et al. reported on a group of 1056 healthy 24-year-old naval aviators who were followed until age 61 for development of coronary artery disease. The men had resting cardiograms obtained at ages 24, 36, 42, and 54 years. T wave flattening and lengthening of the PR interval during ages 24 to 42 appeared predictive of subsequent ischemic heart disease.[133]

Table 1-13   Estimated semiannual incidence of Q-wave myocardial infarction in men and women by age groups*

Age (yrs)	Men† Unrecognized infarctions	Men† All infarctions	Women† Unrecognized infarctions	Women† All infarctions
30-34	0.13	0.64	0.0	0.11
35-44	0.32	1.91	0.13	0.26
45-54	0.83	3.61	0.14	0.65
55-64	1.41	5.40	0.90	2.35
65-74	2.69	7.05	1.06	2.78
75-84	3.01	5.64	1.70	6.42

*These estimates assume constant 10-year incidence. Data derived from 2282 men and 2845 women at risk reported by Kannel and Abbott.[156]
†Numbers refer to incidence per 1000 persons.
From Goldberger AL, O'Konski M: Utility of the routine electrocardiogram before surgery and on general hospital admission, *Ann Intern Med* 105:552, 1986.

Table 1-14   Abnormal findings in 1410 admission ECGs

Abnormality	Number of ECGs
Nonspecific repolarization	435
Left ventricular hypertropy	268
Age indeterminate infarction	197
Arrhythmia	183
Acute ischemia	113
Bundle branch block	56

From Moorman JR, Hlatky MA, Eddy DM et al: The yield of the routine admission electrocardiogram, *Ann Intern Med* 103:590, 1985.

Kannel et al. reported that nonspecific T and ST changes found on routine biannual cardiograms occurred in 14% of asymptomatic and apparently healthy persons in the Framingham population. The incidence of nonspecific changes increased with age and hypertension. During the 30 years of follow-up, coronary heart disease morbidity and mortality occurred at twice the rate among these persons as compared with those who did not have the abnormality. The combination of T wave and ST wave abnormality carried more risk than T wave abnormality alone.[157]

In their literature review, Goldberger and O'Konski concluded that the routine preoperative ECG was unnecessary in asymptomatic adult patients.[116] **While the ECG was acknowledged to be useful in identifying unrecognized myocardial infarction or certain dysrhythmias, the yield increased with age and with positive findings on the history and physical examination.** The authors proposed "new guidelines" for selective ordering of the preoperative ECG. Although clinical judgment is advised in all cases, specific groups to be considered for preoperative ECG include:

- Men over age 40, women over age 55
- Patients with diseases associated with coronary artery disease such as hypertension, diabetes, peripheral vascular disease
- Patients with disease that may have cardiac involvement such as malignancy, collagen vascular disease, or infectious diseases
- Patients using medication such as phenothiazine, antidepressants, doxorubicin
- Patients at risk for electrolyte abnormalities
- Patients having elective intrathoracic, intraperitoneal, aortic surgery, or emergency operations
- Patients having major neurosurgery

Unfortunately, these guidelines are neither new nor selective. Application of these guidelines to Goldman et al.'s surgical population, which was composed of 1001 consecutive patients over 40 years of age who underwent general, urologic, or orthopedic surgery,[119] provides interesting findings. All of the males would have received an ECG. Over 40% of the patients would have been eligible for a ECG on the basis of operative site alone. Over 28% of the patients were hypertensive, and almost 20% of the surgeries were emergent. Thus, while criticizing overuse of ECG, Goldberger and O'Konski's plan would have recommended preoperative electrocardiography for most adult patients in this study!

Hemoglobin/Hematocrit

Loss of blood is an expected occurrence in the surgical patient population. Despite promises to the contrary, blood loss is often more than anticipated and occa-

sionally much more. **Typically, anesthesiologists have recommended that the preoperative hematocrit be such that the patient has adequate reserve for such a possibility.**[4] A "safe" level of preoperative hemoglobin has been classically considered to be about 10 g/dl in the adult[58] (Table 1-15). Recently, recommendations have been proposed to accept lower levels of hemoglobin.[284] Roizen advises that the hematocrit need not even be measured in males under age 60 provided that they are healthy, asymptomatic, and undergoing peripheral surgery, with no excessive blood loss expected.[255]

The question of obtaining a preoperative hematocrit requires information about the causes and incidence of anemia. Anemia can be due to diverticulosis, rectal or other GI bleeding, gastritis, prior small bowel resection, malnutrition, renal disease, African or Mediterranean ancestry, drug reaction, malignancy, or other chronic disease.[18,60,294] **However, persons without known risk factors may also have anemia.** The Second National Health and Nutrition Examination Survey (1976-1980) determined that the incidence of anemia was highest in teenage girls (5.9%), young women (5.8%), infants (5.7%), and elderly men (4.4%). Iron deficiency was the primary cause in infants and young women, whereas inflammatory disease predominated in the elderly.[59] Berwick analyzed the results of 469 Health Fairs, which screened almost 88,703 persons in 1983. Anemia, defined as hematocrit less than 35%, was found in 7.2% of the persons.[17]

It could be argued that a preoperative hemoglobin should be obtained in any "symptomatic" patient. However, in adults, Elwood et al. found no correlation

Table 1-15 Estimated normal values for hemoglobin and hematocrit*

Age/Sex	Hemoglobin g/dl mean (lower limit)	Hematocrit % mean (lower limit)
.5-4 years	12.5 (11.0)	36 (32)
5-10 years	13.0 (11.5)	38 (33)
11-14 years		
Female	13.5 (12.0)	39 (34)
Male	14.0 (12.0)	41 (35)
15-19 years		
Female	13.5 (12.0)	40 (34)
Male	15.0 (13.0)	43 (37)
20-44 years		
Female	13.5 (12.0)	40 (35)
Male	15.5 (13.5)	45 (39)

*Unbracketed numbers are the mean values and those in parentheses are the lower limit of normal.
From Dallman PR: Blood and blood forming tissues. In Rudolph AM, ed: *Pediatrics*, Norwalk, Conn, 1987, Appleton and Lange.

between level of hemoglobin from 8 to 12 g/dl and presence of any of six symptoms commonly attributed to anemia, namely palpitations, fatigue, irritability, dizziness, dyspnea, and headache.[87] Symptoms of fatigue, dyspnea, and ankle edema may not appear until hemoglobin is below 7 g/dl.[328] Findings on physical examination of the chronically anemic patient may also not be striking, but can include pallor, slight edema, bounding pulse, hyperdynamic precordium, systolic ejection murmur, and cervical venous hum. Tachycardia is not prominent because chronic anemia is associated with increased stroke volume rather than heart rate to increase cardiac output. The signs of anemia are also indistinct in pediatric patients. Keyes et al. could find no relationship between level of hematocrit between 19% and 64% and heart rate, respiratory rate, or incidence of bradycardia in a group of premature infants.[166]

Despite a lack of symptoms or signs, anemia has been implicated in morbidity. Infant developmental test scores have improved when iron deficiency anemia was treated adequately with supplemental iron.[192] Low maternal hemoglobin in early pregnancy has been associated with premature births, low birth weights, and perinatal mortality.[217]

When considering whether a preoperative hemoglobin/hematocrit should be measured, it is useful to review the recommendations of others for the general population. The American Academy of Pediatrics recommends screening for anemia at ages 1 to 4 years, 5 to 12 years, and 14 to 20 years.[5] The American College of Obstetricians and Gynecologists recommends prenatal screening for anemia.[6] The National Academy of Sciences Institute of Medicine has recommended screening for anemia once between 40 to 59 years, 60 to 74 years, and over age 75.[222] In their proposal for preventive medicine, Breslow and Sommers recommended screening for anemia every 5 years.[25] The Report of the United States Preventive Services Task Force[327] recommends that all pregnant women and infants be screened for anemia.

What constitutes a safe level of preoperative hemoglobin/hematocrit is a current controversy. The classic "10 g" hemoglobin/dl appears to represent a consensus opinion rather than a product of rigorous study. In a survey of anesthesia departments in the United States, Kowalyshyn in 1972 found that 88% of responders required a hemoglobin of at least 9 g/dl and 44% required a hemoglobin of at least 10 g/dl before anesthesia.[171] In a survey of "expert" opinions, Fabian found controversy with the 10 g/dl figure.[92] Citing examples of successful anesthesia in individuals with chronic anemia because of renal failure, thalassemia, malnutrition, parasitic infection, and sickle cell disease, respondents suggested that lower hematocrits could be acceptable in some circum-stances. More recently, the NIH Consensus Conference on Perioperative Red Cell Transfusion recommended that a value lower than 10 g/dl be used as a "transfusion trigger."[50] Stehling suggested that transfusion is usually indicated when hemoglobin is below 7 g/dl and that widespread use of invasive monitoring, including fiberoptic pulmonary artery catheters to calculate oxygen delivery and extraction ratio, would aid definition of the transfusion trigger for each patient.[298]

When considering these proposals, one must recognize that one major driving force is the risk posed by blood transfusion for the development of serious viral illness. To avoid transfusion, tolerance of some anemia may well be justified. Is the risk of transfusion greater than the risk of widespread invasive monitoring with pulmonary artery catheters? The "acceptable level" of hemoglobin represents a trade-off of relative risks rather than pure physiology. In other words, if blood transfusion was *100% safe,* would experts still advocate a hemoglobin level of 7 g?

Central to all arguments favoring low hemoglobin levels is the assertion that compensatory mechanisms are available to maintain adequate oxygen delivery.[102] These include increases in cardiac output, lowered systemic resistance, increased 2,3 DPG,[301] and increased oxygen extraction ratio.[322] Is utilization of these mechanisms physiologically desirable? First consider the increase in cardiac output, mediated by peripheral vasodilation plus increased sympathetic stimulation. The heart is required to do more work but is supplied with anemic blood. Hoffman has illustrated that in anemia, coronary vascular reserve is utilized to maintain oxygen balance.[145] Murray et al.[218] demonstrated in dogs that when hematocrit was lowered by 50%, the cardiac output doubled but the coronary blood flow nearly tripled. Severe chronic anemia stimulates interarterial coronary anastomoses in pigs and dogs, and Eckstein demonstrated that restoration of a normal hematocrit led to their disappearance.[84] Coronary atherosclerosis would be expected to impair the necessary coronary vascular reserve. Hagl et al.[130] in dogs demonstrated that isovolemic hemodilution caused hypokinesis in a region of restricted coronary flow, but not in the unrestricted zone. This is particularly pertinent to hemodialysis patients who are known to have increased risk of premature atherosclerosis.[187]

Distribution of blood flow within the myocardium is also a concern in anemia. Buckberg and Brazier considered that decreased oxygen delivery and perfusion pressure, plus tachycardia jeopardized subendocardial blood flow. They found that moderate degrees of hemodilution with hemoglobin equaling 5 to 10 g, were well tolerated in dogs but when moderate aortic stenosis was added, subendocardial ischemia occurred. They cautioned that **the margin of safety for acute hemodilution may be compromised by circumstances of: (1) increased oxygen requirements such as hypertension, valvular heart disease, fever; (2) decreased coronary reserve in atherosclerosis; (3) hypoxemia.**[27] These findings raise a question regarding the appropriateness of vasopressor agents in the anemic patient.

Questions also arise concerning other compensatory mechanisms. In the chronic anemic state, increased 2,3 DPG facilitates oxygen unloading. Operative blood loss of this "high efficiency" blood will result in marked decrease in oxygen delivery because stored bank blood[309] has virtually no 2,3 DPG. The "extraction ratio" compensatory mechanism also has limitations. It is true that the overall extraction is only 25% of the carried oxygen, resulting in a mixed venous O_2 saturation of 75%. Why not simply extract more? Physics of oxygen-hemoglobin binding are such that dissociation becomes more difficult at lower levels of Po_2. Further, mixed venous oxygen saturation represents global body oxygen extraction. Some organs e.g., heart, brain, and liver extract more, whereas some organs like skin, kidney, and resting muscle extract less. Thus, **measurement of mixed venous Po_2 cannot be equated with individual organ well-being.** Levine et al. used isovolemic hemodilution to lower hematocrit to 15% in healthy baboons. Hematocrit of 15% was considered safe because all animals survived, and measurement of renal and liver function 4 weeks later was normal.[184] A different conclusion was reached by Nagao et al., who studied somatosensory and visual-evoked potential in healthy baboons subjected to isovolemic hemodilution. At similar hematocrits, evidence of peripheral nerve and spinal cord hypoxia was noted.[221]

The few outcome studies of anemic surgical patients fail to provide convincing evidence that anemia is entirely safe. Morbidity and mortality do tend to be higher in the anemic patients, the authors' biases notwithstanding. Rawstron concluded after a retrospective study of anemic surgical patients:

> While there appeared to be an increase in cardiac arrests or death during surgery or in the early postoperative period in the anemia patients, it is doubtful whether this finding is significant.[244]

Gapalro concluded that transfusion was unnecessary in compensated chronic anemia after presenting details of only four uremic surgical patients, despite the fact that one suffered intraoperative cardiac arrest.[121] Carson et al. studied 125 surgical patients who declined blood transfusions for religious reasons. Operative mortality was inversely related to preoperative hematocrit and directly related to operative blood loss (Table 1-16). In patients who experienced

Table 1-16 Operative mortality according to preoperative hematocrit

Preoperative hemoglobin (g/dl)	Mortality (%)
0-6.0	8/13 (61.5%)
6.1-8.0	3/9 (33.3%)
8.1-10	0/18 (0)
>10	6/85 (7.1%)

From Carson JL, Poses RM et al: Severity of anemic and operative mortality and morbidity, *Lancet* 2:727, 1988.

the lowest blood loss (less than 500 ml), operative mortality was still 35% if preoperative hemoglobin was less than 8 g/dl.[35]

Stehling recently reported a better outcome in a 1-year study of 340 anemic patients who underwent 473 procedures. Cardiac arrest occurred in two patients (incidence 4.2 arrests/1000 anesthetics) and death occurred in six patients.[297] It might be argued that these anemic patients suffered increased morbidity because they were already suffering from life-threatening disease, but there is evidence that ability to survive life-threatening disease is related to capacity to supply oxygen to the body. Shoemaker et al. demonstrated that therapy specifically directed to maximize oxygen delivery increased survival compared with control patients.[280]

The optimal level of hemoglobin is that which provides a reasonable reserve for unanticipated stress. Anemia represents not only a deficiency in blood reserve, but a depletion of compensatory mechanisms. Ideally, hemoglobin should be measured weeks before an elective operation to allow time for diagnosis and therapy of anemia, or possibly autologous blood donation.[233] **The common practice of screening for anemia the night before surgery severely limits these options.** The idea of postoperative erythropoietin therapy is not valid: Levin et al. have demonstrated that increases in reticulocyte count and hematocrit are not seen for the first 5 postoperative days.[183] This is beyond the time of peak incidence of postoperative myocardial infarction (i.e., postoperative day 3). The best strategy to avoid blood transfusion is adequate advance preoperative planning.

Other Blood Tests

One approach to decide whether asymptomatic patients should have preoperative blood tests is to review the recommendations of others. Several authors have addressed the utility of specific tests, such as bleeding time,[11] prothrombin and partial thromboplastin times,[85,90] complete blood count, and leukocyte differential count.[276] The authors concluded that most

Table 1-17   Indications for preoperative tests

Test	Indications
Prothrombin time/partial thrombo- plastin time	Known coagulation disorder, anti- coagulant therapy, hemorrhage, anemia, liver disease, malab- sorption, malnutrition, or other potentially relevant diseases (e.g., systemic lupus erythema- tosus)
Platelet count	Known platelet abnormality, hem- orrhage, purpura, hyper- splenism, hematologic malig- nancy (e.g., leukemia), radiation/chemotherapy, throm- bosis, some anemias (e.g., aplastic), other potentially rele- vant diseases (e.g., systemic lu- pus erythematosus, paroxysmal nocturnal hemoglobinuria, or renal transplant rejection)
Hemoglobin	Potentially bloody operation (de- termined by need for preopera- tive crossmatch), chronic renal failure, known anemia, bleeding disorder, hemorrhage, hemato- logic malignancy, radiation/ chemotherapy, or other poten- tially relevant diseases (e.g., some infections, liver diseases, or malnutrition)
White blood cell count and differ- ent cell count	Infection, diseases of white blood cells, including leukemia, radiation/chemotherapy, immu- nosuppressive therapy, hyper- splenism, aplastic anemia, or other potentially relevant dis- eases (e.g., rheumatoid arthritis)
Six-factor automated multiple analysis	Age 60 yr or over, diuretic usage, renal disease, other fluid/ electrolyte abnormalities (e.g., diarrhea, syndrome of inappro- priate secretion of antidiuretic hormone, diabetes insipidus, or severe liver disease), or other potentially relevant diseases (e.g., convulsions)
Glucose level	Diabetes mellitus, hypoglycemia, steroid treatment, pancreatic disease (e.g., pancreatitis, carci- noma, or glucagonoma), pitu- itary disease (e.g., acromegaly), hypothalamic disease, or adre- nal disease

From Kaplan EB, Sheiner LB, Boeckmann AJ et al: The usefulness of preoperative laboratory screening, *JAMA* 253(24):3576, 1985.

Table 1-18   Results of routine blood tests in 1000 patients

Test	Abnormal	New diagnosis
Elevated bilirubin or aspar- tate amino transferase	71	43
Hematocrit or leukocyte count	43	28
Electrolytes (Na, K, Cl)	26	8
Blood sugar	21	18
BUN	14	8

From Korvin CC, Pearce RH, and Stanley J: Admissions screening: clin- ical benefits, *Ann Int Med* 83:197, 1975.

tests were not indicated, and even when abnormalities were found, no increased morbidity occurred. Unfor- tunately, not one of the authors was an anesthesiol- ogist, and **potential usefulness of a prolonged bleeding time, low platelet count, or prolonged coagulation times in planning for anesthesia (e.g., regional block) was not addressed.** Kaplan et al. proposed that 60% of preoperative blood tests were done for no recog- nizable condition, contributed little to patient care, and could reasonably be eliminated.[159] Table 1-17 lists the medical conditions for which these authors *did* find indications for obtaining preoperative tests. It should be noted that "other potentially relevant diseases" is included for almost every test.

Korvin et al. studied results of 20 routine admis- sion blood tests in 1000 patients. Only 30% of the abnormalities were predictable by chart review, whereas 70% were unexpected.[169] Those tests most frequently leading to new diagnoses are listed in Table 1-18. Blood tests of liver function were the most frequent abnormality and also the most fre- quent cause of new diagnosis. **Screening for unsus- pected liver dysfunction is controversial. Incidence of unsuspected hepatic dysfunction found by blood tests has been noted to be approximately 1 in 700 pa- tients.**[268,333] **Some patients may be at increased risk for elevated liver enzymes, including patients with obesity, malignancy, excessive alcohol intake,[337] his- tory of hepatitis or known exposure, drugs associated with hepatocellular damage, and mononucleosis.** Antepartum screening for hepatitis B and C has been considered for all pregnant patients.[310] Several au- thors indicate that during the acute phase of liver disease, anesthesia and surgery may be contraindi- cated because of increased risk.[77,137,302] Postoperative elevation of liver function tests has been noted for patients undergoing abdominal surgery who received a variety of anesthestics including halothane, enflu- rane, and isoflurane.[148,303,330]

Chest Radiograph

Pulmonary complications account for a significant proportion of postoperative morbidity.[223] Healthy patients can be expected to experience decreased vital capacity and functional residual capacity after an upper abdominal operation.[57] Other problems include blunted responses to hypoxia and hypercapnia.[168] Stein et al.[299,300] demonstrated that patients with preoperative respiratory compromise fare less well. **The rationale for the routine preoperative chest radiograph has been to identify those patients at increased risk and to provide a baseline study should postoperative complications arise.**[213] **However, the routine chest radiograph has been questioned for infants,**[95] **children,**[26,277,345] **patients under age 20,**[259] **patients under age 30,**[246] **gynecologic patients,**[326] **pregnant patients,**[22] **the elderly,**[21,32] **preoperative patients,**[253,313,314,340] **and others.**[1,223] Are abnormalities simply nonexistent on a routine chest radiograph? Is a normal chest radiograph of no value? Has the determination of "usefulness" been made by the internist, the surgeon, or the anesthesiologist, and by what criteria? Because anesthesiologists bear the responsibility for preserving respiratory function, these questions should address our concerns.

Arguments against the preoperative chest radiograph often quote internal medicine studies in which routine admission films yielded few new findings or altered therapy. However this does not mean that the radiographs were *normal*. In the study by Hubbell et al., routine chest radiographs from 294 patients admitted to internal medicine wards demonstrated abnormalities in 36% of the cases.[147] Sagel et al. evaluated 6063 routine chest radiographs done on medical and surgical patients and noted abnormalities in 16.5% of the cases.[259] Fink et al. evaluated 113 chest radiographs taken for patient admission to Veterans Hospitals and found abnormalities in 46% of the cases.[103] Rucker et al. evaluated 905 surgical admission chest radiographs and found abnormalities in 13% of the cases.[258] Unfortunately, **what constitutes an important abnormality may depend on the author's perspective.** Hubbell et al. judged that, although abnormalities occurred in 106 routine chest radiographs, the findings were new in only 20 cases and treatment was changed in only 12 cases (4%).[147] **From an anesthesiologist's perspective, *most* of these abnormalities should be of interest** (Table 1-19). The demonstration that congestive heart failure is stable would be useful information. The presence of pulmonary infiltrate, whether new or chronic, is important. It is of interest that 6 out of 19 cases of congestive heart failure and 5 out of 6 cases of pulmonary infiltrate were new findings, suggesting that a thorough history and physical examination may be less than perfectly sensitive.

Table 1-19   Abnormalities in 106 routine medical chest radiographs

Abnormality	Chronic and/or stable abnormality	New or worsened abnormality
Cardiomegaly only	33	1
Chronic obstructive pulmonary disease	17	0
Congestive heart failure	13	6
Interstitial infiltrate	12	0
Pulmonary infiltrate	6	5
Nodules, masses, hilum	17	4
Pleural effusion	2	2
Bone metastases	2	
Pulmonary artery enlargement	1	1
Cavity disease	1	
Aortic aneurysm	1	
Rib fracture	1	1
TOTAL	106	20

From Hubbell FA, Greenfield S, Tyler JL et al: The impact of routine admission chest x-ray films on patient care, *N Engl J Med* 312(4):209, 1985.

Is there a subgroup of patients who would benefit from a routine chest radiograph preoperatively? Rucker et al. divided patients into two groups on the basis of "risk factors" determined by history, symptoms, or physical examination. Of the 368 patients with no risk factors, only one patient demonstrated an abnormality on chest radiograph. Of the 504 patients with risk factors, 114 (22%) were found to have an abnormality on chest radiograph. Rucker et al. considered age over 60 years to be a risk factor for abnormal chest radiograph [258] (Box 1-4).

The advantage of selective ordering of preoperative chest radiographs has been demonstrated by Charpak et al. in a prospective 1-year study of a protocol for preoperative test ordering.[42] Indications for a preoperative chest radiograph included: any cardiovascular disease, any pulmonary disease, known malignancy, major surgical emergencies, a history of smoking in patients who were over age 50, immunosuppression, and immigration to the United States without a prior health examination. Chest radiographs were ordered in 28% of the 3866 surgical patients. Abnormalities were found in one half of the ordered chest radiographs (Table 1-20).

The usefulness of a chest radiograph may extend beyond the requirement that it must change planned therapy. Although only 5% of the ordered chest radiographs actually modified medical decisions in the study by Charpak et al., 15% of the ordered radio-

---

BOX 1-4
RISK FACTORS FOR ABNORMAL CHEST RADIOGRAPH

History	System review	Physical examination
Cancer	Fever	Fever
Valvular heart disease	Chills	Tachycardia
Stroke	Sweats	Hypertension
Myocardial infarction	Weight loss	Abnormal breath sounds
Chronic obstructive pulmonary disease	Orthopnea	Heart murmur
Angina	PND	S_3
Asthma	Dyspnea	Displaced point of maximal impulse
Tuberculosis	Angina	Ascites
Cigarette use		Abdominal tenderness
Occupational exposure		Organomegaly
Age over 60 years		Tachypnea

From Rucker L, Frye EB, and Staten MA: Usefulness of screening chest roentgenograms in preoperative patients, *JAMA* 250(23):3209, 1983.

---

graphs were considered useful. **In fact, 41 of the chest radiographs were considered useful *because* they were *normal*. "Usefulness" was assessed *by the anesthesiologist* caring for that patient *during* the hospitalization.** This analysis is in marked contrast to the chart review technique of the various negative retrospective studies. Charpak et al. also demonstrated that selective ordering can increase yield without compromising patient safety. Their selection criteria identified patients who had the highest incidence of perioperative complications and thus benefited from preoperative radiography. The authors indicated that their 28% frequency of preoperative chest radiograph ordering was a marked reduction from the 60% rate of preoperative radiographs obtained elsewhere in France.

Urinalysis

Screening urinalysis is frequently used by physicians and insurance companies as an inexpensive means to detect important covert disease. The American Academy of Pediatrics[5] recommends urinalysis during infancy, preschool, late childhood, and early adoles-cence. The report of the United States Preventive Services Task Force 1989[247] finds that it may be clinically prudent to screen preschool children and persons aged 60 and older for asymptomatic bacteriuria, hematuria, and proteinuria. Indications for diagnostic urinalysis suggested by Akin et al.[3] are listed in Box 1-5. Studies in which *screening urinalysis* yielded positive results are listed in Table 1-21.

Preoperative urinalysis may have different indications pertaining to the events of anesthesia and surgery. The kidney may be exposed to unusual stresses such as variations in BP, alteration of renal blood flow, hypovolemia, myoglobin, catecholamine surges, vascular clamping, direct trauma, and potential nephrotoxins such as antibiotics, contrast dye, and

Table 1-20   Selectively ordered chest radiographs in 1101 patients

Result	Number	Percent
Abnormal	568	52%
Unexpected abnormal	133	12%
Modified medical decision	51	5%
Useful to anaesthetist	166	15%

From Charpak Y et al: Prospective assessment of a protocol for selective ordering of preoperative chest x-rays, *Can J Anaesth* 35(3):259, 1988.

BOX 1-5
INDICATIONS FOR DIAGNOSTIC URINALYSIS

History	Physical examination
Dysuria	Fever without other
Frequency	source
Hesitancy	Costovertebral angle
Urethral discharge	tenderness
Flank pain	Generalized edema
History of renal	Abnormal prostate ex-
disease	amination
History of diabetes	Jaundice
History of collagen	
vascular disease	
History of use of	
drug known to	
cause renal	
disease	

Table 1-21   Yield of positive results in screening urinalysis studies

Patients tested	Patients w/ abnormal results	Percentage (%)
3375 maxillofacial surgery preoperative[115]	130	3.85%
2600 screenings of clinic children/adults[96]	182	7%
453 pediatric preoperative patients[231]	73	15%
123 routine screenings in adult admissions to medical service[3]	42	34%

a low but measurable amount of fluoride ion from some anesthetic agents.[203] The kidney may already have been exposed to potential toxins preoperatively in the form of nonsteroidal antiinflammatory agents, gold salts, and ACE inhibitor drugs.[3] The urinalysis may benefit the anesthesiologist and surgeon in ways not appreciated by the internist. Asymptomatic urinary tract infection may pose additional risk if prosthetic devices are surgically implanted. Bladder catheterization may be unanticipated preoperatively but required postoperatively for urinary retention. Urinary tract infection may distort postoperative evaluation by causing abdominal or flank pain, postoperative fever, and leukocytosis. Urine specific gravity is a useful indicator of the patient's hydration status. The presence of glucose raises the question of diabetes and potential hypovolemia from osmotic diuresis. Proteinuria or hematuria may be indicative of significant renal disease.

Whether urinalysis has any specific immediate preoperative benefit to the anesthesiologist in asymptomatic patients is unknown. The above considerations are all quite theoretical. Most anesthesiologists do not, themselves, demand preoperative screening urinalysis on asymptomatic patients.

SUMMARY

This chapter has reviewed preoperative assessment in the "healthy" patient. Ideally, evaluation would include balanced utilization of patient history, physical examination, and laboratory tests, each weighed according to known diagnostic strengths. Economic considerations have redistributed the balance. The history and physical examination are nowadays considered powerful and inexpensive, whereas laboratory tests are criticized as costly expenditures that contrib-

ute little to patient outcome. The truth is less clear cut. The history and physical examination are subject to individual variability and lack sensitivity in important areas. They require considerable expenditure of physician time and thus are not (nor should they be) considered free (although they *are* "free" to the hospital under the DRG system!). Laboratory tests have cost, but, when used selectively, can provide information important to the patient's immediate and long term future. High quality care does cost money. How much is truly necessary? This chapter is not an endorsement of expenditure for every possible preoperative assessment. We do believe that the current vogue of blanket condemnation of all routine lab testing needs tempering.

Much of the quoted literature has not been written by anesthesiologists nor has it addressed our concerns. For example, an internist's finding of hematuria on screening urinalysis has been considered not significant because no "change of therapy" occurred, because "continued observation" was already in progress. The anesthesiologist faced with a new patient for surgery tomorrow does not have this luxury. Continued observation means cancellation of anesthesia and surgery. The same test, the same finding, and the same ongoing therapy translates into different courses of action depending on the physician's perspective. New prospective studies by anesthesiologists would aid our understanding of the cost/efficacy of preoperative assessment.

A second problem is illustrated by the paradox that despite numerous publications, many cost-cutting proposals of medical economists have not gained widespread acceptance. Tierney et al. found that physicians informed of a test's cost at the time of ordering ordered fewer tests.[317] However, after the study ended, differences in behavior disappeared. Goldman explained that *observation of behavior* rather than change in attitude caused the temporary effect.[117] But these findings are not new. Schroeder et al. reported in 1973 that cost audit was an effective means of decreasing laboratory tests.[271] Why have decades of cost-cutting proposals had so little influence? Possibly because the priority of these proposals is saving dollars rather than improving care. Schroeder et al. illustrated this conflict well by stating that their study was "not concerned with measuring quality of care or with correlation of quality to costs." In fact, they found that physicians who ordered more tests also saw their patients more frequently.[271] **When faced with economic choices, physicians tend to be unwilling to compromise care or increase risk for the sake of saving money.**

Can we improve care and make it less expensive? Not long ago controversy raged as to effectiveness and cost of postoperative intermittent positive pressure breathing (IPPB) to prevent atelectasis. The invention of the *effective and inexpensive* incentive spirometer made IPPB an historical issue. Can invention and new developments address cost/quality issues of anesthetic care? **Pulse oximetry and capnography were originally deemed costly but are now mandatory. Mandatory standards by the American Society of Anesthesiologists have established anesthesiologists as leaders in quality assurance. These advancements translate into dollar savings because of the risk reduction.** What new ideas in preoperative assessment can improve care and save money? One proposal of MacPherson et al. is that laboratory tests done during the months before surgery might satisfactorily substitute for tests done immediately before

surgery.[193] By emphasizing usefulness of early preoperative tests, a secondary benefit might be earlier medical work-up for abnormal results, decreasing the number of hasty consultations the night before surgery.

In summary, our recommendation must be to provide the best care possible to each patient. If unnecessary expenditures can be trimmed without affecting care, this is desirable. Shortcuts that compromise safety cannot be recommended no matter what the dollar savings. More selective use of limited resources will be facilitated by prospective studies that specifically address concerns of the anesthesiologist.

KEY POINTS

- The beginning anesthesiologist should study and learn to use the ASA Physical Status Classification.
- If allowed only one medical procedure for preoperative evaluation, the vast majority of anesthesiologists would demand to do a careful medical history.
- The diagnosis of angina pectoris is significantly complicated by the variable presentation of chest pain. Classic angina occurs with exertion and is relieved by rest, yet atypical angina may occur without exertion or during the early morning hours of sleep. It is now understood that much myocardial ischemia is silent.
- Syncope due to a cardiac cause is a significant concern.
- Patients complaining of headaches can be divided into three groups: recent onset, chronic recurrent, and referred or facial pain.
- Fifty-eight million people in the United States are estimated to have hypertension, an important risk factor in coronary artery disease, stroke, congestive heart failure, and renal failure.
- Five major causes of secondary hypertension are renal artery stenosis, primary aldosteronism, Cushing's syndrome, pheochromocytoma, and aortic coarctation.
- The significance of a carotid bruit is markedly influenced by presence of symptoms.

- The question of whether to perform surgery in a patient with an upper respiratory infection is controversial, but, in general, truly elective surgery should probably be postponed.
- One of the most valuable assets in assessing the patient's airway is to review any and all necessary available prior anesthetic records. However, just because the patient could be intubated previously does not mean for certain it can be done again.
- Understanding the essentials of physical examination of the patient's upper and lower airway should be a priority for the beginning anesthesiologist.
- Various neuromuscular diseases seen preoperatively can substantially affect patient anesthetic management.
- The presence of a prior myocardial infarction in the patient's history indicates that the patient may be at increased cardiovascular risk.
- The value of the ECG in preoperative evaluation of patients with suspected or known coronary artery disease is real.
- The lower limit of acceptable preoperative hemoglobin is controversial. The beginning anesthesiologist should study the underlying issues, rather than accept a dogmatic number.
- The yield of preoperative chest radiographs is increased when ordered selectively.

KEY REFERENCES

Consensus Conference: Perioperative red blood cell transfusion, *JAMA* 260(18):2700, 1988.

Goldman L, Caldera DL: Risk of general anesthesia and elective operation in the hypertensive patient, *Anesthesiology* 50:285, 1979.

Goldman L, Caldera DL, Nussbaum SR et al: Multifactorial index of cardiac risk in cardiac surgical procedures, *N Engl J Med* 297(16):845, 1977.

Gronert GA: Malignant hyperthermia, *Anesthesiology* 53:395, 1980.

Keenan RL, Boyan CP: Cardiac arrest due to anesthesia, *JAMA* 253(16):2373, 1985.

MacPherson DS, Snow R, and Lofgren RP: Preoperative screening: value of previous tests, *Ann Intern Med* 113(12):969, 1990.

Mallampati SR, Gatt SP, Gugino RR et al: A clinical sign to predict difficult tracheal intubation: a prospective study, *Can Anaesth Soc J* 32:4, 1985.

1988 Joint National Committee of the National High Blood Pressure Education Program: The 1988 Report of the Joint National Committee on Detection, Evaluation, and Treatment of High Blood Pressure, *Arch Int Med* 148:1023, 1988.

Roizen MF: The compelling rationale for less preoperative testing, *Can J Anaesth* 35(3):214, 1988.

Rucker L, Frye EB, and Staten MA: Usefulness of screening chest roentgenograms in preoperative patients, *JAMA* 250(23):3209, 1983.

Steen PA, Tinker JH, and Tarhan S: Myocardial reinfarction after anesthesia and surgery, *JAMA* 239:2556, 1978.

Stock JGL, Strunin L: Unexplained hepatitis following halothane, *Anesthesiology* 63:424, 1985.

Task Force on Blood Pressure Control in Children (from the National Heart, Lung, and Blood Institute, Bethesda, Md): Report of the Second Task Force on Blood Pressure Control in Children—1987, *Pediatrics* 79(1):1, 1987.

Tisi GM: Preoperative identification and evaluation of the patient with lung disease, *Med Clin N Am* 71(3):399, 1987.

REFERENCES

1. Abrams HL: The "overutilization" of x-rays, *N Engl J Med* 300(21):1213, 1979.
2. Adams HP, Jergenson DP, Kassell NF et al: Pitfalls in the recognition of subarachnoid hemorrhage, *JAMA* 244(8):794, 1980.
3. Akin BV, Hubbell FA, and Frye EG: Efficacy of the routine admission urinalysis, *Am J Med* 82:719, April 1987.
4. Allen JB, Allen FB: *The minimum acceptable level of hemoglobin*, Boston, 1981, Little, Brown.
5. American Academy of Pediatrics Committee on Practice and Ambulatory Medicine: *Recommendations for preventive pediatric health care*, Chicago, Il, 1987.
6. American College of Obstetricians and Gynecologists: *Standards for obstetric-gynecologic services*, ed 6, Washington, DC, 1985, American College of Obstetricians and Gynecologists.
7. Applegate WB: Hypertension in elderly patients, *Ann Intern Med* 110:901, 1989.
8. Artman M, Graham T: Congestive heart failure in infancy: recognition and management, *Am Heart J* 103(6):1040, 1982.
9. Audenaert SM, Schmidt TE: The peril of atlanto-axial subluxation, *Soc Ped Anesth* 3(2):4, 1990.
10. Bannister F, MacBeth RG: Direct laryngoscopy and tracheal intubation, *Lancet* 2:651, 1944.
11. Barber A, Green D, and Galluzzo T: The bleeding time as a preoperative screening test, *Am J Med* 78:761, 1985.
12. Barnes RW, Marszalek PB: Asymptomatic carotid disease in the cardiovascular surgical patient: is prophylactic endarterectomy necessary? *Stroke* 12(4):497, 1981.
13. Barnett HJM, Plum F, and Walton JV: Carotid endarterectomy—an expression of concern, *Stroke* 15(6):941, 1984.
14. Bates B, Yellin JA: The yield of multiphasic screening, *JAMA* 222(1):74, 1972.
15. Bedford RF, Feinstein B: Hospital admission blood pressure: a predictor for hypertension following endotracheal intubation, *Anesth Analg* 59:367, 1980.
16. Beebe HG, Clagett P, DeWeese JA et al: Assessing risk associated with carotid endarterectomy, *Circulation* 79:472, 1989.
17. Berwick DM: Screening in health fairs, *JAMA* 254(11):1492, 1985.
18. Beutler E: The common anemias, *JAMA* 259(16):2433-2437, 1988.
19. Bisno AL, Shulman ST, and Dajani AS: The rise and fall (and rise?) of rheumatic fever, *JAMA* 259(5):728, 1988.
20. Blery C, Charpak Y, Szatan M et al: Evaluation of protocol for selective ordering of preoperative tests, *Lancet* 1:139, 1986.
21. Boghosian SGh, Mooradian AD: Usefulness of routine preoperative chest roentgenograms in elderly patients, *J Am Geriatr Soc* 35(2):142, 1987.
22. Bonebrake CR, Noller KL, and Loehnen CP: Routine chest roentgenography in pregnancy, *JAMA* 240(25):2747, 1978.
23. Braunwald E: Mitral regurgitation: physiological, clinical, and surgical consideration, *N Engl J Med* 281:425, 1969.
24. Bravo EL, Gifford RW: Pheochromocytoma: diagnosis, localization, and management, *N Engl J Med* 311:1298, 1984.
25. Breslow L, Somers AR: The lifetime health-monitoring program, *N Engl J Med* 296(11):601, 1977.
26. Brill PW, Ewing ML, and Dunn AA: The value (?) of routine radiography in children and adolescents, *Pediatrics* 52(1):125, 1973.
27. Buckberg G, Brazier J: Coronary blood flow and cardiac function during hemodilution. In Messmer K, Schid-Schönbein H, eds: Intentional hemodilution, *Biblthca Haemat* 41:173, Karger Basel, 1975.
28. Burrows B, Bloom JW, Traver GA et al: The course and prognosis of different forms of chronic airway obstruction in a sample from the general population, *N Engl J Med* 317:1309, 1987.
29. Burrows B, Martinez FD: Bronchial

responsiveness, atopy, smoking, and chronic obstructive pulmonary disease, *Am Rev Respir Dis* 140:1515, 1989.

30. Calhoun DA, Oparil S: Treatment of hypertensive crisis, *N Engl J Med* 323(17):1177, 1990.

31. Califf RM, Mark DB, Harrell EE Jr et al: Importance of clinical measures of ischemia in the prognosis of patients with documented coronary artery disease, *J Am Coll Cardiol* 11:20, 1988.

32. Canadian Cooperative Study Group: A randomized trial of aspirin and sulfinpyrazone in threatened stroke, *N Engl J Med* 299(2):53, 1978.

33. Caplan LR: Carotid-artery disease, *N Engl J Med* 315(14):886, 1986.

34. Carpenter L, Beral V, Stracham D et al: Respiratory symptoms as predictors of 27 year mortality in a representative sample of British adults, *Br Med J* 299:357, 1989.

35. Carson JL, Poses RM et al: Severity of anemia and operative mortality and morbidity, *Lancet,* April 2, p. 727, 1988.

36. Cass NM, James NR, and Lines V: Difficult direct laryngoscopy complicating intubation for anaesthesia, *Br Med J* 1:488, 1956.

37. Castell DO, O'Brien KD, Muench H et al: Estimation of liver size by percussion in normal individuals, *Ann Intern Med* 70(6):1183, 1969.

38. Cease KB, Nicklas JM: Prediction of left ventricular ejection fraction using simple quantitative clinical information, *Am J Med* 81:429, 1986.

39. Cebul RD, Whisnant JP: Carotid endarterectomy, *Ann Intern Med* 111:660, 1989.

40. Chambers BR, Norris JW: Clinical significance of asymptomatic neck bruits, *Neurology* 35:742, 1985.

41. Chambers RB, Norris JW: Outcome in patients with asymptomatic neck bruits, *N Engl J Med* 315(14):860, 1986.

42. Charpak Y, Bleary C, Chastang C et al: Prospective assessment of a protocol for selective ordering of preoperative chest x-rays, *Can J Anaesth* 35(3):259, 1988.

43. Cheitlin MD, Castro CM, and McAllister HA: Sudden death as a complication of anomalous left coronary origin from the anterior sinus of Valsalva, *Circulation* 50:780, 1974.

44. Chester EM, Agamanolis DP, and Banker EQ: Hypertensive encephalopathy: a clinicopathologic study of 20 cases, *Neurology* 28:928, 1978.

45. Christie LG, Conti CR: Systemic approach to evaluation of angina-like chest pain: pathophysiology and clinical testing with emphasis on objective documentation of myocardial ischemia, *Am Heart J* 102(5):897, 1981.

46. Cohen JA, Kaplan MM: Left-sided heart failure presenting as hepatitis, *Gastroenterology* 74:583, 1978.

47. Cohn PF: Severe asymptomatic coronary artery disease. A diagnostic, prognostic and therapeutic puzzle, *Am J Med* 62:565, 1977.

48. Collen MF: The baseline screening electrocardiogram: is it worthwhile? *J Fam Pract* 25(4);393,'1987.

49. Collen MF, Feldman R, Siegelaub AB et al: Dollar cost per positive test for automated multiphasic screening, *N Engl J Med* 283(9):459, 1970.

50. Consensus Conference: Perioperative red blood cell transfusion, *JAMA* 260(18):2700, 1988.

51. Cook DG, Shaper AG: Breathlessness, lung function, and the risk of a heart attack, *Eur Heart J* 9:1215, 1988.

52. Cooperman LH: Succinylcholine-induced hyperkalemia in neuromuscular disease, *JAMA* 213(11):1867, 1970.

53. Cooperman M, Pflug B, Martin EW Jr et al: Cardiovascular risk factors in patients with peripheral vascular disease, *Surgery* 84:505, 1978.

54. Cormack RS, Lehane J: Difficult tracheal intubation in obstetrics, *Anesthesia* 39:1105, 1984.

55. Corman LC: Clinical spectrum and treatment of rheumatic syndromes in the elderly, *Med Clin N Am* 73(6):1371, 1989.

56. Corrao WM, Braman SS, and Irwin RS: Chronic cough as the sole presenting manifestation of bronchial asthma, *N Engl J Med* 300:633, 1979.

57. Craig DB: Postoperative recovery of pulmonary function, *Anesth Analg* 60(1): 46, 1981.

58. Dallman PR: Blood and blood forming tissues. In Rudolph AM, ed: *Pediatrics,* Norwalk, Conn, 1987, Appleton & Lange.

59. Dallman PR, Yip R, and Johnson C: Prevalence and causes of anemia in the United States, 1976-1980, *Am J Clin Nutr* 39:437, 1984.

60. Danielson DA, Douglas III SW, Herzog P et al: Drug induced blood disorders, *JAMA* 252(23):3257, 1984.

61. Day SC, Cook EF, Funkenstein H et al: Evaluation and outcome of emergency room patients with transient loss of consciousness, *Am J Med* 73:15, 1982.

62. DeGowin EL, DeGowin RL: *Bedside diagnostic examination,* New York, 1976, MacMillan.

63. DelGuercio LRM, Cohn JD: Monitoring operative risk in the elderly, *JAMA* 243:1350, 1980.

64. Delahunt B, Trunball PR: How cost effective are routine preoperative investigations? *N Z Med J* 92:431, 1980.

65. Denny FW, Murphy TF, Clyde WA et al: Croup: An 11-year study in a pediatric practice, *Pediatrics* 71(6):871, 1983.

66. Dermksian G, Lamb LE: Syncope in a population of healthy young adults: incidence, mechanisms, and significance, *JAMA* 168:1200, 1958.

67. DeSoto H, Patel RI, Solimon IE et al: Changes in oxygen saturation following general anesthesia in children with upper respiratory infection signs and symptoms undergoing otolaryngological procedures, *Anesthesiology* 68(2):276, 1988.

68. Detsky AS, Naglie G: A clinician's guide to cost-effectiveness analysis, *Ann Intern Med* 113(2):147, 1990.

69. Detsky AS, Abrams HB, Forbath N, et al: Cardiac assessment for patients undergoing noncardiac surgery, *Arch Intern Med* 146:2131, 1986.

70. DiCarlo LA, Morady F: Evaluation of the patient with syncope, *Cardiol Clin* 3(4):499, 1985.

71. Diehr P, Wood RW, Barr V et al: Acute headaches: presenting symptoms and diagnostic rules to identify patients with tension and migraine headaches, *J Chronic Dis* 34:147, 1981.

72. Dienstag JL, Alter HJ: Non-A, non-B hepatitis: evolving epidemiological and clinical perspectives, *Semin Liver Dis* 6:67, 1986.

73. DiMarco JP, Garan H, Harthorne JW et al: Intracardiac electrophysiologic techniques in recurrent syncope of unknown cause, *Ann Intern Med* 95:542, 1981.

74. Dingle JH, Badger GF, and Jordon WS: *Illness in the home: a study of 25,000 illnesses in a group of Cleveland families,* Cleveland, 1964, Western Reserve University.

75. Dresner MS: Ocular manifestations of hyperlipidemia, *Hosp Physician* 26(5):15, 1990.

76. Dunn M, Rinkenberger RL: Clinical aspects of acute pericarditis, *Cardiovasc Clin* 7(3):131, 1976.

77. Dykes MHM, Walzer SG: Preoperative postoperative hepatic dysfunction, *Surg Gynecol Obstet* 124;747, 1967.

78. Eagle KA, Black HR, Cook EF et al: Evaluation of prognostic classifications for patients with syncope, *Am J Med* 79:455, 1985.

79. Eagle KA, Quertermous T, Singer DE et al: Left ventricular ejection fraction: physician estimates compared with gated blood pool scar measurements, *Arch Intern Med* 148:882, 1988.

80. Easton JD, Sherman DG: Stroke and mortality rate in carotid endarterectomy: 228 consecutive operations, *Stroke* 8(5):565, 1977.

81. Ebi-Kryston KL, Hawthorne VM, Rose G et al: Breathlessness, chronic bronchitis, and reduced pulmonary function as predictors of cardiovascular disease mortality among men in England, Scotland and United States, *Int J Epidemiol* 18:84, 1989.

82. Eckberg DW: Carotid baroreflex function in young men with borderline blood pressure elevation, *Circulation* 59(4): 632, 1979.

83. Eckman MH, Beshansky JR, Durand-Zaleski I et al: *JAMA* 263(11):1513, 1990.

84. Eckstein RW: Development of intraarterial coronary anastomoses by chronic anemia: disappearance following correction of anemia, *Circ Res* 3:306, 1955.

85. Eisenberg JM, Clarke JR, and Sussmann SA: Prothrombin and partial thromboplastin times as preoperative screening tests, *Arch Surg* 117:48, 1982.

86. Ellis FR: Neuromuscular disease and anaesthesia, *Br J Anaesth* 46:603, 1974.

87. Elwood PC, Waters WE, Greene WTW et al: Symptoms and circulating blood level, *J Chron Dis* 21:615, 1969.

88. Empey DW, Laitinen LA, Jacobs L et al: Mechanisms of bronchial hyperreactivity in normal subjects after upper respiratory tract infection, *Am Rev Resp Dis* 113:131, 1976.

89. Epstein SE, Maron BJ: Sudden death and the competitive athlete: perspectives on preparticipation screening studies, *J Am Coll Cardiol* 7(1):220, 1986.

90. Erban SB, Kinman JL, and Schwartz S: Routine use of the prothrombin and partial thromboplastin times, *JAMA* 262(17):2428, 1989.

91. Ewing DJ, Campbell IW, and Clarke BF: Assessment of cardiovascular effects in diabetic autonomic neuropathy and prognostic implications, *Ann Intern Med* 92(part 2):308, 1980.

92. Fabian LW: The experts opine, *Surv Anesth* 15:180, 1971.

93. Fagius J, Karhuvaara S: Sympathetic activity and blood pressure increases with bladder distension in humans, *Hypertension* 14:511, 1989.

94. Fairbairn AS, Wood CH, and Fletcher CM: Variability in answers to a questionnaire on respiratory symptoms, *Br J Prev Soc Med* 13:175, 1959.

95. Farnsworth PB, Steiner E, Klein RM et al: The value of routine preoperative chest roentgenograms in infants and children, *JAMA* 224(6):582, 1980.

96. Faser CG, Smith BC, and Peake MJ: Effectiveness of an outpatient urine screening program, *Clin Chem* 23(12):2216, 1977.

97. Feldman T, Borow KM, Sarne DH et al: Myocardial mechanics in hyperthyroidism: importance of left ventricular loading conditions, heart rate, and contractile state, *J Am Coll Cardiol* 7(5):967, 1986.

98. Fell RH: Migraine and surgery, *Anaesthesia* 35:1006, 1980.

99. Ferris BG, Speizer FE, Worcester J et al: Adult mortality in Berlin, NH, from 1961 to 1967, *Arch Environ Health* 23:434, 1967.

100. Fessu WJ: High uric acid as an indicator of cardiovascular disease: independence from obesity, *Am J Med* 68:401, 1980.

101. Fields WS, Lemak NA, Frankowski RF et al: Controlled trial of aspirin in cerebral ischemia, *Stroke* 8(3):301, 1977.

102. Finch CA, Lenfant C: Oxygen transport in man, *N Engl J Med* 286(8):407, 1972.

103. Fink DJ, Fang M, and Wyle FA: Routine chest x-ray films in a veterans hospital, *JAMA* 245(10):1056, 1981.

104. Fisher M, ed.: *Screening for cerebrovascular diseases in Guide to Clinical Prevention Services: an assessment of the effectiveness of 169 interventions,* Report of the U.S. Prevention Services Task Force, Baltimore, 1989, Williams & Wilkins.

105. Fox JP, Cooney MK, Hall EC et al: Rhinoviruses in Seattle families, 1975-1979, *Am J Epidemiol* 122:830, 1985.

106. Frank BB: Clinical evaluation of jaundice, *JAMA* 262(21):3031, 1989.

107. Friedman LS, Maddrey WC: Surgery in the patient with liver disease, *Med Clin N Am* 71(3):453, 1987.

108. Garber AM, Sox HC, and Littenberg B: Screening asymptomatic adults for cardiac risk factors: the serum cholesterol level, *Ann Intern Med* 110:662, 1989.

109. Gass DG, Olsen GM: Preoperative pulmonary function testing to predict postoperative morbidity and mortality, *Chest* 89(1):127, 1986.

110. Gerson MC, Hurst JM, Hertzberg VS et al: Prediction of cardiac and pulmonary complications related to elective abdominal and noncardial thoracic surgery in geriatric patients, *Am J Med* 88:101, 1990.

111. Glezen WP, Denny FW: Epidemiology of acute lower respiratory disease in children, *N Engl J Med* 288(10):498, 1973.

112. Glick G, Plauth WH, Braunwald E et al: Role of the autonomic nervous system in the circulatory response to acutely induced anemia in unanesthetized dogs, *J Clin Inves* 43(11):2112, 1964.

113. Gluck R, Munoz E, and Wise L: Preoperative and postoperative medical evaluation of surgical patients, *Am J Surg* 155:730, 1988.

114. Godfrey S, Edwards RHT, and Campbell EJM: Repeatability of physical signs in airways obstruction, *Thorax* 24:4, 1969.

115. Gold BD, Wolfersberger WH: Findings from routine urinalysis and hematocrit on ambulatory oral and maxillofacial surgery patients, *Oral Surg* 38:677, Sept 1980.

116. Goldberger AL, O'Konski M: Utility of the routine electrocardiogram before surgery and on general hospital admission, *Ann Intern Med* 105:552, 1986.

117. Goldman L: Changing physicians behavior, *N Engl J Med* 322(21):1498, 1990.

118. Goldman L, Caldera DL: Risk of general anesthesia and elective operation in the hypertensive patient, *Anesthesiology* 50:285, 1979.

119. Goldman L, Caldera DL, Nussbaum SR et al: Multifactorial index of cardiac risk in cardiac surgical procedures, *N Engl J Med* 297(16):845, 1977.

120. Goldman L, Cook EF, Mitchell N et al: Pitfalls in the serial assessment of cardiac functional status, *J Chron Dis* 35:763, 1982.

121. Gopalrao T: Should anemia stop surgery? *Int Surg* 55(4):250, 1971.

122. Gordon SJ, Chatzinoff M, and Peiken SR: Medical care of the surgical patient with gastrointestinal disease, *Med Clin N Am* 71(3):433, 1987.

123. Gordon T, Kannel WB: Multiple risk functions for predicting coronary heart disease: the concept, accuracy, and application, *Am Heart J* 103(6):1031, 1982.

124. Goresky GV: Respiratory complications in patients with upper respiratory tract infections, *Can J Anesth* 34:655, 1987 (letter).

125. Graham DT: Prediction of fainting in blood donors, *Circulation* 23:901, 1961.

126. Greene BA, Berkowitz S: The preanesthetic induced cough as a method of diagnosis of preoperative bronchitis, *Ann Intern Med* 37:723, 1952.

127. Gronert GA: Malignant hyperthermia, *Anesthesiology* 53:395, 1980.

128. Grossman W, Jones D, and McLaurin LP: Wall stress and patterns of hypertrophy in the human left ventricle, *J Clin Invest* 56:56, 1975.

129. Guyton A: Renal function curve—a key to understanding the pathogenesis of hypertension, *Hypertension* 10(1):1, 1987.

130. Hagl S, Hemisch W, Meisner H et al: The effect of hemodilution on regional myocardial function in the presence of coronary stenosis, *Basic Res Cardiol* 72:344, 1977.

131. Hammond JH, Eisinger RP: Carotid bruits in 1,000 normal subjects, *Arch Intern Med* 109:109, 1962.

132. Hampton JR, Harrison MJG, Mitchell JRA et al: Relative contributions of history-taking, physical examination, and laboratory investigation to diagnosis and management of medical outpatients, *Br Med J* 2:486, 1975.

133. Harlan WR, Cowie CC, Oberman A et al: Prediction of subsequent ischemic heart disease using serial resting electrocardiograms, *Am J Epidemiol* 119(2):208, 1984.

134. Harrison DG, Florentine MS, Brooks LA et al: The effect of hypertension and left ventricular hypertrophy on the lower range of coronary autoregulation, *Circulation* 77(5):1108, 1988.

135. Hart RG, Easton JP: Management of cervical bruits and carotid stenosis in preoperative patients, *Stroke* 14(2):290, 1983.

136. Hart R, Hindman B: Mechanisms of perioperative cerebral infarction, *Stroke* 13(6):766, 1982.

137. Harville DD, Summerskill WHJ: Surgery in acute hepatitis, *JAMA* 184(4):257, 1963.

138. Heyman A, Wilkenson WE, Heyden S et al: Risk of stroke in asymptomatic persons with cervical arterial bruits, *N Engl J Med* 302(15):838, 1980.

139. Higgins CB, Vatner SF, Franklin D et al: Effects of experimentally produced heart failure on the peripheral vascular response to severe exercise in conscious dogs, *Circ Res* 31:186, 1986.

140. Higgins MW, Keller JB: Predictors of mortality in the adult population of Tecumseh, *Arch Environ Health* 21:418, 1970.

141. Hill SA, Miller CA, Kosnik EJ et al: Pediatric neck injuries: a clinical study, *J Neurosurg* 60:700, 1984.

142. Hindman BJ: Perioperative stroke: the noncardiac surgery patient. In Hindman BJ, ed: *Neurological and psychological complications of anesthesia and surgery,* vol 24, International Anesthesiology Clinics, Boston, 1986, Little, Brown.

143. Hines S, Houston M, and Robertson D: The clinical spectrum of autonomic dysfunction, *Am J Med* 70:1091, 1981.

144. Hinkle AJ: What wisdom is there in administering elective general anesthesia to children with active upper respiratory tract infection? *Anesth Analg* 68:413, 1989.

145. Hoffman JIE: Maximal coronary vascular reserve, *Circulation* 70(2):153, 1984.

146. Hopkins AU: A neurologist's approach to patients with headache. In Hopkins A, ed: *Headache problems in diagnosis and management,* Philadelphia, 1988, WB Saunders.

147. Hubbell FA, Greenfield S, Tyler JL et al:

The impact of routine admission chest x-ray films on patient care, *N Engl J Med* 312(4):209, 1985.

148. Hussey AJ, Aldridge LM, Ray DC et al: Plasma glutathione S-transferase concentration as a measure of hepatocellular integrity following single general anaesthetic with halothane, enflurane or isoflurane, *Br J Anaesth* 60:130, 1988.

149. Ibrahim MM, Tarazi RC, and Dustan HP: Orthostatic hypotension: mechanisms and management, *Am Heart J* 90(4):513, 1975.

150. Jeffrey CC, Kunsman J, Cullen DJ et al: A prospective evaluation of cardiac risk index, *Anesthesiology* 58:462, 1983.

151. Jenkins LC, McGraw RW: Anaesthetic management of the patient with rheumatoid arthritis, *Can Anaesth Soc J* 16(5):407, 1969.

152. Johanson WG, Peirce AK, and Standord JP: Pulmonary function in uncomplicated influenza, *Am Rev Respir Dis* 100:141, 1969.

153. Jones FL: Frequency characteristics and importance of the cervical venous hum in adults, *N Engl J Med* 267(13):658, 1962.

154. Josephson ME: Antiarrhythmic agents and the danger of proarrhythmic events, *Ann Intern Med* 111(2):101, 1989.

155. Kannel WB: Epidemiological aspects of heart failure, *Cardiol Clin* 7(1):1, 1989.

156. Kannel WB, Abbott RD: Incidence and prognosis of unrecognized myocardial infarction, *N Engl J Med* 311:1144, 1984.

157. Kannel WB, Anderson K, McGee DL et al: Nonspecific electrocardiographic abnormality as a predictor of coronary heart disease: the Framingham study, *Am Heart J* 113:370, 1987.

158. Kannel WB, Feinleib M: Natural history of angina pectoris in the Framingham study, *Am J Cardiol* 729:154, 1972.

159. Kaplan EB, Sheiner LB, Boeckmann AJ et al: The usefulness of preoperative laboratory screening, *JAMA* 253(24):3576, 1985.

160. Kaplan NM: Importance of coronary heart disease risk factors in the management of hypertension, *Am J Med* 86(suppl 1B):1, 1989.

161. Kaplati MM: Liver dysfunction secondary to congestive heart failure, *Prac Cardiol* 6:39, 1980.

162. Kapoor WN, Karpf M, Weiand S et al: A prospective evaluation and follow-up of patients with syncope, *N Engl J Med* 309(4):197, 1983.

163. Kase CS, O'Neal AM, Fisher M et al: Intracranial hemorrhage after use of tissue plasminogen activator for coronary thrombolysis, *Ann Intern Med* 112:17, 1990.

164. Keenan RL, Boyan CP: Cardiac arrest due to anesthesia, *JAMA* 253(16):2373, 1985.

165. Kempczinski R: Discussion of "Carotid endarterectomy in a metropolitan community: the early results after 8535 operations, by Rubin JR et al." *J Vasc Surg* 7:259, 1988.

166. Keyes WG, Donohue PK, Spivak JL et al: Assessing the need for transfusion of premature infants and role of hematocrits, clinical signs, and erythropoietin level, *Pediatrics* 84(3):412, 1989.

167. Kirkendall WM, Armstrong ML: Vascular changes in the eye of treated and untreated patients with essential hypertension, *Am J Cardiol* 9(5):663, 1962.

168. Knill RL, Gelb AW: Ventilatory response to hypoxia and hypercapnia during halothane: sedation and anesthesia in man, *Anesthesiology* 49:244, 1978.

169. Korvin CC, Pearce RH, and Stanley J: Admissions screening: clinical benefits, *Ann Int Med* 83:197, 1975.

170. Koudstaal PJ, Van Gijn J, Staal A et al: Diagnosis of transient ischemic attacks: improvement of interobserver agreement by a check-list in ordinary language, *Stroke* 17(4):723, 1986.

171. Kowalyshyn TJ, Prager D, and Young J: A review of the present status of perioperative hemoglobin requirements, *Anesth Analg* 51(1):75, 1972.

172. Kowey PR, Eisenberg R, and Engel TR: Sustained arrhythmias in hypertrophic obstructive cardiomyopathy, *N Engl J Med* 310(24):1566, 1984.

173. Krakoff LR, Elijovich F: Cushing's syndrome and exogenous glucocorticoid hypertension, *Clin Endocrinol Metab* 10:479, 1981.

174. Lambert EC, Menon VA, and Wagner HR: Sudden unexpected death from cardiovascular disease in children: a cooperative international study, *Am J Cardiol* 34:89, 1974.

175. Lance JW: Headache, *Ann Neurol* 10:1, 1981.

176. Lance JW, Hinterberger II: Symptoms of pheochromocytoma, with particular reference to headache, correlated with catecholamine production, *Arch Neurol* 33:281, 1976.

177. LaPuma J, Lawlor EF: Quality adjusted life-years, *JAMA* 263(21):2917, 1990.

178. Larson AW, Strong CG: Initial assessment of the patient with hypertension, *Mayo Clin Proc* 64:1533, 1989.

179. Lauer MB, Hallowell P, and Goldblatt A: Pulmonary dysfunction secondary to heart disease, *Anesthesiology* 33(7):161, 1970.

180. Lawrence VA, Page CP, and Harris GC: Preoperative spirometry before abdominal operations, *Arch Int Med* 149:280, 1989.

181. Lembo NJ, Dell'Italia LJ, Crawford MH et al: Bedside diagnosis of systolic murmurs, *N Engl J Med* 318:1572, 1988.

182. Leoy RI, Feinleib M: Risk factors for coronary artery disease and their management. In Braunwald E, ed: *Heart disease*, vol 2, Philadelphia, 1984, WB Saunders.

183. Levine EA, Rosen AL, Sehgal LR et al: Treatment of acute postoperative anemia with recombinant human erythropoietin, *J Trauma* 29(8):1134, 1989.

184. Levine E, Rosene A, Sehgal L et al: Physiologic effects of acute anemia: implications for a reduced transfusion trigger, *Transfusion* 30(1):11, 1990.

185. Liberthson RR, Pennington DG, Jacobs ML et al: Coarctation of the aorta: review of 234 patients and clarification of management problems, *Am J Cardiol* 43:835, 1979.

186. Lichstein E, Chapman I, Gupta PK et al: Diagonal ear lobe crease and coronary artery sclerosis, *Ann Intern Med* 85:337, 1976.

187. Lindner A, Charra B, Sherrar DJ et al: Accelerated atherosclerosis in prolonged maintenance hemodialysis, *N Engl J Med* 290(13):697, 1974.

188. Linet MS, Stewart WF, Celentano DD et al: An epidemiologic study of headache among adolescents and young adults, *JAMA* 261:2211, 1989.

189. Linman JW: Physiologic and pathophysiologic effects in anemia, *N Engl J Med* 279(15):812, 1968.

190. Lombard JT, Selzer A: Valvular aortic stenosis: a clinical and hemodynamic profile of patients, *Ann Intern Med* 106:292, 1987.

191. Lowenstein SR, Parrino TA: Management of the common cold, *Adv Intern Med* 32:207, 1987.

192. Lozoff B, Brittenhaun GM, Wolf AW et al: Iron deficiency anemia and iron therapy effects on infant developmental test performance, *Pediatrics* 79:981, 1987.

193. MacPherson DS, Snow R, and Lofgren RP: Preoperative screening: value of previous tests, *Ann Intern Med* 113(12):969, 1990.

194. Mallampati SR, Gatt SP, Gugino RD et al: A clinical sign to predict difficult tracheal intubation: a prospective study, *Can Anaesth Soc J* 32:4, 1985.

195. Mancia G, Bertinieri G, Grassi G et al: Effects of blood pressure measurement by the doctor on patient's blood pressure and heart rate, *Lancet* 2:695, 1983.

196. Maquire JF, Geha RS, and Umetsu DT: Myocardial specific creatine phosphokinase isoenzyme elevation in children with asthma treated with intravenous isoproterenol, *J Allergy Clin Immunol* 78:631, 1986.

197. Marantz PR, Tobin JN, Wassertheil S et al: The relationship between left ventricular systolic function and congestive heart failure diagnosed by clinical criteria, *Circulation* 77(3):607, 1988.

198. Marcus ML, Doty DB, Hiratzka LF et al: Decreased coronary reserve—a mechanism for angina pectoris in patients with aortic stenosis and normal coronary arteries, *N Engl J Med* 307:1362, 1982.

199. Margolis JR, Kannel WB, Feinleib M et al: Clinical features of unrecognized myocardial infarction—silent and symptomatic, *Am J Cardiol* 32:1, 1973.

200. Mark AL, Kioschos M, Abboud FM et al: Abnormal vascular responses to exercise in patients with aortic stenosis, *J Clin Invest* 52:1138, 1973.

201. Maron BJ, Roberts WC, McAllister HA et al: Sudden death in young athletes, *Circulation* 62(2):218, 1980.

202. Martin CE, Shaver JA, and Leonard JJ: Physical signs, apex cardiography, photocardiography and systolic time intervals in angina pectoris, *Circulation* 46:1098, 1972.

203. Mason RA, Arbeit LA, and Giron F: Renal dysfunction after arteriography, *JAMA* 253(7):1001, 1985.

204. Mavler JR: Carotid endarterectomy clinical trials, *Mayo Clin Proc* 64:1026, 1989.

205. Mavra MB, Zerofsky RA: Supraclavicular and carotid bruits in hemodialysis patients, *Ann Neurol* 2:535, 1977.

206. McDowell SA, Dundee JW, and Pandit SK: Para-anaesthetic headache in female patients, *Anaesthesia* 25(3):334, 1970.

207. McFadden ER, Kiser R, and DeGroot WJ: Acute bronchial asthma, *N Engl J Med* 288(5):221, 1973.

208. McGee PA, Castelli WP, McNamara PM et al: The natural history of congestive heart failure: the Framingham study, *N Engl J Med* 26:1441, 1971.

209. McGill WA, Coveler LA, and Epstein BS: Subacute upper respiratory infection in children, *Anesth Analg* 58:331, 1979.

210. Merli GJ, Bell RD: Preoperative management of the surgical patient with neurologic disease, *Med Clin N Am* 71(3):511, 1987.

211. Michelson EL, Morganroth J, Nichols CW et al: Retinal arteriolar changes as an indicator of coronary artery disease, *Arch Intern Med* 139:1139, 1979.

212. Micr-Jedrzejowicz A, Brophy C, and Green M: Respiratory muscle weakness during upper respiratory tract infections, *Ann Rev Respir Dis* 138:5, 1988.

213. Milne ENC: Chest radiology in the surgical patient, *Surg Clin N Am* 60(6):1503, 1980.

214. Monto AS, Ullman BM: Acute respiratory illness in an American community: the Tecumseh study, *JAMA* 227:164, 1974.

215. Moorman JR, Hlatky MA, Eddy DM et al: The yield of the routine admission electrocardiogram, *Ann Intern Med* 103:590, 1985.

216. Morris JF, Koski A, and Johnson LC: Spirometric standards for healthy nonsmoking adults, *Am Rev Resp Dis* 103:57, 1971.

217. Murphy JF, O'Rordon J, Newcombe RG et al: Relation of hemoglobin levels in first and second trimester to outcome of pregnancy, *Lancet* 1:992, 1986.

218. Murray JF, Rapaport E: Coronary blood flow and myocardial metabolism in acute experimental anaemia, *Cardiovasc Res* 6:360, 1972.

219. Murrin KR: Intubation procedures and causes of difficult intubation. In Latto IP, Rosen M, eds: *Difficulties in tracheal intubation,* London, 1985, Bailliere Tindall.

220. Nadeau SE: Stroke, *Med Clin N Am* 73(6):1351, 1989.

221. Nagao S, Roccaforte P, and Moody RA: The effects of isovolemic hemodilution and reinfusion of packed erythrocytes on somatosensory and visual evoked potentials, *J Surg Res* 25:530, 1978.

222. National Academy of Sciences, Institute of Medicine Ad Hoc Advisory Group of Preventive Services: *Preventive services for the well population.* Washington DC, 1978, National Academy of Sciences.

223. Neely WA, Robinson WT, McMullan MH et al: Postoperative respiratory insufficiency, *Ann Surg* 171:679, 1970.

224. Nelson JD: The Marfan syndrome, with special reference to congenital enlargement of the spinal canal, *Br J Radiol* 31:561, 1958.

225. Neuman GG, Weingarten AE, Abramowitz RM et al: The anesthetic management of the patient with an anterior mediastinal mass, *Anesthesiology* 60:144, 1984.

226. Newman DC, Hicks RG: Combined carotid and coronary artery surgery: a review of the literature, *Ann Thor Surg* 45(5):574, 1988.

227. Nichol HC, Zuck D: Difficult laryngoscopy — the "anterior" larynx and the atlanto-occipital gap, *Br J Anaesth* 55:141, 1983.

228. 1988 Joint National Committee of the National High Blood Pressure Education Program: The 1988 Report of the Joint National Committee on Detection, Evaluation, and Treatment of High Blood Pressure, *Arch Intern Med* 148:1023, 1988.

229. Northrip DR, Bohman BK, and Tsrieda K: Total airway occlusion and superior vena cava syndrome in a child with an anterior mediastinal tumor, *Anesth Analg* 65:1079, 1986.

230. Nunn JF, Milledge JS, Chen D et al: Respiratory criteria of fitness for surgery and anesthesia, *Anaesthesia* 43:543, 1988.

231. O'Conner ME, Drasner K: Preoperative laboratory testing of children undergoing elective surgery, *Anesth Analgesia* 70:176, 1990.

232. O'Kelley BF, Massle BM, Tubau JF et al: Coronary morbidity and mortality, pre-existing silent coronary artery disease, and mild hypertension, *Ann Intern Med* 110(12):1017, 1989.

233. Owings DV, Kruskall MS, and Thurer RL: Autologous blood donations prior to elective cardiac surgery, *JAMA* 262(14):1963, 1989.

234. Pardee NE, Winterbauer RH, and Allen JD: Bedside evaluation of respiratory distress, *Chest* 85(2):203, 1984.

235. Parks DP, Ahrens RC, Humphries CT et al: Chronic cough in childhood: approaches to diagnosis and treatment, *J Pediatrics* 115(5 part 2):856, 1989.

236. Pasulka PS, Bistrian BR, Benotti PN et al: The risks of surgery in obese patients, *Ann Intern Med* 106:540, 1986.

237. Patterson RH: Can carotid endarterectomy be justified? Yes, *Arch Neurol* 44:651, 1987.

238. Peiris AN, Sothmann MS, Hoffmann RG et al: Adiposity, fat distribution, and cardiovascular risk, *Ann Intern Med* 110:867, 1989.

239. Perloff JF: The physiologic mechanisms of cardiac and vascular physical signs, *J Am Coll Cardiol* 1:184, 1983.

240. Perloff JK: Neurological disorders and heart disease. In Braunwald E, ed: *Heart disease,* vol 2, Philadelphia, 1984, WB Saunders.

241. Perloff JE et al: Uncommon or commonly unrecognized causes of heart failure, *Prog Cardiovasc Dis* 12:409, 1970.

242. Pickering TG, James GD, Boddie C et al: How common is white-coat hypertension? *JAMA* 259:225, 1988.

243. Raftery EB, Holland WW: Examination of the heart: an investigation into variation, *Am J Epidemiol* 85(3):438, 1967.

244. Rawstron RE: Anemia and surgery: a retrospective clinical study, *N Z J Surg* 39:425, 1970.

245. Rea HH, Sears MR, Beaglehold R et al: Lessons from the National Asthma Mortality Study: circumstances surrounding death, *N Z Med J* 100:10, 1987.

246. Rees AM, Roberts CJ, Bligh AS et al: Routine preoperative chest radiography in noncardiopulmonary surgery, *Br Med J* 1:1333, 1976.

247. *Report from U.S. Preventive Services Task Force,* Baltimore, 1989, Williams & Wilkins.

248. Resnekov L, Fox S, and Selzer A: Task force IV: use of electrocardiograms in practice, *Am J Cardiol* 41:170, 1978.

249. Review Panel on Coronary-Prone Behavior and Coronary Heart Disease: a critical review, *Circulation* 63:1199, 1981.

250. Richter JE, Castell DO: Gastroesophageal reflux — pathogenesis, diagnosis and therapy, *Ann Intern Med* 97:93, 1982.

251. Ries PW: Current estimates from the National Health Interview Survey, United States, 1984: National Center for Health Statistics, 1986, Vital and Health Statistics, series 10, no 156, *Department of Human Services Publication* (PHS) 86-1586.

252. Robbins JA, Mushlin AI: Preoperative evaluation of the healthy patient, *Med Clin N Am* 63(6):1145, 1979.

253. Roberts CJ: Preoperative chest radiology, *Lancet* 2:83, 1979.

254. Roberts WC: Aortic dissection: anatomy, consequences, and causes, *Am Heart J* 101(2):195, 1981.

255. Roizen MF: The compelling rationale for less preoperative testing, *Can J Anaesth* 35(3):214, 1988.

256. Ropper AH, Wechsler LR, and Wilson LS: Carotid bruit and the risk of stroke in elective surgery, *New Engl J Med* 307(22):1388, 1982.

257. Rorsgaard S, Secher NH: Slowing of the heart during hypotension in major abdominal surgery, *Acta Anaesthesiol Scand* 30:507, 1986.

258. Rucker L, Frye EB, and Staten MA: Usefulness of screening chest roentgenograms in preoperative patients, *JAMA* 250(23):3209, 1983.

259. Sagel SS, Evens RG, Forrest JV et al: Efficacy of routine screening and lateral chest radiographs in a hospital-based population, *N Engl J Med* 291:1001, 1974.

260. Salam AA, Davies DM: Acute adrenal insufficiency during surgery, *Br J Anaesth* 46:619, 1974.

261. Salem MR, Mathrubhuthum M, and Bennett EJ: Difficult intubation, *N Engl J Med* 295(16):879, 1976.

262. Sanders JS, Ferguson DW: Profound sympathetoinhibition complicating hy-

povolemia in humans, *Ann Intern Med* 111:439, 1989.

263. Sandler G: The importance of the history in the medical clinic and the cost of unnecessary tests, *Am Heart J* 100:828, 1980.

264. Sandok BA, Whisnant JP, Furlan AJ et al: Carotid artery bruits, *Mayo Clin Proc* 57:227, 1982.

265. Savage DD, Corwin L, McGee DL et al: Epidemiologic features of isolated syncope: the Framingham study, *Stroke* 16:626, 1985.

266. Savage DD, Devereux RB, Garrison RJ et al: Mitral valve prolapse in the general population: 2. Clinical features: the Framingham study, *Am Heart J,* 577, Sept. 1983.

267. Savage DD, Seides SF, Clark CE et al: Electrocardiographic findings in patients with obstructive and nonobstructive hypertrophic cardiomyopathy, *Circulation* 58(3):402, 1978.

268. Schemel WH: Unexpected hepatic dysfunction found in multiple laboratory screening, *Anesth Analg* 55(6):810, 1976.

269. Schildkraut JM, Myers RH, Cupples LA et al: Coronary risk associated with age and sex of parental heart disease in the Framingham study, *Am J Cardiol* 64:555, 1989.

270. Schneider IC, Anderson AE: Correlation of clinical signs with ventilatory function in obstructive lung disease, *Ann Intern Med* 62(3):477, 1965.

271. Schroeder SA, Kenders K, Cooper JK et al: Use of laboratory tests and pharmaceuticals, *JAMA* V225(8):969, 1973.

272. Schwartz PJ, Periti M, and Malliani A: The long Q-T syndrome, *Am Heart J* 89(3):378, 1975.

273. Selzer A: Changing aspect of the natural history of valvular aortic stenosis, *N Engl J Med* 317:91, 1987.

274. Selzer A, Cohn KE: Natural history of mitral stenosis: a review, *Circulation* 45:878, 1972.

275. Semmes BJ, Tobin MJ, Synder JV et al: Subjective and objective measurements of tidal volume in critically ill patients, *Chest* 87(5):577, 1985.

276. Shapiro MF, Greenfield S: The complete blood count and leukocyte differential count, *Ann Intern Med* 106:65, 1987.

277. Shashikant MS, Worsing RA, Wiens CW et al: Value of preoperative chest x-ray examinations in children, *Pediatrics* 60(5):669, 1977.

278. Shim C, Williams HM Jr: Pulsus paradoxus in asthma, *Lancet* 1:530, 1978.

279. Shim CS, Williams MH: Evaluation of the severity of asthma: patients vs. physicians, *Am J Med* 68:11, 1980.

280. Shoemaker WC, Appel RL, Kram HB et al: Prospective trial of trial supranormal values of survivors as therapeutic goals in high-risk surgical patients, *Chest* 94:1176, 1988.

281. Shub C: Heart failure and abnormal ventricular function, *Chest* 96:636, 1989.

282. Shub C: Stable angina pectoris. 1. Clinical patterns, *Mayo Clin Proc* 64:233, 1990.

283. Shub C: Stable angina pectoris. 2. Cardiac evaluation and diagnostic testing, *Mayo Clin Proc* 65:243, 1990.

284. Silberstein LE, Kruskall MS, Stehling LC et al: Strategies for the review of transfusion practices, *JAMA* 262(14):1993, 1989.

285. Silverstein MD, Singer DE, Mulley AG et al: Patients with syncope admitted to medical intensive care units, *JAMA* 248(10):1185, 1982.

286. Sirna S, Biller J, Skorton DJ et al: Cardiac evaluation of the patient with stroke, *Stroke* 21(1):14, 1990.

287. Sleeper JC, Orgain ES, and McIntosh HD: Primary pulmonary hypertension, *Circulation* 26:1358, 1962.

288. Sly MR: Mortality from asthma, *J Allergy Clin Immunol* 84:421, 1989.

289. Snider GL: Changes in COPD occurrence, *Am Rev Respir Dis* 140:S3, 1989.

290. Sox HC, Garber AM, and Littenberg B: The resting electrocardiogram as a screening test, *Ann Intern Med* 111(6):489, 1989.

291. Spagnuolo M, Kloth H, Taranta A et al: Natural history of rheumatic aortic regurgitation, *Circulation* 44:368, 1971.

292. Spodick DH, Quarry VM: Prevalence of the fourth heart sounds by phonocardiography in the absence of cardiac disease, *Am Heart J* 87(2):11, 1974.

293. Staats BA: Dyspnea—heart or lungs? *Int J Cardiol* 19:13, 1988.

294. Stander PE: Anemia in the elderly, *Postgrad Med* 85(2):85, 1989.

295. Stanley A: Migraine treated by inhalation sedation using nitrous oxide and oxygen, *Br Dent J* 149:54, 1980.

296. Steen PA, Tinker JH, and Tarhan S: Myocardial reinfarction after anesthesia and surgery, *JAMA* 239:2556, 1978.

297. Stehling L: Perioperative morbidity in anemic patients, *Transfusion* 29(suppl):S127, 1989.

298. Stehling L, Zauder AL: How low can we go? Is there a way to know? *Transfusion* 30(1):1, 1990.

299. Stein M, Cassara EL: Preoperative pulmonary evaluation and therapy for surgery patients, *JAMA* 211(5):787, 1970.

300. Stein M, Koota GM, Simon M et al: Pulmonary evaluation of surgical patients, *JAMA* 181(9):765, 1962.

301. Stevenson LW, Perloff JK: The limited reliability of physical signs for estimating hemodynamics in chronic heart failure, *JAMA* 261:884, 1989.

302. Stock JGL, Strunin L: Unexplained hepatitis following halothane, *Anesthesiology* 63:424, 1985.

303. Stoelting RK, Blitt CA, Cohen PJ et al: Hepatic dysfunction after isoflurane anesthesia, *Anesth Analg* 66:147, 1987.

304. Strandgaard S: Autoregulation of cerebral blood flow in hypertensive patients, *Circulation* 53(4):720, 1976.

305. Strasberg B, Rechavia E, Sagie A et al: The head-up tilt table test in patients with syncope of unknown origin, *Am Heart J* 118(5 part 1):923, 1989.

306. Strasberg B, Sagie A, Rechavia E et al: The noninvasive evaluation of syncope of suspected cardiovascular origin, *Am Heart J* 117(1):160, 1989.

307. Strauss RA, Eschenroeder RA: Hemiplegic migraine following third molar extractions under intravenous sedation, *J Oral Maxillofac Surg* 47:184, 1989.

308. Stubbing DG, Mathur PN, Roberts RS et al: Some physical signs in patients with chronic airflow obstruction, *Am Rev Respir Dis* 125:549, 1982.

309. Sugerman JH, Davidson DT, Vibur S et al: The basis of defective oxygen delivery from stored blood, *Surg Gyn Obstet* 131:733, 1970.

310. Summers PR, Biswas MK, Pastorek II JG et al: The pregnancy hepatitis B carrier: evidence favoring comprehensive antepartum screening, *Obstet Gynecol* 69(5):701, 1987.

311. Tait AR, Knight PR: The effects of general anesthesia on upper respiratory tract infections in children, *Anesthesiology* 67:930, 1987.

312. Tait AR, Knight PR: Intraoperative respiratory complications in patients with upper respiratory tract infections, *Can J Anaesth* 34(3):300, 1987.

313. Tape TG, Mushlin AI: How useful are routine x-rays of preoperative patients at risk for postoperative chest disease, *J Gen Intern Med* 3:15, 1988.

314. Tape TG, Mushlin AI: The utility of routine chest radiographs, *Ann Intern Med* 104:663, 1986.

315. Tarhan S, Moffitt EA, Taylor WF et al: Myocardial infarction after general anesthesia, *JAMA* 220:1451, 1972.

316. Task Force on Blood Pressure Control in Children (from the National Heart, Lung, and Blood Institute, Bethesda, Md): Report of the Second Task Force on Blood Pressure Control in Children—1987, *Pediatrics* 79(1):1, 1987.

317. Tierney WM, Miller ME, and McDonald CJ: The effect of test ordering of informing physicians of the charges for outpatient diagnostic tests, *N Engl J Med* 322(21):1498, 1990.

318. Tinetti ME, Speechley M: Prevention of falls among elderly, *N Engl J Med* 320:1055, 1989.

319. Tisi GM: Preoperative evaluation of pulmonary function, *Am Rev Resp Dis* 119:293, 1979.

320. Tisi GM: Preoperative identification and evaluation of the patient with lung disease, *Med Clin N Am* 71(3):399, 1987.

321. Törnebrandt K, Fletcher R: Preoperative chest x-rays in elderly patients, *Anaesthesia* 37:901, 1982.

322. Torrance J, Jacobs P, Restrepo A et al: Intraerythrocytic adaptation to anemia, *N Engl J Med* 283(4):165, 1970.

323. Treiman RL, Foran RF, Cohen JL et al: Carotid bruit, *Arch Surg* 114:1138, 1979.

324. Tucker CR, Towles RE, Calin A et al: Aortitis in ankylosing spondylitis: early detection of aortic root abnormalities with two dimensional echocardiography, *Am J Cardiol* 49:680, 1982.

325. Turnball JM, Buck C: The value of preoperative screening investigations in otherwise healthy individuals, *Arch Intern Med* 147:1101, 1987.

326. Umbach GE, Zubek S, Deck HJ et al: The value of preoperative chest x-rays in

gynecological patients, *Arch Gynecol Obstet* 243:179, 1988.

327. U.S. Preventive Services Task Force: Screening for anemia. In Fisher M, ed: *Guide to clinical preventative services,* Baltimore, 1989, Williams & Wilkins.

328. Varat MA, Adolph RJ, and Fowler NO: Cardiovascular effects of anemia, *Am Heart J* 83(3):415, 1972.

329. Veterans Administration Cooperative Study: Role of carotid endarterectomy in asymptomatic carotid stenosis, *Stroke* 17(3):534, 1986.

330. Viegas O, Stoelting RK: LDH$_5$ changes after cholecystectomy or hysterectomy in patients receiving halothane, enflurane, or fentanyl, *Anesthesiology* 54(6):556, 1979.

331. Wallace MR, Garst PD, Papadimos TJ et al: The return of acute rheumatic fever in young adults, *JAMA* 262:2557, 1989.

332. Warlow C: Carotid endarterectomy: does it work? *Stroke* 15(6):1068, 1984.

333. Wataneeyawech M, Kelly KA: Hepatic diseases, *N Y State J Med,* p. 1278, 1975.

334. Weber MA: Antihypertensive treatment, *Circulation* 80(suppl IV):120, 127, 1989.

335. Wedel H: Blood pressure control and mortality: is there a J-shaped curve? *Drugs* 38(suppl 2):9, 1989.

336. Weinberg MH, Grim CE, Hollified JW et al: Primary aldosteronism: diagnosis, localization and treatment, *Ann Intern Med* 90:386, 1979.

337. Westwood M, Cohen MI, and McNamara H: Serum q-glutamyl transpeptidase activity: a chemical determinant of alcohol consumption during adolescence, *Pediatrics* 62(4):560, 1978.

338. Whisnant JP: Epidemiology of stroke: emphasis on transient cerebral ischemic attacks and hypertension, *Stroke* 5:68, 1974.

339. White A, Kander PL: Anatomical factors in difficult direct laryngoscopy, *Br J Anaesth* 47:468, 1975.

340. Wiencek RG, Weaver DW, Bouwman DL et al: Usefulness of selective preoperative chest x-ray films, *Am Surg* 53:396, 1987.

341. Wilkerson DK, Rosen AL, Gould SA et al: Oxygen extraction ratio: a valid indicator of myocardial metabolism in anemia, *J Surg Res* 42:629, 1987.

342. Williams RC: Peridontal disease, *N Engl J Med* 322:373, 1990.

343. Williams RS, Logue EE, Lewis JL et al: Physical conditioning augments the fibrinolytic response to venous occlusion in healthy adults, *N Engl J Med* 302:987, 1980.

344. Wolf PA, Kannel WB, Sorlie P et al: Asymptomatic carotid bruit and risk of stroke, *JAMA* 245(14):1442, 1981.

345. Wood RA, Hoekelman RA: Value of the chest x-ray as a screening test for elective surgery in children, *Pediatrics* 67(4):447, 1981.

346. Working Group on Renovascular Hypertension: Detection, evaluation and treatment of renovascular hypertension, *Arch Intern Med* 147:820, 1987.

347. Wright KE, McIntosh HD: Syncope: a review of pathophysiological mechanisms, *Prog Cardiovasc Dis* 13(6):580, 1971.

348. Yasue H, Omote S, Takizaw A et al: Cardiac variations of exercise capacity in patients with Prinzmetal's variant angina: role of exercise-induced coronary arterial spasm, *Circulation* 59:938, 1979.

349. Younker D, Jones MM, Adenuda J et al: Maternal cortical vein thrombosis and the obstetric anesthesiologist, *Anesth Analg* 65:1007, 1986.

350. Zalzal GH: Stridor and airway compromise, *Ped Clin N Am* 36(6):1389, 1989.

351. Zelis R, Sinoway L, Musch T et al: Vasoconstrictor mechanism in congestive heart failure. 1. *Modern Concepts of Cardiovascular Disease* 58(2):7, 1989.

CHAPTER 2

Premedication

JOHN R. MOYERS

The anesthesiologist should assess both the mental and the physical condition of each patient during the preoperative visit.* Because they are part of and the beginning of the anesthetic process, psychologic preparation and premedication should be based on the same considerations as choice of anesthetic, namely the patient's underlying medical condition, the requirements of surgery, and the skills of the anesthesiologist. Drugs should be prescribed preoperatively with attention given to specific pharmacologic actions and individual patient needs. A proper preoperative visit and premedication can often lead to a smooth anesthetic whereas poor preparation often leads to intraoperative trouble.

_____
* This chapter was adapted in part from Moyers JR: Preoperative medication. In Barash PG, Cullen BF, and Stoelting RK, eds: *Clinical anesthesia,* Philadelphia, 1989, JB Lippincott.

The concept of premedication was well established by the late 1800s. After ether became commonplace, premedication with an anticholinergic ("drying") agent and a sedative became common practice. Unfortunately, as the unwanted properties of anesthetic agents were reduced, the side effects of the premedications themselves became more noticeable.[147,217,218] New premedication drugs were then developed and employed, benzodiazepines being a prime example. Over the years, however, consensus on a reasonable choice for premedication has never been reached. Tradition has dominated with modification coming only as anesthetic agents and techniques have evolved. Anesthesiologists, on the whole, tend to become attached, emotionally and empirically, to a few drugs for premedication.[11,146] Another reason for the lack of consensus regarding premedication has been the fact that different drugs or combinations can accomplish identical goals. Nevertheless, there is general agreement among anesthesiologists that patients should enter the operating room without undue sedation or compromise of safety having had as much relief of anxiety as possible.

PREOPERATIVE VISIT

Equal to or more important than preoperative administration of sedative drugs is good psychologic preparation. Such preparation is accomplished during the preoperative interview when the anesthesiologist explains to the patient and family anticipated events and the proposed anesthetic management in an effort to reduce fear and anxiety. Patients often view surgery as the most significant event in their lives, and they do not want to be treated in an impersonal way.[175]

Preoperative visits should be conducted efficiently, but they must be informative, provide reassurance, and answer all questions.[63] Depending on the type of

Table 2-1 Preoperative visit vs. premedication with pentobarbital (2 mg/kg IM)				
Patient status	Control group	Administration of pentobarbital	Preoperative visit	Preoperative visit and administration of pentobarbital
Felt drowsy	18%	30%	26%	38%
Felt nervous	58%	61%	40%	38%
Adequate preoperative preparation	35%	48%	65%	71%

From Egbert LD, Battit GE, Turndorf H et al: The value of the preoperative visit by the anesthetist, *JAMA* 185:553, 1963.

inquiry, research demonstrates that between 11% and 85% of patients are apprehensive before surgery.[60,140,178] Patients expect that their anxiety will be relieved before they enter the operating room.[131,140] Egbert et al. demonstrated that 57% of patients were anxious preoperatively with the highest levels of anxiety noted in patients scheduled for major genitourologic and cancer surgery.[60] In this study population neither age nor sex differences affected the level of apprehension. Other researchers have found females to be more anxious preoperatively,[53,178] but most investigators found greater levels of anxiety in patients with serious illness with no difference in incidence or severity of anxiety related to age, social status, nature of the operation, or previous hospital experience.[178] Similarly, Domar et al. found anxiety to reflect the patient's personality rather than external factors.[53]

An informative and comforting preoperative visit can effectively substitute for many milligrams of premedication.[172] Egbert et al. demonstrated that more patients were adequately prepared for surgery after a preoperative interview alone than after 2 mg/kg of pentobarbital given intramuscularly an hour before surgery without an accompanying preoperative visit[60] (Table 2-1). In this study, patients were visited in their room the afternoon before surgery by an anesthesiologist. The patient and anesthesiologist discussed the patient's medical condition, the time of the operation, and the planned anesthetic. The patient was informed about perioperative events and questioned about previous anesthetic experiences. Other patients who received pentobarbital for premedication but no interview appeared and felt sedated but were less likely to be relieved of anxiety when compared to the interview group.[60]

Leigh et al. studied adult patients using objective tests of anxiety. They found that a short (10-minute) preoperative visit by the anesthesiologist produced lower anxiety levels in patients compared to anxiety levels in patients who had not been visited at all.[140] Furthermore, they found the preoperative visit was more effective than a booklet given to patients the day before surgery. The booklet was specifically designed to reassure patients about anesthesia, but it was not found to be an adequate substitute for a proper preoperative visit.[140]

Psychologic preparation, however, cannot do everything. It will neither relieve all anxiety nor satisfy all the other goals of preoperative preparation. Amnesia, sedation, or relief of pain cannot be achieved by a preoperative visit alone. In emergent situations there may be little or no time for a preoperative interview, but in nonemergent situations the substitution of depressant premedication for a comforting and tactful preoperative visit may not only prove inadequate in achieving preoperative goals but may even encroach on patient safety.

PHARMACOLOGIC AGENTS USED IN PREMEDICATION

No one drug or combination of drugs provides ideal premedication for all patients in all types of surgical situations. Over the years emphasis has been placed on selecting appropriate goals (Box 2-1) for premedication and, then, based on the patient's physical status and psyche, choosing the proper preoperative drugs to achieve those goals. The choice is made with knowledge of the patient's age, weight, current medications, allergies, and previous response to sedative drugs. In addition to the specific surgery planned, other factors such as duration of surgery and whether it is an emergency or outpatient procedure may affect the choice of premedication. Also, anesthesiologists should select agents with which they are familiar and that can reliably be expected to produce desired effects.

Premedication should fit the requirements of individual patients the same way that anesthetic techniques do. Almost all patients are apprehensive before surgery and require sedation and relief of anxiety. Some patients may also require premedication to increase gastric fluid pH, reduce gastric fluid

Table 2-2   Common drugs used for premedication in adults

Drugs	Dosage
Midazolam	2-5 mg IM, titration of 1-2 mg doses IV
Lorazepam	1-4 mg orally or IV
Diazepam	5-20 mg orally
Pentobarbitol	50-200 mg orally or IM
Droperidol	0.625-2.5 mg IV, 2.5-5 mg IM
Morphine	5-15 mg IM
Fentanyl	Titration of 25-100 μg doses IV
Meperidine	50-150 mg IM
Atropine	0.3-0.6 mg IM or IV
Glycopyrrolate	0.1-0.3 mg IM or IV
Scopolamine	0.2-0.6 mg IM or IV
Cimetidine	150-300 mg orally, IM or IV
Ranitidine	50-200 mg orally
Metoclopramide	5-20 mg orally IM or IV

Modified from Stoelting RK: Psychological preparation and preoperative medication. In Miller RD, ed: *Anesthesia,* New York, 1981, Churchill-Livingstone.

volume, provide analgesia, or dry airway secretions to produce a safer and smoother perioperative course. In a few circumstances prophylaxis against allergic reactions may be needed. Some goals, such as preventing emesis or vagal blockade, however, may best be achieved in the operating room immediately before the anticipated event rather than with earlier premedication. For example, patients with little physiologic reserve (those who are hypovolemic or have head trauma) may be unable to withstand the effects of depressant drugs preoperatively.

Generally, before surgery, the anesthesiologist should try to have the patient enter the operating room free of apprehension and fear, sedated, but arousable and cooperative. The patient should neither display any of the unwanted side effects of premedication nor be overly obtunded. Patients who request to be unconscious before leaving their hospital room should be reminded that reduction in anxiety may be reasonable but to produce general anesthesia on the ward is dangerous.

A list of common preoperative medications is presented in Table 2-2. The timing and route of administration of premedication is important. **As a general rule, oral medications should be given on the ward 60 to 90 minutes before patient arrival in the operating room. For full effect, intramuscular medication should be given at least 20 minutes and preferably 30 to 60 minutes before arrival. Every attempt should be made to have the preoperative medications achieve their peak effectiveness before the patient arrives in the operating room rather than after anesthetic induction. The drug(s), doses, route of administration, and effects should be recorded on the anesthetic record.**

Selection of premedication so far has not been based on extensive scientific data that are either compelling or definitive. Many investigators have examined only a single dose of a drug or single dose of a combination of drugs. In some studies, drugs have been given parenterally while in other cases premedication has been achieved orally or rectally. Different studies have also focused on the effect of the drugs at different times after administration, and patient response as well as observations of responses by investigators have been subjective and difficult to quantify. Furthermore, the actual psychologic preoperative preparation has varied among studies because of the use of hetergeneous groups of subjects. Therefore the choice of premedication is still open to interpretation.

Benzodiazepines

The benzodiazepines are among the most popular agents selected for premedication (Fig. 2-1). They are used to produce sedation, amnesia, and relief of anxiety, but they are not analgetics. Because the site of action of benzodiazepines is on specific receptors in the central nervous system, relatively little depression of the respiratory or cardiovascular system occurs. Although some studies have found significant respiratory depression with benzodiazepines[32,71,163,171,238] and others have not,[146] these drugs certainly would not be expected to cause the profound alterations in respiration that occur with the administration of

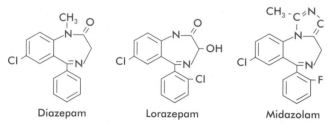

Fig. 2-1. Chemical structures of benzodiazepines commonly used for premedication. (From Reves JG, Fragen RJ, Vinik HR et al: Midazolam: pharmacology and uses, *Anesthesiology* 62:310, 1985.)

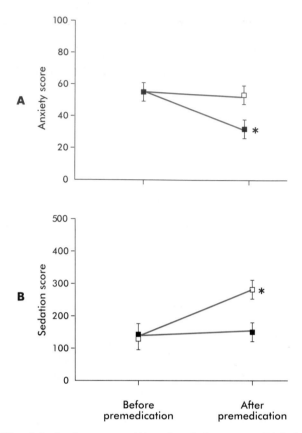

Fig. 2-2. Anxiety scores (**A**) and sedation scores (**B**) before and after premedication with saline placebo (□) or midazolam (■). Values are mean ± SEM; * indicates a significant difference (p < 0.05) between groups. (From Shafer A, White PF, Urquhart ML et al: Outpatient premedication: use of midazolam and opioid analgesics, *Anesthesiology* 71:495, 1989.)

opioids. Benzodiazepines, in general, have wide therapeutic indexes and a low incidence of toxicity. Other than central nervous system depression, few side effects occur so that nausea and vomiting, in particular, are usually not anticipated with use of benzodiazepines for premedication.

Despite careful efforts in prescribing these agents, some unwanted side effects and hazards do exist. With lorazepam, central nervous system depression may be lengthy and profound. After diazepam, pain at the site of intramuscular or intravenous injection may occur as well as phlebitis.[122] Benzodiazepines, also, do not always produce a calming effect but may result in "disinhibition" or agitation. In two studies involving patients during labor and delivery,[111,182] benzodiazepines produced restlessness and delirium in up to one third of the subjects. However, in another study[155] of patients during labor, the combination of benzodiazepines with a narcotic produced satisfactory results.

Specific actions on discrete receptors have been offered as an explanation of the effect of benzodiazepines on the central nervous system.[201,222,232,252] Facilitation or enhancement of inhibitory transmission mediated by gamma-aminobutyric acid (GABA) explains the sedative effect. Anxiolytic actions stem from glycine-mediated inhibition of neuronal pathways in the brain and brainstem. The specific sites or receptors involved in producing amnesia are unknown.

Midazolam

Like the other benzodiazepines, midazolam has sedative, anxiolytic, and amnestic effects (Fig. 2-2). Its physicochemical properties render it a water-soluble, rapidly metabolized drug. Because of its great affinity for the benzodiazepine receptor, midazolam may have three to five times the potency of diazepam. The usual adult intramuscular dose is 0.05 to 0.1 mg/kg. Titration of 1 to 2.5 mg at a time can be done when midazolam is administered to adults. There is no irritation or phlebitis after injection of midazolam and

the incidence of other side effects is low, but large doses or rapid intravenous administration may cause apnea because midazolam is a potent benzodiazepine and rapidly enters the central nervous system. This warning is particularly cogent in dealing with elderly, debilitated patients and those receiving other central nervous system depressants. When midazolam is compared to diazepam, there is a more rapid onset of action, predictability of absorption, and rapid recovery after intramuscular injection. This is probably due to the drug's high lipid solubility, rapid distribution in peripheral tissues, and metabolic biotransformation. The onset after intramuscular injection is 5 to 10 minutes with peak effect occurring after 30 to 60 minutes. The onset of effect after 5 mg is given intravenously should occur in 1 to 2 minutes. Midazolam should usually be given within an hour of anesthetic induction. It is metabolized by hepatic microsomal enzymes to essentially inactive metabolites.[200] Histamine receptor antagonists do not interfere with its metabolism.[94]

The elimination properties of midazolam make it

nearly ideal for short surgical procedures. The elimination half-life of midazolam is approximately 1 to 4 hours, although this may be prolonged in the elderly.[93] Mental function of the patient usually returns to normal within 4 hours after administration,[201] while amnesia after 5 mg is given intravenously lasts from 20 to 32 minutes.[41,55] Lack of recall may be augmented by concomitant administration of scopolamine[74] and is prolonged by administering midazolam intramuscularly.

Lorazepam

The benzodiazepine, lorazepam, is prescribed for **sedation, amnesia, and a calming effect.*** It is approximately 5 to 10 times more potent than diazepam, and, unlike diazepam, **is not associated with phlebitis or pain on injection.** Lorazepam has a shorter elimination half-life than diazepam, but its effects may persist longer because it does not dissociate as rapidly from the benzodiazepine receptor as does diazepam.[251] Because the elimination half-life with lorazepam is 10 to 20 hours, prolonged sedation is a danger; however, this factor can be used to benefit some patients who may require long postoperative periods of sedation (e.g., after cardiac surgery).

After intravenous injection, the maximum effects of lorazepam occur within 30 to 40 minutes.[54] Lorazepam is readily absorbed after both oral and intramuscular doses, but absorption is slow. Bradshaw et al. demonstrated that clinical effects begin 30 to 60 minutes after oral administration.[20] Peak plasma concentrations may not occur until 2 to 4 hours after oral doses. Another study showed amnesia did not occur until 2 hours after intramuscular injection.[16] This necessitates that lorazepam be given well before surgery to ensure the drug will become effective before the patient arrives in the operating room. Lorazepam may also be given sublingually.[78] The usual oral dose in adults is about 25 to 50 μg/kg, not to exceed 4 mg.[54,73,102] The dose may be reduced when combined with other premedications. Using the recommended doses, amnesia may last for up to 4 to 6 hours without excessive sedation. Larger doses lead to prolonged and excessive sedation but not greater amnesia.

Because of its length of action, lorazepam is not useful for outpatient surgery and other short procedures.[81] However, since its metabolism does not depend on microsomal enzymes compared to other benzodiazepines, age or liver disease has less influence on its effect.[134] Lorazepam has no active metabolites and produces little cardiorespiratory depression.† One

study did warn of the danger of unwanted respiratory depression in patients with lung disease.[50]

Diazepam

Diazepam is the standard to which other benzodiazepines are usually compared. The anxiolytic, amnestic, and sedative effects of diazepam make it popular among premedications. However, because it is insoluble in water and must be dissolved in organic solvents, pain often occurs with intramuscular or intravenous injection. In addition, phlebitis can result after intravenous injection. Over 90% of an oral dose is absorbed within 30 minutes to 1 hour in adults and as rapidly as 15 to 30 minutes in children. Patients with low serum albumin levels, such as those with chronic renal failure or with liver disease, may exhibit increased effects of diazepam.[93] It is metabolized by the hepatic microsomal enzyme system to somewhat active metabolites. Prolonged sedation due to these active metabolites is ordinarily a factor only after chronic use rather than following a single administration for premedication. The elimination half-life of diazepam is 21 to 37 hours in healthy volunteers,[123] but this can be prolonged in elderly patients or those with liver cirrhosis.[126] Placental transfer does occur.

Because of the unreliability of absorption after intramuscular injection,[52,105] and the pain that can occur during parenteral administration, many anesthesiologists prefer to give diazepam orally. Diazepam may also be given rectally but may cause local irritation in doses greater than 0.5 mg/kg.[99,154,198] While not as reliable as lorazepam in preventing recall, antegrade amnesia may be enhanced with the addition of scopolamine[77] (Fig. 2-3). As with all other premedication drugs, there is no evidence of retrograde amnesia occurring.[142]

Diazepam has few actions outside the central nervous system and produces little depression of other organ functions. Only slight cardiovascular depression is found after the usual dose of diazepam used for premedication. Indeed, considerably larger intravenous doses without concomitant opioid administration produce little circulatory depression.[155,195] Similarly, little or no effect on ventilation has been demonstrated.[224] In a study by Rao et al.[207] increases in $Paco_2$ were detected only after 0.2 mg/kg of diazepam was given intravenously.[195] The increase in CO_2 was due to a reduction in tidal volume. In another investigation the slope of the carbon dioxide response curve decreased but did not shift to the right after intravenous doses of 0.4 mg/kg.[98] Despite the past record of safety using large intravenous doses of diazepam, respiratory arrest has been reported in some patients given as little as 2.5 mg.[21,47,253] Ventilatory depression may be compounded when other depressant drugs are added, especially narcotics.

---

*References 1, 54, 102, 185, 186, 206, 246, 251.
†References 37, 40, 45, 46, 80, 127.

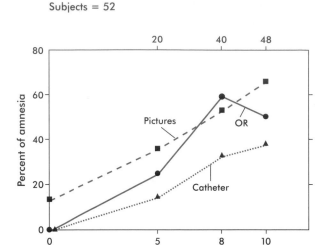

Subjects = 52

Fig. 2-3. Dose-response curves for three tests of memory. Doses of diazepam were 0, 5, 8 and 10 mg/70 kg. All patients received scopolamine (0.5 mg/70 kg) in addition. (From Frumin MJ, Hereker VR, and Jarvick ME: Amnesic actions of diazepam and scopolamine in man, *Anesthesiology* 45:406, 1976.)

In the doses used for premedication, little clinical effect on the neuromuscular junction is evident. There have been attempts to use diazepam to reduce fasciculations and reduce myalgias produced by succinylcholine.[48,241] The effect on fasciculations was variable, but the incidence of myalgias was reduced in a study by Davies.[48] Premedication with diazepam does not reliably prevent increases in intraocular pressure with endotracheal intubation.[66,67,135] Diazepam has reduced the seizure threshold for lidocaine in animals, but this has not been reproduced in humans.[168] Cimetidine delays the hepatic clearance of diazepam due to the inhibition of microsomal enzymes,[92] but there is controversy as to clinical importance of this when diazepam is given in a single dose preoperatively. Diazepam 0.2 mg/kg has been shown to decrease minimum alveolar concentration (MAC) for halothane.[189] The magnitude of reduction in anesthetic requirement using premedication doses of diazepam may or may not be clinically important.

Other benzodiazepines

Oxazepam[7,97] is a pharmacologically active metabolite of diazepam. It is administered orally and is absorbed slowly after administration. Temazepam,* another benzodiazepine, has been given in oral doses of 20 to 40 mg before surgery. This drug is given in capsule form and must be taken well before surgery because its sedative, anxiolytic, and amnestic actions may not occur until 1 or 2 hours after administration. Clinical effects generally last 4 to 5 hours. Triazolam[8,136,169,191,233] is a short-acting benzodiazepine with

---
*References 2, 5, 12, 28, 97, 197.

anxiolytic and good amnestic properties. The adult oral dose of the drug is 0.25 to 0.5 mg, which produces peak plasma concentration after approximately 1 hour. Elimination half-life of triazolam is about 2 to 5 hours. One study of premedication for short surgical procedures did not show shorter duration of action with triazolam compared to diazepam.[191] Other benzodiazepines have been used, namely chlordiazepoxide,[96] for preoperative medication. It is hardly necessary for the anesthesiologist to become familiar with all benzodiazepines when prescribing premedication. Instead, familiarity with a few that can be given orally and parenterally will lead to consistently satisfactory premedication results.

Barbiturates

Barbiturates have been used preoperatively for their sedative effects and have enjoyed a long record of safe use, causing patients little cardiorespiratory depression.[221] They are also inexpensive and may be given orally as well as parenterally. Barbiturates, however, are not analgetic drugs. In fact, in the presence of pain, administration may produce disorientation or even an "antianalgetic" effect. These agents should be avoided in patients with various types of porphyria. Currently, benzodiazepines have largely replaced barbiturates for preoperative sedation because benzodiazepines have a wider therapeutic index and act on specific receptors within the central nervous system.

Secobarbital

The usual adult oral dose for secobarbital is 50 to 200 mg when used for premedication. Onset of sedation occurs 90 minutes afterward and may last 4 hours or longer. Despite the traditional view that secobarbital is a short-acting barbiturate, it can alter consciousness for as long as 10 to 22 hours.[128]

Pentobarbital

Both oral and parenteral forms of pentobarbital are available, and adults usually receive 50 to 200 mg orally. It is not the ideal premedication for short procedures because its elimination half-life is around 50 hours. However, an investigation by Hovi-Viander et al., found pentobarbital equal to diazepam in reducing anxiety preoperatively.[112] In contrast, Dundee et al. found 100 mg of pentobarbital to be no better than a placebo in reducing preoperative apprehension.[147]

Butyrophenones

Droperidol and, very occasionally, haloperidol can be used for premedication. Given intramuscularly or intravenously before surgery, 2.5 to 7.5 mg of droperidol results in the outward appearance of a calm patient. Despite appearances, patients may later complain of dysphoria, restlessness, or even fear of death,[104] with the dysphoria and fear sometimes leading to refusal of surgery.[22,139] Extrapyramidal signs may appear in about 1% of patients after administration of droperidol because of its action as a dopamine antagonist.[187,203] The butyrophenones, in general, can exhibit mild alpha-blocking effects in larger intravenous doses.

Currently, droperidol is most often used for its antiemetic effect rather than its sedative properties (see the section on antiemetics). Small clinical doses of droperidol have been used preoperatively or just before emergence from anesthesia to prevent nausea and vomiting in the recovery room.

Finally, droperidol counters the inhibitory effect of dopamine on the ventilatory response to hypoxia because it is a dopamine antagonist. Therefore it preserves the carotid body response to hypoxia. For these reasons, some researchers have suggested that droperidol may be good premedication for patients dependent on hypoxic ventilatory drive.[247]

Other Sedative-Hypnotics and Tranquilizers
Phenothiazines

Phenothiazines are occasionally used with narcotic analgetic agents for sedative, antiemetic, and anticholinergic effects.[38,124] The most commonly used are promethazine, perphenazine, and promazine.

Hydroxyzine

Hydroxyzine is a nonphenothiazine tranquilizer often used for its purported additive effect to opioids without increasing side effects.[114] It has sedative, calming, antiemetic, and antihistamine properties but does not produce amnesia.[13,157,246,250]

Chloral hydrate

Chloral hydrate has been prescribed as a preoperative medication to relieve apprehension and produce amnesia, especially in elderly patients. Benzodiazepines and other drugs have largely replaced the use of chloral hydrate preoperatively.

Diphenhydramine

Diphenhydramine blocks histamine receptors and has sedative, antiemetic, and anticholinergic properties. Drug effect will persist for 3 to 6 hours after an oral dose of 50 mg in the adult patient. Because of histamine receptor antagonism, diphenhydramine has been used as part of a regimen of prophylaxis before intravenous dye studies or for patients with chronic atopy.[9]

Analgetic Agents

It has been contended that unless pain exists preoperatively, there is no need for opioid premedication.[33] Opioids are not particularly suited for relieving anxiety, producing sedation, or preventing recall of perioperative events.[40,46] Nevertheless, for the patient who is experiencing pain preoperatively, opioids can produce good analgesia and even euphoria. Opioids, as a premedication, have been used to prevent pain that may occur during the insertion of invasive monitoring catheters, during the placing of large intravenous lines, or during needle placement with regional anesthetic techniques. Opioids have also been used in the premedication of narcotic-dependent patients. Morphine and meperidine are the most frequently used opioids for intramuscular preoperative medication; intravenously, the use of fentanyl just before surgery has recently become popular.

Premedication with opioids in other settings is more controversial. They have been administered before nitrous-narcotic anesthesia to achieve a basal state of narcosis when the patient arrives in the operating room and to preview patient response to narcotics. Preoperative administration of opioids can reduce subsequent anesthetic requirement.[208,237] The importance of this varies depending on the patient and anesthetic technique. Some believe that opioid premedication in combination with other drugs facilitates mask induction. This use is especially popular when induction intravenously or rectally is not possible. Opioids decrease respiratory rate during spontaneous breathing and, therefore, increase $Paco_2$. This should decrease the uptake of inhalation anesthetics despite the previous contention that mask inductions may be facilitated. The anesthesiologist may want to consider the use of assisted ventilation after preoperative opioids. Opioids have also been given preoperatively to provide analgesia immediately postoperatively. In contrast, some anesthesiologists have given opioids intravenously during emergence from anesthesia or on patient arrival in the postanesthesia care unit, after assessing levels of pain plus ventilation and consciousness.

Opioid dosage may need to be greatly reduced in elderly or debilitated patients. An elderly patient may have a reduced sensitivity to pain or an increased analgetic response to opioids.[14] Older patients in pain should not be deprived of analgesia, but the effects of aging must be considered.

Premedication with opioids has the potential for several side effects. Opioids, except for large intravenous doses of meperidine, usually exhibit no direct myocardial depressant effects. However, opioids do interfere with the compensatory constriction of the peripheral vascular smooth muscle, which could possibly lead to orthostatic hypotension. Histamine release with morphine may compound the hypotension. Therefore, as with most preoperative medications, it is probably safest to leave the patient resting in bed after premedication with opioids.

The analgetic effects and respiratory depressant properties of opioids are intertwined.[221] The most analgesia achieved, the more depression of ventilation that results. The decreased carbon dioxide response at the medullary respiratory center from opioids may be quite prolonged. In addition, responsiveness to hypoxia is decreased at the carotid body after injection of even small doses of opioids.[249] In general, the opioid agonist-antagonists produce less respiratory depression, but they also provide less analgesia.

Rather than euphoria, opioids may produce dysphoria. This occurs most commonly in patients without preoperative pain who receive opioid premedication. Nausea and vomiting may also follow opioid administration (apomorphine is a good emetic drug). The effect of opioids on the vestibular apparatus, leading to motion sickness and stimulation of the medullary chemoreceptor trigger zone, are postulated as reasons for nausea and vomiting. In addition, stimulation of the chemoreceptor zone has also been proposed as a cause of emesis because a supine position reduces the incidence of nausea and vomiting after opioid administration.

Choledochoduodenal sphincter (sphincter of Oddi) spasm has been reported after opioid injection.[59,193] Opioids can produce smooth muscle constriction of the sphincter, which leads to right upper quadrant pain. Relief of this pain has been achieved with the administration of naloxone and even glucagon.[120] **In the patient with coronary artery disease, pain from choledochoduodenal sphincter spasm may be difficult to distinguish from angina.** An opioid antagonist (e.g., naloxone) should relieve the pain due to spasm of the choledochoduodenal sphincter, whereas nitroglycerine relieves anginal pain. Some anesthesiologists advise against the use of opioid premedication in patients with biliary tract disease. Although all opioids have the potential to induce choledochoduodenal sphincter spasm, meperidine may be less likely to do so than morphine. Opioids may also cause flushing, dizziness, and miosis.

Rather than being used alone, opioids are usually combined with other drugs preoperatively. Sedative-hypnotics and scopolamine[30] are often used with opioids to achieve sedation, relief of anxiety, and amnesia in addition to analgesia. The combination of morphine, a benzodiazepine, and/or scopolamine is a time-tested and popular combination for premedication.

Morphine

Morphine is well absorbed from intramuscular sites with onset of narcotic effect after 15 to 30 minutes. The peak effect after intramuscular injection is seen in 45 to 90 minutes, with effects persisting up to 4 hours. Although morphine is available in an oral preparation, for premedication it is not reliably absorbed through the gastrointestinal tract. It may cause orthostatic hypotension, pruritis, and respiratory depression as do the other opioids. Morphine may also produce nausea and vomiting as a result of its central nervous system actions and may cause decreased motility and increased GI tract secretions. Despite the incidence of side effects, morphine has been used successfully for years when a narcotic is needed as part of premedication.

Fentanyl

Fentanyl is not often given outside the operating room for premedication. It is, however, frequently given intravenously in the operating room shortly before anesthetic induction. Fentanyl is 50 to 125 times more potent than morphine as an analgetic drug. A small (1 to 2 μg/kg) dose given intravenously produces effects within 30 to 60 seconds and usually lasts about 30 to 60 minutes. Its rapid onset and potency compared to morphine probably are due to greater lipid solubility and more rapid redistribution to skeletal muscle and fat (Fig. 2-4). A short duration of action, good

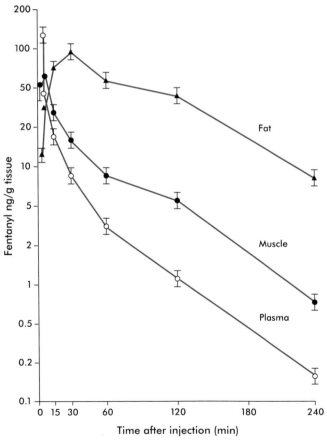

Fig. 2-4. Short duration of action of a single bolus of fentanyl is due to a rapid decline in plasma concentration associated with its redistribution to fat and muscle. (From Hug CC, Murphy MR: Tissue redistribution of fentanyl, *Anesthesiology* 55:372, 1981.)

analgesia, and blunting of circulatory responses to endotracheal intubation are the appeals of using a small dose of intravenous fentanyl immediately before surgery.

Meperidine

Meperidine may be given orally or parenterally. A single dose of meperidine usually lasts 2 to 4 hours. It is about one tenth as potent as morphine. However, the onset after intramuscular injection is unpredictable and there is great variability in time to peak effect.[4] After the administration of meperidine, increased heart rate as well as orthostatic hypotension can occur.

Other opioids

Codeine has been prescribed as a premedication in adults in doses of 50 to 60 mg orally. It can also be given as an intramuscular dose of 120 mg, which is equal to about 10 mg of morphine. If it is given intravenously, histamine release, nausea, and vomiting are relatively likely. Methadone also has the advantage of oral as well as intramuscular administration, but it is a long-acting opioid with an elimination half-life of approximately 35 hours.[89] Hydromorphone is another opioid that may be given orally, as well as intramuscularly.

Opioid agonist-antagonists

The most commonly used opioid agonist-antagonists are pentazocine, butorphanol, and nalbuphine. They have been advocated for premedication in an attempt to reduce the respiratory side effects of pure opioid agonists.[107,137,138,190,239] However, a "ceiling" exists on the amount of analgesia that can be accomplished with these drugs. Their side effects are similar to those produced by the pure opioids, and dysphoria may be even more likely after administration of opioid agonist-antagonists. Another disadvantage is that the opioid agonist-antagonists can reduce the effectiveness of a pure narcotic agonist given later for postoperative pain.

Anticholinergic Agents

The anticholinergic agents used for premedication today include atropine, glycopyrrolate, and scopolamine. Atropine has antisialogogue and strong vagolytic properties. Glycopyrrolate has clinically useful vagolytic and antisialogogue actions, whereas scopolamine has good sedative and antisialogogue effects (Table 2-3).

In the past, anticholinergics were frequently given as a premedication to prevent intraoperative bradycardia and to reduce airway secretions produced by inhalation anesthetics.[95] As newer anesthetic agents have evolved, routine preoperative use of anticholin-

Table 2-3   Comparison of effects of anticholinergic drugs used for premedication

Drugs	Vagolytic action	Antisialagogue effect	Sedation and amnesia
Atropine	3^+	1^+	0
Scopolamine	1^+	2^+	3^+
Glycopyrrolate	2^+	3^+	0

0 = no effect; 3^+ = great effect.
Modified from Stoelting RK: *Pharmacology and physiology in anesthetic practice*, Philadelphia, 1987, JB Lippincott.

ergics for all patients has fallen into disfavor without apparent adverse effects on the conduct or outcome of anesthesia.* Indications for the use of anticholinergics in specific instances do exist: (1) antisialogogue action, (2) sedation and amnesia, and (3) vagolytic effect, especially in very young patients. Some sentiment still exists for using anticholinergic agents as a premedication in the effort to reduce gastric acid secretion and to prevent intraoperative bradycardia in adults as well as in children.

Vagolytic effect

Intravenous atropine is more effective than either scopolamine or glycopyrrolate in increasing heart rate. Tachycardia is produced by blocking the action of acetycholine on the SA node. Bradycardia during surgery from stimulation of the carotid sinus, traction on abdominal viscera or extraocular muscles, or after repeated doses of succinylcholine can be prevented or ameliorated by anticholinergic drugs, especially atropine. Atropine or glycopyrrolate given intravenously just before surgery is more reliable in preventing anticipated intraoperative bradycardia than if given outside the operating room, especially considering the difficulties in timing and dosage of anticholinergic premedication given intramuscularly on the ward.[161] Intravenous glycopyrrolate is equal to atropine in preventing bradycardia after repeated boluses of succinylcholine.[223]

Antisialogogue action

Anticholinergics have been administered specifically to dry upper airway secretions. Falick and Smiler indicated a more satisfactory endotracheal intubation after an anticholinergic drug had been administered preoperatively.[65] The drying effect may be important before extensive instrumentation of the pharynx and airway during bronchoscopy and intraoral surgery. Anticholinergics may also be needed before topical anesthesia to allow the airway mucosal contact with

---

* References 31, 61, 108, 125, 145, 162, 164-166, 219.

the local anesthetic, to avoid dilution with secretions, and to improve visibility during fiberoptic bronchoscopic examination.

Scopolamine is somewhat more effective as an antisialogogue than atropine. It is less likely to increase heart rate and, because it easily crosses the blood-brain barrier, is more likely to produce amnesia and sedation. Glycopyrrolate is a more potent and longer-acting drying agent[207,255] **than atropine and is less likely to increase heart rate or produce dysrhythmias.**[156] **Glycopyrrolate does not cross the blood-brain barrier because it is a quaternary amine. Anticholinergics are not the only drugs that result in reduced oral secretions; other drugs and a placebo may result in a dry mouth.**[70]

Sedative and amnestic properties

Scopolamine is the anticholinergic drug most likely to produce sedation and amnesia. Scopolamine and atropine both cross the blood-brain barrier. Scopolamine is a much more effective sedative and amnestic than atropine. In a study by Conner et al. of patient acceptance of preoperative medication, the combination of morphine and scopolamine was superior to morphine and atropine.[39] Nevertheless, scopolamine cannot be relied on to prevent recall in all patients. It may not be as effective as benzodiazepines in producing amnesia. Frumin et al. showed that the combination of diazepam and scopolamine produced amnesia more often than did diazepam alone, indicating an additive effect[77] (see Fig. 2-3).

Reduction of gastric acid secretion

Histamine receptor blockers and antacids have generally replaced attempts with anticholinergic drugs to raise gastric fluid pH. Even large doses of atropine or glycopyrrolate used in studies by Stoelting[240] and Manchikanti et al.[154] have shown that anticholinergics are unreliable in decreasing gastric hydrogen ion secretion (see section on gastric fluid volume and pH).

Side effects

Scopolamine and atropine can produce central nervous system toxicity manifested as the "central anticholinergic syndrome."[144] This syndrome occurs more commonly after scopolamine but can be seen after large doses (greater than 2 mg) of intravenous atropine. The symptoms of central nervous system toxicity include delirium, confusion, restlessness, and obtundation. Patients experiencing pain and elderly patients[220] appear to be particularly susceptible. Inhalation anesthetics may potentiate the central nervous system toxicity of anticholinergics.[109] Treatment of the syndrome with 1 to 2 mg of intravenous physostigmine is advocated by some anesthesiologists.[57,109]

The anticholinergics also reduce lower esophageal sphincter tone in adults and children.[23,183] Theoretically, after a parenteral dose of anticholinergic premedication, the risk of pulmonary aspiration of gastric contents is greater. This has yet to be proved as an important clinical property of this class of drugs.

Mydriasis and cycloplegia after administration of anticholinergic drugs could theoretically increase intraocular pressure in patients with glaucoma. This appears unlikely with doses used for preoperative medication. Atropine and glycopyrrolate have less potential to cause problems than scopolamine.[79] When ordering premedication for patients with glaucoma, most anesthesiologists feel confident in continuing medications for glaucoma until the time of surgery and in using atropine or glycopyrrolate when necessary.

Atropine is more likely than either glycopyrrolate or scopolamine to cause tachycardia or even dysrhythmias.[166] Unwanted increases in heart rate are much more likely after intravenous rather than intramuscular administration of anticholinergics. As a result of the peripheral agonist effect of anticholinergics, heart rate may actually decrease transiently after intramuscular administration.

Because anticholinergic drugs are vagolytic, relaxation of bronchial smooth muscle occurs and respiratory dead space increases.[213] A dead space increase as large as 25% to 33% has been reported, depending on prior bronchomotor tone. These changes may or may not be of clinical importance. Anticholinergic drugs cause drying and thickening of secretions. Inspissation of secretions and increases in airway resistance may compromise respiratory function in patients with diseases such as cystic fibrosis.

Anticholinergic agents also interfere with cholinergic transmission and the sweating mechanism since sweat glands are innervated by the sympathetic nervous system. A potential for the increase in body temperature after anticholinergic premedication should be considered carefully in the child or adult with a fever.

Agents that Alter Gastric Fluid Volume and pH

In 1946 Mendelson described the syndrome of pulmonary aspiration of gastric contents during obstetric anesthesia.[159] Since then many patients in the operating room or delivery suite have been thought to be at risk for aspiration pneumonitis* (Box 2-2). Based largely on data from studies on experimental animals, critical values for gastric pH (<2.5) and volume (>0.4 ml/kg) have been developed (Fig. 2-5). Similar studies have not and probably could not be ethically done in humans. While gastric acidity may be the

---

* References 15, 42, 88, 121, 159, 182, 184, 240.

BOX 2–2
RISK FACTORS ASSOCIATED WITH
PULMONARY ASPIRATION

Abdominal tumor	Hiatal hernia
Alcohol or other drug overdose	Increased intracranial pressure
Anesthesia	Nasogastric tube
Anxiety	Obesity
Ascites	Outpatient anesthesia(?)
Cardiac arrest	
Cardiovascular accident	Pregnancy
Depression of consciousness	Scleroderma
	Seizures
Diabetes	Trauma
Emergency abdominal surgery	Very young age

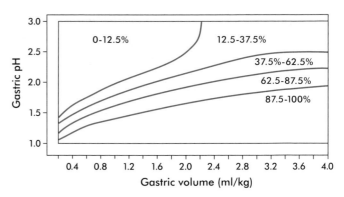

Fig. 2-5. Mortality in the rat as a function of both pH and volume following pulmonary aspiration of gastric contents. (From James CF: Pulmonary aspiration–effect of volume and pH in the rat, *Anesth Analg* 63:667, 1984.)

more important of the two factors, aspiration of material with a pH greater than 2.5 is definitely not always benign. Also, most studies do not address the issue of aspiration and nonacid food particles. Using the preceding rubric for investigation, some researchers have estimated that 20% to 80% of patients coming to surgery may be at risk. Others believe such percentages are overestimated and challenge routine attempts to reduce gastric volume and acid content, emphasizing data that show pulmonary aspiration to be very rare in *elective* surgery in patients without definite risk factors. The NPO status requirement before elective surgery is even being reconsidered, and some adult patients are receiving clear liquids orally up to 2 to 3 hours before anesthesia and surgery.

For emergency surgery and patients at risk, several different classes of pharmaceutical agents have been employed to alter gastric pH and fluid volume. They include histamine receptor–blocking drugs, gastrokinetic agents, clear antacids, and anticholinergics.

Histamine receptor antagonists

The commonly used histamine H_2-receptor antagonists for premedication are cimetidine and ranitidine. Famotidine and nizatidine are also available but are less frequently used in the perioperative setting by anesthesiologists. **These drugs raise gastric fluid pH by reducing secretion of gastric hydrogen ion.** Antagonism in a competitive and selective mode prevents histamine from inducing the secretion of gastric fluid with a high acid content.[15] As with the benzodiazepines, relatively few side effects accompany the use of cimetidine and ranitidine. Because of the many elective surgery patients at risk for aspiration pneumonitis and the few unwanted side effects of histamine H_2-blockers, some researchers have proposed

almost universal use of histamine receptor agonists.[42] Multiple dose regimens[248] beginning the night before surgery are usually more effective in consistently raising gastric pH than a single dose preoperatively given the day of surgery. As with most other drugs, parenteral administration produces a more rapid onset of action than the oral route. **Although these drugs reduce acidity, they should not be expected to decrease gastric fluid volume or emptying time.** Another selected use for cimetidine or ranitidine is if there is the possibility of triggering an allergic response.

Cimetidine. The usual adult dosage of cimetidine is 150 to 300 mg orally or parenterally[42,149,153,228,248] (Fig. 2-6). Giving 300 mg of cimetidine orally 60 to 90 minutes before surgery has been shown by Stoelting to increase the pH of gastric fluid above 2.5 in 80% of patients.[228] No effect on gastric fluid volume in this study was demonstrated. A study by Maliniak et al.[149] reported that cimetidine (300 mg) given intravenously 2 hours preoperatively not only increased gastric fluid pH but also reduced gastric fluid volume. An advantage of cimetidine is that it can also be given intravenously. Cimetidine crosses the placenta, but adverse effects on the fetus are unproved.[106,119] In one multicenter study,[106] 126 patients scheduled for elective cesarean section received either 30 ml antacid 1 to 3 hours preoperatively or 300 mg of cimetidine orally at bedtime and again intramuscularly 1 to 3 hours before surgery. There was a decrease in gastric acid content and gastric fluid volume in the cimetidine group. No differences in neonatal neurobehavioral scores were noted between the two groups. The gastric acid and volume effects of cimetidine last 3 or 4 hours,[43] which must be considered when long procedures are planned. The dose may need to be larger for very obese patients.

As noted, cimetidine has relatively few side effects,

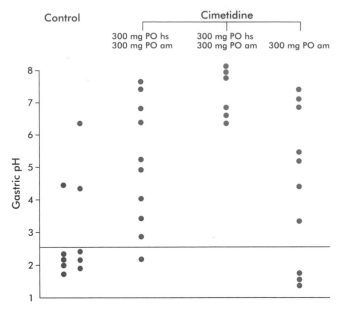

Fig. 2-6. Distribution of gastric aspirate pH values in control patients and in patients receiving cimetidine. (From Manchikanti L, Kraus JW, and Edds SP: Cimetidine and related drugs in anesthesia, *Anesth Analg* 61:595, 1982.)

but some are important. It interferes with the hepatic mixed function oxidase enzyme system and, consequently, has potential for prolonging actions of theophylline, warfarin, chlordiazepoxide, diazepam, propranolol, lidocaine, and other drugs in which action is closely related to metabolism rather than elimination. The clinical significance of this interaction after one or two doses of cimetidine for premedication is uncertain, and significant adverse responses are quite rare. Cimetidine may have prolonged effects in patients with renal insufficiency. Hypotension, dysrhythmias, cardiac arrest, and central nervous system depression have been reported after administration of cimetidine.[34,216] These side effects must be anticipated, especially in elderly and critically ill patients, after rapid intravenous administration. Intravenous administration over 15 to 20 minutes will reduce the likelihood of life-threatening cardiovascular side effects. In theory cimetidine should produce unopposed histamine H_2-receptor–mediated bronchial constriction and cause greater airway resistance in patients with asthma. As mentioned previously, cimetidine has no effect on the pH of fluid already present in the stomach.

Ranitidine. The usual oral dose of ranitidine is 50 to 200 mg. Ranitidine given parenterally in doses of 50 to 100 mg will increase gastric fluid pH within 1 hour.[56,101] It is longer acting, more potent, and has more receptor site specificity than cimetidine. Studies by Zeldis[257] and Gillett[87] show ranitidine reduces the risk of gastric aspiration as well as does cimetidine

while producing fewer cardiovascular or central nervous system side effects. Because the effects of ranitidine last up to 9 hours, it may be superior to cimeditine in reducing the risk of aspiration pneumonitis during extubation and emergence from anesthesia after lengthy surgical procedures.[42]

Gastrokinetic agents

Metoclopramide. **Metoclopramide reduces gastric fluid volume and risk of aspiration because it is a dopamine antagonist that stimulates upper gastrointestinal motility, increases gastroesophageal sphincter tone, and relaxes the pylorus and duodenum.**[23,113,173,256] Metoclopramide hastens gastric emptying but has no known effect on secretion of hydrogen ion and gastric fluid pH. It does have antiemetic features. An oral dose of 10 mg will produce effects within 30 to 60 minutes. A parenteral dose of 5 to 20 mg is usually given 15 to 30 minutes before induction of analgesia. When the drug is injected intravenously in a rapid fashion, addominal cramping can occur; administering the drug over 3 to 5 minutes will usually prevent this. The elimination half-life of metoclopramide is approximately 2 to 4 hours.

Premedication with metoclopramide is beneficial in patients likely to have large gastric fluid volumes preoperatively (e.g., pregnant patients, patients scheduled for emergency surgery, obese patients, outpatients, and diabetic patients. However, giving metoclopramide does not guarantee complete gastric emptying. Significant volumes of gastric fluid may still be present despite its administration.[44] The administration of atropine[24] or prior opioids[177] may reduce the effect of metoclopramide on the upper gastrointestinal tract. Cimetidine may not be effective after the administration of sodium citrate[210] and will not further reduce gastric volume in patients scheduled for elective surgery who already have small gastric volumes.[35] Considering all the drugs available, metoclopramide can be very effective in reducing the risk of pulmonary aspiration of gastric contents when combined with a histamine H_2-receptor–blocker, such as ranitidine, before elective surgery.[150,151,179]

Antacids

Antacids are used to neutralize the acid in fluid already present in the stomach. A single dose of an antacid given 15 to 30 minutes before induction of anesthesia is nearly 100% effective in raising gastric fluid pH above 2.5.[87,152,229,244] **The nonparticulate antacid sodium citrate in an 0.3 M concentration is commonly given preoperatively to reduce gastric acidity.** Colloid antacid suspensions may be even more effective than the nonparticulate type in increasing gastric fluid pH,[76] but aspiration of gastric fluid containing particulate antacids may cause significant and persistent pulmonary damage despite reduction in gastric fluid acidity.[17,85,101,212] The non-particulate antacids do not produce pulmonary damage themselves if aspiration of only gastric fluid containing these antacids occurs.[86]

Antacids work immediately but are effective only on gastric fluid already present. In emergency surgery, this offers a real advantage over other agents used for aspiration prophylaxis since such agents must be administered well before the procedure. Gastric volume is one of the determinants of the severity of aspiration pneumonitis. In contrast to gastrokinetic drugs or histamine H_2-receptor antagonists, antacids increase gastric fluid volume,[72,211,228] especially if repeated doses are given. The issues of effectiveness on partially digested food particles and the completeness of mixing with all gastric fluids are unresolved.

Anticholinergic drugs

Anticholinergic drugs have not been found to be useful in reducing gastric acid production or fluid volume. Stoelting demonstrated that neither intramuscular atropine (0.4 mg) nor glycopyrrolate (0.2 mg) was effective in altering the pH or volume of gastric fluid preoperatively.[229] A similar study using 4 to 5 μg/kg of glycopyrrolate did not reduce the percentage of patients with gastric fluid pH below 2.5 or gastric fluid volume greater than 0.4 mg/kg,[154] and a third study in parturients also found glycopyrrolate (0.3 mg) ineffective.[6] Other studies determined that intravenous doses of anticholinergics may relax the lower esophageal sphincter.[24,183] Therefore, in theory, it is possible for preoperative intramuscular anticholinergic agents to *increase* the risk of aspiration pneumonitis.

As discussed previously, the majority of drugs used to alter gastric volume and pH have relatively few side effects. The risk of unwanted side effects with these drugs is small compared to the benefits of reducing the risk of aspiration of gastric contents. In any case no drug regimen is absolutely reliable in preventing aspiration pneumonitis in all patients and in all circumstances. Drugs do not eliminate the need for skillful airway management to minimize coughing, gastric distension, vomiting, or regurgitation with an unprotected airway.

Antiemetic Agents

Patients scheduled for ophthalmologic or gynecologic surgery, patients with a prior history of vomiting, and obese patients may benefit from antiemetics (Box 2-3). Controversy exists, however, as to the timing of administration of such drugs. Some anesthesiologists incorporate antiemetics into the patient's premedication, whereas others believe they should be given just

---

BOX 2–3
COMMON CAUSES OF POSTOPERATIVE NAUSEA AND VOMITING

Surgical procedures
  Ophthalmologic surgery
  Gynecologic surgery (e.g., laraposcopy, therapeutic abortion)
Drugs
  Opioids
  Etomidate
  N_2O(?)
Medical conditions
  Pregnancy
  Uremia
Gastric inflation from assisted or controlled ventilation
Pain
Hypotension

---

before they are needed or after a demonstrated need at the conclusion of surgery.

Droperidol

Relatively small doses of intravenous droperidol are often effective in preventing or relieving nausea and vomiting.* A study of spinal anesthesia for cesarean section demonstrated the effective antiemetic properties of 2.5 mg of intravenous droperidol.[209] Korttila et al. used 1.25 mg of droperidol IV just before the end of a surgical procedure to reduce the incidence of postoperative nausea and vomiting.[132] Whereas larger doses can lead to undesirable sedation or even alpha-adrenergic blocking actions, small doses may not always be reliable prophylaxis for emesis.[36]

Metoclopramide

In addition to gastrokinetic actions, metoclopramide possesses antiemetic properties.[29,62,215,236] These actions are thought to occur because of the antidopaminergic effects at the fourth ventricle chemoreceptor trigger zone. However, perhaps because of its brief duration of action, metaclopramide has been found inconsistent in preventing postoperative nausea and vomiting.[36,62,215]

Phenothiazines

Prochlorperazine is the most common phenothiazine used to prevent or treat nausea and vomiting. Use of other phenothiazines, such as promethazine, to achieve antiemetic effects is unpopular among some

---

* References 36, 115, 132, 170, 188, 209, 235, 254.

anesthesiologists because of the potential for extrapyramidal effects.

Other drugs

Hydroxyzine[157] and diphenidol[254] have antinausea and antiemetic actions. However, despite antiemetic properties demonstrated in other settings, Korttila et al. did not find domperidone effective in reducing postoperative nausea and vomiting.[132]

Adrenergic-Blocking Agents

There has been some interest in using specific adrenergic-blocking agents for premedication.* The goal is to block sympathetic response and prevent the adverse myocardial effects of perioperative stress. These agents are given to decrease both frequency and severity of perioperative tachycardia and hypertension, both of which may lead to myocardial ischemia. Some of these drugs, such as clonidine, can also decrease the anesthetic requirement. Stone et al.[230] studied the intraoperative electrocardiograms of 128 untreated, mildly hypertensive patients. They found that a single small oral dose of a beta-adrenergic–blocking agent, given with premedication, significantly reduced the risk of myocardial ischemia. The patients in the group given beta-adrenergic–blocking agents with their premedication were much less likely to demonstrate tachycardia and myocardial ischemia during tracheal intubation and emergence from anesthesia. A study by Engelman et al. used oral clonidine (5 μg/kg) for premedication 90 minutes before infrarenal aortic surgery.[64] The study found fewer episodes of tachycardia and of hypertension in patients receiving clonidine compared to a group not receiving clonidine preoperatively. It should be noted that patients receiving adrenergic drugs preoperatively in these studies are more likely to experience bradycardia and hypotension during periods of little stimulation intraoperatively and, postoperatively, in the postanesthesia care unit. Opponents of this type of preoperative premedication do not believe that adrenergic blockade is a substitute for skilled anesthetic care. In addition, they contend that brief periods of stimulation-induced tachycardia or hypertension are not as potentially harmful as a more prolonged period of hypotension during periods of little stimulation during surgery.

PREMEDICATION FOR OUTPATIENT ANESTHESIA

The use of premedication in outpatient anesthesia is controversial because the studies done to date have produced conflicting results.† Some anesthesiologists

avoid it entirely because there is little time for the drugs to work and premedication may prolong the recovery period. Others believe that after proper psychologic preparation, premedication may be used in selected cases. A retrospective analysis of 1553 patients[160] showed that premedication with diazepam or hydroxyzine did not prolong discharge time after outpatient surgery. Both midazolam[194,214] (5 mg IM) and diazepam[117] (0.25 mg/kg orally) have been used successfully in adults to relieve anxiety and produce sedation and analgesia before outpatient surgery. Similarly, opioid analgetics have also been administered in this setting without lengthening recovery time. Investigations using intramuscular meperidine (1.5 mg/kg) with atropine[27] and intravenous fentanyl (100 μg)[110] or oxymorphone (1 mg)[214] concluded that these doses did not adversely affect recovery times. The opioid analgetics may smooth airway management but may also make postoperative nausea and vomiting more likely. As with adults, some investigators have found premedication of pediatric outpatients helpful in anesthetic management.[25,51]

Other researchers see no need for premedication in ambulatory surgery. They reason that outpatients should have lower anxiety levels than inpatients[27] because they remain close to their family and friends, have relatively minor surgical procedures performed; and avoid prolonged recovery time and delayed discharge. Psychomotor skills may be impaired for many hours after the administration of benzodiazepines or opioids.[130] Support for avoiding or minimizing premedication comes from studies of surgical outpatients premedicated with benzodiazepines whose discharge from the hospital was delayed as a result of the premedication.[74,100,199]

In selected outpatients, antiemetic drugs may be desirable before ambulatory surgery[251] (see section on antiemetic drugs). Persistent nausea and vomiting is a major cause of unplanned admission to the hospital following outpatient anesthesia. Small doses of droperidol or the combination of droperidol and metoclopramide may prevent intractable nausea and vomiting after certain procedures and the use of certain anesthetics.

Studies by Ong et al.[181] and Rao et al.[196] suggested that large gastric volumes with high acidic content before anesthetic induction increased the risk of aspiration pneumonitis and made prophylaxis necessary (Fig. 2-7). However, such situations must be weighed against the estimated incidence of aspiration in the risk and cost-benefit ratios of the prophylactic drug regimens themselves. For patients at risk (see section on gastric fluid volume and pH), oral premedication with a histamine H_2-receptor–blocking drug plus metoclopramide can reduce gastric fluid volume, acid content, and the likelihood of postoperative vomiting.

---

*References 64, 68, 82-84, 133, 143, 204, 230.
†References 27, 49, 51, 69, 100, 130, 147, 148, 180, 194, 196, 199, 202.

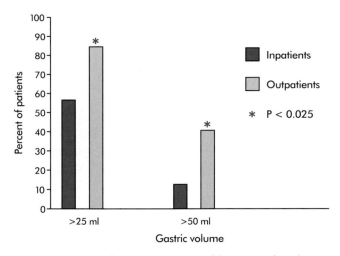

Fig. 2-7. Frequencies of occurrence of large gastric volumes among hospital inpatients and outpatients. (From Ong BY, Pickering BG, Pahalniuk RJ et al: Gastric volume and pH in outpatients, *Can Anaesth Soc J* 25:37, 1978.)

PREMEDICATION FOR PEDIATRIC PATIENTS

In the case of pediatric patients, in contrast to adult patients, premedication needs include aspects of the preoperative visit and psychologic preparation, placing emphasis on oral medications when pharmacologic preparation is needed, and more frequently using anticholinergic agents for their vagolytic activity.[75,129,226] What remains unchanged and critically important is assessing each child and tailoring psychologic preparation and premedication accordingly.

Psychologic Factors

Hospital admission and major surgery can produce long-lasting adverse psychologic effects in some pediatric patients.[26,129,243] For most children, hospitalization evokes stress and apprehension during admission and for a short time afterward although psychologic stress and anxiety are less likely with minor surgical procedures and brief hospitalizations. Contrary to what one might expect, repeated hospitalizations have not been shown to increase incidence of long-lasting psychologic trauma.[118,243] What has an effect on the child is the demeanor, skill, and effort of the anesthesiologist when preparing the child for a visit to the operating room for anesthesia and surgery.

Age is usually the most important aspect when considering the psychologic preparation of the pediatric patient.[227] Others in the health care team can easily substitute when a baby under 6 months of age is separated from its mother. Preoperative preparation in this age group is often directed toward other goals such as obtundation of vagal reflex responses. However, preschool children can be extremely upset when forcibly separated from their parents, and they have a universal fear of needles and operating rooms. This is a time when hospitalization may be the most traumatic.[10,58,243] It is often difficult or impossible to reason with children of this age and to explain forthcoming events. From age 5 years to adolescence it is easier to communicate and even reason with the child. The anesthesiologist offers reassurance and explanation about separation from parents, being away from home, operating room events and fears of surgery and anesthesia. Nevertheless, children older than 5 may already have many of the anxieties inherent in adolescence, especially those related to exposure in the presence of strangers. In addition, they may be apprehensive about loss of consciousness and control, have a fear of death, and worry about what they might say and do following preoperative sedation or during anesthesia. Often it is difficult to identify the fearful child.[19,227] The anesthesiologist should suspect the adolescent who does not talk much during the preoperative interview and who appears calm but uninterested. When these children can be identified preoperatively, they may be candidates for relatively heavy pharmacologic preparation.

Other important psychologic aspects in preoperative preparation of the pediatric patient include the attitude and behavior of parents, the socioeconomic status of the family, the magnitude of the planned surgery, and the hospital environment.[205,234]

Preoperative Visit

It may be even more important with children than with adults to conduct a good preoperative visit that will engender trust and proper psychologic preparation.[18,116,245] This is an art acquired by anesthesiologists through practice and experience. The preoperative visit should be a time of honest and straightforward explanation. Most anesthesiologists will want to include the parents in the preoperative visit when possible. The child will then be able to see parental acceptance of the anesthesiologist. Some hospitals have used films and slide shows to prepare pediatric patients for the operating room.[159,242] The child may want to bring a favorite toy, stuffed animal, or blanket to the operating room for security. It is extremely important that these accompany the child to the postanesthesia care unit and not become misplaced. Some children may want to participate by holding the mask on their faces during induction. Less anxiety and apprehension may be involved if the parents accompany the child to the preanesthetic area and even into the operating room itself. With selected parents and patients, supportive parental presence in the operating room can help dispel separation anxiety, fear of strangers, and apprehension due to lack of control. Nevertheless, the child may be upset despite parental presence, especially if the parents, operating room personnel, or the anesthesiologist exhibits anxiety.

Table 2-4 Premedication for pediatric patients

Medication	Dosage
Atropine	0.02 mg/kg IM or IV
Glycopyrrolate	0.01 mg/kg IM or IV
Scopolamine	0.01 mg/kg IM
Diazepam	0.2-0.5 mg/kg orally
Morphine	0.05-0.02 mg/kg IM
Meperidine	1.0-1.5 mg/kg IM
Pentobarbital	2-4 mg/kg orally, rectally, or IM
Seconal	2 mg/kg IM

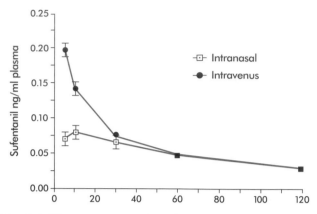

Fig. 2-8. Plasma concentrations (mean ± SEM) after 15 μg intranasal (*n* = 9) and intravenous (*n* = 7) sufentanil absorption and sedation. (From Helmers JH, Noorduin H, Van Peer A et al: Comparison of IV and intranasal sufentanil, *Can J Anaesth* 36:494, 1989.)

Pharmacologic Agents

Choosing drugs for premedication of pediatric patients assumes a proper preoperative visit with good psychologic preparation, a satisfactory operating room environment, and thorough preparation for a skilled, efficient, and timely induction of anesthesia.

Use and choice of premedication in pediatric patients is controversial. No regimen has been proved to prevent adverse psychologic outcome after hospitalization for anesthesia and surgery. Premedication (Table 2-4) may be of benefit if it can aid in smooth induction of anesthesia and reduce the occurrence of psychologic problems postoperatively.[58,214]

Agents for sedation, amnesia, and relief of anxiety

Sedative-hypnotic medications are used in pediatric patients, as in adults, to reduce apprehension and to produce sedation and amnesia. They can also be used to aid in smooth inhalational induction of anesthesia. The child older than 6 to 12 months of age may benefit from a sedative-hypnotic drug before surgery. There is a tendency in the pediatric age group to avoid intramuscular injection because of the child's common fear of needles and the pain of injection. The oral route for preoperative medication is often used in the older child also, while for children less than 3 years old, drugs may be given rectally or even nasally (Fig. 2-8). Many pharmacologic agents from the sedative-hypnotic group, especially benzodiazepines and barbiturates, have been prescribed preoperatively for children. Diazepam and pentobarbital orally seem quite popular for longer surgery. Midazolam can be given orally, intramuscularly, or intranasally. Oral midazolam is not currently available in the United States. It can be prepared by the hospital pharmacy and mixed with fruit juice. The usual oral dose for a child is about 0.5 to 1.0 mg/kg. Perhaps unique in the premedication of children (usually less than 3 years) is the rectal administration of methohexital.[141] Methohexital (20 to 30 mg/kg) may be given immediately

preoperatively while the child remains in the parent's arms. The intramuscular route is also possible.

Anticholinergic drugs

Anticholinergic drugs are especially important in the pediatric age group.[90,125,192,227] Increased vagal tone and bradycardia may result from laryngoscopy, surgical manipulation, or anesthetic drugs such as halothane or succinylcholine. The antisialagogue effect may be important in selected cases. When needed, intravenous atropine can be given immediately after induction of anesthesia. If the intramuscular route is chosen for atropine, the anesthesiologist can administer the drug immediately after unconsciousness during induction of anesthesia. Glycopyrrolate has also been used in children to inhibit vagal activity. Scopolamine has a place in premedication of the pediatric patient to produce sedation, amnesia, and drying of the airway. Finally, one must remember the potential adverse effects of administering anticholinergics to children with inspissated secretions or fevers.

Opioids

There is the occasional need for narcotic premedication in the pediatric age group. Methadone has the advantage of oral administration and is usually prescribed in the 0.1 to 0.2 mg/kg dose range. Opioid analgetics have been given nasally and incorporated into "lollipops" in attempts to avoid intramuscular injection.[103,174,225,231] However, the use of "lollipops" can increase gastric volume, lead to nausea, vomiting, and pruritis and raises the ethical issue of combining opioids with candy. In addition to the unpleasantness of nose drops and the nausea and vomiting associated with nasal sufentanil, decreased lung compliance has been observed. Intramuscular morphine and meperidine are often combined with other sedative drugs. Morphine is often seen as part of the preoperative pharmacologic regimen ordered for the child with congenital heart disease.[158,167] In many hospitals, opioids have been combined with sedative hypnotics and anticholinergic drugs into a "cocktail" that may be given orally for preoperative medication. Nicolson et al. administered meperidine and pentobarbital orally to children older than 1 year and found satisfactory premedication resulted.[176]

SUMMARY

In summary, the anesthesiologist must keep in mind the aspects of premedication, particularly in pediatric patients. These include adjusting psychologic preparation to the age of the child, avoiding intramuscular injections with oral or other routes of administration and using anticholinergic drugs for their vagolytic activity.

KEY POINTS

- Egbert et al. clearly showed that a careful, competent preoperative visit can do wonders in the preoperative "sedation" or "preparation" of the patient. No one has ever really successfully refuted this study. The preoperative visit remains key.

- There are important differences in time of onset and time to peak effect among premedications as well as important effects resulting from possible routes of administration. Recently, researchers have found that oral premedications can often be given with a small sip of water to an otherwise NPO patient without affecting that important NPO status.

- There are detailed differences among states of anxiolysis, analgesia, amnesia, and euphoria in patients. These should be understood thoroughly.

- Patients with preoperative pain, for whatever reason, may benefit from narcotics preoperatively. Whether other patients benefit from narcotics preoperatively is much more controversial, despite the near universal administration of these agents.

- Droperidol is most often used today for its antiemetic effect rather than its sedative properties.

- There is a disparity in the use of similar premedication in younger vs. older patients.

- In the past, anticholinergics were frequently given as premedication because the older anesthetic agents often produced severe salivation. Today, routine preoperative use of anticholinergics for all patients has fallen into disfavor, but there are numerous instances where the anesthesiologist may wish to prevent bradycardia and will give an anticholinergic.

- The commonly used histamine H_2-receptor antagonists, cimetidine and ranitidine, raise gastric fluid pH by reducing secretion of gastric hydrogen ion. They do not decrease gastric fluid volume or emptying time.

- Metoclopramide reduces gastric fluid volume and risk of aspiration because it is a dopamine antagonist that stimulates upper gastrointestinal motility, increases gastroesophageal sphincter tone, and relaxes the pylorus and duodenum.

- A single dose of an antacid (usually sodium citrate) given 15 to 30 minutes before the induction of anesthesia is nearly 100% effective in raising gastric fluid pH above 2.5.

- Many researchers believe that little or no premedication at all is indicated for most patients undergoing true outpatient surgical procedures.

- Anticholinergics are important to consider for pediatric patients because increased vagal tone and bradycardia may result from laryngoscopy, surgical manipulation, or anesthetic drugs such as halothane or succinylcholine. The antisialagogue effect of anticholinergics may also be beneficial in selected cases.

KEY REFERENCES

Egbert LD, Battit GE, Turndarf H et al: The value of the preoperative visit by the anesthetist, *JAMA* 185:553, 1963.

Gibbs CP, Spohr L, and Schmidt D: The effectiveness of sodium citrate as an antacid, *Anesthesiology* 57:44, 1982.

Korttila K, Kauste A, and Auvinen J: Comparison of domperidone, droperidol and metoclopramide in the prevention and treatment of nausea and vomiting after balanced general anesthesia, *Anesth Analg* 58:396, 1979.

Mendelson CL: The aspiration of stomach contents into the lungs during obstetric anesthesia, *Am J Obstet Gynecol* 52:191, 1946.

Reves JG, Fragen RJ, Vinik HR et al: Midazolam: pharmacology and uses, *Anesthesiology* 62:310, 1985.

Stanley TH, Leiman BC, Rawal N et al: The effects of oral transmucosal fentanyl citrate premedication on preoperative behavioral responses and gastric volume and acidity in children, *Anesth Analg* 69:328, 1989.

Steward DJ: Psychological preparation and premedication. In Gregory GA, ed: *Pediatric anesthesia,* New York, 1989, Churchill-Livingstone.

White PF: Pharmacologic and clinical aspects of preoperative medication, *Anesth Analg* 65:963, 1986.

REFERENCES

1. Aleniewski MI, Bulas BJ, Maderazo L et al: Intramuscular lorazepam versus pentobarbital premedication: a comparison of patient sedation, anxiety and recall, *Anesth Analg* 56:489, 1977.
2. Amarasekera K: Temazepam as a premedicant in minor surgery, *Anesthesia* 35:771, 1980.
3. Assaf RAD, Dundee JW, and Gamble JAS: The influence of the route of administration on the clinical action of diazepam, *Anaesthesia* 30:152, 1975.
4. Austin KL, Stapleton JV, and Mather LE: Multiple intramuscular injection — a major source of variability in analgesic response to meperidine, *Pain* 8:47, 1980.
5. Bailie R, Christmas L, Price N et al: Effects of temazepam premedication on cognitive recovery following alfentanil-propofol anaesthesia, *Br J Anaesth* 63:68, 1989.
6. Baraka P, Saab M, Salem MR et al: Control of gastric acidity by glycopyrrolate premedication in the parturient, *Anesth Analg* 56:642, 1977.
7. Barrett RF, James PD, and McLeod KCA: Oxazepam premedication in neurosurgical patients, *Anaesthesia* 39:429, 1984.
8. Baughman VL, Becker GL, Rejan CM et al: Effectiveness of triazolam, diazepam, and placebo as preanesthetic medications, *Anesthesiology* 71:196, 1989.
9. Beaven MA: Anaphylactoid reactions to anesthetic drugs, *Anesthesiology* 55:3, 1981.
10. Beeby DG, Hughes JOM: Behaviour of unsedated children in the anaesthetic room, *Br J Anaesth* 52:279, 1980.
11. Beecher HK: Preanesthetic medication, *JAMA* 157:242, 1955.
12. Beechy APG, Etringham RJ, and Studd C: Temazepam as premedication in day surgery, *Anaesthesia* 36:10, 1981.
13. Bellville JW, Dore Y, Capparell D et al: Analgesic effects of hydroxyzine compared to morphine in man, *J Clin Pharmacol* 19:290, 1979.
14. Bellville JW, Forrest WH, Miller E et al: Influence of age on pain relief from analgesics, *JAMA* 217:1835, 1971.
15. Black JW, Duncan WA, Durant CJ et al: Definition and antagonism of histamine H_2-receptors, *Nature* 236:385, 1972.
16. Blitt CD, Petty WF, Wright WA et al: Clinical evaluation of injectable lorazepam as a premedicant: the effect on recall, *Anesth Analg* 55:522, 1976.
17. Bond VK, Stoelting RK, and Gupta CD: Pulmonary aspiration syndrome after inhalation of gastric fluid containing antacids, *Anesthesiology* 51:452, 1979.
18. Booker PD, Chapman DH: Premedication in children undergoing day-care surgery, *Br J Anaesth* 51:1083, 1979.
19. Bothe A, Galdston R: A child's loss of consciousness: a psychiatric view of pediatric anesthesia, *Pediatrics* 50:252, 1972.
20. Bradshaw EG, Ali AA, Hulley BA et al: Plasma concentrations and clinical effects of lorazepam after oral administration, *Br J Anaesth* 53:517, 1981.
21. Braunstein MC: Apnea with maintenance of consciousness following intravenous diazepam, *Anesth Analg* 58:52, 1979.
22. Briggs RM, Ogg MJ: Patient's refusal of surgery following Innovar premedication, *Plast Reconstr Surg* 51:158, 1973.
23. Brock-Utne JG, Dow TG, Weiman S et al: The effects of glycopyrrolate (Robinal) on the lower esophageal sphincter, *Can Anaesth Soc J* 25:144, 1978.
24. Brock-Utne JG, Rubin J, Downing JW et al: The administration of metoclopramide with atropine: a drug interaction effect on the gastro-esophageal sphincter in man, *Anaesthesia* 31:1186, 1976.
25. Brustowicz RM, Nelson DA, Betts EK et al: Efficacy of oral premedication in pediatric outpatient surgery, *Anesthesiology* 60:475, 1984.
26. Chapman AH, Loeb DG, and Gibbons MJ: Psychiatric aspects of hospitalizing children, *Arch Pediatr* 73:77, 1956.
27. Clark AJM, Hurtig JB: Premedication with meperidine and atropine does not prolong recovery to the street fitness after outpatient surgery, *Can Anaesth Soc J* 28:390, 1981.
28. Clark G, Erwin D, Yate P et al: Temazepam as premedication in elderly patients, *Anaesthesia* 37:421, 1982.
29. Clark MM, Stores JA: The prevention of postoperative vomiting after abortion: metoclopramide, *Br J Anaesth* 41:890, 1969.
30. Clarke RSJ, Dundee JW, and Love WJ: Studies of drugs given before anesthesia. VIII. Morphine 10 mg alone and with atropine or hyoscine, *Br J Anaesth* 37:79, 1965.
31. Clarke RSJ, Dundee JW, and Moore J: Studies of drugs given before anesthesia. IV. Atropine and hyoscine, *Br J Anaesth* 36:648, 1964.
32. Clergue F, Desmonts JH, Duvaidestin D et al: Depression of respiratory drive by diazepam as premedication, *Br J Anaesth* 53:1059, 1981.
33. Cohen EN, Beecher HK: Narcotics in preanesthetic medication — a controlled study, *JAMA* 147:1664, 1951.
34. Cohen J, Weetman AP, Dargie HJ et al: Life-threatening arrhythmias and intravenous injection of cimetidine, *Br Med J* 2:768, 1979.
35. Cohen SE, Jasson J, Talafre HL et al: Does metoclopramide decrease the volume of gastric contents in patients undergoing cesarean section? *Anesthesiology* 61:604, 1984.
36. Cohen SE, Woods WA, and Wyner J: Antiemetic efficacy of droperidol and metoclopramide, *Anesthesiology* 60:67, 1984.
37. Comer WH, Elliott HW, Nomof W et al: Pharmacology of parenterally administered lorazepam in man, *J Int Med Res* 1:216, 1973.
38. Conner JT, Bellville JW, Wender R et al: Morphine and promethazine as intravenous premedicants, *Anesth Analg* 56:801, 1977.
39. Conner JT, Bellville JW, Wender R et al: Morphine, scopolamine and atropine as intravenous surgical premedicants, *Anesth Anal,* 56:606, 1977
40. Conner JT, Katz RL, Bellville JW et al: Diazepam and lorazepam for intravenous surgical premedication, *J Clin Pharmacol* 18:285, 1978.
41. Conner JT, Katz RL, Pagana RR et al: R021-3981 for intravenous surgical premedication and induction of anesthesia, *Anesth Analg* 59:1, 1978.
42. Coombs DW: Aspiration pneumonia prophylaxis, *Anesth Analg* 1983:62: 1055.
43. Coombs DW, Hooper DW: Cimetidine as a prophylactic against acid aspiration at tracheal extubation, *Can Anaesth Soc J* 28:33, 1981.
44. Coombs DW, Hooper DW, and Colton T: Acid aspiration prophylaxis by use of preoperative oral administration of cimetidine, *Anesthesiology* 51:352, 1979.
45. Cormack RS, Milledge JS, and Hanning CD: Respiration and amnesia after

lorazepam or morphine premedication, *Br J Anaesth* 48:813, 1976.

46. Cormack RS, Milledge JS, and Hanning CD: Respiratory effects and amnesia after premedication with morphine or lorazepam, *Br J Anaesth* 49:351, 1977.

47. Dalen JE, Evans GL, Banas JS Jr et al: The hemodynamic and respiratory effects of diazepam (Valium), *Anesthesiology* 30:259, 1969.

48. Davies AO: Oral diazepam premedication reduces the incidence of post-succinylcholine muscle pains, *Can Anaesth Soc J* 30:603, 1983.

49. Dawson B, Reed WA: Anaesthesia for adult surgical outpatients, *Can Anaesth Soc J* 27:409, 1980.

50. Denaut M, Yernault JC, and DeCoster A: Double blind comparison of the respiratory effects of parenteral lorazepam and diazepam in patients with chronic obstructive lung disease, *Curr Med Res Opin* 2:611, 1975.

51. Desjardins R, Ansara S, and Charest J: Preanesthetic medication for paediatric day care surgery, *Canad Anaesth Soc J* 28:141, 1981.

52. Divoll M, Greenblatt DJ, Ochs HR et al: Absolute biavailability of oral and intramuscular diazepam: effect of age and sex, *Anesth Analg* 62:1, 1983.

53. Domar AD, Everett LL, and Keller MG: Preoperative anxiety: is it a predictable entity? *Anesth Analg* 69:763, 1989.

54. Dundee JW, Lilburn JK, Nair SG et al: Studies of drugs given before anaesthesia. XXVI. Lorazepam, *Br J Anaesth* 49:1047, 1977.

55. Dundee JW, Wilson DB: Amnesic action of midazolam, *Anaesthesia* 35:459, 1980.

56. Durrant JM, Strunin L: Comparative trial of the effect of ranitidine and cimetidine on gastric secretion in fasting patients at induction of anesthesia, *Can Anaesth Soc J* 29:446, 1982.

57. Duvoisin RC, Katz RL: Reversal of central anticholinergic syndrome in many by physostigmine, *JAMA* 206:1963, 1968.

58. Eckenhoff JE: Relationship of anesthesia to postoperative personality changes in children, *Am J Dis Child* 86:587, 1953.

59. Economou G, Ward-McQuaid JN: A cross-over comparison of the effect of morphine, pethidine and pentazine on biliary pressure, *Gut* 12:218, 1971.

60. Egbert LD, Battit GF, Turndorf H et al: The value of the preoperative visit by the anesthetist, *JAMA* 185:553, 1963.

61. Eger EI II: Atropine, scopolamine and related compounds, *Anesthesiology* 33:365, 1962.

62. Ellis FR, Spence AA: Clinical trials of metoclopramide (Maxolon) as an antiemetic in anaesthesia, *Anaesthesia* 25:368, 1970.

63. Elsass P, Eikard B, Junge J et al: Psychological effect of detailed preanesthetic information, *Acta Anasthesiol Scand* 31:579, 1987.

64. Engelman E, Lipsaye M, Gilbert E et al: Effects of clonidine on anesthetic drug requirements and hemodynamic response during aortic surgery, *Anesthesiology* 71:178, 1989.

65. Falick YS, Smiler BG: Is anticholinergic premedication necessary? *Anesthesiology* 43:472, 1975.

66. Feneck RD, Cook JH: Failure of diazepam to prevent suxamethonium-induced rise in intra-ocular pressure, *Anaesthesia* 38:120, 1983.

67. Fjeldborg P, Hecht PS, Busted N et al: The effect of diazepam pretreatment on the succinylcholine-induced rise in intraocular pressure, *Acta Anaesthesiol Scand* 29:415, 1985.

68. Flacke JW, Bloor BC, Flacke WE et al: Reduced narcotic requirements by clonidine with improved hemodynamic and adrenergic stability in patients undergoing coronary bypass surgery, *Anesthesiology* 67:11-19, 1987.

69. Forrest P, Galletty DC, and Yee P: Placebo controlled comparison of midazolam, triazolam and diazepam as oral premedicants for outpatient anesthesia, *Anaesth Intensive Care* 15:296, 1987.

70. Forrest WH, Brown CR, and Brown BW: Subjective responses to six common preoperative medications, *Anesthesiology* 47:241, 1977.

71. Forster A, Gardaz J, Suter PM et al: Respiratory depression by midazolam and diazepam. *Anesthesiology* 53:494, 1980.

72. Foulkes E, Jenkins LC: A comparative evaluation of cimetidine and sodium citrate to decrease gastric acidity: effectiveness at time of induction of anesthesia, *Can Anaesth Soc J* 23:29, 1981.

73. Fragen RJ, Caldwell N: Lorazepam premedication: lack of recall and relief of anxiety, *Anesth Analg* 55:792, 1976.

74. Fragen RJ, Funk DI, Avram MJ et al: Midazolam versus hydroxyzine as intramuscular premedicants, *Can Anaesth Soc J* 30:136, 1983.

75. Francis L, Cutler RP: Psychological preparation and premedication for pediatric anesthesia, *Anesthesiology* 18:106, 1957.

76. Frank M, Evans H, Flynn P et al: Comparison of the prophylactic use of magnesium trisilicate mixture B.P.C., sodium citrate or cimetidine in obstetrics, *Br J Anaesth* 56:355, 1984.

77. Frumin MJ, Herekar VR, and Jarvik ME: Amnesic actions of diazepam and scopalamine in man, *Anesthesiology* 45:406, 1976.

78. Gale DG, Galloon S, and Porter WR: Sublingual lorazepam: a better premedication? *Br J Anaesth* 55:761, 1983.

79. Garde JF, Aston R, Endler GC et al: Racial mydriatic response to belladonna premedication, *Anesth Analg* 57:572, 1978.

80. Gasser JC, Kaufman RD, and Bellville JW: Respiratory effects of lorazepam, pentobarbital and pentazocine, *Clin Pharmacol Therap* 18:170, 1975.

81. George KA, Dundee JW: Relative amnesia actions of diazepam, flunitrazepam and lorazepam in man, *Br J Clin Pharmacol* 4:45, 1977.

82. Ghignone M, Calvillo O, and Quintin L: Anesthesia and hypertension: the effect of clonidine on perioperative hemodynamics and isoflurane requirements, *Anesthesiology* 67:3, 1987.

83. Ghignonne M, Noe C, Calvillo O et al: Anesthesia for ophthalmic surgery in the elderly: the effects of clonidine on intraocular pressure, perioperative hemodynamics, and anesthetic requirements, *Anesthesiology* 68:707, 1988.

84. Ghignone M, Quintin L, Duke PC et al: Effects of clonidine on narcotic requirements and hemodynamic response during induction of fentanyl anesthesia and endotracheal intubation, *Anesthesiology* 64:36, 1986.

85. Gibbs CP, Schwartz DJ, Wynne JW et al: Antacid pulmonary aspiration in the dog, *Anesthesiology* 51:380, 1979.

86. Gibbs CP, Schwartz DJ, Wynne JW et al: Antacid pulmonary aspiration, *Anesthesiology* 51:S290, 1979.

87. Gibbs CP, Spohr L, and Schmidt D: The effectiveness of sodium citrate as an antacid, *Anesthesiology* 57:44, 1982.

88. Gorback M: Pulmonary acid aspiration. I. Pathophysiology, clinical settings, consequences and role of proper anesthetic technique, *J Drug Dev* 2(suppl 3):4, 1989.

89. Gourlay GK, Wilson PR, and Glynn CJ: Pharmacodynamics and pharmacokinetics of methadone during the perioperative period, *Anesthesiology* 57:458, 1982.

90. Gravenstein JS, Anton AH: Premedication and drug interaction, *Clin Anesth* 3:199, 1969.

91. Greenblatt DJ, Abernethy DR, Locniskar A et al: Effect of age, gender and obesity on midazolam kinetics, *Anesthesiology* 61:27, 1984.

92. Greenblatt DJ, Abernethy DR, Morse DS et al: Clinical importance of interaction of diazepam and cimetidine, *N Engl J Med* 310:1639, 1984.

93. Greenblatt DJ, Koch-Weser J: Clinical toxicity of chlordiazepoxide and diazepam in relation to serum albumin concentration: a report from the Boston Collaborative Drug Surveillance Program, *Eur J Clin Pharmacol* 7:259, 1974.

94. Greenblatt DJ, Locniskar A, Scavone JM et al: Absence of interaction of cimetidine and ranitidine with intravenous and oral midazolam, *Anesth Analg* 65:176, 1986.

95. Greenblatt DJ, Shader RI: Anticholinergics, *N Engl J Med* 288:1215, 1973.

96. Greenblatt DJ, Shader RI: Benzodiazepines, *N Engl J Med* 291:1239, 1974.

97. Greenwood BK, Bradshaw EG: Preoperative medication for day care surgery: a comparison between oxazepam and temazepam, *Br J Anaesth* 55:933, 1983.

98. Gross JB, Smith L, and Smith TC: Time course of ventilatory response to carbon dioxide after intravenous diazepam, *Anesthesiology* 57:18, 1982.

99. Hansen HC, Harboe H, and Drenck NE: Local irritation after administration of diazepam in a rectal reduction, *Br J Anaesth* 63:287, 1989.

100. Hargreaves J: Benzodiazepine premedication in minor day care surgery: comparison of oral midazolam and

temazepam with placebo, *Br J Anaesth* 61:611, 1988.

101. Harris PW, Morison DH, Dunn GL et al: Intramuscular cimetidine and ranitidine as prophylaxis against gastric aspiration syndrome, *Can Anaesth Soc J* 31:599, 1984.

102. Heisterkamp DV, Cohen PT: The effect of intravenous premedication with lorazepam (Ativan), pentobarbital and diazepam on recall, *Br J Anaesth* 47:79, 1975.

103. Henderson JM, Brodsky DA, Fisher DM et al: Pre-induction of anesthesia in pediatric patients with nasally administered sufentanil, *Anesthesiology* 68:671, 1988.

104. Herr GP, Conner JT, Katz RL et al: Diazepam and droperidol as IV premedicants, *Br J Anaesth* 51:537, 1979.

105. Hillestad L, Hansen T, Melsom H et al: Diazepam metabolism in normal man: serum concentrations and clinical effects after intravenous intramuscular and oral administration, *Clin Pharmacol* 16:479, 1974.

106. Hodgkinson R, Glasserberg R, Joyce TH III et al: Comparison of cimetidine (Tagamet) with antacid for safety and effectiveness in reducing gastric acidity before elective cesarean section, *Anesthesiology* 59:86, 1983.

107. Hofmann RF, Weiler HH: Lorazepam and nalbuphine as local anesthetic ophthalmic surgery premedications, *Ann Ophthalmol* 15:64, 1983.

108. Holt AI: Premedication with atropine should not be routine, *Lancet* 2:984, 1961.

109. Holzgrafe RE, Vondrell JJ, and Mintz SM: Reversal of postoperative reactions to scopolamine with physostigmine, *Anesth Analg* 52:921, 1973.

110. Horrigan RW, Mayers JR, Johnson BH et al: Etomidate vs. thiopental with and without fentanyl—a comparative study of awakening in man, *Anesthesiology* 52:362, 1980.

111. Houghton DJ: Use of lorazepam as a premedicant for cesarean section, *Br J Anaesth* 55:767, 1983.

112. Hovi-Viander M, Kangas L, and Kanto J: A comparative study of the clinical effects of pentobarbital and diazepam given orally as preoperative medication, *J Oral Surg* 38:188, 1980.

113. Howard FA, Sharp DS: Effect of metoclopramide on gastric emptying during labour, *Br Med J* 1:446, 1973.

114. Hupert C, Yacoub M, and Turgeon LR: Effect of hydroxyzine on morphine analgesia for the treatment of postoperative pain, *Anesth Analg* 59:690, 1980.

115. Iwamoto K, Schwartz H: Antiemetic effect of droperiodol after ophthalmic surgery, *Arch Ophthalmol* 96:1378, 1978.

116. Jackson K: Psychological preparation as a method of reducing the emotional trauma of anesthesia in children, *Anesthesiology* 12:293, 1981.

117. Jakobsen H, Wertz JB, Johansen JR et al: Premedication before day surgery: a double-blind comparison of diazepam and placebo, *Br J Anaesth* 61:921, 1985.

118. Jessner L, Blom GE, and Waldfogel S: Emotional implications of tonsillectomy and adenoidectomy on children, *Psychoanal Study Child* 7:126, 1952.

119. Johnston JR, Moore J, McCaughey W et al: Use of cimetidine as an oral antacid in obstetric anesthesia, *Anesth Analg* 62:720, 1983.

120. Jones RM, Riddian-Green R, and Knight PR: Narcotic-induced choleclochoduodenal sphincter spasm by glucagon, *Anesth Analg* 59:946, 1980.

121. Joyce TH: Prophylaxis for pulmonary aspiration, *Am J Med* 83(suppl 6A):46, 1987.

122. Kanto J: Benzodiazepines as oral premedicants, *Br J Anaes* 53:1179, 1981.

123. Kaplan SA, Jack ML, Alexander K et al: Pharmacokinetic profile of diazepam in man following single intravenous and chronic oral administration, *J Pharm Sci* 62:1289, 1973.

124. Keats AS, Telford J, and Kurosu Y: "Potentiation" of meperidine by promethazine, *Anesthesiology* 22:34, 1961.

125. Kessel J: Atropine premedication, *Anaesth Intensive Care,* 2:77, 1974.

126. Klotz U, Avant GR, Hoyumpa A et al: The effects of age and liver disease on the disposition and elimination of diazepam in adult man, *J Clin Invest* 55:347, 1975.

127. Knapp RB, Fierro L: Evaluation of cardiopulmonary safety and effects of lorazepam as a premedicant, *Anesth Analg* 53:122, 1974.

128. Koch-Weser J, Greenblatt DJ: The archaic barbiturate hypnotics, *N Engl J Med* 291:790, 1974.

129. Korsch BM: The child and the operating room, *Anesthesiology* 43:251, 1975.

130. Korttila K, Linnoila M: Psychomotor skills related to driving after intramuscular administration of diazepam and meperidine, *Anesthesiology* 42:685, 1975.

131. Korttila K, Aromaa U, and Tammisto T: Patient's expectations and acceptance of the effects of the drugs given before anaesthesia: comparison of light and amnesic premedication, *Acta Anaesth Scand* 25:381, 1981.

132. Korttila K, Kauste A, and Auvinen J: Comparison of domperidone, droperidol and metoclopramide in the prevention and treatment of nausea and vomiting after balanced general anesthesia, *Anesth Analg* 53:396, 1979.

133. Koukinen S, Pyykko K: The potentiation of halothane anesthesia by clonidine, *Acta Anaesthesiol Scand* 23:107, 1979.

134. Kraus JW, Desmond PV, Marshall SP et al: Effects of aging and liver disease on disposition of lorazepam, *Clin Pharmacol Ther* 24:411, 1978.

135. Kruger AE, Roelofse JA: Precautions against intra-ocular pressure changes during endotracheal intubation—a comparison of pretreatment with intravenous lignocaine and diazepam, *S Afr Med J* 63:887, 1983.

136. Kushner MJ et al: You don't have to be a neuroscientist to forget everything with triazolam—but it helps, *JAMA* 259:350 1988, (letters to the editor).

137. Laffey DA, Kay NH: Premedication with butorphanol: a comparison with morphine, *Br J Anaesth* 56:363, 1984.

138. Lake CL, Duckworth EN, DiFazio CA et al: Cardiorespiratory effects of nalbuphine and morphine premedication in adult cardiac surgical patients, *Acta Anaesthesiol Scand* 28:305, 1984.

139. Lee CM, Yeakel AE: Patients refusal of surgery following Innovar premedication, *Anesth Analg* 54:224, 1975.

140. Leigh JM, Walker J, and Janaganathan P: Effect of preoperative anesthetic visit on anxiety, *Br Med J* 2:987, 1977.

141. Liu LMP, Goudsouzian NG, and Liu PL: Rectal methohexital in children, a dose-comparison study, *Anesthesiology* 53:343, 1980.

142. Liu S, Miller N, and Waye JD: Retrograde amnesia effects of intravenous diazepam in endoscopy patients, *Gastrointes Endosc* 30:340, 1984.

143. Longnecker DE: Alpine anesthesia: can pretreatment with clonidine decrease the peaks and valleys? *Anesthesiology* 67:1, 1989.

144. Longo VG: Behavioral and electroencephalographic effects of atropine and related compounds, *Pharmacol Rev* 18: 965, 1966.

145. Lunn JN, Farrow SC, Fawkes FG et al: Epidemiology in anaesthesia. I. Anaesthetic practice over 20 years, *Br J Anaesth* 54:803, 1982.

146. Lyons SM, Clarke RSJ, and Vulgaraki K: The premedication of cardiac surgical patients, *Anaesthesia* 30:459, 1975.

147. Madej TH, Paasuke RT: Anaesthetic premedication: aims, assessment and methods, *Can J Anaesth* 34:259, 1987.

148. Male CG: Anxiety in day surgery patients, *Br J Anaesth* 53:663P, 1981.

149. Maliniak K, Vakil AH: Pre-anesthetic cimetidine and gastric pH, *Anesth Analg* 58:309, 1979.

150. Manchikanti K, Marrero TC, and Roush JR: Preanesthetic cimetidine and metoclopramide for acid aspiration prophylaxis in elective surgery, *Anesthesiology* 61:48, 1984.

151. Manchikanti L, Colliver JA, Marrero TC et al: Ranitidine and metoclopramide for prophylaxis of aspiration pneumonitis in elective surgery, *Anesth Analg* 63:903, 1984.

152. Manchikanti L, Gnow JB, Colliver JA et al: Sodium citrate and metoclopramide in outpatient anesthesia for prophylaxis against aspiration pneumonitis, *Anesthesiology* 63:378, 1985.

153. Manchikanti L, Kraus JW, and Edds SP: Cimetidine and related drugs in anesthesia, *Anesth Analg* 61:595, 1982.

154. Manchikanti L, Roush JR: The effect of preanesthetic glycopyrrolate and cimetidine in gastric fluid pH and volume in outpatients, *Anesth Analg* 63:40, 1984.

155. McCammon RL, Hilgenberg JC, and Stoelting RK: Hemodynamic effects of diazepam and diazepam-nitrous oxide in patients with coronary artery disease, *Anesth Analg* 59:438, 1980.

156. McCubbin TD, Braun JH, Dewar KN et al: Glycopyrrolate as premedicant:

comparison with atropine, *Br J Anaesth* 51:885, 1979.

157. McKenzie R, Wadhwa RK, Uy NT et al: Antiemetic effectiveness of intramuscular hydroxyzine compared with intramuscular droperidol, *Anesth Analg* 60:783, 1981.

158. McQuiston WO: Anesthetic problems in cardiac surgery in children, *Anesthesiology* 10:590, 1947.

159. Mendelson CL: The aspiration of stomach contents into the lungs during obstetric anesthesia, *Am J Obstet Gynecol* 52:191, 1946.

160. Meridy HW: Criteria for selection of ambulatory surgical patients and guidelines for anesthetic management—a retrospective study of 1553 cases, *Anesth Analg* 61:921, 1982.

161. Meyers EF, Tomeldan SA: Glycopyrrolate compared with atropine in prevention of the ocularcardiac reflex during eye-muscle surgery, *Anesthesiology* 51:350, 1979.

162. Middleton JJ, Zitzer JM, and Urbach KF: Is atropine always necessary before general anesthesia? *Anesth Analg* 46:51, 1967.

163. Mikatti NE: The effects of oral diazepam premedication on blood gases, *Ann R Coll Surg Engl* 63:429, 1981.

164. Mirakhur RA, Clarke RSJ, Dundee JA et al: Anticholinergic drugs in anaesthesia: a survey of their present position, *Anaesthesia* 33:133, 1978.

165. Mirakhur RK: Anticholinergic drugs and anesthesia, *Can J Anaesth* 35:443, 1988.

166. Mirakhur RK: Anticholinergic drugs, *Br J Anaesth* 51:671, 1979.

167. Moffitt EA, McGoon DC, and Ritter J: The diagnosis and correction of congenital cardiac defects, *Anesthesiology* 33:144, 1970.

168. Moore DC, Balfour RI, and Fitzgibbons D: Convulsive arterial plasma levels of bupivacaine and the response to diazepam therapy, *Anesthesiology* 50:454, 1979.

169. Morris HH, Estes ML: Traveler's amnesia: transient global amnesia secondary to triazolam, *JAMA* 258:945, 1987.

170. Mortensen PT: Droperidol (Dehydrobenzperiodol): postoperative antiemetic effect when given intravenously to gynaecologic patients, *Acta Anaesthiol Scand* 26:48, 1982.

171. Morel DR, Forster A, Bachmann M et al: Effect of intravenous midazolam on breathing patterns and chest wall mechanics in humans, *J Appl Physiol* 57:1104, 1984.

172. Moyers J: Anesthesia for cardiac surgery 1949-1956, *J Iowa Med Soc* 47:192, 1957.

173. Murphy DF, Nally B, Gardiner J et al: Effect of metoclopramide on gastric emptying before elective and emergency cesarean section, *Br J Anaesth* 56:1113, 1984.

174. Nelson P, Streisand JB, Mulder SM et al: Comparison of oral transmucosal fentanyl citrate and an oral solution of meperidine, diazepam and atropine, *Anesthesiology* 70:616, 1989.

175. Nicholson MJ: Preanesthetic preparation and premedication. In Hale DE, ed: *Anesthesiology,* Philadelphia, 1954, FA Davies.

176. Nicolson SC, Betts EK, Jobes DR et al: Comparison of oral and intramuscular preanesthetic medication for pediatric surgery, *Anesthesiology* 71:8-10, 1989.

177. Nimmo WS: Drugs, diseases and altered gastric emptying, *Clin Pharmacokinet* 1:189, 1976.

178. Norris W, Baird WLM: Pre-operative anxiety: a study of the incidence and aetiology, *Br J Anaesth* 39:503, 1967.

179. O'Sullivan G, Sear JW, Bullingham RE et al: The effect of magnesium trisilicate, metoclopramide and ranitidine on gastric pH, volume and serum gastrin, *Anaesthesia* 40:246, 1985.

180. Ogg TW: Use of anaesthesia: implications of day care surgery and anaesthesia, *Br Med J* 281:212, 1980.

181. Ong BY, Palahniuk RJ, and Cumming M: Gastric volume and pH in outpatients, *Can Anaesth Soc J* 25:36, 1978.

182. Ong BY, Pickering BG, Palaniuk RJ et al: Lorazepam and diazepam as adjuncts to epidural anesthesia for cesarean section, *Can Anaesth Soc J* 29:31, 1982.

183. Opie JC, Chaye H, and Steward DJ: Intravenous atropine rapidly reduces lower esophageal sphincter pressure in infants, *Anesthesiology* 67:989, 1987.

184. Ostheimer GW: Pulmonary acid aspiration. II. Prevention of complications, *J Drug Dev* 2(suppl 3):18, 1989.

185. Pagano RR, Conner JT, Bellville JW et al: Lorazepam hyoscine and atropine as IV surgical premedicants, *Br J Anaesth* 50:471, 1978.

186. Pandit SK, Heisterkamp DV, and Cohen PJ: Further studies of the antirecall effect of lorazepam: a dose-time-effect relationship, *Anesthesiology* 45:495, 1976.

187. Patton CM: Rapid induction of acute dyskinesis by droperidol, *Anesthesiology* 43:126, 1975.

188. Patton CM, Moon MR, and Dannemiller JT: The prophylactic antiemetic effect of droperidol, *Anesth Analg* 53:361, 1974.

189. Perisho JA, Buechel DR, and Miller RD: The effect of diazepam (Valium) in minimum alveolar anesthetic requirement (MAC) in man, *Can Anaesth Soc J* 18:536, 1971.

190. Pinnock CA, Bell A, and Smith G: A comparison of nalbuphine and morphine as premedication agents for minor gynaecological surgery, *Anaesthesia* 40:1078, 1985.

191. Pinnock CA, Fell D, Hunt PC et al: A comparison of triazolam and diazepam as premedication for minor gynaecologic surgery, *Anaesthesia* 40:324, 1985.

192. Rackow H, Salanitre E: Modern concepts in pediatric anesthesiology, *Anesthesiology* 30:208, 1969.

193. Radnay PA, Brodman E, Mankikor D et al: The effect of equi-analgesic doses of fentanyl, morphine, meperidine and pentazocine on common bile duct pressure, *Anesthetist* 29:26, 1980.

194. Raeder JC, Breivik H: Premedication with midazolam in outpatient general anesthesia, *Acta Anaesthesiol Scand* 31:509, 1987.

195. Rao S, Sherbaniuk RW, Prasad K et al: Cardiopulmonary effects of diazepam, *Clin Pharmacol* 14:182, 1973.

196. Rao TLK, Suseela M, and El-Etr AA: Metoclopramide and cimetadine to reduce gastric pH and volume, *Anesth Analg* 63:264, 1984.

197. Ratcliff A, Indalo AA, Bradshaw EG et al: Premedication with temazepam in minor surgery, *Anaesthesia* 44:812, 1989.

198. Ravnborg M, Hasselstrom L, and Ostergard D: Premedication with oral and rectal diazepam, *Acta Anaesthesiol Scand* 30:132, 1986.

199. Raybould D, Bradshaw EG: Premedication for day care surgery: a study of oral midazolam, *Anaesthesia* 42:591, 1987.

200. Reves JG, Frazen RJ, Vinik HR et al: Midazolam: pharmacology and uses, *Anesthesiology* 62:310, 1985.

201. Richter JJ: Current theories about the mechanisms of benzodiazepines and neurolytic drugs, *Anesthesiology* 54:66, 1981.

202. Rising S, Dodgson MS, and Steen PA: Isoflurane vs. fentanyl for outpatient laparoscopy, *Acta Anaesthesiol Scand* 29:251, 1985.

203. Rivera VM, Keichian AH, and Oliver RE: Persistant parkinsonism following neurolept analgesia, *Anesthesiology* 42:635, 1975.

204. Roizen MF: Should we all have a sympathectomy at birth? Or at least preoperatively? *Anesthesiology* 68:482, 1988.

205. Rothman PE: A note on hospitalism, *Pediatrics* 30:995, 1962.

206. Russell WJ: Lorazepam as a premedicant for regional anaesthesia, *Anaesthesia* 38:1062, 1983.

207. Russell-Taylor WJ, Llewellyn-Thomas E, and Seller EA: A comparative evaluation of intramuscular atropine, dicyclomine and glycopyrrolate using healthy medical students as volunteer subjects, *Int J Clin Pharmacol* 4:358, 1970.

208. Saidman LJ, Eger EI II: Effect of nitrous oxide and of narcotic premedication on the alveolar concentration of halothane required for anesthesia, *Anesthesiology* 25:302, 1964.

209. Santos A, Datta S: Prophylactic use of droperidol for control of nausea and vomiting during spinal anesthesia for cesarean section, *Anesth Analg* 63:85, 1984.

210. Schmidt JF, Jorgensen BC: The effect of metoclopramide on gastric contents after preoperative ingestion of sodium citrate, *Anesth Analg* 63:841, 1984.

211. Schmidt JF, Schierup L, and Banning AM: The effect of sodium citrate on the pH and amount of gastric contents before general anesthesia, *Acta Anaesthesiol Scand* 28:263, 1984.

212. Schwartz J, Wynne JW, Gibbs CP et al: Pulmonary consequences of aspiration of gastric contents at pH values greater than 2.5, *Am Rev Respir Dis* 121:119, 1980.

213. Severinghaus JW, Stupfel M: Respiratory dead space increase following atropine in man, and atropine, vagal or ganglionic blockade and hypothermia in dogs, *J Appl Physiol* 8:81, 1955.

214. Shafer A, White PF, Urquhart ML et al: Outpatient premedication: use of midazolam and opioid analgesics, *Anesthesiology* 71:495, 1989.

215. Shah ZP, Wilson J: An evaluation of metoclopramide (Maxolon) as an antiemetic in anaesthesia, *Br J Anaesth* 44:865, 1972.

216. Shaw RG, Mashford ML, and Desmond PV: Cardiac arrest after intravenous injection of cimetidine, *Med J Aust* 2:629, 1980.

217. Shearer WM: The evolution of premedication, *Br J Anaesth* 32:554, 1960.

218. Shearer WM: The evolution of premedication, *Br J Anaesth* 33:219, 1961.

219. Shutt LE, Bowes JB: Atropine and hyoscine, *Anaesthesia* 34:476, 1979.

220. Smith DS, Orkin FK, Gardner SM et al: Prolonged sedation in the elderly after intraoperative atropine administration, *Anesthesiology* 51:348, 1979.

221. Smith TC, Stephen GW, Zeiger L et al: Effects of premedicant drugs on respiration and gas exchange in man, *Anesthesiology* 28:883, 1967.

222. Snyder SH: Drug and neurotransmitter receptors, *JAMA* 261:3126, 1989.

223. Sorensen O, Eriksen S, Hommelgaard P et al: Thiopental-nitrous oxide-halothane anesthesia and repeated succinylcholine: comparison of preoperative glycopyrrolate and atropine administration, *Anesth Analg* 59:686, 1980.

224. Soroker D, Barzilay E, Konichezky S et al: Respiratory function following premedication with droperidol or diazepam, *Anesth Analg* 57:695, 1978.

225. Stanley TH, Leiman BC, Rawal N et al: The effects of oral transmucosal fentanyl citrate premedication on preoperative behavioral responses and gastric volume and acidity in children, *Anesth Analg* 69:328, 1989.

226. Steward DJ: Experiences with an outpatient anesthesia service for children, *Anesthesiology* 52:877, 1973.

227. Steward DJ: Psychological preparation and premedication. In Gregory GA, ed: *Pediatric anesthesia*, New York, 1989, Churchill-Livingstone.

228. Stoelting RK: Gastric fluid pH in patients receiving cimetidine, *Anesth Analg* 57-675, 1978.

229. Stoelting RK: Responses to atropine, glycopyrrolate and Riopan on gastric fluid pH and volume in adult patients, *Anesthesiology* 48:367, 1978.

230. Stone JG, Foex P, Sear JW et al: Myocardial ischemia in untreated hypertensive patients: effect of a single small oral dose of a beta-adrenergic blocking agent, *Anesthesiology* 68:495, 1988.

231. Streisand JB, Stanley TH, Hagne B et al: Oral transmucosal fentanyl citrate premedication in children, *Anesth Analg* 69:28, 1989.

232. Study RE, Barker JL: Cellular mechanisms of benzodiazepine action, *JAMA* 247:2147, 1982.

233. Thomas D, Tipping T, Halifax R et al: Triazolam premedication, *Anaesthesia* 41:692, 1986.

234. Tisza VB, Angoff K: A play program for hospitalized children: the role of the playroom teacher, *Pediatrics* 28:841, 1961.

235. Tornetta FJ: A comparison of droperidol, diazepam and hydroxyzine hydrochloride as premedication, *Anesth Analg* 56:496, 1977.

236. Tornetta FJ: Clinical studies with the new antiemetic, metoclopramide, *Anesth Analg* 48:198, 1969.

237. Tsunoda Y, Hattori Y, Takasuka E et al: Effects of hydroxyzine, diazepam and pentaxocine on halothane minimum alveolar anesthetic concentration, *Anesth Analg* 52:390, 1973.

238. Utting HJ, Pleuvry BJ: A study of the respiratory effects of oral doses in human volunteers and interactions with morphine in mice, *Br J Anaesth* 47:987, 1975.

239. Vandam LD: Butorphanol, *N Engl J Med* 302:381, 1980.

240. Vaughn RW, Bauer S, and Wise L: Volume and pH of gastric juice on obese patients, *Anesthesiology* 43:686, 1975.

241. Verma RS: Diazepam and suxamethonium muscle pain (a dose response study), *Anaesthesia* 37:688, 1982.

242. Vernon DTA, Bailey WC: The use of motion pictures in the psychological preparation of children for induction of anesthesia, *Anesthesiology* 40:68, 1974.

243. Vernon DTA, Schulman JL, and Foley JM: Changes in children's behavior after hospitalization, *Am J Dis Child* 111:581, 1966.

244. Viegas OJ, Ravindran RS, and Shumacker CA: Gastric fluid pH in patients receiving sodium citrate, *Anesth Analg* 60:521, 1981.

245. Visintainer MA, Wolfer JA: Psychological preparation for surgical pediatric patients: the effect on children's parents' stress responses and adjustment, *Pediatrics* 56:187, 1975.

246. Wallace G, Mindlin LJ: A controlled double-blind comparison of intramuscular lorazepam and hydroxyzine as surgical premedicants, *Anesth Analg* 63:571, 1984.

247. Ward DS: Stimulation of the hypoxic ventilatory drive by droperidol, *Anesth Analg* 63:106, 1984.

248. Weber L, Hirshman CA: Cimetidine for prophylaxis of aspiration pneumonitis: comparison of intramuscular and oral dose schedules, *Anesth Analg* 58:426, 1979.

249. Weil JV, McCullough RE, and Kline JS: Diminished ventilatory response to hypoxia and hypercapnia after morphine in man, *N Engl J Med* 292:1103, 1975.

250. Wender RH, Conner JT, Bellville JW et al: Comparison of IV diazepam and hydroxyzine as surgical premedicants, *Br J Anaesth* 49:907, 1977.

251. White PF: Pharmacologic and clinical aspects of preoperative medication, *Anesth Analg* 65:963, 1986.

252. Whitwam JG: Benzodiazepines, *Anaesthesia* 42:1255, 1987.

253. Wingard DW: Physostigmine reversal of diazepam-induced depression, *Anesth Analg* 56:348, 1977.

254. Winning TJ, Brock-Utne JG, and Downing JW: Nausea and vomiting after anesthesia and minor surgery, *Anesth Analg* 56:674, 1977.

255. Wyant GM, Kao E: Glycopyrrolate methobromide: effect on salivary secretion, *Can Anaesth Soc J* 21:230, 1974.

256. Wyner J, Cohen SE: Gastric volume in early pregnancy: effect of metoclopramide, *Anesthesiology* 57:209, 1982.

257. Zeldis JE, Friedman LS, and Iselbacher KJ: Ranitidine: a new H_2-receptor antagonist, *N Engl J Med* 309:1368, 1983.

CHAPTER 3

The Anesthetic Plan

TOMMY SYMRENG

A satisfactory anesthetic plan cannot be formulated without considering as many different factors as possible that might affect the perioperative care of the patient. **The most important factor must always be patient safety.** During the anesthetic process, whether general, regional, local or some combination, there is significant manipulation of several physiologic patient processes. Often the patient is completely unable to protect himself/herself. **The anesthesiologist, therefore, should have a plan that allows the patient an appropriate level of consciousness, adequate ventilation, and circulation to maintain organ function and protection from the harmful effects of disease, anesthesia, and surgery.**

PATIENT SAFETY

The anesthesiologist must know the pathophysiologic processes for which the patient is coming to surgery as well as be cognizant of any concurrent diseases affecting the patient. To minimize morbidity, the anesthesiologist must ensure preoperatively that the patient is in optimal condition. Each medical problem should be evaluated and vital organ function optimized. For example, a patient with moderate-to-severe chronic obstructive pulmonary disease (COPD) may need pulmonary function tests done preoperatively to ensure that there is no important residual reversible disease. In-depth knowledge of the patient's pathology will enable the physician to predict intraoperative and postoperative problems; for example, determining how a patient with COPD may tolerate an upper abdominal operation. The patient may need to be prepared for waking up with an endotracheal tube in place for several postoperative days, while the effects of surgery on pulmonary function subside. In other cases, an additional 10% to 20% improvement in postoperative lung function may rapidly be regained with adequate pain relief only. Such a patient might be able to be extubated immediately after surgery. Similarly, other organ systems must be optimized preoperatively to minimize problems during and after surgery.

The effect of surgical trauma on fluid and electrolyte balance and stress hormone changes can also be manipulated with anesthetic technique.[31,84] In patients who have marginal organ reserve capacity, morbidity can be decreased by stress reduction measures employed during and after surgery.[99] The anesthetic agents and techniques available today are considerably safer than previously, but they are also more potent. Knowledge of their effects on vital organ physiology (central nervous system, circulatory, respiratory, hepatic, and renal) is essential.

OPTIMAL PREOPERATIVE CONDITIONS FOR ANESTHESIA AND SURGERY

Surgeons should arrange for the best possible operating conditions. The knowledgeable surgeon will inform the anesthesiologist about specific needs that must be met to perform the operation swiftly and safely. Anesthesiologists have the tools to meet most important operating conditions: patient asleep or awake; following commands; normotensive, hypotensive, hypertensive; high muscle tone or relaxed; with or without pain reflexes; and with or without various stress responses. For instance, some surgeons may want a patient to cough at the end of a hernia repair, which is perhaps easiest if the operation is done with the patient under regional anesthesia. Others may want the patient unconscious if they are teaching the residents new surgical techniques. Maintaining a patient in a hypotensive state gives good operating conditions for middle ear surgery and less blood loss in some orthopedic operations. **In any case, sometimes the surgeon's wishes must take a back seat to patient safety and/or desires or comfort, but it is important, whenever possible, to supply the operating team with optimal working conditions.**

PATIENT COMFORT

Patients universally want rapid and pain-free anesthetic induction, optimal care and vigilance during surgery, and a relatively short, pain-free recovery. Pain-free inductions can be accomplished, especially in children, with rectal or inhalation techniques. Nerve blocks involving several needle sticks should be preceded by amnestic drugs intravenously. Drugs should be chosen so that no or only minimal sedation remains if the patient is scheduled to leave the hospital the same day. If the patient is to stay overnight or longer, the patient should still be comfortably sedated postoperatively. Whether general or regional anesthesia is used during surgery, local wound infiltration with bupivacaine considerably decreases postoperative discomfort and morphine requirements.

The most common reason for not wanting regional anesthesia is the patient's wish to be asleep during the operation. This reason is not a real contraindication. A well-functioning regional block does not require supplementation with intravenous drugs, but if the patient or surgeon wishes, some sedation can be given. Inexperienced anesthesiologists tend to oversedate the patient, which can create a situation where the patient is uncooperative and agitated. Such a patient must then be given a general anesthetic to enable the surgeon to finish the operation. In long operations, backache and or stiff joints can be problems, but these respond well to a small intravenous dose of narcotics. These latter problems should encourage, not discourage, the anesthesiologist to perform more regional anesthesia, because these reflexes may protect the patient from ischemic muscle pain postoperatively. Patients should never have to be forced into any kind of anesthetic against their will, but it is the duty of the anesthesiologist to inform them of the choice of anesthetics that are available. Patients should also be advised of what the anesthesiologist believes is the choice of anesthetic in their situation. Safety is more important than comfort.

ABILITY OF THE ANESTHESIOLOGIST

Administering anesthesia is not only a science but also an art. There are anesthesiologists who are quite expert in managing most patients using the inhalational technique. Others are equally successful using regional anesthesia. **It is often the contention that the anesthesiologist who is quite experienced with a given technique and perhaps inexperienced with a technique seemingly advisable on a pharmacologic or physiologic basis actually chooses the technique with which he/she is most familiar. The demand to use a technique with which the anesthesiologist is less familiar may jeopardize the patient. On the other hand, every professional has the obligation to continually learn and judiciously become familiar with new drugs and techniques under elective circumstances.**

INFLUENCE OF TYPE OF SURGERY ON ANESTHETIC CHOICE

The surgical requirements of different procedures differ, and the anesthesiologist's means to meet these requirements can also vary considerably. A brief overview will be offered here for several common areas of surgery.

Abdominal Surgery

Intraabdominal surgery is usually performed with the patient under general anesthesia. Endotracheal intubation is usually indicated to prevent gastric contents from entering the glottis. Good relaxation of the abdominal wall is needed during incision, initial abdominal exploration, and closure of the peritoneum and fascia. Anesthesia induction is commonly intravenous (pentothal, propofol) with relaxation and maintenance with inhalational agents, nondepolarizing relaxants, and/or narcotics. Nitrous oxide is controversial in abdominal surgery because its rapid absorption may distend the bowel. A combination of a light general anesthesia and epidural block is an alternative when bleeding problems are unlikely. However, if there is major bleeding with an extensive sympathetic block during regional anesthesia, profound hypotension can result. High epidural or subarachnoid block alone is sometimes performed for swift abdominal surgery but is not tolerated well by some patients because of the nonblocked diaphragm. An example of this kind of block is the regional anesthesia given for cesarean section. For extensive intraabdominal surgery and in patients with preoperative cardiopulmonary disease, preoperative or intraoperative placement of an epidural catheter for postoperative pain relief should be considered. Intercostal blocks and interpleural catheters should be considered for pain relief after cholecystectomy and kidney surgery. Operations on the abdominal wall can be done under general anesthesia, sometimes without endotracheal intubation or relaxation. However, for hernia repair, coughing while the patient is still intubated should be prevented. Extradural and subarachnoid blocks usually work well for operations on the abdominal wall. The patient can, by surgical request, cough during hernia repair to ensure that tissues and repair are strong enough. Inguinal hernia repair can also be done under ilio-inguinal nerve block plus infiltration of the skin and hernia sac. This latter technique is suitable for same-day surgery and in patients with significant concurrent disease.

Thoracic Surgery

Heart and lung surgical procedures are performed under general anesthesia, with endotracheal intubation and relaxation. Monitoring is often extensive and invasive. Epidural anesthesia can be combined with the general anesthetic intraoperatively and continued for postoperative pain relief.

Urologic Procedures

Nephrectomy is most frequently performed under general anesthesia and with the patient intubated. The lateral position impairs respiration, and use of

the kidney bridge* increases this impairment. Inferior vena cava occlusion leading to hypotension may also occur with use of the kidney bridge in the lateral position.

During suprapubic or retropubic prostatectomy, considerable hemorrhage may occur. Many physicians prefer to give general anesthesia with endotracheal intubation even though extradural or subarachnoid block can be used. Hypotensive technique is sometimes used to decrease blood loss.

Transurethral cystoscopy, bladder tumor excision, and prostatectomy can be performed under general anesthesia with or without endotracheal intubation, but the method of choice is often subarachnoid or extradural anesthesia. If such a regional technique is used, the patient can report symptoms of bladder rupture or "TUR-syndrome," that is, dilutional hyponatremia, and early corrections can be instituted. These problems are discussed in detail in later chapters.

Gynecologic Procedures

Lower abdominal surgery calls for good relaxation to prevent damage to the muscles and peritoneum from abrasion by packs and retractors. Extradural or subarachnoid anesthesia is better tolerated for gynecologic surgery than for upper abdominal surgery, but gynecologic surgery often requires use of the Trendelenburg position, which is poorly tolerated for long periods of time by the awake patient. General anesthesia with endotracheal intubation and relaxation is most commonly used, sometimes in combination with epidural block, which can then be used for postoperative pain relief with local anesthetics or narcotics.

Vaginal surgery can be performed under extradural or subarachnoid block or under general anesthesia. Endotracheal intubation is not necessary unless the Trendelenburg position and/or extensive hemorrhage is likely or possible. For dilatation and curettage, the deepest part of the anesthesia should be at the time of cervical dilatation to avoid reflex laryngeal spasm.

General anesthesia for laparoscopy is a frequently performed procedure. The blind insertion of the trocar, though it leaves only a minimal scar, may have considerable inherent risks. Once the patient is intubated, a possibly distended stomach must be deflated. In addition to watching for the usual anesthetic pitfalls, one must also be vigilant for signs of air embolism, intraabdominal bleeding and dysrhythmias. Laparoscopy can also be performed with

---

* The kidney bridge is a bar built into the operating table, which can be separately extended to push the laterally positioned patient's side upward to improve exposure. This is a compromising surgical position.

epidural anesthesia but tends to be somewhat uncomfortable for the patient.

Vascular Surgery

The general condition of patients undergoing vascular surgery is often poor, and they frequently have other major manifestations of arterial disease. Continuous extradural or subarachnoid block offers good pain relief (with some sympathetic block for peripheral vascular repair) and often is not accompanied by major hemodynamic disturbances. If the procedure extends intraabdominally, a general anesthetic is probably preferable. A high epidural block has more profound hemodynamic effects and aortic repair with cross clamping can be accompanied by major blood loss, correction of which can be impaired by prior regional block–induced sympathectomy. Good muscle relaxation and extensive hemodynamic monitoring are usually needed.

Carotid artery surgery, when performed with the patient under general anesthesia, may cause a hemodynamic roller coaster. With a skilled anesthesiologist-surgeon team, this procedure can be elegantly performed under cervical plexus block anesthesia. The latter allows the patient to be continuously questioned (i.e., using patient cognition as the monitor of adequacy of cerebral perfusion). However, if sudden major neurologic symptoms and signs should occur, the anesthesiologist is not in a very favorable position to intervene.

Orthopedic Surgery

Spinal surgery is performed most frequently with the patient under general anesthesia. Induced hypotension is sometimes used to reduce bleeding. In cases where a "wake-up test" is planned, narcotic supplementation will maintain the patient in a pain-free and cooperative state. Extremity surgery can also be done with the patient under general anesthesia, but regional anesthesia is usually as good or better. Brachial plexus block gives excellent postoperative pain relief in arm and hand surgery. Extradural and subarachnoid blocks depress stress responses, decrease intraoperative blood loss, and reduce risk of thromboembolism associated with lower extremity surgery.

Ear, Nose, and Throat Surgery

In this surgery, many anesthetic problems are related to the fact that the surgery is carried out on the upper respiratory tract itself. The anesthesiologist must preserve a patent airway while providing the surgeon adequate access. Some minor ear, nose, and tonsillar operations can be performed with the patient under local anesthesia, but the majority of procedures are best performed using general anesthesia. Inhalational agents are regarded as safe, since spontaneous breathing can best be maintained, but narcotics give excellent pain relief with less postoperative coughing. Fiberoptic intubation is a good alternative when airway tumors or radiation has made direct laryngoscopy difficult.

Eye Surgery

Many types of eye operations can be performed with local anesthesia, but general anesthesia is also commonly employed. For operations in children and in some adult procedures, general anesthesia is essential. Endotracheal intubation is usually recommended to give the ophthalmologic surgeon access to the eye. Succinylcholine increases intraocular pressure, which can be a problem in penetrating eye injuries, but coughing raises intraocular pressure about three times as much and cannot be tolerated during surgery when the anterior chamber or vitreous body are exposed. Bradycardia and sometimes even cardiac standstill can follow traction on eye muscles or pressure on the eyeball given the oculocardiac reflex. This can be prevented and treated with antimuscarinic drugs.

Neurosurgery

Although it is possible and sometimes necessary to perform craniotomy using regional or local anesthesia, general anesthesia with endotracheal intubation is the most commonly used technique. The highly specialized field of anesthetic practice has many challenges, including use of induced hypotension and, in different circumstances, use of the sitting position with its attendant risks, including air embolism.

PATIENT PREPARATION

Once the patient history, physical examination, interpretation of laboratory tests, and planning for surgery and monitoring have been done, the patient should be informed about pertinent findings. If further workup or therapy is needed, the patient should be told and, as soon as possible, be given a plan. The patient is usually thankful for additional workup and therapy if it is explained that it is intended to improve perioperative safety. On the other hand, it is frustrating for a patient's surgery to be cancelled without offering any further explanation. Most patients are productive members of society and, given a reasonable time plan, they can usually rearrange their schedules to decrease time lost, but respect for *their* schedule must always be shown. When ready for surgery, the patient should be further informed about anesthetic choices, advantages, disadvantages, and risks. For most patients, it is sufficient to describe the anesthesia in relatively general terms. A detailed discussion of the different drugs used may make the patient confused and more anxious. An exception here might be a patient who believes he/she has had a hypersensitivity reaction to a specific anesthetic drug used previously. In these cases, it is important to investigate what drugs the patient reacted to and what kind of reaction occurred. A discussion should be held with the patient about intraoperative and postoperative positioning as well as about a plan for postoperative pain control. The ideal time to discuss this is preoperatively, when the patient has a clear mind, and not postoperatively when the patient is drowsy from anesthetic agents and in pain. Most blocks are easier to perform successfully preoperatively or intraoperatively with a cooperative awake or fully anesthetized patient, as opposed to dealing with an uncooperative patient in pain during the recovery period. The discussion should also include the postoperative period, addressing such issues as waking up, extubation, and perhaps postoperative supportive care.

GENERAL VS. REGIONAL ANESTHESIA

Optimal use of regional or general anesthesia for various surgical procedures is quite controversial.[11] However, with improved specificity of anesthetic agents, anesthesiologists are now able to provide a safe and satisfactory anesthesia with either regional or general anesthesia, and, with both techniques, to provide good pain relief into the postoperative period. Most anesthesiologists seem to prefer regional anesthesia but relatively few regularly practice it.[44]

Advantages of General Anesthesia
Rapid onset of action

Ultra-short-acting intravenous agents (barbiturates, opioids, benzodiazepines) take effect within a few minutes and many in less than 1 minute.[5] The inhalation agents are not as rapid acting unless combined with intravenous drugs. Most local anesthesia techniques require a considerably longer period to take effect. It is rare that a peripheral nerve or even a subarachnoid block results in an adequately anesthetized patient ready for incision within 5 minutes. On the other hand, surgical preparation can be done during this period while the regional anesthesia is "setting up."

Controllable duration of action

It is usually desirable to be able to terminate anesthesia as rapidly as possible after surgery. General anesthetic agents are effective in this regard.[38] Rapid recovery can occur when an ultra-short-acting drug (i.e., alfentanil, propofol, or methohexital) is administered as a slow continuous infusion and then abruptly stopped.[91] Although it is possible to prolong local anesthetic action by adding certain drugs and

using a catheter technique, it is generally difficult to terminate a local (or regional) anesthetic action once the agent is given. A general anesthetic must, of course, be terminated to safely awaken the patient and bring him/her to a recovery period so that the next case can be started. On the other hand, there is usually no need to terminate a regional block exactly at the end of surgery. Indeed, it is common to deliberately prolong the block with "weaker" local anesthetic solutions to provide extended pain relief with less motor block. Therefore, the regionally anesthetized patient is brought to a full recovery some time after the end of surgery and the anesthesiologist is not held up due to airway problems but can immediately proceed to the next case. In outpatient surgery where early ambulation is important, a catheter technique using local anesthetic agents of short duration is very useful.

Technical ease of administration

Intravenous anesthetics are relatively easy to administer especially with today's computerized infusion pumps. Once the intravenous infusion is started, inhalation anesthetics are easily administered after an open airway has been established (with or without an endotracheal tube). More skill is needed to perform various regional blocks with a high success rate, in general, but there are instances where a swift nerve block is sufficient when administration of a general anesthetic would have been much more complicated.

Reliability

General anesthesia can be produced in all patients irrespective of age, whereas local anesthesia can be used only with considerable difficulty in young and uncooperative patients. In addition, even anesthesiologists highly skilled in regional blocks have success rates below 100%. Regional anesthesia is not an option in some cases because of the type of surgery to be performed or because of contraindications, such as bleeding disorders or situations where surgery is to be done in disparate body locations (e.g., a bone graft from the iliac crest used in a reconstructive procedure on an arm). In such cases, general anesthesia should be employed.

Advantages of Regional Anesthesia
Stress response modification

Considerable advances have recently been made in understanding the numerous metabolic effects of anesthesia and surgery.[29] Such effects may result from increased demands on the body caused by the catabolic response after injury/trauma. Techniques that modify this response and maintain organ function may lead to reduced morbidity.[53] Although regional anesthesia in its present form is not ideal, it is currently the most effective method of reducing the stress response.

Specifically, surgical trauma is associated with increases in pituitary hormones (prolactin, growth hormone, ACTH, ADH) as well as adrenal and renal hormones (cortisol, aldosterone, renin, epinephrine, norepinephrine), all of which are inhibited to some extent by epidural block. Metabolic changes, or increases in glucose, lactate hydroxybutyrate, glycerol, free fatty acids, and cyclic AMP seen after surgery/trauma, are also inhibited by epidural block. The mechanism by which epidural anesthesia inhibits endocrine and metabolic alterations during surgery is probably related to blockade of afferent pathways, efferent pathways, or both.

Low mortality

The incidence of death during modern elective surgery is very low, so a large number of patients must be studied before any benefit can be attached to a particular regimen. Pooling 12 controlled mortality studies comparing regional and general anesthesia in patients undergoing acute hip surgery showed a 30% reduction in early mortality in the regional anesthesia group (p < 0.01). Exactly why this finding occurred is unknown. There was no difference in long-term survival, not surprisingly, which depends on factors other than choice of anesthetic.[86] Data from other procedures are few and inconclusive, except for one study that demonstrated significantly reduced mortality in patients undergoing high-risk thoracic, abdominal, or vascular procedures done using general anesthesia combined with epidural analgesia compared to high-dose narcotic-based general anesthesia alone.[99]

Fewer pulmonary complications

Postoperative epidural analgesia seems better than other pain-relieving regimens in minimizing reduction of vital capacity, functional residual capacity, and other parameters of respiratory function.[89] A significant decrease in the incidence of pulmonary infections with regional anesthesia was seen after cholecystectomy,[20] lower limb vascular surgery,[17] and thoracic, abdominal, and vascular procedures.[99] Pooling data from a wide variety of surgical procedures shows that pulmonary infection was observed in 12.8% of regional anesthesia patients compared with 26% in the general anesthesia group (p < 0.0002). Combining results of these controlled trials, each of which had a different design, is not statistically entirely justifiable but should at least encourage further clinical trials.[86] Postoperative pain relief using regional anesthesia may provide a greater margin of safety for avoiding respiratory side effects than does continuous administration of opiates.[13]

Fewer cardiac complications

There is evidence that perioperative cardiac demands are reduced by epidural anesthesia,[81] probably because of diminished catecholamine response to surgery. In high-risk patients undergoing vascular, abdominal, and thoracic procedures, a significant decrease in postoperative cardiovascular failure was found in one study,[99] but data from several other studies showed an insignificant difference in perioperative ischemic changes among the regional anesthesia group (15%) compared to the general anesthesia group (20%).[86]

Fewer gastrointestinal effects

An increase in colonic blood flow from epidural blockade[2] might be expected to have a beneficial effect on the incidence of anastomotic dehiscence, but no solid evidence exists on this point. Epidural blockade does enhance gastric emptying[70] and reduces intestinal transit time,[1] whereas epidural morphine has good pain-relieving properties but does not affect intestinal transit time compared to control patients.[1]

Reduced blood loss

With regional anesthesia, intraoperative blood loss can be significantly reduced by 20% to 50% during orthopedic, vascular, gynecologic, and urologic surgery.[86] The mechanism for the diminished bleeding during regional anesthesia is probably induced hypotension. Interestingly, no decrease in bleeding was found in upper abdominal procedures with the patient under epidural anesthesia.[39]

Lower incidence of thromboembolism

There is a considerable and significant reduction in the incidence of thromboembolism during surgery below the umbilicus performed under epidural anesthesia.[86] The mechanism for the observed reduction in thromboembolism seems to be increased lower extremity blood flow during sympathetic blockade. Reduced platelet aggregation[9] and increased fibrinolytic function may also be responsible. However, thoracic epidural anesthesia for abdominal surgery did not reduce thromboembolic complications,[62] probably because of lack of increased lower limb blood flow.

Improved cerebral function

Immediate postoperative transient mental deterioration, more common after general than regional anesthesia, is not seen later in the postoperative period in most studies on regional anesthesia.[86] Confusion seems to be related more to the use of anticholinergic drugs and to a history of depression than to anesthetic technique alone.[10]

Improved immune function

Recent studies reveal a depressive effect on some immune functions during surgery under general anesthesia, for example, chemotactic migration and phagocytosis of leukocytes.[19,25] Procedures done using regional anesthesia did not show a corresponding depression of leukocyte function.[90] Lymphocyte function and monocyte phagocytosis and cytolysis were depressed after general anesthesia but normal or increased after epidural anesthesia.[41,42] It seems that the immunosuppressive effect of surgery done with general anesthesia is affected through several different mediators whose concentration or half-life may be reduced during epidural anesthesia. These factors could include endocrine stress factors, products from cascade reactions, arachidonic acid metabolites, and perhaps even endorphins and neurotransmitters.

Shortened convalescence

Increased postoperative mobilization and reduced length of hospital stay have also been reported when regional anesthesia is used, but in most studies the differences in these factors compared to the situation with general anesthesia are insignificant.[86]

Conclusions

For certain types of surgery, regional anesthesia may actually reduce perioperative morbidity and mortality and, therefore, is an attractive alternative to general anesthesia. However, the anesthesiologist must be skilled, the block must work, and the postoperative caregiver must be educated in providing the care these extended blocks necessitate. Extended blocks are not without side effects.

PERIOPERATIVE MEDICATION

Premedication involving vagolytic, anxiolytic, and pain-relieving drugs is discussed in other sections of this text and will not be discussed here.

PROPHYLACTIC ANTIBIOTICS

Antimicrobial prophylaxis can decrease the incidence of infection, particularly wound infection after certain types of surgery, but this must be weighed against the risks of allergic and toxic reactions as well as the emergence of resistant bacteria and superinfection.

Classification of Wounds

To evaluate which patients should be given prophylactic antibiotics, a system of classifying surgical procedures based on the probability and the degree of microbial contamination should be used. There is a close correlation between these categories and the incidence of wound infection.[18,43]

Clean wounds

Clean wounds, which constitute approximately 75% of all operations, are those made under ideal operating conditions where no entry is made into the oropharyngeal cavity or the respiratory, alimentary, or genitourinary tract. No inflammation is encountered. These wounds are always primarily closed and seldom drained. The expected incidence of infection is usually less than 5%. However, if antibiotics are used before all clean operations, a large number of persons will be unnecessarily exposed to the risks of adverse drug effects. Routine use of prophylactic antibiotics is, therefore, not recommended in patients undergoing clean operations. In a small number of situations, the use of prophylactic antibiotics may be justified due to the potentially devastating effects that an infection would have.[15] Examples include the insertion of permanent implants,[27] operations performed on patients known to be carriers of pathologic microorganisms, operations on persons known to have an existing infection distant from the operative site; and operations on patients who have a history of rheumatic valvular disease or a previously implanted valve.

Clean-contaminated wounds

Clean-contaminated wounds, present in about 15% of all operations, are those in the oropharyngeal cavity or the respiratory or gastrointestinal tracts but without important spillage. Also included are those in the urinary or lower genital tracts. The incidence of infection after this kind of surgery is approximately 10%. In some operative procedures in this group, the degree of contamination is minimal and the probability of infection not great enough to justify the use of antimicrobial prophylaxis. However, prophylactic antibiotics are useful in patients undergoing operations that require entrance into the oropharyngeal cavity with neck dissection, gastric resection for carcinoma, opening of the lower ileum or colon, intestinal surgery with vascular compromise, entrance into the biliary tract in the presence of contaminated bile, operations on the urinary tract in the presence of obstruction or culture-positive urine, and amputation of an extremity that has had a poor blood supply.

Contaminated wounds

Contaminated wounds are those occurring in the genitourinary or biliary tracts in the presence of infected urine or bile or those in which there is gross gastrointestinal tract spillage. Fresh traumatic wounds are also included in this group. The likelihood of infection in an individual case is about 15% to 20%.

Dirty wounds

Dirty wounds are those that contain devitalized tissue and foreign bodies from old traumatic wounds, other infections, or perforated viscera. Incidence of infection in this group is very high, approaching 100%. Contaminated and dirty wounds account for about 8% of operations, and prophylactic antibiotics are recommended for all these patients.

Chemoprophylaxis
Topical prophylaxis

The rationale for topical antibiotic use in incisional and intraperitoneal infections is that antibacterial activity is delivered directly to the site of contamination in a concentration far exceeding that of systemic administration alone. The ideal topical antimicrobial agent must have a wide range of antimicrobial effects, cause minimal local tissue irritation, have minimal systemic toxic effect, have minimal systemic absorption if toxicity is a hazard, cause minimal allergenicity, and trigger infrequent emergence of resistant microbial forms.[36] For example, surface antimicrobials have significantly increased the survival of patients with large burn injuries.[76]

Studies involving contaminated or potentially contaminated wounds showed that topically applied Neosporin, neomycin, kanamycin, and cephaloridine have substantially reduced the rates of wound infection.[23,77,93]

The use of topical antimicrobial agents in clean wounds is generally not supported by existing data[74,77,78] although there are indications for their use in clean surgery if permanent implants (e.g., vascular grafts, joint prostheses, etc.) are used.[72] The intraperitoneal use of antimicrobial agents to treat peritonitis and prevent septic complications has enjoyed periods of favor and disfavor.[16] Some drugs, like sulfonamides, tetracyclines, and streptomycin, cause severe toxic local and systemic side effects in animals and cannot be recommended for intraperitoneal human use. Emphasis has been placed on agents effective against gram-negative bacteria. The aminoglycosides, (neomycin, kanamycin, cephalothin, bacitracin, and povidone-iodine) may be useful in treating or preventing intraperitoneal infectious complications.[16,32,61,68]

The initial enthusiasm for intraperitoneal aminoglycosides has waned after reports of respiratory arrest due to nondepolarizing neuromuscular blocking effects.[66,80] **The question that remains unanswered is whether local wound therapy is safer and more effective than systemic prophylaxis or, in elective intestinal procedures, whether it is better than oral administration of poorly absorbed antibiotics.**

Systemic prophylaxis

The goal of systemic prophylaxis is to augment local incisional defense mechanisms by wound suffusion and/or perfusion with effective antibiotic concentrations. The agent should have activity against expected pathogens and low systemic toxicity. It should be administered immediately preoperatively and be followed by up to three doses postoperatively. Numerous clinical studies document the usefulness of systemic antibiotic prophylaxis in contaminated and potentially contaminated surgery not only for wound infections[7,14,57,73,94] but also for nonwound postoperative infectious complications.[7] Several different antimicrobial agents have proved useful, but the most common are cephaloridine, cefazolin, and tobramycin-lincomycin. Individuals sustaining penetrating wounds to the abdomen have an increased incidence of infectious complications, which can be significantly reduced when antibiotic therapy is given preoperatively.[30]

Systemic prophylaxis is generally not appropriate in clean operations. The risk of antibiotic side effects in such cases may be greater than the risk of infection. As discussed previously, implantation of foreign bodies and cases where infection causes devastating complications are the exceptions, and antibiotic prophylaxis is indicated.

Enteral prophylaxis

Enteral prophylaxis is an alternative to colon surgery, which has long been associated with a high risk of wound infection. Large numbers of both aerobic and anaerobic bacteria exist in either the normal or the mechanically cleansed colon. Oral antimicrobial therapy produces a 100- to 100,000-fold decrease in the concentration of both aerobic and anaerobic organisms but regularly leaves bacterial densities of 10^4 to 10^6 organisms/gram of feces. The goal is to reduce lumen flora and decrease the number of organisms that reach the incision. The ideal intestinal antiseptic should have a broad spectrum, rapid action, minimal systemic absorption, minimal local and systemic toxicity, stability in the presence of digestive ferments, and the ability to prevent overgrowth of resistant bacteria.[79] The most commonly used drugs with documented effects are neomycin, doxycycline, neomycin-erythromycin, and kanamycin-metronidazole.[34,40,69,79] Enteral and systemic prophylactic results have been compared, and both appear equally protective in preventing infectious complications in patients undergoing elective colon surgery.[58]

Principles and practice of prophylaxis

Timing the administration of prophylactic antibiotics is very important. In elective colonic procedures, oral antibiotics are administered several hours before the procedure. Systemically administered antibiotics need not be given until the start of surgery. Several studies, however, have established that no grace period exists after contamination of the wound.[4,74,75]

So, if low-level contamination occurs continuously throughout the surgical procedure, the period of highest risk for bacterial contamination may most likely be the close, not the beginning, of surgery. Therefore adequate serum and tissue levels of antibiotics should be maintained throughout the surgical procedure,[33] instead of simply giving a bolus dose at the beginning.

Antibiotics given perioperatively for prophylaxis are often continued for 1 to several days into the postoperative period. Several studies comparing short (≤ 48 hours) vs. longer-course prophylaxis have shown no increase in infection rates among the short-course recipients.[33,67,88]

The selection of an appropriate antimicrobial agent must be based on the sensitivity of the expected flora. A major determining factor in successful systemic prophylaxis is the ability to penetrate the tissues in sufficiently high concentrations to exceed the minimum inhibitory concentrations for expected contaminating flora. In gastrointestinal surgery, broad gram-negative coverage is required, but some activity against *Staphylococcus* is also desirable. Doses of cephaloridine and cefazolin given systemically are

Table 3-1   Guidelines for prophylaxis related to type of surgery

Type of surgery	Recommendations
Neurosurgery	Antistaphylococcal antibiotics reduce wound infections after craniotomies[97]; prophylaxis is not indicated in spinal surgery and does not decrease infection rate after cerebrospinal fluid shunt implantation[82]
Ocular surgery	Staphylococci, streptococci, enteric gram-negative bacilli, and *Pseudomonas* can cause devastating endophthalmitis postoperatively[92]; despite limited data on the effectiveness of prophylaxis, antimicrobial eyedrops are commonly used before surgery and subconjunctival injections of antibiotics at the end of the procedure; parenteral antimicrobials penetrate the uninflamed aqueous or vitreous humor too poorly to be useful[92]
Head and neck surgery	Prophylaxis is not indicated in uncontaminated head and neck surgery[50] but is useful when the incision involves oral or pharyngeal mucosa[49]
Cardiac surgery	Prophylaxis is not indicated for pacemaker implantation but decreases the incidence of infection after open heart surgery[98]
Thoracic (noncardiac) surgery	Prophylaxis is not effective after closed tube thoracostomy for chest trauma or spontaneous pneumothorax[56,60]
Vascular surgery	Prophylaxis is not indicated for brachial and carotid artery surgery that does not involve prosthetic material; preoperative cephalosporin is effective for surgery on the abdominal aorta, vascular leg surgery where the groin is involved, and lower extremity amputation for ischemia[37,64,87]; some researchers also recommend prophylaxis for implantation of any vascular prosthetic material
Orthopedic surgery	Prophylactic antistaphylococcal drugs are indicated for prosthetic joint surgery as well as for fractures repaired with nails, screws, and plates[28]
Gastroduodenal surgery	Gastric acidity and motility normally inhibit bacterial growth in the stomach and duodenum; with obstruction, hemorrhage, ulcer, malignancy, or prolonged therapy with H_2-blockers, prophylactic use of a cephalosporin is indicated preoperatively as well as for gastric bypass surgery for obesity[47]
Biliary tract surgery	Patients with an increased risk of infection (age greater than 70 years or those affected with acute cholecystitis, obstructive jaundice, and common duct stones) should have antimicrobial agents perioperatively[59]
Colorectal surgery	Preoperative antibiotics decrease the incidence of infection after colorectal surgery; the regimen should include antimicrobial agents that are effective against both aerobic gram-negative bacteria and anaerobes[71]; for elective operations, oral antibiotics appear to be as effective as parenteral drugs
Gynecologic and obstetric surgery	There is a decreased incidence of infection after vaginal hysterectomy with antimicrobial prophylaxis[24]; prophylaxis is also useful in emergency cesarean section in high-risk situations such as active labor or ruptured membranes[48] and for abortions in women with previous pelvic inflammatory disease[22]
Urologic surgery	Antimicrobial agents are not indicated before urologic surgery on patients with sterile urine; those with positive urine cultures should be treated before surgery or receive a single preoperative dose of an appropriate agent at the time of surgery

supported by well-controlled clinical trials. Topical aminoglycoside antibiotics, Neosporin, and cephaloridine are also effective.

Whether prophylactic regimens should include antibiotics directed against anaerobic bacteria has not yet been determined, but there are indications that successful management of the aerobic component of the mixed aerobic-anaerobic synergistic infection will alter the wound environment sufficiently to also interfere with growth of anaerobic organisms.[95]

Side effects of prophylaxis

The emergence of resistant bacteria has been a main concern in effective prophylaxis but recently seems to be less of a problem, especially in short-course regimens. Pseudomembranous colitis has been noted with several agents, including oral erythromycin and neomycin, parenteral aminoglycosides, metronidazole, cephradine, cephaloridine, and cefoxitin.[8] In view of the extensive use of prophylaxis in the United States, pseudomembranous colitis is an unusual complication. A bleeding disorder occasionally associated with therapeutic use of certain beta-lactam antibiotics represents another potential side effect in prophylaxis.[85] A third potential consequence of prophylaxis is profound hypotension associated with vancomycin prophylaxis, especially with rapid infusion of the antibiotic.[21] Finally, sensitizing patients to antibiotics with resultant anaphylactic reactions after repeated administration is also a well-known risk.

Other Preventive Measures

Antimicrobial agents are not substitutes for preoperative patients showering with a detergent containing an antiseptic and careful surgical technique if at all possible. The preoperative hospital stay should be as short as possible and antibiotics should, if possible, be avoided in the preoperative period. If shaving for hair removal at the operative site is required, it should be performed as close to the time of surgery as possible. Maintenance of adequate perfusion and oxygenation of tissues perioperatively[55] and good nutrition postoperatively are also important aspects of infection prevention. Drains and intravascular devices should be removed as quickly as possible to avoid direct or hematogenous seeding of the operative site.

Selected Surgery and Prophylaxis

Table 3-1 outlines prophylactic guidelines to be observed.

THROMBOSIS PROPHYLAXIS

Prophylaxis for deep venous thrombosis, pulmonary embolism, and deep venous insufficiency is discussed in another chapter of this text.

RELATIONSHIP OF ADRENOCORTICAL MALFUNCTION TO ANESTHESIA AND SURGERY

Acute stress associated with surgery and trauma has profound effects on the homeostasis of the body, and a normal adrenocortic function is of utmost importance for the organism to adequately respond to and survive this stress.

Three kinds of hormones—mineralocorticoids, glucocorticoids, and androgens—are secreted by the adrenal cortex. Insufficient hormone secretion may be caused by primary adrenal insufficiency, not seen until about 90% of the adrenal cortex has been destroyed unless there is an inborn error of metabolism. The most frequent cause is autoimmune destruction of the gland, but other causative factors are bacterial or fungal infections, cancer, or hemorrhage. Insufficient hormone secretion may also be caused by secondary adrenal insufficiency due to hypothalamic or pituitary failure caused by tumor, infection, surgery, or radiation therapy. Secondary adrenal insufficiency can also occur as a result of exogenous administration of glucocorticoids.

Mineralocorticoids

Aldosterone, exerting 95% of the mineralocorticoid activity, is secreted from the zona glomerulosa of the adrenal cortex. The major regulator of aldosterone secretion is the renin-angiotensin system via angiotensin II. Increased potassium concentration and increased adrenocorticotropic hormone (ACTH) levels also cause increased aldosterone secretion.

Glucocorticoids

Cortisol (hydrocortisone) exerts 95% of the glucocorticoid activity in the body and is secreted from the zona fasciculata. Low blood cortisol levels, hyperthermia, hypovolemia, hypoglycemia, and neurogenic stimuli such as stress cause release of corticotropin-releasing hormone (CRH) in the hypothalamus, which in turn stimulates secretion of ACTH and endorphins. ACTH in turn stimulates adrenal cortisol secretion. There is diurnal variation, with the highest blood levels in the morning and the lowest at midnight. Daily production in a healthy man is about 20 to 25 mg/24 hours with an increase to 75 to 150 mg/24 hours during maximal stress.[51] Ninety percent is protein-bound to transcortin and albumin. The plasma half-life of cortisol is 90 minutes. About 70% of cortisol is enzymatically coupled with sulfate or glucuronic acid in the liver to form water-soluble compounds excreted in the urine. Corticosteroids induce a state of well-being through actions on metabolism, electrolyte and water balance, cardiovascular function, the kidneys, skeletal muscle, nervous system, and other organs and tissues. Corticosteroids endow the organism with the capacity to resist many types of noxious stimuli and environmental changes. There is a diabetogenic effect on carbohydrate metabolism, with increased liver glycogen and decreased peripheral glucose utilization. Corticosteroids increase protein degradation and lipolysis. Extracellular volume increases with sodium retention and negative potassium and calcium balance. Capillary permeability, vasomotor response of blood vessels, and cardiac performance all depend on adequate corticosteroid levels.

Clinical Presentation and Preoperative Preparation

In primary adrenal insufficiency (Addison's disease) the symptoms are often longstanding, including weight loss, anorexia, abdominal pain, nausea, vomiting, diarrhea, and constipation.[83] Diffuse hyperpigmentation and hypotension are seen in most patients, mineralocorticoid deficiency is characteristically present, and hyperkalemia may cause cardiac dysrhythmias.

Secondary adrenal insufficiency following anterior pituitary dysfunction is usually associated with fewer fluid balance and electroylye disturbances because aldosterone secretion is maintained. There is no hyperpigmentation, but symptoms resulting from the absence of growth hormone, thyroid-stimulating hormone, and gonadotropins may be seen, as well as manifestations of deficient ACTH secretion.

Adrenal insufficiency secondary to withdrawal of exogenous steroid therapy is uncommon[54,96] **but occurs in patients given corticosteroids for months. A** **rule of thumb is that if 7.5 mg prednisolone or more has been given daily for several months, suppression of the adrenal cortex must be suspected**[3] **and dealt with before anesthesia.** Relative antiinflammatory and sodium-retaining potency of different corticosteroids are described in Table 3-2 as well as their durations of action.

Symptoms of withdrawal are (1) adrenal insufficiency with fever, myalgia, arthralgia, malaise, and hypotension; (2) worsening of the original disease, such as asthma, rheumatoid disease, or colitis; and (3) pseudotumor cerebri with papilledema.

Corticosteroid-induced suppression is effected on a hypothalamic level,[65] but concomitant adrenal cortical atrophy is also important. After discontinuation of steroids, ACTH and cortisol levels in blood are initially low but within 2 to 5 months, ACTH levels increase with continuing low cortisol levels. Six to 9 months after steroids were withdrawn, blood cortisol levels are normalized, and, at 9 to 12 months, the stress response is normal.[35] Patients receiving inhaled or topical steroids may also exhibit pituitary-adrenal suppression following cessation of therapy.[12]

Diagnosis

Biochemical evidence of impaired adrenal or pituitary secretory function will confirm the diagnosis. Plasma concentrations of ACTH are elevated in the presence of primary adrenal insufficiency but reduced in secondary adrenal insufficiency.

A simulated stress response can be performed with synthetic ACTH or insulin-induced hypoglycemia. Patients with adrenal insufficiency will have low baseline plasma cortisol levels and have inadequate or no increased cortisol levels.[35]

Treatment

Patients suspected to have acute adrenal insufficiency should receive immediate therapy, preferably after a plasma cortisol level has been measured. In those patients preoperatively who have been taking steroid medication for several weeks or more, and who are planning to continue postoperatively, perioperative "stress" doses should be given. In those who have no need for postoperative steroids (splenectomy for ITP, colectomy for ulcerative colitis), a preoperative ACTH test will reveal whether steroids can be discontinued immediately postoperatively, minimizing side effects, without any risk of adrenal insufficiency.

The first regimens for corticosteroid replacement in connection with surgery and trauma were empiric. The maximal cortisol production was 75 to 150 mg/24 hours in major surgery[45] and in severely burn-injured patients.[46] A replacement schedule wherein 25 mg hydrocortisone was given at anesthesia induction,

Table 3-2   Comparison of relative effects and duration of action (biologic half-life) for commonly used corticosteroids

Compound	Anti-inflammatory potency	Sodium-retaining potency	Duration of action
Cortisol	1	1	Short
Cortisone	0.8	0.8	Short (8-12 hours)
Prednisone	4	0.8	Intermediate
Prednisolone	4-5	0.8	Intermediate (12-36 hours)
Methylprednisolone	5	0.5	Intermediate
Triamcinolone	5	0	Intermediate
Dexamethasone	25	0	Long
Betamethasone	25-40	0	Long (36-72 hours)
Fludrocortisone	10	125	Short
Aldosterone	0	400-3000	Short

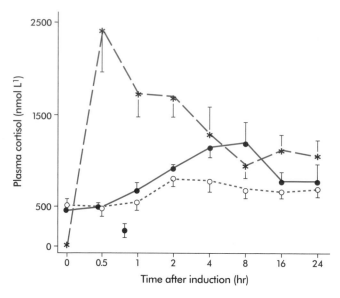

Fig. 3-1. Plasma cortisol response to the stress of anesthesia and surgery. Mean ± SEM. Control patients (●—●), patients receiving long-term corticosteroid treatment with normal response to corticotropin stimulation test but no perioperative substitution (○--○), and patients receiving long-term corticosteroids with a subnormal response to the corticotropin test given low-dose cortisol substitution perioperatively (∗--∗). (From Symreng T, Karlberg BE, Kågedahl B et al: Physiological cortisol substitution of long-term steroid-treated patients undergoing major surgery, *Br J Anaesth* 53:949, 1981.)

followed by 100 mg given continuously over 24 hours (Fig. 3-1), resulted in plasma levels at or above normal stress response levels.[96] These patients, as well as a large group of steroid-treated patients, perioperatively replaced according to this schedule did well clinically with no signs of adrenal insufficiency. There is currently no information that higher doses need to be given. On the contrary, several studies have not indicated the need for an intraoperative stress dose when anesthetic techniques blocking the stress response (preventing cortisol, epinephrine, and norepinephrine production) have been used.[26,31] Anesthetic techniques depressing the stress response have also been shown to be beneficial to the patients, producing less negative nitrogen balance[10] and a decrease in other complications.[99]

Higher doses of steroids cause hyperglycemia and electrolyte disturbances and, if given long term, have numerous other side effects. However, these are usually not seen in a surgical setting.

The need for cortisol replacement usually decreases in the postoperative period, and Kehlet recommends 100 mg/24 hours until the patient is mobilized and the gut is working; thereafter the daily dose should be reduced further.[52] Minor surgery is accompanied by only a minor increase in cortisol production.[54] These patients can take their regular dose in the morning and an additional 25 mg hydrocortisone at induction of anesthesia.[52] Further supplementation is usually not necessary.

In elective surgery there is no evidence favoring preoperative increase in any maintenance dose of corticosteroids.

Patients who have primary adrenal insufficiency usually have neither glucocorticoid nor mineralocorticoid production in sufficient amounts. During replacement with 100 mg hydrocortisone or more, further mineralocorticoid supplementation is not necessary. The mineralocorticoid activity of hydrocortisone is usually enough. However, when the hydrocortisone dose is reduced, mineralocorticoid replacement will be needed. Adequate perioperative blood and fluid replacement are vital in patients with both normal and subnormal adrenal function. In most of the earlier case reports in which patients died of presumed or contended adrenal insufficiency, fluid and/or blood replacement was retrospectively found to be inadequate.

Conclusions

Adrenal insufficiency is a rare disorder, and the question of perioperative stress coverage is most often encountered in preoperatively steroid-treated patients. The evaluation of adrenal function is cumbersome, and the problem is most easily dealt with by giving "physiologic" coverage (see treatment discussed previously) during the stress period.

KEY POINTS

- It sounds mundane, but the anesthesiologist *must* have a plan. This basic rule is often ignored, neglected, or broken.
- Regional anesthesia vs. general anesthesia controversies raise important questions. The issues are numerous and detailed, but the possibility of performing regional anesthesia should always be considered.

- General anesthesia has the obvious advantages of rapid onset of action, controllable duration of action, and relative technical ease of administration.
- Regional anesthesia has the advantage of valid stress response modification, including the possibility that the incidence of deep venous thrombosis in certain kinds of patients may be considerably lessened.

- In the regional vs. general anesthesia controversy, the effect of choice of anesthesia on the incidence of pulmonary complications, incidence of cardiac complications, various gastrointestinal consequences, blood loss, cerebral function, and immune function is the most controversial issue.
- The use of prophylactic antibiotics during surgical procedures is also highly controversial. Usually, surgeons request the administration of antibiotics. Before complying, the anesthesiologist must always thoroughly understand the patient's allergic history, if any.

- The antibiotic vancomycin causes especially serious side effects. Severe, profound, and refractory hypotension can be seen with the apparently innocuous administration of this agent, especially if it is given rapidly.
- The anesthesiologist should understand clearly the various aspects involved in preparing patients for anesthesia and surgery who are or who might be steroid dependent.

KEY REFERENCES

Borg T, Modig J: Potential antithrombotic effects of local anaesthetics due to their inhibition of platelet function, *Acta Anaesthesiol Scand* 29:739, 1985.

Chodak GW, Plaut ME: Use of systemic antibiotics for prophylaxis in surgery: a critical review, *Arch Surg* 112:326, 1977.

Dajee H, Laks H, Miller J et al: Profound hypotension from rapid vancomycin administration during cardiac operation, *J Thorac Cardiovasc Surg* 87:145, 1984.

Kehlet H: The stress response to anaesthesia and surgery: release mechanisms and modifying factors, *Clin Anaesthesiol* 2:315, 1984.

Mellbring G, Dahlgren S, Reiz S et al: Thromboembolic complications after major abdominal surgery: effect of thoracic epidural anesthesia, *Acta Chir Scand* 149:263, 1983.

Pridgen A: Respiratory arrest thought to be due to intraperitoneal neomycin, *Surgery* 40:571, 1956.

Scott NB, Kehlet H: Regional anaesthesia and surgical morbidity, *Br J Surg* 75:299, 1988.

Symreng T, Karlberg BE, Kågedahl B et al: Physiological cortisol substitution of long-term steroid-treated patients undergoing major surgery, *Br J Anaesth* 53:949, 1981.

REFERENCES

1. Ahn H, Bronge A, Johansson K et al: Effect of continuous postoperative epidural analgesia on intestinal motility, *Br J Surg* 75:1176, 1988.
2. Aitkenhead AR: Anaesthesia for bowel surgery, *Ann Chir Gynaecol* 73:177, 1984.
3. Arnoldsson H: Pituitary-adrenocortical function after multennial steroid therapy: significance of dosage and responsiveness to stress. In Bajusz E: *An introduction to clinical neuroendocrinology,* New York, 1967, Karger.
4. Bagley DH, MacLowry J, Beazley RM et al: Antibiotic concentration in human wound fluid after intravenous administration, *Ann Surg* 188:202, 1978.
5. Bailey PL, Stanley TH: Pharmacology of intravenous narcotic anesthetics. In Miller RD, ed: *Anesthesia,* ed 2, New York, 1985, Churchill-Livingstone.
6. Berggren D, Gustafson Y, Eriksson B et al: Postoperative confusion following anesthesia in elderly patients with femoral neck fractures, *Anesth Analg* 66:497, 1987.
7. Bernard HR, Cole WR: The prophylaxis

of surgical infection: the effect of prophylactic antimicrobial drugs on the incidence of infection following potentially contaminated operations, *Surgery* 56:151, 1964.
8. Block BS, Mercer LJ, Ismail MA et al: Clostridium difficile–associated diarrhea follows perioperative prophylaxis with cefoxitin, *Am J Obstet Gynecol* 153:835, 1986.
9. Borg T, Modig J: Potential antithrombotic effects of local anaesthetics due to their inhibition of platelet function, *Acta Anaesthesiol Scand* 29:739, 1985.
10. Brandt MR, Fernandes A, Mordhorst R et al: Epidural analgesia improves postoperative nitrogen balance, *Br Med J* 1:1106, 1978.
11. Bromage PH: Value judgements and choice in regional anesthesia, *Anesthesiol Rev* 9:13, 1981.
12. Carruthers JA, August PJ, and Straughton RCD: Observations on the systemic effect of topical clobetasol propionate (Dermovate), *Br Med J* 4:203, 1975.
13. Catley DM, Thornton C, Jordan C et al:

Pronounced, episodic oxygen desaturation in the postoperative period: its association with ventilatory pattern and analgesic regimen, *Anesthesiology* 63:20, 1985.
14. Chetlin SH, Elliott DW: Preoperative antibiotics in biliary surgery, *Arch Surg* 107:319, 1973.
15. Chodak GW, Plaut ME: Use of systemic antibiotics for prophylaxis in surgery: a critical review, *Arch Surg* 112:326, 1977.
16. Cohn I Jr: Intraperitoneal antibiotic administration, *Surg Gynecol Obstet* 114:309, 1962.
17. Cook PT, Davis MJ, Cronin KD et al: A prospective randomized trial comparing spinal anaesthesia using hyperbaric cinchocaine with general anaesthesia for lower limb vascular surgery, *Anaesth Intens Care* 14:373, 1986.
18. Cruse PJF: Incidence of wound infection on the surgical services, *Surg Clin North Am* 55:1269, 1975.
19. Cullen BF, Heume RG, and Chretien PB: Phagocytosis during general anaesthesia in man, *Anesth Analg* 54:501, 1975.
20. Cuschieri RJ, Morran CG, Howie JC

et al: Postoperative pain and pulmonary complications: comparison of three analgesic regims, *Br J Surg* 72:495, 1985.

21. Dajee H, Laks H, Miller J et al: Profound hypotension from rapid vancomycin administration during cardiac operation, *J Thorac Cardiovasc Surg* 87:145, 1984.

22. Darj E, Strälin EB, and Nilsson S: The prophylactic effect of doxycycline on postoperative infection rate after first-trimester abortion, *Obstet Gynecol* 70:755, 1987.

23. DiVincenti FC, Cohn I Jr: Intraperitoneal kanamycin in advanced peritonitis, *Am J Surg* 111:147, 1966.

24. Duff P: Prophylactic antibiotics for cesarean delivery: a simple cost-effective strategy for prevention of postoperative morbidity, *Am J Obstet Gynecol* 157:794, 1987.

25. Endler M, Endler TA, and Zielinski CH: Influence of hip arthroplasty upon chemotactic behavior of leucocytes, *Acta Orthop Scand* 53:795, 1982.

26. Enggvist A, Brandt MR, Fernandes A et al: The blocking effect of epidural analgesia on the adrenocortical and hypoglycemic responses to surgery, *Acta Anaesthesiol Scand* 21:33, 1977.

27. Ericson C, Lidgren L, and Lindberg L: Cloxacillin in prophylaxis of postoperative infections of the hip, *J Bone Joint Surg (Am)* 55(1):808, 1973.

28. Fitzgerald RH: Infections of hip prostheses and artificial joints, *Infect Dis Clin North Am* 3:329, 1989.

29. Frayn KN: Hormonal control of metabolism in trauma and sepsis, *Clin Endocrinol* 24:577, 1986.

30. Fullen WD, Hunt J, and Altemeier WA: Prophylactic antibiotics in penetrating wounds of the abdomen, *J Trauma* 12:282, 1972.

31. Giesecke K, Hamberger B, Järnberg PO et al: High- and low-dose fentanyl anaesthesia: hormonal and metabolic responses during cholecystectomy, *Br J Anaesth* 61:575, 1988.

32. Gilmore OJ, Sanderson PJ: Prophylactic interparietal povidone-iodine in abdominal surgery, *Br J Surg* 62:792, 1975.

33. Goldman DA, Hopkins CC, and Karchmer AW: Cephalothin prophylaxis in cardiac valve surgery: a prospective, double-blind comparison of two-day and six-day regimen, *J Thorac Cardiovasc Surg* 73:470, 1977.

34. Goldring J, McNaught W, Scott A et al: Prophylactic oral antimicrobial agents in elective colonic surgery: a controlled trial, *Lancet* 2:997, 1975.

35. Graber AL, Ney RL, Nicholson WE et al: Natural history of pituitary-adrenal recovery following long-term suppression with corticosteroids, *J Clin Endocranial Metab* 25:11, 1965.

36. Gray FJ, Kidd E: Topical chemotherapy in prevention of wound infection, *Surgery* 54:891, 1963.

37. Hasselgen PO, Ivarsson L, Risberg B et al: Effects of prophylactic antibiotics in vascular surgery, a prospective, randomized, double-blind study, *Ann Surg* 200:86, 1984.

38. Herbert M, Healy TEJ, Bourke JB et al: Profile of recovery after general anaesthesia, *Br Med J* 1539, 1983.

39. Hjortsø NC, Andersen T, Frøsig F et al: A controlled study of the effect of epidural analgesia with local anaesthetics and morphine on morbidity after abdominal surgery, *Acta Anaestesiol Scand* 29:790, 1985.

40. Höjer H, Wetterfors J: Systemic prophylaxis with doxycycline in surgery of the colon and rectum, *Ann Surg* 187:362, 1978.

41. Hole A, Unsgaard G: The effect of epidural and general anaesthesia on lymphocyte functions during and after major orthopaedic surgery, *Acta Anaesthesiol Scand* 27:135, 1983.

42. Hole A, Unsgaard G, and Breivik H: Monocyte functions are depressed during and after surgery under general anaesthesia but not under epidural anaesthesia, *Acta Anaesthesiol Scand* 26:301, 1982.

43. Howard JM et al: Postoperative wound infections: the influence of ultraviolet irradiation of the operating room and of various other factors, *Ann Surg* 160(Suppl):9, 1964.

44. Hughes TJ, Desgrand DA: Interscalene block for Colles fracture, *Anaesthesia* 38:149, 1983.

45. Hume DM, Bell CC, and Bartter FC: Direct measurement of adrenal secretion during operative trauma and convalescence, *Surgery* 52:174, 1962.

46. Hume DM, Nelson DH, and Miller DW: Blood and urinary 17-hydrocorticosteroids in patients with severe burns, *Ann Surg* 143:316, 1956.

47. Jain NK, Larson DE, Schroeder KW et al: Antibiotic prophylaxis for percutaneous endoscopic gastrostomy: a prospective, randomized, double-blind clinical trial, *Ann Intern Med* 107:824, 1987.

48. Jakobi P, Weissman A, Zimmer EZ et al: Single-dose cefazolin prophylaxis for cesarean section, *Am J Obstet Gynecol* 158:1049, 1988.

49. Johnson JT, Yu VL: Antibiotic use during major head and neck surgery, *Ann Surg* 207:108, 1988.

50. Johnson JT, Wagner RL: Infection following uncontaminated head and neck surgery, *Arch Otolaryngol* 113:368, 1987.

51. Kehlet H: Clinical course and hypothalamic-pituitary-adrenocortical function in glucocorticoid-treated surgical patients, thesis, Copenhagen FADL publication.

52. Kehlet H: A rational approach to dosage and preparation of parenteral glucocorticoid substitution therapy during surgical procedures, *Acta Anaesthesiol Scand* 19:260, 1975.

53. Kehlet H: The stress response to anaesthesia and surgery: release mechanisms and modifying factors, *Clin Anaesthesiol* 2:315, 1984.

54. Kehlet H, Binder C: Adrenocortical function and clinical course during and after surgery in unsupplemented glucocorticoid-treated patients, *Br J Anaesth* 45:1043, 1973.

55. Knighton DR, Halliday B, and Hunt TK: Oxygen as an antibiotic, *Arch Surg* 119:199, 1984.

56. LeBlanc KA, Tucker WY: Prophylactic antibiotics and closed tube thoracostomy, *Surg Gynecol Obstet* 160:259, 1985.

57. Ledger WJ, Sweet RL, and Headington JT: Prophylactic cephaloridine in the prevention of postoperative pelvic infections in premenopausal women undergoing vaginal hysterectomy, *Am J Obstet Gynecol* 115:766, 1973.

58. Lewis RT, Allan CM, Goodall RG et al: Antibiotics in surgery of the colon, *Can J Surg* 21:339, 1978.

59. Lewis RT, Goodall RG, Marien B et al: Biliary bacteria, antibiotic use, and wound infection in surgery of the gallbladder and common bile duct, *Arch Surg* 122:44, 1987.

60. Mandal AK, Montano J, and Thadepalli H: Prophylactic antibiotics and no antibiotics compared in penetrating chest trauma, *J Trauma* 25:639, 1985.

61. McMullan MH, Barnett WO: The clinical use of intraperitoneal cephalothin, *Surgery* 67:432, 1970.

62. Mellbring G, Dahlgren S, Reiz S et al: Thromboembolic complications after major abdominal surgery: effect of thoracic epidural analgesia, *Acta Chir Scand* 149:263, 1983.

63. Miles AA, Miles EM, and Burke J: The value and duration of defense reactions of the skin to the primary lodgement of bacteria, *Br J Exp Pathol* 38:79, 1957.

64. Møller BN, Krebs B: Antibiotic prophylaxis in lower limb amputation, *Acta Orthop Scand* 56:327, 1985.

65. Motta M, Fraschini F, Piva F et al: Hypothalamic and extrahypothalamic mechanism controlling adrenocorticotrophic secretion, *Memoirs Soc Endocrinol* 17:3, 1968.

66. Mullett RD, Keats AS: Apnea and respiratory insufficiency after intraperitoneal administration of kanamycin, *Surgery* 49:530, 1961.

67. Nelson CL, Green TC, Porter RA et al: One day versus seven days of preventive antibiotic therapy in orthopedic surgery, *Clin Orthop* 176:258, 1983.

68. Nelson JL, Kuzman JH, and Cohn I Jr: Intraperitoneal lavage and kanamycin for the contaminated abdomen, *Surg Clin North Am* 55:1391, 1975.

69. Nichols RL, Broido P, Condon RE et al: Effect of preoperative neomycin-erythromycin intestinal preparation on the incidence of infectious complications following colon surgery, *Ann Surg* 178:453, 1973.

70. Nimmo WS, Littlewood DG, Scott DB et al: Gastric emptying following hysterectomy with extradural analgesia, *Br J Anaesth* 50:559, 1978.

71. Norwegian Study Group: Should antimicrobial prophylaxis in colorectal surgery include agents effective against both anaerobic and aerobic microorganisms? a double-blind, multicenter study, *Surgery* 97:402, 1985.

72. Pitt HA, Postier RG, MaGowan WAL et al: Prophylactic antibiotics in vascular surgery, *Ann Surg* 192:356, 1980.
73. Polk HC Jr, Lopez-Mayor JF: Postoperative wound infection: a prospective study of determinant factors and prevention, *Surgery* 66:97, 1969.
74. Polk HC Jr, Miles AA: Enhancement of bacterial infection by ferric iron: kinetics, mechanisms, and surgical significance, *Surgery* 70:71, 1971.
75. Polk HC Jr, Miles AA: The decisive period in the primary infection of muscle by *Escherichia coli, Br J Exp Pathol* 54:99, 1973.
76. Polk HC Jr, Monafo WV, and Moyer CA: Human burn survival: study of efficacy of 0.5 percent aqueous silver nitrate, *Arch Surg* 98:262, 1969.
77. Pollock AV, Froome K, and Evans M: The bacteriology of primary wound sepsis in potentially contaminated abdominal operations: the effect of irrigation, povidone-iodine and cephaloridine on the sepsis rate assessed in a clinical trial, *Br J Surg* 65:76, 1978.
78. Pollock AV, Leaper DJ, and Evans M: Single dose intra-incisional antibiotic prophylaxis of surgical wound sepsis: a controlled trial of cephaloridine and ampicillin, *Br J Surg* 64:322, 1977.
79. Poth EJ: Intestinal antisepsis in surgery, *JAMA* 153:1516, 1953.
80. Pridgen A: Respiratory arrest thought to be due to intraperitoneal neomycin, *Surgery* 40:571, 1956.

81. Reiz S, Bälfors E, Sørensen MB et al: Coronary haemodynamic effects of general anaesthesia and surgery: modification by epidural analgesia in patients with ischemic heart disease, *Reg Anesth* 7(S4):8, 1982.
82. Rieder MJ, Frewen TC, Del Maestro RF et al: The effect of cephalothin prophylaxis on postoperative ventriculoperitoneal shunt infections, *Can Med Assoc J* 136:935, 1987.
83. Rowntree LG, Snell AM: A clinical study of Addison's disease, *Mayo Clin Monographs,* Philadelphia, 1931, WB Saunders.
84. Rutberg H, Håkanson E, Anderberg B et al: Effects of the extradural administration of morphine, or bupivacaine, on the endocrine response to upper abdominal surgery, *Br J Anaesth* 56:233, 1984.
85. Sattler FR, Weitekamp MR, and Ballard JO: Potential for bleeding with the new beta-lactam antibiotics, *Ann Intern Med* 105:924, 1986.
86. Scott NB, Kehlet H: Regional anacsthesia and surgical morbidity, *Br J Surg* 75:299, 1988.
87. Sonne-Holm S, Boeckstyns M, Menck H et al: Prophylactic antibiotics in amputation of the lower extremity for ischemia, *J Bone Joint Surg* 67A:800, 1985.
88. Soper DE, Yarwood RL: Single-dose antibiotic prophylaxis in women undergoing vaginal hysterectomy, *Obstet Gynecol* 69:879, 1987.
89. Spence AA, Smith G: Postoperative analgesia and lung function, a comparison of morphine with extradural block, *Br J Anaesth* 43:144, 1971.

90. Stanley TH, Hill GE, and Hill HR: The influence of spinal and epidural anesthesia on neutrophil chemotaxis in man, *Anesth Analg* 57:567, 1978.
91. Stanski DR, Hug CC Jr: Alfentanil—a kinetically predictable narcotic analgesic, *Anesthesiology* 57:435, 1982.
92. Starr MB: Prophylaxis antibiotics for ophthalmic surgery, *Surv Ophthalmol* 27:353, 1983.
93. Stone HH, Hester TR Jr: Topical antibiotic and delayed primary closure in the management of contaminated surgical incisions, *J Surg Res* 12:70, 1972.
94. Stone HH, Hooper CA, Kolb LD et al: Antibiotic prophylaxis in gastric, biliary, and colonic surgery, *Ann Surg* 184:443, 1976.
95. Stone HH, Kolb LD, and Geheber CE: Incidence and significance of intraperitoneal anaerobic bacteria, *Ann Surg* 181:705, 1975.
96. Symreng T, Karlberg BE, Kågedahl B et al: Physiological cortisol substitution of long-term steroid-treated patients undergoing major surgery, *Br J Anaesth* 53:949, 1981.
97. van Ek B, Dijkmans BA, van Dulken H et al: Antibiotic prophylaxis in craniotomy: a prospective double-blind placebo-controlled study, *Scand J Infect Dis* 20:633, 1988.
98. Wilson APR: Antibiotic prophylaxis in cardiac surgery, *J Antimicrob Chemother* 21:522, 1988.
99. Yaeger MP, Glass DD, Neff RK et al: Epidural anesthesia and analgesia in high-risk surgical patients, *Anesthesiology* 66:729, 1987.

CHAPTER 4

Planning for Monitoring in Healthy Patients

MARK N. GOMEZ

MONITORING IN PERSPECTIVE
Preventable Mishaps, Monitoring, and Outcome

A central question in anesthesia concerns the relationship between clinical monitoring practices and outcomes, especially adverse anesthetic outcomes, in surgical patients. A useful way to frame this question is in the form of a syllogism:

First premise: Preventable anesthetic mishaps result in adverse patient outcomes with major morbidity and mortality and significant costs to society.

Second premise: Improved anesthetic vigilance and monitoring result in fewer preventable anesthetic mishaps.

Conclusion: Improved anesthetic vigilance or monitoring, or both, result in fewer adverse patient outcomes and decreased cost to society.

Although the second premise has not been well tested, the conclusion is widely believed by the anesthetic community. However, relatively unscientific acceptance of this conclusion raises two questions: which anesthetic mishaps can be prevented by adequate monitoring and vigilance, and what constitutes adequate "standard" monitoring for healthy patients undergoing low-risk surgical procedures? **These questions are important; between 2000 and 6000 incidents of anesthesia-related deaths or permanent brain injuries occur every year in the United States, and many of these cases are believed preventable.**[15]

What are the underlying causes of these preventable catastrophies? Studies of anesthetic mortality dating to 1954 show that **hypoxemia, (i.e., insufficient oxygen in the arterial blood to sustain life) is the most common final pathway leading to anesthetic disaster.** Hypoxemia is usually due to failure to ventilate the lungs, which, according to one authority, "almost always results from human error."[19]

Two types of human error lead to preventable hypoxemia: judgment error and error involving failure of vigilance and monitoring.[19] **An example of judgment error is inability to ventilate the lungs after induction of unconsciousness and apnea. More pertinent to this discussion is the second type of error, (i.e., failure of vigilance and monitoring). A common example of this error is failure to detect a breathing circuit disconnection.**

Other types of preventable anesthetic occurrences, in addition to inadequate ventilation, can lead to brain injury or death. Anesthetic drugs have important side effects on the circulatory and respiratory systems. Anesthetic-related death or brain injury can result from relative or absolute anesthetic overdose. Unlike a primary hypoxic event, anesthetic overdosage is not considered *prima facie* evidence of human error. Nonetheless, overdosage can result from error in judgment, or failure in vigilance or monitoring, or both, with regard to known circulatory and respiratory effects of anesthetics. Whatever the initial cause, the final common pathway for all anesthetic disasters resulting in poor outcome involves a simple pathophysiologic principle: loss of cardiopulmonary homeostasis resulting in insufficient oxygen delivery to the brain.

Focus on the Healthy Patient

In an ongoing study of closed malpractice claims against anesthesiologists conducted by the Committee on Professional Liability of the American Society of Anesthesiologists (ASA), 80% of the patients studied, all of whom suffered anesthetic-related injury or death, were classified as ASA physical status I or II (i.e., they were relatively healthy).[42] It is this group of patients, relatively healthy and often undergoing low-risk surgical procedures, in whom preventable anesthetic-related poor outcomes have the greatest impact in terms of personal suffering, tragedy to family, loss of productivity, massive cost to society for long-term care, and consequent jury damage awards.[42]

How do vigilance and monitoring practice relate to adverse anesthetic outcomes in these healthy patients? The answer is not known for certain in every case thus far reviewed, but closed-claims studies show that in the majority of cases, use of additional noninvasive (Box 4-1) and widely available monitors "could have alerted the anesthetist to the danger of the problem and allowed the injury to be prevented."[42]

WHAT SHOULD BE MONITORED AND WHY?
Analysis of Closed Claims

To develop rational and effective approaches to monitoring healthy patients, the pathophysiology of anesthetic-related catastrophies in this group must first be understood. The final common pathway (i.e., the loss of cardiopulmonary homeostasis resulting in insufficient cerebral oxygen delivery) leading to brain injury or death has already been discussed. What events or physiologic derangements lead to this final pathway? Partial answers can be found in the closed-claim studies of the ASA Professional Liability

---

> ### BOX 4-1
> ### INVASIVE CLINICAL MONITORS
>
> **Noninvasive**
>
> Monitor is applied to the skin, as exemplified by electrocardiograph electrodes or blood pressure cuffs.
>
> **Minimally invasive**
>
> Requires breaking the skin, but only for local application of catheters such as intravenous catheters placed in the back of the hand or the crook of the elbow, or abrasion of the skin, (e.g., for placement of cutaneous oxygen electrodes).
>
> **Penetrating**
>
> Requires insertion of a probe into a bodily orifice such as the mouth, bladder, or anus, as is done for the placement of esophageal stethoscopes, temperature probes, and catheters.
>
> **Invasive**
>
> Requires cannulation of an artery or central vein.
>
> **Highly invasive**
>
> Cannulation of a ventricle of the brain or heart, as is done with intracranial pressure monitoring or pulmonary artery catheters.
>
> From Gravenstein JS, Paulus DA: *Clinical monitoring practice*, ed 2, Philadelphia, 1987, JB Lippincott.

Committee. **In 1988 members of the committee reported an in-depth analysis of 14 cases of sudden unexpected cardiac arrest in relatively healthy (ASA physical status I or II) patients during spinal anesthesia.[5] Ten of 14 patients died and 3 of 14 sustained severe neurologic impairment necessitating chronic care.** Using extensive documentation accumulated during the claims review process, the committee constructed a composite picture of the "typical" intraoperative cardiac arrest during spinal anesthesia. In addition to spinal anesthesia, 12 patients received one or more of the following intravenous drugs: fentanyl, diazepam, droperidol, or thiopental. In seven patients this resulted in a "comfortable-appearing, sleeplike" state without spontaneous verbalization. The first sign of impending cardiopulmonary arrest was noticed an average of 12 minutes after the last dose of sedative or narcotic. In each case, cardiopulmonary arrest was signaled by at least two of the following clinical signs: bradycardia, hypotension, cyanosis, loss of consciousness, and asystole. In six of the seven cases where patients exhibited sleeplike states devoid of spontaneous verbalization, *cyanosis* was observed as one of the first adverse signs. The authors acknowledged that respiratory insufficiency may have been present but clinically unrecognized in considerably more patients; it has long been known that cyanosis is difficult to assess clinically.[6] The closed-claims investigators concluded that narcotics and sedatives had not been inappropriately or carelessly used and that anesthetic vigilance appeared adequate. Nonetheless, they strongly recommended the use of a pulse oximeter whenever sedative agents are administered. This first ASA closed-claims report did not address the question of whether the use of additional monitors could have prevented these adverse outcomes. It is possible that the use of pulse oximeters (had they been available) would have prevented the negative outcomes in these cases, because as Knill has shown, administration of narcotics to previously sedated, pain-free patients (e.g., during spinal anesthesia) can cause profound respiratory depression.[21]

A subsequent report from the ASA Closed-Claims Study specifically addressed the impact of additional monitors on outcome. **In 1989 Tinker et al. reported a continuation of the ASA Closed-Claims Study that involved analysis of 1097 insurance claims resulting from injury or death during general or regional anesthesia. In 346 cases (31.5%) the reviewers judged that the injuries or deaths could have been prevented by use of one or more additional monitoring devices. In 305 of the 346 major negative outcomes judged preventable, at least one of the following signs of impending loss of cardiopulmonary homeostasis was noted: cyanosis, bradycardia, hypotension, or asystole. As in the earlier report, cyanosis was common, present in nearly 82% of cases that had preventable negative outcomes. The committee concluded that use of additional monitors, specifically pulse oximetry and capnometry (discussed later), would have prevented 93% of the preventable injuries or deaths.[38]**

The closed-claims studies suggest that improved monitoring or vigilance, or both, should improve patient safety. These studies strongly support the second premise stated earlier. Consequently, it is important to consider which physiologic processes can be safely and should be routinely monitored for signs of impending loss of cardiopulmonary homeostasis.

Monitoring the Basics

Ideally those physiologic processes that depict the overall state of the patient, with special attention focused on the state of the vital organs, should be continuously monitored. Currently the oxygen tensions in the tissues of the vital organs cannot be monitored. However, *inferential* information about vital organ well-being, obtained through clinical monitoring of the state of supply lines to these organs,

can be used to prevent or detect any threats to cardiopulmonary homeostasis. This is accomplished by monitoring adequacy of ventilation, oxygenation, and circulation. Because abnormal body temperature can pose a direct threat to these supply lines or may signal a life-threatening disease process (e.g., malignant hyperthermia), body temperature must be monitored as well.

MONITORING THE ADEQUACY OF VENTILATION

Pulmonary ventilation is defined as the to-and-fro exchange of gas between the lungs (both alveoli and tracheobronchial tree) and ambient air or gas delivery system. Intraoperative monitoring of pulmonary ventilation begins with the preoperative evaluation of the patient. With relatively healthy patients who have normal cardiopulmonary function, the approach to monitoring ventilation is determined mainly by the type of anesthetic to be delivered (regional vs. general), the type of ventilation to be used (spontaneous vs. controlled), and the nature of the surgical procedure (peripheral vs. intraabdominal, intrathoracic, or intracranial).

Awake Patient

One of the basic monitoring standards adopted by the ASA is continuous assessment of ventilation in all patients during anesthesia. Clinical assessment of ventilation begins with auscultation and inspection. For the awake patient undergoing major regional anesthesia (i.e., spinal or epidural anesthesia), a properly positioned stethoscope (precordial, pretracheal, or over any accessible area of the thorax) must be connected to the anesthetist's ear for continuous auscultation of breath and heart sounds whenever physically possible. Even with intercostal muscle paralysis resulting from intrathecally or epidurally administered local anesthetics, resting pulmonary function should be normal[16] and normal breath sounds should be heard. Inspection, though usually not continuous, is also a valuable monitor.

In the awake patient during major regional anesthesia a rhythmically rising and falling rib cage and sternum should be observed.[17] It is important to look for signs of upper airway obstruction such as paradoxical or "rocking" thoracoabdominal motion (i.e., outward motion of the abdomen with indrawing of the intercostal spaces and upper chest), retractions in the jugulum and supraclavicular fossae, and flaring of nasal alae.[14]

Observation of respiratory rate and pattern is extremely important when awake patients are given intravenous sedatives or narcotics during regional anesthesia. These drugs cause slowing of the respiratory rate, less consistently a decrease in tidal volume, central and obstructive apneas, and, occasionally, periodic breathing.[32]

Although capnometry (defined as measurement of CO_2 at the patient's airway during the entire ventilatory cycle[36]) will be discussed later, its use for qualitative assessment of ventilation in awake patients (called "capnography" if there is graphic display of the CO_2 waveform[36]) has been described.[2,12] Capnometry and capnography rely on continuous sampling by gas aspiration through a small tube placed at the patient's airway (e.g., taped under the nose). The aspirating tube conducts the gas to the CO_2 measuring device, usually an infrared spectrometer. Although capnography used in this way is not quantitatively useful, it does provide a graphic, qualitatively useful CO_2 waveform to monitor ventilation in the awake patient whose head and face are covered (e.g., during an ophthalmologic procedure).[2,12]

Unconscious Patient and Spontaneous Ventilation

Virtually all anesthetic agents, intravenous or inhaled, decrease minute ventilation in a dose-dependent manner.[34] This effect, though partially reversed by surgical stimulation, is one of the indicators of the depth of anesthesia.[8] Although volatile anesthetic agents also depress cardiovascular function, profound respiratory depression and apnea usually occur *before* cardiac arrest in a spontaneously breathing patient receiving increasing concentrations of volatile anesthetic agent. For this reason, assessment of ventilation in the unconscious, spontaneously breathing patient may provide an additional safety factor, (i.e., presence of profound respiratory depression) to indicate the need to reduce the dose of volatile agent and avert a cardiac arrest.

In addition to observation and auscultation, assessment of ventilation in the spontaneously breathing patient during general anesthesia can include more sophisticated techniques because the patient's airway is in continuity with the gas delivery system through a tracheal tube or face mask. Several techniques can be used to monitor modern anesthetic delivery systems, and will be discussed in detail in later chapters. However, two methods are particularly relevant to a discussion of monitoring ventilation in the spontaneously breathing patient during general anesthesia, namely spirometry and capnometry.

A spirometer is used to measure the volume of gas flowing through a tube. To measure the volume of gas that has reached the patient's lungs, the spirometer must be located on the expiratory side of the anesthesia breathing system. The most commonly used device is a mechanical spirometer consisting of a turbine in which the number of revolutions (caused by gas flow) are mechanically or electronically transduced and displayed as volume.[16] Other units use pneumotachographs, which work by temperature decreases caused by gas flow or ultrasonic flow meters to provide tidal volumes and minute ventilation.[16] Determination of minute ventilation (the product of respiratory rate and tidal volume) is helpful in monitoring adequacy of ventilation in the anesthetized, spontaneously breathing patient.

Capnometry, or end-tidal CO_2 monitoring, can be thought of as a complement to minute ventilation monitoring. In spontaneously breathing patients subjected to anesthetic-induced respiratory depression, the increased arterial CO_2 tension (Pa_{CO_2}) will be reflected by an increase in end-tidal CO_2 tension, PET_{CO_2}. PET_{CO_2} is normally somewhat lower than Pa_{CO_2}, and this difference is accentuated by general anesthesia, as well as a variety of abnormal conditions such as chronic obstructive lung disease, pulmonary embolism, and low cardiac output or shock states.[32] **Useful information can be obtained from CO_2 waveform monitoring and analysis. Examples of useful information rendered by capnography include location of the breathing tube (trachea vs. esophagus), respiratory rate, evidence of rebreathing of CO_2, expiratory obstruction (i.e., bronchospasm), and disconnection of the gas delivery system (resulting in a low PET_{CO_2} when room air is entrained).**[14]

Unconscious Patient and Controlled Ventilation

Because of the necessity for muscle relaxation during most major surgical procedures, ventilation must be controlled after the airway is secured with a tracheal tube. Ablation of spontaneous ventilation eliminates a useful monitor of anesthetic depth, and just as important, eliminates patient defense against catastrophic hypoventilation. The anesthetized patient breathing spontaneously through an endotracheal tube should be able to breathe room air during the time required to detect and correct a disconnection of the tube from the gas delivery system.

Other hazards, besides disconnection, are present during positive pressure ventilation of the anesthetized, muscle-relaxed patient, and necessitate monitoring the gas delivery system itself. In addition to monitoring adequacy of ventilation by observing the tracheal tube and chest expansion and by auscultating for adventitious breath sounds and leaks around the tracheal tube, the ventilator and inspiratory circuit (airway) pressures must be monitored. A pressure gauge, usually an aneroid manometer, is used to measure the breathing circuit (airway) pressure required to deliver a particular desired tidal volume (the latter measured with spirometry).[14] It is important to monitor trends in peak inspiratory pressure for signs of gradual tracheal tube obstruction or changes in chest compliance because of bronchospasm or extrinsic compression. Airway obstruction and reduced chest compliance result in increasing inspiratory airway pressures. Reduced or absent inspiratory pressure indicates a large circuit leak or complete airway disconnection. Thus the manometer itself functions as a disconnection monitor. Modern anesthesia gas delivery systems have elaborate airway disconnect alarms that will sound when no airway pressure is detected, but the habit of watching the airway pressure manometer is a valuable one.

The spirometer is also useful for detecting airway disconnections. Because it is located in the expiratory limb of the breathing circuit, the spirometer measures the volume of gas leaving the patient's lungs. In the event of a disconnection, the spirometer will indicate no gas returning from the patient's lungs. Again, modern anesthesia equipment has complex circuitry such that no or low gas returning to the spirometer will trigger a separate alarm.

The pulse oximeter can also be used as a "last resort" monitor to detect airway disconnections. Oximeters sound an alarm when oxygen saturation of hemoglobin falls below a critical level. This alarm will occur somewhat later than the "no CO_2" signal by the capnometer and the "no breath detected" signal by the spirometer. The time interval between these alarms and the oximeter's will depend on the oxygen concentration in the patient's lungs. Pulse oximetry will be discussed later in this chapter.

Underlying all the above sophisticated monitors of ventilation is the anesthesiologist's ear. A precordial or esophageal stethoscope in proper position, with the anesthetist *actually listening to every breath*, is a mandatory standard of care unless such monitoring is physically impossible (e.g., a 650 g baby undergoing a patent ductus arteriosus ligation). There is no excuse for not listening to the breathing, whether ventilation is spontaneous or controlled.

MONITORING THE ADEQUACY OF OXYGENATION

There is considerable overlap between strategies for monitoring ventilation and oxygenation because these processes, though by no means the same physiologically, are closely linked. When ventilation is inadequate, usually, but not necessarily, a rapid deterioration in oxygenation follows. Certainly this sequence describes many anesthetic disasters: hypoventilation rapidly followed by arterial hypoxemia and loss of cardiopulmonary homeostasis.

Awake Patient

The awake patient receiving local or regional anesthesia affords the clinician a sensitive monitor of oxygenation (i.e., cerebral function). Given normal cerebral blood flow and blood glucose concentration, progressive hypoxemia results in changes in mental status characterized by loss of judgment, followed by confusion, disorientation, and lethargy.[28] These signs of cerebral dysfunction are not specific for arterial hypoxemia. Local anesthetics, narcotics, and sedatives may cause confusion, disorientation, or lethargy, particularly in elderly patients. It is imperative that arterial hypoxemia be a primary consideration when signs of cerebral dysfunction appear because hypoxemia is the most devastating, yet often the most treatable, cause of cerebral dysfunction.

Although mental status should always be monitored in awake patients, a more specific monitor of oxygenation can now and should also be used in these patients, (i.e., the pulse oximeter). The pulse oximeter is a noninvasive monitor of arterial hemoglobin saturation (Sao_2), and represents a major advance in clinical monitoring of oxygenation. Although pulse oximetry will be discussed in the context of the unconscious anesthetized patient, it is now promulgated as a standard of care by the ASA to monitor oxygenation during general, regional, and monitored local anesthetics.[27] This monitor is increasingly used during nonsurgical diagnostic procedures requiring administration of sedative or narcotic agents (e.g., colonoscopy and bronchoscopy).

Unconscious Patient

In the unconscious anesthetized patient, adequacy of oxygenation must be assessed without direct reliance on vital organ (i.e., brain) function. Clinically, this means obtaining inferential information about vital organ oxygenation by monitoring at peripheral sites using one or more of three methods: observation of skin and blood color, blood gas sampling from a peripheral artery, or pulse oximetry.

Observation of skin color for presence of cyanosis is notoriously unreliable and insensitive for assessment of oxygenation.[6] Cyanosis is difficult to detect in many patients because it requires a near-normal hemoglobin level.[40] Further, when detected, cyanosis is a late-occurring sign of arterial hypoxemia.[40]

Arterial blood gas analysis is the most definitive method for diagnosing arterial hypoxemia and should always be available for use. When the diagnosis of hypoxemia is even a remote possibility, arterial blood gas analysis should be done if at all possible, unless the diagnosis can be readily made via oximetry. Even then, use of blood gas analysis to assess adequacy of therapy is valuable. Arterial blood gas analysis is relatively expensive, requires arterial puncture, and cannot yet be applied continuously (although that technology is under development). Pulse oximetry is noninvasive, is a continuously applied monitor, and is relatively inexpensive for routine use in healthy patients.

The theory and application of pulse oximetry have been extensively reviewed.[19,20,39] The following discussion will summarize the technical aspects, clinical use, and limitations of pulse oximetry.

Pulse Oximetry

The pulse oximeter relies on two physical principles. First, oxyhemoglobin and deoxyhemoglobin each have different absorbances at the two wavelengths of light transmitted and detected by the oximeter. Second, both deoxyhemoglobin and oxyhemoglobin's absorbances, at each wavelength, have pulsatile components because of the fluctuating volume of arterial blood between the light source and detector.

Arterial hemoglobin saturation (Sao_2) is determined by the relative proportions of oxyhemoglobin and deoxyhemoglobin in arterial blood. The pulse oximeter estimates Sao_2 by sensing differences in light absorbances, at two wavelengths, for these forms of hemoglobin. Deoxyhemoglobin absorbs more light in the red band (600 to 750 nm) than does oxyhemoglobin, which has greater absorption in the infrared region (850 to 1000 nm). A pulse oximeter probe contains two light-emitting diodes (LEDs), one producing light at a wavelength in the red band and the other producing light in the infrared band. Any convenient, pulsating vascular bed (e.g., fingertip or earlobe) is placed between the LEDs and the photodetector.

Microprocessors switch the LEDs on and off several hundred times each minute. In this manner, the oximeter samples, at both wavelengths, the amount of light transmitted through the vascular bed many times each second, thus allowing for recognition of the peak and trough of each pulse waveform. The pulsatile waveforms of the absorption spectra result from the fluctuating volumes of arterial blood actually present at that instant, which contain both oxyhemoglobin and deoxyhemoglobin, in the vascular bed. Only the fluctuating components, accounting for 1% to 5% of the total absorbance signal, are processed by an algorithm to estimate Sao_2. These internal algorithms have been empirically derived in studies of healthy volunteers, and so eliminate the need for calibration before each use in clinical practice. Use of this empirical fixed precalibration results in a clinical accuracy within 2% in vivo oximetry in the Sao_2 range of 70% to 100% under ideal conditions.[19] Ideal conditions include absence of motion artifact, venous congestion, electrocautery, and intravenous dyes. Below an Sao_2 level of 70%, no such empirical correlation exists, and the oximeter's accuracy is unknown in this range. Accuracy of pulse oximeters is affected by a variety of factors in addition to those just

mentioned, including severe anemia, dyshemoglobinemias, low-amplitude pulse states, excessive ambient light, and darkly pigmented skin.[19]

One additional caveat should be observed with pulse oximeters. Although the oximeter requires a pulsating vascular bed, it is not designed to monitor the adequacy of peripheral (and certainly not organ) perfusion. In addition to a digital Sao_2 display, most pulse oximeters have a plethysmographic or pulsatile waveform display. This plethysmographic signal and waveform is relatively insensitive to changes in perfusion because as the pulsatile signal decreases, the oximeter amplifies the signal (up to a billion-fold) to estimate Sao_2.[36] The oximeter will detect complete loss of peripheral pulse, but not significant pulse decreases. Lawson et al.[25] showed that pulse oximeters stop detecting finger pulses (and Sao_2) when blood flow decreases to about 8.6% of its control value.

Last, but certainly not least, in monitoring adequacy of oxygenation, is the use of an oxygen concentration monitor in the inspiratory limb of any gas delivery system. These monitors are now incorporated into modern anesthesia gas machines and will be discussed in later chapters.

MONITORING THE ADEQUACY OF CIRCULATION

Perhaps no area of clinical monitoring has experienced as rapid a proliferation of new technologies as the area of hemodynamic monitoring. Despite many current promising developments, including continuous noninvasive cardiac output monitoring, it is unlikely that any single monitor on the horizon will have as great an impact on circulatory monitoring as pulse oximetry has had in the area of oxygenation monitoring. This prediction is based on the following observations.

First, there is no single, ideal monitor of the adequacy of circulation. With the exception of standard 16-lead electroencephalography (EEG), it is not currently possible to monitor adequacy of vital-organ perfusion. Even the EEG, though it is a sensitive monitor of cerebral cortical electrical activity, is not a specific monitor for cerebral perfusion because it is also affected by metabolic, pharmacologic, and hypoxemic insults.[25]

Second, in the traditional approach to monitoring, the circulatory system is intuitively separated into two components, (i.e., cardiac vs. circulation to the tissues). **The heart should be thought of as both the prime mover of the circulation and a vital organ itself dependent on adequate perfusion. Therefore monitoring cardiac function, albeit indirectly, can help detect but not differentiate between primary cardiac problems (e.g., acute left ventricular dysfunction) and**

problems involving the peripheral circulation that affect venous return or myocardial perfusion or both and secondarily compromise heart function.

Third, use of clinical monitoring skills (palpation and auscultation) and routine monitoring technology (electrocardiography and noninvasive blood pressure measurement) in hundreds of millions of anesthetized patients has led to empirical acceptance of these methods and their incorporation into standards of monitoring practice.[13] The careful, knowledgeable use of these traditional "time-tested" (i.e., not statistically tested with regard to clinical outcomes) methods can probably be supplanted only by sensitive and specific monitors of circulatory adequacy that have been shown to improve clinical outcomes.

The following discussion will focus on those circulatory monitors considered basic and yet essential for the conduct of safe anesthesia in healthy patients, (i.e., palpation, auscultation, electrocardiography [ECG], and noninvasive blood pressure measurement).

Palpation and Auscultation

Although the practice of palpating a peripheral artery during anesthesia dates to the time of John Snow in the 1840s,[36] routine auscultation of heart and breath sounds during anesthesia is a relatively recent development.[13] Both palpation and auscultation are universally accepted, practiced, and taught in modern clinical anesthesia. These methods are considered necessary but not sufficient for monitoring the circulation in healthy patients.

Continuous or intermittent palpation of an accessible peripheral artery is part of the qualitative clinical assessment of circulatory homeostasis. The preoperative evaluation should include palpation of one or more peripheral pulses as a baseline for comparison during the anesthetic. Although routine palpation of carotid pulses is not recommended, when there is suspicion of cardiovascular abnormality (preoperatively or intraoperatively), the carotid pulses should be assessed because their contour and volume best reflect cardiac events.[4]

In general, palpation of a peripheral pulse in the anesthetized patient will reveal one of the following states: the pulse will be present and strong, present and weak, or absent. The pulse rate may be fast or slow, regular or irregular. Although the physical determinants of the character of the peripheral pulse (actually a pulse pressure wave) are beyond the scope of this chapter, it must be understood that a diminished pulse amplitude may indicate reduced left ventricular (LV) stroke volume (because of decreased LV filling or depressed contractility) or a marked reduction in systemic vascular resistance, which could occur in the presence of a high cardiac output. Both of these changes are usually accompanied by a reduced arterial blood pressure and perhaps other clinical signs of circulatory compromise, (i.e., a peripheral pulse is only one of several clinical variables used to monitor the circulation). Palpation of a peripheral pulse is a valuable adjunct to commonly used monitoring technologies.

Auscultation is a mainstay of clinical anesthesia monitoring. Continuous use of either a precordial stethoscope or a soft, flexible esophageal stethoscope (considered a "penetrating" monitor, Box 4-1) is a standard of care in clinical anesthesia in the United States.

Auscultatory monitoring is a simple, easy-to-use, continuous qualitative method of assessing cardiac activity and ventilation. Although quantitative assessment of cardiac function is not possible with auscultation, it has been suggested that development of diminished or muffled heart sounds is a relatively late indicator of severe cardiovascular depression.[43]

An important auscultatory finding is the occurrence of a new systolic murmur during anesthesia, which may represent acute mitral regurgitation (MR) secondary to subendocardial and papillary muscle ischemia or because of an acutely dilated LV. The subendocardial region, including the papillary muscles, is particularly prone to ischemia, which may or may not be accompanied by ECG changes.[29] Auscultatory evidence of MR usually represents moderate to severe MR and is neither an early nor a sensitive indicator of ischemia but is considered specific for acute papillary muscle or LV dysfunction.[11]

Electrocardiography

ECG monitoring is standard practice in modern clinical anesthesia. Although the surface ECG only directly monitors the heart's electrical activity, it provides important inferential information about pump function because cardiac dysrhythmias, myocardial ischemia, or electrolyte imbalance, all detectable by ECG, may be associated with significant cardiac dysfunction and compromise of circulatory homeostasis.[18]

Probably the most common anesthesia-related ECG abnormalities seen in apparently healthy patients are dysrhythmias and possible ischemic changes. It has been estimated that over 50% of all patients develop some rhythm disturbance during anesthesia.[14] Factors contributing to the occurrence of dysrhythmias during anesthesia in healthy patients include sympathetic response to tracheal intubation and surgical incision; reflex parasympathetic stimulation caused by visceral traction; acute alterations in arterial blood gas tensions (hypoxemia, hypocarbia, or hypercarbia); hypothermia; and dysrhythmogenic effects of anesthetic agents themselves.[35] Most common rhythm disturbances in healthy patients are well tolerated, but some, particularly atrioventricular junctional rhythms, can result in decreased cardiac output and hypotension resulting from loss of coordinated atrial systole, which results in decreased LV filling.[44] The most useful ECG leads for dysrhythmia detection are those that produce clearly identifiable upright P waves: leads II, MCL_1, and CB_5 (see following discussion) for three-lead systems and precordial lead V_1 for five-lead configurations.[26]

The incidence of actual myocardial ischemia during anesthesia in apparently healthy adults is unknown. There is evidence that a subgroup of these healthy patients, (i.e., males over age 40) does have a significant prevalence of clinically silent coronary artery disease. Studies using exercise ECG screening in asymptomatic men who had no angina or prior myocardial infarction indicate that silent myocardial ischemia (i.e., exercise-induced ischemic ECG changes) occurs in 2.5% to 10% of these patients.[9,24] Therefore it is logical to assume that some apparently healthy males, particularly those with known coronary risk factors such as tobacco use, will demonstrate ischemic ECG changes when subjected to the autonomic stresses of anesthesia and surgery. The relationship between intraoperative ECG evidence of ischemia and perioperative myocardial infarction is not completely understood. There is suggestive evidence from studies of patients known to have severe coronary artery disease that perioperative myocardial infarction is related to intraoperative ischemia.[33] It seems prudent, therefore, to use ECG monitoring to detect myocardial ischemia and to treat ischemia when it occurs.

Elective anesthesia and surgery can perhaps be viewed as the functional equivalent of an exercise ECG test. Two questions arise: (1) how can we maximize the effectiveness of ECG monitoring in detecting intraoperative myocardial ischemia? and (2) what ECG changes are characteristic of myocardial ischemia? If a five-lead ECG system is used, a majority of ischemic events (up to 90% during exercise ECG) can be detected using precordial lead V_5 alone.[1] Sensitivity is further improved when two leads, usually II and V_5, are monitored.[1] A variety of bipolar lead configurations have been developed for three-electrode ECG systems. These modified lead systems have been shown to approach the sensitivity of standard precordial leads in detecting left ventricular myocardial ischemia. These three-electrode systems are described in Table 4-1.[37]

There are few universally accepted ECG criteria for diagnosing myocardial ischemia. The classic patterns of ST segment and T wave changes are relatively nonspecific and labile, reflecting nonuniform myocardial repolarization and effects of altered physiologic states such as exercise.[10] Most cardiologists accept that a critical index of ischemia is 2 mm of ST segment depression (2.0 mV on a voltage-calibrated ECG) at 0.08 seconds after the junction between the QRS complex and ST segment, also called the "J point".[23] Ischemia and infarction can also be signaled by isolated atypical T wave changes. In fact, it has been contended that isolated T wave abnormalities may be

Table 4-1   Bipolar leads for use with three electrodes

Lead system	MCL_1	CS_5	CM_5	CB_5	CC_5
RA electrode	Ground	Under right clavicle $(-)$ (subclavicular)	Manubrium sternum $(-)$	Center of right scapula $(-)$	Right anterior axillary line (V_5R) $(-)$
LA electrode	Under left clavicle	V_5 $(+)$	V_5 $(+)$	V_5 $(+)$	V_5 $(+)$
LL electrode	V_1 $(+)$	Ground	Ground	Ground	Ground
Lead selected	III	I	I	I	I
Advantages and indications	Good P wave and QRS complex; useful for diagnosis of dysrhythmias	Monitoring for anterior ischemia	Monitoring for anterior ischemia	Monitoring for anterior ischemia; good P wave for diagnosis of dysrhythmias	Monitoring for ischemia

From Thys DM, Kaplan JA: Recent advances in electrocardiographic techniques. In Kaplan JA, ed: *Cardiac anesthesia*, ed 2, Philadelphia, 1987, WB Saunders.

the only ECG findings in up to 30% of patients who have acute myocardial infarction.[10] Tall peaked T waves have been observed in early subendocardial ischemia; more often the initial T wave is isoelectric, negative, or biphasic with this type of ischemia.[10]

Computer-assisted ST segment analysis has been reported effective in detecting intraoperative myocardial ischemia.[22] With incorporation of this capability into standard operating room monitors, ST segment analysis may prove a particularly cost-effective, noninvasive method of detecting intraoperative ischemia.

Noninvasive Blood Pressure Monitoring

Although adequate tissue delivery of oxygen is the *sine qua non* of cardiopulmonary homeostasis, the primary variable continuously sensed and regulated by the body's homeostatic mechanisms is not systemic or individual organ blood flow but rather blood pressure. There exists a critical systemic arterial pressure below which perfusion of vital organs is compromised and cardiopulmonary homeostasis is lost. The relatively high pressure maintained in the systemic arteries constitutes a pressure reservoir supplying the driving force propelling blood through the microcirculation.[30]

A useful simplification for this discussion is to consider systemic arterial pressure to be determined by the relationship between two complex variables, cardiac output and systemic vascular resistance.[30] These variables, in turn, are affected by numerous factors, including posture, autonomic nervous system activity, cardiovascular and anesthetic drugs, and reflex and hormonal mechanisms activated or depressed by anesthesia and surgery (Fig. 4-1). Measurement of systemic arterial pressure, a complex and indirect indicator of circulatory well-being, is one of many clinical elements necessary for the safe conduct of anesthesia.

Noninvasive blood pressure measurement can be performed easily and reliably by several methods, provided that some basic technical guidelines are observed. The most commonly used method is manual inflation/deflation of a sphygmomanometer cuff over the upper arm with either palpation of the radial artery or auscultation for Korotkoff sounds over the brachial artery just distal to the cuff. Automated blood pressure cuffs are gaining wide acceptance in operating rooms and recovery rooms.

Automated, noninvasive blood pressure measure-

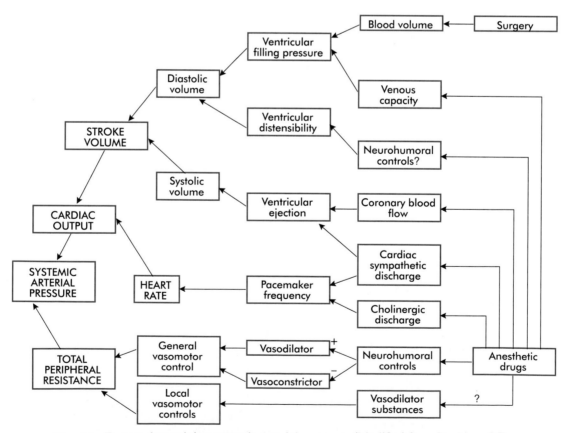

Fig. 4-1. Factors determining systemic arterial pressure. (Modified from Rushmer RF: *Cardiovascular dynamics,* ed 4, Philadelphia, 1976, WB Saunders.)

ment can be performed by mechanical devices that inflate a cuff, then deflate it slowly and record the pressures. Several separate technologies can be used. They may employ microphones, or electronic stethoscopes, for detection of Korotkoff sounds. Other devices use the Doppler principle to detect return of blood flow in the artery. **Most common today is the use of oscillometry to detect magnitude and frequency of oscillations of cuff pressure during deflation as pulsatile flow returns in the artery. Automated oscillometers use electronic microprocessors to calculate blood pressure as follows: the onset of detected oscillations marks systolic blood pressure and the point of maximal pressure oscillation during cuff deflation corresponds to mean arterial pressure.[14] Diastolic pressures are calculated using an algorithm based on the mathematic relationship between mean systolic and diastolic pressures.[14]**

With any of the manual or automated blood pressure measuring methods, the following guidelines should be observed.[14] The cuff should be the proper size for the limb; neither too wide nor too narrow. A proper-sized cuff should be about 20% wider than the diameter of the limb. An overly wide cuff will yield erroneously low pressures; too narrow a cuff gives spuriously high readings (the latter being a very common problem with obese patients). When an ideal cuff fit is not possible, the next wider, rather than the narrower, cuff should be used. The cuff should be snuggly wrapped around the limb because a loose cuff gives an erroneously high pressure (similar to the narrow cuff). Motion of the limb on which the cuff is located may interfere with pressure measurement.

MONITORING TEMPERATURE
Insults: Hypothermia and Hyperthermia

Although healthy patients come to the operating room (OR) for anesthesia and surgery with normal body temperatures, most leave the operating suite with subnormal body temperatures.[7] How does iatrogenic hypothermia occur? Can this be a threat to cardiopulmonary homeostasis? If so, when?

Body heat loss occurs by four physical processes: infrared radiation; conduction of heat to cooler objects in contact with the body; convection or heat transfer to cooler moving air; and water evaporation from skin surfaces.[31] Operating rooms can be considered ventilated refrigerators. They are usually cooled to 18° to 21° C and well-ventilated to reduce airborne contamination. Other factors contributing to hypothermia include infusion of cool (i.e., room temperature) intravenous fluids, surgical exposure of major body cavity surfaces to cool ambient air and irrigating solutions, and cutaneous vasodilation caused by anesthetics.[7] Newer designs of OR lights deliberately

radiate less heat (for added surgeon comfort), thus removing a previous source of heat transfer to the patient during surgery.

Hypothermia alone can depress cerebral function, producing diffuse neurologic signs, including delirium, stupor, or coma.[28] Healthy, awake, unmedicated patients will have at least some clouding of consciousness if their body temperature falls below 32° C.[28] When hypothermia is combined with the pharmacologic and physiologic trespass of anesthesia and surgery, the results can be catastrophic. **With hypothermic patients who have received anesthetic drugs, delayed awakening or prolonged neuromuscular blockade, or both, may occur because of reduced metabolic or renal clearance of these drugs.[7] Postoperative shivering by the awakening hypothermic patient is accompanied by massive increases in oxygen consumption, minute ventilation, and cardiac output.[41] These responses may be deleterious for patients with iatrogenic anemia or hypovolemia, or who have coronary artery disease.**

Intraoperative hyperthermia is less common but certainly can occur. It is usually due to overvigorous warming with heating pads, blankets, heated airway humidifiers, warm ambient temperatures, or occasionally, development of a febrile illness. Malignant hyperthermia (MH) is a genetically determined muscle disease triggered by anesthetics. It produces a true hypermetabolic crisis characterized by hypercapnia, tachycardia, and usually, *but not always,* rapidly rising body temperature.[3] MH has a high death rate if not recognized and treated promptly. Therefore the diagnosis of MH must be considered when body temperature rises during or after anesthesia.

How to Monitor Temperature

Electrical thermometers used intraoperatively most commonly employ either a thermocouple or a thermistor.[7] A thermistor is a metal oxide semiconductor, the resistance of which varies with temperature. A thermocouple is a circuit containing two dissimilar metals. At constant voltage, current in the circuit is directly proportional to temperature difference between the two junctions of the metals.

Temperature can be measured at a number of body sites. Exactly what true "core" temperature means is controversial, but temperatures measured at the nasopharynx, rectum, bladder, and esophagus are often considered core temperatures. The tympanic membrane has also been used to measure core temperature. However, the risk of trauma to the tympanic membrane makes this site unacceptable for routine clinical use. A disposable urethral catheter containing a thermocouple is commercially available to reliably measure urine temperature. In general, for relatively short procedures in healthy patients, mon-

itoring temperature at the nasopharynx, esophagus, or bladder (when these sites are accessible) gives the best combination of accuracy and precision with respect to true core temperature.[7]

SUMMARY

In the United States in 1991 essential monitoring for patients undergoing any type of anesthetic consists of a precordial or esophageal stethoscope, a noninvasive blood pressure measurement, a three- or, preferably, five-lead ECG, a pulse oximeter, either quantitative or qualitative end-tidal CO_2 monitoring, an expiratory spirometer, and an inspiratory airway pressure gauge. Also considered mandatory are the measurement of inspired oxygen concentration and a specific airway disconnection monitor, both of which are now incorporated into anesthesia equipment. None of these monitors is a substitute for constant vigilance and use of clinical skills such as inspection, auscultation, and palpation.

KEY POINTS

- It has been estimated that there are between 2000 to 6000 incidents of anesthesia-related death or permanent brain injury every year in the United States. Further, it is contended that many of these cases are preventable.

- Hypoxemia is the most common final pathway leading to anesthetic disasters, whatever the original causes.

- Human error plays a major role in most anesthesia-related disasters.

- One way of studying anesthesia-related deaths and other disasters is to use closed malpractice claims against anesthesiologists. The ASA Closed-Claims Study should be familiar to the reader.

- The ASA Closed-Claims Study of unexpected sudden cardiac arrest in 14 patients undergoing spinal anesthesia led many to wonder about the "margin of safety" with spinal anesthesia vs. lack of vigilance.

- Another ASA Closed-Claims Study addressed several issues related to monitoring. It concluded that many cases of anesthetic death or permanent brain damage might have been prevented with the application of pulse oximetry and capnometry (although these modalities were not necessarily available at the time the events occurred).

- Virtually all anesthetic agents, intravenous or inhaled, decrease minute ventilation in dose-dependent fashion.

- The capnogram is not a simple monitor. Its proper use requires legitimate understanding of pulmonary physiology and mechanics.

- Most experienced clinicians teach that the anesthesiologist should listen to each breath, no matter how many other devices for monitoring ventilation and/or oxygenation are attached to the patient.

- Waiting for cyanosis means the anesthesiologist waited too long.

- The anesthesia trainee should understand how the pulse oximeter works and its pitfalls. This device has become one of the most valuable monitoring tools.

- The most common ECG abnormalities seen in apparently healthy patients are dysrhythmias.

- The incidence of ischemic ECG changes during anesthesia and surgery and their significance are not known and need to be studied.

- Noninvasive blood pressure monitoring has become routine. The anesthesiologist should know how the various devices work and the relationships between them and intraarterial blood pressure monitoring.

- The width of the cuff considerably affects the indicated blood pressure, whether a manual or automated method is in use.

- Hypothermia can result in delayed awakening, postoperative shivering, and other problems.

KEY REFERENCES

Caplan RA, Ward RJ, Posner K et al: Unexpected cardiac arrest during spinal anesthesia: a closed-claims analysis of predisposing factors, *Anesthesiology* 68:5, 1988.

Comroe JH Jr, Botelho S: The unreliability of cyanosis in the recognition of arterial anoxemia, *Am J Med Sci* 214:1, 1947.

Cullen DJ, Eger EI II, Stevens WC et al: Clinical signs of anesthesia, *Anesthesiology* 36:21, 1972.

Keenan RL: Anesthetic disasters: incidence, causes, and preventability. In Barash PG, ed: *Refresher course in anesthesiology,* vol 16, Philadelphia, 1988, JB Lippincott.

Kelleher JR: Pulse oximetry, *J Clin Monit* 5:37, 1989.

Slogoff S, Keats AS: Does perioperative myocardial ischemia lead to postoperative myocardial infarction? *Anesthesiology* 62:107, 1985.

Tinker JH, Dull D, Caplan RA et al: Role of monitoring devices in prevention of anesthetic mishaps: a closed-claims analysis, *Anesthesiology* 71:541, 1989.

Tremper KK, Barker SJ: Pulse oximetry, *Anesthesiology* 70:98, 1989.

Vaughan MS, Vaughan RW, and Cork RC: Postoperative hypothermia in adults: relationship of age, anesthesia, and shivering to rewarming, *Anesth Analg* 60:746, 1981.

REFERENCES

1. Blackburn H et al: Standardization of the exercise electrocardiogram: a systematic comparison of chest lead configurations employed for monitoring during exercise. In Karvonen MJ, Barry AJ, eds: *Physical activity and the heart,* Springfield, Ill., 1967, Charles C Thomas.
2. Bonsu AK, Tamilarasan A, and Bromage PR: A nasal catheter for monitoring tidal carbon dioxide in spontaneously breathing patients, *Anesthesiology* 71:318, 1989.
3. Britt BA: Malignant hyperthermia. In Orkin FK, Cooperman LH, eds: *Complications in anesthesiology,* Philadelphia, 1983, JB Lippincott.
4. Burnside JW: *Adam's physical diagnosis,* Baltimore, 1974, Williams & Wilkins.
5. Caplan RA, Ward RJ, Posner K et al: Unexpected cardiac arrest during spinal anesthesia: a closed-claims analysis of predisposing factors, *Anesthesiology* 68:5, 1988.
6. Comroe HJ Jr, Botelho S: The unreliability of cyanosis in the recognition of arterial anoxemia, *Am J Med Sci* 214:1, 1947.
7. Cork RC: Temperature monitoring. In Blitt CD, ed: *Monitoring in anesthesia and critical care,* New York, 1990, Churchill-Livingstone.
8. Cullen DJ, Eger EI II, Stevens WC et al: Clinical signs of anesthesia, *Anesthesiology* 36:21, 1972.
9. Erickssen J, Thoulaw E: Follow-up of patients with asymptomatic myocardial ischemia. In Rutishauser W, Roskamm H, eds: *Silent myocardial ischemia,* Berlin, 1984, Springer-Verlag.
10. Fisch C: Electrocardiography and vectorcardiography. In Braunwald E, ed: *Heart disease: a textbook of cardiovascular medicine,* Philadelphia, 1988, WB Saunders.
11. Gahl K, Sutton R, Pearson M et al: Mitral regurgitation in coronary heart disease, *Br Heart J* 39:13, 1977.
12. Goldman JM: Simple, easy, and inexpensive method for monitoring PET_{CO_2} through nasal cannulae, *Anesthesiology* 67:606, 1987.
13. Gravenstein JS: Essential monitoring examined through different lenses, *J Clin Monit* 2:22, 1986.
14. Gravenstein JS, Paulus DA: *Clinical monitoring practice,* ed 2, Philadelphia, 1987, JB Lippincott.
15. Gravenstein JS, Weinger MB: Why investigate vigilance? *J Clin Monit* 2:145, 1986 (editorial).
16. Gravenstein N: Monitoring, *Probl Anesthesia* 1:47-59, 1987.
17. Greene NM: *Physiology of spinal anesthesia,* ed 3, Baltimore, 1981, Williams & Wilkins.
18. Hines RL, Barash PG: Hemodynamic monitoring in the intensive care unit. In Scharf SM, Cassidy SS, eds: *Heart-lung interactions in health and disease,* New York, 1989, Marcel Dekker.
19. Keenan RL: Anesthetic disasters: incidence, causes, and preventability. In Barash PG, ed: *Refresher course in anesthesiology,* vol 16, Philadelphia, 1988, JB Lippincott.
20. Kelleher JR: Pulse oximetry, *J Clin Monit* 5:37, 1989.
21. Knill RL: Cardiac arrests during spinal anesthesia: unexpected? *Anesthesiology* 69:629, 1988 (letter).
22. Kotrly KJ, Kotter GS, Mortara D et al: Intraoperative detection of myocardial ischemia with an ST segment trend monitoring system, *Anesth Analg* 63:343, 1984.
23. Kurita A, Chaitman BR, Bourassa MG: Significance of exercise-induced junctional ST depression in evaluation of coronary artery disease, *Am J Cardiol* 40:492, 1977.
24. Langou RA, Huang EK, Kelly MJ et al: Predictive accuracy of coronary artery calcification and abnormal exercise test for coronary artery disease in asymptomatic men, *Circulation* 62:1196, 1980.
25. Lawson D, Norley I, Korbon G et al: Blood flow limits and pulse oximeter signal detection, *Anesthesiology* 67:599, 1987.
26. McCloskey GF, Curling PE: Electrocardiography. In Barash PG, ed: *Anesthesiology clinics of North America,* vol 6, Philadelphia, 1988, WB Saunders.
27. Orkin FK: Practice standards: the Midas touch or the emperor's new clothes? *Anesthesiology* 70:567, 1989 (editorial).
28. Plum F, Posner JB: *The diagnosis of stupor and coma,* ed 3, Philadelphia, 1980, FA Davis.
29. Roberts WC, Cohen LS: Left ventricular papillary muscles. Description of the normal and a survey of conditions causing them to be abnormal, *Circulation* 46:138, 1972.
30. Rushmer RF: *Cardiovascular dynamics,* ed 4, Philadelphia, 1976, WB Saunders.
31. Ryan JF: Unintentional hypothermia. In Orkin FK, Cooperman LH, eds: *Complications in anesthesiology,* Philadelphia, 1983, JB Lippincott.
32. Sackner MA, Krieger BP: Noninvasive respiratory monitoring. In Scharf SM, Cassidy SS, eds: *Heart-lung interactions in health and disease,* New York, 1989, Marcel Dekker.
33. Slogoff S, Keats AS: Does perioperative myocardial ischemia lead to postoperative myocardial infarction? *Anesthesiology* 62:107, 1985.
34. Stevens WC, Kingston HGG: Inhalation anesthesia. In Barash PG, Cullen BF, and Stoelting RK, eds: *Clinical anesthesia,* Philadelphia, 1989, JB Lippincott.
35. Stevenson RL, Rogers MC: Electrocardiographic monitoring and dysrhythmia analysis. In Blitt CD, ed: *Monitoring in anesthesia and critical care medicine,* ed 2, New York, 1990, Churchill-Livingstone.
36. Swedlow DB, Irving SM: Monitoring and patient safety. In Blitt CD, ed: *Monitoring in anesthesia and critical care medicine,* New York, 1990, Churchill-Livingstone.
37. Thys DM, Kaplan JA: Recent advances in electrocardiographic techniques. In Kaplan JA, ed: *Cardiac anesthesia,* ed 2, Philadelphia, 1987, WB Saunders.
38. Tinker JH, Dull DL, Caplan RA et al: Role of monitoring devices in prevention of anesthetic mishaps: a closed-claims analysis, *Anesthesiology* 71:541, 1989.
39. Tremper KK, Barker SJ: Pulse oximetry, *Anesthesiology* 70:98, 1989.
40. Vandam LD: The senses as monitors. In Blitt CD, ed: *Monitoring in anesthesia and critical care medicine,* ed 2, New York, 1990, Churchill-Livingstone.
41. Vaughan MS, Vaughan RW, and Cork RC: Postoperative hypothermia in adults: relationship of age, anesthesia, and shivering to rewarming, *Anesth Analg* 60:746, 1981.
42. Ward RJ, Lane MJ: Anesthesiology and medicolegal outcome. In Brown DL, ed: *Risk and outcome in anesthesia,* Philadelphia, 1988, JB Lippincott.
43. Webster TA, Petty WC: Do we still need precordial and esophageal stethoscopes? *J Clin Monit* 3:191, 1987.
44. Weinfurt PT: Electrocardiographic monitoring: an overview, *J Clin Monit* 6:132, 1990.

CHAPTER 5

Anticipating Common Intraoperative Problems

ROBERT B. FORBES

ANDREA J. LAYMAN

Common Cardiovascular Problems
    Heart rate and rhythm changes
    Blood pressure changes
Common Respiratory Problems
    Airway problems
    Hypoxemia
    Hypercapnia
    Hypocapnia
    Wheezing
Common Renal Problems
    Oliguria
Common Thermoregulatory Problems
    Hypothermia
    Hyperthermia
Summary

In recent years there has been increasing interest in accurately determining the incidence of serious morbidity and mortality related to anesthesia.[53,59,85,101,102] In addition, many authors have attempted to identify factors that contribute to anesthetic mishaps[23,24] and complications[19,21] and have suggested changes in anesthetic practice or monitoring standards that they believe will diminish risks of catastrophic outcomes.* Although the importance of these serious complications should not be underestimated, they remain rare events. The majority of healthy patients undergoing anesthesia and surgery have excellent outcomes and experience no major complications, either intraoperatively or during their postoperative recovery. In contrast to the low mortality related to anesthesia, there is a high incidence of minor complications, those that cause no long-term sequelae, during the intraoperative period.

In 1986 Cohen et al. described the findings of a large prospective survey that identified major and minor complications in 112,721 patients over a 9-year period.[21] More than 80% of the patients were healthy American Society of Anesthesiologists (ASA) physical status class I or II. All types of surgery and anesthetic techniques were included. The study indicated that 9% of all patients had at least one intraoperative complication. The two most common complications encountered in adults were dysrhythmias (3.9%) and hypotension (2.7%). The next most common were respiratory problems (1%), followed by incidents related to the drugs administered or to the surgical procedure performed. Cardiac arrest was very uncommon. It is of interest that during the period 1975 to 1978, 7.6% of patients experienced some intraoperative complication, whereas during the period 1979 to 1983, the incidence had *increased* to 10.6%. The authors of this study suggested that at least part of this increase was a result of improved monitoring, which permitted better detection of problems, rather than reflecting an actual increase in the overall incidence of intraoperative complications.

In a similar study conducted to determine the incidence of intraoperative anesthetic complications in children, Cohen, Cameron, and Duncan found that 35% of pediatric patients experienced adverse perioperative events, of which 8.5% occurred during the intraoperative period.[19] Although the overall incidence of intraoperative complications was similar to the incidence in adults, the authors did find higher morbidity among neonates that was most frequently

---

* References 23, 24, 32, 40, 52, 100.

related to airway obstruction or other respiratory events.

These studies indicate that a significant number of healthy patients experience some type of adverse event during the course of anesthesia care and that the incidence of complications is increased in neonates[19,102] and the elderly.[101] In addition, adverse events are more common in patients with associated medical problems[19,21] and during emergency surgery.[53,101] Finally, problems related to human errors, including mistakes in drug administration and anesthesia machine mishaps, contribute significantly to the incidence of intraoperative complications.[23,24] By understanding which patients are most likely to experience an adverse event, by being aware of the most common complications, and by recognizing the clinical situations in which these events most frequently occur, clinicians should be able to anticipate and perhaps prevent many of the common intraoperative anesthetic problems that occur in healthy patients.

COMMON CARDIOVASCULAR PROBLEMS
Heart Rate and Rhythm Changes

Cohen et al. identified dysrhythmias as the most common intraoperative complications occurring in the 112,721 patients they studied.[21] During the first 3 years of the study, dysrhythmias were identified in 3.6% of patients, but during the last 4 years the incidence increased to 4.3%. Others have reported perioperative dysrhythmias in more than 60% of surgical patients.[9,107] The majority of these dysrhythmias are benign, particularly if bradycardia (<60 beats/min) and tachycardia (>100 beats/min) are included as dysrhythmias. Nonetheless, the sudden appearance of any abnormal rhythm should be regarded as an indication to seek the underlying event that precipitated the dysrhythmia. It is important that the *cause* of the rhythm disturbance be identified, in addition to initiation of treatment. By seeking a diagnosis, more serious problems may be recognized earlier in their course and major complications avoided. Anesthesiologists must not simply apply reflexive "recipes" (e.g., "hypotension—give ephedrine," or "premature ventricular contractions—give lidocaine").

There are many potential causes of dysrhythmias during anesthesia. The significance of any specific rhythm depends on the clinical situation in which it occurs. Important factors include the patient's medical condition, the measured hemodynamic effect of the dysrhythmias, and the specific rhythm disturbance. Because there are numerous causes of dysrhythmias during anesthesia, an organized approach to determine the cause is required.

Sinus tachycardia

Sinus tachycardia is the most commonly seen dysrhythmia during anesthesia[21] and is defined as heart rate exceeding 100 beats/min with normal P wave morphology. Sinus tachycardia normally does not exceed 180 beats/min, but may occasionally be as high as 200 beats/min in athletes or young children. The upper achievable limit decreases markedly with advancing age. Several common causes should be considered when sinus tachycardia occurs in a patient during anesthesia. Sinus tachycardia may represent a normal response to hypotension or hypovolemia related to blood loss, preoperative fluid deprivation, third-space fluid sequestration, and vomiting or diarrhea. Another common cause of tachycardia, particularly during induction and the early maintenance phase of anesthesia, is the increased level of circulating catecholamines released in response to anxiety, pain, laryngoscopy and intubation, or surgical stimulation at light levels of anesthesia. These common causes of tachycardia can be easily corrected by providing adequate preoperative anxiolysis and analgesia, by repleting existing fluid deficits, or by deepening the level of anesthesia.

Less commonly, sinus tachycardia may be a response to hypoxia or hypercarbia. Careful evaluation of oxygenation and ventilation is necessary in any patient with unexplained tachycardia. More unusual causes of intraoperative sinus tachycardia that should be considered include endocrine disorders such as thyrotoxicosis, pheochromocytoma, and adrenal insufficiency. Fever resulting from excessive extrinsic heating, sepsis, or malignant hyperthermia may also precipitate tachycardia that can be persistent and unresponsive to usual therapy. Myocardial dysfunction, including ischemia, infarction, or pulmonary emboli, can also be associated with tachycardia. Immediate treatment of sinus tachycardia may be necessary if the patient's hemodynamic status is compromised or if myocardial oxygen imbalance is present. There also are many medications that can increase heart rate, including the muscle relaxants gallamine and pancuronium; catecholamines, such as ephedrine, epinephrine, isoproterenol, dobutamine, and dopamine; anticholinergics such as atropine, scopolamine, and glycopyrollate; and the volatile anesthetic agent, isoflurane.

Sinus bradycardia

Sinus bradycardia, similar to sinus tachycardia, is seen frequently in healthy patients during anesthesia. Unless associated with hemodynamic instability, it usually does not require treatment, but **the sudden appearance of sinus bradycardia should provoke a search for the specific precipitating event because**

bradycardia can progress to sinus arrest and even cardiac arrest. Although bradycardia may be associated with specific pathologic conditions, more commonly it occurs in healthy patients in response to surgical manipulation or following administration of a variety of drugs.

Vagally mediated slowing of the heart rate in response to mechanical stimulation may occur during many kinds of surgical procedures.[29,30] Manipulation of the bowel or peritoneum during abdominal or pelvic surgery may cause bradycardia and hypotension, particularly if traction is exerted on the mesentery.[82,91] Sudden bradycardia can occur during dilatation of the cervix.[18,55] Bradycardia is also very common during ophthalmic surgery and occurs in response to pressure on the eye, traction on the extraocular muscles, and following injection of local anesthetic or bleeding into the retrobulbar space. This is called the oculocardiac reflex, and it involves a trigeminovagal reflex arc as follows. The afferent pathway is via the long and short ciliary nerves to the ciliary ganglion, then via the ophthalmic branch of the trigeminal nerve to the sensory nucleus of the fifth cranial nerve. Internuncial fibers connect the nucleus of the trigeminal nerve to the origin of the vagus nerve, the nucleus ambiguus, and the vagus nerve forms the efferent limb of reflex arc, releasing acetylcholine at the sinoatrial and atrioventricular node regions in the heart.

The oculocardiac reflex can produce bradycardia in up to 90% of patients[30]; but many other dysrhythmias, as well as cardiac arrest, have also been reported during ophthalmic surgery.[3,80,94,95] Blanc et al. demonstrated that abrupt, sustained traction on an extraocular muscle was more likely to elicit the reflex than if gentle, progressive traction was applied.[12] It was also demonstrated that vagal escape and fatigue of the reflex occurred, but that the incidence and intensity of the response was unrelated to the muscle that was stimulated, if the same type of stimulus was applied. This is in contrast to other studies, which have suggested that the medial rectus is the most reflexogenic extraocular muscle.[5,30,68] The oculocardiac reflex is augmented in patients who are hypercarbic and, despite some recommendations to the contrary,[10,30] controlled, rather than spontaneous ventilation, is more appropriate for children undergoing strabismus surgery.

Use of anticholinergic agents to prevent the oculocardiac reflex and its associated cardiac dysrhythmias is controversial. It has been shown that use of anticholinergics, including atropine and glycopyrrolate, can decrease the incidence of bradycardia associated with the oculocardiac reflex, but neither drug prevented bradycardia in every patient.[30,49,97] In addition, intravenous atropine is itself associated with a high incidence of ventricular dysrhythmias, which may be as or more serious than the reflex bradycardia. The oculocardiac reflex occurs not only during ophthalmic surgery but can also be seen during repair of a fractured maxilla or zygoma and during temporomandibular joint surgery.[56] Reflex bradycardia should be anticipated whenever the operative procedure involves structures innervated by the ophthalmic branch of the trigeminal nerve. Severe bradycardia has also been reported during electroconvulsive therapy, although other types of dysrhythmias are more common.[4,60,92] Bradycardia also can occur during laryngoscopy and endotracheal intubation, particularly in neonates.[78,97]

Many drugs used in anesthesia can cause bradycardia. Use of succinylcholine[1,71,88] is commonly associated with this problem, but bradycardia can occur with the newer, nondepolarizing neuromuscular blocking agents, vecuronium[25,63] and atracurium,[45] which lack the vagolytic effects of gallamine and pancuronium. Use of narcotics, particularly fentanyl[7] and alfentanil,[6] causes bradycardia. Among the volatile anesthetic agents, use of halothane has been shown to cause bradycardia[64] via an effect on the calcium channel, resulting in slowing of conduction and decreased contractility with a propensity to depress the sinoatrial node. Whenever any of these drugs are used, their effects on heart rate should be considered if bradycardia occurs—the anesthesiologist should not simply assume the bradycardia to be reflexive.

There are many pathologic conditions that may be first noted as intraoperative bradycardia, such as unsuspected ischemic heart disease or increased intracranial pressure. Psychologic stress can also precipitate severe bradycardia[39] or ventricular tachydysrhythmias[15] that can progress to cardiac arrest. It has been suggested that considerable discretion be used when discussing medical problems with conscious patients during the intraoperative period (e.g., during regional or local anesthesia).

Other dysrhythmias

In addition to sinus bradycardia and sinus tachycardia, many other disturbances of cardiac rhythm may be encountered during anesthesia and surgery in apparently healthy patients. Often several factors contribute to the appearance of a dysrhythmia and it can be difficult to determine the primary cause. Several common causes should be considered.

Cardiac dysfunction. Cardiac problems, including ischemic heart disease, mitral valve prolapse,[38] myocarditis,[44] and abnormalities of the conducting system,[89] may exist in patients who appear healthy and are completely asymptomatic. All of these disorders can contribute to intraoperative dysrhythmias. In patients with coronary artery disease, if myocardial oxygen demand exceeds supply as a result of low oxygen-carrying capacity or impaired perfusion, ischemic cells can become sources of abnormal automaticity or reentry phenomena that result in dysrhythmias. Apparently healthy patients in high-risk categories for ischemic heart disease should be carefully monitored for evidence of dysrhythmias.

Electrolyte abnormalities. Abnormal preoperative or intraoperative plasma electrolyte levels may contribute to the appearance of cardiac dysrhythmias in otherwise healthy patients. Acute changes in serum potassium concentration can cause atrial and ventricular dysrhythmias and heart block.[75] Dysrhythmias are more likely to appear when changes in plasma potassium levels occur rapidly. In chronic hypokalemia, the transmembrane potential has time to normalize and it does not appear that chronic hypokalemia is associated with an increased incidence of intraoperative cardiac dysrhythmias, unless there is a history of perioperative dysrhythmias,[106] congestive heart failure, or long-term digoxin therapy.[48]

Acute hyperkalemia can also occur during anesthesia and can precipitate a dysrhythmia. This may occur during rapid intravenous infusion of crystalloid solutions containing substantial amounts of potassium or immediately following use of succinylcholine in patients with burns, severe traumatic injuries, or denervating injuries that have resulted in muscle damage or atrophy. Conduction blocks and ventricular fibrillation may be precipitated when the serum potassium concentration is acutely increased.[96] Low serum magnesium levels often accompany hypokalemia and may contribute to sudden dysrhythmias.[41]

Acute changes, both increases and decreases, in blood carbon dioxide levels can contribute to cardiac irritability. Hypercarbia, whether resulting from hypoventilation or increased carbon dioxide production, stimulates the sympathetic nervous system and increases circulating catecholamines. Hypocarbia results in rapid decreases in extracellular potassium concentration. Both these common clinical situations can contribute to cardiac irritability and should be considered when unexpected cardiac rhythm disturbances occur.

Drug interactions. Many drugs used in anesthesia can be associated with cardiac dysrhythmias in healthy patients, either by direct action on the cardiac conducting system or indirectly via the sympathetic nervous system. Although it has been shown that halothane[8] and isoflurane[14] slow atrioventricular conduction, in healthy patients these volatile anesthetics do not cause significant dysrhythmias, unless they interact with other drugs that have cardiac effects. For example, volatile anesthetics have been shown to increase myocardial sensitivity to the dysrhythmic effects of catecholamines.[50] Dysrhythmias should be anticipated if large doses of epinephrine are administered by the surgeon in an attempt to improve hemostasis during surgery. Other drugs that may interact with the volatile anesthetics and cause dysrhythmias include aminophylline, tricyclic antidepressants, monamine oxidase inhibitors, and cocaine. Toxic doses of local anesthetics, which can occur after inadvertent intravascular injection, can induce ventricular dysrhythmias, conduction blocks, or even cardiac arrest. Numerous other drugs used during anesthesia can alter sympathetic or parasympathetic activity and promote dysrhythmias. These medications include acetylcholinesterase inhibitors, anticholinergics, neuromuscular blockers, ketamine, and sympathetic agonists or antagonists. Because patients receive multiple medications during anesthesia, the occurrence of unexpected drug interactions, resulting in cardiac dysrhythmias, is quite common. This may be further complicated by patients who abuse drugs such as cocaine or amphetamines.[46]

Iatrogenic causes. Cardiac dysrhythmias in healthy patients can also be caused by direct mechanical stimulation of the heart. This most commonly occurs during insertion of central nervous or pulmonary artery catheters, which can precipitate ventricular dysrhythmias or asystole.[26] Direct mechanical stimulation by the surgeon during thoracic surgery may also cause acute cardiac rhythm disturbances that generally disappear when the stimulus is removed. To anticipate the common problems with heart rate and/or rhythm that can occur in healthy patients during anesthesia requires thorough understanding of normal cardiovascular physiology, recognition of clinical situations commonly associated with dysrhythmias, and familiarity with the cardiac effects and drug interactions that can be produced by the anesthetic technique chosen.

Blood Pressure Changes
Hypotension

In the study by Cohen et al., hypotension was the second most frequently encountered intraoperative anesthestic complication; only dysrhythmias occurred more frequently.[21] Transient reduction in arterial pressure of 20% to 30% from preoperative levels is probably not detrimental to healthy patients, but it should be recalled that hypotension was a common clinical sign encountered when a preventable negative anesthetic outcome occurred in the ASA Closed Claims Study.[100] Therefore any unexpected or unexplained hypotension must be seriously considered, its cause identified, and appropriate treatment given.

In awake patients, hypotension may be a manifestation of a vasovagal reaction, which can also result in bradycardia, pallor, sweating, anxiety, and loss of consciousness. Vasovagal syncope occurs most commonly in healthy young males and may be precipitated by an intense emotional experience[39,87] that results in mixed excitatory and inhibitory autonomic responses. Vasodilation in muscle beds causes peripheral blood pooling, which reduces preload and then cardiac output. Increased parasympathetic tone results in profound bradycardia and some depression of myocardial contractility. If cerebral perfusion is impaired by such an abrupt drop in blood pressure and heart rate, the patient may lose consciousness. Appropriate treatment includes administration of intravenous fluids and vagolytics, as well as rapid use of the Trendelenburg position.

Errors in blood pressure measurement may result in an incorrect diagnosis of hypotension. This can occur if the blood pressure cuff is too large or if the transducer for an intraarterial pressure line is improperly placed, poorly calibrated, or if the system is damped (e.g., a partially obstructing clot located at the catheter tip). Although eliminating equipment error is important, an inordinate amount of time should not be spent attempting to repair a malfunctioning device. If hypotension is suspected, but reliable blood pressure readings from a cuff or intraarterial line are difficult to obtain, physical signs may be useful in confirming the diagnosis. The presence of cool, clammy extremities, peripheral cyanosis, and diminution of peripheral pulses are useful clinical signs of inadequate perfusion and hypotension. Auscultation of Korotkoff sounds or use of Doppler blood pressure measurements can usually be easily performed to confirm hypotension.

When hypotension does occur in a healthy patient, several common causes should be first considered. Hypovolemia resulting from prolonged preoperative fasting; bowel preparations; persistent vomiting, diarrhea, or gastrointestinal drainage; acute hemorrhage or insensible losses, particularly in a febrile patient, may result in considerable decreases in blood pressure following anesthesia induction or any time during the procedure. Hypotension may also occur despite adequate intravascular volumes if compression of the inferior vena cava or other large intraabdominal vessels by the surgeon obstructs cardiac venous return. Acute changes in patient position (e.g., rapidly putting the patient into the reverse Trendelenburg or the sitting position) may produce a marked decrease in blood pressure by reducing venous return. Increases in intrathoracic pressure with mechanical ventilation, positive end-expiratory pressure, or pneumothorax can also reduce venous return and cause hypotension.

Direct myocardial depression occurs to some extent with the use of all anesthetic agents, even in healthy patients. Use of barbiturates, volatile anesthetics, propofol, local anesthetics, and even ketamine can reduce myocardial contractility. With the exception (usually) of ketamine, all are common causes of transient hypotension. Adjunct anesthetic medications, such as muscle relaxants or beta-blockers, also may decrease blood pressure. Careful selection of drug dose and slow rates of bolus administration generally avert abrupt changes in blood pressure. Evaluation of hypotension must also consider the intensity of the surgical stimulus, because sudden decreases in surgical stimulation can greatly reduce sympathetic nervous activity and lead to hypotension.

Changes in arteriolar resistance can produce hypotension, and many techniques and medications used during anesthesia affect arteriolar tone. Sympathetic blockade, associated with spinal and epidural anesthesia, can cause hypotension if adequate fluid loading has not occurred. In addition, numerous drugs act directly to reduce tone in resistance vessels, resulting in hypotension. These medications include nitroprusside, hydralazine, labetalol, phentolamine, and other antihypertensive medications. Blood pressure may also be decreased following administration of drugs that cause vasodilation in response to histamine release or ganglionic blockade, such as morphine, *d*-tubocurarine, and atracurium. Although unlikely in healthy patients, pathologic conditions such as septicemia or adrenal insufficiency may also be causes of intraoperative hypotension. By careful consideration of all the potential causes of intraoperative hypotension, those patients who are at increased risk can be identified and steps may be taken to minimize any anticipated decrease in blood pressure.

Initial treatment of systemic hypotension must first include ensuring that the patient's oxygenation and ventilation are adequate. Then, because absolute or relative hypovolemia is a common cause of hypotension, a reasonable fluid bolus can be started while other potential causes of hypotension are evaluated. The blood pressure should be validated and the quality of the pulses, peripheral perfusion, and heart and breath sounds should be assessed. Placing the patient in the Trendelenburg position may be helpful in restoring adequate blood pressure. Electrocardiography may reveal the presence of a cardiac dysrhythmia. Consideration should be given to decreasing the inspired concentration of volatile anesthetic, if one is in use. Administration of cardiovascular depressants should be stopped, if possible, and all drugs being administered should be quickly reviewed. It may be necessary to change the anesthetic technique in an effort to return blood pressure to an acceptable level. Further treatment depends on the cause of hypotension and may include additional fluid administration or use of vasopressors, inotropes, and antidysrhythmics, or repositioning of the patient, retractors, or surgical packs.

Hypertension

A significant increase in blood pressure, exceeding the normal preoperative level, is not uncommon during anesthesia and surgery. When mild to moderate increases in blood pressure occur in healthy patients, it is usually not a matter of great concern. The episodes are generally short lived, easily controlled, and have little impact on the final outome of the surgical procedure. Most commonly intraoperative hypertension in a healthy patient is a normal response to some type of stimulation that results in the release of endogenous catecholamines. The stimulus may be anxiety, excitement, or pain in the immediate preoperative period. Hypertension is also common during induction of anesthesia, especially at the time of laryngoscopy, endotracheal intubation, and initial skin incision. The hypertensive response to endotracheal intubation can be attenuated by ensuring that an adequate depth of anesthesia is achieved before beginning that procedure. Although relatively deep anesthesia is usually well tolerated by healthy individuals, this is generally not acceptable in the elderly or in patients with cardiovascular disease. Supplementing use of barbiturates or a volatile anesthetic with narcotics, beta-blockers, or intravenous lidocaine before intubation can be useful in attenuating the hypertensive reaction to larnygoscopy.

Another cause of hypertension during anesthcsia is the presence of preexisting hypertension that is undiagnosed or has been poorly controlled. Essential hypertension is encountered most frequently, but hypertension related to chronic renal insufficiency, vascular abnormalities, or endocrine diseases, such as pheochromocytomas, hyperthyroidism, or Cushing's syndrome, may be unexpectedly encountered. Toxemia of pregnancy is also a potential cause of intraoperative hypertension in obstetric patients. Therefore, whenever hypertension is encountered and does not respond quickly to deepening the anesthesia, a cause of hypertension other than "light anesthesia" should be considered.

Iatrogenic causes of hypertension may also occur and are often related to the use of vasopressors, such as ephedrine or phenylephrine; vagolytics, such as atropine or pancuronium; or as a result of excessive intraoperative fluid administration. Hypoxia and hypercarbia, by stimulating release of catecholamines, may also cause hypertension. Additional causes that should be considered are malignant hyperthermia, increased intracranial pressure, bladder distension, or prolonged application of a tourniquet used to provide a bloodless surgical field.

When intraoperative hypertension occurs, its cause should be determined and appropriate treatment instituted. Treatment may begin with preoperative sedation of anxious patients and provision of adequate analgesia if the patient has a painful condition. The anesthetic depth should be appropriate for the level of surgical stimulation. This requires knowledge of the specific procedure being performed and anticipation of particularly stimulating events. The hypertensive response to endotracheal intubation may be prevented or minimized by administration of vasodilators, narcotics, or lidocaine before beginning direct laryngoscopy, but there is no evidence that transient, rapidly resolved hypertension during this procedure is harmful to healthy patients. Hypertension in response to hypoxia or hypercarbia is prevented by ensuring adequate oxygenation and ventilation. Volume status should be monitored closely to avoid overhydration. It is also important to consider the potential cardiovascular effects of all drugs that have been administered when intraoperative hypertension is encountered. If the blood pressure does not quickly return to normal by adjusting the depth of anesthesia, the other more uncommon causes of hypertension should be considered.

COMMON RESPIRATORY PROBLEMS
Airway Problems

Airway management is a critical part of the anesthesiologist's role in the care of a healthy patient. A knowledge of the complications associated with securing and maintaining a patent airway is essential, *because airway obstruction can occur at any time during the administration of any anesthetic.* The anesthesiologist must be able to anticipate and diagnose the cause of airway problems and skillfully implement corrective maneuvers to correct complications as they evolve.[35]

Mask ventilation

Establishing an effective seal with a face mask is an important component of airway control during general anesthesia and is necessary to provide positive pressure ventilation. An airtight seal also minimizes loss of anesthetic agent to the atmosphere with subsequent exposure of operating room personnel to trace concentrations of anesthesia. Difficulty in obtaining a precise mask fit should be anticipated in patients who are edentulous; who have anatomic abnormalities, such as a receding jaw or a prominent nose; who have a nasogastric tube or eye patch, which interferes with mask placement; or who have facial abnormalities from previous trauma or surgery.

Before anesthesia induction, an appropriate selection of masks should be immediately available.

Obtaining a good mask fit may be facilitated in some patients by leaving dentures in place, inserting an oral or nasopharyngeal airway, or packing the buccal areas with (counted) gauze sponges. Each of these maneuvers, although potentially effective for improving airway control, may also be complicated by coughing, gagging, laryngospasm, or bleeding, if instituted incorrectly. Placement of any unsecured object in the airway is always a matter of concern.

Airway obstruction

Signs of airway obstruction include either noisy, sonorous breathing or breath sounds that may be decreased. Retraction of the skin over the suprasternal notch, use of accessory muscles of respiration, failure of the reservoir bag to empty or move, and stridor are all important signs of an obstructed airway. A rocking motion of the chest and abdomen may be seen. The signs of airway obstruction can be subtle. With close observation of the patient's chest movement and color, auscultation of breath sounds, and a constant awareness of the movement of gas in the breathing bag, airway obstruction should be quickly recognized. Capnometry is also useful to identify airway obstruction before hypoxia develops but is never a substitute for clinical acumen and vigilance.

The oropharynx is a common site of soft tissue obstruction after induction of anesthesia. Partial or total obstruction of the airway commonly occurs with relaxation of the muscles of the jaw, tongue, and pharynx. Patency of the airway can often be restored by placing the patient in the "sniffing" position by slightly extending the head at the occipital-cervical joint while also flexing the neck on the thorax and applying pressure on the mandible to lift the jaw and tongue forward. Insertion of an oral or nasal airway or gentle application of positive pressure may also alleviate soft-tissue obstruction. Care must be taken to avoid hyperextension of the neck because this may increase airway obstruction.

It is important to remember and anticipate complications that can occur when these maneuvers are used. Soft tissue and mucosa may be injured by insertion of mechanical airways. Laryngospasm may occur if an oral or nasal airway is placed when the patient is only lightly anesthetized. Placement of airways that are too large or too small may result in worsening of airway obstruction.

Complications of intubation

Most healthy patients undergoing general anesthesia have an endotracheal tube placed following induction of anesthesia. This is the most effective method of providing an unobstructed airway, facilitating oxygenation and ventilation. It also provides protection against aspiration of gastric contents. In most patients endotracheal intubation is easily accomplished during direct laryngoscopy. Despite this success, more than 7% of patients have some type of injury related to laryngoscopy and intubation.[13,51] In most patients the injury is minor and does not cause significant morbidity or mortality. Less frequently, patients may sustain significant injury to the larynx or trachea, including vocal cord paralysis, formation of granulomata, polyps, tracheal webs, or subglottic stenosis.[47]

The most common problem attributed to endotracheal intubation is sore throat, which can occur in up to 70% of patients. It is also a common complaint following mask anesthesia; thus the specific factors that influence the occurrence of sore throat following anesthesia are obscure. Other injuries that can occur during intubation include laceration or bruising of the lips, tongue or, oropharynx; epistaxis following nasal intubation or nasal airway insertion; and inadvertent endobronchial or esophageal intubation. After satisfactory endotracheal tube placement, accidental extubation or dislodgment can occur intraoperatively during surgical manipulation or during changes in patient positioning. Kinking or obstruction of the endotracheal tube can also occur, as can other mechanical problems, such as balloon rupture or disconnection from the breathing circuit.

Another problem encountered during laryngoscopy and intubation is dental trauma, which may occur in as many as 1:150 patients.[58,81,83] Trauma includes minor chipping or scratching of enamel, as well as fractures or avulsion of natural teeth or of dental prostheses. Central incisors are most at risk. The factors that contribute to dental injury include extensive dental reconstruction, malocclusion, and periodontal disease. Difficult intubation, whether anticipated or unexpected, that results in multiple attempts at direct laryngoscopy and intubation also increases risk of dental trauma. Careful preoperative assessment of the patient's airway helps predict potentially difficult intubations. **Anatomic characteristics such as a short, muscular neck; prominent central incisors; a receding mandible; a highly arched palate; and limited temporomandibular mobility should alert the anesthesiologist that laryngoscopy may be difficult. Flawless technique during intubation and properly positioning the patient by flexing the lower cervical spine on the thorax (at C7, T1) plus extension of the head at the atlanto-occipital joint should minimize risk of traumatic injuries during intubation.[66]**

In addition to traumatic injuries that can occur during intubation, direct laryngoscopy can also result in a number of physiologic changes that may be problematic even in healthy patients. These responses to laryngoscopy include increased heart rate, blood pressure, intracranial pressure, and intraocular pressure. Measures that can be taken to blunt these responses include use of intravenous lidocaine, narcotics, or antihypertensives before intubation. Ensuring that the patient is adequately anesthetized and avoiding use of succinylcholine during intubation also can help minimize these effects. The type of laryngoscope blade used for intubation does not appear to influence either the physiologic response to direct laryngoscope or the incidence of traumatic injuries.[67,83]

Laryngospasm

Laryngospasm is a common complication encountered during anesthesia, particularly in pediatric patients. Although it usually resolves without serious patient injury, it can result in severe hypoxia with cerebral damage, cardiac arrest, or death.[73] During laryngospasm, airway obstruction occurs for two reasons. First, there is tight approximation of the true vocal cords. In addition, the false cords and supraglottic tissues contribute to the obstruction by acting like a ball valve at the laryngeal inlet (i.e., being thrust into the airway during a negative pressure inspiration). As a result, the degree of obstruction increases as the translaryngeal inspiratory pressure rises.[34]

Several factors contribute to the incidence of laryngospasm. It is more common in children and following airway instrumentation. Direct stimulation of the pharynx or larynx by insertion of an oral airway, suctioning, or extubation can precipitate laryngospasm. Use of barbiturates and volatile anesthetics, particularly isoflurane, has often been associated with laryngospasm.* Of particular importance is the depth of anesthesia when the patient's airway is stimulated. Laryngospasm occurs more commonly at very light levels of anesthesia. Other irritants that can initiate laryngospasm include stimulation of the vocal cords by secretions, blood, or gastric contents; pain; peritoneal traction; and anal dilatation. Clearing the airway of secretions, increasing anesthetic depth in anticipation of painful stimuli, ensuring adequate depth of anesthesia, and using a gentle approach to airway manipulation may reduce the incidence of laryngospasm. Extubation of the patient in a deep level of anesthesia or alternatively when fully conscious are also useful ways of avoiding laryngospasm, but the former approach, especially in children, can be associated with vomiting during emergence when the airway is unprotected in a semiconscious patient.

Laryngospasm can result in partial or complete airway obstruction. If the obstruction is incomplete, ventilation may be accompanied by inspiratory and expiratory vocalization or stridor. As the obstruction becomes more severe the airway noises disappear and the signs of airway obstruction, including indrawing, tracheal tug, and paradoxical movements of chest and abdomen, become more pronounced. If obstruction is incomplete and the patient is not hypoxic, laryngospasm may be terminated by removing the irritant that precipitated the episode, deepening the level of anesthesia, and applying gentle, continuous airway pressure with 100% oxygen. Great care must be taken to avoid sustained application of high airway pressure because this tends to increase obstruction and can force gas into the stomach, further impairing ventilation. Subluxation of the temporomandibular joint to move the jaw anteriorly may also help overcome the obstruction. If the patient begins to become hypoxic or, if airway obstruction is complete, atropine and succinylcholine should be administered to break the spasm and allow ventilation of the patient. If indicated, the patient can be intubated at this time.[84]

Laryngospasm is best avoided by recognizing the clinical situations in which it is most commonly precipitated. Laryngospasm is seen more frequently in children, particularly during induction and emergence during isoflurane anesthesia, and in patients with recent airway infections. It also occurs more frequently in patients in whom the airway has been instrumented and in patients with a nasogastric tube. Although many anesthesiologists recommend that patients be fully awake before extubation, laryngospasm is uncommon if the endotracheal tube is removed when the patient is deeply anesthetized.[76] Nonetheless, patients who are extubated while still anesthetized may be at greater risk for airway obstruction, aspiration, and hypoventilation in the recovery room. Because laryngospasm is relatively common during anesthesia in healthy patients, it is important that the condition be readily recognized and steps be taken to avoid precipitating this potentially serious complication.

Hypoxemia

Changes in pulmonary function are anticipated effects of anesthesia and surgery in healthy patients. They occur with anesthesia induction, and the specific changes seen can often be accurately predicted.[37,62] For most healthy patients these changes in pulmonary mechanics and gas exchange pose little risk, but they can impair a patient's oxygenation ability and can contribute to intraoperative hypoxemia. When intraoperative hypoxemia does occur it is usually mild, easily correctable, and results in no injury. In cases when anesthesia has been judged to contribute to serious perioperative complications, including cardiac arrest, neurologic injury, or death, hypoxemia has been often cited as one of the first clinical signs that indicated deterioration of the patient's condition.*

Hypoxemia ($Pao_2 < 60$ mm Hg) may be difficult to recognize in the operating room for several reasons—anesthesia obtunds the patient's normal cardiorespi-

---

* References 16, 36, 54, 65, 74, 77, 86.

* References 19, 21, 32, 52, 53, 59, 100, 101, 102.

ratory responses to hypoxia; hemoglobin saturation may fall below 85% before cyanosis is clinically apparent to most observers; and hemoglobin levels must be reasonable before it is feasible to visibly detect cyanosis. Other signs of hypoxemia include restlessness or agitation in an awake patient, dark blood in the surgical site, or changes in cardiovascular vital signs. Initially patients may be hypertensive and tachycardic, but with increasingly severe hypoxemia this progresses to hypotension, bradycardia, or other dysrhythmias. In recent years pulse oximetry has become an essential monitor during anesthesia and in most clinical situations accurately reflects arterial oxygenation.[2,103,105] When combined with capnometry, pulse oximetry has been considered extremely useful for avoiding preventable anesthetic mishaps.[100]

There are several mechanisms that can cause intraoperative hypoxemia in healthy patients, including decreased inspired oxygen concentration, hypoventilation, ventilation/perfusion mismatch, diffusion abnormalities, and decreased mixed venous oxygen content. Depending on the severity of the hypoxemia, treatment may be required before specific diagnosis can be made.

Administration of improperly low inspired concentrations of oxygen results in hypoxemia and occurs if the oxygen supply is exhausted, if the wrong gas supply or cylinder has been attached to the anesthesia machine, or if there has been a mechanical failure or gas substitution in the central oxygen supply. Inaccurately set or accidentally altered fresh gas flow may also lead to decreased concentration of inspired oxygen. Accidental disconnection of the breathing circuit from the patient is another potential cause of hypoxemia. Continuous monitoring of inspired oxygen concentration via an in-line oxygen analyzer with an audible alarm set at a predetermined lower limit should prevent administration of a hypoxic gas mixture but will not detect an accidental airway disconnection from the breathing circuit. There are excellent airway disconnect alarms on anesthesia machines, which should also be in use. Decreased alveolar ventilation can also result in hypoxemia, particularly when the inspired oxygen concentration is less than 30%. If a patient has received 100% oxygen for a period of time before a decrease in alveolar ventilation, hypoxemia may be delayed for several minutes even though alveolar ventilation is acutely decreased or completely absent, as occurs with esophageal intubation.[11]

General anesthesia causes complex changes in static lung volumes and pulmonary blood flow, which often results in increasing ventilation/perfusion mismatch. This is probably the most common cause of intraoperative hypoxemia.[61,79] With onset of general anesthesia there is decreased functional residual capacity and increased ventilation-perfusion mismatching. In most healthy patients, increasing inspired oxygen concentration overcomes the effects of mild to moderate ventilation-perfusion defects. Diffusion abnormalities and decreased mixed venous oxygen content are less common causes of significant hypoxemia in healthy patients.[17]

When intraoperative hypoxemia occurs, the inspired concentration of oxygen should be increased to 100% while the specific cause is sought. Adequate oxygen supply pressure should be confirmed by noting the presence of appropriate line pressures for the central oxygen supply and/or the anesthesia machine gas cylinders. Next, oxygen delivery to the patient should be confirmed with a previously calibrated in-line oxygen analyzer. The anesthetic circuit and machine should be checked for disconnections, leaks, line obstructions, and sticking or incompetent valves. The patient should be examined by observing chest wall movement and auscultating heart and lung sounds. Changing to hand ventilation may be a useful technique for assessing compliance of the patient's respiratory system. Correct positioning of the endotracheal tube should also be confirmed by the presence of breath sounds and regular carbon dioxide waveforms on the capnometer. An evaluation of the patient's hemodynamic status may reveal factors that contribute to hypoxemia by producing changes in cardiac output, for example, hypovolemia or surgical compression of major abdominal vessels that reduces venous return. Arterial blood gas analysis may also be helpful in evaluating the cause of hypoxemia and provides accurate information regarding the magnitude of the problem. Hypoxemia related to ventilation-perfusion mismatching can be corrected by increasing the inspired oxygen concentration, whereas hypoxemia caused by right-to-left shunting is not corrected by that maneuver.

If assessment of the patient reveals no specific cause for the hypoxemia, such as esophageal or endobronchial intubation, aspiration of gastric contents, pulmonary edema, pneumothorax, or airway obstruction, then a provisional diagnosis can be made that intraoperative atelectasis may have precipitated the hypoxemic episode. The latter often responds to therapeutic maneuvers to reduce atelectasis, such as airway suctioning followed by hyperinflation of the lungs. Increasing the tidal volume plus the addition of positive end–expiratory pressure may also be effective techniques for correcting intraoperative hypoxemia in healthy patients.

Hypercapnia

Hypercapnia ($PaCO_2$ > 45 mm Hg) occurs during the course of anesthesia when there is imbalance between production of carbon dioxide and its elimination by alveolar ventilation. In most patients, the usual clinical signs of hypercapnia are not seen during anesthesia because the normal physiologic responses to hypercapnia are obtunded. Although hypertension, tachycardia, and the appearance of dysrhythmias can be associated with hypercapnia, they may not appear until the $Paco_2$ is markedly increased, and unfortunately these signs may be entirely absent. Therefore intraoperative hypercapnia can only be reliably detected by continuously monitoring end-tidal carbon dioxide concentration or by intermittent arterial blood gas analysis. When hypercapnia does occur, three basic causes should be considered. First, *elimination* of carbon dioxide may be impaired as a result of inadequate ventilation. Second, *production* of carbon dioxide by the patient may be increased. Finally, *mechanical problems or iatrogenic sources of carbon dioxide* may result in excessive levels of carbon dioxide in the inspired fresh gas supply.

Respiratory depression occurs in response to administration of most anesthetic agents, including opioids,[6,7] volatile anesthetics,[79] barbiturates,[31] and propofol.[90,93] Therefore healthy patients who are allowed to breathe spontaneously during a surgical procedure usually exhibit elevated end-tidal carbon dioxide levels as a result of a decreased response to carbon dioxide. Hypoventilation in spontaneously breathing patients may be exacerbated by the changes in lung volumes and compliance and airway resistance that accompany induction of anesthesia.[31,61,78] Surgical factors such as the patient's position and use of retractors and abdominal packs also may contribute to hypoventilation and carbon dioxide retention.

Many problems associated with hypoventilation in a spontaneously breathing patient can be overcome by using mechanical ventilation, if adequate tidal volume and respiratory rate are chosen. In addition, an appropriate inspiratory/expiratory time ratio must be used to ensure that ventilation is distributed to the most compliant and best perfused alveoli, and that there is adequate exhalation time.

Hypercapnia can also occur if there is increased production of carbon dioxide. This can result from inadvertent patient overheating because of a high environmental temperature or with the use of warming blankets and heated humidifiers. Hypermetabolic states such as shivering, sepsis, malignant hyperthermia, or thyroid storm may result in marked increases in production of carbon dioxide. In a spontaneously breathing patient, this occurrence is accompanied by tachypnea. If the patient is being mechanically ventilated, he/she may begin to overbreathe the ventilator, unless neuromuscular blockade has been used.

Numerous iatrogenic or mechanical sources of carbon dioxide can produce hypercapnia. During insufflation of the abdomen with carbon dioxide before laparoscopy, the end-tidal carbon dioxide concentration is increased. Increased apparatus dead space associated with passive humidifiers, inadequate fresh gas flow during use of nonrebreathing circuits, incompetent valves in a circle system, and exhaustion of the soda lime can all lead to hypercapnia related to rebreathing of carbon dioxide.

When hypercapnia occurs, correction of the problem depends on the cause. Often increasing minute ventilation by decreasing depth of anesthesia in spontaneously breathing patients, or adjusting tidal volume and respiratory rate in patients treated with mechanical ventilation is all that is required. The cause of the problem must then be carefully evaluated by ensuring that the patient is receiving an adequate minute volume and confirming that the anesthetic circuit is intact and functioning appropriately. The patient's cardiorespiratory status, as well as temperature and acid-base status, should be quickly assessed to detect evidence of hypermetabolism and increased carbon dioxide production. The importance of hypercapnia or overbreathing the ventilator should never be underestimated. It is a signal to carefully reassess the patient and the anesthesia apparatus, and the patient should not be treated by deepening the anesthetic or administering a muscle relaxant.

Hypocapnia

Hypocapnia ($Pco_2 < 32$ mm Hg) is commonly noted during anesthesia in healthy patients. Although general anesthesia and hypothermia lead to decreased carbon dioxide production, the most frequent cause of hypocapnia is passive hyperventilation in a patient during mechanical ventilation. Hypocapnia is often dismissed as innocuous and, in healthy patients, mild hypocapnia is unlikely to cause serious injury. Hypocapnia does have important physiologic effects and can result in a variety of problems, particularly if sustained over a long time period.

Hyperventilation and hypocapnia can decrease cardiac output by increasing intrathoracic pressure and decreasing venous return. In addition, hypocapnia decreases the effect of sympathetic nervous activity on the myocardium. It causes cerebral vasoconstriction, leading to decreased cerebral blood flow. Respiratory alkalosis increases affinity of hemoglobin for oxygen, shifting the oxygen-hemoglobin dissociation curve to the left. This can inhibit tissue delivery of oxygen. Hypocapnia also inhibits hypoxic pulmonary vasoconstriction and increases bronchoconstriction.[72] If hyperventilation is maintained for an extended time, body stores of carbon dioxide may be markedly depleted. This can result in prolonged apnea at the end of surgery. The best treatment of hypocapnia is avoidance of the problem. When a patient is treated with mechanical ventilation, the tidal volume and respiratory rate should be chosen carefully and the end-tidal or arterial partial pressure of carbon dioxide should be monitored to ensure appropriate minute ventilation.

Wheezing

Wheezing during anesthesia is not uncommon and can become a major problem, even in healthy patients. Because airway resistance is affected not only by bronchomotor tone but also by lung volume, the decreased functional residual capacity that occurs with onset of anesthesia can contribute to increased airway resistance and result in wheezing.[61,79] Although intraoperative wheezing most commonly results from reactive bronchospasm, other important conditions must be considered when wheezing develops in a healthy patient. Conditions that must be considered in the differential diagnosis of wheezing include endobronchial intubation, mechanical obstruction of the tube related to bleeding, and secretions or kinking. Pulmonary edema, pulmonary embolus, aspiration of gastric contents, and pneumothorax also may present with wheezing. Histamine release associated with administration of numerous medications can cause bronchospasm, as can allergic or anaphylactic reactions to medications, contrast media, or blood products. Each of these potential causative factors must be considered and evaluated whenever wheezing occurs, before a diagnosis of reactive bronchospasm is made.

Careful preoperative evaluation may identify patients who are at risk for developing bronchospasm. Although it is well accepted that acute bronchospasm in response to upper respiratory tract infections (URI) may develop in patients with chronic obstructive pulmonary disease, it should be remembered that otherwise healthy patients may also be prone to bronchospasm during anesthesia for up to 4 weeks after an acute URI.[33,57] Whether asymptomatic patients who have had recent URIs should have their surgical procedures delayed until they have been free of symptoms for at least 4 weeks remains controversial.[20,28,98,99]

When wheezing is detected, the inspired concentration of oxygen should be increased until the cause is determined and the problem is corrected. Many episodes of intraoperative wheezing result from passive bronchoconstriction without increased smooth muscle constriction. These causes of wheezing should be ruled out first. The placement and patency of the endotracheal tube should be confirmed by examining the patient and passing a suction catheter through the endotracheal tube to remove secretions. If the abdomen is distended, a nasogastric tube can be passed to decompress the stomach. Adequate depth of anesthesia and muscle relaxation should be assured

because active expiratory efforts and/or abdominal muscle rigidity can increase airway obstruction and wheezing. Experienced anesthesiologists know that inadequate muscle relaxation in mechanically ventilated patients can often be the cause of wheezing. If all these causes of wheezing and increased airway resistance are eliminated, specific treatment for bronchospasm should be initiated.

Treatment of bronchospasm includes administration of high concentration of oxygen and deepening anesthesia. All the volatile anesthetics cause bronchodilation and can reduce wheezing. Lidocaine and anticholinergics may be useful bronchodilators, if the bronchospasm is not severe. Steroids can also be used but the onset of their effect is delayed. Inhalation therapy with beta-agonists, such as albuterol, is often effective. Theophylline also may be useful in the treatment of intraoperative bronchospasm but its interaction with halothane and sympathomimetic bronchodilators may precipitate cardiac dysrhythmias. Mechanical ventilation should be adjusted to minimize peak airway pressure. Some authors recommend use of low inspiratory flow rates to decrease peak airway pressure and improve the distribution of inspired gas.[27] Others recommend high inspiratory flow rates to allow prolonged expiratory time and reduce hyperinflation.[22] Treatment of wheezing or bronchospasm must be accompanied by vigilant monitoring of vital signs and should include pulse oximetry and capnometry. Wheezing is an indication of significant, dynamic changes in pulmonary function. When it occurs in the intraoperative period the cause must be determined and appropriate treatment initiated. Wheezing must never be "treated expectantly"; wheezing may easily progress to bronchospasm so severe that ventilation is nearly impossible. Wheezing is therefore a true "red flag" to the anesthesiologist.

COMMON RENAL PROBLEMS
Oliguria

Intraoperative oliguria is not uncommon in healthy surgical patients. Marked reduction or cessation of urine output may occur abruptly or develop gradually over several hours and can be related to several pathophysiologic processes. Accurate assessment and diagnosis of oliguria with early treatment may prevent deterioration in postoperative renal function. Hemodynamic changes and urine output are the two parameters generally monitored to assess renal function, but neither is ideal because they are indirect measures. Anesthetic agents affect renal function directly and indirectly to cause oliguria. Inhalation agents decrease renal blood flow, glomerular filtration rate, and renal tubular function. When combined with surgical stress, they may stimulate release of antidiuretic hormone (ADH) and activate the renin-angiotensin system. Anesthesia and mechanical ventilation alter renal function through their effects on the cardiovascular system, if the patient's cardiac output is reduced sufficiently to cause decreased renal blood flow.

Oliguria is usually defined as urine output less than 20 ml/hr in a normal adult. Oliguria can be diagnosed intraoperatively only via use of an indwelling urinary catheter. Lengthy surgical procedures or procedures that require deliberate hypotension, aortic cross-clamping, or cardiopulmonary bypass are all indications for placement of a bladder catheter. If substantial blood loss is anticipated, or if the potential for ureteral damage is high, a catheter should be used.

When oliguria occurs, an effective approach to diagnosis is to consider the causes of prerenal, renal, and postrenal oliguria. Intraoperative oliguria in healthy surgical patients is most commonly prerenal—it is caused by inadequate renal perfusion. When oliguria occurs, the first step in management is to determine if renal blood flow and glomerular filtration rate are decreased. Renal blood flow may be decreased by inhalation anesthetics, low cardiac output, hypoxia, hypercapnia, and positive pressure ventilation. Perhaps the most common cause of renal hypoperfusion is intravascular volume depletion related to intraoperative blood loss and/or dehydration. Rapid infusion of balanced salt solution is a useful diagnostic and therapeutic step during initial evaluation of oliguria. Characteristic changes in urine chemistry may also be useful. Additional fluids should be administered if an appropriate response to the initial bolus occurs and anesthetic-induced changes in renal blood flow can be reversed by discontinuing the agent. In addition to accurately measuring urine output, placement of a central venous pressure monitor may be necessary to assess fluid therapy. If fluid replacement is not successful in reversing oliguria, impaired renal perfusion resulting from cardiovascular depression should be considered as a possible explanation for the oliguria. Use of an inotropic agent, such as dopamine, can increase cardiac output and thereby improve renal blood flow. Use of diuretics in patients with oliguria secondary to hypovolemia is contraindicated, because further reduction in intravascular volume that results may aggravate changes in the kidney.

Oliguria related to renal causes may occur after administration of nephrotoxic drugs, including aminoglycosides and radiocontrast dyes. In addition, oliguria may follow release of free hemoglobin during a hemolytic transfusion reaction or rhabdomyolysis after severe trauma.

Postrenal oliguria is usually caused by urinary tract obstruction or extravasation of urine following ureter damage. Urine flow can be blocked by obstruction of the catheter with mucus, blood, or bladder tissue or after inadvertent ureteral ligation by the surgeon. Also, patients in steep head-down positions may not show adequate drainage of urine from the bladder. Each of these possible sites of obstruction must be evaluated when attempting to determine the cause of oliguria.

There is little evidence that diuretics are useful in the management of intraoperative oliguria. Administration of mannitol may provide some beneficial effects in patients with hemoglobinuria or myoglobinuria, but loop diuretics should not be used unless there is clear evidence that intravascular volume has been adequately replaced and that cardiac output is normal.[43]

COMMON THERMOREGULATORY PROBLEMS

Thermoregulation is the mechanism by which patients are able to maintain constant body temperatures during changing environmental conditions. Temperature receptors in the skin and hypothalamus respond to changes in internal or external environment and initiate a variety of neural and humoral responses to either conserve or dissipate heat. General anesthesia interferes with these mechanisms and patients in the operating room may be unable to maintain normal body temperatures. Use of narcotics and neuromuscular blocking agents interferes with the patient's ability to generate heat by shivering. Volatile agents and anticholinergics interfere with central control of temperature. Regional anesthesia can also interfere with temperature regulation by blocking a portion of the sympathetic nervous system, thus impairing vasoconstriction in anesthetized areas. All these factors render patients at risk for problems with temperature control during surgery. It is essential that the patient's temperature be monitored throughout the procedure.

The transfer of heat either to or from the patient takes place in four basic ways: radiation, conduction, evaporation, and convection. Each factor can be an important mechanism for controlling a patient's temperature in the operating room. To some extent, each mechanism can be influenced by the anesthesiologist. Although hypothermia is the more common problem, aggressive attempts to conserve body temperature or rewarm a patient can actually result in intraoperative hyperthermia.

Hypothermia

Studies have suggested that more than 50% of all patients are significantly hypothermic ($< 35°$ C) when admitted to the recovery room. There are several risk factors that help identify patients most likely to become cool during surgery.[104] Infants and the elderly are at increased risk for heat loss. Young children, particularly neonates, have large surface areas and relatively small body mass, resulting in rapid loss of body temperature, and have limited abilities to generate heat. Geriatric patients have reduced metabolic rates and decreased ability to generate heat. Patients having prolonged surgical procedures that involve opening body cavities and exposing bowel, or those who require significant blood or fluid replacement are also at risk for heat loss and hypothermia. Heat can also be lost if the operating room is cool, if patients are exposed to drafts or air currents, or if they are in contact with cold or wet objects.[69,70]

The adverse effects of cooling may become most apparent in the recovery room and include shivering, peripheral vasoconstriction, and increased myocardial oxygen consumption. During hypothermia the oxygen-hemoglobin dissociation curve is shifted to the left, increasing the affinity of hemoglobin for oxygen. As a result, delivery of oxygen to the tissues may be impaired. Plasma volume is decreased as body temperature decreases. Hypothermia also affects the function of platelets and other clotting factors. As the patient's body temperature decreases, the basal metabolic rate decreases by approximately 7% per degree centigrade. This is associated with decreased cardiac output, and decreased hepatic and renal blood flow. As a result, urine output declines and metabolism and elimination of drugs may be impaired. Hypothermia decreases requirements for volatile anesthetic agents and therefore may lead to delayed awakening if a relative overdose has occurred.

Prevention of hypothermia is easily achieved in the majority of healthy patients. First, the operating room should be warmed to 23° to 24° C until the patient is fully draped. This must often be done despite the objections of operating room nurses and surgeons, and can lead to considerable acrimony if the reasons are not well articulated by the anesthesiologist. Higher room temperatures may be required to maintain body temperature in young children. As much as possible, the patient should be kept covered, especially the patient's head. Use of insulated "space blankets" may help. Preparation solutions, intravenous and irrigating fluids, and blood for transfusions should all be warmed and their temperatures monitored insofar as possible before use. Heated humidifiers can be used to warm anesthetic gases. In very small children, overhead radiant warmers and heating blankets are also effective in preventing heat loss during anesthesia induction and surgery or they can be used to rewarm hypothermic patients. Hypothermia is a common problem during anesthesia but with careful temperature monitoring and aggressive treatment to avoid heat loss, it is a complication that can be avoided.

Hyperthermia

Although less common than hypothermia, hyperthermia ($>38.5°$ C) can also be a problem during anesthesia in healthy patients. It occurs when heat production exceeds the patient's ability to dissipate heat. A patient may gain heat through a variety of internal and external mechanisms, so it is important that body temperature be monitored in all patients. Hyperthermia can result from overly aggressive attempts to warm the operating room or it can occur if the patient's metabolic rate is abnormally increased, as in cases of malignant hyperthermia or thyroid storm. Catecholamines can also stimulate heat production. This is a particularly important source of heat in infants because release of catecholamines stimulates nonshivering thermogenesis via brown fat metabolism. Sepsis and allergic reactions to blood products or drugs can also produce intraoperative hyperthermia.[42]

Hyperthermia increases oxygen consumption, cardiac output, and minute ventilation. Hyperthermia also stimulates lipolysis, gluconeogenesis, and lactate production. Fluid and electrolyte abnormalities can also occur as a result of increased sweating and subsequent dehydration. At temperatures above 40° C, seizures may occur in the awake patient, although this sign may be blocked during general anesthesia. At temperatures above 42° C, central nervous system hypoxia and acidosis develop and may result in irreversible tissue damage or death.

Treatment of hyperthermia depends on its cause. If the cause is specific, such as malignant hyperthermia, thyroid storm, pheochromocytoma, sepsis, and allergic reactions, then very specific therapeutic steps must be taken. These are discussed as separate topics elsewhere in the text. General measures to control hyperthermia include promoting heat loss by exposing the patient to cool fluids or fans, using ice packs, and encouraging sweating. Administration of antipyretics may also be helpful. When intraoperative hyperthermia occurs, the outcome depends on the cause of the hyperthermia, the peak temperature reached, plus the promptness of diagnosis and initiation of treatment.

SUMMARY

Although the majority of patients suffer no major complications that result from their anesthetic care, many do experience some intraoperative morbidity. In most cases these common anesthetic problems can be anticipated. By recognizing the types of patients and the clinical situations in which adverse events are most likely to occur, many of the common intraoperative anesthetic problems that occur in healthy patients can be avoided.

KEY POINTS

- A significant number of healthy patients experience some sort of adverse event during anesthesia. Most do not result in permanent damage, but that fact does not lessen the responsibility of prevention.
- Sinus tachycardia is the most common dysrhythmia during anesthesia.
- Bradycardia should immediately provoke a search for causes. The anesthesiologist should not be content to treat bradycardia with "a touch of atropine."
- Use of many drugs, most certainly including succinylcholine, can cause severe, life-threatening bradycardia. The anesthesiologist should be familiar with these pharmacologic bradycardias.
- Hypotension is the second most frequently encountered intraoperative anesthetic complication; dysrhythmias are the most common.
- The anesthesiologist should progress through a differential diagnosis list for hypotension that includes hypovolemia related to prolonged fasting, bowel preparations, vomiting, or gastrointestinal drainage. Hypovolemia can also result from acute hemorrhage or insensible losses. Hypotension can be caused by decreased venous return because of vena caval compression by the surgeon. Hypotension can be caused by faulty patient positioning. There are many other less common causes, including pneumothorax and other reasons for increases in intrathoracic pressure.
- Commonly encountered airway problems include numerous problems with mask fit and mask ventilation, soft-tissue obstruction in the upper airway, and laryngeal and bronchial spasm.
- The anesthesiologist should thoroughly understand laryngospasm, not only its treatment but also its prevention. Intraoperative hypoxemia can be caused by inspired oxygen concentration, hypoventilation, intrapulmonary ventilation/perfusion mismatch, diffusion abnormalities, and various causes of decreased mixed venous oxygen content.
- Correction of hypercapnia depends on the cause, which should be diligently sought.
- Hypocapnia is not benign.
- Wheezing, bronchospasm, cardiogenic pulmonary edema, and lower airway obstructions may present similar clinical pictures.
- The experienced anesthesiologist does not treat "a little wheezing" expectantly. "A little wheezing" should serve as a "red flag."
- Intraoperative oliguria can be prerenal, renal, or postrenal.
- It is not valid or sufficient to simply treat intraoperative oliguria with diuretics.
- The adverse effects of cooling are numerous; they are better prevented than treated.
- Operating room temperatures must be balanced between patient needs (first) and the very real decreases in efficiency of the gowned personnel when the operating room is too warm.

KEY REFERENCES

Atlee JL: *Perioperative cardiac dysrhythmias: mechanisms, recognition, management,* ed 2, Chicago, 1989, Year Book Medical Publishers.

Cohen MM, Cameron CB, and Duncan PG: Pediatric anesthesia morbidity and mortality in the perioperative period, *Anesth Analg* 70:160, 1990.

Cohen MM, Duncan PG, Pope WDB et al: A survey of 112,000 anaesthetics at one teaching hospital (1975-83), *Can J Anaesth* 33:22, 1986.

Doyle DJ, Mark PWS: Reflex bradycardia during surgery, *Can J Anaesth* 37:219, 1990.

Finucane BT, Santora AH: *Principles of airway management,* Philadelphia, 1988, FA Davis.

Marshall BE, Wyche MQ: Hypoxemia during and after anesthesia, *Anesthesiology* 37:178, 1972.

McIntyre JWR: The difficult tracheal intubation, *Can J Anaesth* 34:204, 1987.

Tinker JH, Dull DL, Caplan RA et al: Role of monitoring devices in prevention of anesthetic mishaps: a closed claims analysis, *Anesthesiology* 71:541, 1989.

REFERENCES

1. Abdul-Rasool IH, Sears DH, and Katz RL: The effect of a second dose of succinylcholine on cardiac rate and rhythm following induction of anesthesia with etomidate or midazolam, *Anesthesiology* 67:795, 1987.
2. Alexander CM, Teller LE, and Gross JB: Principles of pulse oximetry: theoretical and practical considerations, *Anesth Analg* 68:368, 1989.
3. Alexander JP: Reflex disturbances of cardiac rhythm during ophthalmic surgery, *Br J Ophthalmol* 59:518, 1975.
4. Anton AH, Uy DS, and Redderson CL: Autonomic blockade and the cardiovascular and catecholamine response to electroshock, *Anesth Analg* 56:46, 1977.
5. Apt L, Isenberg S, and Gaffney WL: The oculocardiac reflex in strabismus surgery, *Am J Ophthalmol* 76:533, 1973.
6. Arndt JO, Bednarski B, and Parasher C: Alfentanil's analgesic, respiratory, and cardiovascular actions in relation to dose and plasma concentration in unanaesthetized dogs, *Anesthesiology* 64:345, 1986.
7. Arndt JO, Mikat M, and Parasher C: Fentanyl's analgesic, respiratory and cardiovascular actions in relation to dose and plasma concentration in unanesthetized dogs, *Anesthesiology* 61:355, 1984.
8. Atlee JL, Alexander SC: Halothane effects on conductivity of the AV node and His-Purkinje system in the dog, *Anesth Analg* 56:378, 1977.
9. Atlee JL: *Perioperative cardiac dysrhythmias: mechanisms, recognition, management,* ed 2, Chicago, 1989, Year Book Medical Publishers.
10. Berler DK: The oculocardiac reflex, *Am J Ophthalmol* 56:954, 1963.
11. Birmingham PK, Cheney FW, and Ward RJ: Esophageal intubation: a review of detection techniques, *Anesth Analg* 65:886, 1986.
12. Blanc VF, Hardy JF, Milot J et al: The oculocardiac reflex: a graphic and statistical analysis in infants and children, *Can Anaesth Soc J* 30:360, 1983.
13. Blanc VF, Tremblay NAG: The complications of endotracheal intubation: a new classification with a review of the literature, *Anesth Analg* 53:202, 1974.
14. Blitt CD, Raessler KL, Wightman MA et al: Atrioventricular conduction in dogs during anesthesia with isoflurane, *Anesthesiology* 50:210, 1979.
15. Brodsky MA, Sato DA, Iseri LT et al: Ventricular tachyarrhythmia associated with psychological stress. The role of the sympathetic nervous system, *JAMA* 257:2064, 1987.
16. Cattermole RW, Berghese C, Blair IJ et al: Isoflurane and halothane for outpatient dental anesthesia in children, *Br J Anaesth* 58:385, 1986.
17. Cheney FW, Colley PS: The effect of cardiac output on arterial blood oxygenation, *Anesthesiology* 52:496, 1980.
18. Clayton D: Asystole associated with vecuronium, *Br J Anaesth* 58:937, 1986.
19. Cohen MM, Cameron CB, and Duncan PG: Pediatric anesthesia morbidity and mortality in the perioperative period, *Anesth Analg* 70:160, 1990.
20. Cohen MM, Cameron CB: Should you cancel the operation when a child has an upper respiratory tract infection? *Anesth Analg* 72:282, 1991.
21. Cohen MM, Duncan PG, Pope WDB et al: A survey of 112,000 anaesthetics at one teaching hospital (1975-83), *Can J Anaesth* 33:22, 1986.
22. Connors AF, McCaffree RD, and Gray BA: Effect of inspiratory flow rate on gas exchange during mechanical ventilation, *Am Rev Respir Dis* 124:537, 1981.
23. Cooper JB, Long CD, Newbower RS et al: Critical incidents associated with intraoperative exchanges of anesthesia personnel, *Anesthesiology* 56:456, 1982.
24. Cooper JB, Newbower RS, and Kitz RJ: An analysis of major errors and equipment failures in anesthesia management: consideration for prevention and detection, *Anesthesiology* 60:34, 1984.
25. Cozanitis DA, Proutt J, and Rosenberg PH: Bradycardia associated with the use of vecuronium. A comparative study with pancuronium with or without glycopyrronium, *Anaesthesia* 42:192, 1987.
26. Damen J, Bolton D: A prospective analysis of 1400 PA catheterizations in patients undergoing cardiac surgery, *Acta Anesthesiol Scand* 30:386, 1986.
27. Darioli R, Perret C: Mechanically controlled hypoventilation in status asthmaticus, *Am Rev Respir Dis* 129:385, 1987.
28. DeSoto H, Patel RI, Soliman IE et al: Changes in oxygen saturation following general anesthesia in children with upper respiratory tract infection signs and symptoms undergoing otolaryngological procedures, *Anesthesiology* 68:276, 1988.
29. Doyle DJ, Mark PWS: Laparoscopy and vagal arrest, *Anaesthesia* 44:448, 1989.
30. Doyle DJ, Mark PWS: Reflex bradycardia during surgery, *Can J Anaesth* 37:219, 1990.
31. Drummond GB: Factors influencing the control of breathing. In Jones JG, ed: Effects of anesthesia and surgery on pulmonary mechanics and gas exchange, *Int Anesthesiol Clin* 22(4):59, 1984.
32. Eichhorn JH: Prevention of intraoperative anesthesia accidents and related severe injuries through safety monitoring, *Anesthesiology* 70:572, 1989.
33. Empey DW, Laitinen LA, Jacobs L et al: Mechanism of bronchial hyperreactivity in normal subjects after upper respiratory tract infections, *Am Rev Respir Dis* 113:131, 1976.
34. Fink BR: The etiology and treatment of laryngeal spasm, *Anesthesiology* 17:569, 1956.
35. Finucane BT, Santora AH: *Principles of airway management,* Philadelphia, 1988, FA Davis.
36. Fisher DM, Robinson S, Bretl CM et al: Comparison of enflurane, halothane and isoflurane for diagnostic and therapeutic procedures in children with malignancies, *Anesthesiology* 63:647, 1985.
37. Foltz B, Benumof J: Mechanisms of hypoxemia and hypercapnia in the perioperative period, *Crit Care Clin* 3(2):269, 1987.
38. Forbes RB, Morton GH: Ventricular fibrillation in a patient with unsuspected mitral valve prolapse and a prolonged Q-T interval, *Can Anaesth Soc J* 2:424, 1979.
39. Frerichs RL, Campbell J, and Bassell GM: Psychogenic cardiac arrest during extensive sympathetic blockade, *Anesthesiology* 68:943, 1988.
40. Gaba DM, Maxwell M, and DeAnde A: Anesthesia mishaps: breaking the chain of accident evolution, *Anesthesiology* 66:670, 1987.
41. Gambling DR, Birmingham CL, and Jenkins LC: Magnesium and the anaesthetist, *Can J Anaesth* 35:644, 1988.
42. Greenberg C: Diagnosis and treatment of hyperthermia in the postanesthesia care unit. In Shapiro G, ed: Postanesthesia care unit problems, *Anesthesiol Clin* 8(2):377, 1990.
43. Halperin BD, Feeley TW: The effect of anesthesia and surgery on renal function. In Priebe HJ, ed: The kidney in anesthesia, *Int Anesthesiol Clin* 22(1):157, 1984.
44. Hanson CW: Asymptomatic cardiomyopathy presenting as cardiac arrest in the day surgical unit, *Anesthesiology* 71:982, 1989.
45. Hardy PAJ: Atracurium and bradycardia, *Anaesthesia* 40:88, 1985.
46. Herschman Z, Aaron C: Prolongation of cocaine effect, *Anesthesiology* 74:631, 1991.
47. Hirsch IA, Reagan JO, and Sullivan N: Complications of direct laryngoscopy, *Anesthesiol Rev* 17:34, 1990.
48. Hirsch IA, Tomlinson DL, Slogoff S et al: The overstated risk of preoperative hypokalemia, *Anesth Analg* 67:131, 1988.
49. Hunsley JE, Bush GH, and Johnes CJ: A study of glycopyrrolate and atropine in the suppression of the oculocardiac reflex during strabismus surgery in children, *Br J Anaesth* 54:459, 1982.
50. Johnston RR, Eger EI, and Wilson C: A comparative interaction of epinephrine with enflurane, isoflurane and halothane in man, *Anesth Analg* 55:709, 1976.
51. Kambic V, Radsel Z: Intubation lesions of the larynx, *Br J Anaesth* 50:587, 1978.
52. Keats AS: Anesthesia mortality in perspective, *Anesth Analg* 71:113, 1990.
53. Keenan RL, Boyan P: Cardiac arrest due to anesthesia. A study of incidence and causes, *JAMA* 253:2373, 1985.
54. Kingston HGG: Halothane and isoflurane anesthesia in pediatric outpatients, *Anesth Analg* 65:181, 1986.

55. Kirkwood I, Duckworth RA: An unusual case of sinus arrest, *Br J Anaesth* 55:1273, 1983.
56. Lang S, Lanigan DT, and van der Wal M: Trigeminocardiac reflexes: maxillary and mandibular variants of the oculocardiac reflex, *Can J Anaesth* 38:757, 1991.
57. Little JW, Wall WJ, Douglass RG et al: Airway hyperreactivity and peripheral airway dysfunction in influenza infection, *Am Rev Respir Dis* 118:295, 1978.
58. Lockhart PB, Feldbau EV, Gabel RA et al: Dental complications during and after tracheal intubation, *J Am Dent Assoc* 112:480, 1986.
59. Lunn JN, Mushin WW: Mortality associated with anaesthesia, *Anaesthesia* 37:856, 1982.
60. Mark RJ: Electroconvulsive therapy: physiological and anaesthetic considerations, *Can Anaesth Soc J* 31:541, 1984.
61. Marsh HM, Southorn PA, and Rehder K: Anesthesia, sedation and the chest wall. In Jones JG, ed: Effects of anesthesia and surgery on pulmonary mechanisms and gas exchange, *Int Anesthesiol Clin* 22(4):1, 1984.
62. Marshall BE, Wyche MQ: Hypoxemia during and after anesthesia, *Anesthesiology* 37:178, 1972.
63. May JR: Vecuronium and bradycardia, *Anaesthesia* 40:710, 1985.
64. Maze A, Mason DM: Aetiology and treatment of halothane induced arrhythmias. In Mazze RI, ed: Inhalation anaesthesiology, *Clin Anesthesiol* 1(2):301, 1983.
65. McAteer PM, Carter JA, Cooper GM et al: Comparison of isoflurane and halothane in outpatient paediatric dental anaesthesia, *Br J Anaesth* 58:390, 1986.
66. McIntyre JWR: The difficult tracheal intubation, *Can J Anaesth* 34:204, 1987.
67. McIntyre VWR: Laryngoscope design and the difficult adult tracheal intubation, *Can J Anaesth* 36:94, 1989.
68. Moonie GT, Rees DL, and Elton D: The oculocardiac reflex during strabismus surgery, *Can Anesth Soc J* 11:621, 1964.
69. Morley-Forster PK: Unintentional hypothermia in the operating room, *Can Anaesth Soc J* 33:516, 1986.
70. Morrison RC: Hyperthermia in the elderly. In: Nielsen CH, Owens WD, eds: Anesthesia in the geriatric patient, *Int Anesthesiol Clin* 26(2):124, 1988.
71. Nigrovic V: Succinylcholine, cholinoceptors and catecholamines: proposed mechanism of early adverse haemodynamic reactions, *Can Anaesth Soc J* 31:382, 1984.
72. Nunn JF: *Applied respiratory physiology,* ed 2, Boston, 1977, Butterworths.
73. Olsson GL, Hallen B: Laryngospasm during anaesthesia. A computer-aided incidence study in 136,929 patients, *Acta Anaesthesiol Scand* 28:567, 1984.
74. Pandit VA, Steude GM, and Leach AB: Induction and recovery characteristics of isoflurane and halothane anaesthesia for short outpatient operations in children, *Anaesthesia* 40:1226, 1985.
75. Papademetriou V: Diuretics, hypokalemia, and cardiac arrhythmics: a critical analysis, *Am Heart J* 111:1217, 1986.
76. Patel RI, Hannallah RS, Norder J et al: Emergency airway complications in children: a comparison of tracheal extubation in awake and deeply anesthetic patients, *Anesth Analg* 73:266, 1991.
77. Phillips AJ, Brimacombe JR, and Simpson DL: Anaesthetic induction with isoflurane or halothane, *Anaesthesia* 43:927, 1988.
78. Podolakin W, Wells DG: Precipitous bradycardia induced by laryngoscopy in cardiac surgical patients, *Can J Anaesth* 34:618, 1987.
79. Rehder K: Anaesthesia and the respiratory system, *Can Anaesth Soc J* 26:451, 1979.
80. Rhode J, Grom E, Bajares AC et al: A study of electrocardiographic alterations occurring during operations on the extraocular muscles, *Am J Ophthalmol* 46:367, 1958.
81. Risk Management Foundation. Anesthesia claims analysis shows frequency low, losses high, *Risk Management Foundation* 4:1, 1983.
82. Rocco AG, Vandam LD: Changes in circulation consequent to manipulation during abdominal surgery, *JAMA* 164:14, 1957.
83. Rosenberg MB: Anesthesia-induced dental injury. In Lebowitz PW, ed: Anesthesia for dental and oral surgery, *Int Anesthesiol Clin* 27(2):120, 1989.
84. Roy WL, Lerman J: Laryngospasm in paediatric anaesthesia, *Can J Anaesth* 35:93, 1988.
85. Salem MR, Bennett EJ, Schweiss JF et al: Cardiac arrest related to anesthesia. Contributing factors in infants and children, *JAMA* 233:238, 1975.
86. Sampaio MM, Crean PM, Keilty SR et al: Changes in oxygen saturation during inhalation induction of anaesthesia in children, *Br J Anaesth* 62:199, 1989.
87. Sapire DW, Casta A: Vagotonia in infants, children, adolescents and young adults, *Int J Cardiol* 9:211, 1985.
88. Schieber R: Cardiovascular physiology in infants and children. In Motoyama EK, Davis PJ, eds: *Smith's anesthesia for infants and children,* St Louis, 1990, Times Mirror/Mosby College Publishing.
89. Schmeling WT, Warltier DC, McDonald DJ et al: Prolongation of the QT interval by enflurane, isoflurane, and halothane, *Anesth Analg* 72:137, 1991.
90. Sebel PS, Lowdon JD: Propofol: a new intravenous anesthetic, *Anesthesiology* 71:260, 1989.
91. Seltzer JL, Ritter DE, Starsnic MA et al: The hemodynamic response to traction on the abdominal mesentery, *Anesthesiology* 63:96, 1985.
92. Selvin BL: Electroconvulsive therapy — 1987, *Anesthesiology* 67:367, 1987.
93. Skues MA, Prys-Roberts C: The pharmacology of propofol, *J Clin Anesth* 1:387, 1989.
94. Smith RB, Douglas H, and Petruscak J: The oculo-cardiac reflex and sino-atrial arrest, *Can Anaesth Soc J* 19:138, 1972.
95. Sorenson EJ, Gilmore JE: Cardiac arrest during strabismus surgery — a preliminary report, *Am J Ophthalmol* 41:748, 1956.
96. Springman SR, Atlee JL: The etiology of intraoperative arrhythmias, *Anesth Clin North Am* 7(2):293, 1989.
97. Steward D: *Manual of pediatric anesthesia,* ed 3, New York, 1990, Churchill-Livingstone.
98. Tait AR, Knight PR: Intraoperative respiratory complications in patients with upper respiratory tract infections, *Can J Anaesth* 34:300, 1987.
99. Tait AR, Knight PR: The effects of general anesthesia on upper respiratory tract infections in children, *Anesthesiology* 67:930, 1987.
100. Tinker JH, Dull DL, Caplan RA et al: Role of monitoring devices in prevention of anesthetic mishaps: a closed claims analysis, *Anesthesiology* 71:541, 1989.
101. Tiret L, Desmonts JM, Hatton F et al: Complications associated with anaesthesia — a prospective survey in France, *Can Anaesth Soc J* 33:336, 1986.
102. Tiret L, Nivoche Y, Hatton F et al: Complications related to anaesthesia in infants and children, *Br J Anaesth* 61:263, 1988.
103. Tremper KK, Barker SJ: Pulse oximetry, *Anesthesiology* 70:98, 1989.
104. Vaughan MS, Vaughn RW, and Cork RC: Postoperative hypothermia in adults: relation of age, anesthesia and shivering to rewarming, *Anesth Analg* 60:746, 1981.
105. Verhoeff F, Sykes MK: Delayed detection of hypoxic events by pulse oximeters: computer simulations, *Anaesthesia* 45:103, 1990.
106. Vitez TS, Soper LE, Wong KC et al: Chronic hypokalemia and intraoperative dysrhythmias, *Anesthesiology* 63:130, 1985.
107. Wingard DW: What is a normal heart rate prior to surgery? *Anesthesiology* 72:1102, 1990.

CHAPTER 6

Clinical Implications of the Stress Response to Surgery

MICHAEL J. BRESLOW

Surgical trauma elicits a large number of neural and hormonal responses that result in predictable physiologic alterations. Many of these neuroendocrine changes have been recognized for quite some time, and they have generally been regarded as appropriate responses to injury.[12,70] However, data supporting the compensatory nature of the "stress response" is limited, particularly in the setting of controlled surgical trauma. Furthermore, changes in modern surgical practice have increased the number of patients with significant coexisting medical problems undergoing extensive surgical procedures. An emerging body of literature suggests that the physiologic perturbations that predictably accompany such procedures can have untoward effects in these patients, and that interventions to minimize these alterations may be beneficial. This chapter will review the growing literature in this area and try to correlate specific neurohumoral alterations with discrete physiologic events. Literature examining potential beneficial and deleterious effects of the stress response will be discussed, as will newer studies of methodologies to modulate surgically induced physiologic alterations.

SURGICALLY INDUCED NEUROHUMORAL ALTERATIONS

Surgery results in diffuse alteration of endocrine and autonomic nervous system function. Table 6-1 summarizes the more important changes.

Pituitary Alterations

Secretion of most anterior pituitary hormones, including adrenocorticotropic hormone (ACTH),[79] growth hormone,[58] prolactin,[3] and beta-endorphin,[22] is increased during surgery. The pattern of anterior pituitary hormone secretion may also be altered; recent data indicate that secretion of ACTH, which is normally pulsatile, becomes constant postoperatively.[81] The physiologic significance of this alteration is unknown. Thyroid-stimulating hormone (TSH), which may be transiently elevated with surgery, returns to the low-normal range postoperatively and

Table 6-1 Perioperative neurohormonal changes

System/organ	Change
Pituitary	Increased adrenocorticotropic hormone
	Increased prolactin
	Increased, then decreased thyroid-stimulating hormone
	Increased growth hormone
	Increased beta-endorphin
	Increased vasopressin
Autonomic nervous system	Increased plasma norepinephrine
Adrenal gland	Increased adrenal catecholamine secretion
	Increased cortisol
	Increased aldosterone
Pancreas	Increased glucagon
	Decreased insulin
Thyroid	Increased, then decreased T_4, free T_4, free T_3
	Increased rT_3
Miscellaneous	± Renin
	Decreased testosterone
	Increased prostaglandins

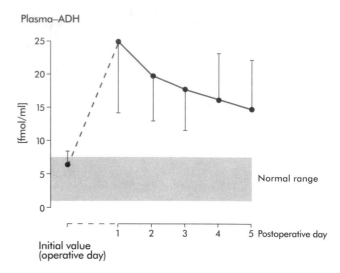

Fig. 6-1. Plasma ADH levels in 51 patients undergoing a variety of abdominal and thoracic surgical procedures. (From Bormann BV, Weidler B, Dennhardt R et al: Influence of epidural fentanyl on stress-induced elevation of plasma vasopressin (ADH) after surgery, *Anesth Analg* 62:727, 1983.)

persists at this level for several days despite reduced circulating levels of thyroid hormone.[15] Leutinizing hormone and follicle-stimulating hormone are unchanged postoperatively.[1]

Secretion of vasopressin (AVP) from the posterior pituitary is markedly increased.[6] Fig. 6-1 shows plasma AVP levels before and for 5 days following a variety of thoracic and abdominal surgical procedures. Plasma AVP levels in these patients increased markedly and remained in excess of levels normally associated with control of plasma osmolality (0 to 8 fmol/ml) **for as long as 5 days following surgery. Because this rise in AVP levels occurs independently of changes in plasma osmolality, postoperative patients are at risk for development of hyponatremia.**[93] Urine and plasma chemistry studies of such patients meet standard criteria for establishing a diagnosis of the Syndrome of Inappropriate Secretion of Antidiuretic Hormone (SIADH). The magnitude and duration of the AVP response to surgery appear to be proportional to the extent of the surgical procedure.[6,20]

Autonomic Nervous System Alterations

Plasma catecholamine levels increase two- to six-fold almost immediately following surgical incision[40] **(Fig. 6-2) and remain elevated for up to 5 days postoperatively.**[17] For reasons that are not understood, plasma epinephrine (EPI) levels begin to return to normal levels 6 to 12 hours postoperatively, whereas plasma norepinephrine (NE) levels remain elevated longer[9] (Fig. 6-3). Dissociation of adrenal medullary and peripheral sympathetic nervous system (SNS) activity responses to a variety of physiologic stresses has been described in other settings,[92] and it must be concluded that SNS activation in response to surgery may not be diffuse. Whether peripheral SNS activity increases similarly in all organs (i.e., heart, kidney) is unknown and of potential physiologic relevance.

The nature of the surgical procedure appears to be the major determinant of both the magnitude and the duration of the increase in NE levels, with more extensive operations resulting in bigger and more prolonged increases.[17]

Fig. 6-4 shows perioperative plasma NE data from the 31 patients included in this study. Patients were segregated according to the extent of the surgical procedure. Group 1 patients who underwent minor surgical procedures (i.e., inguinal hernia repair) had no increase in NE levels. Group 2 patients (moderate stress, [i.e., cholecystectomy]) had three- to fourfold increases in NE at 1 and 24 hours postoperatively but normal levels at 5 days. In contrast, group 3 patients (major stress, [i.e., colectomy]) had sixfold increases in NE that persisted for up to 5 days. Tracer studies using tritiated NE have clearly established that plasma levels are elevated as a result of increased release from peripheral sympathetic nerves and not because clearance mechanisms are altered.[43] Limited data exist on perioperative changes in parasympa-

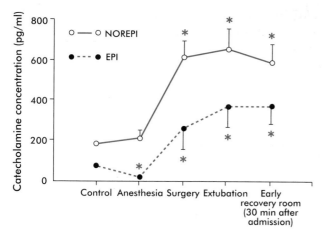

Fig. 6-2. Plasma norepinephrine (NOREPI) and epinephrine (EPI) levels before, during, and immediately following abdominal surgery. * = p ≤ 0.05 compared with control. Data are mean of 8 patients ± SE. (From Halter JB, Pflug AE, and Porte D: Mechanisms of plasma catecholamine increases during surgical stress in man, *J Clin Endocrinol Metab* 45:936, 1977.)

thetic nervous system activity. Vagal stimuli can result in occasional episodes of bradycardia intraoperatively. However, heart rate is consistently increased postoperatively and often cannot be slowed below 80 beats/min by beta-adrenergic receptor antagonists. These observations suggest that **parasympathetic activity, which is dominant over SNS activity in control of heart rate,[53] is reduced postoperatively.**

Thyroid Changes

Although transient increases in total and free T_4 and in free T_3 have been noted during surgery, levels of

these thyroid hormones are substantially reduced postoperatively, often for several days.[15] Increases in reverse T_3 levels parallel the reduction in active thyroid hormone levels,[15,68] a situation analogous to the sick euthyroid syndrome observed in patients with chronic illness.[88] Because plasma TSH levels are not increased at the same time, these perioperative alterations in thyroid hormone homeostasis appear to be centrally mediated. Maintenance of normal thyroid hormone levels during starvation by administration of exogenous hormone exacerbates protein catabolism,[31] prompting some investigators to hypothesize that stress-induced hypothyroidism acts to oppose other catabolic forces activated in response to illness.

Adrenal Effects

Adrenal cortisol[69] and aldosterone[14] secretion is markedly increased following surgery, a response that persists for several days. Whereas this adrenocortical response is largely attributable to augmented ACTH secretion, there are data indicating that adrenal sensitivity to ACTH is also increased, at least intraoperatively.[81] Adrenal catecholamine secretion is also increased (see previous discussion). Presumably other chromaffin granule constituents, such as enkephalins and adenosine, are also released, although studies documenting these changes are not available.

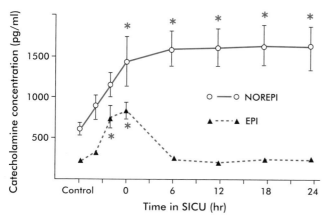

Fig. 6-3. Plasma norepinephrine (NOREPI) and epinephrine (EPI) levels before induction of anesthesia (control), at two points during surgery, and 0, 6, 12, 18, and 24 hours following aortic surgery. *SICU,* Surgical intensive care unit. * = p < 0.05 compared to preinduction value. Data are mean of 12 patients ± SE.

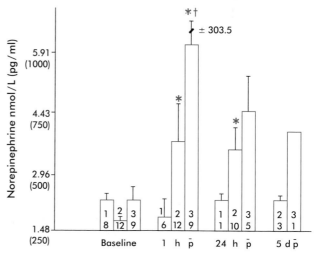

Fig. 6-4. Plasma norepinephrine values for three groups of patients who have undergone surgery (grades 1, 2, and 3) before (baseline), and 1 hour, 24 hours, and 5 days after surgery. Numbers within bars reflect "n" at each time point for each group. Statistical comparisons for each time point were performed between various "grades" and also against baseline values for each group. * = p < .05 compared with baseline. † = p < .05 compared with grade 1. Data are mean ± SE of 31 points. (From Chernow B: Hormonal responses to graded surgical stress, *Arch Intern Med* 147:1273, 1987.)

Pancreatic Changes

Plasma glucagon levels are substantially elevated following surgery[34] **and are believed to contribute to perioperative hyperglycemia. In contrast, insulin levels are often subnormal,** considering that plasma glucose levels are increased.[39] Consistent with these findings, researchers have demonstrated impaired insulin secretory responses to exogenous glucose infusion in surgical patients[39] (Fig. 6-5). Intraoperative changes in insulin secretion may be partially due to pancreatic effects of certain anesthetic agents. However, adrenergic agonists also inhibit insulin release from islet cells,[60] and **surgically induced changes in plasma catecholamines act to suppress insulin secretion throughout the perioperative period.**

Miscellaneous

Despite increased SNS activity, plasma renin activity is not consistently elevated in the perioperative period.[41,66,85] Increases in renin/angiotensin appear to be correlated with intravascular volume depletion and not surgical trauma.[66] Cardiopulmonary bypass, however, has been reported to increase angiotensin levels.[89] Plasma levels of interleukins and tumor necrosis factor do not appear to be elevated following surgery. Data on these potentially important mediators is admittedly scarce at this time and may reflect the relatively low sensitivity of older assay systems or, alternatively, a paracrine type of effect. Levels of testosterone are reduced,[87] suggesting the reordering of organismal priorities in the face of significant injury. Although alterations of other hormonal systems, including prostaglandin metabolites,[82] have been described, these reports come from very selective surgical populations, and their physiologic implications are poorly understood.

POSTOPERATIVE PHYSIOLOGIC CHANGES
Cardiovascular System

Increases in arterial blood pressure, heart rate, and cardiac output are seen routinely after surgical trauma. The actual incidence of postoperative hypertension depends on the nature of the surgical procedure, with major vascular operations often resulting in elevations requiring treatment.[4,36,85] Although postoperative hypertension can result from a variety of causes, **SNS activity (as reflected by plasma catecholamine levels) correlates highly with blood pressure elevations**[40] (Fig. 6-6). In contrast, plasma angiotensin and AVP levels correlate poorly with postoperative increases in blood pressure.[84] Sinus tachycardia is also common in the postoperative period, and other tachydysrhythmias are occasionally seen.[35,51] The efficacy of beta-adrenergic receptor antagonists in controlling heart rate in this setting indicates that increased cardiac SNS activity contributes to these rhythm disturbances.

Although careful studies of cardiac function (preload and afterload maintained constant) are not available, cardiac output is elevated postoperatively in most patients in which it is measured, usually as a

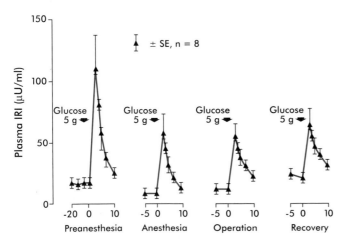

Fig. 6-5. Arterial plasma immunoreactive insulin (IRI) levels before and after administration of glucose (5 g/IV) measured before and after induction of inhalation anesthesia, during surgery, 90 minutes after discontinuation of anesthesia. Data are mean of 8 patients ± SE. (From Halter JB, Pflug AE: Relationship of impaired insulin secretion during surgical stress to anesthesia and catecholamine release, *J Clin Endocrinol Metab* 51:1093, 1980.)

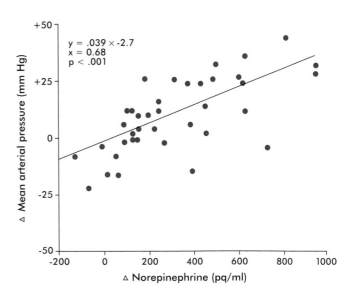

Fig. 6-6. Regression analysis of changes in mean arterial blood pressure from baseline vs. changes in plasma norepinephrine levels for 8 patients having abdominal surgery. Data obtained after induction of anesthesia, during surgery, at extubation, and 30 and 120 minutes postoperatively. (From Halter JB, Pflug AE, and Porte D: Mechanisms of plasma catecholamine increases during surgical stress in man, *J Clin Endocrinol Metab* 45:936, 1977.)

result of increases in both heart rate and stroke volume. **Whole body oxygen consumption is increased by up to 25% postoperatively.**[65,68] Much of this excess oxygen utilization can be attributed to elevated body temperature. The mediators of postoperative increases in body temperature are unknown. Presumably, myocardial oxygen consumption is also increased postoperatively because myocardial work appears to be significantly increased. There remain several unanswered questions concerning perioperative changes in cardiovascular function. For example, catecholamine-induced adrenergic-receptor down-regulation has been described in nonsurgical hyper-adrenergic states[76]; whether this occurs postoperatively is not known. This receptor down-regulation could potentially result in a relative hypoadrenergic state later in the postoperative period when SNS activity returns to basal levels. There are insufficient data concerning perioperative changes in venous compliance and organ blood flow distribution to permit meaningful comment.

Metabolic System

Surgical trauma consistently results in increases in blood sugar,[34] **lipolysis,**[37,77] **and protein catabolism.**[77,80] Blood sugar increases are principally mediated by elevated plasma levels of catecholamines, glucagon, cortisol, and growth hormone. **When infused individually they have a minimal effect on blood sugar, but**

co-administration of epinephrine, glucagon, and cortisol produces significant hyperglycemia[71] (Fig. 6-7). This synergism is apparently the result of differential effects of these agents on glucose uptake (epinephrine) and glucose synthesis (glucagon, cortisol).[25] Breakdown of fat is principally due to epinephrine but is enhanced by cortisol. In addition to providing additional substrate for gluconeogenesis, lipolysis provides an additional source of substrate via beta-oxidation. **Protein catabolism provides additional substrate for gluconeogenesis; however, considerable nitrogen wasting occurs in most patients, suggesting that this process is inefficient.** Increases in nitrogen excretion can be reduced (but not eliminated) by analgesic techniques that attenuate postoperative neuroendocrine changes[80] (Fig. 6-8). They can also be induced in nonsurgical patients by simultaneous infusion of epinephrine, glucagon, and cortisol.[5] Interleukin-1 and tumor necrosis factor can replicate many of these changes. However, a clear-cut etiologic role for these cytokines in postoperative patients has not been established. More work is needed in this area.

Renal/Electrolyte Function

Evaluation of perioperative fluid balance is difficult because of trauma-induced interstitial edema and "third space" fluid losses. However, infusion of

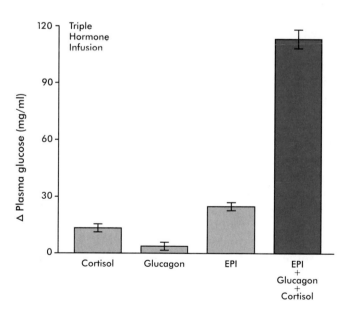

Fig. 6-7. Demonstration of the synergistic effect on blood glucose levels in human subjects when cortisol, epinephrine (EPI), and glucagon are infused simultaneously, compared with the effect of single hormone infusions when these hormones are infused separately. (From Shamoon H, Hendler R, and Sherwin RS: Synergistic interactions among antiinsulin hormones in the pathogenesis of stress hyperglycemia in humans, *J Clin Endocrinol Metab* 52:1235, 1981.)

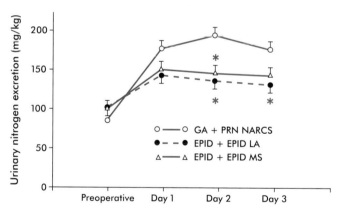

Fig. 6-8. Daily urinary nitrogen excretion obtained before upper abdominal surgery and on the first 3 postoperative days. Thirty patients had the procedure performed under general anesthesia and received parenteral narcotics for postoperative analgesia *(GA + PRN NARCS)*. The remaining patients had the procedure performed using a continuous epidural anesthetic (0.5% bupivicaine) for intraoperative analgesia, and either had an epidural bupivicaine infusion continued postoperatively *(EPID + EPID LA,* n = 20) or had morphine 4 mg every 12 hours administered through the epidural catheter *(EPID + EPID MS,* n = 20). * = p < 0.05 compared to general anesthesia group. (From Tsuji H, Shivasaka C, Asch T et al: Effects of epidural administration of local anaesthetics or morphine on postoperative nitrogen loss and catabolic hormones, *Br J Surg* 74:421, 1987.)

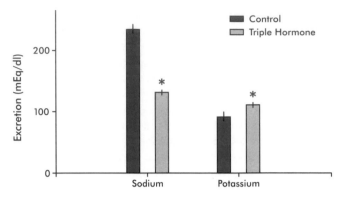

Fig. 6-9. Twenty-four hour sodium and potassium excretion before *(control)* and during combined infusion of cortisol, glucagon, and epinephrine *(triple hormone)*. * = p ≤ 0.05 compared to control. Data are mean of 9 male volunteers ± SE. (From Bessey PA, Walters JM, Aoki TT et al: Combined hormonal infusion simulates the metabolic response to injury, *Ann Surg* 200:264, 1984.)

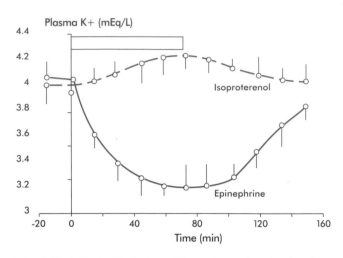

Fig. 6-10. Effect of infusion of isoproterenol and epinephrine on plasma potassium concentration. Epinephrine effect is prevented by beta-specific antagonists. (From Brown MJ, Brown DC, and Murphy MB: Hypokalemia from beta$_2$-receptor stimulation by circulating epinephrine, *N Engl J Med* 309:1414, 1983.)

exogenous cortisol into healthy volunteers to replicate levels seen in surgical patients results in sodium retention[5] (Fig. 6-9). In addition, increased renal sympathetic nerve activity increases proximal tubular sodium absorption, and elevated AVP levels cause free water retention. Thus there are several factors acting to retain fluid following surgical trauma. **Clinically significant problems related to hypervolemia, however, are not common and are usually easily treated with diuretics.**

Hypokalemia occurs commonly in the perioperative period and often cannot be explained by intraoperative fluid therapy or preoperative hypokalemia.[57] Recent demonstration of substantial decreases in serum potassium concentrations in healthy volunteers during beta-adrenergic agonist infusion suggests that **catecholamine-mediated transcellular shifts are probably responsible for perioperative hypokalemia.**[10] Fig. 6-10 illustrates the decrease in plasma potassium concentration these researchers observed with infusion of EPI. There appears to be a similar high incidence of postoperative hypomagnesemia,[18] perhaps reflecting similar transcellular movement of this predominantly intracellular cation.

Miscellaneous

Recent data suggest that postoperative patients are hypercoagulable. Increased levels of Factor VIII, prothrombin, fibrinogen, and decreased levels of antithrombin III have been reported in surgical patients.[7,63] Fibrinolysis appears to be inhibited, perhaps as a result of reduced levels of plasminogen activator and increased levels of antiplasmin globulin.[56] Little data exist concerning platelet function in the perioperative period. Elevated plasma catecholamines, however, can affect platelet aggregation[72] and

may contribute to perioperative hypercoagulability.

Changes in cell-mediated immunity, including reduced lymphocyte count, impaired blastogenic response of lymphocytes to mitogen, and decreased lymphokine production have been observed following surgery.[45,90] These changes are not seen when surgery is performed under epidural anesthesia. Despite data demonstrating significant attenuation of stress-induced suppression of lymphocyte function in adrenalectomized animals,[49] the exact mediators are not known. Whether perioperative alterations in cell-mediated immunity are of clinical importance is questionable because most postoperative infections are bacterial in nature. Unfortunately, data on surgically induced alterations in other, potentially more relevant, aspects of immunocompetence are not available.

Perioperative changes in pulmonary function depend on the location of surgery and do not represent predictable effects of surgical trauma. Finally, it has been recognized for many years that hepatic synthesis of fibrinogen, haptoglobin, and orosomucoid, the so-called acute phase reactants, are increased following surgery.[64] The clinical relevance of these compounds is largely unknown, but some may act as opsonizing agents and thus help in combating infection.

PHYSIOLOGIC ROLE OF THE STRESS RESPONSE

Following major trauma, priorities of the injured organism are to prevent additional injury (fight or flight), minimize blood loss, maintain vital organ blood flow, restore intravascular volume, deliver adequate fuel substrates for wound healing, and prevent infection. In 1929 Cannon first hypothesized an important physiologic role of hormonal secretion during stress.[12] In 1950 Selye expanded on the observations of Cannon and advanced his concept of the "general adaptation responds."[70] He proposed that the body responds to "threats to survival" by increasing catecholamine release from both sympathetic nerves and the adrenal medulla and by secreting cortisol and antidiuretic hormone (AVP). He postulated that catecholamine release acts to improve organ blood flow by increasing blood pressure and cardiac output whereas cortisol and AVP alter fluid balance, fuel homeostasis, and immune function.

Studies performed over the past 30 years have shown that many additional systems are activated (or suppressed) following injury and have clarified their relative contributions to blood pressure support and metabolic alterations. **Three different mediator systems, the catecholamines (from sympathetic nerves and adrenal medulla), AVP, and angiotensin II act to maintain central blood pressure by decreasing blood flow to nonessential organs.** Venous capacitance decreases, and cardiac contractility is augmented. In addition, **arteriolar vasoconstriction decreases capillary hydrostatic pressure, which in turn increases vascular uptake of extracellular water. Further fluid loss is prevented by augmented sympathetic outflow to the kidney and by increased secretion of AVP and aldosterone. Plasma osmolality rises, partially as a result of increased plasma glucose concentrations, and brings intracellular water into the extracellular space.** Circulating levels of fuel substrates are increased as a result of secretion of catecholamines, cortisol, and glucagon. Clotting activity increases, and endogenous enkephalins diminish pain.

Although there can be little doubt about the value of many of the previously mentioned responses, it is important to keep in mind that these compensatory mechanisms evolved before the development of advanced medical care delivery systems. Whereas we can confidently conclude that the stress response is beneficial following extensive trauma or when injury occurs far from a modern medical facility, there are considerably less data available concerning the importance of these physiologic alterations following controlled surgical trauma. In this latter setting, hypotension and hypovolemia should be avoidable, high circulating levels of metabolic substrates can be easily maintained by administration of intravenous alimentation regimens, and pain can be controlled with potent analgesic medications. Whether other unappreciated, or as yet unrecognized, aspects of the stress response may be important for wound healing and prevention of infection is not known.

Coincident with development of improved anesthetic and surgical techniques, the population of patients coming to the hospital for elective surgery has changed markedly. The past decade has seen large increases in the numbers of elderly patients and patients with significant coexisting medical illnesses having elective surgical procedures. **An emerging body of literature suggests that stress-induced physiologic changes may not be well tolerated in some of these patients** and can result in significant morbidity and even, occasionally, mortality. The next section reviews some of these potential complications.

POTENTIAL ADVERSE EFFECTS OF THE STRESS RESPONSE

Potential adverse effects of the stress response are listed in Box 6-1.

Hypertension

Intraoperative hypertension is most often caused by a relative imbalance between anesthetic depth and surgical stimulation and can usually be corrected by deepening the level of anesthesia. Sympathetic hyperactivity appears to be responsible for hypertension in this setting.[40] Anesthetics probably reduce blood pressure by decreasing sympathetic outflow, blunting cardiovascular actions of catecholamines, and by direct effects on cardiac function and vascular tone. In most instances intraoperative hypertension is of little clinical significance.

Substantial increases in afterload can adversely affect cardiac output in patients with poor ventricular function, but such effects, if recognized, are usually easily managed. Increases in blood pressure affect myocardial oxygen consumption and can precipitate ischemic episodes. However, **recent animal studies suggest that relative hypotension, which decreases coronary perfusion pressure, is more frequently associated with myocardial ischemia during anesthesia.**[11] Although there are reports that postoperative neurologic deficits following carotid endarterectomy

---

BOX 6-1
POSSIBLE ADVERSE EFFECTS OF THE STRESS RESPONSE

Hypertension
Myocardial ischemia
Dysrhythmias
Hyperglycemia
Fluid/electrolyte abnormalities
Malnutrition

are more common in patients developing hypertension,[4,75] hypertension has not been shown to increase risk for cerebral ischemic events and may only be a marker of neurologic injury.

A recently published study found a correlation between intraoperative hypertension, which persisted for more than 30 minutes, and the development of postoperative renal dysfunction.[16] It seems unlikely that hypertension affected renal function in this study. Perhaps prolonged intraoperative hypertension reflects generalized increases in sympathetic tone with accompanying renal vasoconstriction. Additional studies are required to confirm these findings. **Finally, the level of arterial blood pressure may affect surgical blood loss. Although reports of hypertension exacerbating bleeding are rare and poorly controlled,[55,83] deliberate hypotension has clearly been demonstrated to reduce blood loss.[2,24,50]** However, it is unlikely that transient intraoperative hypertension will substantively affect transfusion requirements.

Postoperative hypertension is more problematic. Following completion of the surgical procedure, patients must be allowed to awaken, assume responsibility for maintenance of their airway, and begin to ambulate and take deep breaths. Deepening the plane of anesthesia is not an acceptable means to correct hypertension in this setting. When postoperative hypertension requires treatment, potent parenteral antihypertensive agents are frequently used. Often such therapy must be closely monitored, necessitating ICU admission. **The incidence of postoperative hypertension is approximately 5% in a general recovery room population[26,30] and exceeds 50% in patients having aortic,[36] carotid,[4,52] and coronary surgery.[29,85]** Thus, in addition to rare complications related to hypertension, considerable money is spent trying to control postoperative hypertension.

As described earlier, changes in plasma catecholamines correlate well with perioperative increases in blood pressure whereas plasma AVP and angiotensin II levels do not. Furthermore, attenuation of postoperative increases in sympathetic nervous system activity decreases the incidence of hypertension following aortic surgery.[9] These data suggest that rather than resorting to potent antihypertensive drugs, perhaps **more attention should be devoted to interventions that decrease the sympathetic response to surgical trauma.** Hypertension following cardiac surgery, however, is not clearly caused by sympathetic nervous system hyperactivity. Clonidine can decrease plasma catecholamines during cardiac surgery without altering blood pressure,[42] whereas stellate ganglion blockade prevents hypertension without altering catecholamine levels.[29] Further work is required in this area.

Myocardial Ischemia

Myocardial ischemia and infarction continue to account for considerable perioperative morbidity and mortality. Despite reports in the literature indicating improved outcomes in some patient subsets,[61] other studies indicate that **ischemia occurs frequently, even in patients identified preoperatively as being at increased risk.**[23] Our inability to substantially reduce the incidence of perioperative ischemic complications, despite improved diagnostic techniques, extensive use of advanced monitoring modalities, and aggressive interventions, is frustrating. There is still considerable uncertainty about the factors responsible for perioperative ischemic events.

Heart rate, blood pressure, and cardiac output are consistently elevated postoperatively. All three are associated with increased myocardial oxygen consumption, and, in patients with fixed coronary lesions, the potential exists for an imbalance between myocardial oxygen supply and demand. It is interesting to note that in nonoperative settings, small-to-moderate increases in heart rate rarely result in ischemia.[21] In contrast, **heart rate changes appear to be highly correlated with postoperative ischemic events, and beta-adrenergic antagonists have been shown to reduce the incidence of perioperative ischemic episodes.**[74]

It may be that postoperative changes in heart rate closely reflect overall sympathetic tone, whereas many other factors affect heart rate in nonoperative settings. Although it seems likely that increases in sympathetic tone produce ischemia by altering myocardial oxygen consumption, alternate mechanisms are possible, including alpha-adrenergic receptor–induced coronary vasoconstriction. Finally, **acute coronary thrombosis as a result of perioperative changes in coagulation may account for some episodes of ischemia/infarction.** This latter mechanism may help to explain the occasional patient without a prior history of ischemic symptoms who develops severe ischemia postoperatively. These patients often have occluded coronary vessels at catheterization or autopsy.

Dysrhythmias

Tachydysrhythmias and ventricular ectopy are common in the perioperative period. Sinus tachycardia is most frequent but is rarely of concern except in patients with underlying ischemic heart disease. **Accelerated junctional rhythms, which are uncommon in the general medical population, are frequently observed during anesthesia, particularly when inhalational anesthetics are used.**[51,54] They appear to be due to increased sensitivity of the AV nodal pacemaker cells to sympathetic tone and may be treated successfully with beta-adrenergic antagonists.[8] Although usually of little hemodynamic significance, they can result in large decreases in cardiac output in patients with poor left ventricular compliance in whom atrial contraction contributes substantially to ventricular filling.[38]

Atrial fibrillation, reciprocating AV nodal tachycardia, and ventricular ectopy also occur in surgical patients, most commonly in the postoperative period. They occur most often in patients with underlying cardiac and/or pulmonary disease and are more common after extensive surgical procedures and after intrathoracic surgery. Although rarely fatal, these dysrhythmias may be associated with a substantial decrease in cardiac output and can precipitate myocardial ischemia. Admission to an ICU is often required for monitoring and treatment. **These rhythm disturbances are multifactorial in origin, but increased sympathetic activity appears to contribute to their high incidence in the perioperative period.** Beta-adrenergic antagonists are useful in controlling these dysrhythmias in many patients. Beta blockers, in addition to having direct myocardial antidysrhythmic effects, may also be beneficial because they prevent and/or treat catecholamine-induced intracellular shifts of potassium and possibly magnesium.

Hyperglycemia

As discussed earlier, blood glucose levels rise substantially during surgery in both healthy patients and patients with diabetes. This rise in blood sugar is mediated by increased levels of epinephrine, glucagon, and cortisol, which act synergistically to increase gluconeogenesis and inhibit peripheral glucose utilization. Although mild transient hyperglycemia is of little concern, when surgical stress results in significant hyperglycemia in diabetic patients, it can complicate management and increase morbidity. **Potential problems associated with hyperglycemia include glucosuria-induced osmotic diuresis, obtundation, impaired leukocyte function,[59] increased cerebralsensitivity to ischemic injury,[73] and hypoglycemiafrom overzealous insulin therapy.** The magnitude of the neurohumoral response to surgery varies with the extent of the procedure and the type of anesthetic and thus may be difficult to predict. Also, there is significant variability in patients' hormonal responses to surgical stress. Although simple regimens exist for perioperative management of patients with diabetes, they do not provide adequate control of blood sugar in many patients and can also occasionally result in hypoglycemia.[34,86] The inadequacies of these regimens have increased the use of continuous insulin infusion techniques. Although these methodologies offer superior glycemic control, they require frequent blood sugar determinations and are labor intensive.

Fluid/Electrolyte Disturbances

As mentioned earlier in this chapter, AVP levels are substantially elevated for several days following most surgical procedures. **This increase in AVP levels, which occurs regardless of plasma osmolality, impairs free water excretion and results in hyponatremia if hypotonic fluids are administered.** The surgical literature contains several reports of severe hyponatremia, seizures, and death in postoperative patients, indicating the potentially serious consequences of this hormonal response to surgery.[93] This complication can be avoided by appropriate fluid therapy. Hypokalemia is common in postoperative patients and often cannot be attributed to either preoperative potassium deficiency or perioperative fluid management. Catecholamine-mediated intracellular shifts of potassium have been suggested as a possible cause of this hypokalemia. Increased renal loss of potassium as a result of high aldosterone levels may also be contributory. Transient postoperative hypokalemia is rarely of major clinical significance; however, considerable effort is often expended trying to correct this abnormality.

Significant weight gain commonly occurs following major surgical procedures. This weight gain is due primarily to increased extracellular water. **Most of this excess water is located near the site of surgical trauma and represents increased interstitial fluid and so-called third space losses.** This fluid accumulation varies with the site of surgery, the amount of tissue trauma, and the nature of replacement fluids administered. In most instances perioperative fluids are administered to maintain normal intravascular volume, and this weight gain does not represent hypervolemia. However, **failure to excrete this excess fluid when it reenters the vascular system can result in clinically significant hypervolemia.**

Most patients with normal cardiac and renal function are able to eliminate this fluid without problem; however, this is not always the case. Careful balance studies suggest that sodium and water retention occurs in most patients postoperatively. This is probably mediated by increases in renal sympathetic nerve activity, which results in augmented proximal tubular sodium avidity, and by elevated levels of cortisol, aldosterone, and AVP. In support of this hypothesis, administration of cortisol, EPI, and glucagon to healthy volunteers results in sodium and water retention. **This tendency toward fluid retention requires close attention to perioperative fluid status, and some patients may require diuretic therapy to avoid and/or treat hypervolemia.**

Malnutrition

Surgical trauma results in increases in protein catabolism and nitrogen excretion. In most well-nourished patients this transient loss of nitrogen is of no clinical importance. However, **in patients who are either nutritionally depleted before surgery or who develop complications that result in a prolonged stress response, hormonally mediated nitrogen wasting following surgery can contribute to malnutrition.** Because nutritional depletion is associated with an increased incidence of postoperative complications and excess mortality,[19,62] this problem is important. Although improved analgetic regimens can attenuate nitrogen loss following surgery, these methodologies do not prevent catabolism. Accordingly, nutritionally depleted patients scheduled for extensive operative procedures should be considered for preoperative nutritional support. Similarly, high-risk patients who have prolonged postoperative catabolism should receive aggressive nutritional therapy.

AFFERENT MECHANISMS RESPONSIBLE FOR PERIOPERATIVE NEUROHORMONAL CHANGES

Many physiologic disturbances capable of eliciting diffuse neurohormonal changes can occur during surgery, including hypotension, hypoxia, hypercarbia, and hypothermia. Most of these abnormalities are uncommon during elective surgery and thus cannot adequately account for the stress response that is routinely noted in surgical patients. Considerable animal and human data suggest that **afferent neuronal signals from the site of the wound account for many perioperative changes in sympathetic activity and hormonal secretion.** Denervation prevents limb-scald injury–induced hormonal alterations in animals.[46] Similarly, studies in paraplegic patients suggest that intact neural pathways are required for expression of the stress response.[47] However, studies using regional anesthetic techniques to prevent afferent sensory traffic have provided inconsistent results.

When inguinal herniorrhaphy is performed with the patient under spinal anesthesia, no increase in ACTH and growth hormone is observed (Fig. 6-11).[58] Variable results have been reported in patients receiving epidural anesthesia for hysterectomy. Data from Enquist et al. indicate that this inconsistency may be due to differences in the level of the block.[27] As shown in Fig. 6-12, the authors noted that suppression of the cortisol response to laparotomy required a sensory block up to the level of T6. Although adequate postoperative analgesia was reported with the lower blocks, cortisol still increased. These data suggest that **neural pathways other than spinal thalamic sensory tracts must also be blocked to prevent complete expression of the stress response.** With more extensive surgical procedures such as gastrectomy, it is possible to attenuate, but not completely prevent, increases in cortisol using epidural anesthetic techniques (Fig. 6-13), even when these

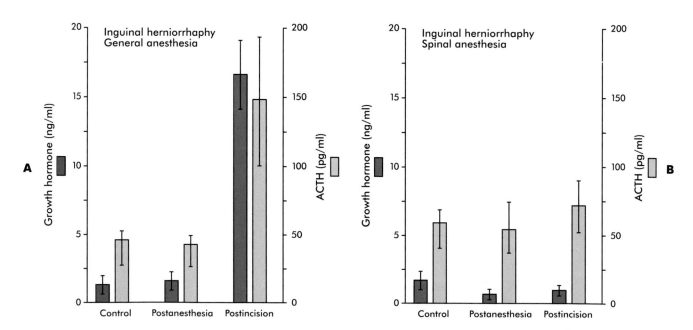

Fig. 6-11. Plasma growth hormone and ACTH levels before surgery, after induction of anesthesia, and 1 hour after skin incision. **A,** Data from nine patients undergoing inguinal herniorrhaphy with general anesthesia. **B,** Data from seven patients undergoing the same procedure with spinal anesthesia. Data shown are means ± SE. (From Newsome HH, Rose JC: The response of human adrenocorticotrophic hormone and growth hormone to surgical stress, *J Clin Endocrinol* 33:481, 1971.)

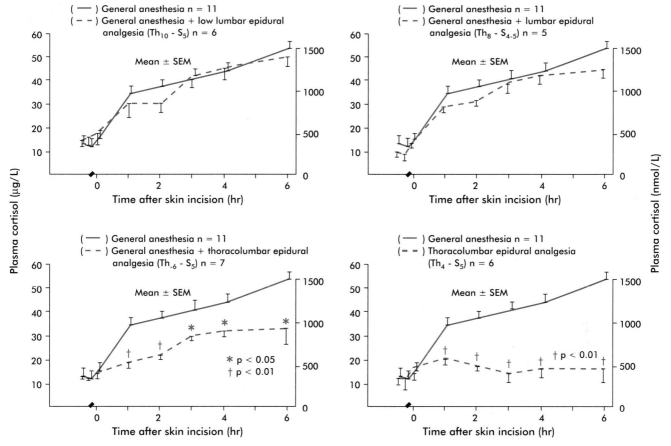

Fig. 6-12. Influence of epidural analgesia on the adrenocortical response to hysterectomy in six patients under low lumbar epidural analgesia and general anesthesia (group II, *upper left*), in five patients under lumbar epidural analgesia and general anesthesia (group III, *upper right*), in seven patients under thoracolumbar epidural analgesia and general anesthesia (group IV, *lower left*), and in six patients under thoracolumbar epidural analgesia without general anesthesia (group V, *lower right*). Included in all figures are 11 control patients (group I) receiving only general anesthesia. Plasma cortisol increased significantly (p < 0.01) in all groups, except in patients exclusively under thoracolumbar epidural analgesia including the fifth thoracic dermatome (group V). * indicates significant difference from control group. (From Engquist A, Brandt MR, Fernandes A et al: The blocking effect of epidural analgesia on the adrenocortical and hyperglycemic responses to surgery, *Acta Anaesthesiol Scand* 21:330, 1977.)

are combined with vagal or splanchnic nerve blockade.[78,79] Increases in plasma catecholamines, however, can be prevented with epidural block.[67]

Fig. 6-14 compares plasma noradrenaline and adrenaline levels following cholecystectomy for patients receiving general anesthesia and parenteral narcotics and for patients in whom 0.25% to 0.5% bupivicaine was used to produce segmental blockade from T4 to L3 throughout the study period. **Patients in the epidural local anesthetic group had complete attenuation of the usual catecholamine response. Serum cortisol levels in this study were lower in patients receiving epidural anesthesia/analgesia but were still elevated above preoperative levels.** Differences in the efficacy of regional anesthesia on these two systems may be due to local anesthetics blocking efferent sympathetic nerve activity.

Because some elements of the stress response following extensive surgical procedures appear to occur independently of afferent neural signals, an alternative mechanism involving humoral mediators must be invoked. Consistent with this hypothesis, Carr et al. report increased secretion of ACTH/cortisol in response to burn injury in animals subjected to prior forearm transplantation of the pituitary.[13] The most likely agents responsible for such effects are inflammatory mediators, such as the interleukins, released by white blood cells at the site of tissue injury. These potent agents, in addition to initiating release of ACTH and similar hormones, also cause fever and increased synthesis of acute phase reactants. Neither of these later phenomena are replicated by infusion of stress hormones into normal volunteers, nor are they blocked by regional anesthetic techniques (Fig. 6-15).[63]

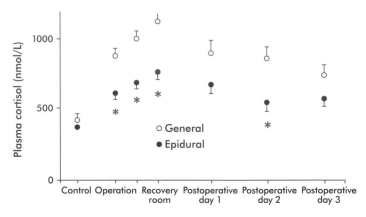

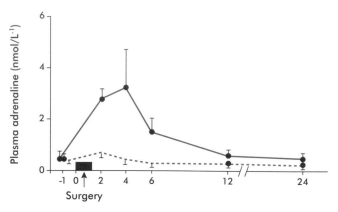

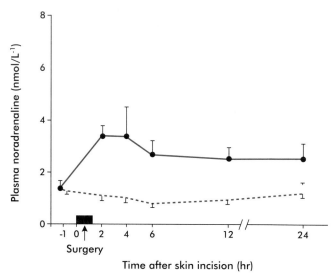

Fig. 6-13. Plasma cortisol levels before, during, and following gastrectomy. Patients (n = 15) in the epidural group received epidural bupivicaine intraoperatively and for postoperative analgesia. (From Tsuji H, Asoh T, Takeuchi Y et al: Attenuation of adrenocortical response to upper abdominal surgery with epidural blockade, *Br J Surg* 70:122, 1983.)

Fig. 6-14. Plasma adrenaline and noradrenaline concentrations (mean ± SEM) before and after cholecystectomy with general anesthesia (●——●); general anesthesia and extradural local anesthesia (●– – –●). (From Rutberg H, Hakanson E, Anderberg B et al: Effects of the extradural administration of morphine, or bupivacaine, on the endocrine response to upper abdominal surgery, *Br J Anaesth* 56:233, 1984.)

To date, however, studies of systemic interleukin levels following surgery have not been able to demonstrate significant elevations. Whether this failure is due to insensitive assays or variable leakage of mediators into the systemic circulation depending on the magnitude of the operation is not known. However, it is possible that white cells activated at the site of injury may travel to distant sites and stimulate some of these processes in a paracrine fashion. Much work remains to be done in this area, including identification of mediators, definition of the time course of mediator-induced changes and the determinants of the magnitude of the response, and elucidation of which systems are activated and their physiologic role in the reaction to tissue injury.

MODIFYING THE STRESS RESPONSE

The introduction of high-dose narcotic techniques for patients undergoing cardiac surgery has markedly altered anesthetic care of the unstable cardiac patient. The profound analgesia induced by large doses of narcotics greatly obviates the need for inhalational anesthetics and thus provides a means to avoid adverse hemodynamic effects of fluorinated hydrocarbons. Furthermore, studies indicate that **high-dose narcotic techniques result in an attenuated hormonal response to surgery.**[32] Fig. 6-16 shows marked suppression of plasma cortisol responses to open heart surgery but normal adrenocortical responses to exogenous ACTH when patients receive large amounts of morphine. This effect of high-dose narcotics on the stress response was recognized as being potentially advantageous and became the center of a major advertising campaign for the manufacturer of fentanyl, a potent synthetic narcotic.

Endocrine effects of high-dose narcotic techniques are widely attributed to superior analgesia; however, other possible mechanisms, such as direct CNS effects of opiates on pathways that mediate aspects of the stress response, have not been excluded. Although intraoperative neurohumoral changes can be suppressed with high dose narcotics, large increases in stress hormones occur as opiate levels fall. Because maintenance of anesthesia for several days is rarely desirable, these agents are of little value in modifying perioperative changes in autonomic nervous system activity and endocrine secretion in most patients.

Regional anesthetic techniques are also capable of attenuating the stress response. When an indwelling catheter is available for readministration of local

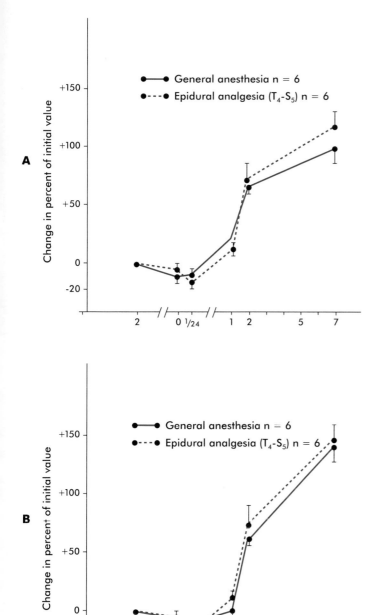

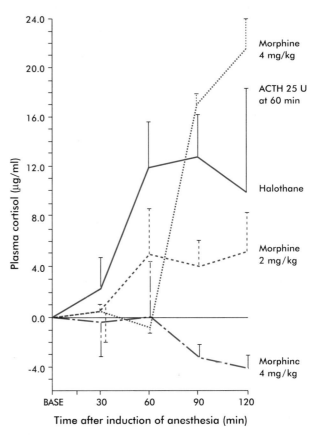

Fig. 6-16. Patients had open heart surgery with either halothane or morphine in varying doses as the anesthetic agent. In one of the two groups of patients receiving 4 mg/kg morphine anesthesia, ACTH 25 U was given intravenously after the 60-minute blood sample was drawn. Plasma cortisol was determined at intervals after induction of anesthesia and was expressed as change from the average of two values (baseline) obtained before induction.
Mean ± SEM. (From George JM, Reier CE, Lanese RR et al: Morphine anesthesia blocks cortisol and growth hormone response to surgical stress in humans, *J Clin Endocrinol Metab* 38:736, 1974.)

Fig. 6-15. Influence of epidural analgesia on postoperative changes in plasma orosomucoid (**A**) and plasma haptoglobin (**B**) following hysterectomy (mean ± SEM). (From Rem J, Nielson OS, Brandt MR et al: Release mechanisms of postoperative changes in various acute phase proteins and immunoglobulins, *Acta Chir Scand* 502:51, 1980.)

anesthetics, these blocks can be maintained for several days. Long-term maintenance of regional blocks is easier and safer than prolonged maintenance of general anesthesia; however, the nonselective neural blockade induced by local anesthetics limits the applicability of this practice. Specifically, motor

blockade often interferes with early ambulation, and sympathetic blockade results in postural hypotension. Although prolonged postoperative use of regional anesthetics has been reported by some investigators, it requires considerable personnel, must be performed in an ICU setting, and represents a considerable expense. This practice is usually reserved for clinical research projects.

Several studies have reported that axial narcotics attenuate some aspects of the stress response, although there are some inconsistencies in the data. Epidural opiates have been reported to decrease postoperative plasma cortisol levels and urinary cortisol excretion in some studies[67,91] but not in others.[44,48] **Sympathetic nervous system activity, however, appears to be consistently reduced in patients receiving epidural opiates.** Fig. 6-17 compares plasma

Fig. 6-17. Arterial plasma concentrations of norepinephrine *(top)*, epinephrine *(center)*, and arginine vasopressin *(bottom)* before induction of anesthesia *(control);* at two points during surgery; and 0, 6, 12, 18, and 24 hours following aortic surgery. *SICU,* surgical intensive care unit; *OR,* operating room *(shaded area).* * = p > 0.5 compared with preinduction value. Data are mean ± SE *(vertical bars).* (From Breslow MJ, Jordan DA, Christopherson R et al: Epidural morphine decreases postoperative hypertension by attenuating sympathetic nervous system hyperactivity, *JAMA* 261[24]:3577, 1989.)

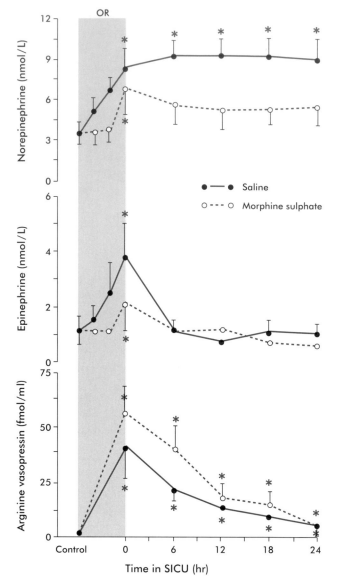

NE, EPI, and AVP levels following aortic surgery in patients randomized to receive either epidural morphine or parenteral morphine for postoperative analgesia. **NE levels in patients receiving epidural morphine were substantially lower than in patients receiving only parenteral narcotics.** Furthermore, patients receiving epidural morphine had a reduced incidence of postoperative hypertension. Although this study found no effect of epidural opiates on plasma AVP levels, other investigators have observed attenuated AVP responses to abdominal and thoracic surgery in patients receiving epidural fentanyl.[6]

Potential explanations for the discrepant findings of these two studies include diferent types of surgical procedures and reduced cephalad spread of fentanyl as a result of greater lipophilicity. This latter possibility raises questions as to the mechanism by which axial narcotics affect stress hormone secretion. If the attenuated response is secondary to the superior analgesia of these techniques, then other analgetic options that offer improved pain relief compared with parenteral narcotics may similarly decrease the hormonal response to surgery. However, if these effects

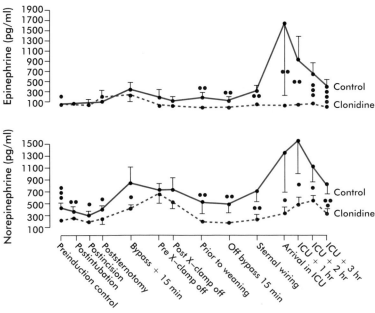

Fig. 6-18. Comparison of plasma epinephrine and norepinephrine levels in control patients (n = 10) and in patients receiving clonidine before and during coronary artery bypass grafting (n = 10). (From Flacke JW, Bloor BC, Flacke WE et al: Reduced narcotic requirement by clonidine with improved hemodynamic and adrenergic stability in patients undergoing coronary bypass surgery, *Anesthesiology* 67:11, 1987.)

are due to stimulation of central opiate receptors, they are specific for the axial narcotics. Despite the widespread use of axial narcotics for postoperative analgesia, little data exist concerning their effects on autonomic nervous system activity and hormonal excretion. Further work in this area should be of considerable interest and may provide additional rationale for use of these techniques in high-risk patients.

Recently, several reports have appeared that suggest that **clonidine, an alpha$_2$-adrenergic agonist, can attenuate the sympathetic nervous system response to surgery.**[28,42] Fig. 6-18 shows EPI and NE levels from 20 patients undergoing coronary artery bypass, half of whom received preoperative and intraoperative clonidine. Catecholamine levels were clearly lower in patients receiving clonidine. Hypertensive and tachycardic responses to noxious stimuli also appear to be reduced by these agents.[28,33] Although hypotension and bradycardia appear to be uncommon, more experience with these drugs is required to establish their safety. Data on the effect of alpha$_2$ agonists on other components of the stress response is limited, and reported effects on selected hormonal systems such as ACTH and cortisol are inconsistent. Finally, no data exist examining the safety and efficacy of these drugs in the postoperative period. Use of alpha$_2$ agents for modulating the stress response has the potential advantage that these agents probably directly modulate central pathways and thus may be titrated to effect. At the current time their use is investigational.

CONCLUSIONS

Surgical trauma elicits a variety of neuronal and endocrine changes that in turn result in substantial physiologic effects. Although the survival benefit of this response is obvious when injury occurs far from medical care, a clear-cut beneficial role for these changes following elective surgery has not been established. Furthermore, physiologic changes resulting from the stress response have the potential to produce complications in patients with underlying medical problems. Several components of the stress response can be attenuated using regional anesthetic techniques, axial narcotics, and alpha$_2$-adrenergic agonists. Results of studies utilizing prolonged postoperative epidural blockade suggest that attenuating surgery induced neurohormonal changes is probably safe.[91] However, at this time, little data exist concerning the clinical utility of such interventions. This is likely to be an area of active investigation in the future.

KEY POINTS

- Surgical trauma results in altered regulatory mechanisms for the secretion of many hormones. AVP increases independent of plasma osmolality changes for up to 5 days. NE is increased for up to 5 days, depending on the magnitude of the procedure. Perioperative hyperglycemia is the result of elevated glucagon levels and subnormal insulin secretion, because of catecholamine suppression.

- Postoperative tachycardia, hypertension, and augmented cardiac output appear to be primarily related to increased sympathetic nervous system activity.

- Hyperglycemia, lipolysis, and protein catabolism, which result from surgical trauma, are the results of epinephrine, glucagon, and cortisol. Lipolysis and protein catabolism provide substrate for further gluconeogenesis.

- Multiple components of the stress response contribute to postoperative interstitial edema; however, problems with hypervolemia are uncommon and easily treated.

- The physiologic role of the stress response, as mediated by catecholamines, AVP, and angiotensin II, is to maintain central perfusion. Cardiac contractility is increased, venous capacitance is decreased, and the extracellular/intravascular compartments are expanded. These physiologic changes may not be well tolerated by the sick or the elderly.

- Sympathetic activity appears to be the major contributor to the adverse cardiovascular effects of this response, which are hypertension, ischemia, and dysrhythmias. Heart rate changes are highly correlated with postoperative ischemia. Beta-adrenergic blockade is effective in modifying these effects.

- The SIADH that results from increased AVP levels postoperatively causes the expansion of extracellular water. Failure to excrete this fluid load as it returns to the vasculature may result in hypervolemia in those patients with impaired renal or cardiac function.

- The protein catabolism and nitrogen excretion mediated by the stress response may result in malnutrition. Those at risk include patients who are nutritionally depleted preoperatively and those with a prolonged stress response. Malnutrition is associated wth an increased incidence of postoperative complications and mortality.

■ The attenuated hormonal response during high-dose narcotic anesthesia may be the result of direct CNS effects and superior analgesia. Sympathetic nervous system activity is consistently reduced in patients receiving epidural opiates compared with parenteral narcotics. This may reflect stimulation of central receptors specific for axial opiates.

■ The physiologic changes resulting from the stress response may not be beneficial to the patient undergoing elective surgery. Components of this response can be modified using regional anesthetics, axial narcotics, and alpha$_2$-adrenergic agonists.

KEY REFERENCES

Bessy PA, Watters JM, Aoki TT et al: Combined hormonal infusion simulates the metabolic response to injury, *Ann Surg* 200:264, 1984.

Eigler N, Sacca L, and Sherwin RS: Glucagon, epinephrine, and cortisol in the dog, *J Clin Invest* 63:114, 1979.

Flacke JW, Bloor BC, Flacke WE et al: Reduced narcotic requirement by clonidine with improved hemodynamic and adrenergic stability in patients undergoing coronary bypass surgery, *Anesthesiology* 67:11, 1987.

Rutberg H, Hakanson E, Anderberg B et al: Effects of the extradural administration of morphine, or bupivacaine, on the endocrine response to upper abdominal surgery, *Br J Anaesth* 56:233, 1984.

Tsuji H, Shirasaka C, Asoh T et al: Effects of epidural administration of local anaesthetics or morphine on postoperative nitrogen loss and catabolic hormones, *Br J Surg* 74:421, 1987.

REFERENCES

1. Adashi EY, Rebar RW, Ehara Y et al: Impact of the acute surgical stress on anterior pituitary function in female subjects, *Am J Obstet Gynecol* 138:609, 1980.
2. Ahlerling TE, Henderson JB, and Skinner DJ: Controlled hypotensive anesthesia to reduce blood loss in radical cystectomy for bladder cancer, *J Urol* 129:953, 1983.
3. Arnetz BB, Lahnborg G, Eneroth P et al: Age-related differences in the serum prolactin response during standardized surgery, *Life Sci* 35:2675, 1984.
4. Asiddao CB, Donegan JH, Whitesell RC et al: Factors associated with perioperative complications during carotid endarterectomy, *Anesth Analg* 61:631-637, 1982.
5. Bessey PA, Watters JM, Aoki TT et al: Combined hormonal infusion simulates the metabolic response to injury, *Ann Surg* 200:264, 1984.
6. Bormann BV, Weidler B, Dennhardt R et al: Influence of epidural fentanyl on stress-induced elevation of plasma vasopressin (ADH) after surgery, *Anesth Analg* 62:727, 1983.
7. Bredbacka S, Blomback M, Hagnevik K et al: Pre- and postoperative changes in coagulation and fibrinolytic variables during abdominal hysterectomy under epidural or general anaesthesia, *Acta Anaesthesiol Scand* 30:204, 1986.
8. Breslow MJ, Evers AS, and Lebowitz P: Successful treatment of accelerated junctional rhythm with propranolol: possible role of sympathetic stimulation in the genesis of this rhythm disturbance, *Anesthesiology* 62:180, 1985.
9. Breslow MJ, Jordan DA, Christopherson R et al: Epidural morphine decreases postoperative hypertension by attenuating sympathetic nervous system hyperactivity, *JAMA* 261:3577, 1989.
10. Brown MJ, Brown DC, and Murphy MB: Hypokalemia from beta$_2$-receptor stimulation by circulating epinephrine, *N Engl J Med* 309:1414, 1983.
11. Buffington CW: Hemodynamic determinants of ischemic myocardial dysfunction in the presence of coronary stenosis in dogs, *Anesthesiology* 63:651, 1985.
12. Cannon WB: *Bodily changes in pain, hunger, fear, and rage*, ed 2, New York, 1934, D Appleton.
13. Carr DB, Ballantyne JC, Osgood PF et al: Pituitary-adrenal stress response in the absence of brain-pituitary connections, *Anesth Analg* 69:197, 1989.
14. Casey JH, Bickel EY, and Zimmerman B: The pattern and significance of aldosterone secretion in the postoperative patient, *Surg Gynecol Obstet* 105:179, 1957.
15. Chan V, Wang C, and Yeung RT: Pituitary-thyroid responses to surgical stress, *Acta Endocrinol* 88:490, 1978.
16. Charlson ME, MacKenzie CR, Gold JP et al: Postoperative renal dysfunction can be predicted, *Surg Gynecol Obstet* 169:303, 1989.
17. Chernow B: Hormonal responses to graded surgical stress, *Arch Intern Med* 147:1273, 1987.
18. Chernow B, Bamberger S, Stoiko M et al: Hypomagnesemia in postoperative intensive care patients, *Chest* 95:391, 1989.
19. Christou NV, Meakins JL, and MacLean LD: The predictive role of delayed hypersensitivity in preoperative patients, *Surg Gynecol Obstet* 2:297, 1981.
20. Cochrane JPS, Forsling ML, Gow NM et al: Arginine vasopressin release following surgical operations, *Br J Surg* 68:209, 1981.
21. Deanfield JE, Maseri A, Selwyn AP et al: Myocardial ischaemia during daily life in patients with stable angina: its relation to symptoms and heart rate changes, *Lancet* 2:753, 1983.
22. Dubois M, Pickar D, Cohen MR et al: Surgical stress in humans is accompanied by an increase in plasma beta-endorphin immunoreactivity, *Life Sci* 29:1249, 1981.
23. Eagle KA, Singer DE, Brewster DC et al: Dipyridamole-thallium scanning in patients undergoing vascular surgery, *JAMA* 257:2185, 1987.
24. Eerola R, Eerola M, Kukinen L et al:

Controlled hypotension and moderate haemodilution in major hip surgery, *Chir Gynaecol* 69:109, 1979.

25. Eigler N, Sacca L, and Sherwin RS: Glucagon, epinephrine, and cortisol in the dog, *J Clin Invest* 63:114, 1979.

26. Eltringham RJ: Complications in the recovery room, *J R Soc Med* 72:278, 1979.

27. Engquist A, Brandt MR, Fernandes A et al: the blocking effect of epidural analgesia on the adrenocortical and hyperglycemic responses to surgery, *Acta Anaesthesiol Scand* 21:330, 1977.

28. Flacke JW, Bloor BC, Flacke WE et al: Reduced narcotic requirement by clonidine with improved hemodynamic and adrenergic stability in patients undergoing coronary bypass surgery, *Anesthesiology* 67:11, 1987.

29. Fouad FM, Estafanous FG, Bravo EL et al: Possible role of cardioaortic reflexes in postcoronary bypass hypertension, *Am J Cardiol* 44:866, 1979.

30. Gal TJ, Cooperman LH: Hypertension in the immediate postoperative period, *Br J Anaesth* 47:70, 1985.

31. Gardner DF, Kaplan MM, Stanley CA et al: Effect of triolodothyronine replacement on the metabolic and pituitary responses to starvation, *N Engl J Med* 300:579, 1979.

32. George JM, Reier CE, Lanese RR et al: Morphine anesthesia blocks cortisol and growth hormone response to surgical stress in humans, *J Clin Endocrinol Metab* 38:736, 1974.

33. Ghignone M, Calvillo O, and Quintin L: Anesthesia and hypertension: the effect of clonidine on perioperative hemodynamics and isoflurane requirements, *Anesthesiology* 67:3, 1987.

34. Goldberg NJ, Wingert TD, Levin ST et al: Insulin therapy in the diabetic surgical patient: metabolic and hormone response to low-dose insulin infusion, *Diabetes Care* 4:279, 1981.

35. Goldman L: Supraventricular tachyarrhythmias in hospitalized adults after surgery, *Chest* 73:450, 1978.

36. Goldman L, Caldera DL: Risks of general anesthesia and elective operation in the hypertensive patient, *Anesthesioogy* 50:785, 1979.

37. Hakanson E, Rutberg H, Jorfeldt L et al: Effects of the extradural administration of morphine or bupivacaine on the metabolic response to upper abdominal surgery, *Br J Anaesth* 57:394, 1985.

38. Haldeman G, Schaer H: Haemodynamic effects of transient atrioventricular dissociation in general anesthesia, *Br J Anaesth* 44:159, 1972.

39. Halter JB, Pflug AE: Relationship of impaired insulin secretion during surgical stress to anesthesia and catecholamine release, *J Clin Endocrinol Metab* 51:1093, 1980.

40. Halter JB, Pflug AE and Porte D Jr: Mechanism of plasma catecholamine increases during surgical stress in man, *J Clin Endocrinol Metab* 45:936, 1977.

41. Hawkins S, Forsling M, Treasure T et al: Changes in pressor hormone concentrations in association with coronary artery surgery, *Br J Anaesth* 58:1267, 1986.

42. Helbo-Hansen S, Fletcher R, Lundberg D et al: Clonidine and the sympaticoadrenal response to coronary artery bypass surgery, *Acta Anaesthesiol Scand* 30:235, 1986.

43. Hilsted J, Christensen NJ, and Madsbad S: Whole body clearance of norepinephrine, *J Clin Invest* 71:500, 1983.

44. Hjortso NC, Christensen NJ, Andersen T et al: Effects of the extradural administration of local anaesthetic agents and morphine on the urinary excretion of cortisol, catecholamines, and nitrogen following abdominal surgery, *Br J Anaesth* 57:400, 1985.

45. Hole A, Unsgaard G: The effect of epidural and general anaesthesia on lymphocyte functions during and after major orthopaedic surgery, *Acta Anaesthesiol Scand* 27:135, 1983.

46. Hume DM, Egdahl RH: The importance of the brain in the endocrine response to injury, *Ann Surg* 150:697, 1959.

47. Hume DM, Bell CC, and Bartter F: Direct measurement of adrenal secretion during operative trauma and convalescence, *Surgery* 52:174, 1962.

48. Jorgensen BC, Andersen HB, and Engquist A: Influence of epidural morphine on postoperative pain, endocrine-metabolic, and renal responses to surgery: a controlled study, *Acta Anaesthesiol Scand* 26:63, 1982.

49. Keller SE, Weiss JM, Schleifer SJ et al: Stress-induced suppression of immunity in adrenalectomized rats, *Science* 221:1301, 1983.

50. Kerr AR: Anaesthesia with profound hypotension for middle ear surgery, *Br J Anaesth* 49:447, 1977.

51. Kuner J, Enescu V, Utsu F et al: Cardiac arrhythmias during anesthesia, *Dis Chest* 52:580, 1967.

52. Lehv MS, Salzman E, and Silen W: Hypertension complicating carotid endarterectomy, *Stroke* 1:307, 1970.

53. Levy MN, Zieske H: Autonomic control of cardiac pacemaker activity and atrioventricular transmission, *J Appl Physiol* 27:465, 1969.

54. Lindgren L: ECG changes during halothane and enflurane anaesthesia for ENT surgery in children, *Br J Anaesth* 53:653, 1981.

55. Mara JE, Baker JL Jr: Hypertesion and haematomas: prophylaxis with apresoline, *Br J Plastic Surg* 30:169, 1977.

56. Modig J, Borg T, Bagge L et al: Role of extradural and of general anaesthesia in fibrinolysis and coagulation after total hip replacement, *Br J Anaesth* 55:625, 1983.

57. Morgan DB, Young RM: Acute transient hypokalemia: new interpretation of a common event, *Lancet* 2:751, 1982.

58. Newsome HH, Rose JC: The response of human adrenocorticotropic hormone and growth hormone to surgical stress, *J Clin Endocrinol* 33:481, 1971.

59. Nolan CM, Beaty JM, and Bagdade JD: Further characterization of the impaired bactericidal function of granulocytes in patients with poorly controlled diabetes, *Diabetes* 27:889, 1978.

60. Porte D Jr, Robertson RP: Control of insulin secretion by catecholamines, stress, and the sympathetic nervous system, *Fed Proc* 32:1792, 1973.

61. Rao TLK, Jacobs KH, and El-Etr AA: Reinfarction following anesthesia in patients with myocardial infarction, *Anesthesiology* 59:499, 1983.

62. Reinhardt GF, Myscofski JW, Wilkens DB et al: Incidence and mortality of hypoalbuminemic patients in hospitalized veterans, *JPEN* 4:357, 1980.

63. Rem J, Fedderson C, Brandt MR et al: Postoperative changes in coagulation and fibrinolysis independent of neurogenic stimuli and adrenal hormones, *Br J Surg* 68:229, 1981.

64. Rem J, Nielsen OS, Brandt MR et al: Release mechanisms of postoperative changes in various acute phase proteins and immunoglobulins, *Acta Chir Scand* 502:51, 1980.

65. Renck H: The elderly patient after anaesthesia and surgery, *Acta Anaesthesiol Scand* 34:1, 1969.

66. Robertson D, Michelakis AM: Effect of anesthesia and surgery on plasma renin activity in man, *J Clin Endocrinol Metab* 34:831, 1972.

67. Rutberg H, Hakanson E, Anderberg B et al: Effects of the extradural administration of morphine, or bupivacaine, on the endocrine response to upper abdominal surgery, *Br J Anaesth* 56:233, 1984.

68. Rutberg H, Kakanson E, Anderberg B et al: Thyroid hormones, catecholamine, and cortisol concentrations after upper abdominal surgery, *Acta Chir Scand* 150:273, 1984.

69. Sandberg AA, Eik-Nes K, Samuels LT et al: The effects of surgery on the blood levels and metabolism of 17-hydroxycorticosteroids, *J Clin Invest* 33:1509, 1954.

70. Selye H: Stress and the general adaptation syndrome, *Br Med J* 1:1383, 1950.

71. Shamoon H, Jacob R, and Sherwin RS: Epinephrine induces platelet fibrinogen receptor expression, fibrinogen binding, and aggregation in whole blood in the absence of other excitatory agonists, *Diabetes* 29:875, 1980.

72. Shattil SJ, Budzynski A, and Scrutton MC: Epinephrine induces platelet fibrinogen receptor expression, fibrinogen binding, and aggregation in whole blood in the absence of other excitatory agonists, *Blood* 73:150, 1989.

73. Sieber FE, Smith DS, Traystman RJ et al: Glucose: a reevaluation of its intraoperative use, *Anesthesiology* 67:72, 1987.

74. Stone JG, Foex P, Sear JW et al: Myocardial ischemia in untreated hypertensive patients: effect of a single small oral dose of a beta-adrenergic blocking agent, *Anesthesiology* 68:495, 1988.

75. Towne JB, Bernhard VM: The relationship of postoperative hypertension to complications following carotid endarterectomy, *Surgery* 88:575, 1980.

76. Tse J, Powell JR, Baste CA et al: Isoproterenol-induced cardiac hypertrophy: modification in characteristics of β-adrenergic receptor, adenylate cyclase, and ventricular contraction, *Endocrinology* 105:246, 1979.

77. Tsuji H, Asoh T, Shirasaka C et al: Inhibition of metabolic responses to surgery with β-adrenergic blockade, *Br J Surg* 67:503, 1980.

78. Tsuji H, Asoh T, Takeuchi Y et al: Attenuation of adrenocortical response to upper abdominal surgery with epidural blockade, *Br J Surg* 70:122, 1983.

79. Tsuji H, Shirasaka C, Asoh T et al: Influences of splanchnic nerve blockade on endocrine-metabolic responses to upper abdominal surgery, *Br J Surg* 70:437, 1983.

80. Tsuji H, Shirasaka C, Asoh T et al: Effects of epidural administration of local anaesthetics or morphine on postoperative nitrogen loss and catabolic hormones, *Br J Surg* 74:421, 1987.

81. Udelsman R, Norton JA, Jelenich SE et al: Responses to the hypothalamic-pituitary-adrenal and renin-angiotensin axes and the sympathetic system during controlled surgical and anesthetic stress, *J Clin Endocrinol Metab* 64:986, 1987.

82. Utsunomiya T, Krausz MM, Dunham B et al: Maintenance of cardiodynamics with aspirin during abdominal aortic aneurysmectomy (AAA), *Ann Surg* 194:602, 1981.

83. Viljoen JF, Estafanous FG, and Tarazi RC: Acute hypertension immediately after coronary artery surgery, *J Thorac Cardiovasc Surg* 71:548, 1976.

84. Vital and Health Statistics: *Heart disease in adults, United States 1960-62,* series II, no 6, Washington DC, 1964, US Dept of Health, Education and Welfare.

85. Wallach R, Karp RB, Reves JG et al: Pathogenesis of paroxysmal hypertension developing during and after coronary bypass surgery: a study of hemodynamic and humoral factors, *Am J Card* 46:559, 1980.

86. Walts LF, Miller J, Davidson MB et al: Perioperative management of diabetes mellitus, *Anesthesiology* 55:104, 1981.

87. Wang C, Chan V, and Yeung RT: Effect of surgical stress on pituitary-testicular function, *Clin Endocrinol* 9:255, 1978.

88. Wartofsky L, Burman KD: Alterations in thyroid function in patients with systemic illness: the euthyroid-sick syndrome, *Endocrine Rev* 3:164, 1982.

89. Watkins L, Lucas SK, Gardner TJ et al: Angiotensin II levels during cardiopulmonary bypass: comparison of pulsatile and non-pulsatile flow, *Surg Forum* 30:229, 1979.

90. Whelan P, Morris PJ: Immunological responsiveness after transurethral resection of the prostate: general versus spinal anaesthetic, *Clin Exp Immunol* 48:611, 1982.

91. Yeager MP, Glass DD, Neff R et al: Epidural anesthesia and analgesia in high-risk surgical patients, *Anesthesiology* 66:729, 1987.

92. Young JB, Rosa RM, Landsberg L: Dissociation of sympathetic nervous system and adrenal medullary responses, *Am J Physiol* 247:35, 1984.

93. Zimmerman B, Wangensteen OH: Observations of water intoxication in surgical patients, *Surgery* 31:654, 1952.

CHAPTER 7

Thrombosis Prophylaxis

TOMMY SYMRENG

Deep venous thrombosis (DVT) and pulmonary embolism (PE) constitute major health problems resulting in significant morbidity and mortality. It is estimated that in the United States DVT and PE are associated with 300,000 to 600,000 hospitalizations a year and that as many as 50,000 persons die each year as a result of PE. In addition, the number of individuals suffering from deep venous insufficiency (DVI) following DVT is estimated at 0.1% to 0.2% of the population and a much larger fraction of the elderly.

Fully **25% of all cases of symptomatic DVT and PE occur postoperatively.** The remaining cases of DVT are associated with nonsurgical conditions such as cardiopulmonary diseases, immobilization, obesity, cancer, stroke, coagulation and fibrinolytic disorders, pregnancy, alcohol and drug abuse, and unknown causes.

A relationship between DVT and PE was identified in the 1840s by Rudolf Virchow. The modern pathophysiology of DVT emanates from Virchow's work that concluded with the famous triad: (1) changes in blood vessel walls, (2) blood flow changes, and (3) changes in the blood.

DVT as a postoperartive complication was first reported in 1894 by von Strauch.[56] DVT prophylaxis was initially mechanical[19,41] via early mobilization, but later heparin,[15] oral anticoagulants,[30] and dextran[27] were used.

DIAGNOSTIC CONSIDERATIONS
Deep Venous Thrombosis

Any vein in the body can thrombose, but postoperative and posttraumatic thrombosis usually occur in the lower extremities. Clinical diagnosis of DVT is unreliable and is wrong about half of the time.

Venography is the "gold standard," because it gives an anatomic and morphologic diagnosis and also a prognostic hint regarding pulmonary embolus because the risk for PE is greater for proximal thrombi, and DVI is more likely if the valves in the popliteal vein are engaged. Disadvantages are variability in film interpretation (10%) and thrombosis associated with the venogram itself.[5]

The fibrinogen uptake test is sensitive in detecting small thrombi, and its correlation with venography is high.[25] Unfortunately, it is not useful for thrombus detection in the pelvis because of high levels of background radioactivity. Moreover, false positive tests are seen with hematoma and inflammatory activity.[25] The clinical relevance of a positive test has also been questioned.[9] Plethysmography and thermography are noninvasive but are relatively insensitive. Doppler ultrasound is also noninvasive, and with newer technology the sensitivity has improved significantly.

Pulmonary Embolism

Clinical diagnosis is very uncertain. The classical symptoms of dyspnea, pleuritis, and hemoptysis are infrequently all seen together. Pulmonary angiography is the most reliable method for detection of PE but is obviously invasive and cumbersome. Ventilation-perfusion scan is less invasive but specificity is lower, especially in the presence of concurrent lung disease.

Other methods including chest radiograph, ECG, and various biochemical tests including arterial Po_2 and fibrinogen degradation product are too nonspecific to be of much diagnostic value.

PREVALENCE

Deep Venous Thrombosis and Pulmonary Embolism

DVT is most commonly caused by factors other than surgery and trauma. DVTs may be present preoperatively. In a mixed surgical population, Laaksonen et al. found 8% of fibrinogen tests positive preoperatively in 107 patients.[28] In hip fractures 8% of patients had DVT verified by preoperative phlebography on day 3 and 15% by day 7.[51]

In general surgery patients over age 40, the incidence of DVT has been reported to be 20% (range 10% to 40%). PE occurred in 1.6% of a general surgical population and lethal PE in almost 1%.[12]

Any patient undergoing orthopedic surgery on a lower extremity is at risk for postoperative development of DVT. The risk is greatest for knee reconstruction and hip surgery, ranging from 45% to 70%. Clinically important PE is reported in up to 20% of patients undergoing hip surgery, with a 1% to 3% incidence of fatal PE.[12]

The incidence of DVT in urologic surgery varies with the procedure. Transurethral surgery had a reported 10% rate, and transvesical prostatectomy had an approximate 40% DVT rate.[12]

The overall risk of DVT in gynecologic surgery was reported as similar to general surgery (7% to 45%), with a similar rate of fatal PE (1%). Patients less than 40 years old undergoing short procedures are considered at low risk with an incidence of DVT less than 3%. Patients 40 to 70 years old are at moderate risk with a 10% to 40% incidence of DVT. The high-risk patients, 40 years or older with added risk factors (varicose veins, infection, malignancy, estrogen therapy, obesity, prolonged surgery or prior DVT/PE), were reported to have a 40% to 70% risk of DVT and 1% to 5% risk of fatal PE.

The incidence of DVT in neurosurgical patients ranged from 9% to 50%. Fatal PE has been seen in 1.5% to 3%. In stroke patients the risk of DVT has been reported to be 75% in the paralyzed leg but only 7% in the nonparalyzed leg.

The risk of thromboembolic disease and PE varies in trauma patients. It was estimated that the incidence of DVT in the young patient with multiple trauma was about 20%. Two subgroups of patients have a significantly higher risk of thrombosis. The elderly patient with a hip fracture and the patient with acute head or spinal cord injury have incidences of DVT about 40% and fatal PE exceeding 4% and 1% respectively.

Deep Venous Insufficiency

DVT and destruction of the popliteal valves are closely related to the development of deep venous insufficiency (DVI). After DVT, symptoms of venous insufficiency gradually increase over time. Tissue induration is seen in 3% of patients 1 year after DVT but is seen in 45% and 72% of patients after 5 and 10 years. Leg ulcers are rare 1 year after DVT but can be seen in 20% and 52% of patients after 5 and 10 years respectively.

FORMATION OF THROMBUS

Fibrinogen uptake studies have indicated that about 50% of the DVTs developed on the day of surgery and an additional 10% to 15% were present after 4 days.[38] Renal transplant patients and patients with malignancies showed later development of DVT.[8,24] Postoperative infection actually seems to delay the onset of DVT. After elective hip surgery two onset peaks for DVT have been noted, one immediately postoperatively and one after 1 week.[7]

The highest incidence of PE appears to be within 24 hours postoperatively. Within 2 weeks, 72% of the patients had evident PE.[14] Lethal PE can be seen weeks postoperatively, and 35% of the patients with lethal PE were seen 3 weeks posttrauma.[47]

PATHOGENESIS OF THROMBOSIS

Thrombosis disease is multifactorial. Several factors seem to cooperate for development of DVT. *Change in the vessel wall* is one known factor in the development of DVT. The endothelial cell is a complex cell that controls permeability and somehow prevents thrombotic buildup. It synthesizes several important products including prostaglandins, bradykinin, angiotensin, plasminogen activators, factor VIII, etc. Venous thrombosis usually develops around valves even in the absence of extensive blood vessel damage, contrary to arterial thrombosis where vessel damage is significant. The oldest part of the clot is composed of fibrin and erythrocytes, whereas platelet aggregation is seen in the growth areas.

Change in blood flow is another factor important for development of DVT. Slowed blood flow will not necessarily cause thrombosis alone but can do so in combination wth other factors (e.g., activation of coagulation factors). Several circumstances during anesthesia and surgery affect venous flow. Positive pressure ventilation decreases venous leg flow.[29] The valve pockets empty slowly with the legs in a horizontal (supine) position. In addition, during anesthesia the calf muscle pumps are not functioning. Any intraoperative reduction of arterial perfusion also contributes to the decreased volume flow. This is partly a result of lowered pressure but more because of zero exercise of the muscles. On the other hand, during epidural anesthesia the arterial flow may be increased, but there still is no muscle exercise.

There are several *changes in the blood* perioperatively. There is a postoperative increase in platelets and also an increased ADP-induced platelet aggregation. Medications modifying platelet function have not had success in DVT prophylaxis, so these changes may not be important in DVT development. There are also postoperative increases in several coagulation factors, including fibrinogen, factor VIII, II, V and VII. These changes are probably not important etiologic factors for thrombosis but may be important for subsequent growth of thrombi. Antithrombin III, an inhibitor for thrombin and activated factor X, is decreased postoperatively, but this has no correlation to postoperative thrombosis.[1] Fibrinolytic activity is increased perioperatively but decreases postoperatively correlating with the increased risk for thrombosis.[40]

These multiple changes in blood vessels, blood flow, and the blood together somehow cause the changes necessary for a thrombus to form. The initiating factors are still unknown in any specific detail.

RISK FACTORS

From epidemiologic and clinical investigations, as well as postmortem findings, numerous risk factors have been identified:

- Age, especially above 40 years[26]
- Surgery (see earlier)
- Multiple trauma
- Prolonged surgery[43]
- Prolonged immobilization[22]
- Previous thromboembolic disease[26]
- Varicose veins[26]
- Malignant disease[26]
- Obesity[26]
- Heart disease, myocardial infarction, heart failure[49]

- Infection[53]
- Pregnancy and postpartum[23]
- Estrogen medication, oral contraceptives[3]

Epidural anesthesia improves venous flow compared with general anesthesia.[29] Modig et al. found that patients undergoing elective hip surgery with epidural anesthesia had significantly less proximal DVT and fewer PE compared with the group that had general anesthesia.[36]

Nutritional factors are somehow linked. DVT is more common in industrialized countries compared with Third World countries.

METHODS FOR THROMBOSIS PROPHYLAXIS

Mechanical Measures

Compressive stockings with decreasing compression proximally do increase leg venous flow.[31] Some have found stockings useful for DVT prophylaxis,[11] whereas others have not.[39]

External pneumatic compression causes intermittent increase in volume flow with washout of different thrombogenic substances. There may also be some activation of the fibrinolytic system. It has proved useful for DVT prophylaxis in nonorthopedic patients undergoing surgery for nonmalignant diseases.[54]

There are indications that external pneumatic compression may have some PE prophylactic effect[42] but controlled studies are few. It is useful only perioperatively and less so postoperatively when the patient is being mobilized. It has a low rate of side effects, but pain, a warm feeling, blistering, and paresthesia along the peroneal nerve have been described.

Interruption of Vena Cava

Numerous methods of interruption of the vena cava have been used in patients with high risk for PE. Ligature of the vena cava causes lower limb edema. Shock can develop secondary to decreased blood return, resulting in some mortality.[58] The newer transvenous cava filters are safer and more efficient in preventing PE and have fewer side effects.[20]

Oral Anticoagulants

Vitamin K is essential for synthesis of coagulation factors II, VII, IX, and X in the liver (prothrombin complex). Oral anticoagulants inhibit synthesis of the active component of the four factors. DVT rates were significantly decreased in orthopedic,[48] surgical,[55] and thoracic surgery patients[52] by oral anticoagulants, as was the rate of lethal PE.[34] The effects of oral anticoagulants are better the earlier the treatment is started. Ideally the patient should be anticoagulated during surgery. Five days of treatment is necessary to reach therapeutic level. Oral anticoagulants are contraindicated with severe bleeding, malignant hypertonia, neurosurgery or eye surgery, and severe liver and kidney disease.

The half-life for different drugs varies from 5 hours for fenindion, 42 hours for warfarin, and 24 to 100 hours for dicumarol. Oral anticoagulants interact with several medications. Some increase the anticoagulant effect (cimetidine, tricyclic antidepressants, steroids), whereas others decrease it (barbiturates, diuretics, diazepam, heparin).

Bleeding is the major side effect of thrombosis prophylaxis, but skin necrosis may also occur. Oral anticoagulants also cross the placenta and can have a teratogenic effect. The anticoagulant effect can be reversed in 6 to 36 hours with vitamin K and even faster with fresh frozen plasma.

Heparin
Low-dose heparin

Heparin can be given in such low doses that regular coagulation tests are not affected. These low doses have thrombosis prophylactic properties if given before surgical trauma occurs. The effect on coagulation depends on molecular weight. Heparin with low molecular weight potentiates the specific inhibition of activated factor X, but heparin with higher molecular weight affects the whole coagulation system.[2] The low molecular fractions are advantageous as thrombosis prophylaxis, and theoretically the risk for bleeding should be less. Commercial heparins are heterogenous and hold several components with molecular weights between 6000 and 30,000. Recently, more homogenous low molecular weight heparin (LMWH) has become available for clinical use.

Heparin binds to antithrombin III to exert its anticoagulation activity. The main reservoir for heparin is the mast cells where it is produced, but heparin can also be found in the basophilic granulocytes.

In addition to its effects on hemostasis, heparin has antilipemic activity and causes complement inhibition. Small amounts of heparin activate lipoprotein lipase and stimulate the reticuloendothelial system, resulting in increased phagocytosis.

Heparin is removed from the circulation through the reticuloendothelial system. The mean half-life is 90 minutes with a range of 23 to 360 minutes.

Heparin accelerates serine proteinase neutralizing effects of antithrombin III. The proteinases that are inhibited are thrombin, plasmin, kallikrein, C1-esterase, urokinase, and the activated coagulation factors VII, IX, X, XI and XII. Because the coagulation system is a multiplicating cascade, a few molecules of factor XIIa eventually activate a large number of thrombin molecules. Hence, fewer antithrombin III molecules are needed to inhibit factor Xa than thrombin. For the same reason heparin

should be given before surgical trauma, before the activation of factor X, and later thrombin.

Prophylactic use of therapeutic doses of heparin postoperatively[16] was not widely used before because of the risk of bleeding.

Low-dose heparin administered subcutaneously every 8 or 12 hours started preoperatively reduces the rate of DVT by about 60% on proximal thrombi and PE by about 50% in general surgery, urology, moderate-to-high risk gynecologic surgery, and neurosurgery but is less beneficial in orthopedic patients. When begun within 2 days after trauma, the DVT rate is also decreased.[12] Low-dose heparin has been used in two different regimens, 5000 IU every 8 or every 12 hours. There does not seem to be a difference between the two regimens with respect to a DVT prophylactic effect, but there are more bleeding complications if the drug is given every 8 hours. The prophylaxis should be continued for a week or until the patient leaves the hospital because the prophylactic effect comes to an end as the heparin is discontinued.

Some recommend that epidural analgesia should be avoided in patients receiving low-dose heparin,[50] but several studies report no problems with the combination.[4,6,8,35,46]

Bleeding is the most common side effect. Wound hematoma is somewhat more common (5% to 10%) in patients on low-dose heparin. In most studies there was, however, no difference in the number of transfusions or the decrease in hemoglobin between control patients and heparin-treated patients.

Heparin rarely causes thrombocytopenia. This is probably of immunologic origin and can also be seen after low-dose heparin administration. Thrombocytopenia occurs after 2 days to 3 weeks of heparin treatment. The reaction is reversible when heparin is discontinued.

Low molecular weight heparin

Low molecular weight heparin (LMWH) has recently been introduced for clinical use. It has a favorably high antifactor Xa:antifactor IIa activity ratio, which implies an improved antithrombotic potential with fewer bleeding side effects. In recent studies LMWH compared favorably with regular heparin 5000 IU administered every 8 hours after abdominal surgery. The LMWH group had significantly fewer DVTs (distal and proximal) and significantly fewer PEs.[18] The bleeding complications were similar in both groups. In another study LMWH was significantly better than dextran for DVT prophylaxis in total hip replacement,[17] and there was even a lower blood loss in the LMWH group. Further studies are needed to verify its usefulness under different clinical circumstances.

Heparin and Other Agents
Dihydroergotamine and low-dose heparin

Dihydroergotamine (DHE) is an alpha-adrenergic receptor stimulant but also causes an increase in venous smooth muscle tone. Its effect on resistance vessels is much less than its venous effect. This results in increased venous flow. DHE alone has some DVT prophylactic effect, but the combination with low-dose heparin has proved quite effective as DVT prophylaxis[32] and PE prophylaxis[21] in orthopedic surgery. DHE is contraindicated in pregnant women.

Low-dose heparin and dextran

Low-dose heparin and dextran lead to two simultaneous but different hemostatic defects,[10] and more bleeding complications were seen after vascular surgery.[37]

Dextran

Dextran, a polysaccharide, was introduced as a plasma substitute in the 1940s. It has several effects on different physiologic systems. Dextran has a colloid osmotic effect. A gram of dextran binds 20 to 25 ml water (1 g albumin binds 18 ml water) and thereby causes effective volume expansion. Low molecular weight dextran (dextran 40) causes disaggregation of erythrocytes, resulting in decreased viscosity. Dextran causes improvement in blood flow through decreased erythrocyte aggregation, hemodilution, and passive capillary dilatation secondary to the colloid osmotic effect. It decreases platelet adhesiveness to vascular endothelium and to foreign material. Coagulation factor VIII decreases with dextran infusion, but the other coagulation factors and the fibrinolytic system are not affected. Clots formed in the presence of dextran are more easily lysed than control clots.[57] Dextran decreases the rate of DVT and PE in general and orthopedic surgery, gynecology, and trauma.[12] It is somewhat less effective in preventing small lower leg thrombi compared with low-dose heparin but is more effective than the latter in orthopedic surgery. Dextran is equal to the oral anticoagulants in DVT and PE.

BOX 7-1
RING AND MESSMER'S GRADED REACTIONS

Grade I: Skin manifestations, lumbar pain, low grade
Grade II: Mild-to-moderate hypotension, respiratory distress
Grade III: Severe hypotension, shock, severe bronchospasm
Grade IV: Cardiac/respiratory arrest

The recommended dose is 500 ml dextran intraoperatively and 500 ml postoperatively. Another 500 ml is given the first postoperative day, and in hip surgery another 500 ml should be given days 3 and 5 as well. There is some risk for volume overload in older patients with cardiac failure, but this can usually be avoided if the infusion is given slowly.

Bleeding time is most prolonged 3 to 9 hours after the infusion. Dextran doses of less than 1 g/kg body weight do not seem to interfere with hemostasis. Increased bleeding can be seen in individual patients especially if large amounts of dextran have been given, but several studies found no increased bleeding compared to control patients.[8]

Severe anaphylactic reactions to colloid volume substitutes occur in 0.003% of plasma infusions; 0.006% with hetastarch; 0.008% with dextran; and 0.038% with gelatin.[45]

Reactions of this type are usually graded according to Ring and Messmer (Box 7-1).[44]

The reaction always occurs during the initial part of the dextran infusion, but the earlier the reaction, the more serious the symptoms. There is a correlation between titer of antibodies to dextran and severity of the reaction. Very low molecular weight dextran (dextran 1) used for hapten inhibition in dextran anaphylaxis has successfully reduced the severe reactions (Grades III and IV) by 95%[33] and should consequently always be given before other dextran preparations are administered.

Substances Affecting Platelets
Acetylsalicylic acid

Epinephrine, collagen, and thrombin cause release of numerous substances from platelets (e.g., adenosine driphosphate [ADP], platelet factor 4, serotonin, and adenosine triphosphate [ATP]). Acetylsalicylic acid (ASA) inhibits release of these factors induced by epinephrine and collagen, but thrombin-induced release is inhibited much less. The blocked ADP release results in inhibited platelet aggregation lasting up to 1 week after a single dose of ASA. Bleeding time is prolonged. There have been conflicting results of the effect of ASA on DVT and PE, probably dependent on dose variations. With low doses, thromboxane A_2 inhibition is achieved with inhibition of platelet aggregation. Higher doses also inhibit prostacycline (PGI_2) and thereby reverse the prolonged bleeding time. Unfortunately, several studies have shown no beneficial effect of ASA on DVT or PE, and it cannot be currently recommended for DVT prophylaxis in connection with surgery or trauma.

Dipyridamole

Dipyridamole was initially used as a vasodilator but it also inhibits ADP-induced platelet aggregation. Some effects have been shown on both arterial and venous experimental thrombosis. Clinically, reductions of embolus rate from artificial heart valves and in small vessel occlusion in transplanted kidneys were seen, but no effect with respect to thrombosis prophylaxis for hip surgery could be documented.

Hydroxychloroquine

Hydroxychloroquine, an antimalaria preparation that is also used in rheumatology, inhibits ADP-induced aggregation of platelets. Several studies have documented its usefulness for DVT prophylaxis[59] in general surgery.

Other Methods
Fibrinolytic stimulation

The combination fenformine-ethyloestronol stimulates blood-spontaneous fibrinolytic activity. This method has been tried for DVT prophylaxis without success.

Lidocaine

Lidocaine, a local anesthetic, suppresses adhesion of leukocytes to venous endothelium, but the coagulation and fibrinolytic systems are not affected. Lidocaine given perioperatively decreased the rate of DVT compared with control patients without increasing bleeding complications.[13]

CLINICAL APPLICATIONS OF THROMBOSIS PROPHYLAXIS

Both PE and DVI are relatively common, the former often lethal, the latter resulting in long-term suffering for the patient. In lethal PE there is a time problem. Within 15 minutes after the onset of symptoms, 39% of the patients are dead and 57% of the patients die within 1 hour. Untreated, PE has 30% mortality. These circumstances make the discussion of prophylaxis very important because time for diagnosis and treatment is short. On the other hand, the time course for DVI is so long that the pathogenesis is not completely known.

The most important risk factors are age, obesity, extent of surgery, earlier thromboembolic disease, and malignancy. The lower age limit for general prophylaxis should be 40 to 50 years.

In general surgery, available data justify routine prophylaxis of all high-risk surgical patients (see preceding discussion). Low-dose heparin with or without DHE, LMWH, and dextran are all effective. Both external pneumatic compression and gradient elastic stockings are effective especially if combined with heparin or dextran.[12]

In orthopedic surgery, patients undergoing hip surgery or knee reconstruction are at high risk, and oral anticoagulants, dextran, low-dose heparin-DHE, and LMWH can be used for prophylaxis. For hip fracture surgery, low-dose heparin is an inadvisable choice because it cannot be given before the trauma that activates factor X. Mechanical methods may also be used if feasible for other patients.

In urology, patients over the age of 40 undergoing transvesical surgery should have DVT prophylaxis. The use of low-dose heparin and dextran are well documented. Pneumatic compression offers an attractive alternative although more trials are necessary in urologic patients.

In gynecologic and obstetric surgery graduated-compression stockings and early ambulation are satisfactory in low-risk patients. Patients at moderate and high risk can be managed with low-dose heparin or dextran with or without external pneumatic compression. The latter is suggested for patients with malignancies. Oral anticoagulants are also useful in high-risk patients. Oral contraceptives and estrogen therapy should be discontinued before elective surgical procedures.

In neurosurgical patients undergoing extracranial surgery such as laminectomy, low-dose heparin and external pneumatic compression are effective either alone or in combination. For intracranial surgery a bleeding complication could be devastating; consequently, external pneumatic compression is recommended.[12] In multiple trauma patients, anticoagulants should be used with caution until the injuries have been assessed and bleeding controlled. Low-dose heparin or dextran is effective if initiated early.[12]

KEY POINTS

- Many anesthesiologists either do not know about or choose to minimize the importance of DVT in PE, both as a major public health problem and also as a significant perioperative problem. A full 25% of all cases of symptomatic DVT and PE occur postoperatively.

- The "gold standard" for the diagnosis of DVT is venography.

- In general surgery patients over age 40, the incidence of deep venous thrombosis postoperatively has been reported to be approximately 20%, with pulmonary embolus 1.6%, and lethal pulmonary embolus in approximately 1%. The incidence is worse in orthopedic surgery and probably in post-trauma patients.

- The anesthesiologist should understand the complications of low-dose heparin therapy, which is administered to many surgical patients at risk for DVT.

- Patients taking aspirin clearly do have prolonged bleeding times, but this drug does not necessarily have a salutary effect on DVT or PE.

- The anesthesiologist should have a clear idea, based on the literature, about whether or not various kinds of regional anesthesia are indicated in patients who are taking various anticoagulants.

KEY REFERENCES

Blaisdell FW: Low-dose heparin prophylaxis of venous thrombosis, *Am Heart J* 97:685, 1979 (editorial).

Consensus Conference: Prevention of venous thrombosis and pulmonary embolism, *JAMA* 256:744, 1986.

Gruber UF, Glattli S, Kradolfer S et al: Fatal postoperative embolism in trauma and orthopedic surgery, *Eur Surg Res* 12(suppl 1):69, 1980.

Kakker VV, Howe CT, Nicolaides AN et al: Deep vein thrombosis of the leg: is there a "high-risk" group? *Am J Surg* 120:527, 1970.

Laaksonen VS, Arola MKJ, Kivisaari A et al: Effect of different modes of operative anaesthesia on the clearance time of ^{125}I-fibrinogen from calf veins, *Ann Chir Res* 6:356, 1974.

Modig J, Hjelmstedt A, Sahlstedt B et al: Comparative influences of epidural and regional anaesthesia on deep venous thrombosis and pulmonary embolism after total hip replacement, *Acta Chir Scand* 14:125, 1981.

Special report: Prevention of venous thromboembolism in surgical patients by low-dose heparin. Prepared by the Council on Thrombosis by the American Heart Association, *Circulation* 55:423, 1977.

REFERENCES

1. Åberg M, Nilsson IM, and Hedner U: Antithrombin III after operation, *Lancet* II:1337, 1973.
2. Andersson LO, Barrowcliffe TW, Holmer E et al: Molecular weight dependency of the heparin potentiated inhibition of thrombin and activated factor X. Effect of heparin neutralization in plasma, *Thromb Res* 15:531, 1979.
3. Åstedt B, Bernstein K, Casslén B et al: Estrogens and postoperative thrombosis evaluated by the radioactive iodine method, *Surg Gynecol Obstet* 151:372, 1980.
4. Ballard RM, Bradley-Watson PJ, Johnstone FD et al: Low doses of subcutaneous heparin in the prevention of deep vein thrombosis after gynaecological surgery, *J Obstet Gynaecol Br Commonw* 80:469, 1973.
5. Berge T, Bergquist D, Efsing Ho et al: Local complications to ascending phlebography, *Clin Radiol* 29:691, 1978.
6. Bergqvist D, Efsing HO, Hallböök T et al: Thromboembolism after elective and posttraumatic hip surgery—a controlled prophylactic trial with dextran and low-dose heparin, *Acta Chir Scand* 145:213, 1979.
7. Bergqvist D, Elvelin R, Eriksson U et al: Thrombosis following hip arthroplasty: a

study using phlebography and ^{125}I-fibrinogen test, *Acta Orthop Scand* 47:549, 1976.
8. Bergqvist D, Hallböök T: Prophylaxis of postoperative venous thrombosis in a controlled trial comparing dextran 70 and low-dose heparin: a study with the ^{125}I-fibrinogen test, *World J Surg* 4:239, 1980.
9. Blaisdell FW: Low-dose heparin prophylaxis of venous thrombosis, *Am Heart J* 97:685, 1979 (editorial).
10. Bloom WL, Brewer S: The independent yet synergistic effects of heparin and dextran, *Acta Chir Scand* 387(suppl):53, 1968.
11. Bolton J: The prevention of postoperative deep venous thrombosis by graduated compression stockings, *Scott Med J* 23:333, 1978.
12. Consensus Conference: Prevention of venous thrombosis and pulmonary embolism, *JAMA* 256:744, 1986.
13. Cooke ED, Bowcock S, Lloyd MJ et al: Intravenous lignocaine in prevention of deep venous thrombosis after elective hip surgery, *Lancet* II:797, 1977.
14. Coon WW, Coller FA: Some epidemiological considerations of thromboembolism, *Surg Gynecol Obstet* 109:487, 1959.
15. Crafoord C: Preliminary report on postoperative treatment with heparin as a

preventive of thrombosis, *Acta Chir Scand* 79:407, 1936.
16. Crafoord C, Jorpes E: Heparin as a prophylaxis against thrombosis, *JAMA* 116:2832, 1941.
17. Eriksson BI, Zachrisson BE, Teger-Nilsson AC et al: Thrombosis prophylaxis with low molecular weight heparin in total hip replacement, *Br J Surg* 75:1053, 1988.
18. The European Fraxiparin Study (EFS) Group: Comparison of a low molecular weight heparin and unfractionated heparin or the prevention of deep vein thrombosis in patients undergoing abdominal surgery, *Br J Surg* 75:1058, 1988.
19. Frykholm R: Om ventrombosens patogenes och mekaniska profylax, *Nord Med* 4:3534, 1939.
20. Fullen WD, Miller EH, Steele WF et al: Prophylactic vena caval interruption in hip fractures, *J Trauma* 13:403, 1973.
21. Gruber UF, Glättli S, Kradolfer S et al: Fatal postoperative embolism in trauma and orthopedic surgery, *Eur Surg Res* 12(suppl 1):69, 1980.
22. Heatley RV, Hughes LE, Morgan A et al: Preoperative or postoperative deep-vein thrombosis, *Lancet* I:437, 1976.
23. Henry M: Pulmonary embolism and maternal mortality 1966-1973, *J Irish Med Assoc* 68:175, 1975.

24. Joffe SN: The incidence of postoperative deep vein thrombosis, *Thromb Res* 7:141, 1975.
25. Kakkar VV, Corrigan TP, Fossard DP et al: Prevention of fatal postoperative pulmonary embolism by low doses of heparin: reappraisal of results, Int Multicentre Trial, *Lancet* I:567, 1977.
26. Kakkar VV, Howe CT, Nicolaides AN et al: Deep vein thrombosis of the leg: is there a "high-risk" group? *Am J Surg* 120:527, 1970.
27. Koekenberg LJL: Experimental use of macrodex as a prophylaxis against postoperative thromboembolism, *Exp Med Amst* 40:123, 1961.
28. Laaksonen VO, Arola MKJ, Hannelin M et al: Effect of anesthesia on the incidence of postoperative lower limb thrombosis, *Ann Chir Gynaecol* 62:304, 1973.
29. Laaksonen VO, Arola MKJ, Kivisaari A et al: Effect of different modes of operative anaesthesia on the clearance time of ^{125}I-fibrinogen from calf veins, *Ann Chir Res* 6:356, 1974.
30. Lehmann J: Thrombosis (treatment and prevention with methyl-bishydroxycoumarin), *Lancet* I:611, 1943.
31. Lewis C, Antoine J, Mueller C et al: Elastic compression in the prevention of venous stasis: a critical reevaluation, *Am J Surg* 132:739, 1976.
32. Lindblad B, Bergqvist D, and Hallböök T: Tromboemboliprevention med dextran 70, dihydroergotaminheparin samt en sulfaterad polysaccarid. Slutrapport, *Sv Läkaresällsk Handl* 88:KI 150, 1979.
33. Ljungström KG, Renck H, Hedin H et al: Hapten inhibition and dextran anaphylaxis, *Anaesthesia* 43:729, 1988.
34. Matis P: Postoperative anticoagulant therapy, *Clin Obstet Gynecol* 11:281, 1968.
35. McCarthy TG, McQueen J, Johnstone FD et al: A comparison of low-dose subcutaneous heparin and intravenous dextran 70 in the prophylaxis of deep venous thrombosis after gynaecological surgery, *J Obstet Gynaecol Br Commonw* 81:486, 1974.
36. Modig J, Hjelmstedt Å, Sahlstedt B et al: Comparative influences of epidural and regional anaesthesia on deep venous thrombosis and pulmonary embolism after total hip replacement, *Acta Chir Scand* 147:125, 1981.
37. Morrison ND, Stephenson CBS, Maclean D et al: Deep vein thrombosis after femoropopliteal bypass grafting with observations on the incidence of complications following the use of dextran 70, *N Z Med J* 84:233, 1976.
38. Nicolaides AN: Prevention of deep vein thrombosis, *Geriatrics* 28:69, 1973.
39. Nillius A, Nylander G: Deep vein thrombosis after total hip replacement: a clinical and phlebographic study, *Br J Surg* 55:324, 1979.
40. Nilsson IM: Coagulation, fibrinolysis, and venous thrombosis, *Triangle* 16:19, 1977.
41. Ochsner A, DeBakey MD: Therapy phlebothrombosis and thrombophlebitis, *Arch Surg* 40:208, 1940.
42. Pedegana L, Burgess E, Moore J et al: Prevention of thromboembolic disease by external pneumatic compression in patients undergoing total hip arthroplasty, *Clin Orthop* 128:190, 1977.
43. Rakoczi I, Chamone D, Verstraete M et al: The relevance of clinical and hemostasis parameters for the prediction of postoperative thrombosis of the deep veins of the lower extremity in gynecologic patients, *Surg Gynecol Obstet* 151:225, 1980.
44. Ring J, Messmer K: Anaphylaktoide reaktionen nach infusion kolloidaler volumenersatzmittel, *Chir Praxis* 21:1, 1976.
45. Ring J, Messmer K: Incidence and severity of anaphylactoid reactions to colloid volume substitutes, *Lancet* I:466, 1977.
46. Schöndorf T, Weber U: Heparin prophylaxis combined with DHE or dextran in hip operations, *Thromb Diathes* 42:249, 1979.
47. Sevitt S: Venous thrombosis and pulmonary embolism: their prevention by oral anticoagulants, *Am J Med* 33:703, 1962.
48. Sevitt S, Gallagher NG: Prevention of venous thrombosis and pulmonary embolism in injured patients, *Lancet* II:981, 1959.
49. Simmons AV, Sheppard MA, and Cox AF: Deep venous thrombosis after myocardial infarction: predisposing factors, *Br Heart J* 35:623, 1973.
50. Special report: Prevention of venous thromboembolism in surgical patients by low-dose heparin. Prepared by the Council on Thrombosis by the American Heart Association, *Circulation* 55:423, 1977.
51. Stevens J, Fardin R, and Freeark R: Lower extremity thrombophlebitis in patients with femoral neck fractures: a venographic investigation and a review of the early and late significance of the findings, *J Trauma* 8:527, 1968.
52. Storm O: Anticoagulant protection in surgery, *Thromb Diathes Haemorrh* 2:484, 1958.
53. Törngren S, Hägglund G, Molin K et al: Postoperative deep venous thrombosis and infectious complications: a clinical study of patients undergoing colorectal surgery, *Scand J Infect Dis* 12:123, 1980.
54. Turpie A, Hirsh J: Prophylaxis and therapy of venous thromboembolism, *Crit Rev Clin Lab Sci* 10:247, 1979.
55. van der Linde DL: Het voorkomen an postoperative diepe venueze thrombose. Thesis, Nijmegen 1975.
56. von Strauch M: Über Venenthrombose der unteren Extremitäten nach Koliotomien bei Bechenhochlagerung und Aethernarkose, *Zentralbl Gynakol* 18:304, 1894.
57. Wallenbeck I, Tangen O: On the lysis of fibrin formed in the presence of dextran and other macromolecules, *Thromb Res* 6:75, 1975.
58. Wheeler CG, Thompson JE, Austin DJ et al: Interruption of the inferior vena cava for thromboembolism, *Ann Surg* 163:199, 1966.
59. Wu T, Tsapogas M, Jordan R: Prophylaxis of deep venous thrombosis by hydroxychloroqine sulfate and heparin, *Surg Gynecol Obstet* 145:714, 1977.

CHAPTER 8

Recovery Management of the Healthy Patient

DAVID L. DULL

Transport
PACU Care
Complications in the PACU
  Pain
  Hypothermia and postoperative tremors
  Nausea and vomiting
  Agitation and delirium
  Obtundation
Neuromuscular Complications
Respiratory Complications
  Airway obstruction
  Hypoxia
  Hypoventilation
Cardiovascular Complications
  Hypotension
  Hypertension
  Dysrhythmias
Renal Complications
  Oliguria
  Polyuria
Postoperative Bleeding

The immediate postoperative period is a time when patients undergo many rapid changes. It is a period of vulnerability even for relatively healthy patients. Studies of anesthetic morbidity and mortality have identified the immediate postoperative period as a time when patients are at significant risk of experiencing anesthetic and/or surgical complications.* Despite the well-documented risk, specialized care

*References 27, 63, 66, 93, 96, 100, 130, 151, 155.

during the immediate postoperative period is a relatively new development.

Before 1950, patients were usually cared for in an ill-defined postoperative unit or on the hospital ward. Patients were frequently transferred from the operating room directly to the ward where they were placed close to the nursing station, or a private duty nurse was employed to maximize postoperative care. **In 1947 the U.S. Anesthesia Study Commission published the results of an 11-year study of anesthetic mortality. They concluded that nearly one third of the anesthetic deaths were a result of inadequate postoperative monitoring.**[130] **These findings, along with a critical nursing shortage, stimulated widespread development of recovery rooms.**[164]

Today, despite the routine use of recovery rooms, the immediate postoperative period continues to be a time when patients are at risk for developing complications.[27,153] This chapter will examine common difficulties experienced by healthy patients in the recovery room and discuss their evaluation and management.

TRANSPORT

Care of the postoperative patient begins in the operating room when the patient is transferred to the gurney for transport. Patients should be transported in the lateral position to the postanesthesia care unit (PACU) to help prevent aspiration unless they are wide awake or there are compelling surgical reasons not to do so. Whenever possible, patients should be transported with the gurney side rails up. Care must be taken to ensure that all extremities are within the side rails. During transport to the PACU, the patient must be observed for evidence of vomiting or airway obstruction secondary to the accumulation of blood or

secretions in the pharynx. **If airway obstruction from these causes is likely, the patient can be transported in a head-down position to facilitate clearance of the secretions from the airway; however, such a position makes oxygenation and ventilation more difficult.**

Ventilation should be monitored during transport by observing the patient's chest and abdomen and by feeling the movement of air during inspiration and exhalation. If ventilation is marginal, the patient should remain intubated and ventilation assisted or controlled during transport. Development of hypoxia during transport has been well described in both adult[141,153] and pediatric patients.[23,72,107,122] **It has also been demonstrated that clinical assessments of oxygenation are unreliable for identification of hypoxia during transport[122] and that apparent recovery from anesthesia does not protect the patient from transport hypoxia.**[142] These findings have been used to justify the routine use of supplemental oxygen during transport.[115,142] It has not been demonstrated that transient, usually mild hypoxia experienced by patients during transport is detrimental. Costs and complications associated with routine use of supplemental oxygen during transport from the operating room to the PACU have not been explored. It is possible that transport with oxygen delivered through an opaque mask may increase the incidence of unrecognized aspiration or laryngospasm. We believe it is reasonable to preoxygenate the patient before transport[157] and then to transport expeditiously. If inadequate oxygenation is likely during transport of the patient, such as during lengthy transports or in patients with severe pulmonary or chest wall abnormalities, transport with pulse oximetry and supplemental oxygen is advisable.

PACU CARE

On entry into the PACU any patient who has received general anesthesia or sedation should be given supplemental oxygen. Once this has been provided the patient should be connected to appropriate monitoring devices and assessed by the caregiver. Following assessment of the patient, a complete report should be given to the PACU caregiver by the responsible anesthesiologist.

The specific method of administration and quantity of oxygen administered depends on patient pathology and clinical circumstances (see hypoxia section). In older children and adult patients who are otherwise healthy, therapy can usually be initiated with 2 to 4 L/min of oxygen by nasal cannula. In young pediatric patients, humidified "blow by" oxygen is usually sufficient. Modification of the initial therapy is based on the oxygen saturation as measured by the pulse

oximeter. After the patient has recovered from the immediate effects of the anesthetic, oxygen therapy can be discontinued while monitoring for desaturation. Should desaturation occur, it is advisable to transfer the patient to the regular patient care unit on oxygen therapy sufficient to maintain satisfactory oxygen saturations.

Monitoring should include measurements of temperature, heart rate, blood pressure, respiratory rate, and oxygen saturation on PACU admission. Thereafter, ECG should be monitored continuously and vital signs measured and recorded at least every 15 minutes. Continuous monitoring of patients with pulse oximeters will soon become the standard of care because significant hypoxia has been demonstrated frequently in healthy patients in the PACU.[102]

Once the initial PACU assessment has been obtained and oxygen administered, a report including the patient's name, operation, diagnosis, a list of allergies and preoperative medications, and pertinent findings from the history and physical examination should be given to the PACU care provider. The anesthesiologist should briefly describe the anesthetic administered, including whether muscle relaxants and reversal agents were given, the method used to ascertain adequacy of reversal, and the use of narcotics. The anesthesiologist should also report the time of administration of any antibiotics, the amount of intraoperative urine output, any intravenous fluids given, and estimated blood loss.

Readiness for discharge from the PACU should be assessed by an anesthesiologist after the patient has remained stable in the unit for a reasonable period of time. **Patients can be considered for transfer out of the PACU once vital signs are stable; temperature is normal; they are easily awakened and respond appropriately for their age; adequate urine output is present; and they are free of uncontrolled surgical or anesthetic complications. In addition, patients should not have received sedatives or narcotics less than 30 minutes before discharge.** Patients recovering from major regional anesthesia (axial blocks) must meet additional criteria. It has been suggested that the sympathetic block has receded sufficiently for safe discharge from the PACU if patients are able to move their legs and flex their knees and are able to recognize touch in the area previously anesthetized. One recent investigation has suggested that hemodynamic stability may return before sensory or motor function returns. These authors suggested that it is safe to discharge patients from the PACU following spinal anesthesia if the blood pressure decreases less than 10% when the patient is moved from the supine position to the sitting position with legs down on two measurements more than 30 minutes apart.[4] These authors concluded that use of their criteria results in decreased duration of PACU stay. These results, however, await independent verification.

Patients who will be discharged home must be able to meet the preceding criteria and also be able to ambulate with assistance, take oral fluids, have voided, and have a responsible adult present to care for them during the first 24 hours after discharge. The responsible adult must be present when the patient receives postoperative and discharge instructions.

COMPLICATIONS IN THE PACU
Pain

Pain in the PACU is by far the most commonly encountered patient care problem. The reported incidence of pain requiring intervention with analgetics ranges from a high of 95% to a low of 20.5%[90,113] **Inadequately treated pain may cause splinting of respiratory muscles resulting in inadequate ventilation and an unwillingness or inability to cough and breath deeply, leading to atelectasis and pneumonia. Postoperative pain may also be a factor in the development of postoperative combativeness, which can lead to patient injury. Inadequate analgesia and the anxiety associated with pain results in the release of catecholamines, resulting in tachycardia, dysrhythmias, increases in blood pressure, and increases in oxygen consumption.**[109] **Many factors affect the patient's perception of pain, including age, preoperative personality, fear of postoperative pain preoperatively, and preoperative psychologic preparation (Box 8-1).** Elderly patients tend to have a higher pain threshold. Preoperative medications also affect the degree of discomfort experienced in the PACU. Premedications such as barbiturates, which lower the pain threshold,

---

BOX 8-1
FACTORS IN POSTOPERATIVE PAIN

Patient factors
Patient age
Preoperative personality
Psychologic preparation

Anesthetic factors
Preoperative medications
Anesthetics administered

Surgical factors
Surgical site
Extent of surgery
Postoperative complications

---

tend to increase the patient's pain in the recovery room, whereas analgetics such as narcotics given preoperatively may at least delay the onset of pain in the PACU.[56,125] In the PACU pain is also affected by the anesthetic given. Administration of narcotics intraoperatively, as adjuncts to anesthesia, delays the first dose of narcotic postoperatively and results in lower pain scores during the first 2 hours postoperatively compared with a pure inhalation anesthetic.[30,64,95] However, neither the administration of narcotics preoperatively nor their use intraoperatively can be relied on to decrease the total quantity of narcotics administered in the postoperative period.[56,64] Finally, the site and extent of surgery, as well as the development of postoperative complications, affect the incidence and severity of pain experienced by patients in the PACU.[74,148,149]

In the postoperative period, analgesia can be achieved in one of two ways. First, nociceptive impulses can be interrupted before they reach the cerebral cortex. This is frequently accomplished in the operating room by placement of nerve blocks, epidural or spinal anesthetics, or local infiltration of the area surrounding the incision. Second, and most common in the PACU, the cerebral response to noxious stimuli can be modulated. This is accomplished with various narcotic and nonnarcotic analgetics.

Pain therapy in the PACU depends on several interrelated factors. These factors include the patient's age and level of cooperation, the surgical site, and underlying medical conditions. Regional anesthesia can frequently be used with considerable efficacy in patients undergoing extremity or abdominal surgery.* In adult patients these blocks can be placed either immediately preoperatively or intraoperatively and can be used for surgical anesthesia as well as for postoperative analgesia. As an alternative, they can be placed in the recovery room. With children or uncooperative adults these blocks are best placed during anesthesia. Local anesthetics can be used in these blocks, or, in the case of epidural and spinal anesthesia, preservative-free narcotic solutions may also be used. The advantages of regional anesthesia for the production of postoperative analgesia include less sedation and lack of side effects common with systemic narcotics. In addition, some investigators have suggested that regional anesthesia may be associated with decreased postoperative morbidity,[3] improved ventilatory function,[139,146] and improved analgesia[14,21,43] compared with parenteral narcotics. These findings are still not clearly established, as

---

*References 3, 12, 14, 16, 17, 20, 21, 34, 35, 38, 43, 51, 59, 69, 82, 118, 139, 143, 145.

other investigators have failed to confirm the reported advantages.[109,112,118] Also, placement of nerve blocks is associated with inherent risks. Regional analgesia is always associated with the risk of intravascular local anesthetic injection, infection at the injection site, hematoma formation, and trauma to nerve tissue in the area of the block. Epidural or spinal analgesia with local anesthesia risks hypotension from the resultant sympathetic block, motor weakness, urinary retention, and excessive spread of local anesthetic resulting in high or "total" spinal anesthesia. Use of axial narcotics is also associated with pruritus, nausea and vomiting, urinary retention, and delayed respiratory depression.

The second and most common method for providing analgesia in the PACU is with parenteral narcotics. Simplicity, efficacy, and applicability to a wide variety of patients recovering from a wide variety of surgical procedures account for the continued popularity of parenteral narcotics in the postoperative period. Although narcotics can be administered by different routes, titration of small intravenous doses is the most common route in the PACU. In a healthy adult, administration of 1 to 3 mg of morphine, or its equivalent, every 10 to 20 minutes with careful observations of the degree of analgesia and respiratory and cardiac depression will result in satisfactory control of postoperative pain. With children, administration of the equivalent of 0.02 to 0.04 mg/kg of morphine or its equivalent every 10 to 20 minutes, again monitoring for evidence of adequate analgesia and respiratory and cardiac function, will usually result in adequate postoperative pain control. Adequate analgesia can normally be obtained with total doses of <0.15 mg/kg morphine. If larger doses are required, careful reevaluation of the patient should be undertaken. Stimulation from pain does not necessarily protect the patient from narcotic-induced respiratory depression.[75]

Recently, increased awareness has developed that analgesia in the period after discharge from the PACU is frequently less than optimal. As a result, interest has developed in the use of "patient-controlled analgesia" (PCA). This technique has gained rapid acceptance and has also been introduced into the recovery room. It is doubtful that PCA has any advantage in the recovery room where analgetics can be carefully titrated to the patients' needs by caregivers who can be in near-constant attendance. However, it may be useful to administer the initial loading dose in the PACU where the patient is under close observation and responses can be monitored.

Finally, the increased interest in the treatment of pain has led to the introduction of several alternative techniques for providing postoperative analgesia, including interpleural injection of local anesthetics,[123]

topical application of local anesthetic to the surgical wound,[140] and the use of transcutaneous electrical nerve stimulation (TENS).[97] However, the efficacy, applicability, side effects, and complications of these techniques are still under investigation.

Hypothermia and Postoperative Tremors

Hypothermia and shivering in the immediate postoperative period are commonly encountered problems reported in greater than 30% of the patients.[106,144,156] Shivering during the immediate anesthesia recovery period has been commonly ascribed to hypothermia in the operating room, although the evidence of this association is at best inconclusive.[85,136] Numerous studies have demonstrated little correlation between patient temperature in the PACU and presence of postoperative tremors[26,65,87,117] (Fig. 8-1). Other investigators have demonstrated a positive correlation between presence of tremors and emergence from anesthesia[134,144] (Fig. 8-2). Other studies have demonstrated that duration of shivering is related to the temperature on admission to the PACU.[156] These studies also demonstrated that radiant heat

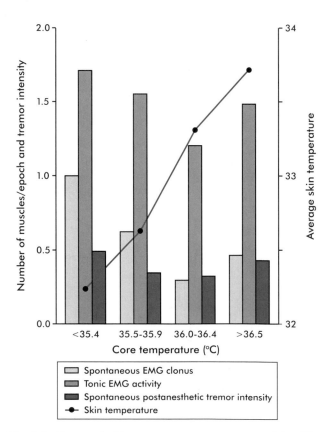

Fig. 8-1. Core and skin temperature vs. tremor activity. The number of muscles/10 min epoch that demonstrated spontaneous EMG clonus and tonic activity plotted against core temperature. (From Sessler DI, Israel D, Pozos RS et al: Spontaneous postanesthetic tremor does not resemble thermoregulatory shivering, *Anesthesiology* 68:843, 1988.)

and heated humidification of the respiratory gases are effective methods of suppressing postoperative tremors.[117,132,138]

Regardless of the mechanism of postoperative shivering, its metabolic consequences may severely harm the patient. Shivering can increase a patient's oxygen consumption by 400% to 500%.[9] Although such increases may be well tolerated in healthy individuals, they have been implicated in the production of postoperative hypoxia, hypercapnia, and increased blood lactate levels.[25,70] In addition, it has been suggested that shivering may increase the risk of postoperative myocardial infarctions[54] and elevations of intraocular pressure.[94] Inhibition of shivering in the postoperative patient has been shown to decrease metabolic requirements,[126,127] but hypothermia in the absence of shivering may still result in increased metabolic requirements compared with normothermic patients because of nonshivering thermogenesis.[105,117] Thus in the postoperative patient it is important to treat both shivering and hypothermia.

Certainly the most effective course of action is to prevent hypothermia in the operating room. First, the patient should be transported to the operating room adequately covered with blankets. Medications given in the preoperative period can result in excessive heat loss, presumably because of vasodilation. The operating room should be kept as warm as possible, at least

until the surgical preparation is complete and the patient is draped. The operating room temperature below which patients will become hypothermic unless additional precautions are taken has previously been determined to be 21° C.[106] Added measures that help in preventing hypothermia include the use of warmed prepping solutions, heating blankets, thermal blankets with reflective surfaces, intravenous fluid warmers, low gas flows through the anesthetic circuit, passive humidifiers ("artificial nose") located in the anesthetic circuit, and actively heated humidifiers in the circuit.* Care should be taken to keep the patient warm during transport from the operating room to the PACU as this is clearly a period when the patient is still at high risk for heat loss.[65] Many of these measures can be continued in the PACU, if despite their use intraoperatively, the patient still arrives in the PACU hypothermic (Box 8-2).

At the completion of surgery, healthy patients with temperatures greater than 33° C can usually be safely extubated.[105] Patients with temperatures below 33° C or elderly and debilitated patients who are hypothermic may benefit from continued ventilatory support until normothermia has returned.[105]

Shivering, whether or not associated with hypothermia, should be treated if it is sufficiently severe or prolonged to cause discomfort or to jeopardize the patient's condition. Current treatment is often only partially successful, and thus many modalities have been suggested. Perhaps the most widely recognized treatment, aside from the previously mentioned warming measures, is the use of small intravenous doses of meperidine.[116] Pauca et al. reported that meperidine 25 mg IV decreased the duration of shivering significantly compared with groups given no narcotics or given morphine or fentanyl. They also reported minimal side effects from meperidine. Recently, small doses of clonidine have been reported

---

* *References 29, 52, 83, 111, 135, 137, 152.

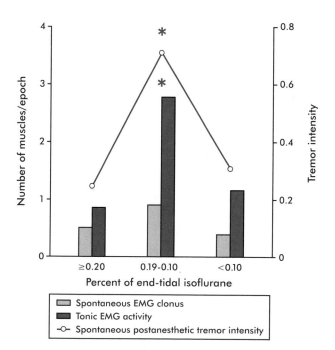

Fig. 8-2. Isoflurane concentration vs. tremor activity. Maximum tremor intensity noted at end-tidal isoflurane concentrations between 0.19% and 0.1%. (From Sessler DI, Israel D, Pozos RS et al: Spontaneous postanesthetic tremor does not resemble thermoregulatory shivering, *Anesthesiology* 68:843, 1988.)

BOX 8-2
TREATMENT OF HYPOTHERMIA AND SHIVERING

Transport patient covered with blankets
Warm the room
Use of heating blankets
Reflective thermal blankets
Intravenous fluid warmers
Passive humidifiers (intubated patients)
Active warming of inspired gases
Radiant warmers
Meperidine

effective in inhibiting postoperative shivering.[53] At present, the intravenous form of clonidine is unavailable in the United States. In addition independent confirmation of its efficacy is currently lacking, but early evidence is promising. The utility of muscle relaxants in preventing postoperative shivering is well documented.[127] This therapy has the obvious disadvantage of requiring postoperative ventilation and sedation. Other pharmacologic means of treating postoperative shivering, including the use of phenothiazines, have been associated with either unacceptable side effects or unverified efficacy.[55,87,126] The application of localized radiant heat has been reported to inhibit postoperative shivering despite continued hypothermia.[132,138] Investigators found that the application of radiant heat to the anterior chest or chest and abdomen inhibited shivering more quickly than was achieved in control groups and resulted in more rapid attainment of normothermia.

Nausea and Vomiting

Postoperative vomiting is a common complication of surgery and anesthesia, although its exact incidence remains controversial. In addition to causing patient discomfort, it is one of the most frequent reasons for unanticipated admission of outpatients following surgery. Postoperative vomiting may also result in electrolyte abnormalities, dehydration, wound disruption, bleeding from the wound, and, perhaps worst of all, aspiration, especially in patients who have depressed levels of consciousness or who have intermaxillary fixation following oral surgery. As with postoperative shivering, no single cause is known and there is no single effective therapy.

It is now generally accepted that there is a vomiting center located in the brainstem that, when stimulated, sends efferent impulses that produce the coordinated action of vomiting. This center receives input from cortical and visual stimuli, the chemoreceptor trigger zone, the vestibular apparatus in the inner ear, the mediastinum, and the gastrointestinal tract. Postoperative vomiting is believed to occur as a result of stimulation of the vomiting center from several of these factors produced during surgery and anesthesia. Treatment is also aimed at inhibiting afferent input from these sites.

The most important factors predisposing a patient to postoperative vomiting, and certainly the most difficult factors for the anesthesiologist to control, are patient factors (Box 8-3). Patients suffering from intraabdominal pathology or those with full stomachs may be more likely to vomit in the postoperative period than other patients. In addition, patients who have increased intracranial pressure or drug-induced or other metabolic disturbances have increased propensities to vomit following surgery. It is often

---

BOX 8-3
FACTORS IN POSTOPERATIVE VOMITING

Patient factors

Intraabdominal pathology
Increased intracranial pressure
Metabolic abnormalities
Preadmission drug ingestion
Gender (female)
Age
Obesity

Surgical factors

Site of operation
Duration of surgery

Anesthetic factors

Premedicants (?)

Other factors

Hypotension
Hypoxia
Postoperative pain

---

contended that female patients are more susceptible to postoperative vomiting than are male patients, especially following intraabdominal surgery.[13,42,77,147] Younger patients are reported to be more likely to vomit postoperatively than are older patients.[128,147] Obesity is also considered a risk factor for postoperative nausea and vomiting.[98] Finally, it appears that there is individual variability that makes certain individuals especially sensitive to the emetic side effects of anesthetic drugs. Patients who vomited following previous anesthetics are more likely to vomit postoperatively with subsequent anesthetics.[80,108] Although most of the literature seems to support these patient factors as important determinants of an individual patient's tendency to vomit postoperatively, some studies have reached the opposite conclusion about their importance.[103,114,158]

In addition to patient factors, there are surgical factors that may influence the incidence of postoperative emetic complications. Chief among these factors is the site of the operation. Surgery involving the extraocular eye muscles; procedures on the ears, nose, or throat; and intraabdominal procedures have consistently had the highest incidences of emetic complications, whereas superficial and extremity surgery have the lowest incidence.[2,15,37,114] Duration of anesthesia and surgery and incidence of postoperative vomiting are also related.[13,15]

Much has been written about the effect of anes-

thetics on postoperative emetic complications. Cyclopropane and ether had undisputed emetic effects, but the effects of currently used anesthetics are less well defined, with studies available to both support and dispute the emetic effects of modern agents and techniques. Premedication with narcotics has long been associated with increased emetic side effects in the postoperative period.[13,124,128] Studies attempting to identify the opiate most likely to cause postoperative vomiting have yielded contradictory results with morphine[18] and meperidine.[13] Consistent among several studies was the finding that antimuscarinic agents capable of crossing the blood-brain barrier used in combination with narcotic premedicants did tend to decrease the emetic potential of the narcotic.[101,124] Of the currently used anesthetics, the potential emetic properties of nitrous oxide have received the most attention. Review of the literature is again inconclusive, although most recent studies fail to implicate nitrous oxide as the cause of postoperative vomiting.* Although premedication with narcotics has been associated with postoperative emesis, there is little evidence that narcotics given during general anesthesia have significant effects on the incidence of emetic complications postoperatively.[114] The same is true for particular volatile agents (i.e., no one agent is clearly more or less likely to cause postoperative emesis).[67] Evidence collected during early clinical trials with propofol suggests that the incidence of emetic side effects may be significantly lower with it than with other agents.[6,40,57] This evidence is far from conclusive, and other studies have failed to show any reduction in emetic complications with propofol-based anesthetics.[36,45]

Although much of the risk of emetic side effects clearly results from patient and operative factors, therapies are available to the anesthesiologist to either prophylactically and/or symptomatically treat emetic side effects. These therapies are all inconsistently effective and are not without side effects themselves. Therefore, in any one patient, multiple agents may be required if vomiting is to be successfully treated.

Prophylactic treatment can be attempted in patients deemed at high risk for nausea and vomiting postoperatively. Droperidol has consistently received the most attention. It has been shown effective in numerous studies when used in high doses (about 0.07 mg/kg).[2,47,86] These large doses have unfortunately been shown to cause sedation sufficient to delay or prevent discharge from the hospital.[28,60] In lower doses droperidol's efficacy is less established.† Additional side effects of droperidol that must be consid-

ered include hypotension, dysphoria, and dystonic reactions.[28,41] In an attempt to balance the side effects of the drug with the potential benefits of prophylactic treatment in patients at risk for postoperative emesis, it seems reasonable to administer a small dose (about 0.02 to 0.03 mg/kg) of the drug intravenously at the beginning of the anesthetic. If the patient develops vomiting in the recovery room and is not unduly sedated, the droperidol can be repeated in recovery. Another agent that has recently received attention is transdermal scopolamine. Initial studies suggest that when placed preoperatively, this form of prophylaxis may be highly effective in preventing nausea and vomiting.[62,81,92] Other agents that have been evaluated for prophylaxis or treatment of postoperative vomiting with only limited success include intravenous metaclopromide,[22,39,88] intravenous lidocaine,[24,161] and intramuscular ephedrine.[120]

In the recovery room, patients should first be evaluated to ensure that hypotension or hypoxia is not responsible for the vomiting. The patient's pain should also be appropriately treated. Nausea and vomiting are often associated with postoperative pain, and if the pain is treated appropriately, the nausea and vomiting often subside, even if narcotics were required for analgesia.[5] Once the pain and/or hypoxia and/or hypotension have been effectively alleviated, pharmacologic measures can be undertaken to symptomatically treat the nausea and vomiting. If possible, intravenous hydration should be continued to prevent dehydration and electrolyte imbalances. Also, attempts at PO intake should be discontinued until the patient is thirsty, at which point gentle attempts to hydrate the patient with oral intake can again be initiated.

Agitation and Delirium

Transient delirium or agitation during the immediate postanesthetic period is not uncommon, particularly in young patients who were significantly anxious preoperatively and in patients who received minimal narcotics intraoperatively and who have undergone painful procedures.[44] Other conditions associated with postoperative agitation include hypoxia, hypercapnia, distension of the stomach or urinary bladder, and the use of barbiturates, antimuscarinics, and phenothiazines as premedication, especially when used without narcotics.[44] Less common conditions that can lead to agitation postoperatively are listed in Table 8-1.[163]

In the recovery room measures must be taken immediately to prevent patients from injuring themselves, and rule out hypoxia and/or hypercapnia. The anesthesiologist must not forget that agitation resulting from hypoxia but "treated" with sedatives or narcotics is a deadly trap that must be avoided. Once

---

*References 80, 91, 99, 108, 114, 133.
†References 1, 28, 47, 60, 120, 125.

Table 8-1 Factors in postoperative delirium

Factors	Specifics	Factors	Specifics
Patient factors		**Environmental and psychosocial factors**	
Factors decreasing cerebral oxygen delivery	Decreased cardiac output Cerebrovascular insufficiency Hypoxemia Hyperviscosity or coagulopathy Increased intracranial pressure	Factors affecting sensory integration	Sleep deprivation Impaired ability to communicate
Factors increasing cerebral oxygen demand	Stress Hyperpyrexia Infection Hyperthyroidism Hypercapnia or acidosis Seizures	Factors that can increase fear and anxiety	Pain and discomfort, including incisional pain; gastric or bladder distension; noise; and frightening activities Bad previous experience in a similar setting Surgical procedure Position Extremes of age Preoperative vocational or retirement-related problems
Factors altering cerebral metabolism or function	Malignant hypertension Hepatic or renal dysfunction Ionic imbalances Endocrine imbalances Drug toxicity, including heavy metals, thiamine or carbon monoxide; ketamine, neuroleptics, opiates, sedatives, anticholinergics, and hallucinogens; withdrawal from alcohol, barbiturates, hallucinogens, opiates, and benzodiazepines; neuroleptic malignant syndrome; and allergic or idiopathic reactions to administered drugs CNS disease, including dementia or organic brain syndrome; Parkinson's disease; and multiple sclerosis Cerebral contusion or injury	Factors that are psychiatric in nature	Underlying psychotic or neurotic (especially paranoid) disorder Endogenous depression Postpartum psychosis Conversion reaction Inadequate preoperative defenses and coping mechanisms Morbid or pessimistic expectations Body image distortion

Modified from Weinger MB, Swerdlow NR, and Miller WL: Acute postoperative delirium and extrapyramidal signs in a previously healthy patient, *Anesth Analg* 67:291, 1988.

hypoxia and hypercarbia are ruled out, small doses of narcotics may be administered if the patient is experiencing discomfort from the procedure. **If, based on the physical examination and review of the anesthetic record, distention of the bladder or stomach is likely, decompression measures should be taken.** If the patient received either scopolamine or atropine preoperatively, small doses of the cholinesterase antagonist physostigmine (0.5 mg) may be effective in terminating the agitation, thought to be secondary to central antimuscarinic actions. If the patient is a child, admission of a parent to the recovery room may be the most effective method of terminating the agitation. Finally, if all else fails, treatment with anxiolytic agents may prove effective.

Obtundation

Persistent obtundation in the PACU is usually the result of the residual effects of premedication and/or anesthetic drugs. Other causes of obtundation in the recovery room include hypoxia, hypercapnia, CNS injury, hypoglycemia, other electrolyte abnormalities, and severe hypothermia. Careful examination and workup of patients who are unexpectedly obtunded is required with particular attention to the neurologic system. Evaluation should be undertaken to rule out hypoxia, hypercapnia, hypoglycemia, hyponatremia, hypocalcemia, hypercalcemia, and hypoosmolar and hyperosmolar states. Once the preceding abnormalities have been ruled out, if large doses of narcotics have been given, small doses (0.04 mg) of intravenous naloxone may be administered incrementally. If narcotic administration is the cause of the depression, some measure of arousal will occur in a minute or less with 0.2 mg of naloxone. If the residual effects of long-acting sedatives are causing postoperative sedation, small doses of physostigmine (0.5 mg/dose, total administration < 3 mg) intravenously often result in rapid improvement in consciousness. If these measures fail to identify the cause of the obtundation, prompt consultation with a neurologist is recommended.

NEUROMUSCULAR COMPLICATIONS

Postoperatively, susceptibility to neuromuscular complications from inordinate pressure on superficial nerves continues until the patient is fully awake. In addition, the patient may sustain injuries during periods of agitation during emergence. When considered together with their intraoperative counterparts, these injuries are among the most common major postoperative complications.[27]

Because of the relative frequency of these injuries, precautions to avoid them should be continued into the immediate postoperative period. During recovery the patient must be protected from trauma. Measures taken may include padding the rails of the gurney and maintaining them in the up position. If agitated, the patient may also need to be restrained. If the patient is somnolent in the PACU or if regional anesthesia has not yet receded, care must be taken to position the patient so that the brachial plexus is not stretched, and pressure is not exerted over the course of a superficial nerve. Areas especially susceptible to injury include the mid-humerus, where the median and ulnar nerve wrap around the bone; the medial

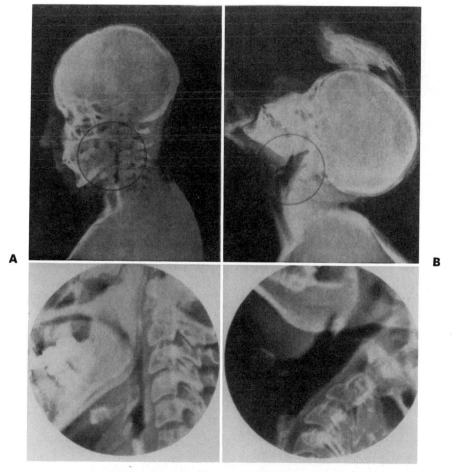

Fig. 8-3. Lateral neck radiographs. **A,** Radiograph with the neck in neutral position. **B,** Radiograph with the neck extended demonstrating increased pharyngeal air space when the neck is extended. (From Ruben HM, Elam JO, Ruben AM et al: Investigation of upper airway problems in resuscitation, *Anesthesiology* 22:271, 1961.)

elbow, where the ulnar nerve courses; and the lateral lower leg, where the perineal nerve crosses the head of the fibula.[89] It is important to assess peripheral nerve function at regular intervals because impingement injuries, such as epidural hematomas, may be readily reversible if identified early during the patient's recovery phase.

RESPIRATORY COMPLICATIONS
Airway Obstruction

Residual effects of drugs employed during general anesthesia often leave the patient with decreased muscle tone and/or a decreased level of consciousness. Both of these can predispose the patient to airway obstruction. The usual proximate cause of airway obstruction in the immediate postoperative period is posterior displacement of the tongue resulting in pharyngeal obstruction.[104] Obstruction can also occur as a result of airway edema from traumatic intubations or surgery in the vicinity of the airway. Laryngospasm can occur in the recovery period and may lead to partial or complete airway obstruction. When a patient is noted or suspected of ineffective attempts to move adequate volumes of air, supplemental oxygen should be administered immediately and the head should be repositioned. Usually extension and flexion of the neck at C1-2 with anterior displacement of the mandible will be effective in opening the airway (Fig. 8-3).[104,129] Attempts to place the patient in the sniffing position (i.e., by adding C7-T1 flexion to C1-2 extension) have not been shown to increase airway patency over simple head tilt and thus may simply waste time when attempting to open an obstructed airway.[104] If pharyngeal obstruction is unrelieved by head tilt in the supine position, repositioning the patient in the lateral position with head extension may help. If these maneuvers are unsuccessful at restoring airway patency, the next step is placement of an artificial airway. In the postoperative period nasopharyngeal airways are more likely to be both successful and tolerated by the patient compared with oropharyngeal airways, but they may result in severe pharyngeal bleeding. On the other hand, they are less likely to cause laryngospasm, gagging, retching, and vomiting than oral airways.

If these measures fail to relieve the obstruction, the airway must be secured by whatever means necessary, including endotracheal intubation and crycothyroidotomy. Laryngospasm resulting in airway obstruction can sometimes be effectively treated with the jaw thrust maneuver.[49] Small amounts of positive airway pressure may be effective in relieving the laryngospasm. If these treatments are ineffective, administration of small amounts of succinylcholine (10 to 20 mg) will relieve the obstruction. Administration of a

muscle relaxant in this situation must be considered only if, despite positive pressure, minute ventilation is inadequate, means of controlling ventilation are immediately available, and the airway was easy to control during the induction of anesthesia. As with pharyngeal obstruction, failure of these therapies to

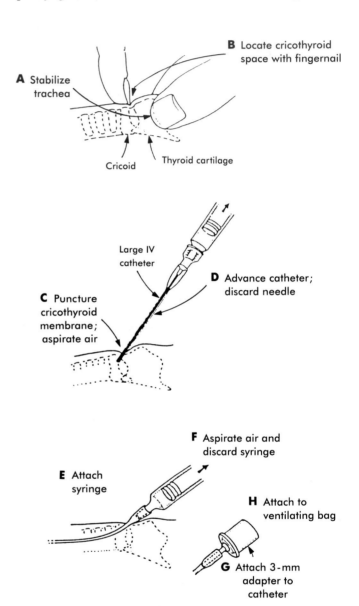

Fig. 8-4. Procedure for cricothyroidotomy with IV catheter. *A,* Identify thyroid cartilage and stabilize with thumb and forefinger. *B,* Locate cricothyroid space with fingernail of other hand. *C,* Insert large bore (14 gauge) IV catheter attached to a syringe through the cricothyroid membrane, aspirating air when catheter stylet enters the trachea. *D* to *F,* Advance catheter to confirm placement for air aspiration. *G,* Attach 3-mm endotracheal tube (ET) adapter to the catheter hut or, for better results, attach ventilator apparatus. *H,* If jet ventilation is not available, connect ET adapter to ventilating bag. (From Cote CJ, Eavey RD, Todres D et al: Cricothyroid membrane puncture: oxygenation and ventilation in a dog model using an intravenous catheter, *Crit Care Med* 16:615, 1988.)

result in adequate ventilation may indicate the need to bypass the obstruction by performing an emergency cricothyroidotomy followed by jet ventilation (Fig. 8-4).[31]

Hypoxia

Hypoxia in the immediate postoperative period is common even in young healthy patients and usually results from multiple factors. The occurrence of hypoxia in the recovery area is of special concern because residual anesthetics plus surgical factors can effectively blunt the response to hypoxia.[78,79,159,162] Thus, in the absence of blood gas analysis and/or pulse oximetry, hypoxia may persist unrecognized.[32]

The differential diagnosis of the cause of hypoxia in the postoperative period is essentially the same as that for hypoxia under other clinical situations. Four broad categories must be considered: hypoventilation (including airway obstruction), ventilation/perfusion mismatch (including shunt), decreased oxygen delivery to the tissues, and increased oxygen consumption.

When faced with hypoxia, airway obstruction must be considered as a likely cause and appropriately and quickly treated. In addition, hypoventilation may occur as a result of residual effects of anesthetics previously administered, excessive administration of narcotic analgetics, and posthypocapnic hypoventilation.[68,131]

Once airway obstruction is ruled out, other causes of hypoxia can be considered. Patients in the postoperative period are at risk for ventilation/perfusion abnormalities and shunting, which produce hypoxia. Factors predisposing a patient to $\dot{V}/\dot{Q}$ abnormalities because of alterations in ventilation include obesity, extremes of age, preexisting pulmonary disease, intraoperative patient position, abdominal distension, restrictive abdominal or thoracic dressings, overhydration, pneumothorax, hemothorax, bronchoconstriction, retained secretions, pulmonary edema, inadequately treated pain, operative site, and surgical approach. These conditions can easily result in the reduction of functional residual capacity (FRC) below the closing capacity of the lung. In patients that are hypoxic because of areas of inadequate, but not absent ventilation, supplemental oxygen will raise the Pao_2 to an acceptable level. The risk of this therapy is minimal, but, if ventilation is severely reduced, increasing the inspired oxygen concentration may speed the development of atelectasis. If the $\dot{V}/\dot{Q}$ ratio is exceedingly low (shunt), supplemental oxygen will be of little efficacy. Once supplemental oxygen has been administered, measures should be taken to reverse the underlying abnormality that created the hypoxia. Patients should recover in a semisitting position, especially if the patient is obese or has significant abdominal distension. Pain should be

adequately treated using regional anesthesia and/or systemic analgetics. Finally, measures aimed at increasing lung volumes must be instituted. These include deep breathing maneuvers, coughing, suctioning, and chest physiotherapy. If these treatments fail to correct the hypoxemia, continuous positive airway pressure (CPAP) may be administered by mask, or the patient may need to be reintubated and CPAP or positive end-expiratory pressure (PEEP) administered.

Decreased oxygen delivery may result from several conditions. In the immediate postoperative period, diffusion hypoxia may occur as a result of the rapid elimination of nitrous oxide from the circulation into the lungs if the patient is breathing room air.[48] Fortunately, nitrous oxide is eliminated quickly after its administration is discontinued. Thus the administration of supplemental oxygen for approximately 5 minutes after discontinuation of the nitrous oxide will eliminate nitrous oxide diffusion as a cause of postoperative hypoxia. Inadvertent delivery of hypoxic gas mixture to a patient is a rare, but not unheard of, cause of hypoxia that must always be considered. Low cardiac output and/or anemia may lead to tissue hypoxia because of inadequate oxygen delivery and/or O_2 carrying capacity. Low cardiac output and anemia may also contribute to hypoxia by causing a decrease in mixed venous Po_2, which, if shunted right to left, will mix with oxygenated blood and decrease Pao_2.[119] Treatment of hypoxia arising from these conditions involves the administration of supplemental oxygen and correction of the underlying defect.

The last causal category of hypoxia is increased oxygen consumption. This is commonly seen in patients with limited cardiac and pulmonary reserves who are hyperthermic or shivering in the recovery room.[9] Again, administration of supplemental oxygen followed by symptomatic and corrective treatment of the underlying cause is essential.

Hypoventilation

Some degree of hypoventilation is present in most patients at some time during recovery from general anesthesia and surgery. Although mild hypoventilation is well tolerated in healthy individuals, marked elevations in arterial $Paco_2$ are harmful to patients, leading to impaired consciousness, agitation, respiratory acidosis, and dysrhythmias. As with hypoxia, the early systemic manifestations of hypercapnia are blunted by the anesthetics, allowing the condition to continue unnoticed until well advanced. In addition, ventilatory responses to hypercapnia are often blunted by the residual effects of anesthetics.[61,68,71,79,162]

In the immediate postoperative period inadequate ventilation may result from two basic causes. First, depressed ventilation with normal or decreased carbon dioxide production occurs either as a result of pharmacologic depression of central respiratory centers from anesthetics and narcotics or as a result of mechanical changes in respiratory parameters resulting from anesthesia and surgery. In the PACU the respiratory depressant effects of the anesthetics usually diminish with time. There have been reports, however, of delayed or recurring respiratory depression following the intraoperative administration of narcotics.[11] The respiratory depressant properties of the anesthetics may become more obvious in the recovery room if levels of noxious stimuli diminish, such as when the endotracheal tube is removed. Respiratory depression as a result of relative narcotic overdose can be antagonized by small, incremental doses of naloxone without completely antagonizing the analgesia produced by the narcotic. Respiratory depression from other medications is best treated with continued controlled ventilation until the drug's effects have dissipated. Although some authors have suggested the use of nonspecific CNS stimulants or respiratory stimulants in this situation, a significant risk of side effects from these agents is present, and their efficacy is at best controversial.[7,84,110,160] Mechanical interference because of splinting from postoperative pain may compromise a patient's ability to adequately ventilate, especially after upper abdominal or thoracic surgery.[46] In this case, administration of narcotics may actually *improve* ventilation in the recovery room. Interference with respiratory muscle function because of inadequate reversal of neuromuscular blockade may also impede ventilation. Muscle relaxant reversal agents are usually effective in restoring adequate ventilation in this situation. If reversal is inadequate after the administration of reversal agents, ventilation should be controlled until spontaneous reversal has occurred. Airway obstruction can lead to hypoventilation *without* hypoxia, especially if supplemental oxygen is administered. Mechanical interference with ventilation may occur as a result of pulmonary edema from any source. Therapy is aimed at treating the cause and eliminating excess lung water while maintaining adequate oxygenation.

A second category of inadequate ventilation is increased carbon dioxide production beyond the point where the body can effectively compensate. This can occur with shivering, hyperthermia, and occasionally with hyperalimentation. Treatment of shivering as outlined earlier will decrease carbon dioxide production. Treatment of hyperthermia requires identifying the underlying cause. Symptomatic measures, including administration of aspirin, removal of blankets, and placement of ice packs, may temporize the situation.

CARDIOVASCULAR COMPLICATIONS

Hypotension

Healthy postoperative patients often experience mild transient decreases in blood pressure. These episodes are usually well tolerated. Decreases of greater than 20% below preoperative values that last more than a few minutes should be aggressively treated because hypoperfusion of vital organs with resulting organ ischemia may rapidly ensue.

In healthy patients without a significant associated disease, the most common cause of postoperative hypotension is hypovolemia. This may result from inadequate fluid and/or blood replacement. It may also result from unrecognized third space losses or excessive urine output because of the presence of osmotic diuretics (including hyperglycemia). Relative hypovolemia may occur as a result of increased venous capacitance, as occurs during spinal or epidural anesthesia. Left atrial hypovolemia can result from a large pulmonary embolus. Other, less likely causes of hypotension in healthy individuals include decreased cardiac output because of myocardial infarction or congestive heart failure and decreased systemic vascular resistance from septic shock.

When a patient is hypotensive, it is important to verify the blood pressure measurement. In a healthy patient without concurrent cardiovascular disease, initial therapy should be aimed at increasing cardiac filling pressures. This is most easily and effectively accomplished by elevating the patient's legs and giving a bolus of intravenous fluids. Controversy surrounds the preferred fluid in this situation. There is little evidence in most clinical situations that colloid holds significant advantages over crystalloid. In addition, crystalloid is significantly cheaper and usually more available. If volume infusion fails to restore arterial pressure, vasoactive agents may be required to stabilize the situation until invasive monitoring can be instituted and the diagnosis established. CVP or pulmonary artery pressure monitoring is useful in this situation to quantitate cardiac filling pressures and adequacy of volume replacement. Pulmonary artery (PA) catheter monitors may more accurately reflect left heart–filling pressures than central venous pressure (CVP) and will allow calculation of systemic vascular resistance. If central pressure monitors indicate that filling pressures are adequate, therapy should include administration of inotropic agents if cardiac output is low, or vasopressors if systemic vascular resistance (SVR) is low during correction of the underlying condition.

Hypertension

The immediate postoperative period is a time when multiple factors interact to provide potent stimuli

Table 8-2   Factors contributing to postoperative hypertension

Factor	Present in patients (%)
Pain	36
Emergence excitement	17
Reaction to endotracheal tube	15
Hypercapnia	2
Excess fluid administration	7
Hypothermia	7
Hypoxia	17
Hypertension by history	58
Uncertain	17

Modified from Gal TJ, Cooperman LH: Hypertension in the immediate postoperative period, *Br J Anaesth* 47:70, 1975.

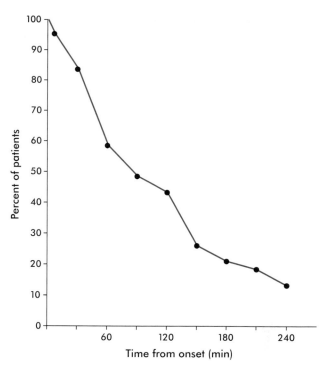

Fig. 8-5. Duration of postoperative hypertension. (From Gal TJ, Cooperman LH: Hypertension in the immediate postoperative period, *Br J Anaesth* 47:70, 1975.)

(Table 8-2) for blood pressure elevations in normal patients and for those with concurrent diseases. In healthy individuals, postoperative hypertension is usually a short term phenomenon that occurs shortly after surgery and persists for less than 3 hours[50] (Fig. 8-5). In these individuals its course is usually benign, with few significant complications reported.

Factors implicated in the development of postoperative hypertension include pain, agitation, airway irritation secondary to an endotracheal tube, hypercapnia, excess fluid administration, hypothermia, and hypoxia.[50] In patients with essential hypertension, acute discontinuation of antihypertensive medications has also been implicated in the development of postoperative hypertension.[73]

In healthy individuals, treatment of hypertension occurring in the PACU should center on identifying and eliminating the factors contributing to it, including narcotics for analgesia and warming measures for hypothermic patients. Specific antihypertensive therapy should only be considered if the patient is on chronic therapy, if the hypertension fails to resolve over a short period of time (not longer than 3 hours), if the hypertension is of severe magnitude, dysrhythmias are initiated, or if the patient develops symptoms as a result of the blood pressure elevations.[50] Patients with histories of hypertension should be treated more aggressively because they are more susceptible to hypertensive complications.[50]

When antihypertensive therapy is instituted in the recovery period it is advisable to treat the patient with relatively short-acting agents. Sodium nitroprusside has been advocated, but it can precipitously decrease blood pressure and cause reflex tachycardia.[150] The drug is also associated with cyanide toxicity if administered in dosages greater than 6 to 8 mg/kg for longer than 1 to 2 hours, for prolonged periods, or in high

doses. Therapy with nitroprusside should ideally be instituted in association with direct arterial pressure monitoring. If the patient is aware and hypertensive with a relatively slow heart rate, sublingual nifedipine 5 to 10 mg may effectively treat the hypertension. The disadvantage of this form of treatment is the somewhat unpredictable response to the therapy and the reflex tachycardia that may result. Labetalol, an alpha/beta antagonist, titrated in 2.5 to 5 mg increments intravenously, lowers blood pressure without significant reflex tachycardia and is the treatment used most commonly in many recovery rooms. Other beta antagonists such as esmolol and propranolol have been advocated but may be ineffective if heart rate is already slow and the hypertension is attributable to vasoconstriction. Finally, it should be remembered that propranolol and labetalol block both $beta_1$ and $beta_2$ receptors and thus may worsen respiratory function in patients with obstructive pulmonary disease.

Dysrhythmias

Dysrhythmias occurring in the postoperative period in healthy patients are usually a result of activation of the sympathetic nervous system. Common dysrhythmias include sinus tachycardia, premature ventricular or atrial contractions, and supraventricular tachycardia. Sinus bradycardia or ventricular tachycardia occur less frequently. Dysrhythmias secondary to sympathetic nervous system activation may be manifestations of hypoxia, hypercapnia, pain, agitation, electrolyte imbalances, or acidosis. The other etiology that must always be considered, but which is less common in healthy patients, is intrinsic myocardial disease. These dysrhythmias usually respond to therapy aimed at correcting the underlying abnormality and rarely require long-term treatment. If the dysrhythmia results in patient compromise or does not respond to treatment of the underlying condition, antidysrhythmic agents appropriate for the particular rhythm abnormality should be given.

RENAL COMPLICATIONS
Oliguria

Oliguria during the postoperative period in a healthy patient is usually a transient condition without long-term sequelae. Oliguria is defined as urine output less than .5 ml/kg/hr.

Postoperative oliguria can be classified into three categories: prerenal, renal, and postrenal (Table 8-3). Prerenal oliguria is the most common category seen in the postoperative healthy patient. It results from kidney hypoperfusion either from hypovolemia or cardiac failure. Hypovolemia is by far the most common etiology for low urine output seen in the PACU. Subclinical cardiac depression may result from residual cardiac depressant effects of the volatile anesthetics but this resolves with recovery from anesthesia. The second most common category of low urine output is postrenal. This category should be

suspected if there is sudden complete absence of urine output. This is due to urinary tract obstruction distal to the kidneys. Common points of obstruction include urinary retention as a result of spinal or epidural anesthesia, obstruction of the urinary catheter with "mucus" or blood, and ureteral edema following removal of a urinary catheter. Less common causes of postrenal oliguria in the recovery room include surgical trauma to the urinary tract, bladder rupture, a retroperitoneal hematoma, intraabdominal or retroperitoneal tumors, and blood clots or stones in the bladder. The least common category of oliguria in the recovery room is renal oliguria. This can be due to ischemic damage to the kidneys, administration of nephrotoxins, or transfusion reactions.

In the healthy patient at low risk for renal or postrenal causes of oliguria, rapid intravenous administration of 5 to 10 ml/kg of a balanced salt solution should be the initial measure taken. If urine output improves, continued aggressive fluid administration should be undertaken. If urine output remains unacceptably low and a urinary catheter has not been placed previously, one should be inserted. The patency of the collection system must also be established at this time. This evaluation depends on the potential causes of obstruction. In patients without intraabdominal pathology, irrigation of the catheter may be all that is necessary. In patients with abdominal pathology, abdominal radiographic studies and ultrasound may be required. If urine output is still low and the patient is at low risk for congestive heart failure, an additional fluid bolus may be administered. At this point continued oliguria necessitates that urinary indices be obtained, including the following measurements: urinary sodium, specific gravity, osmolality, urea, creatinine, and plasma osmolality. Calculation of the fractional excretion of sodium, urinary/plasma osmolality, urinary/plasma urea, and urinary/plasma creatinine will aid in establishing the etiology of the oliguria[10] (Table 8-4). Urine should also be sent for microscopic examination. At this time it is prudent to obtain appropriate surgical and medical consultation. Pulmonary artery catheter placement may also be of value in helping differentiate hypovolemia from cardiac failure to guide further therapy. If oliguria persists with normal or elevated cardiac filling pressures, dopamine in doses of 2 to 5 g/kg/min may be beneficial in restoring urine output by increasing renal blood flow.

Use of diuretics in the presence of oliguria is controversial. Although the ability of diuretics to convert oliguric renal failure to nonoliguric renal failure has been well established, their ability to alter morbidity and mortality from renal failure has not been established.[19,76] Diuretics administered to hypovolemic patients worsen the condition, thus increasing

Table 8-3 Causes of oliguria	
Types of oliguria	**Causes**
Prerenal	Hypovolemia
	Decreased renal perfusion
Renal	Acute tubular necrosis
	Nephrotoxins
	Postischemic
	Transfusion reactions
	Rhabdomyolysis
	Glomerulonephrosis
	Vasculitis
	Papillary necrosis
	Hepatorenal syndrome
	Severe hypercalcemia
Postrenal	Obstruction
	Regional anesthetic—
	induced urinary retention
	Urinary catheter obstruction
	Urethral edema

Table 8-4	Renal function tests		
Tests	Prerenal	Renal	Postrenal
Urine output	0.6-1 L	0.3 L-normal	0-normal
Sediment	1 + -2 + protein	Hyaline, granular casts; many RBC, WBC, and epithelial cells	Frequent-normal
U OSM	>450 mOsm/L	300 mOsm/L	300 mOsm/L
U NA$^+$	<15 mEq/L	30-60 mEq/L	Low, then 30-60 mEq/L*
FE NA$^+$	<1%	>3%	>3%
U : P creatinine	>40 : 1	<20 : 1	<20 : 1
BUN : creatinine	>20 : 1	20 : 1	20 : 1

*For 24 hours after acute obstruction the U Na$^+$ may be less than 10 mEq/L.
From Beck HC: Disordered renal function. In Civett JM, Taylor RW, and Kirby RR, eds: *Critical care*, Philadelphia, 1988, JB Lippincott.

hypotension and the danger of ischemic damage to the kidneys.[154] Osmotic diuretics administered to hypervolemic patients can produce congestive heart failure by further increasing intravascular volume.[8] The administration of diuretics will invalidate urinary indices measured for 12 hours afterward because they interfere with the kidney's ability to absorb and secrete electrolytes. It is prudent, therefore, to delay administration of diuretics until the etiology of the oliguria can be established.

In patients at risk for real failure, oliguria is a much more ominous development. In these patients, aggressive efforts at diagnosis and treatment are required. Those at risk include patients having major vascular or major biliary surgery, those with obstructive jaundice, those requiring massive transfusions and/or who have experienced significant hypotension, elderly patients with prolonged operations, those with preexisting renal disease, patients with major trauma or sepsis, and those receiving nephrotoxic drugs.[33]

Polyuria

Polyuria in the PACU in healthy patients is a condition that requires only careful observation. It is frequently a manifestation of recovery from depressant effects of the anesthetics, which has led to overvigorous intravenous fluid administration intraoperatively. Polyuria may also be a manifestation of hyperglycemia acting as an osmotic diuretic. After checking this possibility, little else needs to be done to treat polyuria in healthy patients except monitoring to ensure that hypovolemia and electrolyte abnormalities do not develop.

POSTOPERATIVE BLEEDING

In the recovery room bleeding must be considered and diagnosis sought any time a patient has evidence of hypovolemia despite reasonable hydration. Postoperative bleeding in the healthy patient is usually because of vascular disruption at the surgical site, although other causes of bleeding including dilutional thrombocytopenia, dilution of coagulation factors, and disseminated intravascular coagulation (DIC) must be considered.

Diagnosis of the cause of the bleeding involves examination of the surgical incision in consultation with the surgeon, examination of the patient for evidence of petechiae, bleeding from IV sites, hematuria, and new bruising. A blood sample from a nonheparinized site should be sent for measurement of hemoglobin, hematocrit, platelet count, prothrombin time (PT), partial thromboplastin time (PTT), and fibrinogen.

Evidence of surgical bleeding will probably require wound exploration. Evidence of coagulopathy requires blood component therapy based on the abnormality identified. Bleeding from thrombocytopenia is correctable by administration of platelet concentrates. Prolongation of the PT or PTT or a low fibrinogen level is corrected by administering fresh, frozen plasma. A decreased fibrinogen level that fails to correct itself with fresh, frozen plasma may indicate DIC. Treatment involves removing the triggering source and replacing the red blood cells, platelets, and coagulation factors until the bleeding is controlled.

KEY POINTS

- Preparation of the patient for a successful recovery period begins in the operating room.
- Clinical assessments of oxygenation are unreliable for identification of hypoxia during transport; apparent recovery from anesthesia does not necessarily protect the patient from hypoxia occurring (or recurring) during transport.
- All patients who are recovering from general anesthesia should be given some form of supplemental oxygen on arrival at the PACU.
- PACU monitoring should include temperature, heart rate, blood pressure, respiratory rate, and oxygen saturation. In addition, the ECG should be monitored continuously and vital signs measured and recorded at least every 15 minutes—often more frequently.
- Continuous monitoring of PACU patients with pulse oximetry will undoubtedly soon become a standard of care.
- Criteria for PACU discharge should be well established in each PACU and should be complied with by all discharging personnel.
- Adequate treatment of pain in the PACU may have other salutary effects, including better ventilation.
- Analgesia in the PACU can be achieved in ways other than always giving parenteral narcotics.
- The best way to deal with postoperative hypothermia and/or shivering is to prevent it. This can be accomplished with proper attention to adequate operating room temperature.

- Postoperative nausea and vomiting is a continuing and major problem, especially in outpatient anesthesia. Whether propofol is better than volatile anesthesia in this regard remains to be proved, although there is early evidence that this is true.
- Small doses of droperidol, administered toward the end of the surgical procedure, have received the most attention with respect to preventing postoperative nausea and vomiting.
- Hypotension and/or hypoxia can cause nausea and vomiting. These conditions should be ruled out before attempting treatment.
- Hypoxia can cause agitation. Pharmacologic treatment of agitation should not be attempted before ruling out hypoxia. Checking the patient's bladder may reveal it to be the cause of agitation.
- The anesthesiologist must be able to recognize and treat airway obstruction in the PACU. Specifically the patient should be objectively assessed to determine whether or not the patient should have been extubated and promptly doing something about it.
- In healthy patients without significant associated disease, the most common cause of postoperative hypotension is hypovolemia.
- Hypertension can be caused by pain, agitation, endotracheal intubation, hypercapnia, etc. Several causes can be interrelated.
- Objective measures must be carefully undertaken in the patient with postoperative oliguria. This usually involves increasing the patient's circulating blood volume as a first step.

KEY REFERENCES

Asgeirsson B, Larsson S, and Magnusson J: Vomiting after pediatric strabismus surgery: comparison of two anaesthetic methods, *Anesthesiology* 71:A1059, 1989.

Cohen MM, Duncan PG, Pope WDB et al: A survey of 112,000 anaesthetics at one teaching hospital (1975-83), *Can J Anaesth* 33:22-31, 1986.

Cohen SE, Woods WA, and Wynder J: Antiemetic efficacy of droperidol and metoclopramide, *Anesthesiology* 60:67, 1984.

Doze VA, Westphall LM, and White PF: Comparison of propofol with methohexital for outpatient anesthesia, *Anesth Analg* 65:1189, 1986.

Holland R: Special committee investigating deaths under anaesthesia: report on 745 classified cases, 1960-1968, *Med J Aust* 2:573, 1970.

Lunn JN, Hunter AR, and Scott DB: Anaesthesia-related surgical mortality, *Anaesthesia* 38:1090, 1983.

Motoyama EK, Glazener CH: Hypoxemia after general anesthesia in children, *Anesth Analg* 65:267, 1986.

Smith DC, Canning JJ, and Crul JF: Pulse oximetry in the recovery room, *Anaesthesia* 44:345, 1989.

Stehling LC, Zauder HL, Fromm B et al: The incidence of postoperative nausea and vomiting, *Anesth Analg* 67:S220, 1988.

Tollosfrud SG, Gundersen Y, and Andersen R: Perioperative hypothermia, *Acta Anaesthesiol Scan* 28:511, 1984.

REFERENCES

1. Abramowitz MD, Elder PT, Friendly DS et al: Antiemetic effectiveness of intra-operatively administered droperidol in pediatric strabismic outpatient surgery, *Anesthesiology* 53:S323, 1980.
2. Abramowitz MD, Oh TH, Epstein BS et al: The antiemetic effect of droperidol following outpatient strabismus surgery in children, *Anesthesiology* 59:579, 1983.
3. Addison NV, Brear FA, Budd K et al: Epidural analgesia following cholecystectomy, *Br J Surg* 61:850, 1974.
4. Alexander CM, Teller LE, Gross JB, et al: New discharge criteria decrease recovery room time after subarachnoid block, *Anesthesiology* 70:640, 1989.
5. Andersen R, Krogh K: Pain as a major cause of postoperative nausea, *Can J Anaesth* 23:366, 1976.
6. Asgeirsson B, Larsson S, and Magnusson J: Vomiting after pediatric strabismus surgery: comparison of two anesthetic methods, *Anesthesiology* 71:A1059, 1989.
7. Barber JG, Ominsky AJ, Orkin FK et al: Physostigmine atropine solution fails to reverse diazepam sedation, *Anesth Analg* 59:58, 1980.
8. Barry KG, Berman AR: The acute effects of the intravenous infusion of mannitol on blood and plasma volumes, *N Engl J Med* 264:1085, 1961.
9. Bay J, Nunn JF, and Prys-Roberts C: Factors influencing arterial Po_2 during recovery from anaesthesia, *Br J Anaesth* 40:398, 1968.
10. Beck C: Disordered renal function. In Civetta JM, Taylor RW, and Kirby RR, eds: *Critical care*, Philadelphia, 1988, JB Lippincott.
11. Becker LD, Paulson BA, and Miller RD: Biphasix respiratory depression after fentanyl-droperidol or fentanyl alone used to supplement nitrous oxide anesthesia, *Anesthesiology* 44:291, 1976.
12. Behar M, Magora F, Olshwang D et al: Epidural morphine in treatment of pain, *Lancet* I:10, 527, 1979.
13. Bellville JW, Bross IDJ, and Howland WS: Postoperative nausea and vomiting IV: factors related to postoperative nausea and vomiting, *Anesthesiology* 21:186, 1960.
14. Blaise G, Roy WL: Postoperative pain relief after hypospadias repair in pediatric patients: regional analgesia vs. systemic analgesics, *Anesthesiology* 65:84, 1986.
15. Bonica JJ, Crepps W, Monk B et al: Postanesthetic nausea, retching, and vomiting. Evaluation of cyclizine (marezine) suppositories for treatment, *Anesthesiology* 19:532, 1958.
16. Bridenbaugh PO, Dupen SL, Moore DC et al: Postoperative intercostal nerve block analgesia vs. narcotic analgesia, *Anesth Analg* 52:81, 1973.
17. Bromage PR: Extradural analgesia for pain relief, *Br J Anaesth* 39:721, 1967.
18. Burtles R, Peckett BW: Postoperative vomiting, *Br J Anaesth* 29:114, 1957.
19. Cantarovich F, Galli C, Benedetti L et al: High dose furosemide in established acute renal failure, *Br Med J* 24:449, 1973.
20. Celleno D, Capogna G: Spinal buprenorphine for postoperative analgesia after cesarean section, *Acta Anaesthesiol Scand* 33:236, 1989.
21. Chayen MS, Rudick V, and Borvine A: Pain control with epidural injection of morphine, *Anesthesiology* 53:338, 1980.
22. Chestnut DH, Vandewalker GE, Owen CL et al: Administration of metoclopramide for prevention of nausea and vomiting during epidural anesthesia for elective cesarean section, *Anesthesiology* 66:563, 1987.
23. Chripko D, Bevan JC, Archer DP et al: Decreases in arterial oxygen saturaton in paediatric outpatients during transfer to the postanaesthetic recovery room, *Can J Anaesth* 36:128, 1989.
24. Christensen S, Farrow-Gillespie A, and Lerman J: Incidence of emesis in postanesthetic recovery after strabismus surgery in children: a comparison of droperidol and lidocaine, *Anesthesiology* 70:251, 1989.
25. Ciofolo MJ, Clergue F, Devilliers C et al: Changes in ventilation, oxygen uptake, and carbon dioxide output during recovery from isoflurane anesthesia, *Anesthesiology* 70:73, 1989.
26. Cohen M: An investigation into shivering following anesthesia, *Proc R Soc Med* 60:752, 1967.
27. Cohen MM, Duncan PG, Pope WDB, et al: A survey of 112,000 anaesthetics at one teaching hospital (1975-83), *Can J Anaesth* 33:22, 1986.
28. Cohen SE, Woods WA, and Wynder J: Antiemetic efficacy of droperidol and metoclopramide, *Anesthesiology* 60:67, 1984.
29. Conahan TJ, Williams GD, Apfelbaum JL et al: Airway heating reduces recovery time (cost) in outpatients, *Anesthesiology* 67:128, 1987.
30. Corssen G, Domeno EF, and Swett RB: Neuroleptanalgesia and anesthesia, *Curr Res Anesth* 43:748, 1964.
31. Coté CJ, Eavey Rd, Todres D et al: Cricothyroid membrane puncture: oxygenation and ventilation in a dog model using an intravenous catheter, *Crit Care Med* 16:615, 1988.
32. Coté CJ, Goldstein EA, Cote MA et al: A single-blind study of pulse oximetry in children, *Anesthesiology* 68:184, 1988.
33. Cousins MJ, Maze RI: Anaesthesia, surgery, and renal function, *Anaesth Intensive Care* 1:355, 1973.
34. Dalens B, Tanguy A, and Haberer JP: Lumbar epidural anesthesia for operative and postoperative pain relief in infants and young children, *Anesth Analg* 65:1069, 1986.
35. Dalens B, Vanneuvlle G, and Dechelotte P: Penile block via the subpubic space in 100 children, *Anesth Analg* 69:41, 1989.
36. DeGrodd PMRM, Melsukuri S, Van Egmund J et al: Comparison of etomidate and propofol for anaesthesia in microlaryngeal surgery, *Anaesthesia* 42:368, 1987.
37. Dent SJ, Ramachandra V, and Stephen CR: Postoperative vomiting: incidence, analysis, and therapeutic measures in 3,000 patients, *Anesthesiology* 16:564, 1955.
38. Desparmet J, Meistelman C, Barre J et al: Continuous epidural infusion of bupivacaine for postoperative pain relief in children, *Anesthesiology* 67:108, 1987.
39. Diamond MJ: Anaesthesia and emesis. Clinical usefulness of metoclopramide, *Can J Anaesth* 32:198, 1985.
40. Doze VA, Westphall LM, and White PF: Comparison of propofol with methohexital for outpatient anesthesia, *Anesth Analg* 65:1189, 1986.
41. Dupre LJ, Stieglitz P: Extrapyramidal syndromes after premedication with droperidol in children, *Br J Anaesth* 52:831, 1980.
42. Dyrberg V: Haloperidol in the prevention of postoperative nausea and vomiting, *Acta Anaesthesiol Scan* 6:37, 1982.
43. Ebert J, Varner PD: The effective use of epidural monitoring sulfate for postoperative orthopedic pain, *Anesthesiology* 53:257, 1980.
44. Eckenhoff JE, Kneale DH, and Dripps RD: The incidence and etiology of postanesthetic excitement, *Anesthesiology* 22:667, 1961.
45. Edelist G: A comparison of propofol and thiopentone as induction agents in outpatient surgery, *Can J Anaesth* 34:110, 1987.
46. Egbert LD, Laver MB, and Bendixen HH: The effect of site of operation and type of anesthesia upon the ability to cough in the postoperative period, *Surg Gynecol Obstet* 115:295, 1962.
47. Eustis S, Lerman J, and Smith DR: Effect of droperidol pretreatment on postanesthetic vomiting in children undergoing strabismus surgery: the minimum effective dose, *J Ped Ophthalmol Strabismus* 24:165, 1987.
48. Fink BR: Diffusion anoxia, *Anesthesiology* 16:511, 1955.
49. Fink BR: Etiology and treatment of laryngeal spasm, *Anesthesiology* 17:569, 1956.
50. Gal TJ, Cooperman LH: Hypertension in the immediate postoperative period, *Br J Anaesth* 47:70, 1975.
51. Glynn CJ, Mather LE, Cousins MJ et al: Peridural meperidine in humans: analgetic response, pharmacokinetics, and transmission into CSF, *Anesthesiology* 55:520, 1981.
52. Goldblat A, Miller R: Prevention of incidental hypothermia in neurosurgical patients, *Anesth Analg* 51:536, 1972.
53. Goldfarb G, Ang ET, Debaene B et al: Effect of clonidine on postoperative shivering in man: a double blind study, *Anesthesiology* 71:A650, 1989.

54. Gonzales ER: Stopping postop shivers eases rewarming, *JAMA* 28:2802, 1982.
55. Goold JE: Postoperative spasticity and shivering, *Anaesthesia* 39:35, 1984.
56. Gravenstein JS, Beecher HK: The effect of preoperative medication with morphine on postoperative analgesia with morphine, *J Pharmacol* 119:506, 1957.
57. Gundwardene RD, White DC: Propofol and emesis, *Anaesthesia* 43:65, 1988.
58. Hammel HT: Anesthetics and body temperature regulation, *Anesthesiology* 68:833, 1988.
59. Hannallah RS, Roadman LM, Belman AB et al: Comparison of caudal and ilioinguinal/iliohypogastric nerve blocks for control of postorchiopexy pain in pediatric ambulatory surgery, *Anesthesiology* 66:832, 834, 1987.
60. Hardy JF, Charest J, Girouard G et al: Nausea and vomiting after strabismus surgery in preschool children, *Can J Anaesth* 33:57, 1986.
61. Harper MH, Hickey RF, Cromwell TH et al: The magnitude and duration of respiratory depression produced by fentanyl and fentanyl pulse droperidol in man, *J Pharm Exp Ther* 199:464, 1976.
62. Harris SN, Sevarino FB, Silverman DG et al: Prophylactic transdermal scopolamine for patients using postoperative patient controlled analgesia (PCA), *Anesthesiology* 71:A690, 1989.
63. Harrison GG: Death attributable to anaesthesia, a 10-year survey (1967-1976), *Br J Anaesth* 50:1041, 1978.
64. Henderson JJ, Parbrook GD: Influence of anaesthetic technique on postoperative pain. A comparison of anaesthetic supplementation with halothane and with phenoperidine, *Br J Anaesth* 48:587, 1976.
65. Holdcroft A, Hall GM: Heat loss during anaesthesia, *Br J Anaesth* 50:157, 1978.
66. Holland R: Special committee investigating deaths under anaesthesia: report on 745 classified cases, 1960-1968, *Med J Aust* 2:573, 1970.
67. Hovorka J, Korttila K, and Erkola O: Nausea and vomiting after general anaesthesia with isoflurane, enflurane, or fentanyl in combination with nitrous oxide and oxygen, *Eur J Anaesthesiol* 5:177, 1988.
68. Hudson HE, Harber PI, and Smith TC: Respiratory depression from alkalosis and opioid interaction in man, *Anesthesiology* 40:543, 1974.
69. Jensen BH: Caudal block for postoperative pain relief in children after genital operations. A comparison between bupivacaine and morphine, *Acta Anaesthesiol Scan* 25:373, 1981.
70. Jones HD, McLaren CAB: Postoperative shivering and hypoxemia after halothane, nitrous oxide, and oxygen anesthesia, *Br J Anaesth* 37:35, 1965.
71. Jordan C: Assessment of the effects of drugs on respiration, *Br J Anaesth* 54:763, 1982.
72. Kataria BK, Harnik EV, Mitchard R et al: Postoperative arterial oxygen saturation in the pediatric population during transportation, *Anesth Analg* 67:280, 1988.

73. Katz JD, Croneau LH, and Barash PG: Postoperative hypertension: a hazard of abrupt cessation of antihypertensive medication in the preoperative period, *Am Heart J* 92:79, 1976.
74. Keats AS: Postoperative pain: research and treatment, *J Chron Dis* 4:72, 1956.
75. Keats AS, Girgis KZ: Respiratory depression associated with reief of pain by narcotics, *Anesthesiology* 29:1006, 1968.
76. Kjellstrand CM: Ethacrynic acid in acute tubular necrosis, *Nephron* 9:337, 1972.
77. Knapp MR: Postanesthetic nausea, vomiting, and retching, *JAMA* 160:376, 1960.
78. Knill RL, Clement JL: Variable effects of anesthetics on the ventilatory response to hypoxemia in man, *Can J Anaesth* 29:93, 1982.
79. Knill RL, Gelb AW: Ventilatory responses to hypoxia and hypercapnia during halothane sedation and anaesthesia in man, *Anesthesiology* 49:244, 1978.
80. Korttila K, Hovorka J, and Erkola O: Nitrous oxide does not increase the incidence of nausea and vomiting after isoflurane anesthesia, *Anesth Analg* 66:761, 1987.
81. Kotelko DM, Rottman RL, Wright WC et al: Transdermal scopolaine decreases nausea and vomiting following cesarean section in patients receiving epidural morphine, *Anesthesiology* 71:675, 1989.
82. Krane EJ, Jacobson LE, Lynn AM et al: Caudal morphine for postoperative analgesia in children: a comparison with caudal bupivacaine and intravenous morphine, *Anesth Analg* 66:647, 1987.
83. Kruse DH: Postoperative hypothermia, *Focus on Crit Care* 10:48, 1983.
84. Larson GF, Hurlbert BJ, and Wingard DW: Physostigmine reversal of diazepam-induced depression, *Anesth Analg* 56:248, 1977.
85. Lawson D, Phillips LH, Harris MM et al: All that quakes does not necessarily shiver, *Anesthesiology* 70:556, 1989.
86. Lerman J, Eustis S, and Smith DR: Effect of droperidol pretreatment on postanesthetic vomiting in children undergoing strabismus surgery, *Anesthesiology* 65:322, 1986.
87. Liem St, Aldrete JA: Control of postanesthetic shivering, *Can J Anaesth* 21:506, 1974.
88. Lin DM, Rodarte A: Metoclopromide prophylaxis against postoperative vomiting in pediatric strabismus patients, *Anesthesiology* 71:A1064, 1989.
89. Lincoln JR, Sawyer JP: Complications related to body positions during surgical procedures, *Anesthesiology* 22:800, 1961.
90. Loan WB, Morrison JD: The incidence and severity of postoperative pain, *Br J Anaesth* 39:695, 1967.
91. Lonie DS, Harper NJN: Nitrous oxide anaesthesia and vomiting, *Anaesthesia* 41:703, 1986.
92. Loper KA, Ready LB, and Dorman BH: Prophylactic transdermal scopolamine patches reduce nausea in postoperative patients receiving epidural morphine, *Anesth Analg* 68:144, 1989.

93. Lunn JN, Hunter AR, and Scott DB: Anaesthesia-related surgical mortality, *Anaesthesia* 38:1090, 1983.
94. Mahajan RP, Grover VK, Sharma SL et al: Intraocular pressure changes during muscular hyperactivity after general anesthesia, *Anesthesiology* 66:419, 1987.
95. Martin SJ, Murphy JD, Colliton RJ et al: Clinical studies with Innovar, *Anesthesiology* 28:458, 1967.
96. Marx GF, Mateo CV, and Orkin LR: Computer analysis of postanesthetic deaths, *Anesthesiology* 39:54, 1973.
97. McCallum MID, Glynn CJ, Moore RA et al: Transcutaneous electrical nerve stimulation in the management of acute postoperative pain, *Br J Anaesth* 61:308, 1988.
98. McKenzie R: Antiemetic effectiveness of intramuscular hydrozyine compared with intramuscular droperidol, *Anesth Analg* 60:783, 1981.
99. Melnick BM, Johnson LS: Effects of eliminating nitrous oxide in outpatient anesthesia, *Anesthesiology* 67:982, 1987.
100. Memery HN: Anesthesia mortality in private practice. A ten year study, *JAMA* 194:1185, 1965.
101. Mirakhur RK, Dundee JW: Lack of antiemetic effect of glycopyroolate, *Anaesthesia* 3:819, 1981.
102. Moller JT, Wittrup M, and Johansen SH: Incidence and duration of hypoxemia in the recovery room (RR) — an observer study, *Anesthesiology* 71:A1181, 1989.
103. Montgomery CJ, Vaghadia H, and Blackstock D: Negative middle ear pressure and postoperative vomiting in pediatric outpatients, *Anesthesiology* 68:288, 1988.
104. Morikawa S, Safar P, and DeCarlo J: Influence of the head-jaw position upon upper airway patency, *Anesthesiology* 22:265, 1961.
105. Morley-Forster PK: Unintentional hypothermia in the operating room, *Can J Anaesth* 33:516, 1986.
106. Morris RH, Wilkey BR: The effects of ambient temperature on patient temperature during surgery not involving body cavities, *Anesthesiology* 32:102, 1970.
107. Motoyama EK, Glazener CH: Hypoxemia after general anesthesia in children, *Anesth Analg* 65:267, 1986.
108. Muir JJ, Warner MA, Offord KP et al: Role of nitrous oxide and other factors in postoperative nausea and vomiting: a randomized and blinded prospective study, *Anesthesiology* 66:513, 1987.
109. Muneyuki M, Ueda Y, Urabe N et al: Postoperative pain relief and respiratory function in man: comparison between intermittent intravenous injections of meperidine and continuous lumbar epidural analgesia, *Anesthesiology* 29:304, 1968.
110. Nagy J, Desci L: Physostigmine, a highly potent antidote for acute experimental diazepam intoxication, *Neuropharmacology* 17:469, 1978.
111. Newman BJ: Control of accidental hypothermia, *Anaesthesia* 26:177, 1971.

112. Nishino T, Hiraga K, Fujisato M et al: Breathing patterns during postoperative analgesia in patients after lower abdominal operations, *Anesthesiology* 69:967, 1988.

113. Parkhouse J, Lambrechts W, and Simpson BRJ: The incidence of postoperative pain, *Br J Anaesth* 33:345, 1961.

114. Pataky AO, Kitz DS, Andrews RW et al: Nausea and vomiting following ambulatory surgery: are all procedures created equal? *Anesth Analg* 67:S163, 1988.

115. Patel R, Norden J, and Hannallah RS: Oxygen administration prevents hypoxemia during postanesthetic transport in children, *Anesthesiology* 69:616, 1988.

116. Pauca AL, Savage RT, Simpson S et al: Effect of pethidine, fentanyl, and morphine on postoperative shivering in man, *Acta Anaesthesiol Scan* 28:138, 1984.

117. Pflug AE, Aasheim GM, Foster C et al: Prevention of postanesthesia shivering, *Can J Anaesth Soc* 25:43, 1978.

118. Pflug AE, Murphy TM, Butler SH et al: The effects of postoperative peridural analgesia on pulmonary therapy and pulmonary complications, *Anesthesiology* 41:8, 1974.

119. Philbin DM, Sullivan SF, Bowman FO et al: Postoperative hypoxemia: contribution of the cardiac output, *Anesthesiology* 32:136, 1970.

120. Poler SM, White PF, Margrabe D et al: Nausea and vomiting in outpatients—use of droperidol prophylaxis, *Anesthesiology* 71:A134, 1989.

121. Pratt JH, Welch JS: Hyabrobal and methadone hydrochloride in preoperative preparation of patients, *J Am Med Assoc* 157:231, 1953.

122. Pullerits J, Burrows FA, and Roy WL: Arterial desaturation in healthy children during transfer to the recovery room, *Can J Anaesth* 34:470, 1987.

123. Reiostad F, Stromskag KE: Interpleural catheter for the management of postoperative pain: a preliminary report, *Reg Anaesth* 11:89, 1988.

124. Riding JE: Postoperative vomiting, *Proc R Soc Med* 53:671, 1960.

125. Rita L, Goodarzi M, and Seleny F: Effect of low dose droperidol on postoperative vomiting in children, *Can J Anaesth* 28:259, 1981.

126. Rodriguez JL, Weissman C, Damask MC et al: Morphine and postoperative rewarming in critically ill patients, *Circulation* 68:1238, 1983.

127. Rodriquez JL, Weissman C, Damask MC et al: Physiologic requirements during rewarming: suppression of the shivering response, *Crit Care Med* 11:490, 1983.

128. Rowley MP, Brown TCK: Postoperative vomiting in children, *Anaesth Intens Care* 10:309, 1982.

129. Ruben HM, Elam JO, Ruben AM et al: Investigation of upper airway problems in resuscitation, *Anesthesiology* 22:271, 1961.

130. Ruth HS, Haugen FP, and Grove DD: Anesthesia study commission. Findings of eleven years' activity, *J Am Med Assoc* 135:881, 1947.

131. Salvatore AJ, Sullivan SF: Postoperative hypoventilation and hypoxemia in man after hyperventilation, *N Engl J Med* 280:467, 1969.

132. Saunders PR, Banish P, Lipton JM et al: Localized regulated radiant heat vs. meperidine in the control of postanesthetic shivering, *Anesthesiology* 71:A184, 1989.

133. Sengupta P, Plantevin OM: Nitrous oxide and day-case laparoscopy: effects of nausea, vomiting, and return to normal activity, *Br J Anaesth* 60:570, 1988.

134. Sessler DI, Israel D, Pozos RS et al: Spontaneous postanesthetic tremor does not resemble thermoregulatory shivering, *Anesthesiology* 68:843, 1988.

135. Sessler DI, Olofsson CI, Rubinstein EH et al: The thermoregulatory threshold in humans during halothane anesthesia, *Anesthesiology* 68:836, 1988.

136. Sessler DI, Pozo RS: In reply to: all that quakes does not necessarily shiver, *Anesthesiology* 70:557, 1989.

137. Sessler DI, Rubinstein EH, and Eger EI: Core temperature changes during N$_2$O fentanyl and halothane/O$_2$ anesthesia, *Anesthesiology* 67:137, 1987.

138. Sharkey A, Lipton JM, Murphy MT et al: Inhibition of postanesthetic shivering with radiant heat, *Anesthesiology* 66:249, 1987.

139. Shuman RL, Peters RM: Epidural anesthesia following thoracotomy in patients with chronic obstructive airway disease, *J Thorac Cardiovasc Surg* 71:82, 1976.

140. Sinclair R, Cassuto J, Hogstrom S et al: Topical anesthesia with lidocaine aerosol in the control of postoperative pain, *Anesthesiology* 68:895, 1988.

141. Smith DC, Canning JJ, Crul JF: Pulse oximetry in the recovery room, *Anaesthesia* 44:345, 1989.

142. Soliman IE, Patel RI, Ehrenpreis MB et al: Recovery scores do not correlate with postoperative hypoxemia in children, *Anesth Analg* 67:53, 1988.

143. Soliman MG, Ansara S, and LaBerge R: Caudal anaesthesia in paediatric patients, *Can Anaesth Soc J* 25:226, 1978.

144. Soliman MG, Gillies DMM: Muscular hyperactivity after general anesthesia, *Can Anaesth Soc J* 19:529, 1972.

145. Soliman MG, Tremblay NA: Nerve block of the penis for postoperative pain relief in children, *Anesth Analg* 57:45, 1978.

146. Spence AA, Smith G: Postoperative analgesia and lung function: a comparison of morphine with extradural block, *Br J Anaesth* 43:144, 1971.

147. Stehling LC, Zauder HL, Fromm B et al: The incidence of postoperative nausea and vomiting, *Anesth Analg* 67:S220, 1988.

148. Swerdlow M, Murray A, Daw RH: A study of postoperative pain, *Acta Anaesthesiol Scand* 7:1, 1963.

149. Swerdlow M, Starmer G, and Daw RH: A comparison of morphine and phenazocine in postoperative pain, *Br J Anaesth* 36:782, 1964.

150. Tinker JH, Michenfelder JD: Sodium nitroprusside, *Anesthesiology* 45:340, 1976.

151. Tiret L, Desmonts JM, Hatton F et al: Complications associated with anaesthesia—a prospective survey in France, *Can J Anesth* 33:336, 1986.

152. Tollofsrud SG, Gundersen Y, and Andersen R: Perioperative hypothermia, *Acta Anaesthesiol Scan* 28:511, 1984.

153. Tyler IL, Tantisira B, Winter PM et al: Continuous monitoring of arterial oxygen saturation with pulse oximetry during transfer to the recovery room, *Anesth Analg* 64:1108, 1985.

154. Ufferman RC, Jaenike JR, Freeman RB et al: Effects of furosemide on low-dose mercuric chloride acute renal failure in the rat, *Kidney Int* 8:362-7, 1975.

155. Utting JE, Gray TC, and Shelley FC: Human misadventure in anaesthesia, *Can J Anaesth* 26:472, 1979.

156. Vaughan MS, Vaugh RW and Cork RC: Postoperative hypothermia in adults: relationship of age, anesthesia, and shivering to rewarming, *Anesth Analg* 60:746, 1981.

157. Vijayakumar HR, Metriyakool K, and Jewell MR: Effects of 100% oxygen and a mixture of oxygen and air on oxygen saturation in the immediate postoperative period in children, *Anesth Analg* 66:181, 1987.

158. Waldmann CS, Verghese C, Short SM et al: The evaluation of domperidone and metoclopramide as antiemetics in day-care abortion patients, *Br J Clin Pharmac* 19:307, 1985.

159. Walsh T, Cheng D, Brown P et al: Are hemodynamic changes a warning of hypoxia during isoflurane anesthesia? *Anesthesiology* 71:A1180, 1989.

160. Walz MA, Davis WM: Experimental diazepam intoxication in rodents: physostigmine and naloxone as potential antagonists, *Drug Chem Toxicol* 2:257, 1979.

161. Warner LO, Rogers GL, Martino JD et al: Intravenous lidocaine reduces the incidence of vomiting in children after surgery to correct strabismus, *Anesthesiology* 68:618, 1988.

162. Weil JV, McCullough RE, Kline JS et al: Diminished ventilatory response to hypoxia and hypercapnia after morphine in normal man, *N Engl J Med* 292:1103, 1975.

163. Weinger MB, Swerdlow NR, and Millar WL: Acute postoperative delirium and extrapyramidal signs in a previously healthy parturient, *Anesth Analg* 67:291, 1988.

164. Wiklund PE: Intensive care units: design, location, staffing ancillary areas, equipment, *Anesthesiology* 31:122, 1969.

CHAPTER 9

Use and Misuse of Consultants

THOMAS H. LEE
LEE GOLDMAN

Role of the Consultant
Logistic Issues in the Performance of a
Consultation
Timing of the preoperative evaluation
Postoperative evaluation
Medicolegal Issues
Factors Associated with the Effectiveness
of Consultations
Summary and Conclusions

In recent years, perioperative consultation has evolved into an increasingly well-defined area of medicine, complete with its own literature.[2,3,13,19] This change is a direct response to clinical needs posed by the aging of the population, which has led to a rise in the prevalence of comorbid illnesses in patients who undergo or are considered for procedures. In one series of preoperative consultations, 47% of patients had two or more chronic diseases.[6] **This trend toward increased risk in the patient population has been complicated by surgical advances that have encouraged the performance of increasingly ambitious procedures and by progress in the fields of anesthesiology and medicine that has made these disciplines so sophisticated that the interfaces between them are areas requiring special skills.**

In addition to the development of a clinical knowledge base,[2,3] an important response to the need for such expertise has been the growth and development of medical consultation services that specialize

in the perioperative evaluation of surgical candidates.[4,6,24,27] Several investigations have shown that such consultations can lead to the detection of important new diagnoses that may warrant preoperative interventions[18,27] or help in arranging followup care.[18] However the effectiveness of consultations provided by such services or by individual physicians is highly variable and is influenced by factors including communication among the surgeon, anesthesiologist, and consultant.[18,20-22,28] When we interviewed consultants and the physicians who requested the consultation in 156 cases at a teaching hospital, we found that they disagreed on both the reason for the consultation and the principal clinical issue in 14% of cases.[22] When communication among physicians is so tenuous, it is not surprising that rates of compliance with the recommendations of consultants are 54% to 77%.[1,17,30]

Furthermore, the period during which such communication can occur is currently being compressed by economic pressures for efficiency that have encouraged increased use of outpatient surgery and the performance of procedures on the day of admission. "Same day" surgery is now routinely being performed at many centers for major procedures such as total joint replacements and cholecystectomies. In such cases, the time during which the surgeon and anesthesiologist must perform a preoperative evaluation, and decide whether to obtain a consultation, is compressed. Even if a consultation is performed, the consultants often are not aware of the specific issues to be addressed,[22] and their recommendations are frequently ignored.[1,17,30]

Thus, although the potential contribution by consultants has never been greater, there are many opportunities for the perioperative consultation process to go awry. This chapter will describe ways in which consultations may be used, and misused, by describing their role, performance, medicolegal issues, and factors associated with effectiveness.

ROLE OF THE CONSULTANT

One of the most common reasons for perioperative consultation is a request for "clearance."[18] For several reasons both the requesting physicians and the consultants should seek to narrow the purpose of the consultation in such cases. "Clearance" implies a guarantee of a good outcome, which is, of course, impossible to provide. Whether it is good judgment from a medicolegal perspective for a consultant to offer such a guarantee is uncertain; furthermore, the impact of consultations aimed at "clearing" patients is usually limited.[7]

All patients, no matter how stable, are at some risk of complications when they undergo anesthesia and surgery, and one of the principal roles of the consultant is to estimate the risk of cardiac and noncardiac complications associated with the planned procedure for the individual patient (Box 9-1). In addition to identification of high- and low-risk patients, the consultant can help compare the risks associated with surgical and medical therapy and identify management strategies that may help minimize those risks. Finally, the consultant can help anticipate which problems are most likely and when they are likely to occur and follow the patient postoperatively to help prevent, detect, and manage such complications.

In the management of acute or chronic medical conditions that may complicate perioperative management, consultants often play a role analogous to that of a primary care internist. For example, input from an internist may be required when the patient has an unstable medical problem (e.g., acute myocardial infarction), an uncertain medical status (e.g., chest pain of unknown cause), or multiple chronic diseases (e.g., diabetes, hypertension, or alcohol abuse). When the internist has been the primary care physician for that patient, familiarity with the past history and the baseline condition may help management of clinical and social issues.

However, all parties must respect the limits of the consultant's role and expertise. Whereas the consultant must perform thorough evaluations and gather primary data through a history and examination (as opposed to a review of the medical record), the primary physicians are the surgeon and the anesthesiologist. On one hand the consultant should not be delegated responsibility for performing the definitive preoperative evaluation; on the other the consultant must respect the relationships among the patient, surgeon, and anesthesiologist, and be appropriately circumspect in conversations with the patient. For example, a consultant might answer a patient's questions about diabetes mellitus but should not engage in lengthy discussions concerning whether the surgery should be performed or is likely to succeed. Expressing an opinion to the patient or other health care personnel that surgery should be cancelled, without prior discussion with the surgeon and anesthesiologist, would obviously be a serious breech of etiquette. The consultant's obligations to the patient can almost always be met through the consultant's primary relationship with the other physicians (see following discussion).

By extension, the consultant should recognize issues on which his/her expertise is less than that of the anesthesiologist or surgeon. For example, an internist's recommendations on the choice and route of anesthesia are not authoritative and may generate animosity among the health care team. Similarly, trivial recommendations (e.g., "avoid hypotension") are unlikely to improve care but remain distressingly common. In a series of medical consultations to surgeons at one teaching hospital, 122 of 1016 recommendations (12%) were judged to be "insulting."[1]

Finally, consultants may play important roles as teachers, just as they are likely to learn from exposure to colleagues in anesthesia and surgery. This educational role also requires tact and sensitivity to the needs of the other physicians. Opinions should be expressed concisely and without condescension, and references should be provided selectively. The description of a differential diagnosis may be helpful, but a long, intellectual discussion in the medical record is unlikely to be read.

BOX 9-1
FUNCTIONS OF THE CONSULTANT

Estimation of cardiac and noncardiac risk of surgery
Identification of management strategies that minimize risks
Anticipation of complications that may occur during the perioperative period
Postoperative followup to help prevent, detect, and manage complications
Perioperative management of acute and chronic medical conditions
Education—teaching and learning

LOGISTIC ISSUES IN THE PERFORMANCE OF A CONSULTATION

Timing of the Preoperative Evaluation

Because the consultant's role in a case has several possible functions, the consultant should be available or should be contacted at several points in time. The increase in outpatient or "same day" surgery has been accompanied by the development at several institutions of "Pre-Admitting Test Centers," where patients undergo preoperative laboratory work and evaluations by anesthesiologists and other personnel. However, medical consultants have not been integrated into such settings routinely, forcing surgeons and anesthesiologists to arrange consultations, often within a very short time frame. Logistical problems may cause postponement of cases and costly disruptions to the operating room schedule.

In the ideal situation, the surgeon who schedules a patient for elective surgery should perform an evaluation that is sufficiently thorough to determine whether the assistance of a consultant will be appropriate and an elective outpatient consultation should be arranged well in advance of the surgical date. A 1- to 2-week interval before surgery will permit a consultant to obtain prior medical records, electrocardiograms, and radiographs; perform additional tests (e.g., an exercise tolerance test); and make adjustments in the patient's medical regimens, such as the initiation of therapy for hypertension. By seeing a patient before and after admission, the consultant becomes more familiar with the patient's baseline mental status and physical examination.

Unfortunately, the need for such information or intervention is often detected only a few days or hours before surgery, during the anesthesiologist's preoperative evaluation. In such cases, the surgeon or anesthesiologist with good professional relationships with medical colleagues may be able to arrange a consultation on short notice, but institutions will find it advantageous to develop a mechanism by which an internist or cardiologist is available to see the patient on a "walk-in" basis.

It is ironic that technologic advances have both increased the need for these consultations and made their performance easier. Computerized electrocardiography machines now provide preliminary interpretations of the tracing, but the interpretative software is generally written to have a high sensitivity for detecting abnormalities. An unofficial reading of "Poor R-wave progression; cannot exclude anterior myocardial infarction" will often force the evaluating anesthesiologist to request a cardiology consultation. However, the widespread availability of fax machines has eased the difficulty of obtaining prior tracings from other institutions for comparison.

When consultations are not or cannot be per-

formed before admission, the need for the consultation may be recognized the evening before or even the morning that a procedure is scheduled. Although surgeons and anesthesiologists have a responsibility to make timely requests for evaluations, consultants should resist any temptation to punish the other physicians (and the patient) by forcing a postponement in the procedure. Because operating room time is among the most costly of hospital resources, the consultant should make every effort to see the patient before the scheduled procedure time. Afterward, the various members of the health care team should attempt to identify strategies for a more orderly consultative process.

Postoperative Evaluation

The need for consultants to be involved in the management of patients in the operating room arises only occasionally, but because patients are least stable in the immediate postoperative period, consultants should be expected to re-evaluate patients shortly after their admission to the recovery room. For example, postoperative hypertension usually occurs 30 to 60 minutes after the end of anesthesia.[8] Thus consultants (and primary physicians) should evaluate the patient's volume status and fluid orders to avoid marked hemodynamic changes and should consider early performance of an electrocardiogram to detect asymptomatic ischemia. A rule used by many experienced consultants is "never go home before the patient is out of the operating room."

The role of the consultant does not end with the immediate perioperative period. Mobilization of extravascular fluid and high sympathetic tone associated with pain may contribute to cardiovascular complications such as acute myocardial infarction 24 to 48 hours or more after surgery,[9] and ischemic heart disease may be exacerbated by increased activity later in the hospitalization. Other medical conditions may worsen later in the hospitalization; for example, mild renal failure may be unmasked by the volume shifts associated with the perioperative state. **Thus it is recommended that consultants follow patients for at least 3 to 5 days after surgery.**

MEDICOLEGAL ISSUES

Although consultations that are ordered purely for "defensive medicine" purposes may lead to delays and increased resource utilization,[22] several legal decisions have made explicit the duty of primary physicians to request consultations when clinical problems lie outside their expertise.[15] There is no duty to consult when the anesthesiologist or surgeon does not recognize any special problems, but judgments against physicians have been made if the patient's recovery does not progress and no consultation is sought, or if a physician undertakes a procedure beyond his/her training when specialists were available. Furthermore, after a consultant's role in a case has been concluded, the primary physician has an obligation to inform the consultant of any developments that may be relevant to the consultant's expertise.[15]

In practical terms these principles imply that anesthesiologists and surgeons must have a low threshold for requesting the assistance of internal medicine and subspecialty consultants when acute or chronic medical conditions may influence the outcome of the patient's surgery. For example, although anesthesiologists may be comfortable managing common problems such as hypertension or diabetes, cardiology consultations for the purpose of reviewing equivocal electrocardiograms or evaluating a chest pain syndrome are reasonable. Informal consultations, in which the internist or subspecialist does not examine the patient and write a note, are not adequate.[5]

When the anesthesiologist or surgeon requests a consultation, legal and ethical considerations indicate that the primary physician should inform the patient and get his/her consent.[14,31] If the patient does not consent, previous legal decisions have indicated that the patient is not liable for the consultant's fees.[14,15] However, if the patient agrees, the request for a consultation should be made in writing.[5] At that point, the consultant forms a relationship with both the primary physician and the patient.

Nevertheless, the primary physician remains the individual who is responsible for all decisions concerning the patient's treatment. The consultant should be required to write a full report since oral recommendations may not be recognized in any legal proceedings. In general the consultants should not discuss findings directly with the patient unless the primary physician has given permission. It is the duty of the primary physician to convey relevant information to the patient.[5]

FACTORS ASSOCIATED WITH THE EFFECTIVENESS OF CONSULTATIONS

Consultations frequently lead to new diagnoses[27] and management decisions, including changes in medical therapy,[18] triage to a new service,[27] and delay or cancellations of surgery.[6] **However, about half of the recommendations made by consultants in the perioperative setting are ignored,[17] indicating either that the consultants are frequently making unimportant or ill-advised recommendations, that they are not conveying the recommendations appropriately to the primary physicians, or that the primary physicians are ignoring them.**

Effective communication between the consultant and the primary physician who requests a consultation has considerable impact on the value of a consultation. As noted, we found disagreement between the consultant and the primary physician on the issues of a consultation in 14% of internal medicine consultations at a teaching hospital.[22] Similarly, at another teaching hospital no specific question was asked in 24% of preoperative diabetic consultations, and consultants ignored the stated question in another 12%.[29] When such breakdowns in communication occur, the primary physicians have significantly lower opinions of the impact of the consultations than the consultants.[22]

Direct oral communication between the consultant and primary physicians is important to prevent such misunderstandings,[26] and continued direct contact with the primary physicians in the days after the initial contact can enhance the effectiveness of the consultation. However, anesthesiologists and surgeons are frequently difficult to reach; in such instances, written notes in the medical record are essential to communication. In hospitals where such services are available, computer mail or fax can augment communication but should not be relied upon for transmittal of critical information.

In addition to direct interaction after the initial evaluation, the consultant should demonstrate continued involvement in the case after surgery. Several investigations have found that recommendations are more likely to be followed if consultants write periodic followup notes, repeating essential recommendations.[16,23,29] For example, Horwitz et al.[16] found that consultations that included more than one followup note had an effect on diagnosis in 92% of cases and an effect on management in 84% of cases. When one or no followup note was written, effects on diagnosis were found in only 74% of cases (p < 0.001), and effects on management were detected in just 56% of cases (p < 0.001).

Several other factors are associated with increased rates of compliance with the recommendations of consultants (Box 9-2). Sears and Charlson found that compliance decreases as the number of recommendations made by a consultant increases.[30] In a series of 202 consultations, compliance was highest when five or fewer recommendations were made, regardless of the severity of the patient's illness. Similarly, MacKenzie et al. found that a long list of suggestions decreases the likelihood that any of them will be followed, including crucial ones.[23]

Consultants can often reduce the number of recommendations made by eliminating trivial suggestions. As already noted, Ballard found that 122 of

---

BOX 9-2

FACTORS ASSOCIATED WITH COMPLIANCE WITH CONSULTANTS' RECOMMENDATIONS

Direct contact[26]
Continued followup of patients[17,23,29]
Limited number of recommendations[26,30]
Identification of high priority recommendations[30]
Specification of drug dosage, route, and duration[16]

1016 recommendations (12%) that were made by a general medical consultation team were judged to be "insulting" by the reviewer, a surgical chief resident, and an additional 61 (6%) were considered to be nonessential.[1] After the consultants at this teaching hospital were encouraged to use moderation in making recommendations, the mean number of recommendations per consultation dropped from 6.2 per patient to 3.8.

Clear identification of important recommendations also leads to a higher rate of compliance. Pupa et al. found that labelling "crucial" recommendations caused greater than 90% compliance even if they were part of a long list of suggestions.[26] Clarifying the priority of recommendations can be best accomplished in the course of direct oral communication.

Since reducing the number of recommendations may improve the chances that important recommendations will be followed, the consultant should decide which issues can be deferred until after surgery, when thorough evaluations can be conducted without disrupting the surgical schedule. For example, postponing surgery to improve hypertension control in patients with a diastolic blood pressure ≤110 mm Hg does not affect cardiac risk.[11,25] Thus the consultant should not emphasize potential recommendations for the evaluation of new-onset hypertension, such as serum catecholamine levels or major changes in management, before surgery.

The consultant can also help the primary physicians comply with recommendations by making them specific. When suggesting a drug, the dose and duration should be provided so that a surgeon or anesthesiologist who may not be familiar with a drug can copy the recommendations directly into the order book. Horwitz et al. found that all drug therapy recommendations were followed when such details were provided, but compliance decreased to 85% when only one was specified and to 64% when neither was listed ($p < 0.001$).[16]

SUMMARY AND CONCLUSIONS

The importance of the role of the consultant has increased in recent years due to changes in the patient population undergoing procedures, the nature of the procedures that are being performed, and the logistic changes that have accompanied the trend toward outpatient and same-day surgery. Advances in anesthesia and internal medicine have helped define a special area of medicine for the consultants who function at their interface, but the knowledge-base within this area is still early in its development. Major areas of uncertainty will require investigation to assist surgeons, anesthesiologists, and consultants in managing common problems,[10] such as deciding whether a patient with coronary artery disease should undergo surgery.

Even as this knowledge-base develops, both the primary physicians and the consultants must be aware of the medicolegal issues in the consultative process and the impact of communication breakdowns on patient care. Primary physicians must recognize when consultations are needed, inform patients that a

---

BOX 9-3

RESPONSIBILITIES OF THE PRIMARY PHYSICIANS

Care of the patient
Identification of problems beyond their expertise
Obtaining the patient's consent to call a consultation
Making the request for the consultation in writing
Clearly identifying the issues for the consultant to address
Conveying the results of the evaluation to the patient

BOX 9-4

TEN COMMANDMENTS FOR EFFECTIVE CONSULTATIONS

---

1. Determine the question
2. Establish urgency
3. Look for yourself
4. Be as brief as appropriate
5. Be specific
6. Provide contingency plans
7. Honor thy turf
8. Teach . . . with tact
9. Talk is cheap . . . and effective
10. Follow up

From Goldman L, Lee T, and Rudd P: Ten commandments for effective consultations, *Arch Intern Med* 143:1753, 1983.

---

consultation will be called, make the request in writing, and clearly identify the specific issue to be addressed (Box 9-3). Finally, they must convey to the patient the results of the consultation and subsequent discussions and must take responsibility for the patient's care.

The consultant has a responsibility to respond to the physician's request in a timely manner, to provide a written note detailing the evaluation, to respect the primary physician's relationship with the patient, and to strive to transmit his/her recommendations to the physician as effectively as possible.

With these considerations in mind, we have described a list of "Ten Commandments for Effective Consultation"[12] that were directed at medical physicians who perform consultations (Box 9-4). These "commandments" recommend that consultants clarify the issue of the consultation, establish priorities, gather primary data via a history and physical examination (as opposed to a review of the chart), and make concise yet detailed recommendations. Furthermore, the consultants are urged to provide contingency plans so that their notes may provide guidance regardless of how a case develops, respect the primary physicians and their relationships with the patient, and directly communicate with the primary physicians. Finally, the consultants are urged to follow the patient for at least several days postoperatively.

KEY POINTS

- The increasing prevalence of high-risk patients undergoing complex surgical procedures has created an increased need for perioperative medical consultation.
- Anesthesiologists and surgeons must recognize when consultations are needed, notify the patient of the planned consultation, and inform the patient of important consultation findings.
- To ensure the effectiveness of the consultation process, the questions to be answered by the consultant should be clearly stated. Conversely, the consultant should limit recommendations to those of high priority in the perioperative period. Direct communication between the primary physician and the consultant can help avoid misunderstandings and clarify treatment goals.
- In addition to estimating perioperative risk and development of appropriate management strategies, the consultant should follow the patient through the postoperative period.
- The consultant must respect the primary physician's relationships with the patient.

KEY REFERENCES

Goldman L, Lee T, and Rudd P: Ten commandments for effective consultations, *Arch Intern Med* 143: 1753, 1983.

Horwitz RI, Henes CG, and Horwitz SM: Developing strategies for improving the diagnostic and management efficacy of medical consultations, *J Chron Dis* 36:213, 1983.

Kleinman B, Czinn E, Shah K et al: The value to the anesthesia-surgical care team of the preoperative cardiac consultation, *J Cardiothorac Anesth* 3:682, 1989.

Lee TH, Pappius EM, and Goldman L: Impact of inter-physician communication on the effectiveness of medical consultations, *Am J Med* 74:106, 1983.

Sears CL, Charlson ME: The effectiveness of a consultation: compliance with initial recommendations, *Am J Med* 74:870, 1983.

REFERENCES

1. Ballard WP, Gold JP, and Charlson ME: Compliance with the recommendations of medical consultants, *J Gen Intern Med* 1:220, 1986.
2. Bolt RJ: *Medical evaluation of the surgical patient,* Mount Kisco, New York, 1987, Futura Publishing.
3. Breslow MJ, Miller CF, and Rogers M: *Perioperative management,* St Louis, 1990, Mosby–Year Book.
4. Burke GR, Corman LC: The general medicine consult service in a university teaching hospital, *Med Clin North Am* 63:1353, 1979.
5. Cetrulo CL, Cetrulo LG: The legal liability of the medical consultant in pregnancy, *Med Clin North Am* 73:557, 1989.
6. Charlson ME, Cohen RP, and Sears CL: General medicine consultation: lessons from a clinical service, *Am J Med* 75:121, 1983.

7. Choi JJ: An anesthesiologist's philosophy on "medical clearance" for surgical patients, *Arch Intern Med* 147:2090, 1987.

8. Gal TJ, Cooperman LH: Hypertension in the immediate postoperative period, *Br J Anaesth* 47:70, 1975.

9. Goldman L: Cardiac risks and complications of noncardiac surgery, *Ann Intern Med* 98:504, 1983.

10. Goldman L: The art and science of perioperative consultation: where we are and where we should be going, *J Gen Intern Med* 2:284, 1987.

11. Goldman L, Caldera DL: Risks of general anesthesia and elective operation in the hypertensive patient, *Anesthesiology* 50:285, 1979.

12. Goldman L, Lee T, and Rudd P: Ten commandments for effective consultations, *Arch Intern Med* 143:1753, 1983.

13. Gross R, Kammerer W: Medical consultation on surgical services: an annotated bibliography, *Ann Intern Med* 95:523, 1981.

14. Holder AR: Consultants and implied contracts, *JAMA* 226:1497, 1973.

15. Holder AR: Duty to consult, *JAMA* 226:111, 1973.

16. Horwitz RI, Henes CG, and Horwitz SM: Developing strategies for improving the diagnostic and management efficacy of medical consultations, *J Chron Dis* 36:213, 1983.

17. Klein LE, Levine DM, Moore RD et al: The preoperative consultation: response to internists' recommendations, *Arch Intern Med* 143:743, 1983.

18. Kleinman B, Czinn E, Shah K et al: The value to the anesthesia-surgical care team of the preoperative cardiac consultation, *J Cardiothorac Anesth* 3:682, 1989.

19. Kroenke K: Preoperative evaluation: the assessment and management of surgical risk, *J Gen Intern Med* 2:258, 1987.

20. Lee TH, Goldman L: Principles of effective communication in consultative medicine. In Bolt RJ, ed: *Medical evaluation of the surgical patient,* Mount Kisco, New York, 1987, Futura Publishing.

21. Lee TH, Goldman L: Perioperative consultation: the science and the art, *J Cardiothorac Anesth* 3:679, 1989.

22. Lee TH, Pappius EM, and Goldman L: Impact of inter-physician communication on the effectiveness of medical consultations, *Am J Med* 74:106, 1983.

23. MacKenzie TB, Popkin MK, Callies AL et al: The effectiveness of cardiology consultations: concordance with diagnostic and drug recommendations, *Chest* 79:16, 1981.

24. Moore DA, Kammerer WS, McGlynn TJ et al: Consultations in internal medicine: a training program resource, *J Med Educ* 52:323, 1977.

25. Prys-Roberts C: Hypertension and anesthesia—fifty years on, *Anesthesiology* 50:281, 1979 (editorial).

26. Pupa LE, Coventry JA, Hanley JF et al: Factors affecting compliance for general medicine consultations to non-internists, *Am J Med* 81:508, 1986.

27. Robie PW: The service and educational contributions of a general medicine consultation service, *J Gen Intern Med* 1:225, 1986.

28. Rudd P: Contrasts in academic consultations, *Ann Intern Med* 94:537, 1981.

29. Rudd P, Siegler M, and Byyny RL: Preoperative diabetic consultation: a plea for improved training, *J Med Educ* 53:590, 1978.

30. Sears CL, Charlson ME: The effectiveness of a consultation: compliance with initial recommendations, *Am J Med* 74:870, 1983.

31. Siegler M: Medical consultations in the context of the physician-patient relationship. In Agich GJ, ed: *Responsibility in health care,* Dordrecht, Holland, 1982, D Reidel Publishing.

CHAPTER 10

Evaluation of the Hypertensive Patient

ATUL R. HULYALKAR
EDWARD D. MILLER, Jr.

The Joint National Committee on Detection, Evaluation, and Treatment of High Blood Pressure defines hypertension as a systolic blood pressure greater than 140 and a diastolic blood pressure greater than 90.[36] The average of three different readings must meet this definition and be reproducible on three different days to make the diagnosis. Hypertension is classified as being primary (essential or idiopathic) in approximately 95% of cases. In only 5% of cases can an underlying cause of hypertension be identified.[6,20,59] Hypertension is a disease afflicting nearly 60 million Americans.[69] Hypertensive patients have a two- to threefold increased risk of coronary artery disease and an eightfold increased risk of stroke compared with normotensive individuals.[8] Furthermore, lowering of blood pressure in hypertensive patients is associated with a decreased risk of both cerebrovascular and coronary artery disease.[15]

Hypertension is a disease of major consequence to the anesthesiologist, both in terms of its potential for end-organ injury and in terms of the anesthetic implications of medications used to control the disorder. In one series, 29% of patients undergoing noncardiac surgery had a history of hypertension.[26] In this chapter, we will discuss the pathogenesis of essential and secondary hypertension, the effects of hypertension on end-organ function, the pharmacotherapy of hypertension, perioperative considerations for the hypertensive patient, and the management of hypertensive crisis.

PATHOGENESIS OF ESSENTIAL HYPERTENSION

Although the definitive causes of essential hypertension have yet to be identified, it is generally accepted that the sympathetic nervous system is dysfunctional. The role of the sympathoadrenal axis in orchestrating chronic elevations in blood pressure in hypertensive patients has been reviewed elsewhere.[22,35]

In response to an acute fall in blood pressure, detected by central baroreceptors located in the heart and great arteries, adaptive activation of the sympathetic nervous system will occur in the normal organism. Beta-adrenergic stimulation will facilitate compensation by augmenting the rate and force of cardiac contraction and stimulating the secretion of renin by the juxtaglomerular cells in the kidney. Alpha-adrenergic stimulation leads to vasoconstriction. These modifications in the physiologic milieu increase the determinants of blood pressure: preload,

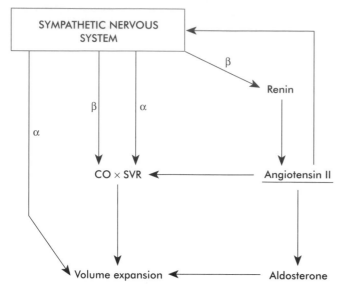

Fig. 10-1. Central position of the sympathoadrenal system in the control of blood pressure. Cardiac output *(CO)* and total systemic vascular resistance *(SVR)* are controlled by various interacting adrenergic receptor influences. Angiotensin II facilitates ongoing sympathoadrenal activity by central and peripheral mechanisms. (From Izzo JL: Sympathoadrenal activity, catecholamines and the pathogenesis of vasculopathic hypertensive target organ damage, *Am J Hypertens* 2:305S, 1989.)

stroke volume, heart rate, cardiac output, and systemic vascular resistance (Fig. 10-1).

In patients with hypertension, these mechanisms become maladaptive. In some patients, augmentation in cardiopulmonary baroreflexes may occur, leading to inappropriate sympathetic nervous system activation.[57,73] Chronic sympathoadrenal activation may lead to downregulation of the beta receptor[22] and abnormal endothelium-dependent vascular relaxation[50]; as a result the hypertensive patient exists in a state of chronic vasoconstriction. Furthermore, norepinephrine may contribute to medial hypertrophy in blood vessels and atherogenesis via direct injury to vascular endothelium.[35] Both of these mechanisms will contribute to the elevated peripheral vascular resistance seen in hypertensive patients.

The kidney plays a major role in the pathogenesis of high blood pressure. The sympathoadrenal axis and renin-angiotensin axis are intimately intertwined. Renin is secreted by the kidney in response to hypotension-induced beta-adrenergic stimulation. Subsequently, it facilitates the conversion of angiotensinogen to angiotensin I. In turn, angiotensin I is converted to angiotensin II. This reaction takes place in the lung, and is catalyzed by angiotensin-converting enzyme (ACE). Angiotensin II mediates an increase in blood pressure in two ways: (1) by its potent vasoconstrictor effects and (2) by stimulating the

production of aldosterone by the zona glomerulosa of the adrenal cortex. Patients with hypertension may be classified as having high, normal, or low renin levels. Patients with high renin levels will respond to ACE inhibitors with a normalization in their blood pressures. It is interesting to note that patients with high renin levels are at significantly increased risk for myocardial infarction than are patients with normal or low renin levels.[2]

The normal kidney will respond to an increase in blood pressure by increasing excretion of sodium and water. This phenomenon of "pressure-natriuresis" is disrupted in hypertensive kidneys. In hypertensive patients, a given sodium load is excreted at higher pressures compared with normotensive patients.[27] Potential mediators of abnormal pressure-natriuresis in hypertensive patients include the renin-angiotensin axis, atrial natriuretic factor, and efferent sympathetic activity.[21,27]

In summary, abnormal activity of the sympathetic nervous system, vasculature, and kidneys have all been observed in clinical and experimental hypertension. The challenge will be to discriminate perpetrators from perpetuators and to identify genetic substrates at increased risk. Insights into these basic questions will enable us to better care for hypertensive patients in the perioperative period.

SECONDARY HYPERTENSION

In several major series, secondary hypertension was estimated to account for about 4% to 5% of all patients with elevated blood pressure.[6,20,59] **The major disorders causing secondary hypertension are renal and endocrine in origin.** These are the only categories that will be discussed for the purposes of this review. More comprehensive discussions of the other causes of secondary hypertension may be found elsewhere.[40]

Renal disease may cause hypertension in one of two ways: as a result of inability to excrete sodium and water or as a consequence of the excessive elaboration of renin. In the first instance, circulating volume will increase, leading to elevations in blood pressure. In the second case, high levels of renin will result in increased circulating levels of angiotensin II and aldosterone, resulting in vasoconstriction and sodium retention. According to Kaplan[40] one or both of these mechanisms may be involved etiologically in the pathogenesis of hypertension in patients with renal disease. In addition, hypertension occurring in patients following organ transplantation may also be a result of sympathetic nervous system activation by cyclosporine.[62]

Renovascular hypertension occurs as a result of atherosclerosis or fibrous dysplasia involving one or both renal arteries. The resulting decreased renal blood flow leads to the secretion of high levels of renin by the involved kidney. As a consequence of the obstruction, the affected kidney will be free from the vasculopathic effects of chronic elevations in blood pressure. The contralateral kidney, however, will suffer the consequences of glomerular hyperfiltration. Paradoxically, such patients may have persistent hypertension even after surgical correction of the renal artery lesion. This is due to the elaboration of renin by the contralateral kidney, a consequence of years of exposure to elevated pressures.[70]

Renovascular hypertension should be suspected if abdominal bruits are noted in young women (as a consequence of fibrous dysplasia), or in elderly patients with peripheral vascular disease (as a consequence of atherosclerosis). Of note, patients with renovascular hypertension should not receive ACE inhibitors because of the risk of precipitating acute renal failure.[33]

The major endocrine causes of secondary hypertension are hyperaldosteronism, Cushing's syndrome, and pheochromocytoma. Together, these three entities account for less than 1% of all causes of hypertension.[40] Each should be considered as a potential cause of secondary hypertension in the proper clinical setting. In patients having hypertension and profound hypokalemia in the absence of diuretic therapy, hyperaldosteronism should be entertained. Cushing's syndrome should be suspected in patients with hypertension, truncal obesity, muscle weakness, striae, and glucose intolerance.

Pheochromocytoma occurs with diaphoresis and paroxysms of hypertension or orthostatic hypotension. It may occur with medullary carcinoma of the thyroid and hyperparathyroidism as part of a multiple endocrine neoplasia complex. **Surgical mortality may be as high as 50% in patients with unsuspected pheochromocytoma who present with intraoperative hypertension.**[5] Preoperative control of blood pressure may be achieved with alpha and beta-adrenergic blockers. Institution of beta blockade without prior alpha blockade may precipitate severe hypertension as a consequence of unopposed alpha activity. Surgical manipulation of the tumor intraoperatively will often result in a rapid increase in blood pressure as a result of release of stored catecholamines into the circulation. Patients with pheochromocytoma often have a reduced blood volume.

EFFECTS OF HYPERTENSION ON CARDIAC FUNCTION

Longstanding hypertension may be directly or indirectly responsible for a spectrum of adverse cardiac sequelae (Box 10-1). In the early stages of mild hypertension, the heart must perform more work to

---

BOX 10-1
SPECTRUM OF CARDIAC ABNORMALITIES ASSOCIATED WITH CHRONIC HYPERTENSION

Abnormalities of diastolic relaxation
Impaired coronary flow reserve
Evolution of coronary artery disease
Left ventricular hypertrophy
Ventricular ectopy and sudden death
Congestive heart failure

---

pump against a constricted vasculature. The first deficits in cardiac function to appear are abnormalities in diastolic relaxation. In hypertensive patients these may not be clinically apparent on history and physical examination. Often diastolic dysfunction may be precipitated during periods of stress such as exercise or surgery. This was demonstrated by Cuoccolo et al. in patients with hypertension and normal left ventricular function at rest. During exercise, patients whose ejection fractions increased by less than 5%, or decreased, were observed to have significant diastolic filling abnormalities.[19]

Pulsed-wave Doppler echocardiography is also useful in identifying patients with diastolic dysfunction. In normal subjects, the velocity of the passive component to ventricular filling (the E wave on the pulsed-wave Doppler profile) will exceed the velocity of the atrial contribution to diastolic filling (the A wave on the pulsed-wave Doppler profile)[47] (Fig. 10-2). In hypertensive patients, there is a greater atrial contribution to diastolic filling. This abnormal diastolic filling pattern develops in patients with hypertensive cardiomyopathy as a consequence of poor left ventricular compliance (Fig. 10-3).[45]

Patients with hypertension often develop angina in the absence of coronary artery disease, probably as a result of impaired vasodilator coronary flow reserve. Houghton et al. have demonstrated impaired coronary flow reserve in patients with hypertension and left ventricular hypertrophy. There was also an association with thallium perfusion defects and impaired coronary flow reserve in these patients without coronary artery disease.[32]

Scheler et al. studied a group of hypertensive patients without coronary artery disease with echocardiography and 24-hour Holter monitor recordings. Transient myocardial ischemia (≥ 1 mm ST segment depression for ≥ 1 minute) was observed in 50% of patients. There was no difference in left ventricular thickness in the group experiencing ischemia compared with the ischemia-free group. Thus myocardial

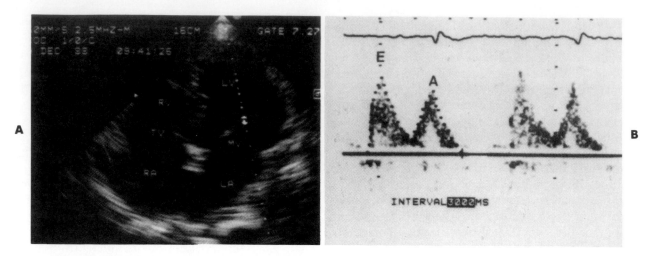

Fig. 10-2. Technique used to record the mitral valve inflow Doppler tracing for evaluation of left ventricular diastolic filling. The apical four-chamber view (**A**) shows the position of the sample volume near the tips of the mitral valve leaflet. The Doppler tracing (**B**) demonstrates the peak velocities at rapid filling (*E*) and during atrial contraction (*A*). *LA,* Left atrium; *LV,* left ventricle; *MV,* mitral valve; *RA,* right atrium; *RV,* right ventricle; *TV,* tricuspid valve. (Scale marks = 20 cm/sec.) (From Missri J: Evaluation of diastolic function. In Missri J: *Clinical Doppler echocardiography,* New York, 1990, McGraw-Hill.)

ischemia occurs commonly in hypertensive patients and is likely due to abnormal coronary flow reserve rather than left ventricular hypertrophy.[61]

In an animal model of hypertensive heart disease, Strauer demonstrated impaired coronary flow reserve and medial hypertrophy. Furthermore, there was regression of the medial hypertrophy and restoration of normal coronary flow reserve following treatment with calcium channel blockers.[68] Harrison et al.

studied coronary autoregulation in a dog model of hypertensive left ventricular hypertrophy. They concluded that hypertension and left ventricular hypertrophy are associated with severely impaired subendocardial perfusion at low perfusion pressures. Subendocardial ischemia may be precipitated during periods of hypotension below the range of coronary autoregulation.[30]

Several studies have addressed the issue of regres-

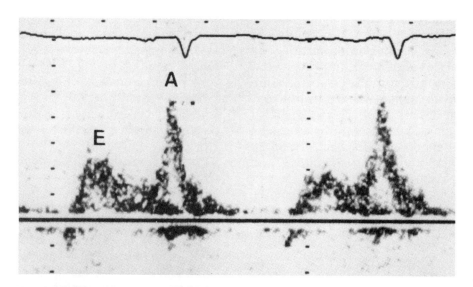

Fig. 10-3. Transmitral flow in a patient with left ventricular hypertrophy and dilated globally hypokinetic ventricle. There is decreased peak early mitral flow velocity *(E),* increased velocity at atrial contraction *(A),* an increased A/E ratio, and a prolonged mitral deceleration time. (Scale marks = 20 cm/sec.) (From Missri J: Evaluation of diastolic function. In Missri J: *Clinical Doppler echocardiography,* New York, 1990, McGraw-Hill.)

sion of left ventricular hypertrophy during antihypertensive therapy. Schulman et al. compared verapamil and atenolol in an elderly population. Both agents achieved effective blood pressure control without compromising systolic function. However, only verapamil caused regression of left ventricular hypertrophy and improvement in indices of diastolic filling.[63] Julien et al. studied a group of hypertensive patients resistant to therapy with metoprolol and furosemide. The patients were randomized to the addition of either captopril or minoxidil and followed prospectively in a blinded manner. Although blood pressure decreased to normal levels in both groups, regression of left ventricular hypertrophy occurred only in the captopril-treated group.[37]

Diuretics and vasodilators can cause a fall in blood pressure independent of effects on regression of left ventricular hypertrophy. Methyldopa can cause regression of left ventricular hypertrophy out of proportion to its effect on blood pressure. Calcium channel blockers can cause both regression in left ventricular hypertrophy and a decrease in blood pressure. These differences in response may be determined by differences in effects on the sympathetic nervous system or the renin-angiotensin system.[46]

Patients with hypertensive cardiomyopathy are at risk for ventricular dysrhythmias and sudden death.[43,44,65] Possible mechanisms include myocardial ischemia secondary to diminished coronary flow reserve and increased myocardial oxygen demand.

One of the hallmarks of hypertensive cardiomyopathy is the poorly compliant ventricle. In the end stages, systolic function is also severely impaired. The histopathologic sequence of events has been reviewed by Weber et al.[74] In the early stages, left ventricular end diastolic pressure will gradually increase. The heart will adapt by first undergoing a process of reactive fibrosis and hypertrophy. This process is unaccompanied by cell necrosis and is a compensatory response allowing for decreased wall tension (recall the Laplace relation, $T = PR/h$ where T denotes wall tension, P denotes left ventricular end diastolic pressure, and h denotes wall thickness). The trade-off is increased diastolic stiffness. If the pressure load is maintained on the heart for an extended period, myocyte necrosis and reparative fibrosis will ensue. Certain antihypertensive agents such as ACE inhibitors may provide prophylaxis against reactive fibrosis. Reparative fibrosis, however, is more extensive and is more difficult to reverse. Necropsy studies have shown that mean heart weight is greatest and fibrosis is most extensive in patients with both hypertension and diabetes. Diabetic hearts are intermediate, whereas hypertensive hearts show the least amount of fibrosis.[72]

EFFECTS OF HYPERTENSION ON THE BRAIN

The role of hypertension in the genesis of stroke[4,8,15,38] is as strong as the evidence that lowering blood pressure in hypertensive patients protects the brain from cerebrovascular events.[15,18,64] Strokes may be ischemic (thrombotic, embolic, or hypotensive) or hemorrhagic in origin. A history of hypertension predisposes to both ischemic and hemorrhagic strokes.

Chronic elevations in blood pressure can cause damage to the vascular endothelium. Endothelial injury triggers localized platelet aggregation, thrombus formation, and eventual generation of an atheromatous plaque. As the plaque grows in size, blood flow distal to the lesion is gradually compromised. As the vessel cross-sectional area narrows, flow also becomes turbulent, thus predisposing to further vessel injury. Additionally, hypertension can cause smooth muscle hypertrophy of the media, further compromising the integrity of the artery.[14,41] This degree of vascular disease involving a major artery to the brain is a precursor to a variety of scenarios culminating in a stroke.

Thrombotic stroke will occur if acute thrombus forms at the site of the flow-limiting lesion. If a portion of the thrombus becomes dislodged distally, embolic stroke can occur. Patients with hypertension are susceptible to rhythm disturbances such as atrial fibrillation. As a result, cardiac thrombi may form and may embolize to the cerebral circulation. Watershed infarcts can occur distal to occlusion involving a major vessel if blood pressure falls precipitously below the range of cerebral autoregulation.[54] Of note, in the setting of longstanding hypertension, the cerebral autoregulatory curve is shifted to the right. In other words, the blood pressure below which cerebral autoregulation fails is higher in hypertensive patients compared with normal subjects.[34]

Hypertension is thought to predispose to hemorrhagic stroke because of damage to the vessel wall.

EFFECTS OF HYPERTENSION ON RENAL FUNCTION

Longstanding hypertension can result in chronic renal injury characterized by intimal hyperplasia, sclerosis of the afferent arterioles, and parenchymal fibrosis. The parenchymal injury arises from decreased blood flow. The clinical course may be one of gradual deterioration in renal function (benign nephrosclerosis) or a more fulminant decline culminating rapidly in irreversible renal failure (malignant nephrosclerosis).[76]

In benign nephrosclerosis, the subsequent deterioration in renal function is thought to be due to compensatory hyperfiltration of normal glomeruli. As a result, glomerular pressure will increase and proteinuria will ensue.[51] In benign hypertensive nephrosclerosis, proteinuria usually does not exceed 500 mg/24 hr. Hyperfiltration results in the propagation of sclerosis to previously normal glomeruli.[31] The progression of nephrosclerosis and insidious decline in renal function may be delayed or even avoided by controlling blood pressure at an early stage.[34]

Malignant nephrosclerosis is associated with hypertensive crisis. Histologically, fibrinoid necrosis of vessel walls is the most prominent feature. The course of malignant nephrosclerosis is such that renal failure will ensue within days to weeks unless blood pressure is rapidly controlled.

PERIOPERATIVE CONSIDERATIONS

Two decades ago the issue of whether to withhold antihypertensive medications preoperatively in patients with hypertension was a subject of controversy.[24,55] At the time, the rauwolfia alkaloids were popular antihypertensive agents. Patients treated with these drugs experienced intraoperative hemodynamic lability. Subsequently, the practice of withholding antihypertensive medications before surgery became popular. Several studies surfaced in the midseventies establishing that intraoperative blood pressure changes were significantly greater in untreated hypertensive patients than in treated patients.[56,60] **In an effort to ensure a more stable perioperative course, practice now dictates that antihypertensive medications be administered on the day of surgery. The exception to this rule is that diuretics should usually be withheld on the day of surgery,** as discussed below.

The next question to be addressed was whether elective surgery should be cancelled in patients discovered to be hypertensive on the day of surgery. Goldman and Caldera tackled this issue in a prospective study of 676 patients undergoing noncardiac surgery. The study groups included normotensive patients, patients with hypertension controlled on medication, patients with hypertension poorly controlled by medication, and untreated hypertensive patients. Of the patients in this series, 29% had hypertension. Greater intraoperative decreases in blood pressure were noted in patients with persistent hypertension compared with patients with controlled hypertension. Despite this, the severity of preoperative hypertension and successful control of blood pressure preoperatively did not correlate with incidence of perioperative cardiac morbidity. The authors concluded that elective surgery in patients with inadequately controlled hypertension was not associated with increased risk of perioperative cardiac morbidity provided preoperative diastolic blood pressure was ≤110 mm Hg and perioperative blood pressure was closely monitored.[26]

Immense growth has occurred in the past decade in the preoperative approach to the patient with cardiovascular disease. The coming-of-age of drugs such as the beta-blockers and the emergence of new hemodynamic monitoring modalities have facilitated many of the recent advances in the field. In this new clinical context, the preoperative approach to the hypertensive patient has been reexamined. Stone et al. concluded that patients with untreated hypertension, or hypertension controlled with diuretics, had an increased risk of intraoperative myocardial ischemia compared to patients treated with atenolol. The latter group included patients who were receiving atenolol chronically and newly discovered hypertensive patients who were started on atenolol on the morning of surgery.[67] In a subsequent study, they concluded that ischemia occurred during times of stress such as intubation or emergence from anesthesia. Myocardial ischemia was associated with tachycardia but not with acute changes in blood pressure.[66]

Charleson et al. compiled clinical criteria associated with postoperative morbidity in patients with hypertension and diabetes who were undergoing noncardiac surgery.[9-12] Preoperative cardiomegaly by chest radiograph or preoperative history of myocardial infarction were predictors of postoperative myocardial ischemia or infarction. Intraoperative hypotension (≥20 mm Hg decrease in mean arterial pressure for ≥1 hr) or hypertension (≥20 mm Hg increase in mean arterial pressure for ≥15 min) alternating with hypotension was associated with an increased incidence of postoperative renal and cardiac morbidity.

Hypertension occurs frequently in patients following organ transplantation. This subset of patients is of particular interest because of the known adverse effects of hypertension on the transplanted heart[23] and kidney.[13] Hypertension predisposes to progression of renal failure in the transplanted kidney. Treatment of hypertension in kidney transplant recipients does not improve graft survival, however.[13]

In patients with transplanted hearts, renal function deteriorates more quickly in recipients who have, or who develop, hypertension.[23] Left ventricular hypertrophy occurs in both normotensive and hypertensive patients following heart transplantation. Fractional shortening decreases in normotensive patients after heart transplantation but remains elevated in hypertensive patients.

Hypertension in patients following organ transplantation probably develops as a consequence of the immunosuppressive therapy. Glucocorticoids are known to have sodium and fluid retentive effects. Cyclosporine increases sympathetic nervous system discharge, which may also culminate in hypertension in the recipient.[62] From an anesthetic standpoint, one of the major goals of perioperative management in the organ transplant recipient is to maintain adequate perfusion to the graft. Autoregulation to the grafted organ is likely to be shifted to higher pressures.

The perioperative management of the patient with cerebrovascular disease presents other challenges. In patients with aneurysmal subarachnoid hemorrhage, treatment of elevated blood pressures may prevent rebleeding. Conversely, antihypertensive therapy in this setting is associated with an increased risk of cerebral infarction.[75] Following surgery for aneurysmal subarachnoid hemorrhage, patients with a preoperative history of hypertension are at increased risk for seizures.[48] Ideally, diastolic pressure should be maintained in the range of 95 to 105 mm Hg. In this setting, nimodipine, a calcium antagonist, is useful in the prevention of cerebral vasospasm in patients with aneurysmal subarachnoid hemorrhage.[3]

ANESTHETIC MANAGEMENT

The approach to the patient with newly discovered hypertension or treated, uncontrolled hypertension should be as follows. **Patients with an elevation of the diastolic pressure >115 mm Hg should have their elective surgery deferred until further evaluation and therapy may be instituted.** If patients with hypertension have evidence of renal dysfunction, ischemic heart disease, or cerebrovascular disease, the adequacy of antihypertensive therapy should be assessed. If this assessment suggests that therapy is adequate, surgery should be performed. On the other hand, urgent surgery for the uncontrolled hypertensive patient should not be cancelled. Blood pressure may be adequately controlled with short-acting parenteral agents such as nitroglycerine, nitroprusside, or esmolol.

In the controlled hypertensive patient it is useful to administer an anxiolytic premedication. Diazepam 0.07 to 0.15 mg orally or midazolam 0.04 mg intramuscularly work well. Patients receiving diuretics should not receive their diuretic on the day of surgery. Usually these patients are volume depleted, and one could make a case for gentle hydration of selected diuretic-treated hypertensive patients before they are brought to the operating room. The patient should otherwise receive the usual antihypertensive regimen on the morning of surgery.

The types of monitors required depend on the nature of the patient's coexisting disease and the type of surgery. In general, for major vascular or abdominal cases in patients with significant cardiac, renal, or neurologic disease, invasive hemodynamic monitoring is essential.

Induction of anesthesia and emergence from anesthesia are periods of great hemodynamic variability in the hypertensive patient. During these periods, adjunctive therapy with short-acting beta-blockers or lidocaine may add to hemodynamic stability. Esmolol, a short-acting selective beta-blocker, is effective in the treatment of sinus tachycardia and hypertension in both cardiac[58] and noncardiac[25] surgery. The authors recommend an initial bolus of 80 mg with subsequent infusion of 12 mg/min. At these doses, there is no significant hemodynamic deterioration. Smaller doses will be necessary in unstable patients. Another agent that has shown promise in the treatment of perioperative hypertension is the parenteral calcium channel blocker, nicardipine.[17,28,29,39]

Any of the agents in the anesthetic armamentarium may be used in the maintenance of anesthesia, with the exception of ketamine. Since hypertension, tachycardia, and increased intracranial pressure are commonly associated with ketamine, the use of this agent is best avoided in the hypertensive patient.

It is important to emphasize one caveat: in addressing acute increases in blood pressure intraoperatively, the vigilant anesthesiologist must rule out correctable problems associated with ventilation, oxygenation, and circulation. Reflexly treating elevations in blood pressure with anesthetics or antihypertensive agents can be catastrophic.

HYPERTENSIVE CRISIS

The management of hypertensive crisis has been reviewed recently.[7,49] Hypertensive crisis occurs when the diastolic blood pressure exceeds 130 mm Hg. Malignant hypertension with evidence of end-organ injury constitutes a medical emergency, and diagnosis and treatment should begin immediately. If there is no evidence of end-organ injury, treatment should proceed in an expeditious, though nonemergent manner. In general, patients with malignant hypertension will require admission to an intensive care unit and invasive monitoring of blood pressure with an arterial line. Noninvasive monitoring of blood pressure should suffice in the absence of end-organ injury. Although parenteral therapy is usually indicated to correct malignant hypertension, sublingual and oral agents are acceptable options for patients without end-organ injury. Potential causes of hypertensive crisis may be neurologic, cardiovascular, or renal.

From a neurologic standpoint, any lesion causing an abrupt increase in intracranial pressure may precipitate a rapid rise in systemic pressure. Teleologically, this reflex allows cerebral perfusion pressure to be maintained in the face of a raised intracranial pressure. Potential neurologic causes of hypertensive crisis include intracranial hemorrhage, subarachnoid hemorrhage, head trauma, CNS tumor, or thromboembolic stroke. Hypertensive crisis usually occurs on a substrate of chronic, stable hypertension. The goal of therapy is to avoid rapid changes in blood pressure without compromising cerebral perfusion. To this end, antihypertensive therapy is not recommended in any patient with hypertensive crisis or in any neurosurgical patient unless there is severe (> 200/130) hypertension.[49] Sodium nitroprusside may be instituted cautiously although it is associated with the theoretic disadvantage of increasing intracranial pressure in patients with compromised intracranial compliance.[71] Beta-blockers have been associated with cerebral vasospasm and should be avoided. Centrally acting agents such as clonidine and methyldopa can cloud the sensorium and also should not be used in treating hypertensive crisis of neurologic origin.

The major cardiovascular causes of hypertensive crisis include myocardial infarction and dissecting aortic aneurysm. Therapy should center on decreasing blood pressure by 20% to 25% to a diastolic pressure of approximately 100 mm Hg. The time course of decreasing the blood pressure should be dictated by the clinical circumstances. In dissecting aortic aneurysm, an additional goal is to decrease dP/dT to help prevent aneurysmal rupture. The combination of sodium nitroprusside and beta-blockade is effective in this setting. In acute myocardial infarction, coronary perfusion should be maintained while systemic pressure is lowered to balance the myocardial supply–demand inequity. Nitroglycerin, calcium channel blockers, and beta-blockers may be used individually or in concert to effectively lower the pressure.

Renal causes for hypertensive crisis include renal artery stenosis and parenchymal renal disease. The aims of therapy are to decrease the blood pressure to prevent fibrinoid necrosis while maintaining renal perfusion. Modulation of renal blood flow occurs as a result of vasoregulation of afferent and efferent arterioles. In patients with renal causes of hypertensive crisis, control of blood pressure may be achieved by using nitroprusside or calcium channel blockers. If the patient's volume status is ambiguous and acute renal failure is imminent, pulmonary artery catheterization may assist with therapeutic decision-making. In some patients with renal failure and malignant hypertension, emergent hemodialysis may be necessary.[49] When using nitroprusside in patients with renal failure, thiocyanate levels should be monitored. In patients with suspected bilateral renal artery stenosis, ACE inhibitors may precipitate renal failure and should be avoided.[33]

Other potential causes of hypertensive crisis include preeclampsia, recreational drugs, tyramine crisis in patients treated with monoamine oxidase inhibitors, pheochromocytoma, and hyperautonomic syndromes associated with chronic spinal cord dysfunction.[7] A summary of the pharmacologic agents available for the treatment of hypertensive crises is presented in Table 10-1.

PHARMACOTHERAPY OF HYPERTENSION
Centrally Acting Sympatholytics

This family of antihypertensive agents includes methyldopa, guanethidine, reserpine, and clonidine. Methyldopa acts by centrally inhibiting sympathetic outflow. Adverse effects associated with methyldopa include sedation, hemolysis, hepatitis, rash, and arthralgias.

Clonidine is an alpha$_2$-adrenergic agonist that acts centrally to inhibit release of catecholamines. The major drawback to the use of clonidine as an antihypertensive agent is the profound rebound hypertension associated with its acute withdrawal. In addition to effects on blood pressure, there is evidence that clonidine and other alpha$_2$ agonists have significant anesthetic, sedative, and anxiolytic effects. The analgesic properties of clonidine appear to be a result of adrenergic modulation of descending pain pathways at the level of the dorsal horn.[42] As we learn more about the neurophysiology of pain, alpha$_2$ agonists will no doubt assume an increasingly important role in the perioperative management of the hypertensive patient.

Peripherally Acting Sympatholytics

Beta blockers have a long and safe track record in the treatment of hypertension. They act by blocking beta-adrenergic receptors in the heart resulting in decreased heart rate, force of contraction, and decreased cardiac output. Both nonselective and beta$_1$-selective agents are available, the selective antagonists having limited effects on bronchial or vascular smooth muscle. The use of beta-blockers as antihypertensive agents may provide prophylaxis against nonfatal myocardial infarction.[53] The emergence of a new, ultra short–acting selective beta-blocker, esmolol, has allowed the anesthesiologist to treat intraoperative hypertension and tachycardia in the unstable patient.[25,58]

The side effect profile of the beta-blockers is vast and includes congestive heart failure in patients with borderline left ventricular function, bronchospasm,

Table 10-1 Parenteral medications used in the treatment of hypertensive emergencies

Drug	Administration*	Onset	Duration of action	Dosage	Adverse effects and comments
Sodium nitro-prusside	IV infusion	Immediate	2-3 min	0.5-10 μg/kg/min (initial dose, 0.25 μg/kg/min for eclampsia and renal in-sufficiency)	Hypotension, nausea, vomiting, apprehension; risk of thiocyanate and cyanide toxicity is increased in renal and hepatic insufficiency, respectively; levels should be monitored; must shield from light
Diazoxide	IV bolus IV infusion	1-5 min	6-12 hr	50-100 mg every 5-10 min, up to 600 mg 10-30 mg/min	Hypotension, tachycardia, nausea, vomiting, fluid retention, hyperglycemia; may exacerbate myocardial ischemia, heart failure, or aortic dissection; may require concomitant use of a beta-antagonist
Labetalol	IV bolus IV infusion	5-10 min	3-6 hr	20-80 mg every 5-10 min, up to 300 mg 0.5-2 mg/min	Hypotension, heart block, heart failure, broncho-spasm, nausea, vomiting, scalp tingling, paradoxical pressor response; may not be effective in patients receiving alpha- or beta-antagonists
Nitroglycerin	IV infusion	1-2 min	3-5 min	5-100 μg/min	Headache, nausea, vomiting; beta tolerance may develop with prolonged use
Phentolamine	IV bolus	1-2 min	3-10 min	5-10 mg every 5-15 min	Hypotension, tachycardia, headache, angina, para-doxical pressor response
Trimethaphan	IV infusion	1-5 min	10 min	0.5-5 mg/min	Hypotension, urinary retention, ileus, respiratory arrest, mydriasis, cycloplegia, dry mouth; more effective if patient's head is elevated
Hydralazine (for treatment of eclampsia)	IV bolus	10-20 min	3-6 hr	5-10 mg every 20 min (if no effect after 20 mg, try another agent)	Hypotension, fetal distress, tachycardia, headache, nausea, vomiting, local thrombophlebitis; infusion site should be changed after 12 hr
Nicardipine	IV infusion	1-5 min	3-6 hr	5 mg/hr, increased by 1-2.5 mg/hr every 15 min, up to 15 mg/hr	Hypotension, headache, tachycardia, nausea, vomiting

*IV denotes intravenous.

From Calhoun DC, Oparil S: Treatment of hypertensive crisis, *N Engl J Med* 323:1177, 1990.

vasoconstriction, depression, and hyperkalemia. Abrupt withdrawal can cause tachycardia, rebound hypertension, and acute coronary ischemia.

Alpha adrenergic blockers currently used as antihypertensive agents include phentolamine and phenoxybenzamine. These agents are useful in the treatment of pheochromocytoma. Prazosin is an $alpha_1$-adrenergic blocker, useful as a vasodilator. However, reflex tachycardia and tachyphylaxis are associated with prazosin, thereby limiting its effectiveness.

Calcium Channel Blockers

These agents act by binding antagonistically to slow inward calcium channels in heart and vascular smooth muscle. The end result is a spectrum of events including peripheral vasodilation, decreased force of cardiac contraction, and decreased heart rate. In addition, there is evidence that nifedipine may have an additional antihypertensive effect by facilitating sodium excretion.[52] The three most commonly used calcium antagonists are nifedipine, verapamil, and diltiazem. Nifedipine is the most potent vasodilator of the three; verapamil has the most significant chronotropic and inotropic effects. Diltiazem has a pharmacologic profile intermediate between nifedipine and verapamil. A new parenteral calcium antagonist, nicardipine, has shown promise in the treatment of perioperative hypertension.[17,28,29,39] In combination with beta-blockers or inhaled anesthetics, calcium channel blockers can cause myocardial depression or heart block.

ACE Inhibitors

ACE inhibitors confer their antihypertensive effects via at least two mechanisms. By blocking the conversion of angiotensin I to angiotensin II, they indirectly interfere with the elaboration of aldosterone from the adrenal gland. In so doing, they diminish fluid and sodium retention. Furthermore, angiotensin II is a potent vasoconstrictor. Blocking its production will result in a decrease in peripheral vascular resistance. ACE is also a kininase that catalyzes the breakdown of bradykinin. Vasodilation from increased availability of bradykinin in response to ACE inhibition may also occur although the clinical significance of this is questionable. In one study, the use of enalapril as a premedication was studied in nonhypertensive patients undergoing abdominal hysterectomies.[77] The group receiving enalapril preoperatively were hemodynamically more stable during induction compared with the placebo group. In patients undergoing coronary artery bypass surgery, preoperative treatment with captopril did not prevent hypertension following cardiopulmonary bypass.[16] Pharmacologic blockade of the renin-angiotensin system may evolve into an important tool for perioperative hemodynamic manipulations; especially if a short-acting intravenous ACE inhibitor is developed.

Side effects of ACE inhibitors include rash, proteinuria, cough, bronchospasm, and interstitial nephritis. In patients with bilateral renal artery stenosis, ACE inhibitors can precipitate acute renal failure.[33]

Diuretics

Several types of diuretic agents are available, but those most commonly used to treat hypertension include the thiazides, loop diuretics, and potassium-sparing diuretics. The thiazides inhibit the reabsorption of sodium in the proximal and distal tubule and the cortical portion of the loop of Henle. The loop diuretics inhibit sodium reabsorption in the medullary portion of the loop of Henle. The potassium-sparing diuretics prevent potassium secretion in the distal tubule and collecting duct. The diuretics lower blood pressure by decreasing circulating volume. Thus patients receiving diuretics will be chronically volume depleted. Side effects of the thiazides include hyperuricemia, hyperglycemia, hyperlipidemia, hypokalemia, hypermagnesemia, and metabolic alkalosis. The use of thiazides as antihypertensive agents has been questioned by some in light of their adverse metabolic profile. Nonetheless, they remain popular because of their low cost and antihypertensive efficacy. Furthermore, clinical significance of the metabolic side effects of diuretics has been questioned.[1] The loop diuretics can cause hypokalemia, hypomagnesemia, hyperglycemia, metabolic alkalosis, and deafness. The potassium-sparing diuretics can cause hyperkalemia and gynecomastia. They are commonly used with either a thiazide or a loop diuretic to attenuate the degree of potassium wasting associated with the latter two agents.

KEY POINTS

- Hypertension is a chronic disorder that may be idiopathic or secondary to renal, endocrine, or neurologic disease.
- Hypertensive heart disease is characterized by a spectrum of abnormalities ranging from mild diastolic dysfunction to overt congestive heart failure.
- Neurologic dysfunction secondary to hypertension occurs as a consequence of injury to the large and

small arteries supplying blood to the brain. Autoregulation of cerebral blood flow occurs over a higher range of pressures in the hypertensive patient compared with a normal individual.

- Anesthetic management of hypertensive patients consists of ensuring that antihypertensive therapy (with the exception of diuretics) is administered on the day of surgery, avoiding agents such as ketamine that may cause hypertension and tachycardia, using short-acting beta-blockers and calcium channel blockers, and anticipating and guarding against

surgical stimulation that may induce a stress response.

- Reflexly treating hypertension and tachycardia can be catastrophic if therapy with antihypertensive agents or anesthetics is instituted without first checking adequacy of ventilation, oxygenation, and circulation.
- Hypertensive crisis is a syndrome of acute and severe elevations in blood pressure associated with extensive end-organ injury. The prognosis is poor unless therapy is instituted at an early stage.

KEY REFERENCES

Buhler FR, Laragh JM, eds: *The management of hypertension,* New York, 1990, Elsevier.

Calhoun DC, Oparil S: Treatment of hypertensive crisis, *N Engl J Med* 323:1177, 1990.

Goldman L, Caldera DL: Risks of general anesthesia and elective operation in the hypertensive patient, *Anesthesiology* 50:285, 1979.

Izzo JL: Sympathoadrenal activity, catecholamines and the pathogenesis of vasculopathic hypertensive target organ damage, *Am J Hypertens* 2:305, 1989.

Kaplan NM: Systemic hypertension: mechanisms and diagnosis. In Braunwald E, ed: *Heart disease: a*

textbook of cardiovascular medicine, Philadelphia, 1988, WB Saunders.

Nishimura RA, Abel MD, Hatle LK et al: Assessment of diastolic function of the heart: background and current application of Doppler echocardiography, *Mayo Clin Proc* 64:181, 1984.

Price TR, Wollam GL, Grady PA: Hypertensive cerebrovascular disease. In Wollam GL, Hall WD, eds: *Hypertension management: clinical and therapeutic dilemmas,* Chicago, 1988, Year Book Medical Publishers.

REFERENCES

1. Alcazar JM, Rodicio JL, and Ruilope LM: Long term diuretic therapy and renal function in essential arterial hypertension, *Am J Cardiol* 65(17):51H, 1990.
2. Alderman MH, Madhavan S, and Ooi WL: Association of renin-sodium profile with the risk of myocardial infarction in patients with hypertension, *N Engl J Med* 324:1098, 1991.
3. Allen GS, Ahn HS, Preziosi TJ et al: Cerebral arterial spasm: a controlled trial of nimodipine in patients with subarachnoid hemorrhage, *N Engl J Med* 308:619, 1983.
4. al Roomi KA, Heller RF, and Olodarczyk J: Hypertension control and the risk of myocardial infarction and stroke: a population based study, *Med J Australia* 153: 595, 602, 1990.
5. Apgar V, Papper EM: Pheochromocytomas: anesthetic management during surgical treatment, *Am Med Assoc Arch Surg* 62:634, 1951.
6. Berglund G, Andersson O, and Wilhelmsen L: Prevalence of primary and secondary hypertension: studies in a random population sample, *Br Med J* 2:554, 1976.
7. Calhoun DC, Oparil S: Treatment of hypertensive crisis, *N Engl J Med* 323: 1177, 1990.

8. Castelli W, Anderson K: A population at risk. Prevalence of high cholesterol levels in hypertensive patients in the Framingham study, *Am J Med* 80(suppl 2A):23, 1986.
9. Charleson ME, MacKenzie CR, Gold JP et al: Postoperative renal function can be predicted, *Surg Gynecol Obstet* 169:303, 1989.
10. Charleson ME, MacKenzie CR, Gold JP et al: The preoperative and intraoperative hemodynamic predictors of postoperative myocardial infarction or ischemia in patients undergoing noncardiac surgery, *Ann Surg* 210:637, 1989.
11. Charleson ME, MacKenzie R, Gold JP et al: Intraoperative blood pressure. What patterns identify patients at risk for postoperative complications? *Ann Surg* 212:567, 1990.
12. Charleson ME, MacKenzie CR, Gold JP et al: Preoperative characteristics predicting intraoperative hypotension and hypertension among hypertensives and diabetics undergoing noncardiac surgery, *Ann Surg* 212:66, 1990.
13. Cheigh JS, Haschmeyer RH, Wang JCL et al: Hypertension in kidney transplant recipients. Effect on long-term renal allograft survival, *Am J Hypertens* 2:341, 1989.

14. Chobanian AV: Adaptive and maladaptive responses of the arterial wall to hypertension, *Hypertension* 15(6 pt 2):666, 1990.
15. Collins R, Peto R, Macmahon S et al: Blood pressure, stroke, and coronary heart disease, Part 2. Short term reductions in blood pressure: overview of randomized drug trials in their epidemiologic context, *Lancet* 335(8693):827, 1990.
16. Colson P, Grolleau D, and Chaptal P: Effect of preoperative renin-angiotensin system blockade on hypertension following coronary artery surgery, *Chest* 93: 1156, 1988.
17. Cook E, Clifton GG, and Vargas R: Pharmacokinetics, pharmacodynamics and minimal effective clinical dose of intravenous nicardipine, *Clin Pharmacol Ther* 47:706, 1990.
18. Coope J, Warrender TS: Randomized trial of treatment of hypertension in elderly patients in primary care, *Br Med J* 293:1145, 1986.
19. Cuoccolo A, Sax FL, Brush JE et al: Left ventricular hypertrophy and impaired diastolic filling in essential hypertension. Diastolic mechanisms for systolic dysfunction during exercise, *Circulation* 81: 978, 1990.

20. Danielson M, Dammstrom B: The prevalence of secondary and curable hypertension, *Acta Med Scand* 209:451, 1981.
21. DiBona GF: Neural control of renal function: cardiovascular implications, *Hypertension* 13:539, 1989.
22. Egan BM: Neurogenic mechanisms in initiating essential hypertension, *Am J Hypertens* 2:357S, 1989.
23. Farge D, Julien J, Amrein C et al: Effect of systemic hypertension on renal function and left ventricular hypertrophy in heart transplant recipients, *J Am Coll Cardiol* 15:1095, 1990.
24. Foex P, Prys-Roberts C: Anaesthesia and the hypertensive patient, *Br J Anaesth* 46:575, 1974.
25. Gold MI, Sacks DJ, Grosnoff DB et al: Use of esmolol during anesthesia to treat tachycardia and hypertension, *Anesth Analg* 68:101, 1989.
26. Goldman L, Caldera DL: Risks of general anesthesia and elective operation in the hypertensive patient, *Anesthesiology* 50:285, 1979.
27. Hall JE, Mizelle L, and Hildebrandt DA: Abnormal pressure natriuresis. A cause or a consequence of hypertension? *Hypertension* 15:547, 1990.
28. Halpern NA, Alicea M, Krakoff LR et al: Postoperative hypertension: a prospective, placebo-controlled, randomized, double-blind trial with intravenous nicardipine hydrochloride, *Angiology* 41 (11 pt 2):992, 1990.
29. Halpern NA, Sladen RN, Goldberg JS et al: Nicardipine infusion for postoperative hypertension after surgery of the head and neck, *Crit Care Med* 18:950, 1990.
30. Harrison DG, Florentina MS, Brooks LA et al: The effect of hypertension and left ventricular hypertrophy on the lower range of coronary autoregulation, *Circulation* 77:1108, 1988.
31. Hostetter TH, Olson JL, Rennke HG et al: Hyperfiltration in remnant nephrons: a potentially adverse consequence to renal ablation, *Am J Physiol* 241:F85, 1981.
32. Houghton JL, Frank MJ, Carr AA et al: Relations among impaired coronary flow reserve, left ventricular hypertrophy and thallium perfusion defects in hypertensive patients without obstructive coronary artery disease, *J Am Coll Cardiol* 15:43, 1990.
33. Hricik DE, Browning PJ, Kopelman R et al: Captopril-induced functional renal insufficiency in patients with bilateral renal-artery stenoses or renal-artery stenosis in a solitary kidney, *N Engl J Med* 308:373, 1983.
34. Ibsen H: Target organ damage and planning therapy. In Buhler FR, Laragh JH, eds: *The management of hypertension,* New York, 1990, Elsevier.
35. Izzo JL: Sympathoadrenal activity, catecholamines and the pathogenesis of vasculopathic hypertensive target organ damage, *Am J Hypertens* 2:305S, 1989.
36. Joint National Committee on Detection, Evaluation, and Treatment of High Blood Pressure: the 1984 Report of the Joint National Committee on Detection, Evaluation, and Treatment of High Blood Pressure, *Arch Int Med* 144:1045, 1984.
37. Julien J, Dufloux M, Prasquier R et al: Effects of captopril and minoxidil on left ventricular hypertrophy in resistant hypertensive patients: a 6 month double blind comparison, *J Am Coll Cardiol* 16:137, 1990.
38. Julius S, Jamerson K, Mejia A et al: The association of borderline hypertension with target organ changes and higher coronary risk. Tecumseh Blood Pressure Study, *JAMA* 264:354, 1990.
39. Kaplan JA: Clinical considerations for the use of intravenous nicardipine in the treatment of postoperative hypertension, *Am Heart J* 119 (2 pt 2):443, 1990.
40. Kaplan NM: Systemic hypertension: mechanisms and diagnosis. In Braunwald E, ed: *Heart disease: a textbook of cardiovascular medicine,* Philadelphia, 1988, WB Saunders.
41. Kaplan NM: Arterial protection: a neglected but crucial therapeutic goal, *Am J Cardiol* 66:36C, 1990.
42. Maze M: Cardiovascular pharmacology in the 1990's: the role of alpha$_2$ adrenergic agonists in anesthesia. In *International Anesthesia Research Society 1991 Review Lectures.*
43. McLenachan JM, Dargie HJ: A review of rhythm disorders in cardiac hypertrophy, *Am J Cardiol* 65:42G, 1990.
44. McLenachan JM, Henderson E, Morris KI et al: Sudden death in hypertension: a possible mechanism (abstr), *Br Heart J* 57:572, 1987.
45. Missri J: Evaluation of diastolic function. In Missri J: *Clinical Doppler echocardiography,* New York, 1990, McGraw-Hill.
46. Motz WH, Strauer BE: Differential therapy of hypertensive heart disease, *Am J Cardiol* 65:60G, 1990.
47. Nishimura RA, Abel MD, Hatle LK et al: Assessment of diastolic function of the heart: background and current application of Doppler echocardiography, *Mayo Clin Proc* 64:181, 1989.
48. Ohman J: Hypertension as a risk factor for epilepsy after aneurysmal subarachnoid hemorrhage and surgery, *Neurosurgery* 27:578, 1990.
49. Opie LH: Treatment of severe hypertension. In Kaplan NM, Brenner BM, Laragh JH, eds: *New therapeutic strategies in hypertension,* New York, 1989, Raven Press.
50. Panza JA, Quyyumi AA, Brush JE et al: Abnormal endothelium-dependent vascular relaxation in patients with essential hypertension, *N Engl J Med* 323:22, 1990.
51. Parving HH, Mogensen CE, Jensen HE et al: Increased urinary albumin excretion rate in benign essential hypertension, *Lancet* 1:1190, 1974.
52. Pevahouse JB, Markandu ND, Cappuccio FP et al: Long term reduction in sodium balance: possible additional mechanism whereby nifedipine lowers blood pressure, *Br Med J* 301:580, 1990.
53. Praty BM, Koepsell TD, Wagner EH et al: Beta blockers and the primary prevention of nonfatal myocardial infarction in patients with high blood pressure, *Am J Cardiol* 66(16):12G, 1990.
54. Price TR, Wollam GL, and Grady PA: Hypertensive cerebrovascular disease. In Wollam GL, Hall WD eds: *Hypertension management: clinical and therapeutic dilemmas,* Chicago, 1988, Year Book Medical Publishers.
55. Prys-Roberts C: Hypertension and anesthesia—fifty years on, *Anesthesiology* 50:281, 1979.
56. Prys-Roberts C, Meloche R, Foex P: Studies on anesthesia in relation to hypertension. I. Cardiovascular responses of treated and untreated patients, *Br J Anaesth* 43:122, 1971.
57. Rea RF, Hamdan M: Baroreflex control of muscle sympathetic nerve activity in borderline hypertension, *Circulation* 82:856, 1990.
58. Reves JG, Croughwell ND, Hawkins E et al: Esmolol for treatment of intraoperative tachycardia and/or hypertension in patients having cardiac operations: bolus loading technique, *J Thorac Cardiovasc Surg* 100:221, 1990.
59. Rudnick KV, Sackett DC, Hirst S et al: Hypertension in family practice, *Can Med Assoc J* 117:492, 1977.
60. Ryhanen P, Hollman A, and Horttonen L: Blood pressure changes during and after anaesthesia in treated and untreated hypertensive patients, *Ann Chir Gyn* 67:180, 1978.
61. Scheler S, Motz W, Vester J et al: Transient ischemia in hypertensive heart disease, *Am J Cardiol* 65:51G, 1990.
62. Scherrer V, Vissig SF, Morgan BJ et al: Cyclosporin-induced sympathetic activation and hypertension after heart transplantation, *N Engl J Med* 323:693, 1990.
63. Schulman SP, Weiss JL, Becker LC et al: The effects of antihypertensive therapy on left ventricular mass in elderly patients, *N Engl J Med* 322:1350, 1990.
64. SHEP Cooperative Research Group: Prevention of stroke by antihypertensive drug treatment in older persons with isolated systolic hypertension. Final results of the systolic hypertension in the elderly program, *JAMA* 265:3255, 1991.
65. Siegel D, Cheitlin MD, Black DM et al: Risk of ventricular arrhythmias in hypertensive men with left ventricular hypertrophy, *Am J Cardiol* 65:742, 1990.
66. Stone JG, Foex P, Sear JW et al: Myocardial ischemia in untreated hypertensive patients: effects of a single small oral dose of a beta adrenergic blocking agent, *Anesthesiology* 68:495, 1988.
67. Stone JG, Foex JW, Sear L et al: Risk of myocardial ischemia during anesthesia in treated and untreated hypertensive patients, *Br J Anaesth* 61:675, 1988.
68. Strauer BE: Significance of coronary circulation in hypertensive heart disease for development and prevention of heart failure, *Am J Cardiol* 65:34G, 1990.
69. Subcommittee on definition and prevalence of the 1984 Joint National Committee: Hypertension prevalence and the status of awareness, treatment, and control in the United States, *Hypertension* 7:457, 1985.

70. Thal AP, Grage TB, and Vernier RL: Function of the contralateral kidney in renal hypertension due to renal artery stenosis, *Circulation* 27:36, 1963.

71. Turner JM, Powell D, Gibson RM et al: Intracranial pressure changes in neurosurgical patients during hypotension induced with sodium nitroprusside or trimethaphan, *Br J Anaesth* 49:419, 1977.

72. van Hoeven KH, Factor SM: A comparison of the pathological spectrum of hypertensive, diabetic, and hypertensive-diabetic heart disease, *Circulation* 82:848, 1990.

73. Victor RG, Morgan BS: Baroreceptors and hypertension, *Circulation* 82:1057, 1990.

74. Weber KT, Jalil JE, Janicka JS et al: Myocardial collagen remodeling in pressure overload hypertrophy: a case for interstitial heart disease, *Am J Hypertens* 2:931, 1989.

75. Wijdicks EF, Vermeulen M, Murray GD et al: The effects of treating hypertension following aneurysmal subarachnoid hemorrhage, *Clin Neurol Neurosurg* 92:111, 1990.

76. Wollam GL, Gifford RW: Benign and malignant nephrosclerosis. In Buhler FR, Laragh JH, eds: *The management of hypertension,* New York, 1990, Elsevier.

77. Yates AP, Hunter DN: Anaesthesia and angiotensin-converting enzyme inhibitors: the effect of enalapril on perioperative cardiovascular stability, *Anaesthesia* 43:935, 1988.

CHAPTER 11

Evaluation of the Adult Patient with Cardiac Problems

ALAN F. ROSS
JOHN H. TINKER

Perioperative cardiac risk has interested and concerned anesthesiologists for many years. Early work identified clinical risk factors and predictors of outcome. Advances in monitoring techniques facilitated precise perioperative pharmacologic interventions. New anesthetic drugs eliminated many undesirable characteristics of older agents, and "stress-free" anesthesia has become a valid possibility.[43,105] Recent innovations, such as dipyridamole-thallium

scanning, ambulatory electrocardiography, and transesophageal echocardiography, have further sharpened clinicians' abilities to detect the patient at serious cardiac risk. At this stage, it is worth recalling the comments of Steen et al[156]:

In the years following 1968, new anesthetic agents and techniques, including enflurane and neuroleptanesthesia, have been introduced, major changes in medical management have come about, and high-risk patients are more often monitored in intensive care units. It has been suggested that reinfarction rates should be declined . . . .

However, as Steen et al. found in 1978, no decline had occurred. In fact, the rates were remarkably similar to those seen a decade earlier. One wonders if our "advancements" since Steen's report have had any better real impact than those of previous years.

Despite our enthusiasm for progress, many expectations of acute cardiovascular medicine remain unfulfilled. Antihypertensive therapy has not demonstrably reduced the incidence of myocardial infarctions,[2,169] therapy for ventricular dysrhythmias has not greatly reduced sudden death,[76] and coronary artery bypass graft surgery may not appreciably prolong life in many patients.[87,99] Can lack of progress be attributed to our willingness to accept the convictions of others? Does a narcotic technique with pulmonary artery catheterization and close attention to hypertension and tachycardia really reduce the risk of a perioperative cardiac event? If so, why do the studies *still* identify adverse outcomes?[97,101-103] This chapter addresses both issues: preoperative risk factor assessment and therapeutic approaches to decrease risk. The first subject is well mapped, but the latter is largely unexplored.

CLINICAL ASSESSMENT OF CARDIAC RISK
Early Studies

Early reports of perioperative cardiac risk have had an important impact on present conceptions (and misconceptions) regarding cardiac risk. Most of the risk factors used by the Goldman Cardiac Risk Index were identified years earlier. Likewise, the admonishment to "avoid hypotension and hypoxemia" has roots in early studies.[49]

In 1930 Butler et al. recognized that patients with acute infarction who underwent surgery had an exceedingly high mortality.[19] When an infarction occurred postoperatively, mortality was also high. In 1935 Saphir et al.[145] noted the correlation between surgery and increased incidence of coronary events. In 1937 and 1938 Master et al. analyzed 35 patients with postoperative myocardial infarction (MI) and determined that age over 60 years, prior coronary disease, cardiac enlargement, and preoperative electrocardiographic (ECG) abnormalities were predictive findings in patients who later experienced perioperative infarctions.[107,108,171] They noted that most such events occurred within 3 days of surgery and that mortality was 65%. Neither type of anesthesia nor its duration was clearly implicated, as demonstrated by infarctions in patients who received general, spinal, or local anesthesia for major and minor surgeries. In 1939 Brumm and Willius of the Mayo Clinic reported a remarkably low operative mortality of 4.3% in a group of 257 patients who had "severe coronary disease."[17] This accomplishment was attributed to "careful preoperative study and judicious selection, expert administration of anesthetic agents, and skillful surgical technic and judgment." Another possibility was that the coronary disease was less severe than contended, as suggested by the incidence of prior MI in only 12.4% of patients. In 1955 Etsten and Proger emphasized that a *recent* MI increased the operative risk by 20 times and that anesthetic management for such a patient was preferably "light," with controlled respiration to avoid hypoxemia and hypercarbia.[50]

Early surgical literature was primarily concerned with long-term success of surgical procedures. Thus, although De Bakey et al. in 1964 acknowledged that coronary disease was present in almost one third of their series of 1449 patients who underwent abdominal aneurysm repair, 91% survived the procedure (remarkable results considering that in 8% of patients the aneurysm had ruptured).[36] In 1960 Lown et al. recommended prophylactic preoperative digitalization for a variety of cardiac problems, although this

drug's efficacy would not be studied until years later.[51,98] **In contrast, early anesthesia literature contended that preoperative atherosclerosis predisposed patients to postoperative complications.** Knapp et al. in 1962 and Topkins and Artusio in 1964 demonstrated that a history of MI or cerebrovascular accident (CVA, stroke) greatly increased the chances of a postoperative myocardial reinfarction or CVA.[89,164] In 1964 Arkins et al. found that recent MI, poor physical condition, and emergency surgery increased the incidence of postoperative myocardial reinfarction. The latter patients had a mortality of 69%.[4]

A remarkable report by Skinner and Pearce in 1964 evaluated 25 cardiac parameters in patients who underwent 857 surgeries.[155] Characteristics associated with increased mortality included intraperitoneal and intrathoracic surgery; severe hypertension; aortic valve disease; cor pulmonale; poor functional class; increased age (highest mortality in those over age 75); ECG abnormality, including atrial fibrillation, atrial flutter, and bundle branch block; and multiple surgical procedures. Neither type of anesthesia nor its duration was considered associated with poor outcome. Higher mortality was noted in patients whose systolic blood pressures were less than 100 mm Hg, probably because patients were brought to surgery already in shock. Many of these factors would be reevaluated by Goldman et al.[65,67,68] more than a decade later.

This literature contained considerable conflicting information. For example, Fraser et al. in 1967 recognized that a recent MI greatly increased the risk of surgery.[56] However, their recommendation that elective surgery be postponed until 3 months after the MI is contrary to most subsequent studies.[57] Mauney et al. in 1970 prospectively studied 365 general surgery patients who had abnormal preoperative ECGs.[110] Acute perioperative MIs occurred in 89% of patients, but surprisingly a previous MI had no bearing on the incidences. The authors' major conclusion was based on retrospective analysis of the anesthetic record, whereby it was determined that intraoperative hypotension and length of anesthesia were associated with more adverse outcomes.

Before the 1970s, many reports suggested a correlation between preoperative cardiac disease and perioperative cardiac events. Most studies concerned small numbers of patients, and the definition of preoperative cardiac disease was often not specified. **Data from the Mayo Clinic in 1972 helped clarify the picture by analyzing the outcome of 422 patients who had experienced an MI before noncardiac surgery.**[159] Postoperative infarctions were more likely following upper abdominal and intrathoracic surgery, most frequent on the third postoperative day, associated with high mortality, and not related to type or duration of anesthesia. **An important contribution was the verification that recent MI significantly increased risk of reinfarction. Specifically, surgery within 3 months of an MI was associated with a 37% reinfarction rate, surgery 3 to 6 months after an MI carried a 16% reinfarction risk, and surgery 6 months or more after an MI carried a 4% to 5% risk of reinfarction.**[159,162] Thus, by the late 1970s, preoperative cardiac disease was known to increase the risk for perioperative cardiac events.

Attempts to Predict Cardiac Risk Using Preoperative Factors

Whether or not the Cardiac Risk Index, first published by Goldman et al. in 1977, is an accurate predictor of cardiac risk, it undoubtedly has had an important impact on the subject.[65,67,68] **In 1977 a retrospective analysis of 1001 patients over 40 years old who underwent major noncardiac surgery was performed.**[67] **Nine statistically independent preoperative variables were contended to correlate with the incidence of postoperative cardiac events, such as MI, pulmonary edema, and ventricular tachycardia** (Table 11-1). Goldman et al. attempted to assign relative weight to each factor to facilitate summation of factors and calculation of "overall cardiac risk."[67] Because the Goldman Cardiac Risk Index was an easy-to-use point scale, it received widespread adoption and use by internists in their preoperative cardiac consultations. **This adoption came despite no confirmation of actual predictive validity.** A more complicated scheme also using multivariate analysis was proposed by Cooperman et al. at approximately the same time.[31] This analysis has received little attention,

perhaps because calculation of cardiac risk required solution of a logarithmic equation.

The Goldman data[67] has several limitations. Some assessments were based on small numbers of patients. For example, the strongest statistical predictor of a postoperative cardiac complication was preoperative third heart sound or jugular venous distension. However, these variables were present in only 35 patients (3.5% of the patient population) preoperatively. Valvular aortic stenosis was present in 23 patients and resulted in complications in only four. Recent MI was present in only 22 patients. **A second limitation of the Goldman study is that detection of some predictive findings depended on individual physical examination skills.**[67] **The authors acknowledged that assessment of jugular venous distension and the differentiation of aortic stenosis from a benign systolic ejection murmur might be difficult in some patients.** Additionally, presence of premature ventricular contractions was assessed without ECG monitoring.

The analysis of Goldman probably underestimated the actual number of complications because a postoperative ECG and cardiac enzyme studies were not routinely obtained but only when patients complained of suspicious chest pain or the managing physician considered that signs suggested a cardiac problem.[25] **These qualitative assessments have been demonstrated to significantly underestimate actual frequency of cardiac events.**[42,167,176] **For example, diabetic patients may not experience chest pain with ischemia. Postoperative narcotic analgetics may mask symptoms. Tarhan et al. demonstrated that about 25% of the postoperative reinfarctions were not heralded by chest pain.**[159] In contrast, patients in the Goldman

---

Table 11-1 Goldman variables arranged by "point" value relative weight

Variable	Point value	Life-threatening but nonfatal complications*	Cardiac deaths*
Third heart sound or jugular venous distension	11	5/35	7/35
Recent myocardial infarction	10	3/22	5/22
Nonsinus rhythm or premature atrial contractions on ECG	7	11/112	10/112
More than five premature ventricular contractions	7	7/44	6/44
Age > 70 years	5	19/324	16/324
Emergency surgery	4	16/197	10/197
Poor general medical condition	3	25/362	13/362
Intraperitoneal intrathoracic or aortic surgery	3	32/437	11/437
Important valvular aortic stenosis	3	1/23	3/23

Total number of patients with cardiac complications was 58, or 5.8% of the group of 1001 patients.
*Numerator indicates number of patients with a complication; denominator indicates number of patients with the risk factor. Nonfatal complications included myocardial infarction, pulmonary edema, and ventricular tachycardia. Nineteen patients died from cardiac problems.
Data from Goldman L, Caldera DL, Nussbaum SR et al: Multifactorial index of cardiac risk in noncardiac surgical procedures, *N Engl J Med* 297:845, 1977.

study who received continuous postoperative monitoring (e.g., because of intensive care placement) may have been relatively overassessed for complications such as ventricular tachycardia.

A look at the Goldman predictive classifications (Table 11-2) reveals that the point ranges for classes I and II are rather narrow.[67,68] It is impossible for a patient to have more than one risk factor and be in class I. Likewise, it is unlikely that a patient could have a prior MI (10 points) or jugular venous distension or third heart sound (11 points) and be in class II. Thus, although the Cardiac Risk Index did separate the healthy patients from the sick ones, it did not prove much more discriminating than that. Patients with several minor risk factors probably fall into class II, which predicts 7% cardiac complications. This was also the frequency of complications when all 1001 patients were pooled, reflecting the average complication rate.

Of note also were the preoperative factors that did *not* correlate to postoperative cardiac events (Table 11-3). Among variables considered "conspicuously insignificant" by Goldman et al. were smoking, diabetes, hypertension, stable angina, peripheral atherosclerotic vascular disease, bundle branch blocks, and congestive heart failure in the absence of a third heart sound or jugular venous distension.[67]

In 1978 Steen et al. reported on a large series of patients from the Mayo Clinic. Of more than 73,000 patients who underwent noncardiac surgery during 1975 to 1976, 587 had a prior history of MI.[156] Factors associated with increased incidence of reinfarction included preoperative hypertension, intraoperative hypotension, and duration of anesthesia and surgery. None of these had correlated with the outcome in the Goldman et al. study.[67] In agreement with Goldman et al., **risk was increased by intrathoracic, intraabdominal, or great vessel surgery but was not increased by preoperative angina, diabetes, or anesthetic technique. The mortality from reinfarction was high. An**

important contribution of this large series was substantiation that surgery following *recent* MI greatly increases the risk of reinfarction.[156] Combining the data of Steen et al. with those of Tarhan et al. from the same institution provides a series of more than 1000 patients illustrating this finding[156,159] (Table 11-4).

Of note is the relatively high percentage of reinfarctions, 10.8%, occurring in patients in whom the *time* of previous MI was either unknown or "old." These data may reflect patients whose most recent infarct was not the "old" one in the history, but rather a recent infarct that was not clinically recognized. Up to one fourth of all MIs have been demonstrated to be clinically silent and are recognized only from the ECG. An interesting coincidence is that the 160 "old or unknown" previous infarctions made up one fourth of the total preoperative infarctions.

Factors similar to those reported by Steen et al. were also noted for a small series of 89 Finnish* patients reported by Eerola et al. in 1980.[48] Retrospective analysis of the six patients who suffered reinfarction revealed risk factors that included age over 60 years, anemia, hypertension, abdominal surgery, dysrhythmias, and intraoperative hypotension. Although these findings echoed those of Steen et al., the presence of a recent MI (less than 4 weeks) was *not* found associated with high reinfarction rate. The small number of patients reported probably account for this discrepancy since most studies have linked *recent* prior MI to high perioperative reinfarction risk.

---

* Finland is acknowledged to have a high incidence of coronary artery disease.

Table 11-3   Preoperative characteristics noted to be insignificantly correlated to postoperative cardiac event (data from Goldman et al. 1977)

Variable	Patients with variable present
Hypertension	280
ST or T wave changes on electrocardiogram	211
Previous old myocardial infarction by history or ECG	119
Cardiomegaly on chest radiograph	117
Stable angina	69
Mitral valve disease	68
Hyperlipidemia	58

Data from Goldman L, Caldera DL, Nussbaum SR et al: Multifactorial index of cardiac risk in noncardiac surgical procedures, *N Engl J Med* 297:845, 1977.

Table 11-2   Goldman predictive classes

Class	Patients with complications*	Point range	Cardiac complication
I	5/537	0-5	1%
II	21/316	6-12	7%
III	18/130	13-25	14%
IV	14/18	>26	78%
TOTAL	58/1001		6%

*Numerator indicates the number of patients with a complications; denominator indicates number of patients in the class.
Data from Goldman L, Caldera DL, Nussbaum SR et al: Multifactorial index of cardiac risk in noncardiac surgical procedures, *N Engl J Med* 297:845, 1977.

Table 11-4 Myocardial reinfarction according to time of surgery after previous infarction

Time of surgery after infarct (months)	Tarhan et al.[159] (1967-1968) (422 patients)*	Steen et al.[156] (1974-1975) (587 patients)	Combined Mayo Clinic (1009 patients)*	Reinfarction
0-3	8 (3)	15 (4)	23 (7)	30%
4-6	19 (3)	18 (2)	37 (5)	13%
7-12	42 (2)	31 (2)	73 (4)	5.5%
13-18	27 (1)	30 (1)	57 (2)	3.5%
19-24	21 (1)	17 (1)	38 (2)	5.3%
25 +	232 (11)	383 (15)	615 (26)	4.2%
Old or unknown	73 (7)	93 (11)	166 (18)	10.8%

*Number alone represents patients with preoperative infarct, and number in parentheses represents number of reinfarctions.

While medical consultants widely used the Goldman Cardiac Risk Index to predict cardiac risk, prospective analysis demonstrated its predictive capacity to be less than expected. **In 1981 Waters et al. applied the Goldman index prospectively to a large series of patients who underwent noncardiac surgery at a different but comparable university hospital.[168] The Goldman index was no better than the ASA Physical Status Classification in predicting adverse cardiac outcomes.** This is important because Goldman et al. had reported that the American Society of Anesthesiologists* classification was not as accurate as the Cardiac Risk Index in identifying these high-risk patients.[67,68] In addition, Waters et al. found that abdominal aortic aneurysm surgery was associated with an increased risk of cardiac complications.[168] Domaingue et al. in 1982 prospectively applied the Goldman index to peripheral vascular surgery patients and found that it significantly underestimated the cardiac complication rate.[41]

Jeffrey et al. in 1983 demonstrated this important weakness of the Goldman index by prospectively applying it to 99 patients who underwent abdominal aortic aneurysm surgery.[80] Patients prospectively categorized by the Goldman classes had many more perioperative cardiac events than predicted by the Goldman scheme. Although these patients came from the same hospital as Goldman's original series and patient management would have been expected to be similar, the study was done several years later. Instead of expected "improvement," these patients did not fare nearly as well as the Goldman Cardiac Risk Index predicted. Jeffrey et al. concluded that the Goldman index was not useful for estimating cardiac risk in patients undergoing abdominal aortic aneurysm re-

---

*Mistakenly referred to as the American Surgical Association Classification by Goldman et al., a mistake ruefully noted in several subsequent letters to the editor.

Table 11-5 Prospective evaluation of Goldman Index in patients undergoing abdominal aortic surgery (data from Jeffrey et al. 1983)

Goldman class	Patients	Goldman prediction of number of events*	Actual events found*
I	56	0-1 (1%)	4 (7%)
II	35	2-3 (7%)	4 (11%)
III	8	1 (14%)	3 (38%)

*Number in parentheses is percentage of patients for each Goldman class who had a cardiac event.
From Jeffrey CC, Kunsman J, Cullen DJ, and Brewster DC: A prospective evaluation of cardiac risk index, *Anesthesiology* 58:462, 1983.

pair and called for further prospective evaluation of the Goldman index[80] (Table 11-5).

Zeldin in 1984 prospectively applied the Goldman index to 1140 consecutive patients for whom he was the primary surgeon.[178] Patients classified into Goldman classes I, II, and III had perioperative cardiac complication rates similar to those predicted by Goldman et al., but the highest-risk class IV patients had only *half* the cardiac events predicted. **Zeldin postulated that awareness of the high cardiac risk of these patients may have created a bias for *better* care that resulted in fewer complications.** An alternative explanation for their unexpectedly superior results may be that patients were excluded if they had *low cardiac output states* associated with noncardiac postoperative conditions such as sepsis or respiratory failure. However, sepsis and adult respiratory distress syndrome (ARDS) are often associated with *high* cardiac output states. Low output states in these circumstances may have represented primary cardiac dysfunction. The exclusion of these patients is another bias toward better results.

Detsky et al. prospectively applied the Goldman index to 268 patients for whom preoperative medical consultation was requested.[39,40] One could argue that this group of patients was selected for consultation because of a perceived increased surgical risk. However, if the Goldman risk factors were accurately weighted and are really predictive, the index should function no matter what patient population is assessed. In this study, although the Goldman index separated high-risk from low-risk patients, Detsky et al. found more cardiac complications than the Goldman analysis predicted. The only accurate predictor of the number of cardiac complications was class II.

These results led Detsky et al. to propose a modified cardiac risk index in 1986.[39,40] Changes included additional risk factors of clinical angina, history of pulmonary edema, and old myocardial infarction. "Significant aortic stenosis" was changed to "critical aortic stenosis" requiring a history of syncope, angina, or congestive failure in addition to the characteristic murmur. The risk factors of jugular venous distension and third heart sound were highly significant in the Goldman analysis[67,68] but were dropped from the modified Detsky index.[39,40] Also dropped was the risk factor of intraabdominal, intrathoracic, or aortic surgery. Important changes were also made in the relative weights of the risk factors. Whereas Goldman assigned the lowest point value to significant aortic stenosis and gave no significance to angina, Detsky assigned both factors the highest point values of the modified index. Goldman's strongest variable, evidence for congestive heart failure, is given only moderate weight in the Detsky index.

Overall the Detsky modified index depends more on *historic information* than physical findings and is *substantially different* from the Goldman index despite a superficial resemblance (Table 11-6). Whether the changes truly improve predictive accuracy remains to be verified. It should be noted that the Goldman index used statistical multivariate analysis to identify and weight the various risk factors, whereas the Detsky index assigned significance based on consensus opinion of their cardiology consultation team. Further, the Detsky index requires a knowledge of "pretest probability" and use of a "likelihood ratio nomogram" that has sacrificed the simplicity that was a major benefit of the Goldman index.[39,40]

Gerson et al. in 1985 applied Goldman criteria, ASA Physical Status Classification, and the results of bicycle exercise and radionucleotide ventriculograms to 100 patients age 65 years or more scheduled for elective abdominal or noncardiac thoracic surgery. Thirteen of these patients had perioperative cardiac complications, including six deaths. By multivariate analysis, the inability to perform 2 minutes of supine

Table 11-6   Detsky's Modified Multifactorial Index arranged according to point value

Variables	Points
Class 4 angina*	20
Suspected critical aortic stenosis	20
Myocardial infarction within 6 months	10
Alveolar pulmonary edema within 1 week	10
Unstable angina within 3 months	10
Class 3 angina*	10
Emergency surgery	10
Myocardial infarction more than 6 months ago	5
Alveolar pulmonary edema ever	5
Sinus plus atrial premature beats or rhythm other than sinus on last preoperative electrocardiogram	5
More than five ventricular premature beats at any time before surgery	5
Poor general medical status†	5
Age over 70 years	5

*Canadian Cardiovascular Society classification for angina.
†Oxygen tension (Po_2) < 60 mm Hg; carbon dioxide tension (Pco_2) > 50 mm Hg; serum potassium < 3.0 mEq/L; serum bicarbonate < 20 mEq/L; serum urea nitrogen > 50 mg/dl; serum creatinine > 3 mg/dl; aspartate aminotransferase abnormality; signs of chronic liver disease; and/or patients bedridden from noncardiac causes.
Data from Detsky AS, Abrams HB, Forbath N et al: Cardiac assessment for patients undergoing noncardiac surgery, a multifactorial clinical risk index, *Arch Intern Med* 146:2131, 1986; and Detsky AS, Abrams HB, McLaughlin JR et al: Predicting cardiac complications in patients undergoing noncardiac surgery, *J Gen Intern Med* 1:211, 1986.

bicycle exercise sufficient to increase the heart rate above 99 beats/min provided predictive data that were not available from the clinical or radionucleotide information[60] (see also later section on stress test).

The many risk indices and conflicting findings deserve comment. **A unifying explanation is provided by Charlson et al., who analyzed reasons why prognostic indices of cardiac risk perform less well when subjected to prospective testing.**[24] **Differences in (1) eligibility criteria, (2) surveillance strategies,**[25] **and (3) outcome criteria may greatly alter results.** Charlson et al. analyzed a population of 232 patients for postoperative cardiac events. All the patients were evaluated daily by clinical examination, ECG, creatine kinase (CK), and creatine kinase isoenzymes (CKMB) for 6 postoperative days. In this way the four different strategies of Goldman, Jeffrey, Detsky, and Gerson could be compared for their capacity to predict adverse cardiac events (Table 11-7). First, eligibility criteria differed such that Goldman et al. would have enrolled all Charlson's prospective population, whereas Jeffrey would have enrolled only 13%.[24]

	Goldman et al.[67]	Jeffrey et al.[80]	Detsky et al.[39]	Gerson et al.[60]
Table 11-7 **Differences in eligibility criteria and surveillance method (data from Charlson et al. 1987)**				
Patient eligibility	All ward patients	Abdominal aneurysm surgery	Suspected cardiac disease	Elderly; abdominal or thoracic surgery
Survey method	Symptoms plus	Symptomatic patients only	Symptoms plus	Symptoms plus
	ECG on day 5		ECG for 2 days CKMB for 2 days	ECG for 3 days CKMB for 3 days

ECG, Electrocardiogram; *CKMB*, creatine kinase isoenzymes.
Data from Charlson ME, Ales KL, Simon R et al: Why predictive indexes perform less well in validation studies, *Arch Intern Med* 147:2155, 1987.

The surveillance method used to identify potential cardiac complications also varied from the least intensive method of Jeffrey et al. to the most intensive method of Gerson et al.[24] Finally, the criteria for diagnosing MI influenced results. The most restrictive criteria was that of Detsky, who required persistent ST-T wave changes for 72 hours plus a CKMB level greater than 5%. The least restrictive criteria was that of Gerson et al., who defined any increase in CKMB to indicate infarction. Combining the factors of different (1) eligibility, (2) surveillance, and (3) outcome criteria greatly influenced the incidence of cardiac complications found. **Using the patients of the Charlson et al. prospective population, only 2.6% cardiac complications were noted if eligibility was unrestricted, surveillance was least intensive, and criteria for infarction most strict. In contrast, when eligibility was selective, surveillance intense, and criteria for infarction the least restrictive, cardiac complications were found in 31% of the population.**[24]

A comment here may clarify the picture. Most of these investigators have used a premise greatly simplified as follows:

If we know enough about → Then we could accu-
the *patient* preopera-   rately predict peri-
tively (e.g., disease,   operative *outcome*
medications, other
medical problems,
past medical history,
allergies)

Perhaps this *premise* is wrong. We suggest modifying the premise as follows:

Preoperative + Perioperative → Much more
knowledge   *process* prob-   accurate un-
about the   lems (see   derstanding
patient   below for   of reasons
                definitions)   for outcome
                                   variability

Perioperative *process* problems include inadvertencies, errors, delays, wrong drugs, airway disconnections, lack of vigilance, equipment malfunction, and many other "nightmares" that, however else they might be linked, are not likely to be predictable preoperatively.[18,27,44,84] Therefore, recently, the past attention given to use of preoperative predictors to try to help improve patient selection and therefore outcome has given way to an increased awareness of *process* and its great effect on outcome and quality.

TECHNOLOGY AND CARDIAC RISK
Simple Electrocardiogram

In this age of ever-increasing sophisticated technology, the simple ECG may seem archaic. It does not require a special camera or radioactive substance. Most physicians are able to perform an ECG and interpret the basic results, making the test and results available at all hours. Finally, the ECG is inexpensive and reproducible, which facilitates comparison over time. Moorman et al. studied the yield of admission ECGs in medical patients and concluded that they are "as cost effective as many accepted medical practices" and that yield is increased with patient age and presence of a clinically evident cardiac abnormality.[121]

The preoperative ECG can provide useful information regarding prediction of cardiac risk. First, the resting ECG may provide firm evidence that a patient has coronary artery disease by "Q waves" indicating a previous MI. This is particularly important because up to one fourth of MIs may have been clinically silent. Although it is unlikely that a preoperative ECG would indicate an acute or recent MI, such a finding would be extremely significant for the patient. Goldberger and O'Konski point out that the semiannual incidence of unrecognized Q wave MIs occurs more often in the elderly.[64] A recent MI is the most important risk factor for patients having noncardiac surgery, a finding documented by almost all cardiac risk-outcome studies.

Other ECG findings have been used to help predict outcome in patients undergoing noncardiac surgery. **A nonsinus rhythm and greater than five premature ventricular contractions (PVCs) were each determined to be independent predictors of cardiac outcome in the study by Goldman et al.**[67] Premature atrial contractions (PACs) were ominous signs in patients who were elderly, having major surgery, and characterized as medically or surgically unstable. The presence of PVCs did not correlate with the incidence of ventricular tachycardia, but rather suggested severe heart disease, since nearly all patients with frequent PVCs had other signs of significant cardiac disease. According to relative weighting by Goldman et al., each ECG risk factor was more important than any other factor except recent MI or signs of congestive heart failure. Together, these two ECG factors accounted for one fourth of the potential risk in the study by Goldman et al.[67] (14 out of 53 possible points). Thus the ECG provided risk assessment data that were certainly comparable with those obtained by the history and physical examination. Further, these ECG risk factors have been incorporated in subsequent investigations of cardiac risk by Detsky et al.,[39,40] Gerson et al.,[60,61] Cooperman et al.,[31] and Eagle et al.[46,47]

Carliner et al. found that the preoperative ECG provided important information to predict outcome of noncardiac surgery.[20,21] Specifically, patients with abnormal preoperative ECGs were 3.2 times more likely to have a cardiac event than patients with normal ECGs. Important ECG abnormalities were intraventricular conduction delays and ST-T abnormalities. Goldman et al. also found some correlation for these variables.[68]

The significance of bundle branch block on the preoperative ECG is controversial. Several authors have indicated that bundle branch block does not increase the risk of developing complete heart block during anesthesia and surgery. Berg and Kotler reported no perioperative episodes of heart block in 20 patients with bilateral bundle branch block.[9] Rooney found no episodes of perioperative heart block in 27 patients with right bundle branch block (RBBB) and left axis.[139] Pastore et al. reported one episode of documented perioperative complete heart block in 44 patients with RBBB and left axis.[130] That episode occurred during intubation and responded to temporary pacing. In the population of Goldman et al., 164 patients had preoperative conduction abnormalities, which included 45 patients with bifascicular block.[68] However, the only episode of *documented* perioperative complete heart block occurred in a patient whose preoperative ECG showed no conduc-

tion disturbance. These considerations may not apply to the patient whose conduction abnormality was recently acquired as a result of an MI. For example, in the population of Goldman et al., a patient with a new bifascicular block and prolonged PR interval *after a recent reinfarction* died even though a prophylactic pacemaker was present. When all patients with QRS abnormalities were considered together, the incidence of postoperative infarction was not increased, but the overall incidence of cardiac death was greater compared with patients who did not have the abnormality.[68] Finally, left bundle branch block (LBBB) on the ECG is useful information because of the reported increased risk of developing complete heart block during placement of a pulmonary artery catheter. Recently the incidence of this has been studied and found to be low.[123]

Stress Test

Common sense dictates that exercise stress testing would be useful to identify the patient with cardiac risk.[174] Early reports were favorable. In 1981 Culter et al. reported strong correlation between exercise test results and postoperative cardiac problems in patients having vascular surgery.[34] McCabe et al. in 1981 found that 80% of patients undergoing vascular surgery with abnormal exercise tests preoperatively had perioperative cardiac problems. Unfortunately the definition of "cardiac problem" was so liberal that it included intraoperative need for vasodilator drugs, inotropic agents, or antidysrhythmic drugs as positive findings.[111] **In contrast, Carliner et al. in 1985 studied 200 patients having vascular surgery and found that neither the exercise test nor the Goldman index were good predictors of postoperative cardiac events, including death, MI, ECG change, or rise in CK.**[20] **Cardiac events occurred more often in patients over age 70, but an abnormal preoperative ECG was the only statistically significant independent predictor of cardiac risk.** Limitations of the study were acknowledged and included the observed complication rate being lower than expected. The study would have required 1000 patients instead of 200 to unequivocally demonstrate their conclusions. The low complication rate was probably influenced by the eligibility criteria, which excluded patients with recent MI, unstable angina, decompensated congestive failure, significant aortic stenosis, significant ventricular dysrhythmias, and uncontrolled hypertension. Carliner et al. suggested that exercise testing may be more predictive in particular subgroups, such as patients over age 70 or those with an already abnormal ECG.[20] A significant concern has been whether patients will be able to perform sufficient exercise for a valid test. In a study of patients having vascular surgery by Gage et al., almost one fourth of the patients could not perform an adequate test, requiring coronary angiography to delineate their cardiac disease.[59]

In 1985 Gerson et al. had identified that the ability to perform supine bicycle was a useful predictor of perioperative cardiac events in geriatric patients undergoing noncardiac surgery.[60] In 1990 a second study by Gerson et al. investigated the predictive use of bicycle exercise in a group of 177 patients aged 65 years or older who were scheduled for elective abdominal or noncardiac thoracic surgery.[61] Presence of one or more Goldman factors or inability to exercise successfully identified 88% of patients with cardiac complications and 92% of patients with pulmonary complications. By multivariate analysis, inability to exercise on a supine bicycle for 2 minutes at heart rates greater than 99 beats per minute was the best predictor of perioperative cardiac and pulmonary complications. Elderly patients able to exercise for at least 2 minutes at a heart rate greater than 99 beats per minute had six times fewer cardiac complications and five times fewer pulmonary complications. Gerson et al.[61] considered that lack of any Goldman risk factors and ability to perform sufficient supine bicycle exercise accurately identified a group of low-risk elderly patients. They emphasized that no evidence indicated that this exercise threshold applied to younger patients (Table 11-8).

Radionucleotide Ejection Fraction

Studies have indicated that preoperative ejection fraction (EF) is a useful predictor for patients undergoing cardiac surgery.[29] The preoperative EF might also be a prognostic guide for *noncardiac* surgery.[92] Pasternack et al. in 1984 investigated predictive capacity of resting gated blood pool EF for 50 patients with abdominal aortic aneurysm.[128] No

cardiac events occurred in patients who had an EF of 56% to 85%. The group with EF of 36% to 55% had a 20% postoperative MI rate; the group with EF of 27% to 35% had an 80% MI rate. Although the authors concluded that the radionucleotide EF was a better predictor than clinical risk factors, only past history of MI and angina were considered. Pasternack et al. next enlarged the study to 100 patients in 1985 with similar results and conclusions.[129]

Despite these studies, the relationship between EF and outcome, especially MI, is not clear. Normal EF does not indicate absence of coronary disease. Many patients who need coronary artery bypass graft (CABG) surgery for triple-vessel disease have normal EFs preoperatively.[122] Upton et al. also demonstrated that a patient with coronary disease can have either a normal or an abnormal EF depending on whether ischemia is present at the time of the scan.[165] Reduced EF may be caused by previous MI and scarring rather than active ischemia. Finally, it is unclear whether the group with a low EF could have been identified by clinical evidence for congestive heart failure.

When radionucleotide techniques have been compared with other methods of estimating cardiac risk, superior results have not been verified. Gerson et al. studied rest and exercise radionucleotide ventriculograms in 155 patients aged 65 or older who also underwent clinical evaluation and bicycle exercise before elective abdominal or noncardiac thoracic surgery.[60] They found that radionucleotide studies of regional wall motion were costly and added little to the predictive information provided by inability to exercise. Gerson et al. considered that advanced age may have influenced the radionucleotide test because an abnormal exercise EF has been shown to be nonspecific for detection of coronary disease in the elderly.

In 1989 Franco et al. confirmed these findings by preoperative study of resting gated blood pool EFs in 85 patients having vascular surgery.[55] Patients were classified into three groups depending on EF. **MIs occurred with similar frequencies in each group, although cardiac deaths occurred only in the group with a low EF (Table 11-9). The authors concluded that normal EF does not preclude risk of postoperative cardiac events. Their findings do suggest that low EF may portend poor outcome.**

Thallium

Although some studies continue to report preoperative and intraoperative risk factors, recent cardiac risk studies are primarily characterized by a new technologic application, that is, thallium cardiac imaging with dipyridamole administration.[16] The landmark study by Boucher et al. in 1985 began this contempo-

---

Table 11-8 Outcome prediction by inability to exercise or Goldman indicators in 177 elderly patients (data from Gerson et al. 1990)

	High risk (102 patients)	Low risk (75 patients)
Preoperative		
Ability to exercise	No	Yes
Goldman indicators	One or more	None
Outcomes		
Pulmonary complications	22 (22%)	2 (3%)
Cardiac complications	22 (22%)	3 (4%)
Deaths	6 (6%)	0

Data from Gerson MC, Hurst JM, Hertzberg VS et al: Prediction of cardiac and pulmonary complications related to elective abdominal and noncardiac thoracic surgery in geriatric patients, *Am J Med* 88:101, 1990.

rary era.[15] An acknowledged problem in risk assessment of vascular surgery was the relatively high incidence of asymptomatic coronary artery disease. Because of vascular limitations on exercise ability, exercise treadmill testing often could not be performed. **Boucher et al. used dipyridamole-thallium imaging to determine patients at risk for ischemic cardiac events. Of 54 patients imaged, thallium redistribution was a strong predictor of perioperative cardiac events (Table 11-10).** Importantly, Boucher et al. had excluded patients with recent MI, congestive heart failure, high-grade ventricular ectopy, unstable angina, severe chronic obstructive pulmonary disease (COPD), and severe renal disease. Thus the 54

Table 11-9   Incidence of cardiac events in patients undergoing vascular surgery according to preoperative ejection fraction (EF) (data from Franco et al. 1989)

	Group I (EF = .56-.92)	Group II (EF = .36-.55)	Group III (EF = .20-.35)
Patients	50	20	15
Myocardial infarctions	9 (18%)	3 (15%)	3 (20%)
Deaths	0	0	2 (13%)

Data from Franco CD, Goldsmith J, Veith FJ et al: Resting gated pool ejection fraction: a poor predictor of perioperative myocardial infarction in patients undergoing vascular surgery for infrainguinal bypass grafting, *J Vasc Surg* 10:656, 1989.

Table 11-10   Patient characteristics and surgical outcome according to results of dipyridamole-thallium test (data from Boucher et al. 1985)

	Normal scan (20 patients)	Persistent defect (12 patients)	Thallium redistribution (22 patients*)
History of chest pain	11 (55%)	8 (67%)	9 (56%)
Prior myocardial infarction	6 (30%)	11 (92%)	11 (69%)
Intraabdominal procedure	13 (65%)	7 (63%)	7 (44%)
Ischemic cardiac events	0	0	8 (50%)

*At discretion of managing physician, 6 of the 22 patients with redistribution were removed to cardiac catheterization, which demonstrated multivessel disease in all.
Data from Boucher CA, Brewster DC, Darling RC et al: Determination of cardiac risk by dipyridamole-thallium imaging before peripheral vascular surgery, *N Engl J Med* 312:389, 1985.

patients studied *would not have been identified as high-risk patients by the Goldman classification.*

Eagle et al. in 1987 reported that in 61 patients having major aortic surgery, a reversible defect on dipyridamole-thallium scan was the most significant predictor of postoperative ischemic events.[47] Historic variables, including Q wave on ECG, congestive heart failure, diabetes, angina, and prior MI were also related. The authors contended that absence of historic risk factors identified a low-risk population for whom dipyridamole-thallium scanning would be unnecessary, but that one or more historic risk factors identified a high-risk population that would benefit from scanning. Eagle et al. tested this hypothesis on 50 other patients undergoing vascular surgery and found it accurate in identifying patients at risk.

In 1989 Eagle et al. further modified their approach. The outcomes of 200 patients having vascular surgery revealed seven factors as independent predictors of postoperative cardiac events.[46] Five risk factors were clinical: advanced age, Q wave ECG, diabetes, angina, and history of ventricular dysrhythmias. Two factors involved the dipyridamole-thallium scan: thallium redistribution and ischemic ECG changes during dipyridamole infusion. **Patients with no clinical risk factors had cardiac events only rarely, suggesting that dipyridamole-thallium scanning was probably unnecessary. Scanning was also deemed unnecessary in patients who had three or more clinical risk factors, since a high incidence of ischemic events was already predicted by clinical characteristics. The major use of the dipyridamole-thallium scan was in the intermediate-risk group, characterized by one or two clinical risk factors.** This group could be successfully divided into high-risk and low-risk subgroups on the basis of the scan. Benefits of this algorithm include more economic use of dipyridamole-thallium scanning.

It should be emphasized that this algorithm (Table 11-11) also substantially improves the purported accuracy of the dipyridamole-thallium scan. For example, in the group with high clinical risk, Eagle et al. determined that the scan was unnecessary because clinical factors had already sufficiently identified the high-risk patients. Another interpretation is that in this high-risk group, the dipyridamole-thallium scan had a false-negative rate of 33%. Despite the lack of thallium redistribution, 3 of 9 patients had ischemic cardiac events. If scans are only obtained in the intermediate-risk group, as recommended by the algorithm, the false-negative rate becomes only 3.2% because only 2 of 62 patients whose scans did not show redistribution had ischemic cardiac events.

The current enthusiasm for the dipyridamole-thallium scan should also include an appreciation of the risks of the procedure. Ventricular ectopy has

Table 11-11 **Algorithm illustrating combination of clinical factors and dipyridamole-thallium scan for cardiac risk prediction in 200 patients (data from Eagle et al. 1989)**

	Low clinical risk (64 patients)	Intermediate clinical risk (116 patients)		High clinical risk (20 patients)
Clinical factors	None	1 or 2		3 or more
Thallium scan results	*	No thallium redistribution	Thallium redistribution	*
Ischemic events	2/64 (3.1%)	2/62 (3.2%)	16/54 (29.6%)	10/20 (50%)

*Indicates that dipyridamole-thallium scan was not recommended. In low-risk group, scan was not recommended because of expected low incidence of cardiac disease. Likewise, scan was deemed unnecessary in high-risk group, in whom a high incidence of cardiac disease was expected on the basis of clinical risk factors.
Eagle KA, Coley MC, Newell JB et al: Combining clinical and thallium data optimizes preoperative assessment of cardiac risk before major vascular surgery, *Ann Intern Med* 110:859, 1989.

been noted to occur during the procedure,[8] and one patient with ventricular fibrillation has been reported. Symptoms of angina have been noted in 16% to 41% of patients, although angina has been promptly relieved with intravenous aminophylline.[85] Blumenthal and McCauley recently have reported acute cardiac arrest and MI in a patient who received oral dipyridamole for thallium imaging.[12] Subsequent coronary angiography revealed complete occlusion of the left anterior descending coronary artery. The mechanisms proposed for dipyridamole exacerbation of ischemia include "coronary steal"[173] and peripheral vasodilation causing hypotension. Overall, however, many dipyridamole-thallium scans have been performed with relatively few reported complications, suggesting the procedure's safety.[77]

Of greater concern is whether the early enthusiasm for the test's predictive capacity will be sustained. Fleisher et al. recently reported three patients undergoing noncardiac surgery in whom the preoperative dipyridamole-thallium scan failed to predict high cardiac risk.[52] Specifically the preoperative dipyridamole-thallium scans were either normal or indicated "fixed" defects but no reperfusion abnormality. Each patient still suffered a postoperative MI. Interestingly, although characteristics such as age over 70, diabetes, vascular surgery, hypertension, prior MI, and ventricular ectopy were present, the Goldman index was not high for any patient. Postoperative epidural anesthesia did not prevent MI in the two patients in whom it was used. Two of the MIs occurred on the third postoperative day.

Recently, Mangano et al. prospectively studied the predictive capacity of the dipyridamole-thallium scan in 60 patients undergoing vascular surgery.[104] Results of the scans were "blinded" so as to avoid influencing patient care or cancellation of the surgery. Thirteen patients had adverse cardiac outcomes, including three MIs (one fatal), five cases of severe ischemia or

unstable angina, and five cases of congestive heart failure. The risk of having an adverse cardiac outcome was not associated with redistribution defects on the preoperative dipyridamole-thallium scan, since 54% of the adverse outcomes occurred in patients without redistribution defects (Table 11-12). The authors concluded that preoperative dipyridamole-thallium imaging has a lower negative predictive value than previously appreciated and that use of the test for preoperative screening of patients undergoing vascular surgery may not be warranted.[104]

Quite a different view was expressed by Pohost in an editorial accompanying the report of Mangano et al.[132] Criticisms of the study by Mangano et al. excluded patients with unstable heart disease, inclusion of "soft" events such as unstable angina or congestive failure, and a limited number of "hard" events, specifically, death or MI. Interestingly, similar criticisms can be made of the classic study by Boucher et al. that originally inspired the enthusiasm for the dipyridamole-thallium test.[15] Pohost acknowledges that to make the test most "cost effective," it should be applied to patients with an *intermediate* probability of severe disease.[132] This recommendation is not clear after criticizing the exclusion of patients with unstable heart disease. Not addressed in the editorial was the specific cost in dollars, which has been estimated at $700 to $1300/test.[104] Despite these concerns, the editorial answers whether dipyridamole-thallium imaging is useful for predicting coronary events after vascular surgery with "an unqualified 'yes'."[132] Undoubtedly the controversy will continue.

Recent Advances

Recently it has been appreciated that a significant amount of myocardial ischemia may be asymptomatic but detectable by *ambulatory ECG*.[86] **This method was explored in 1989 by Raby et al.** who prospectively evaluated ambulatory (Holter) ECG monitoring in

Table 11-12   Adverse cardiac outcomes* according to preoperative dipyridamole-thallium scan test (data from Mangano et al. 1991)

	Redistribution defect (22 patients)	Fixed defect (18 patients)	No defect (20 patients)
Myocardial infarction	1	1	1†
Severe ischemia/ unstable angina	3	1	1
Congestive heart failure	2	2	1

*When multiple events occurred, only the most serious is listed.
†Fatal myocardial infarction.
Data from Mangano DJ, London MJ, Taubaw JF et al: Dipyridamole thallium-201 scintigraphy as a preoperative screening test, a reexamination of its predictive potential, *Circulation* 84:493, 1991.

Table 11-13   Correlation of preoperative ambulatory ischemia to postoperative cardiac events (data from Raby et al. 1989)

	Preoperative ischemia on ambulatory ECG?	
	Yes (32 patients)	No (144 patients)
Postoperative cardiac event	12 (38%)	1 (1%)
No event	20 (63%)	143 (99%)*

*Absence of preoperative ambulatory ischemia was associated with lack of cardiac event in 99% of patients.
Data from Raby KE, Goldman L, Creager MA et al: Correlation between preoperative ischemia and major cardiac events after peripheral vascular surgery, *N Engl J Med* 321:1296, 1989.

176 consecutive patients scheduled for elective vascular surgery.[135] Ambulatory ECG monitoring for 24 to 48 hours within 9 days of surgery demonstrated ischemia in 18% of patients. The ischemia was asymptomatic in almost all patients and more common in those who had characteristics of age 70 or older, hypertension, prior carotid surgery, congestive heart failure, angina, MI, prior coronary bypass surgery, or any coronary disease. Postoperative cardiac events defined as MI, unstable angina, or ischemic pulmonary edema occurred in 38% of patients who had preoperative ischemia. **Preoperative Holter ischemia was the most significant correlate with postoperative events. Hypertension, hypercholesterolemia, and cardiovascular surgery other than carotid endarterectomy had borderline significance. Absence of preoperative ischemia predicted a good outcome** (Table 11-13).[135]

Raby et al. also attempted preoperative exercise testing, but it could only be completed satisfactorily in some patients because of symptomatic vascular disease or amputation. Although dipyridamole-thallium scanning has been demonstrated as effective in assessing exercise-limited patients with vascular problems, Raby et al. noted that ambulatory ECG may cost one-fifth as much. In addition, patients would not be subjected to possible ischemic events from the dipyridamole.

Muir et al. in 1991 reported the use of ambulatory ECG to detect silent myocardial ischemia in 156 surgical patients.[124] Silent ischemia was more prevalent in vascular (18.2%) than nonvascular (7.6%) surgical patients. It was also more likely in patients who had a history of ischemic heart disease or an ECG that suggested a previous MI (28%) than in patients who lacked these characteristics (9%). However, a significant amount of silent myocardial ischemia was detected in patients who did not possess risk factors. The importance of silent ischemia diagnosed by ambulatory ECG has also been reported by Ouyang et al.[127]

Another mode of cardiac assessment is *echocardiography*. The transthoracic technique has been used for years to assess valvular heart disease and ventricular function. **More recently, echocardiography has been combined with exercise, pacing, dobutamine infusion,[5,146] or dipyridamole infusion[13] to facilitate the diagnosis of coronary artery disease. The hypothesis of *stress echocardiography* is that stress-induced ischemia will cause regional wall motion abnormalities that can be imaged.**

Recently, Lane et al.[90] reported the use of dobutamine stress echocardiography in 57 patients scheduled for vascular, intraabdominal, or major orthopedic surgery. Most patients had some cardiac risk factor, including prior MI in 40%. All patients had conditions that prevented traditional exercise testing, but none had unstable angina or severe heart failure. Dobutamine was administered beginning at a dose of 2.5 µg/kg/min and increased to a maximum of 40 µg/kg/min. Three groups were distinguished by echocardiography: group 1, normal wall motion at rest and during dobutamine; group 2, resting wall motion abnormality but no new abnormality with dobutamine; group 3, patients who developed new abnormal wall motion during dobutamine in regions that had been normal at rest. In the 38 patients who underwent surgery, no adverse postoperative cardiac events occurred in groups 1 or 2 but occurred in 21% of group 3 patients. In the 19 patients who did not undergo surgery, apparent cardiac events occurred in four, with three in group 3 patients but also a sudden death in a group 1 patient. Since these techniques are new, their safety and accuracy compared with existing methodology require study.

Might *transesophageal echocardiography* (TEE) offer some advantages for preoperative cardiac assessment? The first consideration is a practical issue of patient acceptance and safety. A recent multicenter survey provides some insight.[35] Fifteen European centers performed 10,218 TEE examinations in *awake* patients over 1 year and concluded that risk is acceptably low. The examination had to be interrupted for reasons such as patient intolerance of the TEE probe (64 cases), bronchospasm (6), vomiting (5), nonsustained ventricular tachycardia (3), transient atrial fibrillation (3), hypoxia (2), bleeding complications (2), third-degree heart block (1), and severe angina pectoris (1). In this survey, mortality was approximately 1/10,000 examinations, which was comparable to the incidence of 0.4/10,000 gastroduodenal examinations.

CARDIAC RISK IN SPECIAL GROUPS

Congestive Heart Failure

Congestive heart failure (CHF), has been recognized by many authors to increase the risk of surgery. Master et al. noted in 1938 that longstanding cardiac enlargement was important in patients with adverse cardiac outcomes after surgery.[108] Skinner and Pearce in 1964 noted that the New York Heart Association (NYHA) functional classification directly correlated with postoperative mortality from noncardiac surgery.[155] Patients taking digitalis or diuretics fared less well than nonmedicated patients in the same functional class, causing Skinner et al. to speculate that this reflected more limited underlying cardiac function.

Goldman et al. determined by multivariate analysis that two signs of CHF, third heart sound or jugular venous distension, were the best predictors of adverse cardiac outcome.[65,67,68] The specific complication of postoperative pulmonary edema could be related to several preoperative factors (Table 11-14). **A good predictor of postoperative failure was preoperative failure according to the NYHA functional classification (Table 11-15).**[3] Goldman et al. also noted that 20% to 25% of patients who had mitral stenosis or regurgitation, or aortic stenosis or regurgitation, developed new or worsened postoperative CHF.

Preoperative CHF was also a significant predictor of myocardial reinfarction by Rao et al. in 1983. Despite widespread invasive monitoring and use of inotropic and vasodilator drugs, preoperative CHF was associated with a significant number of reinfarctions (Table 11-16).[136] Eagle et al. noted that CHF was a useful predictor of postoperative outcomes and an important supplement to the dipyridamole-thallium test.[46,47]

The recent report by Mangano in 1990 addressed CHF as a perioperative complication.[101] Using multivariate analysis, perioperative CHF was associated with history of dysrhythmia, diabetes, duration of anesthesia and surgery, vascular surgery, and some anesthetic techniques. Mangano noted that the relationship of CHF to narcotic vs. isoflurane anesthetics reflected anesthesiologists' appreciation of ventricular dysfunction. Mangano also noted that periopera-

---

Table 11-14 Correlation between preoperative signs of congestive heart failure (CHF) and perioperative pulmonary edema (data from Goldman et al. 1983)

Preoperative variable	Patients with variable	Percent developing pulmonary edema
S$_3$ gallop	17	35%
Jugular venous distension and signs of left-sided heart failure	23	30%
NYHA functional class IV for CHF	17	25%
History of pulmonary edema	22	23%
Left-sided heart failure by preoperative physical examination or chest radiograph	66	16%
History of left-sided heart failure but not evident on preoperative examination or chest radiograph	87	6%
NYHA functional class for CHF		
III	34	6%
II	15	7%
I	935	3%
No history of CHF	853	2%

NYHA, New York Heart Association.
From Goldman L: Cardiac risks and complications of noncardiac surgery, *Ann Intern Med* 98:504, 1983.

tive CHF has a more benign long-term prognosis, in contrast to ischemic outcomes.[101]

Valvular Heart Disease

The presence of valvular heart disease has implications for choice of anesthetic monitoring techniques and requirement for endocarditis prophylaxis. Each lesion has specific characteristics and goals for perioperative management. In terms of outcome from noncardiac surgery, only valvular aortic stenosis has been implicated in postoperative adverse cardiac outcomes. This is in contrast with surgical results concerning valve replacement itself.[88] Junod et al. in 1987 and earlier authors have reported higher mortality rates for mitral (MVR) than aortic valve replacement (AVR).[81] When combined valve replacement and CABG is undertaken, operative mortality for MVR and CABG is substantially higher than for AVR and CABG. **Nonetheless, for *noncardiac surgery*, only aortic stenosis has been identified as a factor that increases cardiac risk.**

Early work by Skinner and Pearce in 1964 evaluated 111 patients with rheumatic heart disease who underwent noncardiac surgery.[155] In general, patients with aortic valve disease did less well than patients with mitral valve lesions, with mortality rates of 10%

and 6%, respectively. When undergoing intrathoracic and intraabdominal surgical procedures, the distinction was even more pronounced; patients with mitral valve disease had no mortality, whereas those with aortic valve disease had a 20% mortality. It is difficult to distinguish between stenotic and insufficiency lesions in the Skinner et al. study. Nine patients with syphilitic aortic insufficiency had noncardiac surgery without mortality, but only one procedure was intraabdominal. Overall, the authors noted that patients with valvular heart disease tolerated surgery better than patients with atherosclerotic heart disease.[155]

In 1977 Goldman et al. found that aortic stenosis was the only valvular lesion associated with adverse cardiac outcomes by multivariate analysis.[67] Twelve patients with aortic insufficiency, 14 with mitral stenosis, and 54 with mitral regurgitation were included in the study. Approximately 20% to 25% of patients with mitral stenosis or regurgitation or aortic regurgitation did develop new or worsening postoperative CHF. **Although aortic stenosis was a stronger predictor than other valvular heart lesions, Goldman et al. ranked it only seventh of the nine multivariate factors.**

In contrast, the Detsky et al. modified cardiac risk index attributed a major prognostic role to preoperative aortic stenosis.[39,40] The authors assigned aortic stenosis the highest predictive valve in the modified index, twice the value assigned to recent MI or history of recent pulmonary edema. The distinction was that Goldman used "important valvular aortic stenosis" as a criterion, whereas Detsky required "suspected critical aortic stenosis" for inclusion. The difference in assigned weighting likely reflects the disease's natural history.[149] Aortic stenosis is characterized by a

---

Table 11-15   New York Heart Association functional classification

Class	Patient description
I	Patients with cardiac disease but without resulting limitations of physical activity. Ordinary physical activity does not cause undue fatigue, palpitation, dyspnea, or anginal pain.
II	Patients with cardiac disease resulting in slight limitation of physical activity. They are comfortable at rest. Ordinary physical activity results in fatigue, palpitation, dyspnea, or anginal pain.
III	Patients with cardiac disease resulting in marked limitation of physical activity. They are comfortable at rest. Less than ordinary physical activity causes fatigue, palpitation, dyspnea, or anginal pain.
IV	Patients with cardiac disease resulting in inability to carry on any physical activity without discomfort. Symptoms of cardiac insufficiency or of the anginal syndrome may be present even at rest. If any physical activity is undertaken, discomfort increases.

From American Heart Association: New York Heart Association functional classification. In Braunwald E, ed: *Heart disease*, ed 2, Philadelphia, 1984, WB Saunders.

Table 11-16   Congestive heart failure (CHF) as persistent risk factor (data from Rao et al. 1983)

Preoperative risk factor	Percent reinfarctions	
	1973-1976	1977-1982*
Recent MI (0-3 months)	36%	5.8%
Recent MI (4-6 months)	26%	2.3%
CHF	18%	11%

*Note that the period of 1977-1982 showed more than a sixfold decrease in rate of reinfarction for patients who had a prior MI. Patients with preoperative CHF had less than a twofold decrease in reinfarction rate. Data from Rao TLK, Jacobs KH, and El-Etr AA: Reinfarction following anesthesia in patients with myocardial infarction, *Anesthesiology* 59:499, 1983.

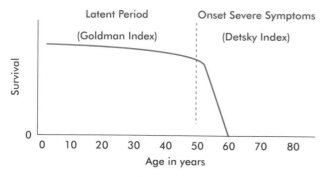

Fig. 11-1. Natural history of aortic stenosis and perioperative cardiac risk indices. Relatively low risk attributed to aortic stenosis by the Goldman index can be explained by latent period and high risk of the Detsky index by symptomatic phase. Cardiac risk index labels have been added. (Redrawn from Ross J Jr, Braunwald E: The influence of corrective operation on the natural history of aortic stenosis, *Circulation* 37(suppl V):61, 1968.)

BOX 11-1
PROCEDURES INDICATING
ENDOCARDITIS PROPHYLAXIS

All dental procedures that may cause gingival bleeding
Respiratory tract procedures, including tonsillectomy, adenoidectomy, biopsy, and bronchoscopy
Incision and drainage of infected tissue
Genitourinary and gastrointestinal procedures such as cystoscopy, colonoscopy, urethral catheterization, gallbladder surgery, and esophageal dilatation

Data from Committee on Rheumatic Fever and Infective Endocarditis, Council on Cardiovascular Disease in the Young, American Heart Association: Prevention of bacterial endocarditis, *Circulation* 70:1123A, 1984.

---

long asymptomatic latent period during which concentric left ventricular hypertrophy compensates for increasing valvular obstruction. Symptoms become manifest in the sixth decade of life and consist of angina, syncope, and CHF. Survival without surgery is limited to approximately 5 years after appearance of angina, but only 2 years after onset of failure.[141] Thus the low weight assigned by Goldman et al. probably reflects younger, asymptomatic patients, whereas the higher weight of Detsky et al. reflects appreciation of the symptomatic period (Fig. 11-1).

The Goldman et al. study had too few patients to access the significance of mitral valve prolapse or idiopathic hypertrophic subaortic stenosis (IHSS). In 1985 Thompson et al. reported 35 patients with IHSS who underwent 56 procedures.[67] Of the four procedures performed under spinal anesthesia, one patient developed an MI and CHF.[161]

Patients with structural heart disease are recommended to receive antibiotic prophylaxis against endocarditis when exposed to circumstances expected to cause bacteremia. **In 1984 the Committee on Rheumatic Fever and Infectious Endocarditis of the American Heart Association**[30] **published revised guidelines for endocarditis prophylaxis.** Some procedures for which antibiotics are indicated are listed in Box 11-1. The report specifically *excludes* simple endotracheal intubation as an indication for antibiotic prophylaxis but specifically *includes* urethral catheterization. Specific drugs and dosages are described for respiratory/dental procedures and genitourinary/gastrointestinal (GI) procedures in adults (Table 11-17). Alternative regimens, including oral antibiotics and pediatric dosages, are specifically listed in the report.

The subject of preoperative antibiotic prophylaxis is controversial.* The 1984 American Heart Association guidelines are a revision of previous guidelines that had poor compliance due to the rigorous regimens. Questions remain regarding mitral valve prolapse[91], as well as procedures such as barium enema, vaginal delivery, and upper GI endoscopy in patients with valvular heart disease. No controlled prospective clinical studies have documented that prophylactic antibiotics actually prevent endocarditis. Because of ethical problems, such a study is unlikely.

Hypertension

Longstanding hypertension clearly has systemic effects, including cardiac hypertrophy, carotid baroreflex alteration, and changes in cerebral blood flow autoregulation and renal function. All these conditions may influence risk. Antihypertensive medications may also influence risk by causing electrolyte abnormalities. Many studies have reported hypertensive responses to various stresses during anesthesia and surgery, and various drugs and techniques have been proposed to blunt these responses. Although this practice seems common sense, evidence that preoperative hypertension increases postoperative cardiac risk is not clear. Several studies have correlated intraoperative hypertension with increased postoperative cardiac complications. **In the multivariate analysis by Goldman et al., however, hypertension did not correlate to adverse postoperative cardiac events despite its presence in more than 25% of the study population.**[67] The question was specifically

---

*References 1, 10, 79, 82, 83, 153, 170.

Table 11-17   Summary of Recommended Antibiotic Regimens for Prevention of Bacterial Endocarditis in Adults

Dental/respiratory tract procedures		Gastrointestinal/genitourinary procedures	
Standard Regimen			
For dental procedures that cause gingival bleeding and for oral/respiratory tract surgery	Penicillin V 2 g orally 1 hour before, then 1 g 6 hours later For patients unable to take oral medications: 2 million units of aqueous penicillin G IV or IM 30-60 minutes before a procedure and 1 million units 6 hours later may be substituted	For genitourinary/gastrointestinal tract procedures	Ampicillin, 2 g IM or IV **plus** gentamicin 1.5 mg/kg IM or IV, given ½ to 1 hour before procedure; 1 follow-up dose may be given 8 hours later
Special Regimens			
Parenteral regimen for use when maximal protection is desired (e.g. for patients with prosthetic valves)	Ampicillin 1-2 g IM or IV **plus** gentamicin 1.5 mg/kg IM or IV, ½ hour before procedure, followed by 1 g oral penicillin V 6 hours later; alternatively, the parenteral regimen may be repeated once 8 hours later	Oral regimen for minor or repetitive procedures in low-risk patients	Amoxicillin 3 g orally 1 hour before procedure and 1.5 g 6 hours later
Oral regimen for pencillin-allergic pateints	Erythromycin 1 g orally 1 hour before, then 500 mg 6 hours later	Parenteral regimen for penicillin-allergic patients	Vancomycin 1 g IV *slowly* over 1 hour, **plus** gentamicin 1.5 mg/kg IM or IV, given 1 hour before procedure; may be repeated once 8-12 hours later
Parenteral regimen for penicillin-allergic patients	Vancomycin 1.0 g IV *slowly* over 1 hour, starting 1 hour before; no repeat dose is necessary		

Modified from Committee on Rheumatic Fever and Infective Endocarditis, Council on Cardiovascular Disease in the Young, American Heart Associaton: Prevention of bacterial endocarditis, *Circulation* 70:1123A, 1984.

addressed with the same patient database by Goldman and Caldera, who found no increased risk of MI when patients with *moderate* hypertension underwent anesthesia and surgery.[66] Stone et al. studied untreated hypertensive patients undergoing anesthesia and surgery. Patients had no obvious signs of coronary artery disease, but those who received beta blockers perioperatively had fewer ischemic episodes than the group of patients receiving placebos. No difference occurred in overall outcome, but this study illustrates that hypertension is a marker for coronary artery disease.[158]

Vascular Surgery

Patients undergoing vascular surgery have long been recognized as having increased risk for cardiac problems. As much as half the perioperative mortality of patients having vascular surgery has been attributed to ischemic myocardial events. In 1982 Hertzer reported a 6- to 11-year follow-up on 273 consecutive patients who had undergone lower extremity revascularization. Half the early postoperative deaths resulted from fatal MIs. The 5- and 11-year mortalities were 20% and 40%, respectively. Again, half the deaths were caused by coronary artery disease.[72] In

1988 White et al. determined that long-term survival after abdominal aneurysm surgery was worse in Goldman classes 3 and 4 patients than in 1 and 2.[172]

To better define the incidence of coronary disease in patients undergoing vascular surgery, routine coronary angiography was employed by Tomatis et al. in 100 consecutive patients before surgery in 1972.[163] Severe coronary disease, defined as 75% to 100% occlusion of any major vessel, was found in approximately 50% of patients who had aortoiliac or femoropopliteal disease and in approximately 75% of patients who had abdominal aortic aneurysm disease. **Severe coronary disease was found in 16% of patients who had no history of angina, MI, CHF, or an abnormal ECG.** Waters et al. in 1981,[168] Domaingue et at. in 1982,[41] and Jeffrey et al. in 1983[80] demonstrated that vascular surgical patients were a high-risk group.[168]

In 1984 Hertzer et al. confirmed the high incidence of coronary disease by reporting a series of 1000 patients who had undergone coronary angiography before elective vascular surgery.[73] A 70% stenosis of at least one coronary vessel was found in more than half the patients. Correctable coronary disease occurred most often in patients with clinically suspected cardiac disease, such as prior MI, angina, or ECG abnormality, but was also found in 14% of patients who had *none* of these markers. Coronary disease was relatively evenly distributed among patients with abdominal aortic aneurysm, lower extremity ischemia, and cerebrovascular disease.[73] A high incidence of coronary artery disease was also found when routine coronary angiography was performed on 506 patients with extracranial cerebrovascular disease.[74] Thompson et al. in 1978 reported that 72% of late deaths after carotid endarterectomy resulted from cardiac problems.[160] In 1986 Chambers and Norris[23] reported on a 4-year follow-up of 500 patients with asymptomatic carotid bruits. Although the study endpoints were transient ischemic attack (TIA) or CVA, most of the adverse events were MIs (Table 11-18). Deaths from MI and CVA occurred in 27 and 3 patients, respectively. In 1990 Sirna et al. concluded that MI is the leading cause of death in patients with asymptomatic bruits, TIA, and ischemic CVA.[154] **Careful assessment for underlying coronary artery disease is warranted in all patients with ischemic cerebrovascular disease.**

Because of lower extremity ischemia, patients undergoing vascular surgery may have limited abilities to exercise; therefore functional status may be difficult to assess.[114-116] The dipyridamole-thallium scan described as a "pharmacologic stress test" has facilitated noninvasive assessment of coronary artery disease. The test is sensitive but not sufficiently specific. Recently the dipyridamole-thallium scan has been combined with clinical markers for coronary

Table 11-18   Outcome in 500 patients with asymptomatic carotid bruit according to initial degree of stenosis (data from Chambers and Norris, 1986)

Event	0%-29% stenosis	30%-84% stenosis	75%-100% stenosis
TIA only	2	6	16
CVA	3 (1)*	3	6 (2)
Nonfatal MI	4	8	4
Fatal MI/sudden deaths	7	8	12

TIA, Transient ischemic attack; *CVA,* cerebrovascular accident (stroke); MI, myocardial infarction.
*Number in parentheses is CVA that was fatal.
Data from Chambers BR, Norris JW: Outcome in patients with asymptomatic neck bruits, *N Engl J Med* 315:860, 1986.

disease—age, angina, ECG Q wave, diabetes, and history of ventricular ectopy requiring treatment—to improve predictive capacity.[46,47] Other tests (e.g., radionucleotide ejection fraction) have not been demonstrated to have the power of the dipyridamole-thallium scan. Some have recently raised controversy regarding the dipyridamole-thallium test.[104]

Prior Coronary Bypass

One might expect that bypass of coronary lesions would protect a patient from adverse cardiac outcome during subsequent elective surgery.[75] Hertzer et al. described improved outcome when patients with severe coronary disease underwent coronary bypass before the vascular surgery.[73] **Unfortunately, repeat coronary revascularization is sometimes required for graft occlusion or stenosis. Thus patients with prior bypass procedures may still be at increased risk for a postoperative cardiac event. Also, an important risk of morbidity surrounds the CABG itself.** In general, authors have reported a reduction in risk by a prior CABG. Scher and Tice[147] in 1976, McCollum et al.[112] in 1977, Mahar et al.[100] in 1978, and Schoeppel et al.[148] in 1983 reported that no postoperative MIs occurred after noncardiac surgery in patients who had a prior CABG.

In 1978 Crawford et al. described 358 patients with prior CABG who underwent 484 noncoronary procedures.[32] MIs occurred in six patients and noncardiac death in four. Most of these complications occurred when the surgery was performed within 30 days of CABG surgery. Mahar et al. compared outcomes from noncardiac surgery in patients who had prior CABG vs. patients with medically treated, angiographically proven coronary disease. Patients with prior CABG had no MIs, whereas those with medically treated coronary disease had a 5% infarction

Table 11-19   Outcome of noncardiac surgery in 1600 patients from CASS registry

Variable	Group I: no coronary disease (399 patients)	Group II: prior CABG (743 patients)	Group III: angiographic coronary disease (458 patients)
Operative mortality	2 (0.5)	7 (0.9)	11 (2.4)
Cardiac deaths*	1 (0.25)	4 (0.54)	8 (1.7%)
Myocardial infarction	0	5 (0.7)	5 (1.1)
Heart failure	3 (0.8)	10 (1.3)	8 (1.8)
Rhythm disturbance	13 (3.3)	25 (3.4)	14 (3.1)

*Included are deaths the authors considered directly related to cardiac causes and deaths to which cardiac causes contributed.
Data from Foster ED, Davis KB, Carpenter JA et al: Risk of noncardiac operation in patients with defined coronary artery disease: The Coronary Artery Surgery Study (CASS) registry experience, *Ann Thorac Surg* 41:42, 1986.

rate.[100] **The authors concluded that coronary bypass lowered the risk of postoperative MI following noncardiac surgery in coronary patients, whatever the mechanism.** In the medically treated group, all the patients with MIs had triple-vessel disease, preoperative chest pain, and relatively long periods of anesthesia time.

In 1986 Foster et al. used data from the Coronary Artery Surgery Study (CASS) registry to identify 1600 patients who underwent major noncardiac surgery[53] (Table 11-19). The patients were classified into three groups: I, no angiographic evidence of coronary disease; II, patients with prior CABG; and III, patients with angiographically verified coronary disease. After the noncardiac surgery, no statistical difference was found in the incidence of MI, heart failure, or rhythm disturbance. Overall mortality and cardiac deaths were higher in the group with coronary disease but without CABG. These data might mean that a patient further out from successful CABG may reassume the high-risk position of a patient with severe coronary artery disease (CAD) coming for noncardiac surgery.

Does this answer the question, should a patient with coronary disease have CABG surgery before noncardiac surgery? Unfortunately, no. **The problem is that patients who receive CABG surgery but die during or after the procedure are never considered for subsequent noncardiac surgery.** Consider that the CASS registry found an average operative mortality of 2.3% for patients undergoing CABG surgery.[22] Thus the overall mortality from CABG surgery plus noncardiac surgery may be comparable to more than noncardiac surgery alone.

THERAPEUTIC OPTIONS FOR HIGH-RISK PATIENTS

Much study of cardiac risk has focused on preoperative diagnosis and prediction of patients at risk.[102,104,106,115] Clinical factors, exercise testing, ECG, thallium scans, and ambulatory monitoring have improved the ability to distinguish high-risk from low-risk patients. However, when a high-risk patient must have surgery, what therapeutic options are available?

One option for the high-risk coronary patient is to undergo coronary revascularization before noncardiac surgery.[58] Hertzer et al. have routinely recommended coronary arteriography to patients scheduled for elective lower extremity revascularization at the Cleveland Clinic since 1978.[72] Patients found to have severe, surgically correctable coronary stenosis have been referred to undergo coronary revascularization surgery before lower extremity revascularization. In a large series, Hertzer et al.[72] considered this successful in reducing morbidity and mortality from vascular surgery. **The option of cardiac catheterization and coronary revascularization is not without risk.** Leppo et al. reported on 100 patients undergoing vascular surgery whose risk was assessed by dipyridamole-thallium scanning and exercise testing.[95] Because high risk was suggested, 11 of the patients had cardiac catheterization. Adverse outcomes associated with cardiac catheterization, subsequent myocardial revascularization, or subsequent vascular surgery occurred in 6 patients (54%) and included CVA (1), MI (1), and death (4). Percutaneous transluminal coronary angioplasty (PTCA) before noncardiac surgery would seem a reasonable alternative.[38]

For patients with severe valvular heart disease, consideration may be given to surgical correction of the heart valve before the noncardiac surgery. Because this option entails considerable risk to the patient, some interest has been shown in percutaneous valvuloplasty techniques.[94,152,157] Levine et al.,[96] Roth et al.,[142] and Hayes et al.[71] have reported their experiences with aortic valvuloplasty before noncardiac surgery (Table 11-20). The results are not uniformly favorable. The patients described by Levine

---

Table 11-20 Percutaneous balloon valvuloplasty of critical aortic stenosis before noncardiac surgery

Author	Number of patients	Valvuloplasty adverse outcomes	Surgical adverse outcomes
Levine et al.[96]	7	None	1 with hemodynamic instability
Roth et al.[142]	7	None	None
Hayes et al.[71]	15	1 with transient congestive heart failure 3 with left ventricular perforations resulting in 1 death	None*

*Of the 14 patients who survived valvuloplasty, six underwent diagnostic procedures only rather than the originally intended surgery. Two of these patients subsequently underwent surgical aortic valve replacement before the originally proposed surgery.

---

et al. and Roth et al. had mostly successful outcomes, whereas Hayes et al. described a relatively high incidence of cardiac tamponade following perforation of the left ventricle. **The Mansfield Valvuloplasty Registry underscored this issue by reporting that the 1-year survival after aortic valvuloplasty in 492 severely symptomatic elderly patients was 64%.**[113,126] Patients with better ventricular function, larger valve areas, and less incidence of MI *before valvuloplasty* appeared to fare better. Unfortunately, therefore, aortic valvuloplasty may be a risky rather than a reasonable option for the poor-risk aortic stenosis patient.[133] None of these studies used a control group to characterize the risk of noncardiac surgery in patients with uncorrected aortic stenosis. **Recently, O'Keefe et al. reported that 48 patients with aortic stenosis underwent a variety of surgical or diagnostic procedures successfully without valvuloplasty intervention.**[125] Although no intraoperative or early postoperative deaths occurred, a significant incidence of hypotension was found during general anesthesia.

A second option for a high-risk cardiac patient is simply to cancel the proposed surgery or substitute a less stressful procedure. This option has been illustrated by Del Guercio and Cohn, who studied 148 patients over 65 years of age who had been "cleared" for surgery by an internist.[37] Pulmonary artery catheterization determined cardiac function and classified patients into one of four groups, depending on whether a functional deficit was present or could be corrected by fluid management, pharmacologic support, and so on. Based on the functional classification, recommendations were made regarding surgery (Table 11-21). Outcome correlated to the preoperative assessment. Group I patients with no deficit underwent surgery with no mortality. Patients in groups II and III underwent surgery with hemodynamic monitoring and had a 8.5% mortality. Group IV patients who did not have surgery or underwent a lesser alternative procedure all survived, whereas group IV patients who underwent the originally proposed surgery *all died.*[37]

Table 11-21 Recommendations for surgery based on preoperative hemodynamic assessment in elderly patients (data from Del Guercio and Cohn, 1980)

Group	Recommendation
I: No functional deficit	Proceed to surgery
II: Mild functional deficit	Perform surgery with hemodynamic monitoring
III: Moderate, correctable deficit	Delay surgery for optimization
IV: Advanced, uncorrectable deficit	Choose alternate treatment

Data from Del Guercio LRM, Cohn JD: Monitoring operative risk in the elderly, *JAMA* 243:1350, 1980.

An important concept of the study by Del Guercio and Cohn is that *preoperative medical optimization* **of a patient's cardiovascular status can improve outcome.** A review by Goldman noted that several identified risk factors are potentially amenable to preoperative intervention.[65] Specifically mentioned strategies were postponement of elective surgery until 6 months after MI, control of CHF by diuresis, and optimization of general medical problems, such as electrolyte abnormalities, anemia, and pulmonary conditions. **Although these are common-sense issues and have been mentioned before, none of these "recommendations" was actually tested by Goldman because this study was retrospective.** A recent study of Berlauk et al. randomized 89 patients having vascular surgery to either receive or not receive a pulmonary artery catheter for preoperative adjustment of hemodynamics.[11] Interventions included fluid loading, vasodilator, and inotropic therapy. Patients who had received the pulmonary artery catheter fared better than the control group in terms of intraoperative problems and postoperative cardiac events. Because the pulmonary artery catheter may have influenced intraoperative management, specific conclusions regarding *preoperative* interventions are obscured.[12] Other accepted preoperative strategies include continuation of the patient's beta-blocker, antihypertensive, and antianginal medications.[65,119]

A longstanding debate is whether general anesthesia vs. regional anesthesia is safer for patients with recognized cardiac risk factors.* Overall, most studies have not found that either technique is superior. Unfortunately the question is often obscured by uncontrolled data. For example, Goldman noted that heart failure developed for the first time or worsened in patients who received general anesthesia but did not occur in patients who had received spinal anesthesia "presumably because spinal anesthetics are not direct myocardial depressants, whereas general anesthetics are."[65] **Another explanation is that regional techniques were used for less extensive peripheral surgery, whereas general anesthesia was used for the intraabdominal, intrathoracic, and aortic procedures, in which patients have significantly greater fluid requirements.** In 1987 Yaeger et al. found that a regional technique *plus* light general anesthesia compared favorably with a "cardiac" general anesthetic in terms of morbidity and length of hospital stay.[177] Recently, however, Baron et al. did not confirm these results.[7] In their study, 173 patients were randomized to receive either combined epidural *plus* light general anesthesia vs. general anesthesia for abdominal aortic surgery. No difference in incidence of MI, CHF, prolonged myocardial ischemia, ventricular tachydysrhythmia, respiratory complications, renal failure, sepsis, GI bleeding, or overall postoperative mortality was noted between the groups. Patients in the combined epidural and general anesthesia group were extubated earlier but intraoperatively required more ephedrine than the general anesthesia group.

An interesting and important study was that of Rao et al., who reported in 1983 that *intraoperative* invasive monitoring, vasoactive drugs, and *postoperative* intensive care could reduce the incidence of myocardial reinfarction after elective surgery.[136] They retrospectively determined the perioperative reinfarction rate for 364 patients who had surgery during 1973 to 1976, before widespread use of pulmonary artery catheterization. These were compared with 733 patients who had surgery during 1977 to 1981 and who received invasive monitoring and pharmacologic optimization. **The authors reported a dramatic reduction in myocardial reinfarction rates overall and for each interval of recent MI compared with all existing literature.** These results still stand alone as the "world record."[162] How were they achieved? Can a group of

physicians focus on one group of diseases or complications and dramatically improve results? That is a possible explanation. Another is that the *practice* might have been different. If patients with recent MIs were not routinely turned down for elective or semielective surgery, a very different population of patients with recent infarcts (i.e., healthier ones) may have received surgery than in prior studies. This is because the prevailing practice has been not to perform surgery on such patients unless no alternatives exist. The Rao et al. study remains controversial.[162]

Several authors have contended that invasive pulmonary artery catheterization may contribute to *worse* outcomes.[137,138] Robin argued that the pulmonary artery catheter was overused and contributed little to therapeutic interventions.[137] Gore et al. concluded that patients with acute MI who received pulmonary artery catheters had higher mortality than those not catheterized.[69] Others contend that many physicians do not even understand this "heart device."[78,175] Because of the potential morbidity associated with the pulmonary artery catheter, in 1988 Robin called for a moratorium on its use.[138] **Other authors report that in experienced hands the pulmonary artery catheter provides important information and that serious complications are rare.**[109,151]

Another strategy involves the use of mechanical devices to assist the circulation when the high-risk cardiac patient requires noncardiac surgery.[93,131] Intraaortic balloon counterpulsation has been applied to cardiac surgical patients and patients with complications of acute MI.[63] Recently, Grotz and Yeston reported the successful use of the intraaortic balloon pump in three high-risk cardiac patients who required urgent noncardiac surgery.[70] Two patients had suffered an MI in the preceding several weeks, and one patient had crescendo angina. The surgical procedures were subtotal gastrectomy for bleeding adenocarcinoma, laparotomy for incarcerated hernia, and craniotomy for resection of symptomatic tumor. Intraaortic balloon pumping was initiated preoperatively and discontinued on postoperative days 1, 2, and 3. No ECG evidence of postoperative MI was found. Epidural catheters were placed for postoperative analgesia in the abdominal surgeries. Others have reported intraaortic balloon pump use in high-risk cardiac patients undergoing gastrectomy, nephrectomy, subtotal colectomy, and thoracotomy.[14,28,54,118]

Future therapeutic options will depend on clinical trials to determine impact on outcome. **Recent work by Mangano has indicated that continuous postoperative ECG can provide an early warning for patients at risk of ischemic events.**[101] **If "anti-ischemia" therapy such as beta blockade could stop an impending MI, outcomes would be improved.** However, definitive therapies, such as coronary bypass grafting,

---

* References 6, 7, 65, 68, 120, 177.

angioplasty,[143] or thrombolytic therapy, may not be desirable in the immediate postoperative period. Also, it would not be desirable to administer such therapies to the many patients with postoperative ischemic episodes (41% of all patients) to prevent an adverse outcome in only a few (3% of all patients).

RECENT VIEWS OF CARDIAC RISK

After so much study, one would expect some consensus regarding characteristics that define patients at increased cardiac risk for surgery. The two most recent reports suggest that the topic is still wide open.

A remarkable finding of many past large cardiac risk studies was that angina was *not* an independent predictor of increased cardiac risk. The reasons, such as more intraoperative or postoperative intensive care, were not clear. Angina was present in many preoperative patients but did not predict adverse outcome.[67,68] **Shah et al. in 1990, reporting on 688 patients undergoing noncardiac surgery, indicated that angina was an important predictor of postoperative MI and cardiac death.**[150] The authors noted that "79% predictive accuracy could be achieved by using the three most important parameters—i.e., chronic stable angina, previous MI and ECG ischemia." These findings may be considered long overdue because clinicians have usually considered angina a risk marker.

Rather than embrace this as a verification of common sense, one might wonder why these results differ from so many earlier studies. One reason that Shah et al.'s findings differ from other risk studies may be population selection. Early studies have examined all patients or specific subgroups, such as the elderly or patients having vascular surgery. Shah et al. studied patients "with cardiac diseases or who were older than 70 years of age." The definition of cardiac disease was not specified. If chronic angina alone was sufficient to gain study eligibility, this may have contributed to its citation as an outcome predictor. Also, angina and ECG signs of ischemia were not the strongest predictors found in this study. The model proposed for predicting adverse cardiac outcomes used eight risk factors.[150] Patients with hypokalemia or emergency surgery had a *higher* incidence of adverse outcomes than patients with ECG signs of ischemia or chronic stable angina. It is interesting to speculate that the patients with hypokalemia might have been those who required diuretics to prevent signs and symptoms of CHF (Table 11-22).

However, a more important question is raised by this work. The study population included 24 patients with recent MIs and 259 patients with diagnosis of previous MI by history or ECG criteria. **Four of the**

Table 11-22 Incidence of adverse cardiac outcomes for risk factors (data from Shah et al. 1990)

Characteristics	Adverse outcomes per patients with risk factor	Percent adverse outcome
Hypokalemia (K$^+$ < 3.5 mEq/L)	2/7	28.6%
Emergency	18/100	18%
ECG ischemia	18/122	14.8%
Chronic stable angina	18/158	11.4%
Abdominal, thoracic, aortic, or major vascular surgery*	28/341	8.2%
Previous myocardial infarction	19/259	7.3%
Age > 70 years	24/349	6.9%

*In the equation proposed by Shah et al., aortic or peripheral vascular surgery was considered separate from abdominal or thoracic surgery.
Data from Shah KB, Kleinman BS, Rao TLK et al: Angina and other risk factors in patients with cardiac diseases undergoing noncardiac operations, *Anesth Analg* 70:240, 1990.

Table 11-23 Incidence of adverse cardiac outcome in patients with preoperative myocardial infarction

	1973–1976[136]	1977-1982[136]	1990[150]
Recent infarction (0-3 months)	36%	5.8%	16.7%
Prior infarction*	6.8%	1.6%	7.3%

*For 1973-1976 and 1977-1982 data of Rao TLK et al., prior infarction includes all previous infarctions except those occurring between 0 to 3 months before surgery.
Data for 1973-1976 and 1977-1982 from Rao TLK, Jacobs, and El-Etr AA: Reinfarction following anesthesia in patients with myocardial infraction, *Anesthesiology* 59:499, 1983; and data for 1990 from Shah KB, Kleinman BS, Rao TLK et al: Angina and other risk factors in patients with cardiac diseases undergoing noncardiac operations, *Anesth Analg* 70:240, 1990.

recent MI patients had reinfarctions or cardiac death (16.7%). Nineteen of the previous MI patients had reinfarction or cardiac death (7.3%).[150] **These figures are considerably worse than those reported by Rao et al. in 1983 from the same institution and do not support early optimisim regarding the value of invasive monitoring and intensive postoperative care** (Table 11-23).[136] Differences between the studies may have influenced results. Rao et al. counted only postoperative MIs, whereas Shah et al. counted postoperative MIs and other cardiac deaths. Rao et al.'s eligibility criteria excluded patients who had ECG evidence of preoperative infarction but lacked a clinical history. Shah et al.'s eligibility criteria included these patients. Earlier work by Tarhan et al.[159] and Steen et al.[156] demonstrated that such patients do constitute a group at risk for reinfarction.

The second recent addition to the literature was provided in 1990 by Mangano et al., who studied 474 men with known or suspected coronary disease undergoing elective noncardiac surgery. Postoperative continuous Holter monitoring was used to detect postoperative cardiac events.[103] Outcomes were classified separately as ischemia-related outcomes, CHF, or ventricular tachycardia. **Multivariate analysis demonstrated that postoperative ischemia detected by Holter monitoring was the only variable that was independently associated with ischemic outcomes, defined as cardiac death, nonfatal MI, and unstable angina.** The authors concluded that no other clinical, historic, or perioperative variable, including the Cardiac Risk Index, was independently associated with ischemic events. Important new information added by this study includes:

- Most postoperative myocardial ischemia is clinically silent.
- A very high-risk population could be identified by presence or suspicion of coronary disease.
- Almost all patients with ischemic outcomes had transient episodes on the first day after surgery, suggesting that a window exists for therapeutic intervention.
- Postoperative ventricular tachycardia was found associated with preoperative use of digoxin for CHF.

However, some important findings are at odds with earlier studies. Consider the long-held concept that a recent MI constitutes a greatly increased risk for surgery. A recent MI was present in 15 patients in this study but was not found predictive of adverse outcomes. Is it now safe to anesthetize and operate on a patient with a recent MI? Will application of a postoperative Holter monitor in such a patient prevent the expected high rate of reinfarction and mortality? Again, before embracing these results, one must try to understand why they are so different from past findings.

One difference may be related to selection criteria. Prior risk studies enrolled consecutive patients without regard to presence of coronary disease. The patients who possessed risk factors (e.g., recent MI) stood apart from the large group of low-risk patients in the analysis. In contrast, Mangano et al. required presence or high suspicion of ischemic heart disease for enrollment.[103] Their population was thus a high-risk group who had an 18% overall incidence of postoperative cardiac events. How high is this risk? Consider the earlier finding by Steen et al., who demonstrated that an MI within 4 to 6 months of

surgery resulted in reinfarction in 11% of patients.[156] Conceivably, therefore, several meaningful cardiac risk variables were obscured by the overall high incidence of events in the Mangano et al. population.[103]

A second important issue raised by Mangano et al. is whether ischemic outcomes should be considered together or separate from outcomes of CHF or ventricular tachycardia, as had been the practice of prior studies. Mangano et al. suggested that ischemic outcomes have different associated variables and different prognoses and thus should be considered separately.[103] The decision has important implications. If ischemic outcomes are considered separately and the multivariate model is used, only the *single,* multivariate predictor of postoperative Holter ischemia is identified. If the 83 cardiac outcomes were considered together, *four* multivariate variables are associated with adverse outcomes: (1) history of dysrhythmia, (2) preoperative digoxin use for CHF, (3) vascular surgery, and (4) postoperative Holter ischemia. Further, when the univariate model was used and the 83 outcomes considered together, *16* variables were correlated to adverse outcomes. This list of variables bears resemblance to the classic risk factors, including prior MI, identified by earlier studies.

Thus conclusions of Mangano et al. may depend somewhat on the definitions employed. Some evidence suggests that the outcomes of infarction, CHF, and ventricular tachycardia should be considered together as "ischemia related." Specifically, postoperative ischemia detected by Holter monitoring was associated with CHF outcomes and dysrhythmia outcomes in univariate analyses. In addition, the original patient population was selected only on the criteria of coronary artery disease, suggesting that the separate outcome entities of dysrhythmia and CHF also had original ischemic etiologies.

SUMMARY

Despite years of study, the recent report by Mangano et al. demonstrates that adverse cardiac outcomes continue to occur.[103] The report indicates that anesthesiologists are using the new anesthetic techniques for high-risk patients but that the promise of a "stable cardiovascular course" remains unfulfilled. Advancements such as dipyridamole-thallium scanning and ambulatory electrocardiography have occurred. However, the initial enthusiasm for the new tests has given way to the realization that predictive accuracy may be less than originally hoped. When differences in methodology are sorted out, the recent and past studies of perioperative cardiac risk seem more alike than different. Most importantly the numerous studies identifying the high-risk cardiac patient *have not* translated into effective therapies to improve outcome. It is time to acknowledge that *it is possible to identify the patient who is at increased risk for periop-* *erative cardiac complications.* Attention now needs to be directed toward therapy to reduce adverse outcomes. Our progress in diagnostic accuracy should facilitate this search. Until therapeutic advancements occur, we will continue to count the complications.

KEY POINTS

- The literature regarding cardiac risk and various attempts at constructing indices may present conflicting information due to differences in study design. An additional problem is that outcomes do not depend solely on the patient's preoperative risk status. Many other factors, including vigilance problems, wrong drugs, wrong dosages, drug/drug interactions, allergies, and other risk factors, complicate an already complex picture. Despite this, several important considerations are common to nearly all studies: (1) a prior myocardial infarction (MI), especially a recent one, increases the cardiac risk of a preoperative patient; and (2) if the patient also has a reduced cardiac functional capacity, this greatly increases cardiac risk.

- Many cardiac tests are available. It is not the anesthesiologist's role to decide which tests are appropriate for a given patient, any more than it is the cardiologist's role to prescribe the type of anesthesia that might be most appropriate for a given patient. Understanding of these separate roles might make the daily practice of anesthesia easier in many institutions.

- One must differentiate between *final outcome* (e.g., whether the patient lived or died, whether a perioperative MI occurred) from *process outcome* (e.g., ischemia in the operating room, hypotension, tachycardia during surgery). With respect to process, it seems logical that minimization of these various physiologic perturbations during anesthesia and surgery might be best for the patient. Usually, one cannot prove that minimizing such perturbations actually improves final outcome. One must carefully understand that because final outcome differences have not yet been demonstrated regarding anesthetic A vs. anesthetic B, this does *not* mean that such differences do not exist. They may exist, but a very large population study may be needed to demonstrate relatively small but important differences. For most anesthesia-related outcomes, such multicenter trials do not exist. Therefore one must carefully guard against the currently popular pronouncement "because there are no outcome studies that clearly show a difference between technique A or B or drug A or B, there must not be any difference between these various techniques or drugs." This is specious reasoning at best.

- The anesthesiologist should be familiar with the details of how ejection fractions, thallium scanning, coronary angiography, and other procedures apply to cardiac testing.

- The ejection fraction has pitfalls, and the anesthesiologist should not assume that the ejection fraction is the best indicator of the patient's preoperative cardiac physical condition. Unless bone or joint or vascular problems exist, the history of exercise tolerance may be the single best predictor of difficulty with anesthesia with respect to the heart (although it is not necessarily a predictor of outcome).

- Special conditions of great importance to anesthesia and preoperative cardiac evaluation include presence or absence of congestive heart failure, dysrhythmias, and valvular lesions, each of which has a specific risk group. To a somewhat lesser extent, presence and control of hypertension is significant. Prior peripheral vascular disease indicates that severe coronary disease may be present.

- Prior coronary bypass, especially if relatively recent, may actually lower perioperative cardiac risk for subsequent noncardiac surgery. Despite this, studies have not determined whether it is reasonable to perform coronary bypass surgery before needed but elective noncardiac surgery if the preoperative cardiac workup reveals extensive coronary disease but the patient's chief complaint is originally elsewhere.

- Most studies have not indicated that angina is a predictive risk factor. This may be related to the finding that a significant amount of myocardial ischemia is silent.

- Mangano et al. have recently and competently addressed the issue of whether perioperative myocardial ischemia is a predictor of negative outcome.[103] Postoperative ECG ischemia was most significant in this report in contrast to the study by Raby et al[135] in which *preoperative* ischemia was the important factor.

KEY REFERENCES

Boucher CA, Brewster DC, Darling RC et al: Determination of cardiac risk by dipyridamole-thallium imaging before peripheral vascular surgery, *N Engl J Med* 312:389, 1985.

Charlson ME, Ales KA, Simon R et al: Why predictive indexes perform less well in validation studies, *Arch Intern Med* 147:2155, 1987.

Committee on Rheumatic Fever and Infective Endocarditis, Council on Cardiovascular Disease in the Young, American Heart Association: Prevention of bacterial endocarditis, *Circulation* 70:1123A, 1984.

Del Guercio LRM, Cohn JD: Monitoring operative risk in the elderly, *JAMA* 243:1350, 1980.

Detsky AS, Abrams HB, Forbath N et al: Cardiac assessment for patients undergoing noncardiac surgery, a multifactorial clinical risk index, *Arch Intern Med* 146:2131, 1986.

Eagle KA, Coley CM, Newell JB et al: Combining clinical and thallium data optimizes preoperative assessment of cardiac risk before major vascular surgery, *Ann Intern Med* 110:859, 1989.

Foster ED, Davis KB, Carpenter JA et al: Risk of noncardiac operation in patients with defined coronary disease: the Coronary Artery Surgery Study (CASS) registry experience, *Ann Thorac Surg* 41:42, 1986.

Freeman WK, Gibbons RJ, and Shub C: Preoperative assessment of cardiac patients undergoing noncardiac surgical procedures, *Mayo Clin Proc* 64:1105, 1989.

Gerson MC, Hurst JM, Hertzberg VS et al: Prediction of cardiac and pulmonary complications related to elective abdominal and noncardiac thoracic surgery in geriatric patients, *Am J Med* 88:101, 1990.

Goldman L, Caldera DL, Nussbaum SR et al: Multifactorial index of cardiac risk in noncardiac surgical procedures, *N Engl J Med* 297:845, 1977.

Mangano DT: Perioperative cardiac morbidity, *Anesthesiology* 72:153, 1990.

Mangano DT, Browner WS, Hollenberger M et al: Association of perioperative myocardial ischemia with cardiac morbidity and mortality in men undergoing noncardiac surgery, *N Engl J Med* 323:1781, 1990.

O'Keefe JH, Shub C, and Rettke SR: Risk of noncardiac surgical procedures in patients with aortic stenosis, *Mayo Clin Proc* 64:400, 1989.

Raby KE, Goldman L, Creager MA et al: Correlation between preoperative ischemia and major cardiac events after peripheral vascular surgery, *N Engl J Med* 321:1296, 1989.

Rao TLK, Jacobs KH, and El-Etr AA: Reinfarction following anesthesia in patients with myocardial infarction, *Anesthesiology* 59:499, 1983.

Steen PA, Tinker JH, and Tarhan S: Myocardial reinfarction after anesthesia and surgery, *JAMA* 239:2566, 1978.

REFERENCES

1. Abramowicz M, ed: Antimicrobial prophylaxis in surgery, *Med Lett* 31(806):105, 1989.
2. Alderman, MH, Ooi WL, Madhaven S et al: Treatment-induced blood pressure reduction and the risk of myocardial infarction, *JAMA* 262:920, 1989.
3. American Heart Association: New York Heart Association functional classification. In Braunwald E, ed: *Heart disease,* Philadelphia, 1984, WB Saunders.
4. Arkins R, Smessaert AA, and Hicks RG: Mortality and morbidity in surgical patients with coronary artery disease, *JAMA* 190:485, 1964.
5. Armstrong WF: Stress echocardiography for detection of coronary artery disease, *Circulation* 84(suppl I):I-43, 1991.
6. Backer CL, Tinker JH, Robertson DM et al: Myocardial reinfarction following local anesthesia for ophthalmic surgery, *Anesth Analg* 59:257, 1980.
7. Baron J-F, Bertrand M, Barré E et al: Combined epidural and general anesthesia *versus* general anesthesia for abdominal aortic surgery, *Anesthesiology* 75:611, 1991.
8. Bayliss J, Pearson M, and Sutton GC: Ventricular dysrhythmias following intravenous dipyridamole during "stress" myocardial imaging, *Br J Radiol* 56:686, 1983.
9. Berg GR, Kotler MN: The significance of bilateral bundle branch block in perioperative patients, *Chest* 59:62, 1971.
10. Bergquist EJ, Murphey SA: Prophylactic antibiotics for surgery, *Med Clin North Am* 71(3):357, 1987.
11. Berlauk JF, Abrams JH, Gilmour IJ et al: Preoperative optimization of cardiovascular hemodynamics improves outcome in peripheral vascular surgery: a prospective, randomized clinical trial, *Ann Surg* 214:289, 1991.
12. Blumenthal MS, McCauley CS: Cardiac arrest during dipyridamole imaging, *Chest* 93(5):1103, 1988.
13. Bolognese L, Sarasso G, and Bongo AS: Dipyridamole echocardiography test, *Circulation* 84:1100, 1991.
14. Bonchek LI, Olinger GN: Intra-aortic balloon counter pulsation for cardiac support during non-cardiac operations, *J Thorac Cardiovasc Surg* 78:147, 1979.
15. Boucher CA, Brewster DC, Darling RC et al: Determination of cardiac risk by dipyridamole-thallium imaging before peripheral vascular surgery, *N Engl J Med* 312:389, 1985.
16. Brown KA: Prognostic value of thallium-201 myocardial perfusion imaging, *Circulation* 83:363, 1991.
17. Brumm HJ, Willius FA: The surgical risk in patients with coronary disease, *JAMA* 112:2377, 1939.
18. Buck N, Devlin HB, and Lunn JN: *The report of a confidential enquiry into perioperative deaths,* London, 1987, Nuffield Provincials Hospitals Trust and the Kings Fund for Hospitals.
19. Butler S, Feeney N, and Levine SA: The patient with heart disease as a surgical risk, *JAMA* 95:85, 1930.
20. Carliner NH, Fisher ML, Plotnick GD et al: Routine preoperative exercise testing in patients undergoing major

noncardiac surgery, *Am J Cardiol* 56:51, 1985.
21. Carliner NH, Fisher ML, Plotnick GD et al: The preoperative electrocardiogram as an indicator of risk in major noncardiac surgery, *Can J Cardiol* 2:134, 1986.
22. CASS Principle Investigators and Their Associates: Myocardial infarction and mortality in the Coronary Artery Surgery Study (CASS) randomized trial, *N Engl J Med* 310:750, 1984.
23. Chambers BR, Norris JW: Outcome in patients with asymptomatic neck bruits, *N Engl J Med* 315:860, 1986.
24. Charlson ME, Ales KA, Simon R et al: Why predictive indexes perform less well in validation studies, *Arch Intern Med* 147:2155, 1987.
25. Charlson ME, MacKenzie CR, Ales K et al: Surveillance for postoperative myocardial infarction after noncardiac operations, *Surg Gynecol Obstet* 167:407, 1988.
26. Charlson ME, MacKenzie CR, Gold JP et al: The preoperative and intraoperative hemodynamic predictors of postoperative myocardial infarction or ischemia in patients undergoing noncardiac surgery, *Ann Surg* 210:637, 1989.
27. Cohen MM, Duncan PG, Pope WDB et al: A survey of 112,000 anesthetics at one teaching hospital (1975-1983), *Can Anaesth Soc J* 31:22, 1986.
28. Cohen SI, Weintraub RM: A new application of counterpulsation: safer laparotomy after recent myocardial infarction, *Arch Surg* 110:116, 1975.
29. Cohn PF, Gorlin R, Cohn LH et al: Left ventricular ejection fraction as a prognostic guide in surgical treatment of coronary and valvular heart disease, *Am J Cardiol* 34:136, 1974.
30. Committee on Rheumatic Fever and Infective Endocarditis, Council on Cardiovascular Disease in the Young, American Heart Association: Prevention of bacterial endocarditis, *Circulation* 70:1123A, 1984.
31. Cooperman M, Pflug B, Martin EW et al: Cardiovascular risk factors in patients with peripheral vascular disease, *Surgery* 84:505, 1978.
32. Crawford ES, Morris GC, Howell JF et al: Operative risk in patients with previous coronary artery bypass, *Ann Thorac Surg* 26:215, 1978.
33. Cutler BS, Leppo JA: Dipyridamole-thallium 201 scintigraphy to detect coronary artery disease before abdominal aortic surgery, *J Vasc Surg* 5:91, 1987.
34. Cutler BS, Wheeler HB, Paraskos JA et al: Applicability and interpretation of electrocardiographic stress testing in patients with peripheral vascular disease, *Am J Surg* 141:501, 1981.
35. Daniel WG, Ervel R, Kasper W et al: Safety of transesophageal echo cardiography, a multicenter survey of 10,419 examinations, *Circulation* 83:817, 1991.
36. De Bakey ME, Crawford ES, Morris GC et al: Late results of vascular surgery in the treatment of arteriosclerosis, *J Cardiovasc Surg* 5:473, 1964.
37. Del Guercio LRM, Cohn JD: Monitoring operative risk in the elderly, *JAMA* 243:1350, 1980.
38. Deron SJ, Kotler MN: Noncardiac surgery in the cardiac patient, *Am Heart J* 116:831, 1988.
39. Detsky AS, Abrams HB, Forbath N et al: Cardiac assessment for patients undergoing noncardiac surgery, a multifactorial clinical risk index, *Arch Intern Med* 146:2131, 1986.
40. Detsky AS, Abrams HB, McLaughlin JR et al: Predicting cardiac complications in patients undergoing noncardiac surgery, *J Gen Intern Med* 1:211, 1986.
41. Domaingue CM, Davies MJ, and Cronin KD: Cardiovascular risk factors in patients for vascular surgery, *Anaesth Intensive Care* 10:324, 1982.
42. Driscoll AC, Hobika JH, Etsten BE et al: Clinically unrecognized myocardial infarction following surgery, *N Engl J Med* 264:633, 1961.
43. Dry TJ: The surgical risk of patients with heart disease, *Surg Gynecol Obstet* 95:120, 1952 (editorial).
44. Duncan PG, Cohen MM: Postoperative complications: factors of significance to anaesthetic practice, *Can J Anaesth* 34:2, 1987.
45. Eagle KA, Boucher CA: Cardiac risk of noncardiac surgery, *N Engl J Med* 321:1330, 1989.
46. Eagle KA, Coley CM, Newell JB et al: Combining clinical and thallium data optimizes preoperative assessment of cardiac risk before major vascular surgery, *Ann Intern Med* 110:859, 1989.
47. Eagle KA, Singer DE, Brewster DC et al: Dipyridamole-thallium scanning in patients undergoing vascular surgery, *JAMA* 257:2185, 1987.
48. Eorola M, Eorola R, Kaukinen S et al: Risk factors in surgical patients with verified preoperative myocardial infarction, *Acta Anaesth Scand* 24:219, 1980.
49. Ernstene AC: The management of cardiac patients in relation to surgery, *Circulation* 4:430, 1951.
50. Etsten B, Proger S: Operative risk in patients with coronary heart disease, *JAMA* 159:845, 1955.
51. Falk RH, Leavitt JI: Digoxin for atrial fibrillation: a drug whose time has gone? *Ann Intern Med* 114:573, 1991.
52. Fleisher LA, Nelson AH, and Rosenbaum SH: Failure of negative dipyridamole thallium scans to predict perioperative myocardial ischaemia and infarction, *Can J Anaesth* 39:179, 1992.
53. Foster ED, Davis KB, Carpenter JA et al: Risk of noncardiac operation in patients with defined coronary disease: the Coronary Artery Surgery Study (CASS) registry experience, *Ann Thorac Surg* 41:42, 1986.
54. Foster ED, Olsson CA, Rutengurg AM et al: Mechanical circulatory assistance with IABC for major abdominal surgery, *Ann Surg* 183:73, 1976.
55. Franco CD, Goldsmith J, Veith FJ et al: Resting gated pool ejection fraction: a poor predictor of perioperative myocardial infarction in patients undergoing vascular surgery for infrainguinal bypass grafting, *J Vasc Surg* 10:656, 1989.
56. Fraser JG, Ramachandran PR, and Davis HS: Anesthesia and recent myocardial infarction, *JAMA* 199:96, 1967.
57. Freeman WK, Gibbons RJ, and Shub C: Preoperative assessment of cardiac patients undergoing noncardiac surgical procedures, *Mayo Clin Proc* 64:1105, 1989.
58. Fudge TL, McKinnon WMP, Schoettle GP et al: Improved operative risk after myocardial revascularization, *South Med J* 74:799, 1981.
59. Gage AA, Bhayana JN, Balu V et al: Assessment of cardiac risk in surgical patients, *Arch Surg* 112:1488, 1977.
60. Gerson MC, Hurst JM, Hertzberg VS et al: Cardiac prognosis in noncardiac geriatric surgery, *Ann Intern Med* 103:832, 1985.
61. Gerson MC, Hurst JM, Hertzberg VS et al: Prediction of cardiac and pulmonary complications related to elective abdominal and noncardiac thoracic surgery in geriatric patients, *Am J Med* 88:101, 1990.
62. Gill JB, Ruddy TD, Newell JB et al: Prognostic importance of thallium uptake by the lungs during exercise in coronary artery disease, *N Engl J Med* 317:1485, 1987.
63. Gold HK, Leinbach RC, Sanders CA et al: Intraaortic balloon pumping for ventricular septal defect or mitral regurgitation: complicating acute myocardial infarction, *Circulation* 47:1191, 1973.
64. Goldberger AL, O'Konski M: Utility of the routine electrocardiogram before surgery and on general hospital admission, *Ann Intern Med* 105:552, 1986.
65. Goldman L: Cardiac risks and complications of noncardiac surgery, *Ann Intern Med* 98:504, 1983.
66. Goldman L, Caldera DL: Risks of general anesthesia and elective operation in the hypertensive patient, *Anesthesiology* 50:285, 1979.
67. Goldman L, Caldera DL, Nussbaum SR et al: Multifactorial index of cardiac risk in noncardiac surgical procedures, *N Engl J Med* 297:845, 1977.
68. Goldman L, Caldera DL, Southwick FS et al: Cardiac risk factors and complications in non-cardiac surgery, *Medicine* 57:357, 1978.
69. Gore JM, Goldberg RJ, Spodick DH et al: A community-wide assessment of the use of pulmonary artery catheters in patients with acute myocardial infarction, *Chest* 92:721, 1987.
70. Grotz RL, Yeston NS: Intra-aortic balloon counterpulsation in high-risk cardiac patients undergoing noncardiac surgery, *Surgery* 106:1, 1989.
71. Hayes SN, Holmes DR, Nishimura RA et al: Palliative percutaneous aortic balloon valvuloplasty before noncardiac operations and intensive diagnostic procedures, *Mayo Clin Proc* 64:753, 1989.
72. Hertzer NR: Fatal myocardial infarction following peripheral vascular operations—a study of 951 patients followed

6-11 years postoperatively, *Cleve Clin Q* 49:1, 1982.

73. Hertzer NR, Beven EG, Young JR et al: Coronary artery disease in peripheral vascular patients—a classification of 1,000 coronary angiograms and results of surgical management, *Ann Surg* 199:233, 1984.

74. Hertzer NR, Young JR, Beven EG et al: Coronary angiography in 506 patients with extracranial cerebrovascular disease, *Arch Intern Med* 145:849, 1985.

75. Hillis LD, Cohn PF: Noncardiac surgery in patients with coronary artery disease, *Arch Intern Med* 138:972, 1978.

76. Hine LK, Laird NM, Hewitt P et al: Meta-analysis of empirical long-term antiarrhythmic therapy after myocardial infarction, *JAMA* 262:3037, 1989.

77. Homma S, Gilliland Y, Guiney TE et al: Safety of intravenous dipyridamole for stress testing with thallium imaging, *Am J Cardiol* 59:152, 1987.

78. Iberti TJ, Fischer EP, Leibowitz AB et al: A multicenter study of physicians knowledge of the pulmonary artery catheter, *JAMA* 264:2928, 1990.

79. Imperiale TF, Horwitz RI: Does prophylaxis prevent postdental infective endocarditis? A controlled evaluation of protective efficacy, *Am J Med* 88:131, 1990.

80. Jeffrey CC, Kunsman J, Cullen DJ et al: A prospective evaluation of cardiac risk index, *Anesthesiology* 58:462, 1983.

81. Junod FL, Harlan BJ, Payne J et al: Preoperative risk assessment in cardiac surgery: comparison of predicted and observed results, *Ann Thorac Surg* 43:59, 1987.

82. Kaplan EL: Bacterial endocarditis prophylaxis—tradition or necessity? *Am J Cardiol* 57:478, 1986.

83. Kaye D: Prophylaxis for infective endocarditis: an update, *Ann Intern Med* 104:419, 1986.

84. Keenan RL, Boyan PC: Cardiac arrest due to anesthesia: a study of incidence and causes, *JAMA* 253:2373, 1985.

85. Keltz TN, Innerfield M, Gitler B et al: Dipyridamole-induced myocardial ischemia, *JAMA* 257:1515, 1987.

86. Kennedy HL, Wiens RD: Ambulatory (Holter) electrocardiography and myocardial ischemia, *Am Heart J* 117:164, 1989.

87. Killip T: Twenty years of coronary bypass surgery, *N Engl J Med* 319:366, 1988.

88. Kirklin JW, Pacifico AD: Surgery for acquired valvular heart disease (2nd of 2 parts), *N Engl J Med* 288:194, 1973.

89. Knapp RB, Topkins RJ, and Artusio JF: The cerebrovascular accident and coronary occlusion in anesthesia, *JAMA* 182:332, 1962.

90. Lane RT, Sawada SG, Segar DS et al: Dobutamine stress echocardiography for assessment of cardiac risk before noncardiac surgery, *Am J Cardiol* 68:976, 1991.

91. Lavie CJ, Khandheria BK, Steward JB et al: Factors associated with the recommendation for endocarditis prophylaxis in mitral valve prolapse, *JAMA* 262(23):3308, 1989.

92. Lazor L, Russell JC, DaSilva J et al: Use of the multiple uptake gated acquisition scan for the preoperative assessment of cardiac risk, *Surg Gynecol Obstet* 167:234, 1988.

93. Lefemine AA, Kosowsky B, Madoff I et al: Results and complications of intraaortic balloon pumping in surgical and medical patients, *Am J Cardiol* 40:416, 1977.

94. Lefèvre T, Bonan R, Serra A et al: Percutaneous mitral valvuloplasty in surgical high risk patients, *J Am Coll Cardiol* 17:348, 1991.

95. Leppo J, Plaja J, Gionet M et al: Noninvasive evaluation of cardiac risk before elective vascular surgery, *J Am Coll Cardiol* 9:269, 1987.

96. Levine MJ, Berman AD, Safian RD et al: Palliation of valvular aortic stenosis by balloon valvuloplasty as preoperative preparation for noncardiac surgery, *Am J Cardiol* 62:1309, 1988.

97. London MJ, Mangano DT: Assessment and perioperative risk, *Adv Anesth* 5:53, 1988.

98. Lown B, Black H, and Moore FD: Digitalis, electrolytes and the surgical patient, *Am J Cardiol* 6:309, 1960.

99. Luchi RJ, Scott SM, Deupree RH et al: Comparison of medical and surgical treatment for unstable angina pectoris results of a Veterans Administration cooperative study, *N Engl J Med* 316:977, 1987.

100. Mahar LJ, Steen PA, Tinker JH et al: Perioperative myocardial infarction in patients with coronary artery disease with and without aorta–coronary artery bypass grafts, *J Thorac Cardiovasc Surg* 76:533, 1978.

101. Mangano DT: Perioperative cardiac morbidity, *Anesthesiology* 72:153, 1990.

102. Mangano DT, ed: *Preoperative cardiac assessment,* Philadelphia, 1990, JB Lippincott (Society of Cardiovascular Anesthesiologists monograph).

103. Mangano DT, Browner WS, Hollenberger M et al: Association of perioperative myocardial ischemia with cardiac morbidity and mortality in men undergoing noncardiac surgery, *N Engl J Med* 323:1781, 1990.

104. Mangano DT, London MJ, Taubau JF et al: Dipyridamole thallium-201 scintigraphy as a preoperative screening test, a reexamination of its predictive potential, *Circulation* 84:493, 1991.

105. Marvin HM: The heart during anesthesia and operative procedures, *N Engl J Med* 199:547, 1928.

106. Masey SA, Burton GW: Preoperative management, *Br J Hosp Med,* 30:386, 1987.

107. Master AM, Dack S, and Jaffe HL: Factors and events associated with onset of coronary artery thrombosis, *JAMA* 109:546, 1937.

108. Master AM, Dack S, and Jaffe HL: Postoperative coronary artery occlusion, *JAMA* 110:1415, 1938.

109. Matthay MA, Chatterjee K: Bedside catheterization of the pulmonary artery: risks compared with benefits, *Ann Intern Med* 109:826, 1988.

110. Mauney FM, Ebert PA, and Sabiston DC: Postoperative myocardial infarction, *Ann Surg* 172:497, 1970.

111. McCabe CJ, Reidy NC, and Abbott WM: The value of electrocardiogram monitoring during treadmill testing for peripheral vascular disease, *Surgery,* 1981, p 183.

112. McCollum CH, Garcia-Rinaldi R, Graham JM et al: Myocardial revascularization prior to subsequent major surgery in patients with coronary artery disease, *Surgery* 81:302, 1977.

113. McKay RG: The Mansfield scientific aortic valvuloplasty registry: overview of acute hemodynamic results and procedural complications, *J Am Coll Cardiol* 17:485, 1991.

114. McPhail N, Calvin JE, Schariatmadar A et al: The use of preoperative exercise testing to predict cardiac complications after arterial reconstruction, *J Vasc Surg* 7:60, 1988.

115. McPhail NV, Ruddy TD, Calvin JE et al: A comparison of dipyridamole-thallium imaging exercise testing in the prediction of postoperative cardiac complications in patients requiring arterial reconstruction, *J Vasc Surg* 10:51, 1989.

116. McPhail NV, Ruddy TD, Calvin JE et al: Comparison of left ventricular function and myocardial perfusion for evaluating perioperative cardiac risk of abdominal aortic surgery, *Can Soc Vasc Surg* 33:224, 1990.

117. Merli GJ, Weitz HH: The medical consultant, *Med Clin North Am* 71(3):353, 1987.

118. Miller MG, Hall SV: Intra-aortic balloon counterpulsation in a high-risk cardiac patient undergoing emergency gastrectomy, *Anesthesiology* 42(1):103, 1975.

119. Miller RR, Olson HG, Amsterdam EA et al: Propranolol-withdrawal rebound phenomenon: exacerbation of coronary events after abrupt cessation of antianginal therapy, *N Engl J Med* 293:416, 1975.

120. Modig J, Borg T, Karlström G et al: Thromboembolism after total hip replacement: role of epidural and general anesthesia, *Anesth Analg* 62:174, 1983.

121. Moorman JR, Hlatky MA, Eddy DM et al: The yield of the routine admission electrocardiogram—a study in a general medical service, *Ann Intern Med* 103:590, 1985.

122. Moraski RE, Russell RO, Smith M et al: Left ventricular function in patients with and without myocardial infarction and one, two, or three vessel coronary artery disease, *Am J Cardiol* 35:1, 1975.

123. Morris D, Mulvihill D, and Wilbur YWL: Risk of developing complete heart block during bedside pulmonary artery catheterization in patients with left bundle-branch block, *Arch Intern Med* 147:2005, 1987.

124. Muir AD, Reeder MK, Foex P et al: Preoperative silent myocardial ischaemia: incidence and predictors in a general surgical population, *Br J Anaesth* 67:373, 1991.

125. O'Keefe JH, Shub C, and Rettke SR: Risk of noncardiac surgical procedures

in patients with aortic stenosis, *Mayo Clin Proc* 64:400, 1989.

126. O'Neill WW: Predictors of long-term survival after percutaneous aortic valvuloplasty: report of the Mansfield scientific balloon aortic valvuloplasty registry, *J Am Coll Cardiol* 17:193, 1991.

127. Ouyang P, Gerstenblith G, Furman WR et al: Frequency and significance of early postoperative silent myocardial ischemia in patients having peripheral vascular surgery, *Am J Cardiol* 64:1113, 1989.

128. Pasternack PF, Imparato AM, Bear G et al: The value of radionuclide angiography as a predictor of perioperative myocardial infarction in patients undergoing abdominal aortic aneurysm resection, *J Vasc Surg* 1:320, 1984.

129. Pasternack PF, Imparato AM, Riles TS et al: The value of radionuclide angiogram in the prediction of perioperative myocardial infarction in patients undergoing lower extremity revascularization procedures, *Circulation* 72(suppl II):II-13, 1985.

130. Pastore JO, Yurchak PM, Janis KM et al: The risk of advanced heart block in surgical patients with right bundle branch block and left axis deviation, *Circulation* 57:677, 1978.

131. Pennington DG, Swartz BA, Codd JE et al: Intraaortic balloon pumping in cardiac surgical patients: a nine year experience, *Ann Thorac Surg* 36(2):125, 1983.

132. Pohost GM: Dipyridamole thallium test: is it useful for predicting coronary events after vascular surgery? *Circulation* 84:931, 1991 (editorial comment).

133. Powers ER: Percutaneous balloon valvuloplasty for critical aortic stenosis: a bridge to safer noncardiac surgical procedures, *Mayo Clin Proc* 64:871, 1989 (editorial).

134. Puech P, Wainwright B: Clinical electrophysiology of atrioventricular block, *Cardiol Clin* 1:209, 1983.

135. Raby KE, Goldman L, Creager MA et al: Correlation between preoperative ischemia and major cardiac events after peripheral vascular surgery, *N Engl J Med* 321:1296, 1989.

136. Rao TLK, Jacobs KH, and El-Etr AA: Reinfarction following anesthesia in patients with myocardial infarction, *Anesthesiology* 59:499, 1983.

137. Robin ED: The cult of the Swan-Ganz catheter, *Ann Intern Med* 103:445, 1985.

138. Robin ED: Defenders of the pulmonary artery catheter, *Chest* 93:1059, 1988.

139. Rooney SM: Relationship of right bundle branch block and marked left axis deviation to complete heart block during general anesthesia, *Anesthesiology* 44:64, 1976.

140. Rose SD, Corman LC, and Mason DT: Cardiac risk factors in patients undergoing noncardiac surgery, *Med Clin North Am* 63:1271, 1979.

141. Ross J Jr, Braunwald E: The influence of corrective operations on the natural history of aortic stenosis, *Circulation* 37(suppl V):61, 1968.

142. Roth RB, Palacios IF, and Block PC: Percutaneous aortic balloon valvulo-plasty: its role in the management of patients with aortic stenosis requiring major noncardiac surgery, *J Am Coll Cardiol* 13:1039, 1989.

143. Roth S, Shay J, and Chua KG: Coronary angioplasty following acute perioperative myocardial infarction, *Anesthesiology* 71:300, 1989.

144. Sapala JA, Ponka JL, and Duvernoy WFC: Operative and nonoperative risks in the cardiac patient, *J Am Geriatr Soc* 23:529, 1975.

145. Saphir O, Priest WS, Hamburger WW et al: Coronary arteriosclerosis, coronary thrombosis and the resulting myocardial changes, *Am Heart J* 10:567, 762, 1935.

146. Sawada SG, Segar DS, Ryan T et al: Echocardiographic detection of coronary artery disease during dobutamine infusion, *Circulation* 83:1605, 1991.

147. Scher KS, Tice DA: Operative risk in patients with previous coronary artery bypass, *Arch Surg* 3:807, 1976.

148. Schoeppel SL, Wilkinson C, Waters J et al: Effects of myocardial infarction on perioperative cardiac complications, *Anesth Analg* 62:493, 1983.

149. Selzer A: Changing aspects of the natural history of valvular aortic stenosis, *N Engl J Med* 317:91, 1987.

150. Shah KB, Kleinman BS, Rao TLK et al: Angina and other risk factors in patients with cardiac diseases undergoing noncardiac operations, *Anesth Analg* 70:240, 1990.

151. Shah KB, Rao TLK, Laughlin S et al: A review of pulmonary artery catheterization in 6.245 patients, *Anesthesiology* 61:271, 1984.

152. Sheikh KH, Davidson CJ, Honan MB et al: Changes in left ventricular diastolic performance after aortic balloon valvuloplasty: acute and late effects, *J Am Coll Cardiol* 16:795, 1990.

153. Shulman ST, Amren DP, Bisno AL et al: Prevention of bacterial endocarditis, *Circulation* 70(6):1123A, 1984.

154. Sirna S, Biller J, Skorton DJ et al: Cardiac evaluation of the patient with stroke, *Stroke* 21:14, 1990.

155. Skinner JF, Pearce ML: Surgical risk in the cardiac patient, *J Chron Dis* 17:57, 1964.

156. Steen PA, Tinker JH, and Tarhan S: Myocardial reinfarction after anesthesia and surgery, *JAMA* 239:2566, 1978.

157. Stoddard MF, Vandormael MC, Pearson AC et al: Immediate and short-term effects of aortic balloon valvuloplasty on left ventricular diastolic function and filling in humans, *J Am Coll Cardiol* 14:1218, 1989.

158. Stone JG, Foëx P, Sear JW et al: Myocardial ischemia in untreated hypertensive patients: effect of a single small oral dose of a beta-adrenergic blocking agent, *Anesthesiology* 68:495, 1988.

159. Tarhan S, Moffitt EA, Taylor WF et al: Myocardial infarction after general anesthesia, *JAMA* 220:1451, 1972.

160. Thompson JE, Patman RD, and Talkington CM: Asymptomatic carotid bruit: long-term outcome of patients having endarterectomy compared with unoperated controls, *Ann Surg* 188:308, 1978.

161. Thompson RC, Liberthson RR, and Lowenstein E: Perioperative anesthetic risk of noncardiac surgery in hypertrophic obstructive cardiomyopathy, *JAMA* 254:2419, 1985.

162. Tinker JH: Perioperative myocardial infarction, *Semin Anesth* 1:253, 1982.

163. Tomatis LA, Fierens EE, and Verbrugge GP: Evaluation of surgical risk in peripheral vascular disease by coronary angiography: a series of 100 cases, *Surgery* 71:429, 1972.

164. Topkins RJ, Artusio JF: Myocardial infarction and surgery: a five year study, *Anesth Analg* 43:716, 1964.

165. Upton M, Rerych S, Newman G et al: Detecting abnormalities in left ventricular function during exercise before angina and ST-depression, *Circulation* 62:341, 1980.

166. von Knorring J: Postoperative myocardial infarction: a prospective study in a risk group of surgical patients, *Surgery* 90:55, 1981.

167. Wasserman F, Bellet S, and Saichek RP: Postoperative myocardial infarction: report of 25 cases, *N Engl J Med* 252:967, 1955.

168. Waters J, Wilkinson C, Golmon M et al: Evaluation of cardiac risk in noncardiac surgical patients, *Anesthesiology* 55: A343, 1981.

169. Weber MA: Antihypertensive treatment—considerations beyond blood pressure control, *Circulation* 80(suppl IV):IV-120, 1989.

170. Weinstein L: Life threatening complications of infective endocarditis and their management, *Arch Intern Med* 146:953, 1986.

171. Wenger NK: A 50 year old useful report on coronary risk for noncardiac surgery, *Am J Cardiol* 66:1375, 1990.

172. White GH, Advani SM, Williams RA et al: Cardiac risk index as a predictor of long-term survival after repair of abdominal aortic aneurysm, *Am J Surg* 156:103, 1988.

173. Wilcken DEL, Paoloni HJ, and Eikens E: Evidence for intravenous dipyridamole (Persantin) producing a "coronary steal" effect in the ischemic myocardium, *Aust NZ J Med* 1:8, 1971.

174. Wilson RF, Marcus ML, Christensen BV et al: Accuracy of exercise electrocardiography in detecting physiologically significant coronary lesions, *Circulation* 83:412, 1991.

175. Winslow R: Many doctors not fully familiar with heart device, survey shows, *The Wall Street Journal*, Dec 12, 1990.

176. Wróblewski F, LaDue JS: Myocardial infarction as a postoperative complication of major surgery, *JAMA* 150:1212, 1952.

177. Yeager MP, Glass DD, Neft RK et al: Epidural anesthesia and analgesia in high-risk surgical patients, *Anesthesiology* 66:729, 1987.

178. Zeldin RA: Assessing cardiac risk in patients who undergo noncardiac surgical procedures, *Can J Surg* 27:402, 1984.

CHAPTER 12

Evaluation of the Patient with Vascular Disease

JEFFREY KATZ

Two major factors distinguish vascular surgery from other specialties. These same two factors obligate the anesthesiologist to pay special attention to them because failure to do so can result in disastrous complications. First, **this is the only type of surgery in which the vascular supply to a major organ or group of organs is totally interrupted during surgery. Second, vascular surgical patients are among those with the highest mortality and morbidity in the United States today** (i.e., these patients have generalized occlusive cardiovascular disease). Despite the ana-tomic location involved, studies have repeatedly indicated that mortality and morbidity from vascular surgery is related to a great extent to myocardial ischemia, failure, and/or infarction.

Although coronary artery disease is part of the same pathophysiologic process as major vascular disease, coronary artery bypass surgery is traditionally discussed in a separate section. Nevertheless, it is fundamental to realize that this is the same group of patients, and therefore a similar level of conccrn and expertise is required in their care. Major vascular surgery usually includes surgcry on the carotid arteries, the aorta, and the peripheral major arteries supplying viscera or the limbs.

It is also important to be aware that danger exists at all phases of surgery, whether it is designed to bypass or to open occluded vessels. Complications occur during clamping, unclamping, or shunting, and result from interruption and/or restoration of blood flow to vital organs. Although it has traditionally been thought that speed of surgery and, therefore, limitation of clamp time (ischemic time) are fundamental to prevention of perioperative complications, it is now understood that meticulous operative technique plays a major role in preventing embolic and thrombotic sequelae.[5]

Since the goal of all surgery should be to restore normal function with minimal patient morbidity and mortality, the success rates of vascular surgery should always be weighed against the incidence of ischemia/infarction in the natural history of the disease. If the complication rate of surgery approaches the infarction rate without surgery, the benefit to the patient is extremely doubtful. Indeed, indications for surgery have become controversial since Winslow et al. analyzed the indications for carotid endarterectomy and estimated that up to 60% of operations are undertaken for wrong or doubtful indications.[126] Available data indicate that despite the crucial surgical manipulations conducted during major vascular surgery, mortality and morbidity are related to the heart and cardiac function. This should not be surprising, because we know that atherosclerosis is a generalized disease and that the heart is a major target organ. Despite the fact that we know that the atherosclerotic process begins early in life, we do not understand how cardiac vessels are spared in some patients whereas carotid or aortic vessels are spared in others. Since these patients come from the same population and develop similar complications, it is obvious that anesthetic preparation, technique, monitoring, and postoperative management should be similar. However, the anatomic location of the surgery does introduce some specific features that will be discussed in this chapter and in Chapter 75.

PATHOPHYSIOLOGY

Goldman attributes the decline in death rates from coronary artery disease (CAD) over the last 25 years to a major decrease in the number of middle-aged men who smoke.[45a] Despite this encouraging news, CAD is still the major cause of death in the United States. More than a half million people die of coronary atherosclerosis each year, many of whom are relatively young.[11] There have been several other changes in life-styles and nutritional habits that have already had an impact on the incidence of CAD.[48] These include better methods for diagnosis and therapy for hypertension, a major increase in leisure-time physical activity, reduced consumption of saturated fats, especially from red meats, eggs, cheese, butter, and cream, and a considerably elevated level of awareness that tobacco use, obesity, and inactivity are proven risk factors in the development and progress of atherosclerosis. It is not clear how important improved medical therapy, coronary care units, better surgical and anesthetic techniques, and new pharmacologic agents have been in the declining death rate. The trend toward a reduced death rate from CAD was evident before the advent of coronary bypass surgery.

Since we know that atherosclerosis is a slowly progressive disease initiated in childhood, it will be a number of years before the full impact of these changes in life-style and diet will be realized. Atherosclerosis involves medium and large muscular arteries such as the coronaries, carotids, basilar, vertebral, aorta, iliacs, and femorals. The more common and therefore most-studied lesions of atherosclerosis are the fatty streak and the artheromatous (fibrofatty) plaque.

Fatty Streak

These lesions are microscopically visible, slightly raised yellow areas that are longitudinally oriented on medium- and large-sized arteries. Many fatty streaks are laid down before the age of 10 years. By the first decade, 10% of the internal surface of the aorta may be covered with fatty streaks.[85] The relationship between fatty streaks, atheromatous plaques, and clinical symptoms is unclear.[86]

Macrophages and smooth muscle cells predominate when fatty streaks are seen under the microscope. These cells are filled with droplets of lipid, mostly cholesterol and cholesteryl esters, which impart the yellow color.[1] There is little extracellular lipid material in fatty streaks.

A reproducible relationship between fatty streaks and their development into fibrofatty (atheromatous) plaques has not been demonstrated. Fatty streaks may appear in anatomic locations where plaques are very rarely found[84] and at sites that commonly develop atheromatous lesions (e.g., the coronary arteries).[110] A current working hypothesis suggests that fatty streaks in the aorta appear early and either disappear or remain harmless, but that fatty streaks in other locations such as the coronaries are able to evolve further into fibrofatty plaques. Fatty streaks are not thought to contribute to actual narrowing of vital nutrient arteries.

Atheromatous Plaque

The fibrofatty (atheromatous) plaque actually impinges on the size of the lumen of arteries and is the site of thrombosis, calcification, and wall weakening that leads to occlusion, aneurysmal dilatation, dissection, or rupture. These atheromatous lesions are frequently rounded, raised, near-white in color, and a centimeter or more in diameter. When the disease is more advanced, the lesion may exude a yellow, thick liquid that has been likened to gruel or porridge. These lesions may become confluent with each other.

The fundamental findings on microscopy include a fibrofatty cap containing many smooth muscle cells lying in a dense, connective tissue matrix that contains leukocytes, elastin, collagen, and proteoglycans. Beneath the cap is a core region made up of macrophages and smooth muscle cells, many of which are full of lipid droplets, called *foam cells.* Still deeper, there are also abundant extracellular elements such as lipid droplets, cholesterol crystals, and collagen. Frequently, T lymphocytes can be seen throughout the plaque. There are also signs of neovascularization, especially on the periphery of the lesions. The relative proportions of fibrous vs. fatty tissue in the plaques vary.

The presence of macrophages, T lymphocytes, fibrous connective tissue, and neovascularization tends to liken the atheromatous plaque to areas of inflammation. This linkage between atherogenesis and inflammation is currently being studied to further elucidate the pathogenesis of atherosclerosis, its prevention, and its treatment.

Shear stresses or disturbed flow might play a role in the distribution of atheromatous plaques.[45,70] Most often, they are found in the lower descending aorta (especially at the ostia of the major branches), in the first 3 inches of the coronary arteries, the arteries of the legs, the descending aorta, the internal carotids, and the circle of Willis. There is still no viable explanation for what makes some individuals more liable to develop lesions in the coronaries vs. the carotids, etc.

Prevention and treatment of atherosclerosis will depend on the ultimate pathogenesis of these lesions. A comprehensive theory of pathogenesis must explain: (1) smooth muscle proliferation in the plaques, (2) the presence of lipid material, (3) the distribution and focal nature of the lesions, and (4) the connection between the already identified major risk factors and the disease.

In 1976 Ross and Glomset proposed a mechanism of pathogenesis based on a theory of vascular response to injury.[100] They had observed that smooth muscle proliferation and plaque-like lesions could be induced experimentally following endothelial denu-

dation and that platelets that become adherent to endothelial faults can secrete a factor that induces smooth muscle growth (i.e., platelet-derived growth factor [PDGF]). Since that time this theory has evolved into the following beliefs: (1) endothelial cells can become dysfunctional for a variety of reasons, (2) platelets are not the only cells that secrete PDGF, and (3) macrophages and monocytes play a role in the vascular response to injury and are major cellular components of fibrofatty plaques[101] (Fig. 12-1).

It is likely that the major risk factors, especially hyperlipidemia, hypertension, and smoking, affect more than one step in atherogenesis. It is well known that some cigarette smoking products adversely affect platelet function, and it has been claimed that they cause experimental endothelial injury.[52,106] Smoking is known to increase the extent of atherosclerosis.[113]

It should not be surprising that hypertension has been shown to cause endothelial damage. Changes in flow and perfusion pressure have been implicated in the atherosclerosis that has been found in venous grafts used for coronary bypass.[111]

The relationship between hyperlipidemia and atherosclerosis has been well documented.[111] Several processes that promote and aggravate the formation and growth of fibrofatty plaques are stimulated and fueled by increased serum levels of low-density lipoproteins, which are the major carriers of choles-

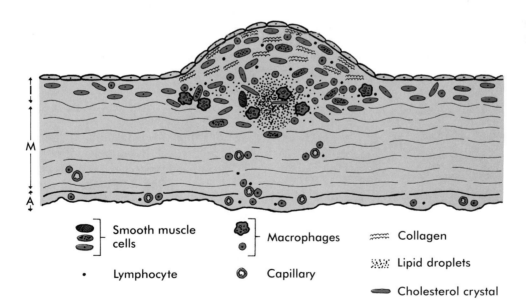

Fig. 12-1. Schematic representation of a cross section through an atherosclerotic plaque (*I,* intima; *M,* media; *A,* adventitia; medial smooth muscle cells not drawn in). Overlying endothelium is intact in this example. Note "cap" with smooth muscle cells and collagenous bands. Underneath this is the core region with abundant extracellular lipid and foam cells. Macrophages are widely distributed, and lymphocytes can be seen in the cap and to the sides of the core. Adventitial capillaries are gravitating toward the intimal lesion. (From Munro MJ, Cotrand RS: Biology of disease, the pathogenesis of atherosclerosis: atherogenesis and inflammation, *Lab Invest* 58[3]:250, 1988.)

terol in plasma. It is also the molecule most closely linked to coronary artery disease in epidemiologic studies.[3,20,79] These mechanisms have been extensively reviewed in a recent summary by Munro and Cotran.[89]

In summary, it is thought that hyperlipidemia and other risk factors can cause endothelial injury, which results in adhesion of platelets and other monocytes; the resulting release of PDGF leads to smooth muscle proliferation and the formation of fibrofatty plaques, fatty streaks, and narrowing of middle- and large-sized arteries.

RISK FACTORS FOR ATHEROSCLEROSIS

Large epidemiologic and outcome studies have recently shed light on the variety of major and minor risk factors involved in ischemic heart disease. The Framingham Study described several risk factors for coronary artery disease (CAD), including hypercholesterolemia, hypertension, and tobacco smoking. Diabetes mellitus and low levels of high-density lipoproteins are also recognized factors. Other alterable risk factors include hypertriglyceridemia, personality type, physical activity, obesity, glucose intolerance, and alcohol use[65] (Box 12-1).

Major Risk Factors
Hypercholesterolemia

In Japan and the Mediterranean countries, which have low CAD rates compared with the United States, Finland, and the Netherlands, people consume foods with much lower serum cholesterol concentrations. In 1986 Simons reported on the relationship between lipids, lipoproteins, and coronary artery disease mortality in 19 countries.[107] Including the Framingham

---

BOX 12-1
MAJOR RISK FACTORS
FOR ATHEROSCLEROSIS

Hypercholesterolemia
Hypertriglyceridemia
Tobacco smoking
Hypertension
Physical inactivity
Obesity
Fat distribution
Platelets
Family history
Psychosocial factors
Stress, type A personality
Diabetes mellitus (glucose intolerance)
Estrogens and gender
Alcohol use

Study, he found an irrefutable relationship between atherosclerotic deaths and serum cholesterol levels.

Although the evidence for a causal relationship between serum cholesterol and atherogenesis is overwhelming, it is not as widely accepted that a reduction in cholesterol concentration can either slow or reverse the process. To elucidate these relationships, many ongoing studies have been designed to answer these questions. One such trial established that a 9% reduction in cholesterol reduced "hard endpoints" of ischemic heart disease (myocardial infarction and coronary disease deaths) by 19% in a 7-year to 10-year follow-up.[80] In a 30-year follow-up of Framingham subjects, those in lower cholesterol groups had a considerable reduction in all-cause mortality without evidence of adverse effects, including malignant diseases. It is generally accepted that people with lower serum levls of low-density lipoprotein cholesterol have a significantly reduced risk of a coronary ischemic death.[91,92]

Hypertriglyceridemia

It is unclear whether hypertriglyceridemia (HTGD) is an independent risk factor for coronary disease. The Framingham Study indicates that HTGD is an independent risk factor in women.[21] A strong correlation exists between HTGD and low levels of high-density lipoproteins and therein may lie the connection. Cabin and Roberts, studying the relationship between serum cholesterol, triglyceride levels, and the severity of coronary narrowing by atherosclerotic plaques at necropsy found a positive relationship between HTGD and the percentage of severely narrowed 5-mm segments.[17] This study indicates that triglycerides may have a more important role in fatal coronary heart disease than serum cholesterol concentrations.

Tobacco smoking

Established effects of tobacco smoking on the cardiovascular system include the following: (1) sympathetic stimulation by nicotine, (2) displacement of oxygen from hemoglobin by carbon monoxide, (3) a significant increase in platelet adhesiveness, and (4) a potential immunologic reaction in vessel walls. Tobacco smoking is recognized as the single most preventable risk factor for cardiovascular disease. The incidence of death from myocardial infarction increases in a linear fashion with an increase in cigarettes smoked.[64] Peripheral vascular disease is particularly aggravated by tobacco smoking. The risk for cerebral vascular disease is 1.5 times higher in smokers.[48] In Framingham subjects, a reduction in myocardial infarction rate was demonstrated within 2 years of smoking cessation.[63] Reductions in myocardial infarction of up to 50% have been reported in individuals who stop smoking.[32,46] Further, those who

smoke more than 25 cigarettes a day have lower high-density lipoprotein levels and higher very low-density lipoproteins, cholesterol, and triglycerides than do nonsmokers, exsmokers, and those who smoke less than 25 cigarettes a day.[13,30] **There are still between 40 and 50 million cigarette smokers in the United States today, and smoking is on the increase in teenage females.**

Hypertension

Hypertension has been demonstrated to be a major risk factor for atherosclerosis in either sex and in a broad range of age groups and races. Approximately 10% to 20% of the population suffers from raised blood pressure. If hypertension is superimposed on other risk factors, the risk is further increased. There has been considerable emphasis on the detection and therapy of hypertension in the United States in the past 20 years. Consequently, it is now estimated that 75% of the hypertensive population are under reasonable control, whereas in the 1960s it was thought that only 12% to 15% were on adequate therapy.[62,66]

In the Australian Therapeutic Trial,[82] hypertensive patients were randomly assigned to placebo or therapeutic groups. The study was abandoned within 3 years because of a 30% difference in mortality between the two groups. The trial demonstrated significant protection against cardiovascular, mainly cerebrovascular, complications by a reduction in diastolic pressure of 5 to 6 mm Hg. This was not true for men under 50 years of age or for women.

Physical activity

Long-term physical activity is known to help maintain body weight and muscle tissue, to lower blood pressure and triglyceride levels, and to raise high-density lipoprotein levels.[48] Subjects who exercise frequently have a considerably lower incidence of sudden death.[34] There is also an inverse relationship between coronary heart disease and caloric intake/kilogram of body mass, which is thought to be related to physical exercise. Experimental evidence in primates[69] indicates that aerobic exercise reduces the severity of atherosclerosis despite an atherogenic diet.

Exercise may decrease atherosclerosis by lowering blood pressure, reducing serum cholesterol concentrations, reducing body fat (weight loss), improving glucose tolerance, and increasing fibrinolytic activity.[5]

Obesity

Although the precise role of obesity in atherosclerosis and coronary heart disease is unclear, the Framingham Study data indicate that in men and women obesity is an independent risk predictor. In these subjects, weight was positively and independently associated with coronary artery disease, stroke, con-gestive heart failure, and cardiovascular deaths. Some of the studies are difficult to interpret because the definition of what constitutes obesity is obscure.

In the United States, 20% of men and 15% of women aged 45 to 54 are estimated to be obese. Approximately 16% of women are thought to be 20% or more overweight. It is widely accepted that obesity correlates positively with other risk factors, such as hypertension, HTGD, hyperinsulinemia, and lack of exercise, and that it varies inversely with serum high-density lipoprotein cholesterol. There is no established level of obesity (i.e., percent over ideal body weight) at which these correlations become relevant.

Fat distribution

In several reports a positive relationship between increased ratio of waist-to-hip circumference and coronary artery disease has been demonstrated in the absence of similar correlation with body mass index and skinfold thickness.[73,75] Thus a masculine pattern of adipose tissue distribution appears to increase the risk of coronary disease in men and women.

Platelets

Platelets are known to secrete PDGF, a factor that inhibits endothelial cell regeneration. It is also likely that platelets play a part in coronary vasospasm and, with endothelial cells, may contribute to vessel wall changes after angioplasty and fibrinolytic therapy. These are all functions independent of intrinsic coagulation activity. Rao et al. have reported that patients with coronary artery disease have increased platelet coagulant activity compared with controls.[94]

Family history and aggregation

Many of the known major risk factors tend to aggregate in families. It is well known that hypercholesterolemia, elevated blood pressure, diabetes, and obesity occur with greater frequency in certain families. Familial aggregation of factors also interact with other factors such as diet, salt intake, and physical activity.

Homocystinuria is another familial disease linked to vascular disease. Shea and Nichols have studied the importance of family history and coronary artery disease.[104] Their findings indicate that family history is of great importance in populations with a high incidence of cardiovascular disease, but is also likely to be more of an independent predictor in populations with lower rates of cardiovascular disease or mortality. Friedlander et al., in an Israeli study, found that a positive family history for myocardial infarction was a predictor independent of other variables.[40] Neufield and Goldbourt have emphasized the importance of genetics in determining degree, time, course, and severity of atherosclerosis and symptoms of disease.[90] They stress the importance of family history in intervention strategy in high-risk individuals.

Psychosocial and behavioral factors

Several studies indicate that emotional distress precedes the development of the symptoms of coronary heart disease. No such evidence is present for myocardial infarction. In a study conducted by Liu et al., educational background had an inverse relationship to blood pressure and cigarette smoking in middle-aged men from Chicago.[81] Likewise, this study indicated an inverse relationship between educational level and cardiovascular disease and death. In a study of DuPont Company employees, educational level was related to ability to modify behavior and change other major risk factors.[26] Although studies do not specifically deal with future prevention, it is clear that education is a major component of a successful reduction of risk factors in all strata of society.

Stress and type A personality

Type A persons are highly competitive, ambitious, impatient, and are perceived to be in a constant struggle with their environment.[41] Current evidence suggests a positive correlation between type A behavior and coronary heart disease.[96] This relationship appears to be independent of other major risk factors. The type A effect is thought to be even more significant in the female population in the Framingham Study. This relationship was also more intense in white collar than in blue collar workers. Jenkins has concluded from available evidence indicating an increased risk of between 2:1 and 3:1 that type A behavior is an independent risk factor as strong as tobacco smoking, elevated blood pressure, or serum cholesterol.[61] Conversely, in the Aspirin Myocardial Infarction Study, type A behavior bore no correlation to the risk of reinfarction or coronary death.[29] The mechanism of type A behavior modulation for risk of myocardial ischemia is unclear. There are no data to support the idea that type A behavior is associated with chronic hypertension. Other possibilities include increased sympathetic stimulation and exaggerated levels of catecholamines in the blood. Future studies of the influence of behavior on the risk of atherosclerotic disease will hopefully provide definitive evidence to enable physicians to reduce the risk by behavior modification.

Glucose intolerance

Diabetes mellitus, or impaired glucose tolerance, has been reported to occur in up to 20% of the population. The relationship between diabetes and coronary artery disease is well established.[41] The Framingham Study found diabetes to be a major risk factor with an overwhelming association with hypertension, obesity, and lipid abnormalities. Further adverse effects may be derived from altered platelet functions and increased red blood cell adhesion. Critical review of the available studies does not support a close relationship between ischemic heart disease and asymptomatic hyperglycemia. The protection afforded females by virtue of their serum concentrations of estrogen does not protect premenopausal women from the risk associated with diabetes mellitus.

Estrogens and sex

It is well known that females have a decreased incidence of atherosclerosis compared to males. In the United States white males are 10 times more likely to suffer myocardial infarction than females.[48] Because a profound increase in coronary artery disease takes place after menopause, it was deduced that estrogen protects against atherosclerosis. A Harvard Medical School study[109] established that the incidence of myocardial infarction was 50% less in postmenopausal women who used estrogen than in those who did not. On the other hand, the Framingham Study found evidence concluding that postmenopausal women who use estrogen have a 50% elevated risk of developing ischemic heart disease and cerebrovascular disease. The Framingham Study is the only such review that comes to this conclusion. In general, it is believed that estrogen does provide some measure of protection against atherosclerosis.

Alcohol use

Several multinational studies have demonstrated an inverse relationship between *moderate alcohol consumption* and ischemic heart disease.[76,114] It is thought that alcohol imparts this protection by increasing high-density lipoprotein cholesterol.[6] However, it is known that drinking two or more drinks a day is associated with elevated blood pressure. *Heavy drinking* is known to increase mortality from many causes, including coronary artery disease. It is extremely unlikely that patients at risk for atherosclerosis will be advised to consume more alcohol, considering the other social and medical implications of excessive alcohol intake.

Minor Risk Factors
Vasectomy

This is a highly controversial issue. In experimental models of atherosclerosis, including that of the rhesus monkey, vasectomy has been demonstrated to increase the severity of diet-induced atherosclerosis.[25] However, in humans, vasectomy has not to date given rise to hypercholesterolemia, myocardial infarction, or hypertension. Although the follow-up time is relatively short, there are no established relationships between vasectomy and atherosclerosis in humans.

Coffee

Several studies have raised the possibility of a relationship between heavy coffee drinking and coronary artery disease. LaCroix et al. have documented a twofold to threefold increase in coronary artery disease among medical students who were heavy coffee drinkers.[72] There is also evidence that coffee drinking raises serum cholesterol concentrations.[117] It is possible that because of their life-style, coffee drinkers may also be prone to increased cigarette smoking. It is still unclear whether heavy coffee drinking is an independent risk factor in atherosclerosis.

Hyperuricemia

The Framingham Study documented a relationship between serum uric acid concentration and hypertension. There is also a positive correlation between uric acid and HTGD. Serum uric acid is a predictor of myocardial infarction but not as an independent factor. Hyperuricemia is viewed as a marker for metabolic disturbance associated with a predisposition for myocardial ischemia.

Fibrinogen

Since it is known that a considerable component of coronary occlusion involves thrombosis and that 90% of myocardial infarctions exhibit a coronary thrombosis, it should be expected that increased fibrinogen would be associated with coronary artery disease. The Framingham Study has documented a positive relationship between increased fibrinogen levels and serum cholesterol and triglycerides. Therefore, fibrinogen is considered a risk factor for coronary artery disease. Thrombi can be part of the actual plaque and are found in cerebral and peripheral vessels that occlude acutely.

Hypercalcemia

Chronic hypercalcemia is associated with accelerated deposition of calcium in coronary arterial intima, in cardiac annuli and valve cusps, and in myocardial fibers. Roberts and Waller suggest that hypercalcemia is a risk factor for accelerated coronary atherosclerosis.[97]

Water hardness

Leoni et al. studied cardiovascular mortality in Italy in relation to water hardness.[77] They found an inverse relationship. Magnesium, selenium, and zinc may be responsible for conferring some protection, whereas

---

BOX 12-2
MINOR RISK FACTORS
FOR ATHEROSCLEROSIS

Vasectomy
Coffee drinking
Hyperuricemia
Fibrinogen
Hypercalcemia
Water hardness
Trace minerals

---

manganese, lead, and cadmium seem to increase the risk.

Trace minerals

Klevay has proposed that a deficiency of copper or an excess of zinc predisposes to hypercholesterolemia and atherosclerosis[68] (Box 12-2).

CEREBROVASCULAR DISEASE

No adequate explanation for the distribution of atherosclerosis exists. Therefore, whatever the reason for the predilection to atheromatous lesion formation, a patient who has suffered any of the clinical symptoms that exemplify cerebrovascular insufficiency has had his/her life forever changed. The disabilities of a stroke are so fearsome that an intense emotional component has muddied the waters of rational indications for surgical intervention. In no branch of vascular disease is the principle that the potential complications of surgery should not outweigh the expected morbidity from the natural course of the disease more relevant. As in all intensely researched areas, there is considerable debate about the importance of cardiac dysfunction or neurologic deficit in the outcome of surgery. The available evidence clearly implicates myocardial ischemia as the determining factor governing survival. Therefore, in the care of these patients, a reasonable goal for anesthesiologists would be to prevent myocardial ischemia first and neurologic events second.

Indications for Carotid Endarterectomy

Although the mortality for carotid endarterectomy (CEA) has decreased from a 6-day rate of 25% in the mid-1960s to about 2% today,[98] considerable doubt still exists over the appropriate indications for surgery. Winslow et al. in 1988 conducted a thorough investigation of the indications, complications, and outcome in CEA in three major geographic areas.[2]

These results indicated a considerable degree of variation between major centers and smaller hospitals regarding what was an appropriate indication for surgery and the complication rate. They estimated, based on their data, that up to one third of CEAs were done for doubtful indications and a further one third for inappropriate reasons. They also determined that approximately 50% of the operations were done for asymptomatic bruits (a condition with a 4% stroke rate/year without surgery), at a complication rate of greater than 9%. Although this study suffered from being retrospective and nonrandomized, it nevertheless threw into doubt a proportion of the 160,000 CEAs performed each each in the United States.

The argument over surgery for asymptomatic bruits also continues. Proponents for surgery in this group present data on the natural history of asymptomatic bruits indicating that a major stroke ensues within 5 years in 15% to 20% of patients.[119] Others, who favor a less invasive approach, insist that the annual rate of stroke in patients with asymptomatic bruits is less than the 2.5% average stroke rate in patients undergoing surgery.[23,43] Whatever the risk, if Winslow's data are applicable to the whole nation, then 40% to 50% of CEAs will continue to be done for asymptomatic bruits, and indications for surgery will continue to be less important than outcome. In fact the only real indication for CEA, other than emergencies, is to prevent a future stroke. It is commonly recognized that any of the syndromes that portend cerebral ischemia, such as a transient ischemic attack (TIA) or a reversible ischemic neurologic deficit (RIND), are warnings of impending stroke and demand a cerebrovascular workup with a view to corrective surgery. Further, even if it is asymptomatic, most surgeons would agree that an occlusion of the internal carotid artery of 75% or greater is associated with a greater risk of stroke than the rate of ischemic complications from surgery and would proceed to CEA.[22,56] In their observations of 500 patients, Chambers and Norris found that 36 had cerebral events and 51 had cardiac events.[22] Only eight patients had frank strokes and they were more likely to have coronary artery disease. It has been suggested that the presence of coronary artery disease contributes to cerebral ischemia by dysrhythmias, hypotension, or embolization. In another study, consistent with Chambers and Norris, Roederer et al. observed 167 patients for up to 3 years and found an incidence of stroke of 4% annually in patients with asymptomatic bruits.[98]

In those medical centers that have become referral centers for patients with ischemic cerebrovascular disease, there is a prevailing sense that, following TIA, patients will do better if they undergo CEA.

In one study 46% of patients who had a stroke previously suffered at least one TIA.[38] The risk of

---

> ### BOX 12-3
> ### POSSIBLE INDICATIONS FOR EXTRACRANIAL CAROTID ARTERY SURGERY
>
> Acute carotid injuries
> Spontaneous carotid dissection
> Fibromuscular hyperplasia
> Extracranial carotid aneurysms
> Carotid "kinks" and "loops"
> Carotid body tumor
>
> From Ferguson G: *Clinical neurosurgery*, vol 29, Baltimore, 1982, Williams & Wilkins.

---

stroke in patients who have had a TIA varies between 4% and 6%/year (higher than asymptomatic bruits) and between 24% and 37% overall.[47] In a review of previous surgical reports West et al. calculated a combined stroke and mortality rate of 9.1%, up to 1979.[123] In the same period nonoperated patients with TIAs would have had a risk of stroke or death in excess of 25%. In contrast, Shaw et al. terminated their study after three deaths and five strokes occurred in the first 20 surgical patients.[105]

A summary of available data indicates that TIAs, other forms of cerebral vascular ischemia, RIND, stroke in progress, and asymptomatic bruits with greater than 75% occlusion are reasonable indications for surgery, whereas asymptomatic bruits with smaller lesions are handled better with medical therapy and continued observation.

Other indications for carotid surgery include trauma, spontaneous dissection, loops and kinks, acute occlusion, and intimal tears (Box 12-3). Since a recent but completed stroke carries with it the risk of reperfusion injury or hemorrhagic extension of the infarction if operated on, surgery is contraindicated (Box 12-4).

Factors Affecting Outcome
Degree of carotid disease

The incidence of postoperative stroke and morbidity from cerebral ischemia is related to the severity of the cerebrovascular disease.[58] Fode et al. demonstrated this in 1986 in a multicenter review where those with a stroke in progress had a mortality/morbidity from stroke of 21.1%, whereas those with only TIAs or asymptomatic bruits had combined mortality/morbidity rates of less than 6.5%.[39] Acute carotid occlusion with a profound deficit is the most severe of the preoperative neurologic diagnoses, and these patients have postoperative mortalities in excess of 20%. However, when surgeons are able to restore flow, there is a good chance of improving neurologic

<table>
<tr><td colspan="3">

BOX 12-4
CONTRAINDICATIONS TO
CAROTID ENDARTERECTOMY

</td></tr>
</table>

BOX 12-4
CONTRAINDICATIONS TO
CAROTID ENDARTERECTOMY

Acute infarction
"Stroke-in-evolution" with infarction
Occlusion of the internal carotid artery
Severe ipsilateral carotid siphon lesion
Limited life expectancy
Major operative risk

From Ferguson G: *Clinical neurosurgery*, vol 29, Baltimore, 1982, Williams & Wilkins.

Table 12-1   Mortality after carotid endarterectomy

		Percent of patients with serious morbidity or mortality	
Reference	Number of patients studied	Cardiac causes	Central nervous system causes
Sundt et al.[114]	1145	50	31
Hertzer et al.[57]	355	60	17
Ennix et al.[35]	1546	60	30
Burke et al.[14]	1141	67	33
Graham et al.[49]	105	100	0
Smith et al.[108]	60	0	100

Modified from Roizen MF: Anesthesia for vascular surgery. In Barash PG, Cullen BE, Stoelting R, eds: *Clinical anesthesia*, Philadelphia, 1989, JB Lippincott.

outcome in up to 58% of patients.[87] Acute carotid occlusion, if untreated, has a mortality of up to 55%. This represents a significant success in therapy and establishes without doubt the value of CEA in acute carotid occlusion.[91]

Age

In an extensive analysis of nonfederal hospitals in California, Glaser et al. have concluded that all mortality in CEA results from factors directly related to age.[44] He found an exponential correlation between increasing age and mortality in all patients 50 years and older. Mortality rose from 0.8% for patients 50 to 60 years, to 4.17% for patients 90 years and older. Therefore, to achieve a meaningful reduction in perioperative mortality in CEA, physicians need to concentrate on the diseases and degenerative changes associated with aging. These changes are particularly related to the cardiovascular, cerebrovascular, and renal systems.

Hypertension and carotid disease

Apart from the fact that as many as 75% of patients needing CEA are also hypertensive, it is known that patients who are hypertensive preoperatively have an increased incidence of postoperative hypertension and also have an increased rate of neurologic deficits after surgery.[4] Postoperative hypertension occurs in 20% of patients having CEA and in 10% of patients suffering neurologic deficits post-CEA. Towne and Bernhard observed that neurologic deficit occurred in 3.4% of normotensive patients and in 10.2% of hypertensive post-CEAs.[120] Hypertension has also been implicated in hemorrhagic cerebral infarction,[19] presumably because after removal of an obstructive plaque, previously protected fragile vessels are exposed to the increased perfusion pressures. Hypertension itself may occur as a result of a cerebral ischemic event, and it is not always possible to

implicate elevated blood pressure as an associated factor affecting outcome.

Diabetes mellitus

Although diabetics may be immunosuppressed and have impaired wound healing, there is only a small difference in complications following CEA. In 1984 Campbell et al. reviewed 156 patients undergoing CEA, two thirds of whom were diabetic.[18] In those patients who were asymptomatic preoperatively, 2.6% of the diabetics and 0% of the nondiabetics had postoperative neurologic deficits. Long-term follow-up indicated that diabetics did have increased long-term death rates, but these were largely attributable to fatal myocardial infarction.

Morbidity and Mortality After Carotid Endarterectomy

In 1981 Hertzer and Less reported on the cause of death within 60 days of CEA. In their series 60% of deaths were caused by myocardial infarction; only 17% died of neurologic causes.[57] Other studies by Ennix et al.,[35] Sundt et al.,[114] Burke et al.,[14] and Graham et al.[49] indicate that myocardial disease is primarily responsible for mortality after CEA. In only one study, by Smith et al., was death primarily related to neurologic causes.[108] These authors believed that this occurred because special efforts were expended to protect myocardium (Table 12-1). In this study, 34% of patients had myocardial ischemia, but none actually died of myocardial infarction during that hospital stay. In the Ennix et al. study, patients were classified according to preexisting coronary disease.[35] Group 1 had no history or symptoms; Group 2 had history of angina, congestive heart failure, or serious ventricular dysrhythmias; Group 3 had coronary disease but had undergone coronary artery bypass surgery. Group 2 had significantly increased mortality including increased rates of cerebrovascular mortality. Similarly, patients with asymptomatic bruits were more likely to have strokes if coronary disease was also present.[31] The patients in Group 3 had lower incidences of mortality and morbidity from myocardial infarction and cerebrovascular incidents. It has been suggested that those patients who were more likely to die or have myocardial or cerebral infarction did so at the time of coronary artery grafting.

Because it became obvious that coronary disease was so important in CEA, the possibility of undergoing coronary artery bypass before or simultaneously with CEA arose. Although Ennix et al.[35] demonstrated improved outcome in patients who had undergone bypass surgery preoperatively (Group 3), if the number of patients who died during and after the surgery is considered, the results are no better. Patients with symptomatic cerebrovascular disease also have a much greater chance of having a stroke during coronary bypass surgery.[67] For patients having simultaneous CEA and coronary bypass, the morbidity and serious mortality rates have never been lower than 10%.[58]

Stroke and myocardial infarction, the two major causes of serious morbidity and mortality from carotid endarterectomy, can occur during or after surgery. Another intraoperative complication that has received attention is damage to a cranial nerve. In one study the authors found an incidence of 12% to 17% for some form of cranial nerve injury.[30] Liapis et al. recently evaluated speech function following CEA.[78] They found a 20% incidence of hypoglossal injury and a 27.5% incidence of cricothyroid or thyroarytenoid dysfunction. They also found that 33% of patients with hypoglossal injury were asymptomatic and could be identified only by direct laryngoscopy. Hypoglossal injury is usually the result of coagulation of the plexus of veins that surround the nerve. Injuries to the vagus and facial nerves have also been described, but many of these may be temporary.

Carotid occlusion is the most serious of the immediate postoperative complications and is the primary cause of postoperative stroke. It is most commonly the result of some technical error during surgery. Occlusions of the external and common carotid arteries may also occur. External carotid flow can be assessed by palpation of the superficial temporal pulse. If external carotid flow is absent after CEA, immediate surgical exploration is indicated. Common carotid occlusion usually follows occlusion in the internal or external branches and is only rarely a primary event.

Hemorrhage from the carotid artery is another potentially lethal complication in the postoperative period. These cases not only have the threat of interrupted flow to the brain, but also carry the danger of airway occlusion owing to rapid bleeding into the neck. These represent true emergencies and require immediate surgical intervention.

Other causes of postoperative complications include infections at the operative site, most often with *Staphylococcus epidermidis;* wound hematomas, especially if patients have taken aspirin before surgery; false aneurysm; and postoperative emoblization following thrombus formation at the arteriotomy site.[37]

Extracranial-to-Intracranial Bypass

When symptoms of cerebrovascular insufficiency (TIA, RIND, etc.) are present and no surgically accessible lesion extracranially (CEA) exists, an extracranial-to-intracranial bypass (EC-IC) procedure may be considered. The most common indicators for this procedure include TIAs and total occlusion of the internal carotid artery. In this procedure the pedicle of the ipsilateral superficial temporal artery (STA) is anastomosed to a branch of the middle cerebral artery.

Although the Mayo Clinic group reported a measure of satisfaction with this technique, several other studies have failed to demonstrate any reason to continue using it.[115] Sundt et al. report that neurologic function was equal to or better than preoperatively in 95% of survivors.[114] They also achieved a 99% bypass pedicle patency at 6 months. Of 54 deaths, 27 were cardiogenic and only 6 were from a stroke. Three other studies have reported less optimistic results.[33,55,105] In one study,[53] disability was greater after surgery than before. Because of these disappointing results, the surgery is rarely done today and is reserved for very focused and specific indications.

VISCERAL AND PERIPHERAL VASCULAR INSUFFICIENCY

Vascular disease of the major arteries in the abdomen and lower limbs is based primarily on atherosclerosis. Since atherosclerosis causes fibrofatty plaques and fatty streaks, the vascular walls can be weakened or loaded with lesions that occlude the lumen. Clinically, this is expressed as aneurysmal or occlusive disease, respectively. Both may become clinically relevant by causing ischemia, but usually the symptoms, signs, prognosis, and outcome are different and should be discussed separately.

As in cerebrovascular disease, the overwhelming cause of major morbidity and mortality is myocardial dysfunction. However, persistent ischemia of intraabdominal organs or the lower limbs can lead to profound disability, severe pain, and failure of major organ functions (e.g., renal) and demands medical attention. Because many of these patients have severe

Table 12-2 Percentages of perioperative mortality related to cardiac events		
Aortic reconstruction series	Deaths/total number of patients	Percent of mortality caused by cardiac dysfunction
Szilagyi et al.[116]	59/401	48
Young et al.[131]	7/144	100
Hicks et al.[59]	19/225	53
Thompson et al.[118]	6/108	83
Mulcare et al.[88]	14/140	79
Whittemore et al.[124]	1/110	100
Crawford et al.[27]	41/860	54
Hertzer[54]	22/523	64
Yeager et al.[130]	4/97	100
Benefiel et al.[7]	3/96	67

Modified from Roizen MF: Anesthesia for vascular surgery. In Barash PG, Cullen BE, and Stoelting R, eds: *Clinical anesthesia*, Philadelphia, 1989, JB Lippincott.

coronary artery disease, hypertension, diabetes, advanced age, and are smokers, the morbidity and mortality are high. Further, because of the nature of the surgery, these patients are subjected to considerable physiologic changes, fluid shifts, variations in cardiac preload and afterload, and tend to be difficult to manage in the postoperative period.

Outcome in vascular surgery is largely determined by the nature of the surgery, the relative urgency of surgery, the severity of coronary disease, and age (Table 12-2).

OCCLUSIVE PERIPHERAL VASCULAR DISEASE

Occlusive peripheral vascular disease traditionally has been divided into three major groups that describe the pathophysiology of the disease, give some clue to the distribution of atherosclerosis, and influence prognosis and outcome considerably.[51]

Type 1

This is a local form of major vascular disease (MVD), which is limited to the aortic bifurcation and the common iliacs. This form of PVD is prevalent in male smokers between 40 and 55 years of age. It usually presents with claudication of the hips and thighs. The 5-year survival for this type of MVD is 90%. It is not well understood why coronary artery disease is rare in this group of patients, but the high 5-year survival is related to the lack of coronary and cerebrovascular diseases and the relatively young age at which it presents.

Type 2

These patients typically have diffuse aortoiliac disease at multiple levels. There is a high coexistence of coronary and cerebrovascular diseases, and patients commonly are smokers, diabetics, and persons with hypertension and hyperlipidemia. These patients have severe claudication and ischemic ulcers of the lower extremities. The 5-year survival after surgery in these patients is 80%, largely because of the increased incidence of coronary and cerebrovascular disease and the relatively advanced age.

Type 3

These patients have only a 65% 5-year survival rate, largely because of extensive small vessel disease. Typical distribution is in the femoral-popliteal and tibial vessels. This disease is more common in females than males and is frequently associated with diabetes mellitus. Patients present with foot ulcers and/or gangrene and have complicated courses because of concomitant systemic disease.

In a study at the Cleveland Clinic, mortality in Type 1, 2, and 3 patients was 28%, 33%, and 41%, respectively.[93] Myocardial infarctions were responsible for 11%, 15%, and 20% of deaths, respectively. Because type 3 patients have more small vessel involvement, the results of surgery are functionally less satisfying than the other types. Small vessels are not accessible to the surgeon, and the disease continues to progress despite the better inflow achieved after vascular surgery.[83]

Several researchers have reviewed the causes of morbidity and mortality in occlusive vascular disease. Regardless of whether the nature of the MVD is occlusive or aneurysmal, mortality has been primarily related to cardiac dysfunction. In two studies focusing on occlusive disease,[54,89] mortality was related to cardiac dysfunction in 79% and 64% of cases respectively. Whereas the overall mortality for CEA ranges between 2% and 3%, the mortality associated with surgery for occlusive MVD is commonly reported to be equal to or greater than 4%, although one group has now achieved a mortality of 2.5%.[27]

Aneurysmal Vascular Disease

Once it was realized that the mortality of surgery for ruptured abdominal aortic aneurysm (AAA) was very high (equal to or greater than 50%), surgeons became more aggressive in the diagnosis and surgical treatment of AAA. Despite the similarity of the patients and their diseases, the mortality from elective AAA surgery is still double that of occlusive MVD (8%).[93] For example, one reported median length of survival was 5.8 years for AAA repair and 10.7 years for aortoiliac revascularization.[15]

The cause for this high mortality is once again

largely related to myocardial dysfunction. In four thorough reviews,[15,124,130,131] mortality was related to cardiac disease in 100% of the noted deaths. Many have stated that since the mortality is so high following surgery for AAA, patients with smaller (< 6 cm) asymptomatic aneurysms should be observed and treated expectantly. It is widely recognized that aneurysms grow at roughly 0.5 cm/year. Proponents of conservative therapy believe that because of the improvements in imaging it is possible to closely monitor the progress of aneurysms and plan to operate when rupture appears to be imminent. To date, this view has not prevailed because perioperative mortality rates have dropped in the last decade; there is continued high mortality (45% to 90%) associated with emergency surgery for ruptured AAA; and predictions regarding which patients are more likely to suffer an aneurysmal rupture are unreliable. In a recent review of 182 autopsies for ruptured AAA, 18.1% were less than 5 cm in diameter.[28] Another factor that worsens the outcome of aneurysm surgery vs. aortic revascularization is that the average age of AAA patients is as much as 10 years older than that of patients for revascularization. Even when patients of comparable age are studied, the life expectancy of aneurysm patients tends to be shorter.

Other Factors Affecting Outcome

Apart from the distinction between aneurysmal and occlusive MVD and the differences in outcome in the various types of occlusive disease, other factors have a distinct influence on outcome.

Cardiovascular disease

Many studies have attested to the dominant role cardiac disease plays in perioperative morbidity and mortality of vascular surgery.[55,89,124,130,131] In a study from the Cleveland Clinic, 62% of patients undergoing aortic reconstruction had some clinical evidence of coronary artery disease.[31] In a review from Europe, in patients undergoing peripheral vascular surgery, 50% had coronary disease.[10] Myocardial infarction is responsible for roughly 40% of mortality after aortic aneurysmectomy and 70% of operative mortality after aortic reconstruction for occlusive disease.[55,60] Long-term mortality was 20% for patients with coronary disease and only 4% for those without coronary problems.[60] This dominant negative effect has encouraged surgeons to consider simultaneous coronary bypass with aortic reconstruction or at least to correct the coronary disease before peripheral vascular surgery is contemplated. Reul reviewed 1093 patients who had coronary bypass surgery before peripheral vascular surgery.[95] In this study no deaths were recorded in 120 patients undergoing AAA surgery. Increasing evidence indicates that patients who un-

dergo coronary bypass before vascular surgery fare better although no randomized studies exist to provide firm data.

Age

As would be expected, increased age carries with it a profoundly worse prognosis. In one study that analyzed the data for age, there was a 1% mortality for patients under 60 and an 8% mortality for patients 60 and over.[31] Age had a greater effect on mortality than the presence of coronary disease or the history of aortic aneurysm rupture. In the study led by Glaser et al. in California there was an exponential relationship between increasing age and mortality in aortic reconstruction patients.[44] With careful selection and preparation of patients, many surgeons believe that perioperative mortality can be reduced considerably and are still prepared to operate on some of these patients despite the poor prognosis.

Renal disease and failure

In the past three decades, deaths from renal failure have declined from 25% to less than 1%.[102,124] Renal physiology and blood supply can be severely impaired by the application of cross clamps to facilitate aortic reconstruction. When postoperative renal failure is severe enough to require dialysis, mortality is considerably higher.[16] Preexisting renal disease increases the risk. Since anesthesiologists have had the technology to assess intravascular volume more accurately, better fluid management has contributed to the reduction of mortality attributed to renal disease.

Smoking and pulmonary diseases

Although it is widely recognized that smoking adversely affects peripheral vascular disease, coronary artery disease, and anesthesia in general, no firm data define the role of smoking on outcome of vascular surgery. Wilson and Fuchs have demonstrated that smokers have decreased 2-year patency rates after femoral artery balloon angioplasty.[125] Smoking has been shown to increase respiratory complications after coronary bypass surgery.[122] If patients are able to stop smoking 8 weeks before surgery, they may be able to reduce respiratory complications to one third that of those patients who stop less than 8 weeks before surgery. Because smoking has a considerable effect on long-term respiratory complications and long-term vessel patency, it seems wise to encourage patients to stop smoking as soon as a diagnosis is made.

Diabetes mellitus

More patients in the type 3 group are diabetic. As a result, diabetics have a worse prognosis than nondiabetics in general. Diabetics have an increased incidence of wound complications.[50]

Miscellaneous

Several other factors contribute to the ultimate outcome of vascular surgery. Nutritional status affects outcome by influencing wound healing and the patient's ability to recover because of general debility. Other factors include graft infections, hepatic failure, and spinal cord ischemia, resulting in varying levels of paraplegia.

REGRESSION OF ATHEROSCLEROSIS

Although atherosclerosis has a multifactorial cause, considerable attention has been given to the reversal of hyperlipidemia and the possibility of inducing regression of atherosclerotic plaques. In the past, cessation of smoking, control of hypertension, exercise, weight loss, and control of blood sugar have enabled physicians to at least retard, if not arrest, the process of atherosclerosis. However, actual regression of the disease would be a major step in the therapy of general occlusive arterial disease and, if reproducible, could herald a new era in the fight against the biggest killer of Americans.

Several workers have been able to create animal models of typical hypercholesterolemia, in which swine or primates have developed severe atherosclerotic lesions after prolonged ingestion of lipid-rich diets. Most of the studies were conducted in monkeys that developed fatty streaks and fibrofatty plaques in a progressive fashion in concert with increasing time on high-fat, high-cholesterol diets. Faggioto et al. noted that within 1 month of returning to a normal diet, the monkeys showed complete regression of the lesions, along with return of serum cholesterol levels to normal.[36] Some studies have also claimed that they have observed reduction in size of the lesions characterized by smooth muscle proliferation. These impressive results have been reproduced in several laboratories.[2,129]

Clarkson et al. demonstrated that regression occurred especially in the abdominal aorta and coronaries rather than the carotid bifurcation.[24] The carotid arteries were observed to develop lesions independent of plasma lipid concentrations. When regression occurred and plasma cholesterol levels returned to normal, the lesions became smaller, contained less lipid, and content of cholesterol and cholesteryl esters were reduced. Regressive changes have also been observed in the connective-tissue proteins with reductions in collagen and elastin elements. These findings would appear to indicate that even chronic, well-established atherosclerotic lesions can regress if meaningful reductions in serum lipids can be achieved.

The literature abounds with studies wherein reductions in consumption of lipid-rich foods and ingestion of cholesterol-lowering drugs have resulted in variable reductions in serum cholesterol and improvements in the high-density lipoproteins to total cholesterol ratio. In these studies, some have demonstrated modest reductions in the rate of myocardial ischemic events compared with control groups that have remained on normal diets. However, many of these studies suffer from poor design and widely criticized statistical methodology and have been treated contemptuously by those who remain skeptical about the potential beneficial effects of dietary change.

Recently, Blankenhorn reviewed three angiographic trials that demonstrated stabilization of lesions in 317 subjects.[8] Although these studies contained patients who had regression of coronary lesions, there also appeared to be lesions that had progressed in the same patients (during the same time as regression).[12] In the most impressive human data to date, Blankenhorn et al. showed that 16.2% of a group on combined colestipol-niacin therapy had documentable regression of coronary lesions versus 3.6% of control patients.[9] This regression accompanied a 43% reduction in the LDL cholesterol and a 26% reduction in total serum cholesterol. In the Leiden Intervention Trial, 3 of 39 subjects on a low-fat vegetarian diet had considerable regression of atherosclerotic plaques, 18 had no progression of atherosclerosis, while 21 had lesions that had progressed.[3]

In a curious study from the University of Chicago, Vesselinovitch et al. found that rhesus monkeys experienced predictable regression when put on low-lipid diets or drug therapy, but cynomolgus monkeys were resistant to this therapy, showing no regression.[121] To explain this, they have postulated that the difference is due to the presence of circulatory immune complexes in the cynomolgus monkey[127] that can adversely influence endothelial integrity, with resultant damage and inflammation in the vessel wall. Wissler et al. also discuss the possibility of toxic reactions in the vessel wall that sustain injury by means of oxidation and peroxidation of low-density lipoprotein and free radical formation, thereby suppressing regression of atheromatous lesions.[128] Progression of lesions is perpetuated, too, by increasing endothelial damage related to size of the lesions and the continual proliferation of smooth muscle cells. Both of these processes are rapidly suppressed when blood lipids are reduced, either by diet or drug therapy.

Still other researchers have concentrated on the capacity of fish oils in omega-3 fatty acids to reduce plasma cholesterol levels,[76] thereby facilitating regression of lesions in hyperlipidemic patients. It is also thought that omega-3 fatty acids might have a beneficial affect by influencing the balance between thromboxane A$_2$, a platelet proaggregating factor, and prostacyclin (PGI$_2$), a potent antiaggregant and vasodilator. Recently, the theory of omega-3 fatty acid efficacy has been questioned since the sale of pills containing omega-3 has reached astronomic levels without convincing data supporting any beneficial effect.

In summary, there is ample evidence that regression of atherosclerotic lesions is possible in human and nonhuman subjects and can be induced by reduction of circulatory blood lipids. When this happens, there is loss of lipid (from the necrotic center and cells), healing of damaged endothelium, remodeling and condensation of cellular elements, and a general reduction in cellularity that indicates less mitotic activity in the arterial smooth muscle cells.

CONCLUSION

The patient undergoing major vascular surgery presents the anesthesiologist with a well-defined array of clinical problems rooted in the atherosclerotic process. Advanced technology has recently enabled researchers to further elucidate the factors that predispose patients to this disease and the mechanism whereby they interfere with normal physiology. Whereas we now understand the actual pathophysiologic process, we still have little indication of how individual distributions of occlusive lesions are selected. Several groups of clinicopathologic symptoms have been defined in peripheral vascular disease, but no explanation for how the carotid arteries, coronary arteries, or aorta are chosen as the target organ is yet available.

Intense attention has been focused on the major risk factors for atherosclerosis and how they can be changed. Based on a wealth of knowledge derived from the Framingham Study, and several smaller epidemiologic reviews, the natural history of atherosclerotic cardiovascular disease has been clearly characterized. Researchers most recently have presented persuasive arguments for modification of the disease process by changes in diet, life-style, behavior modification, and the cessation of tobacco smoking. Although skeptics still criticize the design and interpretation of research protocols, the literature now abounds with convincing evidence of attenuation, retardation, and even reversal of the expected progression of fibrofatty plaques causing arterial occlusion. Indeed, workers in the field of blood lipids have demonstrated considerable regression of fatty lesions generated in experimental models of hyperlipidemias. By combining diet modification and drug therapy, internists are able to effect sizable reductions in blood lipids that are implicated in the generation of obstructive fatty lesions in the peripheral arteries. Some studies have demonstrated reductions in myocardial infarction rates in these groups of patients. Atherosclerotic cardiovascular disease is now being thought of as a reversible disease in many cases; epidemiologists expect the incidence of the related disease syndromes to continue to abate.

Certain facts are, however, undeniable. Morbidity and mortality in the perioperative period is related overwhelmingly to cardiac causes. Because the last 10 years have witnessed considerable improvement in the anesthetic intraoperative management of hemodynamics and myocardial oxygen supply and demand, it is predictable that perioperative morbidity and mortality will be improved in future clinical reviews. Monitoring of pulse oximetry has drastically reduced the incidence of major hypoxic episodes in the operating room. Therefore it is likely that future improvements in clinical care will be accomplished in the postoperative management of these patients. It is also true that the rate of serious morbidity and mortality rises in direct relationship with advancing age. Many studies have documented this phenomenon, and as the aged population swells, we can expect this aspect to become increasingly important when assessing successful outcome.

The anesthetic management of these patients should be seen in the same light as that of patients for open heart surgery.

ACKNOWLEDGEMENT

The author wishes to express his deepest appreciation to Stancia Hottman without whom this manuscript could not have been completed.

KEY POINTS

- Vascular surgery is the only type of surgery in which the vascular supply to a major organ or group of organs is totally interrupted during surgery.
- Vascular patients are among those with the highest mortality and morbidity.

- Atherogenesis is a complex process about which much is known. The Ross and Glomset theory of vascular response to injury has been amplified and added to for many years and, in fact, although atherogenesis is by no means completely understood, it is far better understood than many physicians choose to believe (especially those who continue to smoke).

- Major risk factors for atherosclerosis include hypercholesterolemia, hypertriglyceridemia, tobacco smoking, hypertension, and poor levels of physical activity. Other risk factors include obesity, fat distribution, platelet aggregation, and family history.

- Although there is controversy regarding carotid endarterectomy as an efficacious treatment for carotid atherosclerosis and its known complications, the anesthesiologist must understand that we are generally presented with patients who have decided, upon advice, to have this surgery.

- Some factors that are known to affect outcome from carotid endarterectomy include degree of carotid disease, age, magnitude of hypertension, and diabetes mellitus.

- Factors that affect outcome from abdominal major vascular surgery include concomitant presence of cardiac vascular disease, age, and preoperative presence of renal disease. Concomitant pulmonary disease is usually related to smoking.

- Considerable effort is being expended in the arena of a nonsurgical approach to prevention or regression of atherosclerosis. It appears that regression of these lesions is possible in human subjects and can be induced by reduction of circulatory blood lipids.

KEY REFERENCES

Castelli P: Framingham Heart Study update: cholesterol, triglycerides, lipoproteins, and the risk of coronary heart disease, *Perspect Lipid Dis* 3:20, 1986.

Gotto AM, Farmer JA: Risk factors for coronary disease. In Braunwald E: *Heart disease—a textbook of cardiovascular medicine*, ed 3, Philadelphia, 1988, WB Saunders.

Munro JM, Contran RS: The pathogenesis of atherosclerosis: atherogencsis and inflammation, *Lab Invest* 58(3):249, 1988.

Roizen MF: Anesthesia for vascular surgery. In Barash PG, Cullen BE, Stoelting R, eds: *Clinical anesthesia,* Philadelphia, 1989, JB Lippincott.

Winslow CM, Solomon DT, Chassin RM et al: The appropriateness of carotid endarterectomy, *N Engl J Med* 318(12):721, 1988.

REFERENCES

1. Agle NM, Ball RY, Waldman H et al: Identification of macrophages and smooth muscle cells in human atherosclerosis using monoclonal antibodies, *J Pathol* 146:197, 1985.
2. Armstrong ML, Warner ED, and Connor WE: Regression of coronary atheromatosis in rhesus monkeys, *Circ Res* 27:59, 1970.
3. Arntzenius AC, Kromhout D, Barth JD et al: Diet, lipoproteins, and the progression of coronary atherosclerosis. The Leiden Intervention Trial, *N Engl J Med* 312:805-811, 1985.
4. Asiddao CB, Donegan JH, Whitsell RC et al: Factors associated with perioperative complications during carotid endarterectomy, *Anesth Analg* 61:631, 1982.
5. Baker WH: Management of stroke during and after carotid surgery. In Bergan JJ, Yao JST, eds: *Cerebrovascular insufficiency,* New York, 1983, Grune & Stratton.
6. Barboriak JJ, Anderson AJ, and Hoffman RG: Interrelationships between coronary artery occlusion, high density lipoprotein cholesterol, and alcohol intake, *J Lab Clin Med* 94:348, 1979.

7. Benefiel DJ, Roizen MF, Lampe GH et al: Morbidity after aortic surgery with sufentanil versus isoflurane anesthesia, *Anesthesiology* 65:A516, 1986.
8. Blankenhorn DH: Can atherosclerotic lesions regress? Angiographic evidence in humans, *Am J Cardiol* 65:41F, 1990.
9. Blankenhorn DH, Johnson RL, Nessin SA et al: The Cholesterol Lowering Atherosclerosis study (CLAS): design, methods, and baseline results, *Controlled Clin Trials* 8:354, 1987.
10. Bohmart F, Horkenbach G: Spezielle anaesthesiologische probleme bei esassoperationen, *Anesthesiol Wiederbelebung* 20:8, 1967.
11. Braunwald JPW: *Arteriosclerosis: Report of Working Group on Arteriosclerosis of the National Heart, Lung, and Blood Institute,* vol 2, Washington, DC, 1981, US Department of Health and Human Services.
12. Brensike JF, Levy RI, Kelsey SF et al: Effects of therapy with cholestyramine on progression of coronary atherosclerosis: results of the NHLBI Type II Coronary Intervention Study, *Circulation* 69:313, 1984.

13. Brischetto CS, Connor WE, and Connor SL: Plasma lipid and lipoprotein profiles of cigarette smokers from randomly selected families: enhancement of hyperlipidemia and depression of high density lipoprotein, *Am J Cardiol* 52:675, 1983.
14. Burke PA, Callow AD, O'Donnell TF Jr et al: Prophylactic carotid endarterectomy for asymptomatic bruit, *Arch Surg* 117:1222, 1982.
15. Burnham SJ, Johnson G Jr, and Gurri JA: Mortality risks for survivors of vascular reconstructive procedures, *Surgery* 92:1072, 1982.
16. Bush HL Jr: Renal failure following abdominal aortic reconstruction, *Surgery* 93:107, 1983.
17. Cabin HS, Roberts WC: Relationship of serum total cholesterol and triglyceride levels to the amount and extent of coronary arterial narrowing by atherosclerotic plaque in coronary heart disease, *Am J Med* 73:227, 1982.
18. Campbell DR, Hoar CS Jr, and Wheelock FC: Carotid artery surgery in diabetic patients, *Arch Surg* 119:1405, 1984.

19. Caplan LR, Mohr JP: Intracerebral hemorrhage following carotid endarterectomy: a hypertensive complication? *Stroke* 9:457, 1978.

20. Carlson LA, Ericsson M: Quantitative and qualitative serum lipoprotein analysis. Part 2, Studies in male survivors of myocardial infarction, *Atherosclerosis* 21: 435, 1975.

21. Castelli P: Framingham Heart Study update: cholesterol, triglycerides, lipoproteins, and the risk of coronary heart disease, *Perspect Lipid Dis* 3:20, 1986.

22. Chambers BR, Norris JW: Outcome in patients with asymptomatic neck bruits, *N Engl J Med* 315:860, 1986.

23. Clagett GP, Youkey JR, and Brigham RA: Asymptomatic cervical bruit and abnormal ocular pneumoplethysmography: a perspective study comparing two approaches to management, *Surgery* 96: 823, 1984.

24. Clarkson TB, Bond MG, Bullock BC et al: A study of atherosclerosis regression in *Macaca mulatta* v. changes in abdominal aorta and carotid and coronary arteries from animals with atherosclerosis induced for 38 months and then repressed for 24 or 48 months at plasma cholesterol concentrations of 300 or 200 mg/dl, *Exp Mol Pathol* 41:96, 1984.

25. Clarkson TB, Alexander NJ: Long-term vasectomy: affects on the occurrence and extent of atherosclerosis in rhesus monkeys, *J Clin Invest* 65:15, 1980.

26. Colbourn AW: The decline in coronary heart disease mortality: the DuPont experience, *Del Med J* 58:351, 1986.

27. Crawford ES, Saleh SA, Babb JW III et al: Infrarenal abdominal aortic aneurysm. Factors influencing survival after operation performed over a 25-year period, *Ann Surg* 193:699, 1981.

28. Darling RC: Ruptured artherosclerotic abdominal aortic aneurysms. A pathologic and clinical study, *Am J Surg* 119:397, 1970.

29. de Backer G, Kornitzer M, Kittel F et al: Behavior, stress, and psychosocial traits as risk factors, *Prev Med* 12:32, 1983.

30. De Weese JA, Rob CG, Satran R et al: Results of carotid endarterectomy for transient ischemic attacks five years later, *Ann Surg* 178:258, 1973.

31. Diehl JT, Cali RF, Hertzer MR et al: Complications of abdominal aortic reconstruction. An analysis of perioperative risk factors in 557 patients, *Ann Surg* 197:49, 1983.

32. Doll R, Peto R: Mortality in relation to smoking: 20 years observations on male British doctors, *Br Med J* 2:1525, 1976.

33. EC-IC Bypass Study Group: Failure of extracranial-intracranial arterial bypass to reduce the risk of ischemic stroke. Results of an international randomized trial, *N Engl J Med* 313:1991, 1985.

34. Ekelund LG, Haskell WL, Johnson JL et al: Physical fitness as a predictor of cardiovascular mortality in asymptomatic North American men. The Lipid Research Clinics Mortality Follow-up Study, *N Engl J Med* 319:1379, 1988.

35. Ennix CL Jr, Lawrie GM, Morris GC Jr et al: Improved results of carotid endarterectomy in patients with symptomatic coronary disease: an analysis of 1546 consecutive carotid operations, *Stroke* 10:122, 1979.

36. Faggiotto A, Ross R, Harker L: Studies of hypercholesterolemia in the nonhuman primate. I. Changes that lead to fatty streak formation, *Arteriosclerosis* 4:323, 1984.

37. Ferguson G: *Clinical neurosurgery,* vol 29, Baltimore, 1982, Williams & Wilkins.

38. Fields WS, Maslenikov V, Meyer JS et al: Joint study of extracranial arterial occlusion. V. Progress report of prognosis following surgery or nonsurgical treatment for transient cerebral ischemic attacks and cervical carotid arterial lesions, *JAMA* 211:1993, 1970.

39. Fode NC, Sundt TM, Robertson JT et al: Multicenter retrospective review of results and complications of carotid endarterectomy in 1981, *Stroke* 17:370, 1986.

40. Friedlander Y, Kark JD, and Stein Y: Family history of myocardial infarction as an independent risk factor for coronary heart disease, *Br Heart J* 53:328, 1985.

41. Friedman M: *Pathogenesis of coronary artery disease,* New York, 1969, McGraw-Hill.

42. Garcia MI, MacNamara PM, and Gordon T: Morbidity and mortality in diabetics in the Framingham population, *Diabetes* 23:105, 1976.

43. Glaser RB: Anesthesia for vascular surgery. In Roizen MF, ed: *Morbidity and mortality from major vascular surgery,* New York, 1990, Churchill-Livingstone.

44. Glaser RB, Feigal D: Age-specific surgical morbidity and mortality. An analysis of the California hospital discharge date tapes from the Office of Statewide Health Planning and Development (unpublished 1983).

45. Glasgov S: The pathogenesis of atherosclerosis: hemodynamic risk factors. In Wissler RW, Geer JC, eds: *Mechanical stress, moral architecture, medial nutrition, and the vulnerability of arteries to atherosclerosis,* Baltimore, 1972, Williams & Wilkins.

45a. Goldman L, Cook EF: The decline in ischemic heart disease mortality rates: an analysis of the comparative effects of medical interventions and changes in lifestyle, *Ann Intern Med* 101:825, 1984.

46. Goldner JD, Whisnant JP, and Taylor WF: Long-term prognosis of transient cerebral ischemic attacks, *Stroke* 2:160, 1971.

47. Gordon T, Kannel WB, and McGee D: Death and coronary attacks in men after giving up cigarette smoking, *Lancet* 2:1345, 1974.

48. Gotto AM, Farmer JA: Risk factors for coronary disease. In Braunwald E: *Heart disease—a textbook of cardiovascular medicine,* ed 3, Philadelphia, 1988, WB Saunders.

49. Graham AM, Gewertz BL, and Zarins CK: Predicting cerebral ischemia during carotid endarterectomy, *Arch Surg* 121: 595, 1986.

50. Gurri JA, Burnham SJ: Effect of diabetes mellitus on distal lower extremity bypass, *Ann Surg* 48:75, 1982.

51. Hallet JW Jr: Trends in revascularization of the lower extremity, *Mayo Clin Proc* 61:369, 1986.

52. Hawkins RI: Smoking, platelets, and thrombosis, *Nature* 236:450, 1972.

53. Haynes RB, Mukherjee J, Sackett DL et al: Functional status changes following medical and surgical treatment for cerebral ischemia. Results of the Extracranial-Intracranial Bypass Study, *JAMA* 257:2043, 1987.

54. Hertzer NR: Myocardial ischemia, *Surgery* 93:97, 1983.

55. Hertzer NR, Beven EG, Young JR et al: Coronary artery disease in peripheral vascular patients. A classification of 1000 coronary angiograms and results of surgical management, *Ann Surg* 199:223, 1984.

56. Hertzer NR, Flanagan RA Jr, Beven EG et al: Surgical versus nonoperative treatment of asymptomatic carotid stenosis. 290 patients documented by intravenous angiography, *Ann Surg* 204:163, 1986.

57. Hertzer NR, Lees CD: Fatal myocardial infarction following carotid endarterectomy. Three hundred thirty-five patients followed 6-11 years after operation, *Ann Surg* 194:212, 1981.

58. Hertzer NR, Loop FD, Taylor PC et al: Combined myocardial revascularization and carotid endarterectomy. Operative and late results in 331 patients, *J Thorac Cardiovasc Surg* 85:577, 1983.

59. Hicks GL, Eastland MW, Deweese JA et al: Survival improvement following aortic aneurysm resection, *Ann Surg* 181: 863, 1975.

60. Jamieson WRE, Janusz MT, Miyagishima RT et al: Influence of ischemic heart disease on early and late mortality after surgery for peripheral occlusive vascular disease, *Circulation* 66(Suppl 1):1-92, 1982.

61. Jenkins CD, Zyzanski SJ, and Rosenman RH: Risk of new myocardial infarction in middle-aged men with manifest coronary heart disease, *Circulation* 53: 342, 1976.

62. The Joint National Committee for Detection, Evaluation and Treatment of High Blood Pressure: the 1980 report, *Arch Intern Med* 140:1280, 1980.

63. Kannel WB: Hypertension, blood lipids, and cigarette smoking as co-risk factors for coronary heart disease, *NY Acad Sci* 304:128, 1978.

64. Kannel WB: Update on the role of cigarette smoking in coronary artery disease, *Am Heart J* 101:319, 1981.

65. Kannel WB, Gordon T: *The Framingham Study. An epidemiological investigation of cardiovascular disease.* Section 30: Some characteristics related to the incidence of cardiovascular disease and death: The Framingham Study, 18-year follow-up, Pub No (NIH) 74-599, Washington DC, 1974, Department of Health, Education, and Welfare.

66. Kaplan NM: *Clinical hypertension,* ed 3, Baltimore, 1982, Williams & Wilkins.

67. Kartchner MM, McRae LP: Carotid occlusive disease as a risk factor in major cardiovascular surgery, *Arch Surg* 117: 1086, 1982.

68. Klevay LM: Copper and ischemic heart disease, *Biol Trace Elem Res* 5:245, 1983.

69. Kramsch DM, Aspen AJ, Abramowitz BM et al: Reduction of coronary atherosclerosis by moderate conditioning in monkeys on an atherogenic diet, *N Engl J Med* 305:1483, 1981.

70. Ku DN, Giddens DP, Zarins CK et al: Pulsatile flow and atherosclerosis in the human carotid bifurcation. Positive correlation between plaque location and low end oscillating shear stress, *Atherosclerosis* 5:293, 1985.

71. Reference deleted in proofs.

72. LaCroix AZ, Mead LA, Liang KY et al: Coffee consumption and the incidence of coronary heart disease, *N Engl J Med* 315:977, 1986.

73. Lapidus L, Bentsson C, Larsson B et al: Distribution of adipose tissue and risk of cardiovascular disease and death: a 12-year follow-up of participants in the population study of women in Gothenberg, Sweden, *Br Med J* 289:1257, 1984.

74. La Porte RE, Cresanta JL, and Kuller LH: The relationship of alcohol consumption to atherosclerotic heart disease, *Prev Med* 9:22, 1980.

75. Larsson B, Svardsudd K, Welin L et al: Abdominal adipose tissue distribution, obesity, and the risk of cardiovascular disease and death: a 13-year follow-up of participants in the study of men born in 1913, *Br Med J* 288:1401, 1984.

76. Leaf A, Weber PC: Cardiovascular effects of n-3 fatty acids, *N Engl J Med* 318:549, 1988.

77. Leoni V, Fabiani L, and Ticchiarelli L: Water hardness and cardiovascular mortality rate in Abruzzo, Italy, *Arch Environ Health* 40:274, 1985.

78. Liapis CD, Satiani B, Florance CL et al: Motor speech malfunction following carotid endarterectomy, *Surgery* 89:56, 1981.

79. Lipid Research Clinics Program: The Lipid Research Clinics' coronary primary prevention trial results. I. Reduction in incidence of coronary heart disease, *JAMA* 251:365, 1984.

80. Lipid Research Clinics Program: The Lipid Research Clinics' coronary primary prevention trial results. II. The relationships of reduction in incidence of coronary heart disease to cholesterol lowering, *JAMA* 251:351, 1984.

81. Liu K, Cedres LB, and Stamler J: Relationship of education to major risk factors and death from coronary heart disease, cardiovascular diseases and all causes. Findings of three Chicago epidemiologic studies, *Circulation* 66:1308, 1982.

82. Management Committee: The Australian therapeutic trial in mild hypertension, *Lancet* 1:1261, 1980.

83. Martinez BD, Hertzer NR, and Beven EG: Influence of distal arterial occlusive disease on prognosis following aortofemoral bypass, *Surgery* 88:795, 1980.

84. McGill HC Jr et al: Several findings of the International Atherosclerosis Project, *Lab Invest* 18:498, 1968.

85. McGill HC Jr: Fatty streaks in the coronary arteries and aorta, *Lab Invest* 18:560, 1968.

86. McGill HC Jr: Persistent problems in the pathogenesis of atherosclerosis, *Arteriosclerosis* 4:443, 1984.

87. Meyer FB, Sundt TM Jr, Piepgras DG et al: Emergency carotid endarterectomy for patients with acute carotid occlusion and profound neurological deficits, *Ann Surg* 203:82, 1986.

88. Mulcare RJ, Royster TS, Lynne RA et al: Long term results of operative therapy for aortoiliac disease, *Arch Surg* 113:601, 1978.

89. Munro JM, Cotran RS: The pathogenesis of atherosclerosis: atherogenesis and inflammation, *Lab Invest* 58(3):249, 1988.

90. Neufield HN, Goldbourt U: Coronary heart disease: genetic aspects, *Circulation* 67:943, 1983.

91. Norrving B, Nilsson B: Carotid artery occlusion: acute symptoms and long-term prognosis, *Neurol Res* 3:229, 1981.

92. Pekkanen J, Linn S, Heiss G et al: Ten-year mortality from cardiovascular disease in relation to cholesterol level among men with and without preexisting cardiovascular disease, *N Engl J Med* 322:24, 1700, 1990.

93. Plecha FR, Avellone JC, Bevan EG et al: A computerized vascular registry: experience of the Cleveland Vascular Society, *Surgery* 86:826, 1979.

94. Rao AK, Mintz RD, and Lavine SJ: Coagulant activities of platelets in coronary artery disease, *Circulation* 69:15, 1984.

95. Reul GJ Jr, Cooley DA, Duncan JM et al: The effect of coronary bypass on the outcome of peripheral vascular operations in 1093 patients, *J Vasc Surg* 3:788, 1986.

96. Review Panel on Coronary-Prone Behavior and Coronary Heart Disease: Coronary-prone behavior and coronary heart disease. A critical review, *Circulation* 63:1199, 1981.

97. Roberts W, Waller BF: Chronic hypercalcemia as a risk factor for coronary atherosclerosis, *Cardiovasc Res Rep* 4:1275, 1983.

98. Roederer GO, Langlois YE, Jager KA et al: The natural history of carotid arterial disease in asymptomatic patients with cervical bruits, *Stroke* 15:605, 1984.

99. Roizen MF: Anesthesia for vascular surgery. In Barash PG, Cullen BE, Stoelting R, eds: *Clinical anesthesia*, Philadelphia, 1989, JB Lippincott.

100. Ross R: The pathogenesis of atherosclerosis: an update, *N Engl J Med* 314:488, 1986.

101. Ross R, Glomset JA: The pathogenesis of atherosclerosis, *N Engl J Med* 295:369, 1976.

102. Sabawala PB, Strong MJ, and Keats AS: Surgery of the aorta and its branches, *Anesthesiology* 33:229, 1970.

103. Samson DS, Boone S: Extracranial-intracranial (EC-IC) arterial bypass. Past performance and current concepts, *Neurosurgery* 3:79, 1978.

104. Shea S, Nichols A: The clinical importance of family history of ischemic heart disease, *Cardiovasc Rev Rep* 4:1343, 1983.

105. Shaw DA, Venables GS, Cartlidge NE et al: Carotid endarterectomy in patients with transient cerebral ischemia, *J Neurol Sci* 64:45, 1984.

106. Sieffert GF, Keown K, and Moore SW: Pathologic effect of tobacco smoke inhalation on arterial intima, *Surg Forum* 32:333, 1981.

107. Simons LA: Interrelations of lipids and lipoproteins with coronary artery disease mortality in 19 countries, *Am J Cardiol* 57:5G, 1986.

108. Smith JS, Roizen MF, Cahalan MK et al: Does anesthetic technique make a difference? Augmentation of systolic blood pressure during carotid endarterectomy: effects of phenylephrine versus light anesthesia and of isoflurane versus halothane on the incidence of myocardial ischemia, *Anesthesiology* 69:846, 1988.

109. Stampfer MJ, Willett WC, Colditz GA et al: A prospective study of postmenopausal estrogen therapy and coronary heart disease, *N Engl J Med* 313:1044, 1985.

110. Stary IIC: Atheroma arises in eccentric intimal thickening from concurrent fatty streak lesions, *Fed Proc* 46:418, 1987 (abstract).

111. Steinberg D: Hypercholesterolemia and atherosclerosis. In Steinberg D, Olefsky JM, eds: *Pathogenesis and prevention, current theories of the pathogenesis of atherosclerosis,* New York, 1987, Churchill-Livingstone.

112. St Leger AS, Cochrane AL, and Moore F: Factors associated with cardiac mortality in developing countries with particular reference to the consumption of wine, *Lancet* I:1017, 1979.

113. Strong JP, Richards ML: Cigarette smoking and atherosclerosis in autopsied men, *Atherosclerosis* 23:451, 1976.

114. Sundt TM Jr, Sharbrough FW, Piergras DG et al: Correlation of cerebral blood flow and electroencephalographic changes during carotid endarterectomy, with results of surgery and hemodynamics of cerebral ischemia, *Mayo Clin Proc* 56:533, 1981.

115. Sundt TM Jr et al: Techniques, results, complications and follow-up in superficial temporal artery to middle cerebral artery bypass pedicles. In Sundt TM Jr, ed: *Occlusive cerebrovascular disease: diagnosis and surgical management,* Philadelphia, 1987, WB Saunders.

116. Szilagyi DE, Smith RF, Derusso FJ et al: Contribution of abdominal aortic aneurysmectomy to prolongation of life, *Ann Surg* 164:678, 1966.

117. Thelle DS, Arnesen E: The Tromso Heart Study: coffee consumption and

serum lipid concentrations in men with hypercholesterolemia: a randomized intervention study, *Br Med J* 290:893, 1985.

118. Thompson JE, Hollier LH, Patman RD et al: Surgical management of abdominal aortic aneurysms: factors influencing mortality and morbidity—a 20-year experience, *Ann Surg* 181:654, 1975.

119. Thompson JE, Patman RD, and Talkington CM: Asymptomatic carotid bruit: long term outcome of patients having endarterectomy compared with unoperated controls, *Ann Surg* 188:308, 1978.

120. Towne JB, Bernhard VM: The relationship of postoperative hypertension to complications following carotid endarterectomy, *Surgery* 8:575, 1980.

121. Vesselinovitch D, Wissler RW: Reversal of atherosclerosis: comparison on non-human primate models. In Gotto AM Jr, Smith LC, and Allen B, eds: *Atherosclerosis V* (Proceedings of the Fifth International Symposium), New York, 1980, Springer-Verlag.

122. Warner MA, Diventie MB, and Tinker JH: Preoperative cessation of smoking and pulmonary complications in coronary artery bypass patients, *Anesthesiology* 60:380, 1984.

123. West H, Burton R, Roon AJ et al: Comparative risk of operation and expectant management for carotid artery disease, *Stroke* 10:117, 1979.

124. Whittemore AD, Clowes AW, Couch NP et al: Aortic aneurysm repair. Reduced operative mortality associated with maintenance of optimal cardiac performance, *Ann Surg* 192:414, 1980.

125. Wilson AR, Fuchs JCA: Percutaneous transluminal angioplasty. The radiologists contribution to the treatment of vascular disease, *Surg Clin North Am* 64:121, 1984.

126. Winslow CM, Solomon DH, Chassin MR et al: The appropriateness of carotid endarterectomy, *N Engl J Med* 318:12, 721, 1988.

127. Wissler RW, Vesselinovitch D, and Davis HR et al: A new way to look at atherosclerotic involvement of the artery wall and the functional effects, *Ann NY Acad Sci* 454:9, 1985.

128. Wissler RW, Vesselinovitch D: Can atherosclerotic plaques regress? Anatomic and biochemical evidence from non-human animal models, *Am J Cardiol* 65:33F, 1990.

129. Wissler RW, Vesselinovitch D: Studies of repression of advanced atherosclerosis in experimental animals and man, *Ann NY Acad Sci* 275:363, 1976.

130. Yeager RA, Weigel RM, Murphy ES et al: Application of clinically valid cardiac risk factors to aortic aneurysm surgery, *Arch Surg* 121:278, 1986.

131. Young AE, Sandberg GW, and Couch NP: The reduction of mortality of abdominal aortic aneurysm resection, *Am J Surg* 134:585, 1977.

CHAPTER 13

Evaluation of the Patient with a Difficult Airway

ROBERT T. DONHAM

Then the LORD God formed man of dust from the ground, and breathed into his nostrils the breath of life; and man became a living being.

Genesis 2:7

The preoperative assessment should seek to identify conditions that will dictate or modify the anesthesia plans. In patients with a "difficult" (difficult-to-manage) airway, the objective and problem is to identify, before induction and a failed attempt to intubate, those whose airway changes preclude safe endotracheal intubation by one of the standard techniques. **Failure to identify potential airway problems properly can lead to a paralyzed patient who can be neither intubated nor ventilated.** In addition, in some series, up to 50% of aspiration incidents associated with anesthesia arise from problems of managing difficult airways.[43] **The triad of aspiration, severe hypoventilation, and hypoxemia, with their sequelae, constitutes the more serious complications associated with management of problematic airways.** Benumof and Scheller[5] have quoted other investigators who assert that 50% to 75% of cardiac arrests following the induction of anesthesia result from inadequate ventilation and oxygenation. Further-more, depending on the series quoted, 55% to 93% of patients with intraoperative cardiac arrest either die or have brain death.

How does the anesthesiologist prevent a patient from becoming one of these significant negative outcome (SNO) statistics? The causes of problematic airways may be camouflaged within seemingly innocent information. SNO avoidance calls for individualized management of patients based on carefully obtained and analyzed information (Box 13-1).

To identify patients with potentially difficult-to-manage airways, the history should focus on basic "alert" items: dyspnea or dyspnea on exertion; dysphagia; shortness of breath; hoarseness or stridor; trauma, radiation therapy, or prior surgery of the head and/or neck; or prior difficulty with intubation. If a positive response is obtained for an alert item, both the medical history and the physical examination need to be more extensively explored.

During the basic physical examination, the patient should be viewed from both a frontal and a profile view to assess mandibular size and mobility, mental–alveolar process and mental–hyoid bone or mental–thyroid cartilage distance, and neck rotation and flexion-extension mobility. The neck should be palpated for evidence of masses, tracheal deviation, size of tracheal and cricoid cartilage, and tissue plasticity. One should also check for loose, missing, or overly large teeth; degree of overbite or protrusive occlusion; size of the tongue; visibility and size of faucial structures; patency and size of the nares; or deviation of nasal septum.

During the interview and examination, the quality of the patient's voice and respiratory pattern should be noted. **"Alert" factors for possible airway difficulties include shallow respiration, increased frequency of respiration, retraction, increased effort or use of accessory muscles, shortness of breath or breathlessness, stridor, weak voice, or hoarseness.**

Once the potential problems with a patient's airway are identified, an approach can be devised for the maintenance of adequate airway control and appropriate ventilation. However, such a management plan also requires further crucial evaluation: determination of the patient's level of understanding and cooperation. Lack of patient cooperation can cause a moderately difficult but potentially manageable situation to degenerate into an insurmountable problem. The necessary cooperation is based on the patient thoroughly understanding several details: the nature of the problems, the need to achieve airway control before inducing anesthesia, the implications and the potential complications of alternative management schemes, and the degree of discomfort he/she is likely to experience during each stage of the procedure. Some steps required to achieve a successful intubation while the patient is awake can be highly uncomfortable. For example, application of topical anesthesia can be intensely unpleasant for some patients. For others, anxiety and discomfort during intubation procedures may result in marked vasovagal reactions. Also, noxious sympathetic responses can result from the pressure of passing a tube through the nose or from the severe cough stimulus elicited by a fiberoptic bronchoscope being introduced into an nonanesthetized trachea.

The anesthesiologist should predetermine which emergency approach is most likely to ensure satisfactory ventilation if difficulties negate the initial plans. Beyond this backup plan, a *failed intubation algorithm,* or protocol, should exist (see Fig. 13-5 and later discussion under emergency management techniques). If airway management problems are anticipated, the surgical team should be informed and the options discussed. Plans may need to include having a surgeon and the instruments ready for an emergency tracheostomy.

Potential airway management problems can be classified in many ways. For example, as in this chapter, one could list problems as congenital vs. acquired. Alternatively, classification could be by anatomic region, but infectious, traumatic, neurogenic, allergic, and congenital processes involve multiple anatomic sites. Overall, classifications establish artificial groupings that tend to focus on certain aspects rather than maintain the more global view, which recognizes the poorly defined boundaries of groupings. Serious airway management problems resulting from infectious processes and from congenital anomalies are primarily limited to the pediatric patient population and are discussed in Chapter 26, except as applicable here.

SPECIFIC AIRWAY MANAGEMENT PROBLEMS

For convenience, acquired conditions that can effect airway management are subdivided here into nerve dysfunction, adverse reflexes, infections, trauma, morbid obesity, pregnancy, intrathoracic lesions, and skeletal axis conditions. The congenital conditions are divided into anatomic and enzymatic abnormalities and tumors in different anatomic regions.

Acquired Problems
Nerve dysfunction

In some patients, vocal cord paralysis may be almost totally masked by the use of compensatory mechanisms such as the false cords and the external laryngeal muscles. Symptoms may vary from almost normal speech to aphonia, depending on whether one or both cords are paralyzed, the degree of paresis, and the resultant position of the paralyzed cord(s).[27,29,36,46,93] **Although vocal cord paresis rarely may be caused by a central lesion, it most frequently results from injury to the recurrent laryngeal nerve, the major motor nerve to the larynx.** Less often, injury to the superior laryngeal nerve, which supplies the cricothyroid muscle, causes significant compromise of vocal cord function.

The left recurrent laryngeal nerve is uniquely disposed to injury from diverse causes because of its long path down under the arch of the aorta and back up to the larynx (Box 13-2).

Bilateral (and sometimes unilateral) vocal cord paresis can complicate airway management. **Three features concerning vocal cord paresis are especially important: (1) unilateral paralysis results in a rotation of the cricoid cartilage toward the nonparalyzed side; (2) with positive pressure ventilation the para-**

BOX 13-2
COMMON CAUSES OF INJURY TO LEFT
RECURRENT LARYNGEAL NERVE

Stretching by aortic aneurysm
Stretching by masses in left hilum
Stretching by enlargement of left atrium
Invasion by thyroid carcinomas
Destruction of neck or chest areas by radiation
  therapy
Surgical injury during thymus, thyroid, or neck
  surgery
Trauma to the neck

---

lyzed cord(s) may adduct, resulting in partial or even total occlusion of the airway; and (3) the paralyzed cord(s) may aggravate problems of endotracheal intubation.

Pharyngeal or laryngeal sensory nerve damage, leading to a decrement in the airway protective reflexes, may lead to intermittent or chronic aspiration problems. Since this may put the patient at risk during induction of anesthesia, the preoperative analysis must determine the advisability of a rapid sequence of induction and intubation vs. intubation while the patient is awake.

Other nerve injuries can also add to the complexities of airway management and must therefore be fully evaluated preoperatively. Examples include abnormal or unpredictable reflexes in response to manipulation of nerves that have become entrapped or invaded by tumors of the neck or mediastinum. Nerves may also have been injured during surgery, radiation therapy, or trauma. This evaluation of nerves, which may become important during management of a problematic airway, should encompass the cervical plexus, stellate ganglion, carotid sinus, vagus, hypoglossal, and phrenic nerves. In some instances, even a relatively minor change in head position may elicit an abnormal response. Frequently, the patient recognizes that certain motions evoke peculiar reactions. Patients may have changes in heart rate or rhythm, fluctuations in blood pressure, alterations in breathing pattern, or variation in mentation or level of consciousness.

Adverse reflexes

In addition to unusual or unexpected reflexes from dysfunctional nerves, expected responses to instrumentation or procedures in managing a difficult airway also may cause problems. This may be particularly true in patients with marginal cardiovascular or respiratory reserve, in whom basically "normal" or

intact nerve reflex activity may constitute an SNO-evoking event. Therefore management of the preoperative problematic airway must also consider the stresses inherent to each technique. The incidence of adverse reactions is related to the physical force involved, the anatomic site involved, the duration of the noxious stimuli, and the relative adequacy of the anesthesia.

Insertion of a foreign body into the airway (e.g., endotracheal tube) or surgical manipulation of the airway (e.g., tracheostomy, laryngectomy) may elicit bronchospasm in patients with no prior history of asthma. Autonomic nervous system reflex activity secondary to airway manipulation during surgery can result in delayed onset of bronchospasm. In addition, bronchospasm can be induced by various drugs that release histamine, including muscle relaxants such as succinyldicholine.[35,64] When the patient is under insufficient anesthesia, stimulation of the posterior pharynx or the glottic structures frequently results in a vocal cord spastic closure (laryngospasm) reflex. This reflex can also be elicited by mucus, emesis, or blood on the vocal cords. **Fink**[36] **has defined laryngospasm as the persistent spastic closure of the glottis beyond the termination of an eliciting stimulus. The reflex, mediated by motor fibers of the superior laryngeal nerve, involves the cricoarytenoid, thyroarytenoid, and cricothyroid muscles.**[84] Fortunately, laryngospasm can be stopped by use of muscle relaxants, since the involved musculature is composed of striated (voluntary) muscles. Alternatively, the initiating stimulus can be suppressed with topical anesthesia of the posterior pharynx and larynges or by deep general anesthesia.

Serious cardiovascular reflexes may also accompany instrumentation or manipulation of the airway in a patient with inadequate local or general anesthesia. Thus one may see bradycardia or tachycardia, hypotension or hypertension, or cardiac dysrhythmia.[26,100] Atropine given to halt or prevent vagal manifestations resulting from airway manipulation[26] may lead to tachycardia, which may be detrimental in patients with advanced heart disease. Topical anesthesia of the oropharynx and larynges together with local anesthesia may eliminate sympathetic reflexes.[100] However, the use of lidocaine or procaine may cause other adverse reactions[24,58] or be contraindicated because of cardiac dysrhythmia.[44]

Infections

Infection-related airway compromise is perhaps the major airway management problem in patients under age 10 years. Mortality statistics from a Canadian report of 90 deaths secondary to airway obstruction in children showed that 40.5% of these deaths in children under age 10 were related to infections compromising the airway.[85] The site of infection frequently determines which airway management protocol should be used.

Although infectious processes serious enough to compromise or obstruct the airway are found primarily in children and infants, I have seen and consulted on infections in adults. Most have been advanced or fulminant peritonsillar or retropharyngeal abscesses. Likewise, a few patients with acute epiglottitis have been noteworthy because of the rapid development of serious airway compromise. Several patients with advanced Ludwig's angina had an upward thrusting immobilization of the tongue by the noncompressible "woody" edema of the mouth floor that seriously diminished oropharyngeal size. The airway in these patients with Ludwig's angina is secured via emergency tracheostomy with patients awake under local anesthesia, since laryngoscopy was thought to be impractical and contraindicated.

One should act according to protocols, similar to those used for children and infants, when evaluating and planning anesthesia for adults with airway-compromising infectious processes. **Adults as well as children with epiglottitis are adverse to vocalization and do so only in a whisper. They tend to exhibit systemic toxicity, to resist lying down, and to breathe with their tongues forward and mouth open.** With a presumptive diagnosis of epiglottitis, the patient should be attended by anesthesia and otolaryngology personnel until the airway is secured. I believe that these patients, adults as well as children, should be moved on an emergency basis to an operating room (OR) setting. If the diagnosis is uncertain, and the patient's condition permits, radiographs can be obtained in the OR. **Before attempting an endotracheal intubation over a laryngoscope, equipment and personnel for emergency tracheostomy should be ready.**

For children, one normally induces the patient in the sitting position with an inhalational agent, usually halothane, increasing the depth of anesthesia as tolerated until the patient can be placed supine and intravenous access established. At this point in most children, the airway can be maintained with minimal difficulty. The depth of anesthesia is increased until laryngoscopy is feasible. Then the most skilled member of the team should attempt an oral endotracheal intubation, with the surgeons ready to perform a tracheostomy or cricothyroidotomy if necessary.

In adults the airway often cannot be maintained once the patient is supine. Therefore the choice must be made between preoxygenating the patient in the sitting position and then attempting to intubate following rapid anesthesia induction or trying the more controlled approach generally used in children. With either approach, the surgical team should be fully scrubbed and gowned and ready to perform an emergency tracheostomy or cricothyroidotomy.

When patients have peritonsillar or retropharyngeal abscesses, anesthesiologists are most frequently consulted when intubation and anesthesia are required for an incision and drainage procedure. The preanesthesia evaluation should include judicious, careful examination of the oropharynx and of radiographs of the lateral neck soft tissue to determine the extent of the prevertebral thickening and narrowing of the oropharynx. If indurative or suppurative inflammation of the soft tissue severely reduces oropharyngeal patency, tracheostomy with the patient awake may be the only feasible option. Laryngoscopy, if judged practical, is ideally performed under deep general anesthesia with an inhalational agent and 95 + % oxygenation. **For adults, during induction and intubation and with adequate suction available, a moderate Trendelenburg's position is preferred to prevent aspiration of infected materials should the abscess rupture.** As for patients with epiglottitis, the surgical team must be prepared to undertake an emergency tracheostomy or cricothyroidotomy.

Trauma

Data from the previously mentioned Canadian report on mortality statistics in children[85] indicate that trauma (including the aspiration of food or a foreign body under this definition) has become the major cause of mortality from airway obstruction if the patient population is extended to include patients through 14 years of age. By 1980, trauma in general became the preeminent cause of death for persons 1 to 38 years old.[104] When working in a trauma center or in a large urban hospital with primary trauma service, caring for trauma patients can become a difficult, stressful part of an anesthesiologist's practice. Often, the trauma patient arrives at night when ancillary personnel and diagnostic and treatment facilities are curtailed. Frequently, these patients are mentally and physiologically impaired from injury, shock, or chemical abuse. **Also, all trauma patients should be considered to have a full stomach.** Increasingly, trauma patients are being found to have hepatitis or to test positive for the human immunodeficiency virus (HIV).[3]

Hoarseness, stridor, subcutaneous emphysema, or tracheal deviation should trigger an emergency examination of the airway for evidence of injury. Whether blunt or penetrating, direct trauma to the facial bones, larynx, cervical trachea, or the hyoid suspension apparatus can result in complex, difficult-to-manage airway problems.* Such patients should be under continuous close observation for signs of ensuing obstruction. **In patients who require intubation before ruling out cervical spine injuries, a cervical collar should be left in place or axial traction established.**[31]

---

*References 14, 18, 23, 37, 74, 95.

Fiberoptic intubation techniques may be the preferred method of establishing airway control in patients with head or neck trauma.[70,74,87,110] Alternative techniques include "blind" nasotracheal intubation with the patient awake, retrograde catheter techniques, cricothyroidotomy, transtracheal jet ventilation, and tracheostomy.* (See later section on Airway Management Techniques.)

In patients with facial injury, rapid but thorough evaluation for airway involvement is essential. Many airway injuries are life threatening and yet preclude direct visualization and oral endotracheal intubation. For example, in patients with Le Fort II and III fractures of the maxillae, the fractured bones and overlying soft tissues may become impacted into the posterior nasopharynx or oropharynx.[56] Radiography usually confirms a compromised faucial isthmus.

When limited motion of the jaw is associated with facial trauma, one should not expect to be able to open the patient's mouth further after giving a muscle relaxant, since true mechanical trismus may be present in patients with mandibular fractures.[88] In other patients, swelling or edema may result in immobility of the neck or loss of plasticity of the soft tissues, thereby making direct laryngoscopic visualization of the vocal cords and subsequent orotracheal intubation essentially impossible. Emergency fiberoptic endotracheal intubation, if possible, or cricothyroidotomy membrane tracheotomy with transtracheal jet ventilation may be required as a lifesaving measure.[18,23,74] (See later section on Airway Management Techniques.)

Cerebrospinal fluid (CSF) rhinorrhea or otorrhea is an indicator of patent communication with the calvarial vault. Thus, when assessing airway and anesthesia management problems in patients with ongoing or recent CSF leaks, it is essential that plans be made to avoid positive pressure ventilation until after endotracheal intubation or tracheostomy has provided control of the airway. **Otherwise, positive pressure via a mask may reverse the pressure gradient across the site of the CSF leak, resulting in a pneumocephalus.**†

With either strangulation or direct trauma to the front of the neck, the larynx can be crushed, the cricoid or other tracheal cartilages can be fractured, and the larynx or trachea may be severed.[18,23,37,88,95] One must be aware that these injuries may prevent direct laryngoscopy and endotracheal intubation, fiberoptic bronchoscopic–assisted intubation, or cricothyroidotomy as a means of securing the airway. Tracheostomy below the site of injury is required as an emergency procedure to ensure airway integrity. **With incisional wounds (e.g., knife, glass) that transect the trachea, direct tracheal intubation via the wound may be lifesaving.**

Even without neurologic evidence of cervical cord injury or obvious head and neck injuries, cervical spine radiographs or computed tomographic (CT) scans are indicated during the assessment of most trauma patients who have experienced sudden excessive acceleration, abrupt deceleration, or high-impact forces. Sudden shifts in the moment of inertia may compromise cervical spine stability, which in turn can result in potentially serious complications with intubation.[39] In general, the most common subluxations and unstable fractures can be diagnosed from lateral radiographs, which allow visualization of all seven cervical vertebra (C1 to C7).[8,47] **Three features should be carefully analyzed when assessing the radiographs. First, replacement of the normal cervical spine lordotic curvature with kyphotic flattening or kyphosis may indicate muscular spasm secondary to injury. Second, increases in soft tissue thickness beyond the normal 4 to 7 mm at C3 and a relatively smooth tapering to 18 to 20 mm at C7 may result from hemorrhage or emphysema caused by trauma. Third, variations in the thickness of disc interspace or variations in the smooth progression of the prevertebral, postvertebral, or anterior spinal canal alignments indicate compromise of cervical spine integrity.** Although it may complicate emergency tracheal intubation, the neck should remain splinted or under axial traction until injury to the cervical spine has been ruled out.[31]

Anesthetic management of a patient with a foreign body (FB) in the subglottic airway is complex because of the competition between the surgeon and the anesthesiologist for airway access and control. Also, any positive pressure ventilatory assistance may serve to impact the FB further or drive it further peripherally. When possible, radiographic studies should be undertaken to establish the nature and site of the FB. Unfortunately, aspirated blood, mucus, and gastric contents are not radio-opaque. Also unfortunately, in this age of plastics, many aspirated foreign bodies are radiolucent. Fiberoptic bronchoscopy with the patient awake may be the only means of identifying the presence, location, and nature of an FB.

Surgical incisions, tissue destruction from chemotherapy, or the development of dense, hardened, fibrotic scarring following radiotherapy are not generally considered trauma. However, these iatrogenic processes may result in sufficient limitation of neck mobility and jaw opening to seriously impair the ability to directly visualize any portion of the glottic structures. Airway control from above may also be seriously impaired by tracheal scarring, webs, strictures, or granulomas related to prior intubation, tracheostomy, or laser surgery in the airway. Additionally, surgery or radiotherapy in the head and neck

---

*References 5, 28, 50, 56, 86, 111.
†References 48, 49, 60, 72, 79, 90.

area may result in nerve damage that alters airway reflexes and function. Fiberoptic visualization during fiberoptic nasal or oral intubation techniques with the patient awake may permit diagnosis and evaluation of the degree of airway compromise, as well as minimize the likelihood of additional intubation-related trauma.

Morbid obesity

Airway assessment in morbidly obese patients may be a complex challenge, since both respiratory function and the airway can be greatly altered by relatively minor changes in patient position. The pathophysiologic changes in respiratory and cardiovascular function can be life-threatening when the patient moves from the sitting to the supine position.[80] Even with a shift to the semirecumbent position, soft tissues may intrude on the airway and diaphragm. In the supine position, alterations in chest compliance, total lung volume, and vital capacity make adequate, unassisted, spontaneous ventilation almost impossible. Even with local or regional anesthesia, the work of breathing may become excessive and necessitate ventilatory support. **To complicate airway management further, one study found that 86% of morbidly obese but otherwise healthy patients have a gastric pH of 2.5 or less and residual gastric volumes of 25 ml or greater.**[107] Since an increased incidence of hiatal hernia is also associated with obesity, these patients are at serious risk for aspiration pneumonitis. **Therefore, even with preanesthetic treatment with antacids or H$_2$-blockers, the anesthesiologist must consider endotracheal intubation and controlled ventilation even for relatively short procedures.**

Therefore, under most previous protocols, a rapid sequence of anesthesia induction and intubation would be required to prevent aspiration. In morbidly obese patients, however, this is considered impractical if not impossible. Indeed, controlled oral or nasal endotracheal intubation with a standard laryngoscope is usually difficult. Even if it had not been proved to be a contraindication because of the risks of aspiration, control of the airway with a mask would be next to impossible. Also, in most of these patients, emergency tracheostomy or cricothyroidotomy has been regarded as being so difficult mechanically that neither could be accomplished rapidly enough to prevent severe hypoxia. Therefore, until recently, when one could not visualize the glottic structures on direct laryngoscopy under local anesthesia, "blind" nasal intubation with the patient awake was attempted. Now, using a fiberoptic technique, intubation can be accomplished with the patient awake and in a sitting position.

Thus the preanesthetic assessment problem in the obese patient is to decide whether the patient can still

safely tolerate a rapid sequence of induction and intubation. Can the mouth be opened at least 4.5 cm? Is the genial-hyoid distance more than 4.5 cm and less than 9 cm? Is the tongue so large that it will be difficult to push from the visual field during intubation? Since the jaw may be heavily padded and thus difficult to lift, if the anatomy is further distorted by hypognathia, hypergnathia, or macroglossia, it is unlikely that the glottic opening can be seen with a standard laryngoscope. Is the neck so short and the chest so fat that even a half-handle laryngoscope cannot be inserted into the mouth? With the patient semirecumbent or supine, will folds of fat from the neck or chest impede opening of the jaw? On oral examination, do the cheeks, faucial soft tissues, or pharyngeal walls impinge on the oropharyngeal space? Can the glottic opening be visualized by indirect laryngoscopy? Are excess or encroaching folds of soft tissue seen during indirect laryngoscopy?

Any compromise to the oropharyngeal space or faucial isthmus can be aggravated by loss of supporting tissue tone with anesthesia. Even fiberoptic endoscopy may be significantly impaired by soft tissues collapsing into the airway. Since positioning for induction and intubation greatly alters cardiovascular and pulmonary dynamics,[80] the preanesthetic assessment should also include sufficient laboratory studies to determine the extent of the obese patient's reserve.

Generally, one is dealing with a continuum when discussing obese patients. **Once a patient has reached the morbidly obese category, prudence suggests that a fiberoptic endotracheal intubation with the patient awake in the sitting position is the technique of choice for airway management.** This technique also allows for administration of high flows of supplemental oxygen while avoiding the dramatic, life-threatening alterations in cardiovascular and respiratory physiology that accompany position changes. Therefore this approach is the most conservative, safest, and least stressful choice for such patients.

Pregnancy

In a healthy parturient patient, no inherent airway issues are associated with being pregnant. However, pregnancy can impose special problems in the management of patients with difficult airways. In several ways, airway control considerations in anesthesia for patients undergoing cesarean section parallel the concerns in caring for the obese patient. The physiologic effects of pregnancy on the cardiovascular and respiratory systems can lead to marked alterations in function when the patient changes from a sitting to a supine position. Similar to excessive rolls of fat, breast enlargement may complicate the insertion of a laryngoscope.[63] Airway anatomy may become distorted, since prolonged labor or pathologic states such as toxemia can lead to edematous soft tissue encroachment into the upper airway.[13,51] **Also, as with the obese patient, the obstetric patient must be considered to have a full stomach and therefore to be at serious risk for aspiration.**[43]

Unlike morbid obesity, pregnancy per se does not preclude emergency tracheostomy or cricothyroidotomy. However, neither of these emergency measures is protective against aspiration unless done with the patient awake. In cases of fetal distress or maternal hemorrhage, **time is of the essence.** Therefore intubation with the patient awake and under topical anesthesia, by way of direct visualization with a laryngoscope, must be considered the method of choice for rapid, effective placement of the endotracheal tube. **Nasal approaches, particularly "blind" ones, should be avoided, since mucous membranes become increasingly friable during late pregnancy.**[10] When evaluating alternatives, one might consider the oral fiberoptic technique of Rogers and Benumof[87] or the retrograde methods described by Waters,[111] Powell and Ozdil,[82] and King et al.[54]

Intrathoracic lesions

Various lesions can compromise airway integrity in the mediastinum through compression of the lung parenchyma or the tracheobronchial tree or by invasion of the trachea or bronchi (Box 13-3). Pulmonary function studies frequently elucidate the severity of airway limitation. However, careful analysis of CT scans is essential to planning airway control in patients with mediastinal compromise of the airway. Several groups have advocated the development of an algorithm for airway management in patients with mediastinal masses.[2,77] However, very innovative techniques may be required to establish and maintain airway integrity.

Skeletal axis conditions

Mesenchymal diseases and abnormalities involving the skeletal system can lead to serious and difficult-to-manage airway compromise. In patients with rheumatoid arthritis, scoliosis, lordosis, or kyphosis, airway management is frequently a significant test of the anesthesiologist's expertise.

Rheumatoid arthritis. Rheumatoid arthritis (RA) should be listed under a heading that acknowledges it as a multisystem disease. It is presented here under the skeletal pathologies, since the cervical spine, temporomandibular joint, and cricoarytenoid joint changes may be the pathologic alterations of primary importance to the anesthesiologist. However, during the preanesthetic evaluation of the airway, one must remain alert to the probability of concurrent RA involvement of the immunologic, cardiovascular, respiratory, renal, and hematologic systems.

"Alert" symptoms in patients with RA include recent signs of changes in voice, dysphagia, dysarthria, hoarseness, stridor, stridorous snoring, and a sense of fullness in the oropharynx. A positive history should initiate a careful fiberoptic or indirect laryngoscopic examination of the orpharynx and, more particularly, of the glottic structures. **With two opposing cartilages and a synovial membrane–lined joint space and capsule, the cricoarytenoid is a true diarthric joint, the type often involved in the arthritic process.** Visualization shows edematous, hyperemic arytenoid mucosa with swollen aryepiglottic folds and false cords. The patient's phonation during this examination may reveal a pronounced decrease in mobility of the vocal cords.[41] Endotracheal intubation frequently requires a smaller tube. Fiberoptic bronchoscopic intubation with the patient awake is recommended if cricoarytenoid joint ankylosis is present. **During anesthesia, abrupt airway obstruction may be precipitated by the anesthetic agent or by adjunctive drug-induced dimunition in tone of the laryngeal musculature.**[42]

Airway management in RA patients can also be frustrated by temporomandibular joint ankylosis, which may preclude orotracheal intubation. Therefore preanesthetic airway evaluation must include

---

BOX 13-3
COMMON LESIONS OF THE MEDIASTINUM

Anterosuperior mediastinum (near thoracic inlet)	Posterosuperior mediastinum
Aneurysms	Esophageal diverticulae
Thymic hyperplasia or tumors	Aneurysms
Lymphomas	Neurogenic tumors
Intrathoracic thyroid tumors	Neurinomas
Intrathoracic goiter	Neurofibromas
Anterior middle and middle superior mediastinum	Neuromas
Dermoids	Sympathogoniomas
Teratomas	Posterior middle mediastinum
Midthoracic mediastinum	Neurogenic tumors (see above)
Dermoids	Bronchial defects
Teratomas	Enteric cysts
Lymphomas	Inherent to tracheobronchial tree
Metastatic tumors	Rhabdomyosarcomas
Lymph nodal inflammations (e.g., sarcoid and tuberculosis)	Hemangiomas

determination of the maximal opening of the mouth and the ability to view the fauces. In addition, since hypognathism frequently accompanies juvenile RA, a profile inspection is important in estimating the genial-glottal distance.

Besides the problems just presented, the progressive cervical spondylosis associated with RA frequently leads to even more serious impediments to establishing and maintaining airway control during anesthesia.[52] In the earlier stages of RA, synovial destruction and vertebral erosion, along with ligamentous changes, lead to instability of the cervical spine. Instability of the atlas/odontoid or of subaxial vertebral alignments may lead to subluxation and cord compression. Knowledge of the degree of instability thus becomes critical, particularly with attempts to rotate, extend, or flex the neck forcibly, either during attempts to maintain the airway or during surgery, when the patient must be moved to a position other than supine. Because of the immobility and shortening of the neck associated with advanced cervical spondylosis, the trachea becomes increasingly rotated with an anterolateral displacement, which rotates and tilts the larynx forward.[52]

Even without discernible anatomic changes, a history of neck pain radiating to the occiput associated with decreased neck mobility and upper extremity radiculopathy suggests cervical spine arthritis.[81] **The preceding discussion indicates that the preanesthetic physical examination of the RA patient should include testing for active flexion, extension, and rotation as well as careful palpation of the larynx and trachea for evidence of deviation.** Cervical spine flexion and extension radiographs may be required for evaluation of instability and the potential for spinal cord compression.[52,81] With increasingly severe cervical spine deformity and tracheal distortion, preanesthetic fiberoptic laryngoscopy may be required to determine whether airway management via fiberoptic bronchoscopic intubation or tracheostomy with the patient awake is needed before the administration of sedatives, tranquilizers, narcotics, or anesthetic agents. The objective of the preanesthetic airway assessment of the RA patient is to decide which technique will be the most protective and successful without risk of aspiration or hypoxia.

Scoliosis, lordosis, and kyphosis. As with RA, spinal abnormalities leading to scoliosis, lordosis, and kyphosis can also lead to profound airway management dilemmas when they involve the upper thoracic or cervical vertebra.

Severe cervical spine deformity, instability, subluxation, and ankylosis, along with marked distortion of the rib cage and the tracheobronchial tree, can occur with any of the diseases listed in Box 13-4. Laryngeal deviation may include marked twisting, rotation, or

---

BOX 13-4

ETIOLOGIES OF SCOLIOTIC, LORDOTIC, AND KYPHOTIC SPINAL DEFORMITIES

Idiopathic
  Infantile
  Juvenile
  Adolescent
  Adult
Congenital
Neuropathic
  Nerve dysfunction
  Neurofibromatosis
Myopathic
Congenital mesenchymal disorders
  Dwarfism (e.g., Morquio's syndrome and
    others)
  Marfan's syndrome
  Osteogenesis imperfecta
Acquired mesenchymal disorders (e.g., rheumatoid
  arthritis)
Scheuermann's disease
Trauma

Data from Keim HA, Hensinger RN: Spinal deformities: scoliosis and kyphosis, *Clin Symp* 41:4, 1989.

---

angulation. Chest wall distortion may result in a critical decrease in total lung volume and vital capacity. Thus pulmonary function tests may provide information essential to assessing the uncertain status of ventilatory homeostasis. Furthermore, the anesthesiologist must decide whether the extent of neck deformity and tracheal deviation will preclude a safe, rapid emergency tracheostomy or cricothyroidotomy if intubation is uncertain following induction of anesthesia and use of muscle relaxants. Thus the guidelines presented for preanesthetic airway assessment in RA patients with cervical spine deformity apply to these patients as well.

Congenital Problems

This subject is more fully developed elsewhere in this text, but it is briefly presented here to reinforce the potential for problems in airway management that arise secondary to congenital abnormalities. These problems may first be presented to the anesthesiologist the day before surgery, when the patient (in late childhood, adolescence, or young adulthood) arrives for palliative, reconstructive, cosmetic, or reparative surgery.

Upper airway and laryngeal problems

During preoperative evaluation of patients with congenital defects, one must remember that, as often stated, the existence of one congenital abnormality means that others exist until proved otherwise. Anomalies of the cardiovascular, nervous, musculocutaneous, or excretory systems may be accompanied by abnormalities of the head and neck or upper airway, and vice versa. The preoperative assessment must include appropriate diagnostic procedures to delineate the existence (or absence) and severity of additional anomalies. Compilations of congenital anomalies appear in most pediatric and pathology texts. Rosenberg and Rosenberg[89] have devised an excellent tabulation of and bibliography for the syndromes most often accompanied by aberrations of the upper airway.

Several syndromes of congenital anomalies are particularly notable for grossly abnormal anatomy, which complicates the establishment and maintenance of an airway.[88] Examples include Crouzon's syndrome, Goldenhar's syndrome, Pierre Robin's syndrome and Treacher Collins' syndrome, all of which cause aberrations in varying degrees of severity. Such anomalies include congenital subglottic stenosis, tracheoesophageal or tracheocutaneous fistulas, blind pouches, laryngoceles, congenital webs, spurious membranes, relative macroglossia, agnathia, micrognathia, and hypergnathia.[53,71,81,89,114]

The *whistling face syndrome*[40,108] (craniocarpotarsal dysplasia) is a good example of a congenital anomaly syndrome that can challenge the anesthesiologist. These patients frequently require repeated anesthetics for the surgical correction of multiple musculoskeletal and soft tissue deformities.[32] A particular problem for the anesthesiologist is the severe microstomia, which is anatomic and cannot be significantly improved by deep general anesthesia or muscle relaxants. As the children grow older and begin to evolve teeth, the already meager oral aperture becomes even more crowded and inadequate. Other musculoskeletal anomalies of the thorax severely restrict pulmonary volume and tidal volumes,[62] making these children particularly prone to life-threatening pulmonary or ventilatory dysfunction during the postanesthesia period.[40,62] Until surgical procedures correcting the oral deformities have been accomplished, these patients should probably be considered candidates for either endotracheal intubation while awake or fiberoptic nasal endotracheal intubation.[6] At the minimum, one should strongly consider a laryngoscopic examination with the patient awake as part of the preoperative evaluation.

Wells et al.[113] recently reported that several congenital abnormality syndromes are associated with a shortened trachea. **Their findings indicate fewer tracheal rings and shorter glottal-carinal length of the trachea in a significant percentage of patients with several congenital malformation syndromes associated with cardiovascular anomalies and skeletal dysplasia.** These authors suggest that infants at risk for a shortened trachea should have preoperative radiographic studies to help avoid the complications of bronchial intubation. As an alternative, one could plan to have an appropriate fiberoptic bronchoscope available to check tube placement after intubation. These authors note that the problem tends to improve with growth and maturation.

Congenital malformation syndromes may also be associated with varying degrees of acute, progressive, or chronic airway obstruction. The presence of stridor and retraction or nasal flaring may provide evidence about both the site and the severity of an obstruction.[29] **Severe glossopharyngeal, glottic, and upper tracheal occlusions produce retraction and nasal flaring as well as stridor. Several corollaries are related to inspiratory and expiratory stridor: (1) stridor during inspiration generally indicates obstruction at or above the larynx; (2) expiratory stridor is most often associated with intrathoracic or subglottic obstruction; and (3) obstruction associated with the larynx or immediate glottic region may give rise to a biphasic stridor, although either inspiratory or expiratory sounds may predominate. In an adult, stridor at rest indicates a serious degree of obstruction with a cross-sectional opening less than 4 mm or an irregularly narrowed airway several centimeters in length.[29]**

Although not usually considered congenital anomalies, congenital tumors or cysts may invade or obstruct the airway (Box 13-5). During the preoperative assessment, specifically by physical examination and radiographic studies, one must determine the site of tumor involvement and the extent of obstruction or distortion of the normal anatomy. This information is critical in planning an airway management scheme

---

BOX 13-5
CONGENITAL TUMORS WITH PROPENSITY
FOR INVADING OR OBSTRUCTING
THE AIRWAY

Throughout respiratory tract
  Angiofibromas
  Hemangiomas
  Lymphangiomas
  Cystic hygromas
  Neurofibromas
Nasopharyngeal and oropharyngeal
  Craniopharyngiomas
  Meningoceles
  Meningoencephaloceles
  Gliomas

that will not traumatize the tumor and thus cause a life-threatening hemorrhage or acute swelling and complete obstruction. With tumors of nervous system origin, trauma may result in meningeal infection. Contingency plans for emergency airway management should be well prepared before induction of anesthesia to preclude a crisis should accidental trauma to the tumor occur.

Lower airway or intrathoracic problems

Mediastinal lesions can also lead to life-threatening airway obstructions and may be found in neonates, infants, children, or adults.[2,11,20,78] Congenital mediastinal lesions include some tumors, aberrant vasculature, pulmonic malformations, and abnormalities arising from the esophagus. Congenital tumors or tumors that can arise in early infancy or childhood include hemangiomas, lymphangiomas, cystic hygromas, teratomas, dermoids, rhabdomyosarcomas, neurofibromas, neuromas, and thymic hyperplasia or tumors. The differential diagnosis is frequently aided by the anatomic location (see previous section and Box 13-3).

Perhaps the most significant vascular malformations from the standpoint of airway compromise and control are *trachea-encircling vascular rings,* usually of double aortic arch origin. Mediastinal pulmonary tree abnormalities that seriously threaten airway integrity include tracheomalacia, congenital stenosis, shortened trachea, and bronchogenic cysts. These patients with mediastinal lesions may present the unique challenge of requiring anesthesia for the diagnostic procedures that will delineate the extent and nature of the lesion.

Therefore patients with airway-compromising mediastinal lesions should be evaluated on the basis of a protocol or algorithm that includes the strategy for both elective and emergency airway management, as well as a diagnostic outline.[2,77] The guidelines presented in the section on acquired mediastinal lesions are equally pertinent to the preoperative airway evaluation of patients with congenital intrathoracic lesions.

Cardiovascular defects

In developing an anesthesia management plan for patients with congenital abnormalities of the head and neck or airway, contingencies must be established for handling all the inherent pathophysiologic variations associated with a given syndrome. This may be particularly difficult when the associated anomalies include cardiac septal defects, aberrant aortic arch and pulmonary vasculature, or other malformations leading to significant shunts and the potential for rapid desaturation with even minor changes in cardiac or ventilatory function. Thus, when evaluating pa-

tients with anomalous airways and associated congenital abnormalities, one must determine as precisely as possible the extent and nature of cardiovascular and respiratory anomalies, as well as the airway malformations, through CT scans, radiographs, and physical examination.

The cardiovascular and respiratory function variations likely to arise as side effects of the anesthetic agents may seriously limit the options relative to induction and maintenance of anesthesia. **During the preanesthesia evaluation, one must consider the probability of tachycardia or bradycardia, hypotension or hypertension, and bronchial constriction or laryngospasm as related to a given agent or combination of agents.** Then, within the framework of these limitations, the anesthesiologist must weigh adverse or uncommon reflexes likely to occur with the various intubation techniques in the awake patient vs. reflexes likely to be associated with intubation using various anesthetics. Preoperative preparations may include having a surgical team, technicians, and equipment on immediate standby to institute emergency cardiopulmonary bypass or extracorporal membrane oxygenation (ECMO) support, should this be required (see Chapters 11 and 37).

Malignant hyperthermia

Some patients with congenital anomalies of mesodermal origin are at increased risk for malignant hyperthermia (MH) reactions in association with anesthesia. It is beyond the scope of this chapter to present the genetics and pathophysiology of MH; the natural history, physiology, and treatment of this disease have been well summarized and referenced by Britt[12] and more recently in the *British Journal of Anaesthesia.*[101] However, several features frequently found in patients at risk for MH should be reviewed for emphasis: (1) familial history of adverse reactions to anesthetics; (2) incidence of muscle abnormalities with hypertrophic muscle groups and localized weakness in other groups; (3) muscle imbalances giving rise to lordosis, kyphosis, or scoliosis; (4) a history of non-exercise-related muscle cramps; (5) squint or ptosis; and (6) hypermobile joints. **One must remember that a family history is not an absolute prerequisite, since incomplete penetrance and variable expressivity make it possible for a "normal" parent to pass on the disease genetically.**[12]

In addition to patients with grossly evident malformations of mesodermal origin, others have more subtle conditions that involve mesodermal enzymatic abnormalities. Patients with a higher incidence of MH include those with myopathies such as myotonia congenita,[55,92] central core disease,[25,34,38] Duchenne's muscular dystrophy, Evans' syndrome, and King's syndrome.[66,73]

The correlation of MH episodes in patients who have trismus following administration of succinyldicholine (SDC) has led some to suggest that masseter muscle spasm may herald the onset of trismus.* Muscle biopsy testing of patients with trismus after SDC administration has shown that 50% to 80% of the patients are susceptible to MH on the basis of calcium uptake tests.[30,33,94] However, these results are difficult to interpret, since the testing protocols have not been standardized among the various testing centers.[59,68] In addition, several investigators have suggested that masseter muscles vary from striated twitch muscles in their response to SDC.[105,106] The patients in these latter studies, however, had increased masseter muscle tone, not trismus, and creatine phosphokinase levels were not measured. At present, the true implication of trismus' association with SDC administration is uncertain.

Strategies for the imminent treatment of MH should be incorporated when planning anesthesia for patients with multiple congenital anomalies. The drugs and equipment required under the institution's MH treatment protocol should be readily available and checked for completeness before anesthesia is started.[73]

AIRWAY MANAGEMENT TECHNIQUES

Various techniques have been developed to manage airways when congenital or acquired anatomic features create a "difficult airway."

Mask and Pharyngeal Airways

Control with a mask and airway is inappropriate in patients at risk for aspiration. Every trauma patient, obstetric patient, morbidly obese patient, and patient with hiatal hernia symptoms must be considered to have a full stomach. In addition, the same adverse conditions that result in a problematic intubation frequently make it difficult or impossible to maintain airway integrity with a mask and oral or nasal pharyngeal airway. This may be particularly true when facial or upper airway anatomy is seriously distorted by malformation, trauma, prior surgery, or radiation therapy.

When no contingency plan or equipment is available and the patient has been induced and paralyzed but cannot be intubated, temporary management via *Safar's triple airway maneuver*[91] may be lifesaving. **In this maneuver, with the fingers behind the mandibular rami, the patient's jaw is thrust forward; augmented by pressure from the heels of the hands on the forehead; this extends the head on the neck. Using the face mask, strong downward pressure is exerted on the mental prominence. The resultant forces on the temporomandibular joint result in the condyles moving forward, sometimes to the point of subluxation, and the mouth being held open. This maneuver also stretches taut the geniohyoid and omohyoid musculature and the ligamentous support structures of the larynx, thereby straightening the airway and lifting the tongue and epiglottis.**

However, since Safar's maneuver requires both hands to manage the mask and the required translational forces, a second individual is required to provide assisted or positive pressure ventilation via the reservoir bag in the apneic patient. The insertion of an oropharyngeal airway aids in holding the mouth open and generally improves the patency of the airway. Alternatively, the insertion of a nasopharyngeal airway may obviate the need for forcing the jaw open and may decrease the cervical extension required. In addition, extending the cervical spine and lifting the patient's head forward by placing a pillow behind it decreases the severity of the head extension required to lift the epiglottis from the back of the pharynx.[9]

It is critical to remember that Safar's maneuver is likely to result in severe spinal cord injury in patients with unstable cervical vertebra, whether this instability arises from trauma, from congenital malformation, or from disease processes such as rheumatoid arthritis.

Intubation Techniques with Awake Patients
Direct laryngoscopy

Various techniques exist for intubation of the conscious patient. However, direct laryngoscopy and intubation are normally preferred,[57,103] since this may be the fastest, most effective technique and results in visual confirmation of correct endotracheal tube placement. To avoid undue patient discomfort and abnormal neurologic reflexes, some form of anesthesia of the airway should be provided, even in the patient with a full stomach. Transoral topical application is relatively easy, is effective, and has minimal potential for complications.[21,109,112] Walts[109] argues against the use of translaryngeal, transtracheal, or superior laryngeal nerve blockade. Others believe that superior laryngeal nerve block is safe, since it does not interfere with the tracheal cough reflex.

Numerous laryngoscope blades have been designed to facilitate intubation of problematic airways. **However, the laryngoscope blade of choice is the one with which the anesthesiologist has the most experience.** At most institutions this choice of blades includes the Miller no. 1, 2, 3, and 4 blades and the Macintosh no. 3 and 4 blades mounted on a standard laryngoscope handle or on a Datta-Briwa[22] (half) handle for use in obese patients. Complex or specialty blades should

---

*References 7, 30, 33, 94, 105, 106.

not be used in a crisis situation unless one has developed and maintains true proficiency with them in elective cases.

Nasal fiberoptic endotracheal intubation

The development of small-diameter, flexible fiberoptic bronchoscopes has added a very powerful tool to the armamentarium for management of the difficult airway.[75,83,102] Having decided that direct laryngoscopy and intubation is impractical or contraindicated, one should consider fiberoptic nasotracheal intubation with the patient awake as a first alternative. With the patient under light sedation (if deemed safe), and following careful nasal passage and nasopharyngeal and oropharyngeal topical anesthesia with a lidocaine-vasoconstrictor combination, the nares and nasal passages are progressively dilated with soft nasal airways. The fiberoptic bronchoscope is threaded through an appropriate nasotracheal tube, and both are then passed through the nose into the oropharynx. The bronchoscope is then advanced separately into the trachea and subsequently serves as the stylet over which the endotracheal tube is introduced. Once the tube position and depth have been ascertained, the bronchoscope is removed and anesthesia commenced.

Fiberoptic nasotracheal intubation is of particular value in patients with trismus, marked hypognathism with real or relative macroglossia, tracheal deviation, and cervical spine instability, ankylosis, or kyphosis. However, facial trauma or congenital malformation may so severely compromise or distort the nasal passages that a nasal endotracheal intubation becomes infeasible. **In addition, nasal endotracheal intubation carries the hazard of profuse and difficult-to-control iatrogenic hemorrhage, particularly in patients with small or distorted nasal passageways, nasal polyps or tumors, craniopharyngiomas or angiofibromas, or increased tissue friability, as occurs with pregnancy.** The next logical alternative in such patients is to consider fiberoptic orotracheal intubation.

Oral fiberoptic endotracheal intubation

As described by Rogers and Benumof,[87] an oral fiberoptic intubation technique employing a specialized oral airway has proved exceptionally useful, particularly when nasal endotracheal intubation appears to be impractical. As with direct oral laryngoscopic endotracheal intubations (see preceding sections), fiberoptic oral endotracheal intubations with the patient awake require careful patient preparation and adequate topical analgesia of the mouth, oropharynx, and glottic structures.[21,109,112] Following topical anesthesia, one inserts an oral airway that serves as both a bite block and a smooth central passage for the endotracheal tube. With the fiberoptic bronchoscope inserted through an endotracheal tube, the scope and tube combination is introduced through the oral airway into the pharynx. The fiberoptic bronchoscope is then advanced into the trachea and becomes the stylet for intercalating the endotracheal tube.

If the glottic opening is greatly displaced or the glottic anatomy is severely distorted, fiberoptic endotracheal intubation may not be possible. However, these preparations also apply to intubation via the retrograde technique, which one should consider as the next most rational approach to nasal or oral intubation with the patient awake.

Retrograde method

Although several variations exist, the retrograde technique involves intubation along a guide wire that has been introduced in retrograde fashion through the cricothyroid membrane, upward, and out the glottic opening into the oropharynx.[1,28,54,86,111] Perhaps, as King et al.[54] suggest, a more appropriate name would be *translaryngeal guided intubation*. **This maneuver calls for percutaneous insertion of a needle, aimed superiorly, through the cricothyroid membrane into the trachea, which one identifies by the uninhibited withdrawal of air (Fig. 13-1). A guide wire (or catheter) is passed into the trachea via the needle and is advanced upward through the glottic opening into the oropharynx. Perorally, one visualizes the pharynx, identifies the guide wire, and, with an appropriate instrument (e.g., hemostat), brings the wire forward and out the mouth (Fig. 13-2). (With additional steps, the wire can be brought out through the nose.) The**

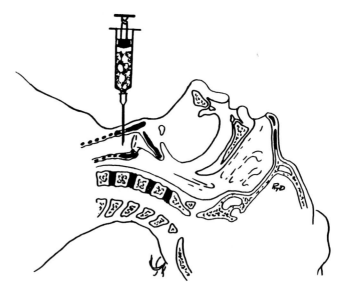

Fig. 13-1. Retrograde intubation method (translaryngeal guided intubation). Placement of transtracheal needle tip in lumen of trachea is verified by uninhibited aspiration of air.

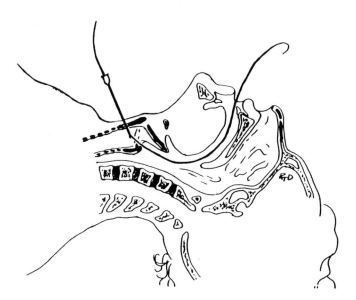

Fig. 13-2. Guide wire through transtracheal needle is passed retrograde into the oropharynx and then brought out through the mouth.

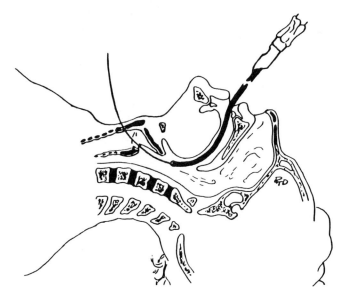

Fig. 13-3. With transtracheal needle removed, guide wire is inserted into instrument channel of fiberoptic scope and serves to guide scope/endotracheal tube combination into trachea.

wire can now be used as a guide for the oral introduction of a catheter into the larynx. Following removal of the transcricothyroid membrane wire and further advancement of the catheter, an endotracheal tube is introduced into the trachea over the catheter. This procedure has been reported to be very successful.

A further variation of the retrograde technique permits visualization of the glottic structures, the larynx, and the cricothyroid membrane puncture site before endotracheal intubation.[15,61] By placing an endotracheal tube high on the shaft of a fiberoptic bronchoscope and then inserting the guide wire into the distal end suction or instrument channel of the bronchoscope, the wire can guide the scope, with visualization of the pathway, into the larynx (Fig. 13-3). The wire is then removed, and the fiberoptic endoscope is advanced until the carina is identified. At this point, the fiberoptic scope becomes the guide over which the endotracheal tube is moved downward and inserted into the trachea (Fig. 13-4).

As an ethical matter, it would be difficult to justify use of the retrograde technique in patients with normal airways or patients in whom less invasive techniques would typically be expected to be equally successful. However, since this technique may eliminate the need for tracheostomy in some patients, one should consider practicing the procedure in an animal laboratory while acquiring expertise in the use of transtracheal jet ventilation (see later discussion). Specialized kits have been designed to facilitate initiation of the retrograde guided intubation maneuver.

The retrograde technique requires reasonable

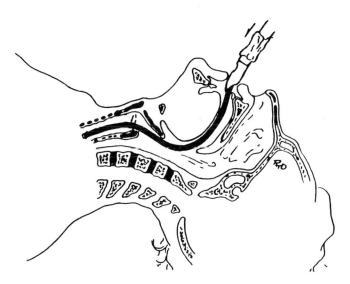

Fig. 13-4. After removing guide wire, fiberoptic scope is advanced until carina is identified. Then the endotracheal tube is inserted into trachea using the scope as a guide.

visualization of the oropharynx beyond the fauces. One would therefore expect the maneuver to be difficult, if not futile, when temporomandibular joint motion is compromised by ankylosis or soft tissue changes. One also should probably not attempt this procedure when the glottic area, faucial isthmus, or oropharynx is grossly distorted by tumor, trauma, or infectious processes.

Tracheostomy

As Colice[19] has noted, tracheostomy has been used to reestablish airway patency since its mention in the

Rig-Veda, 2000 to 1000 BC, and Eber's Papyrus, about 1550 BC. If each of the techniques just discussed proves ineffective or is considered inappropriate, tracheostomy with the patient awake and under local anesthesia becomes obligatory for elective management of difficult airways. In a controlled environment, with a cooperative patient, relatively few contraindications exist to elective surgical tracheostomy.[76] Although anesthesiologists should be capable of performing a tracheostomy or cricothyroidotomy in an emergency, these procedures are normally considered to be in the purview of the surgeon. Therefore the surgeon must be consulted.

A technique for *percutaneous dilatational tracheostomy*[17] has gained variable acceptance. In this system a guide wire is inserted percutaneously into the trachea, between the cricoid and first tracheal cartilages, via a needle. The tracheostomy opening is then created by passing progressively larger dilators over a heavy guide wire.

Under emergency or less than ideal circumstances, the complication rate associated with tracheostomy may approach 45%.* Additionally, the procedure may be technically difficult in obese patients or in patients with very large goiters. Also, a cervical tracheostomy may be almost impossible in patients with deformities in which the neck is severely shortened, flexed, or deformed or in which the mandible is essentially resting on the lower trachea. However, tracheostomy may be the only means of effective airway control in patients with major trauma to the face, jaw, or upper throat or with large tumors of the face, nose, mouth, and throat.

Emergency Techniques

The techniques for dealing with difficult airways discussed in the previous section are predicated on having ample time for staging an elective, controlled procedure. If the preoperative airway evaluation has been sufficiently meticulous and definitive, the need for emergency management techniques in elective situations should seldom arise. However, plans for coping with potential airway crises must be formulated. The patient's well-being does not always allow one to employ the most sophisticated methods just presented.

Failed intubation algorithm

Particularly in emergencies, the many combinations of distorted tissues and disrupted support structures that can compromise the airway defy description. Acute loss of airway integrity in a patient with a difficult airway may occur in the intensive care unit or emergency room as well as in the operating room. As

---

*References 16, 19, 45, 67, 71, 76, 99.

in chess, one must have multiple alternative plans well developed and ready for immediate use should circumstances require.

Designing a rapid-analysis algorithm and presenting it as a flow chart is particularly useful in organizing, presenting, and remembering the failed intubation protocol. I developed the strategy presented in Fig. 13-5. Such strategies for managing airway exigencies are effective only to the extent that the essential equipment is readily available and the necessary personnel are present and ready to provide immediate assistance. Lack of preparedness results from failure to properly assess the potential for airway control difficulties.

Repeated, futile, but traumatic attempts to intubate are inadvisable; the resulting hemorrhage or tissue edema can only complicate the failed intubation/cannot ventilate impasse. Emergency airway management techniques must be instituted to ensure the patient's safety. Thus, given a cannot intubate/cannot ventilate situation, and following my scheme, the next logical alternative is to attempt transtracheal jet ventilation (TTJV) (see following discussion). If it is possible to maintain adequate ventilation via TTJV, more controlled ancillary intubation maneuvers such as nasal or oral fiberoptic intubation or a retrograde guided intubation (see earlier section) should be chosen. If TTJV proves inadequate, little alternative other than an emergency cricothyroidotomy or tracheostomy remains.

Tracheostomy and cricothyroidotomy

For centuries, tracheostomy was the procedure of choice for emergency relief of airway obstruction.[19,45,99] More recently, cricothyroidotomy has become the technique of choice in acute airway emergencies when endotracheal intubation cannot be accomplished.[45] As discussed in this text, emergency tracheostomy may be lifesaving in patients with facial or upper airway trauma. Other chapters present emergency tracheostomy as still being the primary backup method in procedural protocols for various problematic acute infectious processes threatening the integrity of the upper airway, such as quinsy, lingual quinsy, epiglottitis, or advanced Vincent's angina.

The potential for damage to the cricothyroid complex, leading to dysphonia and/or stenosis, has made cricothyroidotomy strictly an emergency procedure. Also, cricothyroidotomy may not be possible in patients with laryngeal or neck injuries. **In addition, the technique clearly represents a more risky procedure in infants or small children.**

Since they are major consultants on emergency airway control for trauma patients, and on airway management during cardiopulmonary resuscitation,

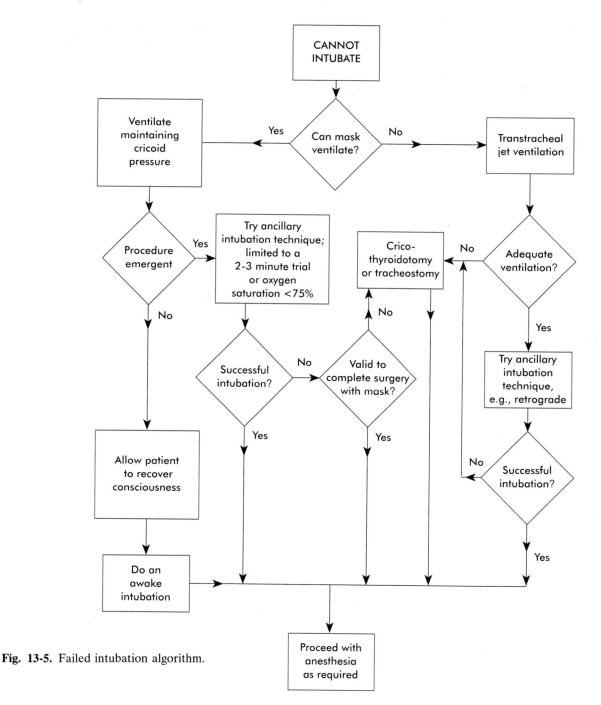

Fig. 13-5. Failed intubation algorithm.

anesthesiologists should be able to perform either an emergency tracheostomy or a cricothyroidotomy. Description of these surgical procedures is beyond the scope of this chapter, particularly since they are well described in many recent articles (e.g., Heffner and Sahn[45]) and surgery texts. Over the past several decades, several kits to facilitate emergency cricothyroidotomy have been marketed, but they have found only limited acceptability. More recently, Melker has developed a maneuver in which the airway catheter stationed on a dilator is interjected into the trachea over a stiff guide wire. The wire is previously positioned percutaneously through the cricothyroid membrane into the trachea via an introducer needle. Such a kit may indeed facilitate airway control by emergency room personnel or paramedic crews at the trauma scene. In the operating room or intensive care setting, one would hope that careful airway assessment and failed intubation algorithms would permit alternative means of effective airway control until a more classic tracheostomy can be performed.

Transtracheal jet ventilation

One such alternative means of effective airway control in emergency situations in the hospital environment is the use of TTJV.[5,50,56,98] Although a few specific situations exist in which TTJV might be ineffective or even contraindicated, if the essential equipment is immediately available, this is perhaps the simplest and fastest way to provide ventilation in most crisis situations. **The TTJV technique calls for the percutaneous antegrade insertion of a large (12 to 16 gauge) cannula through the cricothyroid membrane into the trachea as a route for the periodic injection of a jet of oxygen (O$_2$).** Since the development of intravenous catheters over integral introducer needles, these have become the typically used cannula for TTJV. The cannula is connected to a source of triggerable high-pressure O$_2$ (about 50 psi), preferably with a secondary regulator that can lower injection pressures, if this is deemed necessary to lower the risk of barotrauma. Ventilation is achieved by periodic (15 to 30/minute) injections of a jet of O$_2$ down the trachea. The adequacy of ventilation results from (1) the cannula size (diameter and length), (2) the diameter and length of the trachea and the lung and the patient's chest compliance, (3) the TTJV driving pressure and inspiratory dwell time, and (4) the extent of tracheal outflow compromise.

A relative contraindication to the use of TTJV is loss of structural integrity of the respiratory tract below the distal orifice of the transtracheal catheter, particularly in patients with trauma to the lower trachea or proximal bronchial tree. In such circumstances, injection of pressurized jets of air, which can raise airway pressures to 50 cm H$_2$O or greater,[98] significantly increases the probability of a tension pneumothorax or soft tissue emphysema. Significant tracheal outflow resistance also greatly increases the potential for barotrauma. In patients with trauma to the larynx, distortion or disruption of the tissues in the cricothyroid region may frustrate safe placement of the catheter.

Elective use of TTJV in awake (or anesthetized[4,65]) patients with difficult airways may ensure adequate ventilation while a more stable airway is created by other means. **TTJV is suitable for use with any of the intubation techniques with awake patients discussed earlier, including elective tracheostomy.** In addition, with an appropriate secondary regulator to control the jet injection pressure, the technique can be used in pediatric patients, as well as adults.

An excellent review of the technique, the alternative requisite TTJV equipment assemblies, and the pertinent literature has been presented by Benumof and Scheller.[5] As these authors state, "... TTJV is indeed an effective, simple, and inexpensive solution to the cannot ventilate/intubate problem, and, therefore, can be and should be immediately available in every anesthetizing location."

A note of caution: it is important to be absolutely certain that a adequate length of the cannula is within the tracheal lumen and is not impinging on the posterior wall (checked by unimpeded withdrawal of air with a syringe). The pressures generated at the distal tip of the catheter during injection of O$_2$ are sufficient to force gas submucosally.[97]

CONCLUSION

Reevaluation of the previous discussions reveals several common, complicating anatomic features associated with problematic airways—the "Dozen Draconic Demons of Airway Management" (Box 13-6).

These anatomic variants may help to predict which patients could have difficult-to-control airways. Management becomes progressively more complex with increasing severity in the deviation of a given feature from the norm. Also, as discussed, these complicating variants frequently appear in diverse combinations. Thus the detection of even one of these attributes should initiate close scrutiny and analysis of the airway. In the absence of contravening or negating circumstances, the definitive assessment is direct laryngoscopy. A long-held belief states that, if the glottic structures can be visualized using direct laryngoscopy and topical anesthesia with the patient awake, one can safely proceed with a routine laryngoscopic intubation following induction of anesthesia.[103] Recent evidence may disprove this previously sacrosanct adage. **Sivarajan and Fink**[96] **observed two patients in whom larynges could be visualized with the patient awake under local anesthesia, but not after the patient had general anesthesia and muscle paralysis.**

BOX 13-6
ANATOMIC FEATURES ASSOCIATED WITH DIFFICULT AIRWAYS

Short, heavy, or muscular, "fireplug" neck, with full complement of teeth
Receding, hypognathic jaw
Real or relative macroglossia
Protruding "buck" teeth, particularly upper or lower incisors, or multiple loose or "snag" teeth
Limited temporomandibular joint motion
Long, high-vaulted palate
Increased mandibular alveolar-mental distance
Decreased genial-hyoid or genial-thyroid cartilage distance
Cervical spine instability, ankylosis, or kyphotic curvature
Deviated trachea
Marked diminution of fauces or difficulty in visualizing faucial structures, particularly the uvula
Extreme obesity (morbid)

Regional anesthesia, when possible, is sometimes considered to be a viable alternative to having to manage a troublesome airway. However, I would warn that this constitutes an open invitation to catastrophe. Inadequate anesthesia or complications of regional anesthesia (e.g., total spinal anesthesia, seizures, anaphylaxis) may mandate a crisis intubation that, at best, will be done under precarious circumstances. Therefore a careful preanesthetic assessment of each patient's airway is obligatory. For patients with a potentially difficult airway, the anesthesiologist must determine both a plan of choice for airway control and one or more logical alternatives to use should contingencies require.

KEY POINTS

■ The triad of aspiration, severe hypoventilation, and hypoxemia constitutes the more serious complications associated with management of "difficult" airways.

■ Infection-related airway compromise is the major airway management problem in patients under age 10 years.

■ In an adult, stridor at rest indicates a serious degree of obstruction with a cross-sectional opening less than 4 mm or an irregularly narrowed airway several centimeters in length.

■ Transtracheal jet ventilation is suitable for use with any of the intubation techniques with the patient awake, including an elective tracheostomy.

■ Patients have had larynges that could be visualized with the patient awake under local anesthesia but not after the patient had general anesthesia and muscle paralysis.

KEY REFERENCES

Benumof JL, Scheller MS: The importance of transtracheal jet ventilation in the management of the difficult airway, *Anesthesiology* 71:769, 1989.

Fink BR: *The human larynx: a functional study,* New York, 1975, Raven Press.

Heffner JE, Sahn SA: The technique of tracheostomy and cricothyroidotomy: when to operate—and how to manage complications, *J Crit Illness* 2:79, 1987.

Rex M: A review of the structural and functional basis of laryngospasm: nerve pathways and clinical significance, *Br J Anaesth* 42:891, 1970.

Rogers SN, Benumof JL: New and easy techniques for fiberoptic endoscopy aided tracheal intubation, *Anesthesiology* 59:569, 1983.

Rosenberg H, Rosenberg H: Airway obstruction and causes of difficult intubation. In Orkin FK, Cooperman LH, eds: *Complications in anesthesiology,* Philadelphia, 1983, JB Lippincott.

Saunders WH: The larynx, *Ciba Found Symp* 16:35, 1964.

Stoelting RK: Blood pressure and heart rate changes during short duration laryngoscopy for tracheal intubations: influence of viscous or intravenous lidocaine, *Anesth Analg* 57:197, 1978.

REFERENCES

1. Akinyemi OO: Complications of guided blind endotracheal intubation, *Anaesthesia* 34:590, 1980.
2. Azizkhan RG, Dudgeon DL et al: Life-threatening airway obstruction as a complication to the management of mediastinal masses in children, *J Pediatr Surg* 20:816, 1985.
3. Baker JL, Kelen GD, Silverston KT et al: Unsuspected immunodeficiency virus in critically ill emergencies, *JAMA* 257:2609, 1987.
4. Baraka A: Transtracheal jet ventilation during fiberoptic intubation under general anesthesia, *Anesth Analg* 65:1091, 1986.
5. Benumof JL, Scheller MS: The importance of transtracheal jet ventilation in the management of the difficult airway, *Anesthesiology* 71:769, 1989.
6. Berthelsen P, Prytz S, and Jacobsen E: Two-stage fiberoptic nasotracheal intubation in infants: a new approach to difficult pediatric intubation, *Anesthesiology* 63:457, 1985.
7. Bloom DH, Fonkalsrud EW, and Reynolds RC: Malignant hyperpyrexia during anesthesia in childhood, *J Pediatr Surg* 11:185, 1976.
8. Bohlman HH: Acute fractures and dislocations of the cervical spine, *J Bone Joint Surg* 61A:1119, 1979.
9. Boiden MP: Airway patency in the unconscious patient, *Br J Anaesth* 57:306, 1985.
10. Bonica JJ: *Principles and practice of obstetric analgesia and anesthesia,* Philadelphia, 1967, FA Davis.
11. Bower RJ, Kiesewetter WB: Mediastinal masses in infants and children, *Arch Surg* 112:1003, 1977.
12. Britt BA: Altered temperature regulation: malignant hyperthermia. In Orkin FK, Cooperman LH, eds: *Complications in anesthesia,* Philadelphia, 1983, JB Lippincott.
13. Brock-Utne JG, Downing JW, and Seedat F: Laryngeal oedema associated

with preeclampsia toxemia, *Anaesthesia* 32:556, 1977.

14. Campbell FC, Robbs JV: Penetrating injuries of the neck: a prospective study of 108 patients, *Br J Surg* 67:582, 1980.

15. Carlson CA, Perkins HM, and Veltkan PS: Solving a difficult intubation, *Anesthesiology* 64:537, 1986.

16. Chew JY, Cantrell RW: Tracheostomy: complications and their management, *Arch Otolaryngol* 96:538, 1972.

17. Ciaglia P, Firsching R, and Syniec C: Elective percutaneous dilatational tracheostomy: a new bedside procedure; preliminary report, *Chest* 87:715, 1985.

18. Clarke RSJ: Trauma to face and neck. In Morrow WFK, Morrison WD, eds: *Anesthesia for eye, ear, nose and throat surgery,* Belfast, 1975, Churchill-Livingstone.

19. Colice GL: Prolonged intubation versus tracheostomy in the adult, *J Intensive Care Med* 2:85, 1987.

20. Conklin WS: Tumors and cysts of the mediastinum, *Dis Chest* 17:715, 1950.

21. Curran J, Hamilton C, and Taylor T: Topical analgesia before tracheal intubation, *Anaesthesia* 30:765, 1975.

22. Datta S, Briwa J: Modified laryngoscope for endotracheal intubation of obese patients, *Anesth Analg* 60:120, 1981.

23. Davies RM, Scott JG: Anesthesia for major oral and maxillofacial surgery, *Br J Anaesth* 40:202, 1968.

24. DeJong RH: *Physiology and pharmacology of local anesthetics,* Springfield, Ill, 1970, Charles C Thomas.

25. Denborough MA, Dennet X, and Anderson RM: Central core disease and malignant hyperpyrexia, *Br Med J* 1:272, 1973.

26. Devault M, Griefenstein FE, and Harris LC: Circulatory responses to endotracheal intubation in light general anesthesia: the effect of atropine and phentolamine, *Anesthesiology* 21:360, 1960.

27. DeWeese DD, Saunders WH, eds: *Textbook of otolaryngology,* ed 5, St Louis, 1977, CV Mosby.

28. Dhara SS: Guided blind endotracheal intubation, *Anaesthesia* 35:81, 1980.

29. Donlon JV: Anesthesia for eye, ear, nose, and throat surgery. In Miller RD, ed: *Anesthesia,* New York, 1981, Churchill-Livingstone.

30. Donlon JV, Newfield P, Sreter F, et al: Implications of masseter spasm after succinylcholine, *Anesthesiology* 49:298, 1978.

31. Doolan LA, O'Brien JF: Safe intubation in cervical spine injury, *Anaesth Intensive Care* 13:319, 1985.

32. Duggar RG, DeMars PD, and Bolton VE: Whistling face syndrome: general anesthesia and early postoperative caudal analgesia, *Anesthesiology* 70:545, 1989.

33. Ellis FR, Halsall PJ: Suxamethonium spasm: a differential diagnosis conundrum, *Br J Anaesth* 56:381, 1984.

34. Eng AD, Epstein BS, Engel WK et al: Malignant hyperthermia and central core disease in a child with congenital dislocating hips, *Arch Neurol* 35:189, 1978.

35. Fellini AA, Bernstein RL, and Zauder HL: Bronchospasms due to suxamethonium, *Br J Anaesth* 35:657, 1963.

36. Fink BR: The *human larynx: a functional study,* New York, 1975, Raven Press.

37. Flood LM, Astley B: Anaesthetic management of acute laryngeal trauma, *Br J Anaesth* 54:1339, 1982.

38. Frank JP, Harah Y, Butler IJ et al: Central core disease and the malignant hyperthermia syndrome, *Am J Hum Genet* 30:51A, 1978.

39. Fraser A, Edmonds-Seal J: Spinal cord injuries: a review of the problems facing the anaesthetist, *Anaesthesia* 37:1084, 1982.

40. Freeman EA, Sheldon JH: Craniocarpo-tarsal dystrophy: an undescribed congenital malformation, *Arch Dis Child* 13:277, 1938.

41. Funk D, Raymon F: Rheumatoid arthritis of the cricoarytenoid joints: an airway hazard, *Anesth Analg* 54:742, 1975.

42. Gardner DL, Holmes F: Anaesthetic and postoperative hazards in rheumatoid arthritis, *Br J Anaesth* 33:258, 1961.

43. Gibbs CP: Gastric aspiration: prevention and treatment, *Clin Anesthesiol* 4:47, 1986.

44. Gupta PK, Lichstein E, and Chadda KD: Lidocaine-induced heart block in patients with bundle branch block, *Am J Cardiol* 33:487, 1974.

45. Heffner JE, Sahn SA: The technique of tracheostomy and cricothyroidotomy: when to operate—and how to manage complications, *J Crit Illness* 2:79, 1987.

46. Hochman RA, Martin JT, and Devine KD: Anesthesia and the larynx, *Surg Clin North Am,* 1965, p 1031.

47. Holdsworth F: Fractures, dislocations and fracture-dislocations of the spine, *J Bone Joint Surg* 52A:1534, 1970.

48. Hybels RL: Venous air embolism in head and neck surgery, *Laryngoscope* 90:946, 1980.

49. Jacobs JB, Persky MS: Traumatic pneumocephalus, *Laryngoscope* 90:515, 1980.

50. Jacoby JJ, Hamelburg W, Ziegler CH, et al: Transtracheal resuscitation, *JAMA* 162:625, 1956.

51. Jouppila R, Jouppila P, and Hollmen A: Laryngeal oedema as an obstetric anaesthesia complication, *Acta Anaesthesiol Scand* 24:97, 1980.

52. Keenan MA, Siles CM, and Kaufman RL: Acquired laryngeal deviation associated with cervical spine disease in erosive polyarticular arthritis, *Anesthesiology* 58:441, 1983.

53. Keim HA, Hensinger RN: Spinal deformities: scoliosis and kyphosis, *Clin Symp* 41:4, 1989.

54. King HK, Wang LF, Kahn AK et al: Translaryngeal guided intubation for difficult intubation, *Crit Care Med* 15:869, 1987.

55. King JO, Denborough MA, and Zapf P: Inheritance of malignant hyperthermia, *Lancet* 1:365, 1972.

56. Klain M, Keszler H, and Brader E: High frequency jet ventilation in CPR, *Crit Care Med* 9:421, 1981.

57. Kopman AF, Wollman SB, Ross K et al: Awake endotracheal intubation: a review of 267 cases, *Anesth Analg* 54:323, 1975.

58. Kunkel MD, Rowland M, and Scheinman MM: The electrophysiologic effects of lidocaine in patients with intraventricular conduction defects, *Circulation* 49:894, 1974.

59. Larach MG: Standardization of the caffeine halothane muscle contracture test, *Anesth Analg* 69:511, 1989.

60. Lawson W, Kessler S, and Biller HF: Unusual and fatal complication of rhinoplasty, *Arch Otolaryngol* 109:164, 1983.

61. Lechman MJ, Donahoo JS, and Macuvauch H: Endotracheal intubation using percutaneous retrograde guidewire insertion followed by antegrade fiberoptic bronchoscopy, *Crit Care Med* 14:589, 1986.

62. MacLeodd P, Patriquin H: The whistling face syndrome—cranio-carpo-tarsal dysplasia, *Clin Pediatr* 13:184, 1974.

63. Mallampati SR, Gatt SP, Gugino LD et al: A clinical sign to predict difficult intubation: a prospective study, *Can Anaesth Soc J* 32:429, 1984.

64. Mandappa JM, Chandrasekhara PM, and Nelvigi RG: Anaphylaxis to suxamethonium, *Br J Anaesth* 47:523, 1975.

65. McLellan I, Gordon P, Khawaja S et al: Percutaneous translaryngeal high frequency jet ventilation as an aid to difficult intubation, *Can Anaesth Soc J* 35:404, 1988.

66. McPherson EW, Taylor CA Jr: The King syndrome: malignant hyperthermia, myopathy, and multiple anomalies, *Am J Med Genet* 8:159, 1981.

67. Meade JW: Tracheostomy: its complications and their management; a study of 212 cases, *N Engl J Med* 265:519, 1961.

68. Melton AT, Martucci RW, Kien ND et al: Malignant hyperthermia in humans—standardization of contracture testing protocol, *Anesth Analg* 69:437, 1989.

69. Meschan I: *Roentgen signs in clinical diagnosis,* Philadelphia, 1956, WB Saunders.

70. Messeter KH, Petterson KI: Endotracheal intubation with the fiberoptic bronchoscope, *Anaesthesia* 35:294, 1980.

71. Miller JD, Kapp J: Complications of tracheostomies in neurosurgical patients, *Surg Neurol* 22:186, 1984.

72. Moore GF, Nissen AJ, and Yonkers AJ: Potential complications of unrecognized cerebrospinal fluid leaks, *Am J Otol* 5:317, 1984.

73. Mueller RA: How to identify malignant hyperthermia, *Probl Anesth* 1:233, 1987.

74. Mulder DS, Wallace DH, and Woodhouse FM: The use of the fiberoptic bronchoscope to facilitate endotracheal intubation following head and neck trauma, *J Trauma* 15:638, 1975.

75. Murphy P: A fibre-optic endoscope used for nasal intubation, *Anaesthesia* 22:489, 1967.

76. Neal GD, Gates GA: Complications of tracheostomy and intubation. In Johns ME, ed: *Complications in otolaryngology–head and neck surgery,* Philadelphia, 1986, BC Decker.

77. Neuman GC, Weingarten AE et al: The anesthetic management of the patient with an anterior mediastinal mass, *Anesthesiology* 60:144, 1984.
78. Oldham HN: Mediastinal tumors and cysts, *Ann Thorac Surg* 11:246, 1971.
79. Park JI, Strelzow VV, and Friedman WH: Current management of cerebrospinal fluid rhinorrhea, *Laryngoscope* 93:1294, 1983.
80. Paul DR, Hoyt JL, and Boutros AR: Cardiovascular and respiratory changes in response to change of position in the very obese, *Anesthesiology* 45:73, 1976.
81. Pellici PM, Ranawat CS, Tsairis P et al: A prospective study of the progression of rheumatoid arthritis of the cervical spine, *J Bone Joint Surg* 63A:342, 1981.
82. Powell WF, Ozdil T: A translaryngeal guide for tracheal intubation, *Anesth Analg* 46:231, 1967.
83. Raj PP, Forestner J, Watson T et al: Techniques for fiberoptic laryngoscopy in anesthesia, *Anesth Analg* 53:708, 1974.
84. Rex M: A review of the structural and functional basis of laryngospasm: nerve pathways and clinical significance, *Br J Anaesth* 42:891, 1970.
85. Rhine EJ, Johnson GG: Upper airway obstruction in paediatrics, *Clin Anesth* 3:721, 1985.
86. Riou B, Barriot P, Bodenan P et al: Retrograde tracheal intubation in trauma patients, *Anesthesiology* 67:A130, 1987.
87. Rogers SN, Benumof JL: New and easy techniques for fiberoptic endoscopy aided tracheal intubation, *Anesthesiology* 59:569, 1983.
88. Rosenberg H, Rosenberg H: Airway obstruction and causes of difficult intubation. In Orkin FK, Cooperman LH, eds: *Complications in anesthesiology,* Philadelphia, 1983, JB Lippincott.
89. Rosenberg H, Rosenberg H: Syndromes associated with upper airway abnormalities. In Orkin FK, Cooperman LH, eds: *Complications in anesthesiology,* Philadelphia, 1983, JB Lippincott.
90. Rowe LD, Miller E, and Brandt-Zawadzki M: Computed tomography in maxillofacial trauma, *Laryngoscope* 91:745, 1981.
91. Safar P: *Cardiopulmonary cerebral resuscitation,* London, 1981, Laerdal.
92. Saidman W, Havard ES, and Eger EI: Hyperthermia during anesthesia in a patient with myotonia congenita, *JAMA* 190:1029, 1964.
93. Saunders WH: The larynx, *Ciba Found Symp* 16:35, 1964.
94. Schwartz L, Rockoff MA, and Koka BV: Masseter spasm with anesthesia: incidence and implications, *Anesthesiology* 61:772, 1984.
95. Seed RF: Traumatic injury to the larynx and trachea, *Anaesthesia* 26:55, 1971.
96. Sivarajan M, Fink BR: The position and the state of the larynx during general anesthesia and muscle paralysis, *Anesthesiology* 72:439, 1990.
97. Smith BR, Babinski M, Klaim M et al: Percutaneous transtracheal ventilation, *J Am Coll Emerg Physicians* 5:765, 1976.
98. Spoerel WE, Narayanan PS, and Singh NP: Transtracheal ventilation, *Br J Anaesth* 43:923, 1971.
99. Stauffer JL, Silvestri RC: Complications of endotracheal intubation, tracheostomy, and artificial airways, *Respir Care* 27:417, 1982.
100. Stoelting RK: Blood pressure and heart rate changes during short duration laryngoscopy for tracheal intubations: influence of viscous or intravenous lidocaine, *Anesth Analg* 57:197, 1978.
101. Symposium of malignant hyperthermia, *Br J Anaesth* 60:251, 1988.
102. Taylor PA, Towley RM: The bronchofiberscope as an aid to endotracheal intubation, *Br J Anaesth* 44:611, 1972.
103. Thomas JL: Awake intubation: indications, techniques, and a review of 25 patients, *Anaesthesia* 24:28, 1969.
104. Trunkey DD: Trauma, *Sci Am* 249:28, 1983.
105. Van Der Spek AFL, Fang WB, Ashton-Miller JA et al: The effects of succinylcholine on mouth opening, *Anesthesiology* 67:459, 1987.
106. Van Der Spek AFL, Fang WB, Ashton-Miller JA et al: Increased masticatory muscle stiffness during limb muscle flaccidity associated with succinylcholine administration, *Anesthesiology* 69:11, 1988.
107. Vaughn RW, Bauer S, and Wise L: Volume and pH of gastric juice in obese patients, *Anesthesiology* 43:686, 1975.
108. Vnek J, Janda J, Amblerova V et al: Freeman-Sheldon syndrome: a disorder of congenital myopathic origin? *J Med Genet* 23:231, 1986.
109. Walts LF: Anesthesia of the larynx in the patient with a full stomach, *JAMA* 192:121, 1965.
110. Wang JF, Reves JG, and Gutierrez FA: Awake fiberoptic laryngoscopic tracheal intubation for anterior cervical fusion in patients with cervical cord trauma, *Int Surg* 64:3:69, 1979.
111. Waters DJ: Guided blind endobronchial intubation, *Anaesthesia* 18:158, 1963.
112. Webster AC: Anesthesia for operations of the upper airway, *Int Anesthesiol Clin* 10:110, 1972.
113. Wells AL, Wells TR, Landing BH et al: Short trachea, a hazard in tracheal intubation of neonates and infants: syndromal associations, *Anesthesiology* 71:367, 1989.
114. Wilson RD, Putnam L, Phillips MT et al: Anesthetic problems in surgery for varying levels of respiratory obstruction in infants and children, *Anesth Analg* 53:878, 1974.

CHAPTER 14

Evaluation of the Patient with Pulmonary Disease

PHILIP G. BOYSEN

Pulmonary Function Testing
Chronic Obstructive Pulmonary Disease
  Emphysema
  Chronic bronchitis
  Asthma
Pulmonary Function and Chronic Obstructive
  Pulmonary Disease
Gas Exchange Abnormalities
Bronchodilator Therapy
Preoperative Evaluation
Conclusions

Chronic pulmonary disease, especially chronic obstructive pulmonary disease (COPD), continues to be a major cause of morbidity and mortality,[2] particularly for the surgical patient in whom underlying pulmonary compromise may pose additional risk in the immediate postoperative period. The identification and treatment of COPD are essential to improving outcome.[23,30] Therefore it is useful to review the typical clinical presentations of the various types of COPD and outline the preoperative, intraoperative, and postoperative management techniques that are used to improve physiologic function. Furthermore, a discussion of the objective tests that define limitation of pulmonary function is appropriate.

PULMONARY FUNCTION TESTING

Spirometric testing is simple in concept but often difficult for the patient with chronic lung disease.[25] It involves measuring the amount of gas exhaled over time, as the patient forces air from the lungs from total lung capacity (TLC) to residual volume (RV).[22] In the tracing (Fig. 14-1) several parameters are of interest, including the forced vital capacity (FVC), the forced expiratory volume at 1 second (FEV_1), the ratio of FEV_1/FVC, and measurement of midflows (i.e., the forced expiratory flow from 25% to 75% of the vital capacity (FEF_{25-75}) and the exhaled flow at 50% of the vital capacity (FEF_{50}).[17]

From these data, certain judgments can be made. Reduction of the FVC is characteristic of restrictive physiology, which can be either extrinsic (paralyzed diaphragm, obesity, kyphoscoliosis, and so on) or intrinsic (interstitial fibrosis). The FEV_1 and FEV_1/FVC are generally well preserved. **The patient with chronic obstructive lung disease usually does not show a reduction in FVC until late in the natural history of the disease. Reduction of the FEV_1 and FEV_1/FVC is characteristic of chronic airway obstruction.** Both the patient with asthma and the patient with chronic bronchitis will show an immediate improvement after bronchodilator therapy, especially the patient with asthma.[6,34] An improvement in exhaled midflows (FEF_{25-75} and FEF_{50}) is also important in presurgical patients. It is this group who most benefits from preoperative therapy to maximize pulmonary function.

A more sophisticated way of representing the forced vital capacity maneuver is to plot the changes in exhaled or inhaled gas flow and the relationship to lung volume.[29] If an inspiratory maneuver back to TLC follows forced exhalation, a *flow-volume loop* is inscribed. Similar data can be extracted from these loops, including the FVC, FEV_1, PEFR, FEF_{25-75} and FEF_{50} (Fig. 14-2). The technique is a sensitive means of detecting early chronic obstructive lung disease because the final decrement in flow (i.e., at low lung

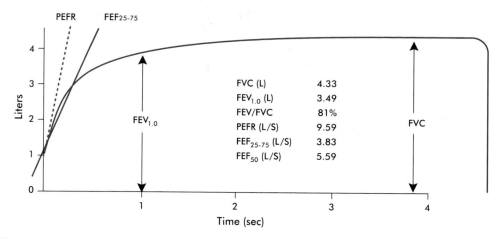

Fig. 14-1. A spirogram plots volume vs. time during a forced exhalation. Several patient attempts are made to achieve the best effort. The forced vital capacity *(FVC)*, forced expiratory volume at 1 second *(FEV$_{1.0}$)*, FEV/FVC ratio, peak expiratory flow rate *(PEFR)*, forced expiratory flow between 25% and 75% of vital capacity *(FEF$_{25-75}$)*, and forced expiratory flow at 50% of vital capacity *(FEF$_{50}$)* are then calculated. Spirometry is repeated after bronchodilator therapy.

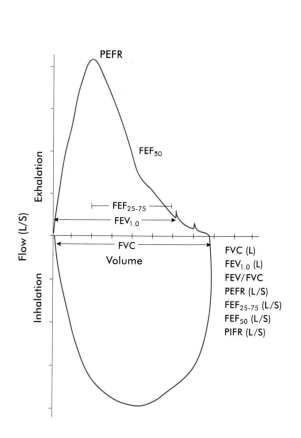

Fig. 14-2. The same forced exhalation shown in Fig. 14-1 is represented on a flow vs. volume graph, and a deep inspiration closes the loop. The FEV$_{1.0}$, FVC, PEFR, FEF$_{25-75}$, and FEF$_{50}$ can also be obtained. Note the coven shape of the last half of the exhalation curve suggesting early airflow obstruction in small airways despite apparently normal FEV$_{1.0}$ and FVC.

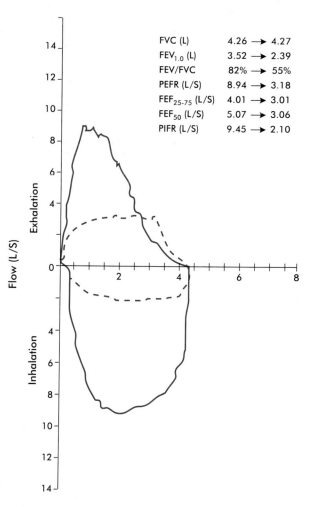

Fig. 14-3. The normal flow-volume loop *(solid line)* is superimposed on a box-shaped loop *(dashed line)* characteristic of fixed upper airway obstruction. Major limitations in peak flow and midflow are recorded.

volume) is independent of effort, and decreased flows are evident before changes in the FEV_1 or FEV_1/FVC are obvious. This results in a "coven-shaped" change in the exhalation portion of the flow-volume loop.

Chronic airflow obstruction of the distal airways can be differentiated from upper airway obstruction by analyzing flow-volume loops.[39] Obstruction of the upper airway anatomy, larynx or trachea, is of particular interest to the anesthesiologist. Such lesions often result in fixed but limited airflow through the obstructing lesion (Fig. 14-3). **When the obstruction is extrathoracic, changes are most obvious during inhalation on the flow-volume loop. The clinical correlate is inspiratory stridor. When the lesion is intrathoracic, exhalation is affected. Fixed obstruction in the upper airway affects the entire loop.**

CHRONIC OBSTRUCTIVE PULMONARY DISEASE

Obstructive pulmonary disease by definition implies that flow resistance is increased during the respiratory cycle. For the most part, chronic obstructive pulmonary disease (COPD) is characterized by resistance to airflow during exhalation. Inspiration during COPD, unlike that during obstruction of the upper airway or pharyngeal obstruction, is usually normal and thus does not contribute to additional respiratory work during ventilation. Several factors may contribute to this increased flow resistance, including changes within the lumen of the airway, in the wall of the airway, or in the peribronchial structures. Intraluminal changes include increased secretions that tend to pool in the airway, aspiration of liquid contents from the pharynx or stomach, and chronic conditions that may also increase airway secretions. **Changes in the lumenal wall are specifically seen with hypertrophy and bronchospasm of bronchial smooth muscle, such as observed in those with asthma and chronic bronchitis.** In addition, edema or inflammation of the wall of the airway may cause airflow obstruction during exhalation. Changes outside the lumen associated with airflow obstruction include loss of lung parenchyma and the concomitant structural support, external compression of the airway such as by lymph nodes or tumors, and peribronchial, perivascular edema impinging on the wall of the airway. Any of these changes or a combination of these changes may be observed in patients with COPD.

Physiologic abnormalities seen in those with COPD include emphysema, chronic bronchitis, and chronic asthma.[5] Each of these three alterations in physiologic structure is accompanied by typical changes in the clinical presentation, history, physical examination, and routine pulmonary function tests. Asthma is usually thought of as an episodic alteration of bronchial smooth muscle tone with normal pulmonary function and a complete absence of symptoms during remission. Many patients, however, have chronic asthma and are usually in a compromised state due to increased smooth muscle tone; they may also have exacerbations that cause acute worsening of their pulmonary function and symptomatology. Because these patients are at increased risk when anesthetized for surgical procedures, they are included under the classification of COPD.

Emphysema

Emphysema is often referred to as Type A COPD in the nomenclature of chronic obstructive lung disease.[14] Many patients have presenting symptoms that indicate a diagnosis of pure emphysema, some show a clinical and physiologic picture consistent with chronic bronchitis, and still others show a mixture of these two clinical conditions. **Emphysema is characterized by destruction of the lung parenchyma with a loss of effective surface area for gas transfer and a loss of radial traction necessary to support the thin, filamentous, anatomic surfaces used for gas exchange.** These patients, however, are referred to as "pink puffers," because they may have relatively advanced disease with preservation of arterial oxygen tensions and no tendency toward arterial oxygen desaturation. In addition, they usually do not retain carbon dioxide so that an increase in alveolar and arterial carbon dioxide tensions is not usually evident until very late in the course of the disease, when death may be imminent. **Spirometry is characterized by diminished airflow at all lung volumes with a decrease in the FEV_1/FVC ratio, the hallmark of chronic air flow obstruction.**[14] **There is also a tendency toward hyperinflation and gas trapping,** which is evident by an increase in the residual volume to total lung capacity (RV/TLC) ratio and by specific changes in the chest radiograph.[16] These include low, **flat diaphragms** and extremely **hyperlucent lung fields,** consistent with both gas trapping and the loss of lung parenchyma. Because of these changes, **the heart usually appears small on the chest radiograph** and there is evidence of decreased pulmonary vasculature along with the destruction of alveolar septae. Most of these patients do not suffer from repeated episodes of respiratory failure, they have scant or insignificant production of sputum, and **they do not manifest signs of right heart failure and cor pulmonale.**

Chronic Bronchitis

Chronic bronchitis is referred to as Type B COPD. It is also characterized by anatomic changes that include **proliferation and hypertrophy of the bronchial glands and reactive bronchial smooth musculature.** Because of the change in glandular anatomy and structure, there is also an increase in se ..ions that tend to inspissate and occlude the airways. **Chronic cough** is characteristic, usually productive, and often purulent, due to colonization of the airway with a variety of gram-positive and gram-negative bacteria. **Unlike the emphysematous patient, there is an early tendency toward arterial oxygen desaturation.** In addition, the alveolar and arterial carbon dioxide tensions often increase, so that **hypoxia and hypercarbia are characteristic** in those with chronic bronchitis. Because of arterial oxygen desaturation, they are often cyanotic and are thus referred to as "blue bloaters" as opposed to the emphysematous "pink puffers." Resting pulmonary function is also characterized by a fall in the FEV_1/FVC ratio; however, **lung volumes are usually near normal unless there is an exacerbation of infection and bronchospasm,** in which case there is also a tendency toward hyperinflation and gas trapping.[14] Consistent changes are observed on the chest radiograph and with measurement of lung volumes. Successful treatment of these acute episodes usually results in a return to baseline of these lung volumes. Thus the course of chronic bronchitis is characterized by multiple episodes of respiratory failure, often with acute and episodic bronchospasm, an increase in secretions, a change to a more purulent productive cough, and a febrile state.[16] During these episodes, hypoxia and hypercarbia may worsen. These patients do not usually do well if it is necessary to intubate the trachea and begin mechanical ventilation. For this reason, recent therapeutic approaches have concentrated on pharmacologic management and low-flow oxygen therapy to preserve oxygen delivery during the acute episode. Finally, these patients **often have an increase in pulmonary vascular resistance,** which is probably due to the changes in arterial oxygen saturation. This is especially noteworthy as the disease progresses, because the work of the right side of the heart often increases, which **can result in right-sided heart failure and cor pulmonale,** manifested by increased hepatojugular reflux and peripheral edema.

Asthma

As already mentioned, asthma is usually characterized in the younger patient by long periods of remission during which time the patient is usually free of symptoms, and measured pulmonary function data are normal or near normal. During exacerbations of chronic airflow obstruction and constriction of bronchial smooth muscle, changes in the FEV_1/FVC ratio are noted. At this time there may also be an increase in secretions that occlude the airway, further compromising exhaled gas flow.[38] These secretions are often thick and tenacious. If they occlude the airway they are referred to as Curschmann's spirals. Exam-

ination of these secretions may reveal hypereosinophilia consistent with the fact that there is often an allergic process either initiating or complicating episodes of airflow obstruction.

The mechanisms of the changes in the airway and the bronchial smooth muscle are not fully elucidated but are now better appreciated. **A series of intracellular events modulates smooth muscle function through the production of cyclic AMP or cyclic GMP. These two compounds antagonize each other such that an increase in cyclic AMP results in relaxation of bronchial smooth muscle, whereas an increase in cyclic GMP results in constriction of bronchial smooth muscle.** This is further modulated by reaction to specific antigens, which is initiated when IgE is released in the presence of antigenemia and fixes itself to plasma cells in the bronchial smooth muscle in the wall of the airway. Once this occurs there is release of mediators from granules in the mast cell. Some of these mediators include histamine, slow-releasing substance of anaphylaxis (SRSA), eosinophilic chemotactic factor (ECF-A), and bradykinins. All of these compounds increase the tone of bronchial smooth muscle, thereby causing bronchospasm.

The autonomic nervous system also plays a factor in control of bronchial smooth muscle tone. **There is a balance between the sympathetic and parasympathetic nervous systems, which results in the alteration of the caliber of the airways. Stimulation of the sympathetic nervous system causes bronchial relaxation or bronchodilation, whereas parasympathetic stimulation causes bronchoconstriction or increased bronchomotor tone.** The latter mechanism is particularly sensitive in patients who tend to have bronchospasm due to emotional stress, nonallergic irritants, inhalation of cold air, or exercise. For this reason, a therapeutic approach has been advised that includes stimulation of the sympathetic nervous system using sympathomimetic agents, or blockade (i.e., parasympatholysis), of the parasympathetic nervous system. Because activation of this system tends to be vagally mediated, there are good reasons to use this therapy in the patient about to receive a general anesthetic. This is because manipulation and intubation of the upper airway may cause bronchospasm.

PULMONARY FUNCTION AND CHRONIC OBSTRUCTIVE PULMONARY DISEASE

Early in the course of chronic bronchitis or emphysema, the forced vital capacity (FVC) is usually normal. However, both conditions are diagnosed by a history, physical examination, and a decrease in the FEV_1/FVC ratio, as noted previously. Because of airflow obstruction, the maximal voluntary ventilation (MVV) also decreases. **The lung volume measure-**

ments are near normal in the patient with chronic bronchitis unless they are measured during an acute exacerbation of this disease.[11] For the emphysematous patient, there is usually an increase in the total lung capacity, but a more marked increase in the functional residual capacity (FRC) and residual volume (RV). Thus most pulmonary function laboratories will report the RV/TLC ratio or the FRC/TLC ratio, which are evidence of the aforementioned hyperinflation and increased gas trapping. The diffusing capacity for carbon monoxide is usually normal or near normal for the patient with chronic bronchitis[12,16] because the anatomic changes are in bronchial smooth muscle and not in lung parenchyma.[28] However, because the emphysematous patient has loss of effective surface area for gas transfer, he/she will have a decrease in the diffusing capacity for carbon monoxide. When either disease progresses, there may be additional changes consistent with each. For example, the patient with chronic bronchitis may manifest changes in lung volumes and diffusing capacity similar to those in the patient with emphysema. The severely affected emphysematous patient may become so compromised and hyperinflated that his/her vital capacity is restricted due to these changes in lung volumes. When this occurs, there is a severe prolongation of the FEV_1 and a decrease in the forced vital capacity consistent with severe hyperinflation.

The patient with asthma also tends to have rather specific pulmonary function abnormalities, especially during exacerbations of the disease. In addition to the decrease in the FEV_1/FVC ratio, there is also a decrease in airflow throughout the range of vital capacity. Tests used to describe these changes include the maximal mid-expiratory flow rate (MMEFR), maximal midflow rate (MMF), and the FEF_{50}, (the forced expiratory flow of 50% of the vital capacity). In addition, during acute attacks of bronchospasm the RV/TLC and the FRC/TLC ratios may increase.[49] The diffusing capacity for carbon monoxide may be abnormal and varies depending on the way it is measured. Many investigators have suggested correcting the diffusing capacity for the alveolar volume or the inhaled gas volume using the single breath technique.[3] This D_L/V_A or the K_{CO} or specific diffusing capacity is a technique meant to normalize the measurement for the alveolar gas volume.[46] This measurement is usually normal, especially during disease remission. In addition, the patient with asthma may evidence a significant response to bronchodilators when spirometry is repeated. In the untreated asthmatic patient it has been suggested that administration of a nebulized bronchodilator, such as isoproterenol, will result in an improvement in airflow and, if the obstruction is severe enough, an increase in the vital capacity. The degree of improvement in

airflow is debatable, but in general a 20% to 25% increase in either the FEV_1 or the FVC is considered a significant response to the bronchodilator consistent with a diagnosis of asthma.

The patient with chronic bronchitis will also tend to respond immediately to a nebulized bronchodilator. In this case there may be anatomic changes in the airway, but also some degree of bronchospasm is evident. It is rare, however, for the patient with chronic bronchitis to manifest a 25% improvement in spirometric function. However, a change in the range of 5% to 10% is consistent with the clinical diagnosis of chronic bronchitis.[6]

It should be reemphasized that spirometric testing is useful only in demonstrating physiologic abnormalities or the degree of impairment. As an example, the patient with chronic bronchitis is diagnosed by history and physical examination. If such a patient produces sputum 2 months out of a year 2 years in a row and has the stigmata and evident history of wheezing cyanosis and so on, this diagnosis is confirmed.[14] The response to bronchodilators has been studied as a technique to determine which patient may benefit from a preoperative regimen of bronchopulmonary toilet that usually includes bronchodilators. This response, when seen in a patient with a consistent history and physical examination, indicates the need to administer preoperative therapy. Particularly when there is improvement in the flows and these can be sustained pharmacologically, both the intraoperative and postoperative courses improve. It is becoming more apparent that not only morbidity decreases but also mortality, particularly after upper abdominal surgery.

GAS EXCHANGE ABNORMALITIES

Gas exchange abnormalities occur in concert with changes in pulmonary mechanics. Where there is bronchospasm and uneven ventilation, there is a subsequent mismatching between ventilation and perfusion. During bronchospasm, perfusion is altered in an attempt to maintain matching between ventilation and blood flow. This is successful to some degree, but the low ventilation/perfusion (V/Q) state particularly consistent with chronic bronchitis and asthma results in arterial oxygen desaturation and hypoxemia. Elegant six gas techniques have been used to document areas of low V/Q and the efficacy of administered bronchodilators; conversely, bronchial provocation tests have also been measured.[1,41] It has been shown that the bronchodilator improves not only airflow obstruction and lung mechanisms but also gas exchange and other abnormalities. A transient decrease in arterial oxygen saturation has sometimes been noted with the administration of a bronchodilator. This is presumably because there is also some effect on vascular smooth muscle that may be more immediate than the subsequent relaxation of bronchial smooth muscle and dilatation of the airways. This fall in the arterial oxygen tension is usually not clinically significant, is transient, and is followed by an immediate rise as bronchial smooth muscle begins to relax.

In most patients with acute bronchospasm, carbon dioxide elimination is normal, even though hypoxemia may be severe. This is because—unlike the oxyhemoglobin association curve—the carbon dioxide dissociation curve is linear, and carbon dioxide is a readily diffusible gas. The ability to eliminate carbon dioxide is fairly well preserved until V/Q abnormalities and bronchospasm are severe. At this point the arterial carbon dioxide tension begins to rise, a particularly ominous sign in the acutely ill asthmatic patient. Chronic carbon dioxide retention, as seen in the patient with chronic bronchitis, is usually observed as the disease progresses and occurs so slowly that a compensated respiratory acidosis is noted on arterial blood gas analysis. The reason for the rise in carbon dioxide tension is not well defined but is probably due to the increased respiratory muscle work that occurs late in the course of the disease.[47] At some point the ability to maintain normal carbon dioxide tension is apparently overwhelmed by a significant increase in respiratory muscle work such that a new baseline must be accepted, and a new steady state then evolves.

BRONCHODILATOR THERAPY

Bronchodilator therapy is efficacious in patients who tend to have bronchospasm and increased intraluminal secretions. As noted previously, there seems to be a system of checks and balances that makes **combined therapy** to achieve desired therapeutic results particularly useful. Therapy is usually begun with an inhaled bronchodilator, specifically a beta$_2$ agonist. These agents are designed to be specific for beta$_2$ receptor sites that modulate changes in smooth muscle tone. The newer drugs are relatively free of the alpha$_1$ and beta$_1$ side effects, tachycardia and an increase in blood pressure. Metaproterenol, orciprenaline, and albuterol are the newer agents of choice. **The second approach is to stimulate the production of c-AMP by the administration of methylxanthines.** Whereas other sympathomimetics are delivered by a metered dose aerosol, these agents are given either intravenously or orally. Aminophylline (85% theophylline) is the agent of choice, and its effect is caused by inhibition of the phosphodiesterase enzyme, which causes the breakdown of cyclic AMP. Thus sympathomimetics increase the intracellular concentration of cyclic AMP, and methylxanthines are phosphodiesterase inhibitors, which impair the breakdown of

this compound. In addition, atropine and its analogs are useful in alleviating bronchospasm by causing **parasympatholysis.** Atropine often has troublesome side effects so that the **atropine analog, ipratropium bromide,** has been recently introduced as an adjunct to bronchodilator therapy. It is also given by metered dose inhaler and has been remarkably free of side effects. **Cromolyn sodium and corticosteroids** are useful in preventing bronchospasm in the asthmatic **patient in remission** but are not particularly useful during acute episodes. Cromolyn sodium tends to **stabilize the mast cell** and prevent release of mediators, and the corticosteroids are inhaled and nonabsorbable. Beclamethasone dipropionate and triamcinolone acetohexamide are examples of these drugs.

PREOPERATIVE EVALUATION

If a patient is suspected of having compromised pulmonary function, it is reasonable and cost-effective to measure baseline spirometry—both before and after the administration of a nebulized bronchodilator—and the maximal voluntary ventilation (MVV). Arterial blood gas analysis further provides a baseline assessment of gas exchange and identifies the patient who is chronically hypoxemic or hypercarbic. Additional studies, such as the measurement of lung volumes and diffusing capacity, further define abnormal physiology and are helpful for the patient being assessed for thoracotomy. For the patient about to undergo an abdominal surgical procedure, there are no clear indications that additional testing is helpful. In addition, whether to extend testing to patients who are elderly or obese or who smoke is controversial. Tisi recommends an approach to preoperative pulmonary function testing, which is listed in Box 14-1.[53]

It is important to recognize the physiologic abnormalities, particularly after abdominal or thoracic surgery, that are superimposed on baseline pulmo-

---

BOX 14-1
CANDIDATES FOR PREOPERATIVE
EVALUATION OF PULMONARY FUNCTION

Patients having thoracic surgery
Patients having upper abdominal surgery
Patients with history of heavy smoking and cough
Obese patients
Elderly patients (> 70 years old)
Patients with documented pulmonary disease

From Tisi GN: *Pulmonary physiology in clinical medicine*, Baltimore, 1980, Williams & Wilkins.

nary function in the immediate postoperative period.[33] **Because of a combination of factors, including abnormal diaphragmatic function,[20,52] there is a loss in lung volume (FRC and TLC), an increase in respiratory rate, a decrease in tidal volume, and a widening of the alveolar-to-arterial oxygen tension gradient.** The latter change is due to the fall in lung volume (often referred to as microatelectasis) and is a manifestation of right-to-left shunt in the lung. In essence, the abnormalities in pulmonary function are characteristic of a transient, superimposed, restrictive physiologic process that is most evident on the first postoperative day (Fig. 14-4). Recovery of 80% of preoperative function is usually evident by the third day after surgery. An underlying chronic change in physiology—either restriction or airway obstruction—may combine with acute changes, resulting in the patient's inability to sustain spontaneous ventilation. Intraoperative and postoperative monitoring, combined with preoperative assessment, are essential to assist recovery during this crucial time. Recovery of lung volume and thus lung function is the goal of postoperative therapy. Inspiratory maneuvers designed to increase FRC include active regimens such as incentive spirometry, deep-breathing exercises, or passive lung inflation by intermittent positive pressure breathing. If FRC increases as a result of these measures, lung mechanics and gas exchange are improved. This improvement is manifested as increased tidal ventilation, decreased respiratory rate, and improved arterial oxygen saturation and oxygen tension. Adequate management of postoperative pain is an integral part of postoperative therapy but will not totally reverse the abnormalities. Furthermore, narcotic therapy may unmask a tendency to retain carbon dioxide in patients with COPD.

Unfortunately, no pulmonary function test specifically relates to postoperative outcome or the occurrence of postoperative pulmonary complications. In addition, it is difficult to assign a specific value for each test or reduction in function that defines risk. Some guidelines are useful, however, and these are represented in Box 14-2. If a given patient fails to meet any of these parameters, the risk of postoperative pulmonary complications is increased. How to respond to these abnormalities depends on the type of surgery being considered. For the patient about to undergo an abdominal procedure, adequate attention should be focused on a regimen of preoperative therapy. This regimen should include the administration of a nebulized beta$_2$ agonist for bronchodilation, an oral theophylline preparation, and antibiotic therapy if there is productive cough and purulent sputum. Consideration should be given to the addition of nebulized atropine or an atropine analog to achieve parasympatholysis and thus facilitate anesthetic induction, especially if there is clinical evidence of reactive bronchospasm.[24]

The patient about to undergo thoracotomy and lung resection who fails to pass these criteria is also at considerable risk.[8,21,35,40] If a pneumonectomy is required, remaining lung tissue may be inadequate to sustain life. Severe hypoxemia and cor pulmonale leading to imminent death may result.[26] An analysis of the total contribution of each lung to overall function, or split lung function studies, is necessary. This has been accomplished by bronchospirometry,[42] the lateral position test,[27,36,48,55] balloon occlusion studies,[13,32,54] and V/Q lung scanning.[9,31,43,44]

Bronchospirometry, an early method of measuring split lung function, is the most direct technique.[42] An **awake patient** is prepared with topical anesthetics and then a **double lumen tube** is passed into the patient's airway. Since the distal portion of the tube allows endobronchial intubation, inflation of appropriately positioned cuffs allows collection of exhaled gas from each lung. Flow resistance through these orifices is

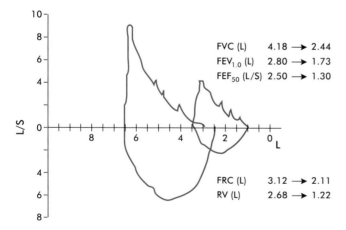

FVC (L)	4.18 → 2.44
FEV$_{1.0}$ (L)	2.80 → 1.73
FEF$_{50}$ (L/S)	2.50 → 1.30

FRC (L)	3.12 → 2.11
RV (L)	2.68 → 1.22

Fig. 14-4. A flow-volume loop measured before cholecystectomy *(left),* and another the first postoperative day after coaching and pain medication *(right).* The shift to the right indicates a fall in lung volumes. The smaller, but similarly shaped, loop indicates a restrictive process.

BOX 14-2
PULMONARY FUNCTION CRITERIA INDICATING INCREASED RISK

FVC < 50% of predicted
FEV$_1$ < 50% of predicted or < 2.0 L
MVV < 50% of predicted or < 50 L/min
D$_{co}$ < 50% of predicted
RV/TLC > 50%

From Tisi GN: *Pulmonary physiology in clinical medicine,* Baltimore, 1980, Williams & Wilkins.

markedly increased, but exhaled volume can be measured and the total FVC appropriately partitioned into right vs. left components.

The **hemodynamic correlate** of the ventilatory measurement achieved by bronchospirometry is **temporary unilateral balloon occlusion of the pulmonary artery of the lung about to be resected.** Interruption of flow to that lung causes a temporary pneumonectomy with subsequent shift of ventilation away from the occluded lung. A rise in the proximal pulmonary artery pressure or a decrease in oxygen tension or saturation indicates lessened likelihood of survival with one lung remaining. **If the arterial oxygen tension falls below 45 mm Hg during occlusion or the mean pulmonary artery pressure rises above 30 mm Hg, the occurrence of cor pulmonale postpneumonectomy is likely.**[54] The results of these studies are combined with those found during low levels of exercise. For general exercise tolerance studies, the usefulness of various protocols have yielded conflicting results.* However, **if low levels of exercise cause the arterial oxygen saturation to fall by more than 2% from resting baseline, the prognosis is serious.**[37]

Less invasive methods of achieving similar information are available, including the lateral position test and V/Q lung scanning. The latter test is now widely available. Lung scanning data can be combined with preoperative pulmonary function data to predict postoperative level of function. The less expensive **perfusion scan can** be used alone with technetium or iodine isotopes,[45] but **radioactive xenon provides information for both ventilation and perfusion with one study.**[31] The total number of counts over both lungs are obtained, and each lung is scanned separately through a split function crystal and collimator. Ventilation and perfusion are reported in the percent of overall function in each lung relative to the total number of radioactive counts taken over a specified

---

* References 4, 7, 10, 15, 18, 19, 50, 51.

period. Predictive formulas usually involve the FEV_1 as follows[43]:

Predicted postoperative FEV_1
$$= \text{Preoperative } FEV_1 \times \% \text{ FNC remaining lung}$$

The predicted postoperative FEV_1 must exceed 800 cc for the patient to survive pneumonectomy after curative surgical resection. Calculations are made for pneumonectomy in all patients since it may be necessary to remove the entire lung once the opened chest is examined during surgery. In the event that less resection is adequate, postoperative function can also be predicted using anatomic information. For example, right upper lobectomy involves removal of 3 of the 10 bronchopulmonary segments on the right side. Therefore,

Predicted postoperative FEV_1
$$= \text{Preoperative } FEV_1 \times \% \text{ FCN remaining lung} + \frac{7}{10} \times \% \text{ FCN operative lung}$$

Pain relief and postoperative therapy are important to recover function in the remaining 70% of lung tissue on the operative side because the lung has usually been collapsed during surgery and may be edematous due to manipulation.

CONCLUSIONS

Preoperative assessment of the patient with pulmonary compromise is based on sound physiologic principles. Knowledge of chronic pulmonary disease and pathophysiologic alterations in pulmonary function is integral to preanesthetic evaluation. Changes in function intraoperatively and postoperatively depend on the site of surgical incision, duration of operation, and underlying pulmonary function. An adequately designed regimen for anesthetic management is designed to maximize pulmonary function during the preoperative, intraoperative, and postoperative periods.

KEY POINTS

- Patients with chronic obstructive lung disease usually do not show reduction in FVC until late in the course of the disease.
- Hallmark of chronic airflow obstruction: decreased FEV/FVC ratio.
- Flow volume loops can differentiate among extrathoracic, intrathoracic, and fixed obstructions.
- Asthma and chronic bronchitis lead to such changes in the bronchial lumen wall as hypertrophy or bronchospasm.

- Emphysema is characterized by destruction of lung parenchyma and loss of surface area for gas transfer.
- Chronic bronchitis is characterized by proliferative hypertrophy of bronchial glands and smooth muscle.
- In asthma the balance between (1) c-AMP → bronchial relaxation and c-GMP → bronchoconstruction and (2) sympathetic nervous system → bronchial relaxation and parasympathetic nervous

system bronchoconstriction is mediated, as well, by antigen/IgE and mediators from mast cells, (e.g., SRSA, ECFA, bradykinin, and histamine).

- Lung volume in (1) chronic bronchitis is near normal, except during acute exacerbation, and in (2) emphysema is usually increased TLC with increased FRC and increased RV.

- Bronchodilator therapy improves airflow obstruction, lung mechanism, and gas exchange (e.g., beta-agonist, methylxanthines, ipratroprium bromide and corticosteroids, and, for the patient in remission, cromolyn sodium).

- Carbon dioxide dissociation curve is linear and the gas is readily diffusible; hence the ability to eliminate carbon dioxide is well preserved until V/Q abnormalities and bronchospasm are severe.

- Physiologic changes are seen in pulmonary function, particularly during abdominal and thoracic surgery: (1) diaphragmatic dysfunction, (2) FRC decreased, (3) TLC decreased, (4) decreased TV, (5) RR increased, (6) A-a gradient increased.

- For the patient about to undergo thoracotomy and lung resection, an analysis of the total contribution of each lung to overall function or split lung function studies is necessary (e.g., V/Q lung scanning). The predicted postoperative FEV must exceed 800 cc for the patient to survive pneumonectomy.

KEY REFERENCES

Gracey DR, Divertie MB, and Didier EP: Preoperative pulmonary preparation of patients with chronic obstructive pulmonary disease, *Chest* 76:123, 1979.

Tisi GN: *Pulmonary physiology in clinical medicine,* Baltimore, 1980, Williams & Wilkins.

REFERENCES

1. Alberts WM, Goldman AC: Clinical use of methacholine bronchial challenge testing, *South Med J* 80:827, 1987.
2. Anthonisen NR, Wright FC, and Hodgkin JE: Prognosis in chronic obstructive pulmonary disease, *Am Rev Respir Dis* 133:14, 1986.
3. Ayers LN, Ginsberg MC, Fein J et al: Diffusing capacity, specific diffusing capacity and interpretation of diffusion defects, *West J Med* 123:255, 1975.
4. Bagg LR: The 12-minute walking distance: its use in the preoperative assessment of patients with bronchial carcinoma before lung resection, *Respiration* 46:342, 1984.
5. Becklake MR: Concepts of normality applied to the measurement of lung function, *Am J Med* 80:1158, 1986.
6. Berger R, Smith D: Acute postbronchodilator changes in pulmonary function parameters in patients with chronic airway obstruction, *Chest* 93:541, 1988.
7. Berggren H, Ekroth R, Malmberg R et al: Hospital mortality and long-term survival in relation to preoperative function in elderly patients with bronchogenic carcinoma, *Ann Thorac Surg* 38:633, 1984.
8. Boushy SF, Billig DM, North LB et al: Clinical course related to preoperative and postoperative pulmonary function in patients with bronchogenic carcinoma, *Chest* 59:383, 1971.
9. Boysen PG, Block AJ, Olsen GN et al: Prospective evaluation for pneumonectomy using the Tc99 quantitative perfusion lung scan, *Chest* 72:422, 1977.
10. Boysen PG, Clark CA, and Block AJ: Graded exercise testing and postthoracotomy complications, *J Cardiovasc Anes* 4:68, 1980.
11. Brugman TM, Morris JF, and Temple WP: Comparison of lung volume measurements by single breath helium and multiple breath nitrogen equilibration methods in normal subjects and COPD patients, *Respiration* 49:52, 1986.
12. Burrows B, Kasik JE, Niden AN et al: Clinical usefulness of the single breath diffusing capacity test, *Am Rev Respir Dis* 84:789, 1961.
13. Carlens E, Hanson HE, and Nordenstrom B: Temporary unilateral occlusion of the pulmonary artery, *J Thorac Surg* 22:527, 1951.
14. Cherniack RM, Cherniack L, and Naimark A: *Respiration in health and disease,* ed 2, Philadelphia, 1972, WB Saunders.
15. Coleman NC, Schraufnagel DE, Rivington RN et al: Exercise testing in evaluation of patients for lung resection, *Am Rev Respir Dis* 125:604, 1982.
16. Cotes JE: *Lung function: assessment and application in medicine,* ed 4, Oxford, 1979, Blackwell Scientific Publications.
17. Crapo RO, Morris AH, and Gardner RM: Reference spirometric values using techniques and equipment that meet ATS recommendations, *Am Rev Respir Dis* 123:659, 1981.
18. Eugene J, Brown SE, Light RW et al: Maximum oxygen consumption: a physiologic guide to pulmonary resection, *Surg Forum* 33:260, 1982.
19. Fee JH, Holmes EC, Gerwirtz HS et al: Role of pulmonary resistance measurement in preoperative evaluation of candidates for lung resection, *J Thorac Cardiovasc Surg* 75:519, 1975.
20. Ford GT, Whitelaw WA, Rosenal TW et al: Diaphragm function after upper abdominal surgery in humans, *Am Rev Respir Dis* 127:431, 1983.
21. Gaensler EA, Cusell DW, Lindgren I et al: The role of pulmonary insufficiency in mortality and invalidism following surgery for pulmonary tuberculosis, *J Thorac Cardiovasc Surg* 29:163, 1955.
22. Gardner RM (chairman): ATS statement—Snowbird workshop on standardization of spirometry, *Am Rev Respir Dis* 119:831, 1979.
23. Ginsberg RJ, Hill LD, Eagan RT et al: Modern 30-day operative mortality for surgical resections in lung cancer, *J Thorac Cardiovasc Surg* 86:654, 1983.
24. Gracey DR, Divertie MB, and Didier EP: Preoperative pulmonary preparation of patients with chronic obstructive pulmonary disease, *Chest* 76:123, 1979.
25. Hankinson JL, Gardner RM: Standard waveforms for spirometric testing, *Am Rev Respir Dis* 126:362, 1982.
26. Harrison RW, Adams WE, Long ET et al: The clinical significance of cor pulmonale in the prediction of cardiopulmonary reserve following extensive pulmonary resection, *J Thorac Surg* 36:352, 1958.
27. Jay SJ, Stonehill RB, Kiblani SO et al: Variability of the lateral position test in normal subjects, *Am Rev Respir Dis* 121:165, 1980.

28. Knudson RJ, Kalterborn WT, Knudson DE et al: The single breath carbon monoxide diffusing capacity: reference equations derived from a healthy non-smoking population and the effects of hematocrit, *Am Rev Respir Dis* 135:805, 1987.

29. Knudson RJ, Lebowitz MD, Hobberg CJ et al: Changes in the normal maximal expiratory flow-volume curve with growth and aging, *Am Rev Respir Dis* 127:725, 1983.

30. Kohman LJ, Meyer JA, Ikins PM et al: Random versus predictable risks of mortality after thoracotomy for lung cancer, *J Thorac Cardiovasc Surg* 91:551, 1986.

31. Kristerrson S, Lindell S, and Stranberg L: Prediction of pulmonary function loss due to pneumonectomy using ^{133}Xe-radiospirometry, *Chest* 62:694, 1972.

32. Laros CD, Swierenga J: Temporary unilateral pulmonary artery occlusion in the preoperative evaluation of patients with bronchial carcinoma, *Med Thorac* 24:269, 1967.

33. Latimer RG, Dickman M, Day WC et al: Ventilatory patterns and pulmonary complications after upper abdominal surgery determined by preoperative and postoperative computerized spirometry and blood gas analysis, *Am J Surg* 122:622, 1971.

34. Light RW, Conrad SA, and George RB: The one best test for evaluating effects of bronchodilator therapy, *Chest* 72:512, 1977.

35. Lockwood P: Lung function test results and the risk of postthoracotomy complications, *Respiration* 30:529, 1973.

36. Marion JM, Alderson PO, Lefrak SS et al: Unilateral lung function: comparison of the lateral position test with radionuclide ventilation-perfusion studies, *Chest* 69:5, 1976.

37. Markos J, Mullin BP, Hillman DR et al: Preoperative assessment as a predictor of mortality and morbidity after lung resection, *Am Rev Respir Dis* 139:092, 1989.

38. McKenzie DK, Gandevia SC: Strength and endurance of inspiratory, expiratory and limb muscles in asthma, *Am Rev Respir Dis* 134:999, 1986.

39. Miller RD, Hyatt RE: Evaluation of obstructing lesions of the trachea and larynx by flow-volume loops, *Am Rev Respir Dis* 108:475, 1973.

40. Mittman C: Assessment of operative risk in thoracic surgery, *Am Rev Respir Dis* 84:197, 1961.

41. Myers JR, Carrow WM, and Braman SS: Clinical applications of methacholine inhalational challenge, *JAMA* 246:225, 1981.

42. Neuhaus H, Cherniak NS: A bronchospirometric method of estimating the effect of pneumonectomy on the maximum breathing capacity, *J Thorac Cardiovasc Surg* 55:144, 1968.

43. Olsen GN, Block AJ, and Tobias JA: Prediction of postpneumonectomy pulmonary function using quantitative macroaggregate lung scanning, *Chest* 66:13, 1974.

44. Olsen GN, Block AJ, Swenson EW et al: Pulmonary function evaluation of the lung resection candidate: a prospective study, *Am Rev Respir Dis* 111:379, 1975.

45. Reichel J: Assessment of operative risk of pneumonectomy, *Chest* 62:570, 1972.

46. Rosenberg E, Ernso P, Leech J et al: Specific diffusing capacity (DLNA) as a measure of the lung diffusing charact-eristics: predictor formulas for young adults, *Lung* 164:207, 1986.

47. Roussos C: Function and fatigue of respiratory muscles, *Chest* 88:124, 1985.

48. Schoonover GA, Olsen GN, Habibian MR et al: Lateral position test and quantitative lung scan in the preoperative evaluation for lung resection, *Chest* 86:854, 1984.

49. Short S, Metic-Emili J, and Martin JG: Reassessment of body plethysmographic techniques for measurement of thoracic gas volumes in asthmatics, *Am Rev Respir Dis* 126:515, 1982.

50. Smith TP, Kinasewitz GT, Tucker WY et al: Exercise capacity as a predictor of post-thoracotomy morbidity, *Am Rev Respir Dis* 129:730, 1984.

51. Soderholm B: The hemodynamics of the lesser circulation in pulmonary tuberculosis: the effect of exercise, temporary unilateral pulmonary artery occlusion, and operation, *Scand J Clin Lab Invest* 26:1, 1957.

52. Tahir AH, George RB, Weill H et al: Effects of abdominal surgery upon diaphragmatic function and regional ventilation, *Int Surg* 58:337, 1973.

53. Tisi GN: *Pulmonary physiology in clinical medicine,* Baltimore, 1980, Williams & Wilkins.

54. Uggla LG: Indication for and results of thoracic surgery with regard to respiratory and circulatory function tests, *Acta Chir Scand* 111:197, 1956.

55. Walkup RH, Vossel LF, Griffin JP et al: Prediction of postoperative pulmonary function with the lateral position test: a prospective study, *Chest* 77:24, 1960.

CHAPTER 15

Evaluation of the Patient with Neurologic Disease

JEFFREY R. KIRSCH

MICHAEL N. DIRINGER

This chapter is designed to facilitate understanding of the pathophysiology of disease of the central nervous system (CNS) and suggest an informed approach to preoperative evaluation of such patients. The principal components follow:

- A short review of the normal anatomy and physiology of the intracranial vault, including concepts useful in the management of elevated intracranial pressure (ICP)
- A description of specific neurologic conditions and pathophysiology that is important to consider during a preoperative evaluation
- The pathophysiology of central nervous system trauma (both brain and spinal cord) and how such pathophysiology affects anesthetic management

Patients with neuromuscular diseases are discussed in Chapter 16.

INTRACRANIAL VAULT PHYSIOLOGY

The intracranial vault has three components: brain parenchyma, cerebrospinal fluid (CSF), and blood. Foreign bodies (e.g., tumors, bullets, bone) may add an additional component to intracranial contents. In adults the skull is a rigid structure and does not expand in response to increases in intracranial contents related to physiologic or pathophysiologic processes. The relationship between ICP and intracranial volume is such that, under normal physiologic conditions, the intracranial vault can tolerate increases in volume with only a small rise in pressure. However, at higher intracranial volumes, cerebral compliance is diminished and a small increase in volume results in a dramatic rise in ICP (Fig. 15-1). Although the skull

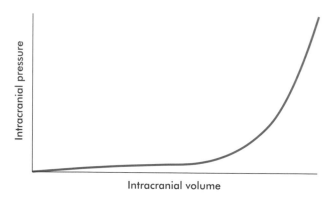

Fig. 15-1. Graph demonstrates the effect of increasing intracranial volume on intracranial pressure.

of an infant before closure of the cranial sutures is much more compliant than that of an adult, it is still subject to intracranial hypertension.

Parenchyma

In adults the brain parenchyma occupies approximately 1400 ml, or about 90% of the intracranial contents. The entry of blood constituents into the parenchyma is strictly regulated by the blood-brain barrier. This barrier excludes endogenous and exogenous blood constituents based on size, lipid solubility, and charge. Concentration gradients of electrolytes across cellular membranes are maintained by selective permeability and continuous action of ionic pumps throughout the brain. Parenchymal edema may result from failure of ionic pumps (cytotoxic edema) and/or breakdown of intracellular components, or leakage of fluid from damaged vasculature endothelium (vasogenic edema).

Cerebrospinal Fluid

The cerebrospinal fluid (CSF) occupies an intracranial volume of approximately 75 ml and accounts for 5% of the intracranial contents. Cerebrospinal fluid is produced by the choroid plexus located in the lateral and fourth ventricles and via bulk movement of fluid through the interstitial space. Under normal circumstances the choroid plexus produces CSF at a rate of 14 to 36 ml/hr.[14] From the fourth ventricle the CSF flows down a pressure gradient through the foramina of Magendie and Luschka, through perimedullary and perispinal subarachnoid spaces, over the brainstem to the cisternae basalis and ambiens. Cerebrospinal fluid then flows over the superior and lateral surfaces of the cerebral hemispheres and down the spinal canal. Reabsorption of CSF occurs in arachnoid villi that are found over the superior surfaces of the cerebral hemispheres, at the base of the brain, and around the spinal nerve roots. Increased CSF volume may result from obstructed flow or reabsorption, or rarely from excessive production.

Blood Volume

The blood volume within the intracranial vault is determined by the cerebral blood flow (CBF) and the size of the capacitance vessel within the brain. **The major capacitance vessels within the brain are veins and sinuses that contain 80% of the intracranial blood volume.** Therefore any factor that affects either CBF or capacitance of cerebral veins will alter cerebral blood volume. **The main physiologic determinants of CBF are cerebral perfusion pressure, arterial oxygen tension (Pao$_2$), arterial carbon dioxide tension (Paco$_2$), and cerebral metabolic rate.** Thus any pharmacologic agent or physiologic intervention that alters one of these four factors, or acts directly on the diameter of cerebral capacitance vessels, will alter cerebral blood volume.

Cerebral perfusion pressure is defined as the difference between mean arterial pressure and the greater of either ICP or cerebral venous pressure. **In normal adults CBF remains constant despite changes in cerebral perfusion pressure from 50 to 150 mm Hg (Fig. 15-2).** This range of autoregulation is shifted to the left in newborns and to the right in patients with chronic hypertension. Cerebral perfusion pressures that exceed the limits of autoregulation increase CBF and therefore cerebral blood volume. In addition, they promote the formation of cerebral edema.

To maintain constant oxygen delivery, the brain responds to a decrease in arterial oxygen content with a compensatory rise in CBF (Figs. 15-3 and 15-4). Cerebral blood flow normally increases when arterial oxygen content falls to approximately half that of normal (Pao$_2$ < 40 mm Hg with a hematocrit of 40% ml/dl). The increase of CBF from decreased arterial oxygen content increases cerebral blood volume and, depending on intracranial compliance, may increase ICP. When arterial oxygen content decreases, brain extraction increases. If the rise in CBF and increase in extraction cannot meet metabolic needs, oxygen consumption (uptake) decreases (Fig. 15-5). Normal oxygen extraction is 30% to 40%; under extreme conditions it may approach 100%. Severe hypoxia that cannot be corrected with an increase in CBF or oxygen extraction leads to direct tissue injury.

Increasing Paco$_2$ produces brain acidosis, which results in vasodilation, increased CBF, and increased cerebral blood volume (see Fig. 15-4). **Decreasing Paco$_2$** produces the opposite response. This relationship is often used clinically to reduce intracranial volume and thus decrease ICP.

Cerebral metabolism and CBF are closely linked. Therefore any drug (e.g., amphetamines) or clinical situation (e.g., fever) that increases metabolism will increase CBF and volume. Drugs that reduce cerebral metabolism (e.g., barbiturates) reduce CBF. Cerebral blood volume is also increased by obstruction of

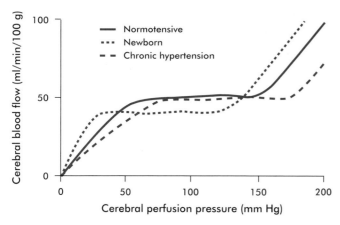

Fig. 15-2. Illustration of changes in cerebral perfusion pressure on cerebral blood flow. The range of autoregulation is shifted to the left in newborns, who have a chronically low cerebral perfusion pressure, and to the right in patients with chronic hypertension.

cerebral venous drainage. Venous drainage can be facilitated by elevating the head of the bed to 30 to 45 degrees and maintaining the head in midline position to avoid jugular compression. In patients with suspected elevation of ICP, anesthesiologists should refrain, if possible, from central venous cannulation via the jugular veins to avoid potential obstruction of cerebral venous drainage.

Increased Intracranial Pressure

Information from the patient history and physical examination may be useful in determining the risk of increased ICP. Historical data help define the nature and extent of the injury. For example, **head trauma with a period of clarity followed by a sudden decline in level of consciousness suggests an epidural hematoma, often secondary to laceration of the middle meningeal artery.** Although headache is usually a benign disorder, when associated with nausea and vomiting or diminished level of consciousness, it suggests increased ICP. The new onset of seizures in an adult may be the first sign of a brain tumor.

The physical examination may reveal diffuse or focal signs of cerebral dysfunction. In the acute setting, global cerebral dysfunction can be quantified with the Glasgow Coma Scale (GCS). This scale, which ranges from scores of 3 to 15, is based on best eye opening and verbal and motor responses (Table 15-1). As ICP rises, the level of consciousness falls, progressing through lethargy, stupor, and finally coma. This may be followed by Cushing's triad (hypertension, bradycardia, and abnormal respiration). This triad is thought to represent severe brainstem dysfunction; however, it is often not seen in its full form. Cranial nerve dysfunction may also be observed in patients with globally increased ICP. **The abducens (VI) nerve, because of its course over the**

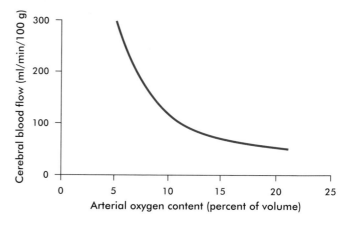

Fig. 15-3. The effect of changes in arterial oxygen content on cerebral blood flow. Arterial oxygen content (CaO_2) can be measured directly or estimated from the hemoglobin concentration (HGB), percent saturation of hemoglobin with oxygen (% sat), and partial pressure of oxygen in arterial blood (PaO_2). $CaO_2 = (1.39)$ HGB (% sat) $+ 0.003$ (PaO_2).

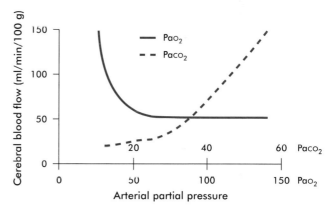

Fig. 15-4. Graph demonstrates the effect of a change in arterial partial pressure of oxygen *(PaO_2)* or carbon dioxide *(PaCO_2)* on cerebral blood flow.

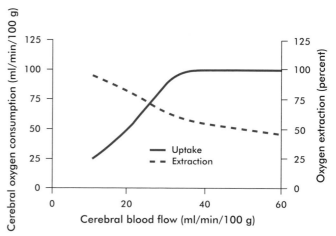

Fig. 15-5. The effect of a change in cerebral blood flow on percent extraction of oxygen from arterial blood *(right axis and dashed line)* and cerebral oxygen consumption *(left axis and solid line)*.

Table 15-1	Glasgow coma scale	
Test	Finding	Score
Eye opening	No response	1
	Response to pain	2
	Response to voice	3
	Spontaneously	4
Verbal response	No response	1
	Incomprehensible sounds	2
	Inappropriate words	3
	Disoriented conversation	4
	Oriented and appropriate	5
Motor response	No response	1
	Decerebrate posturing	2
	Decorticate posturing	3
	Flexion withdrawal	4
	Localizes pain	5
	Obeys commands	6
	Maximum total score	15

Table 15-2	ICP monitoring techniques	
Device	Advantage	Disadvantage
Intraventricular catheter	Potentially most accurate measure	Risks: bleeding, infection, tissue damage
Subarachnoid bolt	Ease of placement Decreased potential for tissue damage Low infection rate	Potential for loss of pressure wave because of microleaks Easily obstructed No removal of CSF Readings may not reflect global ICP
Counter-pressure systems (Ladd ICP monitor)	Low infection rate	No observable waveform Difficult to zero and calibrate in vivo
Fiberoptic ICP device (Camino monitor)	Continuous waveform available Can record pressures from any intracranial location In vivo calibration possible	In vivo zeroing out not possible Monitor failure occurs with damage to optic fibers

edge of the tentorium, may be compromised in the presence of globally elevated ICP and downward shift of the brainstem. Dysfunction of the abducens limits lateral gaze. Focal increases in ICP resulting from mass lesions (tumor, hematoma, or abscess) usually present as progressive focal deficits, which are eventually followed by obtundation, coma, and compartmental herniation. Focal increases in ICP (especially in the temporal lobe) may cause third nerve dysfunction secondary to uncal herniation. This may be manifest by limited vertical and medial gaze, increased pupil gaze with diminished or absent reactivity, and/or ptosis.

Monitoring of patients with increased ICP

Patients with a GCS score of less than eight should have direct monitoring of ICP begun as soon as possible. Monitoring techniques (Table 15-2) include direct measurement via a ventricular catheter, epidural screw, or fiberoptic transducer.*[7,56] The ventricular catheter allows for accurate monitoring of ICP and for drainage of CSF to lower ICP. It poses a significant risk of infection and is limited to patients who have ventricular spaces that are of either normal or increased size. The epidural screw tends to underestimate ICP and is not useful for drainage of CSF. The Camino fiberoptic transducer has the advantage of accurately determining ICP when placed in either tissue or CSF; however in vivo calibration is cumbersome and transducer failure occurs if optical fibers are damaged.

The jugular bulb catheter is another monitor that

---

*Camino Laboratories, San Diego, California.

may be useful in critically ill patients. This catheter is placed into the internal jugular vein and advanced retrograde into the jugular bulb. At this site, the oxygen content of cerebral venous effluent (C_vO_2) can be measured and compared to arterial blood (C_aO_2) samples. **When oxygen extraction ($C_aO_2 - C_vO_2/C_aO_2$) exceeds 60%, total oxygen delivery is presumed to be marginal.** This information may be used to devise a treatment strategy designed to optimize not only ICP but also delivery of oxygen to meet cerebral metabolic demands. For example, in a patient with high ICP and high extraction, barbiturates, which lower cerebral metabolism, may be preferred over hyperventilation, which may further lower cerebral oxygen delivery. Caution must be exercised with use of this catheter since obstruction of cerebral venous outflow may occur and increase ICP. This risk can be minimized by using small-gauge catheters.

Initial medical management

It is important to optimize the medical condition of patients suspected of having elevated ICP before

Table 15-3   Management of elevated ICP

Goal	Method	Disadvantages
Decrease CSF volume	CSF drainage	Placement of ventricular catheter may result in direct brain injury and infection
		Drainage from lumbar space may result in downward herniation if mass lesion present
	Decrease in CSF production with Diamox (acetazolamide)	Slow, small response
Decrease blood volume	Decrease in Pa_{CO_2}	Requires intubation, metabolic consequences, alkalosis
	Decrease in cerebral metabolism with barbiturates	Hypothermia and barbiturates cause myocardial depression
	Avoidance of seizures with anticonvulsants	
	Head in midline position	
	Avoidance of internal jugular catheters if possible	
	Maintenance of $Pa_{O_2} > 100$ mm Hg	
Decrease brain volume	Diuretic therapy	Osmotic diuretics may transiently increase intracranial volume and ICP
	Osmotic therapy	
	Steroids	Only effective for patients with brain tumors; causes catabolism throughout body

surgery. If the patient is awake and alert, no additional therapy may be needed. Conversely, the patient with a depressed level of consciousness may benefit from preoperative measures to reduce ICP (Table 15-3). Several therapeutic options may be used to reduce elevated ICP before anesthesia and surgery, including decreasing CSF volume, blood volume, or brain volume.

Methods of decreasing CSF volume. Methods of decreasing CSF volume are often used in patients with obstruction of CSF circulation or reabsorption but can be used in those with increased ICP from other causes. In an emergency situation drainage is the most expeditious way to decrease CSF volume. Before draining CSF from the lumbar space, a CT scan should be performed to determine if there is an obstruction to CSF flow or a mass lesion. **In patients with obstruction of CSF circulation or a mass lesion, drainage must be done via a catheter inserted into a lateral ventricle by a surgeon.** In other patients drainage can be achieved either via the ventricle or via the lumbar subarachnoid space.

Medical measures to decrease CSF volume have limited efficacy but are occasionally used in patients with either mild elevations of ICP or as a temporizing measure before surgery. Production of CSF can be diminished by a number of agents that may decrease CSF production. Digitalis can decrease the production of CSF but is rarely used clinically. Mannitol, hyperventilation, glucocorticoids, and diuretics (e.g., furosemide, acetazolamide, and ethacrynic acid) decrease CSF production, but they also act via other mechanisms to decrease ICP (see the following sections).

Methods of decreasing cerebral blood volume. Although the blood compartment represents a small portion of the intracranial volume, it is the easiest compartment to manipulate physiologically. The overall goal of management of elevated ICP is to decrease CBF in the normal brain to the lowest level that does not induce ischemia. Decreasing CBF will decrease cerebral blood volume and therefore ICP. However, doing so sacrifices the margin of the safety provided by high CBF and low extraction fraction. Specifically, management includes control of ventilation to avoiding hypoxia ($Pa_{O_2} > 100$ mm Hg) and use of hyperventilation (Pa_{CO_2} 25 to 30 mm Hg). If the patient has a jugular bulb catheter in place, the degree of hyperventilation should be decreased if oxygen extraction exceeds 50%.

Because CBF is so closely linked to cerebral metabolism, suppression of metabolic rate can pro-

duce a marked decrease in CBF. Metabolic suppression can be achieved either pharmacologically (e.g, barbiturates) or physiologically (e.g., hypothermia) and results in reduction in CBF as much as 50% and a significant fall in ICP. Both fever and seizures can increase cerebral metabolic rate and CBF with a consequent rise in ICP. To prevent a rise in ICP, the source of fever should be treated aggressively. Furthermore, when appropriate, anticonvulsant drugs (e.g., phenytoin) should be administered prophylactically or as primary therapy and therapeutic levels maintained.

Methods of decreasing brain volume. Elevated ICP may occur in conjunction with brain tumors, intracerebral hematomas, and head trauma. Large, slow-growing tumors may not increase ICP because of compensatory mechanisms within the intracranial vault. Specifically, CSF can exit the cranium into the spinal canal or be reabsorbed through the arachnoid granulations. Reduction in the size of the blood compartment also occurs by shifting venous blood to extracranial sites. Conversely, in patients with fast-growing tumors, hematomas, or head trauma increased ICP usually develops because the mass rapidly overwhelms the compensatory mechanisms. The edema surrounding these lesions often accounts for a large portion of the mass effect and thus the rise

in ICP. Edema surrounding brain tumors (vasogenic edema) is caused by increased capillary permeability and is the type of edema that responds best to steroids. Preoperatively, patients may be taking as much as 20 to 100 mg/day of dexamethasone in an attempt to reduce edema. Osmotic agents such as mannitol increase serum osmolarity and draw free water from the interstitial and intracellular spaces of normal brain, thus reducing overall brain volume. Mannitol may be administered in a dose of 1 g/kg every 6 to 8 hours. Smaller, more frequent doses produce a smoother reduction in ICP. **The decrease in ICP with mannitol may be preceded by a transient rise in ICP as total intravascular volume, and therefore, the cerebral blood volume rises acutely. This undesirable effect may be minimized by prior hyperventilation or prior administration of a loop diuretic.** Prolonged use of mannitol may be less effective since mannitol may leak into the interstitial space in regions with a defective blood-brain barrier, which decreases the osmolar gradient between the tissue and the vascular space. Fluid restriction and diuretics such as furosemide aid in dehydration of the brain, with a concomitant decrease in brain volume and ICP.

Neurosurgical patients taking steroids preoperatively may have adrenal suppression. To avoid the potential for hemodynamic instability in patients

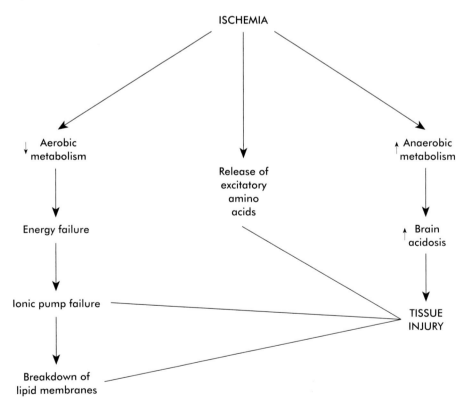

Fig. 15-6. A schematic representation of the hypothesized biochemical sequelae of cerebral ischemia and reperfusion.

taking steroids, most authors now suggest that steroid supplementation is required during the perioperative period.[95] There is some evidence that steroid supplementation is not required if steroids are discontinued within as little as 3 days before surgery.[63] However, because many such patients may still have adrenal suppression, perioperative supplementation with at least physiologic doses of corticosteroids is recommended if the patient has received steroids within the past 6 months.

CAROTID ARTERY ATHEROSCLEROTIC DISEASE

The potential for devastating sequelae from cerebral ischemia led to early enthusiasm for surgical intervention to alter the natural history of carotid atherosclerotic disease. Atheroma of the carotid artery may cause ischemia by producing hemodynamically significant stenosis, or ulcerations in the atheroma may serve as a nidus for emboli. This section addresses the pathophysiology of cerebral ischemia, the potential role of surgical intervention in the setting of carotid artery disease, and preanesthetic considerations in patients undergoing carotid endarterectomy.

Pathophysiology of Cerebral Ischemia

During cerebral ischemia, oxygen delivery to brain tissue is inadequate to meet its needs. The brain is unable to tolerate reduced oxygen delivery because of its high metabolic rate, insufficient stores of metabolic substrates and high-energy phosphates, and inability to obtain sufficient energy from anaerobic metabolism (Fig. 15-6). **When CBF is reduced to less than 15 ml/min/100 g, failure of electrical activity occurs within several minutes.** CBF less than 10 ml/min/100 g results in ionic pump failure and cells die if this state is prolonged beyond 10 to 20 minutes.[6] During ischemia, anaerobic metabolism of glucose produces lactic acid, which causes direct tissue damage and further inhibits substrate utilization.[66] Compared to aerobic metabolism, energy production from anaerobic metabolism of glucose is much less efficient. As a result of insufficient energy supply, ATP-dependent pumps fail, leading to loss of cellular potassium and influx of sodium, chloride, and calcium.[76] Influx of calcium uncouples oxidative phosphorylation (additional energy failure), causes spasm of cerebral blood vessels (additional ischemia), and stimulates phospholipases (breakdown of lipid membranes).[102] Ischemia also causes transmitter release from neurons.[8] The release of excitatory amino acids increases sodium and calcium permeability and metabolic needs in the setting of reduced substrate supply.[25] Increased sodium permeability causes cell swelling and lysis.

Ischemia and reperfusion

It is important to differentiate the biochemical effects of permanent ischemia (e.g., thrombotic stroke) from those of transient ischemia with subsequent reperfusion (e.g., arterial embolus that breaks up, successfully treated vasospasm, transient elevation of ICP, hypotension). **Although reperfusion is necessary for tissue survival, it also contributes to additional brain damage.** Reperfusion is initiated with a transient period of hyperemia followed by a prolonged period of hypoperfusion (Fig. 15-7). **Oxygen-derived free radicals are likely mediators of brain injury during reperfusion.** The pathways involved in the production of oxygen-derived free radicals during reperfusion are actually initiated during ischemia. There is also an accumulation of adenine nucleotides and free fatty acids. When blood flow is restored, adenosine may be reconverted to ATP or be metabolized to uric acid. The production of uric acid involves enzymatic degradation by xanthine oxidase, which produces superoxide anions as a by-product. Similarly, reoxygenation during reperfusion stimulates the lipoxygenase and cyclooxygenase pathways to metabolize free fatty acids that were produced during ischemia and yields free radicals as by-products. Free radicals produce vascular paralysis and tissue damage by breakdown of lipid membranes.[100,107]

Surgical Intervention
Asymptomatic carotid bruit

Approximately 14% of patients 60 years and older have asymptomatic carotid bruits.[92] Patients with asymptomatic carotid bruits have a 1% to 2% per year incidence of stroke[17] and, overall, strokes eventually occur in approximately 19% of patients with asymp-

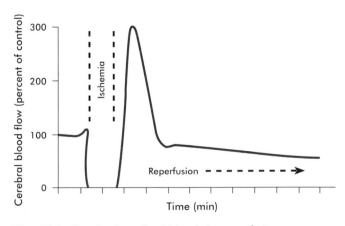

Fig. 15-7. Graph of cerebral blood changes that occur during ischemia and reperfusion. Reperfusion is initiated with a period of hyperemia followed by a period of delayed hypoperfusion.

tomatic carotid bruits.[41,89] Most patients with asymptomatic carotid bruits have transient ischemic attacks (TIAs) before stroke occurs.[17] In addition, **patients with asymptomatic carotid bruits do not appear to have an increased risk of stroke during major noncardiac surgery.**[92] Therefore prophylactic carotid endarterectomy is not recommended in patients with asymptomatic carotid bruits because the risk of surgery exceeds the long-term risk from carotid disease.[90]

After a TIA the incidence of stroke is approximately 10% per year for at least the first 3 years.[15] Caution must be exercised when evaluating the potential benefit of carotid endarterectomy because all published studies to date have been retrospective in analysis. However, these studies do suggest that carotid endarterectomy in patients with TIA may decrease the long-term risks of stroke.[91] In patients who have completed strokes with mild neurologic deficits, carotid endarterectomy may reduce the risk of recurrent stroke and death.[70] Because the surgical procedure is associated with significant morbidity and mortality, studies fail to show any short-term benefits of carotid endarterectomy. The break-even point depends on the morbidity and mortality rate of surgery, which varies considerably from surgeon to surgeon. Recent estimates suggest that only after 3 to 6 years do the benefits from surgery become apparent when compared with medically treated patients.[91]

In patients with surgically inaccessible atherosclerotic disease, there have been attempts to improve perfusion by creating an anastomosis between the extracranial and intracranial circulations. Unlike the studies of carotid endarterectomy, there has been a prospective study of the efficacy of extracranial to intracranial arterial bypass in patients with atherosclerotic cerebrovascular disease.[30] Although the study demonstrated that bypass was not effective in decreasing the risk for stroke or TIA for the entire group, methodologic questions have been raised regarding patient selection for the study. This procedure may be beneficial for carefully selected patients, and it is still performed by some neurosurgeons.

Emergency carotid endarterectomy

In the setting of acute focal ischemia related to carotid stenosis or occlusion, some authors advocate emergency carotid endarterectomy.[24] All studies to date have been retrospective in design. Early studies of patients subjected to emergency carotid endarterectomy demonstrated an increased risk of cerebral hemorrhage and neurologic deterioration.[16] However, later studies suggested that good results could be obtained from emergency carotid endarterectomy if postoperative hypertension is avoided.[24] Indications for surgery include angiographic evidence of severe stenosis with delayed perfusion, thrombus in the lumen distal to stenosis, or carotid occlusion with reflux down to the intrapetrous segment of the carotid artery. Medical management is more appropriate in patients with intraluminal thrombi,[11] decreased level of consciousness, or stenosis in which the residual lumen diameter is greater than 2.0 mm. Patients with carotid occlusion and intracranial extension of the thrombus are not candidates for surgery.

Preoperative Considerations

Patients with atherosclerotic disease of the carotid artery usually have diffuse atherosclerotic disease. Therefore, although many may have a history of coronary artery disease, even those without such a history should be considered prone to coronary ischemia. In addition, many patients undergoing carotid endarterectomy have associated hypertension and the autoregulatory curve is shifted to the right. Often patients scheduled for carotid surgery take anticoagulants or antiplatelet agents. The anesthesiologist should be aware of the patient's coagulation status and take appropriate measures.

CEREBRAL ANEURYSMS

Subarachnoid hemorrhage occurs with a frequency of 11/100,000 persons[44] and has an extraordinarily high morbidity and mortality. The most common diagnosis in patients presenting with subarachnoid hemorrhage (50% to 75%) is that of ruptured intracranial berry aneurysm.[71,72] **Aneurysm rupture occurs most often in otherwise healthy adults in the third to seventh decades of life, with a slight predominance in females.** Survival statistics for patients with untreated aneurysmal subarachnoid hemorrhages indicate that fewer than 50% are alive at 30 days.[71,72] The progressive improvements in treatment strategies over the last three decades have increased the outlook for many patients with this illness.

Although intracranial aneurysms have been noted in up to 9% of routine autopsies, more conservative estimates suggest that **berry aneurysms are found in about 2% of the population.**[81] Cerebral aneurysms may produce brain damage via several mechanisms. Before rupture, an aneurysm may act as a mass lesion and produce tissue damage from direct compression, or it may serve as a source of emboli. Primary injury occurs as a result of aneurysm rupture. Potential mechanisms of secondary injury include increased ICP, rebleeding, seizures, and cerebral vasospasm.

Clinical Presentation

Before rupture, most aneurysms are asymptomatic (Box 15-1). In the relatively few cases in which an aneurysm has been diagnosed before rupture, the risk

---

BOX 15-1
CLINICAL PRESENTATION OF PATIENTS
WITH BERRY ANEURYSMS

Most are asymptomatic
Rupture
Embolic events
Cranial nerve compression

BOX 15-2
HUNT-HESS CLASSIFICATION
FOR ANEURYSMS

Grade I: Asymptomatic or with slight headache
Grade II: Moderate-to-severe headache and
            nuchal rigidity but no focal or lateral-
            izing neurologic signs
Grade III: Drowsiness, confusion, and mild focal
            deficits
Grade IV: Stupor, hemiparesis, early decerebrate
            rigidity, and vegetative disturbances
Grade V: Deep coma and decerebrate rigidity

---

of rupture appears to be related to the size of the aneurysm. **Aneurysms less than 3 mm in diameter have a relatively low risk of rupture;** those greater than 10 mm in diameter should be surgically clipped.

Occasionally patients with aneurysms may have symptoms of an intracranial mass. Because of their large size, giant aneurysms are more likely to present in this fashion. For example, posterior communicating artery aneurysms may cause third cranial nerve compression that produces ipsilateral ptosis, pupillary dilatation, and limited vertical and medial gaze. Similarly carotid artery aneurysms in the vicinity of the cavernous sinus may compress the optic nerve or chiasm, third, fourth, sixth or ophthalmic division of the fifth cranial nerve. Signs attributable to compression of these structures include visual field cuts, limitation of extraocular movements, and eye or facial pain.

Another symptom of an unruptured aneurysm may be that of transient ischemia. Ischemia may result from direct compression of blood vessels adjacent to the aneurysm, or the aneurysm may serve as a source of thromboembolic material. When this material embolizes it can produce ischemiae in a vascular territory distal to the aneurysm. Because giant aneurysms (>2.5 cm diameter) appear to grow by accretion of blood clots within their lumen, they may be more prone to this type of cerebral ischemia.

It has been reported that up to 70% of patients with intracranial aneurysms have a "warning leak" (sentinel bleed)[98] that usually presents as a headache alone. **Aneurysm rupture is almost always associated with a sudden severe headache. Patients often report that this is the worst headache of their life.** The diagnosis can be made by CT scan in approximately 90% of cases. The remainder can be detected by lumbar puncture. The headache is frequently accompanied by nausea and vomiting. **Approximately 45% of patients who survive the initial hemorrhage have a transient loss of consciousness.**[99] This is probably related to either a transient increase in ICP or cardiac dysryth-mia. The final common pathway for both events is a critical reduction in CBF with subsequent compromise of brain function. Aneurysm rupture may be

associated with extensor posturing or seizure activity. A stiff neck develops shortly after the headache. After the acute rupture, there may be focal neurologic deficits, such as hemiparesis, or a global impairment in level of consciousness. Several grading systems have been described to evaluate patients with aneurysmal subarachnoid hemorrhage. Common grading systems are the Hunt-Hess classification (Box 15-2) and the World Federation of Neurologic Surgeons scale (WFNS SAH scale; Table 15-4).

Mechanisms of Primary Neurologic Injury

Aneurysm rupture may cause immediate damage by disrupting adjacent tissue with a jet of blood under arterial pressure, from a local increase in pressure, or from a global increase in ICP. Extravasation of blood into the cortex may cause focal neurologic deficits such as hemiparesis, whereas extravasation of blood into the brainstem may cause apnea, cardiovascular instability, and death. Patients with small hemorrhages may have only headache, but large amounts of subarachnoid blood are often accompanied by lethargy. Overall, approximately 50% of patients die as a result of the first bleed.[71,72]

Table 15-4   World Federation of Neurological Surgeons SAH scale

WFNS grade	GCS score	Motor deficit
I	15	Absent
II	13-14	Absent
III	13-14	Present
IV	7-12	Present or absent
V	3-6	Present or absent

WFNS, World Federation of Neurological Surgeons; *SAH*, subarachnoid hemorrhage; *GCS*, Glasgow Coma Scale.

An increase in ICP after subarachnoid hemorrhage may occur for one of several reasons. When the ruptured aneurysm does not immediately reseal, the pressure in the noncompliant intracranial vault quickly equilibrates with systemic arterial blood pressure and the patient dies. Immediate death is more common in patients who have aneurysm ruptures directly into the subarachnoid space than in patients who have a component of parenchymal hemorrhage, possibly related to tamponade of the aneurysm by the parenchymal hematoma. Both the hemorrhage itself, as well as the associated increased ICP, increase central sympathetic outflow. **High sympathetic tone increases the incidence of cardiac dysrhythmias, large T waves, prolonged QT intervals, and ST segment abnormalities that may be associated with hypotension or fatal dysrhythmias.** Hypotension further decreases cerebral perfusion pressure and increases the risk of cerebral ischemia.

Delayed Neurologic Injury
Rebleeding

The risk of rebleeding is highest in the first day after hemorrhage and declines thereafter (Fig. 15-8). The most effective means of preventing rebleeding is to surgically clip the aneurysm as soon as possible. **Without aneurysm clipping, the overall risk of rebleeding is 50% within the first 6 months after hemorrhage and 3% per year thereafter.**[105] Rebleeding rates are highest in patients with poor clinical grade at presentation, patients in overall poor medical condition, those with high systolic blood pressure, and women.[90] Rebleeding is thought to occur because of increased tension in the aneurysm wall. Wall tension is determined by the radius of the aneurysm and the pressure gradient across the wall (law of Laplace: $T = [P_{in} - P_{out}] \times$ radius) and the wall thickness. Therefore tension in the wall (T) would increase with an increase in arterial blood pressure (P_{in}) or a decrease in the pressure around the aneurysm, which is the ICP (P_{out}) (Fig. 15-9). This relationship helps explain the increased incidence of rebleeding in patients with high arterial blood pressure (high P_{in}) or those who have had rapid decompression of ICP by draining cerebrospinal fluid (low P_{out}) (e.g., during lumbar puncture, or ventricular or lumbar drain placement).

Most clinicians agree that elevations in blood pressure should be avoided immediately following aneurysm rupture (Table 15-5). Physiologic verification is lacking, but there is a strong suggestion that arterial hypertension and swings of arterial, venous,

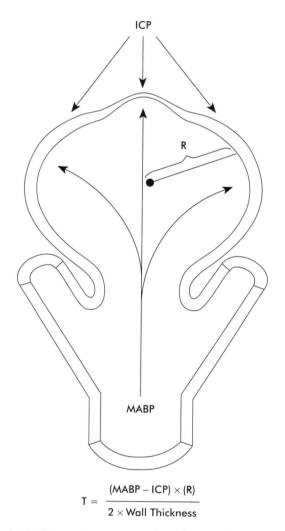

$$T = \frac{(MABP - ICP) \times (R)}{2 \times Wall\ Thickness}$$

Fig. 15-9. Schematic representation of a saccular aneurysm. The tension in the wall of the aneurysm *(T)* is determined by the pressure gradient across the wall of the aneurysm (mean arterial blood pressure *[MABP]* − intracranial pressure *[ICP]*), radius of the aneurysm *(R)*, and thickness of the aneurysm wall.

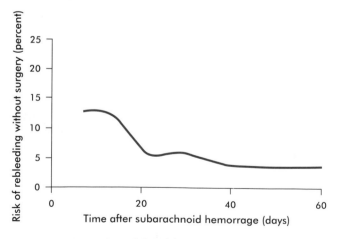

Fig. 15-8. Illustration of the risk of rebleeding from an unclipped aneurysm as a function of time following the initial hemorrhage. In patients with unclipped aneurysms the risk of rebleeding remains at 3% per year after 6 months have elapsed.

and intracranial pressures may provoke hemorrhage. For this reason, bed rest in a darkened room, stool softeners, anticonvulsants, and light-to-moderate levels of sedation are common orders for patients with unclipped aneurysms. Patients with an impaired level of consciousness are at risk of airway obstruction. They must be treated cautiously while securing an artificial airway to avoid hypertension. Steroids (e.g,. dexamethasone sodium phosphate [Decadron]) are used to minimize the symptoms of meningeal irritation and therefore may decrease anxiety and blood pressure but do not reliably reduce brain edema in patients with subarachnoid hemorrhage.

Although it is important to treat hypertension, it is essential to consider the cause of rises in blood pressure because they may represent a homeostatic response to increasing ICP (Cushing's response). Appropriate agents must be used to lower the blood pressure when ICP is elevated. Decreasing arterial blood pressure with vasodilators (e.g., nitroprusside, nitroglycerin) may actually increase ICP. This occurs because the vasodilatory effect of these drugs increases cerebral blood volume. Thus, despite a reduction in cerebral perfusion pressure, there is a net increase in cerebral blood volume[37] (see Fig. 15-2). This rise in ICP further reduces cerebral perfusion pressure.

Antifibrinolytic agents have been used to inhibit the degradation of the clot that forms around aneurysms in an attempt to stabilize the aneurysm wall and prevent rebleeding. Compression of the aneurysm bulb by the clot also decreases the aneurysm size, which reduces wall tension and decreases the tendency to rebleed. In several well-controlled clinical studies it has been clearly shown that **antifibrinolytic agents decreased the incidence of rebleeding after aneurysmal subarachnoid hemorrhage.**[1,58] Unfortunately, inhibition of clot lysis appears to promote vasospasm and hydrocephalus. Use of antifibrinolytic agents increased the incidence of delayed ischemic events and hydrocephalus such that the overall morbidity and mortality rate are not improved.

Increased ICP

After the initial hemorrhage patients may experience global neurologic deterioration without obvious cause. The patient may be noted to be less interactive or to become lethargic. **This deterioration may be related to an increase in ICP that results from an obstruction of CSF flow.** For example, a clot in the aqueduct of Sylvius or basilar cisterns may result in acute obstructive hydrocephalus, which may occur within hours of the subarachnoid hemorrhage. If the hydrocephalus is associated with neurologic deterioration, many clinicians recommend ventricular drainage even with an unclipped aneurysm (Table 15-5). Drain placement may result in an acute decrease in ICP and an increase in transmural pressure that may result in rebleeding. Because of this possibility, some surgeons avoid placing ventricular drains at the bedside; these patients are instead taken to the operating room in preparation for aneurysm clipping and an intraventricular catheter is placed under controlled conditions.

Thick accumulations of red blood cells in the cisterns and arachnoid villi may inhibit reabsorption of CSF and produce communicating hydrocephalus. The most common explanation for delayed increases in ICP seems to be that an inflammatory response to blood in the subarachnoid space[45] occurs and inhibits CSF reabsorption. Following subarachnoid hemorrhage, most of the blood is removed within 1 to 2 weeks, but fibrosis and arachnoid granulation continue to occur for weeks to months. Fibrosis and thickening along with arachnoid granulations obstruct the free flow of CSF and lead to a chronic increase in ICP. This chronic hydrocephalus is corrected with ventriculoperitoneal or lumboperitoneal shunting.

Cerebral vasospasm

The practice of early aneurysm clipping has reduced the incidence of rebleeding markedly; therefore cerebral vasospasm has become a major cause of mortality and morbidity in patients with subarachnoid hemorrhage. **At 7 days after a subarachnoid hemorrhage, angiographic evidence of vasospasm occurs in approximately 60% of patients.**[103] Clinical signs of **vasospasm appear in approximately 30% of patients.** Although vasospasm peaks at 7 days, it may begin as

Table 15-5   Treatment goal for patients before aneurysm surgery

Goals	Comment
Prevent rebleeding	Avoid any activity that may increase pressure; use of controlled sedation and stool softeners is recommended
Prevent seizures	Seizures are frequently associated with rebleeding and may not be preventable with anticonvulsants
Administer prophylaxis for vasospasm	Initiate hydration with 0.9% normal saline; begin oral nimodipine
Treat hydrocephalus	Drainage may precipitate rupture

early as 4 days and last for 2 to 3 weeks.[47,58] When vasospasm is present, blood flow may be reduced in a large vascular distribution with subsequent cerebral ischemia. Although early reports suggested that surgery should be delayed in the setting of vasospasm, these data are not supported by more recent observations using improved surgical techniques.[20]

Diagnosing clinical vasospasm. The neurologic examination is an excellent monitoring technique for early identification of vasospasm-induced ischemia. Although ischemia from vasospasm is more likely in the vascular territory distal to the aneurysm, it may involve any brain region. Two general patterns of clinical symptoms occur: focal deficits and a global decline of level of consciousness. These deficits may occur suddenly or gradually. Vasospasm is considered the cause of a neurologic deterioration only after rebleeding, increased ICP, edema, subdural or epidural hematoma, and/or toxic or metabolic encephalopathy have been ruled out. Arteriographic demonstration of luminal irregularities in large conducting vessels is helpful in confirming the diagnosis of vasospasm. Similarly, transcranial Doppler may demonstrate increased velocity profile for blood flow in major intracranial arteries or ^{133}Xe blood flow measurements may indicate a decrease in flow or lack of autoregulation.

Vascular pathology of vasospasm. **The amount of blood in the subarachnoid space and the degree of vessel narrowing are closely correlated.**[33] It has been hypothesized that morphologic changes, in combination with other contractile mechanisms, produce prolonged vasoconstriction. However, no consensus yet exists on which particular factor in blood initiates the reduction in vessel diameter. In animal models there is evidence that histologic changes are directly related to the proximity of the vasculature to red blood cells in the subarachnoid space. Morphologic changes that have been described include intraluminal platelet and white blood cell accumulation, intimal swelling, proliferation, degeneration, and desquamation; damage to endothelium with subendothelial fibrosis; migration, proliferation, and necrosis of smooth muscle cells with medial infiltration of lymphocytes, plasma cells, and macrophages; degranulation of perivascular nerve terminals; and degeneration of perivascular nerves.

Some of the substances suggested to be important chemical mediators in the cause of vasospasm include serotonin, hemoglobin (oxyhemoglobin and methemoglobin), norepinephrine, bradykinin, angiotensin, prostaglandins, thrombin, fibrin degradation products, thromboxanes, calcium, and oxygen-derived free radicals. Other investigators have hypothesized that vasospasm results from inadequate concentrations of naturally occurring vasodilators (e.g., adenosine, prostacyclin, endothelial-derived relaxation factor).

Neural mechanisms have also been implicated in the pathophysiology of vasospasm.

Regardless of the exact mechanism, reduced vascular diameter probably occurs in vessels down to the arteriolar level. Despite this vasoconstriction and reduction in CBF, cerebral blood volume and ICP may actually increase during vasospasm. The increase in cerebral blood volume may result from compensatory dilatation of cerebral capacitance vessels (veins). Intracranial pressure may increase because of the increase in cerebral blood volume and tissue edema secondary to cerebral ischemia. In addition, **vasospasm is associated with impaired autoregulation.**[97] Although some authors think that the risk of hypotension and additional cerebral ischemia during surgery argues for delaying surgery until vasospasm has subsided, others believe that early surgery decreases the chance of rebleeding and allows for aggressive medical treatment of vasospasm (e.g., hypertension, hypervolemia, free radical scavengers, calcium channel blockers, angioplasty). **We think that the potential benefits of early surgery outweigh the risks and therefore we strongly advocate early surgery.**

Although there is only a loose correlation between clinical grade and CBF at presentation, patients who present with higher CBF values appear to have a better outcome.[46] Some authors have used a low CBF measurement at presentation to justify early aneurysm clipping and prophylactic treatment for vasospasm. When caring for patients with vasospasm, it is important to remember that these blood vessels may not respond normally to carbon dioxide, oxygen, or changes in perfusion pressure.

Treatment of vasospasm. Three types of treatment for vasospasm are currently under investigation: blood volume augmentation, calcium antagonists, and tissue plasminogen activator. Blood volume augmentation is of particular importance in patients in whom hyponatremia develops, which occurs in between 10% and 33% of patients. The incidence of hyponatremia is highest in patients with large subarachnoid clots, thus it often appears concomitantly with vasospasm. **Hyponatremia may rarely be related to the syndrome of inappropriate secretion of antidiuretic hormone, (SIADH); however, metabolic studies have more frequently demonstrated that the hyponatremia is associated with negative sodium balance and intravascular volume contraction.** After subarachnoid hemorrhage patients with hyponatremia who are fluid restricted are at significantly increased risk of ischemia from vasospasm and have an increased incidence of cerebral infarcts.[104] This observation serves as a strong clinical impetus to recommend volume augmentation therapy in patients with aneurysmal subarachnoid hemorrhage.

Similarly, the well-known dependence of vascular smooth muscle on calcium for contraction led to productive trials of calcium antagonists in the prevention of the vasospasm syndrome.[4] The mechanism of action of these agents is not clear; however, the success of initial trials has led to their routine use in patients with subarachnoid hemorrhage.

Treatment of an acute neurologic deterioration resulting from vasospasm is usually accomplished with volume expansion and induced hypertension. Whereas **prophylactic volume expansion is advocated preoperatively, induced hypertension is usually reserved for patients with clipped aneurysms.** Vasospasm that is unresponsive to hypervolemic, hypertensive therapy may respond to arterial dilatation by transluminal angioplasty.

Although these treatments are effective, they have clear drawbacks and are not always successful. Volume replacement and augmentation in the setting of an unclipped aneurysm may increase the likelihood of rerupture. Calcium antagonists have a broad set of actions on smooth muscle and other tissues whose activities are regulated by ion-selective membrane channels. They are often associated with hypotension, a factor known to precipitate cerebral ischemia in patients with increased cerebral vascular resistance. These drugs are usually administered orally, which complicates dosing in uncooperative patients and makes the titration of blood pressure effects more difficult. Furthermore, calcium antagonists significantly limit the efficacy of vasopressor drugs.

New potential prophylactic treatments are currently being investigated. When tissue plasminogen activator is administered intrathecally to animals early after subarachnoid hemorrhage, there is reduction in vasospasm and ischemic deficits are reduced. Clinical trials are currently underway in which tissue plasminogen activator is administered into the subarachnoid space during surgery, after the aneurysm is clipped. It is anticipated that rapid clot lysis will reduce the incidence of vasospasm and prevent ischemic deficits.

ARTERIOVENOUS MALFORMATIONS

It is estimated that **arteriovenous malformations (AVMs) are about one tenth as common as cerebral aneurysms.**[60] Arteriovenous malformations are thought to be congenital and result from arrested development of the capillary beds.[57] A hereditary pattern for these lesions has not been clearly established.[59] A common feature of AVMs is the presence of a shunt or fistula that allows a direct communication between arteries and veins. Because it lacks a capillary network, blood entering the AVM remains at arterial pressure and does not nourish the surrounding tissue. As growth and development occur, the AVM acquires more arterial input and venous distension follows. **More than 90% of AVMs are found in the anterior fossa.**[60]

Most posterior fossa AVMs are found in the cerebellum. As with anterior fossa AVMs, most patients with posterior fossa AVMs present with rupture. However, unlike anterior fossa AVMs, there appears to be a slight female predominance for AVMs of the posterior fossa. It is not surprising that brainstem AVMs tend to be smaller at the time of presentation than those found in the cerebellum.[28]

Classification of AVMs

Several different systems have been developed for grading and classification of AVMs. One common grading system considers size, pattern of venous drainage, and neurologic eloquence of the brain regions adjacent to the AVM.[78] In this system AVMs are rated as grades I through VI. Grade I AVMs are small, superficial, and located in noneloquent cortex; grade V lesions are large, deep, and situated in neurologically critical areas; grade VI lesions are inoperable. Arteriovenous malformations can also be classified by their morphologic characteristics as capillary telangiectasias, cavernous angiomas, and venous angiomas. Capillary telangiectasias usually occur deep in the brain, are generally of no clinical significance, and are associated with Osler-Weber-Rendu disease.[65] Cavernous angiomas are distinguished by their dilated sinusoid channels. They are usually silent and are detected incidentally by computed tomography or at autopsy.[67] These lesions are seen equally in males and females, can be found at any age, and occur most frequently in the supratentorial compartment.[96] Venous angiomas are similar to cavernous angiomas but they lack an arterial contribution. Venous angiomas are usually silent clinically and are the most common type of vascular malformation found at autopsy, occurring in almost 3% of subjects.[74] Because venous angiomas are thought to have a low risk of bleeding or causing other symptoms, those discovered by accident are usually treated conservatively.[67] **Classic AVMs usually receive arterial input from at least two and sometimes all three major cerebral vessels.** Histologically, AVMs are composed of arteries with medial hypertrophy, endothelial thickening, hyaline change, thrombosis, and occasionally, degeneration of the arterial wall with aneurysm formation. Veins are thin-walled vascular channels that have poorly developed elastica, muscularis, and areas of calcification.[82] AVMs that drain in the galenic system are termed aneurysms of the great vein of Galen.

Clinical Presentation

Patients with AVMs often present for medical attention with an intracranial hemorrhage.[42,94] Other common presentations include seizures, headache, nausea, hemiparesis, sensory deficit, bruit, aphasia, and psychosis.[59] Patients usually present between the ages of 20 and 40 years, with an approximately equal sex distribution. Rupture of AVMs is usually not associated with strenuous activity; fewer than 25% of hemorrhages occur during exertion, and up to 36% occur during sleep.[61] The initial management of a hemorrhage is described later in the section on hypertensive hemorrhages. Small and deep-seated AVMs tend to present with hemorrhage, but there is no difference in rebleeding rates for small and large AVMs.[23,36,42] Early reports suggested a relationship between pregnancy and rupture of AVMs; however, more recent studies have not supported this observation. Some believe that pregnant patients with AVMs have an increased risk of bleeding.[69]

Natural History

In general, AVMs that have not previously bled have approximately a 2% to 3% per year risk of bleeding. Rebleeding occurs in approximately 6% of patients during the first year and then the risk of bleeding returns to 2% to 3% per year.[36] Fifteen years after the first hemorrhage, rebleeding rates decrease to less than 1% per year.[42] The first episode has been associated with up to 30% mortality and 80% morbidity.[40] However, more conservative reports estimate 10% mortality and 30% morbidity. After the age of 40, the incidence of bleeding and the risk of death or neurologic injury from a hemorrhage markedly declines. At 50 years of age, the risks of surgery may exceed the risks of spontaneous bleeding.[49] If left untreated, approximately equal numbers of patients will have AVMs that enlarge, get smaller, or remain unchanged.[82] Hemorrhage from AVMs is rarely associated with angiographic vasospasm.[59,84]

Normal Perfusion Breakthrough

Brain regions adjacent to AVMs are often atrophic. This atrophy is presumed to be related to ischemia caused by a vascular steal phenomenon that redistributes blood flow from normal brain to the AVM. As a result of this redistribution, the perfusion pressure in surrounding normal tissue is markedly decreased. When the AVM fistula is occluded, the perfusion pressure to the surrounding normal brain suddenly increases. Even though the perfusion pressure may be "normal" for other brain regions, this region is accustomed to much lower perfusion pressures. The increase in perfusion pressure may be sufficient to produce breakdown of the blood-brain barrier, cerebral edema, and hemorrhage. This phenomenon, termed "normal perfusion pressure breakthrough," has been described both clinically and experimentally following ablation of an AVM.[55,79] To decrease the likelihood of normal perfusion pressure breakthrough, some surgeons have advocated staged resection of large AVMs.[55]

Treatment

AVMs can be managed conservatively with symptomatic treatment of headaches and seizures. Some clinicians recommend intervention only if headaches are intractable, seizures are very difficult to control, or there has been a hemorrhage. The patient's age and location of the AVM also influence the decision to intervene. Recently, in addition to surgical resection, other means of obliterating AVMs have become available. Embolization with particles or glue can completely obliterate some AVMs. Stereotaxic radiosurgery has become available to treat small lesions. In addition, embolization can be used to reduce the size of a lesion and make it more amenable to surgery or radiosurgery.

INTRACEREBRAL HEMORRHAGE

Chronic hypertension is the most common cause of intracerebral hemorrhage. Other rare causes are listed in Box 15-3. Occasionally "normotensive" patients experience a hemorrhage without a demonstrable cause. The most common sites of hypertensive hemorrhages include the thalamus, basal ganglia, cerebellum, and pons. Lobar hemorrhages are usually not associated with hypertension. Hypertensive hemorrhages usually arise from small penetrating arteries that undergo segmental lipohyalinosis caused by long-standing hypertension.

Clinical Presentation

In general, patients experience the sudden onset of a neurologic deficit that may be associated with physical exertion. The patient often experiences a headache, and there may be an associated seizure. The nature of

---

BOX 15-3
CAUSES OF INTRACRANIAL HEMORRHAGE

Primary (hypertensive) intracerebral hemorrhage
Saccular aneurysm
Arteriovenous malformation
Trauma
Hemorrhagic disorders (e.g., leukemia, aplastic anemia, thrombocytopenic purpura, liver disease, complication of anticoagulant therapy)
Hemorrhage into brain tumors
Hemorrhage into infarctions
Inflammatory disease of arteries and veins
Arterial amyloidosis
Miscellaneous (e.g., herpes simplex encephalitis, acute necrotizing hemorrhagic encephalopathy)
Anticoagulation
Undetermined cause

the neurologic deficit is determined by the locus of the hemorrhage. Patients with basal ganglia hemorrhages often present with contralateral hemiparesis, which may be spastic. Thalamic hemorrhages usually produce contralateral sensory loss and, because of compression of the internal capsule, flaccid hemiparesis affecting the face, arm, and leg equally. Both basal ganglia and thalamic hemorrhages may be associated with a gaze preference toward the side of the lesion. Patients may have extension of blood into the ventricular system with resulting hydrocephalus. Pontine hemorrhage presents with the sudden onset of coma, pinpoint pupils, quadriparesis, and ocular palsies; it carries a poor prognosis.[73] The presentation of cerebellar hemorrhage ranges from headache and gait ataxia to obtundation with cranial nerve palsies to coma and death. Cerebellar hemorrhage is considered a surgical emergency. The deficits caused by lobar hemorrhages are determined by the lobe involved and may be accompanied by seizure activity.

Initial Management

Acute management of intracerebral hemorrhage focuses on airway management, control of elevated ICP, therapies to limit the effects of delayed cerebral edema, and cautious control of blood pressure. Patients may be obtunded and require airway protection. Controlled hyperventilation may also be necessary to control ICP. Intubation should be performed so that it does not exacerbate potentially elevated ICP. The same principles for lowering ICP previously described are useful in treating ICP elevations associated with hypertensive hemorrhage. Hyperventilation and active dehydration with mannitol and/or loop diuretics are used most often. The hematoma and surrounding edema often compress the lateral ventricle and make placement of an intraventricular catheter difficult. Edema surrounding the hematoma develops over 2 to 4 days. Initiation of dehydration therapy immediately after the hemorrhage helps limit the detrimental effects of the edema. This may be accomplished through the use of diuretics to raise serum osmolality to 310 to 320 mOsmol. Use of steroids has not proven efficacious in this setting.[86]

Appropriate management of blood pressure must be tailored to the clinical situation. Cerebral hematomas are often associated with a rise in blood pressure, a rise thought by many clinicians to be a homeostatic response to increased ICP in an attempt to maintain adequate cerebral perfusion pressure. In chronically hypertensive patients the autoregulatory curve is shifted to the right. In addition, most have atherosclerotic disease that may produce focal narrowing of the cerebral vessels. For all these reasons, **acute lowering of blood pressure to "normotensive" levels can exacerbate cerebral ischemia.** Many clinicians recommend lowering blood pressure to 170 to 190/90 to 110 mm Hg. Centrally acting vasodilators should be avoided.

Indications for Surgical Evacuation of Hematoma

The indications for surgical evacuation of intracerebral hematomas are controversial. In general, patients with very large hematomas were not previously considered candidates for evacuation because early reports indicated that surgery did not alter their outcome.[54] However, more recent evidence suggests improved neurologic outcomes in patients with large hemorrhages after early surgical evacuation.[43,83] Patients with amyloid angiopathy usually do not benefit from surgery because of a high rate of recurrent postoperative hemorrhage.[12] The location of the hematoma may also be important in determining definitive management. Those that are superficial and in the nondominant hemisphere can be evacuated with minimal disruption of normal brain or impact on language function. However, hemorrhages smaller than 3 cm in diameter in noncomatose patients usually respond well to medical therapy alone. Some neurosurgeons consider surgical intervention only if the patient's condition deteriorates and medical management produces no response. Recently interest has grown in stereotaxic aspiration of acute hematomas, but there is little experience with this approach.

Cerebellar hemorrhage, however, is considered a surgical emergency. Because of the high risk of brainstem compression and obstructive hydrocephalus and the fact that the cerebellum can be resected without producing significant neurologic deficits, emergency evacuation of most cerebellar hematomas is indicated.[12]

SPINAL CORD INJURY
Acute Spinal Cord Injury

Trauma is the most common cause of acute spinal cord injury. Other causes include tumors, infection, and vascular malformations. Approximately 11,000 patients present each year with acute spinal cord injury[50]; most are young men. In 25% to 60% of cases there are other injuries.[3] The most common location for cord injury is in the cervical region. The pathophysiology of traumatic spinal cord injury is thought to be similar if not identical to that for traumatic brain injury (see later discussion). Acute interruption of central input results in loss of control of movement, respiration, and cardiovascular regulation. Preoperative evaluation of such patients should concentrate on changes in respiratory and cardiovascular function, as well as changes in gastrointestinal motility and temperature homeostasis (Table 15-6).

Table 15-6 Sequelae of acute cervical cord injury	
System	**Major findings**
Neurologic	Weakness and loss of sensation below lesion
Respiratory	Loss of diaphragmatic function with lesions above C4; loss of intercostal muscles with lesions above T1
Cardiovascular	Initial spinal shock produces hypotension followed by autonomic hyperreflexia
Metabolic	Gastric atony; delayed hypercalcemia; exaggerated hyperkalemia may occur with use of succinylcholine; abnormal thermal regulation

Clinical presentation

Patients with complete transection of the spinal cord present with flaccid paralysis and complete loss of sensation below the level of injury. Because of overlap of sensory input, the sensory level may be lower than the motor level. Compression at the C7 level or higher results in upper extremity weakness. To determine if the damage to the spinal cord is complete, the function of the sacral segments must be assessed. This is done by determining if perianal sensation or sacral reflexes, such as anal wink, bulbocavernosus, and cremasteric reflexes, are preserved. **Preservation of sacral function demonstrates that the lesion is incomplete and indicates better prognosis.** Early decompression, use of high-dose steroids, and local cooling may be effective in improving outcome from spinal cord compression.

Neurologic deficits from an acute spinal cord compression may also follow a vascular distribution. The anterior spinal artery supplies the central gray, anterior, and lateral columns, but not the posterior columns. Spinal cord compression or vascular pathologic conditions may produce ischemia limited to regions supplied by the anterior spinal artery. The clinical manifestations of this type of injury include paralysis and loss of pain and temperature sensation below the level of injury, with preservation of joint position sense. Some clinicians think that therapies designed to augment blood flow, such as fluid administration and elevation of blood pressure, may be efficacious in this type of injury.

Compression of one side of the spinal cord produces a Brown-Séquard syndrome. In this syndrome patients have ipsilateral weakness and loss of position sense, as well as contralateral loss of pain and temperature sensation. This type of injury is more often related to penetrating trauma but may result from asymmetric cord compression.

Respiration. The degree of respiratory embarrassment is determined by the level of spinal cord injury. **The phrenic nerve is composed of fibers primarily from C4 with contributions from C5 and C3.** If injury occurs above C4, all respiratory musculature is denervated and the patient requires full ventilatory support. Depending on the exact level, lesions below C5 maintain diaphragmatic function and preserve varying degrees of intercostal innervation. The intercostal muscles are innervated by the intercostal nerves, which arise from the first 11 thoracic spinal nerves. **Patients with diaphragmatic innervation alone have vital capacities that are only 20% to 25% of normal.**[80] These patients exhibit **paradoxical respiration, with the chest moving inward during inspiration.** The need for mechanical ventilation is best determined by assessment of respiratory rate, negative inspiratory force, and forced vital capacity.

Ventilation may also depend on patient position. In the upright position, diaphragmatic movement decreases, whereas, in the supine position, elastic recoil of the abdominal wall facilitates maximal diaphragmatic excursion. With decreased cough and expiratory reserve volume, secretions are not cleared efficiently and lead to atelectasis and hypoxia. Factors that may further embarrass respiratory function include ascent of the spinal level because of swelling, aspiration, pulmonary emboli (secondary to immobilization), and pulmonary edema (resulting from overhydration in an attempt to support blood pressure). Interestingly, pulmonary emboli are most common during the first month after injury and then become a rare cause of morbidity or mortality.[106]

Cardiovascular changes. Although studies in animals demonstrate transient hypertension immediately after acute spinal cord compression,[5] this has not been described in humans. The only evidence that hypertension may occur in humans following cervical cord compression comes from observations of hypertension during cervical or thoracic spinal surgery.[64] Most patients with spinal cord compression are hypotensive by the time they reach medical care. This constitutes the hemodynamic consequence of "spinal shock," which may last hours to weeks.[75]

Hypotension following spinal cord compression is a result of ablation of sympathetic tone caused by loss of the sympathetic efferents that exit the spinal cord at the thoracic and lumbar levels. In addition, if hypotension is related to blood loss and the level of spinal cord injury is above T4, reflex tachycardia will be absent. Finally, patients cannot compensate for hypovolemia because of an inability to affect sympathetically induced constriction of arterioles or venous capacitance vessels. Bradycardia may be accentuated in patients with spinal shock because of concomitant hypothermia related to peripheral vasodilation.

Impaired left ventricular function is common after cervical spinal cord compression.[51] The patient is unable to respond to hypovolemia with sympathetically induced tachycardia and increased contractility. Therefore, if not adequately monitored, patients who are given large volumes of fluid to treat hypotension are more likely to have pulmonary edema.[93] Impairment of left ventricular function makes the use of peripheral vasocontrictors to treat hypotension unwise because they lead to increased cardiac afterload, cardiac work, and oxygen consumption. Instead, initial use of volume resuscitation for treatment of hypotension has been advocated, while monitoring pulmonary artery pressure and cardiac output to prevent the formation of pulmonary edema.[51] When fluid administration alone does not produce an adequate response, inotropic agents should be used before resorting to peripheral vasoconstrictors.

Several authors have described cases of pulmonary edema without aggressive fluid resuscitation and have attributed the edema to massive neural discharge (neurogenic pulmonary edema). This discharge is thought to produce increases in systemic and pulmonary vascular pressure, central blood volume, and capillary permeability that lead to extravasation of fluid into the lung.[62,87] The clinical relevance of this syndrome remains controversial. Hemodynamic instability can be exacerbated by a number of problems that often confront the patient with cervical cord injury. These include changes in position, hypoxia, hypercarbia or hypocarbia, high airway pressures from mechanical ventilators, and excessive parasympathetic stimulation from nasopharyngeal or tracheal suctioning.

Metabolic effects. **Gastric atony accompanies spinal shock in many patients.** As a result, gastric distension, which may compromise respiration by elevation of the diaphragm, develops in these patients. When the anesthesiologist is managing airways in such patients, they must all be considered to have a full stomach. In addition, these patients are commonly in a catabolic state. Therefore nutritional support with postpyloric feeding tubes or parenteral nutrition may be necessary to avoid development of a malnourished state.

Patients with spinal cord injuries have a marked inability to maintain thermal regulation.[9,68] Their defect in temperature regulation is twofold. Afferent information from peripheral thermoreceptors in skin, viscera, and spinal cord travel via the autonomic nervous system to the hypothalamus. Afferent neural information is interrupted in patients with high spinal cord compression. The hypothalamus communicates

with the effectors via the autonomic nervous system and endocrine system. With high spinal cord compression, efferent information cannot reach the effector; therefore peripheral vasodilation persists regardless of the ambient temperature. Thus the body **temperature of the patients reflects the atmospheric temperature and they are therefore considered to be poikilothermic.**[19]

Initial management

Acute spinal cord compression is a medical emergency. Assessment and stabilization of respiratory and hemodynamic function should be performed rapidly. During this process it is essential to avoid maneuvers that could potentially extend the spinal injury. The neck should be stabilized immediately. Tachypnea, shallow respirations, forced vital capacity of less than 8 ml/kg or a negative inspiratory force of less than 20 cm H_2O are indications for intubation. When planning the intubation, the physician should choose a technique that will not move the neck and takes into account the patient's full stomach, lack of sympathetic tone, potential for excessive vagal tone, and possible decreased blood volume from other associated injuries. Intubation should be done by an experienced physician with continuous in-line axial traction. **There is no ideal intubation technique for patients with spinal cord injury.** Rapid-sequence induction risks hemodynamic instability and the possibility that adequate visualization cannot be achieved. Awake nasal intubation (blind or fiberoptic) risks excessive nasal bleeding and head movement from coughing after the tube is in the trachea. Laryngeal blocks may be used to decrease cough with tube placement, but they make the patient more likely to aspirate secretions. Awake oral intubation (direct laryngoscopy or fiberoptic) may be difficult without local anesthesia if the patient has a strong gag reflex. The airway may also be secured surgically by cricothyrotomy or formal tracheostomy with the patient under local anesthesia. **We prefer awake intubation (oral or nasal) with local anesthesia above the vocal cords.**

Hypotension should initially be treated with volume resuscitation. Central venous pressure or pulmonary artery pressure monitoring is helpful in avoiding pulmonary edema. Blood pressure should be maintained at a level that ensures adequate urine output and cerebral function. Some clinicians think that higher blood pressures may be helpful in reversing spinal cord ischemia, but there is no compelling evidence to support this notion. Inotropes should be added if fluid administration is insufficient to maintain adequate blood pressure. Vasoconstrictors should be used only if all other measures fail. **Large doses of steroids may be helpful in decreasing neurologic injury from spinal cord trauma if they are**

administered within 8 hours of injury.[13] Although opioid antagonists appear to be efficacious in decreasing spinal cord injury in animal models, they have not been shown to be efficacious in patients.[13]

Chronic Spinal Cord Injury

Whereas the major cause of death in patients with acute spinal cord injury is respiratory failure,[77] the major cause of death in patients with chronic spinal cord injury is renal failure from recurrent urinary tract infections.[27] In most patients with spinal cord injury, spasticity of the intercostal muscles develops by approximately 10 months following injury. This results in better support of the rib cage, preventing its collapse with inspiration[10] and facilitates better ventilation. Because of improved ventilation, patients with chest wall spasticity tend to tolerate changes in position without hypoxia or hypercarbia, which occurs frequently in patients with acute spinal cord injury.[35] Patients with poor intercostal strength also lack the ability to sigh or cough and therefore have an increased incidence of atelectasis with ventilation-perfusion mismatching and hypoxia.

Following the stage of spinal shock, patients with spinal cord compression are at risk for development of autonomic hyperreflexia. Autonomic hyperreflexia occurs in approximately 85% of patients with a sensory level above T6 but is **unlikely to occur in patients with lesions below T10.**[88] Afferent impulses from peripheral sensory fibers normally produce reflex activation of those efferent sympathetic fibers that arise in the spinal cord. Autonomic hyperreflexia results when there is interruption of the cortical fibers that tonically inhibit these spinal reflexes. In patients with spinal cord lesions below T10, stimulation of these reflexes causes vasoconstriction below this level. However, hypertension does not develop as a result of compensatory vasodilation above the level of the lesion. This results in flushing, pilomotor erection, sweating, and congestion of mucous membranes above the level of injury. In patients with lesions above T7, the vascular territory available for dilatation is limited and stimulation of these reflexes results in hypertension. In these patients bradycardia and dysrhythmias induced by stimulation of the carotid sinus by hypertension may also develop. Hypertension may be severe enough to result in loss of consciousness, convulsions, and cerebral hemorrhage and therefore should be treated as a medical emergency.

The best management is prevention. Many patients with high spinal lesions give a history consistent with autonomic hyperreflexia in response to cutaneous stimulation or distension of bowel or bladder. The stimuli should be determined historically and then avoided. Patients should also be given adequate analgesia in anticipation of any invasive procedure.

Treatment of autonomic hyperreflexia involves removing the stimulus, treating the afferent limb of the response (i.e., provide adequate analgesia), and treating the efferent limb of the reflex (i.e., ganglionic-blocking drugs, alpha-adrenergic antagonists, or direct-acting vasodilators). **Electrolyte abnormalities are common in patients with spinal cord injuries.** Although baseline serum potassium concentrations tend to be normal, because of denervation supersensitivity these patients may have exaggerated potassium release from cells in response to succinylcholine. **Hypercalcemia related to immobility** begins approximately 10 days after injury and peaks at approximately 10 weeks.[21] Hypercalcemia is associated with nausea and vomiting and may predispose the patient to ventricular dysrhythmias.

Additional problems for patients with chronic spinal cord injury include gastrointestinal bleeding, muscle spasm, contractures, osteoporosis, emotional and psychologic instability, chronic pain syndrome, drug addiction, urinary calculus formation, and decubitus ulcers.

HEAD TRAUMA

As with spinal cord injury, the incidence of head trauma is highest in males 15 to 30 years old. Aggressive management of problems associated with severe head injury has improved overall mortality.[29] Anesthesiologists care for patients with head injury as part of the team approach to initial stabilization in the emergency room and intensive care unit and for evaluation before surgery.

Pathophysiology of Brain Injury

The pathophysiology of brain injury following trauma is twofold. First, direct cerebral injury results from penetration of skull by projectiles or bone fragments that damage brain and vasculature at the time of impact. Closed head trauma also may result in direct tissue damage by mechanical shearing of axons and rupture of bridging veins.[2] Secondary injury is thought to result from changes in tissue cations and the release of potentially toxic metabolites (e.g., opioids, excitotoxins, oxygen-derived free radicals, biogenic amines) that may lead to increased ICP and cerebral ischemia (see previous sections).

Among the changes in cations that occur after trauma, the increase in intracellular calcium and decrease in intracellular free magnesium levels appear to be best correlated with severity of injury. However, whereas magnesium supplementation attenuates posttraumatic neurologic deficits after brain injury,[53] calcium channel antagonists fail to decrease neurologic injury following spinal cord injury.[34]

Accumulation of the endogenous opioids is

thought to be an important mediator of brain injury following trauma. In particular, dynorphin accumulation in areas of brain subjected to trauma correlates with the degree of secondary neurologic injury.[52] Similarly, treatment with specific antibodies to dynorphin limits posttraumatic neurologic deficits.[31] This same correlation does not exist for other endogenous opioids.

The hypothesis that excitotoxins play a role in the pathophysiology of traumatic brain injury is supported by the finding that excitotoxins are released following trauma. Similarly, several receptor antagonists have been found to decrease neurologic, histologic, and biochemical changes after trauma.[32]

The role for oxygen-derived free radicals in the pathophysiology of brain injury has been studied extensively.[38,39] Free radical generation occurs for up to an hour after the injury.[18,48] Consistent with free radical production is the formation of lipid peroxidation by-products following traumatic injury. Oxygen-derived free radicals are also thought to be important in the production of edema following trauma. Because posttraumatic abnormalities of cerebral physiology can be prevented by pretreatment with cyclooxygenase inhibitors, it has been concluded that the production of free radicals after head trauma is probably related to accelerated arachidonate metabolism via the cyclooxygenase pathway.[101] From a therapeutic perspective, oxygen-derived free radical scavengers (e.g., superoxide dismutase) and antioxidants have been found to decrease neurologic injury following head trauma in laboratory animals.[18,39]

Initial Management

Patients should be rapidly evaluated so that lifesaving therapy can be initiated quickly. Initial evaluation involves assessment of airway, breathing, and circulation. In patients with head injury there are frequently other injuries. If left untreated, these other injuries may result in hypoxia or hypotension and worsen the outcome from head trauma. Patients may have neurologic deterioration ranging from a mild interruption of normal neurologic function (concussive syndrome) to profound coma. Initial management of such patients depends on the simultaneous use of diagnostic tests and therapeutic maneuvers. Assessing the patient with a history and physical examination helps provide the information needed to determine the necessity of immediate invasive therapy (e.g., intubation and hyperventilation). **Serial use of the GCS (see Table 15-1) has been used as a quick method of documenting the level of consciousness in patients with head trauma.** This scale relies on specific assessments of motor, verbal, and eye opening responses. Severe head injury is defined as a **score of 9 or less and is associated with a substantial risk of**

elevated ICP.[26] It is also important to evaluate brainstem reflexes independently because they are not assessed by the GCS. Drug or alcohol intoxication, hypoxia, hypotension, or hypothermia may depress initial GCS scores.

Airway management may be needed in patients with head injury for airway protection because of a decreased level of consciousness and for therapeutic intervention. **A score of less than 9 on the GCS is associated with decreased ability to protect the airway and is a situation in which hyperventilation may be indicated to control or prevent elevated ICP.** Other indications for intubation include brainstem injury with evidence of impaired airway reflexes, cough or ventilatory drive, cervical cord injury, or worsening neurologic condition.

Endotracheal intubation should be performed quickly with an awareness of the potential difficulties in patients with head trauma. Laryngoscopy, hypoventilation, struggling, and use of succinylcholine all may raise ICP. All patients with acute head injury must be considered to have a full stomach and, until radiographs of their cervical vertebrae are available, they must be considered to have cervical spine injuries. Similarly, associated blood loss may make their volume status marginal. Hypotension can worsen neurologic injury if cardiac depressant drugs (e.g., barbiturates, ketamine) are given to facilitate intubation. Many patients can be safely intubated after rapid-sequence induction with an appropriately reduced dose of an amnesic/anesthetic and muscle relaxant. We continue to use succinylcholine as the muscle relaxant of choice because of its rapid onset, despite a controversial association with elevated ICP. Other options for airway control, including tracheostomy, can be used safely in patients with head injury provided the technique is tailored to the patient's individual problems. Regardless of the technique used, once airway control has been achieved, the patient should be hyperventilated to a $PaCO_2$ **of approximately 25 mm Hg and supplemental oxygen should be added to avoid hypoxia (maintain PaO_2 > 90 mm Hg). Patients with head injury may require surgical intervention for intracranial lesions or other associated injuries. Rapid evacuation of clot is the treatment of choice for subdural and epidural hematomas associated with severe head injury.**[22] **Surgical intervention is also appropriate in patients with intraparenchymal hematomas when midline shift is present or if ICP cannot be maintained at less than 20 mm Hg with medical therapy.**[85] **Other common indications for surgery in patients following head trauma include elevation of depressed skull fractures, fractures of long bones, and injury to the viscera.**

Significant increases in ICP occur in 50% of

patients with GCS scores of less than 9 during the first 72 hours after injury.[26] **Institution of ICP monitoring before any surgical procedure that requires use of a general anesthetic should be considered in head trauma patients who have a GCS score of 9 or less.** Different techniques available for the measurement of ICP were presented earlier. In patients with severe head injury without surgical lesions, ICP monitoring should be used as a guide to initiating, increasing, and discontinuing therapy. Monitoring should be continued as long as ICP remains elevated (greater than 20 mm Hg), during active management of ICP, or for 3 days in the absence of significant ICP elevation.[55]

SUMMARY

This chapter reviews important preoperative issues that the anesthesiologist should be familiar with before evaluating patients with neurologic disease. These include intracranial vault physiology, mechanisms and prevention of ischemic brain injury, pathophysiology of tissue injury following subarachnoid hemorrhage, ruptured AVM, hypertensive hemorrhage, spinal cord trauma, and head trauma. It is hoped that the description has filled gaps in knowledge and that there are sufficient references for those who would like further information in any particular area.

KEY POINTS

- The main physiologic determinants of cerebral blood flow are cerebral perfusion pressure, arterial oxygen tension, arterial carbon dioxide tension, and cerebral metabolic rate.

- In normal adults cerebral blood flow remains constant despite changes in cerebral perfusion pressure from 50 to 150 mm Hg.

- Patients with a Glasgow Coma Scale score of less than 8 should have direct monitoring of ICP begun as soon as possible.

- Oxygen-derived free radicals are likely mediators of reperfusion brain injury.

- Patients with asymptomatic carotid bruits do not appear to have an increased risk of stroke during major noncardiac surgery.

- Aneurysm rupture occurs most often in otherwise healthy adults in the third to seventh decades of life, with a slight female predominance.

- Berry aneurysms, found in about 2% of the population, are usually asymptomatic.

- Aneurysms less than 3 mm in diameter have a relatively low risk of rupture.

- Without aneurysm clipping, the overall risk of rebleeding is 50% within the first 6 months after hemorrhage and 3% thereafter.

- Vasospasm after subarachnoid hemorrhage peaks on day 7, with about 60% of patients affected.

- Potential benefits of early surgery for cerebral aneurysms outweigh the risks and, therefore, we advocate early surgery.

- Arteriovenous malformations are about one tenth as common as cerebral aneurysms. More than 90% of AVMs are found in the anterior fossa. Patients usually present between the ages of 20 and 40 years, with an approximately equal sex distribution.

- Hemorrhage from AVMs is rarely associated with angiographic vasospasm.

- The most common cause of acute spinal cord injury is trauma.

- Hypotension following spinal compression is a result of ablation of sympathetic tone related to loss of the sympathetic efferents.

- Preservation of sacral function demonstrates that the spinal cord lesion is incomplete and indicates better prognosis.

- Large doses of steroids may be helpful in decreasing neurologic injury from spinal cord trauma if they are administered within 8 hours of injury.

- The major cause of death in patients with chronic spinal cord injury is renal failure from recurrent urinary tract infections.

- Following the stage of spinal shock, patients with spinal cord compression above T6 are at risk for development of autonomic hyperreflexia.

KEY REFERENCES

Allen GS, Ahn HS, Preziosi TJ et al: Cerebral arterial spasm: a controlled trial of nimodipine in patients with subarachnoid hemorrhage, *N Engl J Med* 308:619, 1983.

Benveniste H, Drejer J, Schousboe A et al: Elevation of the extracellular concentrations of glutamate and aspartate in rat hippocampus during transient cerebral ischemia monitored by intracerebral microdialysis, *J Neurochem* 43:1369, 1984.

Bracken MB, Shepard MJ, Collins WF et al: A randomized, controlled trial of methylprednisolone or naloxone in the treatment of acute spinal-cord injury: results of the second national acute spinal cord injury study, *N Engl J Med* 32:1405, 1990.

Chan PH, Longar S, and Fishman RA: Protective effects of liposome-entrapped superoxide dismutase on posttraumatic brain edema, *Ann Neurol* 21:540, 1987.

Perret G, Nishioka H: Report on the cooperative study of intracranial aneurysms and subarachnoid hemorrhage. Section VI: Arteriovenous malformations: an analysis of 545 cases of craniocerebral arteriovenous malformations and fistulae reported to the cooperative study, *J Neurosurg* 25:467, 1966.

Rehncrona S, Rosen I, and Siesjo BK: Brain lactic acidosis and ischemic cell damage. I. Biochemistry and neurophysiology, *J Cereb Blood Flow Metab* 1:297, 1981.

Siesjo BK: Cerebral circulation and metabolism, *J Neurosurg* 60:883, 1984.

Udelsman R, Ramp J, Gallucci WT et al: Adaptation during surgical stress: a reevaluation of the role of glucocorticoids, *J Clin Invest* 77:1377, 1986.

Wei EP, Christman CW, Kontos HA et al: Effects of oxygen radicals on cerebral arterioles, *Am J Physiol* 248:H157, 1985.

Weir B, Grace M, Hansen J et al: Time course of vasospasm in man, *J Neurosurg* 48:173, 1978.

REFERENCES

1. Adams HP: Antifibrinolytic therapy for prevention of recurrent aneurysmal subarachnoid hemorrhage, *Semin Neurol* 6:309, 1986.
2. Adams JH, Graham DJ, and Gennarelli TA: Contemporary neuropathological considerations regarding brain damage in head injury. In Becker DP, Povlishock JT, eds: *Central nervous system trauma status report,* 1985, National Institutes Health.
3. Albin MS: Resuscitation of the spinal cord, *Crit Care Med* 6:270, 1978.
4. Allen GS, Ahn HS, Preziosi TJ et al: Cerebral arterial spasm: a controlled trial of nimodipine in patients with subarachnoid hemorrhage, *N Engl J Med* 308:619, 1983.
5. Alexander S, Kerr FWL: Blood pressure responses in acute compression of the spinal cord, *J Neurosurg* 21:485, 1964.
6. Astrup J, Symon L, Branston NM et al: Cortical evoked potential and extracellular K^+ and H^+ at critical levels of brain ischemia, *Stroke* 8:51, 1977.
7. Barnett GH, Chapman PH: Insertion and care of intracranial pressure monitoring devices. In Ropper AH, Kennedy SF, eds: *Neurological and neurosurgical intensive care,* Rockville, MD, 1988, Aspen Publishers.
8. Benveniste H, Drejer J, Schousboe A et al: Elevation of the extracellular concentrations of glutamate and aspartate in rat hippocampus during transient cerebral ischemia monitored by intracerebral microdialysis, *J Neurochem* 43:1369, 1984.
9. Benzinger TH: Heat regulation: homeostasis of central temperature in man, *Physiol Rev* 49:671, 1969.
10. Bergofsky EH: Mechanism for respiratory insufficiency after cervical cord injury—a source of alveolar hypoventilation, *Ann Intern Med* 61:435, 1964.
11. Biller J, Adams HP Jr, Boarini D et al: Intraluminal clot of the carotid artery. A clinical-angiographic correlation of nine patients and literature review, *Surg Neurol* 25:467, 1986.
12. Borges LF: Management of nontraumatic brain hemorrhage. In Ropper AH, Kennedy SF, eds: *Neurological and neurosurgical intensive care,* Rockville, MD, 1988, Aspen Publishers.
13. Bracken MB, Shepard MJ, Collins WF et al: A randomized, controlled trial of methylprednisolone or naloxone in the treatment of acute spinal-cord injury: results of the second national acute spinal cord injury study, *N Engl J Med* 322:1405, 1990.
14. Bruce DA: *The pathophysiology of increased intracranial pressure,* Kalamazoo, Mich, 1978, Upjohn.
15. Canadian Co-operative Study Group: A randomized trial of aspirin and sulfinpyrazone in threatened stroke, *N Engl J Med* 299:53, 1978.
16. Caplan LR, Skillman J, Ojemann R et al: Intracerebral hemorrhage following carotid endarterectomy: a hypertensive complication? *Stroke* 9:457, 1978.
17. Chambers BR, Norris JW: The case against surgery for asymtomatic carotid stenosis, *Stroke* 15:964, 1984.
18. Chan PH, Longar S, and Fishman RA: Protective effects of liposome-entrapped superoxide dismutase on posttraumatic brain edema, *Ann Neurol* 21:540, 1987.
19. Cheshire DJE, Coats DA: Respiratory and metabolic management in acute tetraplegia, *Paraplegia* 3:178, 1965.
20. Chyatte D, Fode NC, and Sundt TM Jr: Early versus late intracranial aneurysm surgery in subarachnoid hemorrhage, *J Neurosurg* 69:326, 1988.
21. Clause-Walker JL, Carter RE, Lipscomb HS et al: Daily rhythms of electrolytes and aldosterone excretion in men with cervical spinal cord section, *J Clin Endocrinol Metab* 29:300, 1969.
22. Cooper PR: Traumatic intracranial hematomas. In Wilkin RH, Rengachary SS, eds: *Neurosurgery,* New York, 1985, McGraw-Hill.
23. Crawford PM, West CR, Chadwick DW et al: Arteriovenous malformations of the brain: natural history in unoperated patients, *J Neurol Neurosurg Psychiatry* 49:1, 1986.
24. Crowell RM, Jafar JJ: Surgical revascularization for acute occlusion: theoretical and practical considerations. In Weinstein PR, Faden AI, eds: *Protection of the brain from ischemia,* Baltimore, 1990, Williams & Wilkins.
25. Curtis DR, Phillis JW, and Watkins JC: Chemical excitation of spinal neurones, *Nature* 183:611, 1959.
26. Dearden NM: Management of raised intracranial pressure after severe head injury, *Br J Hosp Med* 36:94, 1986.

27. Desmond J: Paraplegia: problems confronting the anesthesiologist, *Can Anaesth Soc J* 17:435, 1970.

28. Drake CF, Freidman AH, and Peerless SJ: Posterior fossa arteriovenous malformations, *J Neurosurg* 64:1, 1986.

29. Duffy KR, Becker DP: State-of-the-art management of severe closed-head injury, *J Int Care Med* 3:291, 1988.

30. EC/IC Bypass Study Group: Failure of extracranial-intracranial arterial bypass to reduce the risk of ischemic stroke: results of an international randomized trial, *N Engl J Med* 313:1191, 1985.

31. Faden AI, Jacobs TP, and Holaday JW: Endorphin-parasympathetic interaction in spinal shock, *J Auton Nerv Syst* 2:295, 1980.

32. Faden AI, Simon RP: a potential role for excitotoxins in the pathophysiology of spinal cord injury, *Ann Neurol* 23:623, 1988.

33. Fisher CM, Kistler JP, and Davis JM: Relation of cerebral vasospasm to subarachnoid hemorrhage visualized by computerized tomographic scanning, *Neurosurgery* 6:1, 1980.

34. Ford WJ, Malm DN: Failure of nimodipine to reverse acute experimental spinal cord injury, *CNS-Trauma* 2:9, 1985.

35. Goldman AL, George J: Postural hypoxemia in quadriplegic patients, *Neurology* 26:815, 1976.

36. Graf CJ, Perret GE, and Torner JC: Bleeding from cerebral arteriovenous malformations as part of their natural history, *J Neurosurg* 58:331, 1983.

37. Gupta B, Cottrell JE, Rappaport H et al: Intracranial pressure during nitroglycerin-induced hypotension, *J Neurosurg* 53:309, 1980.

38. Hall ED: Free radicals and CNS injury, *Crit Care Clin* 5:793, 1989.

39. Hall ED, Yonkers PA, McCall JM et al: Effects of the 21-aminosteroid U74006 on experimental head injury in mice, *J Neurosurg* 68:124, 1988.

40. Heros RC, Tu Y-K: Is surgical therapy needed for unruptured arteriovenous malformation? *Neurology* 37:279, 1987.

41. Heyman A, Wilkinson WE, Heyden S et al: Risk of stroke in asymptomatic persons with cervical arterial bruits: a population study in Evans County, Georgia, *N Engl J Med* 302:838, 1980.

42. Itoyama Y, Uemura S, Ushio Y et al: Natural course of unoperated intracranial arteriovenous malformations: study of 50 cases, *J Neurosurg* 71:805, 1989.

43. Kaneko M, Koba T, and Yokokama T: Early surgical treatment for hypertensive intracerebral hemorrhage, *J Neurosurg* 46:579, 1977.

44. Kassell NF, Torner JC: Epidemiology of intracranial aneurysms, *Int Anesthesiol Clin* 20:13, 1982.

45. Kibler RF, Couch RSC, and Crompton MR: Hydrocephalus in the adult following spontaneous subarachnoid hemorrhage, *Brain* 84:45, 1961.

46. Knuckey NW, Fox RA, Surveyor I et al: Early cerebral blood flow and computerized tomography in predicting ischemia after cerebral aneurysm rupture, *J Neurosurg* 62:850, 1985.

47. Kodama N, Mizoi K, Sakurai Y et al: Incidence and onset of vasospasm. In Wilkins RH, ed: *Cerebral arterial spasm,* Baltimore, 1980, Williams & Wilkins.

48. Kontos HA, Wei EP: Superoxide production in experimental brain injury, *J Neurosurg* 64:803, 1986.

49. Luessenhop AJ, Rosa L: Cerebral arteriovenous malformations: indications for and results of surgery, and the role of intravascular techniques, *J Neurosurg* 60:14, 1984.

50. Luce JM: Medical management of spinal cord injury, *Crit Care Med* 13:126, 1985.

51. Mackenzie CF, Shin B, Krishnaprasad D et al: Assessment of cardiac and respiratory function during surgery on patients with acute quadriplegia, *J Neurosurg* 62:843, 1985.

52. McIntosh TK, Hayes RL, DeWitt DS et al: Endogenous opioids may mediate secondary damage after experimental brain injury, *Am J Physiol* 253:E565, 1987.

53. McIntosh TK, Faden AI, Yamakami I et al: Magnesium deficiency exacerbates and pretreatment improves outcome following traumatic brain injury in rats: ^{31}P magnetic resonance spectroscopy and behavioral studies, *J Neurotrauma* 5:17, 1988.

54. McKissock W, Richardson A, and Taylor J: Primary intracerebral hemorrhage: controlled trial of surgical and conservative treatment in 180 unselected cases, *Lancet* 2:221, 1961.

55. Morgan MK, Johnston I, Besser M et al: Cerebral arteriovenous malformations, steal, and the hypertensive breakthrough threshold: an experimental study in rats, *J Neurosurg* 66:563, 1987.

56. Narayan RK, Kishore PR, Becker DP et al: Intracranial pressure: to monitor or not to monitor? A review of our experience with severe head injury, *J Neurosurg* 56:650, 1982.

57. Newton TH, Troost BT: Arteriovenous malformation and fistula. In Newton TH, Potts DG, eds: *Radiology of the skull and brain: angiography,* vol 2, book 4, St Louis, 1974, CV Mosby.

58. Nibbelink DW, Torner JC, and Henderson WG: Intracranial aneurysms and subarachnoid hemorrhage: a cooperative study. Antifibrinolytic therapy in recent onset subarachnoid hemorrhage, *Stroke* 6:622, 1975.

59. Parkinson D, Bachers G: Arteriovenous malformations: summary of 100 consecutive supratentorial cases, *J Neurosurg* 53:285, 1980.

60. Perret G, Nishioka H: Report on the cooperative study of intracranial aneurysms and subarachnoid hemorrhage. Section VI: Arteriovenous malformations: an analysis of 545 cases of craniocerebral arteriovenous malformations and fistulae reported to the cooperative study, *J Neurosurg* 25:467, 1966.

61. Perret GE: Conservative management of inoperable arteriovenous malformations. In Pia HW, Gleave JRW, Grote E et al, eds: *Cerebral angiomas: advances in diagnosis and therapy,* New York, 1975, Springer-Verlag.

62. Poe RH, Reisman JL, and Rodenhouse TG: Pulmonary edema in cervical spinal cord injury, *J Trauma* 18:71, 1978.

63. Plumpton FS, Besser GM, and Cole PV: Corticosteroid treatment and surgery: an investigation of the indication for steroid cover, *Anaesthesia* 24:3, 1969.

64. Rawe SE, Perot PL Jr: Pressor response resulting from experimental contusion injury to the spinal cord, *J Neurosurg* 50:58, 1979.

65. Reagan TJ, Bloom WH: The brain in hereditary hemorrhagic telangiectasia, *Stroke* 2:361, 1971.

66. Rehncrona S, Rosen I, and Siesjo BK: Brain lactic acidosis and ischemic cell damage. I. Biochemistry and neurophysiology, *J Cereb Blood Flow Metab* 1:297, 1981.

67. Rengachary SS, Kalyan-Roman UP: Other cranial intradural angiomas. In Wilkins RH, Rengachary SS, eds: *Neurosurgery,* New York, 1985, McGraw-Hill.

68. Richards SA: Temperature regulation. In Mott N, Noakes GR, and Yapp WB, eds: *The Wykeham Science Series,* London, 1973, Wykeham.

69. Robinson JL, Hall CS, and Sedzimir CB: Arteriovenous malformation, aneurysms, and pregnancy, *J Neurosurg* 41:63, 1974.

70. Rubin JR, Goldstone J, McIntyre KE Jr et al: The value of carotid endarterectomy in reducing the morbidity and mortality of recurrent stroke, *J Vasc Surg* 4:443, 1986.

71. Sahs AL, Perret G, Locksley HB et al: *Intracranial aneurysms and subarachniod hemorrhage: a cooperative study,* Philadelphia, 1969, JB Lippincott.

72. Sahs AL, Nibbelink DW, and Torner JC: *Aneurysmal subarachnoid hemorrhage: report of the cooperative study,* Baltimore, 1981, Urban and Schwarzenberg.

73. Sano K, Ochiai C: Brainstem hematomas: clinical aspects with reference to indications for treatment. In Pia HW, Lanjmaid C, and Zierski J, eds: *Spontaneous intracerebral hematomas,* New York, 1980, Springer-Verlag.

74. Sarwar M, McCormick WF: Intracerebral venous angioma: case report and review, *Arch Neurol* 35:323, 1978.

75. Schneider RC, Crosby EC, Russo RH et al: Traumatic spinal cord syndromes and their management, *Clin Neurosurg* 20:424, 1973.

76. Siesjo BK: Cerebral circulation and metabolism, *J Neurosurg* 60:883, 1984.

77. Silver JR, Moulton M: The physiological and pathological sequelae of paralysis of the intercostal and abdominal muscles in tetraplegic patients, *Paraplegia* 7:131, 1969.

78. Spetzler RF, Martin NA: A proposed grading system for arteriovenous malformations, *J Neurosurg* 65:476, 1986.

79. Spetzler RF, Wilson CB, Weinstein P et al: Normal perfusion pressure breakthrough theory, *Clin Neurosurg* 25:651, 1978.

80. Stauffer ES, Bell GD: Traumatic respiratory quadriplegia and pentaplegia, *Orthop Clin North Am* 9:1081, 1978.
81. Stehbens WE: The pathology of intracranial arterial aneurysms and their complications. In Fox JL, ed: *Intracranial aneurysms*, vol I, New York, 1983, Springer-Verlag.
82. Stein BM, Wolpert SM: Arteriovenous malformations of the brain. I. Current concepts and treatment, *Arch Neurol* 37:1, 1980.
83. Suzuki J, Sato T: Grading and timing of operation. In Pia HW, Langmaid C, and Zierski J, eds: *Spontaneous intracerebral hematomas,* New York, 1980, Springer-Verlag.
84. Taveras JM, Pool JL, and Fletcher TM: The incidence of and significance of cerebral vasospasm in 100 consecutive angiograms of intracranial aneurysms, *Trans Am Neurol Assoc* 83:100, 1959.
85. Teasdale G, Galbraith S, and Jennett B: Operate or observe? ICP and the management of "silent" traumatic intracranial hematoma. In Shulman K: *Intracranial pressure IV,* Berlin, 1980, Springer-Verlag.
86. Tellez H, Bauer RB: Dexamethasone as treatment in cerebrovascular disease. 1. A controlled study in intracerebral hemorrhage, *Stroke* 4:541, 1973.
87. Theodore J, Robin ED: Speculations on neurogenic pulmonary edema (NPE), *Am Rev Respir Dis* 113:405, 1976.
88. Thompason CE, Witham AC: Paroxysmal hypertension in spinal cord injuries, *N Engl J Med* 239:291, 1948.
89. Thompson JE, Patman RD, and Talkinton CM: Asymptomatic carotid bruit: long-term outcome of patients having endarterectomy compared with unoperated controls, *Ann Surg* 188:308, 1978.
90. Torner JC, Kassell NF, Wallace RB et al: Preoperative prognostic factors for rebleeding and survival in aneurysm patients receiving antifibrinolytic therapy: report of the cooperative aneurysm study, *Neurosurgery* 9:506, 1981.
91. Toronto Cerebrovascular Study Group: Risks of carotid endarterectomy, *Stroke* 17:848, 1986.
92. Treiman RL, Foran RF, Cohen JL et al: Carotid bruit: a follow-up report on its significance in patients undergoing an abdominal aortic operation, *Arch Surg* 114:1138, 1979.
93. Troll GF, Dohrmann GJ: Anaesthesia of the spinal cord-injured patient: cardiovascular problems and their management, *Paraplegia* 13:162, 1975.
94. Troupp H, Marttila I, and Halonen V: Arteriovenous malformations of the brain: prognosis without operation, *Acta Neurochir (Wien)* 22:125, 1970.
95. Udelsman R, Ramp J, Gallucci WT et al: Adaptation during surgical stress: a reevaluation of the role of glucocorticoids, *J Clin Invest* 77:1377, 1986.
96. Voigt K, Yasargil MG: Cerebral cavernous haemangiomas or cavernomas: incidence, pathology, localization, diagnosis, clinical features and treatment. Review of the literature and report of an unusual case. *Neurochirurgia (Stuttg)* 19: 59, 1976.
97. Voldby B, Enevoldsen EM, and Jensen FT: Cerebrovascular reactivity in patients with ruptured intracranial aneurysms, *J Neurosurg* 62:59, 1985.
98. Waga S, Ohtsubo K, and Handa H: Warning signs in intracranial aneurysms, *Surg Neurol* 3:15, 1975.
99. Walton JN: *Subarachnoid haemorrhage,* Edinburgh, 1956, E & S Livingstone.
100. Wei EP, Christman CW, Kontos HA et al: Effects of oxygen radicals on cerebral arterioles, *Am J Physiol* 248: H157, 1985.
101. Wei EP, Kontos HA, Dietrich WD et al: Inhibition by free radical scavengers and by cyclooxygenase inhibitors of pial arteriolar abnormalities from concussive brain injury in cats, *Circ Res* 48:95, 1981.
102. Weiloch T, Siesjo BK: Ischemic brain injury: the importance of calcium, lipolytic activities, and free fatty acids, *Pathol Biol* 30:269, 1982.
103. Weir B, Grace M, Hansen J et al: Time course of vasospasm in man, *J Neurosurg* 48:173, 1978.
104. Wijdicks EFM, Vermeulen M, Hijdra A et al: Hyponatremia and cerebral infarction in patients with ruptured intracranial aneurysms: is fluid restriction harmful? *Ann Neurol* 17:137, 1985.
105. Winn Hr, Richardson AE, and Jane JA: Long-term prognosis in untreated cerebral aneurysms. II. Late morbidity and mortality, *Ann Neurol* 4:418, 1978.
106. Wolman L: The disturbance of circulation in traumatic paraplegia in acute and late stages: a pathological study, *Paraplegia* 1:213, 1965.
107. Yamamoto M, Shima T, Uozumi T et al: A possible role of lipid peroxidation in cellular damages caused by cerebral ischemia and the protective effect of α-tocopherol administration, *Stroke* 14: 977, 1983.

CHAPTER 16

Evaluation of the Patient with Neuromuscular Disease

CECIL BOREL

Perioperative care of patients with neuromuscular diseases is challenging. These diseases result from a variety of pathologic processes that affect spinal cord, peripheral nerve, neuromuscular junction, or muscle. **Although the cause is distinct, these disease processes all adversely affect respiratory, cardiovascular, and nutritional balance.** Acute illness, anesthesia, and surgery often overwhelm the residual capacity of these organ systems and result in unanticipated complications, especially if the severity of the underlying neuromuscular disorder is underestimated preoperatively.

ORGAN SYSTEM DYSFUNCTION IN NEUROMUSCULAR DISEASE

Respiratory System

Ventilatory performance depends entirely on skeletal muscle activity. **Respiratory insufficiency is the major cause of death in patients with neuromuscular disorders.**[29,48] Although the extent of respiratory system involvement depends on the type, distribution, and duration of neuromuscular disease, respiratory function does not directly parallel the extent of general muscle weakness.[85] Thus essential respiratory functions such as inspiratory ventilatory effort, forced expiratory effort (cough), and maintenance of airway patency require careful assessment.[72]

The insidious loss of ventilatory reserve and inability to increase minute ventilation on demand are often the initial effects of impaired respiratory function in neuromuscular disease.[29] Perioperative changes in lung function and increased metabolic rate frequently increase the work of breathing and result in muscle fatigue and ventilatory insufficiency.[15] **Early responses to increased inspiratory work include (1) frequent changes in respiratory pattern to alternate work between fatiguing muscles and accessory respiratory muscles**[35,78] **and (2) increasing respiratory rate to allow more efficient use of weakened muscles,**[12,79] **resulting in increased inspiratory time and an increased ratio of dead space to tidal volume. Both responses decrease ventilatory efficiency and increase the risk of ventilatory failure.**

Ventilatory muscle fatigue is associated with impaired ventilatory responses to hypercapnia and hypoxia.[48,64,65,87] Central drive mechanisms may be further decreased during sleep in these patients.[76] The altered responses may not directly correlate with static pressures and other assessments of ventilatory muscle strength. These patients often have a baseline hypercapnia that is worse at night, but can be corrected by voluntary hyperventilation. Although some patients have complaints of daytime somnolence and early morning headaches, many are asymptomatic.[29,33,64,65]

Expiratory muscle dysfunction in neuromuscular disease impairs the ability to cough and further exacerbates reductions in forced expiratory capacity observed after abdominal and thoracic procedures.[7,33,72] Impaired cough and retained secretions lead to the collapse of lung segments and predispose the patient to bacterial contamination and pneumonia. Continued perfusion of nonventilated lung regions results in arterial hypoxemia. Microatelectasis has been implicated in the reduced lung compliance, decreased functional residual capacity, and increased work of breathing observed in patients with neuromuscular disease who have respiratory muscle dysfunction.[18,26,33]

Impaired laryngeal and glottic muscle function occurs in patients with neuromuscular disease[48,84] and, when severe, results in recurrent aspiration and airflow obstruction.[29] **Airway muscles, including those of the tongue, jaw, retropharynx, glottis, and larynx, may be affected by any neuromuscular disease process that affects respiratory muscles.** In addition, cranial nerves may be affected by disease processes specific to the brainstem or lower cranial nerves. The ninth, tenth, and twelfth cranial nerves supply most of the motor innervation to the airway, whereas sensory stimuli are mediated through the ninth and tenth cranial nerves. A unilateral lesion of the vagus nerve leads to difficulty in coughing, clearing the voice, and swallowing. Bilateral lesions of the vagus nerves result in difficulty swallowing, regurgitation of food, and positional airway obstruction. The gag reflex constricts and elevates the pharynx and is mediated by the sensory fibers of the glossopharyngeal nerve synapsing in the nucleus ambiguous, sending efferent fibers to the striated muscles of the pharynx. Loss of the gag reflex leads to recurrent aspiration of pharyngeal contents. Residual anesthesia and persistent effects of muscle relaxants administered intraoperatively exacerbate upper airway muscle dysfunction in patients with neuromuscular disease.

Cardiovascular System

Cardiovascular dysfunction is also a common cause of morbidity in patients with neuromuscular illness. **Cardiovascular involvement ranges from autonomic dysfunction with neuropathic diseases (Box 16-1) to myocardial failure with myopathic diseases (Box 16-2).** The cardiovascular response to anesthetics, blood loss, dehydration, and infection will be impeded

---

BOX 16-1
NEUROPATHIES ASSOCIATED WITH DYSAUTONOMIA

Primary peripheral neuropathies with secondary dysautonomia

Guillain-Barré syndrome[16,22]
Acute intermittent porphyria
Heavy metal intoxication and poisoning[47,53]

Systemic diseases with secondary dysautonomia

Diabetes mellitus[42]
Systemic amyloidosis
Uremia
Connective tissue diseases (particularly progressive systemic sclerosis)[51]
Leprosy

---

if the cardiovascular system is impaired by neuromuscular disease. Because of the broad dependence of the cardiovascular system on nerve and muscle function, patients with neuromuscular illness commonly have low cardiac reserve.

The autonomic nervous system regulates heart

BOX 16-2
NEUROMUSCULAR DISEASES ASSOCIATED WITH CARDIAC MUSCLE DYSFUNCTION

Hereditary neuromyopathic disorders

Myotonic muscular dystrophy
Friedrich's ataxia
Progressive muscular dystrophy
    Duchenne's muscular dystrophy
    Becker's muscular dystrophy
    Limb-girdle dystrophy of Erb
    Facioscapulohumeral dystrophy

Other neuromuscular diseases with occasional association

Peroneal muscular atrophy (Charcot-Marie-Tooth)
Humeroperoneal dystrophy
Myotubular myopathy (centronuclear myopathy)
Oculocraniosomatic syndrome (Kearns-Sayre)
Nemaline myopathy
Guillain-Barré syndrome

Neuromuscular disorders presenting as cardiomyopathy

Poliomyelitis
Periodic paralysis
Alcoholic myopathy

rate, inotropic state, venous tone, and systemic vascular resistance. Heart rhythm is balanced by sympathetic and parasympathetic influences: cardiac dysrhythmias ranging from sinus tachycardia to bradycardia and asystole occur when either system is impaired.[67] **Loss of beat-to-beat variability in heart rate is probably the most sensitive indicator of autonomic cardiac involvement.**[70] Resting tachycardia and postural hypotension have been associated with intraoperative hemodynamic instability and need for vasopressor therapy, and unexplained cardiorespiratory arrest during anesthesia has been reported in patients with dysautonomia.[42,57] Vasomotor nerve dysfunction may result in postural hypotension from loss of vasoconstriction, or in hypertension from a disordered response to peripheral vasomotor paresis. **Volume and electrolyte disorders frequently occur in dysautonomic diseases** because the autonomic nervous system controls distribution of systemic blood flow, modulates blood volume by sodium retention through aldosterone release, and limits insensible loss of fluids from the sweat glands. Hypovolemia may be relative, the result of venous pooling; or absolute, the result of increased insensible volume losses. Hypovolemia is a potent stimulus for the release of arginine vasopressin from the pituitary gland, which results in water retention and an increase in venous tone. **Patients with dysautonomia frequently become hyponatremic in the perioperative period from the combination of hypovolemia, arginine vasopressin release, stress, and volume replacement with hyponatremic solutions.**

Diseases of muscle are heterogeneous in expression; cardiac muscle can be directly affected in various myopathies, resulting in congestive heart failure, complex cardiac dysrhythmias, or formation of mural thrombus in the heart.

Patients with neuromuscular diseases, particularly those in whom the autonomic nervous system is involved, need careful monitoring of cardiovascular performance, volume replacement, and sodium metabolism during the perioperative period when fever, dehydration, blood loss, and increased gastrointestinal losses place all patients at risk.

Nutritional Effects

Malnutrition commonly accompanies neuromuscular diseases. Appetite, glutition, gastric emptying, intestinal motility, defecation, and metabolic requirements are affected to some degree in most patients with chronic neuromuscular diseases. Patients avoid eating or drinking when swallowing function is impaired. Paralytic ileus results in the loss of nutrient absorption from the intestine when the autonomic enervation to the gut is impaired. Protein energy malnutrition exacerbates ventilatory dysfunction[71] and proba-

bly increases the risk of wound dehiscence and infection. **The role of preoperative nutritional support is controversial, but repletion therapy is probably beneficial,** since postoperative return to normal dietary intake is likely to be delayed in patients with neuromuscular disease. Nutrients can be delivered in a predigested or "elemental" form so that enteric absorption of nutrient is possible even when dysautonomia causes ileus. Vagal damage during generalized demyelinating neural disorders may lead to delayed gastric emptying and disordered gastric acid secretion during times of perioperative stress.

GENERAL PREOPERATIVE ASSESSMENT
Respiratory System

The preoperative anesthetic evaluation should focus on several key historical aspects in patients suspected of ventilatory muscle involvement from neuromuscular illness. **Breathlessness on exertion is a common feature of neuromuscular disorders,**[74] but patients with more severe skeletal muscle deformities may not be able to generate sufficient exertion to offer this complaint. **Orthopnea is a prominent feature of diaphragmatic weakness** because the weight of the abdominal contents limits the excursion of the diaphragm in the supine position. The patient may offer complaints related to morning headache, snoring, apnea during sleep, or daytime somnolence, suggesting positional airway obstruction or disordered ventilatory drive. A history of difficulty swallowing or aspiration is also important. Finally, the patient may admit to ventilatory failure resulting from a chest infection or prior surgical procedures.

After routine auscultation of the chest, several important findings of ventilatory muscle weakness can be observed during relaxed breathing. **Rapid shallow breathing, the recruitment of accessory muscles of ventilation, an alternating pattern of ventilatory muscle activity between diaphragm and accessory muscles, and ventilatory muscle incoordination are all signs of ventilatory muscle weakness.**[33] Paradoxic upward motion of the abdomen during inspiration suggests profound weakness of the diaphragm (Fig. 16-1), especially when the inspiratory paradox is increased in the supine position.

Preoperative laboratory assessment of respiratory dysfunction in patients with neuromuscular disease requires assessment of oxygenation, ventilatory muscle function, and airway integrity (Table 16-1). Arterial blood gases provide the standard for assessment of arterial oxygenation and carbon dioxide; noninvasive measurement of oxygen saturation by pulse oximetry and carbon dioxide by end-tidal carbon dioxide may suffice in some situations. The chest radiograph is useful for determining the pres-

NORMAL INSPIRATION

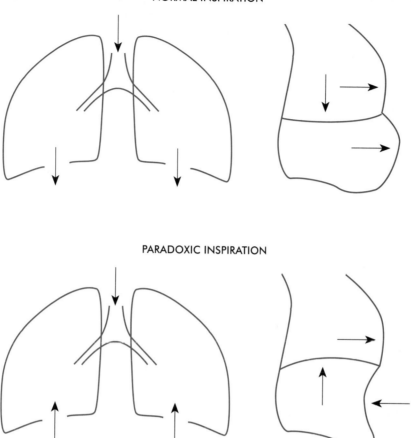

PARADOXIC INSPIRATION

Fig. 16-1. Paradoxic inspiratory motion of the abdomen occurs when the abdomen moves upward and inward during inspiration.

ence of atelectasis or infiltrates. Preoperative pulmonary function studies may be simplified to include forced vital capacity (FVC) and inspiratory force (IF) measurements. Forced vital capacity is a good estimate of ventilatory muscle strength and chest wall compliance in the absence of parenchymal lung disease,[74] although maximal ventilatory effort is required to collect meaningful information. Maximal IF measurements are also useful in assessing ventilatory muscle strength, although general muscle strength, height, and weight make a small contribution to the overall measurement. The combination of both measurements suggests the overall level of ventilatory muscle weakness. Flow-volume loop studies are sensitive measurements of upper airway involvement or ventilatory muscle dysfunction; both reduce peak inspiratory flow rate. Weakness of the bulbar musculature results in fluttering in the loop during expiratory and occasionally inspiratory flow.[84]

Cardiovascular System

The extent and severity of autonomic dysfunction is difficult to assess noninvasively. Orthostatic hypotension, resting tachycardia, paralytic ileus, anhidrosis, and constricted pupils are all clinical signs of generalized autonomic dysfunction.[51] **The presence of clinical signs of dysautonomia may indicate profound hemodynamic instability from adrenergically active anesthetics or blocking drugs.** Assessment of peripheral vascular tone with invasive monitoring may be indicated perioperatively.

Table 16-1 Response to muscle relaxants in neuromuscular disease		
Neuromuscular diagnosis	**Nondepolarizing**	**Depolarizing**
Muscular denervation	Normal	Hyperkalemia
Myasthenia gravis	Increased	Resistant
Myasthenic syndrome	Increased	Increased
Myotonia	Normal-increased	Spasticity
Muscular dystrophy	Normal-increased	Cardiac dysrhythmia

Cardiomyopathy from myopathic illness is relatively common, and preoperative history, assessment of electrocardiogram, echocardiogram, and chest radiographs identify most individuals with serious involvement.[62] **The standard electrocardiogram is the most reliable tool for suspecting cardiac involvement;** tall right precordial R waves and Q waves in leads 1, aV_L, and V_5 to V_6 are most characteristic.[69] Conduction system abnormalities and dysrhythmias are frequent findings, although the implications of these findings for perioperative care are uncertain.[62] Left ventricular dysfunction and mitral valve prolapse are frequently found on echocardiography.[62,88] Determination of creatine phosphokinase has long been used to identify active systemic myopathy, but it may not accurately detect myocardial dystrophy.[69]

Nutritional Effects

A history of weight loss, poor appetite, or difficulty swallowing should be sought in the preoperative period. Laboratory confirmation of hypoalbuminemia, anemia, hypocalcemia, and decreased transferrin levels suggest important preoperative malnutrition that may require repletion therapy to prevent infection and improve wound healing.

Neuromuscular Effects of Anesthetic Agents
General anesthesia

Inhalational anesthetics (halothane, enflurane, and isoflurane) suppress neuromuscular transmission and, **at high concentrations, produce up to 50% diminution in the force of muscle contraction.** As blood anesthetic levels decrease in normal patients, clinically important muscle weakness on emergence from anesthesia is not apparent. However, even low concentrations of residual inhalational anesthetics in patients with neuromuscular disease may prolong return of baseline neuromuscular function postoperatively.

Muscle relaxants

The perioperative effects of depolarizing and nondepolarizing muscle relaxants depend on the type of neuromuscular disease, and each class of drugs must be used cautiously (Table 16-2). **Depolarizing relaxants such as succinylcholine may cause pathologic muscle contracture and lethal hyperkalemia in patients with neuropathic muscle denervation.**[3,30] Abnormal contracture of facial and respiratory musculature in response to depolarizing agents may make orotracheal intubation impossible and impair mechanical ventilatory efforts. Use of succinylcholine increases serum potassium concentrations in normal patients, and the exaggerated release of intracellular potassium may produce lethal hyperkalemia in patients with denervated muscle.[37] **This hyperkalemic response develops approximately 3 weeks after acute denervation injury;** use of depolarizing relaxants should be avoided in all patients with chronic motor neuropathy. **Pretreatment with nondepolarizing relaxants does not prevent succinylcholine-induced hyperkalemia.** Nondepolarizing muscle relaxants have normal effects in patients with denervated muscle,[3] but the clinical response may be prolonged.

The intensity and duration of nondepolarizing relaxants is enhanced in patients with abnormalities of the neuromuscular junction. Although some anesthesiologists avoid use of nondepolarizing agents in these patients, other practitioners use small doses while carefully monitoring the extent of relaxation

Table 16-2 Criteria for ventilatory intervention			
Criteria	**Normal**	**Borderline**	**Failure**
Oxygenation			
Saturation	>97% on room air	>95% on O_2	<95% on O_2
Po_2	>75% on room air	>75 on O_2	<75 on O_2
Chest radiograph atelectasis	None	Subsegmental	Lobar
Ventilation			
Blood gases	Normal Pco_2	$Pco_2 < 50$	$Pco_2 > 50$
	Normal pH	Normal pH	pH <7.37
Inspiratory force (cm H_2O)	<50	<30	>30
Vital capacity (ml)	>15/kg	10-15/kg	<10/kg
Airway			
Swallowing	Liquids and solids	Solids only	Aspirates
Breathing	Unobstructed	Positional obstruction	

with train-of-four electrical stimulation.[3] The effect of depolarizing relaxants in patients with defects of neuromuscular transmission is variable. Some patients are resistant to succinylcholine, whereas in others prolonged noncompetitive (phase II) block develops. It is probably wise to avoid the use of depolarizing relaxants in patients with myasthenia gravis.

Muscle relaxants have variable and unpredictable effects in patients with primary muscle diseases. Relaxants have little effect on the muscle tone of diseased fibers since the site of disease is distal to the neuromuscular junction. However, the response of normal muscle fibers may be exaggerated, and smaller doses of both depolarizing and nondepolarizing agents may be required.[3]

Regional anesthesia

Successful administration of major conduction anesthetics has been reported for a variety of neuromuscular diseases.[45,46] No data exist to indicate that regional techniques with local anesthetics adversely affect the progression of neuromuscular diseases,[83] with the possible exception of amide-type local anesthetics in porphyria. Major conduction blockade also produces sympathectomy, which may exacerbate hypotension in patients with preexisting autonomic dysfunction.[46]

ROLE OF PREOPERATIVE PLASMA EXCHANGE THERAPY

Half of all therapeutic plasma exchanges performed annually in the United States are done in patients with neurologic disorders.[82] Physical separation of plasma from formed elements of the blood and subsequent reinfusion of the formed elements with a plasma replacement permits removal of circulating toxic substances. Plasma exchange is useful in diseases that are mediated by circulating antibodies or other immunologically active substances.[82]

Preoperative plasma exchange in patients with severe myasthenia gravis who are undergoing thymectomy reduces the need for postoperative mechanical ventilation, decreases time to extubation, and decreases the length of stay in intensive care.[17,34] Patients with myasthenia gravis who are difficult to wean from mechanical ventilation postoperatively may benefit from plasma exchange. Plasma exchange improves ventilatory function when used early in the course of patients with Guillain-Barré syndrome.[56] The risks of plasma exchange therapy are probably higher in the perioperative period than at any other time. Bleeding associated with depletion of coagulation factors, regional anticoagulation, citrate-induced hypocalcemia, and activation of either complement or fibrinolytic cascades has been reported.[82] Replacement of coagulation factors with fresh frozen plasma and platelets may reduce the risk of bleeding. Complement activation may result in noncardiogenic pulmonary edema and adult respiratory distress syndrome. Acute changes in plasma volume may aggravate fluid imbalances and require continuous monitoring of ventricular preload and cardiac output.

PREOPERATIVE ASSESSMENT OF SPECIFIC NEUROMUSCULAR DISEASES

Myelopathy

Amyotrophic lateral sclerosis

Amyotrophic lateral sclerosis (ALS) is characterized by degeneration of the lower motor neuron, motor nuclei of the brainstem, and the descending pathway of the upper motor neurons.[9] Progressive muscular atrophy and bulbar muscle weakness with fasciculations are its clinical manifestations.

Atrophy and weakness of respiratory muscles eventually lead to ventilatory failure and death.[9] The impairment of ventilatory musculature, especially airway muscles, affects anesthetic management. Aspiration is a clear danger in the perioperative period when muscular deficits are exaggerated. **Respiratory reserve is reduced from muscle weakness and skeletal deformity, but ventilatory drive is not impaired.** If there is doubt as to the ability of the patient to protect the airway or sustain minute ventilation, ventilatory support should be continued into the postoperative period.

The response to muscle relaxants, either depolarizing or nondepolarizing, is altered in ALS. **There are numerous reports of succinylcholine-induced hyperkalemia, with subsequent cardiovascular collapse.**[21] Motor nerve degeneration and subsequent recruitment by adjacent fibers cause a change in the neuromuscular junction, resulting in increased sensitivity to all nondepolarizing relaxants.[3] Whenever possible, **muscle relaxants should be avoided.** Epidural anesthesia has been safely conducted in several patients.[45]

Multiple sclerosis

Multiple sclerosis (MS) is a demyelinating disease of the brain and spinal cord. Surgery in patients with MS may be required more frequently than in other patients because of the orthopedic, urologic, and neurologic complications of MS. Various stressful situations, particularly those associated with elevated body temperature, may exacerbate the symptoms of MS.[43] **Demyelinization of neural tissue could predispose to local anesthetic neurotoxicity, and patients with MS may have increased autonomic lability.** For these reasons, **spinal anesthesia has generally been**

considered contraindicated. General anesthesia does not appear to pose an additional hazard to patients with MS.[4,46]

Peripheral Neuropathy
Guillain-Barré syndrome

Guillain-Barré syndrome is an inflammatory polyneuropathy that may affect all motor, sensory, autonomic, and cranial nerves.[6] Although this neuropathy most commonly follows acute viral infection, it has been reported in postoperative patients without apparent preceding viral illness. Ascending, symmetric muscle weakness is the major clinical manifestation that evolves over several days. Motor involvement may include ventilatory and facial musculature. Transient paresthesias are common early in the disease. Loss of deep tendon reflexes suggests the diagnosis. Nerve conduction studies differentiate polyneuropathy from high cervical spinal cord lesions or transverse myelitis.[59] Conduction velocities are slowed early as paralysis develops, and denervation potentials appear later with profound disease. Spinal fluid remains acellular, but protein levels increase to maximum levels 4 to 6 weeks after the onset of illness. Other causes of acute polyneuropathy, such as acute intermittent porphyria and heavy metal poisoning, must be excluded.

Respiratory failure in Guillain-Barré syndrome often begins with weakness of forced exhalation and impaired cough.[77] Atelectasis or hypoxemia suggests imminent ventilatory failure. Inspiratory muscle weakness develops later in the disease and is manifested by rapid shallow breathing and decreased FVC and IF. Abnormal inward motion of the abdomen during inspiration and use of accessory inspiratory muscles are often observed. Minute ventilation decreases, and any elevation of carbon dioxide tension portends rapidly progressive ventilatory failure. Abnormal swallowing and glottic dysfunction may occur at any time in the course of Guillain-Barré syndrome. Inability to handle oral secretions, recurrent aspiration, and positional airway obstruction are ominous signs of imminent ventilatory failure.[66] Tracheostomy is indicated early in the course of ventilatory failure, and airway access may be required for management of bulbar muscle weakness long after ventilatory function returns to normal.

Autonomic dysfunction frequently accompanies motor weakness in patients who progress to ventilatory failure.[2,22,27,54,80,81] Sinus tachycardia[32] and repolarization abnormalities are commonly observed on electrocardiogram.[67] Intermittent bradydysrhythmias have resulted in death in some patients, and continuous electrocardiographic monitoring is indicated early in the course of the disease.[38] Episodic hypertension[40,60,89] and profound hypotension regularly occur in patients with severe disease who have quadriparesis and ventilatory failure.[80] Continuous arterial blood pressure monitoring may be indicated for patients with dysautonomia, and pulmonary artery and occlusion pressure measurements may assist in intravascular volume management.[15,41,86] Hypotension may require use of vasoconstrictor agents, volume expansion, or inotropic support.

Acute intermittent porphyria

Acute intermittent porphyria is an inherited disorder of porphyrin metabolism. Increased levels of the breakdown products of porphyrin metabolism cause demyelination and axonal degeneration of peripheral nerves, which result in flaccid paralysis and weakness of skeletal muscle.[6] The ventilatory musculature and autonomic nervous system are often involved by the neuropathic process. Denervation sensitivity to muscle relaxants may also develop. The disease may also be characterized by painful abdominal crises that mimic the acute abdomen.

Use of barbiturates, alcohol, and sulfonamides has been associated with enzyme induction that worsens the syndrome.[6] Although it is rare for any anesthetic drug to induce symptoms during latent porphyria,[63] **anesthesia and surgery both appear to worsen an acute attack. Numerous anesthetics have been shown to induce porphyrin synthesis including barbiturates, etomidate, enflurane, and methoxyflurane.**[21] Ketamine and propofol have been used without adverse sequelae in humans.[5,10,14,61] No harmful effect is expected with opioids, local anesthetics, nitrous oxide, or isoflurane.[43] Regional anesthetic techniques may be appropriate during an acute attack, although major conduction techniques risk interaction with the autonomic neuropathy commonly seen in porphyria.

Neuromuscular Junction Diseases
Myasthenia gravis

Myasthenia gravis is a neuromuscular junction disease that is characterized by weakness and fatigability of skeletal muscles. Autoimmune-mediated reduction of the number of acetylcholine receptors at the neuromuscular junction[19] results in inability to sustain or repeat muscular contractions. Electromyographically, this abnormality corresponds to "fade" of muscle contraction observed during repetitive nerve stimulation after neuromuscular blockade with nondepolarizing muscle relaxants. Muscle strength improves similarly in both myasthenia gravis and nondepolarizing blockade after administration of anticholinesterase drugs.

Prognosis for patients with myasthenia gravis has improved markedly in recent years.[20] Glucocorticoids and regular plasma exchange are particularly effective in patients with severe disease with ventilatory impairment. Although muscle function may initially deteriorate after beginning steroid therapy, improvement of ventilatory function normally occurs after 2 weeks of therapy. Thymectomy improves symptoms in most patients with severe disease, and in some patients results in total remission.[52,68] Median sternotomy for thymectomy initially had a mortality of approximately 25%, and nonlethal respiratory complications were common.[52] However, a recent series of 27 patients reported one perioperative death and 60% of patients were drug-free postoperatively.[31] Improved outcome was attributed to complete resection of thymic tissue and excellent support systems for perioperative care.

Preoperative preparation of patients with myasthenia gravis includes assessment of pulmonary mechanical function such as FVC and IF, arterial blood gases, chest radiographic films, and determination of upper airway competence. If severe abnormalities of these parameters are encountered, surgery should be postponed to allow upward adjustment of anticholinesterase medication or plasma exchange therapy unless the patient is already receiving maximal medical therapy. **Preoperative plasma exchange decreases time on mechanical ventilation and shortens intensive care stay after thymectomy.**[17] **Anticholinesterase medications should be continued until the morning of surgery.**

The goals of anesthetic management include support of respiratory function during operation and return of the patient to preoperative levels of neuromuscular function at the end of the procedure.[48] Use of general anesthesia, endotracheal intubation, and high supplemental oxygen flow usually satisfy the need for respiratory support intraoperatively. **Inhalational agents are ideal because they provide both effective anesthesia and adequate muscle relaxation without administration of supplemental muscle relaxant drugs.** Muscle relaxants should be avoided when possible because patients with myasthenia gravis are 10 to 100 times more sensitive to their effects than normal patients.[20] **If muscle relaxation is required, succinylcholine may be the drug of choice for short-term management, but the onset of "phase II" block occurs at very low doses in these patients.**[3] Return to preoperative neuromuscular function is facilitated by resuming anticholinesterase medication before emergence from anesthesia. Intravenous infusion of prostigmine ($\frac{1}{60}$ of the usual daily oral dose of pyridostigmine over 24 hours) should begin during wound closure. Mechanical ventilatory support should continue postoperatively until all criteria for adequate ventilatory function and airway patency are met. Postoperatively, patients with severe disease may improve muscle strength and ventilatory capacity after plasma exchange, and this therapy may shorten time to tracheal extubation.

Rapid deterioration of neuromuscular and respiratory function (myasthenic crisis) may occur at any time perioperatively as a result of infection, stress, or overdose with anticholinesterase drugs. Endotracheal intubation and mechanical ventilatory support are usually required before the cause of myasthenic crisis can be treated. Although crisis may be the result of inadequate anticholinesterase therapy, satisfactory recovery is not often achieved by increasing the dose of these drugs.[48] Instead, anticholinesterase drugs may be withdrawn after ventilatory support is initiated to avoid precipitating a cholinergic crisis with respiratory and bulbar muscle weakness, excessive salivation, and abdominal cramps. Administration of atropine or glycopyrrolate ameliorates the vagal symptoms of a cholinergic crisis, but muscular strength returns slowly as the anticholinesterase drug is metabolized. Plasma exchange effectively increases muscle strength, facilitates weaning from mechanical ventilation, and allows reintroduction of anticholinesterases at lower dosages during cholinergic crisis.

Myasthenic syndrome (Eaton-Lambert)

Unlike myasthenia gravis, muscles may temporarily increase power during the first few contractions in patients with myasthenic syndrome. Bulbar musculature is less likely to be involved.[75] Preoperative anesthetic considerations are similar to those for myasthenia gravis with regard to respiratory assessment. Also, **unlike myasthenia gravis, the response to neostigmine and pyridostigmine is variable,** although these patients are extremely sensitive to both depolarizing and nondepolarizing muscle relaxants.

Muscular Dystrophies
Duchenne's muscular dystrophy

Muscular dystrophies are a group of primary muscular disorders of unknown cause that often begin in childhood and pursue a rapid and progressive course to death. Duchenne's muscular dystrophy, the most common and severe, is characterized by degeneration of muscle fibers (including diaphragm) and increased content of fat and fibrous tissue.[67] Cardiac muscle is also involved in the dystrophic process.[69] Most patients have detectable cardiac abnormalities, but only 10% of patients have clinically significant abnormalities, and most of these occur in the terminal phases of disease. In a series of 36 patients, **electrocardiographic abnormalities were present in 92% of patients,** decreased diastolic endocardial velocity was observed by echocardiogram in 90%, and ejection fraction was decreased in 21% of patients.[28] Echocardiographic abnormalities did not correlate with the extent of skeletal muscle involvement. **Most patients do not have cardiovascular symptoms, and cardiovascular disease is rarely the cause of death.**

The incidence of serious perioperative complications in patients with muscular dystrophy is low because most surgical procedures are performed early in the course of these diseases. Nondepolarizing muscle relaxants may have either a normal or prolonged response.[3] The response to depolarizing neuromuscular blockade may be normal, but **cardiac arrest possibly related to hyperkalemia has been reported after use of succinylcholine.**[73] Other dysrhythmias unrelated to drug therapy have precipitated cardiac arrest in the immediate postoperative period in patients with muscular dystrophy,[73] and continuous electrocardiographic monitoring may permit early recognition and treatment of this problem. Regional anesthetic techniques have been successfully used to avoid precipitating malignant hyperthermia.

Myotonic dystrophy

Myotonia implies an abnormal persistence of induced or voluntary muscle contractions; increased muscle tone persists even after denervation or paralysis.[21] The increased muscle tone may be the result of a generalized membrane defect in which muscle membranes have normal resting potentials but increased resistance to electrical conduction.

Respiratory and cardiac involvement complicates anesthetic management. Ventilatory dysfunction is characterized by swallowing difficulties and altered ventilatory drive, which may elevate resting P_{CO_2}. **The degree of cardiac involvement does not correlate with the severity of skeletal muscle involvement. Death from cardiac dysrhythmia is common;** the electrocardiogram may reveal bradycardia and delayed intraventricular conduction. Hyperglycemia may result from a membrane-mediated resistance to insulin.

Anesthetic management may be complicated by the sensitivity of the patient to respiratory depressants, and difficulty assisting ventilation because of rigidity of the jaw and chest resulting from respiratory muscle myotonic spasm. Although use of general anesthesia, spinal anesthesia, and depolarizing relaxant drugs cannot prevent a myotonic contracture, the response to nondepolarizing relaxants may be normal.[60] Use of succinylcholine may induce a myotonic response.[21]

Myopathy
Central core disease

It is important to recognize this myopathic disease because of its known association with malignant hyperthermia.[39,44] **All precautions to avoid malignant hyperthermia must be taken** when anesthetizing patients with central core disease.[21]

Proximal muscle weakness is a common feature of this disease and may be associated with secondary skeletal changes such as hip dislocation, kyphoscoliosis, funnel chest, mandibular hypoplasia, and short neck. Bulbar and respiratory musculature is spared. The electrocardiogram is normal.[1]

Mitochondrial Myopathy
Glycogen storage disease

This group of related illnesses is notable for the buildup of glycogen in muscle, resulting in a diffuse pattern of muscle weakness in which proximal muscles are often more involved than peripheral muscles. The muscles of ventilation may be severely involved, resulting in profound diaphragmatic weakness and ventilatory failure. Cardiomyopathy may also be present and limit cardiac reserve. Anesthetic management should be planned to support ventilation in the perioperative period, and not stress cardiac reserve.[13,55]

Familial periodic paralysis

The two forms of familial periodic paralysis are defined by serum potassium levels. In the **hypokalemic form,** weakness is exacerbated by carbohydrate or salt loading, or rest following strenuous exercise. **Flaccid paralysis of voluntary muscle may last up to 36 hours, but bulbar and ventilatory musculatures are spared.**[21] The electrocardiogram may show manifestations of hypokalemia when potassium levels reach 2 to 3 mEq/L, but the severity of skeletal muscle weakness does not correlate well with serum potassium levels. Anesthesia and surgery may initiate an episode of weakness, so that prolonged postoperative monitoring is indicated even after a benign intraoperative course. Because hypothermia or glucose and salt loading can precipitate an attack, careful intraoperative monitoring of temperature, glucose, and electrolytes is important.

Attacks from hyperkalemic periodic paralysis tend to be shorter and are often related to exercise and cold. Increased muscle tone may be present, and patients may have difficulty swallowing or coughing, but **ventilatory musculature is usually spared.** The elevation of serum potassium may be mild and short-lived, and may represent hypersensitivity of the muscle membrane to acetylcholine or mechanical stimulation. Glucose/insulin or calcium infusions may be used to treat the acute attack. Electrocardiographic and temperature monitoring are essential. **Muscle relaxants should be avoided, since use of succinylcholine may induce hyperkalemia,** and neostigmine reversal of nondepolarizing muscle relaxants may induce myotonia from excessive acetylcholine elevation.[21]

Malignant Hyperthermia

Malignant hyperthermia is the feared and often lethal syndrome related to anesthetic drug administration. The mortality from malignant hyperthermia in the

United Kingdom **remains at approximately 24% in diagnosed cases.**[25] Inciting anesthetics trigger a hypermetabolic state that results in temperature elevation and diffuse rhabdomyolysis often associated with muscle rigidity. The underlying defect relates to an increase in the intracellular concentration of calcium ion under basal conditions.[49] An increased rate of calcium delivery to the cytoplasm activates energy-consuming reactions to remove calcium from the contractile proteins. This energy expenditure produces the hypermetabolic state. When calcium delivery exceeds the energy-consuming calcium-sequestering process, the contractile event is prolonged and results in muscle rigidity. The malignant hyperthermic episode represents an imbalance between energy supply and demand. The resultant pathophysiologic condition is identical to that of ischemia.[36] Temperature elevation reflects the magnitude of the hypermetabolic state and may roughly correlate with survival.[58] Rhabdomyolysis follows prolonged muscle rigidity and results in gross elevations in serum creatinine kinase and myoglobin. Acute hyperkalemia and hypocalcemia result from the change in muscle permeability to these ions. Disseminated intravascular coagulation and renal failure may occur during this time.

Malignant hyperthermia may represent a form of inherited myopathy with a mild expression. A susceptible patient may have been previously anesthetized with triggering anesthetic drugs without a clinically apparent reaction. Other neurologic and myopathic illnesses have been associated with malignant hyperthermia, but except for central core myopathy, the association may be coincidental.[8] Nevertheless, **myopathic and neuropathic disorders may share pathogenic mechanisms with malignant hyperthermia, resulting in positive muscle contracture tests and possibly leading to clinical events during anesthesia.**[39] Caution should be exercised during anesthesia with this group of patients.

Any patient who appears to be at increased risk for development of malignant hyperthermia must be the subject of heightened awareness and readiness during anesthetic management. Because of the effectiveness of nontriggering anesthetic techniques in avoiding malignant hyperthermic crisis, pretreatment with dantrolene is probably not needed.[23] A carefully administered nontriggering anesthetic will not induce the clinical syndrome even in a patient with a history of a full-blown crisis. This approach is combined with the expectation that prompt diagnosis and effective treatment with dantrolene are available whenever necessary.

KEY POINTS

- Neuromuscular diseases adversely affect the respiratory and cardiovascular systems; respiratory insufficiency is the major cause of death.
- Early responses to increased inspiratory work include (1) frequent changes in respiratory pattern to alternate work between fatiguing muscles and accessory respiratory muscles and (2) increasing respiratory rate to allow more efficient use of weakened muscles, resulting in increased inspiratory time and an increased ratio of dead space to tidal volume. Both responses decrease ventilatory efficiency and increase the risk of ventilatory failure.
- Cardiovascular involvement ranges from autonomic dysfunction with neuropathic diseases to myocardial failure with myopathic diseases.
- Patients with dysautonomia frequently become hyponatremic in the perioperative period from the combination of hypovolemia, arginine vasopressin release, stress, and volume replacement with hyponatremic solutions.
- Depolarizing relaxants may cause pathologic muscle contracture and lethal hyperkalemia in patients with neuropathic muscle denervation. This hyperkalemic response develops approximately 3 weeks after acute denervation injury.
- The intensity and duration of nondepolarizing relaxants are enhanced in patients with abnormalities of the neuromuscular junction.
- Half of all therapeutic plasma exchanges performed annually in the United States are done in patients with neurologic disorders.
- Demyelinization of neural tissue could predispose patients to local anesthetic neurotoxicity, and patients with MS may have increased autonomic lability.
- Anesthesia and surgery both appear to worsen an acute attack of intermittent porphyria. Numerous anesthetics have been shown to induce porphyrin synthesis, including barbiturates, etomidate, enflurane, and methoxyflurane.
- Myopathic and neuropathic disorders may share pathogenic mechanisms with malignant hyperthermia, resulting in positive muscle contracture tests and possibly leading to clinical events during anesthesia.

KEY REFERENCES

Azar I: The response of patients with neuromuscular disorders to muscle relaxants: a review, *Anesthesiology* 61:173, 1984.

Cohen CA, Zagelbaum G, Gross D et al: Clinical manifestations of inspiratory muscle fatigue, *Am J Med* 73(3):308, 1983.

Gracey D, Howard F, and Divertie M: Plasmapheresis in the treatment of ventilator-dependent myasthenia gravis patients: report of four cases, *Chest* 85(6):739, 1984.

Kytta J, Rosenberg PH: Anaesthesia for patients with multiple sclerosis, *Ann Chir Gynaecol* 73:299, 1984.

McKhann GM, Griffin JW, Cornblath DR et al: Analysis of prognostic factors and the effect of plasmapheresis, *Ann Neurol* 23(4):347, 1988.

Moorsman JR, Coleman RE, Packer DL et al: Cardiac involvement in myotonic muscular dystrophy, *Medicine (Baltimore)* 64:371, 1985.

Mustajoki P, Heinonen J: General anesthesia in "inductible" porphyrias, *Anesthesiology* 53:15, 1980.

Perloff JK: The heart in neuromuscular disease, *Curr Probl Cardiol* 11:509, 1986.

Sethna N, Rockoff M, Worthen M et al: Anesthesia related complications in children with Duchenne muscular dystrophy, *Anesthesiology* 68:462, 1988.

Smith PE, Calverley PM, and Edwards RH: Hypoxemia during sleep in Duchenne muscular dystrophy, *Am Rev Respir Dis* 137:884, 1988.

Utility of therapeutic plamapheresis for neurological disorders, Consensus Conference *JAMA* 256(10): 1333, 1986.

Truax BT: Autonomic disturbances in the Guillain-Barré syndrome, *Semin Neurol* 4(4):462, 1984.

Wintzen AR, Schipperheyn JJ: Cardiac abnormalities in myotonic dystrophy: electrocardiographic and echocardiographic findings in 65 patients and 34 of their unaffected relatives. Relation with age and sex and relevance for gene detection, *J Neurol Sci* 80:259, 1987.

REFERENCES

1. Adams RD, Victor M: *Principles of neurology,* New York, 1981, McGraw-Hill.
2. Appenzekkar O, Marshall J: Vasomotor disturbance in the Landry-Guillain-Barré syndrome, *Arch Neurol* 9:368, 1963.
3. Azar I: The response of patients with neuromuscular disorders to muscle relaxants: a review, *Anesthesiology* 61:173, 1984.
4. Bamford C, Sibley W, and Laguna J: Anesthesia in multiple sclerosis, *Can J Neurol Sci* 5:41, 1978.
5. Bancroft GH, Lauria JI: Ketamine induction for cesarean section in a patient with acute intermittent porphyria and achondroplastic dwarfism, *Anesthesiology* 59: 143, 1983.
6. Bradley WG, Thomas PK: Peripheral nerve diseases. In Walton J, ed: *Disorders of voluntary muscle,* London, 1988, Churchill-Livingstone.
7. Braun N, Arora N, and Rochester D: Respiratory muscle and pulmonary function in polymyositis and other proximal myopathies, *Thorax* 38(8):616, 1983.
8. Brownell AKW: Malignant hyperthermia: relationship to other diseases, *Br J Anaesth* 60:303, 1988.
9. Campbell MJ: Motor neuron diseases. In Walton J, ed: *Disorders of voluntary muscle,* London, 1988, Churchill-Livingstone.
10. Capouet V, Dernovoi B, and Azagra JS: Induction of anaesthesia with ketamine during an acute crisis of hereditary coproporphyria, *Can J Anaesth* 34:388, 1987.
11. Carroll J, Zwillich C, Weil J et al: Depressed ventilatory response in oculocranioisomatic neuromuscular disease, *Neurology* 26(2):140, 1976.
12. Cohen CA, Zagelbaum G, Gross D et al: Clinical manifestations of inspiratory muscle fatigue, *Am J Med* 73(3):308, 1983.
13. Coleman P: McArdle's disease: problems of anaesthetic management for caesarean section, *Anaesthesia* 39:784, 1984.
14. Cooper R: Anaesthesia for porphyria using propofol, *Anaesthesia* 43:611, 1988 (letter).
15. Covert C, Brodie S, and Zimmerman J: Weaning failure due to acute neuromuscular disease, *Crit Care Med* 14(4):307, 1986.
16. Dalos N, Borel C, and Hanley D: Cardiovascular autonomic dysfunction in Guillain-Barré syndrome: therapeutic implications of Swan-Ganz monitoring, *Arch Neurol* 45:115, 1988.
17. d'Empaire G, Hoaglin DC, Perlo VP et al: Effect of prethymectomy plasma exchange in postoperative respiratory function in myasthenia gravis, *J Thorac Cardiovasc Surg* 89:592, 1985.
18. DeTroyer A, Borenstein S, and Cordier R: Analysis of lung volume restriction in patients with respiratory muscle weakness, *Thorax* 35(8):603, 1980.
19. Drachman DB: The biology of myasthenia gravis, *Ann Rev Neurosci* 4:195, 1981.
20. Drachman DB: The present and future treatment of myasthenia gravis, *N Engl J Med* 316(12):743, 1987.
21. Duncan PG: Neuromuscular diseases. In Katz J, Steward DJ, eds: *Anesthesia and uncommon pediatric diseases,* Philadelphia, 1987, WB Saunders.
22. Durscher AG, Senavis B, Caridroix M et al: Autonomic dysfunction in the Guillain-Barré syndrome: hemodynamic and neurological studies, *Intensive Care Med* 6:3, 1980.
23. Eichhorn JH: Testing and pretreatment in malignant hyperthermia, *Wellcome Trends in Anesthesiology* 7:3, 1989.
24. Ellis E, Bye P, Bruder J et al: Treatment of respiratory failure during sleep in patients with neuromuscular disease: positive-pressure ventilation through a nose mask, *Am Rev Respir Dis* 135(1):148, 1987.
25. Ellis RF: The diagnosis of MH: its social implications, *Br J Anaesth* 60:251, 1988.
26. Estenne M, Heilporn A, Selhez L et al: Chest wall stiffness in patients with chronic respiratory muscle weakness, *Am Rev Respir Dis* 128(6):1002, 1983.
27. Faguis J, Wallin BG: Microneurographic evidence of excessive sympathetic outflow in the Guillain-Barré syndrome, *Brain* 106:589, 1983.
28. Farah M, Evans E, and Vignos P: Echocardiographic evaluation of left ventricular function in Duchenne's muscular dystrophy, *Am J Med* 69:248, 1980.
29. Ferguson R, Murphy R, and Lascelles R: Ventilatory failure in myasthenia gravis, *J Neurol Neurosurg Psychiatry* 45:217, 1982.
30. Ferguson R, Wright D, Willey R et al: Suxamethonium is dangerous in polyneuropathy, *Br Med J* 282:298, 1981.

31. Fischer JE, Grivalski HT, Nussbaum MS et al: Aggressive surgical approach for drug-free remission from myasthenia gravis, *Ann Surg* 205(5):496, 1987.

32. Fresin JC, Sanchez L, Garnacho A et al: Heart rate variations in the Guillain-Barré syndrome, *Br Med J* 281:649, 1980.

33. Gibson G, Pride N, Davis J et al: Pulmonary mechanics in patients with respiratory muscle weakness, *Am Rev Respir Dis* 115(3):389, 1977.

34. Gracey D, Howard F, and Divertie M: Plasmapheresis in the treatment of ventilator-dependent myasthenia gravis patients: report of four cases, *Chest* 85(6): 739, 1984.

35. Grinman S, Whitelaw W: Pattern of breathing in a case of generalized respiratory muscle weakness, *Chest* 84(6):770, 1983.

36. Gronert GA, Mott J, and Lee J: Aetiology of malignant hyperthermia, *Br J Anaesth* 60:253, 1988.

37. Gronert G, Theyre R: Pathophysiology of hyperkalemia induced by succinylcholine, *Anesthesiology* 43(1):89, 1975.

38. Haymaker W, Kernohan J: The Landry-Guillain-Barré: a clinicopathologic report of fifty fatal cases and a critique of the literature, *Medicine* 28:59, 1949.

39. Heiman Patterson TD, Rosenberg H et al: Halothane-caffeine contracture testing in neuromuscular diseases, *Muscle Nerve* 11:453, 1988.

40. Hobday JD, Baker AJ: Guillain-Barré complicated by hypertension and ileitis, *Med J Aust* 2:536, 1968.

41. Hodson A, Hurwitz BJ, and Albrecht R: Dysautonomia in Guillain-Barré syndrome with dorsal root ganglioneuropathy, Wallerian degeneration, and fatal myocarditis, *Ann Neurol* 15:88, 1984.

42. Kahn JK, Sisson JC, and Vinik AI: Prediction of sudden cardiac death in diabetic autonomic neuropathy, *J Nucl Med* 29:1605, 1988.

43. Kadis LB: Neurological disorders. In Katz J, Benumof J, and Kadis LB, eds: *Anesthesia and uncommon diseases: pathophysiologic and clinical correlations,* Philadelphia, 1981, WB Saunders.

44. Koch BM, Bertorini TE, Eng GD et al: Severe multicore disease associated with reaction to anesthesia, *Arch Neurol* 42: 1204, 1985.

45. Kochi T, Oka T, and Mizuguchi T: Epidural anesthesia for patients with amyotrophic lateral sclerosis, *Anesth Analg* 68:410, 1989.

46. Kytta J, Rosenberg PH: Anaesthesia for patients with multiple sclerosis, *Ann Chir Gynaecol* 73:299, 1984.

47. Le Quesne PM, Fowler CJ: Quantitative evaluation of toxic neuropathies in man, *Electroencephalogr Clin Neurophysiol* 39 (suppl):347, 1987.

48. Loh L: Neurological and neuromuscular disease, *Br J Anaesth* 58:190, 1986.

49. Lopez JR, Alamo L, Caputo C et al: Intracellular calcium concentration in muscles from humans with malignant hyperthermia, *Muscle Nerve* 8:355, 1985.

50. MacIntyre NR: Respiratory function during pressure support, *Chest* 89:677, 1986.

51. Low P: Autonomic neuropathy, *Semin Neurol* 7(1):49, 1987.

52. Maggi G, Giaccone G, Donadio M et al: A review of 169 cases, with particular reference to results of surgical treatment, *Cancer* 58(3):765, 1986.

53. Matikainen E, Juntunen J: Autonomic nervous system dysfunction in workers exposed to organic solvents, *J Neurol Neurosurg Psychiatry* 48:1021, 1985.

54. Matsuyama H, Haymaker W: Distribution of lesions in the Landry-Guillain-Barré syndrome, with emphasis on involvement of the sympathetic system, *Acta Neuropathol* 8:230, 1967.

55. McFarlane HJ, Soni N: Pompe's disease and anaesthesia, *Anaesthesia* 41:1219, 1986.

56. McKhann GM, Griffin JW, Cornblath DR et al: Analysis of prognostic factors and the effect of plasmapheresis, *Ann Neurol* 23(4):347, 1988.

57. McLeod ME, Creighton RE: Anesthesia for pediatric neurological and neuromuscular diseases, *J Child Neurol* 1:189, 1986.

58. Meuller RA: How to identify malignant hyperthermia, *Prob Anesth* 1:233, 1987.

59. Miller R: Guillain-Barré syndrome: current methods of diagnosis and treatment, *Postgrad Med* 77:57, 1985.

60. Mitchell P, Meilman E: The mechanism of hypertension in the Guillain-Barré syndrome, *Am J Med* 42:986, 1967.

61. Mitterschiffthaler G, Theiner A, Hetzel H et al: Safe use of propofol in a patient with acute intermittent porphyria, *Br J Anaesth* 60:109, 1988.

62. Moorman JR, Coleman RE, Packer DL et al: Cardiac involvement in myotonic muscular dystrophy, *Medicine (Baltimore)* 64:371, 1985.

63. Mustajoki P, Heinonen J: General anesthesia in "inductible" porphyrias, *Anesthesiology* 53:15, 1980.

64. Newsom DJ, Goldman M, Loh L et al: Diaphragm function and alveolar hypoventilation, *Q J Med* 177:87, 1976.

65. Newsom DJ, Loh L: Alveolar hypoventilation and respiratory muscle weakness, *Bull Eur Physiopathol Respir* 15:45, 1979.

66. Newton JH: Prevention of pulmonary complications in severe Guillain-Barré syndrome by early assisted ventilation, *Med J Aust* 142(8):444, 1985.

67. Oakley CM: The heart in Guillain-Barré syndrome, *Br Med J* 288:94, 1984.

68. Papatestas A, Genkins C, Kornfeld P et al: Effects of thymectomy in myasthenia gravis, *Ann Surg* 206(1):79, 1987.

69. Perloff JK: The heart in neuromuscular disease, *Curr Probl Cardiol* 11:509, 1986.

70. Person A, Solders G: R-R variations in Guillain-Barré syndrome: a test of autonomic dysfunction, *Acta Neurol Scand* 67:294, 1983.

71. Rochester D: Malnutrition and the respiratory muscles, *Clin Chest Med* 7(1):91, 1986.

72. Rochester D: Respiratory effects of respiratory muscle weakness and atrophy, *Am Rev Respir Dis* 134(5):1083, 1986.

73. Sethna N, Rockoff M, Worthen M et al: Anesthesia related complications in children with Duchenne muscular dystropy, *Anesthesiology* 68:462, 1988.

74. Shneerson J: *Disorders of ventilation,* Boston, 1988, Blackwell Scientific.

75. Simpson JA: Myasthenia gravis and related syndromes. In Walton J, ed: *Disorders of voluntary muscle,* London, 1988, Churchill-Livingstone.

76. Smith PE, Calverley PM, and Edwards RH: Hypoxemia during sleep in Duchenne muscular dystrophy, *Am Rev Respir Dis* 137:884, 1988.

77. Sunderrajan EV, Davenport J: The Guillain-Barré syndrome: pulmonary neurologic correlations, *Medicine* 64(5): 333, 1985.

78. Tobin MJ, Guenther SM, Perez W et al: Konno-Mead analysis of ribcage-abdominal motion during successful and unsuccessful trials of weaning from mechanical ventilation, *Am Rev Respir Dis* 135:1320, 1987.

79. Tobin MJ, Perez W, Guenther SM et al: The pattern of breathing during successful and unsuccessful trials of weaning from mechanical ventilation, *Am Rev Respir Dis* 134:1111, 1986.

80. Truax BT: Autonomic disturbances in the Guillain-Barré syndrome, *Semin Neurol* 4(4):462, 1984.

81. Tuck R, McLead J: Autonomic dysfunction in the Guillain-Barré syndrome, *J Neurol Neurosurg Psychiatry* 44:983, 1981.

82. Utility of therapeutic plasmapheresis for neurological disorders, Consensus Conference, *JAMA* 256(10):1333, 1986.

83. Vandam L: Neurological sequelae of spinal and epidural anesthesia, *Int Anesthesiol Clin* 24:231, 1986.

84. Vincken W, Elleker G, and Cosio MG: Detection of upper airway muscle involvement in neuromuscular disorders using the flow-volume loop, *Chest* 90:52, 1986.

85. Vincken W, Elleker MG, and Cosio MG: Determinants of respiratory muscle weakness in stable chronic neuromuscular disorders, *Am J Med* 82:53, 1987.

86. Weintraub M: Autonomic failure in Guillain-Barré syndrome — value of Swan-Ganz catheterization, *JAMA* 242: 513, 1979.

87. Weng TR, Schultz GE, Chang CH et al: Pulmonary function and ventilatory response to chemical stimuli in familial myopathy, *Chest* 88:488, 1985.

88. Wintzen AR, Schipperheyn JJ: Cardiac abnormalities in myotonic dystrophy: electrocardiographic and echocardiographic findings in 65 patients and 34 of their unaffected relatives. Relation with age and sex and relevance for gene detection, *J Neurol Sci* 80:259, 1987.

89. Yao H, Fukiyama K, Takada Y et al: Neurogenic hypertension in Guillain-Barré syndrome, *Jpn Heart J* 26(4):593, 1985.

CHAPTER 17

Evaluation of the Patient with Endocrine Disease and Diabetes Mellitus

FREDERICK E. SIEBER

Although it is not as obvious as a physical deformity, a disturbance in endocrine function may increase the complexity of an anesthetic and the risk to the patient. The anesthesiologist must be attuned to the issues of endocrine abnormalities to ensure that the patient is optimally managed preoperatively. This chapter focuses on the issue of proper preoperative management of patients with specific endocrine abnormalities with an emphasis on minimizing anesthetic-related complications.

THYROID DISEASE

Tunbridge et al. surveyed the community of Whickham to obtain an estimate of thyroid disease incidence in Great Britain.[109] Overt hyperthyroidism had a prevalence rate of 19/1000 women, rising to 27/1000 when "possible" cases were included. For men the range was 1.6 to 2.3/1000. **The risk of developing hyperthyroidism is greatest in females 30 to 39 years of age. The primary cause of hyperthyroidism is Graves' disease, whose prevalence closely parallels the overall prevalence of hyperthyroidism.** Hyperthyroidism in patients over the age of 60 accounts for 10% to 17% of the thyrotoxic population.[18] Hypothyroidism is also a common disorder, with a prevalence of 14 to 19/1000 in women and less than 1/1000 for males. In Tunbridge's cohort, elevated thyroid-stimulating hormone (TSH) levels (>6 mu/L) were recorded in 7.5% of women and 2.8% of males. Depressed serum thyroxine (T_4) concentrations have been observed in approximately half of all patients exhibiting an elevated TSH.[87] The majority of patients with hypothyroidism have iatrogenic hypothyroidism or autoimmune thyroiditis. **Also, 95% of all cases of hypothyroidism are primary in nature and are more common in the elderly.** The most severe form of hypothyroidism, myxedema coma, is extremely rare.

Physiology

The synthesis and release of thyroid hormone occur as a result of the interaction of thyroid hormone, the thyroid gland, and the hypothalamic-pituitary axis. The hypothalamus acts to control the release of thyrotropin-releasing hormone (TRH), which is secreted by the hypothalamic neurons and delivered to the adenohypophysis via the hypophyseal portal system. Within the pituitary gland TRH may stimulate the secretion of TSH, which acts at the thyroid gland to control the synthesis and secretion of the thyroid hormones. A negative feedback loop is present between the pituitary and the thyroid in which elevated levels of thyroid hormone inhibit the secretion of TSH from the pituitary. Thyroid hormone levels are the primary determinants of TSH secretion, and elevated thyroid hormone levels can override TRH-mediated hypothalamic influences.[20]

The important physiologically active forms of thyroid hormone are T_4 and its diiodinated form, triiodothyronine (T_3). Thyroxine is synthesized in the thyroid gland. In the systemic circulation T_4 may undergo metabolic conversion to T_3 (35%) or the inactive metabolite reverse T_3 (rT_3) (40%). The secretion of T_4 from the thyroid gland is 80 to 100 μg/day and the half-life of T_4 in the serum is 6 to 7 days. Triiodothyronine is formed primarily by peripheral conversion of T_4 in the liver and kidney (80%) and secondarily by thyroid synthesis (20%). Triiodothyronine is the primary hormone responsible for the effects of the thyroid gland and is approximately three times as potent as T_4. With stress, the level of T_3 may increase. The half-life of T_3 is 24 to 30 hours. The thyroid hormones are bound in the bloodstream by three types of binding proteins: T_4-binding globulin (TBG), thyroxine-binding prealbumin, and albumin. Most thyroid hormone is bound to TGB. About 0.04% T_4 and 0.4% T_3 circulate in free form. **The free hormone concentration is the active component, which determines a patient's metabolic state.**

Numerous tests are available to assess thyroid function. With the advent of radioimmunoassay and dialysis techniques, serum T_3 and T_4 levels are now routinely measured. However, T_4 and T_3 (this measurement includes both bound and unbound) measurements fail to consider the TBG levels that influence free hormone levels. This assumes importance in states associated with elevated levels of TBG, such as pregnancy.[9] To obtain an indication of TBG binding, either TBG or serum-binding capacity can be measured. An alternative approach to estimating free thyroid hormone is the T_3 resin uptake test, which is used to provide an estimate of the unoccupied binding sites on TBG. The T_3 resin uptake does not reflect serum T_4 binding in all clinical states, especially at extremely high or low TBG levels. The product of the T_3 resin uptake test times total T_4 provides an estimate of unbound T_4 known as the "free T_4 index." Similar formulas have been derived for estimating a free T_3 index. Direct measurements of free T_4 and free T_3 require dialysis techniques and are not available in all hospitals. Other thyroid tests include serum TSH concentration, which can be helpful in the diagnosis of hypothyroidism. The hypothalamic-pituitary-thyroid axis can be assessed using the TRH stimulation test, thyroid suppression test, and TSH stimulation test.

Initial screening tests for hyperthyroidism may include T_4 and free T_4 concentrations or, if these are not available, T_4 and T_3 resin uptake. Screening tests for hypothyroidism may include total serum T_4 concentration, some index of free T_4 concentration, and serum TSH. The combination of low serum T_4 concentration and elevated TSH provides evidence of primary hypothyroidism. Serum T_4 and TSH levels are diagnostic in more than 90% of cases with either subclinical or overt hypothyroidism.[69] However, a low serum T_4 or T_3 level alone is not diagnostic of hypothyroidism. In determining the adequacy of the thyroid replacement dose, measurement of serum T_3 is not reliable. Serum T_4 can be used as a guide to replacement therapy although the levels vary depending on the relative T_4 and T_3 content of the thyroid preparation and its absorption. **Serum TSH is probably the most sensitive indicator of the adequacy of thyroid replacement dose.** For more information concerning the uses of various thyroid function tests, there are several excellent texts on this subject.[107]

Thyroid hormones have several important roles in growth and metabolism. Thyroid hormones stimulate calorigenesis and metabolism by increasing metabolic rate and oxygen consumption. In addition to regulating cellular respiration, these hormones cause an increase in body protein turnover and adipocyte lipolysis. Although growth hormone is the primary determinant of linear growth, in human fetal development, thyroid hormone is necessary for skeletal maturation prenatally and for brain development during infancy,[90] as demonstrated by the effects of thyroid hormone depletion in cretinism. Thyroid hormones exert their effects on development through somatomedins, erythropoietin, and epidermal and nerve growth factors.[28] Catecholamine responsiveness is influenced by the thyroid. Although use of propranolol reverses the cardiac effects of thyrotoxicosis, these effects are not secondary to increased catecholamine secretion. Several clinical studies have shown that plasma epinephrine and norepinephrine levels, as well as urinary catecholamine excretion, are unaltered during hyperthyroidism and hypothyroidism.[19] The cardiovascular changes with thyroid disease could also be explained by interactions between thyroid hormone and the beta-adrenergic system. Thyroxine increases the speed of shortening of the contractile elements of the heart.[19] Catecholamine responsiveness of the heart may depend on thyroid integrity whereby thyroid hormone increases the number of beta-adrenergic receptors in the heart.[6]

Changes in thyroid physiology during the perioperative period complicate thyroid function assessment and make total serum T_4 and T_3 unreliable in evaluating thyroid function postoperatively. Generally, when compared with preoperative levels, T_4 increases while T_3 may decrease postoperatively.[86] In particular, the "sick euthyroid syndrome" should be considered in conjunction with surgery and acute illness. **"Sick euthyroid syndrome" occurs with advancing age and systemic nonthyroid illness.** It causes variable changes in total T_4, but the free T_4 level is often normal. Circulating T_3, both free and total, is decreased and reverse T_3 may be elevated. Thyroid-stimulating hormone levels may not be elevated and the usual clinical signs of hypothyroidism are absent. **During sick euthyroid syndrome the rate of T_4 to T_3 conversion is decreased and reverse T_3 elevations may be secondary to either an increased T_4 to rT_3 metabolism or decreased rT_3 degradation. Mortality during surgery is high in patients with reduced T_3 in association with a low total T_4 level.**[65] However, the role of thyroid hormone in this subset of patients with sick euthyroid syndrome has not been determined.

Pharmacology

There are five drugs used primarily to treat hypothyroidism. The thyroid preparations (Table 17-1) are used for thyroid hormone replacement in the treatment of hypothyroidism. These drugs may also be used to suppress TSH, for example, when attempting to decrease the size of a diffuse nontoxic goiter. Because of differences in absorption and peripheral conversion of T_4 to T_3, serum levels of T_4 and T_3 will vary among patients. **Therefore clinical symptoms and serum TSH suppression are better indicators of adequacy of thyroid replacement when evaluating the patient with hypothyroidism.**

There are several drugs used primarily for hyperthyroidism. **The thioamides, which inhibit thyroid hormone synthesis,** are antithyroid drugs and consist of methimazole (tapazole) and propylthiouracil (PTU). Propylthiouracil also decreases peripheral conversion of T_4 to T_3; however, the clinical significance of this effect is unknown. The initial daily doses are PTU, 300 to 600 mg, and methimazole, 15 to 30 mg followed by titration until a euthyroid state is achieved. With the thioamides, clinical and laboratory improvement occurs within 1 to 2 weeks and by 4 to 6 weeks the serum T_4 and T_3 levels may be within the normal range. Side effects are unusual but may include hypersensitivity, serum sickness, and agranulocytosis.

Iodide inhibits thyroid hormone release and synthesis via the Wolff-Chaikoff effect, in which iodide organification is prevented. It also decreases thyroid vascularity. Iodide's effects occur within 24 hours, maximize in several days, and last approximately 14 days. Therefore it is primarily an adjunct rather than a primary mode of therapy for hyperthyroidism. The usual dose is approximately 500 mg/day; however, a dose of 100 to 200 mg probably is sufficient to produce these effects. Iodide is given in conjunction with the antithyroid drugs and propranolol in the treatment of thyrotoxicosis. During preoperative preparation for thyroid surgery, iodine may be given for 7 to 10 days before surgery. Hyperthyroidism can be treated with radioactive iodine and in many cases is the therapy of choice.

Propranolol is useful in controlling the peripheral effects of hyperthyroidism. It consistently reduces heart rate at rest and during exercise as well as reducing cardiac output in thyrotoxicosis.[44] The usual oral dose is 80 to 160 mg daily in divided doses with an adjustment according to heart rate. Administration of atropine counteracts many of the cardiovascular effects of propranolol and should be omitted from preoperative medication regimens in patients with thyrotoxicosis. Other drugs used to alter the sympathetic nervous system during treatment of thyrotoxicosis include guanethidine and reserpine.[12,34] Use of diltiazem has been shown to decrease heart rate and the number of premature ventricular contractions in patients with thyrotoxicosis.[82] Calcium channel block-

Table 17-1 Thyroid hormones

Preparation	Generic name	Brand name	T_4	T_3	Usual dose
Desiccated thyroid	Thyroid tablets	Thyrar	X	X	90-120 mg
Pig thyroid extract	Thyroglobulin	Proloid	X	X	90-120 mg
Synthetic L-thyroxine	Levothyroxine sodium	Synthroid; Levoxine	X		0.1-0.2 mg
Synthetic T_3	Liothyronine sodium	Cytomel		X	50-70 µg
Synthetic T_4, T_3 mixture	Liotrix	Euthroid; Thyrolar	X	X	100-200 µg

ers may provide adjuvant therapy for thyrotoxicosis in the presence of cardiac disease. Use of amiodarone, an iodine-containing antiarrhythmic agent, can control symptoms of thyrotoxicosis through an iodine-induced inhibition of T_4 and T_3 release.[91] However, amiodarone has no advantages over equivalent doses of iodine.

Preoperative Evaluation

All patients with thyroid disease should undergo a careful airway examination, especially when a goiter is present. **Airway compromise in the form of recurrent laryngeal nerve compression, tracheal deviation, or displacement can occur with large goiters.** A preoperative neck CT scan may be efficacious as a further diagnostic tool.

Hyperthyroidism

It is important to assess both the degree of thyrotoxicosis as well as end organ manifestations. Although laboratory tests are used to determine a definitive diagnosis, they do not necessarily reflect the clinical severity of disease. Unfortunately, no scale to assess clinical severity of thyroid disease is in common use, probably because thyrotoxicosis is not one but many syndromes. **The clinical spectrum of hyperthyroidism ranges from asymptomatic mild elevations in laboratory values to thyroid storm. The intraoperative risk increases with severity of disease.** The clinical signs and symptoms of hyperthyroidism are shown in Box 17-1. Two symptoms are closely associated with hyperthyroidism: heat intolerance and weight loss despite increased food intake.[62] Thyrotoxic syndromes are commonly associated with Graves' disease (diffuse toxic goiter), toxic nodular goiter, exogenous hormone or iodine administration.[62] Less common causes of thyrotoxicosis include malignancy and pituitary disorders. Goiter occurs with most of the common causes of thyrotoxicosis except exogenous

---

BOX 17-1
SYMPTOMS AND SIGNS OF
HYPERTHYROIDISM

Symptoms	Signs
Nervousness	Thyroid enlargement
Increased sweating	Tachycardia
Heat intolerance	Atrial fibrillation
Palpitations	Hyperkinesis
Dyspnea	Eye signs
Fatigue and weakness	
Weight loss or gain	
Increased appetite	
Hyperdefecation	

---

thyroid hormone. It is important to note the presence of proptosis so that proper eye protection is undertaken during the intraoperative period. **Thyrotoxicosis can be difficult to recognize in the elderly because the typical hyperkinetic picture is often absent.**[18] Laboratory diagnosis is confirmed by elevations of free T_3, free T_4, or the free hormone index.

Hyperthyroidism causes alterations of the cardiovascular system. McDevitt et al. have shown that the thyroid has a role in regulation of the resting heart rate, with hyperthyroidism causing heart rate elevations compared to normal individuals.[64] Thyrotoxicosis is also associated with increases in stroke volume, cardiac output, and pulse pressure as well as premature ventricular contractions and atrial fibrillation. Forfar et al. showed that atrial fibrillation occurring in elderly patients without an underlying cause is associated with a 13% incidence of hyperthyroidism.[29] It is not clear if hyperthyroidism causes congestive heart failure, but elderly patients with thyrotoxicosis frequently have congestive heart failure. Because of rapid diastolic filling, a third heart sound may be heard and peripheral edema and neck vein engorgement can occur even in the absence of failure. It is difficult to diagnose cardiac pathologic conditions in patients with thyrotoxicosis although symptoms in younger patients may disappear after treatment of the thyroid condition.[19] Death from hyperthyroidism usually occurs from cardiovascular events secondary to emboli or myocarditis.[5,73] Weakness of the respiratory muscles can occur, leading to reductions in vital capacity and compliance, whereas increased carbon dioxide production secondary to hypermetabolism is associated with an increase in minute ventilation. Myopathy has an incidence ranging from 55% to 80% in various series. Electromyographic abnormalities occur in more than 90% of patients with thyrotoxicosis.[78] A familial hypokalemic periodic paralysis may occur in association with thyrotoxicosis in Oriental males.[79] In addition, Graves' disease with its immunoglobulin G derivatives may be associated with myasthenia gravis. Hyperthyroidism may be associated with negative nitrogen balance secondary to hypermetabolic increases in protein synthesis and catabolism.

The diagnosis of thyroid storm is a clinical one characterized by exaggerated thyrotoxic manifestations of gastrointestinal and cardiovascular signs and symptoms, including nausea, vomiting, pain, pulmonary edema, and cardiac failure. The central nervous system manifestations vary but terminate in coma. The signs and symptoms of thyroid storm tend to be more intense and involve more organ systems than thyrotoxicosis.[114] Thyroid storm is rare and usually seen in undiagnosed or incompletely treated patients with complications of major illness (infections, trauma, diabetic ketoacidosis) or surgery.[59] Laboratory studies cannot consistently differentiate thyroid storm from less severe hyperthyroidism. However, Mazzaferri et al. believe that reasonably clear diagnostic criteria exist, including temperature > 100° F; marked tachycardia; exaggerated manifestations of thyrotoxicosis; and central nervous system, cardiovascular, or gastrointestinal dysfunction.[61] In addition, they report elevated levels of protein-bound iodine in comparison to uncomplicated thyrotoxicosis. **The need for diagnosis and aggressive therapy in thyroid storm is emphasized by older studies showing mortality ranging from 28% to 100%[114] that improves to less than 10% with early diagnosis and management.[61]**

Preoperative preparation of the patient with hyperthyroidism depends on the urgency of the surgery and the severity of the thyroid disease. **For elective surgery the patients should be euthyroid.** Optimal preoperative preparation consists of 1 to 2 months of treatment with an antithyroid drug. Approximately 1 to 2 weeks before surgery, iodide may be added to the regimen. Alternatives to this approach have included the use of propranolol in combination with iodine[27] or propranolol alone.[108] Both of these regimens may be more efficacious, since they shorten the preoperative preparation time. However, use of propranolol alone may not prevent thyroid storm.[25] **In patients requiring emergency surgery, a combination of antithyroid drugs, propranolol, and sodium iodide is administered.** Vigorous hydration is provided as well as cooling blankets to decrease heat and fluid loss. Intravenous glucose and oxygen must also be provided because of the increased catabolic state. A suggested approach in emergency situations includes PTU, 600 to 1000 mg orally, in conjunction with intravenous administration of propranolol to control heart rate (1 to 10 mg). Sodium iodide is administered, either intravenously or by mouth, depending on the urgency of the situation, approximately 1 hour after PTU has been given so that iodine is not incorporated into thyronine before hormone synthesis is blocked.[100] Corticosteroids should also be administered because the adrenal reserve is decreased and cortisol decreases peripheral conversion of T_4 to T_3. An alternative regimen for emergency surgery includes propranolol, 1 to 10 mg IV, and sodium iodide, 1 g IV 1 to 2 hours preoperatively.[94] The preferred antipyretic is acetaminophen since salicylates displace thyroid hormones from their serum-binding proteins.

Thyroid storm is treated with similar regimens. When surgery is not imminent, PTU can be given in a dose of 600 to 1000 mg orally followed by 300 mg four times a day or, alternatively, tapazole is given in a dose of 30 to 60 mg daily. Sodium iodide is then administered in a dose of 1 g every 8 to 12 hours IV, starting 1 hour after antithyroid drug administration.

Peripheral manifestations of thyroid storm may be treated with intravenous propranolol, and 2 to 8 mg dexamethasone is given daily. If propranolol is contraindicated, reserpine or guanethidine can be given, although their onset is slow. Alternative treatments include plasmapheresis or peritoneal dialysis.[59] Supportive measures mentioned previously are also undertaken.

The treatment of severe thyrotoxicosis takes precedence over all but the most life-threatening surgical conditions, with the risk of delaying surgery weighed against the risk of precipitating thyroid storm.

Hypothyroidism

Hypothyroidism is characterized by numerous signs and symptoms (Box 17-2). With severe hypothyroidism myopathy occurs and may cause enlargement of the tongue, as well as changes in the voice. Serum creatine phosphokinase activity can increase up to eightfold in patients with hypothyroidism even in the absence of muscle symptomatology.[70] Myocardial contractility may be decreased during even mild hypothyroidism and is reversed following treatment.[7,37] It is controversial whether myxedema causes heart failure. McBrien and Hindle, using the pulse pressure response to the valsalva maneuver, provided evidence that myxedema alone probably does not cause heart failure.[63] In addition, congestive heart failure is unusual in patients with hypothyroidism because both metabolic rate and cardiac output

---

BOX 17-2
SYMPTOMS AND SIGNS OF HYPOTHYROIDISM

Symptoms	Signs
Cold intolerance	Weight gain (or loss)
Dyspnea	Bradycardia
Anorexia	Diastolic hypertension
Constipation	Cardiac rub or soft
Decreased libido	heart tones caused by
Menorrhagia, amen-	pericardial effusion
orrhea	Ileus
Oliguria	Galactorrhea
Arthralgias	Urinary retention
Myalgia, muscle stiff-	Loss of brow and scalp
ness, and cramps	hair
Dryness	Yellow (carotinemic)
Fatigue	skin
Depression	Psychosis
Irritability	Coma
Impaired concentration	Carpal tunnel syndrome
and memory	
Paresthesia	
Pallor	

decrease in parallel. However, other investigators have shown that even short periods of hypothyroidism lead to decreases in response to exercise and cardiac reserve, probably as a result of decreased metabolism.[22] **Patients with hypothyroidism may have bradycardia and decreased ECG voltage.** They are sensitive to digitalis preparations, and care must be taken when treating congestive heart failure. Myxedema does not predispose patients to coronary artery disease, but long-standing hypothyroidism associated with hypertension may be a risk factor for coronary artery disease.[103] Despite decreases in myocardial contractility, angina frequently occurs with hypothyroidism.[72] The pulmonary system may be affected by myxedematous infiltration of the respiratory muscles, and depression of the respiratory responses to hypoxia and carbon dioxide can occur.[123] Wilson and Bedell showed that myxedema decreases maximal breathing capacity and lung diffusion capacity.[120] Laboratory studies can demonstrate bleeding tendencies, hyponatremia secondary to inappropriate antidiuretic hormone (ADH), and hypoglycemia. The decrease in basal metabolic rate can lead to hypothermia.

When treating hypothyroidism in the elderly, the initial dose of L-thyroxine is approximately 25 μg/day, to be increased by 25 μg every 2 to 4 weeks. An alternative regimen for rapid correction of myxedema would be T_3 50 μg/day IV for 1 week.[51] **The dose of thyroxine should be decreased for patients with angina or coronary artery disease. This recommendation comes from the observation that patients with angina and myxedema can have severe coronary artery disease with exacerbations of angina precipitated by rapid replacement of their thyroid doses.**[72] The question remains whether patients with hypothyroidism and angina should undergo coronary artery bypass surgery prior to instituting thyroid replacement therapy. Several series have substantiated the contention that adequate thyroid replacement in these patients can aggravate angina or induce myocardial infarction.[53] Consequently, no or only subtherapeutic replacement doses have been used in these patients before bypass procedures.[72] **The results in untreated or subtherapeutically treated patients with hypothyroidism have shown no increased morbidity and mortality following coronary artery bypass grafting, with full thyroid replacement possible in the postoperative period.**[39,53,72] Therefore the preoperative evaluation of these patients should focus more on treatment of the underlying cardiac condition than on ensuring a euthyroid state. In hypothyroidism secondary to panhypopituitary disease, thyroid replacement is usually superseded by corticosteroid therapy because of problems with adrenal reserve.

Myxedema coma is rare, occurring in less than 0.1% of hospitalized patients.[110] **If untreated, myxedema coma has an 80% mortality.**[43] These patients are often elderly, female, and hypothyroid with coma precipitated by stress. **Important complications that occur with myxedema coma include carbon dioxide retention, gastrointestinal bleeding, severe hyponatremia, and hypotension that is poorly responsive to vasoactive agents.** The pathophysiology of coma in myxedema is unknown. Treatment involves the administration of either T_4, 400 to 500 μg IV followed by 50 to 200 μg IV daily,[43] or as an alternative T_3 can be given as a 500- to 200-μg intravenous bolus followed by maintenance doses. Because of unpredictable absorption, both drugs should be given IV. Triiodothyronine has a faster onset of action but is riskier because precipitous increases in metabolism and oxygen consumption may occur. When administering T_3 or T_4 IV, ECG monitoring for dysrhythmias is mandatory.[110] With myxedema coma, normothermia must be maintained and the airway managed because airway obstruction and decreases in ventilation are common. Underlying electrolyte and metabolic problems such as hyponatremia and hypoglycemia should also be corrected, and body temperature maintained.

Emergency surgery in a patient with hypothyroidism is treated with intravenous L-thyroxine, 300 to 500 μg, in conjunction with hydrocortisone. Because of the long half-life of thyroxine (7 days), this drug may be withheld preoperatively in patients currently stable with their maintenance thyroid replacement therapy.

Assessment of risk

In assessing the surgical risk in patients with hypothyroidism, Weinberg et al. have shown no increased risk with hypothyroidism.[116] In a series of 40 patients with hypothyroidism, Ladenson et al. showed an increased incidence of intraoperative hypotension, perioperative gastrointestinal hypomotility, and neuropsychiatric disturbance.[52] In addition, cardiac surgery in patients with hypothyroidism may be associated with a higher risk of heart failure. Such complications require anticipatory management, but do not dictate cancelling surgery except in cases of severe hypothyroidism.[52] **Patients with hypothyroidism may be divided into four groups depending on disease severity.**[69] Group 1 consists of patients with elevated TSH levels and normal thyroid hormone levels. These patients have subclinical hypothyroidism and provide no additional risk and may undergo elective surgery at any time. Thyroxine replacement therapy is probably not indicated in subclinical hypothyroidism.[3] Patients in group 2 have decreases in thyroid hormone and elevated TSH. These patients may have mild systemic symptoms without cardiovascular, respiratory, or neurologic symptomatology. Patients in group 2 require additional replacement therapy; however, they may have surgery with no additional risk. Group 3 consists of individuals with hypothalamic-pituitary disease and evidence of decreased TSH as well as thyroid hormone levels. Patients in group 3 can undergo surgery without additional risk; however, they will need corticosteroid coverage in addition to replacement therapy perioperatively. **In group 4, patients are overtly hypothyroid with cardiovascular and respiratory functional impairment. These patients are not candidates for elective surgery because there is a risk of precipitating myxedema coma.** Thyroid replacement therapy should be instituted in patients in group 4 before elective procedures, with some correction of hypothyroid symptomatology. Although a clinical end point is difficult to clearly delineate, the clinician's goal should be to correct laboratory abnormalities as much as possible preoperatively.

DISORDERS OF CALCIUM METABOLISM SECONDARY TO PARATHYROID DISEASE

Hypercalcemia secondary to parathyroid disease is a common condition. With the advent of routine chemical screening there has been a marked increase in the incidence of hyperparathyroidism, with approximately 50,000 new cases of primary hyperparathyroidism diagnosed each year in the United States.[54] Of these cases, 25% to 50% are asymptomatic with calcium levels less than 11 mg/dl. The disease primarily affects elderly women. **The most common cause of primary hyperparathyroidism is a parathyroid adenoma (80% to 90%), followed by parathyroid hyperplasia (15%). Parathyroid carcinoma is uncommon.** Secondary hyperparathyroidism is usually not associated with hypercalcemia. However, in patients with renal failure with secondary hyperparathyroidism, hypercalcemia may occur following correction of the renal failure (tertiary hyperparathyroidism). At the other end of the spectrum, hypocalcemia may occur secondary to parathyroid hormone (PTH) deficiency/resistance or vitamin D deficiency. Hypocalcemia secondary to hypoparathyroidism is most commonly caused by surgical ablation, although in the pediatric population one must be cognizant of DiGeorge's syndrome.

Physiology

Calcium exists in three compartments within plasma: protein-bound; complexed to ions such as bicarbonate, phosphate, or citrate; and in the free ionized form. Blood levels of calcium are regulated within a range of 9 to 10.5 mg/dl. **Three hormones interact to provide calcium homeostasis (PTH, calcitonin, and vitamin D) among sources of calcium, including the**

bone and GI absorption, and loss of calcium through bone formation or renal excretion. Parathyroid hormone is secreted from the parathyroid gland and raises serum calcium levels while promoting bone resorption. Vitamin D and its active metabolites 25-hydroxycholecalciferol and 1,25-dihydroxycholecalciferol act in conjunction with PTH to stimulate bone resorption. In the kidney PTH increases the renal absorption of calcium, while increasing the excretion of phosphate, bicarbonate, potassium, sodium, and some amino acids. Parathyroid hormone also promotes the conversion of 25-hydroxycholecalciferol to 1,25-dihydroxycholecalciferol, which increases intestinal Ca^{++} absorption. This latter action allows PTH to indirectly affect Ca^{++} absorption. **Parathyroid hormone release is increased by hypocalcemia and steroids and inhibited by Mg^{++} and vitamin D.** Steroids increase PTH secretion by inhibiting bone resorption and calcium absorption in the gut. Vitamin D inhibits PTH secretion by increasing serum calcium. Hypermagnesemia may inhibit PTH; however, severe hypomagnesemia causes paradoxical hypocalcemia secondary to both inhibition of PTH secretion and end organ response.

Calcitonin is secreted by the thyroid gland in response to hypercalcemia. Calcitonin inhibits bone resorption, and promotes renal excretion of phosphate, sodium, and potassium. In humans, calcitonin is of little physiologic significance.[54]

Preoperative Evaluation

Hyperparathyroidism

When evaluating patients with hypercalcemia, the first step is to repeat the test. **It is preferable to obtain ionized calcium because this is the portion that exerts the primary physiologic effects.** However, if this is unavailable, the calcium level should be interpreted in light of the serum protein concentration. As a rough guide, a 1-g/dl increase in albumin will increase total serum calcium by 0.8 mg/dl. In addition, acidosis may provoke hypercalcemia by decreasing calcium binding. Clinical manifestations of hypercalcemia vary (Box 17-3). **Hyperparathyroidism may be a manifestation of the multiple endocrine neoplasia syndromes type II (MEN II), which include pheochromocytoma, hyperparathyroidism, and medullary thyroid carcinoma.** Patients are usually asymptomatic with calcium levels up to 12 mg/dl. At levels between 12 and 14 mg/dl, mild symptoms occur, which are often associated with hypercalcemia and osteitis fibrosa cystica. Calcium levels greater than 16 mg/dl may be life threatening.

Laboratory abnormalities in hyperparathyroidism usually include hypercalcemia, hypophosphatemia, hypercalciuria, elevations in serum uric acid, and chloride with a decreased serum bicarbonate. The

---

BOX 17-3
SYMPTOMS AND SIGNS OF HYPERCALCEMIA

Symptoms	Signs
Hypertension	Constipation
Dysrhythmias	Anorexia
Digitalis sensitivity	Nausea/vomiting
Catecholamine resistance	Weakness, atrophy
QT shortening	Depression
Nephrocalcinosis	Personality change
Nephrolithiasis	Psychomotor retardation
Tubular dysfunction	Memory impairment
Renal tubular	Psychosis
acidosis	Disorientation
Impaired Na	Obtundation
reabsorption	Coma
Free water loss	Pruritus
Glomerular disorders	
Interstitial nephritis	
Peptic ulcers	
Pancreatitis	
Hyporeflexia	
Seizures	
EEG abnormalities	
Osteopenia	
Osteitis fibrosa cystica	
Skin necrosis	
Corneal calcification	
Conjunctivitis	
Decreased bronchial clearance of secretions	
Hypomagnesemia	

diagnosis is best supported by an elevated PTH level associated with hypercalcemia.

The primary risk in anesthetizing patients with hypercalcemia is cardiac dysrhythmias. Hypercalcemia decreases the refractory period and increases ventricular excitability. However, these effects may depend on Ca^{++} level. Gunst and Drop found no increased incidence of intraoperative ventricular dysrhythmias in patients with a total Ca^{++} level of approximately 11.6 mg/dl.[36] In addition, QT interval changes are an unreliable indicator of hypercalcemia.[83] Digitalis should be administered with caution, because these patients may show increased sensitivity to the drug.

When treating hypercalcemia preoperatively, reversible complications such as dehydration, mental obtundation, and electrolyte disorders should be corrected. Patients with calcium levels less than or equal to 12 mg/dl require no intervention (except possibly preoperative hydration); however, the cause of the hypercalcemia should be sought. Treatment of more severe hypercalcemia may include pharmacologic intervention or hydration with diuresis. Saline hydration and furosemide rapidly decrease the serum calcium level by 2 to 3 mg/dl. Complications of this therapy include hypokalemia, hypomagnesemia, and congestive heart failure. Mithramycin, which acts directly on bone to block calcium resorption, can be used as a secondary line of therapy. The effects occur in 6 to 12 hours and the dose is 25 μg/kg over 4 hours. Use of mithramycin is effective for all types of hypercalcemia associated with increased bone resorption. It should only be given if clotting studies are normal and the platelets are adequate because bleeding diathesis can occur. A combination of calcitonin and steroids can be administered for hypercalcemia associated with hyperphosphatemia. The dose of synthetic salmon calcitonin is 4 IU/kg every 12 hours, subcutaneously. Calcitonin lasts 6 to 12 hours, with onset of action in 1 to 2 hours. Steroids help to prolong the effect of calcitonin. Intravenous phosphates have a rapid onset of action in managing hypercalcemia. However, they are associated with risks of hypotension, pulmonary edema, hypocalcemia, and metastatic calcification and are contraindicated in renal failure. Intravenous phosphate is given in a dose of 1500 mg phosphorus over 6 to 8 hours. Glucocorticoids can decrease serum calcium levels; however, they have a slow onset of action. Indomethacin, which is used for prostaglandin-associated hypercalcemia, also has a slow onset of action.

Hyperparathyroidism in the pregnant patient deserves special mention. Maternal hypercalcemia may have profound effects on the fetus and newborn, leading to neonatal hypocalcemia or tetany.[48] Literature reports suggest that maternal hyperparathyroidism is associated with significant fetal morbidity and mortality. Because the primary treatment for symptomatic hyperparathyroidism is surgery, it would not be unusual for the anesthesiologist to be presented with the pregnant patient for parathyroidectomy.

Hypoparathyroidism

The signs and symptoms of hypocalcemia are shown in Box 17-4. **The cardinal sign of hypocalcemia is tetany.** On laboratory examination, the ECG may exhibit a prolonged QT interval, predisposing patients to ventricular dysrhythmias. Primary hypoparathyroidism is often associated with hypocalcemia, hyperphosphatemia, and depressed levels of PTH. In assessing the degree of hypocalcemia, low serum albumin levels may not be associated with symptoms if the ionized Ca^{++} level is normal. Alkalosis may also predispose patients to hypocalcemia. Magnesium should be determined for all patients with hypocalcemia, especially in cases of alcohol abuse, malabsorption, or poor nutrition.

BOX 17-4
SYMPTOMS AND SIGNS OF HYPOCALCEMIA

Symptoms	Signs
Hypotension	Paresthesias
Cardiac insufficiency	Weakness
Bradycardia	Anxiety
Dysrhythmias	Dementia
Insensitivity to catechol-	Depression
amines and digitalis	Irritability
QT- and ST-interval	Psychosis
prolongation	Confusion
T-wave inversion	
Laryngeal spasm	
Apnea	
Bronchospasm	
Tetany	
Chvostek's and Trous-	
seau's signs	
Muscle spasm	
Seizures	
Extrapyramidal manifes-	
tations	
Coarse, dry, scaly skin	
Brittle nails	
Thin, brittle hair	
Cataracts	

The major anesthetic risks of hypocalcemia are cardiac dysrhythmias, decreased contractility, development of tetany (especially with hyperventilation), and altered response to muscle relaxants. Such patients may be resistant to digitalis.[14]

It is important that the clinical signs of hypocalcemia be controlled before surgical procedures are performed. Hypocalcemia is treated chronically by dietary calcium and vitamin D supplement. For emergency treatment of hypocalcemia, 10 to 20 ml of intravenous 10% calcium gluconate is given over 10 minutes followed by infusion of 0.5 to 2 mg Ca^{++}/kg/hr with monitoring of Ca^{++} levels. Magnesium levels can be restored acutely by 1 to 2 g of 10% magnesium solution IV.

ADRENAL DISORDERS

For the anesthesiologist, disorders of the adrenal gland present one of three problems: excess secretion of corticosteroids (Cushing's syndrome), excess secretion of aldosterone, or insufficient corticosteroid secretion.

Physiology

Adrenal corticosteroid secretion is controlled via a negative feedback loop with the hypothalamic-pituitary axis. Corticotropin-releasing factor from the hypothalamus stimulates the release of adrenocorticotropic hormone (ACTH) from the pituitary, which in turn stimulates the release of adrenal corticosteroids. Within the negative feedback loop, elevated corticosteroid levels depress the ACTH secretion. In addition to the influences of corticosteroids and corticotropin-releasing factor, ACTH release is modulated by stress and diurnal variation. Peak secretion occurs in the morning, with an evening nadir. Therefore random plasma cortisol levels are of marginal benefit in diagnosing the integrity of the adrenal pituitary axis, and various stimulation and suppression tests such as an overnight dexamethasone suppression test are used.

After surgery, plasma cortisol increases 5 to 10 times by 6 hours postoperatively, with levels falling by 24 hours postoperatively unless the stress continues.[75] Epidural anesthesia delays the cortisol stress response; however, it does not prevent it.[8]

Glucocorticoids have several functions. Steroids increase hepatic gluconeogenesis and decrease fatty acid, nucleic acid, and protein synthesis. They also suppress the inflammatory reaction and inhibit vitamin D by reducing calcium absorption from the gut. Steroids antagonize the effects of ADH and enhance catecholamine vasoconstriction. High doses of glucocorticoids can exhibit a mineralocorticoid effect, causing sodium and water retention with potassium loss.

Aldosterone is secreted by the adrenal cortex in response to hyperkalemia and is inhibited by increases in plasma volume. Aldosterone secretion is controlled by the renin-angiotensin system and circulating levels of ACTH. **Aldosterone works in the distal convoluted tubules of the kidney to promote sodium retention and potassium excretion.** It is the major regulator of extracellular fluid volume and potassium balance.

Pharmacology
Corticosteroids

Adrenocorticotropic hormone is primarily used as a diagnostic agent to establish the presence of adrenal insufficiency. Adrenocorticotropic hormone stimulation tests are performed over many periods of time ranging from rapid (IV bolus) to long term (more than 48 hours of administration), and plasma cortisol responses are measured. Intravenous boluses of ACTH may be used to determine adrenal aldosterone secretion in addition to glucocorticoid levels.

The major effects of corticosteroids can be quantified as a relative potency. In general, the relative potencies of each corticosteroid effect closely parallel each other except for the sodium-retaining property. This leads to a natural division among these drugs between those with increased sodium retention po-

Table 17-2   Potency and dosing of several commonly used corticosteroids

Generic name	Brand name	Biologic half-life	Glucocorticoid potency	Mineralocorticoid potency	Relative dose (mg)
Cortisol	Hydrocortone, Solu-Cortef	8-12 hr	1	1	20
Prednisone	Deltasone	12-36 hr	4	0.8	5
Prednisolone	Delta-Cortef	12-36 hr	4	0.8	5
Methylprednisolone	Solu-Medrol	12-36 hr	5	0.5	4
Cortisone	Cortone Acetate	8-12 hr	0.8	0.8	25
Dexamethasone	Decadron	36-72 hr	25	0	0.75
Fludrocortisone	Florinef	8-12 hr	10	125	—

tencies (mineralocorticoids) and those with increased hepatic glycogen production potencies (glucocorticoids). Table 17-2 shows the relative potencies and equivalent doses of several commonly used corticosteroids. Glucocorticoid replacement ranges from 12.5 to 50 mg/day of cortisone with usual doses between 25 and 37.5 mg/day. For mineralocorticoid effect, fludrocortisone is given in doses of 0.05 to 0.1 mg daily. The doses of these drugs vary with ongoing stress.

Steroid toxicity may arise during withdrawal or continued administration. Adrenal insufficiency following the withdrawal of corticosteroids is characterized acutely by fever, myalgia, arthralgias, and malaise and may be averted with numerous tapering regimens.[10] After discontinuation of corticosteroids, adrenal reserve is usually altered. **Adrenocortical recovery of function following steroid withdrawal lags that of the pituitary and may not be restored for up to 1 year.**[55] Both dosage and duration of therapy must be considered in predicting a patient's response to stress. High-dose steroid therapy (25 mg prednisone twice daily) for only 5 days can affect adrenal pituitary function.[106] With alternate-day therapy, depending on the steroid administration, adrenal response to ACTH is better preserved.[38] The suppression can be minimized by using the lowest possible dose in alternate-day therapy. Both inhaled and topical steroids may impair the pituitary-adrenal axis response, depending on the dose.[13] **Patients receiving the equivalent of 30 mg/day of cortisol for longer than 1 or 2 weeks may have impairment for up to 1 year.**[95] **With this in mind, steroid supplementation should be considered in any surgical patient who has undergone high-dose steroid therapy for at least 1 week within the previous year.** Patients who have had short-term administration, alternate-day therapy, or replacement therapy within the previous year should be assessed on an individual basis.

Use of metyrapone blocks the enzyme 11-β-hydroxylase and decreases cortisol production. It is used to test the integrity of the hypothalamic-pituitary-adrenal axis and to differentiate Cushing's disease from Cushing's syndrome. Metyrapone may also be used in the treatment of Cushing's syndrome.

Other adrenolytic drugs include mitotane, aminoglutethimide, trilostane, and ketoconazole. Mitotane is used for the treatment of inoperable adrenal tumors and takes weeks to months for its effects to occur.[2]

Spironolactone is an aldosterone antagonist used in conjunction with other diuretics for treatment of refractory edema. Its administration can result in hyperkalemia.

Preoperative Evaluation

Patients with excess corticosteroids (either exogenous or endogenous) may display manifestations of Cushing's syndrome (Box 17-5). Cushing's syndrome has many causes, including adrenal hyperplasia, adrenal carcinoma, and pituitary hypersecretion. The most common cause is exogenous steroid administration. The presence of hypertension, metabolic and electrolyte disorders, specifically hypokalemia and uncontrolled diabetes mellitus, should be corrected preoperatively. Fluid status and the presence of muscle wasting and compression fractures should be assessed.

All patients with Cushing's syndrome secondary to exogenous steroid administration require perioperative steroid coverage. The dose is controversial. **Many authorities recommend an equivalent dose of cortisol 300 mg/day perioperatively, with gradual tapering postoperatively.** This regimen is based on the measured maximum stress-induced output of 200 to 300 mg/day cortisol.[117] This dose is given only as a guideline and may be tailored to the surgery. The aim of perioperative steroid coverage is to prevent acute adrenal insufficiency and crisis. The perioperative steroid dose can be decreased, but no study has shown detrimental effects from giving the recommended dose of 200 to 300 mg cortisol/day. If sodium retention is a concern, then a glucocorticoid with decreased

---

BOX 17-5
SYMPTOMS AND SIGNS OF CUSHING'S SYNDROME

Symptoms	Signs
Weakness/proximal myopathy	Centripetal obesity
Psychiatric changes	Hypertension
Impotence	Skin changes
Backache	Thin skin/bruising
Thirst/polyuria	Acne, greasy skin
Headache	Hirsutism
Abdominal pain	Plethora
	Abdominal striae
	Infection (e.g., tinea versicolor)
	Pigmentation
	Oligomenorrhea/amenorrhea
	Osteoporosis
	Vertebral collapse
	Pathologic fracture
	Glucose intolerance
	Ankle edema
	Renal calculi
	Exophthalmos

---

mineralocorticoid activity such as dexamethasone can be used. Patients with Cushing's disease secondary to endogenous production do not require coverage intraoperatively, but will require it postoperatively.

Primary hyperaldosteronism (Conn's syndrome) is characterized by diastolic hypertension, hypokalemic alkalosis, inability to concentrate urine, and skeletal muscle weakness. A normal serum K^+ level in a hypertensive patient will rule out this syndrome unless the patient is on a sodium-restricted diet or taking spironalactone. The preoperative preparation is aimed at improving fluid and electrolyte balance. Spironolactone is given in a dose of 25 to 100 mg every 8 hours for at least 1 week preoperatively with concurrent potassium replacement.[40]

Primary adrenal insufficiency is usually iatrogenic secondary to bilateral adrenalectomy, inadequate steroid administration, or unilateral adrenalectomy for a hyperfunctioning adrenal tumor. Primary adrenal insufficiency presenting as Addison's disease usually exhibits hypoaldosteronism. Signs and symptoms of Addison's disease are shown in Box 17-6. In secondary adrenal insufficiency related to a suppressed hypothalamic pituitary axis, aldosterone secretion remains intact and hyperkalemia does not occur. An additional syndrome of isolated hypoaldosteronism occurs secondary to renin deficiency in patients with normal cortisol secretion, but unexplained hyperkalemia. Patients with suspected adrenal insufficiency should undergo systemic evaluation to assess function before surgery. Suggestive laboratory results include low plasma cortisol levels and impaired ACTH stimulation. Additional testing may include metyrapone, insulin-induced hypoglycemia, or corticotropin-releasing hormone. In addition to adequate steroid coverage, volume status replacement, electrolyte management, and correction of hypotension should occur preoperatively.

When adrenal insufficiency develops acutely, the symptoms may be severe and dramatic (Box 17-7). This may occur in a trauma setting in patients with previously unsuspected inadequate adrenal reserve.[45] The dose of glucocorticoids given depends on the urgency and severity of the clinical situation. Mineralocorticoid properties must be provided if primary adrenal insufficiency exists.

BOX 17-6
SYMPTOMS, SIGNS, AND LABORATORY ABNORMALITIES IN ADDISON'S DISEASE

Symptoms	Signs	Laboratory abnormalities
Weakness, tiredness, fatigue	Skin hyperpigmentation	Hyponatremia
Weight loss	Hypotension	Hyperkalemia
Anorexia	Buccal or tongue pigmentation	Azotemia
Nausea, vomiting	Calcification of the pinnae	Fasting or reactive hypoglycemia (infrequent in adults)
Unspecified gastrointestinal complaints	Vitiligo	Hypercalcemia
Abdominal pain	Hyperthermia or hypothermia	
Diarrhea	Loss of axillary hair in females	
Muscle pain		
Salt craving		
Orthostatic hypotension, dizziness, or syncope		
Lethargy, disorientation		

BOX 17-7
SYMPTOMS AND SIGNS OF ACUTE
ADRENAL INSUFFICIENCY

Symptoms	Signs
Severe clinical deterioration	Fever
Nausea, vomiting	Hypotension
Abdominal or flank pain	Abdominal distension
Lethargy, obtundation	Hyponatremia
	Hyperkalemia

PHEOCHROMOCYTOMA

Pheochromocytomas are tumors of chromaffin tissue origin and are members of the family of amino precursor uptake and decarboxylation (APUD) tumors. **Massive amounts of catecholamines are released by these tumors, causing their characteristic signs and symptoms. They are rare, occurring in 0.5% of all hypertensive patients.**[58] Although usually located unilaterally near the adrenal gland, pheochromocytomas may be found in a variety of locations, including urinary bladder or bilaterally in both the chest and abdomen. From 2% to 3% of these growths constitute neck and/or thoracic masses.[89] Most tumors occur in adults. Children with pheochromocytomas have fewer malignant tumors but tend to have a greater incidence of bilaterality, extraadrenal location, and associated multiple endocrine neoplasia.[49] Pheochromocytoma can be a manifestation of the genetic disorder of multiple endocrine neoplasia syndromes type II (MEN type II). Familial pheochromocytoma is associated with the neuroectodermal dysplasias, including neurofibromatosis, tuberous sclerosis, Sturge-Weber syndrome, and von Hippel-Lindau disease.

Physiology

Pheochromocytomas secrete predominantly norepinephrine. Both the acute effects of catecholamine bursts and their chronic end organ sequelae may influence postoperative outcome. Studies examining the effects of surgery and anesthesia on catecholamine secretion have shown marked increases in norepinephrine during surgery.[111] Dysrhythmias,[101] as well as catecholamine-induced cardiomyopathies, have been estimated to occur in 20% to 30% of these patients.[33] Pulmonary artery pressure monitoring in patients with pheochromocytomas has found a poor relationship between right atrial pressure and pulmonary artery wedge pressure.[66] In addition, chronic vasoconstriction secondary to elevated catecholamine levels may lead to decreases in intravascular volume as well as insensitivity of alpha-receptors to normal levels of catecholamine.[99] These effects are thought to contribute to postoperative hypotension commonly observed in inadequately prepared or undiagnosed patients.

In most cases diagnosis usually rests on documentation by laboratory tests. **High circulating levels of catecholamines or presence of their urinary breakdown products is sufficient diagnostic confirmation.** Often a 24-hour urine collection for measurement of the catecholamine breakdown products of metanephrine, vanillylmandelic acid (VMA), normetanephrine, and catecholamines is used as a screening test. However, tests to find elevated levels of urinary metabolites may give a false-positive result and can result from various medication regimens and alterations in renal function. The relative sensitivity and specificity of various tests for pheochromocytoma are given in Table 17-3. Alternatively, pharmacologic tests (e.g., clonidine suppression) may be used if catecholamine levels are equivocal.

Pharmacology

Phenoxybenzamine is the drug of choice for long-term alpha-blockade.[104] **Preoperative treatment with phenoxybenzamine results in a significantly smoother course than untreated patients.**[104] This drug has a long half-life (approximately 12 hours) and is highly lipid soluble. However, it has unpredictable absorption

---

Table 17-3   Sensitivity and specificity of various tests for pheochromocytoma

Test	Reference values	Sensitivity	Specificity
Plasma NE + E (after clonidine)	>500 pg/ml*	0.97	0.99
Plasma NE + E	>950 pg/ml†	0.94	0.97
Urinary MN	>1.8 mg/24 hr†	0.79	0.93
Urinary VMA	>11 mg/24 hr†	0.42	1.00

NE + E denotes norepinephrine plus epinephrine; *MN* metanephrines; *VMA*, vanillylmandelic acid.
*Upper 95% confidence limits of basal values in 47 normotensive control patients.
†Upper 95% confidence limits of basal values in 70 patients with essential hypertension.
From Bravo EL, Gifford RW Jr: Pheochromocytoma: diagnosis, localization and management, *N Engl J Med* 311:1302, 1984.

through the gut. Its primary side effect is orthostatic hypotension. The starting dose is 20 mg daily in two doses. Every 3 to 4 days the dose is increased, depending on the patient's symptoms and tolerance, with a final dosage range of 40 to 100 mg/day. Preoperative preparation should include 1 to 2 weeks of alpha-adrenergic blocker therapy. Volume replacement is important when instituting alpha-blocker therapy, and often patients have a decreased hematocrit level after the institution of therapy. If the tumor has not been located before exploratory surgery, partial, instead of complete, alpha-blockade may be required by the surgeon to allow for an intraoperative pressor response during tumor palpation. If required, either full blockade should not be instituted, or phenoxybenzamine should be withdrawn 2 to 3 days before surgery. However, these intraoperative concerns may no longer be valid with the advent of CT scanning, which locates pheochromocytoma in 90% of cases.[105] Other alpha-blockers, such as prazosin, have been used with success in such patients. The use of phentolamine is limited because of its short duration.

Beta-blockers (propranolol) are administered for persistent tachycardia and to control other peripheral beta-adrenergic effects of catecholamine excess. These drugs should never be given before alpha-blockade, as serious hypertensive sequelae may result.

The drug α-methyltyrosine inhibits the synthesis of norepinephrine. It is a well-tolerated drug that does not produce hypotension in these patients when given in the dosage of 500 to 2000 mg four times daily. This drug preserves the tissue responsiveness to adrenergic agents. Adequate blockade is achieved in 1 or 2 weeks. Case reports have emphasized that use of α-methyltyrosine without concurrent alpha-adrenergic blocking agents does not prevent hypertensive crisis.[112] Calcium channel blockers can inhibit peripheral catecholamine release. Several case reports have noted the successful use of nifedipine preoperatively, and nicardipine intraoperatively.[1] Further experience is needed with these drugs.

Preoperative Evaluation

Surgical mortality is 1% to 3% in patients with pheochromocytomas.[60] A 10% mortality has been assessed in patients who are untreated and undergo routine surgical procedures.[46]

The adequacy of preoperative preparation may be assessed by determining if ongoing symptoms of catecholamine excess are occurring. Signs and symptoms of pheochromocytoma should be specifically sought (Box 17-8), and the length of preoperative preparation should be determined. When using alpha-blockers, Roizen et al. have used the following

---

> **BOX 17-8**
> **SYMPTOMS AND SIGNS OF PHEOCHROMOCYTOMA**
>
> **Symptoms**
> Headache (severe)
> Excessive sweating (generalized)
> Palpitations with or without tachycardia
> Anxiety or nervousness
> Pain in chest, abdomen, lumbar regions, lower abdomen, or groin
> Nausea and vomiting
> Weakness, fatigue, prostration
> Weight loss (severe)
> Dyspnea
> Warmth with or without heat intolerance
> Visual disturbances
> Dizziness or faintness
> Constipation
> Paresthesia or pain in arms
> Bradycardia (noted by patient)
>
> **Signs**
> Blood pressure changes
> Hypertension with wide fluctuations
> Hypertension induced by physical maneuver such as exercise, postural change, or palpation and massage of flank or mass elsewhere
> Orthostatic hypotension
> Paradoxical blood pressure response to some antihypertensive drugs and marked pressor response with induction of anesthesia
> Hyperhidrosis
> Tachycardia or reflex bradycardia; very forceful heartbeat; dysrhythmia
> Pallor of face and upper part of body
> Anxious, frightened, troubled appearance
> Hypertensive retinopathy
> Leanness or underweight
> Tremor
> Raynaud's phenomenon
> Fever
> Dilated pupils

---

end points for determining optimal dosage: no marked symptoms of catecholamine excess, blood pressure ≤ 160/90 mm Hg on more than two measurements in the 36 hours preceding surgery, systolic blood pressure decreasing ≥ 15% from supine to standing, but blood pressure not lower than 80/45 mm Hg, and the ECG free of ST- and T-wave changes for 2 weeks.[80] These criteria should only be used as a basic guide because some end points, especially the latter, may take several months to achieve. The preoperative cardiovascular examination should seek signs of orthostasis, reveal evidence of heart failure or cardiomyopathy, and determine volume status.

Preoperative preparation should be performed

with the surgeon and internist, depending on the operative requirements. Steroid coverage should be considered if bilateral adrenalectomy is contemplated.

PITUITARY DISORDERS

Most pituitary diseases do not provide special considerations for the anesthesiologist except those that might cause secondary metabolic alterations or diabetes insipidus.

Hypopituitarism

The pituitary gland is composed of the anterior portion (adenohypophysis) and the posterior portion (neurohypophysis). The adenohypophysis responds to hypothalamic release factors by secreting ACTH, TSH, growth hormone (GH), and gonadotropin. The neurohypophysis secretes vasopressin and oxytocin. Hormone deficiencies leading to hypopituitarism may be caused by lesions in the brain, trauma, irradiation, or granulomatous disease. Gonadotropin deficiency is not of major significance to anesthetic management. Patients with hypopituitary disorders may present with hypothyroidism and inadequate ACTH secretion. Steroid coverage and/or thyroid replacement may be required; however, mineralocorticoid therapy is usually not necessary in these cases. **Diabetes insipidus (DI) (decreased vasopressin secretion) requires special consideration because volume status and electrolytes may be affected.** Diabetes insipidus is an uncommon disease and is usually secondary to hypothalamic disease, primary neoplasm, head trauma, or pituitary surgery.

Diabetes insipidus is associated with large volumes of urine (> 250 ml/hr), polydipsia, and a low urine specific gravity (1.000 to 1.005) accompanied by serum osmolarity > 295 mOsm/kg and serum Na^+ > 145 mEq/L. The preferred diagnostic test is the administration of exogenous ADH following fluid restriction of sufficient length to produce no further increases in urine osmolarity. Fluid-deprived patients with DI will increase their urine osmolarity after ADH adminis-

tration. With diabetes insipidus, careful preoperative assessment of volume status, renal function, electrolytes, and plasma osmolarity is important. Partial DI is treated with chlorpropamide (200 to 500 mg/day) clofibrate (2000 mg/day), or carbamazepine (400 to 600 mg/day).[32] Hypoglycemia is a possible side effect with use of chlorpropamide. Complete DI can be treated with vasopressin or desmopressin. Vasopressin constricts all parts of the vascular bed and must be used with caution in patients with coronary artery disease. The doses of vasopressin are given in Table 17-4.

Hyperpituitarism

Hypersecretion by the pituitary gland presents specific issues to the anesthesiologist. **Patients with acromegaly may have glucose intolerance secondary to growth hormone, as well as an elevated metabolic rate. Patients with acromegaly may present with myopathy, neuropathy, arthritis, cardiomegaly, and hypertension. Macroglossia and prognathism in this condition may be associated with airway management problems and difficulty with intubation.**

Inappropriate ADH secretion is associated with hyponatremia and can occur with tumors (e.g., extrapituitary sources such as oat cell), head trauma, and in association with the stress response. Inappropriate ADH secretion may require fluid restriction and treatment of hyponatremia with hypertonic saline solution and furosemide. Demeclocycline, a tetracycline, antagonizes the renal effects of ADH and is used as adjunct therapy.

DIABETES MELLITUS

The majority of patients with diabetes have either type I, juvenile onset, insulin-dependent diabetes, or type II, adult-onset, noninsulin dependent diabetes. **More than 90% of all diabetic patients are type II and are not prone to ketoacidosis.** In the United States, type II diabetes has a 1% to 5% incidence and type I diabetes has a 0.5% incidence, with perhaps an equal percentage of undiagnosed patients of both types. In addition, over 200,000 new cases of diabetes are diagnosed each year in the United States. It is estimated that 50% of all diabetic patients will require an operation during their lifetime.[81]

Diabetes mellitus is considered a risk factor for surgery and anesthesia. This view is based on both the metabolic alterations and the long-term complications of this disease. However, whether diabetes mellitus is a risk factor as opposed to its long-term complications is debatable. Surprisingly, there is a paucity of data concerning the subject. This controversy is illustrated by surgical studies concerning cholecystectomy in diabetics. Older studies showed an

Table 17-4   Dose of vasopressin or desmopressin in treatment of moderate-to-severe diabetes insipidus

Drug	Route	Dose
Aqueous vaso-pressin	Subcutaneous, IM	5-10 U every 4-6 hr
Vasopressin	IV infusion	0.1-0.2 U/hr
Desmopressin	Intranasally	5-25 μg/day
Desmopressin	Subcutaneous	1-4 μg/day

increase in postoperative mortality following acute cholecystitis in patients with diabetes. These results led to recommendations for gallstone screening in asymptomatic diabetic patients.[68,88] Sandler et al. showed an increased incidence of postoperative complications associated with biliary tract surgery and diabetes, but when the long-term complications of diabetes are accounted for, diabetes does not appear to present a greater risk to patients.[85] Walsh et al. found that morbidity and mortality in patients with acute cholecystitis was independent of diabetes and determined primarily by the presence of vascular or renal disease.[115] **To date, no study has shown that diabetes under reasonable control significantly contributes to morbidity/mortality during surgery rather than the patient's underlying complications or metabolic problems.** This point is worth emphasis because the anesthesiologist presented with a diabetic patient must pay close attention to the complications of diabetes rather than the intraoperative management of blood glucose alone.

Nonetheless, it is important to recognize that in certain surgical populations intraoperative management of diabetes may assume critical importance in influencing surgical outcome. For instance, there is increasing evidence that hyperglycemia occurring before and during a neurologic event may contribute to a poor neurologic outcome. The evidence in animal studies is convincing; however, human data are less definitive. Studies by Longstreth et al. showed a correlation between hyperglycemia and poor neurologic outcome following out-of-hospital cardiac arrest.[57] However, the authors subsequently refuted this study, showing that the hyperglycemia exhibited in patients with a poor neurologic outcome was secondary to the length and difficulty of resuscitation.[56] Therefore poor neurologic outcome was better predicted by the difficulty of the resuscitation rather than the hyperglycemia per se. Pulsinelli et al. found a correlation between hyperglycemia and poor stroke outcome in patients with moderately elevated initial blood glucose levels after stroke.[77] In addition, hyperglycemia has been correlated with greater cerebral edema on head CAT scan following stroke.[4] However, it is not clear whether the hyperglycemia is a stress response to a large stroke or whether hyperglycemia contributes to the poor stroke outcome. **In the surgical setting, patients who incur strokes as a result of carotid endarterectomy have an elevated blood glucose level in association with a poor neurologic outcome.**[98] Whether hyperglycemia in the diabetic patient has similar detrimental effects on neurologic outcome is controversial. However, most authorities believe that diabetes presents a similar scenario, and higher blood glucose levels in the diabetic patient may influence neurologic outcome. Therefore it may be

prudent to tightly control blood glucose in situations when neurologic insults may occur.

Blood glucose in the diabetic mother is important in determining neonatal outcome during labor and delivery. Neonatal hypoglycemia (defined as a blood glucose level < 40 mg/dl in the first 12 hours of life) may be influenced by both maternal glucose control during the latter half of pregnancy and maternal glycemic control during labor and delivery. **Maternal glucose levels > 90 mg/dl during delivery significantly increase the frequency of neonatal hypoglycemia.**[102] Therefore glucose boluses should be avoided in the peripartum period and strict blood glucose control should be initiated. In addition, episodes of hypotension in the diabetic mother during regional anesthesia may be associated with lower pH and base excess in the neonate.[17]

Hypoglycemia is more frequent in the patient with diabetes and may be associated with neurologic complications. Recent animal studies have shown that moderate hypoglycemia not associated with EEG changes may cause profound changes in cerebral blood flow and metabolism during hyperventilation or hypotension.[97] **Nuclear magnetic resonance studies have demonstrated that hypoglycemia in combination with hyperventilation may lead to rapid depletion of high-energy phosphates in the brain, leading to a flat EEG and inability of the brain to vasoconstrict.**[21] Moderate hypoglycemia also interferes with brain autoregulation at lower blood pressures.[96]

Poorly controlled diabetes may cause severe metabolic abnormalities, and patients can present with diabetic ketoacidosis or hyperglycemic hyperosmolar nonketotic coma. Perioperative management strongly influences outcome in such patients.

Other theoretic risks of diabetes in the surgical setting are based on diabetic animal models that show defects in wound healing that were partially corrected by the administration of insulin even without the restoration of euglycemia. However, the importance in humans has not been determined. In addition, the patient with diabetes may be prone to infections during the perioperative period.

Physiology

The alterations that occur in glucose physiology in diabetic patients are associated with the stresses of fasting and surgery.

Normal fasting physiology

During fasting, adaptive changes occur that cause the mobilization of endogenous energy sources to maintain the metabolic rate. During a 24-hour fast the brain preferentially oxidizes glucose at a rate of 110 to 200 g/day and in the absence of exogenous glucose, glycogenolysis and gluconeogenesis of approximately

180 g/day helps to meet this need.[11] During the initial 24 hours of starvation, liver glycogenolysis occurs at high rates to produce this glucose. Other tissues such as heart, skeletal muscle, and renal cortex use free fatty acids or ketone bodies as their primary fuel source, accounting for some of the triglyceride mobilized.

Perioperative changes in glucose metabolism

The major influence causing the immediate postoperative catabolic state is the stress response. The surgical stress response is characterized by increases in sympathetic tone, glucagon levels, pituitary hormone levels (notably ACTH and growth hormone), and interleukin-1. During the perioperative period, elevations of plasma norepinephrine and epinephrine levels occur. Epinephrine and norepinephrine stimulate liver glycogenolysis and gluconeogenesis[93] and inhibit glucose uptake by insulin-dependent tissues. Both the alpha and beta effects of the catecholamines may influence glucose metabolism. For instance, epinephrine increases metabolic rate through its beta effects.[119] The alpha and beta effects also have profound influences on pancreatic function. Beta-receptor stimulation enhances insulin and glucagon release, whereas alpha-receptor stimulation inhibits the release of insulin. During the intraoperative and immediate postoperative course, alpha effects predominate, causing suppression of insulin secretion. Decreased insulin levels coupled with increased gluconeogenesis and insulin resistance cause hyperglycemia and glucose intolerance, prompting the term "diabetes of injury." During the following convalescent stage, the hormonal milieu maintains the elevated levels of gluconeogenesis while glucose uptake by the peripheral tissues is normalized and insulin secretion increases. The pancreas is also able to respond normally to excess glucose loads. One of the contributing factors to this change in glucose kinetics is the hormonal shift from alpha to beta catecholamine effects.[118] Plasma glucagon levels rise after surgery and promote hepatic amino acid uptake, gluconeogenesis, and glycogenolysis.[84] However, the increase in splanchnic glucose production with glucagon is a transient phenomenon, and it is only with the combined effects of all the stress hormones that the level of hepatic gluconeogenesis is maintained.[92] Increased pituitary release of ACTH leads to elevated glucocorticoid levels, which can produce a moderate glycemic response as well as a sustained nitrogen loss.[31] Postoperative elevations in growth hormone have an anabolic effect, causing nitrogen retention, protein synthesis, lipolysis, and decreased peripheral glucose uptake.[121] The net effects of the neuroendocrine response on metabolism during the convalescent stage of tissue injury include blood sugar elevations,

stimulation of lipolysis, and increased rate of gluconeogenesis, resulting in increased protein breakdown and nitrogen excretion.

During surgery, blood glucose concentrations in nondiabetic patients may increase to as high as 60 mg/dl above preoperative levels.[15] The amount of surgical stress is the primary determinant of the absolute increase in glucose values. Inadequate insulin secretion, coupled to the stress hormone milieu and the preoperative fasting state, makes the diabetic patient more susceptible to hyperglycemia, hypovolemia, osmotic diuresis, ketosis, and possible changes in the patient's acid-base balance. Hyperglycemia may have detrimental effects if it is untreated. Osmotic diuresis secondary to the osmotic activity of glucose occurs when the patient's blood glucose exceeds the renal glucose threshold (approximately 180 to 250 mg/dl). This osmotic diuresis can result in dehydration and electrolyte abnormalities. Although hyperglycemia per se does not have direct effects on the patient's acid-base status, the ketone bodies that result from inadequate insulin therapy can elicit such effects. Acetoacetic acid and beta-hydroxybutyric acid may alter pH status by the accumulated dissociation of hydrogen ions.

Pharmacology

Several pharmacologic issues are important in the perioperative management of the diabetic.

Steroids

Steroid-induced diabetes may occur during procedures when high doses of glucocorticoids are given. If there is the possibility of hyperglycemia causing problems in this setting, the approach to these patients can be modified by avoiding intraoperative glucose administration. **If the anesthesiologist elects to use insulin in this setting, there are no conclusive studies that have shown that steroid-induced hyperglycemia increases surgical morbidity.**

Beta-blockers

Beta-blockers inhibit the beta catecholamine effects on carbohydrate and fat metabolism. Propranolol can prevent the rise in plasma free fatty acids as well as selectively inhibit the lipolytic action of catecholamines. In addition, the hyperglycemic response to epinephrine is reduced by beta-adrenergic blockers. In normal individuals use of propranolol does not affect the rate or magnitude of the fall in plasma after insulin. However, it does slow the recovery from hypoglycemia. **Because of the interference with the hypoglycemic response, diabetic patients who are taking beta-blockers and undergoing surgery must have their blood glucose concentrations carefully monitored whenever insulin is administered.**

Preoperative Evaluation

The preoperative evaluation of the diabetic surgical patient should assess for end organ disease.

Cardiac disease

The most common cause of death in patients with diabetes mellitus is coronary artery disease, which accounts for one third of all deaths in diabetic patients older than 40 years of age. In addition, the diabetic patient is more than twice as prone to having heart disease as the general population. It is controversial whether the diabetic patient has a greater incidence of coronary artery disease than the general population. However, when compared with age-matched controls, the patient with diabetes has more atherosclerotic vessel involvement, more myocardial infarctions, and greater coronary collateralization.[113] The severity and extent of coronary artery lesions are not related to the severity of the diabetes. Therefore some common factor among diabetic patients, such as hyperglycemia, and not the length or severity of diabetes may be the underlying factor causing accelerated atherosclerosis. This emphasizes that coronary artery disease should be sought and expected even in cases of mild, easily controlled diabetes.

Myocardial infarction is more common in the diabetic population. Because of the autonomic neuropathy that occurs with long-standing diabetes, it has been assumed that there is an increased incidence of silent myocardial infarctions in diabetic patients. Electrocardiographic studies of diabetic patients show multiple abnormalities despite lack of symptoms. Exercise stress testing has shown that although 26% of a control population will exhibit ST-segment abnormalities, more than 50% of diabetic patients may show ST-segment abnormalities during stress testing, with the incidence increasing with long-standing diabetes.[122]

The diabetic population has a greater incidence of congestive heart failure. **In the Framingham study, a 20-year follow-up demonstrated that diabetic males had two times the risk and diabetic females had five times the risk for congestive heart failure.**[47] When coronary artery disease, hypertension, age, and other risk factors were considered, the diabetic population still was at increased risk for congestive heart failure, especially females. Persons with diabetes exhibit a range of cardiac abnormalities. The young asymptomatic person may have subclinical abnormalities of left ventricular function, the incidence of which is unknown. During early diabetes a noncompliant ventricle may be observed when the patient has an abnormal exercise tolerance and dyspnea secondary to elevated filling pressures and diastolic dysfunction.[67] With progression of diabetes, systolic dysfunction gradually develops as well as elevated filling pressures and decreased ejection fraction.[16] It is important to note that congestive heart failure can exist in the absence of hypertension or coronary artery disease.

The prevalence of hypertension in the diabetic population is increased twofold and the incidence may vary among races. It is known from the Framingham Study that diabetes associated with hypertension compounds the risk of cardiovascular events. For example, hypertensive diabetic patients have an increased risk of stroke and transient ischemic attacks when compared to nonhypertensive diabetics.

Sudden cardiac death has an elevated incidence in diabetic patients although the exact cause of these events currently is not clearly delineated.[71]

Urologic disorders

Voiding dysfunction has an estimated incidence of 25% to 87% in diabetic patients.[26,50] The incidence correlates with the duration and severity of illness. Voiding dysfunction may lead to urosepsis and subsequent postoperative complications.

Renal disorders

Kidney disease with or without hypertension is common in the diabetic population, with renal insufficiency eventually developing in almost half of insulin-dependent diabetic patients.[50] In addition, renal failure is a significant contributor to the cause of death in type 1 diabetics. It is important to maintain adequate hydration and good urine output during surgical procedures in diabetic patients. This point should be emphasized during radiologic procedures when injected contrast agents may contribute to renal insufficiency.

Diabetic neuropathy

Because of the increased frequency of peripheral neuropathy, a careful neurologic evaluation should be performed preoperatively, especially if regional anesthesia is considered. Attention must be paid to intraoperative positioning and padding of all pressure points to prevent ulceration and postoperative infection.

The autonomic neuropathies may involve one of several organ systems, including cardiovascular, gastrointestinal, and genitourinary. The genitourinary problems have been described previously. Within the cardiovascular system, subclinical autonomic dysfunction is probably very common in the diabetic patient. Although patients are often asymptomatic, the earliest signs are impaired vagal innervation of the heart, as demonstrated by the absence of heart rate variation during respiration.[74] With progression of autonomic dysfunction a fixed resting tachycardia and abnormal cardiac response to postural changes or exercise may be evident. The presenting clinical symptoms may include decreased exercise tolerance, orthostatic hypotension, and palpitations, syncope, or weakness on assuming an upright posture. The decrease in exercise tolerance has been attributed to a blunted increase in heart rate at low levels of exercise secondary to an impaired ability to withdraw vagal tone. Similarly, an increase in heart rate may be blunted at high exercise levels secondary to impaired sympathetic tone. Orthostatic symptoms in diabetic patients may be secondary to a blunted rise in norepinephrine levels that occurs when the patient assumes the upright posture. However, before ascribing any postural hypotension to diabetes, it is important to rule out other causes. The occurrence of autonomic cardiovascular dysfunction in the diabetic patient may be important in light of reports of unexplained cardiac arrest in young patients with severe autonomic neuropathies.[71]

Gastroparesis (gastroparesis diabeticorum) and impaired esophageal motility are common diabetic autonomic neuropathies. Although overt symptoms of esophageal dysfunction are rare, a study by Hollis et al. of 50 diabetic patients showed a 56% incidence of abnormal esophageal motility.[42] Delayed gastric emptying in diabetic patients has a 20% to 30% incidence. These patients are usually asymptomatic or intermittently symptomatic, with a clinical presentation consisting of gastric reflux, nausea, vomiting, and anorexia.[35] Poor control of diabetes or hyperglycemia can contribute to poor gastric emptying. Metoclopramide may be useful in these patients in doses of 10 mg IV approximately 30 minutes before induction. In addition, **aspiration precautions must be taken when anesthetizing these patients.**

During hypoglycemic episodes, glucagon and epinephrine are released to increase the blood glucose level. However, the release of these hormones may be impaired in diabetics secondary to impaired epinephrine secretion and blunted hypoglycemic symptomatology.[76]

Laryngoscopy and intubation

Diabetes may be associated with a higher incidence of difficult laryngoscopy and intubation. In patients with type 1 diabetes, stiff joint syndrome may occur, affecting all joints including those of the cervical and thoracic spine. Often such patients are of short stature and do not present before puberty.[23] Hogan et al. have described a 40% incidence of difficult laryngoscopy in a group of patients with severe diabetes.[41] Several other investigators have reported similar findings although at lower incidences.[24]

The important consideration in preoperative evaluation of the diabetic patient is that the major cause of morbidity and mortality is cardiovascular events.[30] Therefore, although the degree of glucose control is important to assess, the end organ pathology should play an equal or greater role in formulating the anesthetic plan.

SUMMARY

Preoperatively the anesthesiologist must carefully ascertain both the degree of autonomic neuropathy, particularly that involving the heart, and the severity of cardiovascular disease. With this approach anesthetic morbidity and mortality in the diabetic population will continue to decrease.

KEY POINTS

- The risk of developing hyperthyroidism is greatest in females 30 to 39 years of age, with the primary cause being Graves' disease.
- The preoperative preparation of a patient with hyperthyroidism depends on the urgency of the surgery. Elective surgery should be withheld until the patient is euthyroid. The risks of delaying emergency surgery must be weighed against the risks of precipitating a thyroid storm.
- Hypothyroidism is more common in the elderly, with 95% being idiopathic cases.
- Serum TSH is the most sensitive indicator of hypothyroidism and should be monitored along with clinical signs during thyroid replacement.
- Patients with large goiters should have careful airway examination to exclude recurrent laryngeal nerve compression or tracheal deviation.

- Systemic nonthyroidal illness may alter thyroid function.
- Myxedema coma, although rare, can have up to an 80% mortality if untreated. Important complications include carbon dioxide retention, gastrointestinal bleeding, hyponatremia, and hypotension that responds poorly to vasoactive drugs.
- The primary risk of anesthetizing patients with hypercalcemia is cardiac dysrhythmia.
- The major risks of hypocalcemia are cardiac dysrhythmias, decreased contractility, tetany (especially with hyperventilation and alkalosis), and altered response to muscle relaxants.
- Pheochromocytoma accounts for approximately 0.5% of all hypertensive patients. If not appropriately treated, it carries a 10% mortality among routine surgical procedures.

- Patients with acromegaly may have glucose intolerance and may present with myopathy, neuropathy, arthritis, cardiomegaly, and hypertension. Macroglossia and prognathism associated with this condition can result in airway management problems.
- More than 90% of all diabetic patients are type II and are not prone to ketoacidosis.
- A poor neurologic outcome has been found among patients with an elevated blood glucose level who incur strokes as a result of a carotid endarterectomy.

- Blood glucose control in the diabetic mother during labor and delivery is important in determining neonatal outcome.
- The diabetic patient is more than twice as prone to having heart disease than the general population, with the most common cause of death being coronary artery disease. Although the degree of glucose control is important to assess, the end organ pathology should play an equal or greater role in formulating the anesthetic plan.

KEY REFERENCES

Byyny RL: Preventing adrenal insufficiency during surgery, *Postgrad Med* 67:219, 1980.

Feek CM, Sawers JS, Irvine WJ et al: Combination of potassium iodide and propranolol in preparation of patients with Graves' disease for thyroid surgery, *N Engl J Med* 302:883, 1980.

Gunst MA, Drop LJ: Chronic hypercalcemia secondary to hyperparathyroidism: a risk factor for anesthesia? *Br J Anaesth* 52:507, 1980.

Ladenson PW, Lewin AA, Ridgway EC et al: Complications of surgery in hypothyroid patients, *Am J Med* 77:261, 1984.

Levine HD: Compromise therapy in the patient with angina pectoris and hypothyroidism, *Am J Med* 69:411, 1980.

Mazzaferri EL: Thyrotoxicosis: clinical syndromes and laboratory diagnosis, *Postgrad Med* 73:85, 1983.

Murkin JM: Anesthesia and hypothyroidism: a review of thyroxine physiology, pharmacology, and anesthetic implications, *Anesth Analg* 61:371, 1982.

Paine TD, Rogers WJ, Baxley WA et al: Coronary arterial surgery in patients with incapacitating angina pectoris and myxedema, *Am J Cardiol* 40:226, 1977.

Roizen MF, Hunt TK, Beaupre PN et al: The effect of alpha-adrenergic blockade on cardiac performance and tissue oxygen delivery during excision of pheochromocytoma, *Surgery* 94:941, 1983.

Sandler RS, Maule WF, Baltus ME et al: Factors associated with postoperative complications in diabetics after biliary tract surgery, *Gastroenterology* 91:157, 1986.

Walsh DB, Eckhauser FE, Ramsbargh SR et al: Risk associated with diabetes mellitus in patients undergoing gallbladder surgery, *Surgery* 91:254, 1982.

REFERENCES

1. Arai T, Hatano Y, Ishida H et al: Use of nicardipine in the anesthetic management of pheochromocytoma, *Anesth Analg* 65:706, 1986.
2. Becker D, Schumacher DP: ø, p' DDD therapy in invasive adrenocortical carcinoma, *Ann Intern Med* 82:677, 1975.
3. Bell GM, Todd WT, Forfar JC et al: End-organ responses to thyroxine therapy in subclinical hypothyroidism, *Clin Endocrinol Oxf* 22:83, 1985.
4. Berger L, Hakim AM: The association of hyperglycemia with cerebral edema in stroke, *Stroke* 17:865, 1986.
5. Bhasin S, Wallace W, Lawrance JB et al: Sudden death associated with thyroid hormone abuse, *Am J Med* 71:887, 1981.
6. Bilezekian JP, Loeb JN: The influence of hyperthyroidism and hypothyroidism on α- and β-adrenergic receptor systems and adrenergic responsiveness, *Endocr Rev* 4:378, 1983.
7. Bough EW, Crowley WF, Ridgway C et al: Myocardial function in hypothyroidism: relation to disease severity and response to treatment, *Arch Intern Med* 138:1476, 1978.
8. Bromage PR, Shibata HR, and Willoughby HW et al: Influence of prolonged epidural blockade on blood sugar and cortisol responses to operations upon the upper part of the abdomen and the thorax, *Surg Gynecol Obstet* 132:1051, 1971.
9. Burrow GN: Hyperthyroidism during pregnancy, *N Engl J Med* 298:150, 1978.
10. Byyny RL: Preventing adrenal insufficiency during surgery, *Postgrad Med* 67:219, 1980.
11. Cahill GF Jr, Owen OE, and Morgan AP: The consumption of fuels during prolonged starvation, *Adv Enzyme Regul* 6:143, 1968.
12. Canary JJ et al: Effects of oral and intramuscular administration of reserpine in thyrotoxicosis, *N Engl J Med* 257:435, 1957.
13. Carruthers JA, August PA, and Staughton RC et al: Observations on the systemic effect of topical clobetasol proprionate (Dermovate), *Br Med J* 4:203, 1975.
14. Chopta D et al: Insensitivity to digoxin with hypocalcemia, *N Engl J Med* 296:917, 1977.
15. Clarke RSJ: The hyperglycemic response to different types of surgery and anaesthesia, *Br J Anaesth* 42:45, 1970.
16. D'Elia JA, Weinrauch LA, Healy RW et al: Myocardial dysfunction without coronary artery disease in diabetic renal failure, *Am J Cardiol* 43:193, 1979.
17. Datta S, Brown WU: Acid-base status in diabetic mothers and their infants following general or spinal anesthesia for cesarean section, *Anesthesiology* 47:272, 1977.
18. Davis PJ, Davis FB: Hyperthyroidism in patients over the age of 60 years: clinical features in 85 patients, *Medicine* 53:161, 1974.

19. Degroot LJ: Thyroid and the heart, *Mayo Clin Proc* 47:864, 1972.

20. Demeester-Mirkine N, Dumont JE: The hypothalamo-pituitary-thyroid axis. In DeVisscher M, ed: *The thyroid gland,* New York, 1980, Raven Press.

21. Derrer SA et al: Effect of hypoglycemia and hypocarbia on brain pH, ATP, phosphocreatine and blood flow, *J Neurosurg Anesthesiol* 1:166, 1989.

22. Donaghue K, Hales I, Allwright S et al: Cardiac function in acute hypothyroidism, *Eur J Nucl Med* 11:147, 1985.

23. Duby S et al: Limited joint mobility in an adult diabetic population. Proceedings of the Seventh Pan-American Congress of Rheumatology, Washington, DC, 1982.

24. Eleborg L, Norberg A: Are diabetic patients difficult to intubate? *Acta Anaesthesiol Scand* 32:508, 1988.

25. Eriksson M, Rubenfeld S, Garber AJ et al: Propranolol does not prevent thyroid storm, *N Engl J Med* 296:263, 1977.

26. Fagerberg SE, Kock NG, Peterén I et al: Urinary bladder disturbance in diabetics, *Scand J Urol Nephrol* 1:19, 1967.

27. Feek CM, Sawers JS, Irvine WJ et al: Combination of potassium iodide and propranolol in preparation of patients with Graves' disease for thyroid surgery, *N Engl J Med* 302:883, 1980.

28. Fisher DA, Huath S, and Lakshmanan J: The thyroid hormone effects on growth and development may be mediated by growth factors, *Endocrinol Exp* 16:259, 1982.

29. Forfar JC, Miller HC, and Toft AD et al: Occult thyrotoxicosis: a correctable cause of "idiopathic" atrial fibrillation, *Am J Cardiol* 44:9, 1979.

30. Galloway JA, Shuman CR: Diabetes and surgery: a study of 667 cases, *Am J Med* 34:177, 1963.

31. Gelfand RA, Mathews DE, Bier DM et al: Role of counterregulatory hormones in the catabolic response to stress, *J Clin Invest* 74:2238, 1984.

32. Germon K: Fluid and electrolyte problems associated with diabetes insipidus and syndrome of inappropriate antidiuretic hormone, *Nurs Clin North Am* 22:785, 1987.

33. Gilsanz FJ, Luengo C, Conejero P et al: Cardiomyopathy and phaeochromocytoma, *Anaesthesia* 38:888, 1983.

34. Goldstein S, Killip T III: Catecholamine depletion in thyrotoxicosis: effect of guanethidine on cardiovascular dynamics, *Circulation* 31:219, 1965.

35. Goyal RK, Spiro HM: Gastrointestinal manifestations of diabetes mellitus, *Med Clin North Am* 55:1031, 1971.

36. Gunst MA, Drop LJ: Chronic hypercalcemia secondary to hyperparathyroidism: a risk factor for anesthesia? *Br J Anaesth* 52:507, 1980.

37. Hamolski MW et al: The heart in hypothyroidism, *J Chronic Dis* 14:558, 1961.

38. Harter JG, Reddy WJ, and Thorn GW: Studies on an intermittent corticosteroid dosage regimen, *N Engl J Med* 269:591, 1963.

39. Hay ED et al: Thyroxine therapy in hypothyroid patients undergoing coronary revascularization: a retrospective analysis, *Ann Intern Med* 95:456, 1981.

40. Henig RE: Primary aldosteronism. In Streak WF, Lockwood DH, eds: *Endocrine diagnosis: clinical and laboratory approaches,* Boston, 1983, Little, Brown.

41. Hogan K, Rusy D, Springman SR et al: Difficult laryngoscopy and diabetes mellitus, *Anesth Analg* 67:1162, 1988.

42. Hollis JB, Castell DO, and Braddom RL: Esophageal function in diabetes mellitus and its relation to peripheral neuropathy, *Gastroenterology* 73:1098, 1977.

43. Holvey DN, Goodner CJ, Nicoloff JT et al: Treatment of myxedema coma with intravenous thyroxine, *Arch Intern Med* 113:189, 1964.

44. Howitt G, Rowlands DJ: β-Sympathetic blockade in hyperthyroidism, *Lancet* 1:628, 1966.

45. Hubay CA, Weckesser EC, and Levy RP: Occult adrenal insufficiency in surgical patients, *Ann Surg* 181:325, 1975.

46. Izenstein B et al: Pheochromocytoma. In Vandam LD, ed: *To make the patient ready for anesthesia,* Menlo Park, Calif, 1980, Addison-Wesley.

47. Kannel WB, Hjortland M, and Castelli WP: Role of diabetes in congestive heart failure: the Framingham study, *Am J Cardiol* 34:29, 1974.

48. Kaplan EL, Burrington JD, Klementschitsch P et al: Primary hyperparathyroidism, pregnancy, and neonatal hypocalcemia, *Surgery* 96:717, 1984.

49. Kaufman BH, Telander RL, van Heerden JA et al: Pheochromocytoma in the pediatric age group: current status, *J Pediatr Surg* 18:879, 1983.

50. Kussman MJ, Goldstein H, and Gleason RE: Clinical cause of diabetic nephropathy, *JAMA* 236:1861, 1976.

51. Ladenson PW, Goldenheim PD, and Ridgway EC: Rapid pituitary and peripheral tissue responses to intravenous L-triiodothyronine in hypothyroidism, *J Clin Endocrinol Metab* 56:1252, 1983.

52. Ladenson PW, Lewin AA, Ridgway EC et al: Complications of surgery in hypothyroid patients, *Am J Med* 77:261, 1984.

53. Levine HD: Compromise therapy in the patient with angina pectoris and hypothyroidism, *Am J Med* 69:411, 1980.

54. Levine MA: Disorders of bone and mineral metabolism. In Harvey AM, Johns RJ, and McKusick VA, eds: *The principles and practice of medicine,* Norwalk, Conn, 1988, Appleton & Lange.

55. Livanau T et al: Recovery of hypothalamo-pituitary-adrenal function after corticosteroid therapy, *Lancet* 2:856, 1957.

56. Longstreth WT Jr, Diehr P, Cobb LA et al: Neurologic outcome and blood glucose levels during out-of-hospital cardiopulmonary resuscitation, *Neurology* 36:1186, 1986.

57. Longstreth WT, Inui TS: High blood glucose level on hospital admission and poor neurological recovery after cardiac arrest, *Ann Neurol* 15:59, 1985.

58. Ludmerer KM, Kissane JM: Micturition-induced hypertension in a 58-year-old woman, *Am J Med* 78:307, 1985.

59. MacKin JF, Canary JJ, and Pittman CS: Thyroid storm and its management, *N Engl J Med* 291:1396, 1974.

60. Manger WM, Gifford RW Jr: Current concepts of pheochromocytoma, *Cardiovasc Med* 3:289, 1978.

61. Mazzaferri EL et al: Thyroid storm: a review of 22 episodes with special emphasis on the use of guanethidine, *Arch Intern Med* 124:684, 1969.

62. Mazzaferri EL: Thyrotoxicosis: clinical syndromes and laboratory diagnosis, *Postgrad Med* 73:85, 1983.

63. McBrien DJ, Hindle W: Myxedema and heart-failure, *Lancet* 1:1066, 1963.

64. McDevitt DG et al: The role of the thyroid in the control of heartrate, *Lancet* 1:998, 1968.

65. McLarty DG, Ratcliffe WA, McColl K et al: Thyroid hormone levels and prognosis in patients with serious nonthyroidal illness, *Lancet* 1:275, 1975.

66. Mihm FG: Pulmonary artery pressure monitoring in patients with pheochromocytoma, *Anesth Analg* 62:1129, 1983.

67. Mildenberger RR, Bar-Shlomo B, Druck MN et al: Clinically unrecognized ventricular dysfunction in young diabetic patients, *J Am Coll Cardiol* 4:234, 1984.

68. Mundth ED: Cholecystitis and diabetes mellitus, *N Engl J Med* 267:642, 1962.

69. Murkin JM: Anesthesia and hypothyroidism: a review of thyroxine physiology, pharmacology, and anesthetic implications, *Anesth Analg* 61:371, 1982.

70. Nevins MA, Saran M, Bright M et al: Pitfalls in interpreting serum creatine phosphokinase activity, *JAMA* 224:1382, 1973.

71. Page MM, Watkins PJ: Cardiorespiratory arrest and diabetic autonomic neuropathy, *Lancet* 1:14, 1978.

72. Paine TD, Rogers WJ, Baxley WA et al: Coronary arterial surgery in patients with incapacitating angina pectoris and myxedema, *Am J Cardiol* 40:226, 1977.

73. Parker JLW, Lawson DH: Death from thyrotoxicosis, *Lancet* 2:894, 1973.

74. Pfeifer MA, Cook D, Brodsky J et al: Quantitative evaluation of cardiac parasympathetic activity in normal and diabetic man, *Diabetes* 31:339, 1982.

75. Plumpton FS, Besser GU: The adrenocortical response to surgery and insulin-induced hypoglycemia in corticosteroid-treated and normal subjects, *Br J Surg* 55:857, 1968.

76. Polonsky K, Bergenstal R, Pons G et al: Relationship of counterregulatory responses to hypoglycemia in type I diabetics, *N Engl J Med* 307:1106, 1982.

77. Pulsinelli WA, Levy DE, Sigsbee B et al: Increased damage after ischemic stroke in patients with hyperglycemia with or without established diabetes mellitus, *Am J Med* 74:540, 1983.

78. Ramsay EI: Muscle dysfunction in hyperthyroidism, *Lancet* 2:931, 1966.

79. Robson NJ: Emergency surgery complicated by thyrotoxicosis and thyrotoxic periodic paralysis, *Anaesthesia* 40:27, 1985.

80. Roizen MF, Hunt TK, Beaupre PN et al: The effect of alpha-adrenergic blockade on cardiac performance and tissue oxygen delivery during excision of pheochromocytoma, *Surgery* 94:941, 1983.

81. Root HF: Preoperative care of the diabetic patient, *Postgrad Med* 40:439, 1966.

82. Roti E, Montermini M, Roti S et al: The effect of diltiazem, a calcium channel–blocking drug, on cardiac rate and rhythm in hyperthyroid patients, *Arch Intern Med* 148:1919, 1988.

83. Rumancik WM, Denlinger JK, Nahrwold ML et al: The QT interval and serum ionized calcium, *JAMA* 240:326, 1978.

84. Russell RCG, Walker CJ, Bloom Sr et al: Hyperglucagonaemia in the surgical patient, *Br Med J* 1:10, 1975.

85. Sandler RS, Maule WF, Baltus ME et al: Factors associated with postoperative complications in diabetics after biliary tract surgery, *Gastroenterology* 91:157, 1986.

86. Sara CA, Joasoo A, and Goldie JE: Changes in the circulating thyroid hormones during anesthesia and thyroid surgery, *Med J Aust* 2:241, 1977.

87. Sawin CT, Chopra D, Azizi F et al: The aging thyroid: increased prevalence of elevated serum thyrotropin levels in the elderly, *JAMA* 242:247, 1979.

88. Schein CJ: Acute cholecystitis in the diabetic, *Am J Gastroenterol* 51:511, 1969.

89. Schutz W, Vogel E: Pheochromocytoma of the urinary bladder—a case report and review of the literature, *Urol Int* 39:250, 1984.

90. Schwartz HL: Effect of thyroid hormones on growth and development. In Oppenheimer JH, Samuels HH, eds: *Molecular basis of thyroid hormone action,* New York, 1983, Academic Press.

91. Sheldon J: Effects of amiodarone in thyrotoxicosis, *Br Med J* 286:267, 1983.

92. Sherwin R, Wahren J, Felig P et al: Evanescent effect of hypo- and hyperglucagonemia on blood glucose homeostasis, *Metabolism* 25:1381, 1976.

93. Sherwin RS, Sacca L: Effect of epinephrine on glucose metabolism in humans: contribution of the liver, *Am J Physiol* 247:E157, 1984.

94. Siddiq YK, Gebhart SSP: Disorders of the thyroid gland. In Lubin MF, Walker HK, and Smith RB, eds: *Medical management of the surgical patient,* Boston, 1988, Butterworths.

95. Siddiq YK, Watts NB: Disorders of the adrenal gland. In Lubin MF, Walker HK, and Smith RB, eds: *Medical management of the surgical patient,* Boston, 1988, Butterworths.

96. Sieber FE et al: Hypoglycemia and cerebral autoregulation, *Anesthesiology* 71:A605, 1989.

97. Sieber FE, Koehler RC, Derrer SA et al: Effect of hypoglycemia on cerebral metabolism and carbon dioxide responsivity, *Am J Physiol* 256:H697, 1989.

98. Sieber FE, Toung TJK: Hyperglycemia and stroke outcome following carotid endarterectomy, *Anesthesiology* 71:A1136, 1989.

99. Sjoerdsma A et al: Pheochromocytoma: current concepts of diagnosis and treatment, *Ann Intern Med* 65:1302, 1966.

100. Slap GB: The surgical patient with thyroid disease. In Goldmann DR et al, eds: *Medical care of the surgical patient,* Philadelphia, 1982, JB Lippincott.

101. Solares G, Ramos F, Martin-Duran R et al: Amiodarone, phaeochromocytoma and cardiomyopathy, *Anaesthesia* 41:186, 1986.

102. Soler NG, Soler SM, and Malins JM: Neonatal morbidity among infants of diabetic mothers, *Diabetes Care* 1:340, 1978.

103. Steinberg AD: Myxedema and coronary artery disease—a comparative autopsy study, *Ann Intern Med* 68:338, 1968.

104. Stenstrom G, Haljamae H, Tisell LE et al: Influence of preoperative treatment with phenoxybenzamine on the incidence of adverse cardiovascular reactions during anaesthesia and surgery for phaeochromocytoma, *Acta Anaesthesiol Scand* 29:797, 1985.

105. Stewart BH, Bravo EL, Haoga J et al: Localization of pheochromocytoma by computed tomography, *N Engl J Med* 299:460, 1978.

106. Streck W, Lockwood DH: Pituitary-adrenal recovery following short-term suppression with corticosteroids, *Am J Med* 66:910, 1979.

107. Green WL, ed: *The thyroid,* New York, 1987, Elsevier.

108. Toft AD, Irvine WJ, Sinclair I et al: Thyroid function after surgical treatment of thyrotoxicosis, *N Engl J Med* 298:643, 1978.

109. Tunbridge WMG, Evered DC, Hall R et al: The spectrum of thyroid disease in the community: the Whickham survey, *Clin Endocrinol* 7:481, 1977.

110. Urbanic RC, Mazzaferri EL: Thyrotoxic crisis and myxedema coma, *Heart Lung* 7:435, 1978.

111. Vater M, Achola K, Smith G et al: Catecholamine responses during anaesthesia for phaeochromocytoma, *Br J Anaesth* 55:357, 1983.

112. Venkata C et al: Failure of α-methyltyrosine to prevent hypertensive crisis in pheochromocytoma, *Arch Intern Med* 145:2114, 1985.

113. Vigorita VJ, Moore GW, Hutchins GM et al: Absence of correlation between coronary arterial atherosclerosis and severity or duration of diabetes mellitus of adult onset, *Am J Cardiol* 46:535, 1980.

114. Waldstein SS, Slodki SJ, Kaganiec I et al: A clinical study of thyroid storm, *Ann Intern Med* 52:626, 1960.

115. Walsh DB, Eckhauser FE, Ramsbargh SR et al: Risk associated with diabetes mellitus in patients undergoing gallbladder surgery, *Surgery* 91:254, 1982.

116. Weinberg AD, Brennan MD, Gorman CA et al: Outcome of anesthesia and surgery in hypothyroid patients, *Arch Intern Med* 143:893, 1983.

117. Williams GH, Dluhy RG: Diseases of the adrenal cortex, In Braunwald E et al: *Principles of internal medicine,* New York, 1987, McGraw-Hill.

118. Wilmore DW: Carbohydrate metabolism in trauma, *Clin Endocrinol Metab* 5:731, 1976.

119. Wilmore DW: Hormonal responses and their effect on metabolism, *Surg Clin North Am* 56:999, 1976.

120. Wilson WR, Bedell GN: The pulmonary abnormalities in myxedema, *J Clin Invest* 39:42, 1960.

121. Wright PD, Johnston IDA: The effect of surgical operation on growth hormone levels in plasma, *Surgery* 77:479, 1975.

122. Zoneraich S: Cardiac pathology, peripheral vascular disease, and hypertension. In Sussman KE, Draznin B, and James WE, eds: *Clinical guide to diabetes mellitus,* New York, 1987, Alan R Liss.

123. Zwillich CW, Pierson DJ, Hofeldt FD et al: Ventilatory control in myxedema and hypothyroidism, *N Engl J Med* 292:662, 1975.

CHAPTER 18

Evaluation of the Patient with Renal Disease

CLAIR F. MILLER

Dialysis Patients with End-Stage Renal Failure
   Perioperative outcome
   Preoperative assessment and management
Patients with Renal Dysfunction not Requiring Dialysis
   Outcome of perioperatively acquired renal dysfunction
   Causes of perioperatively acquired renal dysfunction
   Preoperative assessment and management

When compared with patients who have normal renal function, perioperative morbidity and mortality are greater in patients with (1) end-stage renal failure on dialysis, (2) preexisting but stable renal insufficiency, or (3) any deterioration of renal function before, during, or after anesthesia and surgery. To improve perioperative outcome, preoperative assessment of patients with end-stage renal disease is aimed at the identification and management of the many physiologic abnormalities that are common to all functionally anephric patients. In contrast, preoperative evaluation of patients with less than normal (but not end-stage) renal function is aimed at preservation of existing renal function and prevention of further renal injury in the perioperative time. This chapter, therefore, discusses preoperative assessment and management of two distinctly different patient populations: dialysis patients with end-stage renal failure and patients with renal dysfunction not requiring dialysis.

DIALYSIS PATIENTS WITH END-STAGE RENAL FAILURE

Dialysis patients probably undergo more surgical procedures in their lifetimes than any other group of patients. Of the operations performed, 80% to 90% are required to establish vascular access for dialysis.[68] However, gastrointestinal, cardiac, and major vascular procedures are increasingly common in patients with chronic renal failure.[62] The anesthesiologist is frequently confronted not only with the disease that caused the kidneys to fail but also with the physiologic complications of chronic renal failure itself.

Many diseases that cause end-stage renal failure (Table 18-1) remain active after dialysis therapy is started and may themselves adversely affect perioperative outcome. Hypertension and diabetes in dialysis patients, for example, require the same careful preoperative assessment and management as in patients with normal renal function. Preoperative evaluation of these diseases is discussed in Chapters 10 and 17.

To highlight the increased risk of surgical intervention in these patients, this section reviews the perioperative morbidity and mortality that is associated with anesthesia and surgery in dialysis patients. The physiologic complications of end-stage renal failure are then discussed in detail.

Perioperative Outcome
Mortality

Procedures to establish vascular access for dialysis are usually well-tolerated, and operative mortality is rare regardless of the type of anesthesia used.[44,64,67] In contrast, **invasive procedures performed with the**

Table 18-1 Causes of end-stage renal failure in 16,000 patients	
Causes	Percent of cases
Glomerulonephritis	28
Pyelonephritis/interstitial nephritis	20
Unknown causes	13
Hereditary/congenital	12
Diabetes	10
Miscellaneous known	9
Vascular/hypertensive	8

Modified from Broyer M et al: Demography of dialysis and transplantation in Europe, 1984, *Nephrol Dial Transplant* 1:1, 1986.

Table 18-2 Perioperative mortality in dialysis patients after surgery under regional or general anesthesia		
Procedure	Number of patients	Deaths	Mortality rate (%)
Cardiac surgery	104	8	7.7
Aortocoronary bypass	64	3	4.7
Valve replacement	40	5	12.5
Emergency	7	4	57.1
Elective	33	1	3.0
General surgery	334	14	4.2
Nephrectomy (pretransplant)	457	15	3.3

Data compiled from references 9, 18, 34, 35, 49, 53, 68, 78, 86, 91, and 93.

Table 18-3 Postoperative complications for dialysis patients undergoing surgical procedures		
Complications	Number of occurrences	Percent of occurrences
Hyperkalemia	138	29
Shunt thrombosis	55	11
Pneumonia	52	11
Wound infections	45	10
Hypotension	41	9
Hypertension	36	8
Hemorrhage	25	5
Hypoventilation	17	4
Sepsis	12	3

Complications observed after 585 surgical procedures in 334 dialysis patients. Data from references 9, 34, 35, 49, and 68. Some patients had more than one complication.

patient under general or regional anesthesia are associated with greater perioperative mortality in dialysis patients than are similar procedures in patients with normal renal function. From the studies reviewed in Table 18-2, overall mortality after major procedures in dialysis patients is 5.6%. **Cardiac surgical procedures have the highest mortality, especially emergency valve replacement.** Of the 14 deaths in the general surgical group, six (43%) occurred in patients undergoing emergency laparotomy for sepsis or gastrointestinal bleeding. Although pretransplant nephrectomy is no longer performed routinely,[78] this group is included for discussion to illustrate the substantial risk of death in dialysis patients who undergo major elective subdiaphragmatic procedures. Causes of death in the 29 patients who died in the general surgical and nephrectomy groups combined include the following: septic complications in 12 patients (41%), excessive postoperative bleeding in 6 patients (21%), cardiovascular dysfunction such as congestive heart failure or unexplained hypotension in 6 patients (21%), and hyperkalemia in 3 patients (10%). Deaths attributed to bleeding, cardiovascular dysfunction, and hyperkalemia tended to occur within the first 24 hours after operation, whereas deaths caused by sepsis usually occurred 2 or more days postoperatively. **Thus dialysis patients who are undergoing invasive procedures, especially emergency operations, are at increased risk for perioperative death.** The role of anesthesia in contributing to some of these deaths or in preventing death cannot be ascertained from the existing literature.

Morbidity

Complications that reflect the physiologic abnormalities of chronic renal failure occur frequently in dialysis patients after anesthesia and surgery (Table 18-3). The complications listed in Table 18-3 were observed in 334 dialysis patients who had either general or regional anesthesia for 585 general surgical procedures not including vascular access and endoscopic procedures. **Hyperkalemia occurred more frequently than any other complication and was the primary reason for which dialysis was required within the first 24 hours after surgery in 36% of cases.** Cardiovascular instability such as hypotension and hypertension appeared to reflect changes in intravascular volume status, and these abnormalities occurred most commonly during the first 24 hours postoperatively. Shunt thrombosis related to either malpositioning of the affected extremity or periods of hypotension postoperatively was discovered at intervals throughout the first postoperative week. Septic complications involving the lungs, wound, and blood developed later in the postoperative course than other complications. Many of these complications may be eliminated or their effects attenuated by careful preoperative assessment and management of each of

BOX 18-1
ABNORMALITIES OF END-STAGE RENAL FAILURE THAT MAY ALTER PERIOPERATIVE MANAGEMENT

Anemia
Bleeding abnormalities
Cardiovascular and blood volume abnormalities
Electrolyte and metabolic disturbances
Infectious complications
Pharmacologic alterations

Table 18-4   Outcome of acute postoperative renal failure requiring dialysis

Procedure	Number of patients	Deaths	Mortality rate (%)
General trauma	177	115	65
Major vascular	96	71	74
Cardiac surgery	47	30	64

Data from references 1, 2, 8, 15, 31, 59, and 60.

the expected physiologic abnormalities of chronic renal failure.

Preoperative Assessment and Management

Complete cessation of renal function regularly and predictably results in physiologic abnormalities that adversely alter perioperative outcome (Box 18-1). These complications are remarkably similar regardless of the immediate cause of renal failure. For each abnormality listed in Table 18-4, suggested guidelines for preoperative assessment are followed by a discussion of the respective abnormality.

Anemia

Recommendations. The following steps should be taken in managing patients with anemia:

- Measure serum hematocrit and red blood cell indexes. Check these values against dialysis records to ensure that no acute changes have occurred. Preoperative hematocrit levels that do not differ significantly from those on dialysis records suggest that the patient is able to tolerate any existing anemia.
- Acutely decreased hematocrit values and/or indexes that suggest other than a normochromic-normocytic anemia should trigger an investigation for other causes of anemia before surgery proceeds.
- Routine red blood cell transfusions are not indicated if the anemia is chronic and well tolerated. However, if indicated (acutely decreased or poorly tolerated hematocrit value), there is no need to withhold red cell transfusions for fear of sensitization to histocompatibility antigens.[66]

Evaluation of data. Serum hematocrit values of less than 30% are commonly encountered in functionally anephric patients. **The kidney is normally the major site of production of erythropoietin, and inadequate production of erythropoietin to sustain red blood cell production is the primary cause of the normochromic-**

normocytic anemia of end-stage renal failure.[24,28] Endogenous erythropoietin levels and serum hematocrit values increase to normal after successful renal transplantation.[83] Exogenous administration of human recombinant erythropoietin also corrects the anemia of chronic renal failure.[23-26,47]

Erythropoietin is currently available for use, but widespread use is not customary. Anemia is therefore regularly encountered in preoperative patients who depend on dialysis for survival. **Hematocrit values of 25% to 30% appear to be well tolerated, and routine transfusion of blood preoperatively is not recommended.** In dialysis patients with hematocrit values averaging 25%, treadmill exercises that significantly increase systolic arterial blood pressure and heart rate (from approximately 120 to 150 mm Hg, and 75 to 150 beats/min, respectively) are not associated with significant changes in arterial pH, lactate, or electrolyte levels.[51] These findings suggest that the compensatory limits for cardiac output, oxygen delivery, and tissue oxygen extraction are not exceeded in patients with the anemia of chronic renal failure at levels of hemodynamic stress that are common in the perioperative time.

Bleeding abnormalities

Recommendations. The following steps should be taken in managing patients with bleeding abnormalities:

- Laboratory investigation is unlikely to alter clinical concerns or plans; a tendency for increased bleeding is assumed. If measured, bleeding time may be slightly prolonged and platelet count will be mildly depressed. Prothrombin and partial thromboplastin times are normal in patients with uremia. Any deviation from this pattern should be investigated before surgery.
- Question the patient and check previous anesthesia records, if available, about excessive bleeding. Consider the use of desmopressin throughout the perioperative period if the patient has a history of bleeding and/or the planned procedure is normally associated with excessive blood loss. Desmopressin may be the agent of

choice when unexpected bleeding is encountered in the perioperative time.

- Make sure that dialysis is done 24 hours or less before surgery; abnormal platelet function in uremia is partially corrected by effective dialysis.
- Use gastrointestinal cytoprotective agents (histamine$_2$-receptor blocking drugs, antacids, or sucralfate) throughout the perioperative period to decrease the incidence of stress ulcer bleeding.

Evaluation of data. The cause of excessive bleeding in patients with chronic uremia remains unexplained. **Bleeding time prolongation is the most common clotting abnormality observed.** Although platelet count and thrombopoietic activity are decreased mildly in chronic renal failure,[30] abnormal platelet function appears to be responsible for the increase in bleeding time and tendency for excessive bleeding.[19,70] **Dialysis partially corrects platelet dysfunction in uremia,[19,70] and dialysis within 24 hours before surgical intervention remains the standard preoperative hemostatic therapy in patients with chronic renal failure.** Additional hemostatic options in cases of uremia include use of desmopressin (1-[3-mercaptoproprionic acid]-8-D arginine vasopressin),[55] cryoprecipitate,[39] and conjugated estrogens.[50] Through unknown mechanisms, each of these agents shortens the bleeding time and may decrease blood loss during surgical procedures in dialysis patients. Desmopressin is probably the agent of choice in uremia because it is safe and well tolerated. It has a more rapid onset of action than estrogen therapy and, unlike cryoprecipitate, is not associated with infectious complications of human blood product administration. **Administration of desmopressin shortens bleeding time, increases circulating levels of factor VIII/von Willebrand antigen, and may decrease perioperative blood loss in patients with uremia.**[40] These effects of desmopressin are not unique to patients with uremia because similar effects are observed in patients with normal renal function who are treated with desmopressin during procedures that are associated with large blood losses, such as cardiac surgery[75] and placement of Harrington rod procedures.[42]

Radiographic and endoscopic studies in dialysis patients document a high incidence of mucosal inflammatory changes in the esophagus, stomach, and duodenum.[56] Although ulcerative lesions are not a feature of these changes, dialysis patients should be considered to be at high risk for gastrointestinal bleeding during the stress of the perioperative time. Because histamine$_2$-receptor blocking drugs, antacids, or sucralfate are probably equally effective alternatives for prophylaxis against stress ulcer bleeding,[80,88] therapy with one of these agents is indicated in dialysis patients who require surgical intervention.

Cardiovascular and blood volume abnormalities

Recommendations. The following steps should be taken in managing patients with cardiovascular and blood volume abnormalities:

- Assume that clinically important coronary artery disease exists. Interview the patient and review old records to evaluate the extent, stability, and present therapy for ischemic disease and congestive heart failure. Depending on these findings and the nature of the proposed surgical procedure, invasive hemodynamic monitoring may be indicated perioperatively.
- Obtain a recent ECG tracing and carefully compare to previous tracings. Recent myocardial infarctions carry the same prognostic significance as in any other patient with coronary artery disease. See the chapter on preoperative assessment of the patient with coronary artery disease.
- From a review of dialysis records, correlate body weight changes with changes in arterial blood pressure and heart rate before and after dialysis to provide a noninvasive index by which to gauge the adequacy of intravascular volume status throughout the perioperative time. This information will also provide knowledge regarding the levels of hypertension, hypotension, and heart rate that the patient is able to withstand without adverse sequelae.
- As with any surgical patient, maintenance of intravascular volume is mandatory. Use a normal saline solution that is free of potassium supplements. Invasive hemodynamic monitoring may be necessary to guide volume repletion therapy. Preoperative ultrafiltration may leave the patient hypovolemic; this deficit must be replaced preoperatively.
- Note the location and patency of the arteriovenous fistula or shunt that is presently used for dialysis and avoid use of that extremity for blood pressure recordings, venipuncture, and placement of intravascular catheters. Be careful throughout the operative time to protect the fistula site and verify its patency at intervals, especially intraoperatively when the patient may not be able to communicate that a problem exists.

Evaluation of data. **In nonsurgical settings, ischemic heart disease is the most common cause of death in patients with chronic renal failure.**[11] The high incidence of ischemic heart disease in dialysis patients is attributed to the nearly uniform presence of multiple risk factors such as hypertension, hyperlipidemia, and abnormal carbohydrate metabolism[72] rather than to an accelerated atherosclerotic process peculiar to uremia.[48] It is remarkable that ischemic complications are not prominent features in the perioperative morbidity and mortality data for dialysis patients that were reviewed in the referenced studies.

Blood volume repletion and cardiovascular management in general are difficult in dialysis patients undergoing surgery because of preexisting myocardial dysfunction, presence of coronary artery disease, arteriovenous shunts, autonomic dysfunction, and the unpredictable effects of uremia, acidosis, and adrenergic stimuli on the cardiovascular system.[22,29,41] However, as in patients with normal renal function, maintenance of adequate left ventricular preload is mandatory for perioperative hemodynamic stability. Intraoperatively, blood, evaporative, and "third-space" losses must be replaced with blood and potassium-free normal saline solutions. The volume of evaporative losses and third-space sequestration may be large; 10 to 15 ml/kg/hr may be required during intraabdominal or retroperitoneal procedures. Limiting either salt or volume administration because of anuric renal failure invariably results in hyponatremia and intravascular volume contraction. Postoperatively, mobilization of third-space fluid sequestration requires careful monitoring for early signs of intravascular fluid overload. Volume restriction and frequent dialysis treatments may be required to avoid congestive heart failure, pulmonary edema, respiratory failure, and precipitation of myocardial ischemia in susceptible patients. Invasive intravascular monitoring is often needed to guide cardiovascular therapy throughout the perioperative period in patients who require procedures that are normally associated with large intravascular fluid shifts.

Electrolyte and metabolic abnormalities

Recommendations. The following steps should be taken in managing patients with electrolyte and metabolic abnormalities:

- Arrange for dialysis treatment within 24 hours before planned surgical procedure.
- Check serum potassium concentration immediately preoperatively and compare to usual predialysis potassium levels to determine the level of hyperkalemia that is normally tolerated without untoward sequelae. If elevated, another dialysis treatment may be indicated or some other form of antihyperkalemic therapy may be required.
- Check serum electrolytes. An "anion-gap" acidosis is normal, but a serum bicarbonate concentration below 12 to 15 mEq/L should prompt an immediate investigation for other causes such as ketoacidosis or lactic acidosis.

- Further laboratory evaluation is unlikely to alter anesthetic plans. Hypermagnesemia may be present even with effective dialysis therapy, but mildly elevated magnesium levels do not appear to result in clinically important hypotension, central nervous system depression, or potentiation of nondepolarizing muscle relaxants.[89] Total serum calcium concentrations are decreased, but ionized calcium levels are normal.

Evaluation of data. Dialysis therapy must be continued in the perioperative time to remove toxic waste products, control metabolic acidosis, remove excess sodium and body water, and control hyperkalemia. Platelet dysfunction and bleeding tendencies are also improved by dialysis. Before dialysis therapy was available to treat patients with chronic renal failure, surgical intervention was accomplished at great cost. In 24 nondialyzed patients (blood urea nitrogen (BUN), mean value = 124; range = 41 to 300 mg/dl), major surgical procedures with the patients under general anesthesia resulted in two intraoperative deaths from cardiac arrest, and another patient died in the immediate postoperative period from uncontrolled hypotension; mortality for this series was 12.5%. **Patients with BUN values greater than 100 mg/dl had a 50% incidence of serious perioperative bleeding; patients with BUN values less than 100 mg/dl had a 12% incidence of bleeding.**[76]

It is reasonable to insist that all dialysis-dependent patients receive a dialysis treatment within 12 to 24 hours prior to anesthesia and surgery. **Hyperkalemia is the most immediately life-threatening problem encountered postoperatively in dialysis patients, and it is also the most common reason for which approximately 36% of cases require dialysis within the first 24 hours postoperatively.** Dialysis is the most definitively effective means to manage perioperative hyperkalemia. Use of kayexalate with sorbitol is also effective, but colonic instillation of these agents by enema has been associated with colonic necrosis, especially in renal transplant recipients.[46,90] Other techniques to treat hyperkalemia, including insulin in glucose infusions, bicarbonate administration, and infusion of epinephrine, effectively promote rapid translocation of extracellular potassium to the intracellular space during hyperkalemic emergencies in anephric patients, but definitive therapy with dialysis will eventually be required.

Preoperative hemodialysis may be logistically difficult to achieve in patients who require vascular access procedures. However, alternative dialysis techniques including peritoneal dialysis and hemodialysis via specialized venous catheters are available and should be used preoperatively, especially in patients with hyperkalemia, advanced uremia, or severe metabolic acidosis. There is no need to subject any patient with uncontrolled complications of end-stage renal failure to the risks of anesthesia and surgery for an elective procedure.

Infectious complications

Recommendations. The following steps should be taken in managing patients with infectious complications:

- *Protect the patient.* Uncompromising adherence to aseptic techniques is mandatory during all intravascular cannulations. Line sepsis that results from nonsterile techniques on insertion is an infectious complication that can be eliminated.
- *Protect yourself.* Wear gloves and protective eyewear, avoid recapping needles, and discard all needles in appropriate containers immediately after use. Infectious hepatitis remains a common problem in dialysis patients.

Evaluation of data. Infectious complications are a leading cause of death in dialysis patients who require anesthesia and surgery. Precise mechanisms to account for the increased susceptibility to bacterial infections in end-stage renal disease are not known, but protein calorie malnutrition,[92] cutaneous anergy,[4] and functional abnormalities of neutrophils, monocytes, and macrophages[45,73] have been implicated in dialysis patients. The need for frequent intravascular instrumentation provides a portal for inoculation of infectious agents unless aseptic techniques are rigorously used.

Blood-borne infections with hepatitis B and C viruses are more common in dialysis patients than in the population at large.[81,94] To avoid self-inoculation of these infectious agents, anesthesiologists must protect themselves from exposure to contaminated blood and secretions. Protective eyewear, gloves, and proper handling of needles should be routine; these measures are especially important when caring for dialysis patients.

Pharmacologic alterations

Recommendations. The following steps should be taken in managing patients with pharmacologic alterations:

- Standard dosages of many drugs that are commonly used in the perioperative time may have exaggerated and/or prolonged effects in anephric patients. Premedicants, analgesics, and nondepolarizing muscle relaxants should be titrated to the desired effects rather than according to recommended dosage schedules (including dosing guidelines that account for the effects of end-stage renal disease).

- Although it is not absolutely contraindicated, use of succinylcholine increases serum potassium concentration and is best avoided in dialysis patients.
- Choice of anesthetic technique should be dictated by the requirements of the surgical procedure, desires of the patient, and skills of the anesthesiologist rather than by the physiologic abnormalities of renal failure itself.

Evaluation of data. **Pharmacologic management of the anephric surgical patient must consider the loss of renal mechanisms for drug elimination, the biochemical abnormalities of uremia that alter drug bioavailability, and the effects of dialysis on drug removal.** Because dialysis patients normally take a variety of medications, possible adverse drug interactions and signs and symptoms of drug toxicity must be investigated and treated preoperatively. Regularly published guidelines for drug dosing in chronic renal failure should be consulted in these investigations and in planning for subsequent anesthetic management.[7]

There is no ideal anesthetic regimen that applies to patients with chronic renal failure. Premedicants should probably be withheld until the patient is under the direct observation of the anesthesiologist. Use of benzodiazepines and barbiturates may cause excessive sedation in end-stage renal disease because of relative hypoproteinemia, decreased protein binding (increased free drug available), and impaired renal elimination of active metabolites.[7,21,33] Similarly, narcotic analgesics are associated with excessive sedation and respiratory depression in renal failure because of impaired elimination of active metabolites.[7,14,20] **Benzodiazepines, barbiturates, and narcotics can be safely administered if they are titrated in small and incremental doses to the desired effect under direct observation.** Patients undergoing vascular access procedures can be safely managed with local infiltration anesthesia, general inhalation anesthesia, or brachial plexus blockade. Brachial plexus blockade and local techniques cause less hemodynamic instability intraoperatively than general anesthesia; brachial plexus blockade is associated with higher blood flows in newly created arteriovenous fistulas than general or local techniques, but this effect is not significant enough to recommend one technique over another.[64] The duration of brachial plexus block in cases of renal failure is similar to that in patients with normal renal function.[57]

Procedures other than vascular access operations are also safely managed with a variety of techniques. For example, spinal or epidural anesthesia has been advocated for renal transplantation,[89] but the superiority of these techniques over general anesthesia has not been demonstrated. General inhalational anesthetics are eliminated from the body through the lungs independent of renal mechanisms. **Atracurium may be the nondepolarizing neuromuscular–blocking agent of choice in renal failure because it is eliminated by nonenzymatic degradation independent of renal function, and duration of action is not prolonged in renal failure.**[27] Vecuronium is 80% to 90% excreted in the bile,[85] but the duration of neuromuscular blockade is longer in patients with renal failure than in patients with normal renal function.[52] Although other nondepolarizing neuromuscular–blocking agents such as gallamine, metocurine, pancuronium, or *d*-tubocurarine can be safely used with careful neuromuscular monitoring, these drugs depend 50% to 100% on the kidney for elimination.[10,85] Regardless of the agent used, each drug should be titrated slowly to achieve the level of relaxation desired, and recovery from neuromuscular blockade should be carefully monitored. **Use of succinylcholine, a depolarizing neuromuscular relaxant, increases serum potassium concentrations by 0.5 mEq/L in patients with or without renal failure and should probably be avoided in anephric patients.**[43]

PATIENTS WITH RENAL DYSFUNCTION NOT REQUIRING DIALYSIS

Preoperative assessment of patients with end-stage renal disease who require dialysis for survival is directed toward identification of the physiologic complications of the anephric state and planning for supportive management of these abnormalities. In contrast, **preoperative planning for patients with renal dysfunction (but not end-stage disease) is aimed at strategies to preserve existing renal function.** Prevention of renal injury is a more challenging problem than supportive management of established end-stage disease because the factors responsible for mediating the development of perioperative renal dysfunction are incompletely understood. This section reviews the outcome of patients in whom renal injury develops in the perioperative time, discusses the proposed causes of perioperatively acquired renal dysfunction, and presents recommendations that may prevent this serious perioperative complication. **The anesthesiologist provides the first and perhaps the most important line of defense against the development of renal injury in the perioperative period.**

Outcome of Perioperatively Acquired Renal Dysfunction

Whether preexisting renal function is normal or impaired, the prognosis for patients in whom acute renal deterioration develops in the perioperative time is worse than for patients who maintain stable indexes of renal function before, during, and after anesthesia and surgery. In patients in whom renal dysfunction develops, the prognosis is worse for patients who require dialysis than for those who do not require dialysis.

Mortality for patients with renal failure severe enough to require dialysis after a variety of surgical procedures is shown in Table 18-4. These dismal mortality statistics are similar regardless of the type of surgical procedure. The overall incidence of renal failure after anesthesia and surgery is not known. Postoperative renal failure requiring dialysis develops in 0.5% to 1.5% of trauma patients,[79] in 1.5% to 2.5% of patients after cardiac surgery,[31,37] and in 2.0% to 2.5% of patients after abdominal aortic reconstructive procedures.[59]

Perioperative mortality is also increased in patients with renal impairment that is not severe enough to require dialysis, and mortality appears to increase in parallel with the level to which renal function deteriorates. In one large series of cardiac surgical patients, for example, mortality increased from 0.8% in patients with normal renal function after anesthesia and surgery, to 10.6% in patients with postoperative creatinine levels of 1.5 to 2.5 mg/dl, to 23.5% in patients with postoperative serum creatinine concentrations between 2.5 and 5.0 mg/dl. The incidence of perioperative renal deterioration was higher in patients with preexisting chronic renal insufficiency than in patients with normal preoperative renal function.[1]

The overall incidence of development of renal dysfunction after anesthesia and surgery is not known. However, hospital-acquired renal insufficiency develops in 2% to 5% of adult patients who are admitted to the general medical and surgical services of large university hospitals.[38,82] Development of acute renal insufficiency during hospitalization (defined as an increase of serum creatinine concentration of at least 0.9 mg/dl when admission creatinine level is less than 2.0 mg/dl, or an increase of at least 1.5 mg/dl when the baseline level is greater than 2.0 mg/dl) is associated with a hospital mortality of 35%, compared to 3.5% in patients with unchanged serum creatinine concentrations throughout their hospitalizations.[82]

Causes of Perioperatively Acquired Renal Dysfunction

Deterioration of renal function is a common perioperative complication that is more lethal than is generally appreciated. Failure of modern supportive measures such as dialysis to prevent mortality in surgical patients in whom complete cessation of renal function develops suggests that the underlying causes of perioperatively acquired renal dysfunction mediate severe and widespread systemic injury that is often irreversible and lethal; impaired renal function appears to be a marker for the severity of the initiating insult. To preserve existing renal function and prevent renal injury in the perioperative time, the anesthesiologist must identify and effectively manage the factors that increase the risk for developing perioperative renal dysfunction.

Causes of perioperative renal dysfunction fall into two main categories: decreased renal perfusion and exposure to nephrotoxic agents (Box 18-2). Abnormalities of renal perfusion are probably more common and more important causes of renal deterioration in surgical patients than nephrotoxic exposures. In a careful case-controlled study of hospital-acquired renal insufficiency, the presence of either intravascular volume depletion or myocardial failure increased the risk of developing renal impairment tenfold, whereas aminoglycoside or radiocontrast exposure each increased the risk approximately fivefold.[82] It is common in the perioperative time for many of these causes to occur simultaneously, and the interactive effect of one variable on another may substantially increase the risk of renal deterioration. Aminoglycoside nephrotoxicity, for example, is enhanced in the presence of either volume depletion or arterial hypotension.[61,63] Radiocontrast exposure in patients with chronic stable renal insufficiency often causes further reversible decreases in renal function in patients with either myocardial failure or diabetes mellitus.[77,84] **Diabetic patients have a tenfold greater risk for renal deterioration during hypovolemic episodes than patients without diabetes.**[82]

Thus patients who are at increased risk for development of renal dysfunction in the perioperative time include: (1) patients exposed to deliberate and complete interruption of renal blood flow during procedures that require suprarenal aortic cross-clamping; (2) patients exposed to partial renal ischemia during cardiopulmonary bypass procedures; (3) patients with chronic stable renal insufficiency, especially diabetics; and (4) patients with poor myocardial function. Preoperative evaluation and planning in these patients are aimed at strategies to prevent renal deterioration during surgery.

Preoperative Assessment and Management

Recommendations. The following steps should be taken in preoperative assessment and management:

- Measure serum BUN and creatinine concentrations and check against previously measured values to determine whether there has been a recent decrease in renal function. Further laboratory assessment is not likely to alter anesthetic management.
- If acute deterioration of renal function is documented preoperatively, the cause and potential reversibility must be assessed before proceeding with anesthesia and surgery. There is no need to expose a patient with reversible acute renal injury (such as may occur after aminoglycoside or radiocontrast exposure) to an elective procedure during which numerous other nephrotoxic insults are likely to develop.
- Discuss with medical and/or cardiology consultants about the adequacy of the present medical management of patients with myocardial dysfunction. Before proceeding with elective procedures, the anesthesiologist should be unequivocally convinced that optimal medical management is already being administered and that further delay for additional treatment is unlikely to substantially improve myocardial performance.
- Plan for aseptic placement of intravascular catheters for intravascular volume repletion and/or for assessment of the adequacy of ventricular preload and arterial perfusion pressure according to the physiologic requirements of the patient.
- Choose anesthetic techniques that satisfy the requirements of the surgical procedure, the desires of the patient, and the physiologic requirements of the patient rather than by avoidance of a particular anesthetic drug or technique. Because of the potential for fluoride nephrotoxicity, enflurane is probably the only anesthetic agent that should be avoided in patients with preexisting renal dysfunction or in patients who require renal blood flow interruption during their surgical procedure.
- Consider use of "renal protective agents" such as dopamine, furosemide, and/or mannitol in patients having aortic cross-clamping or cardiopulmonary bypass procedures.

Evaluation of data. Serum BUN and creatinine concentrations should be measured within 12 to 24

BOX 18-2
CAUSES OF PERIOPERATIVE RENAL FAILURE

Decreased renal perfusion
    Intravascular volume contraction
    Congestive heart failure
    Cardiopulmonary bypass
    Aortic cross-clamping
Nephrotoxin exposure
    Aminoglycosides
    Radiocontrast agents
    Anesthetic agents

hours before anesthesia and surgery, and these values must be compared with admission values. If acute deterioration of renal function has developed preoperatively, reversible causes such as volume contraction, acute myocardial dysfunction, or nephrotoxin exposure should be treated; return of BUN and creatinine concentrations to baseline values should be documented before proceeding with anesthesia and surgery in elective cases. **Because the acutely ischemic kidney is more vulnerable to subsequent ischemic insults than the normal kidney,[65] and because many risk factors for development of renal injury coexist in the perioperative time, it is unreasonable and potentially dangerous to proceed with elective anesthesia and surgery in patients with acute elevations of BUN and creatinine that are discovered in the immediate preoperative period.**

Maintenance of effective intravascular volume throughout the perioperative time is probably the most definitive strategy to preserve renal perfusion and to prevent development of renal impairment in surgical patients. Preoperative fluid deficits that result from NPO status, bowel preparations, diseases that promote fluid loss such as vomiting or diarrhea, and the osmotic diuretic effects of radiocontrast agents must be replaced. Intraoperative blood loss, evaporative losses from exposed serosal surfaces, and extravascular sequestration of fluid must also be replaced. The beneficial effects of maintaining intravascular volume have been amply demonstrated in many clinical studies. The lower incidence of death from oliguric renal failure in soldiers who were wounded in Vietnam compared to Korean War casualties is largely attributed to prompt and vigorous fluid, blood, and electrolyte resuscitation after injury in Vietnam.[87] Civilian trauma patients have a markedly lower incidence of death from oliguric renal failure if intravascular volume repletion is not restricted.[79] Optimal volume loading in a variety of other surgical procedures is associated with higher urine flow rates, lower incidence of development of renal impairment, and improved perioperative outcome.[5,12,13,36] Because intraoperative urinary output is not necessarily an accurate indicator of renal perfusion,[3] assessment of the adequacy of intraoperative volume repletion therapy may require replacement of central venous or pulmonary artery catheters with frequent determinations of cardiac output, especially in patients with impaired myocardial function. Generally it is preferable to err on the side of overhydration intraoperatively rather than to restrict fluids; the consequences of fluid overload, including pulmonary edema and respiratory failure, can be easily reversed, but ischemic renal failure that results from intravascular volume contraction is a highly lethal disease.

Anesthetic agents do not appear to be important mediators of renal injury, even in patients with preexisting renal dysfunction. The direct nephrotoxic effect of inorganic fluoride ion historically associated with the use of methoxyflurane is rarely encountered. Of the halogenated agents in common use today (halothane, enflurane, isoflurane), only enflurane is appreciably defluorinated metabolically.[16,58] Serum fluoride concentrations of 20 to 30 μmol/L are commonly encountered after enflurane anesthesia, but renal deterioration at these levels is rarely observed, even in patients with renal insufficiency.[17] Serum concentrations of 50 to 80 μmol/L appear to be necessary to initiate the often irreversible, polyuric, vasopressin-resistant renal failure that is associated with fluoride ion accumulation.[17] **As with all potentially toxic agents, it is wise to avoid their use in settings where equally effective and nontoxic alternatives are available. Thus use of enflurane is probably best avoided in patients in whom renal preservation is a primary anesthetic goal.**

Renal function is adversely affected during spinal or epidural anesthesia only to the extent to which sympathetic nervous system blockade results in arterial hypotension and renal hypoperfusion.[17] Similarly, the vasodilatory and myocardial depressant effects of inhaled anesthetics may decrease renal blood flow, but primary effects of these agents on the renal vasculature have not been described. Renal blood flow is normally autoregulated over a wide range of arterial blood pressures at high and low concentrations of inhaled halogenated agents.[6,69] Normal renal tubular cells are not damaged by exposure to halothane or isoflurane.[71] Although urine flow rates are frequently decreased during anesthetic administration, this effect is probably related to avid salt and water retention associated with stress-induced neurohumoral activation that is common in the perioperative time rather than to adverse effects of anesthetic agents on the kidney. Anesthetic management is thus directed at the physiologic requirements of the patient rather than at avoidance of one or another drug or technique that may have adverse effects on the kidney.

Patients undergoing procedures that require interruption of renal blood flow may benefit from administration of "renal-protective agents" before and after the ischemic insult. The normal kidney is able to withstand up to 50 minutes of total renal ischemia during suprarenal aortic cross-clamping and up to 150 minutes of partial ischemia during cardiopulmonary bypass before the incidence of irreversible renal damage markedly increases. Patients with chronic renal insufficiency are probably more susceptible to these ischemic insults than patients with normal renal function and may benefit from administration of dopamine, mannitol, and/or furosemide. The benefit of these agents in maintaining urine flow, supporting glomerular filtration rate, and preventing renal failure in animal models of renal ischemia has been repeatedly demonstrated,[54] and use of these agents in humans is virtually universal during aortic cross-clamping and cardiopulmonary bypass procedures.[32] Although not widely used in surgical settings, calcium antagonists also appear to prevent and reduce the severity of ischemic renal injury when given before and after an ischemic insult.[74] These agents may soon be used for renal protection in surgical patients.

KEY POINTS

- Dialysis patients undergoing invasive procedures, especially emergency operations, are at increased risk for perioperative death.

- Stable normochromic-normocytic anemia associated with chronic renal failure appears to be well tolerated with hematocrit values between 25% and 30%. Routine preoperative transfusion is not recommended.

- Dialysis can partially correct bleeding time prolongation commonly seen in chronic uremia due to abnormal platelet function and remains the standard preoperative hemostatic therapy for patients with chronic renal failure.

- Ischemic heart disease in dialysis patients is the most common cause of death and is attributed to the nearly uniform presence of multiple risk factors present such as hypertension, hyperlipidemia, and abnormal carbohydrate metabolism.

- Hyperkalemia is the most common and immediately life-threatening problem encountered postoperatively in dialysis patients.

- Pharmacologic management of the anephric surgical patient must take into account the loss of renal mechanisms for drug elimination, the biochemical abnormalities of uremia that alter drug bioavailability, and the effects of dialysis on drug removal.

- Atracurium may be the nondepolarizing neuromuscular–blocking agent of choice in renal failure due to elimination completely independent of renal function.

- Although the overall incidence of developing renal dysfunction after anesthesia and surgery is not known, the perioperative mortality is directly proportional to the degree of acute deterioration in renal function compared to those maintaining stable indices.

- The two major causes of perioperative renal dysfunction are situations leading to decreased renal perfusion and exposure to nephrotoxic agents, both of which can be enhanced with underlying medical conditions such as diabetes mellitus and myocardial dysfunction.

- Because the acutely ischemic kidney is more vulnerable to subsequent ischemic insults than the normal kidney, any acute deterioration in renal function preoperatively should be investigated before proceeding with anesthesia and surgery in elective cases.

- Patients having aortic cross-clamping or cardiopulmonary bypass procedures may benefit from the use of "renal-protective agents" such as dopamine, furosemide, and/or mannitol.

- Because of potential fluoride nephrotoxicity, it is probably best to avoid enflurane use, even though the risk appears small.

KEY REFERENCES

Abel RM et al: Etiology, incidence, and prognosis of renal failure following cardiac operations: results of a prospective analysis of 500 consecutive patients, *J Thorac Cardiovasc Surg* 71:323, 1976.

Alpert RA et al: Intraoperative urinary output does not predict postoperative renal function in patients undergoing abdominal aortic revascularization, *Surgery* 95:707, 1984.

Barry KG, Mazze RI, and Schwartz FD: Prevention of surgical oliguria and renal-hemodynamic suppression by sustained hydration, *N Engl J Med* 270:1371, 1964.

Bastron RD et al: Autoregulation of renal blood flow during halothane anesthesia, *Anesthesiology* 46:142, 1977.

Cousins MJ et al: Metabolism and renal effects of enflurane in man, *Anesthesiology* 44:44-52, 1976.

Eschbach JW et al: Correction of the anemia of end-stage renal disease with recombinant erythropoietin: results of a combined phase I and II clinical trial, *N Engl J Med* 316:73, 1987.

Eschbach JW et al: Recombinant human erythropoietin in anemic patients with end-stage renal disease: results of a phase III multicenter clinical trial, *Ann Intern Med* 111:992, 1989.

Fahey MR et al: The pharmacokinetics and pharmacodynamics of atracurium in patients with and without renal failure, *Anesthesiology* 61:699, 1984.

Kobrinsky NL et al: 1-Desamino-8-D-arginine vasopressin (Desmopressin) decreases operative blood loss in patients having Harrington rod spinal fusion surgery: a randomized, double-blinded, controlled study, *Ann Intern Med* 107:446, 1987.

Koide M, Waud BE: Serum potassium concentrations after succinylcholine in patients with renal failure, *Anesthesiology* 36:142, 1972.

Mannucci PM et al: 1-Desamino-8-D-arginine vasopressin shortens the bleeding time in uremia, *N Engl J Med* 308:8, 1983.

Martin R, Beauregard L, and Tetrault JP: Brachial plexus blockade and chronic renal failure, *Anesthesiology* 69:405, 1988.

Mazze RI, Calverley RK, and Smith NT: Inorganic fluoride nephrotoxicity: prolonged enflurane and halothane anesthesia in volunteers, *Anesthesiology* 46:265, 1977.

REFERENCES

1. Abel RM et al: Etiology, incidence, and prognosis of renal failure following cardiac operations: results of a prospective analysis of 500 consecutive patients, *J Thorac Cardiovasc Surg* 71:323, 1976.
2. Abreo K, Moorthy AV, and Osborne M: Changing patterns and outcome of acute renal failure requiring hemodialysis, *Arch Intern Med* 146:1338, 1986.
3. Alpert RA et al: Intraoperative urinary output does not predict postoperative renal function in patients undergoing abdominal aortic revascularization, *Surgery* 95:707, 1984.
4. Bansal VK et al: Protein-calorie malnutrition and cutaneous anergy in hemodialysis maintained patients, *Am J Clin Nutr* 33:1608, 1980.
5. Barry KG, Mazze RI, and Schwartz FD: Prevention of surgical oliguria and renal-hemodynamic suppression by sustained hydration, *N Engl J Med* 270:1371, 1964.
6. Bastron RD et al: Autoregulation of renal blood flow during halothane anesthesia, *Anesthesiology* 46:142, 1977.
7. Bennett WM et al: *Drug prescribing in renal failure: dosing guidelines for adults,* Philadelphia, 1987, American College of Physicians.
8. Berne TV, Barbour BH: Acute renal failure in general surgical patients, *Arch Surg* 102:594, 1971.
9. Brenowitz JB, Williams CD, and Edwards WS: Major surgery in patients with chronic renal failure, *Am J Surg* 134:765, 1977.
10. Brotherton WP, Mattes RS: Pharmacokinetics and pharmacodynamics of metocurine in humans with and without renal failure, *Anesthesiology* 55:273, 1981.
11. Broyer M et al: Demography of dialysis and transplantation in Europe, 1984, *Nephrol Dial Transplant* 1:1, 1986.
12. Bush HL et al: Prevention of renal insufficiency after abdominal aortic aneurysm resection by optimal volume loading, *Arch Surg* 116:1517, 1981.
13. Carlier M et al: Maximal hydration during anesthesia increases pulmonary arterial pressures and improves early function of human renal transplants, *Transplantation* 34:201, 1982.
14. Chauvin M et al: Morphine pharmacokinetics in renal failure, *Anesthesiology* 66:327, 1987.
15. Cioffi WG, Ashikaga T, and Gamelli RL: Probability of surviving postoperative acute renal failure: development of a prognostic index, *Ann Surg* 200:205, 1984.
16. Cousins MJ, Skowronski G, and Plummer JL: Anaesthesia and the kidney, *Anaesth Intensive Care* 2:292, 1983.
17. Cousins MJ et al: Metabolism and renal effects of enflurane in man, *Anesthesiology* 44:44-52, 1976.
18. Deutsch F. et al: Coronary artery bypass surgery in patients on chronic hemodialysis: a case-control study, *Ann Intern Med* 110:369, 1989.
19. DiMinno G et al: Platelet dysfunction in uremia: multifaceted defect partially corrected by dialysis, *Am J Med* 79:552, 1985.
20. Don HF, Dieppa RA, and Taylor P: Narcotic analgesics in anuric patients, *Anesthesiology* 42:745, 1975.
21. Dundee JW, Richards R: Effect of azotemia upon the action of intravenous barbiturate anesthesia, *Anesthesiology* 15:333, 1954.
22. Endou K et al: Hemodynamic changes during hemodialysis, *Cardiology* 63:175, 1978.
23. Erslev A: Erythropoietin coming of age, *N Engl J Med* 316:101, 1987.
24. Eschbach JW et al: Correction of the anemia of end-stage renal disease with recombinant erythropoietin: results of a combined phase I and II clinical trial, *N Engl J Med* 316:73, 1987.
25. Eschbach JW et al: Treatment of the anemia of progressive renal failure with recombinant human erythropoietin, *N Engl J Med* 321:158, 1989.
26. Eschbach JW et al: Recombinant human erythropoietin in anemic patients with end-stage renal disease: results of a phase III multicenter clinical trial, *Ann Intern Med* 111:992, 1989.
27. Fahey MR et al: The pharmacokinetics and pharmacodynamics of atracurium in patients with and without renal failure, *Anesthesiology* 61:699, 1984.
28. Fisher JW: Mechanisms of the anemia of chronic renal failure, *Nephron* 25:106, 1980.
29. Fraser CL, Arieff AA: Nervous system complications in uremia, *Ann Intern Med* 109:143, 1988.
30. Gafter U et al: Platelet count and thrombopoietic activity in patients with chronic renal failure, *Nephron* 45:207, 1987.
31. Gailiunas P et al: Acute renal failure following cardiac operations, *J Thorac Cardiovasc Surg* 79:241, 1980.
32. Gamulin Z et al: Effects of infrarenal aortic cross-clamping on renal hemodynamics in humans, *Anesthesiology* 61:394, 1984.
33. Ghoneim MM, Pandya H: Plasma protein binding of thiopental in patients with impaired renal or hepatic function, *Anesthesiology* 42:545, 1975.
34. Haimov M et al: General surgery in patients on maintenance hemodialysis, *Ann Surg* 179:863, 1974.
35. Hampers CL et al: Major surgery in patients on maintenance hemodialysis, *Am J Surg* 115:747, 1968.
36. Hesdorffer CS et al: The value of Swan-Ganz catheterization and volume loading in preventing renal failure in patients undergoing abdominal aneurysmectomy, *Clin Nephrol* 28:272, 1987.
37. Hilberman M et al: Acute renal failure following cardiac surgery, *J Thorac Cardiovasc Surg* 77:880, 1979.
38. Hou SH et al: Hospital-acquired renal insufficiency: a prospective study, *Am J Med* 74:243, 1983.
39. Janson PA et al: Treatment of the bleeding tendency in uremia with cryoprecipitate, *N Engl J Med* 303:1318, 1980.
40. Kentro TB, Lottenberg R, and Kitchens CS: Clinical efficacy of desmopressin acetate for hemostatic control in patients with primary platelet disorders undergoing surgery, *Am J Hematol* 24:214, 1987.
41. Kinet J et al: Hemodynamic study of hypotension during hemodialysis, *Kidney Int* 21:868, 1982.

42. Kobrinsky NL et al: 1-Desamino-8-D-arginine vasopressin (Desmopressin) decreases operative blood loss in patients having Harrington rod spinal fusion surgery: a randomized, double-blinded, controlled study, *Ann Intern Med* 107:446, 1987.

43. Koide M, Waud BE: Serum potassium concentrations after succinylcholine in patients with renal failure, *Anesthesiology* 36:142, 1972.

44. Lawton RL, Gulesserian HP, and Rossi NP: Surgical problems in patients on maintenance dialysis, *Arch Surg* 97:283, 1968.

45. Lewis SL, Van Epps DE: Neutrophil and monocyte alterations in chronic dialysis patients, *Am J Kidney Dis* 9:381, 1987.

46. Lillemoe KD et al: Intestinal necrosis due to sodium polystyrene (Kayexalate) in sorbital enemas: clinical and experimental support for the hypothesis, *Surgery* 101:267, 1987.

47. Lim VS et al: Recombinant human erythropoietin treatment in pre-dialysis patients: a double-blind placebo-controlled trial, *Ann Intern Med* 110:108, 1989.

48. Linder A et al: Accelerated atherosclerosis in prolonged maintenance hemodialysis, *N Engl J Med* 290:697, 1974.

49. Lissoos I et al: Surgical procedures on patients in end-stage renal failure, *Br J Urol* 45:359, 1973.

50. Livio M et al: Conjugated estrogens for the management of bleeding associated with renal failure, *N Engl J Med* 315:731, 1986.

51. Lundin AP et al: Fatigue, acid-base and electrolyte changes with exhaustive treadmill exercise in hemodialysis patients, *Nephron* 46:57-62, 1987.

52. Lynam DP et al: The pharmacodynamics and pharmacokinetics of vecuronium in patients anesthetized with isoflurane with normal renal function or with renal failure, *Anesthesiology* 69:227, 1988.

53. Malek GH, Kisken WA, and Taylor CA: The management of patients undergoing bilateral nephrectomy, *Surg Gynecol Obstet* 131:973, 1970.

54. Mann HJ, Fuhs DW, and Hemstrom CA: Acute renal failure, *Drug Intellig Clin Pharm* 20:421, 1986.

55. Mannucci PM et al: 1-Desamino-8-D-arginine vasopressin shortens the bleeding time in uremia, *N Engl J Med* 308:8, 1983.

56. Margolis DM et al: Upper gastrointestinal disease in chronic renal failure: a prospective evaluation, *Arch Intern Med* 138:1214, 1978.

57. Martin R, Beauregard L, and Tetrault JP: Brachial plexus blockade and chronic renal failure, *Anesthesiology* 69:405, 1988.

58. Mazze RI, Calverley RK, and Smith NT: Inorganic fluoride nephrotoxicity: prolonged enflurane and halothane anesthesia in volunteers, *Anesthesiology* 46:265, 1977.

59. McCombs PR, Roberts B: Acute renal failure following resection of abdominal aortic aneurysm, *Surg Gynecol Obstet* 148:175, 1979.

60. Merino GE, Buselmeier TJ, and Kjellstrand CM: Postoperative chronic renal failure: a new syndrome? *Ann Surg* 182:37, 1975.

61. Meyer RD: Risk factors and comparison of clinical nephrotoxicity of aminoglycosides, *Am J Med* 80(Suppl 6B):119, 1986.

62. Miller CF: Renal failure. In Breslow MJ, Miller CF, and Rogers MC, eds: *Perioperative management*, St Louis, 1990, Mosby–Year Book.

63. Moore RD et al: Risk factors for nephrotoxicity in patients treated with aminoglycosides, *Ann Intern Med* 100:352, 1984.

64. Mouquet C et al: Anesthesia for creation of a forearm fistula in patients with endstage renal failure, *Anesthesiology* 70:909, 1989.

65. Myers BD, Moran SM: Hemodynamically mediated acute renal failure, *N Engl J Med* 314:97, 1986.

66. Opelz G: Blood transfusion: current relevance of the transfusion effect in renal transplantation, *Transplant Proc* 27:1015, 1985.

67. Palder SB et al: Vascular access for hemodialysis: patency rates and results of revision, *Ann Surg* 202:235, 1985.

68. Pinson CW et al: Surgery in long-term dialysis patients: experience with more than 300 cases, *Am J Surg* 151:567, 1986.

69. Priano LL: Effect of halothane on renal hemodynamics during normovolemia and acute hemorrhagic hypovolemia, *Anesthesiology* 63:357, 1985.

70. Remuzzi G et al: Bleeding in renal failure: altered platelet function in chronic uraemia only partially corrected by haemodialysis, *Nephron* 22:347, 1978.

71. Rice MJ, Hjelmhaug JA, and Southard JH: The effect of halothane, isoflurane, and verapamil on ischemic-isolated rabbit renal tubules, *Anesthesiology* 71:738, 1989.

72. Rostand SG et al: Ischemic heart disease in patients with uremia undergoing maintenance hemodialysis, *Kidney Int* 16:600, 1979.

73. Ruiz P, Gomez F, and Schreiber AD: Impaired function of macrophage Fc receptors in end-stage renal disease, *N Engl J Med* 322:717, 1990.

74. Russell JD, Churchill DN: Calcium antagonists and acute renal failure, *Am J Med* 87:306, 1989.

75. Salzman EW et al: Treatment with desmopressin acetate to reduce blood loss after cardiac surgery: a double-blind randomized trial, *N Engl J Med* 314:1402, 1986.

76. Schreiner GE, Maher JF: The patient with chronic renal failure and surgery, *Am J Cardiol* 12:317, 1963.

77. Shafi T et al: Infusion intravenous pyelography and renal function: effect in patients with chronic renal insufficiency, *Arch Intern Med* 138:1218, 1978.

78. Sheinfeld J et al: Selective pre-transplant nephrectomy: indications and perioperative management, *J Urol* 133:379, 1985.

79. Shin B et al: Postoperative renal failure in trauma patients, *Anesthesiology* 51:218, 1979.

80. Shuman RB, Schuster DP, and Zuckerman GR: Prophylactic therapy for stress ulcer bleeding: a reappraisal, *Ann Intern Med* 106:562, 1987.

81. Shusterman N, Singer I: Infectious hepatitis in dialysis patients, *Am J Kidney Dis* 9:447, 1987.

82. Shusterman N et al: Risk factors and outcome of hospital-acquired acute renal failure: clinical epidemiologic study, *Am J Med* 83:65-71, 1987.

83. Sun CH et al: Serum erythropoietin levels after renal transplantation, *N Engl J Med* 321:151, 1989.

84. Taliercio CP et al: Risks for renal dysfunction with cardiac angiography, *Ann Intern Med* 104:501, 1986.

85. Upton RA et al: Renal and biliary elimination of vecuronium (ORG NC 45) and pancuronium in rats, *Anesth Analg* 61:313, 1982.

86. Viner NA et al: Bilateral nephrectomy: an analysis of 100 consecutive cases, *J Urol* 113:291, 1975.

87. Whelton A, Donadio JV: Post-traumatic acute renal failure in Vietnam: a comparison with the Korean War experience, *Johns Hopkins Med J* 124:95, 1969.

88. Wilcox CM, Spenney JG: Stress ulcer prophylaxis in medical patients: who, what, and how much? *Am J Gastroenterol* 83:1199, 1988.

89. Wong KC, Liu WS: Anesthesia for urologic surgery, *Adv Anesth* 3:349-392, 1986.

90. Wootton FT et al: Colonic necrosis with kayexelate-sorbitol enemas after renal transplantation, *Ann Intern Med* 111:947, 1989.

91. Yarimizu SN et al: Mortality and morbidity in pretransplant bilateral nephrectomy: analysis of 305 cases, *Urology* 12:55, 1978.

92. Young GA et al: Anthropometry and plasma valine, amino acids, and proteins in the nutritional assessment of hemodialysis patients, *Kidney Int* 21:492, 1982.

93. Zamora JL et al: Cardiac surgery in patients with end-stage renal disease, *Ann Thorac Surg* 42:113, 1986.

94. Zeldis JB et al: The prevalence of hepatitis C virus antibodies among hemodialysis patients, *Ann Intern Med* 112:958, 1990.

CHAPTER 19

Evaluation of the Patient with Liver Disease

ELIZABETH L. ROGERS

Anesthesia administration to patients with liver disease is associated with mild-to-catastrophic alteration of hepatic function. Mortality can be high from otherwise simple procedures, especially if the liver disease is unrecognized, or if the liver disease is acute or is acutely deteriorated. Sophistication in the understanding, diagnosis, and treatment of liver disease over the past quarter century can affect the liver-related mortality of surgery. **To this end, members of the treatment team should demonstrate critical thinking in their approach to (1) the patient's history, physical, and diagnostic studies, (2) preoperative assessment of the cause and activity of the liver problem, (3) preoperative optimization of the patient's hepatic function, and (4) perioperative avoidance of factors known to cause deterioration of liver function.**

Failure of physicians to recognize and diagnose liver disease is a recurring theme in medical literature. Sometimes this results from failure to ask simple questions or to look for obvious findings on physical examination. At other times, insufficient attention is paid to data clearly available in the chart or there is failure to pursue clues until a diagnosis is clearly delineated. However, even with careful attention to detail, some cases of liver disease can be misdiagnosed, even by experts. Most frequently, however, the cause of misdiagnosis is lack of information or attention on the part of the responsible team preoperatively.

If the patient presents with jaundice or evidence of liver disease, a diagnosis should be made preoperatively, if time permits. It is useful to review, then, the common causes of jaundice and liver disease that may be present in a surgical patient of any type.

COMMON FORMS OF LIVER DISEASE

Common causes of jaundice are outlined in detail in Box 19-1; **these causes of jaundice can be condensed into four major categories: nonhepatic jaundice, acute parenchymal jaundice, obstructive jaundice, and chronic liver disease.** By such classification, the

---

**BOX 19-1
COMMON CAUSES OF JAUNDICE**

Nonhepatic

Hemolysis
Gilbert's syndrome

Acute parenchymal

Infectious diseases
   Hepatitis A
   Hepatitis B
   Hepatitis C and non-A, non-B
   AIDS-related
      Cytomegalovirus
      Herpes
      Tuberculosis
   Parasites
   Reye's syndrome
Trauma
Budd-Chiari syndrome

Obstructive

Metabolic obstruction
   Rotor's syndrome
   Dubin-Johnson syndrome
Congenital lesions of biliary tract
   Biliary aplasia
   Caroli's disease
   Polycystic disease
Primary biliary cirrhosis
Extrahepatic obstruction
   Acute cholecystitis with common duct
      obstruction
   Choledocholithiasis
   Pancreatic carcinoma
   Cholangiocarcinoma
   Sclerosing cholangitis

Chronic liver disease

Metabolic
   Wilson's disease
   α_1-antitrypsin deficiency
   Hemochromatosis
   Amyloidosis
Drug-induced idiosyncratic reactions
Granulomatous hepatitis
Sarcoidosis
Chronic persistent hepatitis
Chronic active hepatitis
Alcoholic hepatitis and Laënnec's cirrhosis
Cirrhosis
Tumors
   Hepatocellular carcinoma
      Metastatic disease
      Lymphoproliferative disorders

---

physician is more likely to remember causes of jaundice, such as hemolysis without overt liver failure, and that there are patients, such as those with compensated cirrhosis, who have significant distortion of hepatic architecture and function but who may not be clinically jaundiced.

Patients with jaundice secondary to the hemolysis of sickle cell disease frequently have been diagnosed before presentation for surgery. Patients with other forms of hemolysis, such as those with glucose-6-phosphate dehydrogenase (G6PD) deficiency and those with Coombs'-positive hemolytic anemias, may not have had previous recognition of their problems. Other prehepatic causes of bilirubin overload can be seen in patients with trauma or other reasons for large hematomas and in patients with so-called shunt hyperbilirubinemia from ineffective erythropoiesis. Patients with hemolysis or other causes of prehepatic jaundice are asymptomatic with regard to liver disease and have no physical findings of liver disease. Laboratory studies reveal an increased indirect hyperbilirubinemia and show no abnormality of transaminase, alkaline phosphatase, prothrombin time, or albumin. Imaging studies of the liver and liver biopsy are completely normal.

Approximately 7% of sampled populations may have a congenital benign hyperbilirubinemia known as Gilbert's syndrome. With stress, such as fasting, lack of sleep, exertion, or surgery, such patients demonstrate a partial deficiency of one of the enzymes necessary for conjugation of bilirubin. The importance in recognizing these patients is to avoid expensive and invasive diagnostic procedures or avoid delay in treating other problems because of the otherwise benign jaundiced condition. A history of recurrent scleral icterus with stress is helpful, as is the lack of symptomatology for or physical findings of liver disease, the lack of abnormal laboratory studies other than the unconjugated hyperbilirubinemia, and the absence of evidence for hemolysis. Arias reviews other inheritable and congenital hyperbilirubinemias.[4] The presence of Gilbert's syndrome should not affect decisions regarding surgery.

Acute parenchymal disease is the most important type of liver disease to diagnose because it is the most frequently missed and the most likely to be associated with unexpected significant morbidity and mortality. The most common reasons for acute parenchymal liver disease include infectious diseases, trauma, and acute venoocclusive disease. Acute viral hepatitis can be the result of viruses such as hepatitis A, hepatitis B, hepatitis C, and other forms of non-A, non-B hepatitis as well as viruses found mainly in immunodeficient neonates and adults. Mortality risks from surgery in patients with acute viral hepatitis are as high as 10% and will be discussed later.

Hepatitis A, with a short incubation of 15 to 45 days, appears with sudden onset and is frequently spread epidemically throughout schools, restaurants, and social organizations. Spread through fecal-oral contamination, the symptoms range from flulike symptoms such as headache, low-grade fever, malaise, and anorexia, to significant jaundice, nausea, and vomiting. Because chronic liver failure does not occur after infection with the hepatitis A virus, symptoms and severe derangement of liver function usually resolve within 2 months. Some derangements of hepatic function can continue for up to a year.

Hepatitis B, or serum hepatitis, appears after 30 to 180 days of incubation and is spread venereally, by sharing of contaminated needles during intravenous drug abuse, by accidental needlestick in a health care facility, or by transfusions. As in hepatitis A, there are a wide range of symptoms, from the asymptomatic patient, to moderate fatigue, malaise (95% of cases), anorexia (90%), nausea with vomiting (80%), and vague right upper-quadrant discomfort (60%).[94] Arthralgias and urticaria can sometimes also be found. Acute fulminant hepatic failure occurs in 10% of patients and can then be associated with hepatic encephalopathy, bleeding diathesis, hepatorenal syndrome, and death. Chronic active hepatitis with eventual cirrhosis is seen in another 10% of people infected with hepatitis B virus. Significant derangement of hepatic function can be expected for 3 to 4 months, with continued metabolic derangements observable for a year or longer, even if chronic disease does not ensue.

Despite the ability to test for hepatitis A and hepatitis B, there is still a 10% chance of hepatitis after blood transfusion, venereal contact, or other blood-borne modes of contamination. Previously known as non-A, non-B hepatitis, it is recognized to have presentation and complications similar to that of hepatitis B. Recently, it has become possible to reproducibly identify some of the offending organisms. It has been shown that the majority of post-transfusion hepatitis is caused by hepatitis C. Clarification of the remainder of non-A, non-B hepatitis should evolve quickly.

Cytomegalovirus, Epstein-Barr, measles, coxsackie, and herpes virus infections of the liver have long been described in neonates and have served as the source of neonatal hepatitis. With the advent of acquired immunodeficiency syndrome (AIDS), these endemic viruses are now responsible for hepatic disorders in children and adults. Hepatic tuberculosis, until recently thought to be a disease of Third World countries or the past, has again become prevalent both in patients with AIDS, and in elderly, institutionalized nursing home patients. Miliary tuberculosis is present in the liver 70% of the time and is frequently associated with renal involvement and sterile pyuria. Diagnosis can be made of opportunistic involvement of the liver by viral serology and liver biopsy. Toxoplasmosis and cryptococcal hepatitis, especially in immunodeficient patients, is now being seen. Patients present with a primarily cholestatic status, which may be diagnosed by serology and liver biopsy. In cryptococcal disease, noncaseating granulomas with positive fungal stains on light microscopy and positive fungal cultures occur.

Entamoeba histolytica, most frequently contracted in Third World areas, can lead to large asymptomatic cysts in the liver that present as space-occupying lesions; sometimes patients also have elevated alkaline phosphatase levels. Plain radiographs or CT scans may show a rim of calcium surrounding a low-density center. Acute rupture of a cyst may result in an acute condition in the abdomen with shock.

Reye's syndrome of hyperbilirubinemia, microvesicular fatty liver, and severe encephalopathy occurs in young children after a viral upper respiratory infection. Thought to be aggravated by administration of aspirin during the course of the infection, it is a disease process that seems to be decreasing in frequency.

Budd-Chiari syndrome, or venoocclusive disease of the hepatic veins, is frequently misdiagnosed. It is most frequently seen in patients with cirrhosis or in patients who have recently undergone bone marrow transplantation. Classic presentation of Budd-Chiari syndrome involves acute abdominal swelling, right upper quadrant discomfort, and hepatomegaly. Red blood cells and high protein ascites can be determined by paracentesis. Liver spleen scan shows acute enlargement of the cordate lobe of the liver. In a study of Powell-Jackson, Greenway, and Williams, Budd-Chiari syndrome as a cause of hepatomegaly and rapidly developing ascites was dismissed as abdominal malignancy, without the appropriate diagnostic studies being performed; therefore inappropriate interventions were made.[80]

Obstructive liver disease is termed cholestatic, from *chole,* meaning bile, and *statis,* meaning not moving. Both intrahepatic and extrahepatic causes of cholestasis occur. Common causes of intrahepatic cholestasis include metabolic disorder, congenital anomalies, primary biliary cirrhosis, alcoholic fatty liver, viral cholestasis, drug-induced cholestasis, granulomatous hepatitis, amyloidosis, sarcoidosis, leukemic infiltrates, and solid tumors in the liver. Extrahepatic obstruction, conversely, can be related to common duct obstruction by stone, benign stricture of the common duct, sclerosing cholangitis, tumor of the common duct, and carcinoma of the pancreas.

Metabolic causes of cholestatic jaundice include Rotor's and Dubin-Johnson syndromes; both are benign disorders characterized by chronic nonhemolytic, predominantly conjugated hyperbilirubinemias. Liver biopsy reveals histologically normal liver, except for the deposition of a melaninlike pigment within hepatocytes in patients with Dubin-Johnson syndrome. Refer to an excellent review of cholestasis by Javitt[47] for further information.

Three congenital structural anomalies that can result in cholestatic jaundice include choledochal cyst, Caroli's disease, and congenital hepatic fibrosis. Choledochal cysts usually occur along the common duct and can present with unexplained recurrent cholangitis. Both Caroli's disease and congenital hepatic fibrosis show intrahepatic bile ductal ectasia with recurrent intrahepatic infection and inflammation. Therapy is aimed toward reduction of pruritus by binding of bile acids with sequestering agents such as cholestyramine and avoidance of fat-soluble vitamin malnutrition. Treatment with azathioprine, steroids, and penicillamine have not been reproducibly successful.

A more frequent cause of intrahepatic cholestasis is primary biliary cirrhosis, an idiopathic disease of females in the 40- to 60-year age range. The disease usually starts as pruritus or asymptomatic elevation of alkaline phosphatase, with hepatosplenomegaly, hypercholesterolemia, and hyperphospholipidemia. Progression of intrahepatic cholestasis results in insufficient excretion of bile salts; steatorrhea, fat-soluble vitamin deficiency, hypocalcemia, and hypercholesterolemia may also be seen. Diagnosis is suspected with the findings of high alkaline phosphatase, positive antimitochondrial antibody, and elevated IgM antibody levels. Ultrasonography and endoscopic retrograde cholangiopancreatography (ERCP) should rule out extrahepatic obstruction or dilatation of any bile ducts. Liver biopsy results then become conclusive, showing periportal infiltration with mononuclear cells and loss of bile ductules. Treatment programs with penicillamine, steroids, and other antiinflammatory agents are frequently unrewarding. Liver transplant may eventually be necessary.

Intrahepatic cholestasis related to sarcoidosis should be considered in patients with erythema nodosum, arthralgias, and bilateral hilar adenopathy shown on chest radiographs. The liver is involved in the majority of patients with sarcoidosis, but the involvement may not cause symptomatology.[50] Liver abscess, granulomas of tuberculosis or brucella, and amebic liver disease can also cause cholestatic symptoms.

Drug-induced hepatitis with cholestasis is most frequently related to use of chlorpromazine (Thorazine), prochlorperazine maleate (Compazine), methyltestosterone, and oral contraceptives. Use of tetracycline, especially in pregnant women, can cause fatty vacuolization of the hepatocytes.

Alcohol abuse can lead to alcoholic hepatitis, with right upper-quadrant pain, fever, leukocytosis, and jaundice. Transaminase levels are rarely greater than fivefold elevated, and may be very low, despite significant liver damage. The presence of hyperbilirubinemia greater than 12 mg/dl, elevation of prothrombin time by greater than 3 seconds, and leukocytosis of greater than 12,000 cells/mm^3 with the findings of alcoholic hepatitis on biopsy is associated with a mortality of 30% before and without the trauma of surgery. Abstention from alcohol, fluid and electrolyte maintenance, treatment of encephalopathy and concurrent infections, and avoidance of hepatorenal syndrome can be associated with slow resolution of hepatic damage. Correction of prothombin time prolongation may take 6 months to a year if abstention continues.

Sclerosing cholangitis is a progressive inflammatory disease of the bile ducts that can involve either intrahepatic or extrahepatic ducts. Although it can be seen in association with ulcerative colitis or scleroderma, it is most frequently idiopathic in origin. It occurs in both men and women but is not associated with antimitochondrial, antismooth muscle, or antinuclear antibodies. Sclerosing cholangitis is usually slowly progressive, with elevation of alkaline phosphatase for years before the bilirubin level becomes elevated. After hyperbilirubinemia occurs, the clinical course usually rapidly deteriorates. Sclerosing cholangitis remains poorly responsive to steroids, antibiotics, and chelating agents. When the disease is primarily extrahepatic, percutaneous stents may be useful in prolonging life. Liver transplantation may be the only satisfactory treatment for intrahepatic sclerosing cholangitis; however, the transplanted liver may also be affected by this idiopathic process.

Carcinoma of the pancreas is frequently asymptomatic until weight loss and bone metastases are obvious. When pancreatic carcinoma is associated with pain, it is epigastric, radiating to the back, relieved by raising the knee to the chest, and worse if the patient lies on the back or right side.

Chronic hepatitis can be caused by viruses, drugs, and unknown factors. Chronic active hepatitis is a progressive disorder, tends to occur in young women, and is often associated with the systemic features of fatigue, anemorrhea, febrile episodes, arthralgias, acne, and striae. There is often a persistent elevation of transaminase levels and a marked increase in gamma globulin levels. Active necrosis of hepatic cells occurs, with formation of fibrous septae, and with ultimate development of cirrhosis and liver failure in a high percentage of patients. Drugs that most frequently cause chronic active hepatitis include methyldopa (Aldomet), isoniazid, and halothane.

Chronic persistent hepatitis may involve similar

symptomatology but milder transaminasemia, but with little hepatic focal necrosis and no development of cirrhosis. Biopsy is frequently required to differentiate chronic active from chronic persistent hepatitis and to rule out other causes of the chronic liver failure.

Metabolic causes of chronic liver disease include hemochromatosis, Wilson's disease, and α_1-antitrypsin deficiency. Hemochromatosis is associated with the deposition of large amounts of iron in the hepatic parenchymal cells with eventual periportal destruction and cirrhosis. Hemochromatosis occurs more frequently in men between the ages of 40 and 60 years. Iron deposition in the pancreas, heart, and pituitary is associated with diabetes mellitus in 50% of patients, congestive heart failure in 15%, and impotence in 15%. Deposition of iron and stimulation of melanin in the skin results in the classic bronze discoloration. Cirrhosis eventually develops in untreated patients, and development of hepatoma is common. Avoidance of iron intake, recurrent phlebotomy, and chelation therapy can prevent disease progression. Another common chronic metabolic disorder, Wilson's disease, is associated with defective excretion of copper into the bile and depression or absence of serum ceruloplasmin. The disease usually appears in those aged 10 to 30 years old and presentation includes the findings of chronic liver disease, hemolytic anemia, and neurologic symptoms of tremors, gait disturbance, or personality changes. Chelation therapy and administration of D-penicillamine and azathioprine therapy have been used to treat Wilson's disease.

Another congenital defect that leads to chronic liver disease is α_1-antitrypsin deficiency. Seen in the homozygous state in children and in the heterozygous state in adults, it is a rare cause of progressive cirrhosis. Diagnosis is made by liver biopsy and is suspected by the absence of α_1-globulin on serum protein electrophoresis. Further review of other causes of chronic liver disease and cirrhosis, with approaches to treatment, can be found in a review by Gregory.[37]

RECOGNITION OF PATIENTS WITH LIVER DISEASE

Recognition of liver disease requires attention to the symptoms, physical examination, and commonly ordered laboratory tests.[29] A review by Powell-Jackson, Greenway, and Williams of 36 patients referred to a liver unit, after unsuspected liver disease was found at laparotomy, revealed that **misdiagnosis resulted from insufficient attention to the history and physical signs in 31 patients and omission or misinterpretation of liver function tests in the remaining five patients.**[80]

This study is important because it occurred when the "high-tech" testing listed in a later section should have been easily available to define the liver disease and avoid an exploratory laparotomy, if the history and physical examination had been carefully analyzed.

History and Symptoms as Diagnostic Tools

A carefully taken history is unlikely to miss clinically significant disease,[29] **unless the physician is not looking for clues of liver disease. A previous history of jaundice should be investigated to exclude the suspicion of chronic active hepatitis or anesthetic-related jaundice.** Information indicating symptoms commonly associated with liver disease, such as malaise, anorexia, pruritus, and jaundice, should be solicited. Reference to drugs known to be associated with liver disease, such as alcohol, methyldopa, isoniazid, chlorpromazine, and sulfonamides, should be pursued. The physician should also inquire regarding previous operations and anesthetics, blood transfusions, allergies, and drug sensitivities as well as current use of medications.

Age alone may provide a diagnostic clue. Infants are more likely to have congenital disorders, neonatal hepatitis, or biliary atresia, whereas young adults are more likely to have viral hepatitis, and the elderly are more likely to suffer from obstructive jaundice or tumor.

Patients with Gilbert's disease or hemolysis, not unexpectedly, are notable for lack of symptoms referable to the liver. The sudden development of clinically detectable jaundice in such patients is frequently associated with a history of fasting, trauma, sepsis, or other stress.

The diagnosis of acute viral hepatitis should be suggested by a history of prodromal symptoms including malaise, fatigue, and anorexia, followed by acute onset of nausea, aversion to food (especially meats), loss of taste for cigarettes, and the presence of dark urine and clay-colored stool. Low-grade fever may be present although shaking chills are rare. The finding of darkened urine is most commonly caused by the presence of excess conjugated bilirubin in the serum (since unconjugated bilirubin is not water soluble, it does not appear in the urine). Similar symptoms may also be found in patients with early liver disease secondary to drug hypersensitivity or alcohol; careful investigation for these causes is indicated when such symptoms are present.

Patients with chronic active hepatitis may experience symptoms of extreme malaise, anorexia, mild jaundice, and mild right upper-quadrant discomfort. Extrahepatic manifestations of arthralgias, neuropathy, glomerulonephritis, amenorrhea, and gynecomastia, among others, may also be found.[37]

Alcoholics usually have a history of alcohol abuse, that is, more than six drinks/day for a prolonged period of time. For the purpose of semiquantification of liver damage, one shot of whiskey is equal to one bottle of beer, which is equal to one glass of fine wine. Patients with alcoholic liver disease may also complain of anorexia and/or pruritus. Alcoholism should be excluded when patients present with fever, leukocytosis, and right upper-quadrant pain.

Patients with hepatic obstruction may be asymptomatic, but more frequently present with epigastric or right upper-quadrant pain and pruritus. The itching of cholestasis is thought to be related to bile acid accumulation in the skin, and can occur before clinically detectable jaundice is present. Acute onset of jaundice, the right upper-quadrant pain of biliary cholic, fever with shaking chills, nausea, and vomiting with leukocytosis are typical of cholecystitis or cholangitis. A history of prior biliary tract surgery plus cholangitis suggests a common duct stone or biliary stricture.[29] Patient with prolonged cholestasis are usually free of the symptoms of viral hepatitis; however, weight loss or steatorrhea may be present with long-lasting obstruction.

A history of drug use, including phenothiazines, sulfonamides, oral hypoglycemics, antithyroid drugs, thiazides, oral contraceptives, chlordiazepoxide, phenylbutazone, testosterone derivatives, azathioprine, or 6-mercaptopurine, should raise the possibility of drug-induced cholestatic liver disease.[93]

Patients with neoplasms in the liver tend to complain more of weight loss, general weakness, and fatigue than of symptoms directly referable to the liver. Patients with hepatoma can also note loss of taste for cigarettes and meat.

Physical Findings as Diagnostic Tools

The hallmark of liver disease is jaundice with scleral icterus. If carefully looked for, jaundice can usually be detected in patients with bilirubin levels of greater than 3 mg/dl. The best places to check for jaundice include the sclera, mucous membranes, and the skin. The next step in physical examination is to determine if the liver disease is acute or chronic.

Signs of chronic liver disease should be sought and excluded. The findings or stigmata indicative of chronic disease include spider telangiectasias, gynecomastia, palmar erythema, and Dupuytren's contractures. These findings are frequently present in patients with chronic active hepatitis, alcoholic liver disease, and cirrhosis regardless of cause. Patients with chronic active hepatitis almost always have hepatosplenomegaly. The findings of splenomegaly, ascites, esophageal varices, and prominent collateral veins on the abdominal wall with an ascending blood flow (caput medusae) are suggestive of portal hyper-

Table 19-1	**Recognition of encephalopathy**
Classification	Characteristics
Grade I:	Altered sleep habits
	Altered affect
	Loss of spatial orientation
Grade II:	Slurred speech
	Drowsy but responsive to simple commands
	Asterixis present
Grade III:	Stuporous, responds only to noxious stimuli
Grade IV:	Unresponsive
	Decerebrate or decorticate posturing

From Rogers E, Rogers MC: Fulminant hepatic failure and hepatic encephalopathy, *Pediatr Clin North Am* 27(3):701, 1980.

tension. Xanthelasmas, zanthomas, Kayser-Fleischer rings, bronze discolorations of the skin, and hyperpigmentation are found with various specific causes of chronic liver disease. The finding of a bruit on auscultation over the liver implies a vascular tumor, most frequently hepatoma. Prolonged protein-calorie malnutrition in patients with chronic liver disease can be associated with limb muscle atrophy and loss of subcutaneous fat. It should be noted, however, that as many as 50% of patients with well-compensated inactive cirrhosis may have none of the classic stigmata of chronic liver disease.[80] Absence of these findings, therefore, does not rule out the presence of liver disease.

In patients with liver disease, regardless of the cause, the liver may be mildly enlarged. A firm, scalloped border suggests cirrhosis, whereas hard nodules indicate neoplasm. Extreme hepatic tenderness suggests an acute severe hepatic process, obstruction with inflammation, or pancreatitis.

The finding of a palpable gallbladder in a patient with jaundice is known as Courvoisier's sign, and occurs when there is slow distension of the gallbladder in a patient with carcinoma of the head of the pancreas. This is an especially useful finding when the jaundice is painless and there is evidence of occult blood–positive stool.

Asterixis, or liver flap, is a sign of encephalopathy, regardless of the origin of the liver disease. It is elicited by having the patient hold his/her arms straight out in front, with the wrists cocked back at right angles to the arms. Attempts to hold this position against gravity result in intermittent loss of extensor tone, with the "flap" occurring. Other causes of asterixis include carbon dioxide retention, severe congestive heart failure, and severe renal failure.

Asterixis is only one manifestation of hepatic encephalopathy. **Evaluation of the depth of enceph-**

alopathy is one of the most reliable means of assessing and following the severity of hepatic failure.[87] A suggested grading system for encephalopathy is included in Table 19-1 because many practitioners fail to test for asterixis and because many of the findings are wrongly attributed to aging or other excuses, when in fact previously unidentified liver disease may be present. If encephalopathy is suspected on physical examination, an EEG and blood ammonia test may be helpful in demonstrating whether a metabolic encephalopathy is indeed present.

Diagnostic Techniques

Mass screening of large populations in Britain has found that liver disease, diabetes, and hypercholesterolemia are the conditions found most frequently as a result of investigating subjects previously thought to be "normal."[58] **Unsuspected liver disease in that study was found to occur in 1% of the subjects studied. Unrevealed alcoholism and unknown acute viral hepatitis were the most frequent liver problems identified.**

Although many tests have been proposed to evaluate the liver, **the common battery of tests includes determinations of serum bilirubin, transaminases (aminotransferases), alkaline phosphatase, albumin, total protein, and prothrombin time.** Additional common studies that are routinely performed in some laboratories include gamma glutamyltransferase (GGT), 5'-nucleotidase, serum bile acids, and lactate dehydrogenase. All of these tests may be influenced by pathologic processes outside the liver and therefore are not absolutely specific to the liver. When ordered as a battery of tests, however, improved specificity and sensitivity can occur.

The only commonly used tests just mentioned that actually reflect liver function include bilirubin, albumin, and prothrombin time. Other tests that are infrequently used because of complexity and cost, but which have been developed to better characterize hepatic function, include bile acid clearance, aminopyrine breath test, and excretion of the markers indocyanin green (ICG) and bromsulphalein (BSP).

Immunologic abnormalities found with liver disease include positive fluorescent antinuclear antibody and lupus erythematosus cell preparation in some patients with chronic active hepatitis, and positive antimitochondrial antibodies in patients with primary biliary cirrhosis.

Nonspecific laboratory abnormalities that may be found in patients with liver disease include a leucocytosis with obstruction and alcoholic hepatitis, and a lymphocytosis with chronic active hepatitis. Mild anemia and thrombocytopenia are common with many forms of liver disease. Elevated gamma globulin levels are usually associated with chronic liver disease,

especially chronic active hepatitis and alcoholic hepatitis. Serum cholesterol elevation during obstructive disease, and altered cholesterol metabolism in end-stage liver disease may also be useful.

Tests that measure liver function

Bilirubin. Bilirubin is formed from red blood cell degradation. With destruction of the red blood cell, biliverdin is released into the bloodstream and is converted to unconjugated bilirubin. The bilirubin is conjugated in the liver and thus made water-soluble. The conjugated bilirubin is excreted into the bile ducts and into the intestine, where it undergoes enterohepatic recirculation. Therefore increase in bilirubin can occur at a number of sites:

- With increased red blood cell destruction, as seen in patients with hemolysis or hematoma, there is increased unconjugated, indirect bilirubin, usually with only mild (1 to 3 mg/dl) elevations
- Increased indirect bilirubin can also be seen if there is disturbance of transport into or through the liver cell as is seen in Gilbert's syndrome and Crigler-Najjar syndrome
- Disruption of transport out of the liver cell as in Dubin-Johnson syndrome, with increased conjugated, direct bilirubin
- Blockage of the biliary tree, as in extrahepatic obstruction, with increased conjugated, direct bilirubin

Therefore primarily unconjugated hyperbilirubinemia implies prehepatic impairment. This usually indicates hemolysis, a congenital deficiency, or the action of certain drugs that impair the activity of glucuronide transferase.

Most diseased hepatocytes have impaired ability to both conjugate and excrete bilirubin. Therefore an increase of both indirect and direct bilirubin is usually seen in most viral, cholestatic, and drug hepatitic processes when the bilirubin is greater than 3 mg/dl.

Javitt stated that "the major stumbling block to the clinical recognition of cholestasis is the mistaken belief that if there is no jaundice, there is no liver disease."[47] In early cholestasis hyperbilirubinemia may not occur. Common duct stones usually increase bilirubin slowly, 1 to 2 mg/dl/day, and rarely increase bilirubin to greater than 10 mg/dl. Sudden increase of bilirubin is most frequently the result of hemolysis or hepatitis. Bilirubin levels greater than 10 mg/dl are usually related to neoplasm, alcoholic hepatitis, or severe end-stage chronic liver disease. For more information on the formation and elimination of bilirubin, refer to the reference by Bissell.[8]

Albumin. Serum albumin is synthesized only in the rough endoplasmic reticulum of the liver. Synthesis of serum albumin is decreased in patients with cirrhosis and prolonged severe acute liver failure. Because turnover of albumin requires 14 to 20 days, changes in serum albumin do not occur quickly. In severe, prolonged viral hepatitis and cirrhosis, slow improvement of serum albumin levels may reflect response to therapy and prognosis. Parenteral addition of albumin, however, does not improve prognosis.

Prothrombin time. The liver is the source for production of blood clotting factors V, VII, IX (Christmas factor), and X. With liver disease, prolongation of prothrombin time correlates with the functional severity of the disease, response to therapy, and prognosis. It is one of several reasons for the bleeding diathesis seen in patients with liver failure. Only patients with obstructive jaundice respond to parenteral vitamin K administration.

Common indicators of liver problems

Alkaline phosphatase. Alkaline phosphatase is manufactured in the liver bile canaliculus. It increases whenever there is increased pressure within the bile canaliculus from any source. Thus the alkaline phosphatase level is elevated with any form of bile stasis including extrahepatic obstruction, biliary tract disease, space-occupying lesions, such as tumors or abscesses, infiltrative or inflammatory diseases, such as amyloid or sarcoid, and hepatocyte enlargement, as seen in fatty liver.

Alkaline phosphatase levels are high in 2% to 5% of apparently healthy adults, most frequently the result of unsuspected alcoholism or unsuspected Paget's disease of the bone. Fractionation of alkaline phosphatase can differentiate liver from bone fractions. The typical pattern in extrahepatic biliary obstruction shows a twofold to threefold elevation of alkaline phosphatase with serum glutamic-oxaloacetic transaminase (SGOT) less than six times normal. Other enzymes released during cholestasis include 5'-nucleotidase, gamma-glutamyl transpeptidase (GGTP), and leucine aminopeptidase (LAP).

Ammonia. Ammonia is a simple nitrogenous substance synthesized by gut bacteria and metabolized by the normal liver.[49] Elevated serum levels can occur with increased absorption from the gut, shunting around the liver, or ineffective extraction from the liver. Venous and arterial levels are higher in patients with cirrhosis than in normal subjects, and tend to be higher in patients with encephalopathy. Although the level of ammonia does not correlate with the level of encephalopathy in population studies, serial ammonia measurements may be useful. For those individuals with an elevated ammonia level with encephalopathy, the ammonia level decreases as the encephalopathy improves and rises as the encephalopathy worsens. Properly collected, arterial ammonia measurements more closely correlate with the clinical state[43] than venous ammonia measurements.

Bile acid levels. Measurement of serum bile acids has been made in several research laboratories across the country. Although such tests are not widely used, studies have shown that elevation of postprandial bile acids is associated with reduced ability of the hepatocyte to transport bile acids, implying a reduction in bile flow and cholestasis.[48] Serum bile acid concentrations have been shown to increase in patients with histologic evidence of alcoholic hepatitis or cirrhosis.[61] In this study, chenodeoxycholic acid was usually the predominant serum bile acid elevated, with elevation seen in 93% of the patients with hepatic necrosis or connective tissue change, whereas serum bilirubin levels were elevated in only 43% of the same individuals, thus suggesting that serum bile acids may be a more sensitive indicator of disease process.

Hepatitis virus panels. Patients with symptoms or physical findings suggestive of acute viral hepatitis can have the diagnosis confirmed serologically. Hepatitis A is caused by an RNA virus. Surveys have shown that 30% of healthy adults in the United States have been exposed to hepatitis A at some point in their life. Because there is no known carrier state or chronic disease from hepatitis A, it is important to rule out the presence of acute hepatitis from this virus. The presence of IgM antibodies to hepatitis A virus (anti-HAV) signifies acute disease. After a year, IgM anti-HAV disappear, leaving lifelong protective titers of IgG anti-HAV.

Hepatitis B is caused by a DNA virus. The presence of hepatitis B surface antigen (HBsAG) can be easily determined by radioimmunoassay. For patients with hepatitis B infection, the presence of HBsAG and hepatitis B e antigen (HBeAG) usually precedes the appearance of jaundice and transaminasemia. HBsAG usually disappears during convalescence from the illness. Antibodies to hepatitis B (anti-HBs and anti-HBc) indicate previous infection with the appropriate development of antibodies, but may be present in those with chronic active or chronic persistent hepatitis. Testing for hepatitis C (a form of non-A, non-B hepatitis) is now available in commercial laboratories.

Viral screening for coxsackie, measles, and Epstein-Barr viruses can also be ordered if results of the more common viral studies are negative and clinical suspicion is high.

Transaminases. The commonly tested transaminases are released during hepatocellular injury regardless of etiology. SGOT, or aspartate aminotransferase (AST), is seen with both hepatic and obstructive problems, whereas serum glutamic-pyruvate transaminase (SGPT), or alanine aminotransferase (ALT), is more frequently elevated with hepatic problems. The amount of increase of the enzyme levels per se does not correlate with the severity of the liver damage, but in any individual patient, the trend of the enzyme elevation does correlate with activity of the process.

Elevation of AST is found in 2% to 6% of apparently healthy adults, but evidence of liver disease develops in only a small number. Elevation of SGOT (serum aminotransferase) to greater than 400 usually implies liver disease as the cause of the elevation. The highest values of SGOT are seen in toxic hepatitis, such as carbon tetrachloride poisoning, where values as high as 27,000 IU/L can be seen. Acute viral hepatitis is associated with elevations from 500 to 2500 IU/L, and such elevations form the most reliable biochemical markers of the disease.[94] Alcoholic hepatitis rarely is associated with SGOT elevations greater than 250 IU/L, despite the histologic and functional evidence of severe hepatocellular damage. The finding of very rapid elevation of SGOT and SGPT (10-fold to 15-fold), followed by a sharp decline in 48 hours is associated with passage of a common duct stone.[29]

In chronic persistent hepatitis, transaminase elevations are mild, usually not exceeding 250 IU/L. Conversly, in chronic active hepatitis, elevations in excess of 400 IU/L are common.

The major value of testing for GGTP is in the management of the alcoholic patient whose GGTP levels may rise with drinking before liver damage from the alcohol becomes clinically apparent. One third of heavy drinkers, however, show no elevation of GGTP; thus it is not a sensitive screening test for alcoholism.[58]

Table 19-2 reviews the likely enzyme changes seen with liver disease. Recognition of obstructive jaudice should occur if the alkaline phosphatase is elevated, the SGOT is moderately elevated and is higher than the SGPT, and the hyperbilirubinemia if present, is primarily direct. Urinary urobilinogen should be present except when there is total obstruction, a high degree of liver failure (as in submassive hepatic necrosis), or when antibiotics have been administered.

Other function studies

The liver has a remarkable ability to perform a wide variety of synthetic, storage, excretory, and metabolic activities. Studies have shown that removal of almost half of its mass results in only transient changes in the liver function tests usually measured. As a result, alteration of liver function must be reasonably severe before usual studies begin to deviate from normal. Attempts to develop more sensitive indicators of hepatic function have revolved around identifying compounds that are metabolized only in the liver, whose metabolism is not affected by changes in blood flow seen with portal hypertension or shunting alone, whose use is safe, and whose findings are reproducible and reflective of functional hepatic mass.

Table 19-2   Enzyme changes with liver disease

Disease	SGPT	SGOT	Alkaline phosphatase
Hemolysis	Normal	Normal	Normal
Viral	10-fold	5-fold to 10-fold	Almost normal
Cholestatic	Almost normal	2-fold	Increased 2-fold to 10-fold
Alcoholic	Normal	1-fold to 5-fold	Increased 1-fold to 3-fold
Neoplasms	1-fold to 2-fold	1-fold to 2-fold	Increased 2-fold to 10-fold
Drugs			
Hepatitic	2-fold to 10-fold	Increased 2-fold to 10-fold	Almost normal
Cholestatic	Almost normal	Almost normal	Increased 2-fold to 5-fold

One of the best markers of functional status of the liver is indocyanine green (ICG), a relatively safe organic anionic dye, originally introduced for the measurement of cardiac output, which is taken up by the liver following Michaelis-Menton kinetics. Because ICG does not undergo extrahepatic removal, intrahepatic conjugation, or enterohepatic circulation, it serves as a measure of hepatic protein receptor mass and indicates hepatic uptake function when administered in doses of 1.0 to 5.0 mg/kg body weight.[62] The maximal rate of uptake, R_{max}, correlates closely with functional liver mass. In smaller doses, the limiting factor in removal is liver blood flow rather than hepatocellular function. Competitors for hepatic binding sites, such as bilirubin, bromsulphalein (BSP), and rifampin, do not change the R_{max}. The only condition that has been shown to affect R_{max} is hypothermia; thus its use during various surgical procedures may be compromised.[82]

BSP was used for many years to estimate hepatic function. Measurement of BSP retention 45 minutes after intravenous administration has been a sensitive index of hepatocyte function. Its use, however, has been curtailed in many centers because of the risk of anaphylactic reactions, local toxicity, the tendency toward extrahepatic removal as liver disease progresses,[62] and the substitutability of ICG.

The ^{14}C labeled aminopyrine breath test is a measure of hepatic microsomal function and N-demethylation. It is a sensitive and quantitative indicator of liver dysfunction. Studies have shown that aminopyrine breath tests predict short-term survival, clinical improvement, and histologic severity better than conventional liver function tests in patients with alcoholic hepatitis. It also is useful in detecting patients with unsuspected cirrhosis. A study by Gill et al. has shown that the aminopyrine breath test can predict those patients with extremely high surgical mortality.[32] It also demonstrated that some patients with compensated cirrhosis and normal breath tests tolerate elective surgery well.

Other serum markers

In appropriate situations, diagnostic markers of disease may help when specific diseases are suspected in the jaundiced patient. Antismooth muscle antibodies can be elevated in women with chronic active hepatitis. Antimitochondrial antibody elevation is seen in primary biliary cirrhosis. Serum ceruloplasmin determination can be helpful in Wilson's disease. Alpha-fetoprotein can be elevated in hepatocellular carcinomas. As discussed earlier, detection of antibodies to hepatitis A and hepatitis B can be very useful clinically. Cytomegalovirus and Epstein-Barr virus antibody titers can also be useful in certain situations.

Imaging studies

I firmly support the warning of the American Gastroenterological Association that the importance of "thoughtful interpretation of bedside clues and simple laboratory tests" should not be forgotten "in the race to apply newly developed high-technology diagnostic modalities."[29] Careful history and physical examination, attention to common laboratory tests, and judicious use of modalities developed over the past 20 years, however, should prevent the inadvertent operation on the patient with undiagnosed liver disease.

Cholestatic jaundice, whether related to infiltrative disease, viral infection, or extrahepatic obstruction, has a similar biochemical presentation. The widespread use of ultrasonography, computerized axial tomography (CT), percutaneous transhepatic cholangiography (PTC), and endoscopic cholangiopancreatography (ERCP) has facilitated the differentiation of intrahepatic from extrahepatic obstruction.[13]

Real-time linear ultrasonography has been called the equivalent of the stethoscope for the modern hepatologist.[71] It allows immediate detection of dilatation of the biliary tree, thus differentiating between obstructive and hepatitic processes. Ultrasonography has been suggested in preference to CT scan because of its lack of radiation exposure, lower cost, and similar diagnostic accuracy.[29] Ultrasonography is useful in identifying dilated bile ducts and stones in the gallbladder. Evidence of dilated ducts on ultrasonography is a highly reliable sign of extrahepatic ductal obstruction in patients who have not had previous

biliary surgery. Absence of ductal dilatation, however, can be found in incomplete or intermittent biliary obstruction, tumor encasement of the ducts, sclerosing cholangitis, or cirrhosis.[29] Ultrasonography is also useful in detecting parenchymal echogenicity, as might be seen in a patient with intrahepatic metastases or abscesses, but is falsely negative in 20% to 40% of patients with stones low in the common bile duct.[29] One study has shown that half of patients with the combination of gallstones and biliary dilatation can have obstruction from a cause other than the gallstones.[11] When evidence of obstruction is found, ERCP or PCT should be undertaken to futher delineate the pathologic nature of the process. It may be difficult to obtain an adequate ultrasound study in patients with an acute abdominal condition, because of increased intraabdominal air in these patients, which interferes with the study. In general, a normal ultrasound "may be sufficient to permit a conservative watch and wait approach, thus avoiding an exhaustive search for extrahepatic obstruction or even surgical intervention with its increased morbidity and mortality in acute hepatitis."[29]

The CT scan, on the other hand, is sensitive for detecting dilated intrahepatic ducts, mass lesions within the liver, cirrhosis, and hemochromatosis, as well as showing surrounding organs and the retroperitoneum. Its accuracy in extrahepatic obstruction is 78% to 90%.[29] The CT scan has a major advantage over ultrasound in that it requires less operator expertise to obtain quality images. In the area of intraductal stones causing biliary obstruction, ultrasonography has repeatedly fared less well than the CT scan,[11] because common duct stones can produce biliary obstruction with minimal ductal dilatation. In other areas, however, the CT scan has not been found to be more sensitive or specific for the detection of most focal lesions than is ultrasound in experienced hands, and the technology is considerably more expensive.[96]

Magnetic resonance imaging (MRI) may be helpful in suggesting the diagnosis of hemochromatosis and may prove to be useful in assessing hepatic blood flow.

Either PTC or ERCP of the biliary tree can be performed to definitively outline the biliary tree, precisely define the anatomic area of obstruction, and differentiate between stone and tumor as the reason for obstruction.[17] Both procedures can be performed in patients with dilated bile ducts, are relatively safe when performed by experienced physicians, and correctly visualize the disease process in 80% to 100% of the cases. Regardless of technique, if high-grade extrahepatic obstruction is found, the visualization should be followed by biliary decompression, or sepsis may quickly follow. Decompression can occur through percutaneous or endoscopic techniques for patients with cancer as the cause of the obstruction. Endoscopic papillotomy or surgery is usually performed if obstruction is caused by an impacted stone. ERCP provides a higher chance of visualization for patients with little or no evidence of intrahepatic duct dilatation, and is the first choice for a distal lesion or a lesion suspected below the hepatic hilum. PTC, combined with drainage, is useful in a patient with dilated intrahepatic bile ducts as a result of a proximal lesion.

Oral cholecystography is used infrequently since the advent of ultrasonography, and is of no value in patients with hyperbilirubinemia or liver disease. Similarly, performance of intravenous cholangiograms has given way to use of radionucleotide studies. Use of oral cholecystography or intravenous cholangiograms in patients with unsuspected liver disease may result in technically unsatisfactory results or may be misinterpreted as showing a nonfunctioning gallbladder.

Blood pool markers. Slope analysis of hepatic radionuclide vascular flow has been used to generate an index of relative portal flow that has been shown to corrleate well with angiographic classification of portal perfusion.[89] Using described techniques, this has been referred to as radionuclide angiography, and has been shown to have good reproducibility and to correlate well with interventional visceral angiography. This is most useful in assessment of portal venous flow before consideration for shunt surgery.

Metabolic or functional markers. Visualization of the biliary system can be clinically useful in patients with suspected biliary tract disease. Rose bengal sodium ^{131}I was the first radiopharmaceutical used to image the hepatobiliary system. When administered intravenously, the material binds to plasma proteins, is absorbed by the hepatocytes, is secreted into the biliary system, concentrates in the gallbladder, and is excreted through the common duct into the duodenum. Difficulties were encountered in clinical use of this compound because of poor imaging, a relatively high radiation dose, and its slow concentration in the biliary system, which made it less useful in disorders such as acute cholecystitis.

Technetium-labeled radiopharmaceuticals are superior to rose bengal because of their higher counting rate, short half-life (6 hours), relatively low dose of radiation to the patient, and satisfactory imaging of the biliary tree and gallbladder.[95] Scintigraphy using technetium sulfur colloid, or the "liver spleen scan," was useful in delineating space-occupying lesions in the liver before the advent of more sensitive means such as CT and MRI. Approximately 15% of liver/spleen scans are equivocal.[96] This is related to difficulty interpreting the difference between regenerating nodules and tumors, and interpreting defects

in certain anatomic locations such as the tip of the right or left lobes of the liver, the porta hepatis, and the right renal and gallbladder fossae, which may be the result of an impression from normal contiguous organs or may be related to tumor.

Nuclear medicine cholescintigraphy is a useful noninvasive means to confirm diagnosis of cystic duct obstruction during acute cholecystitis. It has proved to be as useful as ultrasonography in the diagnosis of low common duct stones, which may not cause common duct obstruction. Contrary to traditional teaching, obstruction in the absence of dilatation and dilatation in the absence of obstruction are not uncommon.[11] With use of transit time, clearance time, and washout curves, it can detect normal clearance and thus good functional compensation in patients with bile duct dilatation from prior stone passage or previous biliary surgery but with no active obstruction.[11]

In the interest of using the most practical test first, however, the guidelines of the Patient Care Committee of the American Gastroenterological Association suggest that when jaundice is present, ultrasonography followed by visualization of the ducts by ERCP or PTC is recommended if duct obstruction is suspected.[29]

Role of liver biopsy in preoperative assessment

Certain types of liver disease are associated with increased perioperative morality, as discussed in the next section. For that reason, **patients with suspected or unexplained liver disease might well be advised to undergo liver biopsy and purposeful decision making before elective surgery. Improved survival has been clearly shown in patients with alcoholic hepatitis who have evidence of alcoholic hyaline bodies on initial biopsy.** In such situations, it has been recommended that liver biopsies be performed before contemplated surgery, especially if there is a suspicion that there has not been a sufficient period of abstinence from alcohol.[51] Because delay of elective surgery for drug-associated hepatitis, acute hepatitis, and alcoholic hepatitis may result in considerable reduction in surgical morbidity, liver biopsy to confirm these diagnoses and thus appropriately delay elective surgery may be beneficial to these patients.

Liver biopsy may also be useful to differentiate cirrhosis from fatty infiltration of the liver in patients with alcoholism, since the presence of cirrhosis might alter the plan for surgery, whereas the finding of fatty liver might suggest that surgery could be done after short-term abstinence. When cholestatic disease is suspected but imaging does not show dilated ducts, liver biopsy may show intrahepatic cholestasis of viral, drug, alcohol, or primary biliary cirrhosis causes, thus showing that surgery could be avoided. Liver biopsy may also be indicated in preoperative assessment when a mass lesion is suspected. In those cases, ultrasonographic or CT scan–guided biopsy may yield the desired diagnosis without the risk of laparotomy.

FACTORS ASSOCIATED WITH LIVER DISEASE THAT AFFECT MORTALITY

Dye retention studies show that **half of all patients with even mild preoperative liver function abnormalities experience up to a 30% loss of liver function postoperatively.**[15] **The risk of anesthesia and surgery in patients with liver disease is associated with (1) the risk of aggravating the underlying liver disease, (2) the risk associated with extrahepatic complications of liver disease, (3) the risk associated with alteration of hepatic synthetic functions, and (4) the risk related to altered drug disposition.**[34] **In general, the risk of postoperative liver dysfunction is not affected by the specific route or type of anesthesia selected, but rather by the degree of preoperative hepatic disease activity and the development of hypoxia, altered hepatic flow during surgery, or other noxious factors during the perioperative period.** The mortality from surgery and anesthesia may be higher when the risk of liver disease is not suspected. Powell-Jackson, Greenway, and Williams reported a 31% mortality and 61% significant morbidity when liver disease was present but ignored or not suspected before laparotomy.[80] All patients in that series with viral or alcoholic hepatitis died. Patients with asymptomatic preoperative liver biochemical abnormalities are also advised to postpone elective surgery until a thorough evaluation for liver disease is conducted and the course of the disease is observed.[30] Patients with a distant history of viral hepatitis who now feel well and who have normal bilirubin, transaminase, globulin, and albumin levels and prothombin time are not likely to be at higher risk during surgery than the normal population.[60]

Acute viral hepatitis has been reported by Harville and Summerskill to carry a surgical mortality of 9.5% and a morbidity of 11.9%.[40] **This is a high enough rate to discourage many from elective surgical procedures in patients with known acute viral hepatitis.** As discussed earlier, however, identification of patients with early acute viral hepatitis can be difficult because of the nonspecific history, atypical symptoms, or misinterpretation of laboratory studies. When acute viral hepatitis is suspected, medical supervision for 3 to 4 weeks may clarify the situation and allow the liver disease to run its course, without significantly prejudicing the benefits of operation for suspected gallstones or cancer. Many clinicians recommend that patients with acute viral hepatitis not undergo elective surgery until liver function tests have returned to normal.[93]

Patients undergoing hip fracture repair who have acute drug hepatitis may carry a mortality as high as 10% to 80%. The decision to perform elective hip surgery on a patient with suspected drug hepatitis should therefore be carefully weighed against the benefits of the surgery and the need for the surgery to occur without delay. Limited experience with patients who have symptomatic chronic active hepatitis suggests that surgical mortality is increased. Therefore if there is evidence of HBsAG or e antigen detected in the serum, or if there is any abnormality in liver function tests in a patient with a distant history of jaundice, development of chronic liver disease is possible, and the absolute need for surgery should be carefully contemplated.

Evidence of acute alcoholic hepatitis clinically, or evidence of Mallory's hyaline bodies on biopsy (a feature of alcoholic hepatitis), is associated with increased mortality disproportionate to biochemical or other clinical markers. A frequently quoted paper by Greenwood, Leffler, and Minkowitz[36] showed that the mortality after laparotomy with open biopsy in patients with alcoholic hepatitis was 58%. Similar patients being followed up medically with closed biopsies had a mortality of 10%.[36] These authors concluded that laparotomy should be avoided if possible in chronic alcoholics with the clinical features of alcoholic hepatitis. Another study on the significance of hyaline necrosis in liver biopsies of patients with cirrhosis undergoing portacaval shunt surgery for bleeding varices revealed an immediate postoperative mortality of 37% in patients with hyaline necrosis, compared to only 9% in similar patients with cirrhosis without hyaline necrosis.[51] Many recommend, therefore, that patients with alcoholic hepatitis should be treated with rest and nutritional therapy, with abstinence from alcohol, until fever resolves and bilirubin and white blood cell counts approach normal levels.[60] This may require 6 to 12 weeks or longer before the acute insult resolves. If there is any doubt, liver biopsy should be performed to ensure that acute necrosis and Mallory's bodies are no longer present.

Review of the literature by Thaler and Gellis shows that laparotomy on neonates with neonatal hepatitis raised the mortality and morbidity to six times that of similar infants who did not have surgery.[97] That study showed that the incidence of cirrhosis also increased threefold in infants with neonatal hepatitis who had surgery for possible biliary atresia, regardless of the specific anesthetic agent or technique.

The magnitude and duration of postoperative hepatic dysfunction is greater in patients with chronic liver disease than in patients with normal preoperative liver function having similar operations with similar types of anesthesia.[103] Between 4% and 16% of previously unidentified patients with cirrhosis, presumably with compensated liver function, die after an operation.[45] A study frequently quoted on the incidence of postoperative complications is that by Lindenmuth and Eisenberg, in which complications developed in 25% of patients with chronic liver disease.[52] The risk of developing complications in that study appeared related to the degree of preoperative dysfunction. Patients with increased BSP retention and low serum albumin had a complication rate of 35% compared to 16% with well-compensated cirrhosis. In patients with advanced chronic liver disease, such as severe cirrhosis, regardless of the cause, the risk of postoperative liver function deterioration and thus mortality increases with the degree of preoperative functional deterioration of the liver and may exceed 90%.

The most useful classification of risk of surgery for patients with liver disease has been that developed originally for shunt surgery and known as the Child's classification.[15] Although only semiquantitative and subjective in part, it has proved to be as accurate a predictor as recent sophisticated measurements and analysis. Table 19-3 provides a modification of Child's assessment, which can be used for initial risk assessment of patients undergoing any major surgical procedure.[84]

Using a somewhat different modification of Child's classification, Pugh et al. developed a point scoring system for each abnormality and determined that patients in the "minimum" category had a 71% 6-month survival, whereas patients in the "moderate" category had only 36% survival.[81] No patients in the severe category survived 6 months. Regression analysis of the factors listed in Table 19-3 compares favorably to clinical judgments on nonoperative survivability for patients with biliary cirrhosis,[69] especially when strong emphasis is placed on serum bilirubin. Comparison of the Pugh weighting system with more sophisticated systems using pharmacokinetic parameters, such as indocyanine green clearance, has revealed by linear regression analysis that the clinical Pugh score remains the best predictive variable for survival.[79]

Similar variables were found in a more recent study by Doberneck, Sterling, and Allison.[25] Mortality in 80 patients was 20%, with a complication rate of 47%. Factors significantly associated with increased postoperative mortality included a bilirubin concentration greater than 3.5 mg/dl, an alkaline phosphatase concentration greater than 70 IU/dl, an increase in prothrombin time longer than 2 seconds, and an increase in parital thromboplastin time longer than 2 seconds. Additional factors that significantly increased postoperative mortality included emergency operation, alimentary tract operation, the presence of ascites, operative blood loss of more than 1000 ml, and

Table 19-3　Child's assessment of clinical risk			
Factors	**Minimal**	**Moderate**	**Severe**
Encephalopathy	None	Provoked	Grade 2-4
Ascites	None	Controlled	Uncontrolled
Nutrition	Good	Good	Poor
Bilirubin (mg/dl)	2	2-3	3
Bilirubin (μmol/L)	34	34-50	50
Prothrombin time prolongation (sec)	2	2-3	3
Albumin (mg/dl)	3.5	3-3.5	3
Albumin (g/L)	35	30-35	30

Modified from Rogers EL: Emergency anesthesia in patients with liver disease. In Adams T, ed: *Emergency anesthesia*, London, 1986, Edward Arnold.

postoperative complications.[25] The mortality increased to 41% by the time that jaundice could be clinically detected (i.e., when serum bilirubin was greater than 3.5 mg/dl). In that study, the sum of the unfavorable factors present in each patient was significantly associated with mortality, ranging from 5% for zero factors to 66% for six or more factors.

A similar study, using multivariate analysis of 100 consecutive patients with cirrhosis undergoing nonshunt surgery, was able to predict mortality with 89% accuracy if coagulopathy, presence of active infection, and low serum albumin were present. Similarly, with few operative transfusions, absence of postoperative ascites, pulmonary failure, or gastrointestinal bleeding, survival was predicted with 100% accuracy. Overall mortality was 30%, with additional morbidity of 30%. Sepsis with multisystem organ failure was the most common cause of death.[31] Of patients who underwent surgical treatment on an urgent basis, 57% died compared to only 10% mortality for patients who had elective surgery. Aranha and Greenlee found an even higher risk with emergency surgery; 86% of 29 patients who underwent surgery under emergency conditions died.[3]

Recent studies of patients undergoing orthotopic liver transplantation revealed that risk factors for early major bacterial infection during hospitalization were white blood cell count and polymorphonuclear cell count, IgG, and plasma creatinine levels, all of which were statistically higher in patients who developed major early bacterial infections. The strongest risk factor in that study was the serum creatinine level, which achieved an accuracy of 69% when the creat-

---

**BOX 19-2
ASSOCIATED COMPLICATIONS IN
LIVER DISEASE**

Hyperkinetic cardiovascular system
Hypoxia related to venous admixture
Dysrhythmias
Increased intraabdominal pressure
Poor temperature control
Susceptibility to infection
Anemia
Coagulopathy
Electrolyte imbalance
Susceptibility to renal failure

---

inine level was greater than 1.5 mg/dl.[18] By stepwise discriminant analysis, it was shown in that study of 93 consecutive patients that the variables associated with a significantly increased risk of death were ascites, hepatic encephalopathy, elevated white blood and polymorphonuclear cell count, decreased helper/suppressor T cell ratio, and elevated plasma creatinine and bilirubin levels. Of these, the elevated serum creatinine level was the greatest risk factor for mortality.

Risk of surgery in patients with liver disease is related both to the ability of the liver to continue functioning adequately during and after surgery as well as to the associated complications found in liver disease (Box 19-2). A number of cardiopulmonary changes have been shown in patients with chronic liver disease.

Cardiovascular hemodynamic changes are seen in patients with chronic liver disease who may need to undergo various surgical procedures.[66] Evidence of cardiovascular alterations is seen in patients with chronic liver disease. Multiple pulsating spider angiomatas, warm palmar erythema, and bounding pulse are all associated with decreased circulation time and widened pulse pressure related to decreased peripheral resistance.[20] The increased cardiac output related to decreased total peripheral resistance may be the result of decreased tissue stores of norepinephrine.[20]

Survival after elective surgery was thought by Greenspan and Del Guercio to be predicated on sufficient ventricular reserve to tolerate the hyperdynamic cardiac state.[35] In a 6-year study of patients with cirrhosis who underwent shunt surgery, they demonstrated persistent elevation of cardiac index, postoperative decrease in peripheral resistance, and an increase in mean ejection rate over preoperative values, all reflecting the hyperdynamic state that develops in the postoperative period. These changes

may persist for as long as 2 years postoperatively. Patients with hyperdynamic patterns preoperatively maintained high levels of stroke work even during hypothermic anesthesia. The patients who had a stormy postoperative course or died after elective surgery were those with an elevated preoperative cardiac index. Preoperative cardiac index was slightly below normal in the patients who survived with no serious postoperative complications.[20] High mean systolic ejection rate and/or high central blood volume were also found to indicate a poor prognosis.

Displacement of the oxygen affinity curve to the right in patients with severe liver disease suggests reduced affinity of hemoglobin for oxygen. This shift of the oxygen dissociation curve to the right in patients with cirrhosis is thought to be the result of the increased concentration of sodium within red blood cells,[20] associated with the renal metabolic electrolyte alterations seen in patients with liver disease. Preoperative metabolic alkalosis, as demonstrated by elevated pH without statistical alteration in Po_2 or Pco_2, was more frequently seen in those who died postoperatively. Continued deterioration of the patient was demonstrated by continued elevation of pH during the postoperative period. Similar findings of pH elevation were noted in the group of patients who needed emergency surgery, all of whom died.[20]

Del Guercio et al. also noted the high degree of venoarterial admixture. High values of mixed venous Po_2 reflected peripheral arteriovenous shunting preoperatively, and further increase in pulmonary arteriovenous admixture occurred in the postoperative period.[20] Severe arterial hypoxemia secondary to pulmonary arteriovenous admixture was not uncommon.[20] Cardiac ventricular dysrhythmias have also been noted to be more common in patients with liver failure. Whether this is related to the hypoxia, the hyperdynamic state, or other factors, is not known.

Endotoxemia has been shown to be present in 92% of patients with cirrhosis in the absence of sepsis.[7] Studies have shown that increasing levels of endotoxemia are associated with hepatic failure, encephalopathy, and death.[54]

Increased intraabdominal pressure found in patients with enlarged livers and ascites can increase the risk of aspiration of gastric contents during induction of anesthesia, requiring appropriate precautions.

Because the liver is the site of nonshivering thermogenesis, accidental hypothermia can be a problem in patients with liver disease. Altered reticuloendothelial activity in the liver, protein calorie malnutrition, and altered leukocyte function can all be seen in patients with severe liver disease; all these conditions predispose patients to an increased susceptibility to infection.

Endotoxemia

Endotoxins have been implicated in bleeding associated with disseminated intravascular coagulopathy (DIC) as well as gastritis. Endotoxins have been shown to increase gastric secretion and alter gastric endothelial integrity, leading to the stress gastritis. Although administration of antibiotics to animals prevents stress-induced ulceration, this effect has not been proved in humans.

Attempts to reduce the development of endotoxemia before and during surgery have included administration of oral bile salts, cholestyramine, and kaolin to absorb gut endotoxin. Use of cimetidine has been suggested to prevent endotoxin absorption. Oral lactulose has been suggested to alter bacterial flora and abolish endotoxemia associated with encephalopathy and renal failure in patients with cirrhosis or obstructive jaundice.[74] Use of bowel preparations to reduce bowel flora preoperatively have not proved beneficial, and may increase the amount of endotoxin released.

The complications of anemia, coagulopathy, electrolyte imbalance, renal failure, and perhaps endotoxemia may have reversible components that should be addressed before elective surgery in patients with liver disease, and are discussed later in this chapter.

HEPATOBILIARY SURGERY IN PATIENTS WITH LIVER DISEASE

Gallstones occur frequently in patients with cirrhosis, and are sometimes the source of symptomatology and infection.[1] Although cholecystectomy is frequently undertaken with little to no morbidity or mortality in patients without liver disease, similar findings do not apply to patients with cirrhosis. A study by Bloch, Allaben, and Walt showed a mortality of 23% when Child's C classification patients were operated on. Intraperative blood loss, amount of blood transfused, and mortality correlated with the Child's classification system. These authors therefore have recommended that although elective surgical intervention for Child's class A and B patients with symptomatic cholelithiasis may be warranted, every attempt should be made to avoid operation on Child's class C patients if there is a chance that they could be increased to a class B category with medical management.[10] Newer techniques with percutaneous endoscopic cholecystectomy may reduce the morbidity in high-risk liver patients.

Patients with liver disease who undergo biliary tract surgery appear to be at particularly high risk of complications or death from surgery. Even in patients without other reasons for liver disease, **the degree of jaundice found in patients undergoing surgery for extrahepatic obstruction has been correlated with the operative mortality.**[77,78] Increased morbidity and mortality may be related to cholangitis, which is present in a significant porportion of patients undergoing biliary tract surgery. Malignancy and malnutrition, both associated with obstruction of the biliary tree, may contribute to depression of cell-mediated immunity, increased susceptibility to infection, and delayed wound healing. Although anemia in some studies has also been shown to correlate with morbidity, correction of anemia by blood transfusions does not change mortality statistically, indicating that some of the mortality associated with anemia may be related to associated malnutrition.

Doberneck, Sterling, and Allison have shown a 35% mortality for biliary operations in patients with chronic liver disease.[25] Pitt et al. reviewed 155 consecutive patients to provide an assessment of operative risk that can be determined within 48 hours of admission.[78] Their findings of risk included advanced age, presence of underlying malignancy, fever, or leukocytosis at the time of surgery, reduced serum albumin, anemia, elevated creatinine, hyperbilirubinemia, or elevated alkaline phosphatase levels; all were associated with poor results in these patients. As also found in other studies, the number of risk factors present in an individual correlates with the mortality and with the development of postoperative complications, including renal failure, bacteremia, and upper gastrointestinal hemorrhage. Pain, Cahill, and Bailey reviewed the literature on 929 patients with obstructive jaundice; between 1980 and 1985 mean postoperative mortality was 13%. The presence of anemia, hyperbilirubinemia, and malignancy raised this to a 60% mortality. The high morbidity may also be related to endotoxemia, which results from an increased absorption of gut-derived endotoxins and a reduction in their clearance by the liver.[74]

The association of renal failure and obstructive jaundice is well known, and accounts for one third of deaths in patients operated on for obstructive jaundice. From 60% to 75% of patients with obstructive jaundice experience a decrease in glomerular filtration rate after surgery, with overt renal failure occurring in 9%.[74] After renal failure occurs, mortality exceeds 50%. Factors that have been implicated in this correlation include hypovolemia and hypotension during the perioperative period, bile salt effects on the kidney (the so-called hepatorenal syndrome), and endotoxins. After surgery, endotoxins can be demonstrated in the peripheral blood in at least 50% of jaundiced patients. Renal failure is rarely seen in those without demonstrable postoperative endotoxin.

The protective effect of mannitol has also been demonstrated in patients with obstructive jaundice.[19]

Perioperative use of mannitol diuresis is therefore regularly used in many surgical centers. Working as an osmotic diuretic, it causes volume expansion, retains renal blood flow at low perfusion pressures, and prevents endothelial cell swelling and tubular obstruction. Although renal functional preservation is greater with use of mannitol than without use of mannitol, maintenance of renal function does not always occur despite use of mannitol.

Coagulopathy resulting from malabsorption of vitamin K is seen in obstructive jaundice, and is probably one of the few situations when administration of parenteral vitamin K results in normalization of prothrombin time. Another reason for perioperative bleeding in patients with biliary obstruction is the occurrence of DIC, most frequently seen with biliary tract infection and endotoxemia.

Biliary surgery frequently is complicated by postoperative wound infection and other septic complications. Use of parenteral antibiotics effective against both the coliforms commonly found in bile plus the staphylococci found in wound infections is therefore recommended.

Because mortality is approximately 30% in those with bile duct obstruction and an initial hematocrit of 30% or less, an initial plasma bilirubin greater than 200 μmol/L, and a malignant obstructing lesion, it has been recommended that this group of high-risk patients be considered for nonoperative biliary drainage via PTC or ERCP rather than submitting them to surgery.[24] Surgery in most of these patients is palliative, and because few survive longer than 8 months, drainage with an internal biliary stent appears to offer palliation similar to operative bypass without the risk of operative mortality.

Hepatic Lobectomy

Twenty years ago partial hepatectomy carried with it a mortality of 20% to 50%. Experienced liver surgeons now report a mortality of 0 to 10% when surgery is performed for single lesions.[22,39] Higher mortality is found with multiple lesions, lesions crossing lobes, and cirrhosis. Diagnostic advances such as CT scan–directed liver biopsies, MRI, and duplex scanning have facilitated preoperative diagnosis, definition of hepatic anatomy, and blood flow with hepatic arteriography.[26] Especially important has been the ability to define portal and hepatic vein flow characteristics and patency of vasculature. ICG has been used to determine the preoperative hepatic functional reserve and to determine the parenchymal resection rate, thus predicting survival.[70]

An extensive review of a 25-year experience with hepatic resections revealed an operative mortality of 10.9%, with intraabdominal sepsis occurring in 17%,

biliary leak in 11%, hepatic failure in 8%, and hemorrhage in 6% of cases. However, seven of 26 patients with hepatocellular carcinoma died within a month of operation. Poor survival followed resections for cholangiocarcinoma and mixed tumors. Hepatic resection was most valuable in the management of some patients with hepatic trauma, Caroli's disease, liver cysts, and intrahepatic stones.[98]

Important factors for the development of hepatic failure after hepatic resection are the disproportionately elevated levels of alkaline phosphatase relative to the serum bilirubin, presence of large tumor, preoperative administration of chemotherapy, presence of hepatoma rather than metastatic carcinoma, and intraoperative blood loss.[22] It has been hypothesized that the initial high alkaline phosphatase in these patients is related to regenerating hepatic tissue around the tumor. With resection of the tumor and the immediately surrounding area, this rapidly regenerating tissue is removed, with subsequent development of hepatic failure.

Patients who require hepatic resection frequently exhibit significant hepatic dysfunction postoperatively.[73] Intensive preoperative evaluation and preparation to achieve optimal conditions before surgery are recommended.[99] Survival is promoted by hepatic regeneration, which is marked by decreasing bilirubin levels associated with increasing alkaline phosphatase levels in the early postoperative period. A consistent postoperative pattern of increasing bilirubin with subnormal alkaline phosphatase levels corresponds to lack of hepatic regeneration on repeated CT scans.

Cirrhosis is considered a relative contraindication to major hepatic resection by many surgeons, because of the increased problems with hemostasis found during the liver transection, bleeding from the liver remnant, and defects in the functional hepatic reserve of the remnant,[26] all contributing to increased operative mortality. Recent studies by Japanese researchers, however, have shown that hepatomas can be resectable even in the presence of liver cirrhosis, provided they are discovered at a relatively early stage.[67] For patients without cirrhosis, modern surgical equipment such as Nd-Yag laser and the Cavitron Ultrasonic Aspirator allow surgery to progress with better control of bleeding. Use of cell savers helps recirculate the blood lost.

With hepatic lobectomy or segmentectomy, elderly patients with cirrhosis face a mortality of 89% related to intraperitoneal sepsis, compared to a rate of 25% for elderly patients without cirrhosis. It has therefore been suggested that elderly patients with cirrhosis should be considered for only limited hepatic resections if surgery must be performed.[105]

Table 19-4 Common diagnoses and indications for liver transplantation	
Diagnoses	**Indications**
Fulminant hepatic failure	Ascites refractory to
Viral	therapy
Drug	Severe hepatic encepha-
	lopathy
Reye's syndrome	Recurrent variceal
	bleeding
Massive trauma	Recurrent spontaneous
	bacterial peritonitis
Cirrhosis	Hepatorenal syndrome
	Liver-related:
Sclerosing cholangitis	Severe malnutrition
	Osteodystrophy
Budd-Chiari syndrome	Chronic fatigue
	Coagulopathy
Hepatocellular carcinoma	Intractable pruritus

From Munoz SJ, Friedman LS: Liver transplantation, *Med Clin North Am* 73(4):1011, 1989.

BOX 19-3
CONTRAINDICATIONS TO TRANSPLANTATION

Absolute contraindications

Extrahepatic hepatic malignancy
Active sepsis outside hepatobiliary tree
Severe cardiopulmonary disease
Acquired immunodeficiency syndrome (AIDS)
Thrombosis of the portal and superior mesenteric veins

Relative contraindications

Age older than 60 years
Hypoxemia related to intrapulmonary shunts
HIV-positivity without clinical AIDS
HBsAg positivity
Prior complex hepatobiliary surgery
Active alcoholism or drug abuse
Inability to understand magnitude of the undertaking

Portocaval or Mesocaval Shunts

Variceal bleeding continues as a major problem in patients with chronic liver disease. It has been shown that varix size increases with the increased severity of the liver disease, and the frequency of hemorrhage increases with increase of varix size. Previously the most frequently used option to treat patients with recurrent variceal bleeding was shunt surgery. High surgical mortality and evidence that 2-year survival was not improved by shunt surgery,[46] however, decreased the frequency of its use. Today many patients with bleeding varices are treated with endoscopic sclerotherapy. Prophylactic sclerotherapy has been shown to diminish the frequency of variceal bleeding from 57% to 9% in controlled studies. Overall 2-year mortality has also been shown to decrease from 55% to 23% with sclerotherapy compared to controls.[104]

Survival after shunt surgery has improved dramatically over the past 40 years, since the original studies.[9,53] Much of the reduction in mortality has occurred because of rejection for surgery of patients in Child's classification C. If patients are selected who continue to bleed despite sclerotherapy, but who show no activity of progression of liver disease as proved by biopsy, adequate portal perfusion as shown on sequential scintigraphy, adequate liver size of 1000 to 2500 ml on ultrasound, and suitable anatomy, then operative mortality rates are 8% to 10%.[75] A history of pancreatitis, preoperative treatment for refractory ascites, and demonstration of hepatofugal portal flow are considered relative contraindications to the performance of the shunt.[75] After patients have met the rigorous selection criteria, control of modifiable risk factors as discussed becomes crucial. With accomplishment of low mortality, the Warren shunt has been recommended as the treatment of choice for the long-term management of hemorrhagic portal hypertension.

Transplantation

As for other major surgical conditions in patients with liver disease, preoperative evaluation of a patient for transplant focuses on establishing a well-supported diagnosis, determining the severity of the liver failure, and identifying coexisting complications. Principal diagnoses and indications for liver transplantation are listed in Table 19-4.[65] When present, they imply that the patient has begun a downhill course from liver failure. These indications are reviewed in depth by Dindzans, Schade, and Van Thiel.[23]

Although listed in Table 19-4, it is now recognized that recurrence of hepatitis B virus–positive disease as well as Budd-Chiari syndrome, hepatocellular carcinoma, and cholangiolar cancer in the allograft is frequent. Contraindications to transplantation have been decreasing over the past decade (Box 19-3). Patients with chronic renal disease can undergo transplant if they receive a kidney graft or undergo dialysis after liver transplantation. Patients older than age 60 may qualify for transplant if they have adequate cardiopulmonary function. The current

Table 19-5   Mortality risk factors with liver transplantation

Risk factor	Value	Accuracy
Creatinine	> 1.7 mg/dl	79%
Bilirubin	> 18.7 mg/dl	76%
Encephalopathy		76%
Ascites		76%
WBCs	> 7632 WBC/mm³	76%
PMN leukocytes	> 1300 WBC/mm³	76%

From Cuervas-Mons V, Millan I, Gavaler JS et al: Prognostic value of preoperatively obtained clinical and laboratory data in predicting survival following orthotopic liver transplantation, *Hepatology* 6(5):922, 1987.

upper age for liver transplant is 76 years of age. Chronic alcoholism formerly was an absolute contraindication, but now may serve as a relative finding if there is evidence of significant abstention.

Because patients with previous right upper-quadrant surgery are more difficult to operate on safely, it has been suggested that the decision to undertake elective procedures, such as cholecystectomy, be evaluated against the possibility that the patient may require transplant in the future.

Patients undergoing liver transplantation have a lower mortality than those with similar liver disease undergoing less massive surgery, because the transplanted liver then available for postoperative recovery is a healthier, more functional liver. In a study on 93 consecutive orthotopic liver transplants, the survival rate was 65%. Higher survival rates were seen for those having surgery for primary biliary cirrhosis than for those undergoing the same operation for postnecrotic cirrhosis or primary hepatic tumors. For the patient with cirrhosis, the principal problems have been the numerous surgical difficulties caused by the presence of both coagulopathy and portal hypertension,[38] the poor condition of the patient with cirrhosis at the time of surgery, and the universal return of the original B virus in those who are HBV carriers.[100] Table 19-5 reviews the result of stepwise discriminant analysis of risk factors for death occurring after liver transplantation.[18]

The results of transplantation for fulminant hepatic failure appear to be better than those with standard medical management, although there has not been a controlled trial. Success rates vary from 0 to 58%, depending on the frequency of transplant for this problem and the relative scarcity of donor organs.[91] Patients with acetaminophen-induced fulminant hepatic failure have an even better prognosis than patients with viral disease.

Approximately 70% of transplant recipients survive for 1 year, and these patients have an excellent

prospect for long-term survival.[102] The most common reasons for liver graft dysfunction postoperatively include ischemic injury at the time of harvesting, hepatic artery thrombosis, biliary obstruction or leaks, recurrence of the original viral infection, and drug-induced liver disease. Other postoperative complications after transplantation include rejection of the liver graft (which can occur in up to 80% of cases), infectious complications (especially within the first 2 months, these are the most frequent causes of mortality), renal dysfunction with oliguria, and neuropsychiatric complications, which can occur in 10% to 40% of patients. Grand mal seizures can occur despite a normal neurologic examination, heat CT scan, and spinal fluid analysis. Hallucinations, paranoid delusion, apathy, agitation, delirium, euphoria, regression, and amnesia also are seen. Despite these complications, for the patients who survive the 6 months immediately following liver transplantation, the long-term prognosis is generally excellent.

MODIFIABLE RISK FACTORS IN LIVER DISEASE

Therapy of the patient with hepatic failure depends on an experienced physician team delivering concentrated medical care, attention to detail, and avoidance of iatrogenic complications. Preoperative control of intravascular volume and administration of glucose before and during surgery are important. Some of the modifiable risk factors sometimes present in the patient with liver failure are further described in the following sections. **When time permits, an effort should be made to allow hepatic function to return toward normal, improve nutrition, control ascites, preserve renal function, control electrolyte abnormalities, and treat encephalopathy.**

Ascites

In addition to the Child and Pugh criteria, which emphasize the role of ascites in survival from surgery, a more recent study by Doberneck, Sterling, and Allison showed that for nonshunt laparotomy in patients with cirrhosis, the presence of preoperative ascites as well as elevated bilirubin could differentiate between probable survivors and nonsurvivors.[25] They showed a mortality of 37% when surgery was performed in the presence of ascites, in contrast to 14% for similar patients with cirrhosis without ascites. Similarly, Powell-Jackson, Greenway, and Williams have shown that bacterial peritonitis, wound dehiscence, and hepatic failure developed in 13 of 15 patients with ascites related to cirrhosis or Budd-Chiari syndrome. Proof in either study that the mortality was related to the severity of the liver disease vs. the simple presence of ascites, however, has not been clarified. Evidence that ascites alone is a grim prognosticator is derived from a study by Arroyo et al., wherein the 1-year survival probability rate was found to be only 56% for a patient needing admission for ascites, even without the insult of surgery.[5]

Ascites forms as a result of portal hypertension, low oncotic pressure due to hypoalbuminemia, and sodium retention.[72] Patients with cirrhosis have a remarkable ability to retain sodium, and their urine may be virtually sodium free. This results in extracellular fluid accumulation, ascites, and edema. Continued accumulation of fluid occurs as long as the dietary sodium exceeds the maximal urinary sodium excretion.

Mechanisms for sodium retention include hyperaldosteronism, inappropriate secretion of antidiuretic hormone, and alteration of prostaglandin metabolism. The renin-angiotensin-aldosterone system, which stimulates sodium reabsorption in the distal nephron, and the sympathetic nervous system, which enhances sodium reabsorption in the proximal tubule, loop of Henle, and distal nephron, arc activated in patients with cirrhosis with ascites.[5] In addition, the release of natriuretic hormones may be reduced in these patients. Renal production of prostaglandin E_2, prostacyclin, prostaglandin $F_{2\alpha}$, and thromboxane B_2 are increased in patients with cirrhosis with ascites. Although the mechanism of this phenomenon is not known, it is probably related to the increased activity of endogenous vasoactive systems present in these patients.[5]

Avoidance of ascites is best achieved by strict maintenance of low sodium intake. Approximately 20% of patients with cirrhosis may lose ascites simply by reducing the sodium content in the diet.[5] Ascites frequently appears or is exacerbated during hospitalization when intravenous administration of fluids high in sodium is ordered. Another common reason for increase in ascites is administration of nonsteroidal antiinflammatory agents, which inhibit cyclooxygenase activity with ensuing enhanced sodium retention.

With new-onset ascites, diagnostic paracentesis to exclude infectious, venoocclusive, pancreatic, or neoplastic causes is recommended. Treatment of the patient waiting for surgery includes sodium restriction to less than 1 g/day, discontinuation of prostaglandin inhibitors, such as aspirin and indomethacin, and administration of spironolactone. Spironolactone is more effective than loop diuretics in nonazotemic patients with cirrhosis and ascites.[5] After it is shown that spironolactone and bed rest alone are not causing diuresis, furosemide in low doses may be used. A therapeutic schedule used in many centers is to start 100 mg/day spironolactone with 40 mg/day furosemide. If there is no response after 5 days of

treatment, the dosage is increased stepwise up to 400 mg/day of spironolactone and 160 mg/day furosemide. Administration of furosemide in initial doses greater than 40 mg/day may be associated with depletion of effective intravascular volume and hepatorenal syndrome. Diuresis of ascitic fluid in a patient who does not have peripheral edema should not exceed 2 pounds per day. Usually 25% of patients with cirrhosis with ascites develop azotemia related to intravascular volume depletion as a result of use of diuretics.[5]

Ordinarily, water restriction is not necessary in the treatment of ascites, but it may be of value in the treatment of dilutional hyponatremia,[46] when plasma antidiuretic hormone concentration becomes increased, leading to impairment of free water excretion.

For the patient whose surgery should not be delayed while waiting for slow diuresis to be successful, repeated large volume paracenteses have been suggested by Arroyo et al.[5] The need for intravenous albumin infusion to maintain intravascular volume after paracentesis is highly recommended. Paracentesis, although a simple procedure, should be performed carefully and under strict sterile conditions; it alone may entail greater than a 7% mortality. Ascites rarely require surgical correction.[56]

Coagulopathy, Anemia, and Bleeding

Bleeding during surgery is a major complication. When bleeding occurs in liver disease, it may be related to the issues listed in Box 19-4. Parenteral vitamin K can be administered as 10 mg/day if prothrombin time prolongation is found. Correction of prothrombin time by vitamin K occurs only in patients with obstructive liver disease. If the prothrombin time does not return to normal, fresh frozen plasma can be used during surgery to reduce the risk of hemorrhage. Low levels of one or more of the factors synthesized in the liver (II, V, VII, IX, and X) are found in 80% of patients with liver disease on presentation to the hospital. The usual reasons for thrombocytopenia are splenic sequestration, alcoholism, folate deficiency, marrow aplasia from viral

---

BOX 19-4
PROBLEMS ASSOCIATED WITH BLEEDING

Decreased synthesis of factors V, VII, IX, X
Thrombocytopenia
Diffuse intravascular coagulopathy
Accelerated fibrinolysis
Increased capillary fragility
Portal hypertension

hepatitis, and consumption secondary to bleeding or DIC. Replacement of platelets and coagulation factors should be postponed until surgery, and may be associated with precipitation of worsened DIC.

Increased endotoxin release in patients with liver disease can be associated with DIC. In general, patients with increased fibrin degradation products (FDP) before operation have a poor prognosis. In a study by Hunt et al., 44% of patients with elevated FDP levels died after surgery, compared with no deaths in those with normal levels of FDP.[44] DIC, which is known to worsen during surgery, can also worsen with bleeding, infection, or any major stress. High levels of FDP can remain elevated for at least 9 days after surgery.

Preoperative stabilization of the patient with gastrointestinal bleeding includes rapid restoration of blood pressure, hematocrit, and renal function, if possible. Preoperative stabilization may improve the outcome of surgery. Undertreatment occasionally occurs when well-intentioned physicians are afraid to pass a nasogastric tube or endoscope because of the suspected presence of varices. Ritter et al. have shown that the risk of variceal bleeding from esophageal instrumentation with nasogastric tubes or esophageal stethoscopes is low.[83]

Coagulopathies occurring during surgery can be recognized quickly by the use of a thromboelastrograph (TEG), which permits rapid diagnosis and indicates appropriate therapy for platelet abnormalities, coagulation factor deficiency, and fibrinolysis.

Electrolyte Abnormalities

Electrolyte abnormalities occur frequently in patients with liver disease. Sodium control is important to prevent exacerbation of ascites. Diets as low as 2 g of sodium can be maintained indefinitely at home, but may not be effective in preventing ascites when urine sodium output decreases to less than 250 mg sodium per day. For the hospitalized patient awaiting surgery who has a tendency toward sodium accumulation, oral sodium intake should be tailored to correspond to urine sodium excretion.

Inappropriate secretion of antidiuretic hormone is responsible for a tendency toward hyponatremia, despite total body sodium overload. The incidence of dilutional hyponatremia in cirrhosis is approximately 35%. Serum sodium levels should be maintained above 130 mEq/L by fluid restriction if necessary. Administration of salt-poor albumin followed by furosemide has been used to increase free water clearance; however, care must be taken to prevent too vigorous a diuresis, and precipitation of hepatorenal syndrome. Decline of serum sodium below 120 mEq/L may be associated with altered mental status and seizure activity. In such situations, administration of hypertonic saline solution may be necessary, but will further complicate ascites and intravascular fluid accumulations.

Secondary hyperaldosteronism can be associated with profound hypokalemia, especially if furosemide has been administered. Decreased dietary intake, negative nitrogen balance, and diarrhea or vomiting are also reasons for hypokalemia in this setting. Use of parenteral glucose, potent diuretics, steroids, or cation exchange resins can also cause severe hypokalemia. Correction of the hypokalemia and the associated dilutional alkalosis is important. Potassium replacement should be particularly vigorous in patients receiving digitalis for cardiac decompensation.

Encephalopathy

Hepatic encephalopathy is a clinical syndrome demonstrated by altered neurologic function in patients with acute or chronic liver disease. It appears to be the result of complex biochemical alterations occurring during hepatic failure, leading to neurotransmitter depression that is related to the degree of hepatic dysfunction present. Encephalopathy implies that hepatic decompensation is present, and it is frequently associated with altered end-organ responsiveness to inhalation anesthetics.[34]

As discussed earlier, encephalopathy is associated with behavioral alterations, altered sleep patterns, loss of spatial orientation, and various degrees of confusion. A hallmark of encephalopathy is asterixis. Deterioration of encephalopathy further can result in coma and decerebrate posturing. Throughout its course, the depth of hepatic encephalopathy is one of the more reliable means of assessing and following the severity of hepatic failure.

Hepatic encephalopathy has been attributed to depression of neural energy metabolism, ammonia intoxication, alteration of neurotransmission across cortical neurons, response to altered serum amino acid profiles, methionine and mercaptan poisoning, short-chain fatty acid intoxication, and excess of the inhibitory neurotransmitter gamma-aminobutyric acid.[6,85]

Precipitating causes of suddenly worsening encephalopathy are shown in Box 19-5. The first step in treatment involves correction of the precipitating causes. After correction of precipitating causes, treatment is focused on suppression of urea-splitting organisms in the gut, reduction in the quantity of protein in the gut, reduction of the interaction time of bacteria and protein, and suppression of the transport mechanism for ammonia across the gut. This can be accomplished by administration of lactulose, oral or rectal neomycin, nasogastric aspiration of blood products during bleeding, low-protein diet, and catharsis to purge bacteria and blood products rapidly through the gut. Lactulose, an unabsorbable disac-

---

BOX 19-5
PRECIPITATING CAUSES OF
HEPATIC ENCEPHALOPATHY

Upper intestinal bleeding
Infection
Electrolyte abnormalities
Metabolic alkalosis
Use of sedatives
Protein intolerance
Hypoxia
Renal failure

BOX 19-6
AMINO ACIDS IN LIVER DISEASE

Decreased	Increased
Valine	Methionine
Leucine	Glutamine
Isoleucine	Tyrosine
	Phenylalanine
	Trytophan

---

charide, reduces colonic pH, reduces the number of urea-splitting colonic organisms that produce ammonium, and traps ammonia (NH_4^+) in the colon. It can also be given as an enema in patients with intestinal ileus or obstipation.

Hyperbilirubinemia

Numerous studies have shown hyperbilirubinemia to be a risk factor for surgery. The advent of percutaneous transhepatic drainage of the biliary tract, which was originally described as treatment for patients with incurable neoplastic obstructions of the biliary, was thought to also be useful as a first step procedure before surgery to allow decrease in serum bilirubin levels. Preoperative decompression of the bilary tree by PTC had been suggested based on studies in Europe, Japan, and the United States.[68] If, indeed, the risk in biliary surgery were related primarily to the hyperbilirubinemia itself, then decompression should result in a lowered mortality. Early nonrandomized studies by Nakayama[68] and Pitt,[78] for example, noted a mortality decrease from 28% to 8%. The theory that jaundice itself led to morbidity was further supported by animal models that showed that cholemia (that is, deep jaundice with minimal liver damage) was associated with impaired left ventricular performance by blunting the myocardial contractile response to sympathomimetic agents.[33]

Complications of PTC, such as cholangitis, sepsis, hemorrhage, and biliary leakage, however, inhibited its generalized acceptance as a preoperative tool. Several randomized studies have subsequently shown that preoperative biliary decompression did not decrease postoperative morbidity or mortality,[41,59] did increase hospital stay without benefit, and did result in a nearly doubled chance of complications.[76] Use of PTC for decompression preoperatively, therefore, is no longer recommended as a routine procedure.[41,76,78,85]

Nutritional Depletion

Malnutrition contributes to the morbidity and mortality of surgical procedures in patients with and without liver disease.[64] People with poor intake as a result of anorexia, chronic disease, or alcoholism ultimately consume fewer calories than are necessary to maintain nutritional status. Chronic hepatic failure can further result in deranged metabolism not only of macronutrients and micronutrients but also of various hormones.[92] Patients are frequently in a catabolic state. During active protein calorie starvation, subcutaneous fat stores are used. Altered hepatic metabolism is associated with hormonal alteration, leading to increased levels of insulin, glucagon, epinephrine, and cortisol, all of which contribute to the catabolic state.[92] With stress, gluconeogenesis uses amino acids acquired from the active turnover of protein in the body cell mass, with a resultant depletion of body muscle mass seen as wasting of the skeletal muscles. Visceral protein levels, such as albumin and transferrin, also decrease as a result of their increased catabolism.[42] This catabolism further exacerbates the decreased protein synthesis found in liver disease.

In addition to a catabolic state, the patient with cirrhosis has additional dysfunctional metabolic consequences of liver disease. Because of impairments of hepatic oxidation of amino acids and defective protein synthesis, there is impairment of protein metabolism, with resultant increased net catabolism of amino acids from the body cell mass. Of the mobilized amino acids, only the branched-chain group is effectively utilized by muscle. This results in a decline in valine, leucine, and isoleucine. Inadequate amino acid degradation by the liver leads to simultaneous elevations of methionine, glutamine, and the aromatic amino acids of tyrosine, phenylalanine, and tryptophan, which begin to accumulate. This results in the hepatic pattern of amino acids in serum and spinal fluid associated with hepatic encephalopathy (Box 19-6).[90] In addition, abnormal concentrations of serotonin, norepinephrine, and dopamine form from the elevated aromatic amino acid precursors.

Long-chain fatty acids are also incompletely metabolized by the failing liver, leading to an accumulation of short-chain fatty acids. A mild degree of steatorrhea may also be seen in up to 50% of patients with cirrhosis.[92]

Clinical evaluation of nutrition revolves around historical evidence of weight loss, change in appetite, anorexia, or vomiting; all could lead to the development of malnutrition. Objective evidence of weight loss, decrease in subcutaneous fat stores with low triceps skinfold measurements, loss of muscle mass with low muscle arm circumference, and temporal wasting are all signs of malnutrition (Box 19-7). In addition, dermatitis, glossitis, cheilosis, and neuromuscular irritability may reflect mineral or vitamin deficiency. Magnesium and zinc deficiency may be particularly prominent in patients with liver disease who are taking diuretics.

Common laboratory studies for malnutrition, such as serum albumin, transferrin, and total lymphocyte count, may also be abnormal from the liver disease. Serum albumin, for example, may be decreased as a result of the liver disease alone. Serum transferrin, as an acute phase reactant, may be high in acute liver disease, but is usually normal in chronic liver disease. Total lymphocyte count may be elevated with tuberculous hepatitis or viremia, but should not be decreased as a result of the liver disease. Indexes to identify patients at risk from malnutrition have been developed by Harvey and by Buzby et al.[12] The Prognostic Nutritional Index (PNI) is based on measurement of serum albumin, serum transferrin, triceps skinfold, and cutaneous delayed hypersensitivity testing. The PNI correlates with morbidity and mortality in gastrointestinal operations[12]; however, it may not have value in patients with liver disease because the variables used to calculate this index are altered by chronic liver disease.[21]

If surgery is not urgent, nutritional supplementation is a major part of the preoperative preparation.[93] When time permits, oral repletion of nutrition is a viable option. Patients with cirrhosis of the liver are almost always able to maintain positive nitrogen balance when a diet adequate in protein is provided, although return to a normal nutritional state may be slow.[106] The diet should be as palatable as possible and tailored to individual tastes. Various low-protein diets, with and without branched-chain amino acid supplementation, are used in the conservative management of cirrhosis based on the inability of some patients to tolerate high-protein intakes without encephalopathy. In general, proteins derived from vegetable sources are better tolerated than those derived from meat. At least 40 g of protein per day is required to meet insensible nitrogen loss. If tolerated, 60 to 70 g per day is necessary to replete lean tissue. The total number of calories, as carbohydrates and fats, should range from 30 to 40 kcal/kg. Trace minerals and fat-soluble vitamins can be supplemented in patients with end-stage liver disease.[21]

The role of branched-chain amino acid formulas has received much attention over the past 10 years.[90] It appears that in select patients with protein intolerance, branched-chain formulations are better tolerated and can achieve positive nitrogen balance.[55] Studies have shown that infusion of hepatamine, or solutions high in branched-chain amino acids, can correct the abnormal plasma amino acid profile; however, for many patients, there has been no clearly proved benefit of use of branched-chain compounds over standard amino acids.

If the patient is unable to eat unaided, enteral alimentation can be given using a small, flexible nasogastric tube with constant flow delivery.[93] When this approach is not feasible because of primary gastrointestinal disease, parenteral alimentation is necessary. Other indications for parenteral alimentation include intolerance to other feeding methods, or high risk for aspiration because of altered mental status.[92] Various guidelines for the use and administration of parenteral alimentation have been developed. There is speculation that intravenous amino acids may be more effective than oral amino acids in promoting hepatic regeneration by stimulating the release of the putative hepatotrophic factors of insulin and glucagon directly into the portal vein; however, this remains to be proved.[2] Hepatomegaly as a result of fatty infiltration with nonspecific periportal inflammation and minor elevation of transaminases can be seen in patients receiving total parenteral nutrition. The high glucose load and altered metabolic ability of the liver are partly responsible for this finding. Jaundice is rare in adults, but can occur in children, as a response to too rapid administration of total parenteral nutrition. Correction of essential fatty acid deficiency with addition of intravenous fat emulsions has decreased the frequency of clinically apparent fatty liver. The benefit of intravenous alimentation must always be weighed against the risk of septic complications. Parenteral albumin should not be used to raise serum albumin levels, because it is quickly metabolized, expensive, and serves little purpose except in the perioperative period when intravascular volume may be critical.

An aggressive nutrition support regimen can induce positive nitrogen balance, promote hepatic protein synthesis, and expand lean body mass, even in patients with end-stage liver disease.[92]

Prerenal Azotemia

A recent study by Cuervas-Mons et al. has shown that one of the highest risk factors for predicting survival or death of patients undergoing orthotopic liver transplantation is the serum creatinine level. A preoperative serum creatinine level less than 1.72 mg/dl accurately predicted survival in 79% of the cases, whereas creatinine levels greater than 1.72 mg/dl were usually not associated with survival.[18]

Patients with liver disease frequently have total body water and sodium overload but, because of the altered flow through the portal system and hormonal alterations, eventually have ineffective intravascular volume and diminished renal function associated with intrarenal shunting. Prerenal azotemia and even hepatorenal syndrome can develop. Recent evidence suggests that alterations in renal prostaglandin metabolism participates in the pathogenesis of this problem. The patient with liver disease has an increased dependence on renal synthesis of prostaglandins for maintenance of normal renal hemodynamics. It has been suggested that the vasoconstriction seen in hepatorenal syndrome is related to the relative concentration of vasodilator to vasoconstrictor prostaglandins.[27] Prostaglandins also appear to inhibit the action of vasopressin, causing a dilution of medullary interstitial tonicity.[27]

The most frequent reason for the development of renal problems in a hospitalized patient is overly aggressive diuresis or administration of nonsteroidal antiinflammatory agents. The diagnosis should be suspected when there is elevation of creatinine and/or blood urea nitrogen with low volume urine and low urine sodium. Elevation of central pressures greater than 8 cm H_2O is associated with increased portal pressures and potentially decreased flow through the liver, without additional benefit to the kidney. Cautious use of a diuretic may therefore be tried to effect continued urination, as long as the central venous pressure is monitored.

Other causes of renal impairment in patients with cirrhosis include drugs. Aminoglycoside nephrotoxicity may occur in 32% of patients with cirrhosis who are receiving aminoglycosides.[63]

Nonsteroidal antiinflammatory drugs (NSAIDs) reduce renal plasma flow and glomerular filtration rate, and induce renal failure, water retention, dilutional hyponatremia, and diuretic resistant ascites[5]; therefore they should be used with care, if at all, in patients with cirrhosis and ascites. It has been shown that indomethacin administered to patients with alcoholic liver disease and ascites caused decreased creatinine clearance of up to 58%.[28] Studies with indomethacin also show that prostaglandin inhibition is associated with a marked reduction of the renal ability to excrete free water. Inhibition of cyclooxygenase activity by NSAIDs therefore can lead to sodium retention, diminished renal plasma flow, and depressed glomerular filtration rate in patients with decompensated cirrhosis.

Hepatorenal syndrome is defined as the occurrence of renal failure without any obvious cause in a patient with severe liver disease. It rarely occurs without other evidence of liver failure, such as ascites or encephalopathy. Hepatorenal syndrome (HRS) almost always develops after the patient with liver disease has been hospitalized,[27] and frequently follows a sudden loss of effective blood volume from gastrointestinal bleeding, paracentesis, or overly vigorous diuretic therapy. The diagnosis of HRS is one of exclusion. Liver disease, oliguria, elevated blood urea nitrogen, normal urinary sediment, and very low urine sodium are found in prerenal azotemia and HRS. Before the grim prognosis associated with HRS is sealed, causes of prerenal azotemia should be ruled out. Renal flow studies have shown renal hypoperfusion with preferential renal cortical ischemia to underlie the renal failure of HRS.[28] Because the kidneys are normal histologically, and function normally if transplanted, the mechanism for the development of HRS is thought to be neurohumoral. Water immersion studies have shown that the peripheral vasodilation and diminished effective intravascular volume of patients with cirrhosis, coupled with renal vasoconstriction, are reversible and probably related to altered prostaglandin activity.[28] The potentially adverse effect of NSAIDs in patients with compromised renal function may be related to this altered prostaglandin activity.

When HRS is suspected, a quick volume challenge can be administered with albumin, blood products, or saline solution. If prerenal azotemia alone is responsible for the renal failure, improvement should occur immediately. Elevation of central venous pressure to 3 to 8 cm H_2O by administration of salt-poor albumin and fluid should be associated with increased urine output if the cause is intravascular depletion. The usefulness of calcium antagonists to overcome the intense renal ischemia of HRS is now being investigated. Intensive hemodialysis has been used to manage HRS complicating acute reversible liver injury. Preoperative presence of HRS, however, is associated with nearly 100% mortality if the surgery is other than liver transplant.

TIMING OF SURGERY IN LIVER DISEASE

For the hip fracture patient with acute drug hepatitis, delay of surgery for even a few days or weeks may be in the best interest of the patient. Similarly, delay of elective surgery in patients with alcoholic hepatitis until the Mallory's bodies and inflammatory changes in the liver can improve is associated with an increased tolerance to surgery. Maximization of hepatic function in patients with viral or alcoholic liver disease, however, can take up to a year before hepatic enzyme function and hepatic functional reserve completely normalize. **When the clinical condition does not warrant waiting the full time until maximum hepatic function can be achieved, at least waiting until evidence of acute liver cell necrosis has disappeared is recommended in all elective cases. For patients with chronic liver disease with cirrhosis, delay to improve correctable factors such as encephalopathy, anemia, metabolic abnormalities, and infection may improve outcome. Mortality in cirrhosis is not improved by further delay of surgery beyond this point.**

After extensive review of their own series, Doberneck, Sterling, and Allison recommended that **no patient with cirrhosis should undergo elective surgery without the same intensive preoperative preparation that a patient with cirrhosis who is to undergo an elective portosystemic shunt operation receives.**[25] Linedenmuth and Eisenberg also comment that patients with severe or moderately severe cirrhosis at the time of admission can improve within a period of days to months with intensive nutritional support, allowing time for liver healing and regeneration as noted by improvement in coagulation defect, and improvement in bilirubin and albumin.[52] Only true emergency operations should be performed without the delay for such preparation.[25]

Progress in treatment can be gauged by the clearing of jaundice, the disappearance of dependent edema and ascites, the return of a clear sensorium, the diminution of flapping tremors, and the development of a positive lean body mass weight gain.[45]

PREOPERATIVE ANESTHETIC CONSIDERATIONS IN LIVER DISEASE

Except for agents that are no longer used in the United States, no anesthetic agent is a direct hepatotoxin. Most anesthetic agents, however, including those administered by the spinal or epidural routes, reduce liver blood flow and result in decreased oxygen uptake by the liver and splanchnic organs. Any anesthetic agent, therefore, may thus increase liver damage. In addition, many anesthetic agents are metabolized by the liver and therefore can behave differently in the patient with liver disease. A major concern in the selection of anesthetic agents is to develop a regimen that minimizes the occurrence of hypotension and hypoxemia. Halothane, enflurane, and nitrous oxide affect liver blood flow the least of the currently used general anesthetic agents, and therefore have been the treatment of choice when a patient with liver disease needs surgery.

Previous history of surgical procedures is important in making a decision on anesthetic approaches. **A history of jaundice occurring after the administration of halothane without other explanation should suggest that alternative anesthetic agents be given this time.** Evidence of hepatitis related to halothane use has been definitely proved, with demonstration of antibodies to the surface of halothane-altered hepatocytes.[101] When there is no history of potential sensitivity to halothane, there is no reason to avoid use of halothane simply because the patient has known liver disease.

In patients with preexisting liver disease, the anesthetic-induced fall in hepatic oxygen uptake, especially in the face of hypotension or hypoxemia, is more likely to result in overt liver dysfunction than in patients without liver disease.[30]

Inadequacy of the supply of oxygen to the liver is the single most important threat to hepatic function during the perioperative period.[14] Any situation that decreases the oxygen in the blood, limits the blood supply to the liver, or increases the liver's need for oxygen can result in hepatic damage.[14] Hepatic hypoxia as a result of altered blood flow through a damaged liver is therefore a major perioperative consideration. The first experimental evidence of the role of hypoxia in hepatic injury during anesthesia was produced in 1928, when extensive hepatic necrosis resulted from hypoxia during nitrous oxide administration.[14] It has been shown that hypercarbia aggravates the liver injury induced by hypoxia.

The liver receives 75% of its oxygen supply through the portal venous system. Oxygen extraction occurs through the hepatic bed; the hepatocytes closest to the exiting central veins are the least well oxygenated. This centrilobular area of the liver is thus most sensitive to reduced oxygen delivery. Distortion of hepatic architecture from liver disease, with altered delivery to the hepatocytes, portal hypertension with reduced portal flow, splanchnic hypoperfusion leading to further reduced portal flow, increased central venous pressure that prevents venous outflow from the liver, and reduced oxygen content of the blood all can worsen hepatic hypoxia. Levels of anesthetic agents that block sympathetic activity may also lower systemic blood pressure and decrease hepatic blood flow. Reduction in systolic blood pressure and decreased hepatic blood flow can be seen with most general and regional anesthetic techniques. The decrease in hepatic perfusion exceeds the decrease in hepatic oxygen consumption, causing a reduction in hepatic vein oxygen tension with decreased margin of safety for splanchnic visceral oxygenation.

During septic shock there is decrease of the oxygen content of blood, decreased perfusion pressure to the liver, and increased hepatic oxygen required as a result of fever. Inadequate hepatic blood flow during shock may be further reduced if vasopressors are used. Studies with halothane have shown that when oxygen tension in the liver is insufficient, a reductive pathway for the metabolism of halothane may generate metabolites that are far more reactive than more usual oxidative intermediates, leading to further hepatic damage.

The liver also functions to metabolically convert inactive medications to their active form, to produce protein carriers, and to convert polar, fat-soluble drugs to water-soluble forms necessary for excretion. In liver disease there is altered biotransformation of drugs, altered protein binding, and decreased excretion.

Hepatic microsomal enzyme activity, especially cytochrome P450 activity, is usually reduced in liver disease, resulting in inhibition of the usual oxidative and reductive processes. Reduced hepatic clearance results in prolonged elimination half-lives for drugs that require extensive metabolism by the liver. Patients with alcoholism, however, may have microsomal enzyme induction secondary to the effects of alcohol on the liver. This induction of cytochrome P450 is responsible for the relative resistance of chronic, nonintoxicated alcoholics to diazepam, when inactivation of the drug may sometimes appear to occur as quickly as it can be administered. A similar phenomenon is also responsible for the increased defluorination of some inhalation anesthetics observed in some chronic alcoholics. The anesthetic agents themselves may also induce hepatic microsomal enzyme activity, thus leading to an additional variable in the patient's response to perioperative medications.

Biotransformation, or metabolism of drugs, in patients with liver disease results in altered drug metabolism and altered excretion of a number of anesthetic agents, including barbiturates, opioids, and muscle relaxants. Because most inhalation anesthetics do not require metabolism for them to produce their effects, the major changes seen are related to dosage required to maintain sedation, and the rate of removal of agents after administration. Inhalation anesthetics in general are lipid-soluble compounds that must be transformed by the liver to a water-soluble compound for excretion in the bile. The degree of metabolism varies from agent to agent—20% for halothane, 3% for enflurane, and 1% for isoflurane. Prolonged action can therefore be seen with reduced hepatic functional metabolism. Reactive intermediate metabolites can also be seen with anesthetic agents. The lipoperoxidases formed, if not quenched by tissue glutathione, are free to cause tissue damage.

Altered binding of drugs to protein occurs with the changes in serum proteins seen in patients with liver disease. Because serum globulin is increased, and serum albumin can be decreased in patients with liver disease, the effect of these changes causes higher or lower binding potential, depending on which protein the drug is bound to. Reduced synthesis of albumin results in reduced plasma-binding sites for drugs such as salicylates, and increase of the free drug fraction. Conversely, effects of pancuronium may be increased if increased globulins are present.

A decreased serum concentration of the particular protein necessary for binding results in an increase in the pharmacologic action at the myoneural junction as a result of the increased availability of free drug. Altered sensitivity to curare-type products therefore can be expected in patients with liver disease. The large doses of such drugs needed in these patients may cause problems in reversing their effects after surgery. Prolonged duration after muscle paralysis may be ameliorated by using agents, such as gallamine or atracurium, that are not metabolized by the liver.[30] Patients with liver disease have increased sensitivity to barbiturates, opiates, and phenothiazines. Evidence of increased duration of response and enhancement of encephalopathy can be seen with all of these agents. In patients with decompensated liver disease, therefore, sedatives (such as diazepam), narcotics (such as meperidine), or induction agents (such as phenobarbital) may cause a prolonged depression of consciousness if used in standard doses.

Increased plasma and extracellular fluid volumes form an increased volume of distribution for water-soluble drugs, and this increased volume of distribution may present as decreased sensitivity to the drug initially.

Altered portal flow or portacaval shunting may increase the bioavailability of orally administered drugs by reducing "first-pass" metabolism usually present.

Generally, drugs tend to produce a more profound and prolonged effect than normal. It is therefore recommended that initial doses should be reduced in proportion to the severity of the liver disease and titrated against the response observed.[57] Heightened sensitivity should be expected from centrally acting agents.

SUMMARY

Because the patient with liver disease is at increased risk for development of intraoperative and postoperative complications, the decisions of whether and when a surgical procedure should be undertaken must be based on the consequences of delaying or avoiding the procedure versus the acuteness and reversibility of the liver process.[86] Of primary importance is the need to recognize that the patient does indeed have liver disease, since the risk of surgery increases when liver disease is unsuspected.

Preoperative assessment of the patient with liver disease requires knowledge of the kinds of liver disease that may be present, especially understanding whether the liver disease is acute and transient, chronic and stable, or chronic and improvable. To this end, evaluation of symptoms, physical findings, and diagnostic techniques available to further define the activity of the disease are necessary. Use of markers of viral hepatitis infection, testing for autoantibodies, diagnostic imaging procedures, and commonly available laboratory tests help define the presence and cause of the liver disease. Liver biopsy is occasionally useful in clarifying the process, and perhaps in avoiding otherwise unnecessary surgery. In addition, knowledge about the anatomic and physiologic changes that occur with liver disease is necessary to properly approach the patient with liver disease with regard to the anesthetic perspective.

Patients with unsuspected liver disease from early acute hepatitis or chronic active hepatitis tend to have a high risk of morbidity and mortality associated with activation of the liver disease and accumulated mild or moderate hepatic insults during surgery. Based on these findings, many have suggested that only patients in the minimum risk category should undergo elective surgery. Patients with severe hepatic dysfunction represent an almost prohibitive risk, regardless of anesthetic agent or technique. Patients in all categories, however, may require emergency surgery.[57] Interestingly, patients with known, stable liver disease undergoing surgery that is careful to minimize hepatic ischemia or hepatotoxicity, may have nearly normal morbidity rates.[88]

As somewhat whimsically stated by Conn, to reduce the high mortality associated with surgery, surgeons can either "shunt better the patients they select, or select better the patients they shunt."[16] In fact, operative risk of patients having surgery during the period from 1985 to 1990 indicated a lower expected mortality of less than 10%, reduced from earlier studies because of better preoperative selection and the availability of other methods of treatment.[76] Complications that led to death in the newer series more frequently were associated with severe concomitant illness, inadequate operation, and technical failure.[76] Most patients with advanced unresectable disease are now diagnosed without laparotomy and are then treated by nonoperative means.[76]

Part of the decision regarding timing of surgery requires understanding of the risk factors that the patient faces with surgery and scrutiny to ensure that modifiable risk factors are controlled before surgery, if possible. Reduction of the morbidity or surgery depends on close attention to detail in the many aspects of management. Optimization of volume and renal status, electrolytes, cardiovascular status, encephalopathy, and nutrition is particularly important. Anesthetic agents that function differently in liver disease and that adversely affect liver function require consideration preoperatively, especially when patients with liver disease are undergoing surgery that may further compromise hepatic function. Of major importance, however, is the need to correct preoperatively any modifiable risk factors and to cautiously maintain the patient perioperatively to avoid hypotension, hypoxia, and further hepatic damage.

For any surgical patient with liver disease, care should be taken to recognize the presence of the liver disease, modify those factors that can be altered before surgery, and then perform the surgery with careful anesthetic techniques (see Chapter 18).

KEY POINTS

- Mortality from surgery and anesthesia in patients with liver disease can be high even with simple procedures, especially if the liver disease is unrecognized or if it is acute or acutely deteriorated.

- Failure to recognize and diagnose liver disease sometimes results from lack of preoperative information or attention on the part of the responsible team.

- If a patient presents with jaundice or evidence of liver disease, the diagnosis should be made preoperatively, if time permits.

- Common causes of jaundice include nonhepatic, obstructive, acute parenchymal jaundice, and jaundice associated with chronic liver disease.

- Acute parenchymal liver disease is the most frequently missed diagnosis and the most likely to be associated with unexpected and significant patient morbidity and mortality.

- A carefully taken patient history should include history of jaundice, reference to drugs known to cause liver disease, symptoms suggestive of liver disease, and evidence of significant alcohol ingestion. Signs of chronic liver disease as well as evidence of acute scleral icterus should be looked for and excluded.

- The LFTs, which measure liver function, include bilirubin, albumin, and prothrombin time. Imaging studies are useful once the presence of liver disease is suspected.

- Risk of anesthesia in patients with liver disease is associated with risk of aggravating the underlying liver disease, risk associated with extrahepatic complications, risk associated with alteration of hepatic synthetic functions, and risk related to altered drug disposition.

- Risk of postoperative liver dysfunction is not affected by the specific route or brand of anesthesia selected but rather by the degree of preoperative hepatic disease activity and the development of hypoxia, altered blood flow, or other noxious factors that occur during the perioperative period itself.

- Risk of surgery during acute viral hepatitis is approximately 10%, such that elective surgical procedures should be delayed in patients with known acute viral hepatitis or in patients with alcoholic hepatitis.

- The presence of cirrhosis, even with normal liver function tests, is associated with increased morbidity.

- The most useful classification regarding risk of surgery in patients with liver disease is Child's classification.

- Patients with liver disease who undergo biliary tract surgery appear to be at particularly high risk of experiencing complications or death from surgery. Although the risk of surgery in obstructive disease increases as the bilirubin increases, preoperative decompression does not reduce that risk.

- The protective effect of mannitol in patients with obstructive jaundice has been repeatedly demonstrated.

- Patients requiring hepatic resection frequently exhibit significant hepatic dysfunction postoperatively. Survival is promoted by hepatic regeneration.

- Patients undergoing liver transplantation have a lower mortality than those with similar liver disease undergoing less massive surgery because the transplanted liver (available for postoperative recovery) is a healthier, more functional liver.

- Modifiable risk factors that should be maximally corrected before surgery include control of ascites, preservation of renal function, control of glucose and electrolyte abnormalities, improved nutrition, and treatment of encephalopathy.

- Anesthetic agents that function differently in liver disease and which adversely affect liver function need preoperative consideration.

KEY REFERENCES

Arroyo V, Gines P, Planas R et al: Management of patients with cirrhosis and ascites, *Semin Liver Dis* 6(4):353, 1986.

Cuervas-Mons V, Millan I, Gavaler JS et al: Prognostic value of preoperatively obtained clinical and laboratory data in predicting survival following orthotopic liver transplantation, *Hepatology* 6(5):922, 1987.

Doberneck RC, Sterling WA, and Allison DC: Morbidity and mortality after operation in nonbleeding cirrhotic patients, *Am J Surg* 146:306, 1983.

Greenspan M, Del Guercio LRM: Cardiorespiratory determinants of survival in cirrhotic patients requiring surgery for portal hypertension, *Am J Surg* 115:43, 1968.

Lindenmuth WW, Eisenberg MM: The surgical risk in cirrhosis of the liver, *Arch Surg* 86:235, 1963.

Powell-Jackson P, Greenway B, and Williams R: Adverse effects of exploratory laparotomy in patients with unsuspected liver disease, *Br J Surg* 69:449, 1982.

Schafer DF, Shaw BW Jr: Fulminant hepatic failure and orthotopic liver transplantation, *Semin Liver Dis* 9(3):189, 1989.

Smith LG, Perez G: Viral hepatitis: the alphabet game, *Postgrad Med* 84(5):179, 1988.

REFERENCES

1. Anciaux ML, Pelletier G, and Atkali P: Prospective study of clinical and biochemical features of sympathetic choledocholithiasis, *Dig Dis Sci* 31:449, 1986.
2. Achord JL: Malnutrition and the role of nutritional support in alcoholic liver disease, *Am J Gastroenterol* 82(1):1, 1987.
3. Aranha GV, Greenlee HB: Intraabdominal surgery in patients with advanced cirrhosis, *Arch Surg* 121:275, 1986.
4. Arias IM: Inheritable and congenital hyperbilirubinemia: models for the study of drug metabolism, *N Engl J Med* 285(25):1416, 1971.
5. Arroyo V, Gines P, Planas R et al: Management of patients with cirrhosis and ascites, *Semin Liver Dis* 6(4):353, 1986.
6. Bernardini P, Fischer JE: Amino acid imbalance and hepatic encephalopathy, *Annu Rev Nutr* 2:419, 1982.
7. Bigatello LM, Broitman SA, Fattori L et al: Endotoxemia, encephalopathy, and mortality in cirrhotic patients, *Am J Gastroenterol* 82(1):11, 1987.
8. Bissell DM: Formation and elimination of bilirubin, *Gastroenterology* 69(2):519, 1975.
9. Blakemore AH: Portacaval anastomosis—observations on technic and postoperative care, *Surg Clin North Am* 28:279, 1948.
10. Block RS, Allaben RD, and Walt AJ: Cholecystectomy in patients with cirrhosis: a surgical challenge, *Arch Surg* 120:669, 1985.
11. Burrell MI, Zeman RK: Of cholescintigraphy, sonography, and great bears: a view on modern biliary imaging, *J Clin Gastroenterol* 10(2):123, 1988.
12. Buzby GP, Mullen JL, Matthews DC et al: Prognostic nutritional index in gastrointestinal surgery, *Am J Surg* 139:160, 1980.
13. Cabrera OA, Van Sonnenberg E, Bowen F et al: Gallstones and a dilated common bile duct on ultrasound: is direct clear cholangiography indicated and what is the etiology of obstruction? *Radiology* 153:108, 1984.
14. Cahalan MK, Mangano DT: Liver function and dysfunction with anesthesia and surgery. In Zakin D, Bager TD, eds: *Hepatology: a textbook of liver disease,* Philadelphia, 1982, WB Saunders.
15. Child CG III: The liver and portal hypertension. In Dunphy JE, ed: *Major problems in clinical surgery,* Philadelphia, 1964, WB Saunders.
16. Conn HO: A peek at the Child–Turcotte classification, *Hepatology* 1(6):673, 1981.
17. Cronan JJ, Mueller PR, Simeone JF et al: Prospective diagnosis of choledocholithiasis, *Radiology* 146:467, 1983.
18. Cuervas-Mons V, Millan I, Gavaler JS et al: Prognostic value of preoperatively obtained clinical and laboratory data in

predicting survival following orthotopic liver transplantation, *Hepatology* 6(5):922, 1986.
19. Dawson JL: Post-operative renal function in obstructive jaundice: effect of a mannitol diuresis, *Br Med J* 1:82, 1965.
20. Del Guercio LRM, Commaraswamy RP, Feins NR et al: Pulmonary arteriovenous admixture and the hyperdynamic cardiovascular state in surgery for portal hypertension, *Surgery* 56(1):57, 1964.
21. DiCecco SR, Wieners EJ, Wiesner RH et al: Assessment of nutritional status of patients with end-stage liver disease undergoing liver transplantation, *Mayo Clin Proc* 64:95, 1989.
22. Didolkar MS, Fitzpatrick JL, Elias EG et al: Risk factors before hepatectomy, hepatic function after hepatectomy and computed tomographic changes as indicators of mortality from hepatic failure, *Surg Gynecol Obstet* 169:17, 1989.
23. Dindzans VJ, Schade RR, and Van Thiel DH: Medical problems before and after transplantation, *Gastroenterol Clin North Am* 17(1):19, 1988.
24. Dixon JM, Armstrong CP, Duffy SW et al: Factors affecting morbidity and mortality after surgery for obstructive jaundice: a review of 373 patients, *Gut* 24:845, 1983.
25. Doberneck RC, Sterling WA, and Allison DC: Morbidity and mortality after operation in nonbleeding cirrhotic patients, *Am J Surg* 146:306, 1983.
26. Edwards WH, Blumgart LH: Liver resection in malignant disease, *Semin Surg Oncol* 3:1, 1987.
27. Epstein M: The hepatorenal syndrome, *Hosp Pract* 24(4):65, 1989.
28. Epstein M: Renal prostaglandins and the control of renal function in liver disease, *Am J Med* 80(Suppl 1A):46, 1986.
29. Frank BB, Members of the Patient Care Committee of the American Gastroenterological Association: Clinical evaluation of jaundice, *JAMA* 262(21):3031, 1989.
30. Friedman LS, Maddrey WC: Surgery in the patient with liver disease, *Med Clin North Am* 71(3):453, 1987.
31. Garrison RN, Cryer HM, Howard DA et al: Clarification of risk factors for abdominal operations in patients with hepatic cirrhosis, *Ann Surg* 199(6):648, 1984.
32. Gill RA, Goodman MW, Golfus GR et al: Aminopyrine breath test predicts surgical risk for patients with liver disease, *Ann Surg* 198(6):701, 1983.
33. Green J, Beyar R, Sideman S et al: The "jaundiced heart": a possible explanation for postoperative shock in obstructive jaundice, *Surgery* 100(1):14, 1986.
34. Greene NM: Anesthesia risk factors in patients with liver disease, *Contemp Anesth Pract* 4:87, 1981.
35. Greenspan M, Del Guercio LRM: Cardiorespiratory determinants of survival

in cirrhotic patients requiring surgery for portal hypertension, *Am J Surg* 115:43, 1968.
36. Greenwood SM, Leffler CT, and Minkowitz S: The increased mortality rate of open liver biopsy in alcoholic hepatitis, *Surg Gynecol Obstet* 134:600, 1972.
37. Gregory P: Chronic hepatitis, *Gastroenterology* 4:1, 1989.
38. Haagsma EB, Gips CH, Wesenhagen H et al: Liver disease and its effect on hemostasis during liver transplantation, *Liver* 5:123, 1985.
39. Hardy KJ: Liver surgery: a revolution, *Aust N Z J Surg* 59(7):519, 1989.
40. Harville DD, Summerskill WHJ: Surgery in acute hepatitis, *JAMA* 184(4):257, 1963.
41. Hatfield AR, Terblanche J, Fataar S et al: Preoperative external biliary drainage in obstructive jaundice, *Lancet* 2(8304):896, 1982.
42. Hehir DJ, Jenkins RL, Bistrain BR et al: Nutrition in patients undergoing orthotopic liver transplant, *J Parenter Enter Nutr* 9(6):695, 1985.
43. Hoyumpa AM, Desmond PV, Avant GR et al: Hepatic encephalopathy, *Gastroenterology* 76(1):184, 1979.
44. Hunt DR, Allison MEM, Prentice CRM et al: Endotoxemia, disturbance of coagulation, and obstructive jaundice, *Am J Surg* 144:325, 1982.
45. Jackson FC, Christophersen EB, Peternel WW et al: Preoperative management of patients with liver disease, *Surg Clin North Am* 48(4):907, 1968.
46. Jackson FC, Perrin EB, Smith AG et al: A clinical investigation of the portacaval shunt. II. Survival analysis of the prophylactic operation, *Am J Surg* 115:22, 1968.
47. Javitt NB: Cholestasis in infancy: status report and conceptual approach, *Gastroenterology* 70(6):1172, 1976.
48. Javitt NB: Cholestatic liver disease: mechanisms, diagnosis, and therapy, *Adv Intern Med* 25:147, 1980.
49. Jones EA: The enigma of hepatic encephalopathy, *Postgrad Med J* 59(Suppl 4):42, 1983.
50. Keeffe EB: Sarcoidosis and primary biliary cirrhosis, *Am J Med* 38:977, 1987.
51. Kern WH, Mikkelsen WP, and Turrill FL: The significance of hyaline necrosis in liver biopsies, *Surg Gynecol Obstet* 129(4):749, 1969.
52. Lindenmuth WW, Eisenberg MM: The surgical risk in cirrhosis of the liver, *Arch Surg* 86:235, 1963.
53. Linton RR: The selection of patients for portacaval shunts, *Ann Surg* 134(3):433, 1951.
54. Locasciulli A, Bacigalupo A, Alberti A et al: Predictability before transplant of hepatic complications following allogenic bone marrow transplantation, *Transplantation* 48(1):68, 1989.
55. McCullough AJ, Mullen KD, Smanik EJ

et al: Nutritional therapy and liver disease, *Gastroenterol Clin North Am* 18(3): 619, 1989.

56. McDermott WV: The double portacaval shunt in the treatment of cirrhotic ascites, *Surg Gynecol Obstet* 110:457, 1960.

57. McEvedy BA, Shelly MP, and Park GR: Anaesthesia and liver disease, *Br J Hosp Med* 34:26, 1986.

58. McIntyre N: The limitations of conventional liver function tests, *Semin Liver Dis* 3(4):265, 1983.

59. McPherson GAD, Benjamin IS, Hodgson HJF et al: Pre-operative percutaneous transhepatic biliary drainage: the results of a controlled trial, *Br J Surg* 71:371, 1984.

60. Matloff DS, Kaplan MM: Gastroenterology. In Molitch ME, ed: *Management of medical problems in surgical patients,* Philadelphia, 1982, FA Davis.

61. Milstein JH, Bloomer JR, and Klatskin G: Serum bile acids in alcoholic liver disease, *Digest Dis* 21(4):281, 1976.

62. Moody FG, Rikkers LF, and Aldrete JS: Estimation of the functional reserve of human liver, *Ann Surg* 180(4):592, 1974.

63. Moore RD, Smith CR, and Lietman PS: Increased risk of renal dysfunction due to interaction of liver disease and aminoglycosides, *Am J Med* 80:1093, 1986.

64. Mullen JL, Buzby GP, Waldman MT et al: Prediction of operative morbidity and mortality by preoperative nutritional assessment, *Surg Forum* 30:80, 1979.

65. Munoz SJ, Friedman LS: Liver transplantation, *Med Clin North Am* 73(4): 1011, 1989.

66. Murry JF, Dawson AM, and Sherlock S: Circulatory changes in chronic liver disease, *Am J Med* 24:358, 1958.

67. Nagasue N, Yukaya H, Ogawa Y et al: Hepatic resection in the treatment of hepatocellular carcinoma: report of 60 cases, *Br J Surg* 72:292, 1985.

68. Nakayama T, Ikeda A, and Okuda K: Percutaneous transhepatic drainage of the biliary tract, *Gastroenterology* 74(3): 554, 1978.

69. Neuberger J, Altman DG, Christensen E et al: Use of a prognostic index in evaluation of liver transplantation for primary biliary cirrhosis, *Transplant* 41(6):713, 1986.

70. Okamoto E, Kyo A, Yamanaka N et al: Prediction of the safe limits of hepatectomy by combined volumetric and functional measurements in patients with impaired hepatic function, *Surgery* 95(5): 586, 1984.

71. Okuda K, Tsuchiya Y, Saotome N et al: How to investigate cholestasis: utility of ultrasound as the first imaging study, *Semin Liver Dis* 3(4):308, 1983.

72. Orloff MJ, Halasz NA, Lipman C et al: Complications of cirrhosis of the liver, *Ann Intern Med* 66:165, 1967.

73. Pack GT, Molander DW: Metabolism before and after hepatic lobectomy for cancer. Studies in twenty-three patients, *Arch Surg* 80:685, 1960.

74. Pain JA, Cahill CJ, and Bailey ME: Perioperative complications in obstructive jaundice: therapeutic considerations, *Br J Surg* 72:942, 1985.

75. Paquet KJ, Mercado MA, Koussouris P et al: Improved results with selective distal splenorenal shunt in a highly selected patient population, *Ann Surg* 210(2):184, 1989.

76. Pellegrini CA, Allegra P, Bongard FS et al: Risk of biliary surgery in patients with hyperbilirubinemia, *Am J Surg* 154: 111, 1987.

77. Pitt HA, Cameron JL, Postier RG et al: Factors affecting mortality in biliary tract surgery, *Am J Surg* 141:66, 1981.

78. Pitt HA, Gomes AS, Lois JF et al: Does preoperative percutaneous biliary drainage reduce operative risk or increase hospital cost? *Ann Surg* 201(5):545, 1985.

79. Pomier-Layrargues G, Huet PM, Infante-Rivard C et al: Prognostic value of indocyanine green and lidocaine kinetics for survival and chronic hepatic encephalopathy in cirrhotic patients following elective end-to-side portacaval shunt, *Hepatology* 8(6):1506, 1988.

80. Powell-Jackson P, Greenway B, and Williams R: Adverse effects of exploratory laparotomy in patients with unsuspected liver disease, *Br J Surg* 69:449, 1982.

81. Pugh RNH, Murray-Lyon IM, Dawson JL et al: Transection of the oesophagus for bleeding oesophageal varices, *Br J Surg* 60:646, 1973.

82. Rikkers LF, Moody FG: Estimation of functional hepatic mass in resected and regenerating rat liver, *Gastroenterology* 67(4):691, 1974.

83. Ritter DM, Rettke SR, Hughes RW et al: Placement of nasogastric tubes and esophageal stethoscopes in patients with documented esophageal varices, *Anesth Analg* 67:283, 1988.

84. Rogers EL: Emergency anesthesia in patients with liver disease. In Adams T, ed: *Emergency anesthesia,* London, 1986, Edward Arnold.

85. Rogers EL: Hepatic encephalopathy, *Crit Care Clin* 1(2):313, 1985.

86. Rogers EL, Perman JA: Gastrointestinal and hepatic failure. In Rogers MC, ed: *Textbook of pediatric intensive care,* Baltimore, 1986, Williams & Wilkins.

87. Rogers EL, Rogers MC: Fulminant hepatic failure and hepatic encephalopathy, *Pediatr Clin North Am* 27(3):701, 1980.

88. Runyon BA: Surgical procedures are well tolerated by patients with asymptomatic chronic hepatitis, *J Clin Gastroenterol* 8(5):541, 1986.

89. Sarper R, Tarcan YA: An improved method of estimating the portal venous fraction of total hepatic blood flow from computerized radionuclide angiography, *Radiology* 147:559, 1983.

90. Sax HC, Talamini MA, and Fischer JE: Clinical use of branched-chain amino acids in liver disease, sepsis, trauma, and burns, *Arch Surg* 121:358, 1986.

91. Schafer DF, Shaw BW Jr: Fulminant hepatic failure and orthotopic liver transplantation, *Semin Liver Dis* 9(3): 189, 1989.

92. Shronts EV, Teasley KM, Thoele SL et al: Nutrition support of the adult liver transplant candidate, *J Am Diet Assoc* 87(4):441, 1987.

93. Siefkin AD, Bolt RJ: Preoperative evaluation of the patient with gastrointestinal or liver disease, *Med Clin North Am* 63(6):1309, 1979.

94. Smith LG, Perez G: Viral hepatitis: the alphabet game, *Postgrad Med* 84(5):179, 1988.

95. Stadalnik RC, Matolo NM: Radionuclide imaging of the biliary tree, *Surg Clin North Am* 61(4):827, 1981.

96. Taylor KHW: Liver imaging by ultrasonography, *Semin Liver Dis* 2(1):1, 1982.

97. Thaler MM, Gellis SS: Studies in neonatal hepatitis and biliary atresia. II. The effect of diagnostic laparotomy on longterm prognosis of neonatal hepatitis, *Am J Dis Child* 116:262, 1968.

98. Thompson HH, Tompkins RK, and Longmire WP Jr: Major hepatic resection, *Ann Surg* 197(4):375, 1983.

99. Trachtenberg HA: Anesthesia for the patient with hepatic disease, *Int Anesthesiol Clin* 8:437, 1970.

100. Van Thiel DH, Makowka L, and Starzl TE: Liver transplantation: where it's been and where it's going, *Gastroenterol Clin North Am* 17(1):1, 1988.

101. Vergani D, Mieli-Vergani G, Alberti A et al: Antibodies to the surface of halothane-altered rabbit hepatocytes in patients with severe halothane-associated hepatitis, *New Engl J Med* 303(2):66, 1980.

102. Wall WJ: Liver transplantation: current concepts, *Can Med Assoc J* 139:21, 1988.

103. Wallach JB, Hyman W, and Angrist AA: Cause of death in patients with Laënnec's cirrhosis, *Am J Med Sci* 234:56, 1957.

104. Witzel L, Wolbergs E, and Merki H: Prophylactic endoscopic sclerotherapy of oesphageal varices, *Lancet* 1(8432): 773, 1985.

105. Yanaga K, Kanematsu T, Takenaka K et al: Hepatic resection for hepatocellular carcinoma in elderly patients, *Am J Surg* 155:238, 1988.

106. Yonemoto RH, Davidson CS: Herniorrhaphy in cirrhosis of the liver with ascites, *New Engl J Med* 255:733, 1956.

CHAPTER 20

Evaluation of the Patient with Anemia and Coagulation Disorders

DAVID J. MURRAY

Diseases of the Erythrocyte
    Anemia
    Primary anemias
    Sickle cell anemia
Bleeding Disorders
    Hemophilia
    Acquired coagulation disorders

DISEASES OF THE ERYTHROCYTE

Anemia

The most common hematologic abnormality in perioperative patients is anemia. In most surgical patients, anemia is secondary to an underlying surgical or chronic medical illness. A smaller proportion of anemias represent primary disorders of the erythrocyte and generally can be identified as a problem with the erythrocyte membrane or with the primary intracellular protein, hemoglobin.

Whether the red cell disorder is a primary or a secondary problem, the decrease in oxygen-carrying capacity that occurs as a result of a decreased circulating red cell mass is the primary perioperative concern. Although the quantity of hemoglobin available for oxygen transport is reduced, hemoglobin function is maintained in most anemias. However, in a few primary anemias, hemoglobinopathies and specifically sickle cell disease, the oxygen-carrying function of the hemoglobin molecule is altered by the underlying abnormality.

A simplistic approach to diagnosing both primary and secondary anemias is the assessment of the three major causes for a smaller than normal red cell mass.

- Are there losses of erythrocytes from the vascular space (blood loss)?
- What role does decreased production of erythrocytes play in the anemia?
- Is there cause for an increased destruction of erythrocytes?

Although treatment of anemia with blood in the immediate preoperative period is rapid and effective, determining which patients would significantly benefit from transfusion is more difficult. At present, indications for blood transfusion in anemic perioperative patients is based more on opinion than on fact. Consensus conferences, general public awareness, the lack of clear evidence of improved outcome, and the infectious as well as immunologic risks of transfusion have led to changes in the transfusion practice of many clinicians.

Definition of anemia

A decreased concentration of hemoglobin and hematocrit in a sample of blood is used to define a patient with a deficit in red cell mass. However, a true estimate of red cell mass cannot be made without an assessment of vascular volume. The first question that must be answered when decreased hemoglobin and hematocrit concentrations are measured is whether this decline reflects a decrease in red cell mass. During pregnancy, plasma volume and red cell mass increase, but plasma volume increases more than red cell mass. A decline in hematocrit exists but the red cell mass is not decreased. Conversely, a normal

Table 20-1   Normal hemoglobin and hematocrit changes with age and sex

Patient	Hemoglobin (g)	Hematocrit (%)
Newborn	16	55
1-month-old	12	38
3-month-old	10	30
12-month-old	12	38
Adult male	14	45
Adult female	12	36

hematocrit measurement in a patient with a deficit in vascular volume secondary to dehydration or acute blood loss may falsely indicate the presence of a normal red cell mass. The normal hemoglobin concentration changes throughout life and differs slightly between males and females. Recognition of age-related differences in hematocrit values is particularly well illustrated in the term infant, who at birth has a hematocrit greater than 50%. During the first 2 months of life hematocrit declines to 30%. Despite the rapid change in normal hematocrit values within a 2-month period, a hematocrit of 30 in a newborn indicates a serious hematologic problem. Immediate investigation and treatment are indicated in the newborn, whereas the same hematocrit is a normal finding in the 2-month-old infant (Table 20-1).

Preoperative preparation

The approach to the anemic patient begins with a search for the underlying condition that has precipitated the decline in red cell mass. Frequently, the actual cause of the anemia may represent a combination of causes. In the patient with a colonic cancer, chronic gastrointestinal blood loss may lead to a deficiency of hemoglobin substrates when iron or folate reserves are exhausted from prolonged over-production of erythrocytes. A chronic underlying illness such as chronic renal disease or rheumatoid arthritis may have an anemia associated with a decreased red cell survival as well as the additional problem with decreased bone marrow production of red cells.

A cause for most anemias will be determined from a careful history and physical examination. Additional laboratory tests may help confirm the diagnosis. The red cell size and shape (red cell indices), reticulocyte count, folate level, serum iron or ferritin levels, serum haptoglobin, bilirubin, or serum iron-binding capacity all may help confirm whether the problem is primarily a result of losses (either extravascular or intravascular), decreased production, or increased destruction of red cells. Additional laboratory and radiologic

tests, including an examination of bone marrow, may be required to define the exact cause of the anemia.

The decision to proceed with the anesthetic care of a patient with anemia depends initially on confirmation of the anemia's etiology. An elective hysterectomy in an otherwise healthy 55-year-old woman who has had a long history of menometrorrhagia and currently has a hematocrit of 26% might be contrasted with an unexplained hematocrit of 30% in an otherwise apparently healthy 18-year-old male who requires an elective inguinal hernia repair. The anesthetic management of the 18-year-old male might not be significantly altered by this mild anemia but the anemia's underlying cause may be of greater importance to his general health than an elective operation.

Physiologic compensation for anemia

Three steps can be taken to maintain tissue oxygen delivery if there is a decline in red cell mass:

- Increase blood flow to tissue
- Enhance oxygen extraction
- Displace the oxygen-dissociation curve to the right

The primary initial mechanism is an increased tissue blood flow that occurs without changing cardiovascular work.[29,64,85] The non-Newtonian flow properties of blood provide an explanation for how flow increases without increased myocardial work or greater myocardial oxygen requirements.[38] In situations of decreased flow or decreased vessel cross-sectional area, blood flow rate decreases more than flow rate of a Newtonian fluid such as water.[13,14,29] As the hematocrit is lowered, blood flow increases in the microvascular bed, and the greater blood flow compensates for the lower oxygen-carrying capacity. Guyton et al. demonstrated that with a stable blood volume, change in hematocrit from 45 to 30 results in an increase in venous return but similar cardiovascular work.[29] At hematocrit values considerably less than 25, additional compensatory mechanisms become operative (i.e., right shift of hemoglobin dissociation curve and increased oxygen extraction redistribution of cardiac output) (Box 20-1).

Healthy patients can tolerate relatively low hemoglobin levels without a measurable decline in oxygen delivery to tissues. A decrease in circulating oxygen content of blood occurs with anemia, but a decrease in blood viscosity that favors microvascular blood flow counters the lowered oxygen content.[13,22,66] The relationship between hematocrit and viscosity provides an explanation of how and why tissue oxygenation can be maintained without a measurable increase in cardiovascular work over a wide range of hematocrit values.[13,29] At some point below a hematocrit of 30%, perhaps 25%, tachycardia and increased contractility lead to higher myocardial oxygen demand, and even

---

BOX 20-1
HOW TISSUE OXYGENATION IS MAINTAINED DURING ANEMIA

Decreased blood viscosity
    Lowered peripheral resistance
    Increased venous return
Autoregulation
    Redistribution of tissue blood flow
Increased cardiac output
    Tachycardia
    Increased contractility
Greater tissue oxygen extraction
Shift of hemoglobin dissociation curve
    Increase in 2,3-diphosphoglycerate

---

greater decreases in hematocrit may be tolerated by patients.[66] Although cardiovascular work is increased, healthy patients may tolerate hematocrits of 20%.[13,22,64,66] For this reason, a hematocrit of 21% was selected as a current recommendation for blood administration in the healthy patient.[12] Just as there were no studies to suggest that a hematocrit of 30% was appropriate in the past,[13,14,46] a carefully controlled outcome study is not available to confirm the validity of the current recommendation for hematocrit levels.[8,12,104]

At the opposite extreme, polycythemia increases cardiovascular work as a result of the increased blood viscosity (hematocrit > 50%).[101] Despite the high oxygen content of fully saturated blood, cardiovascular work is greater at higher hematocrits because of increased blood viscosity and sluggish microvascular blood flow. The actual hematocrit limits at either end of the spectrum, where cardiovascular work becomes increased either because of decreased oxygen-carrying capacity (anemia) or increased viscosity (polycythemia), are not clearly defined and probably change depending on the patient's health. During the catabolic stresses of the postoperative period greater oxygen requirements exist; in addition, increased coagulation protein levels may alter viscosity. Little information is available suggesting whether lower or higher hematocrit values are more favorable in management of patients with perioperative catabolic stress. For this reason, the need to correct an abnormality in red cell mass must be based on the clinical setting and should take into consideration the patient's underlying medical condition, the surgical procedure, and the anticipated perioperative recovery period. For example, a 65-year-old man with a hematocrit of 26% following a total hip replacement should be considered differently than the same patient with the same perioperative hematocrit value

recovering from a thoracoabdominal approach to resect an esophagogastric cancer.

Although decreased blood viscosity in anemia patients is the primary mechanism to maintain oxygen delivery without increased cardiovascular work,[22,64] an additional compensation in anemic patients is increased levels of the organic phosphate ester, 2,3-diphosphoglycerate (DPG), which binds to deoxygenated hemoglobin and decreases oxygen affinity.[70,85] This allows for greater unloading of oxygen in the tissue beds. The increased levels of 2,3-DPG in anemic patients shift the hemoglobin dissociation curve to the right and favor unloading of oxygen to the tissues. This additional mechanism enhances oxygen delivery without increasing cardiovascular work. In many patients with chronic anemia, the decreased hemoglobin concentration also leads to circulatory adaptations that increase cardiac output and vascular volume.[102] The correction of anemia with transfusion not only exposes the patient to the long-term risks of blood transfusion such as viral infection and hemosideroses but also to the acute problems of vascular volume overload.[14,61] In most patients with anemia associated with chronic disease, the use of homologous transfusion provides only a transient benefit. The decision to use a transfusion in a chronically anemic patient often becomes a question of whether the transient benefit of transfusion is needed during the perioperative period.[8,12,104]

Perioperative use of blood transfusions

Whether the current perioperative management of an anemic patient should include blood replacement is a controversial question. The relatively liberal use of blood components in the past[46] has been reconsidered by physicians despite the fact that little new information is available regarding an acceptable perioperative hematocrit value.* The improved sense of well-being of patients and better performance of athletes who have received blood transfusions are evidence that potential benefit does occur with transfusion therapy[27,102]; however, no evidence of more rapid recovery, faster wound healing, or lowered infection rates has been demonstrated in healthy patients who have been maintained at higher hematocrit (values greater than 30%) compared to patients maintained with hematocrit values of less than 25% in the postoperative period.[40,61] The major new information that has changed transfusion practice is the recognition of infectious and immunologic risk.[12]

Primary Anemias

The primary anemias result from a structural abnormality of the red cell. Either the erythrocyte mem-

---

* References 8, 13, 14, 38, 53, 104.

brane (hereditary spherocytosis) or the process of producing the hemoglobin molecule (hemoglobinopathies) is abnormal in these anemias. **The primary abnormalities of the red cell lead to variable degrees of decreased production and increased red cell destruction; a chronic anemia is common to all of these conditions.** In most of the primary anemias, transfusion considerations do not differ from those for patients who have anemia secondary to their underlying medical or surgical disease because the qualitative function of the hemoglobin molecule in oxygen delivery is not altered by the abnormality. The primary anemias will only be transiently improved by homologous transfusion. Unfortunately, the most common cause of primary anemia, sickle cell disease, is characterized by anemia and a qualitative hemoglobin function abnormality. For this reason, oxygen delivery can be impaired and special perioperative preparation is required.[21]

Sickle Cell Anemia

The hemoglobinopathies represent a group of disorders characterized by qualitative or quantitative abnormalities of globin synthesis. After birth, the four different globin chains are synthesized under the control of separate single active gene loci on one of the paired chromosomes.[33,34,69,90] Alpha globin, beta globin, gamma globin, and sigma globin chains are synthesized at different rates in the erythrocyte. When two pairs of globin chains combine with heme, the three different types of hemoglobin result. Each of the three types of hemoglobin (Hgb) contains two alpha globin chains. In Hgb A (97%), the second pair of globin chains are beta globin. Whereas in the adult the combination of two alpha chains with two gamma globin chains accounts for only 2% of the hemoglobin, Hgb F (fetal hemoglobin) is the predominant hemoglobin in utero. Two alpha globin and two sigma globin chains (1% of adult hemoglobin) combine to form Hgb A_2. Two distinct types of hemoglobinopathies occur either as a result of inadequate production of normal globin chains (the thalassemia syndromes) or as a result of qualitative abnormalities of globin synthesis, leading to a structural hemoglobinopathy such as hemoglobin S or C (Table 20-2).

In patients with structural hemoglobinopathy, that is, sickle cell disease or sickle cell trait, the synthesis of beta globin is altered by a substitution of valine for glutamine in the sixth amino acid sequence.[5,16,21,36] When both chromosomes direct abnormal hemoglobin S production (homozygous SS disease), a major disease process occurs since Hgb A accounts for 97% of the circulatory hemoglobin, and Hgb F and Hgb A_2 cannot be increased to compensate for the abnormal Hgb S. Because only one chromosome locus is directing globin synthesis in the red cell, the heterozy-

Table 20-2 Hemoglobin values

Normal	Sickle cell disease	Sickle cell trait
97% Hgb A ($\alpha_2\beta_2$)	70%-80% Hgb S ($\alpha_2\beta_2$)	50%-60% Hgb A
2% Hgb F ($\alpha_2\beta_2$)	10%-15% Hgb F ($\alpha_2\beta_2$)	30%-40% Hgb S
1% Hgb A_2 ($\alpha_2\beta_2$)	5% Hgb A_2 ($\alpha_2\beta_2$)	2% Hgb F
		1% Hgb A_2

gous state (one normal gene locus and one sickle cell locus) results in the production of a population of normal Hgb A and abnormal Hgb S. Fortunately, very few or no clinical problems exist in the patient with sickle trait despite an Hgb S level of approximately 40%.[33] The proportion of Hgb S must be great enough to lead to precipitation in the red cell, which alters the red cell milieu. Sickle cell disease occurs when both chromosomes direct the abnormal S globin synthesis instead of the beta globin synthesis. This homozygous state, known as SS disease, affects about 0.4% of African-Americans in the United States.[10,73] The prevalence of the heterozygous state, which has few or no symptoms, is approximately 6% to 8%[21] (Table 20-3).

The pathophysiologic mechanisms of sickle cell disease (SS disease) encompass the entire spectrum of oxygen delivery to the tissues.* When oxygen binds to hemoglobin, a minor configurational change occurs in the hemoglobin molecule, and each succeeding oxygen molecule added to hemoglobin favors the addition of further oxygen molecule until four oxygen molecules are ultimately carried by the fully saturated

---

*References 11, 16, 34, 69, 70, 81, 83.

Table 20-3 Nomenclature and frequency of the commonest hemoglobinopathies in adult African-Americans*

Hemoglobinopathy	Abbreviated name	Frequency
Sickle cell trait	Hb SA	1:122
Sickle cell anemia	Hb SS	1:708
Sickle cell–hemoglobin C disease	Hb SC	1:757
Hemoglobin C disease	Hb CC	1:4790
Hemoglobin C trait	Hb CA	1:41
Hemoglobin S–β-thalassemia	Hb Sβ-thal	1:1672
Hemoglobin S–high F	Hb S–HPFH	1:3412

*Prevalence data derived from references 21, 33, and 74.

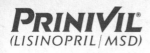

PRINIVIL®
(LISINOPRIL / MSD)

MSD
MERCK
SHARP&
DOHME

Page 344

Table 20-2
20-3

Page 345
Box 20-2
BOX 20-3

L6231-788-3578   PRINTED IN U.S.A.

BOX 20-2
PHYSIOLOGIC PROBLEMS WITH
SICKLE CELL DISEASE

Less pliable, more rigid red blood cell
Greater adhesiveness to endothelium
Shorter half-life
Increased viscosity of blood
More rapid release of oxygen (rightward shift of
 Hgb dissociation curve)

BOX 20-3
STEPS LEADING TO TISSUE INFARCTION
IN SICKLE CELL DISEASE

Deoxygenated hemoglobin SS polymers form in
 red cell
↓
Polymers lead to gel formation in the cell
↓
Interference with erythrocyte membrane function
↓
Red cell volume (sickled cell) lost
↓
Blood viscosity increased because of the viscid
 red cell
↓
Capillary flow decreases
↓
Sickled cells adhere to endothelium
↓
Platelets aggregate
↓
Fibrin is deposited
↓
Tissue infarction occurs

---

oxygenated hemoglobin molecule.[70] This creates the sigmoid shape of the Hgb-O_2 dissociation curve. When oxygen is released from hemoglobin, the process is reversed and each oxygen molecule unloaded alters the structural configuration of hemoglobin. The presence of elevated levels of 2,3-DPG alters the configuration of hemoglobin and favors the unloading of oxygen while further enhancing oxygen release to the tissues.

In sickle cell disease, the configuration change that occurs in the deoxygenated hemoglobin molecule alters the solubility of hemoglobin and leads to the precipitation of hemoglobin in the red cell[69] (Box 20-2). With a quantity of precipitated deoxygenated SS hemoglobin in the erythrocyte, red cell function is altered, and both the intracellular contents and the integrity of the red cell membrane are damaged by the precipitation of sickle hemoglobin.[5,69] The usually pliable, biconcave erythrocyte is transformed by deoxygenation and precipitation of hemoglobin S into a gelated form that is much smaller, less compliant, and viscid.[5,11,19,34,83] This loss of membrane function and intracellular contents leads to the sickled cell that is pathognomonic of the disease.[68,69,86]

The major problem once sickling of red cells occurs relates to the effect of this viscid red cell, which occludes vascular beds and triggers thrombosis and infarction[11,31,34,78] (Box 20-3). The sickled cell is either rapidly removed from the circulation or adheres to the vascular endothelium with other sickled cells. When sickled cells adhere to the vascular endothelium, platelet aggregation and ultimately fibrin formation occurs, leading to thrombus formation and ischemia of the tissue beds. The increased viscosity of blood, particularly in the capillary beds, and the constellation of events that promotes thrombus formation lead to a vasoocclusive crisis.[3,11,30,34,68] This sequence of events is not reversed by oxygenation. Treatment must be aimed primarily at preventing the sickling process.[11,93]

Situations associated with increased oxygen demand (such as fever, exercise, or infection) or decreased or sluggish tissue blood flow (dehydration and cold) can lead to deoxygenation of hemoglobin to the point of sickle cell formation. Tissue beds that have a tenuous oxygen supply as a result of high metabolic demand or limited collateral or stagnant blood flow are at particular risk for vasoocclusion and infarction. The pooling of blood in the spleen produces splenic infarction at an early age in patients with sickle cell disease, and an increased susceptibility to fulminant infection develops, which is a leading cause of death in patients with sickle cell disease.[59,73,74,76,88] Vasoocclusive crisis, particularly in the hip joint, can lead to aseptic necrosis of the femoral head,[43] retinal and vitreous hemorrhage, renal medullary infarctions, and renal papillary necrosis, all of which are prevalent in patients with sickle cell disease.[63] Pulmonary and central nervous system infarctions are common and are probably related to emboli of sickled cells and platelet aggregates that have formed in other tissue beds rather than to a primary process initiated in the lung or brain.*

As a result of the recurrent precipitation of hemoglobin in the red cell, the erythrocytes of the patient with sickle cell disease have a shorter life span (10 to 20 days), and an anemia is present with compensatory changes in increased red cell produc-

---

*References 6, 35, 82, 92, 93, 94, 100.

BOX 20-4
METHODS TO PREVENT VASOOCCLUSIVE CRISIS OF SICKLE CELL DISEASE

Avoid factors leading to lower venous oxygen
  saturation
  Increased oxygen consumption (temperature
    elevation, shivering)
  Decreased tissue blood flow (hypothermia,
    hypovolemia)
  Stagnant circulation (tourniquets)
Lower blood viscosity
  Hyponatremia
  Appropriate vascular volume
Decrease sequelae of increased "adhesiveness"
  of cells
  Antiplatelet drugs
Increase production of other hemoglobin (Hgb F
  and A$_2$)
  Hydroxyurea
Add or substitute normal hemoglobin from
  donor erythrocytes
  Simple transfusion
  Exchange transfusion

---

tion (elevated reticulocyte count). Any disease process (e.g., some viral infections) that impairs the marrow production of red cells, which have a life span of 12 days instead of 120 days, may lead to a second major problem in sickle cell disease, the aplastic crisis. In this process there is marked anemia as a result of the continued destruction of red cells without bone marrow replacement.[55] A third cause of morbidity and mortality in sickle cell disease, sequestration crisis, occurs when blood is pooled in the spleen, particularly in infants with SS disease or in older children with SC disease (splenic infarction is less common in SC disease), resulting in a rapid fall in vascular volume.[33,76,78] The numerous problems associated with sickle cell disease begin in infancy shortly after the decline in Hgb F that occurs after birth[73] (Box 20-4).

Preoperative evaluation

The frequency of sickle cell trait is approximately 6% to 8% in the African-American population. An additional gene pool of sickle cell trait occurs in the individuals from the Mediterranean area as well as from India. The incidence of the homozygous disease state (sickle cell disease) may approximate 2 to 3/1000 African-Americans. A number of important questions must be addressed in the preoperative period for all patients who may have a hemoglobinopathy.

- Does the patient belong to a high-risk group for

carrying sickle cell disease or sickle cell variants (SC or S-thalassemia)?
- Is a rapid screening test for sickle cell disease or sickle cell variants indicated? Will a positive or negative result of the Sickledex screen alter the anesthetic plan or the postoperative plan?
- Does the patient have sickle cell trait (SA)?
- Does the patient have the more serious sickle cell disease or one of the variants?
- If so, what are the results of hemoglobin electrophoresis?
- Is the problem the more common SS disease or is it a variant, SC or S-thalassemia?
- What is the extent of organ dysfunction from the recurrent sickling episodes? Is there evidence of pulmonary disease? Cardiac disease? CNS disease? Renal dysfunction?
- Is the surgery planned urgent or elective?
- If urgent, is the reason for surgery related to an acute complication of sickle cell disease? Priapism? Acute abdominal pain secondary to vasoocclusive crisis? If so, what emergency therapy has been initiated for the problem?
- If the surgery is elective, what preparation has been done?
- Is the preparation for surgery adequate for the intended operative procedure?
- If so, when was the preparation started, what was accomplished? If exchange or simple transfusion is needed, what level of Hgb S is now present?
- What plans have been made for the postoperative care of the patient?

In assessing a patient in a high-risk group for sickle cell disease, the patient history usually indicates whether sickle cell disease or sickle cell trait is present. If the diagnosis is in doubt, physical examination may indicate the presence of sickle cell disease with evidence of end organ involvement of the lung, central nervous system, or renal and cardiovascular systems* or the presence of the more common sickle cell trait, which has no major clinical manifestations. Anemia and mild jaundice are almost always present in sickle cell disease and absent in sickle cell trait.[21,34,73,74] Evidence of secondary sites of erythropoiesis, such as an enlarged maxilla as well as hepatomegaly, likely indicates sickle cell disease rather than sickle cell trait. Cor pulmonale and emphysema may be the sequelae of repeated pulmonary infarctions in patients with sickle cell disease.[6,91] Finally, the peripheral blood smear will be distinctly abnormal in sickle cell disease with sickled red cells, intracellular inclusions, and abnormal red cell indices; these are all absent in sickle cell trait.[21,33,93] Infrequently, the separation of sickle cell trait from the

---

* References 6, 7, 10, 52, 91, 99, 100, 101.

Table 20-4 Hematologic changes in sickle cell disease, sickle cell trait, and sickle cell variants (SC or S-thalassemia)

	Sickle cell disease	Sickle cell trait	Sickle cell variant
Anemia	Normal Hgb level	Mild anemia
Sickle cell on peripheral smear	No sickled erythrocyte in peripheral smear	
Target cells present	Absent	Present
Nucleated red cells	Absent	Present
Elevated reticulocyte count	Normal	Present
Hypochromic, microcytic indices	Normal red cell indices	Hypochromic, microcytic indices

variants of sickle cell disease such as SC or S-thalassemia is difficult on the basis of symptoms and signs.[21] Although patients with these sickle cell variants usually have clinical symptoms and signs, often clinical abnormalities can be mild and anemia may also be absent.[81] For this reason, hemoglobin electrophoresis may be required to separate these uncommon variants of sickle cell disease from sickle cell disease or sickle cell trait[21,33] (Table 20-4).

Screening for sickle cell disease

Rapid screening tests for sickle cell disease are frequently recommended in high-risk populations that require either elective or emergency surgery.[21,67] These tests use various oxidant solutions to establish a sickling tendency in the erythrocytes. A positive Sickledex test provides information that a population of sickle hemoglobin is present but does not differentiate among the heterozygous state (SA) with minimal symptoms or the homozygous state (SS), or a sickle variant (SC, S-thalassemia).[21,67] Without a patient history and physical examination, this sensitive but nonspecific screening test provides little relevant information. The test will also not be helpful in screening during infancy because relatively low Hgb S concentrations are present in early life because of the preponderance of Hgb F[21] (Box 20-5).

In an emergency situation, a history, physical examination, and additional laboratory information may help define the likeliest possibility when the sickle cell screening test is positive.[21] In a healthy adult patient with no prior history or clinical findings

BOX 20-5
FEATURES OF POSITIVE SICKLEDEX TEST

Sensitive but nonspecific test for the presence of hemoglobin S
Positive test occurs in sickle cell disease, sickle cell trait, and sickle cell variants (SC or S-thalassemia)

suggestive of sickle cell disease and a normal hematologic profile on laboratory evaluation, a positive Sickledex result would most likely represent a heterozygous state (Hgb AS disease) although rarely a patient with SC disease and S-thalassemia may also have relatively normal Hgb levels.[21,33] Although the presence of SA disease should not alter the anesthetic plan, it may be worthwhile to avoid the use of tourniquets for orthopedic procedures.

A positive Sickledex result associated with a history of sickle cell symptoms most likely represents a homozygous state or a variant that may require special preoperative preparation. Hemoglobin electrophoresis will be necessary to define any abnormality not already identified.[21] Without a patient history, sickle cell disease can be difficult to differentiate from other sickle cell variants such as SC or S-thalassemia. Vasoocclusive problems associated with the two most common variants of sickle cell disease are in many circumstances less severe than with Hgb SS, partially because of the less severe precipitation of deoxygenated hemoglobin that occurs in these variants and therefore the less severe anemia.[81]

The clinical presentation of the patient with sickle cell disease is frequently altered by the different proportions of hemoglobin S, F, and A_2 that can occur in sickle cell disease.[81] Hemoglobin electrophoresis is valuable in determining the proportion of Hgb F and Hgb A_2 and whether the disease process is the more common SS disease or the less common variants, SC disease or S-thalassemia.[21,33] Hemoglobin C results from a different amino acid substitution on the beta globin chain and also predominately occurs in blacks.[21] An anemia occurs in the homozygous state (hemoglobin C); when combined with Hgb S, SC disease results in a mildly anemic patient who is at risk for sickling episodes.[21,33] Patients with SC disease usually have less severe manifestations than patients with sickle cell disease (SS). A similar situation can occur when β-thalassemia is combined with sickle cell disease. These two variants differ particularly in the degree of anemia as well as in the compensatory changes in the level of Hgb F and A_2 present in the red cell. The left-shifted dissociation curve of Hgb F favors a greater proportion of oxygenated hemoglobin in tissues and therefore a lesser tendency for precipitation and sickling of the Hgb S population. The higher proportion of Hgb F in S-thalassemia results in a disease process with fewer symptoms than SS disease. The presence of Hgb C also tends to decrease the frequency of hemoglobin precipitation and has less severe manifestations than Hgb SS.[21,33,81]

Preoperative preparation

The primary focus of therapy for patients with sickle cell disease who require surgery has been simple transfusion or exchange transfusion to lower the proportion of Hgb S to less than 40%. Because of the shortened red cell life span of the sickle cell compared to the transfused erythrocyte, the therapeutic benefit persists for a number of weeks after transfusion.[24,33,35,64,66] The sickle cell patient with chronic anemia, increased vascular volume, and elevated cardiac output is at greater risk for vascular overload with the use of transfusion and an acute increase in blood viscosity from rapid transfusion of packed red cells. The use of repeated small-volume transfusions or exchange transfusion is the usual approach indicated in anticipation of surgery or for the long-term therapy of patients who have pulmonary or neurologic complications or in the management of pregnancy in patients with sickle cell disease.* This preoperative therapy decreases the frequency of vasoocclusive crisis in these patients but does not alter the higher incidence of infectious complications that occurs in the perioperative period.[32,59,88] The transfusion of one packed red cell unit in an anemic patient with sickle cell disease (hemoglobin 6 to 7 g) who weighs 70 kg should increase Hgb A concentrations by 10% to 15% or more, depending on the severity of the underlying anemia. When red cell transfusion is repeated two or three times on an outpatient basis, the population of sickle hemoglobin decreases to less than 40%. The decision to use simple transfusion or exchange transfusion is based on the preoperative hemoglobin concentration. A patient with sickle cell disease who has a hemoglobin level less than 8 g can probably be managed with simple transfusion, whereas a patient with sickle cell disease with a higher initial hematocrit may require exchange transfusion to avoid polycythemia.

Patients with the disease also present for elective or emergency surgery for problems related to the underlying pathologic changes created by recurrent tissue infarction secondary to vasoocclusion.† This patient population may require elective or urgent surgery more frequently than the general population as a result of the higher turnover of red cells that may lead to bilirubin stones and the need for cholecystectomy.[41,47,79] Genitourinary surgery and orthopedic surgical procedures may be required with greater frequency because of ischemic damage secondary to vasoocclusive episodes that occur in sickle cell disease and that lead to renal papillary infarctions and necrosis of the femoral head.[43,63] Splenectomy is often required in patients who have the disease.[76] The management of the patient with sickle cell disease who requires emergency surgery is based on decreasing the Hgb S percentage by using transfusion.[21,39,47] Exchange transfusion may be indicated since the rapid infusion of two to three units of red cells might otherwise lead to poorly tolerated further increases in blood viscosity and vascular volume overload in the patient with the disease.[10,11,65]

Other factors that are important in maintaining tissue oxygenation require careful attention in this patient population. Adequate hydration in the preoperative, intraoperative, and postoperative periods is extremely important, as well as the avoidance of hypothermia and acidosis.

Many other methods of preventing vasoocclusive crisis in sickle cell disease other than transfusion are being investigated and may offer an alternative to transfusion in the future.* Induced hyponatremia helps prevent the red cell membrane change that leads to sickling of cells. Pharmacologic approaches to increase the production of other globin chains, such as enhancing Hgb F production in sickle cell disease,[18,50,60,71] offer a promising alternative to transfusion therapy, as do selective genetic approaches and bone marrow transplantation for treating the genetic disorder to eliminate the gene loci responsible for Hgb S production.[87]

The postoperative period may be more problematic than the intraoperative period and careful attention to postoperative pulmonary function, hydration, temperature, and pain relief is particularly important in this patient population.

Sickle cell trait, sickle cell disease, and cardiopulmonary bypass

Sickle cell trait has minimal clinical symptoms, and although sickling has been described in this disease, it occurs only with profound desaturation of hemoglobin as may occur during prolonged exertion, dehydration, or situations of profound decreases in tissue blood flow and severe hypoxia. The Po_2 at which irreversible sickling occurs is 20 to 25 mm, compared to 40 to 45 mm in sickle cell disease. Although exchange or simple transfusion is not necessary for even major surgery, the presence of sickle cell trait in

---

*References 10, 21, 24, 35, 65, 76, 81, 82, 100.

† References 6, 7, 30, 43, 51.

---

*References 9, 16, 18, 48, 50, 60, 71, 86, 103.

a patient who requires cardiopulmonary bypass merits special consideration. In anticipation of cardiopulmonary bypass, the actual proportion of Hgb S should be known to ensure that sickle cell trait is indeed the diagnosis. Whereas exchange or simple transfusion has been recommended by some, cardiopulmonary bypass should not result in sickling of erythrocytes, because the severe decrement in Po_2 to 20 to 25 mm that would result in sickling in a patient with sickle cell trait generally does not occur during cardiopulmonary bypass. Hypothermia, when not associated with vasoconstriction and decreased blood flow, actually increases the solubility of Hgb S and prevents the precipitation of Hgb S in the red cell.[19] The induction of hypothermia using a cardiopulmonary bypass circuit should not be associated with decreases in tissue perfusion. When combined with a lower metabolic rate and associated decreased blood viscosity by hemodilution, hypothermia markedly decreases the likelihood of sickling leading to vasoocclusion. Deep hypothermic circulatory arrest may merit special considerations since the severity of the physiologic trespass is profound, and preoperative transfusion is advocated by some who care for patients with sickle cell trait who require deep hypothermic circulatory arrest.

A patient with sickle cell disease (SS) who requires cardiopulmonary bypass will need exchange or simple transfusion to reduce sickle cell Hgb levels to less than 40% in the preoperative period.[17] Although many advocate even lower levels of Hgb S in the perioperative period, the level of Hgb S will further decrease during the initiation of cardiopulmonary bypass as a result of the dilution and decrease in blood viscosity that occurs during bypass. In view of the other beneficial therapeutic interventions (anticoagulation) that occur during cardiopulmonary bypass, decreasing Hgb S levels further in this setting seems unwarranted.

It is not clear whether the perioperative period in the current era of increased monitoring represents a period of increased risk to patients with sickle cell disease.[21,32] With heightened awareness of the increased risk of transfusion therapy and with increased understanding of the causes of sickle cell vasoocclusive crisis, transfusion may not be indicated for all patients in the perioperative period.[21] Certainly use of a properly managed general or regional anesthetic for a minor orthopedic procedure, myringotomy, dental restoration, and inguinal herniorrhaphy may not be associated with a situation that leads to sickling of erythrocytes. Indeed, in most aspects, patients with sickle cell disease should be less likely to experience problems during general or regional anesthetic than in their normal activities of daily life. A decrease in tissue oxygen consumption, increased inspired oxygen concentration, and (in many tissue beds) an increase in blood flow should decrease the likelihood of sickling of erythrocytes during general or regional anesthesia. Use of halothane appears to enhance the solubility of hemoglobin S and theoretically could actually further decrease the incidence of sickle cell formation. Although in many tissue beds a decrease in metabolic rate and an increase in tissue blood flow should decrease sickling, splanchnic and renal blood flow decrease during anesthesia and surgery, particularly during an intraabdominal procedure. Perhaps this setting should be considered differently than minor operative procedures. Successful management of patients with sickle cell disease who require major operations such as cholecystectomy has been reported in some series without a resultant sickle cell crisis, but whether this can be recommended at present awaits a larger controlled clinical trial.[21] The major problem in conducting anesthesia in the patient with levels of hemoglobin S greater than 70% is a vasoocclusive crisis. Prevention of sickling is the only completely effective method to decrease this complication. Preoperative simple or exchange transfusion is recommended. The major cause of mortality in the perioperative period in patients with sickle cell disease is an increased incidence of fulminant infection. The functional asplenia that occurs as a result of splenic infarction in patients with sickle cell disease contributes to this serious problem.

The intraoperative management of a patient with sickle cell disease should be based on a clear understanding of the condition of the patient, pathophysiology of the disease, and operative requirements. No specific anesthetic technique has been indicated to be superior to another in the management of patients for surgery.

BLEEDING DISORDERS

The hemostatic function of blood is a complex interrelated process involving platelets, the fluid phases of blood via coagulation proteins, the vascular endothelium, and the interstitial fluid. Clot formation and clot dissociation are delicately balanced to maintain blood in a fluid phase until a physiologic trespass such as trauma or surgery occurs. The congenital and acquired disorders of coagulation illustrate the importance of the clot formation aspect of this balance, particularly as it relates to hemorrhagic problems during surgery. The less understood problems of deficiency in clot dissociation leading to thrombosis are less studied than clot formation but may be of equal importance since the perioperative period is often associated with an increased thrombotic tendency.[3]

In even the most minor operative procedures, vascular integrity is disrupted and hemostatic function tested. A simplistic explanation of the events surrounding the cessation of bleeding following an opening of the vessel wall involves two events. The platelet events—aggregation, adhesion, and release of platelet contents—followed by the second event—deposition of a fibrin meshwork—result in formation of a hemostatic plug. If the initial events of platelet aggregation, adhesion, or release of vasoactive and chemostatic substances are inadequate secondary to either a quantitative or qualitative platelet defect, hemostasis will not occur. If a problem with coagulation proteins related to either quantity or quality is present in the circulation or if an imbalance exists between clot formation and clot dissolution, a fibrin meshwork will not be incorporated into the plug, and the platelet plug that is formed initially will dissolve and hemostasis will not occur.

In the operating room, increased surgical bleeding is the main manifestation of congenital and acquired types of coagulation defects. The often complicated diagnostic tests and separate therapies required to treat congenital and acquired coagulopathies must be carefully considered preoperatively since diagnosis and treatment during a major surgical procedure associated with pathologic blood loss is difficult and often lethal for the patient.

Fortunately, the patient history and physical examination rarely, if ever, mislead the clinician in assessing whether a surgical patient has significant bleeding risk based on an underlying coagulopathy. In addition, sensitive and specific tests of coagulation further enhance diagnosis and provide a guide to the adequacy and appropriateness of replacement therapy.

The search for problems with hemostasis begins with appropriate patient history questions:

- Is there a family history of coagulopathy? Is there a history of excessive blood loss following other surgeries, dental procedures, during menstruation, or childbirth? Has there been excessive bleeding in response to angiographic procedures or to venipuncture?
- Are there any problems indicating a possible hemostatic problem, such as epistaxis, hematuria, or melena?
- Are there contributing underlying illnesses that could cause bleeding problems? Uremia, malignancy, liver disease, collagen diseases?
- What medications is the patient taking? Could these contribute to a bleeding diathesis?

A physical examination contributes to the diagnosis because the presence of petechiae, purpura, or hematoma without a history of trauma may suggest a hemostatic problem.

Hemophilia

The congenital disorders of coagulation are frequently encountered in anesthesia practice.[62] In patients with congenital coagulation abnormalities, particularly hemophilia A (factor VIII deficiency) and hemophilia B (Christmas disease or factor IX deficiency), acute bleeding problems that require surgical intervention may develop. The deep and often severe tissue bleeding characteristic of these disorders may require emergency fasciotomy of extremities or craniotomy for a rapidly expanding hematoma.[1,23,54] In addition, the recurrent hemarthrosis associated with this coagulopathy may require corrective or palliative orthopedic procedures secondary to the destructive changes in joints caused by the bleeding.[58] The acquired disorders of factor VIII and von Willebrand's disease in females frequently lead to menorrhagia and metrorrhagia and eventually require elective hysterectomy.

Coagulation factor deficiencies

The underlying abnormality of classic hemophilia (factor VIII) is inherited as an X-linked recessive trait and, therefore, males are affected almost exclusively.[28,49,62] The incidence is 1/10,000.[42] The degree of the deficiency of factor VIII coagulation activity is directly related to the severity of bleeding complications (Box 20-6). Because the severe deficiency of factor VIII (coagulation factor activity of less than 3%) leads to spontaneous hemorrhage, these patients may require continuous replacement of coagulation factor activity. Less severe manifestations of the disease occur when coagulation factor activity is greater than 5%, and few manifestations are present when 20% of normal coagulant activity is present. In patients with 30% of normal factor VIII activity, minimal problems occur and even major surgery can be accomplished.

An approach to the patient with hemophilia who requires an operation can be based on the answers to a number of important questions:

- What type of congenital coagulation disorder is present?
- How severe is the coagulation disorder?
- What preparations have been used to manage bleeding problems in this patient in the past?
- Do inhibitors of coagulation factor activity complicate the congenital deficiency?
- What is the nature of the surgical procedure?
- Will blood replacement be required in this patient? If so, for how long? What level should be maintained during the surgical procedure? In the postoperative period?
- What method should be used to monitor the adequacy of replacement?

BOX 20-6
APPROACH TO THE PATIENT
WITH HEMATOLOGIC DISEASE

Current level of coagulation factor
Volume of distribution of factor
Half-life of coagulation factor
Factor level required for anticipated surgery
Concentration of factor in blood component or
 derivative

- How frequently should such monitoring occur to ensure adequate replacement?
- What preparation of coagulation factor would be best for this patient?

The clinical manifestations and diagnosis of hemophilia are rarely in doubt after a history and physical examination are performed. The manifestations of severe hemophilia are present early in life and represent a life-long problem. As with many chronic diseases, the patient has a clear understanding of the requirements and the need for therapy. With the availability of newer factor replacement preparations, many manage their own disease at home.[42]

A prolonged partial thromboplastin time (PTT) is a classic laboratory finding in patients with hemophilia.[25] The PTT, which measures the time for clot formation when plasma is added to a thromboplastin activator such as kaolin, is used to assess the in vitro activity of the intrinsic coagulation factors (VIII, IX, XI, and XIII) and will be abnormal in the various types of hemophilia.[62] Hemophilia A (factor VIII deficiency) is the most common disorder, accounting for 85% of patients with hemophilia. Only 14% of hemophilias are Christmas disease (factor IX), and factor XI deficiency is very uncommon. The abnormality in the PTT test will depend not only on the level of factor VIII present but also on the sensitivity of the test to coagulation factor levels. With improvements in PTT sensitivity, the PTT becomes elevated when factor VIII or factor IX levels are less than 60% of normal. The sensitivity of in vitro coagulation tests makes detection of even minor factor VIII deficiency possible. An elevation of the PTT is not specific for which coagulation factor is decreased in the intrinsic system (VIII, IX, XI); therefore a factor assay is required to determine which intrinsic coagulation factor level is decreased.

Preoperative preparation

The management of a patient who requires surgery in the presence of a coagulation factor deficiency also requires an understanding of (1) the kinetics of the coagulation factor in plasma, (2) the preparations of coagulation components available to treat the disease, (3) the requirements of the surgical procedure, and (4) the interpretation of the tests used to monitor the coagulation factor level.

The approach to replacement of coagulation factor deficits can best be understood by applying pharmacokinetic principles for the missing coagulation protein, much as for pharmacologic agents. To determine the coagulation factor requirements for the perioperative period, an assessment of the current coagulation factor level present, the coagulation level desired for surgery, the volume of distribution of the coagulation factor, and half-life of the coagulation factor are relevant in estimating the initial dose factor replacement and when additional doses will be required to maintain coagulation activity perioperatively.[42]

The standardization of coagulation factor activity based on international units has further aided understanding and initiating therapy for these disorders. For almost all coagulation protein (except fibrinogen), a normal level of coagulation activity is defined as 1 international unit (IU)/ml of plasma.[42] Coagulation factor activity is usually defined in terms of percent of normal activity. Coagulation factor replacement therapy is also conveniently defined in units of coagulant activity. Initial therapeutic intervention can be based on the desired activity level required/milliliter of plasma and the volume of distribution of the coagulation factor.

The most severe forms of hemophilia have relatively low coagulation factor protein levels. For this reason, a plan for replacement might reasonably ignore the current level of circulating factor VIII or IX present in patients with severe deficiency. In the past, requirements for replacement of coagulation factor during a surgical procedure were based on patients with coagulation factor deficits who required major surgery but did not receive factor replacement. A level of 30% factor VIII activity was adequate to prevent serious bleeding during surgery. This coagulation factor activity of 30% factor VIII does not correct abnormalities of the PTT. Many published replacement regimens have focused on the maintenance of at least a 50% and often a 100% coagulation factor level for surgery although current evidence seems to indicate that clinical bleeding does not become apparent until levels fall below 30%. Although the coagulation activity of factor VIII is primarily limited to the plasma, the volume of distribution of factor VIII can extend to the extracellular fluid space. As a rough guide, replacement therapy for the initial dose of factor VIII required can be assumed to distribute in a space slightly larger than the blood volume. A convenient estimate of volume of distribution is 100 ml/kg.

Using the aforementioned information, the requirements for factor VIII replacement can be estimated. Various formulas to guide replacement therapy in essence are based on the preceding pharmacokinetic data. If an assumption of volume of distribution of 100 mg/kg is made for factor VIII and the basis of replacement is to achieve 50% of normal factor VIII activity (0.5 U/ml), then a factor VIII dose of 50 U/kg should be given initially. In a patient weighing 70 kg, this estimate of 50% replacement therapy, if minimal intrinsic coagulation factor activity is present, requires approximately 3500 units of factor VIII activity.

With information regarding the half-life of coagulation factor activity, the need for repeated dosages can also be assessed or perhaps, more appropriately, the requirements for a continuous infusion to maintain coagulation factor levels can be estimated. For factor VIII levels with a half-life of 12 hours, a clearance of factor VIII in a patient weighing 70 kg is approximately 150 U/hr; therefore maintenance of a 50% factor level in such a patient after the initial bolus dose of 3500 units requires a continuous infusion of approximately 150 U/hr or, alternatively, a repeated bolus of 1700 units every 12 hours. This approach to therapy must be monitored with either repeated factor VIII assays or PTT to ensure stable factor VIII levels are present during the perioperative period.

A similar therapeutic plan for all the coagulation factor levels can be made by applying specific pharmacokinetic data for the other coagulation factors. The volume of distribution of the coagulation factors may be slightly lower or the half-life either shorter or longer than factor VIII, and for this reason dosage requirements may need to be adjusted based on these kinetic considerations. There are numerous formulas based on either kilograms of body weight or body surface area to guide therapy of the disease. In all situations the formulas provide a rough guide to replacement that must be adjusted based on patient response and hemostatic monitoring.

Several preparations of factor VIII have been developed since Pool recognized that plasma frozen and then thawed at 4° to 8° C led to a small residual precipitated substance that was rich in factor VIII activity.[72] Cryoprecipitate and other factor VIII preparations were rapidly developed to improve the management of hemophilia. Newer preparations have the advantage of providing the factor VIII levels in smaller total volumes of plasma and are extracted by special processes to limit the transmission of infectious diseases. These preparations are currently the most desirable way to manage patients with the two most common coagulation abnormalities (factors VIII and IX). The current preparations are derived from pooled donors, and, even with treatment processes and newer extraction techniques, a minor risk for transmission of viral diseases still exists. With newer methods of purification and the real possibility of a plasma-free factor VIII manufactured by recombinant DNA techniques, the future therapy for patients with hemophilia A and B may have very few risks in the transmission of infectious disease.

In many patients with the severest deficiencies of factor VIII or IX, the continuous replacement of the missing coagulation factor may be associated with the development of an antibody response to the missing antigen.[97,98] This antibody inhibits exogenous factor VIII or IX activity and complicates replacement. In this setting, large quantities of factor VIII antigen, or alternatively factor VIII, derived from porcine sources may be required. Occasionally an attempt to either bypass the factor VIII activity by providing activated factor IX substances such as Proplex,[54] or concomitant use of drugs that depress the antibody response to antigens such as steroids or antichemotherapeutic agents is required.[37] Occasionally plasmapheresis may be used to decrease the inhibitor antibody level. A small group of patients with autoimmune disorders, particularly systemic lupus erythematosus, may develop antifactor VIII antibodies similar to those observed in patients with hemophilia in whom factor VIII inhibitors develop. For the most part, patients with autoimmune disorders and factor VIII inhibitors have relatively minor symptoms and many tolerate major surgery without factor replacement. The diagnosis of an inhibitor of coagulation can be rapidly accomplished in vitro by a 1:1 mix of fresh plasma with the patient's plasma. A failure to normalize the PTT with the plasma suggests an inhibitor rather than a decreased circulating factor level.[77]

von Willebrand's disease

The interrelationship between the activity of plasma coagulation factors and platelets in hemostasis as well as the complexity of the factor VIII complex has partially been explained by the investigation of patients with von Willebrand's disease.[75,105] The structure-activity relationship of factor VIII can be divided into two protein systems—a smaller active coagulation protein with synthesis directed by a gene loci on the X chromosome and a larger molecular weight–carrier protein referred to as von Willebrand factor.[4] The carrier protein von Willebrand factor prevents the rapid activation and removal of the coagulant protein, factor VIII, from the circulation and also facilitates the activation of platelet activity in response to tissue injury. The role of von Willebrand factor in platelet aggregation can be measured using a platelet test of aggregation to the antibiotic ristocetin (ristocetin aggregation). The absence of von Willebrand factor will lead to platelet aggregation when ristocetin is added. The abnormality in hemostasis created by the absence of von Willebrand factor then is twofold; however, symptoms and signs are less severe than in hemophilia, probably because of von Willebrand's inheritance as an autosomal dominance disorder with only one of two gene loci involved in the abnormality. Replacement of von Willebrand factor with cryoprecipitate containing a large amount of von Willebrand factor results in a relatively prolonged elevation of factor VIII activity, manifest as a decrease in PTT, but only a short-term normalization of platelet function as measured by the bleeding time.

A significant storage pool of factor VIII activity and von Willebrand factor can be released presumably from the sinusoidal endothelial liver stores.[45,57,93] Desmopressin, an analog of vasopressin, when given to patients with mild disorders of hemophilia or von Willebrand's disease, can produce a prompt threefold to fourfold rise in factor VIII or von Willebrand factor activity in an intravenous dose of 0.3 mg/kg.[45,56,57,92] Repeated doses have less profound effect, presumably because storage of factor VIII activity in the endothelium is limited.

Desmopressin has also been given to blood donors to improve the yield of factor VIII activity and has been used to decrease bleeding in patients following complicated as well as uncomplicated cardiopulmonary bypass. The ability of desmopressin to reduce bleeding times in normal patients may be useful in patients who are having major surgery (Harrington rod insertion or cardiopulmonary bypass).[80] This observation of decreased blood loss in patients with previously hemostatic normal status needs more extensive study because an imbalance between clot formation and clot dissolution may result. In addition, decreases in renal blood flow and urine output may be troublesome side effects of the drug.

Acquired Coagulation Disorders
Drug therapy
The use of coumadin in patients with atrial fibrillation, prosthetic heart valves, or thromboembolic disease can prevent the serious thromboembolic consequences of these medical problems.[75,77] Administration of coumadin prevents vitamin K participation as a cofactor in the final stages of synthesis of coagulation factors II, VII, IX, and X. The role of vitamin K in the final structural modification of coagulation factors II (prothrombin), VII, IX, and X probably involves carboxylation of terminal glutamic acid residues. The inhibition of vitamin K by coumadin or the decreased absorption of vitamin K in patients with obstruction of

the common bile duct, severe liver disease, or malabsorption syndromes may lead to a deficiency of vitamin K–dependent coagulation factors. The coagulation factors are still synthesized; however, when decreased vitamin K activity is present, these coagulation factors are not converted rapidly to the activated form in the presence of Ca^{++} and phospholipid. Coumadin pharmacokinetics and pharmacodynamics are also altered by a multitude of pharmacologic agents that either alter metabolism of the drug or, by a secondary effect on the coagulation system (e.g., aspirin on platelets), lead to an undesirable increase in bleeding tendency. When patients are given coumadin for an underlying medical disorder, the desired goal of anticoagulation is a relatively profound degree of decrease in factor activity.

The half-life of coumadin compounds is 24 to 48 hours. Therefore for the patient taking coumadin who requires surgery, preoperative discontinuation of the drug is advised at least 48 hours before surgery. Heparin therapy should be instituted to ensure that anticoagulation is maintained in the immediate preoperative period. Elective operation for the patient taking coumadin is best managed by substituting the shorter half-life anticoagulant heparin for the longer half-life coumadin preoperatively over a period of 2 to 3 days. Postoperatively anticoagulation with heparin is resumed and coumadin is reintroduced. In this manner, anticoagulation is stopped for the shortest period possible during the perioperative period.

Emergency surgery for patients receiving coumadin is occasionally required as a result of a severe bleeding complication or other medical problems. Reversal of anticoagulant therapy must be accomplished rapidly with administration of parenteral vitamin K, which will be effective in 3 to 6 hours. Use of fresh frozen plasma is also recommended, particularly in view of the complications associated with preparations of vitamin K complex factors (Proplex or Konyne).[54,84]

Platelet disorders
Congenital problems with platelet function are rare, but numerous drugs and diseases acquired may alter platelet function or lead to an autoimmune destruction of platelets.[15,20,52,95,96] Clinical management of drug- or disease-related platelet function disorders is best approached by discontinuing the drug if possible (β-lactam antibiotics, nonsteroidal antiinflammatory, quinidine) because most drug effects on platelet function are short lived.[20] However, acetylsalicylic acid's prolonged effect on platelet function does not resolve for 10 days to 2 weeks following discontinuation.[96] The autoimmune destruction of platelets associated with idiopathic thrombocytic purpura and occasionally observed in other autoimmune disorders

is more difficult to treat effectively because exogenous platelets are rapidly destroyed following administration.[2,44] Use of plasmapheresis, high-dose steroids, or immunosuppressive therapy may be required to prepare for splenectomy, which may help resolve severe thrombocytopenia in recalcitrant cases.

KEY POINTS

- Anemia is the most common hematologic abnormality found in preoperative patients and is usually of a secondary, not primary, nature.

- A careful patient history and physical examination will reveal the cause of most anemias although additional laboratory tests may be helpful.

- The old dogma that preoperative elective surgery should be postponed until and unless hematocrit can somehow be increased to above 30% is not valid. The risk/benefit ratio of preoperative transfusions should be carefully understood.

- Sickle cell anemia clearly presents a major challenge to the anesthesiologist. Although it is not commonly encountered in most anesthesia practices, it is the kind of disease that can "blindside" the unprepared anesthesiologist and is common enough, and deadly enough, that a thorough understanding of its pathophysiology is critically important.

- Sickle cell diagnosis as well as preoperative preparation should be understood.

- In a patient with sickle cell disease, the decision to use a simple transfusion vs. the necessity for an exchange transfusion is usually based on actual preoperative hemoglobin concentration. If the preoperative hemoglobin is relatively low, simple transfusion will suffice.

- No specific anesthetic technique has demonstrated conclusively to be superior in patients with sickle cell disease or trait.

- Preoperative history-taking must include a careful assessment of the possibility that there might be either a patient history or family history of various kinds of bleeding disorders or diatheses.

- The approach to the patient with hemophilia must be based on both underlying severity of the coagulation defect and anticipated operative procedure.

- Hemotherapy for hemophilia is really an exercise in complex but relatively straightforward pharmacokinetics. The actual factor deficiencies must be understood as well as the half-lives of the various products available. Understanding hemophilia therapy is helpful in treating other coagulation disorders including DIC.

- Another disease that confronts anesthesiologists frequently in their preoperative patient evaluation is von Willebrand's disease. Replacement of von Willebrand factor and factor VIII in cryoprecipitate results in increasing levels of these factors that last quite a while, but platelet aggregation may not be improved for very long.

- There are also numerous acquired bleeding disorders, the most common of which occur from the use of anticoagulants such as coumadin.

KEY REFERENCES

Bloom AL: Inherited disorders of blood coagulation in hemostasis and thrombosis. In Bloom AL, Thomas DP, eds: *Hemostasis and thrombosis,* New York, 1981, Churchill-Livingstone.

Chien S: Rheology of sickle cells and the microcirculation, *N Engl J Med* 311:1567, 1984.

Consensus Conference: Perioperative red cell transfusion, *JAMA* 260:2700, 1988.

Esseltine DW, Baxter M, and Bevan JL: Sickle cell states and the anaesthetist, *Can J Anaesth* 35:385, 1988.

Honig GR: Sickle cell syndromes, *J Pediatr* 92:556, 1978.

Kasper CK, Dietrich SC: Comprehensive management of hemophilia, *Clin Hematol* 14:489, 1985.

Messmer KF: Acceptable hematocrit levels in surgical patients, *World J Surg* 11:41, 1987.

Perutz MF, Pulsinelli PD, and Ranney HM: Structure and sub-unit interaction of haemoglobin, *Nature* 237:259, 1972.

Weiss JH: Platelet physiology and abnormalities of platelet function (pt 2), *N Engl J Med* 293:580, 1975.

Zauder HL: Preoperative hemoglobin requirement, *Anesthesiol Clin North Am* 8:471, 1990.

REFERENCES

1. Andes WA, Wulff K, and Smith WB: Head trauma in hemophilia: a prospective study, *Arch Intern Med* 144:1981, 1984.
2. Aster RH: Immune thrombocytopenias, *Hosp Pract* 18:187, 1983.
3. Baumgartner HR: The role of blood flow in platelet adhesion, fibrin deposition, and formation of mural thrombi, *Microvasc Res* 5:167, 1973.
4. Bloom AL: Inherited disorders of blood coagulation in hemostasis and thrombosis. In Bloom AL, Thomas DP, eds: *Hemostasis and thrombosis,* New York, 1981, Churchill-Livingstone.
5. Brittenham GM, Schechter AN, and Noguchi CT: Hemoglobin S polymerization: primary determinant of the hemolytic and clinical severity of the sickling syndromes, *Blood* 65:183, 1985.
6. Bromberg PA: Pulmonary aspects of sickle cell disease, *Arch Intern Med* 133:652, 1974.
7. Buckalew VM, Someren A: Renal manifestations of sickle cell disease, *Arch Intern Med* 133:660, 1974.
8. Carron TL, Speare RK, and Poses RM: Severity of anemia and operative mortality and morbidity, *Lancet* 1:727, 1988.
9. Chang H, Ewert SM, Bookchin RM et al: Comparative evaluation of fifteen antisickling agents, *Blood* 61:693, 1983.
10. Charache S: The treatment of sickle cell anemia, *Arch Intern Med* 133:698, 1974.
11. Chien S: Rheology of sickle cells and the microcirculation, *N Engl J Med* 311:1567, 1984.
12. Consensus Conference: Perioperative red cell transfusion, *JAMA* 260:2700, 1988.
13. Crowell JW, Smith EE: Determinant of the optimal hematocrit, *J Appl Physiol* 22:501, 1967.
14. Czer LSC, Shoemaker WC: Optimal hematocrit value in critically ill postoperative patients, *Surg Gynecol Obstet* 147:363, 1978.
15. Day JH, Rao AK: Evaluation of platelet function, *Semin Hematol* 23:89, 1986.
16. Dean J, Schechter AN: Sickle-cell anemia: molecular and cellular bases of therapeutic approaches, *N Engl J Med* 299:752, 804, 863, 1978.
17. deLavar MR et al: Open heart surgery in patients with inherited hemoglobinopathies, red cell depressions and coagulopathies, *Arch Surg* 109:618, 1974.
18. Dover GJ, Charache S, Nora R et al: Progress toward increasing fetal hemoglobin production in man: experience with 5-azacytidine and hydroxyurea, *Ann NY Acad Sci* 445:218, 1985.
19. Eaton WA, Hofrichter J: Hemoglobin S gelatin and sickle cell disease, *Blood* 10:1245, 1987.
20. Eisenstaedt R: Blood component therapy in the treatment of platelet disorders, *Semin Hematol* 23:1, 1986.
21. Esseltine DW, Baxter M, and Bevan JL: Sickle cell states and the anaesthetist, *Can J Anaesth* 35:385, 1988.

22. Fan FC, Chen RY, Schuessler GB et al: Effects of hematocrit variations on regional hemodynamics and oxygen transport in the dog, *Am J Physiol* 238:H545-H552, 1980.
23. Federici A, Mannucci PM, Minetti D et al: Intracranial bleeding in haemophilia: a study of eleven cases, *J Neurosurg Sci* 27:31, 1983.
24. Foster H: Transfusion therapy in pregnant patients with sickle cell disease: a National Institute of Health Consensus Development Conference, *Ann Intern Med* 91:122, 1979.
25. Giddings JC, Peake IR: Laboratory support in the diagnosis of coagulation disorders, *Clin Haematol* 14:571, 1985.
26. Gilchrist GS, Piepgras DG, and Roskos RR: Neurologic complications in hemophilia. In Hilgartner MW, ed: *Hemophilia in the child and adult,* New York, 1982, Masson.
27. Gregg SC, Kern M, and Brooks GA: Acute anemia results in an increased glucose depletion during sustained exercise, *J Appl Physiol* 66:1874, 1989.
28. Grill FM: Congenital bleeding disorders: hemophilia and von Willebrand's disease, *Med Clin North Am* 68:601, 1984.
29. Guyton AC, Richardson TQ: Effect of hematocrit on venous return, *Circ Res* 9:157, 1961.
30. Hebbel RP, Boogaerts MAB, Eaton JW et al: Erythrocyte adherence to endothelium in sickle-cell anemia: a possible determinant of disease severity, *N Engl J Med* 302:992, 1980.
31. Hilgartner MW: Factor replacement therapy. In Hilgartner MW, ed: *Hemophilia in the child and adult,* New York, 1982, Masson.
32. Homi J et al: General anesthesia in sickle cell disease, *Br Med J* 1:1599, 1979.
33. Honig GR: Sickle cell syndromes, *J Pediatr* 92:556, 1978.
34. Horne MK: Sickle cell anemia as a rheologic disease, *Am J Med* 70:288, 1981.
35. Huttenlocher PR et al: Cerebral blood flow in sickle cell cerebrovascular disease, *J Pediatr* 73:615, 1984.
36. Ingram VM: Gene mutations in human hemoglobin: the chemical difference between normal and sickle cell hemoglobin, *Nature* 180:326, 1957.
37. Itultin MB: Studies of factor IX concentrate therapy in hemophilia, *Blood* 62:677, 1982.
38. Jan K-M, Chien S: Effect of hematocrit variations on coronary hemodynamics and oxygen utilization, *Am J Physiol* 233:H106, 1977.
39. Janik J, Seeler RA: Perioperative management of children with sickle hemoglobinopathy, *J Pediatr Surg* 15:117, 1980.
40. Jensen JA, Goodson WH, and Vaconez LO: Wound healing in anemia, *West J Med* 144:465, 1986.

41. Karayalcin G et al: Cholelithiasis in children with sickle cell disease, *Am J Dis Child* 133:306, 1979.
42. Kasper CK, Dietrich SC: Comprehensive management of hemophilia, *Clin Hematol* 14:489, 1985.
43. Keeley KK, Buchanan GR: Acute infarction of long bones in children with sickle cell anemia, *Pediatrics* 101:170, 1982.
44. Kelton JG: Management of the pregnant patient with idiopathic thrombocytopenic purpura, *Ann Intern Med* 99:796, 1983.
45. Kobrinsky NL, Gerrard JM, Watson CM et al: Shortening of bleeding time by DDAVP in various bleeding disorders, *Lancet* 1:1145, 1984.
46. Kowalyshyn TJ, Prager D, and Young J: A review of the present status of preoperative hemoglobin requirements, *Anesth Analg* 51:75, 1972.
47. Kudsk KA et al: Acute surgical illness in patients with sickle cell anemia, *Am J Surg* 142:113, 1981.
48. Kwaku JG et al: Trial of low doses of aspirin as prophylaxis in sickle cell disease, *J Pediatr* 102:781, 1983.
49. Levine PH: The clinical manifestations and therapy of hemophilias A and B. In Coleman RW, Hirsh J, Marder VJ et al, eds: *Hemostasis and thrombosis: basic principles and clinical practice,* Philadelphia, 1982, JB Lippincott.
50. Ley TJ, DeSimone J, Noguchi C et al: 5-Azacytidine increases globin synthesis and reduces the proportion of dense cells in patients with sickle cell anemia, *Blood* 62:370, 1982.
51. Lindsay J et al: The cardiovascular manifestations of sickle cell disease, *Arch Intern Med* 133:643, 1974.
52. Lindsay RM, Clark WF: Platelet destruction in renal disease, *Semin Thromb Hemost* 8:138, 1982.
53. Lundsgaard-Hansen P: Hemodilution: new clothes for an anemic emperor, *Vox Sang* 36:321, 1979.
54. Lusher JM, Blatt PM, Penner JA et al: Autoplex versus proplex: a controlled, double-blind study of effectiveness in acute hemarthroses in hemophiliacs with inhibitors to factor VIII, *Blood* 62:1135, 1983.
55. Mann JR et al: Anaemic crisis in sickle cell disease, *J Clin Pathol* 28:341, 1975.
56. Mannucci PM: Desmopressin: a non transfusional form of treatment for congenital and acquired bleeding disorders, *Blood* 72:1449, 1988.
57. Mannuci PM, Canciani MT, Rota C et al: Response of factor VIII/von Willebrand factor to DDAVP in healthy subjects and patients with hemophilia A and von Willebrand's disease, *Br J Haematol* 47:283, 1981.
58. McCollough NC III, Enis JE et al: Subtotal or total replacement of the knee in hemophilia, *J Bone Joint Surg* 61A:69, 1979.

59. McIntosh S, Ritchey AK: Fever in young children with sickle cell disease, *J Pediatr* 96:199, 1980.
60. Mehta P, Albiol L: Prostacyclin and platelet aggregation in sickle cell disease, *Pediatrics* 70:354, 1982.
61. Messmer KF: Acceptable hematocrit levels in surgical patients, *World J Surg* 11:41, 1987.
62. Miller CH: Genetics of hemophilia and von Willebrand's disease. In Hilgartner MW, ed: *Hemophilia in the child and adult*, New York, 1982, Masson.
63. Minkin SK et al: Urologic manifestations of sickle hemoglobinopathies, *South Med J* 72:23, 1979.
64. Mirhashemi A, Ertefai S, Messmer K et al: Model analysis of the enhancement of tissue oxygenation by hemodilution due to increased microvascular flow velocity, *Microvasc Res* 34:290, 1987.
65. Morrison JC et al: Use of partial exchange transfusion preoperatively in patients with sickle cell hemoglobinopathies, *Am J Obstet Gynecol* 132:59, 1978.
66. Murray JF, Rappaport E: Coronary blood flow and myocardial metabolism in acute experimental anemia, *Cardiovasc Res* 6:360, 1972.
67. Nalbanian RM: Sickledex test for hemoglobin S: a critique, *JAMA* 218:1679, 1971.
68. Nash GB, Johnson CS, and Meiselman HJ: Mechanical properties of oxygenated red blood cells in sickle cell (HbSS) disease, *Blood* 64:73, 1984.
69. Noguchi CT, Schechter AN: The intracellular polymerization of sickle hemoglobin and its relevance to sickle cell disease, *Blood* 58:1057, 1981.
70. Perutz MF, Pulsinelli PD, and Ranney HM: Structure and sub-unit interaction of haemoglobin, *Nature* 237:259, 1972.
71. Platt OS, Orkin SH, Dover GJ et al: Hydroxyurea enhances fetal hemoglobin production in sickle cell anemia, *J Clin Invest* 74:652, 1984.
72. Pool JG, Hershgold EJ, and Pappenhagen AR: High potency antihemophiliac factor concentrate prepared from hemoglobin precipitate, *Nature* 202:316, 1964.
73. Powars D et al: Commentary: infections in sickle cell and SC disease, *Pediatrics* 103:342, 1983.
74. Powars DR: Natural history of sickle cell disease—the first ten years, *Semin Hematol* 12:267, 1975.

75. Prentice CRM: Acquired coagulation disorders, *Clin Haematol* 14:441, 1985.
76. Rao S, Gooden S: Splenic sequestration in sickle cell disease and role of transfusion therapy, *Am J Pediatr Hematol/Oncol* 7:298, 1985.
77. Rizza CR: Management of patients with inherited blood coagulation disorders. In Bloom AL, Thomas DP, eds: *Hemostasis and thrombosis*, New York, 1981, Churchill-Livingstone.
78. Rodgers GP, Schechter AN, Noguchi CT et al: Periodic microcirculatory flow in patients with sickle cell disease, *N Engl J Med* 311:1534, 1984.
79. Rutledge R, Croom RD, Davis JM et al: Cholelithiasis in sickle cell anemia; surgical considerations, *South Med J* 79:28, 1986.
80. Salzman EW, Weinstein WJ, and Weintrave RM: Treatment and desmopressin to reduce blood loss after cardiac surgery: a double blind randomized trial, *N Engl J Med* 314:1402, 1986.
81. Schechter AN, Bunn HF: What determines severity in sickle cell disease? *N Engl J Med* 306:295, 1982.
82. Secler RA, Royal JE: Commentary: sickle cell anemia, stroke, and transfusion, *J Pediatr* 96:243, 1980.
83. Serjeant GR et al: Red cell size and the clinical and haematological features of homozygous sickle cell disease, *Br J Haematol* 48:445, 1981.
84. Sullivan DW, Purdy LJ, Billingham M et al: Fatal myocardial infarction following therapy with prothrombin complex concentrates in a young man with hemophilia A, *Pediatrics* 74:279, 1984.
85. Sunder-Plasmann L, Lovekorn WP, and Messmer K: Perioperative hemodilution basic adaptation mechanisms and limitation of clinical applications, *Anesthetist* 25:124, 1976.
86. Sunshine HR, Hofrichter J, and Eaton WA: Requirements for therapeutic inhibition of sickle hemoglobin gelation, *Nature* 275:238, 1978.
87. Thomas ED: Marrow transplantation for nonmalignant disorders, *N Engl J Med* 312:44, 1985.
88. Topley JM et al: Pneumococcal and other infections in children with sickle cell-hemoglobin C (SC) disease, *J Pediatr* 101:176, 1982.
89. VanHoff J, Ritcher AK, and Shaywitz BA: Intracranial hemorrhage in children with sickle cell disease, *Am J Dis Child* 139:1120, 1985.

90. Walker BK et al: The diagnosis of pulmonary thromboembolism in sickle cell disease, *Am J Hematol* 7:219, 1979.
91. Wall MA et al: Lung function in children with sickle cell anemia, *Ann Rev Respir Dis* 120:210, 1979.
92. Warrier AL, Luscher JM: DDAVP: a useful alternative to blood components in moderate hemophilia A and von Willebrand's disease, *J Pediatr* 102:228, 1983.
93. Wautier JL, Galacteros F, Wautier MP et al: Clinical manifestations and erythrocyte adhesion to endothelium in sickle cell syndrome, *Am J Hematol* 19:121, 1985.
94. Weiss JH: Platelet physiology and abnormalities of platelet function (pt 1), *N Engl J Med* 293:531, 1975.
95. Weiss JH: Platelet physiology and abnormalities of platelet function (pt 2), *N Engl J Med* 293:580, 1975.
96. Weiss JH, Aledort LM, and Kochwa S: The effect of salicylates on the hemostatic properties of platelets in man, *J Clin Invest* 47:2169, 1968.
97. White GC et al: Factor VIII inhibitors: a clinical overview, *Am J Hematol* 13:335, 1982.
98. White GC, McMillan CW, Blatt PM et al: Factor VIII inhibitors: a clinical overview, *Am J Hematol* 13:335, 1982.
99. Williams J et al: Efficacy of transfusion therapy for one to two years in patients with sickle cell disease and cerebrovascular accidents, *J Pediatr* 96:205, 1980.
100. Wood DH: Cerebrovascular complications of sickle cell anemia, *Stroke* 9:73, 1978.
101. Wood JH, Kee DB: Hematology of the cerebral circulation in stroke, *Stroke* 16:768, 1985.
102. Woodson RD, Willis RE, and Lenfewt C: Effect of acute and established anemia in O_2 transport at rest, submaximal and maximal work, *J Appl Physiol* 44:36, 1978.
103. Zago MA et al: Treatment of sickle cell disease with aspirin, *Acta Haematol* (Basel) 72:61, 1984.
104. Zauder HL: Preoperative hemoglobin requirement. *Anesthesiol Clin North Am* 8:471, 1990.
105. Zimmerman TS, Ruggeri ZM: Von Willebrand's disease, *Clin Haematol* 12:175, 1983.

CHAPTER 21

Evaluation of the Patient with Orthopedic Disease

DENIS L. BOURKE

HELEN YATES

Orthopedics is a unique surgical specialty for a number of reasons. Until the early 20th century, orthopedics largely consisted of the use of casts, splints, turnbuckle apparatus, braces, suspension devices, and other mechanical means to effect gradual changes in deformities, most often congenital deformities; hence the name *orthopedics*. In addition, these nonoperative treatments did not require the use of anesthesia. Many of the operative treatments such as fracture repairs, tenotomies, and amputations were performed without the use of anesthesia. The advent of the first practical antibiotic, sulfonamide, in 1935

and the impetus provided by the injuries during World War II in the early 1940s were the catalysts for a great increase in operative orthopedics. Because of the orthopedic surgeon's need for radiographs and electrical equipment, the development of the nonexplosive inhalational anesthetic, halothane, in 1956 removed the last barrier to the growth of orthopedic surgery. Since that time, technologic and other advances have only served to fuel the progress of orthopedic surgery.[6]

The variety of procedures performed by modern orthopedic surgeons ranges from such minor operations as manipulation under anesthesia to a thoracoabdominal retroperitoneal approach to the anterior spine. Orthopedic surgeons operate on virtually every area of the body from the cervical spine to the pelvis to the toes. Patients range from infants to the elderly.

The volume of orthopedic procedures is large and continuously expanding as witnessed by the fact that in the United States alone a single orthopedic procedure, the total hip arthroplasty, accounts for more than 100,000 operations each year.[32,37] For many reasons, the number and types of operations will continue to increase and in all likelihood become a larger proportion of the total number of operations performed. The general aging of the population exposes increasing numbers of people to osteoarthritis and fractures among other orthopedic diseases. Participation in physical fitness activities is causing an increasing number of athletic injuries. Affluence and leisure time, in addition to more drivers in ever-faster cars, lead to new opportunities for injury in the home workshop or around a variety of powerful recreational vehicles. Certain patient groups who are particularly susceptible to orthopedic problems, such as patients with sickle cell disease, chronic renal failure, systemic lupus erythematosus, or cancer, now have longer life expectancies and can be anticipated to require even more orthopedic operations. Technologic advances not only permit more sophisticated orthopedic diagnoses but have vastly expanded the range of treatment options and operations available to the modern orthopedic surgeon. Finally, technologic, physiologic, and pharmacologic advances in anesthesiology allow the orthopedic surgeon to contemplate longer, more extensive, and more innovative operations on older, younger, and sicker patients than previously was possible.

In the future the anesthesiologist can expect to evaluate and anesthetize more orthopedic patients with a wider array of disease processes for a broader range of procedures. However, there is another unique aspect of the orthopedic patient that warrants the anesthesiologist's attention, especially during the preoperative visit. The psychologic attitude and expectations of the orthopedic patient are often quite different from most other surgical patients. With the exception of the patient with massive trauma, the orthopedic patient seldom has either a short- or long-term life-threatening disease process. The most common emotional issues for the orthopedic patient are potential loss of a limb, disfigurement or disability, and/or reduction of the quality of life. The first group of patients are often otherwise healthy individuals who, possibly for the first time in their lives, are medically threatened, usually by an entirely unanticipated accident. Because of the nature of orthopedic problems, their concerns frequently relate to their body image. They seldom have had previous experience or sufficient time to learn to cope with the many fears surrounding their problem. Anxiety results from sudden new uncertainties about pain, deformity, and death.

Concerns among the second group of patients are quite different. These patients' concerns are not related to disfigurement or mortality but rather to the quality of life. They usually hope to reduce discomfort, increase mobility, or improve function. Most have lived with congenital deformities or have had long-term chronic problems with which, in large part, they have learned to cope. They are frequently familiar with hospitals, surgery, and pain. Their anxieties and expectations, based on experience, are generally more realistic.

In the preoperative evaluation and treatment of the orthopedic patient it is important for the anesthesiologist to recognize these special psychologic aspects as well as the usual preoperative concerns for the primary and other disease processes.

ORTHOPEDIC DISEASES

The underlying disease states that require bone and joint surgery range from the most chronic to the most acute in duration. It is important for the treating anesthesiologist to understand not only the most apparent manifestation of the disease state that is the reason for the operation planned but also the sometimes myriad and subtle systemic effects of the same process. The spectrum of chronicity can range from inborn genetic defects, in utero injury, and acquired diseases such as rheumatoid arthritis, to the most acute of disease states, multiple organ system trauma. Some of the more common chronic disease states are compounded by concurrent old age; approximately one in four surgical patients will be older than 65 years of age and about one in 10 over 75 years of age.[53]

The next section attempts to provide an overview of some of the more common orthopedic diseases, with an emphasis on airway, cervical spine, and systemic manifestations that might affect anesthetic management.

Osteoarthritis

Osteoarthritis is the most common of the rheumatologic diseases, affecting between 40 and 60 million Americans.* The hallmark of the disease is the loss of articular cartilage with joint margin and subchondral reactive changes, and there is commonly associated secondary inflammation.[41] **Other common terms** for the same disease process include the more European expression *osteoarthrosis* and the universal equivalent term **degenerative joint disease;** as Mankin points out, the first denies the inflammatory component of the disease, and the second invokes degenerative processes not found to be part of the biologic process.[32]

Osteoarthritis is so common among the elderly that it has long been thought to be a natural concomitant process of aging. The evidence supports increased vulnerability of elderly joint tissues but not aging of the cells per se as a cause of the process.[33] The association with age, however, is very strong epidemiologically. Nearly 40% of people between the ages of 18 and 24 will have some evidence of osteoarthritis and approximately 85% in the 75- to 79-year-old age group.[40] Radiographs of knees reveal osteoarthritis in 27% of people between 65 to 69 years of age and 51% of those over 85 years of age.[55] Similarly, radiographs of hands and feet show that 90% of women and 85% of men have osteoarthritis after age 65.[32,38] Clinical signs will be evident in more than 50% of people over the age of 60.[9,32,38] Differences between male and female patients are generally not significant although

---

* References 25, 32, 33, 40, 41, 55.

women tend to have more symptomatic disease, and racial and ethnic differences are not found in the United States.[23,55] **Osteoarthritis is the presenting disease process for the majority of some 100,000 total hip replacements and a nearly equal number of total knee replacements** in the United States each year.[32,34,40]

Osteoarthritis can be subdivided between primary and secondary osteoarthritis; the first category can also be loosely subdivided between localized and generalized. The differentiation is based on whether there is a clearly recognizable underlying etiology. Confusion over the actual pathogenesis is secondary to osteoarthritis being the "final common pathway" of many processes.[32,55] Excessive or repetitive stresses on the cartilage with a diminished ability of the cartilage to respond causes a breakdown of the joint surface and allows biomechanical and biochemical changes of the articular matrix[33,41]; secondary inflammation and failed reparative attempts result in some of the characteristic changes other than loss of articular surface, such as osteophyte formation (thus the other common phrase for this disease, **hypertrophic arthritis**), subchondral erosion, and cyst formation. Unlike many other rheumatologic diseases to be discussed in this section, there are no recognizable systemic abnormalities.[32,34]

The clinical manifestations of osteoarthritis are pain, crepitance, decreased motion, and finally deformity around the involved joint or joints. Those joints most commonly affected include the hips, knees, and those of the spine, hands, and feet. The associated spurring and swelling of the distal interphalangeal joints are called Heberden's nodes and those of the proximal interphalangeal joint, Bouchard's nodes. Spinal involvement is most common at the L3 to L4 level and can cause symptoms ranging from local pain to even cauda equina syndrome with sphincter dysfunction. Spinal involvement is also common in the cervical spine, and radicular pain from either area can be a cause of diagnostic problems; referred pain in the area of commonly affected joints such as the hips, knees, and shoulders can mask its true source.[32,41,55]

Surgical intervention can take many forms depending on the involved joints. Total joint replacements are now the most common surgical solution to end-stage osteoarthritis of the hips and knees. Arthrodesis is a common surgical procedure for the small joints of the hands and feet, along with interpositional arthroplasty and sometimes replacement of the trapeziometacarpal joint. Spinal procedures are usually decompressive in nature, with stabilization and fusion a secondary consideration for any preexisting or resultant instability.

Although there are no systemic manifestations of osteoarthritis, the anesthesiologist should be aware of some associations, including the more obvious such as age, as well as some less obvious found in some cross-sectional studies such as obesity, hyperuricemia, and diabetes.[23] Multiple procedures are not uncommon, and the anesthesiologist should be cognizant of other major joint replacements and previous spinal procedures with regard to positioning and intubation. Concomitant osteoporosis in the elderly increases the risk of periprosthetic fractures both in the current joint procedure and in previous ones. The patient history and physical examination should be sensitive to radicular signs and symptoms that may be the harbingers of spinal involvement as well as to those positions and motions that might exacerbate discomfort in the involved joints for which surgery is not planned.

The patient's previous history of nonsteroidal antiinflammatory drug use should be carefully taken to elicit the frequent multiplicity of such agents, looking for the not uncommon concurrent use of these medications that put the patient at higher risk for gastric ulcerations and the theoretic risk of delayed clotting time. The risk of such medications inducing reversible renal failure has been recently shown[58]; thus comparison of past with preoperative creatinine and blood urea nitrogen levels is useful if the data are available. Finally, the limitations imposed on this elderly population by their arthritis can mask exertional angina, so patient history and ECG should be examined with a healthy bias toward possible underlying coronary artery disease.

Rheumatoid Arthritis

Although less common than osteoarthritis, **rheumatoid arthritis affects approximately 1% of adults in the United States,** with an estimated 100,000 to 200,000 new cases each year.[21,23] **The disease affects women two to three times more often than men** and increases in incidence with age. Genetic factors are implicated as well, with a known incomplete association with histocompatibility antigen HLA-DR4.[21,23]

Because there is no absolute specific laboratory test for rheumatoid arthritis, it remains a clinical diagnosis supported by serum blood tests and radiographs. Inflammation, polyarticular involvement that is often symmetric, and systemic manifestations are the hallmarks. The small joints of the hand and foot, the wrist, and the knee are most often involved, as well as the elbow, shoulder, and hip less frequently.[3] **The revised 1988 American Rheumatism Association criteria for diagnosis include morning stiffness, arthritis of three or more joints, hand arthritis, symmetry of involvement, rheumatoid nodules, serum rheumatoid factor, and radiographic changes.**[21] This list includes various modifiers not discussed in this chapter; the diagnosis of rheumatoid arthritis is made when four of the above seven criteria are met and when the first four are present for at least 6 weeks. Seronegative patients meet the preceding requirements but test negative for serum rheumatoid factor.

The cervical spine is commonly found to be involved with rheumatoid arthritis. The most frequent presentation is that of anterior subluxation of C1 on C2 secondary to inflammatory erosion of retaining supports. Less common, but even more dangerous, are posterior subluxation and vertical migration at the same joint. Anterior atlantoaxial subluxation has been estimated to occur in 20% to 40% of this patient population, but symptomatic involvement is less frequent. Symptoms will present in one of two common patterns of either progressive myelopathy or intermittent signs and symptoms of medulla compression.[21] Surgical intervention to stabilize these problems has traditionally been restricted to symptomatic patients and/or to those patients with demonstrated long tract signs[29,30]; various researchers, however, have recommended prophylactic fusion of C1 to C2 for patients with anterior subluxation of ≥ 8 mm to avoid the probably irreversible changes that occur with established symptomatic myelopathy.[13,45] Despite controversy over the efficacy of stabilization in asymptomatic patients, it is probably wise to screen such patients if they are scheduled for surgery by obtaining cervical spine radiographs and, if these are not grossly abnormal, flexion-extension films. The prophylactic fusion of the unstable rheumatoid spine before elective surgery possibly requiring general anesthesia has been advocated by some,[46] but this is controversial. Positive findings on screening radiographs allow for at least consultation with a specialist dealing with such procedures and further neuroradiographic workup if indicated. It also allows the anesthesiologist to more rationally plan the safest intubation technique. The thoracic and lumbar spine are typically spared in patients with rheumatoid arthritis.

The systemic, extraarticular manifestations of rheumatoid arthritis are variable and myriad (Table 21-1). It is not uncommon for patients to have low-grade fever, mild lymphadenopathy, and various types of neuritis. The heart can be involved as well; pericarditis is the most common of these expressions of this disease, but it can also cause valvular insufficiency, conduction abnormalities, and myocarditis.[3] Pleural involvement is common but is not so commonly symptomatic and can take the form of pleural effusions, subpleural nodules, and/or present as a diffuse pneumonitis. This patient group can develop Sjogren's syndrome,[3] and the anesthesiologist should be aware of possible iatrogenic corneal injury as a result of dry eyes. The small diarthroidial cricoarytenoid joint can be involved to the point of causing laryngeal obstruction and respiratory stridor; a sign of such involvement is hoarseness.[3] Rheumatoid nodules on the vocal cords seen with laryngoscopy can mimic laryngeal cancer.[21]

Operative procedures for patients with rheumatoid arthritis are varied and are commonly multiple for each patient. Realignment and repair of the hand tendons and replacement of the metacarpophalangeal joints are frequently done all at once for the entire hand and can be a prolonged procedure. Total joint procedures are also common, with total knee replacements probably being the most frequently needed. Open and arthroscopic synovectomies of various joints are also common.

During the preoperative assessment, the history and physical examination should be guided by the previously mentioned systemic aspects of rheumatoid arthritis as well as the more obvious presenting symptom for surgery. Chest pain may represent pericarditis or impending tamponade, shortness of breath may be the symptom representing one of the pulmonary manifestations, and hoarseness may be the clue to cricoarytenoid involvement. The examiner should actively seek the friction rub or even the pulsus paradoxus of pericarditis and possible tamponade; similarly, the fine rales of pneumonitis can be elicited.

Table 21-1   Anesthetic neck and airway problems in connective tissue diseases

Disease	Cervical spine	Airway
Osteoarthritis	Stiffness Radiculopathies	Temporomandibular joint involvement
Rheumatoid arthritis	Axial instability (C1/C2) Vertical instability (C1/C2) Instability at other cervical levels Myelopathy Basilar invagination	Cricoarytenoid joint involvement Vocal cord nodules
Ankylosing spondylitis	Fixed flexion deformity	Fixed flexion deformity

The medication history of this patient population is much more involved than for patients with osteoarthritis. The same caveats concerning nonsteroidal antiinflammatory drugs hold true. In addition to nonsteroidal antiinflammatory drugs, other medications will include gold, penicillamine, and prednisone therapy; prednisone must be considered in terms of the need for perioperative stress coverage with a steroid bolus. The absolute necessity of this is variable in terms of the degree of stress and the patient's history of prednisone use.

Ancillary studies that might reveal the systemic manifestations of rheumatoid arthritis include the ECG, pulmonary function testing, if indicated, and the previously mentioned cervical spine radiographs. Results of blood work may reveal anemia of chronic disease; anemia, thrombocytopenia, neutropenia, lymphadenopathy, and splenomegaly in a patient with rheumatoid arthritis may represent Felty's syndrome.[3] Plans for positioning should allow for the osteopenia of rheumatoid arthritis itself, which can be compounded by prednisone usage, as well as any areas involved with neuritis. As with patients with osteoarthritis, previous procedures should also be considered for positioning.

Spondyloarthropathies

The seronegative spondyloarthropathies represent a broad group of inflammatory arthritides that are distinguished from rheumatoid arthritis by their involvement of the joints of the spine and their asymmetric involvement of the large joints. They include spondylosing ankylosis, psoriatic arthritis, Reiter's syndrome, and the arthritis of chronic inflammatory bowel disease.[22] These diseases have some common overlapping features, including involvement of the sacroiliac joints; changes around the enthesis (the site of ligamentous insertion into bone) more than the synovium; extraskeletal changes affecting the aortic valve, eye, lung, and skin; and a strong tendency toward hereditary factors revolving around the known association with HLA-B27.[11]

Although all of the spondyloarthropathies may have joint involvement requiring orthopedic surgery, **ankylosing spondylitis is the disease entity most likely to cause disability or deformity severe enough to require major surgical intervention.** This is because of its higher prevalence, lack of remission or relapses, and more predictable involvement of the spine and, to a lesser degree, the hips. The prevalence of ankylosing spondylitis is estimated to be around 0.5%, following the prevalence of HLA-B27, which is about 8% in whites, 18% to 50% in American Indians, and 1% in black Africans and Japanese. The risk of the disease developing in a patient with HLA-B27 is 20% although 5% of whites with ankylosing spondylitis will not have the genetic marker. The disease has equal distribution between men and women but has a milder course in the latter, which caused it to historically be thought to be a predominantly male disease.[11,12]

The back pain of ankylosing spondylitis begins insidiously in patients younger than 40 years of age, most typically around age 20; the discomfort's persistence, association with morning stiffness or increased discomfort with rest, and improvement with exercise are characteristic.[11,12] Progression to the fused or bamboo spine appearance on radiographs occurs in the cervical region, but in the thoracolumbar spine this can lead to flexion deformity, including the chin-on-chest deformity. Both the deformities themselves and cord compression or cauda equina syndrome will lead to surgical intervention. Ankylosis of the hips can cause significant disability, which is treated successfully on a regular basis with total hip arthroplasty.[12]

Extraarticular manifestations of the disease are many. Systemic symptoms can include fatigue, weight loss, and low-grade fever; uveitis occurs in 25% of the patients but is usually self-limited.[11,12] Of more significance to the anesthesiologist are the cardiopulmonary effects of the disease. An estimated 20% of patients with ankylosing spondylitis have pathologic changes in the aortic valve, although few have clinical dysfunction presenting as aortic insufficiency, cardiomegaly, and conduction delays. Complete atrioventricular block can develop along with Stokes-Adams attacks.[12] Pulmonary changes are a later problem in this patient group. The changes are typically fibrotic and chronic infiltrative changes in the upper lobes; symptoms include cough, excess sputum, and dyspnea, but, despite the fibrotic changes, ventilation is usually well maintained through the diaphragm. Cystic changes can progress to superinfection with *Aspergillus,* leading to hemoptysis and radiographic changes that mimic tuberculosis.[11,12]

Preoperative attention to the spine, heart, and lung is essential in the patient with ankylosing spondylitis. Signs and symptoms suggesting spinal cord encroachment or cauda equina syndrome should be sought aggressively. Examination of the heart and lungs should focus on aortic valve murmurs and upper lobe changes by auscultation. Previous chest radiographs, if available, can be used to help determine any interval change. The ECG should be studied for conduction delays.

Deformity of the cervical spine, as well as its ankylosis, requires careful evaluation for the use of fiberoptic intubation and careful evaluation of extubation criteria, especially in the patient with chin-on-chest deformity. Attention to ankylosis of the hips and shoulders should be evaluated preoperatively to avoid possible harmful attempts at manipulation for posi-

Table 21-2 Arthritis, primary level of spinal involvement

Disease	Cervical	Thoracic	Lumbar
Osteoarthritis	+ + +	+	+ + + +
Rheumatoid arthritis	+ + + +	−	−
Ankylosing spondylitis	+ + + +	+ + + +	+ + + +
Marfan's syndrome (scoliosis)	−	+ + +	+ + +

tioning while the patient is anesthetized. The degree of ankylosis of the spine can be evaluated both by examination and radiographically and may predict the success of spinal or epidural insertion (Table 21-2).

Communication with the surgeons is essential, especially with spinal procedures. Corrective osteotomies of the spine might entail spinal cord monitoring and wake-up tests, and planning for the procedure should reflect this. Simmons, among others, has more safely performed cervical laminectomy and osteotomy for chin-on-chest deformity with use of local anesthesia in the sitting patient already in fixation.[50] This entails a management challenge to the anesthesiologist in terms of sedation and monitoring; however, it allows a safer, slow correction of the deformity, which is stopped when the patient expresses symptoms or signs of compression.

Systemic Lupus Erythematosus and Other Connective Tissue Diseases

Systemic lupus erythematosus (SLE) and the other connective tissue diseases (CTDs) have crossover symptoms and signs as well certain common epidemiologic features.[23] Some of the CTDs include scleroderma, dermatomyositis, mixed connective tissue disease, and undifferentiated connective tissue disease disorders. Patients with SLE or CTD will seldom have surgery for the disease itself but more commonly as a result of the avascular necrosis that is a side effect of the corticosteroid drugs used to control their ailments. Both because of its greater prevalence and its early onset of severe disease with the concomitant complications of steroid therapy, SLE will be discussed.

SLE has an approximate incidence of 50/100,000 people. The female/male ratio ranges from 8:1 to 13:1, with black women increasingly affected; one study estimated the incidence in black women to be 1/250. Onset peaks between the second and fourth decade, with disease in the elderly being milder.[23,49]

The actual cause of the disease remains unknown; the pathogenesis revolves around chronic inflammation at many sites secondary to autoimmune processes. The destructive behavior of the disease led to the name *lupus,* which is Latin for wolf.[1,51]

The protean manifestations of the disease help to make it difficult to diagnose. There are 11 accepted criteria, and if any four are present, the patient is said to have SLE. Serum tests include LE cell preps, anti-DNA and antinuclear antibody, and a persistent false-positive syphilis (STS) result. Musculoskeletal complaints are the most common and can occur as myalgias, arthralgias, and arthritis; up to 95% of patients with SLE have such symptoms.[2,49] Cutaneous manifestations include the malar butterfly rash.

The anesthesiologist evaluating a patient with SLE should be aware of the effects of the disease on internal vital organs. Cardiac manifestations, including pericarditis, myocarditis, and endocarditis, may be expressed as cardiomegaly; also there are ECG changes (usually ST-T wave abnormalities), resting tachycardia, and even myocardial infarction and valvular lesions. The lungs and pleura are at risk for pleurisy, pleuritis, pleural effusions and, more commonly, acute and chronic lupus pneumonitis; the underlying changes of the disease state and the use of steroids put these patients at risk for superimposed infections as well. Hematologically, the disease may express itself as anemia, thrombocytopenia, leukopenia, lymphadenopathy, and splenomegaly.[2,49] Glomerulonephritis, sometimes bizarre central nervous system manifestations, and various gastrointestinal complications only barely cover some of the other systemic effects of this disorder.

Because of these effects, the preoperative evaluation of the patient with SLE must be more complete than usual for people in the commonly affected second to fourth decade. **A careful history should include questions concerning chest pains, shortness of breath, and cough. The examination should include careful attention to evidence of pleural effusions, pleuritis, or pneumonia, as well as any cardiac manifestations. The ECG tracing and chest radiograph should be scrutinized for any subclinical evidence of disease** that might become problematic with use of anesthesia. An awareness of current renal function helps with intraoperative fluid management, and a good neuropsychiatric history might forewarn the anesthesiologist of possible perioperative behavioral or psychiatric changes that otherwise might be attributed to other causes. Depression in this patient population is understandable as a reactive process but is also recognized as being secondary to both the disease itself and steroid therapy.[2] Sensitivity to this aspect of SLE might help the anesthesiologist in counseling patients through their perioperative course successfully.

Marfan's Syndrome

Although technically a hereditary, congenital disease, Marfan's syndrome is discussed with the rheumatologic disorders because it is so frequently discovered after childhood. Scoliosis and acetabulum protrusio are common orthopedic problems that bring a patient with Marfan's syndrome to the operating room with the diagnosis already known; the ligamentous laxity associated with disease, however, will present as injury without concomitant appreciation of its causes. The cardiovascular effects of the syndrome are potentially life threatening.

The diagnosis of **Marfan's syndrome** should be made with hesitation and only after evaluation by an expert in genetic disorders because such a diagnosis carries potent implications and can affect job and insurance applications adversely. The disease is **autosomal dominant,** but the actual biochemical defect has yet to be discovered. Some of the **skeletal manifestations include above-average height, arachnodactyly (long slender digits),** excessive arm span, pes excavatum, pes planovalgus, and lax and hypermobile joints that can result in repetitive dislocations. Such patients typically have myopia and are at risk for ocular lens dislocation; hernias are also common.[44,54,61]

The **cardiac and pulmonary manifestations of the disease are of prime importance to the anesthesiologist.** Up to 5% of patients with Marfan's syndrome have **apical bullae that lead to pneumothorax**[44]; thus evaluation of the chest radiograph might forewarn the anesthesiologist of this risk before positive ventilation is initiated. Even more life threatening are the cardiovascular aspects of Marfan's syndrome. Patients **often have a defect in the media of the wall of the ascending aorta** that leads to dissecting aortic aneurysms, aortic valve incompetence, and insufficiency of the coronary arteries. **Aortic dissection and aortic valve incompetence are the leading causes of death in this patient group.**[44] **In addition, patients are at risk for mitral valve prolapse and possible subsequent mitral regurgitation.**[44,61] A patient with findings suggestive of Marfan's syndrome warrants further investigation into the family history, with attention to early and sudden death, a careful examination, and probably most importantly, an echocardiogram to rule out any of the aortic or cardiac manifestations.

CONGENITAL AND DEVELOPMENTAL ORTHOPEDIC DISEASES

A myriad of congenital disorders might be present in patients who require bone and joint surgery. Many of these are better discussed in the chapters dealing with pediatric anesthesia, neuromuscular disorders, and endocrine abnormalities. This discussion will be limited to those conditions that more frequently require bone and joint surgery, such as osteogenesis imperfecta, probably the penultimate genetic disease of bone, and scoliosis, a less well-understood process in terms of etiology.

Osteogenesis Imperfecta

Osteogenesis imperfecta (OI) is best defined as a congenital "condition of abnormal fragility and plasticity of bone with recurring fractures on minimal trauma." It was first described by Eckmann in 1788.[52]

Osteogenesis imperfecta is inherited as an autosomal dominant trait although certain rare cases would suggest a recessive mode of inheritance. There are a number of classifications of this disease; the most common division is between the more severe osteogenesis imperfecta congenita and the condition more compatible with life, osteogenesis imperfecta tarda.[47] Osteogenesis imperfecta has an incidence between 1/20,000 and 1/60,000 live births. Defective collagen synthesis is believed to be the underlying biochemical abnormality.[24] The clinical features of OI include blue sclerae and fragile bones and teeth. Associated problems include deafness, abnormal platelet function, elevated thyroxine levels, increased oxygen consumption, increased metabolic rate, cardiovascular anomalies including aortic and mitral regurgitation, premature atherosclerosis, cleft palate, hydrocephalus, and spina bifida.[47] The cause of the hypermetabolism has not been fully elucidated. Progression of OI usually arrests in puberty. It may become reactivated in women after menopause.[15] Scoliosis occurs in about 50% of patients with the severe form of the disease.

Surgical management of OI can include multiple intramedullary nailings, Sofield osteotomies, and corrective surgery for scoliosis.[24] Specific areas in the patient history should focus on any underlying cardiac abnormality or respiratory problems secondary to scoliosis. Any old or concurrent fractures must be documented in the preoperative anesthesia record.[24] These patients tend to become hyperthermic during anesthesia, but this is not believed to be of the malignant variety and usually responds to use of a cooling blanket and administration of cold intravenous fluids. Both a patient history and chart review may be necessary to elicit previous occurrences. It may be wise to avoid use of agents known to trigger malignant hyperthermia. Finally, patient history should address any previous signs of bleeding abnormalities.

The physical examination should especially address the airway. Patients with OI may have short necks, large tongues, and their teeth, jaws, and cervical vertebrae are fragile.[28] Auscultation of their hearts may reveal the presence of a murmur, which may require consultation with the patient's cardiologist. If there is evidence of respiratory involvement secondary to scoliosis, pulmonary function tests should be obtained. There is usually a reduction in vital capacity in patients with scoliosis although other parameters of lung function remain normal.[18] Calculation of normal standards should be revised because of bowed arms and legs. Examination of the forearms for intravenous access is important, as there is a significant incidence of subcutaneous hemorrhage.

Antibiotic prophylaxis must be administered if cardiac lesions are present. Fracture of the humerus may occur with the use of a blood pressure cuff.[28] It may be prudent to cannulate the artery directly for all but very minor surgical procedures. Great care must be taken with positioning the patient in the operating room. The operating room table should be well padded. Extreme caution must also be exercised during intubation because of the known incidence of damaged teeth and fractures of both the mandible and cervical spine. The use of succinylcholine is also relatively contraindicated because of the possibility of a fasciculation-induced fracture.[28]

Many patients with OI require multiple surgeries; this in conjunction with their deafness and with the pain associated with their fractures should alert the anesthesiologist to their possible increased preoperative anxiety and concerns. The differential diagnosis of OI must include the battered child syndrome.

Scoliosis

Spinal deformity was first described by Hippocrates. Scoliosis is derived from a Greek root meaning "crooked." It represents lateral and rotational deformity of the vertebral column.

Scoliosis is loosely classified as congenital, idiopathic, neuromuscular, and osteogenic. The idiopathic form is most common and can be further subdivided into infantile, juvenile, and adolescent variants, the distinction being the age of onset or diagnosis (Table 21-3). Infantile scoliosis occurs up to 4 years of age, juvenile between 4 and 9 years, and the adolescent variety between 10 years and skeletal maturity.[47]

The incidence of scoliosis in North America is 4/1000 live births.[24] Females make up 85% of cases of adolescent scoliosis and usually have a right-sided curve. Juvenile scoliosis occurs equally in both sexes and is also more commonly right-sided in curvature.

Table 21-3 Classification of idiopathic scoliosis

Classification	Age (years)
Infantile	0-4
Juvenile	4-9
Adolescent	10-skeletal maturity

Infantile scoliosis usually occurs in males and is associated with a left-sided curve that may resolve spontaneously; this form of scoliosis is uncommon in North America but is almost as common in Europe as adolescent scoliosis is in North America.[24]

Most patients who present for scoliosis surgery are asymptomatic and otherwise well. The respiratory and cardiovascular systems become involved as the disease progresses. A curvature less than 65 degrees is unlikely to be associated with pulmonary dysfunction. Pulmonary findings are consistent with a restrictive pattern of disease; the most noticeable reduction is in vital capacity. Lesser reductions occur in total lung capacity and functional residual capacity.[47]

Gas exchange abnormalities are related to ventilation/perfusion mismatch. The alveolar-arterial oxygen difference and dead-space/tidal volume ratios are increased. The Pao_2 is usually decreased, with a normal $Paco_2$. Hypercapnia usually implies more severe disease, although the carbon dioxide response is altered early.[47]

Patients with scoliosis associated with neuromuscular disease also have abnormalities in central respiratory control and innervation of the motor neurons of the respiratory muscles.[47] Inability to cough adequately also predisposes such patients to the development of respiratory infections.

Cardiovascular manifestations most often result from pulmonary hypertension, which occurs secondary to chronic hypoxia. This ultimately leads to cor pulmonale and death. Congenital scoliosis may be associated with cardiac anomalies.

Surgical correction should ideally be performed before cardiorespiratory dysfunction occurs. Surgery is unlikely to improve pulmonary function although improvement in gas exchange has been shown.[24] Surgery, however, may prevent further deterioration in pulmonary function. Surgery is reserved for significant and progressive curves, usually greater than 40 degrees. Most curves may be managed with posterior correction and fusion alone; instrumentation varies from the traditional Harrington rod, segmental Luque, and Wisconsin style techniques to Cotrel-Dubouset rods. Curvatures with greater deformity and less flexibility may require a two-stage procedure starting with anterior discectomy, release and fusion, followed by posterior instrumentation and fusion.

Preoperative evaluation should address the cause of the disease and look for associated abnormalities. Pulmonary function studies should be performed in all cases with curvatures of greater than 65 degrees. Vital capacity less than 30% predicted usually implies the need for postoperative mechanical ventilation.[24] Signs of pulmonary hypertension, such as a loud pulmonic second sound, should be sought. Right ventricular enlargement may be seen on the ECG.

Since the majority of the patients who have scoliosis are young and asymptomatic, significant effort is expended to protect the patient from neurologic injury, which has been reported at a rate of 0.72%,[31] hence the need for intraoperative monitoring of spinal cord function. **This may be accomplished by a "wake-up" test or by the use of somatosensory-evoked potentials** (SSEPs). Patients should be informed about the possibility of an intraoperative "wake-up" test preoperatively. If changes occur in the SSEPs, a "wake-up" test may be required. The possibility of mechanical ventilation, the need for aggressive pulmonary toilet, and the use of deep breathing exercises in the postoperative period must be emphasized to the patient before surgery. Avoidance of heavy premedication is advisable in view of the increased susceptibility of these patients to respiratory depression because of the altered carbon dioxide response.

Spinal cord monitoring

There are two methods currently available to monitor the integrity of the spinal cord intraoperatively. The "wake-up" test remains the gold standard and simply means waking up the patient at one or more intervals during surgery after distraction of the spinal cord and asking the patient to move the hands and feet. This method has the advantage of being definitive and simple to perform. The disadvantages are that it is not continuous and it may be associated with excessive movement of the patient, which can result in the endotracheal tube or surgical instruments being dislodged. It also may be psychologically damaging to the patient.

The second method of monitoring spinal cord function is by measuring SSEPs. This type of monitoring is based on the transmission of impulses up and down the spinal cord. The stimulating electrodes are placed over the posterior tibial nerves in the lower extremities, commonly, and over the median nerves in the upper extremities.[42] Recording electrodes are placed over the neck and scalp. A computer supplies a repetitive stimulus that triggers the recording system.

The most common measurements used to interpret the recordings are latency and amplitude. An increase in the latency of 10% or more and a decrease in the amplitude of more than 50% have been generally accepted as cause for serious concern.[42] Measurements are recorded at specific times throughout surgery. If changes in the SSEPs persist for 15 to 20 minutes, a "wake-up" test may be required, and the determining forces applied to the spine must be released.

A number of factors can affect SSEPs, such as temperature, blood pressure, concentration of respiratory gases, and hematocrit. Anesthetic agents can also depress the SSEPs.[19] The use of inhalational agents and nitrous oxide has been implicated.[36] It is important to stimulate each limb separately so that both halves of the spinal cord can be evaluated. Upper and lower extremity monitoring allows the effects of previously mentioned systemic factors to be seen and differentiated from SSEP changes arising from spinal cord distraction.

ORTHOPEDIC TRAUMA

Modern medical facilities, such as extensively equipped surface emergency vehicles, highly trained paramedical personnel, and helicopters, have greatly extended the ability of the victim of massive trauma to survive to reach the hospital and, ultimately, the operating room.[8,35] Therefore the anesthesiologist is faced with violently injured patients who will require extensive emergency surgery.

Orthopedic trauma encompasses a great variety of problems. The degree or severity ranges from problems as minor as simple finger fractures or uncomplicated Colles fractures to such life-threatening problems as cervical vertebral fractures or complicated pelvic fractures. The impact of orthopedic trauma is only hinted at by the fact that hip fractures alone accounted for more than 3 million days of hospital care in 1987.[27] **The urgency of surgery for orthopedic trauma is equally varied. Open fractures of joints, because of the possibility and nature of the infections, are truly emergent. Similarly, fractures causing vascular occlusion that can be limb-threatening require immediate repair.** Simple closed fractures, however, are seldom emergencies and many can almost be considered elective surgery. Trauma is not selective; it strikes male and female, young and old, responsible and derelict, and the healthy as well as extremely sick patients.

Because of the nature of operating room schedules and the triage of other emergency cases, the anesthesiologist is often required to make decisions about the timing of the surgery for these cases.[14] In this capacity the anesthesiologist must have a basic knowledge of the nature of the orthopedic problem and make a thorough preoperative evaluation of the patient. Using knowledge of the orthopedic process and the patient's other diseases, the anesthesiologist must carefully assess the overall risks and benefits to the patient. With this information the anesthesiologist and the orthopedic surgeon must come to a rational decision as to the timing and extent of the surgery to be performed. An intelligent and cooperative approach can best serve the patient.

Paramount to the anesthesiologist's intelligent

decision making is a comprehensive preoperative evaluation. The preoperative evaluation not only guides the choice of anesthetic technique and intraoperative management but aids the surgeon in decisions about the timing and extent of the surgical procedure.[39]

Unfortunately, unlike elective surgery, the preoperative evaluation of the orthopedic trauma patient may have to be abbreviated. Often there is insufficient time to explore the patient's complete medical history or to obtain all the preoperative tests desired. The trauma victim may be unconscious, hysterical, uncooperative, or all too frequently inebriated, making the history unavailable or unreliable. There is seldom an old medical history to consult. Frequently there are no relatives or friends available who can elaborate on the medical history of the patient. The anesthesiologist must do the best possible preoperative evaluation with the information at hand. Intelligence, experience, and common sense play important roles in these situations.[8,16,35,39]

Minor orthopedic trauma is seldom emergent except when there is vascular compromise either by direct obstruction to blood flow or by obstruction related to increased intracompartmental pressures. In most of these cases there is sufficient time to obtain a history and perform an adequate physical examination. Such a patient is often healthy, and the injury is frequently an athletic injury or a household accident. Despite the apperance of the patient and the trivial nature of the accident, a careful preoperative evaluation should be performed. Even minor trauma may delay gastric emptying beyond the normal 4 to 8 hours. In addition, the patient may have received narcotic analgetics before coming to the operating room, which will further delay gastric empyting.[39] Simple methods of evaluating the intravascular volume should be used in all cases since such apparently minor injuries as lacerations to the highly vascular hand can result in significant blood loss. Heart rate, blood pressure, palpation of the pulse, and temperature of the extremities, in addition to hemoglobin and hematocrit studies, can yield valuable clues to intravascular volume status. Whether general or regional anesthesia is used, unanticipated hypovolemia can cause severe hypotension or cardiac arrest when the unsuspecting anesthesiologist does not take proper precautions. Whenever a minor injury results from a motor vehicle accident, the operation of heavy equipment, or similar circumstances, the anesthesiologist should be wary. Despite other physicians' best efforts many major injuries, such as deceleration injury to the aorta, ruptured spleen, and liver laceration, go undiagnosed only to manifest themselves during induction of anesthesia or later during the operation when making an accurate diagnosis can be extremely difficult.[14,35,39]

Major orthopedic trauma infrequently occurs as an isolated event. More often major orthopedic trauma is only one aspect of the polytraumatized patient whose initial surgery is directed at such immediate life-threatening injuries as the repair of major vascular or organ injury. Whenever feasible, however, major fractures should be stabilized during the patient's initial procedure. Surgery for major orthopedic trauma, whether isolated, part of surgery for polytrauma, or performed as a delayed procedure, has several unique aspects that require special attention in the preoperative evaluation.[14]

Obtaining a useful patient history may be extremely difficult in the absence of old medical records or a knowledgeable friend or relative. Although many traumatized patients are unconscious, those who are conscious may be of little help. Patients may not be able to offer useful information because of anxiety or a hysterical reaction.[39] However, the patient without a head injury who seems to be unable to give a useful history may be suffering from cerebral hypoxia or hypoglycemia. Diabetes is fairly common, particularly in the older age group. Trauma and hypovolemia further increase the possibility of hypoglycemia in the diabetic patient. Hypoxia may be related to hypotension secondary to hypovolemia or may be the result of an undiagnosed pneumothorax or fat embolism[17,20,59] (Table 21-4). Confusion in the traumatized patient is often the result of alcohol or drug use. In the United States approximately one half of the motor vehicle trauma victims are intoxicated, and more than 20% of those are simultaneous users of other drugs. Ingestion of alcohol and many abused drugs such as benzodiazepines, barbiturates, and cocaine reduces minimum alveolar concentration (MAC) and may interact with anesthetics in unexpected ways. Alcohol use reduces the patient's ability to withstand hemorrhage as well as increases the likelihood of hypothermia. Intoxicated patients tend to become hypoglycemic and may require glucose, which may be contraindicated if the

Table 21-4 Occurrence of diagnostic features of fat embolism	
Diagnostic feature	**Occurrence (% of patients)**
Fever	95-100
Increased alveolar–arterial oxygen gradient	95-100
Tachypnea	90-100
Tachycardia	80-95
Positive lung scan	70-85
Chest radiograph infiltrates	60-80
Mental status change	50-75
Petechiae	50-75

altered mental status is related to head injury.[8,10,60] The use of nitrous oxide in a patient who has an undiagnosed pneumothorax will exacerbate the condition.

The fat embolism syndrome develops in as many as 15% of patients with long bone or pelvic fractures. Changes in mental state such as drowsiness, confusion, and agitation may be caused by the hypoxia that results from the adult respiratory distress syndrome (ARDS) that accompanies fat embolism. Petechiae may not occur early and may be very transient when they do occur. Although a lung scan almost always confirms the diagnosis of fat embolism, it is seldom possible to obtain a scan in the emergency trauma victim. **The most consistent early signs of fat embolism are temperature elevation, tachycardia, and tachypnea.** These three signs in the presence of the appropriate fractures virtually assure the diagnosis of fat embolism, which can be confirmed with arterial blood gas determination.[17,20,59]

Unconsciousness or an altered mental state, for any of the preceding reasons, will deny the anesthesiologist valuable information that could have been obtained during the usual preoperative evaluation. Such important information as allergies, medications, and other concurrent acute or chronic diseases may be unknown. The anesthetic plan must incorporate this lack of knowledge. Much of the preoperative information may have to be obtained from laboratory studies and monitoring aids. An arterial catheter for direct continuous pressure monitoring as well as blood gas and other blood studies and a central venous or pulmonary artery catheter are invaluable aids in assessing preoperative status. Even when not absolutely indicated preoperatively, the anesthesiologist is wise to consider their placement in the trauma patient, because the unfolding of unanticipated events intraoperatively may necessitate their use at a time when their placement may be distracting and difficult. Insertion of a urinary catheter is virtually always indicated in the trauma patient not only to diagnose oliguria related to hypovolemia or renal trauma, but because many trauma surgeries take considerably longer than originally anticipated.

Except in cases of minor and isolated trauma, any trauma violent enough to cause major fractures should be assumed to have been sufficient to cause neck injuries. Therefore, unless cervical spine radiographs have been taken to confirm the absence of injury, **all trauma patients should be considered to be at risk for cervical spinal cord injury, including those with a clear sensorium and no symptoms.**[14,48] Also, since all trauma patients should be considered to have a full stomach, an awake intubation is mandatory if the cervical spine has not been cleared.

The traumatized patient presents multiple challenges to the anesthesiologist, not the least of which is obtaining a satisfactory preoperative evaluation. At the worst no history will be available and the entire basis of the perioperative evaluation will be based on a physical examination, laboratory studies, and the information gleaned from a careful choice of monitoring devices; caution and experience, therefore, are invaluable aids.

Reimplantation

Most if not all candidates for reimplantation of a digit or a limb are by definition reasonably young and healthy. Generally, reimplantation surgery is too long to expect that a patient can comfortably remain awake during a regional anesthetic. However, it is usually wise during the preoperative evaluation to obtain permission for a continuous regional anesthetic in combination with general anesthesia. **The sympathetic blockade provided by a regional technique makes the surgery technically easier and can be continued into the postoperative period, not only to provide analgesia but also to help ensure perfusion by blocking sympathetically mediated vasospasm.**

METHYLMETHACRYLATE AND TOTAL HIP ARTHROPLASTY

For the first few years after the introduction of total hip arthroplasty, it had the highest mortality associated with any noncardiac elective operation.[7,37] Since that time surgeons and anesthesiologists have become aware of the factors that set this operation apart from most other elective surgical procedures. There are several unique aspects of total hip arthroplasty that must be taken into consideration in the preoperative evaluation of these patients beyond the usual considerations. Most significant is the use of the methylmethacrylate cement to distribute the forces of the femoral and acetabular prosthetic components. Although once used in virtually all total hip arthroplasty procedures, because of improved prosthetic component design, methylmethacrylate is now used only when there is doubt of the ability of the bony seat to withstand the asymmetric stresses without fracturing, for example, in patients older than 70 years.

Methylmethacrylate has had a long history of use in medicine. In addition to its most common use today as the cement for total hip arthroplasty, it has been used as an internal cast for fractures, for prosthetic testicles, as pellets for plombage, to cover cranial defects, to encapsulate cerebral aneurysms, and for prosthetic middle ear ossicles. However, its use during total hip arthroplasty has some unique aspects, in particular, the large volume of the cement used and the fact that much of the curing process takes place within the body. Methylmethacrylate is supplied in two portions, a liquid portion, the monomer, and a powdered portion, prepolymerized methylmethacrylate. The powdered portion contains an activator that, when the two portions are mixed, causes the monomer to polymerize, entrapping the powdered long prepolymerized chains and forming the final cement. The polymerization reaction is exothermic. The cement does not hold the prosthesis in place but is used to distribute forces evenly from the prosthesis to the bone.

Most problems with methylmethacrylate use during total hip arthroplasty relate to the cementing in the femoral prosthesis. After the femoral shaft has been reamed out, incompletely cured methylmethacrylate is forced into the femoral shaft and held firmly in place until the curing process is complete. Unpolymerized monomer is volatile and can be absorbed into the circulation. The monomer, being volatile, can be eliminated through the lungs. The monomer that is not excreted through the lungs is metabolized, primarily in the Krebs cycle. However, while in the circulation the monomer may have cardiovascular effects. Evidence indicates that **the primary pharmacologic effect of the methylmethacrylate monomer is as a direct vasodilator.** The vasodilation usually occurs within the first minute after application and can last as long as 10 minutes.[5,7,26] **A second problem that can occur when the femoral prosthesis is inserted into the femoral canal is venous embolism.** When the prosthesis is forced into the femoral canal, any loose material, particles of methylmethacrylate, clots, fat, bone fragments, and air can be forced into the open venous sinuses of the bone.

It should be noted that when the femoral prosthesis is inserted circulating blood volume may be at its lowest because of unmeasured bleeding into the large muscles around the hip and the recent femoral reaming. Decreases in blood pressure, particularly systolic, frequently accompany the insertion of the femoral prosthesis, presumably primarily as a result of the vasodilating effect of circulating monomer. The magnitude of the decrease in blood pressure is directly related to existing blood pressure, age, blood loss, and inversely related to volume replacement. It is less severe during spinal or epidural anesthesia, especially if the blood pressure is not elevated at the time of prosthesis insertion.[5,7,26] Another consistent finding **at the time of femoral insertion is a decrease in the patient's Pao_2.** The decrease in Pao_2 is most likely related to pulmonary embolism of the various materials just mentioned. Typically a decrease of 20 to 80 mm Hg is seen. This also occurs within the first minute after insertion of the prosthesis and can last for several minutes.

The combination of arterial hypotension caused by circulating monomer and pulmonary hypertension related to pulmonary embolism may cause a reversal in the left-to-right atrial pressure gradient. This is even more likely if general anesthesia and positive pressure ventilation are used. If a paradoxical atrial pressure gradient occurs, it will occur just when embolic material may be passing through the right atrium. Several autopsy reports have confirmed left-sided embolism after deaths during total hip arthroplasty.

These unique features of total hip arthroplasty must be considered during the preoperative evaluation and anesthetic planning. The usual reason for total hip arthroplasty is pain and subsequent loss of function. Osteoarthritis is the most common etiology. Osteoarthritis is more common with advancing age. These patients can be expected to have the usual array of diseases afflicting the older population. Hypertension is a common concurrent disease and will predispose such patients to greater degrees of hypotension because of the circulating monomer when the femoral cement and prosthesis are inserted. For this reason hypertension should be under the best possible control before surgery is scheduled.[5] Cardiac function may also be reduced as a result of the inactivity mandated by the painful hip. Further, this activity limitation can prevent adequate preoperative stress testing. Therefore all cardiac and antihypertensive medications should be carefully reviewed and adjusted if necessary. Because of the painful and chronic nature of the disease, patients with osteoarthritis usually have a long history of analgetic use. Most take nonsteroidal antiinflammatory drugs. The coagulopathy associated with nonsteroidal antiinflammatory drug use may cause increased intraoperative bleeding and, equally important, may preclude the use of spinal or epidural anesthesia. Others may take narcotic analgetics that may alter anesthetic requirements and may complicate postoperative pain management. Older patients may have varying degrees of pulmonary impairment wherein any decrease in Pao_2, as might be expected at the time of prosthesis insertion, may lead to dangerous levels of hypoxia. Most surgeons perform total hip arthroplasty with the patient in the lateral position. Because older patients may have an obstruction to carotid and/or vertebral artery blood flow, they should be checked preoperatively for the development of neurologic symptoms with the head in the various positions that might occur during the operation.

Rheumatoid arthritis is another common cause of hip problems requiring total hip arthroplasty surgery. Although patients in this group may be younger, many are older and deserve the same considerations as patients with osteoarthritis. Patients with rheumatoid arthritis, however, may have a myriad of other problems (mentioned earlier in this chapter) that warrant special attention during the preoperative evaluation. Rheumatoid arthritis may affect a number of joints that can make airway management difficult. Temporomandibular ankylosis will severely restrict mouth opening and may make oral intubation impossible. Mouth opening should always be checked during the preoperative evaluation of patients with rheumatoid arthritis. Arthritis of the cricoarytenoid joints occurs in as many as 40% of patients with rheumatoid arthritis. A history of breathing problems, dyspnea, hoarseness, stridor, or sore throat may indicate acute exacerbations of chronic cricoarytenoiditis. During general anesthesia cricoarytenoiditis may cause airway obstruction and may make intubation difficult or impossible. Trauma during intubation or extubation has caused acute postoperative airway obstruction in patients with chronic cricoarytenoiditis. Ankylosis of the cervical spine can further impair airway maintenance and intubation. Rheumatoid lung involvement, such as cystic honeycombing, rheumatoid nodules, or diffuse interstitial fibrosis, may impair oxygenation and result in dangerous desaturation at the time of prosthesis insertion. Rheumatoid disease of the spine and ribs causing decreased compliance can further aggravate pulmonary problems.

Avascular necrosis of the femoral head, a complication of sickle cell disease, is another source of total hip arthroplasty patients. As discussed elsewhere in this text, patients with sickle cell disease may have multiple organ problems as a result of their disease. Of particular importance to the patient with sickle cell disease who is scheduled for total hip arthroplasty are other joint problems and oxygenation. These patients may have other joints that are fused or deformed because of previous bleeding diastheses. A careful history of other joint problems is essential because special care must be taken in positioning such patients so as not to aggravate preexisting joint problems. Oxygenating, however, is a more critical issue. Pulmonary function may already be decreased as a result of sickle cell lung infarcts. Patients with sickle cell disease invariably have an unrelenting anemia. Impaired pulmonary gas exchange combined with anemia will ensure decreased oxyhemoglobin saturations. In addition, with the potential for abrupt decreases in PaO_2 during femoral prosthesis insertion, care must be taken to avoid a sickle cell crisis.[5] Most, if not all, patients with sickle cell disease should have a preoperative rapid exchange transfusion. Care must also be exercised to prevent an overzealous exchange transfusion that results in too high a hematocrit level that impairs flow characteristics and promotes sludging. Use of a regional anesthesia is clearly the best choice since sympathetic blockade promotes good blood flow and oxygenation, lessens the chance of acute hypotension at the time of prosthesis insertion, and aids in the maintenance of body temperature.

A number of other diseases may be the antecedent cause for total hip replacement. In each instance the specific problems associated with the disease and any other diseases the patient may have must be viewed in light of the unique problems associated with the use of methylmethacrylate and prosthesis insertion during total hip arthroplasty.

Although methylmethacrylate is used during total knee arthroplasties, its use during this operation is not of the same order of concern as during the total hip arthroplasty. Patients have the same antecedent and concurrent diseases; however, the exposure to the uncured cement is much smaller, blood loss is limited and related to the use of a tourniquet, and there is no extensive intramedullary reaming; therefore the risk of embolism is much smaller. If problems occur, they will manifest themselves on release of the tourniquet. Similarly, problems associated with the use of methylmethacrylate during shoulder arthroplasty surgery are seldom of major cardiovascular significance.

INTEGRATING ANESTHESIA AND SURGERY

Orthopedic surgery, because of the variety of procedures and the fact that virtually every area of the body is a potential operative site, requires that the anesthesiologist have a knowledge of the particular surgeon, the operation, the positioning of the patient, and the duration of the operative procedure. In addition, because many orthopedic procedures can be performed with the patient under regional anesthesia, an understanding of the emotional and intellectual state of the patient is essential. A patient's reactions to the circumstances of the surgery may pose problems that are as serious and as important as the medical aspects of the anesthetic itself. It is valuable to integrate all of these aspects of the surgery and the patient with the usual medical information that is obtained during the preoperative evaluation to ensure a successful intraoperative course.

The length of the surgical procedure will affect the choice of anesthetic technique. Although catheters permit most regional anesthetic techniques to last as long as desired, other considerations may dictate use of either general anesthesia or combined regional and general anesthesia. Even in the supine position most patients become very uncomfortable after lying on a flat operating room table for more than several hours. Narcotics for this sort of discomfort unnecessarily depress respiration. In these situations using hypnotics in an attempt to control discomfort often results in a disinhibited, uncontrollable patient when use of a general or a combined regional and general anesthetic would have been preferable. In a patient with a history of myocardial ischemia the respiratory depression from narcotics or the hypertension and tachycardia from disinhibition and confusion secondary to sedatives may outweigh the advantages of regional anesthesia.

Conversely, some orthopedic procedures, such as examination or manipulation under anesthesia, or removal of external fixation devices, cause intense pain but may be so brief that in most cases the duration of regional anesthesia and the possibility of toxic reactions from such misadventures as intravascular injection of local anesthetics would indicate that use of a brief general anesthetic may often be the best choice.

Knowledge and understanding of the patient obtained as part of the preoperative evaluation can prevent what would otherwise have been a perfect regional anesthetic from becoming a painful and frightening experience for the patient and an unsatisfying one for the anesthesiologist and surgeon. Noises from power tools such as drills and saws or the sound of mallet hitting chisel can unnerve some patients. Many common intraoperative manipulations or movements are interpreted by patients as violent. Careful evaluation and patient selection as well as appropriate explanations at the time of the preoperative interview of what can be anticipated during surgery with regional anesthesia will obviate the need for excessive sedation or conversion of a regional anesthetic into an unnecessary general anesthetic.

Positioning of the patient during surgery should be considered at the time of the preoperative evaluation. Various orthopedic procedures are performed with patients in almost every possible position—supine, prone, lateral, and sitting. The issues of proper positioning, support, and padding are discussed in Chapter 38. However, the effects of these positions should be considered during the preoperative evaluation. Many orthopedic patients' diseases or deformities limit the extent to which they can be ideally positioned. Pressure necroses and fractures can result from exceeding these limits unknowingly after either regional or general anesthesia has been instituted. Whenever there is any doubt, the patient should be asked to assume the operative position during the preoperative evaluation. Many older patients who will be in either the lateral or prone position for their surgery may have arteriosclerosis. In these positions the head is often turned to an unusual position. If there is significant carotid obstruction because of arteriosclerosis, unusual head positions may seriously impair already marginal cerebral blood flow. If there is a carotid bruit or other reason to suspect carotid insufficiency, the patient should be asked to hold the head in various positions emulating the possibilities during surgery while the anesthesiologist looks for neurologic symptoms or signs. Typical symptoms that will occur within 1 or 2 minutes are visual obscurations, slurring of speech, lightheadedness, or confu-

sion and possible loss of consciousness. Most of these symptoms may be misinterpreted during use of regional anesthesia if analgetics or hypnotics are used and will go totally unnoticed if general anesthesia is used.

Orthopedists frequently require tourniquets during extremity surgery. Whether the anesthesiologist is primarily responsible for the tourniquet or not, he/she is invariably in a position to monitor proper tourniquet procedure and function. Although tourniquets seldom cause major problems, there are a number of potential problems that warrant attention during the preoperative evaluation. **Tourniquets can cause nerve damage.** It is believed that nerve damage results primarily from pressure and anatomic distortion, not primarily ischemia. Properly placed tourniquets inflated to appropriate pressures for less than 3 hours rarely cause nerve injury. Improper tourniquet sizes, padding, or inflation pressures are usually responsible for nerve damage.[43] Characteristically, excessive tourniquet pressure causes deformation of the nerve at the edges of the tourniquet cuff. Nerves are stretched at these areas. Myelinated nerves may have the paranodal myelin stretched on one side of the node and invaginated on the other side. Because there is no similar movement of the Schwann cell junction, there can be local rupture of the Schwann cell membrane and subsequent nerve damage. The careful anesthesiologist makes notes during the preoperative evaluation of the neurologic status of the limb in question to avoid accusations of negligence in monitoring tourniquet use or the implication that a regional nerve block procedure caused nerve injury.

Tourniquet inflation and deflation can cause hemodynamic changes that must be considered during the preoperative evaluation. Patients with cardiac disease or hypertension, especially during general anesthesia, are at greater risk. Exsanguination of a lower extremity, transfusing the central circulation with as much as 500 ml of blood, followed by the sudden inflation of a tourniquet, causing both pain and an abrupt increase in systemic vascular resistance, will often cause a marked increase in blood pressure.[57] Deflation of a tourniquet also causes a simultaneous decrease in systemic vascular resistance and a decrease in venous return, or a brief relative hypovolemia, while the vascular bed in the extremity fills with blood. In addition, muscle blood flow to the limb will remain 5 to 10 times normal for up to 15 minutes after tourniquet deflation.[56] In patients at risk for these hemodynamic variations preoperative attention to optimizing cardiac and antihypertensive medications is important. The current evidence indicates that these hemodynamic changes can be ameliorated by the use of regional anesthesia techniques either alone or in combination with general anesthesia.[56]

During tourniquet inflation, the operative limb, not being perfused, will decrease in temperature in direct relation to total tourniquet time. Deflation of the tourniquet and reperfusion of the ischemic limb will cool the perfusing blood and subsequently reduce core body temperature. After 1 hour of leg tourniquet time, reperfusion will typically cause core body temperature to decrease by approximately 0.6° C.

Finally, consideration must be given to the effects on arterial blood gases and serum electrolytes that occur when reperfusion of the ischemic limb begins after tourniquet deflation. Some preoperative conditions or laboratory findings that otherwise would be of minor consequence may be considerably more important in view of the changes that can be anticipated following tourniquet deflation. Tourniquet inflation times longer than one half hour result in anaerobic metabolism. Reperfusion after a period of anaerobic metabolism will have systemic effects. Pao_2 may decrease by 20 to 30 mm Hg. $Paco_2$ may increase as much as 20 mm Hg. As a result of a mixed respiratory and metabolic acidosis, pH can decrease by 0.2 units, standard bicarbonate increases, and serum lactate increases. Serum potassium has been observed to increase by more than 0.5 mmol/L. The combination of these changes all occurring at the same time is potentially dangerous, particularly in patients with cardiac and pulmonary disease.[4]

PLANNING THE ANESTHETIC

Although a more complete discussion of the anesthetic management of patients undergoing orthopedic procedures is considered in Chapter 84, many aspects of the anesthetic plan for orthopedic surgery are discussed with the patient, decided on, and instituted during the preoperative evaluation. General issues such as the timing of procedure, the choice of anesthetic techniques, appropriate premedication, monitoring, management of blood loss, and possibilities for postoperative analgesia must be integrated into a coherent plan of perioperative medical and anesthetic management of the patient.

The timing of the orthopedic procedure is usually left to the surgeon; however, there are times when decisions about the appropriate time to perform the planned procedure can be a vexing issue. Safety, convenience, and cost are all matters that must be considered. In today's environment many patients scheduled for major elective surgery are not admitted until the day of surgery. Previously unsuspected medical problems that are discovered just before surgery present real dilemmas to the anesthesiologist; balancing the cost and inconvenience of delaying surgery against the risks of proceeding requires considerable judgment and experience.

Nonelective orthopedic procedures range from absolute emergencies to cases whose urgency can be measured in days. Neurovascular compromise from fractures or dislocations, spinal fractures that cause cord compression, compartment syndromes, and open fractures all require immediate attention. The uncontrollable hemorrhage of unstable pelvic fractures necessitates their immediate fixation and stabilization. Certain unreducible dislocations (shoulder, hip, knee, talus) are emergencies. Likewise, any delay in reimplantation surgery drastically reduces the chances of success. In such absolute emergencies the anesthesiologist must obtain as much preoperative information as possible and simply cope with the problems and the unknowns. Seldom is there sufficient risk to warrant a delay in dealing with these limb-threatening diseases.

A few procedures constitute relative emergencies so that they can be delayed while other lifesaving surgery is performed or while time is taken to treat serious medical conditions that would pose great anesthetic risks. Thoughtful use of time in such instances as femoral neck fractures or skeletal stabilization of multitrauma victims is important since the results deteriorate rapidly with time.

Finally, urgent cases such as open reductions with internal fixation or hip fractures can be safely delayed for 48 to 72 hours if the patient's medical condition or other factors dictate. Even in these urgent cases, however, usually the longer the delay the more difficult for the surgeon to achieve an optimal outcome.

In these cases in which there are varying degrees of surgical urgency and a wide range of anesthetic risks, an intelligent and forthright dialog between the orthopedist and anesthesiologist will always clarify the situation and ensure the best care for the patient.

Anesthetic Technique

More frequently in orthopedic surgery than in most other surgical subspecialties there are several distinctly different anesthetic techniques from which to choose.[54] **Regional techniques are available for the majority of orthopedic operations.** Although sufficient reliable data are lacking, most anesthesiologists believe and there is considerable logic to support the view that, whenever possible, regional anesthetic techniques or combined regional and general anesthetic techniques are safer than general anesthetic alone techniques. The details of the techniques and intraoperative management are discussed in more detail in Chapter 84. However, it is **during the preoperative evaluation that the anesthesiologist, based on the patient's medical condition and the procedure to be performed, decides on the technique to be preferred and discusses this with the patient.**

Many patients are reluctant to have regional anesthesia. It is during the preoperative evaluation that the anesthesiologist establishes a relationship with the patient and gains the patient's confidence in his/her knowledge and abilities. This relationship and confidence allow the anesthesiologist to explain and convince the anxious patient that the technique selected is the appropriate one for the particular patient. This effort is made much easier by the orthopedic surgeon who understands the benefits to the patient of different anesthetic techniques and helps the anesthesiologist with difficult patients.

Premedication

One of the final tasks of the anesthesiologist's preoperative evaluation is the ordering of premedication. Naturally, the choice of premedication depends on a number of factors: age, medical conditions, anxiety, pain, the time of surgery, anesthetic technique, and surgical procedure. Although there are a number of rules of thumb, the anesthesiologist uses experience and his/her feel for the patient, developed during the preoperative interview, to individualize the drugs to be used, dosages to be administered, route of administration, and the timing of administration. Traditionally, three types of drugs, separately or in combination, have been used: antisialogogues, hypnotic/sedatives, and narcotics. More recently, it has become popular to omit premedication altogether and administer premedication-type drugs intravenously just before the beginning of anesthesia. In the case of antisialogogues the latter method is almost always preferred. Currently, the benzodiazepines are used almost exclusively as the drug for preoperative sedation/anxiolysis. They can be administered before the patient comes to the operating area or intravenously in the operating room area. The decision to use a preoperative benzodiazepine is usually based on the need for anxiolysis. The excellent anxiolysis of the benzodiazepines must be balanced against the possibility of oversedation, particularly in the elderly, and consequent uncooperativeness and incoherence of the patient as well as the desirability or undesirability of amnesia. Narcotic premedication, which has fallen from favor with many anesthesiologists, is often the ideal choice for regional anesthetic techniques. Like benzodiazepines, narcotics can be given before the patient comes to the operating room or intravenously after the patient has arrived in the operating room area. Narcotics provide mild sedation and euphoria without impairing cognitive function. Narcotic analgesia lessens the patient's discomfort during the needle placements and the injections that are essential to the performance of a regional anesthetic. This combination of effects allows the patient to be reasonably comfortable during a regional block procedure while also being able to provide the information that the anesthesiologist often needs to confirm accurate needle placement. Narcotics have the additional benefit of having a specific antagonist should the effect be more than desired.

Anticipating Blood Loss

Many orthopedic procedures incur sufficient blood loss to require blood transfusion. The dangers and undesirability of homologous blood transfusions are well known. Although with the encouragement of the surgeon many patients now predeposit several units of their own blood, this may not be sufficient to replace all of the intraoperative and postoperative blood loss or it may simply not be possible for a patient to predeposit blood. With intelligent preoperative planning the anaesthesiologist can reduce the number of or eliminate the need for homologous transfusions. **Among the strategies available to the anesthesiologist to limit the need for blood transfusions are the use of regional anesthetic techniques, deliberate hypotension, hemodilution, and immediate preoperative blood harvesting.** All of these techniques require planning that is part of the preoperative evaluation. Deliberate hypotension requires careful preoperative assessment of renal function and cardiovascular status, particularly in the older patient population. Hemodilution will reduce the red cell mass lost per volume of intraoperative blood loss; however, patients with limited cardiovascular reserve may be at risk as a result of the volume loading required. Immediate preoperative blood harvesting also stresses both renal and cardiovascular systems. These methods can be of great help in minimizing the need for transfusions in many patients; however, careful preoperative assessment and planning are essential to their success.

SUMMARY

The orthopedic surgeon brings to the operating room some of the greatest challenges for the anesthesiologist. The range of various factors, such as age, health status, disease processes, the urgency of surgery, and the type and extent of operative procedures, provide a bewildering list of possible combinations of circumstances with which an anesthesiologist may be asked to cope. This is in contrast to many other surgical specialties in which patient factors and operative procedures are much more predictable from day to day. It is for these reasons that the preoperative evaluation of the orthopedic patient is so important. More frequently than in other operative areas the preoperative planning of anesthetic management for orthopedic surgery requires the integration of many unpredictable factors to formulate an effective and innovative plan for a particular patient and procedure.

KEY POINTS

- Osteoarthritis is the most common rheumatologic disease, accounting for the majority of total hip and total knee replacements in the United States. Its hallmark is the loss of articular cartilage.

- Rheumatoid arthritis affects approximately 1% of adults in the United States; women are affected two to three times more often then men.

- The revised criteria for diagnosis of rheumatoid arthritis include morning stiffness, arthritis of three or more joints, hand arthritis, symmetry of involvement, rheumatoid nodules, serum rheumatoid factor, and radiographic changes. The cervical spine is commonly involved, especially with subluxation of C1 on C2.

- The seronegative spondyloarthropathies are distinguished from rheumatoid arthritis by their involvement of the joints of the spine and their asymmetric involvement of the large joints.

- Preoperative attention to the spine, heart, and lung is essential in the patient with ankylosing spondylitis.

- The patient with systemic lupus erythematosus exhibits effects on internal vital organs, and signs and symptoms include chest pains, shortness of breath, cough, pleural effusions, pleuritis or pneumonia, and cardiac manifestations.

- Marfan's syndrome is an autosomal dominant–inherited disease characterized by above-average height; arachnodactyly; lax, hypermobile joints; and cardiac and pulmonary manifestations such as apical bullae, defects in the media of the wall of the ascending aorta, and risk of mitral valve prolapse.

- Osteogenesis imperfecta is best defined as a congenital "condition of abnormal fragility and plasticity of bone with recurring fractures on minimal trauma"; the physical examination should especially address the airway.

- Preoperative evaluation of the patient with scoliosis should include pulmonary function studies when the curvature is greater than 65 degrees. Vital capacity less than 30% of predicted usually implies the need for postoperative mechanical ventilation.

- Because of the possibility and nature of infections, open fractures of joints are truly emergency situations. Similarly, fractures that cause vascular occlusion or a compartment syndrome can be limb threatening.

- In as many as 15% of patients with long bone or pelvic fractures the fat embolism syndrome develops, characterized by consistent early signs of temperature elevation, tachycardia, and tachypnea.

- All trauma patients should be considered to be at risk for cervical spinal cord injury. Since these patients are also treated as having a full stomach, an awake intubation is mandatory if the cervical spine has not been cleared.

- Sympathetic blockade provided by a regional anesthetic technique makes the surgery for reimplantation technically easier and can be continued into the postoperative period not only to provide analgesia but also to help ensure perfusion by blocking sympathetically mediated vasospasm.

- Among the strategies available to the anesthesiologist to limit the need for blood transfusions are the use of regional anesthetic techniques, deliberate hypertension, hemodilution, and immediate preoperative blood harvesting.

KEY REFERENCES

Calin A: Ankylosing spondylitis. In Kelley WN, Harris ED Jr, Ruddy S et al, eds: *Textbook of rheumatology,* Philadelphia, 1989, WB Saunders.

Harris ED Jr: The clinical features of rheumatoid arthritis. In Kelley WN, Harris ED Jr, Ruddy S et al, eds: *Textbook of rheumatology,* Philadelphia, 1989, WB Saunders.

Mankin HJ: Clinical features of osteoarthritis. In Kelley WN, Harris ED Jr, Ruddy S et al, eds: *Textbook of rheumatology,* Philadelphia, 1989, WB Saunders.

Milne BR, Jenkins MT: Anesthetic considerations in the multiply injured adult. In Meyers MH, ed: *The multiply injured patient with complex fractures,* Philadelphia, 1984, Lea & Febiger.

Salem MR: Anesthesia for orthopedic surgery. In Gregory GA, ed: *Pediatric anesthesia,* New York, 1983, Churchill-Livingstone.

Wilkins KE: Fat embolism. In Zauder HL, ed: *Anesthesia for orthopedic surgery,* Philadelphia, 1980, FA Davis.

REFERENCES

1. Alarcon-Segovia D: Systemic lupus erythematosus: pathology and pathogensis. In Schumacher HR Jr, Kippel JH, Robinson DR et al, eds: *Primer on the rheumatic diseases.* Atlanta, 1988, Arthritis Foundation.

2. Asheron RA, Graham RV: Systemic lupus erythematosus: clinical features. In Schumacher HR Jr, Kippel JH, Robinson DR et al, eds: *Primer on the rheumatic diseases,* Atlanta, 1988, Arthritis Foundation.

3. Bennett JC: Rheumatoid arthritis: clinical features. In Schumacher HR Jr, Kippel JH, Robinson DR et al, eds: *Primer on the rheumatic diseases,* Atlanta, 1988, Arthritis Foundation.

4. Benzon HT, Toleikis JR, Meagher LL et al: Changes in venous blood lactate, venous blood gases, and somatosensory evoked potentials after tourniquet application, *Anesthesiology* 69:677, 1988.

5. Bernstein RL: Anesthesia for total hip replacement. In Zauder HL, ed: *Anesthesia for orthopedic surgery,* Philadelphia: 1980, FA Davis.

6. Betcher AM: Development of anesthesia for orthopedic surgery. In Zauder HL, ed: *Anesthesia for orthopedic surgery,* Philadelphia, 1980, FA Davis.

7. Bourke DL, Lawrence J: Methylmethacrylate and the cardiovascular system, *Anesth Rev* 4:27, 1977.

8. Bourke DL, Rosenberg MB, and Schmidt KF: Anesthesia for the trauma patient. *Orthop Clin North Am* 9:661, 1978.

9. Brandt KD, Fife RS: Aging in relation to the pathogenesis of osteoarthritis, *Clin Rheumatol Dis* 12:117, 1986.

10. Bruce DL: Alcoholism and anesthesia, *Anesth Analg* 62:84, 1983.

11. Calin A: Ankylosing spondylitis and the spondylarthropathies. In Schumacher HR Jr, Kippel JH, Robinson DR et al, eds: *Primer on the rheumatic diseases,* Atlanta, 1988, Arthritis Foundation.

12. Calin A: Ankylosing spondylitis. In Kelley WN, Harris ED Jr, Ruddy S et al, eds: *Textbook of rheumatology,* Philadelphia, 1989, WB Saunders.

13. Clark CR, Goetz DD, and Memezes AH: Arthrodesis in the cervical spine in rheumatoid arthritis, *J Bone Joint Surg [Am]* 71:381, 1989.

14. Claudi BF, Meyers MH: Priorities in the treatment of the multiply injured patient with musculoskeletal injuries. In Meyers MH, ed: *The multiply injured patient with complex fractures,* Philadelphia, 1984, Lea & Febiger.

15. Cropp GV, Meyers DN: Physiological evidence of hypermetabolism in osteogenesis imperfecta, *Pediatrics* 49:375, 1972.

16. Donegan J: Overview of anesthesia for emergency surgery. In Donegan J, ed: *Manual of anesthesia for emergency surgery,* New York, 1987, Churchill-Livingstone.

17. Evarts CM: The fat embolism syndrome. In Meyers MH, ed: *The multiply injured patient with complex fractures,* Philadelphia, 1984, Lea & Febiger.

18. Falvo KA, Klein DB, Krauss AN et al: Pulmonary function studies in osteogenesis imperfecta, *Am Rev Respir Dis* 108: 1258, 1973.

19. Grundy BL: Intraoperative monitoring of sensory-evoked potentials, *Anesthesiology* 58:72, 1983.

20. Guenter CA, Braun TE: Fat embolism syndrome: changing prognosis, *Chest* 79(2):143, 1981.

21. Harris ED Jr: The clinical features of rheumatoid arthritis. In Kelley WN, Harris ED Jr, Ruddy S et al, eds: *Textbook of rheumatology,* Philadelphia, 1989, WB Saunders.

22. Harris ED Jr: Rheumatoid arthritis: pathophysiology and implications for therapy, *N Engl J Med* 322:1277, 1990.

23. Hochberg MC: Epidemiology of the rheumatic diseases. In Schumacher HR Jr, Kippel JH, Robinson DR et al, eds: *Primer of the rheumatic diseases,* Atlanta, 1988, Arthritis Foundation.

24. Holtby HM, Relton JES: Orthopedic diseases. In Katz J, Steward DJ, eds: *Anesthesia and uncommon pediatric diseases,* Philadelphia, 1987, WB Saunders.

25. Hough AJ et al: Aging phenomena and osteoarthritis: cause or coincidence? *Ann Clin Lab Sci* 16:502, 1986.

26. Kim KC, Ritter MA: Hypotension associated with methylmethacrylate in total hip arthroplasties, *Clin Orthop Rel Research* 88(10):154, 1972.

27. LaCroix AZ, Wienpahl J, White LR et al: Thiazide diuretic agents and the incidence of hip fracture, *N Engl J Med* 322(5):286, 1990.

28. Libman RH: Anesthetic considerations for the patient with osteogenesis imperfecta, *Clin Orthop* 159:123, 1981.

29. Lipson SJ: The cervical spine. In Kelley WN, Harris ED Jr, Ruddy S et al, eds: *Textbook of rheumatology,* Philadelphia, 1989, WB Saunders Co.

30. Lipson SJ: Rheumatoid arthritis in the cervical spine, *Clin Orthop* 239:121, 1989.

31. MacEwan GD, Bunnell WP, and Sriram K: Acute neurological complications in the treatment of scoliosis, *J Bone Joint Surg [Am]* 57(3):404, 1975.

32. Mankin HJ: Clinical features of osteoarthritis. In Kelly WN, Harris ED Jr, Ruddy S et al, eds: *Textbook of rheumatology,* Philadelphia, 1989, WB Saunders.

33. Mankin HJ, Brandt KD: Pathogensis of osteoarthritis. In Kelly WN, Harris ED Jr, Ruddy S et al, eds: *Textbook of rheumatology,* Philadelphia, 1989, WB Saunders.

34. Mankin HJ, Brandt KD, and Shulman LE: Workshop on etiopathogenesis of osteoarthritis, *J Rheumatol* 13:1127, 1986.

35. McFee AS, Franklin ME: Evaluation of the patient with multiple injuries. In Zauder HL, ed: *Anesthesia for orthopedic surgery,* Philadelphia, 1980, FA Davis.

36. McPherson RW, Mahla M, Johnson R et al: Effects of enflurane, isoforane, and nitrous oxide on somatosensory evoked potential during fentanyl anesthesia, *Anesthesiology* 62:626, 1985.

37. Melton LJ, Stauffer RN, Chao EYS et al: Rates of total hip arthroplasty, *N Engl J Med* 307:1242, 1982.

38. Mikkelson WN et al: Age-sex specific prevalence of radiologic abnormalities of the hands, wrists, and cervical spine of adult residents of the Tecumseh, Michigan, community health study area, 1962-1965, *J Chronic Dis* 23:151, 1970.

39. Milne BR, Jenkins MT: Anesthetic considerations in the multiple injured adult. In Meyers MH, ed: *The multiply injured patient with complex fractures,* Philadelphia, 1984, Lea & Febiger.

40. Moskowitz WR: Clinical and laboratory findings in osteoarthritis. In McCarty DJ, ed: *Arthritis and allied conditions. A textbook of rheumatology,* Philadelphia, 1989, Lea & Febiger.

41. Moskowitz WR, Goldberg VM: Osteoarthritis. In Schumacher HR Jr, Kippel JH, Robinson DR et al, eds: *Primer on the rheumatic diseases,* Atlanta, 1988, Arthritis Foundation.

42. Nash CL, Brown RH: Current concepts review: spinal cord monitoring, *J Bone Joint Surg [Am]* 71:627, 1989.

43. Ochoa J, Fowler TJ, and Gilliatt RW: Anatomical changes in peripheral nerves compressed by a pneumatic tourniquet, *J Anat* 113(3):433, 1972.

44. Pyeritz RE: Heritable disorders of connective tissue. In Schumacher HR Jr, Kippel JH, Robinson DR et al, eds: *Primer on the rheumatic diseases,* Atlanta, 1988, Arthritis Foundation.

45. Ranawat CS: Cervical spine fusion in rheumatoid arthritis, *J Bone Joint Surg [Am]* 61:1003, 1979.

46. Read CJ, Mennen U: Cervical spine instability in rheumatoid arthritis, *S Afr Med J* 63:116, 1983.

47. Salem MR: Anesthesia for orthopedic surgery. In Gregory GA, ed: *Pediatric anesthesia,* New York, 1983, Churchill-Livingstone.

48. Schaefer SD, Anderson RG, and Carder HM: Management of the upper airway in the injured patient. In Meyers MH, ed: *The multiply injured patient with complex fractures,* Philadelphia, 1984, Lea & Febiger.

49. Schur PR: Clinical features of SLE. In Kelley WN, Harris ED Jr, Ruddy S et al, eds: *Textbook of rheumatology,* Philadelphia, 1989, WB Saunders.

50. Simmons EH: Flexion deformities of the neck and ankylosing spondylitis, *J Bone Joint Surg* 51:193, 1969.

51. Steinberg AD: Management of systemic lupus erythematosus. In Kelly WN, Harris ED Jr, Ruddy S et al, eds: *Textbook of rheumatology,* Philadelphia, 1989, WB Saunders.

52. Stoltz MR et al: Osteogenesis imperfecta perspectives, *Clin Orthop* 242:120, 1989.

53. Anesthesia for orthopedic surgery. In *Orthopedic knowledge,* Park Ridge, Ill,

1990, American Academy of Orthopedic Surgeons.

54. See reference 53.

55. Arthritis. In *Orthopedic knowledge update,* Park Ridge, Ill, 1990, American Academy of Orthopedic Surgeons.

56. Valli H, Rosenberg PH: Effects of three anesthesia methods on haemodynamic responses connected with the use of thigh tourniquet in orthopaedic patients, *Acta Anaesthesiol Scand* 29:142, 1985.

57. Valli H, Rosenberg PH, Kytta J et al: Arterial hypertension associated with the use of a tourniquet with either general or regional anaesthesia, *Acta Anaesthesiol Scand* 31:279, 1987.

58. Whelton A, Stout RL, Spilman PS et al: Renal effects of ibuprofen, piroxicam, and sulindac in patients with asymptomatic renal failure: a prospective, randomized crossover comparison, *Ann Intern Med* 112:568, 1990.

59. Wilkins KE: Fat embolism. In Zauder HL, ed: *Anesthesia for orthopedic surgery,* Philadelphia, 1980, FA Davis.

60. Wolfson B: Acute and chronic alcohol abuse. In Donegan J, ed: *Manual of anesthesia for emergency surgery,* New York, 1987, Churchill-Livingstone.

61. Zaleske DJ, Doppelt SJ, and Mankin H: Metabolic and endocrine abnormalities of the immature skeleton. In Lovell WW, Winter RB, eds: *Pediatric orthopedics,* Philadelphia, 1986, WB Saunders.

CHAPTER 22

Evaluation of the Patient with Oncologic Disease

DAWN P. DESIDERIO
RONALD A. KROSS
ROBERT F. BEDFORD

Modern cancer treatment regimens often incorporate the combined modalities of surgery, radiation, and chemotherapy, all of which may affect the anesthesiologist. Advances in the diagnosis and treatment of various cancers have led to an ever-increasing number of patients with cancer who present for both elective and emergency surgery. Optimal anesthetic management for the cancer patient, however, requires an understanding of the anatomic and pathophysiologic disturbances associated with the patient's malignancy and a knowledge of the potentially adverse effects of prior anticancer treatments.[17,51]

ANATOMIC DISTURBANCES ASSOCIATED WITH CANCER

Airway Problems

Causes of the difficult airway

Airway compromise in the cancer patient is most often associated with upper airway obstruction, hemorrhage, or infection. Indeed, problems with airway management have been identified as the most common cause of anesthesia-related injuries,[10] whether related to primary airway pathologic conditions or to complications of cancer therapy. Upper airway obstruction occurs most often with progressive growth of cancers of the larynx, pharynx, thyroid, and base of the tongue.[81] These lesions are usually slow growing and take weeks to months before reaching sufficient size to produce clinically significant respiratory problems.[18,25] Progressive hoarseness, dysphagia, odynophagia, and speech disturbances are early symptoms that are often overlooked until **increasing dyspnea and inspiratory stridor herald impending respiratory compromise** that requires prompt investigation and treatment. Thus these patients may be scheduled for either curative or palliative surgery and may present either as elective or emergent cases.

Evaluation of the difficult airway

Every patient with head and neck cancer should be considered a difficult intubation case since the primary tumor and previous radiation and surgical therapy all conspire to alter the normal flexibility and anatomic relationships of the airway. Various risk factors have been investigated to predict the difficult

---

BOX 22-1
FACTORS USED TO EVALUATE THE
DIFFICULT AIRWAY

Degree of micrognathia
Cleft, high-arched palate
Protruding teeth
Loose or capped teeth
Prosthetic devices
Temporomandibular joint mobility
Cervical spine mobility
Visualization of soft palate, uvula
Distance between lower border mandible and
  thyroid notch
Palpable neck mass
Tracheal deviation
Scars from previous head and neck surgery
Mobility of larynx after radiation

---

intubation[48,90] (Box 22-1). In brief, a detailed history and physical examination, including indirect laryngoscopy, appropriate radiographic studies, and careful planning by the surgeon and the anesthesia care team are all required.

In assessing the patient with head and neck cancer for difficulty during intubation, the clinician should view the patient in profile so that visible anatomic disturbances such as micrognathia and the degree of incisor prominence are readily detectable. Furthermore, the patient should be requested to open the mouth to document temporomandibular joint mobility, the presence of prosthetic devices, and loose or capped teeth. Voluntary or painful limitation of motion will disappear once anesthesia is induced. Structural defects, however, will remain to plague the anesthetist. Having the patient protrude the tongue helps in visualizing the soft palate, uvula, and faucial pillars. It has been suggested that easy visualization of these structures predicts an easy intubation,[48] whereas a difficult intubation can be anticipated if only the soft palate can be seen.

The distance between the lower border of the mandible and the thyroid notch has also been used to assess the ease of intubation. In adult patients, the rule of 6.5 cm is important to remember: if, in an adult, the distance from the mandible to the thyroid notch is less than 6.5 cm and the patient has a stiff neck and protruding teeth, visualization of the larynx will almost always be difficult. **If the measurement is less than 6 cm, visualization will be virtually impossible with a direct laryngoscope.**[65]

Cervical spine mobility must also be evaluated because extension of the neck is usually required for endotracheal intubation using direct laryngoscopy. The normal range of flexion and extension varies among individual patients and decreases with age. Any type of movement that produces parathesias or motor or sensory deficits should be avoided.

When an oropharyngeal tumor is suspected, the neck should be examined for palpable masses, tracheal deviation, scars from previous surgery, old tracheostomy scars, and mobility of the larynx. Radiation to the head and neck region causes fibrosis, resulting in an immobile larynx and epiglottis, with airway edema and trismus.

The induction of general anesthesia often precipitates airway obstruction and can contribute to a difficult intubation. Use of general anesthesia and muscle paralysis can cause anterior displacement of the larynx, making indirect laryngoscopy more difficult than in the awake state.[74] In the case of supraglottic and oral tumors the surrounding structures provide support for maintaining a patent airway; with the induction of general anesthesia and subsequent relaxation of these supporting tissues, airway obstruction may ensue.

In addition to a detailed assessment of the airway, patients with head and neck cancer often are heavy smokers with a history of ethanol abuse.[18] Pulmonary function studies, arterial blood gas analysis, and flow-volume loops are helpful in assessing the amount of both extrinsic and intrinsic airway obstruction present and the patient's response to bronchodilators.

Management of the difficult airway

The most important aspect of airway management is that a clear plan be developed preoperatively for intubation of patients with possible airway compromise. **The fiberoptic laryngoscope and/or bronchoscope is particularly useful for emergency intubation when patients present with obstructing laryngeal lesions.**[89] **It is most effective when used while the patient is awake, before anesthesia-induced changes in anatomy occur or before blood, secretions, and edema from unsuccessful rigid laryngoscopy obscure airway landmarks.**

A step-by-step procedure should be followed when performing a fiberoptic intubation (Box 22-2). Sedation should be used with caution and may be contraindicated in impending airway obstruction. Transtracheal and superior laryngeal nerve blocks may be difficult or even dangerous if tumor is obstructing nearby anatomic landmarks. It is crucial to have several alternatives available in the event of intubation failure[65] (Fig. 22-1). These might include the use of cricothyroidotomy[70] or the insertion of a large-bore intravenous catheter through the cricothyroid membrane. The large-bore IV catheter can be attached to a breathing circuit by the use of an endotracheal tube adaptor. Alternatively, jet ventilation via a large-bore intravenous catheter has also been used in the emergency situation.[1] These are only temporary maneu-

---

BOX 22-2
CHECKLIST FOR FIBEROPTIC INTUBATION

Preoxygenate the patient
Apply monitoring devices
Apply topical anesthesia (nasal and/or oral)
Perform local blocks if applicable
Check light source
Suction and administer oxygen via three-way stop-
   cock on side port
Focus endoscope
Lubricate endoscope, avoiding lens
Precut endotracheal tube (ETT)
Load endotracheal tube onto endoscope
Insert endotracheal tube into the pharynx
Visualize larynx
Enter vocal cords
Identify tracheal rings above carina
Advance endotracheal tube over endoscope

---

vers, however, until a formal tracheostomy can be performed. To reemphasize, the optimal decision for the safety of a patient with an upper airway tumor often is to intubate with a fiberoptic endoscope before induction of anesthesia.[78]

In patients with bulky, friable lesions of the pharynx and larynx, a tracheostomy is preferable since attempts at nasal or oral intubation may cause hemorrhage and edema that can lead to complete airway obstruction. A tracheostomy should be performed with the patient under local anesthesia in the operating room in a controlled environment, with appropriate hemodynamic monitoring, oxygenation, and the judicious use of sedation. Once the airway is secured, then general anesthesia can be safely induced for further surgical resection.

Treatment for patients with airway tumors

The use of laser resection for cancer of the airway presents a particular concern for the anesthesiologist.[59] Use of the carbon dioxide laser affords precise excision of small superficial lesions of the upper airway with minimal edema formation. The neodymium-yttrium-aluminum-garnet (Nd:YAG) laser produces a greater depth of resection and is used primarily for bulky tracheal or bronchial tumors.[15]

Carbon dioxide laser surgery on or above the larynx can be performed with or without insertion of an endotracheal tube. One method for providing ventilation is with a Sanders-type jet injector mounted on the operating laryngoscope. A high-velocity jet of oxygen is oriented toward the glottic opening and room air is entrained via Venturi effect. Inhalational anesthetics are difficult to regulate with this system, and intravenous anesthetics often prove to be more useful.[23] As with all laser surgery, the patient must be immobile to avoid unexpected movement and injury to normal tissues from the laser.

Although the risks of hypoventilation and aspiration are of concern with a nonintubation technique, the use of an endotracheal tube has its own problems: primarily the risk of an airway fire from ignition of flammable endotracheal tube material. The index of flammability of polyvinylchloride endotracheal tubes is higher than that of either red rubber or silicone, making polyvinylchloride tubes less likely to ignite.[91] Although plain unmarked and unwrapped tubes are preferred, many clinicians use metal tape wrapped around the endotracheal tube to decrease the risk of tube ignition. Unfortunately, this increases the risk of reflecting the beam to adjacent structures, with the most likely place for an aberrant laser strike being the endotracheal tube cuff. Because the cuff cannot be wrapped, it represents a vulnerable area for possible

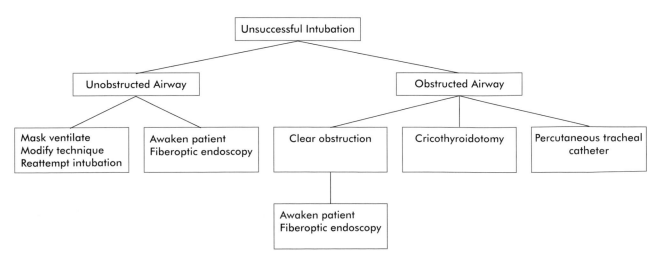

Fig. 22-1. Alternative procedures for the unsuccessful intubation.

ignition. Accordingly, many anesthesiologists choose to inflate the cuff with saline solution so that cuff deflation acts as a fire extinguisher.

Manipulation of inspired gases may also facilitate laser surgery of the airway and reduce the risk of fire. **Use of nitrous oxide, since it supports combustion, should be avoided.** One protocol that has been recommended for laryngotracheal carbon dioxide laser surgery is to **use helium as a diluent gas with oxygen** (Table 22-1). Helium has a high thermal diffusivity and thus prevents high temperatures in materials contacted by the laser.[60] Furthermore, helium permits a higher oxygen concentration than can be used when air alone serves as the diluent gas.

Helium is also useful when airway stenosis is caused by intrinsic or extrinsic tumor encroachment. Helium is a light gas, with a molecular weight of 4 and a density of 0.14 (air = 1). When gas flow is turbulent, as occurs in partial airway obstruction, the pressure gradient required to produce a given flow is proportional to the density of the gas and the square of the flow rate. Under these conditions a greater flow can be achieved with a mixture of 80% helium and 20% oxygen (density = 0.33) as compared with air (density = 1). In addition, the critical velocity required to produce turbulent flow is greater with helium than with air.[44]

Bronchial obstruction is a relatively common complication of bronchogenic carcinoma. It can result in obstructive pneumonitis, atelectasis, hypoxemia, and respiratory distress. It may present as impending airway obstruction or as hemoptysis requiring prompt surgical intervention. The use of the Nd:YAG laser via a rigid or flexible fiberoptic bronchoscope has become the treatment of choice for bleeding endobronchial lesions.[35] Preoperative pulmonary function studies, particularly forced vital capacity and maximal expiratory flow volume curves, can be helpful in distinguishing tumor obstruction of the airway from generalized chronic obstructive lung disease.[45] Equally important in planning the patient's anesthetic management is a preoperative arterial blood gas determination.

When a flexible fiberoptic bronchoscope is used for endobronchial laser resection, the resection can be performed either with topical anesthesia and intravenous sedation or with general anesthesia.[6,88] When general anesthesia is used, the fiberoptic endoscope can be inserted through a large-bore endotracheal tube; during the laser resection, ventilation can be temporarily stopped. Smoke generated by the laser should be suctioned from the proximal airway. Ventilation with the lowest acceptable concentration of inspired oxygen in helium or air diluent is recommended, although safe limits for inspired oxygen and laser power density have not yet been established. Because the laser beam is beyond the endotracheal tube, the fire hazard is mainly related to flaming debris expelled through the endotracheal tube.

If an airway fire does occur with either the carbon dioxide or the Nd:YAG laser (Box 22-3), ventilation should be stopped and the oxygen disconnected to prevent further spread of the fire. The burning tissue and/or endotracheal tube should be removed from the airway and replaced. The extent of pulmonary damage should be assessed before awakening the patient. Pulse oximetry is probably one of the most important monitoring devices during laser surgery since it allows the lowest inspired oxygen concentration to be used so

---

Table 22-1 Helium protocol for laryngotracheal carbon dioxide laser operations

Protocol consideration	Limitation
Gases	
Helium	≥ 60%
Oxygen	$FIO_2 \leq 0.40$
Inhalational anesthetic agents	Enflurane, halothane, or isoflurane, as indicated
Nitrous oxide	Cannot be used for anesthetic maintenance
Endotracheal tube	Plain, unmarked polyvinylchloride, unwrapped
Carbon dioxide	
Power density	≤ 10 W at 0.8-mm spot size (1992 W/cm²)
Exposure	Repeated bursts ≤ 10 sec of 0.5-sec pulsed beam
Monitoring	Standard monitors, oxygen analyzer, pulse oximeter

From Pashayan AG, Gravenstein JS, Cassisi NJ et al: The helium protocol for laryngotracheal operations with CO_2 laser: a retrospective review of 523 cases, *Anesthesiology* 68:801, 1988.

```
BOX 22-3
MANAGEMENT OF A LASER-INDUCED
AIRWAY FIRE

Discontinue ventilation
Disconnect oxygen source
Flood the field with water
Remove burned material from airway
Ventilate patient by mask or reintubate
Assess injury
Monitor patient for at least 24 hours
Administer steroids, antibiotics
Ventilate patient if necessary
Review serial chest radiographs
```

that the risk of fire is minimized while providing adequate oxygenation.

Once an acute upper airway obstruction has been suddenly relieved, acute pulmonary edema may ensue.[75] It has been postulated that the highly negative intrapleural pressures generated while inhaling against an obstructed upper airway lead to increased pulmonary vascular volume and impaired left ventricular ejection. This, in turn, may predispose the patient to postobstructive pulmonary edema.

Anterior Mediastinal Masses

Malignant mediastinal tumors, whether primary or metastatic, may compress or invade surrounding structures. **Obstruction of major airways, the superior vena cava, and the heart is a potential consideration when preparing a patient for anesthesia.**[31] Symptoms include syncope, dyspnea, orthopnea, stridor, and cyanosis. When vena caval obstruction occurs, then venous engorgement, edema of the head and neck, and raised intracranial pressure may also be present (Table 22-2). **The primary concern for the anesthesiologist, however, is the risk of total loss of the airway, cardiac arrest, and death occurring soon after induction of general anesthesia.**[38,47,57,62]

The most common tumors of the anterior mediastinum include thymomas, lymphomas, and germ cell neoplasms, particularly in children 1 to 16 years of age. Primary lung and metastatic carcinoma to mediastinal lymph nodes may also produce the previously discussed clinical problems in adults. Preoperative radiation, chemotherapy, and use of corticosteroids have been recommended for severely symptomatic patients to reduce the size of the tumor before induction of anesthesia. However, optimal treatment for these tumors differs, depending on the histologic cell type; often the pathologist cannot distinguish tumor type in irradiated tissue. Accordingly, it is not uncommon for a patient to have anesthesia for a diagnostic biopsy before the institution of therapy. Because obtaining an adequate tissue specimen for diagnosis is not always possible with use of local anesthesia, anesthesia personnel will continue to be confronted with symptomatic untreated patients who will require general anesthesia.

A thorough preoperative cardiovascular and respiratory evaluation is essential. Computerized tomography (CT scans) and recent radiographic findings are helpful in detecting airway obstruction. Similarly, **pulmonary flow-volume loop studies are a sensitive noninvasive method for evaluating obstructive lesions of the major airways.** Limitations in the inspiratory limb of the loop are used to diagnose extrathoracic airway obstruction, whereas delayed flow in the expiratory limb is indicative of intrathoracic obstruction. These tests should be performed with the patient in both the supine and upright positions since airway obstruction is often made worse during recumbency. In addition, transthoracic or transesophageal echocardiography can be useful in evaluating the size of the tumor, its relationship to vital structures, and the effect of changes in position.[21]

Use of general anesthesia exacerbates extrinsic intrathoracic airway obstruction in several ways. During spontaneous respiration, the larger airways are supported by negative intrathoracic pressure. Thus extrinsic compression is masked in all but the most severe cases. With loss of consciousness and cessation of spontaneous respiration, however, these compensatory mechanisms are removed and airway compression may ensue. Furthermore, positive-pressure ventilation from above a region of compression can lead to total airway occlusion. Therefore when muscle paralysis is used to facilitate endotracheal intubation, all the muscular contribution to chest expansion is lost. Because of this sequence of events, **it is recommended that these patients maintain spontaneous respiration at all times.**[57] Even after successful intubation, hypoxia may still occur, usually as a result of compression of the pulmonary outflow tract, a problem seen most often with right-sided tumors.

Patients are also affected by positioning. **Tumors obstructing venous return can cause cardiovascular collapse in the supine position, when the weight of the tumor falls onto the heart and major vessels. At this time changing the patient to the sitting, lateral, or prone position may be a lifesaving maneuver.** As a last

Table 22-2   Diagnosis of anterior mediastinal mass

	Airway symptoms	Cardiovascular symptoms
History	Stridor	Syncope
	Cough	Headache
	Dyspnea	Exacerbation in supine position
	Cyanosis	
	Orthopnea	
Physical	Wheezing	Venous engorgement
	Decreased breath sounds	Edema of head and neck
		Papilledema
		Pallor
Tests	CT scans	Echocardiography
	Chest radiograph	
	Flow-volume studies	

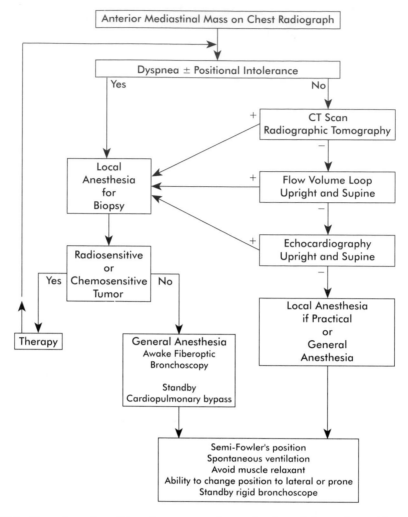

Fig. 22-2. Flow chart describing the preoperative evaluation of the patient with an anterior mediastinal mass; + indicates positive finding; − indicates negative workup. (From Neuman GG, Weingarten AE, Abramowitz RM et al: The anesthetic management of the patient with an anterior mediastinal mass, *Anesthesiology* 60:144, 1984.)

resort, extracorporeal circulation should be considered when total airway occlusion or severe venous admixture is a potential problem.

Fig. 22-2 illustrates one approach to the patient with an anterior mediastinal mass. In those who require use of a general anesthetic for the resection of tumors that are either benign or insensitive to irradiation or chemotherapy, a number of precautions should be taken. First, **awake fiberoptic intubation with the patient in the sitting position is strongly recommended,** unless the patient is totally uncooperative. Once the airway is secured, general anesthesia can be induced with inhalational anesthetics while maintaining spontaneous ventilation. Use of muscle relaxants should be avoided. As an alternative, a mask induction with the patient in the sitting position, maintaining spontaneous ventilation with a volatile anesthetic agent and 100% oxygen, may be used. In cases in which superior vena caval syndrome is

suspected, venous access should be secured in the lower extremities before induction of anesthesia.

Pericardial Effusion and Tamponade
Causes

Metastatic tumor involvement of the heart or pericardium is not uncommon in patients with cancer, particularly in those with leukemia, lymphoma, melanoma, breast, and lung carcinoma.[5,29,61] Cardiac tamponade occurs as the heart is compressed by fluid exuded from malignant cells within the pericardial sac in combination with obstruction of the lymphatic and venous drainage. Normally, 20 to 25 ml of fluid surrounds the heart, whereas the development of symptoms depends on the rate of fluid accumulation, the volume of fluid in the pericardium, and the underlying ventricular function. If it accumulates slowly, 80 to 100 ml of pericardial fluid can collect before signs of tamponade occur. This is a volume greater than the normal stroke volume. When the effusion reaches a critical level, hemodynamic compromise develops, characterized by a decrease in cardiac output and impaired systemic perfusion.

Cardiac tamponade may also follow constrictive pericarditis induced by inflammatory processes or thoracic irradiation. Hemopericardium is also not uncommon with thrombocytopenia and other coagulopathies associated with malignant tumors.

Pathophysiology

Pericardial tamponade results from impaired diastolic filling of the heart related to elevation of the intrapericardial pressure surrounding the heart. This limits the diastolic expansion of the heart chambers, with resultant increases in intraatrial, intraventricular, and pericardial pressures.[42] In addition, total blood volume is increased secondary to renal retention of salt and water. **Ultimately, there is an equalization of the diastolic pressures throughout the heart, resulting in a fixed stroke volume. At this point cardiac output becomes rate-dependent, and adrenergic stimulation results in increased plasma catecholamine levels, vasoconstriction, and tachycardia.** Although these compensatory mechanisms maintain blood flow and arterial pressure initially, they become less effective with time.

Symptoms

Malignant pericardial disease is unpredictable in its presentation (Box 22-4). The classical Beck's triad of quiet heart sounds, increased venous pressure, and decreased arterial pressure may or may not be seen.[83] Symptoms of neoplastic pericardial involvement often include dyspnea, cough, retrosternal or nonspecific chest pain, orthopnea, palpitations, weakness, fatigue, and dizziness. Patients are usually tachypneic and tachycardic, with jugular venous distension, distant heart sounds, and pericardial friction rub. With progressive elevations in right-sided cardiac pressures, venous stasis develops in the liver and splanchnic veins, leading to abdominal discomfort and distension. Higher venous pressures lead to swelling of the face and extremities.

The presence of pulsus paradoxicus may be helpful in making the diagnosis of cardiac tamponade although it is not pathognomonic. Pulsus paradoxicus represents an exaggeration of the normal 6 mm Hg change in systemic arterial pressure that occurs during inspiration and exhalation. Pulsus paradoxicus is an unreliable indicator of pericardial tamponade in patients with cancer because they often have concurrent intravascular depletion and underlying cardiac and pulmonary dysfunction. Electrocardiography usually shows tachycardia and low QRS voltage in all leads. With each contraction the heart changes

---

BOX 22-4
DIAGNOSIS: NEOPLASTIC
PERICARDIAL TAMPONADE

Symptoms

Anxiety; chest pain; dyspnea; upright, forward-leaning posture

Signs

Jugular venous distension, cardiac enlargement, distant heart sounds, pericardial friction rub, tachycardia, hypotension, pulsus paradoxicus, electrical alternans

---

position within the effusion, causing a continuous variation in the electrical axis called electrical alternans. Chest radiographs demonstrate an enlarged cardiac silhouette, with a "water bottle" or globular shape. **The most sensitive tool for making the diagnosis of pericardial effusion is echocardiography,** which can detect as little as 15 ml of fluid. In cancer patients the use of intraoperative transesophageal echocardiography is particularly useful because it can locate persistently loculated posterior effusions during pericardial drainage procedures.

Anesthetic management

Management of patients with pericardial effusion depends on the degree of preexisting hemodynamic compromise. Definitive treatment of tamponade is pericardiocentesis either percutaneously or through a subxiphoid pericardial window. The use of the pericardial window is preferred in those patients who require repeated percutaneous drainage procedures or who are unresponsive to radiation therapy. The subxiphoid approach is considered the procedure of choice for management of malignant effusions. It allows irrigation of the pericardial cavity, lysis of adhesions, placement of a large chest tube for drainage, and avoidance of a formal thoracotomy.

The sequence of anesthesia and surgery depends on the hemodynamic state of the patient. In severely compromised patients, pericardiocentesis or subxiphoid exploration can be performed with the patient under local anesthesia until there is sufficient relief of the pressure to allow general anesthesia to be induced safely. In cases with less cardiovascular impairment, the patient should be prepared and draped for a surgical incision before anesthetic induction, lest the clinical assessment of the degree of compromise be underestimated and rapid surgical intervention is required. In either situation, hemodynamic monitoring should be instituted beforehand, with the patient in the semi-Fowler's position. Monitoring should

---

BOX 22-5
ANESTHETIC MANAGEMENT OF CARDIAC TAMPONADE

Maintain

Vasoconstriction
Tachycardia
Full intravascular volume
Upright position

Avoid

Myocardial depressants
Vasodilation
Bradycardia
Positive pressure ventilation

BOX 22-6
PARANEOPLASTIC SYNDROMES

Neuromuscular disorders

Dermatomyositis and polymyositis
Myasthenic syndromes (Eaton-Lambert)

Hematologic disorders

Anemia associated with cancer
Granulocytosis
Thrombocytopenia and thrombocytosis
Coagulation abnormalities

Endocrinologic disorders

Pheochromocytoma
Carcinoid syndrome
Thyrotoxicosis
Hypercalcemia and parathyroid disease

Fever, anorexia

---

include the placement of an intraarterial catheter and either a central venous or a Swan-Ganz catheter. **It is important to maintain or increase intravascular volume and avoid bradycardia. Vasoconstriction should be maintained to preserve arterial perfusion pressure (Box 22-5). Ketamine is the agent of choice for maintaining hemodynamic stability in this situation.**

Spontaneous ventilation is preferred to preserve venous return. If controlled ventilation is necessary, then rapid rates with small tidal volumes should be used. High inspiratory airway pressures, intermittent positive pressure ventilation, and positive end-expiratory pressure should be minimized since they will further decrease cardiac output.[56]

PATHOPHYSIOLOGIC DISORDERS ASSOCIATED WITH CANCER

Many pathophysiologic disturbances are associated with cancer and may produce signs and symptoms distant from the primary tumor or its metastases. These are often referred to as paraneoplastic syndromes (Box 22-6).

Hematologic Problems
Anemia and blood transfusion

Anemia is a common problem in patients with cancer because a variety of mechanisms, including anemia of "chronic disease," direct bone marrow invasion, bone marrow suppression by chemotherapy or radiotherapy, blood loss as a result of bleeding, shortened red cell survival from hypersplenism, red cell aplasia, autoimmune hemolysis, and vitamin and iron deficiency anemia.[7]

One of the first decisions an anesthesiologist must make in these cases is the need for preoperative transfusion. The indications for blood transfusion have changed dramatically in recent years, partly because of the risk of infectious diseases such as acquired immunodeficiency syndrome (AIDS), hepatitis, and cytomegalovirus,[28] and partly as the result of new information regarding the immunologic effects of blood transfusion.

The indications for blood transfusion are twofold: to increase oxygen-carrying capacity and to maintain intravascular volume. Intravascular volume can be increased by the administration of crystalloid or colloid solutions, with no risk of transmitting disease. Thus maintenance of oxygen-carrying capacity is the only remaining indication for blood transfusion in a patient with anemia. Whereas a hematocrit value of less than 30% or a hemoglobin of less than 10 g/dl was considered an indication for perioperative blood transfusion in the past,[55] the FDA Drug Bulletin for July 1989 suggested that a hemoglobin of 7 g/dl is sufficient for oxygen-carrying capacity when the intravascular volume is adequate and the patient has normal cardiovascular compensatory mechanisms. Indeed, there is evidence that a hematocrit of 20% is well tolerated in this situation.[52]

In a situation of acute blood loss or in patients with coronary artery disease, however, it may not be possible to increase cardiac output to compensate for diminished oxygen-carrying capacity. Currently there is no definitive answer regarding the safe limits for isovolumic hemodilution, particularly in patients with ischemic heart disease who are not undergoing myocardial revascularization. In general, however,

---

BOX 22-7
INDICATIONS FOR PLATELET TRANSFUSION

Active bleeding
Nonsurgical patients with platelet counts < 20,000
Surgical patients with platelet counts < 60,000

No active bleeding
Nonsurgical patients with platelet counts < 10,000
Surgical patients with platelet counts < 50,000

BOX 22-8
CLOTTING FACTOR ABNORMALITIES
ASSOCIATED WITH CANCER

Decreased production
Liver dysfunction, chemotherapy, malignancies, vitamin K deficiency (nutritional or malabsorption)

Dilutional effect
Massive transfusion, plasmapheresis

Immunologic effect
Lupus anticoagulant, dysproteinemias

Consumption effect
DIC, thrombotic disorders

---

the physiology seems unfavorable in this situation when the hematocrit is less than 30%.

The use of autologous blood that is either predonated or autotransfused via a "cell saver" has increased markedly in recent years. These procedures should not be viewed as entirely safe, however, since there is still room for clinical error and consequent transfusion reaction with predonated blood. **In cancer patients concern for disseminating viable cancer cells has limited the use of the "cell saver" during oncologic surgery.** Recent reports, however, suggest that transfused tumor cells have a low theoretic risk of producing hematogenous spread of cancer, particularly since recurrence as a result of intraoperative peritoneal spillage is always a possibility.[36,39] Furthermore, **it appears cancer patients who receive, instead, homologous blood transfusions have an increased risk of immunosuppression, which may enhance the progression of malignant tumors.**[2,8,87] This nonspecific immunosuppressive action of blood transfusions has been found to be therapeutic in kidney transplant patients although it has been suggested that it increases infection rate. Although the exact mechanism by which blood transfusions alter the immune system is unknown, it has been related to increased synthesis of prostaglandin E, decreased interleukin-2 generation, and fibrinogen degradation products found in fresh frozen plasma.[55] Blumberg et al. found that patients with cancer who received packed red blood cell transfusions had an improved survival compared to those who received whole blood transfusions.[4] They theorized that plasma contained some immunosuppressive factor that contributed to the survival difference. Thus it has been recommended that packed red blood cells be used when transfusion is deemed necessary in cancer patients.[2]

Coagulopathies

Thrombocytopenia in patients with cancer is usually related to chemotherapy, radiation therapy, acute leukemia, or disseminated intravascular coagulation

(DIC). Unexplained thrombocytopenia is an indication to search for an occult malignancy. Box 22-7 lists some of the indications for platelet transfusion.

Coagulopathies are among the most common paraneoplastic syndromes (Box 22-8). These abnormalities can be divided into those related to lack of production, immune destruction, and consumption of clotting factors. The majority of the coagulation factors are produced in the liver; abnormalities of liver parenchyma, related either to primary tumor or metastatic disease, are not uncommon in disseminated malignancy or in cancer treatment. In addition to liver disease, various malignancies are associated with a decrease in clotting factors. These include factor V deficiency in chronic myelogenous leukemia and Fletcher factor deficiency in chronic lymphocytic leukemia.[37]

The consumption coagulopathy in DIC may present as a chronic disorder, as an acute hemorrhagic diathesis, or as a coagulation abnormality detected by routine laboratory tests alone. Abnormalities on routine blood coagulation tests have been reported in as many as 92% of patients with cancer.[64] The most common are elevations in fibrin/fibrinogen degradation products, thrombocytosis, and hyperfibrinogenemia. Overt DIC with resultant bleeding, however, is relatively infrequent. Other causes of DIC in patients with cancer include infections, particularly those associated with septicemia; surgical manipulation of neoplastic tissue with intravascular release of thromboplastin; and massive transfusion reactions. Successful treatment of DIC depends on the underlying cause and its reversibility. Infections and septic states can be treated with antibiotics and aggressive management of sepsis; leukocyte-dependent thromboplastic release may be inhibited by use of glucocorticoids. The use of heparin, an inhibitor of activated clotting factors, remains controversial. The liberal use of fresh frozen plasma and platelets and heparin therapy is considered in the face of life-threatening uncontrolled bleeding or in cases of chronic DIC with recurrent thromboembolic episodes.[7]

During radical cancer surgery multiple transfusions are often necessary. Bleeding after massive transfusion may be a result of dilutional thrombocytopenia, deficiency in factors V and VIII, DIC, or hemolytic transfusion reaction. **Dilutional thrombocytopenia is most closely correlated with the coagulopathy seen during massive transfusion, usually greater than 10 to 15 units.** Periodic platelet counts after every 10 units may facilitate a decision regarding timing of platelet transfusion. Platelets should be given empirically at the first clinical signs of a coagulopathy, even if the platelet count is unavailable. **By contrast, factor deficiency related to transfusion of stored blood is less often a problem because only low levels of these factors are actually necessary for clotting.** Disseminated intravascular coagulation after massive transfusion may be related to the release of tissue thromboplastin from acidotic tissues; the diagnosis is made by laboratory findings of a consumption coagulopathy, a decrease in the platelet count, a fibrinogen level below 100 mg/dl (or prothrombin or partial thromboplastin values greater than 1.5 times control), and the presence of fibrin degradation products. Fresh frozen plasma and platelets should be given in this setting.

Neuromuscular Disorders

The Eaton-Lambert or myasthenic syndrome, while rare, is most often associated with carcinoma of the lung.[80] It is characterized by limb-girdle weakness, with symptoms that mimic those of myasthenia gravis. The use of anticholinesterase agents in these patients, however, is not beneficial although they are extraordinarily sensitive to both depolarizing and nondepolarizing muscle relaxants. One common clinical scenario is the use of muscle relaxants during a diagnostic endoscopy, which then results in the requirement for postoperative ventilatory support until the relaxant is almost completely metabolized.

Pheochromocytoma

Pheochromocytomas are catechol-secreting tumors derived from chromaffin tissue, usually the adrenal medulla. Extraadrenal sites, however, are not uncommon, and include the sympathetic chain, the organ of Zuckerkandl at the bifurcation of the aorta, the bladder, the spleen, and in the neck. **Most pheochromocytomas produce both norepinephrine and epinephrine.** Rarely, epinephrine is the sole catecholamine released, resulting in hyperglycemia and increased metabolic rate as the presenting symptoms. Although rarely a primary cause of hypertension, pheochromocytomas can result in fatal hypertensive paroxysms. Pheochromocytomas may be associated with autosomally dominant familial disorders, multiple endocrine neoplasia, types II and III (Box 22-9). Furthermore, a small percentage of these tumors (<5%) are malignant. Thus early detection and surgical excision can cure the hypertension and may reduce the probability of metastatic disease.[14]

The patient with pheochromocytoma usually presents with diaphoresis, tachycardia, and headache. These symptoms, along with the presence of systemic hypertension, are virtually hallmarks of pheochromocytoma (Box 22-10). Less common presentations include myocardial infarction, cerebral hemorrhage, or congestive heart failure secondary to catechol cardiomyopathy.[79]

BOX 22-9
SYNDROMES ASSOCIATED WITH PHEOCHROMOCYTOMA

Multiple endocrine neoplasia, type II

Medullary carcinoma of the thyroid
Primary hyperparathyroidism
Pheochromocytoma

Multiple endocrine neoplasia, type III

Medullary carcinoma of the thyroid
Multiple mucosal neuromas
Pheochromocytoma

BOX 22-10
CLINICAL MANIFESTATIONS OF PHEOCHROMOCYTOMA

Common

Palpitations
Headaches
Diaphoresis

Uncommon

Abdominal pain
Chest pain
GI symptoms
Weakness
Visual symptoms

The diagnosis of pheochromocytoma is confirmed by abnormally high levels of catecholamines or catechol metabolites in blood or urine. Assay of urinary metanephrine remains the most reliable indicator of excess catecholamine secretion. Tumors larger than 1 cm are best localized by use of CT scan. Additional diagnostic tools include selective venous sampling, radioisotope scanning, and rarely, arteriography.

Treatment of pheochromocytoma is surgical excision of the tumor. **Since the introduction of perioperative alpha-adrenergic blockade, mortality from surgery has been reduced from 40% to 60% to 0% to 6%.**[67] **Prazosin or phenoxybenzamine may be used to produce preoperative alpha-adrenergic blockade.**[33] These drugs act by blocking the vasoconstrictive effects of excess catecholamine levels, thus allowing for repletion of the intravascular volume. In patients with dysrhythmias or tachycardia, **beta-blockade may be useful but should only be used with concomitant alpha-blockade to prevent unopposed vasoconstricton.** Labetalol, a mixed alpha- and beta-blocker, has been used in perioperative preparation in pheochromocytoma. It has, however, been associated with pulmonary edema when used in large doses.[49]

Patients are considered to have adequate preoperative treatment when hospital blood pressure remains below 165/95 mm Hg, when orthostatic hypotension occurs with pressures greater than 80/45 mm Hg, when there is absence of ST-T wave changes on ECG tracings for 1 to 2 weeks, and when there is a maximum of one premature ventricular contraction/5 min.[68] Additional criteria for preoperative treatment are summarized in Box 22-11.

During anesthesia and surgery, the primary goal is to avoid massive sympathetic outflow associated with manipulation of the pheochromocytoma or with other painful stimuli. Before insertion of invasive cardiovascular monitoring catheters, the patient should be well sedated before arrival in the operating room. A pulmonary artery catheter may be useful but need not be inserted before anesthetic induction; by contrast, an **intraarterial catheter should definitely be placed and connected to a pressure transducer system before induction.** One or two large-bore intravenous catheters are also desirable, in addition to other standard monitoring devices.

Anesthetic techniques for these patients range from use of general to regional anesthesia or a combination of both. Vasodepressor and vasopressor infusions should be ready when the patient arrives in the operating room. A few anesthetic drugs probably should be avoided, including those that release histamine, which, in turn, causes catecholamine release. Examples are morphine, curare, atracurium, and metocurine. Agents that have sympathomimetic effects or that are vagolytic may potentiate the effects of epinephrine. These include atropine, pancuronium, gallamine, and succinylcholine. Agents that sensitize the myocardium to catecholamines, such as halothane, are not recommended unless their use is strongly indicated for some other reason. Finally, use of drugs as disparate as droperidol, ephedrine, tricyclic antidepressants, chlorpromazine, glucagon, and metoclopramide have all been associated with exaggerated pressor response. Box 22-12 for a more complete listing of drugs that may be problematic in patients with pheochromocytoma.

Once preoperative cardiovascular control has been established, **transient intraoperative blood pressure and heart rate changes may be controlled by the use of short-acting vasodilators such as nitroprusside and rapid-acting beta-blocking drugs such as esmolol.**[32,84,92] The clinician should anticipate that blood volume will need to be maintained by the use of crystalloid or colloid solutions and that these requirements are usually high despite preoperative alpha

---

BOX 22-11
PREOPERATIVE CRITERIA
FOR PHEOCHROMOCYTOMA

Blood pressure < 165/95 mm Hg in hospital
Orthostatic hypotension
No ST-T wave changes on ECG tracing
Maximum of one premature ventricular contraction/5 min

BOX 22-12
DRUGS TO AVOID IN PATIENTS WITH
PHEOCHROMOCYTOMAS

Histamine releasers
Morphine, curare, atracurium, metocurine

Vagolytics, sympathomimetics
Atropine, pancuronium, gallamine, succinylcholine

Myocardial sensitizers
Halothane

Indirect catechol stimulators
Droperidol, ephedrine, tricyclic antidepressants, chlorpromazine, glucagon, metoclopramide

sympatholysis. As previously mentioned, **a pulmonary catheter may be helpful in determining perioperative fluid requirements,** but its use should not be considered mandatory in all circumstances.

Postoperatively, accelerated volume replacement is usually required as sympathetic tone continues to decrease. In addition, hypoglycemia may occur as catecholamine stimulation is withdrawn. Hypertension usually resolves in 1 to 3 days.[66] Postoperative hypertension may be related to pain, volume overload, ligation of the renal artery, or residual unresected tumor.

Carcinoid Tumors

Carcinoid tumors arise most commonly in the gastrointestinal tract (75%) but also have been found in the head and neck, gonads, thymus, bronchus, urinary tract, gallbladder, and heart, where they may present as right-sided valvular disease and myocardial plaque formation. The most frequent site in the gastrointestinal tract is the appendix, and the tumor is often discovered during surgery for "acute appendicitis."[24] Hepatic metastases are usually present when carcinoid syndrome is manifested.

A variety of vasoreactive agents are released by carcinoid tumors, including serotonin, histamine, kallikrein, and prostaglandins. Carcinoid syndrome results from the release of these substances and may cause the patient to present with profound hypotension, bronchospasm, hypertension, and dysrhythmias requiring prompt treatment (Box 22-13). Only 5% of carcinoid tumors result in carcinoid syndrome. Flushing is common in patients with carcinoid but is uncommon in patients with pheochromocytoma. Abdominal pain and diarrhea are additional symptoms; hyperglycemia may also occur as a result of serotonin-stimulated glycogenolysis.

Many stimuli may precipitate the carcinoid syndrome. These include tumor manipulation during surgery, scrubbing of the abdomen before surgery, eating, defecating, or emotional stress.[46] **Pharmaco-logic agents that prevent the release of vasoactive substances include clonidine and alpha- and beta-sympathetic antagonists. Recently, use of somatostatin analog has been reported to avert carcinoid crisis when given intravenously.**[50] Agents that may decrease the symptoms of carcinoid syndrome by blocking the effects of vasoactive agents include ketanserin, a competitive serotonin receptor antagonist; **anthistamines of both the H_1- and H_2-blocking groups;** droperidol; and aminocaproic acid. The latter, while it has antibradykinin effects, may accelerate clot formation and, therefore, be more problematic than helpful.

Bronchospasm occurs during carcinoid syndrome secondary to the release of kinins and histamine and may be prevented with H_1 and H_2 antagonists and steroids. It is best treated, however, with somatostatin analog. Similarly, it has been found that flushing and diarrhea also respond well to somatostatin analog.[41]

Profound hypotension is a major problem intraoperatively, secondary to the effects of vasoactive mediators as well as underlying hypovolemia.[82] Therefore patients should be adequately hydrated before surgery. The presence or absence of carcinoid heart disease may be detected by echocardiography. Preoperative treatment with steroids and antihistamines may be effective in attenuating intraoperative hypotension. Intraoperative hypotension, a condition that is usually unresponsive to fluid and vasopressor therapy once it has occurred, also has been found to be amenable to treatment with somatostatin analog.

Hypertension in carcinoid syndrome is usually related to tumor manipulation and secretion of serotonin. It responds well to conventional antihypertensive therapy although preoperative treatment with ketanserin may prevent or attenuate intraoperative hypertensive events. In general intraoperative carcinoid crisis may be avoided by smooth anesthetic induction, with endotracheal intubation facilitated by agents that minimize cardiovascular stimulation, and by the avoidance of histamine-releasing drugs.

COMPLICATIONS ASSOCIATED WITH CHEMOTHERAPY

Chemotherapy for cancer therapy was first introduced in the 1940s with the alkylating agents. It has become increasingly popular both as a primary treatment for cancer and, more importantly, an adjuvant therapy to be administered in association with surgery and/or radiation therapy. Therefore many patients who present for elective or emergency surgery will be undergoing or have undergone chemotherapy at some point in their treatment. The clinical benefits of chemotherapy often are limited by the toxic effects of these agents on vital organ systems. Accordingly, it is

---

BOX 22-13
CLINICAL PRESENTATION IN PATIENTS WITH CARCINOID TUMORS

Hypotension, hypertension
Bronchospasm
Dysrhythmia
Hyperglycemia
Flushing
Abdominal pain
Diarrhea

Table 22-3   Chemotherapy and associated toxicities

Agents	Major toxicity
Nitrogen mustard	Myelosuppression, local tissue damage
Cyclophosphamide (Cytoxan)	Myelosuppression, hemorrhagic cystitis, water retention, pulmonary fibrosis, plasma cholinesterase inhibition
Methotrexate	Renal tubular injury, hepatotoxicity
5-Fluorouracil (5-FU) and cytosine arabinoside (ARA-C)	Hemorrhagic enteritis, diarrhea, myelosuppression
Vincristine (Oncovin)	Neurotoxicity, dilutional hyponatremia
Vinblastine (Velban)	Myelosuppression
Cis-platinum	Renal toxicity
Nitrosoureas (BCNU, CCNU)	Myelosuppression, renal failure, pulmonary fibrosis
Adriamycin (doxorubicin)	Cardiac toxicity
Bleomycin	Pulmonary toxicity
Mitomycin C	Myelosuppression, pulmonary toxicity

important for the anesthesiologist to have a clear understanding of the various chemotherapeutic agents, their actions, interactions, and toxic effects.[11,13,16,72] A thorough preoperative evaluation is essential, including a knowledge of the exact type and dose of chemotherapy agents used and a detailed examination of the organ systems most likely affected (Table 22-3).

Alkylating Agents

The alkylating agents include some of the most commonly used chemotherapy drugs: cyclophosphamide (Cytoxan), nitrogen mustard, busulfan, melphalan, and chlorambucil. These drugs have a broad spectrum of antitumor activity and are used in the treatment of lymphoma, breast carcinoma, ovarian carcinoma, melanoma, and multiple myeloma. **They can cause a rapid destruction of tumor mass, producing an increase in the purine and pyrimidine breakdown products and potentially leading to uric acid nephropathy.**[69] To prevent this complication, intravenous fluids, alkalization of the urine, and administration of allopurinol are indicated at the initiation of treatment. **Alkylating agents also induce severe bone marrow suppression,** resulting in anemia,

agranulocytosis, and thrombocytopenia. Marrow suppression is the most common dose-limiting factor seen with these drugs. Use of busulfan, chlorambucil, and melphalan has also been associated with pulmonary toxicity, which can lead to fibrosis in extreme cases.

Nitrogen mustard was one of the first agents found to be effective for lymphoma and is now used for a variety of cancers. Because it causes severe local tissue damage when infiltrated, it is used to obliterate the pleural space in patients with chronic malignant pleural effusion. In addition, nitrogen mustards are used for a technique called "isolated limb perfusion" for metastatic melanoma.[40] In this technique the chemotherapy agent is perfused into the arterial circulation of a limb, which has both its arterial inflow and venous outflow cannulated and connected to an extracorporeal pump. This enables the chemotherapeutic agent to be concentrated in the affected limb. Because this procedure is intensely painful and lasts for approximately 3 to 4 hours, general anesthesia must be used for patient comfort. During this procedure there is the possibility that there may not be complete circulatory isolation of the limb, thus allowing both for considerable blood to be lost to the pump from the general circulation and for chemotherapeutic agents to enter the general circulation. For these reasons, central venous volume status assessment is an important element in perioperative monitoring.

Cyclophosphamide (Cytoxan) is another important alkylating agent. Since its excretion products are active, hemorrhagic cystitis and inappropriate water retention are possible complications of its use. The water retention is related to a direct toxic effect on renal tubules. This, in turn, may result in hyponatremia, leading to seizures and coma. Pulmonary fibrosis has also been reported rarely and may affect perioperative pulmonary function. Of further interest is the fact that cyclophosphamide inhibits synthesis of plasma cholinesterase; its use therefore may result in prolonged action of succinylcholine.[30,93]

Antimetabolites

Antimetabolite agents include methotrexate, 5-fluorouracil (5-FU), and cytosine arabinose (ARA-C). They are structural analogs of normal cellular metabolites and thus interfere with cellular function. Although used mainly in patients with gastrointestinal and pulmonary carcinomas, they may also be used as treatment for sarcomas and leukemias.

The major complications of use of antimetabolites are bone marrow suppression, severe diarrhea, nausea, and vomiting. Use of methotrexate is associated with serious renal tubular toxicity in 10% of treated patients. This is characterized by rising BUN and serum creatinine, with a decreasing urine volume.

Hydration and urine alkalization should be initiated at the start of high-dose treatment. **Acute and chronic hepatotoxicity have also been associated with use of these agents.** Liver enzymes rise acutely during high-dose therapy, usually returning to normal within 1 week after termination of treatment. When administered intrathecally for control of central nervous system metastasis, increased cerebral spinal fluid pressure may occur. These renal, liver, and CNS effects should be considered when evaluating a patient for anesthesia, particularly if therapy is ongoing or recently completed.

Plant Alkaloids

Vincristine and vinblastine are commonly used plant alkaloids. **Vinblastine has its major toxic effect on the bone marrow, whereas vincristine has its effect on the neurologic system.**[54] A progressive and disabling neurologic condition develops, with signs of decreased deep tendon reflexes and peripheral paresthesias. Although these paresthesias rarely cause muscle damage, there can be considerable muscle wasting in severely incapacitated patients. Because of the risk of hyperkalemia in this situation, succinylcholine should be used with caution.

Cis-platinum

Use of *cis*-platinum is highly effective against testicular tumors, ovarian carcinomas, bladder carcinomas, and head and neck cancers. **The primary dose-limiting problems are myelosuppression and a 31% incidence of nephrotoxicity.** *Cis*-platinum is usually administered 4 to 6 hours after IV hydration and administration of 25 to 50 g of mannitol IV.[53] Patients receiving systemic antibiotics such as aminoglycosides have an increased risk of renal toxicity.[27] In humans the primary pathologic finding is a coagulation necrosis of the distal renal tubules and collecting ducts. This causes a reduction in renal blood flow and glomerular filtration rate, with concomitant magnesium and potassium wasting. The magnesium loss can lead to symptomatic tetany. Perioperative management of these patients should focus on optimizing renal perfusion, fluid, and electrolyte balance. Appropriate hemodynamic monitoring is essential, and a pulmonary artery catheter may be required for optimal management. Mannitol is the drug of choice for maintaining adequate diuresis once intravascular volume status has been optimized. Anesthetic agents that might be nephrotoxic as a result of free fluoride release should be avoided.

Antibiotics

Antibiotic chemotherapy agents include the anthracyclines (Adriamycin and daunorubicin), bleomycin, and mitomycin C.[22,86]

Anthracyclines are used to treat lymphomas and solid tumors such as breast, lung, thyroid, and ovary. **Cardiotoxicity is the dose-limiting factor during anthracycline therapy. An acute cardiac effect that is unrelated to drug dose occurs hours to days after treatment.** It usually presents as mild and transient ECG disturbances or, in extreme cases, as overt pump failure related to reduced myocardial contractility. Sudden death has been reported in this situation. ECG studies demonstrate benign nonspecific changes in 10% of patients with an increase in supraventricular tachydysrhythmias, heart block, and ventricular dysrhythmias.[34] This usually resolves 1 to 2 months after therapy; its incidence is increased in patients with preexisting heart disease. In some patients a decrease in ejection fraction that may lead to acute congestive heart failure is seen 24 to 48 hours after anthracycline administration.

Chronic cardiotoxicity associated with anthracycline administration is a dose-dependent cardiomyopathy that leads to congestive heart failure in 2% to 10% of patients. Once initiated, this process may be irreversible in up to 59% of patients. The risk factors that seem to be associated with cardiotoxicity are listed in Box 22-14. The pathologic diagnosis can be determined by endocardial biopsy.[3] Adriamycin-induced myocardial injury appears to be the result of oxygen free radical formation. Cardiac tissue is low in catalase, the enzyme that detoxifies free radicals. It is thought that dilatation of the sarcoplasmic reticulum and a buildup of calcium deposits in cardiac myocytes results from free radical–induced injury, which ultimately results in cardiac failure. Patients receiving Adriamycin or daunorubicin are followed by serial ECGs, echocardiograms, and radionucleotide-gated pool studies performed both at rest and with exercise. These tests detect cardiac compromise that may contraindicate additional chemotherapy treatment.

For the anesthesiologist, a thorough preoperative evaluation is needed to determine the degree of cardiac compromise. The clinical signs of congestive heart failure such as dyspnea, inspiratory rales, peripheral edema, pleural effusion, and an S_3 gallop may or may not be present. Patients with overt

---

BOX 22-14
RISK FACTORS ASSOCIATED WITH ADRIAMYCIN TOXICITY

Total cumulative dose > 550 mg/m²
Concomitant cyclophosphamide therapy
Prior history of heart disease
Age over 65 years

anthracycline-induced congestive heart failure may require administration of digoxin, diuretics, and other inotropic support; it is essential that their cardiovascular status be optimized before surgery. Intraoperative management should include monitoring with a pulmonary artery catheter and, if available, transesophgeal echocardiography. Intraoperatively, cardiac function is best preserved with an anesthetic technique that lowers systemic vascular resistance, similar to the recommendations for patients with idiopathic cardiomyopathy.[85]

Bleomycin is a chemotherapeutic agent that is primarily dose-limited by pulmonary toxicity, ocurring in 5% to 10% of patients treated. The antitumor effects of bleomycin and its toxicity are the result of its binding to cellular DNA. When bleomycin binds to DNA, a ferrous ion on the bleomycin undergoes oxidation to the ferric state, liberating electrons. The electrons are accepted by oxygen and form both superoxide and oxygen free radicals.[73] The lungs are the primary target for bleomycin toxicity because they have a high concentration of oxygen, and the lung is low in the enzyme, bleomycin hydrolase, a metabolic inactivator of the drug. The actual mechanism of pulmonary damage is controversial. Experimental models show that the injury occurs in two phases. The first is an exudative phase, occurring 1 week after treatment and characterized by interstitial edema, sloughing of the alveolar lining cells, and hyaline membrane formation. The second phase is characterized by a proliferative period, with interstitial infiltration by inflammatory cells and hyperplasia of type II pneumocytes that eventually results in pulmonary fibrosis.

The clinical signs of bleomycin toxicity include a nonproductive cough, dyspnea, and fever. Symptoms usually begin 4 to 10 weeks following therapy. Pulmonary function studies are used to follow these patients. **With the onset of pulmonary damage a restrictive pattern develops and a decrease in the carbon monoxide–diffusing capacity occurs.**[77] Chest radiographs show a progressive bibasilar infiltrate. Certain risk factors have been associated with the development of the pulmonary toxicity (Box 22-15). Once pulmonary toxicity is recognized, treatment is supportive in nature, with administration of high-dose corticosteroids in an attempt to prevent progression of pulmonary fibrosis.

In addition to the direct pulmonary toxicity seen with bleomycin, **of concern to the anesthesiologist is the possibility of contributing to oxygen toxicity when these patients are exposed to high concentrations of oxygen.** Numerous animal studies have shown that exposure to increased oxygen concentrations results in an increased incidence of pulmonary toxicity and death after bleomycin.[76] Goldiner et al. suggested that

---

BOX 22-15
RISK FACTORS ASSOCIATED WITH BLEOMYCIN TOXICITY

Total cumulative dose > 200 mg
Concomitant thoracic radiation therapy
Possibly increased oxygen concentrations
Age over 65 years

---

an FO_2 greater than 28% enhanced the risk of developing postoperative respiratory distress syndrome in patients treated with bleomycin.[26] Although this observation has been substantiated in other studies,[19,58] the topic remains controversial. In 1984 LaMantia et al. reported a series of patients who received bleomycin therapy and subsequently underwent surgery for testicular carcinoma. Although the patients received 40% oxygen, there was not an increased incidence of postoperative pulmonary complications.[43] Despite this study, it is still our practice to limit the perioperative oxygen concentration to 28% or to use the lowest FIO_2 compatible with maintaining satisfactory arterial oxygenation. This requires continuous monitoring with pulse oximetry and frequent arterial blood gas determinations.

Mitomycin C is a relatively new chemotherapy agent that is active against gastrointestinal, lung, and breast cancers. Originally, its major dose-limiting factor was thought to be myelosuppression. Mitomycin, however, becomes active by undergoing enzymatic reduction; once activated, it inhibits DNA function and causes cell death. During this process **mitomycin forms oxygen radicals,[63] and there have been recent reports of severe interstitial pneumonitis, similar to those associated with use of bleomycin.**[9,20] The lung is the likely target for this toxicity because of its high complement of NADPH cytochrome P-450 reductase. This enzyme, and the increased oxygen tensions found in the lung, are responsible for both activation of mitomycin and for generation of oxygen free radicals. The incidence of pulmonary toxicity is not thought to be dose dependent, but once this complication develops, there is a very high mortality; therapy is, at best, supportive. The use of high-dose corticosteroids at the onset of symptoms, prednisone 60 mg/day for 2 to 3 weeks with a gradual tapering over 4 weeks, has been recommended.[12] As in the case with bleomycin toxicity, the triad of dyspnea, cough, and fever is often seen, and the diagnosis is frequently difficult to distinguish from other disease processes.

Although the issue of increased oxygen concentration and the risk of pulmonary toxicity has been raised with regard to mitomycin-treated patients, our experience has been that the incidence of postoperative pulmonary complications appears to be a function of preoperative pulmonary dysfunction, at least as reflected in impaired diffusing capacity, rather than the result of exposure to elevated FIO_2 intraoperatively.

Interferon

Interferon is used in the treatment of several tumors, including melanoma, Kaposi's sarcoma, leukemia, and lymphoma. Its use has not been found effective in common solid tumors such as lung, breast, and gastrointestinal cancer, except when used at its maximum tolerated dose. Interferon is synthesized by human cells as a normal protective response to viral infections. Use of this agent is based on the theory that some malignancies may be induced by virus-mediated changes in nucleic acids (oncogenes). Most patients treated with interferon require intensive care management because of severe immune deficiency syndromes, hypotension, hyperthermia, and sepsis.[71] These complications are associated with therapy and resolve after discontinuation. The anesthesiologist may be confronted with patients treated with interferon either in the intensive care unit or when they present for emergent surgical complications.

SUMMARY

Proper anesthetic management of patients with cancer requires knowledge of the specific problems associated with various types of tumors and with the chemotherapy agents used to treat them. Many of these drugs have side effects and interactions with anesthetic agents; an understanding of their interactions is essential to adequate preoperative evaluation and intraoperative management of patients with oncologic disease.

KEY POINTS

- Every case of head and neck cancer should be considered a difficult intubation situation.
- An awake fiberoptic intubation is often the technique of choice for securing the airway of a patient with an obstructing laryngeal lesion.
- Laser surgery on the airway can be complicated by airway fires; thus, the use of flammable endotracheal tubes and combustible mass mixtures should be avoided.
- Masses of the anterior mediastinum can obstruct major airways, the superior vena cava, and the heart. This obstruction can thereby cause total loss of the airway, cardiac arrest, or death on the induction of general anesthesia.
- Anesthesia for the patient with pericardial tamponade is focused on the maintenance of sympathetic tone and intravascular volume.

- Anemias and coagulations are common in patients with cancer.
- Most pheochromocytomas produce both norepinephrine and epinephrine; perioperative alpha-adrenergic blockade has dramatically reduced the surgical mortality associated with these lesions.
- Various vasoreactive agents are released by carcinoid tumors, including serotonin, histamine, kallikrein, and prostaglandins.
- Use of alkylating agents, antimetabolites, and *cis*-platinum can cause severe bone marrow suppression; methotrexate and *cis*-platinum administration often causes serious nephrotoxicity; use of Adriamycin and daunorubicin causes cardiotoxicity; and bleomycin and mitomycin C use causes dose-related pulmonary toxicity.

KEY REFERENCES

Biebuyck JF: The possible immunosuppressive effects of perioperative blood transfusion in cancer patients, *Anesthesiology* 68:422, 1988.

Chung F: Cancer, chemotherapy and anesthesia, *Can Anaesth Soc J* 29(4):364, 1982.

Desiderio DP: Cancer chemotherapy: complications and interactions with anesthesia, *Hosp Formul* 25(2):176, 1990.

Ginsberg SJ, Comis RL: The pulmonary toxicity of antineoplastic agents, *Semin Oncol* 9(1):34, 1982.

Goldiner PL: Airway problems in head and neck cancer. In Howland WS, Carlon GC, eds: *Critical care of the cancer patient,* Chicago, 1985, Year Book Medical Publishers.

Hull CT: Pheochromocytoma: diagnosis, perioperative preparation and anesthetic management, *Br J Anaesth* 58:1453, 1986.

Lake CL: Anesthesia and pericardial disease, *Anesth Analg* 62:431, 1983.

Mallampati SR, Gatt SP, Gugino LD et al: A clinical sign to predict tracheal difficult intubation: a prospective study, *Can Anaesth Soc J* 32:429, 1985.

Neuman GG, Weingarten AE, Abramowitz RM et al: The anesthetic management of the patient with an anterior mediastinal mass, *Anesthesiology* 60:144, 1984.

Pashayan AG, Gravenstein JS, Cassisi NS et al: The helium protocol for laryngotracheal operations with CO_2 laser: a retrospective review of 523 cases, *Anesthesiology* 68:801, 1988.

Selvin BL: Cancer chemotherapy: implications for the anesthesiologist, *Anesth Analg* 60(6):425, 1981.

Warner ME, Warner MA, and Leonard PF: Anesthesia for neodymium YAG laser resection of major airway obstructing tumors, *Anesthesiology* 60:230, 1984.

REFERENCES

1. Benumof JL, Scheller MS: The importance of transtracheal jet ventilation in the management of the difficult airway, *Anesthesiology* 71:769, 1989.
2. Biebuyck JF: The possible immunosuppressive effects of perioperative blood transfusion in cancer patients, *Anesthesiology* 68:422, 1988.
3. Billingham M et al: Endomyocardial biopsy findings in adriamycin treated patients, *Proc Am Assoc Cancer Res* 17:281, 1976.
4. Blumberg N, Heal JM, Murphy P et al: Association between transfusion of whole blood and recurrence of cancer, *Br Med J* 293:530, 1986.
5. Brook JL, Kaplan JA: Cardiac disease. In Katz J, Benumof J, and Kadis LB, eds: *Anesthesia and uncommon diseases*, Philadelphia, 1981, WB Saunders.
6. Brutinel WM, McDougall JC, and Cortese DA: Bronchoscopic therapy with neodymium-yttrium-aluminum-garnet laser during intravenous anesthesia, *Chest* 84(5):518, 1983.
7. Bunn PA, Ridgway EC: Paraneoplastic syndromes. In DeVita VT, Hellman S, and Rosenberg SA, eds: *Cancer principles and practice of oncology, ed 3*, Philadelphia, 1989, JB Lippincott.
8. Burrows L, Tartter P: Effect of blood transfusions on colonic malignancy recurrence rate, *Lancet* 2:662, 1982 [letter].
9. Buzdar AU, Legha SS, Luna MA et al: Pulmonary toxicity of mitomycin, *Cancer* 45:236, 1980.
10. Caplan RA et al: Respiratory mishaps: principal areas of risk and implications for anesthetic care, *Anesthesiology* 67:A469, 1987.
11. Chabner BA, Myers CE: Clinical pharmacology of cancer chemotherapy. In DeVita VT, Hellman S, and Rosenberg SA, eds: *Cancer principles and practice of oncology, ed 3*, Philadelphia, 1989, JB Lippincott.
12. Chang AYC, Kuebler JP, Pandya KJ et al: Pulmonary toxicity induced by mitomycin C is highly responsive to glucocorticoids, *Cancer* 57:2285, 1986.
13. Chung F: Cancer, chemotherapy and anesthesia, *Can Anaesth Soc J* 29(4):364, 1982.
14. Cryer PE: The adrenal medulla and the sympathetic nervous system. In Wyngaarden J, Smith L, eds: *Cecil textbook of medicine*, Chicago, 1985, WB Saunders.
15. Dedhia H, Lapp NL, Jain PR et al: Endoscopic laser therapy for respiratory distress due to obstructive airway tumors, *Crit Care Med* 13:464, 1985.
16. Desiderio DP: Cancer chemotherapy: complications and interactions with anesthesia, *Hosp Formulary* 25(2):176, 1990.
17. DeVita VT, Hellman S, and Rosenberg SA, eds: *Cancer principles and practice of oncology, ed 3*, Philadelphia, 1989, JB Lippincott.
18. Donlon JV: Anesthesia for eye, ear, nose and throat surgery. In Miller Rd, ed: *Anesthesia*, New York, 1986, Churchill-Livingstone.
19. Douglas MJ, Coppin CM: Bleomycin and subsequent anesthesia: a retrospective study at Vancouver General Hospital, *Can Anaesth Soc J* 27(5):449, 1980.
20. Doyle LA, Idhe DC, Carney DN et al: Combination chemotherapy with doxorubicin and mitomycin C in non-small cell bronchogenic carcinoma, *Am J Clin Oncol* 7:719, 1984.
21. Ferrari LR, Bedford RF: General anesthesia prior to treatment of anterior mediastinal masses in pediatric cancer patients, *Anesthesiology* 72:33, 1990.
22. Ginsberg SJ, Comis RL: The pulmonary toxicity of antineoplastic agents, *Semin Oncol* 9(1):34, 1982.
23. Godden DJ, Willey RF, Fergusson RJ et al: Rigid bronchoscopy under intravenous general anesthesia with oxygen and Venturi ventilation, *Thorax* 37:532, 1982.
24. Godwin JD: Carcinoid tumors: an analysis of 2837 cases, *Cancer* 36:560, 1975.
25. Goldiner PL: Airway problems in head and neck cancer. In Howland WS, Carlon GC, eds: *Critical care of the cancer patient*, Chicago, 1985, Year Book Medical Publishers.
26. Goldiner PL, Carlon GC, Cvitkovic E et al: Factors influencing postoperative morbidity and mortality in patients treated with bleomycin, *Br Med J* 1:1664, 1978.
27. Gonzalez-Vitale JC, Hayes DM, Cvitovic E et al: Acute renal failure after *cis*-dichlorodiamine platinum II and gentamicin-cephalothin therapies, *Cancer Treat Rep* 95:732, 1978.
28. Gravlee GP: *Blood transfusion and component therapy*, ASA Refresher Course, 1990.
29. Groeger JS: Shock states and cancer. In Howland WS, Carlon GC, eds: *Critical care of the cancer patient*, Chicago, 1985, Year Book Medical Publishers.
30. Gruman GM: Prolonged apnea after succinylcholine in a case treated with cytostatics for cancer, *Anesth Analg* 51:761, 1972.
31. Halpern S, Chatten J, Meadows AT et al: Anterior mediastinal masses: anesthesia hazards and other problems, *Clin Lab Observ* 102(3):407, 1983.
32. Hamilton WF, Forrest AL, Gunn A et al: Beta-adrenergic blockade and anesthesia for thyroidectomy, *Anaesthesia* 39:355, 1984.
33. Hull CT: Pheochromocytoma: diagnosis, perioperative preparation and anesthetic management, *Br J Anaesth* 58:1453, 1986.
34. Jones SE, Ewy GA, and Grove BM: Electrocardiographic detection of Adriamycin heart disease, *Proc Am Soc Clin Oncol* 16:228, 1975.
35. Kaiser LR: Tracheobronchial emergencies: use of the neodymium:YAG laser. In Turnbull ADM, ed: *Surgical emergencies in the cancer patient*, Chicago, 1987, Year Book Medical Publishers.
36. Karczewski DM, Lema MJ, and Glaves-Rapp D: The efficacy of using an autotransfusion system for removal of tumor cells from blood harvested during cancer surgery, *Anesthesiology* 71:A87, 1989.
37. Kempin S, Gould-Rossbach P, and Howland WS: Disorders of hemostasis in the critically ill cancer patient. In Howland WS, Carlon GC, eds: *Critical care of the cancer patient*, Chicago, 1985, Year Book Medical Publishers.
38. Keon TP: Death on induction of anesthesia for cervical node biopsy, *Anesthesiology* 55:471, 1981.
39. Klimberg I, Siroisi R, Wajsman Z et al: Intraoperative autotransfusion in urologic oncology, *Arch Surg* 121:1326, 1986.

40. Krementz ET et al: Hyperthermic regional perfusion for melanoma of the limbs. In Balch CM, Milton GW, eds: *Cutaneous melanoma: clinical management and treatment results worldwide,* Philadelphia, 1985, JB Lippincott.

41. Kvols LK, Moertel CG, O'Connell MJ et al: Treatment of malignant carcinoid syndrome, *N Engl J Med* 315:663, 1986.

42. Lake CL: Anesthesia and pericardial disease, *Anesth Analg* 62:431, 1983.

43. LaMantia KR, Glick JH, and Marshall BE: Supplemental oxygen does not cause respiratory failure in bleomycin-treated surgical patients, *Anesthesiology* 60:65, 1984.

44. Linton RAF: Oxygen and associated gases. In Churchill-Davidson HC, ed: *A practice of anaesthesia,* Chicago, 1984, Year Book Medical Publishers.

45. Lockwood P: Assessment of generalized airway obstruction in patients with carcinoma of the bronchus, *Respiration* 41(4): 252, 1981.

46. Longnecker D, Roizen M: Patients with carcinoid syndrome, *Anesthesiol Clin North Am* June:313, 1987.

47. Mackie AM, Watson CB: Anaesthesia and mediastinal masses, *Anaesthesia* 39: 899, 1984.

48. Mallampati SR, Gatt SP, Gugino LD et al: A clinical sign to predict tracheal difficult intubation: a prospective study, *Can Anaesth Soc J* 32:429, 1985.

49. Marschall K: *Anesthetic management of the patient undergoing resection of pheochromocytoma,* ASA Refresher Course Lectures, 1987.

50. Marsh HM, Martin JK Jr, Kvols LK et al: Carcinoid crisis during anesthesia: successful treatment with somatostatin analogue, *Anesthesiology* 66:89, 1987.

51. McCammon RL: Cancer. In Stoelting RK, Dierdorf SF, eds: *Anesthesia and co-existing disease,* New York, 1983, Churchill-Livingstone.

52. Messmer KFW: Acceptable hematocrit levels in surgical patients, *W J Surg* 11:41, 1987.

53. Midias NE, Harrington JT: Platinum nephrotoxicity, *Am J Med* 65:307, 1978.

54. Miller BR: Neurotoxicity and vincristine, *JAMA* 253:2045, 1985.

55. Miller RD: *Current perspectives on blood transfusions,* IARS Review Course Lectures Suppl, *Anesth Analg,* 57, 1990.

56. Moller CT, Schoonbee CG, and Rosendorff C: Haemodynamics of cardiac tamponade during various modes of ventilation, *Br J Anaesth* 51:409, 1979.

57. Neuman GG, Weingarten AE, Abramowitz RM, et al: The anesthetic management of the patient with an anterior mediastinal mass, *Anesthesiology* 60:144, 1984.

58. Nygaard K, Smith-Erichsen J, Hatlevoll R et al: Pulmonary complications after bleomycin, irradiation, and surgery for esophageal cancer, *Cancer* 41:17, 1978.

59. Pashayan AG: *Anesthesia for laser surgery,* ASA Refresher Course Lectures, 1988.

60. Pashayan AG, Gravenstein JS, Cassisi NS et al: The helium protocol for laryngotracheal operations with CO_2 laser: a retrospective review of 523 cases, *Anesthesiology* 68:801, 1988.

61. Pass HI: Treatment of malignant pleural and pericardial effusions. In DeVita VT, Hellman S, and Rosenberg SA, eds: *Cancer principles and practice of oncology,* Philadelphia, 1989, JB Lippincott.

62. Piro AJ, Weiss DR, and Hellman S: Mediastinal Hodgkin's disease: a possible danger for intubation anesthesia, *Int J Radiat Oncol Biol Phys* 1:415, 1976.

63. Pritsos CA, Sartorelli AC: Generation of reactive oxygen radicals through bioactivation of mitomycin antibiotics, *Cancer Res* 46:3528, 1986.

64. Rickels FR, Edwards RL: Activation of blood coagulation in cancer: Trousseau's syndrome revisited, *Blood* 63:14, 1983.

65. Roberts JT: *Fundamentals of tracheal intubation,* ed 1, New York, 1983, Grune & Stratton.

66. Roizen MF: Anesthetic implications of concurrent disease. In Miller R, ed: *Anesthesia,* New York, 1986, Churchill-Livingstone.

67. Roizen MF, Hunt TK, Beaupre PN et al: The effect of alpha-adrenergic blockade on cardiac performance and tissue oxygen delivery during excision of pheochromocytoma, *Surgery* 94:941, 1983.

68. Roizen MF, Scherider D, and Hassan S: Anesthesia for patients with pheochromocytoma, *Anesthesiol Clin North Am* June:269, 1987.

69. Rundles RW, Wyngaarden JB: Drugs and uric acid, *Annu Rev Pharmacol Toxicol* 9:345, 1969.

70. Schecter WP, Wilson PJ: Management of upper airway obstruction in the intensive care unit, *Crit Care Med* 9:577, 1981.

71. Scott GM, Sechor DS, Flowers D et al: Toxicity of interferon, *Br Med J* 282:1345, 1981.

72. Selvin BL: Cancer chemotherapy: implications for the anesthesiologist, *Anesth Analg* 60(6):425, 1981.

73. Sikic BI: Biochemical and cellular determinants of bleomycin cytotoxicity, *Cancer Surv* 5(1):81, 1986.

74. Sivarajan M, Fink BR: The position and the state of the larynx during general anesthesia and muscle paralysis, *Anesthesiology* 72:439, 1990.

75. Sofer S, Bai-Ziv J, and Scharf SM: Pulmonary edema following relief of upper airway obstruction, *Chest* 86:401, 1984.

76. Sogal RN, Gottlieb AA, Boutros AR et al: Effects of oxygen on bleomycin-induced lung damage, *Cleve Clin J Med* 54(4):503, 1987.

77. Sorensen PG, Rossing N, and Rorth M: Carbon monoxide diffusing capacity: a reliable indicator of bleomycin-induced pulmonary toxicity, *Eur J Respir Dis* 66: 333, 1985.

78. Stehling L: *Fiberoptic intubation of the trachea,* ASA Refresher Course Lecture, 1988.

79. Stoelting RK, Dierdorf SF, and McMamman RC: *Endocrine disease, anesthesia and coexisting disease,* New York, 1988, Churchill-Livingstone.

80. Stoelting RK, Dierdorf SF, and MaCamman RC: *Skin and musculoskeletal disease, anesthesia and coexisting disease,* New York, 1988, Churchill-Livingstone.

81. Strong EW: Head and neck emergencies. In Turnbull ADM, ed: *Surgical emergencies in the cancer patient,* Chicago, 1987, Year Book Medical Publishers.

82. Stone HH, Donnelly CC: The anesthetic significance of serotonin secreting carcinoid tumors, *Anesthesiology* 21:203, 1960.

83. Thomas SJ: Non-coronary heart disease, IARS Review Course Lectures Suppl, *Anesth Analg,* 80, 1986.

84. Thorne AC, Bedford RF: Esmolol for perioperative management of thyrotoxic goiter, *Anesthesiology* 71:291, 1989.

85. Thorne AC, Shah NK, and Matarazzo D: Isoflurane or fentanyl for patients with Adriamycin-induced cardiomyopathy? *Anesthesiology* A58, 1988.

86. Von Hoff DD, Rozencweig M, and Piccart M: The cardiotoxicity of anticancer agents, *Semin Oncol* 9(1):23, 1982.

87. Voogt PJ, van de Velde CJ, Brand A et al: Perioperative blood transfusion and cancer prognosis, *Cancer* 59:836, 1987.

88. Warner ME, Warner MA, and Leonard PF: Anesthesia for neodymium YAG laser resection of major airway obstructing tumors, *Anesthesiology* 60:230, 1984.

89. Wei WI, Siu KF, Lau WF et al: Emergency endotracheal intubation under fiberoptic guidance for malignant laryngeal obstruction, *Otolaryngol Head Nec Surg* 98(1):101, 1988.

90. Wilson ME, Spiegelhalter D, Robertson JA et al: Predicting difficult intubation, *Br J Anaesth* 61:211, 1988.

91. Wolf GL, Simpson JI: Flammability of endotracheal tubes in oxygen and nitrous oxide enriched atmosphere, *Anesthesiology* 67:236, 1987.

92. Zakowski M, Kaufman B, Berguson D et al: Esmolol use during pheochromocytoma: report of three cases, *Anesthesiology* 70:875, 1989.

93. Zsigmond EK, Robins G: The effects of a series of anticancer drugs on plasma cholinesterase activity, *Can Anaesth Soc J* 19:75, 1972.

CHAPTER 23

Evaluation of the Patient with Perioperative Malnutrition

CLIFFORD SCOTT DEUTSCHMAN

As a result of advances in critical care medicine, operative intervention is often being provided for older and sicker patients. These individuals frequently suffer the consequences of disease-induced altered metabolism and nutritional depletion. Today's anesthesiologist, therefore, requires a solid working knowledge of perioperative metabolic abnormalities and their effects on organ function, drug metabolism, and patient outcome. This chapter addresses: (1) the definition of malnutrition, (2) the assessment of malnutrition, (3) the incidence of malnutrition in surgical patients, (4) the effects on organ system function, (5) the consequences of attempted reversal on organ system function, and (6) the association of reversal with improved outcome.

DEFINITION AND SCOPE OF PROTEIN-ENERGY MALNUTRITION

Inadequate intake of macronutrients (carbohydrate, protein, fat) is referred to as protein-energy malnutrition (PEM). The hallmark of this process is a reduction in lean body-cell mass. Original work on PEM centered on children in underdeveloped nations and adults on experimental diets designed to mimic famine or "life-raft" conditions.* Bistrian first advanced the hypothesis that **PEM in sick adults represents a broad spectrum of abnormalities. These result from the interplay of metabolic changes resulting from starvation with those occurring as a result of "stress" (inflammation, infection, surgery, trauma, and neoplasia).**[22] A brief review of these two different states is important, because the **clinical presentation of the two is different** and because **nutritional management principles derived for use in starvation are ineffective (and in fact may lead to complications) in the face of stress.**[45]

In the face of an initial period of fasting, metabolic rate decreases to conserve endogenous substrate, especially nitrogen.[46,58,76,147,182] Glucose is the predominant fuel of early starvation and continues to be made available to those tissues that require it (brain,

---

* References 36, 84, 130, 144, 157, 170.

fibroblasts, red cells, white cells, renal medullary tissue). Glucose is initially derived from glycogen, but following the depletion of stores (about 24 hours following the start of a fast) hepatic and renal gluconeogenesis from amino acids supplied by muscle catabolism predominate.[147,181,182] Insulin secretion decreases because gluconeogenesis is unable to maintain blood glucose concentration at prestarvation levels.[147,182] Low insulin levels promote lipolysis (by activation of a hormone-sensitive lipase) and ketonemia.[87,156] Ketones inhibit pyruvate dehydrogenase and prevent the conversion of pyruvate to acetyl coenzyme A (CoA); utilization of the end-products of glycolysis in the tricarboxylic acid cycle is therefore blocked.[156] As a consequence, the primary fuel for most tissues switches to acetyl CoA derived from fat or ketones. This change is reflected in a decrease in the respiratory quotient (carbon dioxide production/oxygen consumption).[46,147] In addition, the drop in glucose level is associated with secretion of epinephrine, cortisol, and glucagon. The effect of these three "counterregulatory" hormones is stimulation of proteolysis, lipolysis, and gluconeogenesis.[58,87,147,182] Fuel for tissues that are obligate glucose users is supplied by muscle-derived gluconeogenesis. If allowed to continue unchecked, such a process would culminate in rapid depletion of endogenous protein primarily because of high demand by neural tissue. To counter this effect, brain tissue adapts to the use of ketones, permitting a further decrease in glucose demand and sparing lean body mass to some degree.[46,92,181]

Adaptation to exogenous substrate is excellent; when given glucose, a starved individual responds to the increase in serum glucose by increasing insulin secretion and decreasing levels of counter-regulatory hormones. This decreases levels of proteolysis, lipolysis, and gluconeogenesis, spares endogenous tissues, and allows for reliance on the externally supplied glucose.[147] Similar patterns are noted when exogenous fuel is supplied as fat or protein.[46] When demand for energy increases, as in exercise, anaerobic metabolism of glucose also increases.[76] Primary use of branched-chain amino acids by muscle may help meet the new demand.[46,147] Lactate from anaerobiosis and amino acids derived from proteolysis (which are in part driven by increased levels of catecholamines) are released by exercising muscle and are recycled by the liver via a gluconeogenic pathway. The newly synthesized glucose can return to skeletal muscle and again be burned to lactate. These processes make metabolic rate responsive to tissue demand and exogenous substrate availability with only low levels of neuroendocrine modulation.[46,76] **Prolonged fasting metabolism eventually results in a clinical picture similar to the form of PEM described in children as marasmus.**[83,157,159] **This is characterized by uniform loss of** **fat and muscle mass in all tissues and a concomitant loss of water in proportion to nonaqueous mass.**[133]

In contrast, **acute stress metabolism involves high levels of neurohumoral modulation.**[45,46,48] Inflammation, surgery, trauma, or infection activates monokines, lymphokines, prostanoids, hormones, neural pathways, complement, and a host of other endogenous mediators, which in turn "drive" metabolism and increase energy expenditure.[*] Part of the source for this alteration appears to be derived directly from the energy and substrate demands of hepatic macrophages and the white cell infiltrate in wound tissue.[44,164] After a specific injury this **response runs a regulated time course, with a peak in metabolic rate about 3 days after the insult and a gradual decline to baseline by postinjury day 7.**[45,46,48,60,242] The response will run longer if a new activating event occurs or if the source of the initial event (i.e., an undrained abscess) is not removed.[45,48,60,242] The magnitude of the response is proportional to the magnitude of the injury.[45,60,79] Hepatic processes responding to the altered neurohumoral milieu generate substrate for the increased metabolism. Amino acids from proteolysis, lactate from devascularized tissues, and glycerol from lipolysis are directed into gluconeogenetic pathways.[20,60,61,72,185] Amino acids are also used to synthesize enzymes[39] and structural proteins while free fatty acids provide an alternate energy source. Because endogenous mediators stimulated in part by devascularized wound tissue mediate this process, it remains relatively unresponsive to exogenous substrate.[11,56,77,114,151] The hormonal pattern is characterized by elevations of counterregulatory hormones, driven by wound (especially white cell) demands; blood glucose then becomes elevated. The result is an elevation of insulin levels. This pattern of metabolism leads to depletion of visceral protein (in excess of muscle mass) and fat and is associated with an expansion of the extracellular fluid compartment.[81,133,166,222] Physical findings (edema, hypoalbuminemia, fatty liver) are similar to those noted in childhood kwashiorkor.[21,22]

Assessment of the presence and extent of PEM is essential to determine the effect of the process on perioperative physiology. Quantification is best accomplished by direct measurement of body cell mass; unfortunately, this requires the use of multiple isotopic techniques and is often not clinically realistic.[83,119,166] **Alternative methodology has traditionally involved the use of indirect parameters** that are believed to correlate with body-cell mass.[96,244] Anthropometrics, biochemical markers (most often circulating hepatic-derived proteins), and tests of immunologic function have all been used. Unfortunately, all

---

are associated with serious drawbacks that make their validity questionable.

Most anthropometric measures were originally developed for the assessment of malnutrition in childhood PEM.[157,159] Consequently parameters that are of key importance in adults but are negligible in children (frame size, build, fat patterning) are neglected.[22,157,159] Ninety-five percent confidence intervals for these parameters do not exist, reflecting the fact that they were developed to apply to populations and not individuals.* Edema is a prominent characteristic in stress-induced PEM. This factor makes the interpretation of anthropometric measurements difficult. Decreases in specific hepatic-derived transport proteins (albumin, transferrin, prealbumin, retinol-binding protein) are common in any stress state and reflect the interplay of decreased synthesis, tissue extravasation, and extracellular fluid expansion, both from endogenous and exogenous sources.[81] The role of actual depletion of body cell mass on these biochemical markers is unclear. Serum protein concentrations are often only mildly decreased in pure starvation PEM despite significant loss in body cell mass because of the proportional loss of mass and water.[36,123,130,199] In stress states, these markers will decrease irrespective of whether body cell mass is lost to any appreciable degree.[81,93,221] Abnormalities of cell-mediated immunity and absolute lymphopenia have also been touted as indices of PEM.[165] The presence of these abnormalities in such diverse disease states as cancer, collagen-vascular disease, sepsis, uremia, and cirrhosis, as well as the alterations produced by drug administration, make them particularly nonspecific.[25,119,163] Finally, all three of these commonly used measures lack specificity and are derived from population studies that may have little bearing on individual patients.[95,157]

Alternative approaches have been advocated by a number of workers to overcome the deficiencies inherent in the standard assessment of malnutrition. Shizgal et al. have used isotopic techniques to measure the ratio of exchangeable potassium to exchangeable sodium, which should estimate the ratio of extracellular to intracellular mass and thus estimate lean body mass.[83,84,215] The problem with this approach, as pointed out by Moore et al.[166] and Hill[109] is that there may be variability in potassium from tissue to tissue. The cadaver studies necessary to determine normal exchangeable potassium values have never been performed. Other individuals have recommended following multiple parameters over time.[26,45,227] Composite prognostic indices calculated from a series of unrelated variables have been formulated by these workers to classify and stratify the

extent of PEM.[42,103] All these indices lack specificity, however, and although they are indeed prognostic and capable of identifying patients at risk for complications, it is not clear that these complications are related to PEM.[157,159] Several clinicians have advocated a thorough history and physical examination coupled with evidence of weight loss or the presence of a known "catabolic" disease as being as valid as any sophisticated test or technique.[13,66,152,180] Finally, more studies are directed at assessing the role of **indirect calorimetry,** which **directly measures oxygen consumption and carbon dioxide production and uses these values to calculate resting energy expenditure.** Further testing is required to fully assess the usefulness of this modality.[132]

Accurate estimation of the presence and severity of PEM clearly remains problematic, especially for the anesthesiologist whose evaluation of the patient is often brief and who therefore relies on the workup done by his medical and surgical colleagues. The presence of a severe disease producing rapid depletion (i.e., an aggressive malignancy) or a prolonged process involving limited intake or absorption (vomiting, diarrhea, upper gastrointestinal obstruction) makes depletion likely. Indirect calorimetry is useful in evaluating overall metabolic rate with the caveat that these data must be obtained in a reliable and reproducible manner. New developments offer promise. Functional testing of recovery time from isolated twitch in somatic muscle,[120] direct measurement of the size of extracellular compartment size,[83] and quantification of T-cell subpopulations, particularly killer cells,[1] are techniques of promise and may soon be routinely available.

The importance of assessment of PEM to the practicing anesthesiologist lies in awareness that malnutrition, as detailed in a following section, is often present in patients presenting for surgery and has profound implications with respect to organ function and physiology. Therefore the anesthesiologist should suspect the presence of depletion and recognize its potential for precipitating difficulties in perioperative management.

INCIDENCE OF MALNUTRITION IN HOSPITALIZED SURGICAL PATIENTS

Malnutrition in the hospitalized patient does not represent a new concern,[33,187] but true recognition of the presence of a serious nutritional problem can be traced to the work of Bistrian and colleagues. These researchers identified **abnormalities of anthropometrics or biochemical markers consistent with malnutrition in 50% of general surgical patients**[23] **and 44% of general medical patients**[24] in a large urban hospital. Numerous other investigations have confirmed these

---

* References 22, 41, 57, 83, 97, 120, 121, 157, 192, 244.

findings in various hospital settings and patient populations.* However, the use of anthropometrics, biochemical markers, and demonstration of altered delayed hypersensitivity as diagnostic criteria for malnutrition is of uncertain specificity and value and may overestimate the extent of the problem. In a study conducted at a Veterans Administration hospital, an abnormality of one or more of these variables was present in 97% of patients.[168] Such an estimate seems unreasonable. Symreng et al. found that **28% of surgical patients had, on admission to the hospital, three or more abnormalities consistent with depleted body cell mass.**[227] This would appear to be a more valid estimate and is consistent with data reported elsewhere.[110,169] Perhaps of even greater significance is a study noting that in **75% of patients admitted with nutritional indices interpreted as "normal" abnormalities developed over the course of hospitalization.**[238] Together these findings suggest that, although the actual incidence of malnutrition is unclear, the problem exists on a relatively wide scale in hospitalized patients and may develop or worsen over the course of hospitalization. **For the working anesthesiologist, there are two key points. The first is that PEM represents a real and not uncommon problem that alters normal physiology. The second is that PEM acquired over the course of hospitalization may alter a patient's response from one anesthetic to the next.**

EFFECTS OF PROTEIN-ENERGY MALNUTRITION AND NUTRITIONAL REPLETION ON INDIVIDUAL ORGAN SYSTEM FUNCTION

The effects of protein-energy malnutrition and its repletion on individual organ systems are reviewed in this section. When possible, human data will be cited; otherwise appropriate animal studies will be presented. An attempt has been made to separate the effects of starvation from stress; the former is disproportionately represented.

Cardiovascular Changes

Starvation PEM is associated with morphologic, functional, and electrical abnormalities of the cardiovascular system. **Heart size decreases in proportion to loss of body mass**[4,5,30,129,130] and the left ventricular free wall is thinned.[4,95] Histologic examination reveals myocardial atrophy and interstitial edema.[2,47,89] Left atrial, aortic root, and left ventricular end-systolic and end-diastolic dimensions are reduced relative to normal controls[95] and left ventricular compliance is reduced.[4] **Heart rate at rest, blood pressure, and pulse pressure are decreased,**[30,129,130] and a subnormal re-

sponse is noted in these parameters on exercise testing.[95] **Cardiac index and ejection fraction remain at prestarvation levels**[4,95,106] **and appear to increase appropriately with exercise**[95] or beta-adrenergic stimulation.[4] ECG amplitude is diminished, axis shows a rightward deviation, PR and QT intervals are prolonged, T waves are inverted to flattened, ST-T segments are depressed, and nodal escape beats and ventricular tachycardia have been reported.[6,95,118,217,233]

Stress metabolism in cachectic humans is associated with a somewhat different picture than noted in isolated starvation. **Heart rate and indexed ventricular mass** (per kilogram of body weight) **are increased.**[107] **This suggests that stressed myocardium is spared from some of the protein-depleting aspects of PEM and can respond normally to increased demand for work even when other tissues are being wasted.** The heart's ability to use virtually any fuel (glucose, fat, ketones, lactate) may partially account for this. Severe histologic changes have been noted in starvation in animals such as rats, who are believed to exist in a persistent "hypermetabolic" state.[177,183]

Protein and calorie repletion in previously healthy adults subjected to a semistarvation diet **results in a rapid increase in heart size.**[85,95,129,130] Heart rate, blood pressure, and pulse pressures initially increase with repletion to above prestarvation levels and gradually return to baseline. **Ejection fraction and cardiac output/index may actually fall and congestive failure has been reported.** The cause of these abnormalities is unknown[129,130] but may reflect mobilization of interstitial fluid coupled with the inability of depleted cardiac muscle to handle the fluid load. ECG amplitude and QT interval abnormalities persist for variable periods despite repletion.[30,95,129]

Only one study to date has focused on the effects of repletion of stress-induced PEM on cardiac function.[107] Ventricular mass, heart rate, end-diastolic volume, cardiac output, and ejection fraction all increased, but congestive heart failure developed in three of five patients and a pericardial effusion developed in a fourth patient. The true nature of these findings is unknown given the small sample size.

Pulmonary Changes

Lung cell mass (lung weight:body weight) appears to increase in cases of PEM, but overall wet and dry lung weights decrease with depletion.[63,202,203,229] **Morphologic changes similar to those observed in emphysema are characteristic;** distances between alveolar walls are increased, the surface area for gas exchange is decreased, and air space is grossly enlarged as a result of disruption of alveolar septae.[128,204,205] Peripheral lung tissue is more affected than central mass and a significant loss of collagen and elastin is noted.[101,128,202-208] **The phospholipoprotein content of**

---

* References 84, 146, 168, 169, 241, 243.

surfactant is grossly depleted.* In the early stages of depletion, pressure-volume relationships are normal,[86,190,229] but after prolonged starvation surfactant concentrations decrease, active surface forces increase, and exposure of alveolar surfaces leads to an **altered functional residual capacity.**[38,78,172,190]

Diaphragmatic muscle mass decreases in direct proportion to loss of body weight.[9,10,127] As a result, the tension developed in isolated diaphragmatic muscle strips is reduced. Mechanical efficiency, however, appears to be unchanged.[149,193] Observed changes in the time to achieve 50% tension reduction following 20 or 100 Hz tetanus indicate that diaphragmatic fatigability is reduced.[127] Animal studies indicate a selective depletion of fast (glycolytic or oxidative) fibers with sparing of the slow oxidative fibers, a finding that supports the notion of decreased fatigability.[127]

After a period of mild acute starvation in otherwise healthy adult women, forced vital capacity, forced expiratory volume, inspiratory pressure, and maximal voluntary ventilation were normal.[19] A more prolonged course of severe depletion in both human and animal subjects results in decreases in all lung volumes, maximal pressure generation, and maximal ventilatory effort.[9,101,195] **Respiratory rate is decreased, perhaps reflecting altered carbon dioxide production; the ventilatory response to carbon dioxide is preserved but hypoxic ventilatory drive is markedly attenuated.**[12,71] The number of alveolar macrophages and their ability to clear aerosolized *Staphylococcus aureus* is decreased.[98,167,213]

Refeeding in rats leads to return to normal of lung weight and lung hydroxyproline, elastin, and surfactant contents.[203,204] Parenchymal emphysematous changes, however, are incompletely reversed.[204] As body weight is regained so too is diaphragmatic contractile force.[193] Respiratory muscle function, maximal inspiratory pressure,[126] and phagocytic capacity also improve.[213] Abnormalities of hypoxic ventilatory drive, however, are not prevented despite the provision of amino acids formulas sufficient to prevent negative nitrogen balance.[195] The effects of repletion on lung volumes and hypoxic ventilatory drive are unkown.

Renal Changes

In the face of starvation, renal mass is lost in proportion to body mass and renal protein content is reduced.[54,94,231,234,240] **Clearance of creatinine and free water are decreased and effective renal plasma flow, glomerular filtration rate, and filtration fraction fall dramatically.†** However, total renal blood flow is not reduced.[74] **The ability to concentrate the urine in response to water restriction is impaired.**[82,135-138,209] A normal response to exogenous antidiuretic hormone has been reported, indicating that the defect in concentrating ability is most likely related to interstitial urea depletion and is not an intrinsic defect in collecting duct function.[135-138]

Total body water is decreased by starvation PEM but exchangeable sodium remains normal, implying that cellular mass and exchangeable potassium are decreased.[219] Free water clearance and sodium excretion are elevated early in the course of starvation[34,49,211] but decline after several days.[29,31,236] Renin and aldosterone levels are elevated in this early natriuretic period. The role that this plays in sodium homeostasis in the face of PEM is uncertain.[49,90,140,211] Titratable acid excretion is decreased while serum bicarbonate and urinary ammonia concentrations increase.[90,91] Refeeding following starvation PEM improves glomerular filtration rate, filtration fraction, concentrating ability, and free water clearance.[32,135,201,231] Sodium and acid excretion increase as do plasma and extracellular volume.[18,54] After a period of refeeding, accompanied by increasing plasma osmolality, interstitial water moves into the intravascular compartment. This is associated with a diuretic phase.

Surgical or traumatic stress activates renal mechanisms to conserve salt and water[45,166] **and thus expand the vasculature to improve substrate delivery. Both antidiuretic hormone and aldosterone are involved in this response, and plasma volume contraction in this setting can produce a metabolic alkalosis.**[46] The effects of prolonged stress are unknown and no data exist regarding repletion.

Gastrointestinal Changes

Intestinal mass, a rapid turnover tissue, is lost at a proportionately greater rate than body weight in starved rats.[162,224] Small intestine as a whole, and mucosal cells in particular, have decreased contents of DNA, RNA, and nitrogen.* Epithelial cell renewal and migration are reduced[37] and villus size[7] and crypt cell number, size, and mitotic rate[55] are decreased. Gastric ulceration, gastric and intestinal atrophy, and mucosal hemorrhage are all present to a great extent,[130,131] perhaps reflecting mucosal breakdown either as a result of increased lysosomal acid hydrolase[65] or failure to synthesize mucosal glycoproteins. Gastrin concentrations fall.[150] Long-term fasting appears to be required for mucosal changes to occur; Knudsen et al. found normal histologic conditions following a 7-day fast in obese individuals.[139]

Mucosal transport, reflected in decreased uptake of

---

* References 38, 78, 88, 172, 190, 200, 203, 207, 239.
†References 54, 94, 130, 135-138, 188, 201, 209, 234.

* References 112, 113, 130, 162, 224, 226.

oral mannitol, may be impaired.[75] Sucrase and maltase (but not lactase) activities are decreased, with this change being most prominent in the proximal GI tract.[7,28,73,186] Glucose transfer across the mucosa decreases but mucosal-to-serosal transport of both glucose and histidine increase.[111,173] Loss of brush border enzymes impairs absorption and promotes bacterial overgrowth.[131]

Healing of mucosal ulcerations has been reported in depleted patients with Crohn's disease who receive parenteral nutrition. Increased nitrogen retention and improved gastric motility in starved individuals has been noted.[124,130] Cell populations and absorptive capacity improve,[7] activity of brush border enzymes is restored,[65,130,139] and lysosomal enzyme activities decrease to normal.[65,131]

Enteral feeding seems to be more effective than parenteral nutrition in restoring GI function postoperatively.[8,155,210] Mucosal integrity, brush border enzyme levels, and absorptive capacity all improve rapidly in depleted animals refed orally.[80,148,232] Use of glutamine has been implicated in this improvement[220]; it appears that even parenterally administered glutamine (which is not present in most total parenteral nutrition formulations) is of benefit.[179]

Pancreatic Changes

Pancreatic mass decreases in direct proportion to body mass and acinar atrophy; also loss of architecture, fibrosis, and exocrine duct dilatation are all noted in response to starvation PEM.[73,145,147] Rough endoplasmic reticulum and mitochondria are decreased.[27] Amylase and trypsinogen content in the pancreas falls, and lipase is increased.[145,147,184] Duodenal aspirates show a sequential decrease in level of lipase, trypsin, and amylase as PEM progresses. Bicarbonate secretion also decreases in adults.[184] Loss of structural integrity is reflected in increased serum amylase levels and indices of amylase production in patients with anorexia nervosa.[176] The exocrine pancreas following PEM in rats shows decreased responsiveness to carbachol stimulation; in addition, insulin responsiveness to glucose stimulation is attenuated.[70,145] Insulin secretion, exocrine responses to carbachol, and serum amylase and lipase levels return to normal after refeeding.[145,176]

Hepatic Changes

In humans, starvation results in a rapid loss of liver glycogen. Because of defective triglyceride excretion and carnitine-limited uptake, reesterification of free fatty acids in the periportal region occurs.[3,45,134,141,147] Prolonged PEM will eventually deplete even the periportal fat deposits. In chronic protein deficiency in rats, liver mass and rough endoplasmic reticulum are lost.[226] **Loss of RNA, water, fat, and protein as well**

as cellular atrophy have all been reported, but it appears that hepatocytes are remarkably resistant to loss of structure or number.[35,147,158,214] Patients with weight loss as great as 55 kg have had histologically normal liver biopsies although the presence of pigment deposits, fibrosis, and fatty infiltration has also been reported.[147,178] In pure starvation, hepatic enzyme levels and bilirubin may be normal or elevated[14,15,197,198]; albumin synthesis and total albumin content decrease but concentrations may be normal.[134] Urinary nitrogen loss decreases, reflecting activation of amino acid–conserving enzymes and decreased urea cycle activity.[158]

Protein deficiency reduces drug metabolism in many cases as a result of decreased microsomal enzyme activity and altered cytochrome P-450/NADPH–dependent transport mechanisms.[16,17,154] **Thus decreased transformation of compounds that are hepatically detoxified may lead to pathologic responses that require dosage alteration. However, compounds that are biotransformed into toxic metabolites are better tolerated.**[160,161]

Levels of many products of hepatic protein synthesis are altered during stress.[45,185] **The level of mRNA for acute-phase products, such as fibrinogen, or α_1-antiproteases, is increased while synthesis of transport proteins such as albumin is decreased.**[39]

Liver size and function return to normal with refeeding; gross and ultrastructural morphology are restored after several weeks of repletion.[141,226] Hepatocellular enzyme levels in the serum may initially increase with refeeding but eventually normalize.[14,67,144] Effects of repletion on drug metabolism are unknown.

Immunologic Changes

Protein-energy malnutrition is associated with a reduction in the mass of lymphoid tissue in excess of loss of body mass.[69,100] Both small lymphocytes and germinal centers are affected. Total circulating polymorphonuclear (PMN) cell counts are reduced but the fraction of total white cells that are PMNs is increased. Macrophage and PMN chemotaxis, bacterial engulfment, and intracellular killing are impaired.[52,69,100] Serum levels and activity of complement components C3 and C5 are normal in stress, but all other components of both the direct and indirect pathways are reduced in stress and all components are reduced in starvation.[69,100,185]

Circulating B cells are reduced in absolute number but account for an increased percentage of the total lymphocyte count. Serum immunoglobulin levels may be low, normal, or high.[69,102] Impairments of antibody binding and antigen specificity have been reported.[69,100] Impaired cell-mediated immunity is one of the characteristics of the malnourished state.[62,69,100,115,175] Absolute numbers of T cells and the ratio of T cells to total white cells is reduced.[68,100] The proportion of T-helper and T-suppressor cells is normal in starvation but reduced in stress; T-killer cells are reduced in both states.[1]

Lymphoid tissue mass, cell populations, and germinal center populations respond well to nutritional repletion. Phagocytosis and chemotaxis improve but the effects of refeeding on engulfment and intracellular killing are unknown.[68,69,100] Delayed hypersensitivity to skin testing[142] antibody levels (circulating or fixed)[69,142,143] and complement levels[68,69] return to normal with nutritional therapy.[143,174,175] Short-term repletion has no effect on T cell subpopulations in stress or starvation.[1] The effects of longer treatment are unknown.[1]

Nervous System Changes

Peripheral nerves have demonstrated diminished conduction velocity and associated sensory abnormalities have been reported in PEM.[50] In moderate PEM, nerve biopsies are normal, but severe depletion is associated with segmental demyelination.[196,216] Chronic malnutrition may lead to lethargy, confusion, and impaired initiative.[130] Cerebral atrophy, ventricular dilatation, and diffuse EEG slowing have been noted.[64,147] In adult rats deprived of protein the phosphatidylglycerol and sphingophospholipid fractions are low but other myelin components are present in normal quantities.[237] Refeeding appears to restore nerve conduction and structure[196,216] and to improve mental status.[130]

Anesthetic Implications of Systems Dysfunction

The dysfunctions caused by PEM have important implications intraoperatively. **Cardiac reserve may be compromised,** as evidenced by subnormal blood pressure and heart rate responses to stress testing, but appropriate increases in cardiac output in the face of exercise or beta stimulation argue against this. **The potential for myocardial depression by volatile anesthetics** may have important implications for the depleted patient. In addition, the **partially repleted patient may be at risk for pulmonary edema when mobilization of fluid occurs;** this implies that the **cardiac response to fluid challenges may be inadequate** and, coupled with renal abnormalities, has implications for perioperative fluid administration. **Pulmonary disease resembling emphysema may impair gas exchange, whereas respiratory muscle failure may preclude early extubation,** especially in the face of even mild residual paralysis. **The selective depletion of fast fibers, which may alter the ability to effectively excrete an acute load of carbon dioxide, also may have implications for early extubation given the predictable rise in metabolic rate following surgery associ-** ated with moderate-to-high levels of stress.[48] **Resistance to pulmonary infection is normally maintained by bacterial clearance** (ciliary action and coughing) **and macrophage function; both are impaired in PEM** and will be further depressed by use of general anesthesia. **Renal abnormalities may reduce the clearance of both solute and solvent, resulting in retention of water as well as toxic by-products.** Thus fluid loads may be poorly tolerated and clearance of drugs and cellular debris impaired. **Altered gastric motility places patients at risk for aspiration; prophylactic measures may be indicated.** In addition, because of the loss of brush border enzymes and depletion of GI mucosa, **oral absorption of drugs may be altered. Blood sugar levels in stress may need to be monitored given the relatively impaired insulin response to hyperglycemia. Hepatic drug metabolism may also be altered,** with impaired clearance of some drugs (e.g., vecuronium) but increased tolerance for certain others whose toxic metabolites may not be synthesized (e.g., nitroprusside). **Metabolism of inhalational anesthetics may also be decreased.** Perhaps most important, **lower total circulating levels of albumin and other transport proteins have wide implications regarding drug administration and volume of distribution.** A partial list of commonly used agents that may be affected is noted in Table 23-1. **An increased risk of infection mandates the use of careful sterile technique in even routine line placement.** Use of inhalational anesthetics also may have depressant effects on white cell function. Finally, the **peripheral neuropathy has profound implications with respect to the use of conduction anesthesia, and mental status changes may impinge on rapid and total recovery from general anesthesia.**

EFFECTS OF PERIOPERATIVE PROTEIN-ENERGY MALNUTRITION ON OUTCOME IN SURGICAL PATIENTS
Effects of Malnutrition on Mortality

In 1936, Studley reported that if preoperative weight loss exceeded 20% of premorbid weight, the mortality from surgery for peptic ulcer disease was 33%.[225] This early and unsophisticated study first underscored the importance of nutritional status. More recent studies, focusing on alterations in anthropometrics, transport proteins, and white cell parameters have confirmed these data. Reinhardt found that serum albumin levels less than 3.0 mg/dl were associated with a 30-day mortality of 24% and that patients whose levels were below 2.0 mg/dl had a mortality of 62%.[189] Seltzer et al., in a similar study, noted that albumin levels less than 3.5 mg/dl were associated with fourfold increases in mortality and morbidity, whereas lymphocyte counts below 1500 were associated with a

Table 23-1 Commonly used drugs that are plasma-protein bound	
Drug	**Protein bound (%)**
Narcotics	
Morphine	30
Meperidine	60
Fentanyl	84
Sufentanil	92
Alfentanil	92
Barbiturates	
Thiopental	72-86
Phenobarbital	40-60
Benzodiazepines	
Diazepam	96-98
Midazolam	96-98
Lorazepam	96-98
Nonbarbiturate induction agents	
Etomidate	76
Propofol	98
Local anesthetics	
Tetracaine	80
Lidocaine	70
Mepivacaine	77
Bupivacaine	95
Etidocaine	95
Prilocaine	55
Cardioactive drugs	
Digitalis	25
Labetalol	50
Propranolol	90-95
Nadolol	40-60
Pindolol	<50
Captopril	25-30
Others	
Heparin	
Coumadin	
Aspirin	
Phenytoin	90

fourfold increase in mortality alone.[212] Concurrent abnormalities of both albumin and lymphocyte counts were associated with an 18-fold increase in mortality relative to patients with normal indices. Impaired cell-mediated immunity appears to be an important marker for increased mortality.[108] Meakins et al. noted a perioperative death rate of 3.1% in surgical patients with normal delayed hypersensitivity (assessed by intradermal injection of a battery of antigens), while anergy was associated with a mortal-

ity of 35%. The development of anergy following normal initial testing was invariably fatal.[163] A number of studies have confirmed the association of anergy and poor postoperative outcome.* However, anergy is associated with numerous other factors, all of which may increase perioperative risk independent of malnutrition.

In an attempt to improve specificity, Harvey et al. developed a discriminant function that was used to predict the development of sepsis and surgical mortality.[103,104] This function was primarily based on delayed hypersensitivity testing, transferrin, albumin, and total lymphocyte counts. Prospective evaluation of the index has not been reported. Mullen et al. have developed a "prognostic nutritional index" (PNI) based on a number of nutritionally relevant variables.[168,169] Patients identified by this index as high risk had a mortality of nearly 60%; those categorized as low-risk had mortalities of only 3%. Prospective evaluation of this index has confirmed its utility in identifying high-risk patients, but the true relationship between the variables studied and malnutrition is unclear.[13]

Effects of Malnutrition on Complications

Surgical complications have been shown to occur more frequently in patients with markers for PEM. Patients with preoperative anergy and patients in whom anergy developed postoperatively have greatly increased rates of postoperative sepsis.[163] Preoperative anergy was further associated with a doubling of nonseptic postoperative complications[153,163] and is a significant predictor of prolonged hospitalization.[53] Hypoproteinemia in surgical patients was noted by Rhoads and Alexander to be associated with twice the rate of wound infections and an increased incidence of other infectious complications.[191] In both patients and experimental animals, punch biopsies of wound tissue in starvation showed evidence of impaired collagen synthesis[223]; Cruse and Foord concluded that malnutrition increased the incidence of clean wound infections from 1.8% to 16.6%.[59] Abnormalities of plasma proteins and albumin have been associated with an increased incidence of anastomotic dehiscence.[116] Starved rats with low serum proteins and albumin have decreased colonic collagen content and decreased colonic wall–bursting tension as well as loss of tensile anastomotic strength and collagen content.[117] These final findings could not be confirmed by a second group of investigators.[228]

The uniform association of abnormalities of weight loss, serum proteins, and white cell function with mortality and morbidity in the perioperative period is

---

* References 51, 53, 122, 125, 153, 163.

impressive. Animal studies in which dietary manipulation has ensured the presence of PEM have demonstrated similar results. However, human studies have used nonspecific markers that may correlate with PEM but also may correlate with other risk factors not tested for independence. Thus the true impact of PEM as an independent risk factor for surgical outcome is unknown.

Effect of Repletion on Outcome

Although nutritional repletion may reverse many of the abnormalities that develop in individual organ systems as a result of malnutrition, the **overall effect of perioperative alimentation on outcome is unclear.** Most studies addressing the issue are poorly designed—patients are not randomized, investigators are not blinded and patient populations lack uniformity. Of key importance is that most studies compare different alimentation regimens to each other and, therefore, lack a suitable untreated control group. Finally, the end points are not objective measures of outcome. Despite these limitations, some conclusions can be drawn.

Patients with mild-to-moderate preoperative depletion do not appear to benefit from combined preoperative and postoperative alimentation as compared to postoperative support alone.

In comparing unrandomized, mildly depleted patients with gastrointestinal malignancies to undepleted control patients, Thompson et al. were unable to demonstrate that combined preoperative and postoperative repletion altered mortality or morbidity.[230] Buzby et al., Mullen et al., Heatley et al. (in patients with gastric or esophageal cancer and normal preoperative albumin levels) and Smale et al.[43,105,170,218] (in unrandomized low-risk patients with cancer) compared preoperative and postoperative parenteral nutrition to postoperative support alone and also could not demonstrate a difference in mortality or morbidity.

Significantly depleted patients appear to demonstrate different behavior. When comparing combined preoperative and postoperative intravenous alimentation to postoperative support alone, both Mullen et al. and Smale et al. reported reductions in mortality (9% vs. 47%) and morbidity (23% vs. 56%).[170,218] Muller et al. confirmed these findings in a randomized study of patients with cancer.[171] **Outcome is significantly affected by the duration and efficacy of therapy.** Thus Rombeau et al. retrospectively studied patients undergoing surgery for inflammatory bowel disease and noted that 5% of patients who had received hyperalimentation for 5 or more days had complications, but 46% of those receiving less than 5 days of therapy had some morbidity.[194] Grimes et al. noted similar findings in general surgical patients who were

severely depleted.[99] In another study, one patient (4%) who responded to 1 week of repletion had a perioperative complication, whereas nine of 20 (45%) who did not respond had perioperative morbidity.[222] When therapy in nonresponders was continued for an additional 4 to 6 weeks, until a response consistent with improved nutritional status was noted, the complication rate was 13%. It, therefore, appears that **preoperative repletion of appropriate duration to elicit a response consistent with an improved nutritional status is of benefit in improving perioperative outcome.** Questions of methodology in all the studies cited mandate that conclusions be drawn cautiously.

The blueprint for a well-designed randomized prospective trial has been published.[42] Unfortunately the results[236a] were disappointing and the conclusions unjustified. Only 395 patients were studied; this fell short of the original projection. Patients were randomized to receive either 7 to 15 days of preoperative total parenteral nutrition (TPN) followed by 3 days of postoperative TPN or no TPN until the third postoperative day. No difference in major complications or mortality was noted. However, when patients were stratified by degree of pre-existing malnutrition (based on the Prognostic Nutritional Index), severely malnourished patients receiving TPN had a lower complication rate. The problem is that no assessment was made of the efficacy of nutritional support; specifically, the authors did not report on whether or not nutritional status, even as assessed by their own nutritional index, improved before surgery as a result of TPN. Thus the conclusions are difficult to interpret and the role of TPN remains to be fully elucidated.

Finally, there remains the patient with normal preoperative status about to undergo an extremely stressful procedure or who will be unable to eat for a prolonged period after surgery. Despite the myriad of studies addressing nutritional support there exists no reasonably designed, well-performed study that deals with such patients relative to a meaningful control group. Thus, although it seems self-evident that appropriate support of the catabolic patient should improve outcome, no data exist to support this hypothesis.

Implications of Altered Outcome for the Anesthesiologist

The competent anesthesiologist has, as part of his/her duty to the patient, the charge of ensuring that the patient presenting for elective surgery is in the best possible condition to tolerate the operation and postoperative course. **The relatively poor outcome associated with malnutrition, coupled with the apparent benefits of repletion in the severely depleted individual, constitutes one more problem that can be addressed to improve overall patient outcome.** Dealing with the issue by instituting an appropriate course of repletion in a highly malnourished individual may well be necessary, and calling attention to this potential problem and its remedy may also fall to the anesthesiologist.

SUMMARY

As the field of anesthesiology grows and the scope of the anesthesiologist expands, the disease processes with which the sound practitioner needs to be familiar also increase. **Malnutrition constitutes one more area in which patient disease may alter behavior under anesthesia and increase the potential difficulties for the patient and the anesthesiologist. Knowledge of these effects and their reversal with therapy is useful and potentially lifesaving.**

KEY POINTS

- Older and sicker surgical patients frequently suffer consequences of disease-induced altered metabolism and nutritional depletion. The anesthesiologist must be aware of such consequences and the resulting implications with respect to organ function and physiology in the perioperative period.
- Syndromes of inadequate intake of macronutrients are collectively referred to as protein-energy malnutrition (PEM) and include the disease states resulting from starvation and "stress."
- Prolonged fasting metabolism is characterized by uniform loss of fat and muscle mass in all tissues and a concomitant loss of water in proportion to nonaqueous mass.
- Acute stress metabolism involves high levels of neurohumoral modulation and runs a regulated time course with a peak in metabolic rate about 3

days after the insult and a gradual decline to baseline by postinjury day 7.
- Accurate estimation of the presence and the severity of PEM in the perioperative period remains a clinical problem. The anesthesiologist must be aware of potential alterations in normal physiology resulting from PEM during the entire perioperative period.
- Protein-energy malnutrition results in dysfunction in every major organ system and has profound anesthetic and morbidity/mortality implications.
- The relatively poor outcome associated with malnutrition, coupled with the apparent benefits of repletion in the severely depleted individual, are issues that need to be addressed to improve anesthetic management and overall patient outcome.

KEY REFERENCES

Alden PB, Madoff RD, Stahl TJ et al: Left ventricular function in malnutrition, *Am J Physiol* 253:H380, 1987.

Bistrian BR: Interaction of nutrition and infection in the hospital setting, *Am J Clin Nutr* 30:1228, 1977.

Bistrian BR, Blackburn GL, and Hallowell E: Protein status of general surgical patients, *JAMA* 230:858, 1974.

Buzby GP, Knox LS, Crosby LO et al: Study protocol: a randomized clinical trial of total parenteral nutrition in malnourished surgical patients, *Am J Clin Nutr* 47(suppl):366, 1988.

Cerra FB: Hypermetabolism, organ failure and metabolic support, *Surgery* 101:1, 1987.

Chernow B, Alexander HR, Smallridge RC et al: Hormonal responses to graded surgical stress, *Arch Intern Med* 147:1273, 1987.

Cuthbertson D, Tilstone W: Metabolism during the post-injury period, *Adv Clin Chem* 12:1, 1977.

Fleck A: The acute phase response: implications for nutrition and recovery, *Nutrition* 4:109, 1988.

Hill GL, Blackett RL, Pickford I et al: Malnutrition in surgical patients: an unrecognized problem, *Lancet* 2:689, 1977.

Keys A et al: *The biology of human starvation*, Minneapolis, 1950, University of Minnesota Press.

Klahr S, Alleyne GA: Effects of chronic protein calorie malnutrition on the kidney, *Kidney Int* 3:129, 1973.

Lewis M et al: The effects of malnutrition on diaphragmatic contractility and muscle fiber morphometry, *Am Rev Respir Dis* 131:A326, 1985.

McLaren DS: A fresh look at protein-energy malnutrition in the hospitalized patient, *Nutrition* 4:527, 1972.

Moore FD, Oleson KH, McMurrey JD et al: *The body cell mass and its supporting environment*, Philadelphia, 1978, WB Saunders.

Mullen JL, Buzby GP, Matthews DC et al: Reduction of operating morbidity and mortality by combined preoperative and postoperative nutritional support, *Ann Surg* 192:604, 1980.

O'Dwyer ST, Smith RJ, Weng TL et al: Maintenance of small bowel mucosa with glutanine enriched parenteral nutrition, *J Parenter Enter Nutr* 13:571, 1989.

Owen OE, Reichard GA Jr, Patel MS et al: Energy expenditure in feasting and fasting, *Adv Exp Med Biol* 111:169, 1979.

Rochester DF: Malnutrition and the respiratory muscles, *Clin Chest Med* 7:91, 1986.

Sahebjami H: Nutrition and the pulmonary parenchyma, *Clin Chest Med* 7:111, 1986.

Starker PM, LaSala PA, Askanazi J et al: The influence of preoperative total parenteral nutrition upon operative morbidity and mortality, *Surg Gynecol Obstet* 162:569, 1986.

REFERENCES

1. Abbott WC, Tayek JA, Bistrian BR et al: The effect of nutritional support on five lymphocyte subpopulations in protein calorie malnutriton, *J Am Coll Nutr* 5:577, 1986.
2. Abel RM, Grimes JB, Alonso D et al: Adverse hemodynamic and ultrastructural changes in dog hearts subjected to protein calorie malnutrition, *Am Heart J* 97:733, 1979.
3. Addis T, Poo JL, and Lew W: The quantities of protein lost by various organs and tissues of the body during a fast, *J Biol Chem* 115:111, 1936.
4. Alden PB, Madoff RD, Stahl TJ et al: Left ventricular function in malnutrition, *Am J Physiol* 253:H380, 1987.
5. Alexander JK, Peterson KL: Cardiovascular effects of weight reduction, *Circulation* 45:310, 1972.
6. Alleyne GA: Cardiac function in severely malnourished Jamaican children, *Clin Sci* 30:553, 1966.
7. Altmann GG: Influence of starvation and refeeding on mucosal size and epithelial renewal in the rat small intestine, *Am J Anat* 133:391, 1972.
8. Alverdy J, Chi HS, and Sheldon GF: The effect of parenteral nutrition on gastrointestinal immunity: the importance of enteral stimulation, *Ann Surg* 202:681, 1985.
9. Arora NS, Rochester DF: Effect of body weight and muscularity on human diaphragm muscle mass, thickness and area, *J Appl Physiol* 52:64, 1982.
10. Arora NS, Rochester DF: Respiratory muscle strength and maximal voluntary ventilation in undernourished patients, *Am Rev Respir Dis* 126:5, 1982.
11. Asknazi J, Carpentier YA, Elwyn DH et al: Influence of total parenteral nutrition on fuel utilization in injury and sepsis, *Ann Surg* 191:40, 1989.
12. Baier H, Somani P: Ventilatory drive in normal man during semi-starvation, *Chest* 85:222, 1984.
13. Baker JP, Langer B, Wesson DE et al: Nutritional assessment: a comparison of clinical judgment and objective measurements, *N Engl J Med* 306:969, 1982.
14. Baron DN: Serum transaminase and isocitrate dehydrogenase in kwashiorkor, *J Clin Pathol* 13:252, 1960.

15. Barrett PVD: Hyperbilirubinemia of fasting, *JAMA* 217:1349, 1971.
16. Basu TK: Effects of protein malnutrition and ascorbic acid levels on drug metabolism, *Can J Physiol Pharmacol* 61:295, 1983.
17. Basu TK, Dickerson JW, and Parke DV: Effects of protein/energy nutrition on rat plasma corticosteroids and liver microsomal hydroxylase activity, *Nutr Metab* 18:49, 1975.
18. Batuman V, Dreisbach A, Maesa Ka JK et al: Renal and electrolyte effects of total parenteral nutrition, *J Parenter Enter Nutr* 8:546, 1984.
19. Bender PR, Martin BJ: Ventilatory and treadmill endurance during acute starvation, *J Appl Physiol* 60:1823, 1986.
20. Birkhahn RL, Long CL, Fitkin D et al: Effects of major skeletal trauma on whole body protein turnover in man measured by L-[1, 14C]-leucine, *Surgery* 88:294, 1980.
21. Bistrian BR: Anthropometric norms used in the assessment of hospitalized patients, *Am J Clin Nutr* 33:2211, 1980 [letter].
22. Bistrian BR: Interaction of nutrition and infection in the hospital setting, *Am J Clin Nutr* 30:1228, 1977.
23. Bistrian BR, Blackburn GL, and Hallowell E: Protein status of general surgical patients, *JAMA* 230:858, 1974.
24. Bistrian BR, Blackburn GH, Vitale J et al: Prevalence of malnutrition in general medical patients, *JAMA* 2356:1567, 1976.
25. Bistran BR, Sherman M, Blackburn GL et al: Cellular immunity in adult marasmus, *Arch Intern Med* 137:1408, 1977.
26. Blackburn GL, Bistrian BR, Maini BSet al: Nutritional and metabolic assessment of the hospitalized patient, *J Parenter Enter Nutr* 1:11, 1977.
27. Blackburn WR, Rinijchiakul K: The pancreas in kwashiorkor: an electron microscopic study, *Lab Invest* 20:305, 1969.
28. Blair DG, Yakimets W, and Tuba J: Rat intestinal sucrase. II. The effects of rat age and sex and of diet on sucrase activity, *Can J Biochem Physiol* 41:917, 1963.
29. Bloom WL: Fasting as an introduction to

the treatment of obesity, *Metabolism* 8:214, 1959.
30. Bloom WL, Azar G, and Smith EG: Changes in heart size and plasma volume during fasting, *Metabolism* 15:409, 1966.
31. Bloom WL, Mitchell W Jr: Salt excretion in fasting patients, *Arch Intern Med* 106:321, 1960.
32. Boag F, WeeraKoon J, Ginsburg J et al: Diminished creatinine clearance in anorexia nervosa: reversal with weight gain, *J Clin Pathol* 238:60, 1985.
33. Bollet AJ, Owen SO: Evaluation of nutritional status of selected hospital patients, *Am J Clin Nutr* 26:931, 1973.
34. Boulter PR, Hoffman RS, and Arky RA: Pattern of sodium excretion accompanying starvation, *Metabolism* 22:675, 1973.
35. Brass EP, Hoppel CL: Carnitine metabolism in the fasting rat, *J Biol Chem* 253:2688, 1978.
36. Broom J, Fraser MH, and McKenzie K: The protein metabolic response to short-term starvation in men, *Clin Nutr* 5:63, 1986.
37. Brown HO, Levine ML, and Lipkin M: Inhibition of intestinal epithelial renewal and migration induced by starvation, *Am J Physiol* 205:868, 1963.
38. Brown LA, Bliss AS, and Longmore WJ: Effects of nutritional status on the lung surfactant system: food and caloric restriction, *Exp Lung Res* 6:133, 1984.
39. Buchman TG, Cabin DE, Vickers S et al: Molecular biology of circulatory shock. II. Expression of four groups of hepatic genes is enhanced following resuscitation from cardiogenic shock, *Surgery* 108:559, 1990.
40. Buetler B, Cerami A: Cachectin (tumor necrosis factor): a macrophage hormone governing cellular metabolism and inflammatory response, *Endocr Rev* 9:57, 1988.
41. Burgert SL, Anderson CF: An evaluation of upper arm measurement used in nutritional assessment, *Am J Clin Nutr* 31:2136, 1979.
42. Buzby GP, Knox LS, Crosby LO et al: Study protocol: a randomized clinical trial of total parenteral nutrition in malnourished surgical patients, *Am J Clin Nutr* 47(suppl):366, 1988.

43. Buzby GP, Mullen JL, Matthews DC et al: Prognostic nutritional index in gastrointestinal surgery, *Am J Surg* 139:160, 1980.
44. Caldwell MD: Importance of cellular metabolism in the inflammatory response to tissue injury. In Bihari DH, Cerra IB, eds: *Multiple organ failure,* Fullerton, Calif, 1989, Society for Critical Care Medicine.
45. Cerra FB: Hypermetabolism, organ failure and metabolic support, *Surgery* 101:1, 1987.
46. Cerra FB, ed: *Pocket manual of surgical nutrition,* St Louis, 1984, CV Mosby.
47. Chauhan S, Nayak NC, and Ramalingaswami V: The heart and skeletal muscle in experimental protein malnutrition in rhesus monkeys, *J Pathol Bacteriol* 90:301, 1965.
48. Chernow B, Alexander HR, Smallridge RC et al: Hormonal responses to graded surgical stress, *Arc Intern Med* 147:1273, 1987.
49. Chinn RH, Brown JJ, Fraser R et al: The natriuresis of fasting: relationship to changes in plasma renin and plasma aldosterone concentrations, *Clin Sci* 39:437, 1970.
50. Chopra JS, Dhand UK: Effect of protein-calorie malnutrition on peripheral nerves, *Brain* 109:307, 1986.
51. Christou NV, McLean APH, and Meakins JL: Host defense in blunt trauma: interrelationships of kinetics of anergy and depressed neutrophil function, nutritional status and sepsis, *J Trauma* 20:833, 1980.
52. Christou NV, Meakins JL: Neutrophil function in surgical patients: two inhibitors of granulocyte chemotaxis associated with sepsis, *J Surg Res* 26:355, 1979.
53. Christou NV, Meakins JL, and MacLean LD: The predictive role of delayed hypersensitivity in preoperative patients, *Surg Gynecol Obstet* 152:297, 1981.
54. Cizek LJ, Simchon S, and Nocenti MR: Effects of fasting on plasma volume and sodium exchange in male rabbits, *J Proc Soc Exp Biol Med* 154:299, 1977.
55. Clarke RM: The effects of growth and of fasting on the number of villi and crypts in the small intestine of the albino rat, *J Anat* 112:27, 1972.
56. Clowes GH Jr, Heideman M, Lindberg B et al: Effects of parenteral alimentation on amino acid metabolism in septic patients, *Surgery* 88:531, 1980.
57. Collins JP, McCarthy ID, and Hill G: Assessment of protein nutrition in surgical patients—the value of anthropometrics, *Am J Clin Nutr* 32:1527, 1979.
58. Consolazio CF, Matoush LO, Johnson HL et al: Metabolic aspects of acute starvation in normal humans, *Am J Clin Nutr* 20:72, 1967.
59. Cruse PJ, Foord R: A five-year prospective study of 23,649 surgical wounds, *Arch Surg* 107:206, 1973.
60. Cuthbertson D, Tilstone W: Metabolism during the post-injury period, *Adv Clin Chem* 12:1, 1977.
61. Dale G, Young G, Latner AL et al: The effects of surgical operation on venous plasma free amino acids, *Surgery* 81:295, 1977.
62. Daly JM, Dudrick SJ, and Copeland EM: Effects of protein depletion and repletion on cell-mediated immunity in experimental animals, *Ann Surg* 188:791, 1978.
63. D'Amours R, Clerch L, and Massaro D: Food deprivation and surfactant in adult rats, *J Appl Physiol* K55:1413, 1983.
64. Datlof S, Coleman PD, Forbes GB et al: Ventricular dilation on CAT scans of patients with anorexia nervosa, *Am J Psychiatry* 143:96, 1986.
65. Desai ID: Regulation of lysomal enzymes. II. Reversible adaptation of intestinal acid hydrolases during starvation and refeeding, *Can J Biochem* 49:170, 1971.
66. Detsky AS, Baker JP, Mendelson RA et al: Evaluating the accuracy of nutritional assessment techniques applied to hospitalized patients: methodology and comparisons, *J Parenter Enter Nutr* 8:153, 1984.
67. Deutschman CS et al: Transient elevation of hepatic enzymes following resumption of gut feedings in ICU patients. *Nutr Int* 3:42, 1987.
68. Dionigi R, Zonta A, Dominioni L et al: The effects of total parenteral nutrition on immunodepression due to malnutrition, *Ann Surg* 1985:467, 1977.
69. Dionigi R, Gnes F, Bonera A et al: Nutrition and infection, *J Parenter Enter Nutr* 3:62, 1979.
70. Dixit PK, Kuang HLC: Rat pancreatic B cells in protein deficiency: a study involving morphometric analysis and alloxan effect, *J Nutr* 115:375, 1985.
71. Doekel RC, Zwillich CW, Scoggin CH et al: Clinical semi-starvation; depression of hypoxic ventilatory response, *N Engl J Med* 295:358, 1976.
72. Duke JH Jr et al: Contribution of protein to caloric expenditure following injury, *Surgery* 68:174, 1970.
73. Ecknauer R, Raffler H: Effects of starvation on small intestinal enzyme activity in germ-free rats, *Digestion* 18:45, 1978.
74. Edgran B, Wester PO: Impairment of glomerular filtration in fasting for obesity, *Acta Med Scand* 190:389, 1971.
75. Elia M, Goren A, Behrens R et al: Effect of total starvation and very low calorie diets on intestinal permeability in man, *Clin Sci* 73:205, 1987.
76. Elia M, Lammert O, Zed C et al: Energy metabolism during exercise in normal subjects undergoing total starvation, *Hum Nutr Clin Nutr* 38C:355, 1984.
77. Elwyn DH, Kinney JM, Jeevanandam M et al: Influence of increasing carbohydrate intake on glucose kinetics in injured partients, *Ann Surg* 190:117, 1979.
78. Faridy EE: Effect of food and water deprivation in the surface activity of lungs of rats, *J Appl Physiol* 29:493, 1970.
79. Fath JJ, Meguid MM, and Cerra FB: Hormonal and metabolic responses to surgery and stress. In Goldsmith HM, ed: *Practice of surgery,* New York, 1985, Harper & Row.
80. Feldman EJ, Dowling RH, McNaughton J et al: Effects of oral vs intravenous nutrition on intestinal adaptation after small bowel resection in the dog, *Gastroenterology* 70:712, 1976.
81. Fleck A: The acute phase response: implications for nutrition and recovery, *Nutrition* 4:109, 1988.
82. Fohlin L: Body composition, cardiovascular and renal function in adolescent patients with anorexia nervosa, *Acta Paediatr Scand* 268(suppl):6063, 1977.
83. Forse RA, Shizgal HM: The assessment of malnutrition, *Surgery* 88:17, 1980.
84. Forse RA, Crosilla P, Rompre C et al: Efficacy of total parenteral nutrition, *Surg Forum* 30:87, 1979.
85. Freund HR, Holroyde J: Cardiac function during protein malnutrition and refeeding in the isolated rat heart, *J Parenter Enter Nutr* 10:470, 1986.
86. Gal DB, Massaro GD, and Massaro D: Influence of fasting on the lung, *J Appl Physiol* 42:88, 1977.
87. Garber AJ, Menzel PH, Boden G et al: Hepatic ketogenesis and gluconeogenesis in humans, *J Clin Invest* 54:981, 1974.
88. Garbozni R et al: Effects of lipid loading and fasting on pulmonary surfactant, *Respiration* 25:458, 1968.
89. Garnett ES, Barnard DL, Ford J et al: Gross fragmentation of cardiac myofibrils after therapeutic starvation of obesity, *Lancet* 1:914, 1969.
90. Garnett ES, Cohen H, Nahmias C et al: The roles of carbohydrate, renin and aldosterone in sodium retention during and after total starvation, *Metabolism* 22:867, 1973.
91. Gelman A, Sigulem D, Sustovich DR et al: Starvation and renal function, *Am J Med Sci* 263:465, 1972.
92. Gjedde A, Crone C: Induction processes in blood brain transfer to ketone bodies during starvation, *Am J Physiol* 229:1165, 1975.
93. Golden MH: Transport proteins as indices of nutritional status, *Am J Clin Nutr* 35:1159, 1982.
94. Goodman MN, Lowell B, Belur E et al: Sites of protein conservation and loss during starvation; influence of adiposity, *Am J Physiol* 246:E383, 1984.
95. Gottdiener JS, Gross HA, Henry WL et al: Effects of self-induced starvation on cardiac size and function in anorexia nervosa, *Circulation* 58:425, 1978.
96. Grant JP, Custer PB, and Thurlow J: Current techniques of nutritional assessment, *Surg Clin North Am* 61:437, 1981.
97. Gray GE, Gray LK: Validity of anthropometric norms used in the assessment of hospitalized patients, *J Parenter Enter Nutr* 3:366, 1979.
98. Green GM, Kass EK: Factors influencing the clearance of bacteria by the lung, *J Clin Invest* 43:769, 1964.
99. Grimes CJC, Younathan MT, and Lee WC: The effects of preoperative total parenteral nutrition on surgery outcomes, *J Am Diet Assoc* 87:1202, 1987.
100. Gross RL, Newberne PM: Role of nutrition in immunologic function, *Physiol Rev* 60:188, 1980.
101. Harkema JR, Manderly JL, Gregory RE

et al: A comparison of starvation and elastase models of emphysema in the rat, *Am Rev Respir Dis* 129:584, 1984.

102. Harris JA, Cobb CG: Persistent gram-negative bacteria: observations in twenty patients, *Am J Surg* 125:705, 1983.

103. Harvey KB, Moldawer LL, Bistrian BR et al: Biological measures of the formulation of a hospital prognostic index, *Am J Clin Nutr* 34:2013, 1981.

104. Harvey KB et al: Hospital morbidity-mortality risk factors using nutritional assessment, *J Clin Nutr* 26:581A, 1978.

105. Heatley RV, Williams RH, and Lewis MH: Preoperative intravenous feeding—a controlled trial, *Postgrad Med J* 55:5412, 1979.

106. Hexhe JJ: Experimental undernutrition. 1. Its effects on cardiac output, *Metabolism* 12:1086, 1967.

107. Heymsfield SB, Bethel RA, Ansley JD et al: Cardiac abnormalities in cachectic patients before and during nutritional repletion, *Am Heart J* 95:584, 1978.

108. Hiebert JM, McGough M, Rodeheaver G et al: The influence of catabolism on immunocompetence in burned patients, *Surgery* 86:242, 1979.

109. Hill GL: Editorial, *Nutr Int* 4:287, 1988.

110. Hill GL, Blackett RL, Pickford I et al: Malnutrition in surgical patients: an unrecognized problem, *Lancet* 2:689, 1977.

111. Hindmarsh JT, Kilby D, Ross B et al: Further studies on intestinal active transport during semistarvation, *J Physiol* 188:207, 1967.

112. Hirschfield JS, Kern F Jr: Protein starvation and the small intestine. III. Incorporation of orally and intraoperitoneally administered 11-leucine 4,5-3H into mucosal protein of protein-deprived rats, *J Clin Invest* 48:1224, 1969.

113. Hopper AF, Wannemacher RW Jr, and McGovern PA: Cell population changes in the intestinal epithelium of the rat following starvation and protein depletion, *Proc Soc Exp Biol Med* 128:695, 1968.

114. Imamura M, Clowes GH Jr, Blackburn GL et al: Liver metabolism and gluconeogenesis in trauma and sepsis, *Surgery* 77:868, 1975.

115. Ing AFM, Meakins JL, McLean AP et al: Determinants of susceptibility to sepsis and mortality: malnutrition vs anergy, *J Surg Res* 32:249, 1982.

116. Irvin TT, Goligher JC: Aetiology of disruption of intestinal anastomoses, *Br J Surg* 461, 1973.

117. Irvin TT, Hunt TK: Effect of malnutrition on colonic healing, *Ann Surg* 180:765, 1974.

118. Isner JM, Sours HE, Paris AL et al: Sudden unexpected death in avid dieters using liquid-protein modified-fast diet, *Circulation* 60:1401, 1979.

119. Jeejeebhoy KN, Marliss EB: Energy supply in total parenteral nutrition. In Fischer JE, ed: *Surgical nutrition,* Boston, 1983, Little Brown.

120. Jeejeebhoy KN, Meguid MM: Assessment of nutritional status in the oncologic patient, *Surg Clin North Am* 66:1077, 1986.

121. Jeejeebhoy KN, Baker JP, Wolman SL et al: Critical evaluation of the role of clinical assessment and body composition studies in patients with malnutrition and after total parenteral nutrition, *Am J Clin Nutr* 35:1117, 1982.

122. Johnson WC, Ulrich F, Mequid MM et al: Role of delayed hypersensitivity in predicting postoperative morbidity and mortality, *Am J Surg* 137:536, 1979.

123. Jones WP, Hay AM: Albumin metabolism: effect of nutritional state and dietary protein intake, *J Clin Invest* 47:1958, 1968.

124. Ju JS, Nasset ES: Changes in total nitrogen content of some abdominal viscera in fasting and realimentation, *J Nutr* 68:633, 1959.

125. Kaminski MV et al: Correlation of mortality with serum transferrin and anergy, *J Parenter Enter Nutr* 1:27A, 1977.

126. Kelly SM, Rosa A, Field S et al: Inspiratory muscle strength and body composition in patients receiving total parenteral nutrition therapy, *Am Rev Respir Dis* 130:33, 1984.

127. Kelsen SG, Ference M, and Kapoor S: Effects of prolonged undernutrition on structure and function of the diaphragm, *J Appl Physiol* 58:1354, 1985.

128. Kerr JS, Riley DJ, Lanza-Jacoby S et al: Nutritional emphysema in the rat; influence of protein depletion and impaired lung growth, *Am Rev Respir Dis* 131:644, 1985.

129. Keys A, Henschel A, and Taylor HL: The size and function of the human heart at rest in semistarvation and subsequent rehabilitation, *Am J Physiol* 50:153, 1947.

130. Keys A et al: *The biology of human starvation,* Minneapolis, 1950, Uiversity of Minnesota Press.

131. Kim YS, McCarthy DM, Lane W et al: Alterations in the levels of peptide hydrolases and other enzymes in brush-border and soluble fractions of rat small intestine mucosa during starvation and refeeding, *Biochem Biophys Acta* 321:262, 1973.

132. Kinney JM: Indirect calorimetry in malnutrition: nutritional assessment or therapeutic reference? *J Parenter Enter Nutr* 11:905, 1987.

133. Kinney JM, Weissman C: Forms of malnutrition in stressed and unstressed patients, *Clin Chest Med* 7:19, 1986.

134. Kirsch RE, Saunders SJ: Nutrition and the liver, *S Afr Med J* 46:2072, 1972.

135. Klahr S, Alleyne GA: Effects of chronic protein calorie malnutrition on the kidney, *Kidney Int* 3:129, 1973.

136. Klahr S, Tripathy K: Evaluation of renal function in malnutrition, *Arch Intern Med* 118:322, 1966.

137. Klahr S, Tripathy K, Balonos O FT et al: On the nature of the renal concentrating defect in malnutrition, *Am J Med* 43:84, 1967.

138. Klahr S, Tripathy K, and Lotero H: Renal regulation of acid-base balance in malnourished man, *Am J Med* 325, 1970.

139. Knudsen KB, Bradley EM, Lecocq FR et al: Effect of fasting and refeeding on the histology and disaccharidase activity of the human intestine, *Gastroenterology* 55:46, 1968.

140. Kolanowski J, Desmecht P, and Crabbe J: Sodium balance and renal tubular sensitivity to aldosterone during total fast and carbohydrate refeeding in the obese, *Eur J Clin Invest* 6:75, 1976.

141. Kumar V, Deo MG, and Ramalingaswami V: Mechanisms of fatty liver in protein deficiency; an experimental study in rhesus monkeys, *Gastroenterology* 62:445, 1972.

142. Law DK, Dudrick SJ, and Abdou NI: Immunocompetence of patients with protein-calorie malnutrition, The effects of nutritional repletion, *Ann Intern Med* 79:545, 1973.

143. Law DK, Dudrick SJ, and Abdou NI: The effects of dietary protein depletion on immunocompetence. The importance of nutritional repletion prior to immunologic induction, *Ann Surg* 179:168, 1974.

144. Lee PA, Wallin JD, Kaplowitz N et al: Endocrine and metabolic alterations with food and water deprivation, *Am J Clin Nutr* 30:1953, 1977.

145. Lee PC, Books S, and Lebenthal E: Effect of fasting and refeeding on pancreatic enzymes and segretogogue responsiveness in rats, *Am J Physiol* 242:G215, 1982.

146. Letsou AP, Connaughton MC, and O'Donnell TF: Nutritional survey of a university hospital population, *J Parenter Enter Nutr* 1:40A, 1977.

147. Levenson SM, Seifter E: Starvation; metabolic and physiologic responses. In Fischer JE, ed: *Surgical nutrition,* Boston, 1983, Little Brown.

148. Levine GM, Deren JJ, and Steiger E: Role of oral intake in the maintenance of gut mass disaccharide activity, *Gastroenterology* 67:975, 1974.

149. Lewis M et al: The effects of malnutrition on diaphragmatic contractility and muscle fiber morphometry, *Am Rev Respir Dis* 131:A326, 1985.

150. Lichtenberger L, Welsh JD, and Johnson LR: Relationship between the changes in gastrin levels and intestinal properties in the starved rat, *Dig Dis* 21:33, 1976.

151. Long CL, Kinney JM, and Gieger JW: Nonsuppressibility of gluconeogenesis by glucose in septic patients, *Metabolism* 25:193, 1976.

152. MacBurney M, Wilmore DW: Decision-making in nutritional care, *Surg Clin North Am* 61:571, 1981.

153. MacLean LD, Meakins JL, Taguchi K et al: Host resistance in sepsis and trauma, *Ann Surg* 182:207, 1975.

154. Marshall J, McLean AEM: The effects of oral phenobarbitone on hepatic microsomal cytochrome P-450 and demethylation in rats fed normal and low protein, *Biochem Pharmacol* 18:153, 1969.

155. Materese LE: Enteral nutrition. In Fischer JE, ed: *Surgical nutrition,* Boston, 1983. Little Brown.

156. McGarry JD, Foster DW: Regulation of

ketogenesis and clinical aspects of the ketotic state, *Metabolism* 21:471, 1972.

157. McLaren DS: A fresh look at protein-energy malnutrition in the hospitalized patient, *Nutrition* 4:1, 1988.

158. McLaren DS, Bitar JG, and Nassar VH: Protein calorie nutrition and the liver, *Prog Liver Dis* 4:527, 1972.

159. McLaren DS, Meguid MM: Nutritional assessment at the crossroads, *J Parenter Enter Nutr* 7:575, 1983.

160. McLean AE, McLean EK: The effect of diet and 1,1,1-trichloro-2,2-bis-(pchlorophenyl) ethane (DDT) on microsomal hydroxylating enzymes and on sensitivity of rats to carbon tetrachloride poisoning, *Biochem J* 100:564, 1966.

161. McLean AE, Verschuuren HG: Effects of diet and microsomal enzyme induction on the toxicity of dimethylnitrosamine, *Br J Exp Pathol* 50:22, 1969.

162. McManus JP, Isselbacher KJ: Effect of fasting versus feeding on the rat small intestine. Morphological, biochemical and functional differences, *Gastroenterology* 59:214, 1970.

163. Meakins JL, Pietsch JB, Bubenick O et al: Delayed hypersensitivity; indicator at acquired failure of host defenses in sepsis and trauma, *Ann Surg* 186:241, 1977.

164. Mezaros K, Bojta J, Bautisla AP et al: Glucose utilization by Kupffer cells, endothelial cells and gronulocytesin endotoxemic rat liver, *Am J Physiol* 260:G7, 1991.

165. Miller CL: Immunological assays as measurements of nutritional status: a review, *J Parenter Enter Nutr* 2:554,1978.

166. Moore FD, Olesen KH, McMurrey JD et al: *The body cell mass and its supporting environment*, Philadelphia, 1978, WB Saunders.

167. Moriguchu S, Sone S, and Kishino Y: Changes in alveolar macrophages in protein-deficient rats, *J Nutr* 113:40, 1983.

168. Mullen JL et al: Nutritional and immunological status of surgical patients, *J Parenter Enter Nutr* 1:39A, 1977.

169. Mullen JL, Buzby GP, Matthews DC et al: Reduction of operating morbidity and mortality by combined preoperative and postoperative nutritional support, *Ann Surg* 192:604, 1980.

170. Mullen JL, Gertner MH, Buzby GP et al: Implications of malnutrition in the surgical patients, *Arch Surg* 114:121, 1979.

171. Muller JM, Brenner U, Dienst C et al: Preoperative parenteral feeding in patients with gastrointestinal carcinoma, *Lancet* 1:68,1982.

172. Myer BA, Dubick MA, Gerreits J et al: Protein deficiency: effects on lung mechanics and the accumulation of collagen and elastin in rat lung, *J Nutr* 113:2308, 1983.

173. Newey H, Sanford PA, and Smyth DH: Effects of fasting on intestinal transfer of sugars and amino acids in vitro, *J Physiol* 208:705, 1970.

174. Nohr CW, Tchervenkov JI, Meakins JL et al: Malnutrition and homoral immunity: short-term acute nutritional deprivation, *Surgery* 98:769, 1985.

175. Nohr CW, Tchervenkov JI, Meakins JL et al: Malnutrition and homoral immunity: long-term protein deprivation, *J Surg Res* 40:432, 1986.

176. Nordgren L, Von Scheele C: Hepatic and pancreatic dysfunction in anorexia nervosa: a report of two cases, *Biol Psychiatry* 12:681, 1977.

177. Nutter DO, Murray TG, Heymsfield SB et al: The effects of chronic protein calorie undernutrition in the rat on myocardial function and cardiac function, *Circ Res* 45:144,1979.

178. Obeyesekere I: Malnutrition among Ceylonese adults, *Am J Clin Nutr* 18:38, 1977.

179. O'Dwyer ST, Smith RJ, Weng TL et al: Maintenance of small bowel mucosa with glutamine enriched parenteral nutrition, *J Parenter Enter Nutr* 134:571, 1989.

180. Ottow RT, Bruining HA, and Jeekel J: Clinical judgment versus delayed hypersensitivity skin testing for the prediction of postoperative sepsis and mortality, *Surg Gynecol Obstet* 159:475,1984.

181. Owen OE, Felig P, Morgan AP et al: Liver and kidney metabolism during prolonged starvation, *J Clin Invest* 48: 574, 1969.

182. Owen OE, Reichard GA Jr, Patel MS et al: Energy expenditure in feasting and fasting, *Adv Exp Med Biol* 111:169, 1979.

183. Pissaia O, Rossi MA, and Oliveira JSM: The heart in protein-calorie malnutrition in rats: morphological, electrophysiological and biochemical changes, *J Nutr* 110:2035, 1980.

184. Pitchumoni CS: Pancreas in primary malnutrition disorders, *Am J Clin Nutr* 26:374, 1973.

185. Popp MB, Brennan MF: Metabolic response to trauma and infection. In Fischer JE, ed: *Surgical nutrition,* Boston, 1983, Little Brown.

186. Powell GK, McElveen MA: Effect of prolonged fasting on fatty acid esterification in rat intestinal mucosa, *Biochem Biophys Acta* 369:8, 1974.

187. Prevost EA, Butterworth CE: Nutritional care of hospitalized patients, *Clin Res* 22:579, 1974.

188. Pullman TN, Alving AS, Dern RS et al: The influence of protein intake on specific renal functions in normal man, *J Lab Clin Med* 44:320, 1954.

189. Reinhardt GF, Myscofski JW, Wilkins DB et al: Incidence and mortality of hypoalbuminemic patients in hospitalized veterans, *J Parenter Enter Nutr* 4:357, 1980.

190. Rhoades RA: Influence of starvation on the lung; effect on glucose and palmitate utilization, *J Apply Physiol* 38:513, 1975.

191. Rhoads JE, Alexander CE: Nutritional problems of surgical patients, *Ann NY Acad Sci* 63:268,1955.

192. Rich AJ: The assessment of body composition in clinical conditions, *Proc Nutr Soc* 41:389, 1982.

193. Rochester DF: Malnutrition and the respiratory muscles, *Clin Chest Med* 7:91, 1986.

194. Rombeau JL, Barot LR, Williamson CE et al: Preoperative total parenteral nutrition and surgical outcome in patients with inflammatory bowel disease, *Am J Surg* 143:139, 1982.

195. Rosenbaum SH et al: Respiratory patterns in profound nutritional depletion, *Anesthesiology* 51:S366, 1979.

196. Roy S, Singh N, Deo MG et al: Ultrastructure of skeletal muscle and peripheral nerve in experimental protein deficiency and its correlation with nerve condition studies, *J Neurol Sci* 17:399, 1972.

197. Royle GT, Kettlewell MG: Liver function tests in surgical infection and malnutrition, *Ann Surg* 192:192, 1980.

198. Royle GT, Kettlewell MG, Ilic V et al: Galactose and hepatic metabolism in malnutrition and septic man, *Clin Sci Molec Med* 55:199, 1978.

199. Roza AM, Tuitt D, and Shizgal HM: Transferrin—a poor measure of nutritional status, *J Parenter Enter Nutr* 8:523, 1984.

200. Rubin JW, Clowes GH Jr, Macnicol MF et al: Impaired pulmonary surfactant synthesis in starvation and severe nonthoracic sepsis, *Am J Surg* 123:461, 1972.

201. Russell GFM, Bruce JT: Impaired water diuresis in patients with anorexia nervosa, *Am J Med* 40:38, 1966.

202. Sahebjami H: Nutrition and the pulmonary parenchyma, *Clin Chest Med* 7:111, 1986.

203. Sahebjami H, MacGee J: Changes in connective tissue composition of the lung in starvation and refeeding, *Am Rev Respir Dis* 128:644, 1983.

204. Sahebjami H, MacGee J: Effects of starvation and refeeding on lung biochemistry in rats, *Am Rev Respir Dis* 126:483, 1982.

205. Sahebjami H, Vassallo CL: Effects of starvation and refeeding on lung mechanics and morphometry, *Am Rev Respir Dis* 119: 443, 1979.

206. Sahebjami H, Vassallo CL: Influence of starvation on enzyme induced emphysema, *J Appl Physiol* 48:284, 1981.

207. Sahebjami H, Vassallo CL, and Wirman JA: Lung mechanics and ultrastructure in prolonged starvation, *Am Rev Respir Dis* 117:77, 1978.

208. Sahebjami H, Wirman JA: Emphysema like changes in the lungs of starved rats, *Am Rev Respir Dis* 124:619, 1981.

209. Sargent F, Johnson RE: The effects of diet on renal function in healthy men, *Am J Clin Nutr* 4:466, 1956.

210. Schlichtig R, Ayres SM: *Nutritional support of the critically ill,* Chicago, 1988, Year Book Medical.

211. Schloeder FX, Stinebaugh BJ: Renal tubular sites of natriuresis of fasting and glucose induced sodium conservation, *Metabolism* 19:1119, 1970.

212. Seltzer MH, Bastidas JA, Cooper DM et al: Instant nutritional assessment, *J Parenter Enter Nutr* 3:157, 1979.

213. Shennib H, Chiu RC, Mulder DS et al: Depression and delayed recovery of alveolar macrophage function during starvation and refeeding, *Surg Gynecol Obstet* 158:535, 1984.

214. Sherlock S, Walshe V: Effects of undernutrition in man on hepatic structure and function, *Nature* 161:604, 1948.
215. Shizgal HM, Spanier AH, and Kurtz RS: Effects of parenteral nutrition on body composition in critically ill patients, *Am J Surg* 131:156, 1976.
216. Sima A: Studies on fibre size in developing sciatic nerve and spinal roots in normal, undernourished and rehabilitated rats, *Acta Physiol Scand* 406(suppl):3, 1974.
217. Simonson E, Henschel A, and Keys A: The electrocardiogram of man in semi-starvation and subsequent rehabilitation, *Am Heart J* 35:584, 1948.
218. Smale BF, Mullen JL, Buzby GP et al: The efficacy of nutritional assessment and support in cancer surgery, *Cancer* 47:2375, 1981.
219. Smith R, Drenick EJ: Changes in body water and sodium during prolonged fasting for extreme obesity, *Clin Sci* 31:437, 1966.
220. Souba WW, Smith RJ, and Wilmore DW: Glutamine metabolism by the intestinal tract, *J Parenter Enter Neutr* 9:608, 1985.
221. Starker PM, Gump FE, Askanazi J et al: Serum albumin levels as an index of nutritional support, *Surgery* 91:194, 1982.
222. Starker PM, La Sala PA, Askanazi J et al: The influence of preoperative total parenteral nutrition upon operative morbidity and mortality, *Surg Gynecol Obstet* 162:569, 1986.
223. Stein HD, Keiser HR: Collagen metabolism in granulating wounds, *J Surg Res* 11:277, 1971.
224. Steiner M, Bourges HR, Freedman LS et al: Effect of starvation on the tissue composition of the small intestine in the rat, *Am J Physiol* 215:75, 1968.

225. Studley HO: Percentage of weight loss: a basic indicator of surgical risk in patients with chronic peptic ulcer, *JAMA* 106:458, 1936.
226. Svoboda D, Grady H, and Higginson J: The effects of chronic protein deficiency in rats, *Lab Invest* 15:731, 1966.
227. Symreng T, Anderberg B, Kågedal B et al: Nutritional assessment and clinical course in 112 elective surgical patients, *Acta Chir Scand* 149:657, 1983.
228. Temple WJ, Voitk AJ, Snelling CF et al: Effect of nutrition, diet and suture material on long term wound healing, *Ann Surg* 182:93, 1975.
229. Thet LA, Alvarez H: Effect of hyperventilation and starvation on rat lung mechanics and surfactant, *Am Rev Respir Dis* 126:286, 1982.
230. Thompson BR, Julian TP, and Stremple JF: Perioperative total parenteral nutrition in patients with gastrointestinal cancer, *J Surg Res* 30:497, 1981.
231. Thompson CS, Mikailidis DP, Jeremy JY et al: Effect of starvation on biochemical indices of renal function in the rat, *Br J Exp Pathol* 68:767, 1987.
232. Thompson JS, Vaughan WP, Forst CF et al: The effect of the route of nutrient delivery on gut structure and diamine oxidase levels, *J Parenter Enter Nutr* 11:28, 1987.
233. Thurston J, Marks P: Electrocardiographic abnormalities in patients with anorexia nervosa, *Br Heart J* 36:719, 1974.
234. Train VM, Sath BT: Effect of starvation on renal function, *Lancet* 2:620, 1973.
235. Twomey P, Ziegler D, and Rombeau J: Utility of skin testing in nutritional assessment: a critical review, *J Parenter Enter Nutr* 6:50, 1982.

236. Van Liew JB, Eisenbacb GM, Dlouha H et al: Renal sodium conservation during starvation in the rat, *J Lab Clin Med* 91:560, 1978.
236a. The Veterans Affairs Total Parenteral Nutrition Cooperative Study Group. Perioperative total parenteral nutrition in surgical patients, *N Engl J Med* 325:525, 1991.
237. Vrbaski SR: The effects of long-term low protein intake on lipids of rat brain during adulthood, *J Nutr* 113:899, 1983.
238. Weisnier RL et al: Hospital malnutrition: a prospective evaluation of general medical patients during the course of hospitalization, *Am J Clin Nutr* 32:418, 1979.
239. Weiss HS, Jurrus E: Starvation on compliance and surfactant of the rat lung, *Respir Physiol* 12:123, 1971.
240. Widdowson EM, Dickerson JW, and McCance RA: Severe undernutrition in growing and adult animals. 4. The impact of severe undernutrition on the chemical composition of the soft tissues in the pig, *J Parenter Enter Nutr* 1:25A, 1977.
241. Willicuts HD: Nutritional assessment of 1000 surgical patients in an affluent suburban community hospital, *J Parenter Enter Nutr* 1:25A, 1977.
242. Wilmore DW, Long JM, Mason AD Jr et al: Catecholamines: mediators of the hypermetabolic response to thermal injury, *Ann Surg* 180:653, 1974.
243. Yates B, Lopez A, and Jackson SS: Nutritional status of hospitalized patients, *Clin Res* 25:20, 1977.
244. Young GA, Chem C, and Hill GL: Assessment of protein calorie malnutrition in surgical patients from plasma proteins and anthropometric measurements, *Am J Clin Nutr* 31:429, 1978.

CHAPTER 24

Evaluation of the Patient with Acquired Immunodeficiency Syndrome and Other Serious Infections

IVOR D. BERKOWITZ

Despite the introduction of a multitude of antimicrobial agents into clinical medicine during the past several decades, infectious diseases remain a major cause of mortality and serious morbidity. Rather than provide an encyclopedic description of various infections, this chapter will discuss only a limited range of entities that have particular anesthetic implications. Examples include the acquired immunodeficiency syndrome (AIDS), selected because of the importance of understanding the implications of the multisystem nature of the disease in the anesthetic management of such patients. AIDS and the other diseases reviewed (e.g., hepatitis and herpetic infections), are of particular risk to anesthesiologists and other health care workers, and an understanding of the underlying biology and epidemiology is important for safe anesthetic practice.

ACQUIRED IMMUNODEFICIENCY SYNDROME

Acquired immunodeficiency syndrome (AIDS) is a "new" viral-induced disease first described in 1981. Selective destruction of helper T lymphocytes results in cell-mediated immunodeficiency with the clinical development of serious opportunistic infections and otherwise uncommon neoplasms, particularly Kaposi's sarcoma[41] and lymphocytic malignancies.[91] The etiologic agent is a retrovirus variously termed the human immunodeficiency virus (HIV), human T-cell lymphotropic virus (HTLV-III), or the lymphadenopathy-associated virus (LAV).[6,55,72] **HIV infection is now in an epidemic phase, and, because of its multisystem involvement, widespread prevalence in patients of all ages, and uniformly lethal outcome, it behooves the anesthesiologist to know its etiology, epidemiology, diagnosis, spectrum of clinical manifestations, and implications for anesthetic care.**

Etiology

HIV is a member of the lenti virus group, so named because of the protracted nature of the diseases caused by members of this viral genus. Fig. 24-1 illustrates the molecular structure of HIV. The diploid viral RNA strands are covered by proteins (p) p7 and p9 that, together with reverse transcriptase and a core-covering protein, p24/25, make up a disc-shaped core particle. The core is surrounded by a shell of protein components, p17, and a host cell–derived lipid bilayer, the viral envelope. This viral envelope contains glycoproteins gp41 and gp120 that allow the virus to attach to a specific receptor for HIV—the CD4 receptor on the host cell—and thereby initiate infection.[40,58,73] After viral attachment to the CD4 receptor, the viral envelope fuses with the host cell membrane, and the core material is injected into the host cytoplasm. Reverse transcriptase translates genomic viral RNA into double stranded DNA ("provirus") that enters the host cell nucleus to become incorporated into the host genome. The host cell and its progeny now remain permanently infected and the source of synthesis of viral structural proteins and reverse transcriptase that can become incorporated into new viral particles that bud from the surface of the infected cells to subsequently infect other cells.[58] Factors that are not well understood determine the outcome of cellular infection. Persistent infection can remain "silent" without cell damage, but infection may also lead to rapid viral replication followed by cell lysis and death. Infection can also result in the formation of syncytia—a result of fusion of many infected cells.

Pathogenesis

The clinical manifestations and organ dysfunction of HIV infection, can, in part, be accounted for by the specific localization of HIV. **The distribution of infected cells parallels that of the distribution of the CD4 molecule, the cellular receptor that provides**

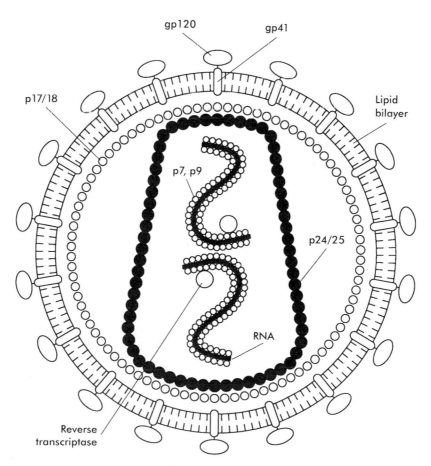

Fig. 24-1. The ultrastructure of the human immunodeficiency virus. (From Gallo RC, Montagnier L: AIDS in 1988, *Sci Am* 259:41, 1988.)

attachment for HIV. The primary target of the virus, however, is the T lymphocyte of the helper/inducer subset identified by the OK T4 (CD4) or Leu-3 phenotypic markers, a cell that plays a central role in both cell-mediated and humoral immunity.[61,79] Lysis and depletion of these T4-helper lymphocytes compromise cell-mediated immunity and components of the humoral immune system to enhance the susceptibility of HIV-infected patients to opportunistic infection with viruses, parasites, fungi, and certain bacteria, e.g., listeria and mycobacteria.[30,53,58] HIV virus not only is lymphotropic but also infects and replicates in cells of other organs, e.g., bowel epithelium, myocardium, adrenal cortex, glial cells, hemopoietic cells, macrophages, and monocytes. Viral infection of these organs may explain in part the multisystem nature of this infection.

Epidemiology

When first described, AIDS appeared confined to particular high-risk groups. These included male homosexuals and bisexuals, heterosexual intravenous drug abusers, recent Haitian immigrants, and persons with hemophilia. Transmission appeared to be via sexual activity and the sharing of needles contaminated by infected blood.[25] Soon thereafter recipients of multiple blood transfusions (before HIV blood testing) and infants of high-risk mothers (intravenous drug abusers, prostitutes, heterosexual mothers with bisexual husbands) were added to the high-risk groups. HIV certainly can be transmitted between heterosexuals, and it is this category of patients that is growing most rapidly in the United States. Recent estimates suggest that there are between 1 and 1.5 million people in the United States infected with HIV and that there will be between a quarter and a half million cases of AIDS diagnosed in the United States by the end of 1991.[42]

Clinical Classification and Course of HIV Infection

The case definition originally proposed by the Centers for Disease Control (CDC)[11] identified patients with AIDS-HIV infection in its most advanced stage, particularly for purposes of surveillance and epidemiologic study. The clinical spectrum of HIV infection is, however, much broader, ranging from an asymptomatic but seropositive patient, through a range of intermediate disease with chronic lymphadenopathy, to frank AIDS with severe life-threatening

---

BOX 24-1
CLASSIFICATION OF HIV INFECTION

Acute infection: Mononucleosis-like syndrome associated with seroconversion.

Asymptomatic infection: Patient is asymptomatic, but with serologic or culture evidence of infection.

Persistent generalized lymphadenopathy:
Palpable lymphadenopathy (>1 cm) at two or more extrainguinal sites for >3 months in absence of concurrent illness other than HIV infection to explain findings.

Other HTLV-III disease.
Subgroup A: Constitutional disease.
One or more of the following: fever or diarrhea >1 month or 10% baseline weight loss in absence of concurrent illness other than HIV infection to explain findings.
Subgroup B: Neurologic disease.
One or more of the following: dementia, myelopathy, or peripheral neuropathy in absence of concurrent illness other than HIV.

Subgroup C: Secondary infectious diseases.
Infectious diseases associated with HIV infection or at least moderately indicative of a defect of cell-mediated immunity (see Table 24-2).
Subgroup D: Secondary cancers.
Diagnosis of one or more cancers known to be associated with HIV infection and at least moderately indicative of a defect in cell-mediated immunity (Kaposi's sarcoma, non-Hodgkin's lymphoma, or primary lymphoma of brain).
Subgroup E: Other conditions in HIV infection.
Clinical findings or diseases not classifiable above that may be attributable to HIV infection and are indicative of a defect in cell-mediated immunity. These include chronic lymphoid interstitial pneumonitis, other infectious diseases, and neoplasms not listed above.

From Centers for Disease Control: Classification system for human T-lymphotropic virus type III/lymphadenopathy-associated virus infections, *MMWR* 35:334, 1986.

opportunistic infections and frequently associated Kaposi's sarcoma[61,82] (Box 24-1). The clinical presentation of HIV-infected patients depends on the functional integrity of the cell-mediated immune system. **The Walter Reed classification of HIV infection defines the course and severity of HIV infection in terms of the degree of immune impairment, reflected primarily by the number of T4 lymphocytes.**[75] Table 24-1 outlines the clinical stages of HIV infection from exposure (WR0) and the onset of infection (WR1), through the stages of progressive immune deficiency, to full-blown AIDS with severe life-threatening opportunistic infections (WR6).

Although most patients infected with HIV do not develop clinical symptoms with the initial infection, a minority develop signs of a mononucleosis-like infection characterized by fever, fatigue, lymphadenopathy, a rash 2 to 3 weeks after the initial infection, and even self-limited central nervous system manifestations.[22,83] These symptoms gradually resolve and the patient becomes asymptomatic in spite of progressive viral replication. **Infection can remain subclinical for many years during this latency period, while the patient is nevertheless infectious and capable of transmitting the infection.** For most patients the next stage is that of chronic lymphadenopathy (stage WR2) attributed to B cell hyperstimulation.[34] Stage 2 usually lasts from 3 to 5 years. Worsening cell-mediated immune deficiency that develops over several years characterizes stages 3 and 4. Complete skin anergy and/or the development of severe viral and fungal infections of skin and mucous membranes (oral and vaginal thrush, herpetic infection, and oral hairy leukoplakia) characterize stage WR5. The onset of a vast array of opportunistic infections (Box 24-2) marks the beginning of stage 6. By this stage

T4 lymphocyte counts are usually less than 100 mm³.

In addition to recurrent severe opportunistic infections, Kaposi's sarcoma and non-Hodgkin's lymphoma frequently develop in HIV-infected patients.[90] **Approximately half of the lymphomas involve the central nervous system, where they present as intracranial mass lesions.** Extra–central nervous system, non-Hodgkin's lymphoma in HIV-infected patients frequently develops in unusual sites, e.g., the orbit, tongue, or rectum. Immunodysregulation and possible Epstein-Barr viral infection rather than a failure of host immune tumor surveillance have been implicated as causes of these lymphomas.

Diagnostic Techniques

The presence of HIV infection can be determined by laboratory techniques that include viral culture and the detection of HIV antigens or antibodies to HIV and its protein and glycoprotein components.[58,81,85] These tests vary in their sensitivity, specificity, and technical sophistication. The most specific test for the diagnosis of HIV infection is viral isolation. Since the degree of viremia depends on the stage of illness, with higher titers present early in the course of the illness, this technique overall reflects poor sensitivity. In addition, viral culture is technically difficult and is not widely available. HIV infection is usually indirectly identified by serologic tests that determine the presence of antibody to the virus. **The enzyme-linked immunosorbent assay (ELISA) detects the presence of antibody to a semipurified extract of HIV grown in tissue culture. It remains the primary screening test for HIV infection because of its high degree of sensitivity (>99%), reproducibility, and low cost. False positives do occur** and are possibly caused by autoantibodies that react against cellular antigens

Table 24-1   The Walter Reed Staging Classification for HIV infection

Stage	HIV antibody and/or virus isolation	Chronic lymphadenopathy	T-helper cells (mm³)	Delayed hypersensitivity	Thrush	Opportunistic infections
WR0	−	−	>400	Normal	−	−
WR1	+	−	>400	Normal	−	−
WR2	+	+	>400	Normal	−	−
WR3	+	±	<400	Normal	−	−
WR4	+	±	<400	Partial anergy	−	−
WR5	+	±	<400	Complete anergy and/or thrush	+	−
WR6	+	±	<400	Partial or complete anergy	±	+

From Redfield RR, Wright DC, and Tramont EC. The Walter Reed Staging Classification for HTLV-III/LAV, *N Engl J Med* 314:131, 1986.

(e.g., HLA and DR4) contaminating the viral reagents. **The Western blot test is the most widely used confirmatory test.** In this test, viral protein antigens are separated by electrophoresis, blotted onto nitrocellulose strips, and incubated with patients' serum. The presence of specific antibodies to viral protein components (e.g., p24, gp41) is determined by the binding of either enzyme-labelled or isotopically labelled antihuman globulin to these protein bands.[28] The cytoplasmic immunofluorescent assay (IFA), a highly specific HIV assay, is another available confirmatory test.[4] Certain viral antigens (e.g., p24) can be detected in patients' serum by commercially available tests. The polymerase chain reaction, an in vitro DNA amplification procedure, can also detect HIV proviral sequences in infected patients.[80]

Preoperative Evaluation

Multisystem involvement by opportunistic infections, secondary tumor development, or direct HIV damage results in altered organ function with implications for the anesthesiologist. Thorough preoperative evaluation and the subsequent planning of an appropriate anesthetic depend on a knowledge of HIV infection and its system-specific complications. In addition, the HIV-infected intravenous drug abuser may already be severely compromised from an anesthesiologist's point of view by coexisting disease, such as cardiac valve damage secondary to endocarditis, pulmonary disease from septic emboli, talc granulomata, or pulmonary hypertension, as well as by renal disease.

Pulmonary system

The pulmonary system is often compromised in patients with AIDS, particularly by opportunistic infections caused by a wide array of viral, protozoal, fungal, and bacterial pathogens, by lymphoid interstitial pneumonitis (LIP) and less frequently by Kaposi's sarcoma or non-Hodgkin's lymphoma.[35,67,68] *Pneumocystis carinii* represents, by far, the most common opportunistic pathogen causing pneumonia. This is followed by cytomegalovirus (CMV) and mycobacterial infection. The typical symptoms of pneumocystis pneumonia include tachypnea, nonproductive cough, and low-grade fever. Whereas pneumocystis infection in non-AIDS patients develops acutely, this infection in AIDS patients can be much more insidious in onset and protracted, developing over several weeks. Some patients with pneumocystis pneumonia can even remain asymptomatic in spite of pulmonary infiltration and abnormal pulmonary function tests. Chest radiographs demonstrate bilateral interstitial infiltrates and restrictive lung disease, and impaired diffusion can be demonstrated by pulmonary function tests. **Since other opportunistic infections and LIP present with indistinguishable clinical** and radiographic findings, fiberoptic bronchoscopy with lavage, transbronchial biopsy, and even open lung biopsy are necessary for histologic and microbiologic diagnosis. Kaposi's sarcoma involvement of the pulmonary system includes infiltration of lung parenchyma, pleura, and tracheobronchial tree.[48] Tracheobronchial involvement with Kaposi's sarcoma and hilar and mediastinal lymphadenopathy from non-Hodgkin's lymphoma can produce tracheobronchial narrowing of obvious concern to an anesthesiologist.

In addition to opportunistic infections, the pulmonary function of the intravenous drug abuser with AIDS may be compromised by pulmonary fibrosis from talc granulomas as well as by secondary pulmonary hypertension.

Appropriate preoperative evaluation of the AIDS patient with pulmonary involvement should include a thorough history and physical examination as well as chest radiograph and arterial blood gas analysis. **If there is concern about possible compression of the trachea from mediastinal masses in patients with non-Hodgkin's lymphoma or tracheobronchial narrowing from Kaposi's sarcoma, obtaining a thoracic CT or MRI scan or even performing fiberoptic bronchoscopy preoperatively is advised to determine the severity of these complications.**[78] Pulmonary function tests, including flow loops, can quantitate the severity of the restrictive disease and tracheobronchial obstruction. Postoperative ventilation may be required for AIDS patients who undergo major surgery.

Cardiovascular system

Cardiac abnormalities in patients with AIDS have until recently received little attention, and studies of myocardial involvement in HIV infection have been largely confined to autopsy investigation. **Cardiac complications in HIV infection include myocarditis (caused by HIV and opportunistic infections, e.g., CMV, *toxoplasma*, and *mycobacteria*), pericarditis with pericardial effusion, and dilated cardiomyopathy.*** AIDS patients with pericardial disease usually have concomitant myocardial disease, e.g., Kaposi's sarcoma or opportunistic myocarditis. Dilated cardiomyopathy characterized by four-chamber enlargement and echocardiographic evidence of poor contractility is the most frequent cardiac disease in patients with HIV infection.[21,43] In general, abnormalities of cardiac function occur late in the course of the disease and occur particularly in patients with low T4-lymphocyte counts and who suffer active opportunistic infection. **Preoperative cardiac evaluation consisting of a physical examination, ECG, and echocardiography is**

---

* References 2, 5, 8, 10, 23, 32, 59.

crucial in the patient with dyspnea and pulmonary infiltrates since the differential diagnosis must include not only opportunistic lung infections but also congestive heart failure. However, echocardiographic evidence of left ventricular dilatation and hypokinesis can be present in asymptomatic AIDS patients even in the early stages of HIV infection.[59]

Central nervous system

Soon after its discovery, HIV was noted to be not only lymphotropic but also neurotropic. A wide spectrum of neurologic diseases that affect anesthetic management of patients affects more than 50% of AIDS patients.[56,76] **Central nervous system (CNS) involvement is due not only to infection of neurons and glia with HIV but also to opportunistic CNS infections and the development of CNS tumors, e.g., primary CNS lymphoma or metastatic Kaposi's sarcoma.** Subacute encephalopathy, an invariably fatal disease that causes AIDS-related dementia or AIDS dementia complex, is the most common CNS disease in patients with HIV infection. Clinical presentation includes dementia, motor weakness, personality changes, dysarthria, tremors, and other movement disorders. The AIDS dementia complex is the initial manifestation of

HIV infection in 10% to 20% of patients. Other neurologic complications of HIV nervous system involvement include peripheral neuropathies,[71] atypical aseptic meningitis with cranial nerve neuropathies, and spinal vacuolar myelopathy with a Guillain-Barré–like syndrome.[71,77] Opportunistic infections, with a host of viral, bacterial, fungal, and parasitic pathogens (see Box 24-2), primary CNS lymphoma, metastatic Kaposi's sarcoma, and AIDS-related cerebrovascular disease produce serious neurologic disease.[29] **Patients with such CNS involvement can demonstrate intracranial hypertension, seizures, dementia, coma, and peripheral nerve damage**—clinical features that must be carefully considered when planning a safe anesthetic.

Preoperative cranial CT or MRI scan of patients with neurologic signs and symptoms[57] will alert the anesthesiologist to the presence of a space-occupying lesion or to evidence of elevated intracranial pressure, factors that strongly influence the choice of anesthetic technique (see Chapter 15).

Hematopoietic system

Hematopoietic abnormalities are almost a sine qua non of HIV infection and include lymphopenia,

---

BOX 24-2
OPPORTUNISTIC INFECTIONS IN PATIENTS WITH
ACQUIRED IMMUNODEFICIENCY SYNDROME (AIDS)

Viral	Fungal	Protozoal	Bacterial
Cytomegalovirus	*Candida albicans*	*Pneumocystis carinii*	*Mycobacteria avium-*
Pneumonia	Oropharyngitis	Pneumonia	*intracellulare*
Chorioretinitis	Esophagitis	*Toxoplasma gondii*	Enteritis
Encephalitis	Disseminated	Encephalitis	Pneumonia
Colitis	*Cryptococcus*	Brain abscess	Meningitis
Myocarditis	*neoformans*	Myocarditis	Disseminated
Pericarditis	Meningitis	*Cryptosporidium*	*Legionella*
Herpes simplex	Pneumonia	Enteritis	Pneumonia
Encephalitis	Disseminated	*Isospora belli*	Infections with "nonopportu-
Mucocutaneous	*Histoplasma*	Enteritis	nistic" bacteria (e.g., *M.*
Disseminated	Disseminated		*tuberculosis, D. pneumoniae,*
Varicella zoster	*Aspergillus*		*H. influenzae, Salmonellae*)
Primary	Pneumonia		
Disseminated	Disseminated		
Epstein-Barr virus			
Oral hairy leukoplakia			
Lymphoid interstitial			
pneumonitis			
Papovavirus			
Progressive multifocal			
leukoencephalopathy			

Modified from Groopman JE: Clinical symptomatology of the acquired immunodeficiency syndrome (AIDS) and related disorders, *Prog Allergy* 37:188, 1986.

neutropenia and, of most concern to anesthesiologists, **anemia, thrombocytopenia, and a bleeding disorder secondary to the presence of a lupus anticoagulant in some patients with AIDS and opportunistic infections.**[9,20] Zidovudine (AZT, Retrovir), the primary HIV antiviral agent, radiation, chemotherapy treatment of non-Hodgkin's lymphoma and Kaposi's sarcoma, and many drugs used in the therapy of opportunistic infections demonstrate hematopoietic side effects that aggravate anemia and thrombocytopenia. A characteristic form of immune thrombocytopenia develops in a proportion of AIDS patients and responds in varying fashion to steroids, high-dose intravenous gamma globulin, danazol,[33] or splenectomy.[1,66] Serious bleeding complications are uncommon in spite of often severe thrombocytopenia. Judicious preoperative administration of packed red cells, platelet transfusions, and, if necessary, fresh frozen plasma must be a part of the preoperative preparation of the patient with AIDS, particularly when major surgery is contemplated.

Gastrointestinal system

Common gastrointestinal manifestations of HIV infection include chronic diarrhea, dysphagia, and esophagitis (candida and herpes). These entities contribute to dehydration, hypovolemia, and electrolyte imbalances, particularly hyponatremia and hypokalemia, that if not appreciated by the anesthesiologist at the preoperative visit might place the patient in jeopardy when receiving an anesthetic.

Renal and endocrine system

Renal involvement and electrolyte disturbances frequently complicate the course of patients with HIV infection and present important preoperative considerations for the anesthesiologist.[38] **Hyponatremia, the most common electrolyte disturbance, occurs in approximately 60% of hospitalized patients with AIDS or AIDS-related complex.** Gastrointestinal fluid loss from diarrhea is the most frequent cause of hyponatremia, but other causes of hyponatremia include the syndrome of inappropriate antidiuretic hormone secretion (secondary to pneumocystis pneumonia or pulmonary lymphoma) as well as AIDS-related adrenal insufficiency, an uncommon complication of HIV infection.[38,64]

Several categories of renal disease that include acute tubular necrosis, a heterogenous group of glomerular and tubulointerstitial nephritides, renovascular diseases, and a unique entity—an HIV associated nephropathy—can complicate the course of the HIV-infected patient and present important anesthetic considerations. Acute renal failure can be toxic in etiology secondary to antibiotic agents, e.g., amphotericin B, acyclovir, pentamidine, and aminoglycosides, or ischemia from septic shock or dehydra-

tion. The heterogenous group of glomerular tubulointerstitial diseases includes glomerulonephritis secondary to bacterial infection and hepatitis B infection, interstitial nephritis secondary to opportunistic infection and drugs, nephrotic syndrome associated with heroin abuse, and a rare form of hemolytic uremic syndrome. HIV nephropathy is a unique, recently described form of renal disease that frequently rapidly progresses to end-stage renal failure.[38,70,74] **Frequent renal involvement and electrolyte disturbances mandate the preoperative evaluation of renal function with urinalysis, BUN, creatinine, and electrolyte determinations as well as close evaluation of the state of hydration.**

Anesthetic Management

The choice of anesthetic techniques for patients is wide and is determined largely by underlying organ involvement and the planned surgical procedure. Local anesthesia, supplemented with sedation by intravenous narcotics such as fentanyl or combined with an intravenous benzodiazepine such as midazolam, provides safe and effective relief of pain and amnesia for many minor procedures. These include fiberoptic bronchoscopy with bronchial brushings, alveolar lavage, transbronchial lung biopsy, Hickman catheter placement, esophagoscopy, sigmoidoscopy, and superficial lymph node and skin biopsies. Droperidol and other drugs with pyramidal side effects should be avoided in patients with AIDS dementia complex who display a parkinsonian-like syndrome, because of the potential for exacerbating the movement disorder. General anesthesia is required for other diagnostic and therapeutic procedures, such as brain biopsy in patients with suspected herpetic or toxoplasma encephalitis, splenectomy for patients with AIDS-associated immune thrombocytopenia, and colectomy for patients with perforated cytomegalovirus colitis. Particular precautions must be taken during anesthetic induction if myocardial dysfunction or intracranial hypertension are present (see Chapters 71 and 72). The choice of muscle relaxants should be made with thorough knowledge of the nature of neurologic involvement and the state of renal function. Succinylcholine should be avoided in patients with severe renal failure, myelopathy, hemiparesis, and peripheral neuropathy because of the risk of life-threatening hyperkalemia. Atracurium is the muscle relaxant of choice in patients with renal failure. Enflurane should be avoided in patients who have seizures because of its epileptogenic potential.

Transmission Precautions for HIV and Hepatitis B

Of great concern to health care providers is the issue of the potential for transmission of a uniformly lethal disease from patients to health care workers. A rational approach to this problem must be based on an understanding of the possible modes of transmission of HIV infection in the hospital setting.

Although HIV has been detected in many body fluids such as blood, semen, vaginal secretions, urine, tears, cerebrospinal fluid, pleural, pericardial, and synovial fluid, and breast milk, **epidemiologic evidence suggests that blood is the single most infectious medium for HIV (as well as hepatitis B) in the medical care setting.**

In 1983 the CDC published *Guidelines for Isolation Precautions in Hospitals,* which recommended blood and body fluid precautions when patients were infected or suspected of being infected with blood-borne pathogens such as HIV or hepatitis B virus. However, as outlined earlier in this chapter, it became apparent that there were many asymptomatic patients who entered the health care system for surgical care who were unknowingly but nevertheless highly contagious for these infections and who posed a risk to health care workers who participated in their care. Ethical, logistic, and financial concerns obviate the possibility of preoperative screening of all patients for HIV or hepatitis B infection.[39,65] In addition, there is no evidence that "extraordinary vigilance" in dealing with such infected patients reduces the risk of needle stick injuries to or blood or body fluid contaminations of health care workers in the perisurgical setting.[51,86] For these reasons, **in 1987, the CDC suggested that every patient be assumed to be contagious for a blood-borne pathogen and recommended that blood and body fluid precautions be consistently adopted for all patients irrespective of whether they were known to be infected or not.** These precautions are known as "Universal Blood and Body Fluid Precautions" or "Universal Precautions."[12-14,18,18a] Although semen and vaginal secretions have not been implicated in the transmission of HIV infection or hepatitis B in the health care setting, they have been implicated in sexual transmission of these infections, and universal precautions should also apply to these secretions. In addition, although the risk of transmission of HIV and hepatitis B virus from CSF and synovial, pleural, pericardial, and amniotic fluid is unknown, universal precautions should be adopted when handling these fluids. These recommendations obviously have implications for the anesthesiologist. Universal precautions, however, do not apply to stool, urine, saliva, nasal secretions, tears, and vomitus unless they are visibly contaminated with blood. The application of these guidelines to operating room and anesthetic practice is outlined later in this chapter.

The most likely potential sources of HIV and hepatitis B infection for the anesthesiologist are either direct parenteral inoculation of blood by accidental needle stick exposure or exposure to mucous membranes and secretions contaminated with blood. **Approximately 80% of accidental occupationally acquired HIV infection results from contaminated needle stick injuries rather than from exposure to infected secretions.**[16,17] Several studies have reported more than 1000 cases of health care workers who sustained **needle stick exposure to HIV-infected blood** over the past several years. The cumulative results of these studies suggest that **the risk of acquiring HIV infection under these circumstances is approximately 1%.**[50,60,63] **The risk is approximately 10 times lower than after similar exposure to hepatitis-B–contaminated blood.**[86,87]

Gloves should be worn during venipuncture or when performing vascular access procedures, intubation, extubation, passage of nasogastric tubes, and oral and nasopharyngeal suctioning. They should be removed after the procedure before handling other noncontaminated articles and equipment. Anesthesiologists must use appropriate "barrier precautions" to prevent skin and mucous membrane contamination by a patient's blood and body fluids. Masks and protective eyewear (e.g., glasses or face shields) should be worn during procedures that generate droplets of blood or body fluids (e.g., major vessel cannulations and fiberoptic bronchoscopy). Gowns should also be used if blood or body fluid contamination of articles of clothing is likely. Hands should be washed after gloves have been removed and if they have been contaminated by a patient's blood or body fluids.[14]

Since parenteral exposure to infected blood by accidental needle stick injury is the overwhelming cause of HIV and hepatitis B infection in health care workers, extraordinary care must be taken to prevent injury to hands from needles, scalpels, and other sharp instruments. If stopcocks are placed in IV lines, the use of needles for injection will be minimized. After use, needles and scalpel blades must be placed in puncture-resistant containers for disposal. **To reduce the hazard of injury, needles must not be recapped, bent, or removed from disposable syringes before being discarded.**[14,18a]

Management of the Health Care Worker Exposed to HIV

Guidelines for the management of health care workers exposed to HIV have been proposed by the CDC. If a health care worker suffers a contaminated needle stick injury or mucous membrane exposure to either blood or other body fluids, or has extensive skin contamination with large amounts of blood, particularly if the skin is not intact (chapped, abraded), the appropriate employee health service should be contacted to initiate evaluation and follow-up.

The source patient should be informed of the incident, and this patient's HIV antibody status determined after appropriate consent. If the source patient has AIDS, is seropositive for HIV antibody, or refuses testing, **HIV antibody testing should be performed on the injured worker immediately after exposure and at 6, 12, and 24 weeks thereafter to determine whether HIV infection has been transmitted.** The health care worker should be advised to report any acute febrile illness, particularly if it is associated with rash or lymphadenopathy, since this might represent acute HIV infection. HIV serologic testing beyond 24 weeks of exposure is not indicated if the source patient is seronegative and is not at high risk for HIV infection.[16]

Sterilization and Disinfection of Anesthesia Equipment

Standard sterilization and disinfection procedures that are currently in use are effective in sterilizing nondisposable items of anesthesia equipment, e.g., laryngoscope blades or fiberoptic bronchoscopes that become contaminated with body fluids or blood. **After thorough cleansing with detergent and water to remove blood and secretions, these instruments should be sterilized or receive "high-level" disinfection with chemical germicides that are registered with the U.S. Environmental Protection Agency as "sterilants."**

VIRAL HEPATITIS

Although many viral agents cause hepatitis, this chapter will review only the diseases produced by the four primary hepatotropic viruses, namely hepatitis A, hepatitis B, non-A, non-B hepatitis; and delta hepatitis. These infectious agents have implications for anesthesiologists because of the relatively high degree of infectivity, the frequency of accidental exposure in health care workers, and the risk of transmission to patients via blood transfusion.[7,27] The preoperative evaluation of patients with hepatitis is reviewed in Chapter 19. The anesthesiologist should be familiar with the epidemiology, mode of transmission, and laboratory diagnosis in order to reduce the risks of accidentally acquiring and transmitting these potentially life-threatening infections.

In general, since the clinical manifestations of acute hepatitis produced by these agents are similar, the specific etiologic diagnosis is based on laboratory tests to identify either specific antigens or patterns of antibody response. The spectrum of illnesses is broad, ranging from asymptomatic disease to fulminant hepatic failure. Chronic disease may similarly be subclinical and persistent or progressive with the development of cirrhosis or hepatocellular carcinoma (Table 24-2).

Table 24-2 Viral hepatitis: comparison of disease entities

Feature	Hepatitis A	Hepatitis B	Non-A, Non-B hepatitis	Delta hepatitis
Virus	27-nm entero-virus	42-nm DNA hepadna virus	?	35-nm defective RNA virus
Incubation period (days)	15-45	30-180	15-160	28-150
Mode of transmission				
Fecal-oral	+ + +	−	Some forms	?
Parenteral	+/−	+ + +	+ + +	?
Sexual/maternal/ neonatal contact	+/−	+ +	+ +	?
Transfusion related*	Rare	5%-10%	90-95%	?
Onset	Acute	Often insidious	Insidious	
Fulminant hepatic failure	Rare	1%	<5%	Coinfection 1%-10% Superinfection 5%-20%
Progression to chronicity	None	5%-10%	5%-10%	Coinfection <5% Superinfection >75%
Carrier state	No	0.1%-3%, varies worldwide	>50%	Coinfection <5% Superinfection >75%
Prophylaxis	Immunoglob-ulin (IG)	HBIG, hepatitis B vaccine	?	Hepatitis B vaccine

*Values are for percentage of cases of transfusion-related hepatitis caused by each type of virus.
Modified from Dienstag JL, Wands JR, and Isselbacher KJ: Acute hepatitis. In Wilson JD et al, eds: *Harrison's principles of internal medicine*, ed 12, New York, 1991, McGraw-Hill.

Hepatitis A

The hepatitis A virus (HAV) is a 27-nm, nonenveloped RNA virus—an enterovirus type 72.

Epidemiology

Hepatitis A accounts for about 40% of hepatitis-like illnesses in the United States.[15] **This infection is almost always acquired by the fecal-oral route,** with outbreaks occurring under conditions of poor hygiene and overcrowding. Outbreaks associated with the ingestion of contaminated food and water have been described. **Only rarely is hepatitis A transmitted by blood transfusion, and acquiring infection from a contaminated needlestick injury is unlikely.**[27]

Patients with hepatitis A are most infectious during the 2 weeks or so before the development of clinical illness, when the virus is present in stools. Usually patients are not contagious during the clinical phase of acute hepatitis, but, because the virus may be shed for a longer period, enteric isolation precautions should be applied to the hospitalized hepatitis A patient.[31] A chronic carrier state does not exist with hepatitis A.

Clinical manifestations and diagnosis

Most patients with acute hepatitis A are, in fact, asymptomatic, with clinically overt disease occurring in only about 5% of cases. The disease, which is usually self-limited with a very low mortality rate, does not produce chronic hepatitis or cirrhosis. Since identification of fecal or serum HAV antigen is not routinely available, the diagnosis of HAV depends on serologic methods. The HAV antibody (anti-HAV) is first detected with the onset of clinical illness. Initially this is of the IgM subclass, but subsequently the HAV IgG titer rises and remains elevated for many years (Fig. 24-2). The diagnosis of acute hepatitis A is therefore confirmed by an elevated HAV IgM titer, whereas increased HAV IgG antibody indicates previous HAV infection and an immune host.[7,27]

Prophylaxis

Commercially available preparations of immune globulin (IG) contain anti-HAV in sufficient titer to prevent the development of clinically overt disease when administered early in the incubation period and even up to 2 weeks after exposure. The efficacy of IG prophylaxis declines to very low levels when administered more than 2 weeks after exposure. Administration to health care workers should be considered only after exposure to feces of infected patients.[47]

Hepatitis B

The etiologic agent of hepatitis B is the hepatitis B virus (HBV), a member of a hepatotropic group of DNA viruses, the hepadnaviruses. Three morpholog-

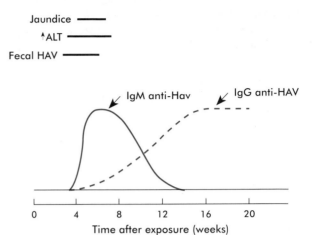

Fig. 24-2. Typical clinical manifestations and serologic course of acute hepatitis A virus *(HAV)*. Lines at upper left represent presence and timing of factors. (Modified from Dienstag JL, Wands JR, and Isselbacher KJ: Acute hepatitis. In Wilson JD et al, eds: *Harrison's principles of internal medicine,* ed 12, New York, 1991, McGraw-Hill.)

ically distinct viral type particles are detected by electron microscopy in a serum of acutely infected patients. The intact virion, a 42-nm sphere, contains the hepatitis B surface antigen (HbsAg) within a surrounding envelope.[7,27,44,84] Several HbsAg subtypes that provide useful epidemiologic markers are described. The 22-nm spheric or filamentous particles that represent excess surface antigen envelope material outnumber intact virions by a factor of 100 to 1000. In the intact virion this envelope surface antigen, HbsAg, surrounds a 27-nm nucleocapsid core, the surface of which expresses the hepatitis core antigen, HbcAg. Uncoated core particles, unlike excess envelope material, do not circulate in infected serum. The hepatitis B "e" antigen, a third hepatitis B antigen, is derived from HBcAg. This antigen contributes to the infectivity of the HBV. The nucleocapsid core also contains the genome of partially double-stranded DNA and a DNA polymerase.

Clinical manifestations and diagnosis

The clinical manifestations of hepatitis B infection resemble those of the other acute viral hepatitis infections. **Of hepatitis B patients, 90% will experience a self-limited disease, most of which will be asymptomatic and resolve without chronic sequelae. Fewer than 1% of patients will develop fulminating liver failure with a high mortality rate. The chronic carrier state develops in 6% to 10% of infected patients, and 25% of these carriers will develop chronic active hepatitis that variably progresses to cirrhosis.** In addition, the incidence of hepatocellular carcinoma is increased by 12 to 300 times in HBV

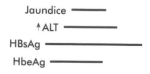

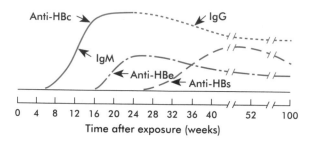

Fig. 24-3. Typical clinical manifestations and serologic course of acute hepatitis B virus. Lines at upper left represent presence, sequence, and timing of factors. (Modified from Dienstag JL, Wands JR, and Isselbacher KJ: Acute hepatitis. In Wilson JD et al, eds: *Harrison's principles of internal medicine,* ed 12, New York, 1991, McGraw-Hill.)

carriers.[7,27,47] The relationship between clinical disease, the appearance of virologic markers, and the serologic response is outlined in Fig. 24-3.

After an average incubation period of 75 days, HBsAg is detectable in serum. This laboratory finding precedes clinical manifestations and transaminase and bilirubin elevations. HBsAg titers fall as the acute illness clears, and HBsAg is usually undetectable within a month or two of resolution of the illness. **Antibody to HBsAg, anti-HBs, becomes measurable in the serum as HBsAg disappears, and anti-HBs persists indefinitely thereafter, a marker of previous hepatitis B infection. Anti-HBs is the antibody primarily responsible for long-lasting immunity.**

HBcAg is detectable only in hepatocytes and not in serum because of its incorporation within the HBsAg coat. However, **antibody to HBcAg, anti-HBc, appears in serum within a week or two of HBs antigenemia, even before the clinical onset of disease. Occasionally a hiatus or window of several weeks may exist between the disappearance of HBsAg and the detection of anti-HBs. Anti-HBc may be the only indicator of acute HBV infection under these circumstances.** Anti-HBc remains detectable indefinitely and together with anti-HBs is indicative of previous infection. It is for this reason that anti-HBc is a component of the surrogate testing of donated blood in order to detect potentially infected units. Characterization of recent vs. remote infection can be made by determining whether anti-HBc is of the IgM or IgG subclass (Fig. 24-3). Such IgM antibodies are detectable for approximately 6 months after infection, after which time they are replaced by IgG anti-HBc.

HBeAg, a third hepatitis B antigen, is indicative of high levels of viral replication and as such correlates with clinical infectivity. HBeAg is detectable in the serum concurrently with or shortly after the rise of HBsAg and disappears with the peak elevation of aminotransferase activity. Anti-HBe correlates with a period of reduced infectivity. **In chronic HBV infection (chronic active hepatitis or chronic persistent hepatitis) HBeAg remains detectable, as does anti-HBc, but antibodies to HBsAg are not present.**[7,27]

Transmission of hepatitis B infection

Carriers of the hepatitis B virus are potentially infectious for the health care worker whether the carriers are acutely ill or asymptomatic chronic carriers. Although the degree of infectivity is related to the presence of HBsAg, individuals who are positive for HBsAg should be regarded as potentially infectious. The concentration of HBV is highest in the blood and serous fluids of infectious patients, but virus is also present in saliva and semen. All these body fluids are potentially infectious.

Anesthesia personnel acquire HBV infection via percutaneous inoculation from contaminated sharp instruments and needles. Transmission probably does not occur through intact skin exposed to contagious blood, saliva, or other body fluid, but HBV may infect such exposed persons through minute clinically insignificant skin breaks.[47]

Prevention

Universal precautions. The prevalence of serologic markers of HBV infection varies throughout the population, ranging from 3% to 5% in healthy U.S. adults to greater than 60% in intravenous drug abusers. Since patients who are HBV carriers cannot practically be routinely identified, the high seroprevalence rates mandate the use of "universal precautions" for the prevention of transmission of hepatitis B.[47] These measures are discussed in detail in the previous section on the prevention of HIV infection.

Since antibodies to HBsAg provide immunity to HBV infection, other preventive strategies involve the administration of immune globulin to provide temporary passive immunity and active immunization with hepatitis B vaccine for long-term immunity.

Hepatitis B immune globulin. **Hepatitis B immune globulin (HBIG) is used for the passive immunization of susceptible individuals (i.e., anti-HBs–negative persons) after significant exposure to blood or secretions of individuals with HBV infection.** HBIG is manufactured from plasma preselected for high anti-HBs titers. The U.S.-manufactured product has anti-HBs titers of greater than 1:100,000. This preparation is 75% effective in preventing HBV infection when a two-dose regimen (first dose postexposure, second dose 1 month later) is administered after percutaneous exposure[47] (see Table 24-2).

Hepatitis B vaccine. At present, two hepatitis B vaccines are licensed for use in the United States. The first, introduced in 1982, is an inactivated purified preparation of 22-nm surface antigen particles. The manufacturing process inactivates all known classes of infectious agents, including HIV. In 1986 a genetically engineered HBsAg vaccine was introduced for clinical use. After a three-injection course of either vaccine, 95% of recipients responded with levels of serum antibody that are protective for at least 5 years. The necessity for booster doses continues to be evaluated but at present they are not recommended.[47]

Since the hepatitis B vaccine is safe and highly effective in preventing HBV infection, immunization of health care workers at high or moderate risk for such infection should be strongly encouraged.

Management of the health care worker exposed to HBV

Since the risk of acquiring hepatitis B infection after needle stick exposure to HBsAg-positive blood ranges between 6% and 30%, the CDC has proposed prophylaxis strategies to reduce the likelihood of infection. These recommendations, outlined in Table 24-3, take several factors into consideration. First, the hepatitis B vaccination status of the injured worker; second, whether the source of the blood can be identified; and third, whether the HBsAg status of the source blood is known.[47]

Delta Hepatitis

Hepatitis delta virus (HDV), the etiologic agent of delta hepatitis, is a "defective" virus that replicates only in the presence of HBsAg. Delta hepatitis, therefore, occurs either as a "coinfection," simultaneous with acute HBV infection, or as "superinfection" with chronic HBV infection. HBV is a 35-nm "hybrid" structure. The outer coat antigen of HBsAg, coded for by the genome of the "helper" HBV, surrounds the internal nucleocapsid containing delta antigen and a small segment of circular RNA.[44,45]

Clinical manifestations and diagnosis

HDV infection resembles HBV infection in that it causes both acute and chronic hepatitis but usually of a more severe course. Acute delta hepatitis occurs in two forms. First, as a "coinfection" (the simultaneous occurrence of both HBV and HDV infection) and second, as a "superinfection" (the development of acute delta infection in a chronic HBV carrier). There is a marked difference in the morbidity, mortality, and serologic response, however, between two forms of delta infection[44,45] (see Table 24-2).

Acute HDV coinfection is usually relatively benign and self-limited. Fewer than 5% of such cases progress to develop chronic hepatitis. During the incubation period, HBsAg, HDVAg and HDV-RNA are detectable first. HDVAg is expressed primarily in hepatic nuclei, and sensitive assays to detect this antigen in serum are not yet routinely available. The titer of anti-HDV, initially of the IgM subclass, rises with the onset of clinical symptoms, and the elevation of bilirubin and serum amino transferase stabilizes. HDV replication and clinical disease resolve with clearance of HBsAg. With self-limited infection, the titer of anti-HDV is usually low and short-lived, becoming undetectable soon after the disappearance of HBsAg and HBVAg. Acute delta coinfection can be distinguished from acute superinfection by detect-

---

Table 24-3   Recommendations for hepatitis B prophylaxis after percutaneous exposure

	Exposed person	
Source	Unvaccinated	Vaccinated
HBsAg-positive	HBIG × 1 immediately Initiate HB vaccine series	Test exposed person for anti-HBs If inadequate antibody, HBIG × 1 immediately plus HB vaccine booster dose
Known source		
High-risk HBsAg-positive	Initiate HB vaccine series Test source for HBsAg; if positive, HBIG × 1	Test source for HBsAg only if exposed person is vaccine non-responder; if source is HBsAg-positive, give HBIG × 1 immediately plus HB vaccine booster dose
Low-risk HBsAg-positive	Initiate HB vaccine series	Nothing required
Unknown source	Initiate HB vaccine series	Nothing required

From Recommendations of the Immunization Practices Advisory Committee, *MMWR* 34:313, 1985.

ing a rise in IgM anti-HBc antibody, a serologic marker of acute HBV infection. **Acute HDV superinfection, i.e., the development of acute HDV infection in an HBV viral carrier, on the other hand, demonstrates a high morbidity with 80% of such infected patients developing chronic hepatitis.** Indeed, most patients with chronic delta hepatitis probably manifest HDV superinfection. HDV superinfection is characterized by an acute elevation of serum ALT levels and anti-HDV titers in a chronic HBsAg carrier. Persistently abnormal liver function tests, a sustained rise in anti-HDV with titers, and the appearance of HDV-RNA characterize the persistent HDV replication of chronic HDV superinfection.[7,27,45]

Epidemiology

Since HDV is "defective" and can only replicate with the "helper" function of HBV, the epidemiology of this disease is inexorably linked with that of HBV infection.[45] Delta hepatitis displays three distinct epidemiologic pictures worldwide. This infection is endemic and particularly widespread in the Mediterranean area, the Mideast, and North Africa, where it is spread by predominantly nonpercutaneous routes, e.g., close personal contact. It is, however, an uncommon infection in the United States and northern Europe, and uncommon even in Southeast Asia and China in spite of a high HBV carrier rate in those areas. In the United States and northern Europe, HDV infection is spread primarily by parenteral blood exposure and as such occurs primarily in the groups at risk for HBV infection, namely intravenous drug abusers and patients who require frequent administration of blood transfusions, e.g., persons with hemophilia.[7,27,45] Venereal transmission probably also occurs. Transmission of HDV to health care workers has only occasionally been described.[54]

Prevention

From an understanding of the pathogenesis of this disease it is clear that patients who are immune to hepatitis B, either from natural infection or from immunization with hepatitis B vaccine, will be immune to HDV infection. However, patients who are HBsAg carriers remain susceptible. At present there is no known immunoprophylactic measure to protect such HBsAg carriers from acquiring HDV superinfection. Such individuals should avoid contact with delta hepatitis agent.[45]

Non-A, Non-B Hepatitis

The development of serologic tests that identified patients with hepatitis A and B made it clear that there remained another type of infectious hepatitis, so called non-A, non-B (NANB) hepatitis. This disease, initially observed in the recipients of blood transfu-

sion, is now responsible for most cases of transfusion-associated hepatitis. **The etiologic virus(es) have not been structurally characterized, but it appears that two distinct agents may be responsible for NANB hepatitis.**[26] **Recently, reports have identified an agent responsible for NANB hepatitis—the hepatitis C virus (HCV).**[19] Indeed, antibodies to this virus were detected in a group of patients who developed posttransfusion NANB hepatitis.[52] Assays to measure anti-hepatitis C antibodies are now commercially available. Whether other agents are also responsible for posttransfusion NANB hepatitis remains to be determined.

Epidemiology

Although originally thought to be an infection acquired only by transfusion, NANB hepatitis is now known to be acquired by other modes of transmission. Most NANB hepatitis in the United States and western Europe resembles hepatitis B in its modes of transmission, in that it is primarily transmitted by percutaneous blood transmission but also by nonpercutaneous routes.[26] Transfusion-associated hepatitis is the most frequent form of NANB infection. **NANB hepatitis represents approximately 20% to 40% of acute viral hepatitis. Approximately 20% of these cases are transmitted by blood transfusion.**[88] **NANB hepatitis accounts for approximately 90% of posttransfusion hepatitis.**[89] Despite the elimination of paid blood donors and screening of blood for HBsAg, **the reported incidence of posttransfusion hepatitis is still of the order of one to six cases/1000 units, and NANB hepatitis develops in 7% to 10% of multitransfused patients.** Although an ELISA anti-hepatitis C test is now in routine use in the screening of donor blood, measurement of ALT in donor blood units remains a surrogate test for NANB hepatitis in blood banks.[91] The risk of transmitting NANB infection depends on the type of blood product administered and, in particular, on the manufacturing process. Albumin and immune and hyperimmune globulin pose no risk since their production entails heat treatment at 60° C and ethanol precipitation. Single unit whole blood, packed cells, platelets, and plasma represent average risks. **The risk of infection with single pooled donor blood products (e.g., factors II, VII to X) approximates 20% to 30%.**[26,27]

NANB virus also causes sporadic cases of hepatitis in IV drug abusers. NANB hepatitis has become the most common cause of acute hepatitis in patients and staff members of dialysis units since effective measures to reduce the spread of HBV have been introduced.[26] Sexual transmission of NANB hepatitis appears to be less than that of HBV infection. NANB infection is not a major risk to the health care worker. Only rare cases have been ascribed to needle sticks.[62]

Clinical disease

The clinical manifestations of NANB hepatitis are similar to the other forms of hepatitis, but the disease is generally less severe and is more likely than the other forms to be anicteric. Fulminant liver failure complicating NANB hepatitis is rare. **However, the long-term sequelae of NANB hepatitis appear more serious than was previously considered, with a substantial proportion of patients progressing to develop chronic hepatitis and cirrhosis.** NANB infection may also be a precursor of hepatocellular carcinoma.

HERPES SIMPLEX INFECTIONS

Herpes simplex infections are of concern to the anesthesiologist for several reasons. First, herpes simplex virus (HSV) is an occasional pathogen causing herpetic whitlow, a self-limited but nevertheless painful infection of the fingers. Second, there is increased incidence of the reactivation of latent HSV labialis infection in women who received epidural morphine for postoperative analgesia after cesarean section.

Epidemiology

HSV infections are widespread and among the most common viral infections of humans. Two serotypes (HSV-I and HSV-II) demonstrate different modes of transmission although both are spread by direct contact. HSV-I is transmitted primarily by nonvenereal contact and is responsible for most herpetic infections above the waistline. HSV-2, on the other hand, is usually spread venereally and involves sites below the waist. Primary infection, which is often subclinical, tends to occur in children, but pharyngitis, gingivostomatitis, and occasionally ocular infections can represent clinically overt primary infections.

HSV infections are characterized by latency—the ability of the virus to lie dormant for many years within sensory neurons innervating the area involved in the primary infection. At intervals thereafter, stimuli such as fever, stress, trauma, surgery, sunlight, epidural morphine, and immunosuppression reactivate the "dormant" virus to produce recurrent or recrudescent infection that develops close to the site of the primary infection. Herpes labialis or "fever blisters" is such an example. These reactivation infections are usually milder than the primary infection because of acquired immunity, but under conditions of immunosuppression, such reactivation infections may become disseminated and life-threatening.[49,69]

Herpetic Whitlow

Herpetic whitlow is an occupational disease of anesthesiologists and other health care workers characterized by painful but self-limited HSV vesicopustular infection of fingers. The infection is usually acquired by health care workers by direct contact with herpetic lesions or by the inoculation of HSV virus contained in contaminated saliva and respiratory secretions through either an inapparent or an overt break in the skin. Health care professionals, e.g., anesthesiologists, dentists, ICU nurses, and respiratory therapists, are at high risk because of constant exposure to potentially contaminated secretions.

The infection is characterized by a prodrome of pain, tingling of the distal phalanges, and the subsequent appearance of numerous 1 to 3 mm diameter vesicles overlying an erythematous base. These vesicles can coalesce to produce large bullous lesions and an exquisitely tender digit. Systemic signs of infections, e.g., fever, malaise, and regional lymphadenopathy, may also occur. **This infection is self-limited, usually resolving within 2 to 3 weeks.**[49,69]

Herpetic whitlow therapy includes conservative measurements such as analgesia and limb elevation. Incision of a tense bullous may help relieve severe pain, but deep incision into the pulp space is contraindicated and may prolong healing. Antibiotics are usually not required unless bacterial superinfection has developed. Topical acyclovir, as a 5% ointment, shortens the clinical course and decreases viral shedding in a primary infection. It is, however, less effective in decreasing shedding with recurrent infections. Oral acyclovir prevents clinical disease when administered at the first signs of recurrence of herpetic whitlow, but skin lesions often develop when the drug is discontinued.[37] Intravenous acyclovir is also effective in the therapy of the acute disease, but as with other herpetic infections, the virus remains latent in the ganglia even after clinical response.

Anesthetic implications

Prevention. Herpetic whitlow is a preventable disease. Since 10% of the population may be asymptomatic carriers of HSV, all patients should be considered infectious. Contact with such potentially infected oral, respiratory, and genital secretions can be prevented by the wearing of gloves when exposure to such secretions is likely. Such precautions are indeed strongly recommended for the prevention of exposure to other more serious infections, namely, HIV and hepatitis B infections. If accidental contact is made with such secretions, hand washing with soap may inactivate the HSV virus and prevent initiation of herpetic whitlow. To avoid transmission of HSV infection to patients under their care, anesthesiologists and other health care professionals with active herpetic lesions must avoid contact with patients, particularly those who are immunosuppressed or who are otherwise susceptible (e.g., neonates and burn patients), until the lesions are encrusted and dried.[49,69]

Epidural morphine and herpes labialis. Recent studies have demonstrated an association between the use of epidural morphine used for postcesarean-section analgesia and the reactivation of latent herpes labialis. **In these studies there was an increased incidence of postcesarean-section herpes labialis in the groups that received epidural morphine for analgesia compared with the groups that received intramuscular morphine.[24,36] The explanation for this finding is unclear but may be related to facial irritation and viral activation caused by the increased itching that occurred in the groups that received epidural morphine.** Although it is unclear whether there is an increase in neonatal herpetic infections in the infants of these patients, caution was urged by these investigators in choosing epidural morphine, particularly in patients with a history of herpes labialis.[35]

TUBERCULOSIS

The progressive decline in the incidence and morbidity of tuberculosis was accelerated in the 1950s by the introduction of effective antituberculous chemotherapy, such that by the beginning of the 1990s, tuberculosis has largely become a disease of the elderly, the homeless, alcoholics, and poor immigrants and refugees. The explosion of the AIDS epidemic has, however, been paralleled by an increase in the incidence of tuberculosis in patients with HIV infec-

tion. **The prevalence of tuberculosis in AIDS patients has increased greatly compared with that of the general population.[17]** The spectrum of tuberculous disease has also changed in the AIDS era. Whereas pulmonary tuberculosis was by far the most frequent manifestation of disease before the 1980s, extrapulmonary tuberculosis involving central nervous system, meninges, liver, gastrointestinal tract, and bone marrow is now observed in greater than 70% of HIV patients with mycobacterial disease. In addition, infection with atypical mycobacteria, particularly mycobacterium avium complex, is recognized with increasing frequency as an opportunistic disseminated infection in patients with AIDS.[46]

Anesthetic Implications

Apart from the organ-specific implications for the anesthesiologist (e.g., restrictive lung disease or massive hemoptysis), the implications for the anesthesiologist are largely those of infection control. High-level disinfection or sterilization will readily decontaminate instruments (e.g., bronchoscopes and laryngoscopes) possibly contaminated with infectious secretions of a tuberculosis patient. **The anesthesia machine does not represent a source of microbial contamination,[3] and no particular precautions need to be taken beyond those of routine cleaning. Breathing circuits and inflating breathing bags should be disposed of or sterilized after possible tuberculosis contamination.**

KEY POINTS

- The clinical spectrum of HIV infection ranges from the asymptomatic seropositive patient, through a range of intermediate disease with chronic lymphadenopathy, to frank AIDS with life-threatening opportunistic infections. Of note is that infection can remain subclinical during its latency period for many years, while the patient is, nevertheless, infectious and capable of transmitting disease.

- Multisystem involvement by opportunistic infections, secondary tumor development, or direct HIV damage results in altered organ function with implications for the anesthesiologist. Specific dysfunction in all major organ systems should be sought preoperatively before planning an anesthetic in the patient with AIDS.

- Opportunistic infections, lymphoid interstitial pneumonitis, and neoplasms often compromise pulmonary function in the patient with AIDS. Both lung parenchyma as well as the tracheobronchial tree can be affected by these pathologic processes.

- Cardiac complications of HIV infection include myocarditis, pericarditis, pericardial effusion, and dilated cardiomyopathy. Preoperative electrocardiogram and echocardiography can be helpful in the diagnosis of cardiac dysfunction.

- Neurologic involvement of HIV infection includes both the central nervous system and the peripheral nervous system. Patients with neurologic compromise can demonstrate intracranial hypertension, seizures, dementia, and peripheral neuropathy.

- HIV infection often causes anemia and thrombocytopenia, and renal damage by HIV infection can lead to electrolyte disturbances and alterations in creatinine clearance.

- Approximately 80% of accidental occupationally acquired HIV infection results from contaminated needle stick injuries rather than from exposure to infected secretions, with 1% of all such needle sticks leading to HIV seroconversion.

- Hepatitis A is acquired primarily by the fecal-oral route and is only rarely transmitted by blood transfusion.
- Of patients with hepatitis B infection, 90% experience a self-limited disease. The chronic carrier state develops in 6% to 10% of infected patients, and only 25% of these carriers will develop chronic active hepatitis with progression to cirrhosis. In addition, 1% of patients will develop fulminating liver failure with a high mortality rate.
- Non-A, non-B (NANB) hepatitis accounts for approximately 90% of posttransfusion hepatitis, with the incidence of posttransfusion hepatitis being about one to six cases/1000 units. NANB hepatitis develops in 7% to 10% of multitransfused patients.
- Herpetic whitlow is an occupational disease of anesthesiologists and other health care workers characterized by a painful but self-limited herpes simplex virus infection of the fingers.
- An association exists between the use of epidural morphine for postcesarean-section analgesia and the reactivation of latent herpes labialis.

KEY REFERENCES

Berry AJ: Viral hepatitis, *Anesth Clin North Am* 7:771, 1989.

Centers for Disease Control: Recommendations for prevention of HIV transmission in health-care settings, *MMWR* 36(suppl 2):229, 1988.

Centers for Disease Control: Update: an acquired immunodeficiency syndrome and human immunodeficiency virus infection among health-care workers, *MMWR* 37:229, 1988.

Centers for Disease Control: Update: universal precautions for prevention of transmission of human immunodeficiency virus hepatitis B virus and other bloodborne pathogens in health-care settings, *JAMA* 260:462, 1988.

Fauci AS, moderator: The acquired immunodeficiency syndrome: an update, *Ann Intern Med* 102:800, 1985.

Gieraerts R: Increased incidence of itching and herpes simplex in patients given epidural morphine after cesarean section, *Anesth Anal* 66:1321, 1987.

Hoofnagle JH: Type D (delta) hepatitis, *JAMA* 261:1321, 1989.

Levy WS et al: Prevalence of cardiac abnormalities in human immunodeficiency virus infection, *Am J Cardiol* 63:86, 1989.

Warner MA, Kunkel SE: Human immunodeficiency virus infection, *Anesth Clin North Am* 7:795, 1989.

Whitsett CF: Infections acquired through blood transfusions, *Anesth Clin North Am* 7:902, 1989.

REFERENCES

1. Abrams DI: HIV-related immune thrombocytopenic purpura. In Cohen PT, Sande MA, and Volberding PA: *The AIDS knowledge base,* Waltham, 1990, The Medical Publishing Group.
2. Acierno LJ: Cardiac complications in acquired immunodeficiency syndrome (AIDS): a review, *JACC* 13:1144, 1989.
3. AORN Recommended Practices Subcommittee: Recommended practices—cleaning and processing anesthesia equipment, *AORN J* 41:625, 1985.
4. Ascher MS, Wilber JC: Immunofluorescence for serodiagnosis of retrovirus infection, *Arch Pathol Lab Med* 114:246, 1990.
5. Baroldi et al: Focal lymphocytic myocarditis in acquired immunodeficiency syndrome (AIDS): a correlative morphologic and clinical study in 6 consecutive fatal cases, *JACC* 12:463, 1988.
6. Barre-Sinnousi F et al: Isolation of a T-lymphocyte retrovirus from a patient at risk for acquired immunodeficiency syndrome (AIDS), *Science* 220:868, 1983.
7. Berry AJ: Viral hepatitis, *Anesth Clin North Am* 7:771, 1989.
8. Bestetti RB: Cardiac involvement in the acquired immunodeficiency syndrome, *Int J Cardiol* 22:143, 1989.
9. Bloom EJ, Abrams DI, and Rodgers GM: Lupus anticoagulant in the acquired immunodeficiency syndrome, *JAMA* 256:491, 1986.
10. Cammarosano C, Lewis W: Cardiac lesions in acquired immunodeficiency syndrome (AIDS), *J Am Coll Cardiol* 5:703, 1985.
11. Centers for Disease Control: Classification system for human T-lymphotropic virus type III/lymphadenopathy-associated virus infection, *MMWR* 35:334, 1986.
12. Centers for Disease Control: Recommendations for preventing possible transmission of human T lymphotropic virus type III/lymphadenopathy associated virus during invasive procedures, *MMWR* 35:221, 1986.
13. Centers for Disease Control: Recommendations for prevention of HIV transmission in health-care settings, *MMWR* 36(suppl 2):15, 1987.
14. Centers for Disease Control: Recommendations for prevention of HIV transmission in health-care settings, *MMWR* 36(suppl 2):229, 1988.
15. Centers for Disease Control: Revision of the CDC surveillance case definition for acquired immunodeficiency syndrome, *MMWR* 36:1, 1987.
16. Centers for Disease Control: Summary of notifiable diseases, United States, *MMWR* 36:54, 1987.
17. Centers for Disease Control: Tuberculosis, United States, 1985, and the possible impact of HTLV-III/LAV infections, *MMWR* 35:74, 1985.
18. Centers for Disease Contol: Update: acquired immunodeficiency syndrome and human immunodeficiency virus infection among health-care workers, *MMWR* 37:229, 1988.
18a. Centers for Disease Control: Update: universal precautions for prevention of transmission of human immunodeficiency

virus, hepatitis B virus and other blood-borne pathogens in health-care settings, *JAMA* 260:462, 1988.

19. Choo QL et al: Isolation of a cDNA clone derived from a blood-borne non A, non B viral hepatitis genome, *Science* 244:359, 1989.

20. Cohen AJ, Philips TM, and Kessler CM: Circulating coagulation inhibitors in the acquired immunodeficiency syndrome, *Ann Intern Med* 104:175, 1986.

21. Cohen IS et al: Congestive cardiomyopathy in association with acquired immunodeficiency syndrome, *N Engl J Med* 315:628, 1986.

22. Coopers et al: Acute AIDS retrovirus infection definition of a clinical illness associated with seroconversion, *Lancet* 1:537, 1985.

23. Corboy JR, Fink L, and Millen WT: Congestive cardiomyopathy in association with AIDS, *Radiology* 165:139, 1987.

24. Crone LAL et al: Herpes labialis in parturients receiving epidural morphine following cesarean section, *Anesthesiology* 73:208, 1990.

25. Curran JW et al: The epidemiology of AIDS: current status and future prospects, *Science* 229:1352, 1985.

26. Dienstag JL, Alter HA: Non A-Non B hepatitis: evolving epidemiologic and clinical perspective, *Semin Liver Dis* 6:67, 1986.

27. Dienstag JL, Wands JR, and Koff RS: Acute hepatitis. In Wilson JD et al, eds: *Harrison's principles of internal medicine*, ed 12, New York, 1991, McGraw-Hill.

28. Dodd Ry, Fang CT: The western immunoblot procedure for HIV antibodies and its interpretation, *Arch Pathol Lab Med* 114:240, 1990.

29. Engstrom JW, Lowenstein DH, and Bresden DE: Cerebral infarctions and transient neurologic deficits associated with acquired immunodeficiency syndrome, *Am J Med* 86:528, 1989.

30. Fauci AS, moderator: The acquired immunodeficiency syndrome: an update, *Ann Intern Med* 102:800, 1985.

31. Favero MS et al: Guidelines for the care of patients hospitalized with viral hepatitis, *Ann Intern Med* 91:872, 1979.

32. Fink L, Reicheck N, and Sutton MG: Cardiac abnormalities in acquired immunodeficiency syndrome, *Am J Cardiol* 54:1161, 1984.

33. Fischl MA et al: Use of danazol in autoimmune thrombocytopenic purpura associated with the acquired immunodeficiency syndrome, *Blood* 64(suppl 1): 2362, abstract, 1984.

34. Fishbein DB et al: Unexplained lymphadenopathy in homosexual men. A longitudinal study, *JAMA* 245:930, 1985.

35. Garay SM et al: Pulmonary manifestations of Kaposi's sarcoma, *Chest* 91:39, 1987.

36. Gieraerts R: Increased incidence of itching and herpes simplex in patients given epidural morphine after cesarean section, *Anesth Analg* 66:1321, 1987.

37. Gill JM et al: Therapy for recurrent herpetic whitlow, *Ann Intern Med* 105:631, 1986.

38. Glassock RJ, moderator: Human immunodeficiency virus (HIV) infection and the kidney, *Ann Intern Med* 112:35, 1990.

39. Hagen MB, Meyer KB, and Parker SG: Routine preoperative screening for HIV: does the risk to the surgeon outweigh the risk to the patient, *JAMA* 260:542, 1988.

40. Haseltine WA, Wong-Staal F: The molecular biology of the AIDS virus, *Sci Am* 259:52, 1988.

41. Heyer DM, Kahn JO, and Volberding PA: HIV-related Kaposi's sarcoma. In Cohen PT, Sande MA, and Volberding PA, eds: *The AIDS knowledge book*, Waltham, Mass, 1990, The Medical Publishing Group.

42. Heyward WL, Curran JW: The epidemiology of AIDS in the U.S., *Sci Am* 259:72, 1988.

43. Himelman RB et al: Cardiac manifestations of human immunodeficiency virus infection: a two-dimensional echocardiographic study, *JACC* 13:1030, 1989.

44. Hoofnagle JH: Type B hepatitis: virology, serology and clinical course, *Semin Liver Dis* 1:7, 1981.

45. Hoofnagle JH: Type D (delta) hepatitis, *JAMA* 261:1321, 1989.

46. Horsburgh RC, Selik RM: The epidemiology of disseminated nontuberculous mycobacterial infections in AIDS, *Am Rev Respir Dis* 139:4, 1989.

47. Immunization Practices Advisory Committee: Recommendations for protection against viral hepatitis, *MMWR* 34:313, 1985.

48. Kaplan LD et al: Kaposi's sarcoma involving the lung in patients with acquired immunodeficiency syndrome, *J AIDS* 1:23, 1988.

49. Klotz RW: Herpetic whitlow: an occupational hazard, *JAAN* 58:8, 1990.

50. Kuhls TL et al: Occupational risk of HIV, HBV and HSV-2 infections in health care personnel caring for AIDS patients, *Am J Public Health* 77:1306, 1987.

51. Kunkel SE, Warner MA: Human T-cell lymphotropic virus type III (HTLV III) infection: how it can affect you, your patients and your anesthesia practice, *Anesthesiology* 66:195, 1987.

52. Kuo G et al: An assay for circulating antibodies to a major etiologic virus of human non A, non B hepatitis, *Science* 244:362, 1989.

53. Lane HC et al: Correlation between immunologic function and clinical subpopulations of patients with the acquired immunodeficiency syndrome, *Am J Med* 78:417, 1985.

54. Lettau LA et al: Nosocomial transmission of delta hepatitis, *Ann Intern Med* 104:631, 1986.

55. Levy J et al: Isolation of lymphocytopathic retroviruses from San Francisco patients with AIDS, *Science* 225:840, 1984.

56. Levy RM, Bredesen DE, and Rosenblum DE: Neurological manifestations of the acquired immunodeficiency syndrome (AIDS): experience at UCSF and review of the literature, *J Neurosurg* 62:475, 1985.

57. Levy RM et al: The superiority of cranial magnetic imaging (MRI) to computed tomography (CT) brain scans for the diagnosis of cerebral lesions in patients with AIDS (abstract). In *National Conference on AIDS,*, Proceedings, p. 37, Paris, 1986.

58. Levy JA et al: Infection by the retrovirus associated with the acquired immunodeficiency syndrome, *Ann Intern Med* 103:694, 1985.

59. Levy WS et al: Prevalence of cardiac abnormalities in human immunodeficiency virus infection, *Am J Cardiol* 63:86, 1989.

60. Marcus R: Surveillance of health-care workers exposed to blood from patients infected with the human immunodeficiency virus, *N Engl J Med* 319:1118, 1988.

61. Masur H, Fauci AS: Acquired immunodeficiency syndrome (AIDS). In Sleisenger MH, Fordtran JS, eds: *Gastrointestinal disease, pathophysiology diagnosis, management*, ed 4, Philadelphia, 1988, WB Saunders.

62. Mayo-Smith MF: Type non A, non B and type B hepatitis transmitted by a single needle stick, *Am J Infect Control* 15:266, 1987.

63. McCray E: Cooperative needlestick group. Occupational risk of the acquired immunodeficiency syndrome among health-care workers, *N Engl J Med* 314:1127, 1986.

64. Membreno L et al: Adrenocortical function in acquired immunodeficiency syndrome, *J Clin Endocrinol Metab* 65:482, 1987.

65. Meyer KB, Parker SG: Screening for HIV: can we afford the false positive rate? *N Engl J Med* 317:238, 1987.

66. Morris L et al: Autoimmune thrombocytopenic purpura in homosexual men, *Ann Intern Med* 96:714, 1982.

67. Murray JF et al: Pulmonary complications of the acquired immunodeficiency syndrome: report of a National Heart, Lung and Blood Institute Workshop, *N Engl J Med* 310:1682, 1984.

68. Murray JF et al: Pulmonary complications of the acquired immunodeficiency syndrome: an update, *Am Rev Respir Dis* 135:504, 1987.

69. Orkin FK: Other viral infections, *Anesth Clin North Am* 7:813, 1989.

70. Pardo V et al: AIDS-related glomerulopathy: occurrence in specific risk groups, *Kidney Int* 31:1167, 1987.

71. Parry GJ: Peripheral neuropathies associated with human immunodeficiency virus infection, *Ann Neurol* 23(suppl):S49, 1988.

72. Propovic M et al: Detection, isolation and continuous production of cytopathic retrovirus (HTLV-III) from patients with AIDS and pre-AIDS, *Science* 224:497, 1984.

73. Rabson AB, Martin MA: Molecular organization of the AIDS retrovirus, *Cell* 40:447, 1985.

74. Rao TK, Friedman EA, and Nicastri AD: The types of renal disease in the acquired immunodeficiency syndrome, *N Engl J Med* 316:1062, 1987.

75. Redfield RR, Wright DC, and Tramont EC: The Walter Reed Staging Classifica-

tion for HTLV-III/LAV, *N Engl J Med* 314:131, 1986.

76. Rosenblum ML, Levy RM, and Bredesen DE: *AIDS and the nervous system,* New York, 1988, Raven Press.

77. Rosenblum et al: Disassociation of AIDS-related vacuolar myelopathy and productive HIV-I infection of the spinal cord, *Neurology* 39:892, 1989.

78. Small PM, Hopewell PC: Respiratory system: techniques for definitive diagnosis. In Cohen PT, Sande MA, Volberding PA, eds: *The AIDS knowledge base,* Waltham, Mass, 1990, The Medical Publishing Group.

79. Smith RD: The pathobiology of HIV infection, *Arch Pathol Lab Med* 114:235, 1990.

80. Sninsky J, Kwok S: Detection of human immunodeficiency viruses by the polymerase chain reaction, *Arch Pathol Lab Med* 114:259, 1990.

81. Steckelberg JM, Cockerill FR: Serologic testing for human immunodeficiency virus antibodies, *Mayo Clin Proc* 63:373, 1988.

82. Streicher H, Schlar L: Human retroviruses and their associated diseases: biology, pathophysiology and clinical consequences of human retroviral infection, *Clin Chest Med* 9:363, 1988.

83. Tindall R et al: Characterization of the acute clinical illness associated with human immunodeficiency virus infection, *Arch Intern Med* 148:945, 1988.

84. Tiollais P, Pourcel C, and Dejean A: The hepatitis B virus, *Nature* 317:489, 1985.

85. Warner MA, Kunkel SE: Human immunodeficiency virus infection, *Anesth Clin North Am* 7:795, 1989.

86. Werner BJ, Grady GF: Accidental hepatitis B surface antigen positive immulations: use of antigen to estimate infectivity, *Ann Intern Med* 97:367, 1982.

87. West D: The risk of hepatitis B in health-care professionals in the United States, *Am J Med Sci* 287:26, 1984.

88. Whitsett CF: Infections acquired through blood transfusions, *Anesth Clin North Am* 7:902, 1989.

89. Wick MR, Moore S, and Taswell HF: Non-A, non-B hepatitis associated with blood transfusion, *Transfusion* 25:93, 1985.

90. Ziegler JL et al: Non-Hodgkin's lymphoma in 90 homosexual men, *N Engl J Med* 311:565, 1984.

91. Zuck TF, Sherwood WC, and Bove JR: A review of recent events related to surrogate testing of blood to prevent non-A, non-B post transfusion hepatitis, *Transfusion* 27:203, 1987.

CHAPTER 25

Evaluation of the Neonate

MYRON YASTER

Physical Examination and Review of Systems
  Head and neck
  Respiratory system
  Circulatory system
  Central nervous system
  Renal function
  Thermoregulation
Evaluation of Metabolism
  Glucose
  Calcium

The newborn presenting for emergency surgery is among the most daunting and challenging patients facing the anesthesiologist. **Critically ill and hemodynamically unstable, these tiny, fragile patients demand a level of specialized knowledge, skill, and attention to detail that is inversely proportional to their size and gestational age.** Providing safe anesthesia is possible only when the specialized equipment and techniques necessary to conduct an anesthetic are in the hands of individuals who understand the anatomic, physiologic, and pathologic differences that characterize these patients during their transition from intrauterine to extrauterine life.

Although the types of surgical procedures in the newborn span a wide variety of life-threatening congenital anomalies, each with its own problems of management, there are, nevertheless, many aspects of preoperative and intraoperative anesthetic management common to all infants of this age. In this chapter, emphasis will be placed on those aspects of preoperative assessment, monitoring, and supportive care that are pertinent to newborn patients in general, with special attention to disease states, anesthetic agents, and surgical interventions that can influence the infant's transition from fetal to newborn existence.

Except for extraordinary circumstances, all newborns require anesthesia for surgery.[5,78] In the past, it had been assumed that newborns neither experienced nor perceived painful stimuli to the same degree that adults do.[2,66] It was believed that the newborn did not have the neurologic substrate necessary for the perception of pain because of lack of myelinization, incomplete pain pathways from the periphery to the cortex, or immaturity of the cerebral cortex. There is absolutely no evidence that any of this is true. **Newborns respond to noxious stimuli with behavioral, physiologic, metabolic, and hormonal responses suggestive of substantial stress.**[1,3,37,77] It is also clear that the neurophysiologic pathways for nociception from the peripheral receptors to the cerebral cortex are developed even in premature infants. Furthermore, the primary pathways of pain transmission involve unmyelinated C and A delta fibers, so postnatal myelination is not required for most pain perception. Finally, failure to provide anesthesia is associated with an increased incidence of circulatory, respiratory, and metabolic complications in newborns.[3] Thus **the preponderance of evidence suggests that newborns not only respond to noxious stimuli but that the failure to provide analgesia and anesthesia significantly increases perioperative morbidity and mortality.**

The parents of critically ill children require substantial support and reassurance that their newborn child will perceive no pain during surgery and will be as safe as is humanly possible. **Parents experience an acute emotional crisis when their newborns face surgery.** Aside from the deprivation of contact with their infant, parents experience anticipatory grief and a profound sense of failure.[30] When their infant faces surgery, parents anticipate the infant's death or mutilation. Many parents undergo a period of mourning for the loss of the perfect infant they were anticipating. The shock of the situation may deafen parents to the clinician's explanations, and one must be prepared to repeat descriptions of the baby's problems two or three times during the preoperative interview. Reassurance is the key. Although a successful outcome cannot be guaranteed, one can promise to do one's best. The child's parents can be reassured that the overwhelming majority of children not only survive surgery but grow up healthy and productive. It is important to emphasize the baby's normal, healthy aspects and use calm and positive statements about the correction to be achieved by surgery. Failure to do this may significantly affect how the parents interact and bond with their child.

The newborn undergoing emergency surgery to correct a congenital anomaly must be optimally prepared for surgery within the constraints of performing an emergency procedure. To do this the clinician must complete a history and physical examination that concentrates on the birth history; the presence of other anomalies; cardiorespiratory function, acid-base balance, glucose, fluid and temperature homeostasis; and coagulation status, because these are of paramount importance.

The presence of one congenital anomaly should always alert the anesthesiologist to the likelihood of others; currently, approximately 2% of live born infants have a congenital anomaly recognized at birth.[27,61,65] Congenital anomalies fall into several broad categories. A **congenital malformation** is a primary structural defect that results from a localized error of morphogenesis (e.g., a cleft lip or a ventricular septal defect). A **malformation syndrome** is a recognized pattern of malformations believed to have the same etiology but not resulting from a single error of morphogenesis (e.g., Down's syndrome or trisomy 21).[27,61,65] When a recognized pattern of malformation is caused by a single localized error of morphogenesis, it is called an **anomalad,** for example, Pierre-Robin syndrome. Finally, patterns of recognized malformations occur in a nonrandomized fashion and are called **associations,** for example, the VATER (Vertebral defects, imperforate Anus, Tracheo Esophageal fistula, and Renal defects) association.

Box 25-1 lists the more common congenital anomalies, syndromes, and associations that present for surgical correction during the first few weeks of life. Comprehensive reviews are available for the more unusual anomalies seen in children (Table 25-1).[27,61,65] The presence of an anomaly or an associated defect can often be inferred from the use of this table and from a history obtained from the child's parents and the referring physician.

Several congenital anomalies either result from

BOX 25-1
COMMONLY ENCOUNTERED LESIONS IN THE NEONATE

I. Airway lesions
   A. Choanal atresia
   B. Pierre-Robin syndrome
   C. Upper airway obstruction
      1. Cystic hygroma
      2. Cleft lip and/or palate
      3. Upper airway cysts and webs
II. Thoracic lesions
   A. Tracheoesophageal fistula (TEF) or atresia
   B. Congenital diaphragmatic hernia
   C. Congenital heart disease
   D. Pneumothorax, pneumomediastinum, pneumopericardium
   E. Lobar emphysema, cystic adenomatoid malformation
   F. Mediastinal masses
III. Abdominal lesions
   A. Omphalocele
   B. Gastroschisis
   C. Intestinal obstruction
   D. Malrotation and volvulus
   E. Imperforate anus
   F. Exstrophy of the bladder or cloaca
   G. Hirschsprung's disease
   H. Biliary atresia
   I. Incarcerated hernia
   J. Necrotizing enterocolitis (NEC)
IV. Neurosurgical lesions
   A. Myelomeningocele
   B. Encephalocele
   C. Craniosynostosis
   D. Intracranial masses
   E. Arteriovenous malformations (vein of Galen)
   F. Skull fractures
   G. Hydrocephalus
   H. Subdural hemorrhage
   I. Spinal tumors

---

abnormal pregnancy or manifest themselves during pregnancy[27,61,65] (Box 25-2). For example, polyhydramnios is associated with high intestinal obstruction and oligohydramnios with renal and lung hypoplasia. Similarly, maternal exposure to alcohol and other teratogens is associated with many congenital malformations. Maternal drug abuse and addiction is of special importance. Infants born to these mothers may have withdrawal symptoms, seizures, and acquired immunodeficiency syndrome (AIDS).

Of equal importance is the delivery history (Box 25-3). Attention must be paid to the duration of pregnancy and labor. Was the delivery traumatic?

BOX 25-2
MATERNAL PREGNANCY HISTORY

I. Polyhdramnios: high intestinal obstruction (e.g., duodenal atresia, congenital diaphragmatic hernia, omphalocele); central nervous system anomalies (e.g., hydrocephalus, spina bifida); respiratory abnormalities (e.g., pulmonary hypoplasia, pleural effusions); genitourinary tract abnormalities (e.g,. posterior urethral valves, urethral stricture; maternal diabetes, Rh-isoimmunization, multiple pregnancy)

II. Oligohydramnios: renal failure; hypoplastic lungs; marked crowding of fetal limbs causing multiple skeletal contractures; neonatal infection (chorioamionitis)

III. Toxemia of pregnancy: frequently associated with decreased placental perfusion and premature separation of the placenta; associated problems include small-for-gestational-age infants, hypoglycemia, and anemia; magnesium used in BP therapy produces neonatal hypotonia and apnea

IV. Diabetes: large-for-gestational-age infants; hypoglycemia despite enormous glucose loading; prematurity (yet > 2500 g birth weight); congenital heart disease; anencephaly; sacral agenesis

V. Seizures: two to three times greater incidence of congenital malformations

VI. Intrauterine infection: prematurity; fetal infection, particularly pneumonia; persistent fetal circulation; heart defects (rubella)

VII. Medication: teratogens (e.g., anticonvulsants, warfarin, antimetabolites); hypoglycemia, floppy infant

VIII. Drug abuse:
   A. Fetal alcohol syndrome: growth retardation, mental deficiency, heart defects, flexion contractures
   B. Opioid withdrawal: seizures; jittery, irritable infants; hypoglycemia; diarrhea
   C. Amphetamines: congenital heart disease

IX. Maternal age: trisomy 13, 18, 21

X. Single umbilical artery: renal malformations

BOX 25-3
DELIVERY HISTORY

I. Prolonged labor
   A. Abnormal fetus (e.g., hydrocephalus, abdominal wall defect, breech presentation)

II. Premature rupture of membranes
   A. Prematurity
   B. Infection, pneumonia
   C. Oligohydramnios or polyhydramnios

III. Traumatic delivery
   A. Intracranial hemorrhage, skull fracture, vocal cord paralysis, brachial plexus injury

IV. General anesthesia
   A. Hypotonia, respiratory distress

V. Prematurity (< 36 weeks postconceptual age or birth weight < 2500 g)
   A. Hyaline lung disease
   B. Hypocalcemia, hypoglycemia, hypomagnesemia
   C. Infection
   D. Necrotizing enterocolitis
   E. Patent ductus arteriosus
   F. Hyperbilirubinemia
   G. Increased risk of oxygen toxicity to the eyes (retinopathy of prematurity or "retrolental fibroplasia")

VI. Postmaturity (> 41 weeks postconceptual age)

Was the presentation abnormal, for example, breech? Was anesthesia used during childbirth? Will residual drugs affect the newborn's anesthetic management? Were the placenta and umbilical cord normal? Finally, what were the child's birth weight and Apgar score?

Infants who were asphyxiated at birth must be identified before surgery. These newborns have de-pressed myocardial function and decreased perfusion to the brain and gastrointestinal system. This is of particular concern in the newborn because these organs are particularly vulnerable to ischemic damage. Additionally, various metabolic derangements, such as hypoglycemia, hypocalcemia, and hyperkalemia, occur in asphyxiated newborns. Other problems seen in these infants are clotting abnormalities, meconium aspiration, and, most ominous of all, intracranial hemorrhage (impaired autoregulation of the cerebral circulation).

PHYSICAL EXAMINATION AND REVIEW OF SYSTEMS
Head and Neck

The newborn is an obligate nose-breather. If both nostrils are obstructed, respiratory distress will occur. Choanal atresia, an anomaly in which there is absence of the nasopharynx bilaterally, is diagnosed by respiratory distress in the delivery room, (which is easily treated by oral intubation), and by an inability to pass a catheter through the nostrils. Occasionally, respiratory distress is caused by obstruction of the nasopharynx by a nasograstric tube and overzealous

Table 25-1   Anesthetic implications of syndromes and unusual disorders

Name	Description	Anesthetic implications
Arthrogryoposis multiplex	Multiple congenital contractures; congenital heart disease	Possible airway problems due to limitations of mandibular movement
Asplenia syndrome	Absent spleen; complex congenital heart disease; malrotation of abdominal organs	Cyanotic heart disease very common; echocardiography essential preoperatively
Beckwith's syndrome	Birth weight >4000 g; macroglossia, visceromegaly	Airway problems due to large tongue; hypoglycemia common
Cherubism	Fibrous dysplasia of the mandible and maxilla	Intubation may be extremely difficult; tracheostomy may be the only way to secure the airway
Congenital hypothyroidism	Goiter; large tongue; respiratory depression; hypoglycemia; hypotension	Airway obstruction secondary to large tongue, particularly in supine position; slow to awaken at the completion of surgery
Crouzon's disease	Craniosynostosis; hypertelorism, hypoplastic mandible	Intubation may be difficult
Dandy-Walker syndrome	Hydrocephalus	Increased intracranial pressure rare in the newborn period; head may be enormously enlarged
DiGeorge's syndrome	Absent thymus and parathyroids; hypocalcemia, immune deficiency; aortic arch abnormalities	All blood products should be irradiated to prevent graft vs. host disease; stridor may be due to hypocalcemia
Down's syndrome (trisomy 21)	Large tongue, unstable cervical spine, small mouth; high incidence of congenital heart disease, particularly AV canal; intestinal obstruction	Intubation may be difficult; ? in line traction during intubation, ? cervical spine radiographs before intubation in older children; echocardiography required before surgery in the newborn
Ehlers-Danlos syndrome	Collagen abnormality-hyperelasticity and fragile tissue; dissecting aneurysm of aorta; bleeding diasthesis; heart, lung, GI problems	Poor tissue and clotting defects may lead to hemorrhage; spontaneous pneumothorax
Ellis–van Creveld syndrome	Ectodermal and skeletal defects; congenital heart disease; cleft lip and palate, mandibular hypoplasia; hepatosplenomegaly	Airway problems; intubation may be difficult; chest wall anomalies cause poor lung function
Epidermolysis bullosa	Skin cleavage at dermal-epidermal junction, minor trauma denudes skin	Do not use adhesive tape of any sort; avoid instrumentation of the airway if possible; use a well-padded mask or apply ointment to rim; secure IV, monitoring devices with Kerlex; sterile technique
Familial dysautonomia (Riley-Day syndrome)	Poor suck and swallow; hypertension and hypotension; insensitivity to pain; absent sweating and lacrimation	Recurrent aspiration and pneumonia; respiratory center insensitive to CO_2; labile intraoperative blood pressure
Fetal alcohol syndrome	Growth retardation; microcephaly, cranio-facial abnormalities; congenital heart disease; renal abnormalities	Intubation is usually not difficult, ventricular septal defects are common and require subacute bacterial endocarditis (SBE) prophylaxis
Glucose-6-phosphate deficiency	Hemolytic anemia caused by drugs and infection	Aspirin, sulfa, methylene blue cause anemia

From Steward DJ: *Manual of pediatric anesthesia*, New York, 1985, Churchill-Livingstone.

Table 25-1   Anesthetic implications of syndromes and unusual disorders—cont'd

Name	Description	Anesthetic implications
Goldenhar's syndrome	Hemifacial microsomia, congenital heart disease	Very difficult intubation, vertebral instability
Hemangioma with thrombocytopenia	May involve the airway; bleeding, anemia	Airway involvement may require radiation therapy; transfuse components as necessary
Jeune's syndrome (asphyxiating thoracic dystrophy)	Severe thoracic malformations, renal failure	Respiratory failure, prolonged mechanical ventilation; care with drugs excreted by kidneys
Klippel-Feil syndrome	Hemivertebra or fused vertebra	Intubation may be difficult
Maple syrup urine disease	Inability to metabolize leucine, isoleucine, and valine	Acid base imbalance; preoperative fasting; glucose early and check frequently
Mucopolysaccharidoses (Hurler's, Hunter's, Morquio's syndrome)	Bony abnormalities, dwarfism, kyphoscoliosis, abnormal facies, congenital heart disease	Very difficult intubations, unstable necks, respiratory failure perioperatively
Myasthenia congenita	Similar to adult form	Avoid muscle relaxants and narcotics
Osteogenesis imperfecta	Pathologic fractures; abnormal platelets, vascular fragility	Extreme caution when positioning and during intubation; blood pressure cuff may cause fractures
Pierre-Robin syndrome	Cleft palate, micrognathia, glossoptosis, congenital heart disease	Very difficult intubation, may require tongue suture or awake tracheostomy; best nursed in prone position
Prader-Willi syndrome	Hypotonia, obesity	Hypoglycemia common; assisted ventilation may be required postoperatively
Prune-belly syndrome	Agenesis of the abdominal musculature, renal failure	Respiratory failure common, postoperative ventilation, avoid respiratory depressants; avoid drugs excreted by the kidneys
Treacher Collins' syndrome	Micrognathia, mid-face hypoplasia, congenital heart disease	Very difficult intubation, may require tongue suture or awake tracheostomy; best nursed in prone position
Thrombocytopenia with absent radius syndrome	Episodic thrombocytopenia precipitated by stress, infection, surgery; congenital heart disease	Platelet transfusion before surgery; SBE prophylaxis
Trisomy 18	Congenital heart disease; micrognathia; renal malformation; most die in infancy	Ethical considerations concerning surgery in a patient with a fatal anomaly; assess cardiac status carefully
Trisomy 21 (see Down's syndrome)		
VATER syndrome	Vertebral defects, imperforate anus, tracheoesophageal fistula, renal and cardiac defects	Examine carefully for associated anomalies

taping that occludes the opposite nostril. The airway must be evaluated for any abnormality that may result in a difficult intubation, such as a small or receding jaw (micrognathia, Pierre-Robin syndrome, Treacher Collins' syndrome) or a large tongue (Beckwith's syndrome, glycogen storage diseases, hypothyroidism, and Down's syndrome).[17] Additionally, lesions that

cause upper airway obstruction, such as hemangiomas, cystic hygromas, and laryngeal webs and cysts, may make intubation difficult or impossible.[38,47] The presence of cutaneous hemangiomas must alert the anesthesiologist to the possibility of an airway lesion (see Table 25-1). Furthermore, some hemangiomas trap and consume platelets, potentially producing a bleeding diathesis. On the other hand, cleft lips and palates usually do not present intubation problems; they may provide more room for the laryngoscope blade and facilitate endotracheal intubation.

Infants with a history of endotracheal intubation who are stridorous or who have a weak cry may have developed subglottic stenosis or subglottic granulomas. **The narrowest part of the adult's airway is at the level of the vocal cords, whereas that of the infant is at the level of the cricoid ring.**[38] The subglottis is very easily injured and explains in part the use of non-cuffed endotracheal tubes for patients in this age group. The trachea of most infants can be intubated with a 3-mm endotracheal tube. Premature infants occasionally require smaller, 2.5-mm tubes. With infants in whom subglottic narrowing is anticipated or who require intubation with tubes smaller than 2.5 mm, tracheostomy and/or bronchoscopy should be considered and discussed with the parents before surgery.

Respiratory System

During fetal life, respiratory gas exchange occurs at the placenta. **The first breath after birth expands the lungs, establishes the residual volume and the functional residual capacity, increases alveolar oxygen content, and causes pulmonary arterial vasodilation.**[4,42,44] Gas exchange in the lungs is maintained by successful removal of the lung fluid from the airways and alveoli. This is achieved by drainage and increased pulmonary lymphatic flow for several hours after birth and by the presence of surface active phospholipids (surfactant). The **increase in arterial oxygen content** that occurs with the successful transition to extrauterine life **decreases pulmonary vascular resistance and leads to the functional closure of the ductus arteriosus and atrial septum.**[42,44]

Respiratory control is very poorly developed in the neonate, particularly the premature.[19,50,51] This can predispose the infant to life-threatening respiratory complications both before and after the administration of anesthesia.[34,36,48] **The respiratory depressant effects of opioids and inhalational agents are profound and long-lasting.**[13,31,32] Morphine penetrates the newborn's brain more easily than that of the adult and achieves levels that are two to four times higher.[33,75] Furthermore, the μ receptor is exquisitely sensitive to respiratory depression in the newborn when compared with that of the adult.[45,80] Thus a history of prematurity and/or apnea must alert the anesthesiologist to possible respiratory compromise in the postoperative period, particularly if a narcotic-based anesthetic is used. Indeed, premature infants are at risk of developing postanesthetic apnea for months after birth (52 to 60 weeks postconceptual age) even when a potent vapor (halothane) is used.[34]

Oxygen consumption in the newborn is two to three times that of older children and adults. Unfortunately, the newborn responds to hypercarbia and hypoxia paradoxically when compared with the adult or older child.* Unlike the adult, **the newborn's response to hypoxia is apnea rather than hyperventilation.** Apnea may also occur in response to hypothermia or when energy reserves are limited (as in the premature).[60,64] Thus a devastating cascade of events may be set in motion. Increased oxygen consumption, depressed respiratory function, and limited reserves lead to hypoxemia. Hypoxemia results in apnea and cardiovascular collapse. Other disadvantages of the newborn include a very compliant rib cage (which tends to collapse the chest wall), inefficient diaphragmatic contraction, and a low percentage of fatigue-resistant type I muscle fibers in the diaphragm.[20,28,29,59,67] The combination of high work of breathing, increased oxygen consumption, and less resistance to muscle fatigue can produce abnormal breathing patterns, such as periodic breathing, apneic episodes, and respiratory failure.

Neonates suffering from respiratory distress syndrome (hyaline membrane disease) have low lung compliance, a diminished functional residual capacity, and diffuse microatelectasis. These infants are often hypoxemic and hypercarbic and exhibit tachypnea, expiratory grunting, and inspiratory retractions. They are often intubated and either positively pressure ventilated or spontaneously ventilated on continuous positive airway pressure (CPAP). Maintaining normal gas exchange in these infants requires careful monitoring and respiratory support. Increased peak inspiratory pressures and positive end-expiratory pressures may be needed to maintain adequate oxygenation. Unfortunately this may lead to pneumothorax, pneumomediastinum, and interstitial emphysema. Indeed, the perioperative development of pulmonary barotrauma should alert the anesthesiologist to the possibility of intraoperative pneumothorax, which will manifest itself by catastrophic and sudden cardiovascular collapse.

Circulatory System

The fetal circulation is characterized by the preferential shunting of "arterialized" placental ("right-sided") blood across the foramen ovale and ductus arteriosus into the systemic ("left-sided") circulation.[11,58] This right-to-left shunting of blood is caused by the increased pulmonary vascular resistance and decreased systemic vascular resistance that characterize the fetal circulation. The combination of breathing room air and clamping the umbilical cord reverses these resistances and results in the functional

---

* References 7, 8, 10, 19, 36, 42, 44, 49-51.

closure of the foramen ovale and the ductus arteriosus. Unfortunately, **arterial hypoxemia, hypercarbia, or acidosis will reverse this transitional circulation and restore the fetal circulatory pattern; this is referred to as "persistent fetal circulation" or "persistent pulmonary hypertension of the newborn."**[11,58,62] It has catastrophic consequences. The increased pulmonary artery hypertension caused by arterial hypoxemia reduces pulmonary blood flow and reopens the foramen ovale and ductus arteriosus. This further exacerbates the hypoxemia and acidosis. Persistent fetal circulation can occur with sepsis, hypotension, meconium aspiration, diaphragmatic hernia, and inefficient ventilation.

On the other hand, closure of the foramen ovale and ductus arteriosus may be detrimental in patients with certain types of congenital heart disease.[24-26,58] Patients with transposition of the great vessels, complete or partial tricuspid or pulmonary valvular obstruction or atresia, and hypoplastic left heart syndrome depend for their very survival on continued flow across these shunts.[24-26,58] Indeed, intravenous infusion of prostaglandin E1, to maintain the patency of the ductus arteriosus, may be life sustaining in these patients.

The newborn's myocardium is less compliant than that of the adult or older child, and **cardiac output depends primarily on heart rate.**[46,57,58,68] The heart has incomplete or decreased sympathetic innervation with reduced catecholamine stores. Furthermore, studies performed in newborns during exchange transfusions have revealed that the newborn has reduced capacity for peripheral vasoconstriction during hypovolemia.[72,73]

Several powerful reflexes control the cardiovascular system of the neonate. The arterial baroreceptor is the most powerful and consists of the carotid sinus and aortic arch baroreceptors.[58] These receptors are stretch receptors stimulated by pressure deformation of the vessel wall tissue in which they reside. An increase in transmural pressure stretches the receptors and increases the rate of baroreceptor firing. Afferent nerves carry these signals to the vasomotor centers of the medulla, and parasympathetic and sympathetic efferent fibers slow the heart rate, strengthen contraction, and reduce venous and arterial resistance. A reduction in arterial blood pressure has the opposite effect, causing a central afferent sympathoadrenal discharge that increases systolic and diastolic blood pressure. The arterial baroreceptor reflex is intact in healthy, full-term newborns but may be significantly depressed in stressed or premature infants. Anesthetic agents, particularly halothane, may also significantly depress this response.[21,76]

The arterial chemoreceptors form the second powerful cardiovascular reflex arc. The carotid and aortic chemoreceptor bodies are responsible for the cardiovascular response to acute hypoxia.[14,35] The primary central response to hypoxia is bradycardia. Once stimulated, the peripheral chemoreceptors cause tachypnea and increased sympathetic discharge to the heart and peripheral tissues. These receptors are stimulated by hypoxic hypoxia (low PaO_2) and decreased cardiac output but not by reduced oxygen content caused by anemia. Once again, the stressed or premature infant or the full-term infant anesthetized with halothane may have a blunted or absent sympathetically mediated response to hypoxia. *The most common cause of bradycardia in the newborn is hypoxia; in the operating room, unexplained bradycardia should always be considered to be caused by hypoxia until proved otherwise.*

Thus it may be dangerous to anesthetize a stressed neonate who is either hypovolemic or dehydrated, particularly with a potent inhalational anesthetic vapor such as halothane. Hypovolemia or dehydration should be assumed in septic patients (necrotizing enterocolitis), ventilated patients who are being treated with diuretics and fluid restriction (hyaline membrane disease, patent ductus arteriosus), and, in the operating room, when hemorrhage occurs.

Central Nervous System

The central nervous system is the least mature major organ system at birth. This structural immaturity predisposes the newborn to certain risks, including **intraventricular hemorrhages, seizures, respiratory depression, and retinopathy.*** Hypoxia, hypercarbia, hypotension, acidosis, and pain may produce any and all of these complications. The stressed premature infant is particularly at risk. Indeed, intraventricular hemorrhage, in which subependymal hemorrhage occurs, is now the leading cause of death and morbidity in these infants and has an incidence as high as 50%.[40,69,71]

Hydrocephalus also occurs frequently in either its noncommunicating form, in which the flow of cerebral spinal fluid is obstructed (aqueductal stenosis, spina bifida), or its communicating form, in which the flow of cerebrospinal fluid is unimpeded but resorption is affected (intraventricular hemorrhage). Increased intracranial pressure secondary to hydrocephalus may or may not be present because the newborn's cranial sutures are open at birth and allow for intracranial decompression. On the other hand, the resulting large head may present very difficult airway management problems. Furthermore, the stretching of cranial nerves that may occur with hydrocephalus or with other intracranial pathology, such as the Arnold-

---

* References 6, 18, 40, 41, 70, 71.

Chiari malformation, may cause vocal cord paralysis and/or stridor.[22,52,79]

Renal Function

The **glomerular filtration rate in newborns is less than a quarter of the adult's.** Furthermore, the newborn's **ability to concentrate urine is significantly reduced.** In fact, the maximum concentrating ability of the newborn's kidney does not exceed 700 mOsm/liter. Thus the newborn requires fluids containing sodium intraoperatively. Not only will these infants lose salt intraoperatively through third space and hemorrhagic losses, but they continue to lose sodium through obligate urinary losses because of a tubular inability to increase sodium reabsorption.

Thermoregulation

The newborn infant, even the premature infant, is quite capable of maintaining a stable core temperature in the face of changing ambient temperatures. This is accomplished by balancing heat production with skin blood flow, sweat production, and changing minute ventilation.[7,15] When exposed to cold, neonatal compensatory mechanisms operate only within a narrow temperature range. For adults, the lower range of thermoregulation is 0° C, whereas for full-term newborns it is 22° C. Premature infants require an even higher ambient temperature to ensure thermal homeostasis. At ambient temperatures of less than 32° to 34° C, the premature infant must significantly increase oxygen consumption to stay warm. The ambient temperature at which a state of thermal equilibrium exists, that is, in which heat loss and heat production are equal and occur without an increase in oxygen consumption, is called the **neutral thermic state.**[7,15,16,64]

After delivery, the newborn infant rapidly loses heat because of a large surface area relative to body mass and a lack of heat-insulating subcutaneous tissue (fat). The infant loses heat by evaporation, convection, conduction, and radiation. **Evaporative heat loss is the major source of heat loss in the perioperative period.**[7,15,54,55] Physical factors that govern evaporative losses include relative humidity, velocity of air flow, and minute ventilation. The driving force for evaporative heat loss is the difference between vapor pressure on the surface of the skin and vapor pressure in the environment. Physiologic factors that affect evaporative loss relate to the infant's ability to sweat and to increase minute ventilation. Premature infants less than 30 postconceptual weeks of age have underdeveloped sweat glands and do not perspire. Preventing or minimizing evaporative heat loss is the primary means of heat control in the perioperative period. Wrapping newborns inside plastic bags and using heated humidifiers are the most effective ways

of minimizing evaporative heat losses and should be used not only in the operating room during surgery but in transport as well.[53,55,56]

Heat production is achieved by voluntary muscle activity, shivering, and nonshivering thermogenesis. Shivering is rarely observed in the newborn and with the small muscle mass present would not be very effective. Nonshivering thermogenesis is a heat-producing and oxygen-consuming mechanism stimulated by cold, in which there is a generalized increase in metabolism and a marked increase in the metabolic activity in certain specialized tissues, most notably in the brown adipose tissue ("fat").[7,15,64] This tissue is located principally in the interscapular region, mediastinum, and tissues surrounding the kidneys and adrenal glands. Unlike white fat, it has a rich blood supply and very high oxygen consumption when metabolically active. Morphologically, brown fat contains multiloculated cells with numerous mitochondria. The mitochondria appear densely packed with cristae and have increased respiratory chain components. The brown adipose tissue is also abundantly enervated by the sympathetic nervous system. In fact, the metabolism of brown fat is stimulated by the local release of catecholamines, particularly norepinephrine.[7,15,64]

Thus **the control of heat-producing mechanisms depends on skin (not central) thermoreceptors.**[9,60,64] When skin temperature falls, central control mechanisms trigger increased metabolic activity in brown adipose tissue. This is mediated by the sympathetic nervous system. Unfortunately, anesthetic agents, particularly halothane, may paralyze these systems and convert the infant's system into a poikilothermic one. Alternatively, hypoxia may interfere with thermoregulation. Hypoxia impairs heat production and heat conservation by producing peripheral vasodilation.

The infant can be protected from unnecessary heat loss quite easily. Aside from wrapping the infant in plastic bags and humidifying the anesthetic vapors, heat can be conserved by warming the operating room to 25° C (85° F); using a warming water mattress; warming intravenous fluids, blood, and irrigation solutions; and using a radiant heater with a servocontrol mechanism.

EVALUATION OF METABOLISM
Glucose

Another physiologic transition that must occur at birth involves glucose and energy homeostasis. Before birth, all of the newborn's nutritional needs are continuously provided by the maternal circulation. After birth, major physiologic and metabolic changes are required to adjust to intermittent enteral feeding.

Glucose is the substrate used for the energy production necessary for the maintenance of body temperature, respiration, and muscular activity.[12,39] Blood glucose concentration is normally maintained at a relatively constant level by a fine balance between hepatic glucose output and peripheral glucose uptake. Hepatic glucose output depends on adequate glycogen stores, sufficient supplies of endogenous gluconeogenic substrate, a normally functioning gluconeogenic and glycogenolytic system, and a normal endocrine system for modulating these processes. The newborn has limited glycogen stores that may be rapidly depleted. On the other hand, endogenous gluconeogenic substrate availability is not a limiting factor nor are the liver's gluconeogenic and glycogenolytic systems.[12,39]

Hypoglycemia is common in the following infants: (1) those born to diabetic mothers, (2) those who required resuscitation, (3) those who are premature, and (4) those who are small-for-gestational age.[7,12,23] By definition, hypoglycemia is a blood glucose level less than 35 mg/dl in the full-term infant or less than 25 mg/dl in the preterm infant during the first 3 days of life. After 3 days, glucose values should be greater than 45 mg/dl.[7,12] The clinical manifestations of hypoglycemia include tremors or jitteriness, apnea, cyanotic spells, convulsions, limpness or lethargy, hypothermia, sweating, refusal to feed, and cardiac failure or arrest. These are nonspecific signs and symptoms and must be differentiated from birth asphyxia, central nervous system abnormalities such as hemorrhage or cerebral edema, congenital heart disease, sepsis, drug withdrawal, apnea, and other metabolic abnormalities such as hypocalcemia, hypomagnesemia, and hyponatremia.[7,12]

Symptomatic babies must be treated rapidly to prevent neurologic damage. Treatment should be started with a 250 to 500 mg/kg bolus of glucose (25% dextrose-containing solution, D25), followed by an infusion of 4 to 6 mg/kg/min (65 to 100 ml/kg/hour) of a 10% to 15% dextrose-containing solution.[7,12] Failure of this regimen to produce blood glucose concentration of 80 to 120 mg/dl should alert the physician of the possibility of hyperinsulinism. Hyperinsulinism occurs in maternal diabetes, erythroblastosis, Beckwith-Wiedemann syndrome, polycythemia, and insulin-secreting tumors (nesidioblastosis).[7,12,17]

Calcium

Calcium in the blood circulates as three fractions: protein bound, complexed, and ionized.[69,74] Ionized calcium is the only physiologically active fraction.[69,74] In fact, if total calcium levels in the blood are reduced as a result of low plasma protein and if the ionized fraction remains normal, there may be no physiologic changes. On the other hand, if total calcium levels are normal but the ionized levels are low, as may occur when chelating agents are used (citrated blood products), significant physiologic effects occur.

During pregnancy, there is rapid transfer of calcium from mother to fetus via an active placenta pump. At birth there is an abrupt termination of this calcium supply. Furthermore, dietary calcium in the first days of life is significantly less than the amount normally received from the mother. A fall in serum calcium is expected to occur. In the sick newborn, even greater deprivation of calcium is common because of the conventional withholding of milk feeding and the substitution of calcium-free intravenous feeding.

Neonatal hypocalcemia is therefore common in the first few days of life.[39,43,74] Definitions vary as to the level of serum calcium required for the diagnosis, but most agree that when the serum calcium level falls below 7 mg/dl, the infant should be considered hypocalcemic. Infants at particular risk include (1) those infants who are born prematurely, (2) those who are born to diabetic mothers, (3) those who are small-for-gestational age, (4) those who have received large volumes of citrated blood products or sodium bicarbonate, (5) those who are alkalotic secondary to hyperventilation, and (6) those who have experienced birth asphyxia.[7,39,43,74]

The classic clinical signs and symptoms of hypocalcemia, namely Chvostek's sign (facial muscle twitching when stimulated) and Trousseau's sign (carpal spasm after constriction of the upper arm), are of little value in the newborn. Rather, nonspecific symptoms occur, namely jitteriness, twitching, convulsions, and, occasionally, hypotension. Symptomatic hypocalcemia is treated by acute intravenous administration of 1 to 2 ml/kg of either 10% calcium gluconate or chloride while the heart rate is monitored continuously.[7,39,43,74] In the newborn the acute administration of calcium can produce significant bradycardia. The other important complication of this therapy is extravasation of calcium into the soft tissues when a peripheral intravenous catheter is used. This extravasation can cause skin sloughing and necrosis.

KEY POINTS

- Newborns respond to surgical stress, and providing anesthesia and analgesia reduces perioperative morbidity and mortality.
- A careful history and physical examination of the newborn are required, with particular attention to the history of asphyxia at birth and to the presence of congenital anomalies affecting the respiratory, cardiovascular, gastrointestinal, genitourinary, or neurologic systems.

- Neonates have limited ability to tolerate perioperative insults, such as drug overdose, hypoxia, hypothermia, or glucose and electrolyte disturbances.
- Parents of critically ill children require considerable emotional support and reassurance during the perioperative period.

KEY REFERENCES

Anand KJ, Hickey PR: Pain and its effects in the human neonate and fetus, *N Engl J Med* 317:1321, 1987.

Anand KJ, Sippell WG, and Aynsley Green A: Randomised trial of fentanyl anaesthesia in preterm babies undergoing surgery: effects on the stress response (published erratum appears in *Lancet,* 1987, Jan 24, 1[8526]:234), *Lancet* 1:62, 1987.

Cowett RM: Pathophysiology, diagnosis, and management of glucose homeostasis in the neonate, *Curr Probl Pediatr* 15:1, 1985.

Gregory GA: The baroresponses of preterm infants during halothane anaesthesia, *Can Anaesth Soc J* 29:105, 1982.

Kurth CD, Spitzer AR, Broennle AM et al: Postoperative apnea in preterm infants, *Anesthesiology* 66:483, 1987.

Maze A, Bloch E: Stridor in pediatric patients, *Anesthesiology* 50:132, 1979.

Menon RK, Sperling MA: Carbohydrate metabolism, *Semin Perinatol* 12:157, 1988.

Pang LM, Mellins RB: Neonatal cardiorespiratory physiology, *Anesthesiology* 43:171, 1975.

Rowe MI, Taylor M: Transepidermal water loss in the infant surgical patient, *J Pediatr Surg* 16:878, 1981.

Schieber RA: Cardiovascular physiology of the fetus and newborn. In Cook DR, Marcy JH: *Neonatal anesthesia,* Pasadena, 1988, Appleton Davis.

Tsang RC, Steichen JJ, and Brown DR: Perinatal calcium homeostasis: neonatal hypocalcemia and bone demineralization, *Clin Perinatol* 4:385, 1977.

Volpe JJ: Intravascular hemorrhage and brain injury in the premature infant: diagnosis, prognosis, and prevention, *Clin Perinatol* 16:387, 1989.

Wear R, Robinson S, and Gregory GA: The effect of halothane on the baroresponse of adult and baby rabbits, *Anesthesiology* 56:188, 1982.

REFERENCES

1. Anand KJ: Neonatal stress responses to anesthesia and surgery, *Clin Perinatol* 17:207, 1990.
2. Anand KJ, Hickey PR: Pain and its effects in the human neonate and fetus, *N Engl J Med* 317:1321, 1987.
3. Anand KJ, Sippell WG, and Aynsley Green A: Randomised trial of fentanyl anaesthesia in preterm babies undergoing surgery: effects on the stress response (published erratum appears in *Lancet,* 1987, Jan 24, 1[8526]:234), *Lancet* 1:62, 1987.
4. Avery ME: The J. Burns Amberson Lecture—in pursuit of understanding the first breath, *Am Rev Respir Dis* 100:295, 1969.

5. Berry FA, Gregory GA: Do premature infants require anesthesia for surgery? *Anesthesiology* 67:291, 1987.
6. Betts EK, Downes JJ, Schaffer DB et al: Retrolental fibroplasia and oxygen administration during general anesthesia, *Anesthesiology* 47:518, 1977.
7. Bikhazi BG, Davis PJ: Anesthesia for neonates and premature infants. In Motoyama EK, Davis PJ, eds: *Smith's anesthesia for infants and children,* St Louis, 1990, Mosby–Year Book.
8. Brady JP, Ceruti E: Chemoreceptor reflexes in the new-born infant: effects of varying degrees of hypoxia on heart rate and ventilation in a warm environment, *J Physiol (Lond)* 184:631, 1966.

9. Ceruti E: Chemoreceptor reflexes in the newborn infant: effect of cooling on the response to hypoxia, *Pediatrics* 37:556, 1966.
10. Chernick V, Avery ME: Response to premature infants with periodic breathing to ventilatory stimuli, *J Appl Physiol* 21:434, 1966.
11. Clyman RI, Mauray F, Heymann MA et al: Influence of increased pulmonary vascular pressures on the closure of the ductus arteriosus in newborn lambs, *Pediatr Res* 25:136, 1989.
12. Cowett RM: Pathophysiology, diagnosis, and management of glucose homeostasis in the neonate, *Curr Probl Pediatr* 15:1, 1985.

13. Davies RO, Edwards MW Jr, and Lahiri S: Halothane depresses the response of carotid body chemoreceptors to hypoxia and hypercapnia in the cat, *Anesthesiology* 57:153, 1982.

14. Davies RO, Lahiri S: Absence of carotid chemoreceptor response during hypoxic exercise in the cat, *Respir Physiol* 18:92, 1973.

15. Davis PJ: Thermoregulation of the newborn. In Cook DR, Marcy JH, eds: *Neonatal anesthesia,* Pasadena, 1988, Appleton Davies.

16. Du JN, Oliver TK Jr: The baby in the delivery room. A suitable microenvironment, *JAMA* 207:1502, 1969.

17. Engstrom W, Lindham S, and Schofield P: Wiedemann-Beckwith syndrome, *Eur J Pediatr* 147:450, 1988.

18. Flynn JT: Oxygen and retrolental fibroplasia: update and challenge [editorial], *Anesthesiology* 60:397, 1984.

19. Frantz ID III, Adler SM, Thach BT et al: Maturational effects on respiratory responses to carbon dioxide in premature infants, *J Apply Physiol* 41:41, 1976.

20. Frantz ID III, Milic Emili J: The progressive response of the newborn infant to added respiratory loads, *Respir Physiol* 24:233, 1975.

21. Gregory GA: The baroresponses of preterm infants during halothane anaesthesia, *Can Anaesth Soc J* 29:105, 1982.

22. Grundfast KM, Harley E: Vocal cord paralysis, *Otolaryngol Clin North Am* 22:569, 1989.

23. Hertel J, Kuhl C: Metabolic adaptations during the neonatal period in infants of diabetic mothers, *Acta Endocrinol Suppl (Copenh)* 277:136, 1986.

24. Heymann MA, Berman W Jr, Rudolph AM et al: Dilatation of the ductus arteriosus by prostaglandin E1 in aortic arch abnormalities, *Circulation* 59:169, 1979.

25. Heymann MA, Rudolph AM: Ductus arteriosus dilatation by prostaglandin E1 in infants with pulmonary atresia, *Pediatrics* 59:325, 1977.

26. Hoffman JI, Rudolph AM, and Heymann MA: Pulmonary vascular disease with congenital heart lesions: pathologic features and causes, *Circulation* 64:873, 1981.

27. Katz J, Steward DJ: *Anesthesia and uncommon pediatric diseases,* Philadelphia, 1987, WB Saunders.

28. Keens TG, Bryan AC, Levison H et al: Developmental pattern of muscle fiber types in human ventilatory muscles, *J Appl Physiol* 44:909, 1978.

29. Keens TG, Ianuzzo CD: Development of fatigue-resistant muscle fibers in human ventilatory muscles, *Am Rev Respir Dis* 119:139, 1979.

30. Kennell JH, Slyter H, and Klaus MH: The mourning response of parents to the death of a newborn infant, *N Engl J Med* 283:344, 1970.

31. Knill RL, Bright S, and Manninen P: Hypoxic ventilatory responses during thiopentone sedation and anaesthesia in man, *Can Anaesth Soc J* 25:366, 1978.

32. Knill RL, Gelb AW: Ventilatory responses to hypoxia and hypercapnia during halothane sedation and anesthesia in man, *Anesthesiology* 49:244, 1978.

33. Kupferberg HJ, Way EL: Pharmacologic basis for the increased sensitivity of the newborn rat to morphine, *J Pharmacol Exp Ther* 141:105, 1963.

34. Kurth CD, Spitzer AR, Broennle AM et al: Postoperative apnea in preterm infants, *Anesthesiology* 66:483, 1987.

35. Lahiri S, Mulligan E, Nishino T et al: Relative responses of aortic body and carotid body chemoreceptors to carboxyhemoglobinemia, *J Appl Physiol* 50:580, 1981.

36. Marchal F, Bairam A, and Vert P: Neonatal apnea and apneic syndromes, *Clin Perinatol* 14:509, 1987.

37. Maxwell LG, Yaster M, Wetzel RC et al: Penile nerve block for newborn circumcision, *Obstet Gynecol* 70:415, 1987.

38. Maze A, Bloch E: Stridor in pediatric patients, *Anesthesiology* 50:132, 1979.

39. Menon RK, Sperling MA: Carbohydrate metabolism, *Semin Perinatol* 12:157, 1988.

40. Ment LR, Ehrenkranz RA, and Duncan CC: Intraventricular hemorrhage of the preterm neonate: prevention studies, *Semin Perinatol* 12:359, 1988.

41. Merritt JC, Sprague DH, Merritt WE et al: Retrolental fibroplasia: a multifactorial disease, *Anesth Analg* 60:109, 1981.

42. Motoyama EK: Respiratory physiology. In Cook DR, Marcy JH, eds: *Neonatal anesthesia,* Pasadena, 1988, Appleton Davies.

43. Noe DA: Neonatal hypocalcemia and related conditions, *Clin Lab Med* 1:227, 1981.

44. Pang LM, Mellins RB: Neonatal cardiorespiratory physiology, *Anesthesiology* 43:171, 1975.

45. Pasternak GW, Zhank AZ, and Tecott L: Developmental differences between high and low affinity opiate binding sites: their relationship to analgesia and respiratory depression, *Life Sci* 27:1185, 1980.

46. Perloff WH: Physiology of the heart and circulation. In Swedlow DB, Raphaely RC, eds: *Cardiovascular problems in pediatric critical care,* New York, 1986, Churchill-Livingstone.

47. Richardson MA, Cotton RT: Anatomic abnormalities of the pediatric airway, *Pediatr Clin North Am* 31:821, 1984.

48. Rigatto H: Apnea and periodic breathing, *Semin Perinatol* 1:375, 1977.

49. Rigatto H, Brady JP: Periodic breathing and apnea in preterm infants. I. Evidence for hypoventilation possibly due to central respiratory depression, *Pediatrics* 50:202, 1972.

50. Rigatto H, Brady JP: Periodic breathing and apnea in preterm infants. II. Hypoxia as a primary event, *Pediatrics* 50:219, 1972.

51. Rigatto H, Brady JP, de la Torre Verduzco R: Chemoreceptor reflexes in preterm infants. I. The effect of gestational and postnatal age on the ventilatory response to inhalation of 100% and 15% oxygen, *Pediatrics* 55:604, 1975.

52. Ross DA, Ward PH: Central vocal cord paralysis and paresis presenting as laryngeal stridor in children, *Laryngoscope* 100:10, 1990.

53. Rowe MI, Arango A: The neonatal response to massive fluid infusion, *J Pediatr Surg* 6:365, 1971.

54. Rowe MI, Marchildon MB: Physiologic considerations in the newborn surgical patient, *Surg Clin North Am* 56:245, 1976.

55. Rowe MI, Taylor M: Transepidermal water loss in the infant surgical patient, *J Pediatr Surg* 16:878, 1981.

56. Rowe MI, Weinberg G, and Andrews W: Reduction of neonatal heat loss by an insulated head cover, *J Pediatr Surg* 18:909, 1983.

57. Rudolf AM: *Congenital diseases of the heart,* Chicago, 1974, Year Book Medical Publishers.

58. Schieber RA: Cardiovascular physiology of the fetus and newborn. In Cook DR, Marcy JH eds.: *Neonatal anesthesia,* Pasadena, 1988, Appleton Davis.

59. Scott CB, Nickerson BG, Sargent CW, et al: Diaphragm strength in near-miss sudden infant death syndrome, *Pediatrics* 69:782, 1982.

60. Sidi D, Kuipers JR, Heymann MA et al: Effects of ambient temperature on oxygen consumption and the circulation in newborn lambs at rest and during hypoxemia, *Pediatr Res* 17:254, 1983.

61. Smith DW: *Recognizable patterns of human malformation,* Philadelphia, 1982, WB Saunders.

62. Soifer SJ, Clyman RI, and Heymann MA: Effects of prostaglandin D2 on pulmonary arterial pressure and oxygenation in newborn infants with persistent pulmonary hypertension, *J Pediatr* 112:774, 1988.

63. Soifer SJ, Morin FC III, Kaslow DC et al: The developmental effects of prostaglandin D2 on the pulmonary and systemic circulations in the newborn lamb, *J Dev Physiol* 5:237, 1983.

64. Stephenson JM, Du JN, and Oliver TK Jr: The effect of cooling on blood gas tensions in newborn infants, *J Pediatr* 76:848, 1970.

65. Steward DJ: *Manual of pediatric anesthesia,* New York, 1985, Churchill-Livingstone.

66. Swafford LI, Allan D: Pain relief in the pediatric patient, *Med Clin North Am* 71:36, 1968.

67. Taeusch HW, Carson S, Frantz ID et al: Respiratory regulation after elastic loading and CO_2 rebreathing in normal term infants, *J Pediatr* 88:102, 1976.

68. Teitel DF, Sidi D, Chin T et al: Developmental changes in myocardial contractile reserve in the lamb, *Pediatr Res* 19:948, 1985.

69. Tsang RC, Steichen JJ, and Brown DR: Perinatal calcium homeostasis: neonatal hypocalcemia and bone demineralization, *Clin Perinatol* 4:385, 1977.

70. Volpe JJ: Intravascular hemorrhage and brain injury in the premature infant: diagnosis, prognosis, and prevention, *Clin Perinatol* 16:387, 1989.

71. Volpe JJ: Intraventricular hemorrhage in the premature infant—current concepts. Part II, *Ann Neurol* 25:109, 1989.

72. Wallgren G, Hanson JS, and Lind J: Quantitative studies of the human neonatal circulation. III. Observations on the

newborn infants' central circulatory responses to moderate hypovolemia, *Acta Paediatr Scand,* 1967.

73. Wallgren G, Lind J: Quantitative studies of the human neonatal circulation. IV. Observations on the newborn infants' peripheral circulation and plasma expansion during moderate hypovolemia, *Acta Paediatr Scand,* 1967.

74. Wandrup J: Critical analytical and clinical aspects of ionized calcium in neonates, *Clin Chem* 35:2027, 1989.

75. Way WL, Costley EC, and Way EL: Respiratory sensitivity of the newborn infant to meperidine and morphine, *Clin Pharmacol Ther* 6:454, 1965.

76. Wear R, Robinson S, and Gregory GA: The effect of halothane on the baroresponse of adult and baby rabbits, *Anesthesiology* 56:188, 1982.

77. Williamson PS, Williamson ML: Physiologic stress reduction by a local anesthetic during newborn circumcision, *Pediatrics* 71:36, 1983.

78. Yaster M: Analgesia and anesthesia in neonates, *J Pediatr* 111:394, 1987.

79. Zalzal GH: Stridor and airway compromise, *Pediatr Clin North Am* 36:1389, 1989.

80. Zhang AZ, Pasternak GW: Ontogeny of opioid pharmacology and receptors: high and low affinity site difference, *Eur J Pharmacol* 73:29, 1981.

CHAPTER 26

Evaluation of Children

RANDALL C. WETZEL

Many obvious differences between adults and children affect anesthetic management. Apart from the obvious differences of size, communication skills, and issues involving parents, there are also multiple, less obvious differences in the physiology, psychology, anatomy, and pharmacology of children. The most characteristic and significant feature of childhood is development. Not only does the child's responsiveness to other people undergo recognized patterns of psychological development that require appropriate responses from the anesthesiologist, but virtually every organ system undergoes distinct, well-described development that is relevant to the anesthetic management of that child. The key to understanding pediatric anesthesiology is to understand the dynamic processes that occur at the various developmental stages of childhood. The sense for this dynamic must be acquired by all of those who wish to anesthetize children. The mind set required is not that of understanding anesthesia that is appropriate for adult physiology and adapting this anesthetic approach to children but rather to flexibly approach the child as he/she grows from fetus to adult. A specific anesthetic plan appropriate to developmental stages must be designed for each child. Because the developmental characteristics of children determine anesthetic management, we will focus on those changes that occur after the neonatal period. For a discussion of neonatal physiology, please see Chapter 25 on neonatal anesthesia. The purpose of this chapter will be to familiarize the anesthesiologist with the anesthetic implications of the transition from the neonatal period to adulthood.

DEVELOPMENTAL IMPLICATIONS

Growth is not simply a process of proportional enlargement. In fact, total body composition, including proportional fluid content, the relationship of head to body size, and cardiorespiratory function, all change disproportionately during development.[71] For example, as the child grows, the head becomes proportionately smaller with relatively little change in the size of the cranial vault after 2 years of age but at the same time significant changes in the facial configuration take place. Most striking is the development of the mandible, which develops from being small and obliquely set to the skull in the infant, to becoming proportionately larger, less obliquely set, and more mobile in the adult.

The development of body composition is important because it is an essential determinant of developmental pharmacology. **In the fetus, 90% of total body composition is water; at full term, 75% is water, but, by a year of age, 60% of total body content is water.**[28] Adult body composition is attained by 1 year of age. There is also a change in the relative proportion of extracellular water over the first years of life. Extracellular water volume demonstrates a greater decrease than intracellular volume, which undergoes a complementary increase. **Intracellular fluid increases** from approximately 20% in the premature infant to 30% in the term infant and 40% in the adult, while extracellular fluid falls from 60% in the premature infant to 45% in the term infant, and 20% in the adult.[98] The percentage of body composition that is muscle in premature infants is less than 20%, becoming greater than 20% at term, and attaining 50% by adulthood.[28] Fat likewise increases with age from 13% in the term infant to 22% of total body weight in adults.[28] There is also an age-dependent change in the relative proportion of blood flow to the various organs. Distribution of blood flow to various organ groups defined by their vascularity (vessel-rich group [VRG], muscle group, [MG], and vessel-poor group [VPG]) also demonstrates significant developmental change[24] (Table 26-1). For example, there is a **decreased percentage of flow going to vessel-rich groups with increasing age.** The vessel-rich group in newborns accounts for 22% of total body volume, whereas in the adult it is only 10%. Thus one would expect a smaller portion of blood flow to vessel-poor groups in infants, and a more rapid attainment of the plateau phase of the F_a/F_i ratio for inhalational anesthetics. This has clear implications for the induction of inhalational anesthesia in children and, not surprisingly, the uptake and distribution of inhalational anesthetics in children.[23]

Respiratory System

The major features of the respiratory system that undergo significant developmental changes are (1) the upper airway, (2) the caliber of the airways, (3) pulmonary mechanics, (4) central respiratory control, and (5) respiratory muscle characteristics. Each of these will be described separately.

The upper airway undergoes significant development (Fig. 26-1). The first developmental difference that is apparent to those who intubate children is that an infant's **tongue is relatively large** compared with the rest of the airway. Intubation may be hampered by the **overlarge tongue situated in the relatively small jaw.** The infant is usually described as having an **anterior, cephalad displaced glottis** with the airway forming an inverse cone (Fig. 26-2). The **narrowest segment of the airway is at the cricoid cartilage,** and this remains true until puberty. These factors have significance for intubation. An endotracheal tube that will be admitted to the glottis may be too tight for the subglottic area. The presence of an **air leak below 30 cm H_2O** airway pressure should always be assured for routine anesthesia.

In the infant, the glottis is actually located at C2, two to three vertebral bodies higher than in the adult, in whom the glottis is generally located at the C4 to C5 level. The cricoid cartilage is at C4 in children and C6 to C7 in adults. The obliquity of the vocal cords also changes with age. In infants these are slanted downward anteriorly, compared with adults. This clearly makes the angle for intubation more acute and more difficult in children and makes blind nasal intubation more difficult. A further difference in the pediatric airway is the nature of the epiglottis. **The epiglottis in** small children is generally relatively larger, longer, more curved (omega shaped), and quite floppy, compared with its adult counterpart. Maturation begins to occur after 2 years of age, and the adult configuration is achieved sometime near puberty, when the epiglottis is shorter, smaller, blunter, and less curved, rather than omega shaped. These anatomic differences in the airway have a major effect on which intubation techniques will be useful in children. For example, **a straight laryngoscope blade that can lift the epiglottis out of the larynx during glottic visualization is useful in children.**

Airway caliber undergoes continuous developmental change, from the nares to the small airways. Although airway branching has been completed by birth, the **caliber of the airways continues to increase.** Airway resistance is inversely proportional to the fourth power of the radius, as seen in the Poiseuille equation:

Table 26-1 Tissue type volume as percent of body volume

Age	Vessel-rich group	Muscle group	Vessel-poor group
Neonate	22	39	13
1 year	17	39	25
4 years	17	41	23
8 years	13	45	21
Adult	10	50	22

Modified from Eger EI II, Bohlman SH, and Munson ES: The effect of age on the rate of increase of alveolar anesthetic concentration, *Anesthesiology* 35:365, 1971.

$$\text{Resistance} = 8 \, Ln/\pi \, r^4$$

L is the airway length, n is the viscosity of the fluid, and r is the radius of the airway. It should be noted that total airway resistance is affected by this consideration of caliber all the way from the nares to the alveoli. **Small airways have quite high resistance. The consideration of size also makes the significance of airway edema greater in younger children.** A proportional increase in mucosal thickness in children increases resistance to a greater extent than it does in adults because equal mucosal thickening proportionately decreases caliber more in children. Airway resistance decreases approximately 15 times from infancy to adulthood, with a dramatic change occurring near the age of 8 years.[36] This **decrease in resistance with increasing age** is largely due to an increase in diameter of the small airways.[103] Infants are **obligate nose-breathers,** and nasal obstruction can cause severe respiratory embarrassment. This is more severe in premature infants.[61]

Respiratory mechanics change dramatically from birth to adulthood. These changes result from **increasing alveolarization, increasing airway size, and changes in the chest wall.** Only as the rib cage ossifies does its configuration change and become more rigid. **In infants, the chest wall is soft and pliable due to its largely cartilaginous structure,** which makes the chest wall highly compliant. The effect of this compliance is

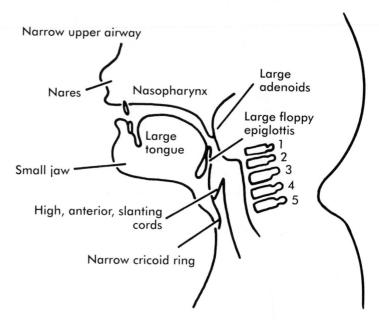

Fig. 26-1. Diagram of a coronal section through the airway of an infant. Areas where there are significant differences from adults are highlighted. (From Wetzel RC: Anesthesia for pediatric trauma. In Stene JK, ed: *Trauma anesthesia,* Baltimore, 1989, Williams & Wilkins.)

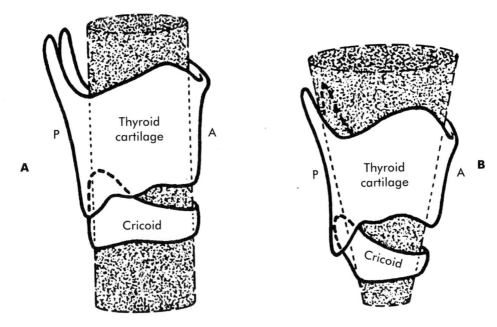

Fig. 26-2. Schematic drawing of an adult (**A**) and infant (**B**) airway. Note the comparison between the cylindrically shaped airway with uniform diameters in the adult as compared to the conically shaped airway of the child with the narrowest region at the cricoid. *P,* posterior; *A,* anterior. (From Cote CJ, Todres ID: The pediatric airway. In Ryan JR, Todres ID, Cote CJ et al, eds: *A practice of anesthesia for infants and children,* Philadelphia, 1986, WB Saunders.)

that **when there is increased work of breathing required with the need for more negative intrathoracic pressure, the chest wall tends to collapse.** The clinical consequences associated with these chest wall factors are seen in infants with respiratory distress. **Marked sternal and subcostal retractions are frequently seen in these children.** The infant's chest wall is at a mechanical disadvantage during breathing because greater pressure is required per unit of tidal volume moved. In addition to the compliance of the chest wall, there is also a decrease in elastic recoil of both the total respiratory system and the chest wall. This low elastic recoil tends to alter the relationship between closing volume, FRC, and residual volume (Fig. 26-3).

The respiratory system also demonstrates significant neuromuscular development. Central respiratory control, muscle fiber makeup (type I vs. type II), and neural innervation of the chest wall all show distinct developmental changes in infants and small children.[44] Most dramatically, central respiratory control undergoes distinct developmental changes. For example, the full and preterm **newborn demonstrates depression of the CO$_2$ response curve and secondary apnea with hypoxia.**[76] This is in contrast to the

characteristic adult response, which is increased CO$_2$ responsiveness in the presence of hypoxia, which results in tachypnea. Clearly the impact of hypoxia in the presence of this paradoxic, immature response can be catastrophic in the newborn.[76] This infantile pattern of respiratory control most certainly is related to the risk of postanesthetic apnea in neonates.[52] Anesthetic effects on the CO$_2$ response curve are similar in infants and adults. The CO$_2$ response curve undergoes depression by potent inhalational anesthetic agents and narcotics in adults as it does also in children.[47]

Respiratory muscle type distribution does not reach the adult pattern until approximately 2 years of age. The pattern of relative **muscle type distribution predisposes the infant to fatigue.** Type II muscle fibers are predominant and do not have the ability to perform repeated exercise against increased workloads as do type I fibers.[44] Type I fibers become predominant around 2 years of age. With regard to neural innervation, reflex responses and spindle innervation of the thoracic cage also undergo developmental changes. In part, this reflects the change in compliance of the thoracic wall. This is reflected by the fact that the Hering-Breuer response is accentu-

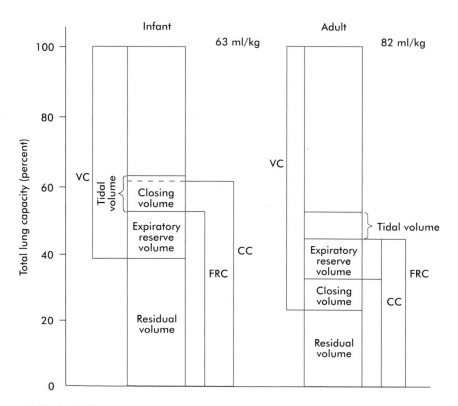

Fig. 26-3. Bar graphs representing proportional lung volumes in both infants and adults. Note the relationship of functional residual capacity *(FRC)* to closing volume and how this changes with age. *VC,* vital capacity; *CC,* closing capacity. (From Smith CA, Nelson NM: *The physiology of the newborn infant,* Springfield, Ill, 1976, Charles C Thomas.)

ated in preterm infants as contrasted with full-term infants.[69] These characteristics have a significant impact on cyclic respiration as can be seen from the immature respiratory pattern of periodic breathing. In addition, changes in respiration from sleep state and REM sleep show distinct developmental differences.[41]

These changes in chest wall recoil, elasticity, compliance, and neural innervation have a significant impact on lung volumes (Fig. 26-3). One of the most important factors is the tendency in younger children toward airway closure and alveolar collapse with atelectasis. As children breathe, tidal respiration is very close to closing volume. Airway closure may occur even during tidal respiration in small infants.[86] Induction of anesthesia is associated with decreased elastic recoil and airway tone as well as decreased

respiratory muscle tone, and, thus, an expected lung volume decrease occurs with tidal respiration falling below closing volumes. These factors and those responsible for the loss of functional residual capacity (FRC) on induction of anesthesia in part account for the rapid occurrence of hypoxemia in apneic infants during induction of anesthesia. The other major factor related to the **rapid occurrence of hypoxemia in apneic infants is their relatively increased oxygen consumption. In newborn infants oxygen consumption is approximately 7 ml/kg/min.**[35] On a consumption/weight basis, this is approximately double that seen in adults. This undergoes a smooth decrease with age. **Although FRC/kg is less (30 ml vs. 34 ml) in infants than adults, increased oxygen consumption is the major factor in the rapidity of desaturation in infants and small children who are apneic.** The developmental differences in respiratory physiology are summarized in Table 26-2.

In addition to oxygenation issues, development of the respiratory system also affects ventilation. **For example, V_d/V_t, the ratio of dead space to tidal volume ventilation, is approximately 33%, as it is in adults. In the newborn with a 7-ml dead space and a 20-ml tidal volume, the relative proportion during spontaneous ventilation without respiratory equipment is the same. However, the addition of just a few milliliters of dead space by the superimposition of anesthetic equipment may increase dead space from 7 to 12 ml and have a serious effect on V_d/V_t and CO_2 clearance in neonates.** For this reason, the dead space of all ventilatory equipment, endotracheal tubes, and especially face masks as well as anesthesia circuitry must be minimized, and the anesthesiologist must be aware of the significance of these changes in dead space in newborns.

Cardiovascular System

The cardiovascular system also undergoes dramatic developmental changes.[27,63] The most obvious and dramatic changes occur perinatally, and these have been detailed in the section on perinatal physiology. **Even in full-term infants there is a perioperative risk of complications related to the transitional circulation. Anything that may contribute to pulmonary hypertension, such as infection, acidosis, hypoxia, hypercarbia, hypothermia, and aspiration, may lead to a serious decrease in cardiac output, hypoxemia, and hypotension.** Obviously these factors must be avoided in the anesthetic plan for any infant. Multiple developmental changes occur in myocardial function. Changes in the proportion of muscle content to connective tissue with developmental stage lead to an alteration in myocardial compliance.[27] In addition, **developing left ventricular dominance also alters ventricular characteristics.** These factors underlie

Table 26-2   Respiratory mechanics

Respiratory frequency (breaths/min)	30-40	12-16
Inspiratory time (sec)	0.4-0.5	1.2-1.4
I:E ratio	1:1.5-1:2	1:2-1:3
Inspiratory flow (L/min)	2-3	24
Tidal volume		
ml	18-24	500
ml/kg	6-8	6-8
Functional residual capacity (FRC)		
ml	100	2200
ml/kg	30	34
Vital capacity		
ml	120	3500
ml/kg	33-40	52
Total lung capacity		
ml	200	6000
ml/kg	63	86
Total respiratory compliance		
ml/cm H_2O	2.6-4.9	100
ml/cm H_2O/ml FRC	0.04-0.06	0.04-0.07
Lung compliance		
ml/cm H_2O	4.8-6.2	170-200
ml/cm H_2O/ml FRC	0.04-0.07	0.04-0.07
Specific airway conductance		
ml/sec/cm H_2O/ml FRC	0.24	0.28
Respiratory insensible water loss		
ml/24 hr	45-55	300

Modified from Gioia FR, Stephenson RL, and Alterwitz SA: Principles of respiratory support and mechanical ventilation. In Rogers MC, ed: *Textbook of pediatric intensive care,* Baltimore, 1987, Williams & Wilkins.

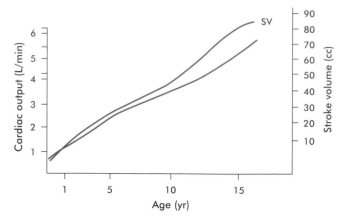

Fig. 26-4. Stroke volume and cardiac output increase with age. (From Wetzel RC, Rogers MC: Pediatric hemodynamic monitoring. In Shoemaker WC, Thompson WL, eds: *Critical care—state of the art,* vol 2, Fullerton, Calif, 1983, The Society of Critical Care Medicine.)

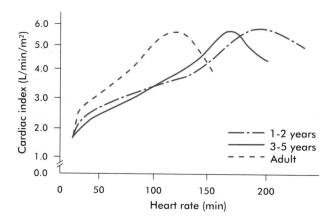

Fig. 26-5. Cardiac output is shown as it relates to heart rate in normal children and adults. (From Wetzel RC, Rogers MC: Pediatric hemodynamic monitoring. In Shoemaker WC, Thompson WL, eds: *Critical care—state of the art,* Fullerton, Calif, 1983, The Society of Critical Care Medicine.)

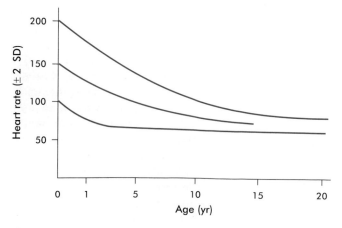

Fig. 26-6. Normal heart rates ± 2 SD shown in relation to age.

differences in how the myocardium responds to volume loading, afterload, and strategies for increasing cardiac output at different ages. The anesthesiologist must be familiar with these normal developmental changes in cardiovascular physiology to design an adequate anesthetic plan. Although myocardial ischemia only rarely plays a role in the anesthetic management of children, these factors and the varying responses to pharmacologic agents can lead to rapid and, occasionally catastrophic, hemodynamic decompensation in children undergoing anesthesia.[79] Virtually every determinant of cardiac output (heart rate,[63] contractility,[74] afterload,[1] and preload relationships[45]) undergoes distinct developmental changes (Fig. 26-4).

In newborns and infants, heart rate is the predominant determinant of cardiac output.[83] The infant's heart is able to sustain greater rates than that of the adult while maintaining preload, contractility, and myocardial oxygenation before there is a fall in cardiac output (Fig. 26-5). Normal heart rates for infants and children are shown in Fig. 26-6. Bradycardia can drastically and seriously decrease the cardiac output in infants and children. **Increasing cardiac output by increasing heart rate should be considered early in responding to intraoperative falls in cardiac output as represented by hypotension.** Bradycardia also results from a predisposition to **parasympathetic hypertonia, which is common in young children** and can be induced by painful stimuli or hypoxia. Laryngoscopy, intubation, eye surgery, airway surgery, abdominal traction, and herniorrhaphy are frequently associated with marked increases in vagal tone and profound bradycardia. Under these circumstances, the cardiac output of the heart-rate–dependent infant heart can significantly decrease. The fact that children adapt to changes in cardiac output by changes in heart rate accounts for the wide ranges in heart rate seen in normal children. This is the usual response in children, and heart rates may vary over a great range in any given healthy child. Anesthetic suppression of atrial conduction and loss of p waves on the ECG with nodal escape rhythms are frequently seen during anesthesia, and the resultant bradycardia can be quite significant. The depression of heart rate by halothane, which may be accompanied by low output, can be readily treated with atropine and is the reason why many anesthesiologists make atropine part of any inhalational anesthetic plan in infants and small children. **Sinus dysrhythmia, a variation in the heart rate with respirations, is so common in children as to be considered normal but frequently can be confused with extra systoles or sinus arrest during anesthesia.**

Changes in contractility also occur with development. As Friedman originally reported in 1973, the myocardial length-tension relationships vary between pediatric and adult hearts and developmental differences in contractility are clearly seen.[27] These differences are explained by changes in muscle mechanics, innervation, myocardial blood flow, and histologic structure, all of which have been implicated in the child's relative inability to increase contractility. Fetal myocardial muscle sarcomeres themselves are quite active and have about the same contractile power as the adult sarcomere.[27] **The fact that neonatal ventricular tissue contains less muscle mass and more noncontractile mass/unit volume than adult tissue accounts for the fact that the neonatal myocardium is less able than the adult to generate adequate force.[93] In addition the neonatal heart is only partially innervated by the autonomic nervous system (although this innervation increases until mid-childhood). Therefore not only is the myocardium less able to develop inotropic force, but sympathetic innervation is also decreased.** The Frank-Starling preload relationship also appears to be altered by difference in the fiber make-up of the infant myocardium, and the relationship of the right ventricle to the left ventricle.[27] These changes in compliance characteristics frequently make the **infant heart preload-insensitive.** Volume load may generate higher filling pressures over a narrower proportional range in infants and small children than in adults.[80] **Normal adult contractility and compliance is generally reached by 1 or 2 years of age.** The final determinant of cardiac output, afterload, also changes with age. At birth, systemic resistance greatly increases with removal of the placenta, while afterload in the pulmonary circuit decreases dramatically.[1,83] Adjustment to this massively increased afterload in the systemic circulation occurs rapidly, but further increases in afterload may be poorly tolerated in the first year of life. Right and left ventricular mass and wall thickness are relatively equal in the newborn. Over the next year or so of life, the left ventricle becomes markedly dominant. In general, as a result of the factors mentioned previously, optimal cardiac output occurs at lower filling pressures in neonates compared with adults.[80]

All of these factors lead to optimal cardiovascular function at higher heart rates and lower blood pressures in infants than in adults (Fig. 26-5). Familiarity with normal range of blood pressures (Table 26-3) is essential. Attempting to maintain a blood pressure of 120/80 in a 1-year-old child during anesthesia may be virtually impossible without risking inadequate anesthesia or the use of pressors and is manifestly unnecessary. Familiarity with the normal range of blood pressures is absolutely essential in order to adequately interpret monitoring, even during routine anesthesia.

Congenital heart defects may affect all of the determinants of cardiac output: heart rate, contrac-

Table 26-3   Normal range of blood pressures

Age	Mean systolic/diastolic
Premature neonates	Systolic 40-60
Full-term neonates	75/50
1-6 months	80/50
6-12 months	90/65
12-24 months	95/65
2-6 years	100/60
6-12 years	110/60
12-16 years	110/65
16-18 years	120/65
Adult	125/75

Approximate ranges: pressure ± 20% = 95% confidence limits. Females are approximately 5% lower than these levels.
Data from Lowry GA: *Growth and development of children,* ed 6, Chicago, 1975, Year Book Medical Publishers; and Report of the Task Force on Blood Pressure Control in Children, National Heart, Lung, and Blood Institute, *Pediatrics* 59(suppl):803, 1977.

tility, preload, and afterload, as well as oxygenation. Left-to-right intracardiac shunting will alter preload, potentially alter contractility, and even alter RV afterload as pulmonary vascular resistance increases. Right-to-left shunting clearly affects systemic oxygenation, and cyanotic lesions frequently require expert anesthetic management. Valvular disease can increase preload (regurgitant lesions), decrease ventricular preload (mitral and tricuspid stenosis), or increase afterload (aortic and pulmonic stenosis). Congenital and surgically acquired lesions may alter conduction and therefore give rise to cardiac dysrhythmias. Thus careful evaluation of all aspects of cardiac function is necessary in assessing children with congenital heart disease.

Hemoglobin content and oxygen affinity also vary with age.[10] These proportional changes need to be borne in mind when designing an anesthetic for children. In the infant born at term, the normal **hemoglobin concentration falls dramatically during the first year of life, reaching a nadir around 2 to 3 months, the so-called physiologic anemia of infancy.**[10] **Although a physiologic hematocrit at this age could dip below 29%, a hemoglobin of <10 g/dl is rare. In the preterm infant, the hemoglobin concentration may fall to between 6 and 8 g/dl within the first 6 to 8 weeks of life.**[90] Although this is usual, it should not be considered "physiologic," and the same concern regarding a hematocrit of <25% in older children is appropriate. The hematocrit slowly increases to adult levels after puberty. Knowledge of these normal levels is necessary to guide blood transfusion and the timing of elective surgery that may be associated with significant blood loss.

Circulating blood volume is greater in newborns

Table 26-4 Intravascular blood volume	
Age	Blood volume/kilogram body weight (ml/kg)
Infants	
Premature	90-100
Full-term	80-90
Less than 1 yr	75-80
1-6 years	70-75
>6 years and adult	65-70

Table 26-5 Development of renal function		
Age	Kidney weight (g)	GFR/1.73 m^2 mean ± SD ml/min
Infants		
Term	27	20 ± 4
6 mo	32	77 ± 18
1 yr	71	115 ± 25
Children		
2 yr	93	127 ± 19
8 yr	149	127 ± 19
12 yr	191	127 ± 19
Adults	290	131 ± 21

Modified from Chantler C: The kidney. In Godfrey S, Baum JD, eds: *Clinical paediatric physiology*, Oxford, 1979, Blackwell Scientific Publications.

than in adults on the basis of body weight. Intravascular volume for a newborn is generally 80 to 90 ml/kg (Table 26-4). Understanding this relative change in total estimated blood volume (body weight times estimated volume/kilogram [EBV]) is necessary when determining the allowable blood loss in children. The following formula is useful for estimating how much blood a child can lose before the hematocrit is unacceptably low (allowable blood loss [ABL]):

$$ABL = EBV \times \frac{Hct_1 - Hct_2}{Mean\ Hct}$$

Hct$_1$ is the starting hematocrit, **Hct$_2$** is the desired or allowable hematocrit, and the mean hematocrit is the simple arithmetic mean of **Hct$_1$ + Hct$_2$**. Thus in a 12 kg, 1-year-old child with an initial hematocrit of 37% in whom a final hematocrit of 25% is acceptable, the allowable blood loss would be:

$$ABL = 12\ kg \times \frac{80\ ml}{kg} \times \frac{.37 - .25}{0.5(.25 + .37)} = 247\ ml$$

A comparison of the estimate of expected intraoperative loss to the estimate of allowable loss should be made before surgery. If possible, preoperative therapy should be designed to decrease the need for blood transfusion. Iron and nutritional supplements may be beneficial.

Renal Function

Renal function changes dramatically with age.[14] This can most easily be seen by referring to Table 26-5, where it can be seen that the **glomerular filtration rate (GFR)/1.73 m^2 changes from less than 40 ml/min at birth to 100 ml/min in the first year of life, which compares with 130 ml/min in the adult.** These changes in renal function and GFR are also accompanied by changes in the ability to regulate salt and water metabolism and by responses to changes in ADH that occur during anesthesia.[5] Although the factors regulating neonatal kidney function are complex in the transitional phase, the net result is that water is

excreted in excess of sodium. It is generally said that the neonatal kidney wastes sodium, and thus there is a tendency toward hyponatremia in the premature and full-term neonate. The kidney of the full-term infant is able to conserve sodium.[88] In contrast, **the ability of the kidney to concentrate urine is limited and maximal osmolarity may be only 700 mOsm/L in an infant.**[5] Thus an excess water load may lead to extra sodium loss, so the infant is also less able to defend intravascular volume against water deprivation. **Complete maturation of renal function usually occurs by about 2 years of age.** Obviously these developmental aspects of renal function have an effect on pharmacology. The effects of these changes are most prominent in the first few months of life and require careful fluid management in neonates, as well as attention to sodium and potassium balance.[3] Blood pressure regulation and the characteristics of hypertensive renal disease also show distinct differences in children.[33] In children with renal disease, hypertension should be looked for; blood pressure regulation, intraoperatively, may be difficult.

Dentition

Although teeth are occasionally present at birth, they may not erupt until nearly a year of age. The mean age for the development of the first tooth, usually a lower incisor, is around 6 months. By a year, children usually have both upper and lower teeth present. **By 6 years of age, permanent teeth begin to appear,** and the average 6-year-old has an intubation gap between his/her front incisors. **The significance of deciduous teeth is that they fall out.** The importance of this is that they should not fall out during anesthesia. All children under the age of

12, but especially those with loose incisors, around 6 years of age, should be questioned and examined for the presence of loose teeth. Loose and carious teeth are at increased risk for dislodgment by the placement of oral airways, laryngoscope blades, and endotracheal tubes. A **history of endotracheal intubation in the neonatal period is associated with subsequent development of abnormal dentition in neonates.**[65] Whether this is a result of direct trauma from the laryngoscope or from long-term placement of endotracheal tubes is, however, not clear.[100] Attention to the child's oropharynx and condition of dentition is an essential part of the anesthetic evaluation of all children.

Gastrointestinal System

The gastrointestinal tract also undergoes distinct developmental stages that may affect a child's response to anesthesia. At birth, gastric pH is alkalotic; however, by the second day of life, a normal physiologic range of gastric pH has been achieved. The secretion and amount of gastric contents in full-term infants is similar to adults. Although fasting gastric contents and pH in children are similar to those in adults, the reflex coordination of swallowing and lower esophageal sphincter (LES) function is not fully mature until 6 months of age.[7] **Slack LES tone with reflux is quite common in this age group.** This is relevant to the question of preoperative fasting. **The maintenance of low residual gastric volumes by NPO regulations (a questionable assumption) must be balanced against the propensity of fasting children to develop hypoglycemia.**[7] This is especially true if the infants/children are premature, small for gestational age (SGA), nutritionally deprived, or have increased metabolic needs because of conditions such as fever, sepsis, increased respiratory effort, or the condition that requires surgery. For these reasons, to assure a suitable period of fasting, especially in small, ill children, preoperative intravenous supplementation with dextrose-containing solutions is indicated.

Development of the gastrointestinal tract is generally complete at birth. Problems caused by congenital malformations or developmental anomalies are generally obvious within the first few days of birth.[7] Upper gastrointestinal obstruction, such as duodenal atresia and malrotation, are indicated by bilious vomiting and regurgitation within the first few days of life. Lower intestinal anomalies, such as volvulus or atresia of the small or large bowel, are manifested by failure to pass stools and by abdominal distension. Another major cause of gastrointestinal dysfunction in the first year of life is pyloric stenosis, which usually occurs between 3 and 6 weeks of age. The major symptoms are failure to gain weight and projectile vomiting.

The liver in neonates and young infants is also functionally immature. This functional immaturity is generally due to two main causes: (1) the development and growth of enzyme systems that, although present at birth, are not fully induced and (2) relatively decreased hepatic blood flow.[96] The ability of the liver to both conjugate and catabolize circulating substrate and pharmacologic substances is diminished at birth. For this reason, drugs tend to have longer half-lives in neonates compared with older children. This functional immaturity of the liver is reflected by **decreased concentrations of products of hepatic synthesis, such as albumin,** in neonates.[38] This leads to **decreased protein binding of many pharmacologic agents,** which may lead to altered pharmacology and pharmacodynamics. Hepatic function reaches adult levels usually within the first few months of life. This **rapid maturation in hepatic function** may be the reason why, in infants and older children, elimination half-lives of drugs may actually be less than in adults.

Thermoregulation

Perhaps no area is of greater concern to the pediatric anesthesiologist than the need to maintain normal body temperature perioperatively. The need for thermoregulatory control is underemphasized in adults but is critical in the management of children. **Defending the thermoneutrality of infants has been a cornerstone of pediatrics since the nineteenth century.** In 1900, Picrre-Constant Boudin demonstrated that there were striking differences in the survival of infants of less than 2000 g, which depended solely on their rectal temperature.[9] The mortality rate for infants with core temperatures less than 35° C was greater than 90% and for those over 35° C was only 23%. Boudin designed an incubator that provided heated air and humidity and then conclusively demonstrated that its use could dramatically improve the survival of children.[9] This observation found its way to Julius Hays Hess who is considered the founder of premature care in North America.[89] He recognized the importance of these observations and in 1922 opened the first premature infant center at the Michael Reese Hospital.

During anesthesia, environmental challenges to temperature integrity must be minimized. Hypothermia increases the demands on the cardiorespiratory system because of an increase in oxygen demand and the need for thermogenesis and alters every basic enzyme system. **Cold stress in neonates can lead to increased oxygen consumption, hypoxia, acidosis, respiratory distress, depletion of glycogen stores, hypoglycemia, pulmonary vasoconstriction, and hypertension with persistence of the fetal circulation, shock, and even disseminated intravascular coagulation.** In addition to this, drug metabolism, emergence from anesthesia, prolongation of the effects of neuromuscular blocking agents, and other pharmacologic effects accent the need for intraoperative thermoregulatory control in children.[89]

Heat loss occurs through four basic mechanisms: conduction, convection, radiation, and evaporation. Each of these, under certain circumstances, can be the major cause of heat loss. Conductive heat losses can be eliminated by minimizing the direct contact of children with surfaces colder than themselves. The use of a warming pad or heating blanket in the operating room can eliminate heat loss to the cold operating room table. In addition, warming of the operating room greatly reduces conductive heat loss. Convective heat losses can be further limited by the use of an incubator as well as by draping and warm blankets for the child. Radiant heat losses must also be minimized. Heat is radiated to objects of lower temperature. Warming objects in the patient's environment will lead to decreased radiant losses. This is the principle that underlies "radiant" neonatal warmers.[20] The use of double-walled incubators significantly decreases radiant losses. Transportation of neonates to the operating room in double-walled isolettes is probably optimal, but the use of radiant warmers that minimize convective loss is also acceptable. Finally, evaporative losses intraoperatively must be curtailed to minimize heat loss.

The use of warmed solutions for skin preparation and irrigation is important. The use of heated humidified air for ventilation also contributes greatly to the thermoregulatory control in children. For these reasons, it is our routine practice to use humidifiers in all pediatric circuits, maintain warm operating rooms with a high humidity, and use heating pads for all children who are anesthetized. For newborns and small neonates the operating room should be maintained at 80° F; for infants to 6 months at 78° F; for those 6 months to 2 years at 76° F always maintaining a minimum of 80% humidity. Warming of all intravascular fluids and rapidly transfused blood is also necessary. **Factors that contribute to infants becoming cold are basically related to their large surface area to mass ratio.** In addition, areas richly supplied with blood, such as the head and cranial vault, are proportionally larger in infants, giving rise to a great deal of heat loss. In premature infants this situation is aggravated by their **decreased subcutaneous tissue.** For these reasons, some method should be used to eliminate heat loss from the skin surface, especially the head, such as the use of plastic wraps and blankets.

Thermoregulation is a complex process, involving peripheral and central thermoreceptors, the CNS, and hypothalamic integration with central thermoreceptors.[32] A complex integration of responses occurs that leads to alterations in cutaneous blood flow and thermogenesis from both shivering and nonshivering sources.[12] This complex system is absolutely necessary to maintain mammalian core temperature within a normal range. Sources of heat production include basal metabolism, movement, shivering thermogenesis, and nonshivering thermogenesis. Basal metabolism is responsible for the greatest amount of baseline heat production. Shivering thermogenesis is the uncontrolled, rapid contraction of skeletal muscles and is frequently active on emergence from anesthesia in older patients. **Nonshivering thermogenesis is under direct control of the autonomic nervous sytem and produces heat by mobilizing fat from muscles, liver, and brain.**[11] **In newborns, both white and brown fat are metabolized, but brown fat is used by newborns to a much greater extent than it is in adults. This is necessary because newborns cannot respond to cold stress with shivering thermogenesis until the age of 6 months to a year.** Brown fat is distributed around the back of the neck, mediastinum, and interscapular regions, as well as around the kidneys and adrenals. **Brown fat is brown due to its high content of mitochondria and rich blood supply, which mirror its metabolic capability.** Brown fat is metabolized to increase heat production under the stimulation of the autonomic nervous system through catecholamine release.[11] Cold stress also leads to norepinephrine secretion, which causes adipocytes to release glycerol and fatty acids from brown fat depots. In the infant who is anesthetized in a cold room, not moving, with decreased metabolic rate, brown fat metabolism provides the only possibility of increasing body temperature. Cardiac output is diverted from other organs to brown fat depots. Vasoconstriction occurs as a result of norepinephrine release in both the systemic and pulmonary circulations. Therefore cold stress can lead to peripheral vasoconstriction, pulmonary vasoconstriction, decreased cardiac output, and shunting of cardiac output away from other organ systems to brown fat depots, all of which may pose a significant threat to newborn infants. Although this system is able to compensate for heat stress, the cost is high. Avoiding cold stress altogether is preferred.

GENERAL PRINCIPLES OF PEDIATRIC PHARMACOLOGY

The developmental differences among neonates, infants, and adults (discussed previously) all have a significant impact on the pharmacology and pharmacokinetics that are seen in children. Until recently our understanding of pediatric pharmacology has been at best, sketchy, and, at worst, incorrect. It must be remembered that the pharmacokinetic principles that govern the distribution and metabolism of anesthetic agents in adults are not directly applicable to children. Pediatric dosages were initially determined by calculating the proportionate amount of an agent on a weight basis. Assumptions about converting adult doses to children's doses on a per kilogram, surface area, or age basis have at times proven incorrect. **Perhaps no other area demonstrates more clearly that children are not small adults.** Scaling down doses on a per kilogram basis does not yield either the same drug concentrations or the same pharmacologic effect. There are many reasons for this. During the development from fetus to adult, factors that affect drug uptake, distribution, metabolism, and sensitivity to drugs all change. Volume of distribution, elimination half-lives, drug sensitivity, side effects, organ immaturity, protein binding, and clearance all undergo significant changes with age. Understanding the developmental aspects of general pharmacologic principles allows a theoretic approach to the use of many agents valuable in treating infants and children.

Complex issues of clinical investigation contribute to the poor knowledge of actual pharmacokinetics in children. Medicolegal and ethical issues affect our ability to obtain data from and, therefore, directly applicable to children. These factors have resulted in a largely empiric approach to pediatric anesthesia. This empiricism has recently been yielding to better-designed, better-informed studies in small children, aided by the advent of microassay techniques that require smaller volumes of blood sampling. Recently there have been several excellent studies of pharmacokinetics of many agents, including local anesthetics, narcotics, and sedatives in children, as well as of the uptake and distribution of inhalational agents. Absence of actual measurements perhaps renders an understanding of basic pharmacokinetic principles even more useful in the practice of pediatric anesthesia. These issues will be specifically addressed in sections dealing with particular pharmacologic agents.

Drug Administration

Anesthetic agents may be delivered orally, rectally, transnasally, percutaneously, conjunctivally, intramuscularly, intravenously, or by inhalation. Administration of drugs across mucous membranes requires passive diffusion, which depends on the concentration and the chemical properties of the agents used as well as the amount of surface area exposed. The fact that agents are absorbed across the mucous membrane in the rectum, for example, has made this route of administration popular for numerous sedatives and induction agents, such as methohexital, midazolam, thiopental, and ketamine.[56] Because the degree of ionization generally depends on pH and surface area, formulation is particularly important. **In general,**

rectal absorption will be enhanced by large volumes of dilute solutions. Drug uptake, and thus effect, will generally be more rapid with large-volume, dilute concentrations, which come in contact with a greater surface area.[25] Analgetic agents can also be administered by this route, allowing mild analgesia without the need for oral administration in the perioperative period. This route is acceptable to most children under 3 to 5 years of age.

Intranasal and transconjunctival administration of benzodiazepines, ketamine, and narcotics have been reported.[2,34,95] Formulation, solubility characteristics, desired end-points, and concentration all affect the rapidity of sedation, its duration and depth, and define an agent's suitability to induce anesthesia. Novel formulations, such as oral transmucosal fentanyl citrate, have been investigated in recent years, but have yet to find a place in routine clinical practice.[6,56]

Intramuscular administration is not popular in pediatric anesthesia because of pain on injection as well as pain after injection, which may last for several days after administration.[66] Induction agents, neuromuscular blocking agents, and analgetic agents may all be administered intramuscularly when the need indicates. When no other route of administration of an induction agent is possible, intramuscular ketamine (5 to 10 mg/kg) may achieve anesthetic induction in an agitated, uncooperative child within 5 to 7 minutes. Intramuscular administration of narcotics is time honored; however, we generally avoid it. Administration of benzodiazepines in the past has been associated with much burning and muscle pain; however intravenous water-soluble midazolam appears to be less irritating than these former formulations. Pain on injection and variable duration make intramuscular administration of drugs a method rarely used in children.[66]

The distribution of drugs administered intravenously depends on many factors, most of which are affected by developmental changes. Degree of binding to circulating blood elements such as proteins and red cells, blood-tissue partition coefficients, distribution of blood flow to various tissue beds, and changes in tissue volumes all affect the distribution of intravenously administered agents.

Drug Distribution

The existence of the free, nonbound, water-soluble moietie in the circulation is required for a drug to cross the endothelium and other cell membranes (where its effect is achieved) as well as for plasma clearance. **The bulk of protein binding is due to albumin; however, α-1-glycoprotein is also a significant circulating protein to which drugs bind.** The concentration of the latter and therefore its contribution to protein binding appear to be greater in children than in adults. Infants have very low concentrations of α-1-glycoprotein; therefore they may have a larger, unbound circulating concentration of certain drugs.[104] Curare, metocurine, propranolol, lidocaine, bupivacaine, digoxin, barbiturates, and narcotics all demonstrate a significant amount of protein binding. Their protein affinities have a significant effect on the pharmacokinetics of drugs in children. **Since the protein-bound fraction acts as a reservoir for the drug to maintain tissue and plasma concentrations, concomitant presence of substances that displace drugs from binding sites, such as bilirubin in the neonate, will alter the pharmacology of highly protein-bound agents.** Substances that reduce protein binding are free fatty acids, maternal steroids, and sulfonamides. Another factor in protein binding is its relation to the volume of distribution. Agents that are poorly protein bound have a larger apparent volume of distribution since they are soluble fractions. **If the free drug is more able to penetrate the tissues, a reduction in plasma protein binding causes an increase in the apparent volume of distribution, and this partially explains the large volume of distribution frequently found in neonates.** For example, nearly twice as much barbiturate and morphine is bound in the neonatal CNS at least in part due to reduced plasma protein binding in neonates.[30] Plasma protein binding also may have a significant effect on determination of blood-gas and blood-tissue partition coefficients and may in part underlie the developmental changes seen in these, which lead to developmental differences in uptake and distribution of anesthetics.[17]

The developmental changes of blood flow to various tissue compartments and body fluid composition not surprisingly cause differences in drug distribution with increasing age. Distribution is altered by the relatively small muscle mass and fat stores in neonates, which results in greater flow to the central organs such as the liver, brain, blood, heart, and kidneys. For example, water-soluble drugs may require a larger initial dose to achieve the desired blood levels. This is relevant for most antibiotics and, most notably, for succinylcholine. The increased volume of distribution may also have an effect on clearance, causing delayed excretion and delayed metabolism, and prolonged half-lives. A further effect of change in body composition is seen with regard to fat-soluble drugs. For example, drugs that rely on redistribution into fat for the termination of their therapeutic effects, such as thiopental, may have a more prolonged clinical effect in younger children. Those that redistribute into muscle, such as narcotics, may also have a prolonged effect.[48]

Other factors may alter the uptake and distribution of anesthetic agents. First is the change in the blood-brain barrier that occurs perinatally.[105] **The integrity of the blood-brain barrier is generally reported to be immature at birth.** Since many anesthetic drugs are lipid soluble, this may lead to a more rapid uptake of anesthetic agents by the neonatal CNS than occurs in the adult. In addition, the proportion of blood flow to the brain is much higher in the neonate than in the adult, and, for highly lipid-soluble drugs, diffusion across the blood-brain barrier will lead to higher brain concentrations in neonates compared with adults and a larger apparent volume of distribution. A second factor that may affect uptake of anesthetic agents arises from differences in dose-response relationships, which may be due to receptor affinities, changes in receptor density, and/or sensitivity with age. For example, with uptake and distribution taken into account, the MAC of inhalational anesthetics, the hypnotic dose of thiopental, and the sensitivity to succinylcholine all have age-related differences that can be explained by potential differences in receptor sensitivity to these agents.

The termination of a drug's effect depends on distribution, metabolism, and excretion. Distribution, as shown previously, varies dramatically with age. Drug metabolism and the enzyme systems responsible, especially cytochrome p450 and hepatic conjugation, also undergo distinct developmental changes.[30,85] Finally, the developmental differences in renal function may also have an effect on the clearance and termination of drug effects.

Myriad developmental differences and multiple factors varying significantly with age determine the uptake, distribution, metabolism, and excretion of anesthetic agents. It is therefore not surprising that there is no simple relationship between age and a dose calculated on a mg/kg basis. For this reason, the effects of various specific agents are discussed where appropriate in other chapters.

PRINCIPLES GUIDING PREOPERATIVE EVALUATION AND PREPARATION

Evaluating and preparing children for anesthesia and surgery requires a specialized approach because of the unique physiologic and psychologic needs of children and their families. The same basic goals of preoperative evaluation that must be achieved in adults are also applicable to children, but, in addition, the emotional and psychologic needs of not only the child but the child's family must be addressed. Familiarity with the specific perioperative needs of children and their families is necessary for the anesthesiologist to obtain an appropriate history, physical examination, and thorough preoperative evaluation from a wailing infant, a hyperactive child, or a shy, frightened 5-year-old, without undue trauma for all concerned. In these situations, although it may be difficult, it is necessary to thoroughly evaluate children. Therefore understanding the physiology and psychology of children is absolutely necessary.

Purpose

The two goals of preoperative evaluation are: (1) for the anesthesiologist to obtain, through interview history and physical examination of the patient, information pertinent to the child's physiologic and emotional preparedness for surgery, and (2) for the patient, to allay the anxieties of both the child and parent and prepare them for surgery. Both of these goals are important and should be viewed as necessarily compatible in the anesthetic management of children. From the outset, both goals should be constantly kept in mind (Box 26-1).

The anesthesiologist's first contact with the child and family necessarily sets the stage for the remainder of the anesthesia management. The information obtained and the interactions that occur during the preoperative evaluation will determine the quality of the intraoperative management and the postoperative recovery. Although this is obvious when evaluating the physiologic status of the child, which will be used to guide the choice of preoperative medication, induction agent, and anesthetic maintenance as well as the postoperative requirements, it is likewise true for addressing the emotional and psychologic needs of both the child and family. Not only should the preoperative evaluation familiarize the anesthesiologist with the child and the parents, but it should also provide an excellent and critical opportunity for the child and family to become comfortable with the anesthesiologist and to understand his/her responsibilities. The preconceived notions of children and their families about the events that will occur in the perioperative period and the personnel with whom they will interact form the background for the preoperative interview. The skilled and experienced anesthesiologist will be aware of these preconceptions and address them whether or not they are mentioned by the child or the family. This anticipatory approach to the child's needs will frequently smooth the path for induction and emergence from anesthesia for the

child, the family and, not unimportantly, the anesthesiologist.

The key to smooth anesthetic management is not only the complete familiarity of the anesthesiologist with the child's medical and psycho-emotional background but also the child's and family's understanding of the procedures associated with anesthesia and surgery. A comfortable, competent anesthesiologist, familiar with all aspects of the perioperative course of surgery in children should be able to optimize this experience for all concerned. This approach applies to infants or older children and to inpatients or outpatients. The exact setting and the child's unique characteristics will determine the specific technique for dealing with each individual circumstance. Whereas it may be necessary in one case to separate the child from the family early and use significant preoperative sedation, in another, parental presence during induction and emergence may be the optimal approach. The knowledge and experience of the anesthesiologist in determining which approach is best for which child are important.

The first objective of preoperative evaluation and preparation is to assure that the child is in his/her optimal status for the procedure planned. The mere question of whether the child can tolerate the anesthetic and surgery has become less relevant today. Pediatric anesthesiologists are quite capable of providing the most advanced physiologic support in virtually any circumstance for children who require complex surgery. It is almost always possible to provide monitored critical care and analgesia for any surgical procedure. What will vary from patient to patient is not the ability of the anesthesiologist to deliver anesthesia care and assure survival but the risk to the child for each set of circumstances. The all-important question of whether the anesthetic and surgical risk to the child is greater than the benefits of the procedure in question must be addressed. Today, concerns of survival are largely replaced by a precise, accurate, and clear evaluation of the risks of anesthesia for each individual child, which can then be realistically compared with the child's surgical needs. The **underlying goal is that for each child, given the circumstances, the best possible preoperative status will be attained for the procedure.** Clearly, this varies tremendously if the child is undergoing decompression of an epidural hematoma after a traffic accident in which he/she has sustained bilateral femoral fractures, a ruptured spleen, pulmonary contusion, and intracranial injury with very little time for preoperative assessment as compared with myringotomy in a child with Down syndrome and a recently diagnosed atrioventricular canal defect who also happens to be wheezing. Certainly both of these children can be anesthetized and are likely to survive

---

BOX 26-1
PURPOSES OF PREOPERATIVE EVALUATION
Prepare the anesthesiologist Prepare the child and family

BOX 26-2
PREPARATION FOR SURGERY

Goal

Optimal physical and mental status for surgery

Contingencies

Medical judgment
Optimization of medical therapy
Timing
Psychoprophylaxis of child and family

BOX 26-3
SOURCES OF PARENTAL ANXIETY

Anesthesia complications

Brain damage
Death

Results of surgery

Disfigurement
Dismemberment
Death

Separation, loss of control

Hostility generated by

Poor information and communication
Apparent lack of due concern

---

at least the anesthetic; however, the wisdom of immediately proceeding varies considerably based on the analysis of the specific risk/benefit relationship.

It is the anesthesiologist's responsibility to ensure that an accurate assessment of the risks and benefits of the anesthesia is as clear as possible to the child, the parents, the surgeon, and the pediatrician. Careful attention to these details is essential in evaluating and preparing children for anesthesia. Questions of preoperative preparation, timing of surgery, specific surgical procedure to undertake, and anesthetic plan are all within the anesthesiologist's purview. These should be addressed by the anesthesiologist in the preoperative evaluation. A thorough and adequate evaluation of the child is essential for identifying and predicting not only physiologic but also psychologic and emotional problems that the child may encounter intraoperatively and postoperatively.[15] The anesthesiologist, armed with this extensive background information, can provide the best intraoperative care and advise on postoperative management (Box 26-2).

General Approach
Preconceptions

It is essential to understand some of the preconceived notions that the child and family may have acquired from society and the surgeon. Virtually all parents think that anesthesia is a source of some risk to their child; the spectrum may vary from fear of postoperative nausea, vomiting, headaches, and behavioral disturbances to fear of a significant threat to the child's life. These notions are almost always present. To recognize, inquire about, and address these issues is important because these preconceptions frequently differ from the anesthesiologist's view.

Whereas the anesthesiologist may view an ASA I child for a unilateral myringotomy as being at extremely low risk and very low on the anxiety scale, parents do not necessarily always appreciate this (Box 26-3). They may frequently demonstrate a parental "moro response" to any perceived threat no matter

how trivial to their child. Any threat to their child may naturally trigger defensive and protective responses and significant levels of anxiety in families. The underlying concerns and anxieties experienced by parents of children undergoing what, to us, may be quite routine surgery frequently do not qualitatively differ from those of parents whose children have been admitted to the pediatric intensive care unit. Although we may consider this parental response inappropriate, it is nevertheless important for us to recognize that the parents of a child undergoing routine surgery may be terribly concerned for their child's well-being. A sympathetic and understanding approach to this parental response is a crucial ingredient of expert management. Ensuring calm, informed, confident parents is frequently the most essential aspect of ensuring calm, cooperative children. Terrified, nervous, defensive, angry, ill-informed parents will be virtually incapable of allaying their child's anxieties for the upcoming procedure.

Areas of childhood anxiety

Childhood anxieties in the perioperative period center on five areas (Box 26-4).[15] The first, fear of injury, is universal; fear of death (even for minor procedures) is often present. Most obviously, fear of pain and the potential for resulting body disfigurement is commonplace. Second, fear of parental separation (separation anxiety) is common in children over 6 months of age and can still be an overriding concern in adolescents. Common sense dictates that the less time the conscious child is separated from the parents the better this is for all concerned. Apart from obvious humanitarian concerns, a calm, comfortable, nonscreaming child is both more aesthetic physiologically and is better able to tolerate anesthesia and surgery than a

---

BOX 26-4
SOURCES OF CHILDHOOD ANXIETY

Fear of pain, injury, and death
Fear of parental separation
Fear of loss of autonomy
Fear of the unknown
Fear of punishment

---

distraught child.[94] The third area of anxiety that correlates with the developmental stage of separation-individuation concerns fears centered on the loss of individuality and autonomy, which may be a source of considerable stress in children. Taking a child who has spent several years learning to walk, who is comfortable away from his/her parents only for short times, and who has independent control of major functions, and suddenly reducing the child to lying on his/her back, surrounded by giants, with no control of the situation whatsoever, clearly can provoke a significant degree of anxiety. Along with this threatened loss of autonomy is the threatened loss of function and loss of control that has been so recently won. Anything that can be done to encourage and enhance the child's autonomy and control of the situation, such as allowing choices; for example, position (sitting, lying, standing), method of induction, which stuffed animal to bring to the operating room, or color of gown, can go a long way in calming the child's fears.

The fourth issue is simply fear of the unknown. Children are often intimidated by the new. Most children will not have undergone either anesthesia or surgery in the past, and this in and of itself generates a great deal of anxiety. Recognition of this issue, followed by frank, honest, and as complete a disclosure as possible of the procedures and occurrences that the child will be required to experience is necessary. The child's knowledge reduces the dark, mysterious areas of ignorance and uncertainty. The phrases "it won't hurt" or, "you have nothing to worry about," can well be some of the most anxiety-provoking words an anesthesiologist can utter. The child knows it is not true and suspects a cover-up.

The final area, and perhaps the least obvious, is the child's fear of breaching behavioral standards and eliciting from authority figures, including parents, a reprimand. The fear of transgression and punishment is a characteristic underlying anxiety of childhood (and frequently extends into adulthood) and may be a major source of concern to the child. Explaining the permissibility of crying appropriately, of expressing anxiety and fear about the procedures, and of having

a negative attitude toward the procedure, and thus validating the child's emotions will decrease the anxiety associated with this particular area of childhood concern.

In general, these areas should be constantly remembered and consciously addressed by the anesthesiologist in his/her approach toward the child.[39] Openness, honesty, and cheerful confidence are the main tools for allaying child and family anxieties and in producing a setting that is most conducive to obtaining information, both by history and by physical examination. Children are quite capable of seeing through fraud and spotting lack of confidence. Once their trust has been lost, the ability to provide them with the best of anesthesia care has also been lost. Honestly telling a child that an IV start may be unsuccessful and will be painful is preferable to saying "it won't hurt" and then repeating this painful procedure unsuccessfully several times. Spending the extra time to gently talk a child through a mask inhalational induction may frequently be more rewarding (although more time consuming) for the child, the parent, and the anesthesologist, than walking into the room and with little preparation, jabbing a needle in the child's thigh. Developing the skills necessary to approach children and their families greatly increases the facility with which the anesthesiologist may provide the best of anesthesia care and increases the rewards of anesthesia practice.[78]

Developmental stage

Just as an adult approach is inappropriate for the child, so is an approach that does not take account the developmental stage of the child. The anesthesiologist's approach to a 6-month-old infant will be quite different from the approach taken with a 14-year-old pubertal adolescent. In general, developmental stage determines approach (Table 26-6).

Newborn and infants less than six months old. Probably because the infant and newborn are unable to express themselves, it has been long assumed that the psychologic ramifications of separation and surgery are minimal. This assumption is just as erroneous as the assumption by earlier medical practitioners that infants were unable to feel pain. Just as we now know the latter is untrue, it is just as likely that there are ramifications of separation for surgery. Although young children do not have the apparent adverse responses to strangers that are seen in older children (greater than 6 months of age) and can be comforted by a nurse or physician, they unquestionably recognize their mother and are comforted by her presence.[49] Therefore it is judicious to minimize the amount of time the child is separated from the parent. For this age group, although direct psychologic preparation of the child is not possible, parental

Table 26-6 Developmental behavior

Age	Stage	Characteristics
0-6 months	Infantile	No expression Passivity Dependence
9 mo-5 yr	Separation Individuation	Communicative Separation anxiety Poor reality per- ception Developing inde- pendence
5 yr-adolescent	Childhood	Imaginative ratio- nale Self-focused Fearful Limited expres- siveness

preparation can form the basis of the approach to the newborn and young infant. Experience indicates that fretful, anxious, uptight parents frequently convey this attitude even to their young infants. Thus psychologic preparation should be directed toward the child's family. Most parents know how sensitive their child is and perceive him/her as quite delicate, especially when under threat by modern medicine. They know that anesthesia and surgery present a threat to an adult and thus reason that surely this is much greater for a frail infant. Specifically addressing this frequent, although false, assumption and pointing out that a robust infant undergoing routine surgery is more likely to recover rapidly from the stress of surgery and anesthesia than a grandparent, or indeed a parent, is important. Frequently such information can alleviate anxiety and remarkably calm the parents, who in turn calm the infant.

Seven months to five years. With older infants and preschool children between approximately 9 months and 5 years of age, a difficult stage has been reached. They are quite aware of their environment and surroundings, are able to perceive a threat, and can remember painful experiences quite well. Unfortunately this is combined with inability to reason and a poor perception of reality. Although they are able to recognize stressful situations, they are unable to express their fears by modes of communication other than crying, regressive behaviors, sullen withdrawal, or other nonspecific responses to stressful situations.[22] Although it may not be possible to determine exactly what is most disturbing to a child, attention to the areas mentioned previously and a specific explanation can somewhat alleviate their concerns. There is value

in explaining what is going to happen and in familiarizing the child with the procedure, even though he/she may not appear to be receptive. If this has no other benefit than to demonstrate the anesthesiologist's concern for the child's well-being to the parents, it is well worthwhile. They can then in turn express to the child what is going on.

Five years to adolescence. This developmental stage of childhood is characterized by an increasing capability of expression and the ability to reason. Gaining control over behavioral and emotional responses is one of the major tasks of this period. The ability to understand and trust adults, even strangers, generally develops during this time. Disclosure of anesthetic procedures and careful, honest, compassionate explanation of events that surround surgery will generally be rewarded in this age group. Again, explaining to the child and parents the anesthesiologist's role and what will be happening, as well as what the child can expect during the perioperative period, goes a long way in decreasing anxiety. In this age group, and throughout adolescence, the child's imagination is well developed. Frequently this imagination, aided and abetted by exposure to the hyperkinetic modern media (television), can lead to vivid and distorted anticipation of what actually goes on inside an operating room. As much realistic exposure to personnel, equipment, methods of dress, procedures, and explanation as possible before the procedure may drive some of these vivid, preconceived, and frequently terrifying notions from the child's (as well as the parents') minds.[73] It is often very informative to ask the child what he/she anticipates, and, if one is fortunate enough to have a communicative child, this may be well worthwhile.

In older children and adolescents, an underlying fear is that of death. This may be reinforced by well-meaning parents, friends, adults, and even medical personnel. For example, saying that the child "will be put to sleep" or the anesthesiologist's reference to "getting him down" may be counterproductive. Unfortunately, these statements may remind little Johnny of what happened to "Bowzer." In adolescence the fear of death can be quite strong, and this, coupled with the loss of control and autonomy that must accompany anesthesia, frequently worries children and teenagers. Talking expectantly and openly about the postoperative period is worthwhile. Discussing how the child will feel and what steps will be taken to wake him/her up and to relieve pain, will confidently lead the child away from any notion that he/she will not wake up after surgery.

A "macho" attitude in teenagers may lead them to be trapped in silence with their fears. In dealing with adolescents, it is therefore worthwhile to specifically ask if the young adult has any fears and specifically ask if there is concern about pain and dying. The frequency with which these questions are answered in the affirmative is quite revealing. Understanding these underlying anxieties and specifically, honestly, and openly addressing them is valuable and certainly rewards the small amount of time required to do it.

Preoperative Psychologic Preparation

Psychologic preoperative preparation begins for the child even before coming to the hospital. Clearly informing the parents that they should explain openly and honestly to the child what is about to occur begins the psychologic preparation at home. Honesty and an open demeanor cannot be overemphasized as the cornerstones of this reassurance.[39,78,94] What will occur with the child should be truthfully discussed with the parents. Many hospitals have programs for both inpatients and outpatients designed to introduce the child and family to the hospital and operative setting in an enjoyable manner. There are many alternatives for accomplishing these goals, including a preoperative film, a puppet show, a coloring book, a tour of the hospital, or a friendly meeting with doctors and nurses.[39,49] Selecting from these options is not as important as implementing a program to ensure that the child's association with the hospital or surgical center begins on a positive note. This provides a significant contribution to the preoperative preparation of children. Younger children and, indeed, occasionally older children should be encouraged to

bring familiar things to the hospital. They should bring their stuffed animals and their own pajamas, arrive in their own clothes, and be allowed to retain them as long as possible. Comforting, familiar books and toys should certainly be encouraged. The parents should be reminded of the importance of this. With older children, encouraging them to be involved in the planning of the surgery can also be quite beneficial. Allowing them to participate in selecting the time of surgery and participating in the planning process can do a lot to raise the young adult's spirits.

At all times during the preoperative evaluation, it must be remembered that the evaluation is a two-way street. Not only does the medical establishment (whether it is a nurse, nurse practitioner, or anesthesiologist) gain information pertinent to the anesthetic management of the child, but the child and family gain information that is useful for confidence-building and anxiolysis about the anesthesiologist and hospital setting. It is useful to remember that throughout the interview with the family, the child is the center of attention. The battle may already be lost with both parent and child if the anesthesiologist interacts only with the parent to obtain information about the child, tells the parent the procedure, and leaves the room. The initial contact should be made with the child, with a cheerful greeting and an attempt made to win his/her confidence before beginning the medical interview (Fig. 26-7). Assuring the child that the main intent is not to inflict injury but to get to know him/her

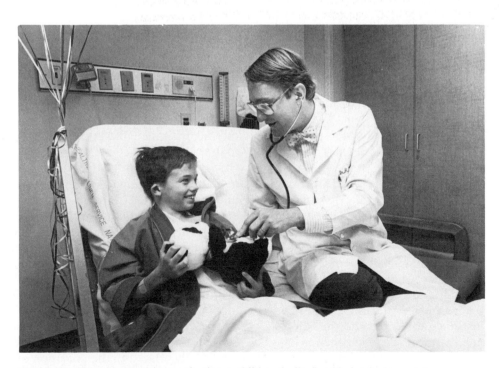

Fig. 26-7. Time invested in comforting a child and allaying his intrinsic anxiety ensures a smooth preoperative evaluation as well as a smooth induction of anesthesia.

is crucial. No one will appreciate this more than the parents. Making it clear to the child and family that the anesthesiologist takes the child's procedure as seriously as the child does and is there to help, not only during the painful times but also during the anxiety-provoking times, is very beneficial. Explanations of how the child will awaken and what will be done to manage pain are well worthwhile.

PREOPERATIVE EVALUATION

Just as psycho-emotional preoperative preparation of the child should begin before the anesthesiologist meets the child, the anesthesiologist also should have prepared before the meeting. The anesthesiologist should be familiar with the surgery that the child requires, the surgeon's needs, and the anesthetic implications of the surgical procedure. In addition to this, the anesthesiologist should be as familiar as possible with the child's medical background as documented in the medical records. Communication with the pediatrician and surgeon before meeting the child and family will reveal areas of particular interest to the anesthesiologist before the interview. In addition, an anesthesiologist who is aware of the child's name, age, general background, medical problems, and surgical procedure, and who has communicated with the child's pediatrician and surgeon, is in a strong position to win the confidence of the child and family. In the case of an extensive previous medical history, it is well worthwhile reviewing old records. Specific attention should be directed to the presence of congenital anomalies and pediatric syndromes that may be associated wtih anomalies that are entirely unrelated to the surgery but that could complicate the anesthetic management. In addition, a review of the drug and allergy history from the chart may provide information critically important to the anesthetic management.

Finally, if there have been any previous anesthetic procedures, careful review of these records may provide an opportunity to improve anesthetic management. Specifically noting whether premedication was necessary, its effect when given, the response to various anesthetic agents, airway management, and emergence may be particularly useful. There may be obvious information on this record the anesthesiologist wishes to have before speaking to the parents. For example, if the child, after what appeared to be a minor procedure, was intubated and ventilated in the ICU for 3 days, the parents would be, not surprisingly, somewhat skeptical should the anesthesiologist be unaware of this. Unnecessarily repeating this sequence would be unacceptable.

It may well be worth discussing areas of concern with the surgeon and the child's physicians before meeting the family so the family can have the most complete information possible at the time of the preoperative assessment. When meeting with the family, the anesthesiologist should determine the child's general health, level of activity, interests, toys, background, and significant mental and medical condition. Knowledge of the parents' nickname for the child may be useful during emergence. Finding out which fingers or thumb the child sucks to guide IV placement may make the difference between a calm patient and an inconsolable patient postoperatively.

A systems review of appropriate depth is always indicated. In addition, a history of both current and recent drugs and a history of allergies should be completed in all cases. Specific questioning about previous anesthetics and a history of siblings or family members who have had prolonged awakening, canceled surgery in the operating room, intraoperative cardiorespiratory catastrophes, or unexplained fevers should be specifically sought in each case. Frequently no one else will have asked questions concerning potential drug allergies, malignant hyperthermia, or adverse anesthetic reactions before this time. Relying solely on the chart or physical examination of the child to reflect these specific anesthetic concerns is a risky and unacceptable practice.

Physical Examination

The examination of the child should begin as soon as the physician enters the room. During the time spent obtaining the history from the parents and where appropriate from the child, important observations can be made. In addition, this period is invaluable for establishing rapport with the child and family. Constant efforts to gain the child's confidence, for example, by getting down to his/her level (sitting down is necessary, Fig. 26-8), offering a toy, or interacting with the child, are of tremendous help. While discussing the child with the family, attempting to interact with the child and thus desensitizing him/her to the close presence of the anesthesiologist is critical. Briskly walking into the room, interrogating the mother, and turning to the child will not yield optimal information from the physical examination. On the other hand, interacting with, humoring, reassuring, and playing with the child during the interview will not only calm the child but may also provide valuable information regarding the child's general health status, respiratory condition, level of activity, state of hydration and perfusion, and level of anxiety concerning hospitalization.

The examination of the child falls into three areas: (1) general health and systems examination, (2) areas specifically related to the provision of anesthesia, and (3) areas related to surgery. Clearly the physical examination will be guided by the findings in the

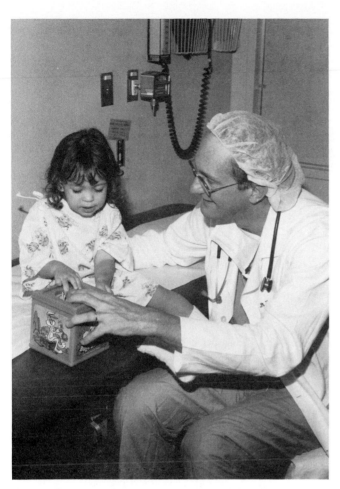

Fig. 26-8. The preoperative evaluation. Play can create a comfortable, friendly atmosphere for the examination.

history and interview and the needs of the surgical procedure. As mentioned previously, the examination begins when the anesthesiologist first meets the child. A great deal can be learned about the patient's perfusion, hemodynamic status, and respiratory status by general observation. Determining the child's growth and weight (e.g., short stature, failure to thrive) are essential as they will guide anesthetic management and may indicate the necessity for closer evaluation (Figs. 26-9 to 26-12).

The airway can be assessed by observing phonation, inspiratory sounds, and respiratory rate; evidence of respiratory distress, such as retractions or tachypnea, can be readily noted without interfering with the child. In addition, coughs, runny noses, and upper respiratory tract infections can be detected without hands-on examination of the child. With specific regard to airway evaluation, determining presence of airway anomalies, such as cleft lip or palate, large tonsils, the state of the child's dentition, loose teeth, or absent teeth is also essential. A small

jaw or a skeletal anomaly that may indicate associated difficult intubation should be noted. It is quite possible to obtain a fairly comprehensive impression of the child's overall status without actually having to physically examine the child.

Familiarity with the surgical procedure is also necessary. The anesthesiologist should have a fair idea of how extensive the surgery is going to be, whether it will affect airway management, what sort of blood loss to expect, and if there are any particular complicating factors concerning anesthesia. Concerns about positioning and duration of surgery should be addressed. The presence of a cystic hygroma, for example, should dictate meticulous examination of the airway, auscultation for upper airway sounds, and determining if any airway involvement may have occurred. Discovery of capillary hemangiomas may also indicate the need to rule out airway involvement.

Systems review

Neuromuscular system. Much will be apparent about the developmental stage of the child's nervous system during the initial contact. Conversely, assessment of anesthetically relevant neurologic conditions will depend on the child's age and developmental status. **Familiarity with the developmental milestones of children** will give the anesthesiologist a background on which to assess the child (Fig. 26-13). There is a wide spectrum of neuromuscular disorders that accompanies various childhood conditions and are of importance to the anesthesiologist. In all children information concerning **mental and developmental stage, gestational age, gross motor function, presence of a seizure disorder, and any pre-existing neurologic sensory deficits should be sought.**

CEREBRAL PALSY/MENTAL RETARDATION. A common problem in children who present for surgery for either multiple congenital anomalies or complications after prematurity is mental retardation and/or cerebral palsy. It should be stressed that not all children with cerebral palsy, even those with severe neuromuscular involvement, are mentally retarded. Incapacitating hypertonicity and spasticity, which may render a child unable to readily express himself/herself, do not necessarily interfere with the ability of the child to understand or the anesthesiologist's responsibility to inform the child about the course of the perioperative period. **The anesthetic implications of mental retardation and cerebral palsy are legion.** The response to a host of anesthetic drugs, including muscle relaxants, sedatives, analgetics, and hypnotics, vary and are far less predictable in these children compared with healthy children. In older children with mental retardation and cerebral palsy there may also be significant **pulmonary** complications. These may arise from musculoskeletal anomalies caused by imbalance of

Text continued on p. 465.

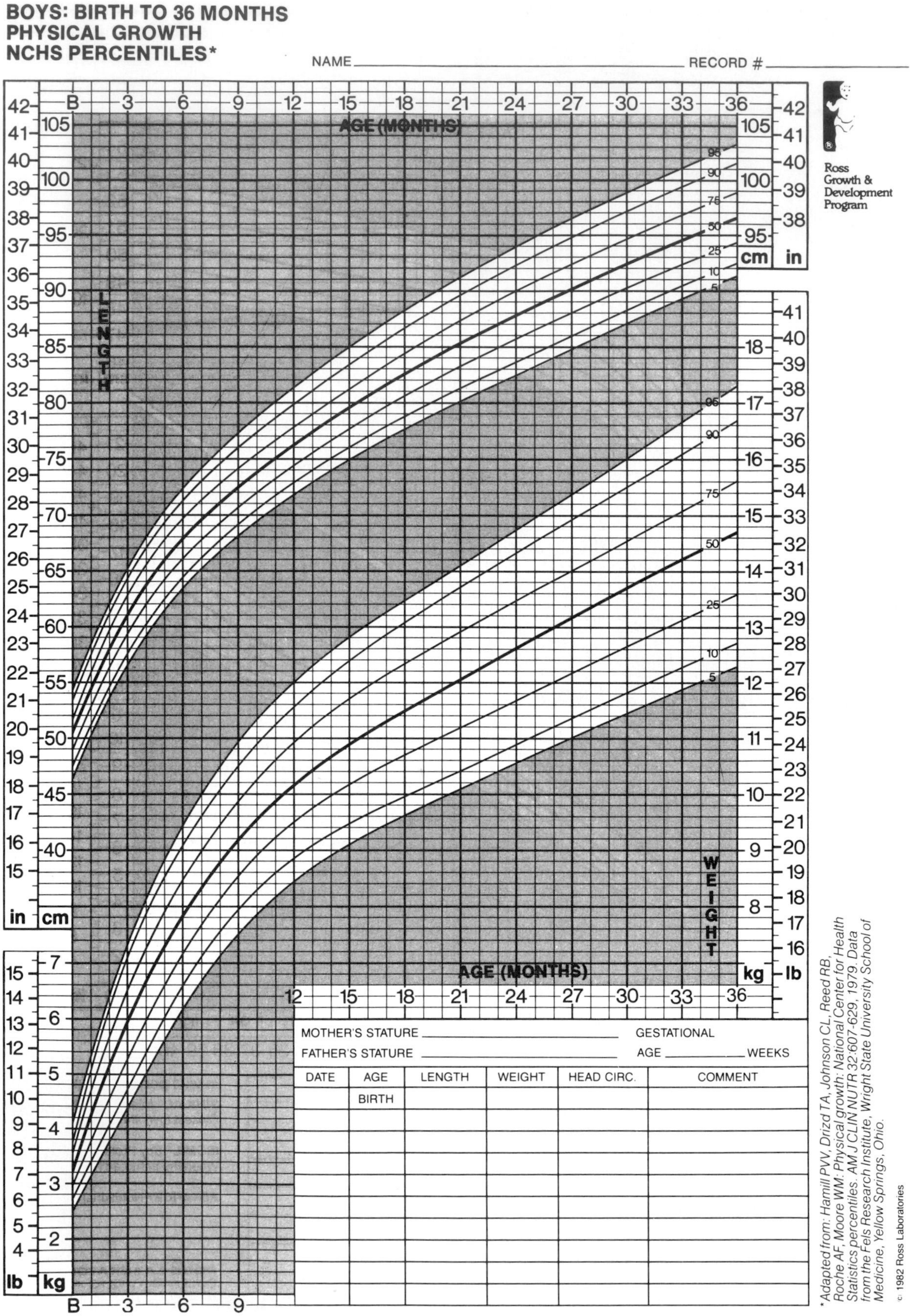

Fig. 26-9. Standard growth curves for both length and weight for newborn to 36-month-old boys. (Courtesy Ross Laboratories, 1982.)

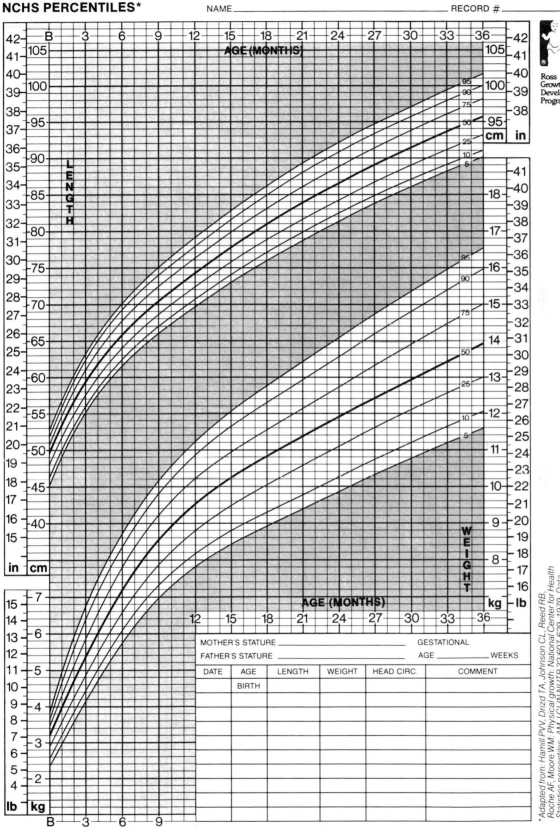

GIRLS: BIRTH TO 36 MONTHS
PHYSICAL GROWTH
NCHS PERCENTILES*

Fig. 26-10. Standard growth curves for both length and weight for newborn to 36-month-old girls. (Courtesy Ross Laboratories, 1982.)

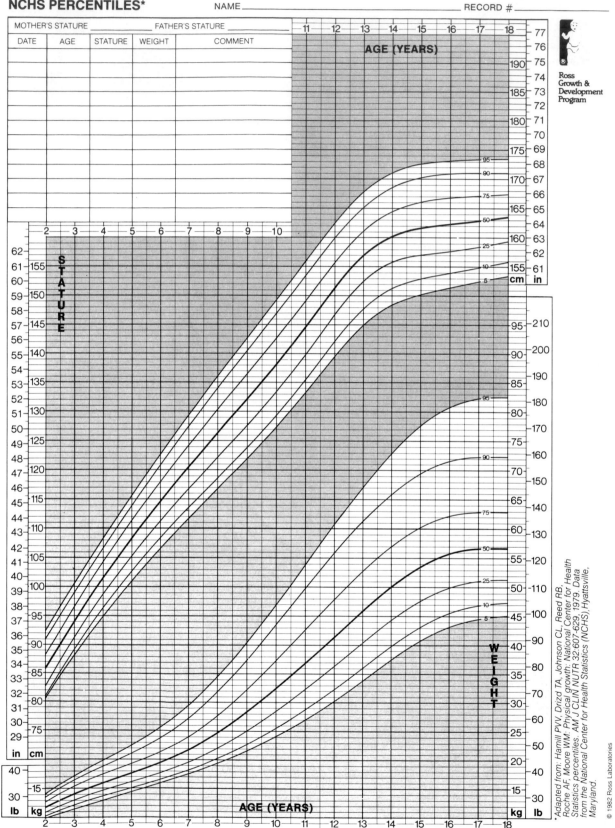

GIRLS: 2 TO 18 YEARS PHYSICAL GROWTH NCHS PERCENTILES*

Fig. 26-11. Standard growth curves for both height and weight for girls 2 to 18 years of age. (Courtesy Ross Laboratories, 1982.)

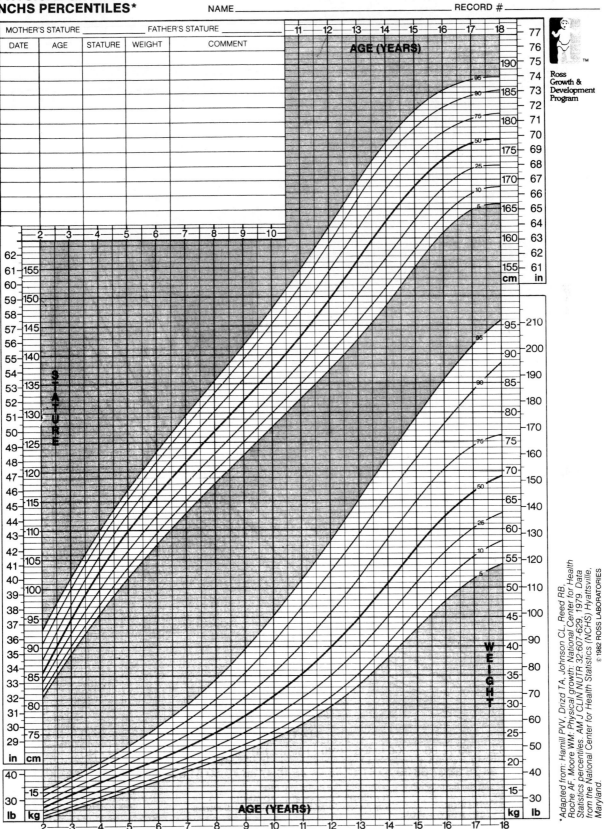

Fig. 26-12. Standard growth curves for both height and weight for boys 2 to 18 years of age. (Courtesy Ross Laboratories, 1982.)

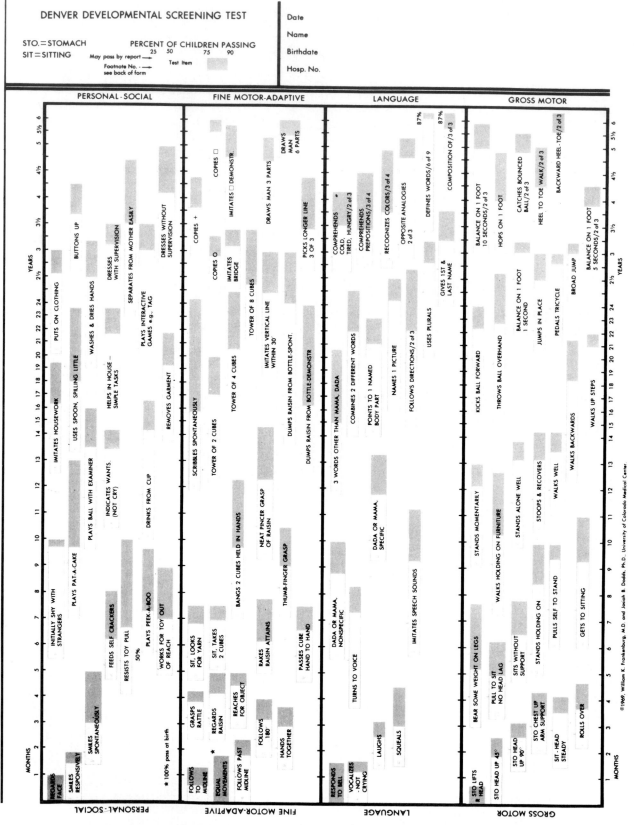

Fig. 26-13. Denver Developmental Screening Test serves as a guide to the development of language, motor, and social skills of children from 1 month to 6 years of age. (Copyright Frankenberg WK and Dodds JB, University of Colorado Medical Center, 1969.)

muscle groups, resulting in **scoliosis** and **kyphosis and leading to restrictive lung pathology.** In addition, **pharyngeal discoordination** and **difficulty with handling secretions,** as well as the not infrequent association of **gastroesophageal reflux** in children with mental retardation and cerebral palsy can lead to **recurrent, chronic pulmonary parenchymal injury,** which may complicate the anesthetic management. The presence of gastroesophageal reflux should always be sought, as it is frequent in this patient population. This may have particular relevance to the NPO precautions and may even indicate the need for histamine receptor (H_2) antagonism, antacids, agents that hasten gastric emptying, and rapid sequence intubation. **Specific questioning about gastroesophageal reflux, recurrent aspiration, recurrent pneumonias, and wheezing** should be directed toward the parents, and the anesthetic altered accordingly.

SEIZURE DISORDERS. Children with a history of epilepsy or seizure disorders are also of concern perioperatively. In the past, problems have resulted from a failure to maintain adequate anticonvulsant levels in the perioperative period. Most oral anticonvulsants can be given on the morning of surgery and have a sufficiently long half-life to assure adequate levels intraoperatively. Sodium valproate and carbamazepine may be exceptions. **It is incumbent on the anesthesiologist to ensure that the optimal serum levels of anticonvulsants are achieved preoperatively and that these are maintained perioperatively.** If a prolonged NPO status postoperatively is anticipated, alteration of anticonvulsant therapy preoperatively may be indicated to include agents that can be given parenterally. A consultation with the child's pediatrician or pediatric neurologist may be required. Obviously preoperative awareness of the child's epilepsy should lead to **avoiding epileptogenic anesthetic agents such as methohexital, ethrane, and possibly etomidate.**

INTRACRANIAL HYPERTENSION. The management of anesthesia for children with intracranial hypertension requires special care. Recognition of the **classic triad of hypertension, bradycardia, and apnea** in children who may require neurosurgical procedures or ventricular peritoneal shunts, or who have suffered acute head injury is crucial in determining the anesthetic management of these children. In addition, **in younger children with chronically elevated intracranial hypertension, the need for perioperative management of intracranial pressure is indicated by complaints of nausea, vomiting, headache, irritability, lethargy, and finding on physical examination of the sunsetting sign.** Careful questioning for an acute change in the child's status may indicate the need preoperatively for measures directed at decreasing intracranial pressure, such as diuresis and osmolar

therapy. In addition, intraoperative use of hyperventilation and barbiturates would be wise.

If the child has an existing decompressive shunt, the anesthesiologist should be aware of this. If it contains a valve and pump mechanism, it should be evaluated to assure that it is functioning. Perioperative fluid shifts may alter CSF function and upset the balance of CSF production and drainage, leading to elevated intracranial pressure and perioperative catastrophe, especially in the anesthetized child. For this reason, **assurance of shunt patency and functional history is necessary.**

MUSCULAR DYSTROPHY. Congenital neuromuscular disease, such as muscular dystrophy, and acquired diseases, such as myositis, dermatomyositis, and collagen vascular diseases, raise questions concerning the use of muscle relaxants. Clearly in patients with myotonic dystrophy, the use of succinylcholine should be avoided.[62] This is less clear in some of the muscular dystrophies; however, the occurrence of rhabdomyolysis and the suspicion of an increased incidence of malignant hyperthermia in patients with Duchenne's muscular dystrophy suggest caution in the use of depolarizing muscle relaxants and inhalational anesthetics in children with muscular dystrophy.[60] The use of nondepolarizing muscle relaxants in children who have muscle weakness and neuromuscular impairment clearly should be guided by meticulous perioperative monitoring and perhaps are best avoided whenever possible (Box 26-5).

The majority of neurologic deficits and impairments will be obvious from review of the patient's record, the parents' interview, and observation of the child. If detailed neurologic examination and docu-

---

BOX 26-5
NEUROMUSCULAR DISEASE IN WHICH NEUROMUSCULAR AGENTS SHOULD BE USED WITH CAUTION

Muscular dystrophy
   Facioscapulohumeral
   Duchenne's

Myasthenia gravis
   Eaton-Lambert (very rare)

Cerebral palsy

Myotonias
   Myotonia congenita

Spinal muscle atrophy
   Spina bifida (thoracic level)

Table 26-7 Common syndromes associated with difficult intubation

Syndrome	Airway	Associated anomalies
Achondroplasia	Small nares and mouth	Hydrocephalus
	Midface hypoplasia	Atlantoaxial instability
	Megacephaly	Atropine sensitivity
Apert	Narrow, occasionally cleft palate	Mental retardation
	Small maxilla	Cardiac anomalies
	Craniosynostosis	Renal anomalies
	Flat facies	Syndactyly, often severe
Arthrogryposis congenita	Small mandible	Scoliosis
	Cleft palate	VSD
	Torticollis, contracture	
	Klippel-Feil syndrome	
Beckwith-Wiedemann	Large tongue	Retardation
	Prognathism	Hypoglycemia
		Exomphalos
		Gigantism
Cornelia de Lange	Micrognathia	Cardiac anomalies
	Short neck	Retardation
	Cleft palate	
	Mandibular spurs	
Crouzon	Small maxilla	Proptosis
	Large tongue	
	Craniosynostosis	
Down	Large tongue	Cardiac
	Small mouth	Atlantoaxial instability
	Small mandible	Hypotonia
Goldenhar	Small mandible and zygoma	Cervical spine defects
	Cleft palate	
	Macrostomia	
Congenital hypothyroidism	Large tongue	Hypothermia
		Retardation, if untreated
		Umbilical hernia
Freeman-Sheldon (whistling face)	Very small mouth	Scoliosis
	High palate	
Klippel-Feil	Short neck, limited extension	Deafness
		Ventricular septal defect (VSD)
Marfan	Narrow face	Cardiac anomalies
	Narrow palate	Scoliosis
		Restrictive lung disease
Möbius	Small mandible	Talipes equinovarus
	Small mouth	Ptosis
	Aspiration	Cranial nerve palsies
Mucopolysaccharidosis	Large tongue	Cardiac anomalies
	Narrow airway	
	Limited opening	
Pierre-Robin	Micrognathia	
Robinow	Small mouth	Hemivertebra
	Micrognathia	Hypertelorism
	Crowded teeth	Atrial septal defect (ASD)
	Large tongue	
Rubinstein-Taybi	Small maxilla	Retardation
	Narrow palate	Cardiac anomalies
		Cervical instability

Data from Smith DW: *Recognizable patterns of human malformation: genetic, embryologic and clinical aspects,* ed 2, Philadelphia, 1976, WB Saunders.

Table 26-7   Common syndromes associated with difficult intubation—cont'd

Syndrome	Airway	Associated anomalies
Russell-Silver	Small stature Small mandible	Hypoglycemia
Treacher-Collins	Facial hypoplasia Mandible, maxilla Cleft palate Choanal atresia	Cardiac disease Cervical vertebral anomalies
Turner	Small narrow maxilla, mandible Short neck	Retardation Coarctation Hypertension
Zellweger	Small mandible Short neck	Cardiac Contractures

mentation is required or the presence of serious CNS disease is suspected, a pediatric neurologist should be consulted. With the increasing use of regional anesthesia, it is wise for the anesthesiologist to search for and clearly document existing neurologic deficits before performing nerve blocks.

Respiratory system. A host of illnesses and congenital abnormalities affect respiratory function in children. **Many congenital anomalies are associated with small, difficult-to-visualize airways, upper airway obstruction perioperatively, and difficult intubation.** All of these conditions should be specifically sought and investigated whenever the suspicion arises. **The relatively small diameter of a child's airway and a child's different anatomic makeup, as well as high oxygen consumption relative to FRC, put children at particular risk for developing hypoxia, and therefore the margin of error is less than in adults.** For these reasons, careful assessment of the child's airway and respiratory system is required (Table 26-7).

Specific questioning about airway obstruction such as snoring, recurring episodes of croup, and tonsil or adenoid hypertrophy, as well as seeking a history of apneas, is part of routine history-taking in pediatric anesthesia. Noticing characteristic facies, such as those associated with Treacher-Collins' syndrome, Pierre-Robin syndrome, or Hunter and Hurler mucopolysaccharidosis is an essential skill of the pediatric anesthesiologist in detecting the potential for difficulty with intubation and upper airway obstruction perioperatively. Careful examination of the nares, of the oropharynx for loose teeth, and for the presence of respiratory distress indicating airway obstruction should be part of every examination. Routine attention to these airway issues will prevent potentially lethal complications in the operating room.

Assessment of children with chronic respiratory disease is also necessary. The frequency of chronic lung disease (bronchopulmonary dysplasia, BPD) in premature infants who required ventilatory support in the neonatal period should be remembered.[46] Evidence should be sought for this in the patient's record, as well as by questioning the parents. BPD may range from mild recurrent wheezing to chronic oxygen requirement and even mechanical ventilation at home. **In children with BPD and asthma, the anesthesiologist should be completely familiar with the child's respiratory status and ensure that therapy has been optimized preoperatively.** The child's exact therapy should be understood, and, when possible, an effort should be made to ensure that the appropriate level of bronchodilator therapy has been achieved, with determination of theophylline levels where indicated. A history of recent steroid use should be sought and consideration given to initiating steroid therapy preoperatively.

Particular attention should be directed to the history of **exercise tolerance** in children with, or suspected of having, chronic lung disease. In patients with musculoskeletal disease, especially kyphosis or scoliosis, one should seek evidence of restrictive lung abnormalities. Preoperative adjunctive investigations in children with chronic lung disease may include determination of blood gases and pulmonary function tests. In addition, a cardiac examination with electrocardiogram and possibly echocardiography may be necessary to discover and define the severity of pulmonary hypertension and cor pulmonale.

In general, evidence of acute lung disease should be sought and, when discovered, is an indication for canceling elective surgery. Pneumonia, croup, and acute asthma all pose significant perioperative threats, not only acutely but also after apparent resolution. For example, **airway reactivity is increased for several weeks after an acute asthmatic attack.**[57] Deteriorating pulmonary status due to viral or bacterial infection, superimposed on BPD, cystic fibrosis, or asthma may well cause serious intraoperative hypoxia, increased secretions with the risk of endotracheal tube obstruction, and difficulty in maintaining airway patency. In addition, postoperative atelectasis and pneumonia are serious complications after surgery. Specific questioning about apneas should be included, as these may be associated with fatal postoperative respiratory difficulties.[50]

RUNNY NOSE PROBLEM. Frequently the problem of the child with a runny nose arises. Rhinorrhea can be caused by an acute viral or bacterial upper respiratory tract infection, allergic rhinitis, or foreign object. **There is evidence that recent upper respiratory tract infections (URIs) increase airway hyperreactivity for 6 to 8 weeks after infection.**[4] Anecdotally, anesthesiologists think that increased secretions, increased incidence of laryngospasm and bronchospasm, increased endotracheal tube obstruction, and intraoperative respiratory difficulties are more common in children with upper respiratory tract infections.[58] Increased incidence of postintubation stridor and intraoperative and postoperative respiratory complications has been reported.[16] On the other hand, experience in recent years has failed to substantiate an increased risk of complications in patients with simple URIs.

When is it appropriate to cancel elective surgery on the basis of rhinorrhea? Again, the patient should be in optimal condition before induction of anesthesia. The recent onset of mucopurulent rhinorrhea, especially if accompanied by pharyngitis and a fever, is an indication for cancellation of elective surgery. The child who always has clear rhinorrhea on the basis of allergic rhinitis probably is at no increased anesthetic risk. Multiple considerations, such as the inconvenience to the family perhaps due to long travel and arranged time off work to accompany the child for elective surgery, the potential of complications from delayed surgery, and the risks of proceeding, all need to be weighed when deciding whether to proceed. In general, with healthy children who are afebrile and have clear rhinorrhea, we proceed with elective surgery. We are more cautious in the face of other respiratory diseases, especially asthma and bronchopulmonary dysplasia.[4,91] **Although this topic remains controversial, whenever possible, surgery and anesthesia should be delayed for at least 2 weeks.**[40]

Cardiovascular system. Due to the multiple cardiovascular effects of anesthetics in children and the frequency with which cardiac anomalies accompany other congenital malformations, particular attention to the cardiovascular system is necessary (Table 26-8).

Table 26-8 Syndromes associated with congenital heart disease

Syndrome	Associated disease
Apert	Pulmonic stenosis, VSD
Asplenia/polysplenia	ASD, VSD
Cornelia de Lange	VSD
DiGeorge	Aortic arch, truncus, VSD, PDA, tetralogy
Down	A-V canal, ASD, VSD
Ellis–van Creveld	ASD
Fetal alcohol	VSD, cardiomyopathy
Holt-Oram	ASD, VSD
Kartagener's	ASD, VSD
Marfan	Aortic and mitral valve diseases, dilated aortic root
Noonan	Pulmonic stenosis, ASD
Opitz	ASD
Robinow	ASD
VATER	VSD
Williams	Pulmonic stenosis

Recognition of the setting in which congenital heart disease may occur, coupled with careful attention to the previous history and questioning of the family, help define the type and severity of the defect. Examination of the child may on occasion lead to discovery of hitherto undiagnosed cardiac defects or at least the presence of a cardiac murmur and demonstrate the need to alter the anesthetic plan and perhaps to seek further pediatric cardiology consultation. The cardiovascular system undergoes significant developmental changes, and reference to normal age-related values is essential in assessing children (see Figs. 26-4 to 26-6).[31]

Poor exercise tolerance, as in adults, is a hallmark of inadequate cardiovascular function. Children who tire easily, become tachypneic, have dyspnea on exertion, or have orthopnea clearly must be carefully evaluated. **In infants the major exercise is feeding.** An irritable child with a history of poor feeding accompanied by diaphoresis and tachypnea may have borderline cardiac function. **In addition, failure to thrive may well indicate compromised cardiac function.** In younger infants, clubbing is never present and cyanosis may be difficult to detect. Palpation and auscultation remain the cornerstones of the cardiology examination. Particular attention should be paid to the **presence of brachial-femoral delay, indicating coarctation,** and for left and right ventricular heaves. Detection of a **new murmur** frequently raises the question of whether it is benign or significant. Differentiating between a venous hum or ventricular

Table 26-9   Innocent asymptomatic murmurs

	Venous hum	Vibratory murmur
Area	Aortic area into neck Pulmonary	Apex to sternum Basal (occasionally mitral) Not transmitted to axilla
Timing	Continuous (ductus murmur) Diastolic accentuation	Systolic
Character	Increased with inspiration	Coarse, low-pitched, scratchy, twang
	Loudest in sitting position	Short, limited area
	Jugular pressure diminishs intensity	Decreased with inspiration
	S_1 and S_2 normal	S_1 may be softened; S_2 normal
	Very common	

BOX 26-6
SBE PROPHYLAXIS

Indications

Congenital or acquired valvular heart disease
Surgically constructed shunts (Waterston, Blalock-Taussig, Potts, etc.)
Subaortic stenosis
Mitral valve prolapse
Rheumatic heart disease
Prostethic valves

Procedures

All genitourinary or gastrointestinal surgery
All dental procedures
Incision and drainage procedures
Adenoidectomy or tonsillectomy
Airway surgery or bronchoscopy

Prophylaxis not necessary for secundum ASD or patent ductus arteriosis repaired > 6 months ago

---

Table 26-10   SBE prophylaxis regimen

	Time	Dosage
Dental and respiratory		
Routine		
Amoxicillin PO or	1 hour before, 6 hours after initial dose	50 mg/kg/ (max 3 g) 25 mg/kg (max 1.5 g)
Penicillin G IV	30-60 min before, 6 hours after initial dose	50,000 units/kg
For maximal protection		
Ampicillin IV and	30 min before, repeat	50 mg/kg
Gentamicin IV	8 hours after initial dose	2 mg/kg
PCN-allergic patients		
Erythromycin PO or	1 hour before, 6 hours after initial dose	20 mg/kg (max 1 g) 10 mg/kg (max 1500 mg)
Vancomycin IV	1 hour before (administer slowly)	20 mg/kg (max 1 g)
Gastrointestinal/genitourinary procedure		
Routine	As for maximal protection above	As for maximal protection above
Minor or repetitive in low-risk children		
Amoxicillin PO	1 hour before, 6 hours after initial dose	50 mg/kg (max 3 g) 25 mg/kg (max 1.5 g)
PCN-allergic patients		
Vancomycin IV and	1 hour before (repeat once)	20 mg/kg (max 1 g)
Gentamicin IV	8-12 hours after initial dose	2.0 mg/kg

outflow murmur and a more serious murmur requires specific attention during examination (Table 26-9). **When in doubt, consultation with a pediatric cardiologist is indicated.** In general, the child with a murmur who is asymptomatic, acyanotic, healthy, and gaining weight along appropriate percentiles, and who has a normal S_1 and S_2 will almost certainly tolerate routine anesthesia without any serious complications. The questions that arise are the need for further cardiology follow up, which may not occur unless brought to the parents' attention by the anesthesiologist, and the question of SBE prophylaxis (Table 26-10 and Box 26-6). When the history and physical examination raise the question of significant cardiac disease, a hematocrit, ECG, chest radiograph, and oxygen saturation (pulse oximetry) form the basis of the laboratory workup. In known significant heart disease, the anesthesiologist is responsible for completely understanding the anatomy and physiology of the defect. Even a hemodynamically inconsequential atrial septal defect, ventricular septal defect, mitral valve prolapse, or the presence of a bicuspid aortic valve may predispose the child to an untoward intraoperative event, and consultation with a pediatric cardiologist may be indicated. For most children with heart disease, it is prudent to obtain a recent consultation with the child's pediatric cardiologist after informing him/her the child requires surgery.

Renal system. Asymptomatic renal disease, apart from asymptomatic bacteruria, is rare in childhood. The likelihood of discovering a new renal lesion during routine physical examination done for the preanesthetic evaluation is close to nonexistent. The presence of hypertension, with reference to normal BP ranges from children (see Table 26-3), should indicate the need for urinalysis and electrolyte analysis.[33] The unexpected presence of anemia may also indicate chronic renal disease. **The anesthetic implications of renal disease in the presence of normal electrolytes, normal growth and development, and normotension are minimal.** In infants, there may be the inability to concentrate urine or to handle a large fluid load, both of which dictate cautious fluid management perioperatively.

In the presence of serious preexisting renal disease, careful attention must be directed to the child's preoperative preparation. If the child requires dialysis (peritoneal dialysis or hemodialysis) to maintain optimal electrolyte levels and growth, then consideration of dialysis on the day before surgery is indicated. Antihypertensive therapy, if required, should be optimized. Electrolytes should be carefully monitored. Particular attention is necessary concerning the serum potassium concentration. Serum potassium greater than 5.5 mEq/L is certainly worrisome in children with renal disease. The propensity of succinylcholine to induce hyperkalemia in patients who may have a concurrent metabolic acidosis puts these patients at particular risk. **Elective surgery should be canceled in the presence of a potassium higher than the acceptable upper level of normal for the individual hospital's lab (5.5 mEq/L, generally).** With regard to hematocrit in chronic renal failure, there is some controversy. It is usual practice to accept a lower hematocrit in these children than would normally be tolerated (20%). This is based on the assumption of chronic adaptation. **The adaptation to lower blood oxygen content includes increased blood volume and increased cardiac output.** These may be compromised during anestheisa. **Although the child may be chronically adapted, it must be remembered that the reserve necessary to tolerate the stresses that may accompany anesthesia and surgery is markedly decreased. There may well be a role for preoperative erythropoietin therapy and even transfusion before surgery, if time will allow.**

Gastrointestinal system. The major anesthetic issues concerning the GI system center on predisposition to aspiration pneumonitis. Children with increased gastric residual volumes and gastroesophageal reflux should be identified preoperatively. Those children who have a history of **tracheoesophageal fistula, mental retardation, cerebral palsy, apnea, and recurrent aspiration pneumonia should always be suspected of having gastroesophageal reflux**[70] (Box 26-7). Careful scrutiny of the medical record and questioning of the parents may indicate that this in fact has been evaluated in the past. Consultation with pediatric colleagues about patients previously uninvestigated for this risk is well worthwhile. Certainly the history of recurrent aspiration pneumonia in a child with a predisposing condition should definitely raise the suspicion of the likelihood of aspiration during anesthesia, and rapid sequence induction is indicated. The management of children with gastroesophageal reflux could include antacids, histamine

---

BOX 26-7
CONDITIONS ASSOCIATED WITH GASTROESOPHAGEAL REFLUX

Apnea	Tracheoesophageal fistula
Prematurity	
Recurrent pneumonia syndromes	Bronchopulmonary dysplasia
Cerebral palsy/mental retardation	Pregnancy
Gross obesity	Recurrent, persistent vomiting

(H$_2$) receptor antagonists, agents that encourage gastric emptying (metoclopramide) and the Sellick maneuver during induction and intubation.[54] **In young infants, awake intubation should be considered.**

Halothane hepatitis developing de novo in children appears to be exeedingly rare, occurring in perhaps less than 1 in 50,000 to 250,000 anesthetic inductions.[13,97] The relationship between the occurrence of halothane toxicity in patients with previous liver damage and resulting hepatitis is unclear. Many premature infants have abnormal liver function tests and elevated bilirubins. Some children may also have hyperbilirubinemia and elevated transaminases. The advisability of using halothane under these circumstances is not clear; however, it is probably best avoided since suitable alternatives are available.

Laboratory Investigations

It may seem surprising that the American Society of Anesthesiologists, the American College of Surgeons, and the American Academy of Pediatrics do not make any specific recommendations for preoperative testing in children. Specific laboratory testing that is indicated by information obtained from the chart review, history, and examination of the child is fairly straightforward. **Routine testing for healthy children remains controversial.** In the past, guidelines that had been developed for adults were applied to children. These included a complete blood count, urinalysis, and chest radiograph. With the streamlining influence prevalent in health care systems today, critical appraisal of the routine need for these examinations has been undertaken. All aspects of the preoperative laboratory investigation have been questioned. Certainly the standard that required a routine chest radiograph in healthy children without symptoms or signs was abandoned years ago.[105] Our recent experience with large numbers of outpatient anesthetics has also raised serious questions about the need for routine performance of other laboratory tests.[72]

Hematology

It is still generally accepted that at minimum a preoperative hematocrit should be obtained in virtually all children. **Although the need to obtain a hematocrit may be accepted, the lower limit of acceptable hemoglobin and hematocrit is less clear.** In addition, the value of a complete blood count with indices and a white blood cell count and whether there is a role for determination of platelets and coagulation studies are far less clear. These decisions should be guided by individual patient consideration. There are developmental differences in the standard level of hematocrit (Table 26-11).[82] For years "normal" hematocrits were required for elective surgery. This standard has been challenged, and the lower limits of normal became

Table 26-11	Mean hematocrit and hemoglobin vs. age	
Age	Hct (SD) %	Hgb (SD) g/dl
1-3 days	56 ± 5	18.5 ± 2.0
2 weeks	53 ± 4	16.6 ± 1.6
1 month	44 ± 5	13.9 ± 1.6
2 months	35 ± 4	11.2 ± 0.9
6 months	36 ± 3	12.6 ± 0.7
6-24 months	36 ± 2	12.0 ± 0.8
2-6 years	37 ± 2	12.5 ± 0.5
6-12 years	40 ± 3	13.5 ± 1.0
12-18 years	43 ± 4	14.5 ± 0.7
Adult	41 ± 2	14.0 ± 1.0

From Rowe PC. Laboratory values. In Oski FA, De Angelis CD, Feigin RD et al, eds: *Principles and practice of pediatrics,* Philadelphia, 1990, JB Lippincott.

acceptable. For surgery, the lower limit of normal, which was defined as a hematocrit of 30% or a hemoglobin of greater than 10 g/dl in nearly all age groups, was the previous requirement. Elective surgery should probably await attaining this level, short of transfusion. Iron and nutritional support are indicated. In the emergent situation, transfusion therapy may be indicated as directed by patient need, such as anticipated blood loss and cardiorespiratory status. Transfusion should not rely on some arbitrary and unsupported boundary of "normal" hemoglobin. With recent concerns about the blood supply, this dogma has become less attractive.[67]

What are the essential considerations? In a healthy child with normal cardiorespiratory function, a fully saturated hemoglobin of 10 g/dl would require a cardiac index of 3.4 L/min/m^2 to provide an oxygen delivery three times the average oxygen consumption. If the child's hemoglobin were 7 g/dl (hematocrit approximately 20%), a cardiac index of 4.8 L/min/m^2 would be required to maintain the same level of oxygen delivery. Clearly in a healthy child this is well within the cardiac reserve and should represent no significant difficulty. The assumptions underlying this are that the child remains 100% saturated, receives no cardiac depressant drugs, and loses little blood. Needless to say, these circumstances frequently cannot be guaranteed during surgery and anesthesia, and this is the key issue. The major concern is not for healthy children having minor surgery, but when surgery will result in blood loss and lower this margin of reserve even further. A child whose hemoglobin drops by 5 g/dl from 10 to 5 g/dl must double cardiac output to around 6.6 L/min/m^2 to maintain oxygen delivery. This remains well within the average child's cardiac reserve. If however, a child's hemoglobin drops by 5 g/dl from 7 to 2 g/dl intraoperatively, he/she would require a cardiac index of nearly 17 L/min/m² to maintain a marginal oxygen delivery, and this is clearly beyond the ability of even the normal child's cardiovascular system to compensate, especially when anesthetized.

A third issue that is frequently raised is **adaptation.** The classic teaching is that children with renal disease tolerate lower hematocrits because they have had time to adapt. There is little evidence to demonstrate this is so; for example, 2-3-DPG may not be increased in children with renal disease, and there is no reason to suggest that they have a shift in the oxyhemoglobin dissociation curve. The concept that they can adapt to lower levels of oxygen delivery and/or consumption is unsupported. In any case, if significant blood loss is expected perioperatively, the margin of safety is considerably less in patients who begin with low hematocrits. As mentioned previously, there are no absolute guidelines for preoperative hematocrit and, at present, each anesthesiologist must decide on a standard for each child. In deciding it is worth noting Motoyama and Glasner's work.[64] In essence a hemoglobin of 7.5 to 8.5 g/dl will deliver equivalent oxygen to the tissues of a child as 10 g/dl will in an adult. In neonates, 12 to 13 g/dl is necessary. This is largely related to shifts in the P_{50}.[64] **It seems reasonable that a hemoglobin of 8 g/dl in an ASA I child may well be acceptable if no significant perioperative blood loss is expected.** On the other hand, a child about to undergo scoliosis repair, with chronic restrictive lung disease, should have a hemoglobin higher than 10 g/dl (at least initially). Obtaining a blood specimen to determine hemoglobin is a simple test, performed either by venipuncture or finger stick in children. It may reveal a significant incidence of anemia, depending on the population studied. Whether this incidence of anemia is relevant to anesthetic practice should be addressed in light of the previous caveats and the broader question of health care screening needs.

Many abnormalities of laboratory testing may be discovered during preoperative screening.[43] These fall into two categories: those that are relevant to the anesthetic management of the child and those that are relevant to the child's general health. Depending on the hospital setting, the degree to which a preanesthesia screening clinic wishes to be responsible for the general health care of children needs to be determined in each hospital. There is clearly a responsibility of ensuring follow-up for abnormal laboratory tests that may be discovered coincidentally with preoperative assessment. In a recent study by O'Connor and Drasner, 17% of children who had a CBC were anemic or had a microcytosis.[68] Only two of these children had surgery canceled due to anemia with hemoglobins less than 10 g/dl.[68] A mechanism to

arrange follow-up with the pediatric clinic should be available for the anesthesia preevaluation clinics, and communication must be assured at this point.

Sickle cell disease. The American Academy of Pediatrics' recommendations for the screening for sickle cell disease **requires that a sickle preparation or other screening test be performed in all black children.** Is it reasonable for the anesthesiologist to insist on receiving the results of a sickle cell preparation in all black children requiring anesthesia and surgery? Does anesthetic management change for those who have sickle trait, as compared with the normal population? Is it necessary to have a sickle cell preparation in nonanemic black children? Clearly, anesthetizing a child with sickle cell disease who is anemic, with 95% sickle hemoglobin, poses a major threat to that child and should never be undertaken without good reason. However, the likelihood of a child greater than 2 years old with a normal hemoglobin having sickle cell disease is extremely low although sickle cell disease is possible. If all children with hemoglobins less than 10 g/dl require further investigation, then among the factors that will be investigated, in addition to iron deficiency, will be sickle hemoglobin status in black children. This, however, may not apply to newborns or infants, who may have hemoglobins greater than 10 g/dl and still have sickle cell disease and significant levels of sickle hemoglobin. In these children, unless a sickle hemoglobin preparation has been performed, cases may be missed in a population particularly at risk for hypoxia and low cardiac output during anesthesia. **Our recommendation is to perform a sickle cell preparation on all black children unless the status is known and to screen for anemia in all other children. In those with positive sickle screen, hemoglobin electrophoresis is required. It should be noted that infants less than 4 months of age have maternal antibodies that interfere with performing a quick sickle index preparation. These children require hemoglobin electrophoresis to determine their sickle cell disease status.**

Does sickle trait pose a threat to older children who may not be anemic but still have some amount of sickle hemoglobin? Although there are some anecdotal stories of sickling and rare vasoocclusive phenomena in children with sickle cell trait during anesthesia with resulting hypothermia, ischemia, and hypoxia, **sickle cell trait is generally associated with less than 40% of hemoglobin S in the circulating blood.[37] This is the target level that is obtained with transfusion protocols for sickle cell disease.** Prudent avoidance of tourniquets that cause blood stasis and hypoxia in the affected limb is probably wise in patients with sickle cell trait. Anesthetic management will not vary, as the routine goals of anesthesia (avoidance of hypoxia, hypothermia, hypovolemia, and hypotension) are as important in routine anesthetic management as they are for patients with sickle cell trait.[37]

In patients with sickle cell disease, preoperative management is directed at reducing sickle hemoglobin to less than 40%. Chronic transfusion, exchange transfusion, and acute blood transfusion have all been reported to be useful in achieving this goal.

White blood cell counts. In a recently published study, white blood cell counts were abnormal only in patients who were ill or otherwise suspected of having an infection.[81] No occult leukocytosis was discovered in 463 preoperative screening evaluations.[68] **When indicated by suspicion of sepsis, infection, fever, or respiratory tract infection, a CBC may be useful in arriving at the diagnosis; however, routine WBC determination does not appear to be warranted.**

Urinalysis

Routine urinalysis has been part of preoperative recommendations in children. Apart from providing an obvious contribution to routine health screening, the relevance to anesthetic management is unclear.[51] Clearly in children who are febrile, have congenital anomalies of the urinary tract, or have suspected renal function anomalies, urinalysis may be beneficial. In otherwise healthy children, where urinalysis is difficult to obtain and unreliable, abnormal results appear to occur in 15% of children and are usually asymptomatic bacteriuria.[68] The majority of these are either false positives, clinically insignificant, or previously known. In only 2 out of 453 cases was surgery canceled, and both of these were due to suspected colonization or asymptomatic bacteriuria, which were of no significant anesthetic relevance. **In afebrile ASA I children with an absence of a history of renal disease, most centers have abandoned routine urinalysis.**

Drug levels

In children receiving therapuetic drugs it is frequently worthwhile to know whether the therapeutic level has been achieved as required. The two major areas where this is of concern is in children with **epilepsy and asthma. Obtaining routine blood levels of theophylline and anticonvulsants to ensure compliance with therapy and adequate levels for the perioperative management appears to be a wise precaution.** It is reassuring to determine that the child is receiving an appropriate therapy at an appropriate level so that the surgery may proceed uneventfully. **It is not so clear, however, what should be done with an abnormal result.** Does an asymptomatic healthy child with a nontherapeutic drug level still require therapy? Should therapeutic levels of indicated drugs be achieved before elective surgery? This decision will clearly involve input from the child's primary care physician and perhaps pediatric neurology in the case of children with epilepsy. Frequently it is worthwhile to inform the primary caretaker that the level is subtherapeutic, and the drug could be discontinued before surgery. There is a caveat to this. Discontinuing anticonvulsants may lead to withdrawal seizures, not a pleasant prospect in the perioperative period. In the case of theophylline, asymptomatic children with low theophylline levels may not be wheezing on the day of evaluation but may well have developed wheezing on the day of surgery and may still have significant underlying bronchial hyperreactivity, which may pose difficulties intraoperatively. Our current practice is as follows: if a child requires theophylline to suppress wheezing episodes, then perioperatively, during a time of stress and a likely time for airway complications, the child requires therapeutic theophylline levels, and care should be taken to achieve therapeutic levels preoperatively if possible. Frequently if this is not possible, **knowing the level will allow the anesthesiologist to specifically direct therapy intraoperatively, if required.** Further tests will be guided by the patient's underlying medical condition.

Preoperative assessment for elective surgery should be done early enough to allow the whole gamut of special investigations to be performed before surgery. Consultation with other services and the performance of other investigative procedures, such as CT scans, ECGs, and echocardiograms, should be timed in a fashion that allows the results to be available to the anesthesiologist before induction of anesthesia. Deciding that such information is important preoperatively but acting before it is adequately obtained clearly sets the stage for medical or legal misadventures.

NPO Status

Of all the shibboleths of pediatric anesthesia, perhaps the one most time honored and also currently most under attack is NPO status. The days of NPO after midnight for all children who require surgery are waning. **For years we have realized that small infants, with their unique glucose and fluid requirements, do not benefit by being NPO for 12 hours before surgery. Significant hypovolemia with intraoperative hypotension and hypoglycemia are the result.** There have been concerns raised about hypoglycemia occurring in older children after a prolonged fast.[42] There are also concerns about comfort and the need for the imposition of starvation on children preoperatively. The goal, of course, is to reduce gastric volume and eliminate the risk of aspiration pneumonia perioperatively. There are many studies looking at factors predisposing to gastric acid aspiration and lung injury and their relationship to gastric residual volumes. Nevertheless, the fact remains that perioperative aspiration pneumonia is remarkably rare (a fact that may attest to the success of severe NPO restrictions or merely to the minimal likelihood of aspiration).

There is little evidence that in a normal child prolonged fasts are required to ensure minimal gastric volumes. Clearly, NPO for solid foods and large meals for 8 hours before surgery should be maintained. After a solid meal, gastric volumes may be increased for up to 6 hours. The question becomes less clear with fluids. Several studies have even demonstrated that ad lib clear liquids up until 2 hours before surgery are actually associated with lower gastric volumes and higher pHs than those in starved patients.[55,84] If this is the case, the recommendation ought to be to encourage PO clear fluids preoperatively rather than to limit them. On the other hand, there are recent studies that demonstrate that not only is there no significant burden of hypoglycemia placed on the normal child by fasting, but that feeding the child clear liquids is associated with increased gastric volumes.[59,99] The final factor that needs to be considered is whether one should change an age-old guideline for a more liberal approach that may be confusing and lead to changes in requirements that are not intended. The guideline of NPO after midnight is perhaps draconian but absolutely clear to all concerned. No solids after midnight and clear liquids up to an hour before surgery ad lib, if the patient is healthy, without gastroesophageal reflux or other significant GI disease, is certainly less clear. These liberal rules are bound to be applied in inappropriate situations, potentially leading to catastrophe. Certainly some major institutions allow clear liquids up until an hour or two before surgery in their outpatients, and a large series reported from the Children's Hospital of Philadelphia reports no incidence of gastric aspiration after years of this approach.[84] Review of all standards of anesthetic care periodically is worthwhile as is setting policy and ensuring quality control. Communication, education, monitoring all current protocols, as well as flexibility in approach, based on known facts, should form the guidelines for anesthesia practice. This is no less true with regard to NPO rules. **It is clear that the trend is toward more liberal NPO restriction for clear liquids.**[18,21]

One final question: What are clear liquids? Water, glucose water, and Pedialyte are all clear. Some institutions consider breast milk a clear liquid and cow's milk a solid food. Some institutions encourage jello (no additives) and fruit juices, including pulp-free orange juice, as perfectly allowable. It is unlikely that there will ever be hard scientific data to aid the anesthesiologist in these decisions. The application of common sense and the provision of clear instructions for families are essential.

EVALUATION OF THE CRITICALLY ILL CHILD

Intraoperative management of critically ill children can present the anesthesiologist with great challenges. The use of cardiovascularly active anesthetic agents in critically ill children can frequently demand the most meticulous anesthesia care. Thorough preoperative evaluation and preparation is essential to assure optimal intraoperative management. A **rigorous, compulsive systematic evaluation of critically ill children is essential,** and, although it follows the basic outline of systems review, the underlying assumption is that the severity of illness in each system is clearly much worse than in the patient for elective surgery.

Establishing a rapport with the child in an intensive care unit can range from difficult to impossible. Clearly an unconscious, heavily sedated, paralyzed child requiring advanced mechanical ventilation and neuroresuscitation will not be communicative. Discussing the anesthesia care with the child's family may often be awkward, as survival is the parents' primary concern. Before contacting the family it is essential that the anesthesiologist be completely familiar with the child's problems so that the parents can be confident that all physicians who are caring for their child are knowledgeable and concerned. In addition, many parents have bonded to the ICU staff and transferring their child's care to other physicians can provoke great anxiety. The anesthesiologist needs to demonstrate concern and clearly state that the intraoperative care and management will be every bit as meticulous as that provided for the child in the ICU. Although it is natural to focus entirely on the child's immediate surgical needs or indication for admission to the ICU, other problems that may have anesthetic import should be sought just as they would be in a routine evaluation. Therefore a systems review, previous drug and allergy history, and family history must not be neglected. Areas of interest that are specifically relevant in the critically ill child should be reviewed.

Neurologic status

The level of consciousness, presence of CNS injury, intracranial pressure, and neurologic deficits must be specifically determined. In addition, psychotropic drugs, sedatives, and other obtunding agents that may supplement, augment, or interact with anesthetic agents should be clearly defined. Some children in the ICU will be nearly totally anesthetized at the time of transfer to the operating room, whereas others may have received little medication. Complete **review of current neurologic status and psychotropic drugs is therefore mandatory.**

Respiratory Status

Respiratory evaluation should be meticulous. **The level of oxygen required, respiratory rate, ventilatory rate, tidal volume, airway pressures, and blood gas form the basis of this information.** If the child is on a ventilator, it is necessary to be familiar with the degree of ventilatory support the child is requiring, including the **FIO_2, mean airway pressure, peak end-expiratory pressure, and respiratory rate.** A **blood gas** just before transfer to the operating room is critical information. Anesthesia machine ventilators, although more than adequate for patients with normal pulmonary function, may be inadequate in advanced stages of lung disease and adult respiratory distress syndrome. In this case, the anesthesiologist must be able to **organize sophisticated ventilatory support in the operating room where indicated.** This should be done before transfer of the child to the operating room in conjunction with respiratory therapy.

Cardiovascular System

Complete familiarity with the child's hemodynamic function is essential. All patients in the critical care unit should be suspected of having compromised cardiovascular function and borderline oxygen delivery. Complete evaluation of perfusion status, temperature, cardiac output and indices, and **hemodynamic information** as obtained from pulmonary artery catheterization, if present, should be reviewed, and, where necessary, preoperatively optimized. **The intravascular volume and fluid replacement status,** as well as the **hematocrit** and **availability of blood products** should be ensured. Finally, a review of **cardiovascular drugs** the child is receiving and optimization where important should be undertaken. It is necessary to ensure that constant, smooth delivery of inotropic and cardiovascular active drugs and infusions be continued during transportation intraoperatively. Finally, an **ECG and review of the child's rhythm history** for the presence of cardiac dysrhythmias or predisposition to cardiac dysrhythmias should be conducted.

Renal Status

Urine output and fluid requirements in the preoperative period should be reviewed. A recent **creatinine and BUN** should be known. Renal function should be assessed and may have important bearing on the use of neuromuscular relaxants, intraoperative fluid requirements, and electrolyte status. **Electrolyte abnormalities** are common in critical illness and may lead to cardiorespiratory failure and cardiac dysrhythmias intraoperatively. This, in general, should be corrected preoperatively.

Gastroenterology

All patients who are ill enough to require admission to an ICU should be suspected of having full stomachs. Acute, critical, and chronic illnesses delay gastric emptying. **Even though the child may have been NPO for a prolonged period of time, hypersecretion and high gastric acid content may predispose the child to aspiration on induction.** Certainly patients who have suffered trauma and for whom no NPO history is available should as a precaution be treated as having full stomachs.

Laboratory Tests

Laboratory investigation should be thoroughly reviewed. **At a minimum, baseline complete blood counts, electrolyte profiles, calcium, and blood gases are essential. Therapeutic levels of drugs such as theophylline or anticonvulsants are indicated if the child is receiving them. A final check to make sure cross-matched blood is available,** where indicated, is prudent.

When it is certain that the anesthesiologist can deliver care equivalent to that being provided to the child in the ICU and that ongoing resuscitation is ensured, then the child can be transferred to the operating room. Selection of induction and anesthetic maintenance agents will critically depend on the child's overall cardiorespiratory function and oxygen delivery status. Every precaution should be taken to optimize and maintain these perioperatively. Thorough preparation will allow applied critical care in the operating room to proceed smoothly, and the safe provision of analgesia and amnesia and, where indicated, akinesia, should be possible even in the most seriously ill children.

KEY POINTS

- The percentage of total body composition that is water decreases with age; intracellular fluid increases and extracellular fluid decreases.

- Fat and muscle mass increase from 13% to 22% and 20% to 50%, respectively, with age.

- The distribution of blood flow varies, with a decreased percentage of flow going to the vessel-rich groups with increased age.

- Infants have an overlarge tongue and relatively small jaw. The infant is usually described as having an anterior/cephalad displacement of the airway with the narrowest segment at the level of the cricoid. The epiglottis is generally large and floppy as compared with the adult.

- Younger children tend to experience airway closure and alveolar collapse with atelectasis because their tidal volume is very close to the closing volume.

- Although the functional residual capacity in milliliters/kilogram is somewhat smaller in infants compared with adults (30 vs. 34), increased oxygen consumption is the major factor in the rapid desaturation in infants.

- The perioperative risk of reversion to a transitional circulation is related to pulmonary hypertension triggered by decreased oxygen, increased carbon dioxide, decreased temperature, acidosis, and increased catecholamines.

- Cardiac output depends on heart rate in the infant and young child. Infants have parasympathetic hypertonia, decreased sympathetic innervation, and a ventricle with less muscle and more noncontractile mass/unit volume. This all leads to a myocardium that is less able to generate adequate force than in the adult.

- Hematocrit nadir of approximately 35 at about 3 months of age is the so-called physiologic anemia of infancy.

- The glomerular filtration rate/1.73 m² increases from 40 to 130 ml/mm with age. Ability to concentrate urine is limited, and maximal osmolarity may be only 700 mOsm.

- Slack LES tone with reflux is common in infants less than 6 months of age, but the maintenance of low gastric volumes by NPO regulations must be countered by risk of hypoglycemia.

- The liver is functionally immature in children, affecting synthetic/metabolic function.

- Defending the thermoneutrality of infants is a cornerstone of pediatrics.

- Cold stress in neonates can lead to increased oxygen consumption and decreased oxygen delivery, leading to increased hydrogen ion concentration and decreased glycogen and glucose. This leads to respiratory distress, disseminated intravascular coagulation, shock, and persistent fetal circulation.

- The large surface-area-to-mass ratio in children and decreased subcutaneous tissue mass lead to increased heat loss via conduction, convection, radiation, and evaporation.

- The large volume of distribution noted in neonates is related to protein binding and greater proportion of extracellular water.

- The integrity of the blood-brain barrier is immature at birth, and an increased percentage of blood flow goes to the vessel rich group.

- In preoperative evaluation, the anesthesiologist must prepare himself/herself, the family, and the child. The primary objective is to ensure that the child is in optimal condition. Evaluation of respiratory status begins with the simple observation of rate, signs of distress, inspiratory sounds, and phonation. Developmental milestones and growth charts should be reviewed to assist in the overall general assessment of well-being. Optimal drug levels (e.g., of anticonvulsants and theophylline) must be ensured. Shunt patency should be ensured, and a functional history should be obtained in children with decompression shunts.

- Many congenital anomalies are associated with airway and cardiac abnormalities.

- In children with known cardiopulmonary disease presently or in the past, it is imperative that the anesthesiologist be completely familiar with the child's status and be assured that therapy has been optimized preoperatively.

- In infants, feeding is the major exercise, and failure to thrive may indicate compromised cardiovascular function.

- The "runny nose" remains a controversial area, but, whenever possible, surgery and anesthesia should be delayed at least 2 weeks when the child has a runny nose associated with lower respiratory or systemic symptoms.

- Routine laboratory testing for healthy children remains controversial and should be dictated by clinical situation.

- The trend of NPO status is toward a more liberal NPO restriction for clear liquids.

- Rigorous, compulsive, and systematic evaluation of critically ill children is essential.

KEY REFERENCES

Davies JM, Davison JS, Nimmo WS et al: The stomach: factors of importance to the anaesthetist, *Can J Anaesth* 37:896, 1990.

Eger EI II, Bohlman SH, and Munson ES: The effect of age on the rate of increase of alveolar anesthetic concentration, *Anesthesiology* 35:365, 1971.

Jacoby DB, Hirshman CA: General anesthesia in patients with viral respiratory infections—an unsound sleep? *Anesthesiology* 74:969, 1991.

Jansen AH, Chernick V: Development of respiratory control, *Physiol Rev* 63:437, 1983.

Kurth CD, Spitzer AR, Broennille AM et al: Postoperative apnea in preterm infants, *Anesthesiology* 66:483, 1987.

Maxwell LG, Wetzel RC: Induction techniques in pediatric anesthesia, *Anesth Rep* 1:110, 1988.

O'Connor ME, Drasner K: Preoperative laboratory testing of children undergoing elective surgery, *Anesth Analg* 70:176, 1990.

Orenstein SR, Orenstein DM: Gastroesophaeal reflux and respiratory disease in children, *J Pediatr* 112:847, 1988.

Stockman JA III: Anemia of prematurity: current concepts in the issue of when to transfuse, *Pediatr Clin North Am* 33:111, 1986.

REFERENCES

1. Adam FH: Fetal and neonatal circulations. In Adams FH, Emmanouilides GC, eds: *Moss' heart disease in infants, children, and adolescents,* ed 3, Baltimore, 1983, Williams & Wilkins.

2. Aldrete JA, Roman-de Jesus JC, Russell LJ et al: Intranasal ketamine as induction adjunct in children: preliminary report, *Anesthesiology* 67:A514, 1987.

3. Aperia A, Zellerstrom R: Renal control of fluid homeostasis in the newborn infant, *Clin Perinatol* 9:523, 1982.

4. Aquilina AT, Hill WJ, Douglas RG et al: Airway reactivity in subjects with viral upper respiratory tract infections, *Am Rev Respir Dis* 122:3, 1980.

5. Arant Jr BS: Renal and genitourinary disease. In Oski FA, DeAngelis CD, Feigin RD et al, eds: *Principles and practice of pediatrics,* Philadelphia, 1990. JB Lippincott.

6. Asburn MA et al: Oral transmucosal fentanyl citrate in paediatric outpatients, *Can J Anaesth* 37:857, 1990.

7. Belknap WM: Developmental disorders of gastrointestinal function. In Oski FA, DeAngelis CD, Feigin RD et al, eds: *Principles and practice of pediatrics,* Philadelphia, 1990, JB Lippincott.

8. Belknap WM: Sucking and swallowing disorders and gastroesophageal reflux. In Oski FA, DeAngelis CD, Feigin RD et al, eds: *Principles and practice of pediatrics,* Philadelphia, 1990, JB Lippincott.

9. Boudin P: *LeNourisson, alementation et hygeine des enfants debeles-enfants nes a Terme,* Paris, A 1900, Dion.

10. Buchanan GR: Hematopoietic diseases. In Oski FA, DeAngelis CD, Feigin RD, et al, eds: *Principles and practice of pediatrics,* Philadelphia, 1990, JB Lippincott.

11. Britt BA: Temperature regulation. In Gregory GA, ed: *Pediatric anesthesia,* ed 2, New York, 1989, Churchill-Livingstone.

12. Cabanac M: Temperature regulation, *Ann Rev Physiol* 37:415, 1975.

13. Carney FMT, Van Dyke RA: Halothane hepatitis; a critical review, *Anesth Analg* 51:135, 1972.

14. Chantler C: The kidney. In Godfrey S, Baum JD, eds: *Clinical paediatric physiology,* Oxford, 1979, Blackwell Scientific Publications.

15. Chapman AH, Loeb DG, and Gibbons MJ: Psychiatric aspects of hospitalizing children, *Arch Paediatr* 73:77,1956.

16. Cohen MM, Cameron CB: Should you cancel the operation when a child has an upper respiratory tract infection? *Anesth Analg* 72:282, 1991.

17. Cook DR, Davis PJ: Pharmacology of pediatric anesthesia. In Motoyama EK, Davis PJ, eds: *Smith's anesthesia for infants and children,* ed 5, St Louis, 1990, Mosby–Year Book.

18. Cote CJ: NPO after midnight for children—a reappraisal, *Anesthesiology* 72:589, 1990.

19. Cote CJ, Todres ID: The pediatric airway. In Ryan JF, Todres ID, Cote CJ, et al, eds: *A practice of anesthesia for infants and children,* Philadelphia, 1986, WB Saunders.

20. Darnall RA Jr, Ariagno RL: Minimal oxygen consumption in infants cared for under overhead radiant warmers compared with conventional incubators, *J Pediatr* 93:283, 1978.

21. Davies JM, Davison JS, Nimmo WS et al: The stomach: factors of importance to the anaesthetist, *Can J Anaesth* 37:896, 1990.

22. Eckenhoff JE: Relationship of anesthesia to postoperative personality changes in children, *Am J Dis Child* 86:587, 1953.

23. Eger EI II: *Anesthetic uptake and action.* Baltimore, 1974, Williams & Wilkens.

24. Eger EI II, Bohlman SH, and Munson ES: The effect of age on the rate of increase of alveolar anesthetic concentration, *Anesthesiology* 35:365, 1971.

25. Forbes RB, Vandewalker GE: Comparison of two and ten per cent rectal methohexitone for induction of anaesthesia in children, *Can J Anaesth* 35:345, 1988.

26. Frankenberg WK, Dodds JB: *Denver developmental screen test,* University of Colorado Medical Center, 1969.

27. Friedman WF: The intrinsic physiologic properties of the developing heart. In Friedman WF, Lesch M, and Sonnenblick EH, eds: *Neonatal heart disease,* New York, 1973, Grune & Stratton.

28. Fries-Hansen B: Body composition during growth. In vivo measurements and biochemical data correlated to differential anatomical growth, *Pediatrics* 47:264, 1971.

29. Gioia FR, Stephenson RL, and Alterwitz SA: In Rogers MC, ed: *Textbook of pediatric intensive care.* Baltimore, 1987, Williams & Wilkins.

30. Gregory G: Pharmacology. In Gregory GA, ed: *Pediatric anesthesia,* ed 2, New York, 1989, Churchill-Livingstone.

31. Greene MG, ed: *The Harriet lane handbook,* Baltimore, 1991, Mosby–Year Book.

32. Hansel H: Thermoreceptors, *Am Rev Physiol* 36:233, 1974.

33. Hanna JD, Chan JCM, and Gill Jr JR: Hypertension and the kidney, *J Pediatr* 118:327-340, 1991.

34. Helmers JH, Noorduin H, VanPeer A et al: Comparison of intravenous and intranasal sufentanil absorption and sedation, *Can J Anaesth* 36:494, 1989.

35. Hill J, Rahintull KA: Heat balance and the metabolic rate of newborn babies in relation to environmental temperature and the effect of age and weight on basal metabolic rate, *J Physiol* 180:239, 1965.

36. Hogg JC, Williams J, Richardson B et al: Age as a factor in the distribution of lower airway conductance and in the pathologic anatomy of obstructive lung disease, *N Engl J Med* 282:1283, 1970.

37. Howells TH, Huntsman RG, Boyes JE et al: Anesthesia and sickle cell hemoglobin, *Br J Anaesth* 44:975, 1972.

38. Hyvarinen M, Zelter P, Oh W et al: Influences of gestational age on serum levels of α 1 feto protein, IgG globulin and albumin in newborn infants, *J Pediatr* 82:430, 1973.

39. Jackson K: Psycholgoical preparation as a method of reducing the emotional trauma of anesthesia in children, *Anesthesiology* 12:293, 1951.

40. Jacoby DB, Hirshman CA: General anesthesia in patients with viral respiratory infections—an unsound sleep? *Anesthesiology* 74:969, 1991.

41. Jansen AH, Chernick V: Development of respiratory control, *Physiol Rev* 63:437, 1983.

42. Jensen BH, Werberg M, and Adersen M: Preoperative starvation and blood glucose concentration in children undergoing inpatient and outpatient anesthesia, *Br J Anaesth* 54:1071, 1982.

43. Kaplan EB, Sheiner LB, Boeckmann AJ et al: The usefulness of preoperative laboratory screening, *JAMA* 253:3576, 1985.

44. Keens TG, Bryan AC, Levinson H et al: Developmental pattern of muscle fiber types in human ventilatory muscles, *J Appl Physiol* 44:909, 1978.

45. Kirkpatrick SE, Pitlick PT, Naliboff J et al: Frank-Starling relationship as an important determinant of fetal cardiac output, *Am J Physiol* 231:495, 1976.

46. Kliegman RM, Behrman RE: Diseases of the newborn infant: premature and full-term. In Behrman RE, Vaughan III VC, eds: *Nelson textbook of pediatrics,* ed 13, Philadelphia, 1987, WB Saunders.

47. Knill RL, Gelb KW: Ventilatory responses to hypoxia and hypercapnia during halothane sedation and anesthesia in man, *Anesthesiology* 49:244, 1978.

48. Koehntop DE, Rodman JH, Brundage DM et al: Pharmacokinetics of fentanyl in neonates, *Anesth Analg* 65:227, 1986.

49. Korsch BM: The child and the operating room, *Anesthesiology* 43:251, 1975.

50. Kurth CD, Spitzer AR, Broennille AM et al: Postoperative apnea in preterm infants, *Anesthesiology* 66:483, 1987.

51. Lawrence VA, Gafni A, and Gross M: The unproven utility of the preoperative urinalysis: economic evaluation, *J Clin Epidemiol* 42:1185, 1989.

52. Liu LMP, Cote CS, Goudsouzian NG et al: Life-threatening apnea in infants recovering from anesthesia, *Anesthesiology* 59:506, 1983.

53. Lowry GA: *Growth and development of children,* ed 2, Chicago, 1975, Mosby–Year Book.

54. Machida HM, Forbes DA, Gall DG et al: Metoclopramide in gastroesophageal reflux of infancy, *J Pediatr* 112:483, 1988.

55. Maltby JR, Sutherland AD, Sale JP, et al: Preoperative oral fluids; is a five-hour fast justified prior to elective surgery? *Anesth Analg* 65:1112, 1986.

56. Maxwell LG, Wetzel RC: Induction techniques in pediatric anesthesia, *Anesth Rep* 1:110, 1988.

57. McFadden ER Jr, Ingram RH: Pulmonary performance in asthma. In Fishman AP, ed: *Pulmonary diseases and disorders,* New York, 1980, McGraw-Hill.

58. McGill WA, Coveler LA, and Epstein BS: Subacute upper respiratory infection in small children, *Anesth Analg* 58:331, 1979.

59. Meakin G, Dingwall AE, and Addison GM: Effects of fasting and oral premedication on the pH and volume of gastric aspirate in children, *Br J Anaesth* 59:678, 1987.

60. Miller ED, Sanders DB, Rowlingson JC et al: Anesthesia-induced rhabdomyolysis in a patient with Duchenne's muscular dystrophy, *Anesthesiology* 48:146, 1978.

61. Miller MJ, Carlo WA, Strohl KP et al: Effect of maturation on oral breathing in sleeping premature infants, *J Pediatr* 109:515, 1986.

62. Mitchell MM, Ali MM, and Savarese JJ: Myotonia and neuromuscular blocking agents, *Anesthesiology* 49:216, 1976.

63. Montague TJ, Taylor PG, Stockton R et al: The spectrum of cardiac rate and rhythm in normal newborns, *Pediatr Cardiol* 2:33, 1982.

64. Motoyama EK: Respiratory physiology in infants and children. In Motoyama EK, Davis PJ, eds: *Smith's anesthesia for infants and children,* ed 5, St Louis, 1990, Mosby–Year Book.

65. Moylan FMB, Selden EB, Shannon DC et al: Defective primary dentition in survivors of neonatal mechanical ventilation, *J Pediatr* 96:106, 1980.

66. Nicolson SC, Betts EK, Jobes DR, et al: Comparison of oral and intramuscular preanesthetic medication for pediatric inpatient surgery, *Anesthesiology* 71:8, 1989.

67. NIH and FDA Perioperative Red Blood Cell Transfusion Consensus Conference, Bethesda, Md, April, 1988.

68. O'Connor ME, Drasner K: Preoperative laboratory testing of children undergoing elective surgery, *Anesth Analg* 70:176, 1990.

69. Olinsky A, Bryan MH, and Bryan AC: Influence of lung inflation on respiratory control in neonates, *J Appl Physiol* 36:426, 1974.

70. Orenstein SR, Orenstein DM: Gastroesophageal reflux and respiratory disease in children, *J Pediatr* 112:847, 1988.

71. Oski FA, DeAngelis CD, Feigin RD et al, eds: *Principles and practice of pediatrics.* Philadelphia, 1990, JB Lippincott.

72. Pasternak LR: Preoperative evaluation of the ambulatory surgery patient, *Anesthes Rep* 3:8, 1990.

73. Peterson L, Ridley-Johnson R, Tracy K et al: Developing cost-effective presurgical preparation, *J Pediatr Psych* 9:439, 1984.

74. Reiminschnieder TA, Breener RA, and Mason DT: Maturational changes in myocardial contractile state of newborn lambs, *Pediatr Res* 15:349, 1981.

75. Report of the Task Force on Blood Pressure Control in Children: National Heart, Lung, and Blood Institute, *Pediatrics* 59(suppl):803, 1977.

76. Rigatto H, Brady JP: Periodic breathing and apnea in the preterm infant. I. Evidence for hypoventilation possibly due to central depression, *Pediatrics* 50:202, 1972.

77. Rigatto H, de la Torre Verduzco R, and Cates DB: Effects of O_2 on the ventilatory response to CO_2 in preterm infants, *J Appl Physiol* 39:896, 1975.

78. Roberts MC, Wurtele SK, Boone RR et al: Reduction of medical fears by use of modelling, *J Pediatr Psych* 6:293, 1981.

79. Rogers MC, Wetzel RC, and Deshpande JK: Unusual causes of pulmonary edema, myocardial ischemia and cyanosis. In Rogers MC, ed: *Textbook of pediatric intensive care,* vol 1, Baltimore, 1987, Williams & Wilkins.

80. Romero TE, Friedman WF: Limited left ventricular response to volume overload in the neonatal period: a comparative study with the adult animal, *Pediatr Res* 13:910, 1979.

81. Rossello PJ, Ramos Cruz A, and Mayol PM: Routine laboratory tests for elective surgery in pediatric patients: are they necessary? *Bol Assoc Med PR* 72:614, 1980.

82. Rowe PC: Laboratory values. In Oski FA, DeAngelis CD, Feigin RD, et al, eds: *Principles and practice of pediatrics,* Philadelphia, 1990, JB Lippincott.

83. Rudolph AM, Heyman MA: Cardiac output in the fetal lamb: the effects of spontaneous and induced changes of heart rate on right and left ventricular output, *Am J Obstet Gynecol* 124:183, 1976.

84. Schreiner MS, Triebwasser A, and Keon TP: Ingestion of liquids compared with preoperative fasting in pediatric outpatients, *Anesthesiology* 72:593, 1990.

85. Sereni F: Principals of developmental pharmacology, *Am Rev Pharmacol* 8:453, 1968.

86. Smith CA, Nelson NB: *The physiology of the newborn infant,* ed 4, Springfield, Ill, 1976, CC Thomas.

87. Smith DW: *Recognizable patterns of human malformation: genetic, embryologic and clinical aspects,* ed 2, Philadelphia, 1976, WB Saunders.

88. Spitzer A: The role of the kidney in sodium homeostasis during maturation, *Kidney Int* 21:539,1982.

89. Stern L: The newborn infant and his thermal environment, *Curr Prob Pediatr* 1:3, 1970.

90. Stockman JA III: Anemia of prematurity: current concepts in the issue of when to transfuse, *Pediatr Clin North Am* 33:111, 1986.

91. Tait AR, Knight PR: Intraoperative respiratory complications in patients with upper respiratory tract infections, *Can J Anaesth* 34:300, 1987.

92. Thomas DKM: Hypoglycaemia in children before operation, *Br J Anaes* 51:161, 1974.

93. Tietel DF, Side D, Chen T et al: Developmental changes in myocardial contractile reserve in the lamb, *Pediatr Res* 19:948, 1985.

94. Visintainer MA, Wolfer JA: Psychological preparation for surgical pediatric patients. The effect of children's and parents' stress responses and adjustment, *Pediatrics* 56:87, 1975.

95. Walbergh EJ, Willis RJ, and Eckhert J: Plasma concentrations of midazolam in children following intranasal administration, *Anesthesiology* 74:233, 1991.

96. Walker-Smith JA: Gut and digestion. In Godfrey S, Baum JD, eds: *Clinical paediatric physiology,* Oxford, 1979, Blackwell Scientific Publications.

97. Wark HJ: Postoperative jaundice in children: the influence of halothane, *Anaesthesia* 38:237, 1983.

98. Weil WB Jr, Bailie MD: *Fluid and electrolyte metabolism in infants and children: a unified approach,* New York, 1977, Grune and Stratton.

99. Wellborn LG, McGill WA, Hannallah RS et al: Perioperative blood glucose concentrations in pediatric outpatients, *Anesthesiology* 65:543, 1986.

100. Wetzel RC: Defective dentition following mechanical ventilation, *J Pediatr* 97:334, 1980.

101. Wetzel RC: Anesthesia for pediatric trauma. In Stene JK, ed: *Pediatric trauma,* Baltimore, 1989, Williams & Wilkins.

102. Wetzel RC, Rogers MC: Pediatric hemodynamic monitoring. In Shoemaker WC, Thompson WL, eds: *Critical care—state of the art,* Fullerton, Calif, 1983, The Society of Critical Care Medicine.

103. Wood L, Prichard S, Weng T et al: Relationship between anatomic dead space and body size in health, asthma, and cystic fibrosis, *Am Rev Respir Dis* 104:215, 1971.

104. Wood M, Wood AJJ: Changes in plasma drug binding and α-1-glycoprotein in mother and newborn infant, *Clin Pharmacol Ther* 29:522, 1981.

105. Wood RA, Hoekelman RA: Value of the chest x-ray as a screening test for elective surgery in children, *Pediatrics* 67:447, 1981.

CHAPTER 27

Evaluation of the Geriatric Patient

JUDITH L. STIFF

It is difficult to define when old age begins because by "old" we generally mean the start of decline in physical condition rather than a specific age. However, regardless of the age one takes to be the beginning of old age, this is the fastest-growing segment of the population in Western countries. In the United States in 1986 there were 29.1 million people over the age of 65, which is 12% of the total population; 1% of the population is over 85. On reaching 65, an individual has a life expectancy of 15 to 20 more years. If we assume that older people have more health problems requiring surgery than the general population, we would expect far more than 12% of our patients to be over 65.

ETHICAL ISSUES IN SURGERY ON GERIATRIC PATIENTS

Because older patients tend to be sicker and require more hospitalization, the health care of the geriatric population is disproportionately more expensive. It is projected that in 50 years 45% of health care expenses will be for care of the elderly.[10] Whether the costs of medical care will be allowed to continue to escalate unchecked is a societal issue, and, if there are to be economic limitations, our society as a whole will need to decide where and to whom those limitations will be applied. Individual physicians must concern themselves with this issue and be aware of the costs of various tests and treatments and choose the most cost-effective measures.

At the level of the individual patient, anesthesiologists more frequently are providing care for these older and sicker patients, and troubling questions arise concerning the goals of any particular operation. These goals should be consistent with societal ethical principles. An obvious goal is that an operation should be beneficial to the patient. Although this goal usually means restoring a patient to health, in older patients the goal may be more limited, perhaps to save some degree of function, to improve the quality of life, to relieve pain, or to avoid increased suffering. Thus an operation might be performed on a terminally ill cancer patient to alleviate pain or enhance mobility for the time that patient has left to live. However, care must be taken with the assumptions about operations. For example, operative repair of a hip fracture is thought to be beneficial because it will enable a patient to get out of bed and probably ambulate. A small study in nursing home patients with hip fractures showed that if patients who had disabilities such that they had little hope of walking again were managed nonoperatively, they had no complications and could get up to a chair within 6 weeks. Even in those with a good chance of becoming ambulatory, operative repair meant a very high risk of complications and death and did not always lead to ambulation.[58]

Therefore another goal of surgery should be to do no harm (nonmalfeasance) or to ensure that the expectation of benefit is much greater than the potential for harm. Cataract extraction is often performed in geriatric patients who may have many other medical conditions. Yet the operation has such a low risk,[3] with the beneficial result being restoration of vision, that it would be exceedingly rare that performing it would not be consistent with goals of benefit and nonmalfeasance.

The case for cataract surgery is straightforward, but many other situations are not. Until fairly recently it was thought that open-heart operations should not be offered to patients over 80 years of age. The reluctance to perform these major operations arose from the thought that an octogenarian had lived his/her life and would lack the will and stamina to endure such an ordeal. However, in a study of 100 such operations, although 29 patients died within 3 months, all the survivors were functionally improved and their survival statistics were equivalent to the expected survival for all persons of the same age.[28]

These goals cannot be viewed only from the vantage point of the physician because an underlying principle in our society is autonomy; the patient must decide what is to be done to his/her body. Thus the decision as to what is beneficial is the patient's, and the patient has the right to decide how to weigh the negative aspects against the potential good. A patient, particularly one who is at a considerably different point in his/her life than the physician, may well place different values on function or pain compared with what he/she must undergo in an operation.

An attempt to quantify benefits vs. risk has been done in the case of prostatectomy for patients with moderate urinary symptoms.[5] Considering the risk of death associated with the operation for a 70-year-old man, the net utility is a loss of 1.01 months of life expectancy. However, assigning a value to the odds of relief of symptoms, a gain of 2.94 quality-adjusted life-months is reached. This analysis is for the "average" patient and cannot address perioperative risks to a specific patient with a set of medical conditions. The conclusion is that the important factor is the patient's preference, how his/her symptomatology is viewed. How to adequately present this kind of information to a patient remains a question.

Occasionally an older patient is incompetent to give consent to surgery. However, physicians need to remember that even though a patient's decision regarding treatment seems medically irrational, the patient is not necessarily incompetent. Before deciding a seemingly demented or delusional patient is incompetent, the physician should treat all reversible causes of the deranged mental state. This can be as simple as stopping psychotropic medications, talking to the patient at the time of day he/she is most lucid,

or making sure that he/she can hear adequately.

In dealing with an incompetent patient, decisions are usually made by the nearest relative, and relatives need the same kind of information concerning risks and benefits that the patient would receive. In emergency situations, contacting relatives is not always possible, and treatment should proceed with notation in the chart concerning the situation. In a situation regarding resuscitation, unless the possibility of "no resuscitation" has been discussed previously with the consenting relative, reasonable treatment should be provided, just as one would resuscitate a competent person unless "no resuscitation" had been decided on by the patient in advance.

Anesthesiologists often think that they have little to do with deciding ethical issues of whether to operate or not and, to a large extent, this is true. However, anesthesiologists frequently know better than surgeons what the true risks of the perioperative period are for a particular procedure and a particular patient with a particular medical condition. Given this knowledge, anesthesiologists should participate in the difficult decisions concerning whether to operate or not.

RISK OF ANESTHESIA AND SURGERY

To consider the risk of anesthesia and surgery for geriatric patients, the question needs to be asked: Is age alone a risk factor for perioperative morbidity and mortality? Certainly many studies show that older patients do have higher perioperative morbidity and mortality (Fig. 27-1 and Tables 27-1 and 27-2). However, to answer that question, data must be obtained that compare younger and older patients having similar disease status. Table 27-1 presents the results of one recent study stratified for disease status

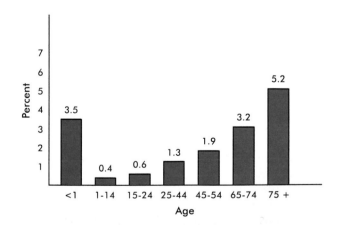

Fig. 27-1. Major anesthetic complications (per 1000) related to age. (Data from Tiret L, N'Doye P, and Hatton F: Complications associated with anaesthesia—a prospective survey in France, *Can Anaesth Soc J* 33:336, 1986.)

Table 27-1 Major anesthesia complications (per 1000) as a function of age and associated disease

| Age | Number of associated diseases | | | |
	0	1	2	3
<34	<1	1	1.5	
35-54	1	1.2	1.5	3
55-74	1	2	4.5	7
>74	1.5	2.5	5.5	13

Modified from Tiret L, N'Doye P, Hatton F et al: Complications associated with anaesthesia—a prospective survey in France, *Can Anaesth Soc J* 33:336, 1986.

Table 27-2 Percent of perioperative morbidity and mortality in patients over 90 as a function of ASA physical status

	II	III	IV
Elective	4.0	8.9	15.8
Emergency	20.0	15.0	26.8

Modified from Hosking MP, Warner MA, Lobdell CM et al: Outcomes of surgery in patients 90 years of age and older, *JAMA* 261:1909, 1989.

at various ages.[90] **This study indicates that for patients without significant disease the risk of anesthesia and operation appears to be unchanged by age. However, when there is preexisting disease, the older patient is at increased risk compared with the younger patient with the same amount of disease.** Looking at an older subset—**patients 90 years and older—the morbidity and mortality do increase even in the healthy ASA II physical status patients** (Table 27-2).[47] However, part of the reason that the risk may be so high in these patients is the type of operation that they need. Operations on the hips or pelvis had an 11% morbidity and mortality in patients over 90, and operations on the digestive system had 29%; these operations accounted for 50% of all operations in this series.[96]

Operation-specific risk data for older patients often exist for only small groups and as such cannot be generalized. However, data for hip fracture repair, prostatectomy, and open-heart procedures in the elderly are available. **In a multihospital group of 698 patients over 65 years of age undergoing operation for hip fracture, there was a 4.3% mortality in hospital.**[59] This study and others report mortality above expected rates for the general population up to 1 year after this operation.[20,99] **Assuming that the majority of prostatic operations are performed on older men, multihospital data showed mortality at 3 months to be 3.5% for transurethral resection and 3.8% for open procedures.**[98] **In patients over 65 years of age in the Coronary Artery Surgery Study, the 30-day mortality was 5.2% and 5-year survival was 83%.**[37] Long-term survival was influenced most by preexisting left ventricular function. In a series of 320 patients, **cardiac valve replacement had an in-hospital mortality of 8.75%.**[48]

Therefore, age in and of itself is not a very significant risk factor, and evaluation of an older patient should proceed much as it would for any

patient. However, in this as in any assessment one is comparing the patient with what is normal, and for older patients normal may well be different. Additionally, in geriatric patients it can be more difficult to obtain a good medical history because of memory and hearing deficits, dementia, or perhaps a more subtle problem in that an older patient may expect a paternalistic approach to his/her problems (i.e., "My doctor takes care of me; I don't need to know about my medical condition."). Also, many geriatric patients have assumed a very sedentary lifestyle that keeps them symptom-free in the face of significant disease. The anesthesiologist needs to have an idea of the prevalence of various disease conditions in the geriatric population and the clues to those conditions so that the probabilities of these conditions can be inferred in the difficult-to-evaluate patient and the appropriate workup can be chosen.

CARDIOVASCULAR SYSTEM

Age causes changes in the cardiovascular system but not decline, for there are compensatory mechanisms that take over to maintain cardiac function although cardiac reserve may not be as great in the elderly. Expected changes in cardiac function at rest and with exercise in individuals without heart disease are presented in Table 27-3. **In older patients, the heart rate tends to be slightly lower and the stroke volume is slightly increased, leading to little or no decrease in cardiac output. This can be likened to a physiologic beta-blockade.** The older heart undergoes a progressive left ventricular hypertrophy, which parallels the increase in arterial systolic blood pressure.[53] Studies do not agree on the mechanism to maintain cardiac output, but the result is that left ventricular filling is slowed initially but enhanced late in the cycle, leading to smaller end-diastolic volume, compensated by an increase in end-diastolic pressure.[23,54] The older heart probably depends more on the atrial contribution to filling.[23]

With exercise the older heart may not show as great an increase in cardiac output, ejection fraction, and

Table 27-3   Cardiovascular function in healthy older individuals

Cardiovascular parameter	Aging effect at rest	Aging effect with exercise
Heart rate	No change or slight decrease	Less increase
Blood pressure		
Systolic	Increased	Greater increase
Diastolic	No change	Slightly greater increase
Cardiac output	No change	Slightly less increase
Ejection fraction	No change	Less increase
Stroke volume	No change or slight increase	Greater increase

Table 27-4   Percent of patients with peripheral vascular disease who also have coronary artery disease

Coronary artery disease	AAA (%)	CVD (%)	Other (%)	Total
Absent	6	10	9	8
Mild to moderate	29	33	32	32
Severe	65	57	59	60

AAA, abdominal aortic aneurysm; *CVD,* cerebrovascular disease; mild to moderate, coronary lesion >70%; severe, greater than 70% stenosis in one or more coronary arteries.
Modified from Hertzer NR, Beven EG, Young JR et al: Coronary artery disease in peripheral vascular patients: a classification of 1000 coronary angiograms and results of surgical management, *Ann Surg* 199:223, 1984.

heart rate but may show a greater increase in stroke volume and blood pressure.[80] The extent of the decline in maximum work capacity of the heart in older individuals is quite variable, depending on the conditioning of the individual.[54]

The vascular system also undergoes changes. The aorta becomes stiffer, which increases the pulse wave velocity and changes the pulse wave contour. This and the loss of distensibility in the rest of the vasculature leads to higher systolic blood pressure.[53] Along with the change in cardiac function and vasculature, **the baroreceptor sensitivity decreases with age in both hypertensive and normotensive individuals.**[86] **Older people show less of a heart rate response to hypotension and thus are at risk for orthostatic hypotension.** Similarly, the cardiopulmonary stretch receptor response to increased or decreased venous return is reduced.[13] It has been hypothesized that during stress the cardiovascular system of the older individual is less responsive to beta-adrenergic effects even though the levels of norepinephrine and epinephrine are higher.[53] A clinical study of the response to laryngoscopy and intubation comes to the same conclusion. Older patients had a lesser response in heart rate yet a greater response in norepinephrine.[9]

Of course, for many elderly patients the cardiovascular system does deteriorate due to heart disease, other diseases, nutritional status, or lifestyle. The chance that a geriatric patient may have cardiovascular disease can be estimated by knowing data for the prevalence of the various diseases. Fig. 27-2 presents data from the National Health Interview Survey that represents patients' knowledge of their health sta-

tus.[70] The true incidence of these conditions is undoubtedly higher.

Careful history may fail to elicit symptoms of coronary artery disease. **The incidence of unrecognized or "silent" myocardial infarction increases with age.** In a series of older patients with a discharge diagnosis of myocardial infarction, 42% of those over 65 years old had had no chest pain.[68] **The percentage of myocardial infarctions that were diagnosed solely by the appearance of new pathologic Q waves or new loss of R-wave potential in patients over 65 was greater than 29% in the Framingham Study and reached a high of 45.5% in women over 85.**[49] In the evaluation of older patients, ECG evidence of an old myocardial infarction, even though the medical history is negative, must be considered as a positive finding.

Silent ischemia is a more difficult problem, and it is rarely found on a routine ECG. It has been shown that silent ischemia with stable angina leads to increased probability of a cardiac event.[78] In the elderly even angina can go undiagnosed because it masquerades as other conditions such as indigestion or musculoskeletal pain. **A patient with risk factors needs to be evaluated for ischemia by either a stress test or 24-hour ambulatory ECG monitoring.**[39] Because of preexisting ECG abnormalities (left ventricular hypertrophy, bundle branch block, Wolff-Parkinson-White syndrome, baseline ST segment abnormalities), ambulatory monitoring is not possible in some patients; however, in the rest it seems to be a very good predictor for high risk.[78]

A significant predictor for the presence of coronary artery disease (CAD) is the presence of other vascular disease. In a study of 1000 patients with peripheral vascular disease, 500 had normal ECGs and 446 had no indication of coronary artery disease.[44] All underwent coronary angiography (Table 27-4). Only 8% of patients in the study were found to be free of CAD,

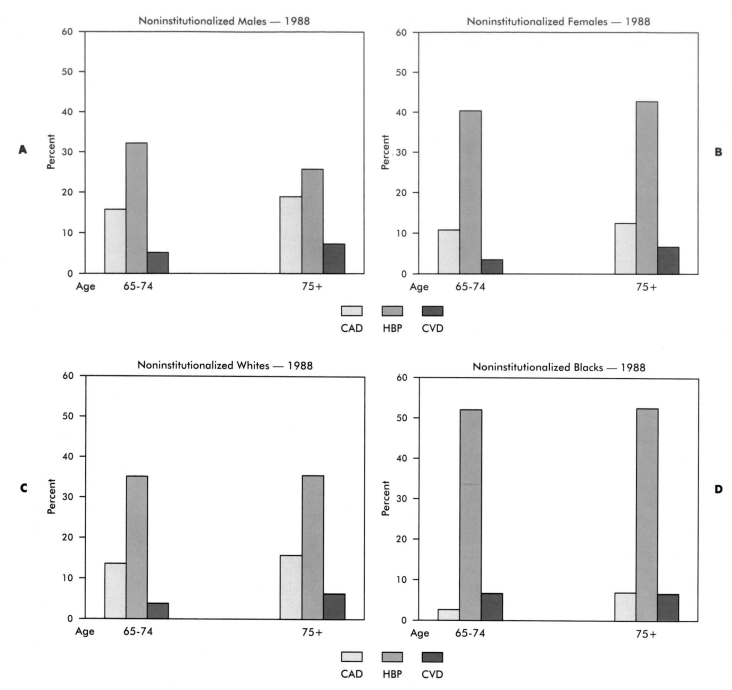

Fig. 27-2. Incidence of cardiovascular disease in older patients. **A,** Noninstitutionalized males. **B,** Noninstitutionalized females. **C,** Noninstitutionalized whites. **D,** Noninstitutionalized blacks. *CAD,* coronary artery disease; *HBP,* high blood pressue; *CVD,* cerebrovascular disease. (From National Center for Health Statistics: Current estimates from the National Health Interview Survey, 1988. Vital and Health Statistics Series 10, No. 173, US Government Printing Office, October, 1989.)

and 60% had severe disease. In a group of 50 patients who were admitted for a transient ischemic attack or a stroke (mild enough to allow testing), although in 34 patients coronary artery disease was not suspected, 14 were found to have a positive test (as well as 15 of the 16 with suspected disease) for an overall incidence of 58%.[81]

A recent study suggests that in patients scheduled for major vascular surgery, presence of as few as two of five risk factors that were significant predictors should lead to testing for coronary artery disease; those factors were age greater than 70, history of angina, Q waves on ECG, diabetes mellitus, and history of PVCs requiring treatment.[27] The appropri-

Table 27-5 Percent of older patients without apparent heart disease who have dysrhythmias		
Ventricular dysrhythmia	> 60	> 80
PVCs > 5/hr	74% (2)	
> 10/hr		46% (3)
> 30/hr	36% (2)	
> 50/hr		14% (3)
Couplets	11% (2)	8% (1)
V-tach	4% (2)	2% (1)

Modified from Fleg JL: Ventricular arrhythmias in the elderly, *Geriatrics* 43:23, 1988; Fleg JL, Kennedy HL: Cardiac arrhythmias in a healthy elderly population; *Chest* 81:302, 1982; and Kantelip JP, Sage E, and Duchene-Marullaz P: Findings on ambulatory electrocardiographic monitoring in subjects older than 80 years, *Am J Cardiol* 57:398, 1986.

Table 27-6 Aging and pulmonary function	
Respiratory factors	Changes
Vital capacity	Decreased (20 ml/yr)
FEV_1	Decreased
FEV_1/FVC	Unchanged to slight decrease
Closing capacity	Increased
FRC	Increased
RV	Increased
TLC	Unchanged to slight decrease
Diffusing capacity	Decreased
Pao_2*	Decreased

*Pao_2 (mm Hg) = 103.7 − (0.24 × age).[75]

ate testing for coronary artery disease is discussed in Chapter 11, but for elderly patients stress tests often need to be modified or be of a type so that the patient can achieve an adequate level of work.

With aging the conduction system undergoes certain changes, including fibrosis of the sinoatrial node, a decrease in the number of pacemaker cells, and atrophy of conducting tissue. There is an increased incidence of dysrhythmia and block, and indeed, sick sinus syndrome and trifascicular block are diseases of the elderly. Older patients have increased bradycardia, slowed conduction through the A-V node, and a shift of the QRS axis leftward.[61] In 24-hour ECG studies of older patients without apparent heart disease, there are considerable occurrences of both supraventricular and ventricular dysrhythmias[33,35,49,50] (Table 27-5).

If dysrhythmias are not unusual in older patients and a patient has no signs or symptoms of coronary artery disease, what ECG findings should lead to further investigation? Evidence of an old MI, as was mentioned previously, is a sign of pathology, as is left bundle branch block, left anterior hemiblock, and intraventricular conduction defects. Right bundle branch block (RBBB) may not be an indicator of cardiac disease. **In a longitudinal study, men with RBBB had no higher incidence of cardiac disease than the control population,** and RBBB did not increase the risk of cardiac problems over the long term.[34] For dysrhythmias, artrial fibrillation or flutter is indicative of the presence of disease. In the Framingham population **only 11% of those with atrial fibrillation did not have coexisting heart disease.**[8] Determining the significance of PVCs is more difficult. Frequent and complex PVCs are seen in healthy older patients. However, in many studies PVCs are factors predicting coronary artery disease or postop-

erative cardiovascular complications.[21,38] The age-related increase in ectopic beats does not constitute a risk in healthy subjects, and, in fact, the institution of dysrhythmia suppression therapy may be a greater risk. However, since dysrhythmias may be a manifestation of coronary artery disease or left ventricular hypertrophy or distenstion that is not obvious on ECG or clinical examination, it is necessary to discover those patients whose PVCs are a manifestation of disease. Left ventricular changes can be demonstrated by echocardiography. If coronary artery disease is suspected, appropriate testing needs to be obtained.

RESPIRATORY SYSTEM

Respiratory changes with aging consist of changes in lung and chest wall function, changes in alveolar gas exchange, and changes in the control of ventilation (Table 27-6). Lung and chest wall mechanics are altered by loss in muscle strength, stiffening of the chest wall, decrease in intervertebral spaces, and decrease in the elastic recoil of the lungs. This leads to a decrease in vital capacity and an increase in residual volume while functional residual capacity tends to remain unchanged. Dynamic lung volumes and capacities decrease with age mainly due to the changes in chest wall mechanics. The decrease in elastic recoil leads to airway closure, and the closing volume or closing capacity increases with age. **Airway closure becomes significant at the point at which closing capacity exceeds functional residual capacity and, although this is more prevalent with advancing age, it depends much more on body habitus than on age.** Large airways increase in diameter while small airways decrease. This leads to an increase in anatomic and physiologic dead space; however, airway resistance is essentially unchanged.[95]

Alveolar gas exchange declines in efficiency with age. This is believed to be due to a ventilation/perfusion mismatch caused by uneven distribution of inspired gas due to airway closure. There is also thought to be an increase in maldistribution of pulmonary blood flow as well as structural changes in the alveolar membrane.[95] These factors lead to a decline in arterial partial pressure of oxygen. An equation for the decline in Pao_2 with age is presented in Table 27-6.

Control of ventilation markedly changes with aging. **The ventilatory responses while awake to hypoxia and hypercarbia are both reduced.**[73] There is reduction in flow but not in tidal volume.[74] During sleep, older individuals have more irregular breathing patterns and more apneas.[73] In view of this, the response of an elderly patient to premedication is of concern. A study that compared the ventilatory response to a single-dose, slow IV push of morphine showed that although both older and younger patients had similar reductions in minute ventilation and frequency and a similar increase in end-tidal carbon dioxide, older patients had increased apneas and periodic breathing.[2]

Evaluation of the respiratory system in a geriatric patient should be undertaken as it would be for any patient (see Chapter 12). However, the geriatric patient with a hip fracture is common and requires careful evaluation. These patients come from a sicker population and, specifically, almost all have hypoxemia. **Control populations of patients have higher Pao_2s than patients scheduled for hip pinning.** In two stud-

ies, the mean values for the control patients were not different from that of the Raine and Bishop formula for prediction of Pao_2 (Table 27-7), but for the **hip fracture patients the Pao_2 values were significantly lower, by approximately 10 mm Hg to 20 mm Hg.**[62,83]

NERVOUS SYSTEM

Brain mass declines by about 2%/decade after age 50. Gross anatomic changes include flattening of the gyri and a slight increase in the size of the ventricles. There is a constant neuronal loss, but this is highly variable among the areas of the brain; the substantia nigra can lose up to 50% of its neurons while the sensory areas lose very little.[46] According to a study of neuronal cell counts in the neocortex, there is virtually no loss in total neuron population. What does happen is a decrease in large neurons, offset by a gain in small neurons, a "neuronal shrinkage."[89] In animals the aged nervous system has been shown to be capable of repair through axon sprouting and stimulus-dependent synapse turnover.[18] These processes are adequate only for minor neuronal loss. Axon sprouting has been observed in Alzheimer's disease, but it appears to be an aberrant process leading to the formation of plaques.[18] All of the morphologic changes of normal aging are exaggerated in patients with Alzheimer's disease. These include neurofibrillary tangles, neuritic plaques, granulovacuolar organelles, and lipofuscin granules. The question is whether Alzheimer's disease is merely an accelerated form of aging becoming more prevalent because of our aging population, or is it a specific pathology. Much of the current research centers on biochemical changes in the brain with aging.

Most of the data about the biochemical changes in the central nervous system with aging are of necessity derived from animal experiments. In normal aging there is a moderate decrease in glycolytic processes. This is accentuated in persons with Alzheimer's disease and is accompanied by impairment of acetylcholine synthesis and a large decrease in choline acetyltransferase.[64] The acetylcholine system has been extensively studied. In normal aging the deficits in both the presynaptic and postsynaptic parts are unevenly distributed but are not extensive in any area.[77] In Alzheimer's disease the area of very diminished acetylcholine activity, like the morphologic changes, is in the hippocampus and temporoparietal associational area.[17] Pharmacologic treatment with cholinesterase inhibitors has had some limited positive results. Undoubtedly other neurotransmitters are involved.

There is a decline in dopamine (D2) receptors in the striatum with aging in humans. Parkinson's disease may be an accelerated aging of the dopami-

Table 27-7 Modification of anesthetic drugs in older patients

Type of Drug	Modifications
Benzodiazepines	(?) Increased receptor sensitivity, decreased clearance
Narcotics	(?) Increased receptor sensitivity, probable decreased clearance
Inhalational agents	Probable increased sensitivity, decreased MAC
Neuromuscular blockers	
Succinylcholine	No change
Nondepolarizing neuromuscular block (except atracurium)	Decreased clearance
Neostigmine	Decreased clearance
Induction agents	(?) Increased sensitivity, smaller initial compartment
Thiopentol	
Etomidate	

nergic system of the brain[67] or a different lesion (i.e., a destruction of the dopaminergic neurons in the substantia nigra).[17] In Alzheimer's disease the dopaminergic system does not differ from that in normal aging. Less is known about other neurotransmitters. The norepinephrine system seems to be unchanged with aging as does the serotonin system.[66] The serotonin system may be involved in some depressive disorders and seems to be compromised in Alzheimer's disease.[66]

Cerebral blood flow has been shown to be lower in the elderly, both at rest and with activity; however, both young and elderly subjects have similar increases in flow with activity.[31] There may be considerable regional differences. Dementia caused by cerebral vascular disease in the elderly is much less common than the Alzheimer's type. Cerebrovascular disease can affect either the large arteries or small ones. Large-vessel disease is usually arteriosclerotic in origin and presents as transient ischemic attacks or strokes with stepwise progression. Small-vessel disease, usually the result of hypertension, can cause scattered bilateral small "lacunar" infarcts and often has a steadily deteriorating course.

Any routine clinical mental state examination, such as the Mini Mental State,[36] **should be normal in the healthy elderly patient, and abnormalities should lead to investigation of the etiology of the disorder.**[46] Dementia can be characterized as a loss of intellectual abilities sufficient to interfere with normal daily function. Mild memory deficits in secondary or short-term memory, minor gait disorders, and loss of muscle power are part of normal aging.

Potential causes of dementia include metabolic derangements, toxicities, vascular disease, head trauma and space-occupying lesions, and infectious or inflammatory conditions. Treatable causes need to be sought, and even a patient with a degenerative dementia may have other factors superimposed. In a small prospective study of acute confusion (delirium) in elderly patients admitted to the hospital, 25% had confusion either on admission or during hospitalization. Of the patients with preexisting dementia, half had episodes of acute confusion. Infections and congestive heart failure were the predominant diagnoses.[79]

Most commonly dementia is degenerative, and over 50% of elderly patients with dementia are thought to have Alzheimer's disease. The diagnosis of Alzheimer's disease is not always clear cut; however, new techniques such as positron emission tomography (PET) and single photon–emission computed tomography (SPECT) are improving diagnostic capability. **In the United States the prevalence of Alzheimer's disease in a noninstitutionalized population was 10.3% in persons over 65 and increased with age to 47.2% in persons over 85. Alzheimer's dementia was nine times more prevalent than dementia due to other causes.**[30]

Although there is little clinical evidence that patients with Alzheimer's disease are more sensitive to sedatives, tranquilizers, and narcotics, many physicians think that this is the case. In dealing with the very easily agitated demented patient, it is best to have a family member who manages the patient well accompany the patient to the operating room where sedation can be safely undertaken.

There are other nervous system changes with aging that affect anesthesia care. **Thermoregulation becomes impaired, and many of the elderly have less insulation from subcutaneous tissue and skin to protect against heat loss.** In a study of postoperative hypothermia, older patients had lower body temperatures than younger patients on arrival in the recovery room.[92]

The special senses undergo decline with aging. In large community populations over 65 years old surveyed for a wide variety of medical conditions, 11% had vision sufficiently impaired so that they could not read a newspaper and 11% had hearing loss significant enough so that they could not hear a voice in a quiet room.[16] A lesser degree of hearing loss is usual in the elderly, and complaints of vertigo are common. The sense of smell becomes less acute, and loss of olfactory sensation is often present in patients with Alzheimer's disease.

Reaction time is slowed in older individuals, and, in repeated trials or more complex tasks, the error rate is higher.[88] The slowing appears to be due to the components of converting the signal into a stimulus and the activation of the muscles in response.[97] Perception of pain is difficult to compare between individuals, but, using thermal stimulation, older individuals did seem to estimate magnitudes of pain similar to the manner younger individuals did.[42]

RENAL FUNCTION AND PHARMACOLOGY

Another aspect of "normal" aging that can affect anesthesia is **renal decline, which seems to be fairly predictable at the rate of about 1%/year or a 1 ml/min/yr decline in creatinine clearance** after age 40. The following formula estimates creatinine clearance based on age from serum creatinine measurement.[14]

$$\text{Creatinine clearance} = \frac{(140 - \text{age}) \times \text{wt (kg)}}{72 \times \text{serum creatinine}}$$

Various aspects of drug handling also change with normal aging. Box 27-1 lists those aspects that need to be considered in predicting whether there will be a change in drug effect in an older patient, and Table 27-7 lists drugs of interest to the anesthesiologist as

---

BOX 27-1
ALTERED DRUG EFFECTS IN
THE OLDER INDIVIDUAL

Pharmacodynamics

Decrease in receptor numbers
Decrease in receptor sensitivity
Increase in receptor sensitivity

Pharmacokinetics

Decrease in absorption—oral
Change in distribution
    Decline in muscle mass, increase in adipose
    tissue
Increased bioavailability—decrease in albumin
Reduced clearance
    Decreased hepatic blood flow
    Reduced hepatic metabolism—oxidative
    Reduced renal clearance

---

related to possible effects of aging. Very little has been actually proved about specific drugs and their pharmacodynamic properties in older patients. As mentioned previously, baroreceptors undergo a decline in sensitivity with age, which may be the reason why older patients have more difficulty with orthostasis with certain antihypertensives. There is some evidence for a decrease in number of dopamine receptors in older persons and for a decline in the sensitivity of benzodiazepine receptors.

The changes associated with aging of most concern are those dealing with pharmacokinetics. Although anesthesiologists deal very little in orally administered drugs, it is significant that absorption is somewhat slowed in older individuals. Changes in distribution seem to be of limited importance, but, because of decline in muscle mass and relative increase in adipose tissue, there can be a larger depot of lipid-soluble drugs. This is probably the case with lidocaine and the benzodiazepines. Bioavailability, again, is not a great cause of changes in drug effect, but, with a decrease in albumin, there might be a slight increase in response to an initial dose of a drug that is highly bound to albumin. More important, however, is the effect this may have on interpretation of laboratory-determined drug levels (e.g., a lower total drug level may well represent the same level of free drug).

The major effect of aging on drug action is in clearance. Hepatic blood flow decreases with age and can reduce first-pass drug extraction, leading to higher blood levels. Propranolol is an example of a drug so affected. The phase I or oxidative metabolic processes of the liver decline with age, whereas the

synthetic or phase II processes show little change. Therefore, drugs such as benzodiazepines and theophylline, whose initial degradation is oxidative, have a prolonged action. The decrease in renal function, as mentioned previously, is obviously very important for drugs being administered chronically, such as digoxin, cimetidine, procainamide, and lithium, but is of lesser importance in drugs briefly administered in the operating room.

The minimum alveolar concentration (MAC) of inhalational anesthetic agents decreases with increasing age and is similar for all agents. An 80-year-old patient will generally require about 25% less agent than a young adult.[41,69,87] EEG studies seem to indicate a pharmacodynamic difference—that older individuals are more sensitive to these agents.[84] However, rigorous pharmacokinetic studies have not been done. Another change is in tissue solubilities. Blood/gas partition coefficients decrease from younger to older adults, and muscle/gas coefficients increase. Coefficients for other tissues show less change.[56] However, even with the decreased blood solubility of the anesthetic gases, uptake is slower in the elderly.[26]

Older patients require smaller doses of both thiopental and etomidate to induce anesthesia, but this is due to pharmacokinetics rather than increased sensitivity. Thiopental has a change in initial distribution, with a smaller central compartment.[45] Etomidate shows a similar change, as well as a decreased clearance.[1] **Older patients also seem to require lower doses of propofol**[24] and have a reduced clearance.[51]

The evidence about the pharmacodynamic and pharmacokinetic changes with age for narcotics is difficult to interpret. Pharmacokinetic studies of a single dose of intravenous morphine[72] and meperidine[43] showed initial plasma levels to be unchanged with aging. However, over time the two drugs differ in that morphine has a smaller volume of distribution but a faster elimination in the elderly, and meperidine has a higher volume of distribution in the elderly. Fentanyl and alfentanil have been shown to be cleared more slowly by older patients.[6,85]

However, a question of greater interest is the effect of these drugs: Are older individuals more sensitive to opioids or do they seem to be more sensitive because of initial distribution effects? A study of fentanyl as an induction agent showed that 30 µg/kg provided an adequate induction in patients over 60 years of age but was not always adequate in younger patients.[4] Using fentanyl or alfentanil to a brain monitoring end point (half maximal spectral edge frequency) showed older patients needed a lower serum concentration and a lower dose.[85] However, another group found that using a continuous infusion of alfentanil regulated to prevent response to surgical stimulation, older patients reached the same plasma levels as younger patients but required less drug to reach these levels.[55] Although the question is not answered, it does seem that in planning an anesthetic using fentanyl and its derivatives, the dose should be lowered, and certainly our clinical experience with morphine and demerol indicates that those doses should also be lowered.

The effects of narcotics in the elderly must also be considered in the postoperative management of these patients. In a comparison of younger and older patients following intravenous morphine, both groups had the same decrease in the slope of the CO_2 response curve and rise in end-tidal CO_2.[19] However, in a comparison of intravenous morphine with regional analgesia with bupivacaine, older patients showed more oxygen desaturation and disordered breathing patterns with the morphine, and older patients had more episodes of apneas and paradoxical breathing than younger patients.[11]

It is thought that older individuals are more sensitive to the benzodiazepines. A study of the dose of diazepam necessary to induce sedation showed that an increase in age from 20 years to 75 years reduced the diazepam requirement by about one half and that there was a strong correlation between dose and plasma levels.[15] Assuming that there is no difference in initial distribution kinetics, **this would indicate that older individuals are more sensitive to intravenous diazepam; this also seems to hold true for midazolam.**[76]

The nondepolarizing neuromuscular blockers all seem to require the same initial dosing in older patients to get the same effect, with plasma levels correlating well with effect.* **With the exception of atracurium, all have slower clearance in older patients.** Atracurium has an unchanged clearance, most likely because of degradation in the plasma by Hoffman elimination taking over where liver metabolism and renal excretion diminish. **Succinylcholine's action and clearance are not age-dependent. Doses of reversal agents need not be modified for older patients.**[100]

Local anesthetics in older patients are cleared less rapidly, leading to a longer duration of regional block.[93,94] **Older patients require the same dose to achieve the same level of subarachnoid block,**[91,94] but **require less in epidural block.**[32,93] In planning an anesthetic, it is often thought that a regional technique will leave a geriatric patient better postoperative mental function. However, in a study comparing general anesthesia with spinal anesthesia, only at 6 hours postoperatively was the Mini Mental State score worse in the general anesthesia patients. At 1,

2, and 3 days there was no difference.[12] **Preexisting depression or antidepressant medications are high-risk factors for postoperative confusion.**[7]

OTHER CONSIDERATIONS

Other areas of homeostasis are affected by the aging process (Box 27-2). The control of water balance is impaired, both by blunting of thirst sensation and by the diminished ability of the kidney to conserve water. Additionally, sodium conservation may be impaired. **All of this leaves an older patient vulnerable to hypovolemia and hyponatremia.**[65]

Geriatric patients often have impaired glucose tolerance, specifically, 36% of those 65 to 74 years of age and 42% of those over 75.[57] This is due to many factors, including decreased insulin synthesis or secretion, insulin resistance, impaired glucose utilization, change in body composition, and change in diet and activity level. In the older patient this can more easily lead to a hyperosmolar, nonketotic state. Adult-onset type diabetes mellitus as well as other factors, such as renal insufficiency, hypothermia, and drugs that decrease insulin secretion or promote dehydration, increase this possibility.[40] General anesthesia and the administration of large quantities of hypertonic solution also add to the risk.

Although geriatric patients have decreased gastric acid secretion, they still are at risk for aspiration. In patients over 65 after a fast of greater than 8 hours, 60% had a gastric pH lower than 2.5 and 12% had a volume of greater than 0.40 ml/kg.[60] Aging causes a decrease in airway reflexes, leading to a greater risk of aspiration when those reflexes are further blunted by drugs.

---

* References 22, 25, 52, 63, 71, 82

> **BOX 27-2**
> **OTHER CHANGES IN HOMEOSTASIS**
> **WITH AGING**
>
> **Impaired glucose tolerance**
>
> Decreased insulin production or secretion
> Insulin resistance or impaired glucose utilization
> Changes in body composition
> Changes in diet and activity level
>
> **Reduction in defense against fluid and electrolyte imbalance**
>
> Decrease in renal concentrating ability
> Decrease in sodium conservation
> Altered thirst perception

CONCLUSIONS

Certainly the anesthesia management of an elderly patient requires an attention to detail that one also associates with the care of a patient at the other extreme of life. Although the goals of surgery toward the end of a natural life span are different, the geriatric patient deserves our best efforts toward making old age a decent and honorable time of life.

KEY POINTS

- Along with a change in cardiac function and vasculature, the baroreceptor sensitivity decreases with age in both hypertensive and normotensive individuals. Older people show less heart rate response to hypotension and thus are at risk for orthostatic hypotension.

- In older patients, the heart rate tends to be slightly lower and the stroke volume is slightly increased, leading to little or no decrease in cardiac output. This can be likened to a physiologic beta-blockade.

- The incidence of unrecognized or "silent" myocardial infarctions increases with age.

- Airway closure becomes significant at the point at which closing capacity exceeds functional residual capacity, and, although this is more prevalent with advancing age, it depends much more on body habitus than on age.

- With age the ventilatory responses while awake to hypoxia and hypercapnia are both reduced.

- There is a decline in dopamine (D2) receptors in the striatum with aging in humans. However, the norepinephrine system seems unchanged as does the serotonin system.

- In the United States the prevalence of Alzheimer's disease in a noninstitutionalized population was 10.3% of persons over 65 and increased with age to 47.2% in persons over 85. Alzheimer's dementia was nine times more prevalent than dementia due to other causes.

- Thermoregulation becomes impaired with age, and many elderly have less insulation from subcutaneous tissue and skin to protect against heat loss.

- Renal function declines at a fairly pedictable rate of about 1%/year or 1 ml/min/year in creatinine clearance.

- The major effect of aging on drug action is in clearance. The phase I or oxidative metabolic processes of the liver decline with age, whereas the synthetic or phase II processes show little change.

- The minimum alveolar concentration (MAC) of inhalational anesthetic agents decreases with increasing age and is similar for all agents. An 80-year-old patient will generally require about 25% less agent than a young adult.

- Older patients require smaller doses of propofol, thiopental, and etomidate to induce anesthesia.

- Older patients seem to be more sensitive to intravenous diazepam and midazolam.

- Nondepolarizing neuromuscular blockers, except atracurium, are cleared more slowly in older patients. Doses of reversal agents need not be modified for these patients.

- Older patients require the same dose of local anesthetics to achieve the same level of subarachnoid block but require less in epidural block.

- Preexisting depression or antidepressant medications are high-risk factors for postoperative confusion.

- The control of water balance is impaired in the elderly, leaving such patients vulnerable to hypovolemia and hyponatremia.

KEY REFERENCES

Horvath TB, Davis KL: Central nervous system disorder in aging. In Schneider EL, Rowe JW, eds: *Handbook of the biology of aging,* ed 3, San Diego, 1990, Academic Press.

Lakatta EG: Heart and circulation. In Schneider EL, Rowe JW, eds: *Handbook of the biology of aging,* ed 3, San Diego, 1990, Academic Press.

Tiret L, Desmonts JM, and Hatton F: Complications associated with anaesthesia—a prospective survey in France, *Can Anaesth Soc J* 33:336, 1986.

Wahba WM: Influence of aging on lung function— clinical significance of changes from age twenty, *Anesth Analg* 62:764, 1983.

REFERENCES

1. Arden JR, Holley FO, and Stanski DR: Increased sensitivity to etomidate in the elderly: initial distribution versus altered brain response, *Anesthesiology* 65:19, 1986.
2. Arunasalam K, Davenport HT, Painter S, et al: Ventilatory response to morphine in young and old subjects, *Anaesthesia* 38:529, 1983.
3. Backer CL, Tinker JH, Robertson DM, et al: Myocardial reinfarction following local anesthesia for ophthalmic surgery, *Anesth Analg* 54:257, 1980.
4. Bailey PL, Wilbrink J, Zwanikken P, et al: Anesthetic induction with fentanyl, *Anesth Analg* 64:48, 1985.
5. Barry MJ, Mulley AG Jr, Fowler FJ, et al: Watchful waiting vs immediate transurethral resection for symptomatic prostatism. The importance of patients' preferences, *JAMA* 259:3010, 1988.
6. Bentley JB, Borel JD, Nenad RE Jr, et al: Age and fentanyl pharmacokinetics, *Anesth Analg* 61:968, 1982.
7. Berggren D, Gustafson Y, Eriksson B, et al: Postoperative confusion after anesthesia in elderly patients with femoral neck fractures, *Anesth Analg* 66:497, 1987.
8. Brand FN et al: Characteristics and prognosis of lone atrial fibrillation. 30-year follow-up in the Framingham Study, *J Am Med Assoc* 254:3449, 1985.
9. Bullington J, Mouton Perry SM, Rigby J, et al: The effect of advancing age on the sympathetic response to laryngoscopy and tracheal intubation, *Anesth Analg* 68:603, 1989.
10. Callahan D: Aging and the ends of medicine, *Ann N Y Acad Sci* 530:125, 1988.
11. Cately DM et al: Pronounced, episodic oxygen desaturation in the postoperative period. Its association with ventilatory pattern and analgesic regime, *Anesthesiology* 63:20, 1985.
12. Chung F, Meier R, Lautenschlager E, et al: General or spinal anesthesia: which is better in the elderly, *Anesthesiology* 67:422, 1987.
13. Cléroux J, Giannattasio C, Bolla G, et al: Decreased cardiopulmonary reflexes with aging in normotensive humans, *Am J Physiol* 257:H961, 1989.
14. Cockcroft D, Gault M: Prediction of creatinine clearance from serum creatinine, *Nephron* 15:31, 1976.
15. Cook PJ, Flanagan R, and James IM: Diazepam tolerance: effect of age, regular sedation, and alcohol, *Br Med J* 289:351, 1984.
16. Cornoni-Huntley J et al: Established populations for epidemiologic study in the elderly, Department of Health and Human Services (NIH) pg. 20 86-2443, Washington.
17. Coté L: Aging of the brain and dementia. In Kandel ER, Schwartz JH, eds: *Principles of neural science,* New York, 1981, Elsevier.
18. Cotman CW: Synaptic plasticity, neurotrophic factors and transplantation in the aged brain. In Schneider EL, Rowe JW, eds: *Handbook of the biology of aging,* ed 3, San Diego, 1990, Academic Press.
19. Daykin AP, Bowen DJ, Saunders DA, et al: Respiratory depression after morphine in the elderly, *Anaesthesia* 41:910, 1986.
20. Davis FM, Woolner DF, Framptom C, et al: Prospective, multi-centre trial of mortality following general or spinal anaesthesia for hip fracture surgery in the elderly, *Br J Anaesth* 59:1080, 1987.
21. Detsky AS, Abrams HB, Forbath N et al: Cardiac assessment for patients undergoing noncardiac surgery. A multifactorial clinical risk index, *Arch Intern Med* 146:2131, 1986.
22. d'Hollander AA, Luyckx C, Barvais L et al: Clinical evaluation of atracurium besylate requirement for stable muscle relaxation: lack of age-related effects, *Anesthesiology* 59:237, 1983.
23. Downes TR, Nomeir AM, Smith KM et al: Mechanism of altered pattern of left ventricular filling with aging in subjects without cardiac disease, *Am J Cardiol* 64:523, 1989.
24. Dundee JW, Robinson FP, McCollum JS et al: Sensitivity to propofol in the elderly, *Anaesthesia* 41:482, 1986.
25. Duvaldestin P, Saada J, Berger JL et al: Pharmacokinetics, pharmacodynamics, and dose-response relationships of pancuronium in control and elderly subjects, *Anesthesiology* 56:36, 1982.
26. Dwyer R: The effect of aging on uptake of halothane, *Anesthesiology* 71:A313, 1989.
27. Eagle KA, Coley CM, Newell JB et al: Combining clinical and thallium data optimizes preoperative assessment of cardiac risk before major vascular surgery, *Ann Intern Med* 110:859, 1989.
28. Edmunds LH Jr, Stephanson LW, Edie RN et al: Open-heart surgery in octogenarians, *N Engl J Med* 319:131, 1988.
29. Reference deleted in proofs.
30. Evans DA, Funkenstein HH, Albert MS et al: Prevalence of Alzheimer's disease in a community population of older persons, higher than previously reported, *J Am Med Soc* 262:2551, 1989.
31. Ewing JR, et al: 133 Xenon inhalation: accuracy in detection of ischemic cerebral regions and angiographic lesions. In Wood JH, ed: *Cerebral blood flow,* New York, 1987, McGraw-Hill.
32. Finucane BT, Hammonds WD, and Welch MB: Influence of age on vascular absorption of lidocaine from the epidural space, *Anesth Analg* 66:843, 1987.
33. Fleg JL: Ventricular arrhythmias in the elderly: prevalence, mechanisms and therapeutic implications, *Geriatrics* 43:23, 1988.
34. Fleg JL, Das DN, and Lakatta EG: Right bundle branch block: long-term prognosis in apparently healthy men, *J Am Coll Cardiol* 1:887, 1988.
35. Fleg JL, Kennedy HL: Cardiac arrhythmias in a healthy elderly population. Detection by 24-hour ambulatory electrocardiography, *Chest* 81:302, 1982.
36. Folstein MF, Folstein SE, and McHugh PR: "Mini Mental State": a practical method for grading the cognitive state of patients for the clinician, *J Psych Res* 12:189, 1975.
37. Gersh BJ, Kronmal RA, Schaff HV, et al: Long-term (5 year) results of coronary bypass surgery in patients 65 years old or older: a report from the Coronary Artery Surgery Study, *Circulation* 68(supp II):190, 1983.
38. Goldman L: Cardiac risks and complications of noncardiac surgery, *Ann Intern Med* 98:504, 1983.
39. Gottlieb SO, Gerstenblith G: Silent myocardial ischemia in the elderly: current concepts, *Geriatrics* 43:29, 1988.
40. Greene DA: Acute and chronic complications of diabetes mellitus in older patients, *Am J Med* 80:39, 1986.
41. Gregory GA, Eger EI, and Munson ES: The relationship between age and halothane requirement in man, *Anesthesiology* 30:488, 1969.
42. Harkins SW, Price DD, and Martelli M: Effects of age on pain perception: thermonociception, *J Gerontol* 41:58, 1986.
43. Herman RJ, McAllister CB, Branch RA et al: Effects of age on meperidine disposition, *Clin Pharmacol Ther* 37:19, 1985.
44. Hertzer NR, Beven EG, Young JR, et al: Coronary artery disease in peripheral vascular patients: a classification of 1000 coronary angiograms and results of surgical management, *Ann Surg* 199:223, 1984.
45. Homer TD, Stnaski DR: The effect of increasing age on thiopental disposition and anesthetic requirement, *Anesthesiology* 62:714, 1985.
46. Horvath TB, Davis KL: Central nervous system disorders in aging. In Schneider EL, Rowe JW, eds: *Handbook of the biology of aging,* ed 3, San Diego, 1990, Academic Press.
47. Hosking MP, Warner MA, Lobdell CM et al: Outcomes of surgery in patients 90 years of age and older, *JAMA 261:1909, 1989.*
48. Jamieson WR, Donner J, Munro AI, et al: Cardiac valve replacement in the elderly: a review of 320 consecutive cases, *Circulation* 64(suppl II):177, 1981.
49. Kannel WB, Abbott RD: Incidence and prognosis of unrecognized myocardial infarction: an update of the Framingham Study, *N Engl J Med* 311:1144, 1984.
50. Kantelip JP, Sage E, and Duchene-Marullaz P: Findings on ambulatory electrocardiographic monitoring in subjects older than 80 years, *Am J Cardiol* 57:398, 1986.

51. Kirkpatrick T: Pharmacokinetics of propofol (Diprivan) in elderly patients, *Br J Anaesth* 60:146, 1988.

52. Kitts JB, Fisher DM, Canfell PC et al: Pharmacokinetics and pharmacodynamics of atracurium in the elderly, *Anesthesiology* 72:272, 1990.

53. Lakatta EG: Heart and circulation. In Schneider EL, Rowe JW, editors: *Handbook of the biology of aging*, ed 3, San Diego, 1990, Academic Press.

54. Lakatta EG, Mitchell JH, Pomerance A et al: Human aging: changes in structure and function, *J Am Coll Cardiol* 10:42A, 1987.

55. Lemmens HJM, Bovill JG, Hennis PJ et al: Age has no effect on the pharmacodynamics of alfentanil, *Anesth Analg* 67:955, 1988.

56. Lerman J, Schmitt-Bantel BI, Gregory GA et al: Effect of age on the solubility of volatile anesthetics in human tissues, *Anesthesiology* 65:307, 1986.

57. Lipson LG: Diabetes in the elderly: diagnosis, pathogenesis and therapy, *Am J Med* 80:10, 1986.

58. Lyon LJ, Nevins MA: Management of hip fractures in nursing home patients: to treat or not to treat? *J Am Geriatr Soc* 32:391, 1984.

59. Magaziner J, Simonsick EM, Kashner TM et al: Survival experience of aged hip fracture patients, *Am J Public Health* 79:274, 1989.

60. Manchikanti L, Colliver JA, Marrero TC, et al: Assessment of age-related acid aspiration risk factors in pediatric, adult and geriatric patients, *Anesth Analg* 64:11, 1985.

61. Marcus FI, Ruskin JN, and Surawicz B: Arrhythmias, *J Am Coll Cardiol* 66A, 1987.

62. Martin VC: Hypoxaemia in elderly patients suffering from fractured neck of femur, *Anaesth* 32:852, 1977.

63. Matteo RS, Backus WW, McDaniel DD et al: Pharmacokinetics and pharmacodynamics of d-tubocurarine and metocurine in the elderly, *Anesth Analg* 64:23, 1985.

64. Meier-Ruge W: Neurochemistry of the aging brain and senile dementia. In Gaetz CM, Samorajski T, eds: *Aging 2000: our health care destiny, vol I*, New York, 1985, Springer-Verlag.

65. Miller M: Fluid and electrolyte balance in the elderly, *Geriatrics* 42:65, 1987.

66. Morgan DG, May PC: Age-related changes in synaptic neurochemistry. In Schneider EL, Rowe JW, eds: *Handbook of the biology of aging*, ed 3, San Diego, 1990, Academic Press.

67. Morgan DG, May PC, and Finch CE: Dopamine and serotonin systems in human and rodent brain: effects of age and neurodegenerative disease, *J Am Geriatr Soc* 35:334, 1987.

68. Muller RT, Gould LA, Betzu R et al: Painless myocardial infarction in the elderly, *Am Heart J* 119:202, 1990.

69. Munson ES, Hoffman JC, and Eger EI II: Use of cyclopropane to test generality of anesthetic requirement in the elderly, *Anesth Analg* 63:998, 1984.

70. National Center for Health Statistics. Current Estimates from the National Health Interview Survey, 1988. Vital and Health Statistics, Series 10, No 173, US Government Printing Office, October, 1989.

71. O'Hara DA, Fragen RJ, and Shanks CA: The effects of age on the dose-response curves for vecuronium in adults, *Anesthesiology* 63:542, 1985.

72. Owen JA, Sitar DS, Berger L et al: Age-related morphine kinetics, *Clin Pharmacol Ther* 34:364, 1983.

73. Pack AI, Millman RP: Changes in control of ventilation awake and asleep, in the elderly, *J Am Geriatric Soc* 34:533, 1986.

74. Peterson RD et al: Effects of aging on ventilatory and occlusion pressure responses to hypoxia and hypercapnia, *Am Rev Respir Dis* 124:387, 1981.

75. Raine JM, Bishop JM: A-a difference in O_2 tension and physiological dead space in normal man, *J Appl Physiol* 18:284, 1963.

76. Reeves JG et al: Midazolam pharmacology and uses, *Anesthesiology* 62:310, 1985.

77. Rinne JO: Muscarinic and dopaminergic receptors in the aging human brain, *Brain Res* 404:162, 1987.

78. Rocco MB, Nabel EG, Campbell S et al: Prognostic importance of myocardial ischemia detected by ambulatory monitoring in patients with stable coronary artery disease, *Circulation* 78:877, 1988.

79. Rockwood K: Acute confusion in elderly medical patients, *J Am Geriatr Soc* 37:150, 1989.

80. Rodenheffer RJ, Gerstenblith G, Becker LC et al: Exercise cardiac output is maintained with advancing age in healthy human subjects: cardiac dilatation and increased stroke volume compensate for a diminished heart rate, *Circulation* 69:203, 1984.

81. Rokey R, Rolak LA, Harati Y et al: Coronary artery disease in patients with cerebrovascular disease: a prospective study, *Ann Neurol* 16:50, 1984.

82. Rupp SM, Castagnoli KP, Fisher DM et al: Pancuronium and vecuronium pharmacokinetics and pharmacodynamics in younger and elderly adults, *Anesthesiology* 67:45, 1987.

83. Sari A, Miyauchi Y, Yamashita S et al: The magnitude of hypoxemia in elderly patients with fractures of the femoral neck, *Anesth Analg* 65:892, 1986.

84. Schwartz AE, Tuttle RH, and Poppers PJ: Electroencephalographic burst suppression in elderly and young patients anesthetized with isoflurane, *Anesth Analg* 68:9, 1989.

85. Scott JC, Stanski DR: Decreased fentanyl and alfentanil dose requirements with increasing age. A simultaneous pharmacokinetic and pharmacodynamic evaluation, *J Pharmacol Exp Ther* 240:159, 1987.

86. Shimada K, Kitazumi T, Ogura H et al: Differences in age-independent effects of blood pressure on baroreflex sensitivity between normal and hypertensive subjects, *Clin Sci 70:489, 1986.*

87. Stevens WC, Dolan WM, Gibbons RT et al: Minimum alveolar concentrations (MAC) of isoflurane with and without nitrous oxide in patients of various ages, *Anesthesiology* 42:197, 1975.

88. Suci GJ, Davidoff MD, and Surwello WW: Reaction time as a function of stimulus information and age, *J Exp Psychol* 640:242, 1960.

89. Terry RD, DeTeresa R, Hansen LA: Neocortical cell counts in normal human aging, *Ann Neurol* 21:530, 1987.

90. Tiret L, N'Doye P, and Hatton F: Complications associated with anaesthesia—a prospective survey in France, *Can Anaesth Soc J* 33:336, 1986.

91. Tuominen M, Pitkänen M, Doepel M et al: Spinal anaesthesia with hyperbaric tetracaine: effect of age and body mass, *Acta Anaesthesiol Scand* 31:474, 1987.

92. Vaughan MS, Vaughan RW, and Cork RC: Postoperative hypothermia in adults: relationship of age, anesthesia, and shivering to rewarming, *Anesth Analg* 60:746, 1981.

93. Veering BT, Burn AG, van Kleef JW et al: Epidural anesthesia with bupivacaine: effects of aging on neural blockade and pharmacokinetics, *Anesth Analg* 66:589, 1987.

94. Veering BTH et al: Spinal anesthesia with glucose-free bupivacaine: effects of age on neural blockade and pharmacokinetics, *Anesth Analg* 66:965, 1978.

95. Wahba WM: Influence of aging on lung function—clinical significance of changes from age twenty, *Anesth Analg* 62:764, 1980.

96. Warner MA, Hosking MP, Lobdell CM et al: Surgical procedures among those >90 years of age. A population-based study in Olmsted County, Minnesota, 1975-1985, *Ann Surg* 207:380, 1988.

97. Welford AT: Reaction time, speed of performance, and age, *Ann N Y Acad Sci* 515:1, 1988.

98. Wennberg JW, Roos N, Sola L et al: Use of claims data systems to evaluate health care outcomes. Mortality and reoperation following prostatectomy, *JAMA* 257:933, 1987.

99. White BL, Fisher WD, and Laurin CA: Rate of mortality for elderly patients after fracture of the hip in the 1980s, *J Bone Joint Surg* 69A:1335, 1987.

100. Young WL, Matteo RS, and Ornstein E: Duration of action of neostigmine and pyridostigmine in the elderly, *Anesth Analg* 67:775, 1988.

CHAPTER 28

Evaluation of
the Pregnant Patient

DAVID H. CHESTNUT

In discussing the approach to the pregnant patient, two considerations should be emphasized—one obvious, the second perhaps not so obvious. First, advances in intrauterine fetal monitoring and fetal therapy have established that the fetus is a patient.

The anesthesiologist who provides care for the pregnant patient actually provides care for two patients—the mother and the fetus. Second, and perhaps less obvious, pregnancy elicits feelings and emotions that often differ from those which accompany other conditions that require the administration of anesthesia. Whereas the nonpregnant patient is primarily concerned with his/her welfare, the pregnant patient typically is more concerned with the welfare of the fetus: "Will my baby be normal and healthy?" "Will labor and delivery be painful?" "Will the anesthetic harm my baby?" "Can I hold my baby immediately after delivery?" "Can my husband remain with me throughout labor and delivery?"

The anesthesiologist who cares for obstetric patients spends considerable time caring for awake, nonsedated patients. Good care of the pregnant patient requires interpersonal skills. The thoughtful obstetric anesthesiologist will not only work to protect maternal-fetal physiology but will also attempt to ensure a pleasant experience for the patient and her husband or support person.

PHYSIOLOGIC CHANGES DURING PREGNANCY

Pregnancy, labor, and delivery are associated with major changes in maternal physiology. The anesthesiologist should understand these changes and their implications for anesthetic management.

Cardiovascular Changes

Maternal blood volume increases 35% to 40% during normal pregnancy. The increase begins early during the first trimester and continues until early in the third trimester. The increase in maternal blood

volume is greater in twin pregnancies than in single-ton pregnancies. Typically, plasma volume increases more than does red blood cell volume, resulting in physiologic anemia. A maternal hemoglobin concentration less than 11 g/dl is abnormal. Pathologic anemia during pregnancy often occurs as a result of iron deficiency.

The increased blood volume during pregnancy allows most parturients to tolerate the normal delivery blood loss (approximately 600 ml during vaginal delivery and 800 to 1000 ml during cesarean section). The uterus contracts at delivery, resulting in an autotransfusion of approximately 500 ml. Blood volume returns to prepregnancy levels within 7 to 14 days postpartum.

Changes in cardiac output parallel changes in blood volume. Cardiac output increases 30% to 50% during normal pregnancy, with most of the increase occurring during the first trimester. The increase in cardiac output allows a 10- to 20-fold increase in uterine blood flow. Cardiac output increases as a result of increased stroke volume and heart rate (i.e., an increase of 10 to 20 beats/min).[20,30] **Mean arterial pressure does not increase during normal pregnancy; rather, it often *decreases* during the second trimester. Healthy pregnant women have a refractory response to the pressor effect of angiotensin II.**[50]

Early studies, performed with pregnant women in the supine position, suggested that cardiac output decreases toward prepregnancy values during the third trimester. But the supine position allows the gravid uterus to compress both the inferior vena cava and aorta. Vena caval compression results in decreased right atrial return and cardiac output. Approximately 10% to 15% of term pregnant women have symptomatic hypotension when they lie supine (i.e., "supine hypotension syndrome").[62] Anesthetic drugs or techniques that cause venodilation will further decrease venous blood return in the presence of vena caval obstruction. Some women who maintain normal brachial artery blood pressures in the supine position may have unrecognized decreases in uteroplacental perfusion. This may occur for two reasons. First, vena caval compression increases uterine venous pressure, which further decreases uterine blood flow. Second, uterine arterial hypotension may occur because the uterine artery is a branch of the hypogastric artery, which emerges distal to the level of aortic compression.

Studies performed with pregnant women in the lateral position have not noted significant decreases in cardiac output near term.[76,122] Thus pregnant women should not lie supine after 20 weeks of gestation; a lateral position is preferred. If the supine position cannot be avoided, the mother's right hip should be elevated approximately 10 to 15 cm to displace the uterus leftward, off the inferior vena cava. The uterus should also be displaced leftward during cardiopulmonary resuscitation.

Cardiac output increases further during labor. Each uterine contraction results in an autotransfusion and thereby transiently increases central blood volume and cardiac output 15% to 30%. The greatest increase (i.e., 80% above prelabor cardiac output) occurs immediately after delivery, resulting from both autotransfusion and relief of vena caval compression. Thus cardiac decompensation is most likely to occur after delivery in parturients who have cardiovascular disease. Ueland and Hansen observed that caudal epidural anesthesia attenuated the cumulative increase in maternal central venous pressure and cardiac output that occurs during labor.[121]

Physical examination of the pregnant woman typically reveals a point of maximal impulse that is displaced cephalad and leftward from its nonpregnant location. One often hears a soft (grade I or II), physiologic systolic murmur across the precordium. This murmur is thought to result from increased cardiac output and decreased blood viscosity and is innocent. Any diastolic murmur is abnormal and requires further evaluation.

Diaphragmatic elevation displaces the heart leftward so that it may appear enlarged on chest radiographs. Similarly, the ECG often shows left axis deviation of approximately 15 degrees. Finally, a small pericardial effusion may occur in healthy, asymptomatic women during the third trimester of pregnancy.[45]

Respiratory Changes

Minute ventilatory volume increases approximately 50% during normal pregnancy. This results primarily from increased tidal volume and secondarily from a small increase in respiratory rate. Typically, Pao_2 increases by 5 to 10 mm Hg, and $Paco_2$ decreases to approximately 32 mm Hg. Decreased serum bicarbonate results in partially compensated respiratory alkalosis. During active labor, painful uterine contractions may cause a 200% increase in minute ventilation over that of nonpregnant women, with accompanying maternal hypocarbia (i.e., $Paco_2$ less than 20 mm Hg) and alkalemia. The parturient may then hypoventilate between contractions, and maternal hypoxemia can occur.

Maternal oxygen consumption increases due to increased maternal and fetal metabolic requirements and work of breathing. Painful uterine contractions further increase oxygen consumption. Despite decreased maternal hemoglobin concentration, maternal and fetal demands for more oxygen are met by (1) increased minute volume of ventilation, which results in slightly increased maternal Pao_2, (2) increased cardiac output, (3) vasodilation and hemodilution, which probably allow increased perfusion of important target organs such as the uterus and kidneys, and

(4) shift of the maternal oxyhemoglobin dissociation curve to the right in healthy pregnant women. In contrast, preeclampsia is associated with leftward shifts in the oxyhemoglobin dissociation curve.[68]

Pregnancy causes little change in maternal lung volume measurements and capacities, and little or no change in vital capacity. Increased transverse and anteroposterior chest diameters compensate for diaphragmatic elevation. Most important is a 15% to 20% decrease in functional residual capacity (FRC) by term. This results from increased tidal volume, with attendant reduction of expiratory reserve volume. Diaphragmatic compression further reduces FRC when the pregnant woman lies supine. This may result in airway closure and increased alveolar-arterial oxygen gradient during normal tidal ventilation. As many as 50% of normal pregnant women develop airway closure during normal tidal ventilation.[15,109] Increased oxygen consumption, decreased FRC, and increased alveolar-arterial oxygen gradient lead to more rapid development of hypoxemia during apnea in pregnant women.[4] This risk is aggravated by increased oxygen consumption during labor. Altogether, these risk factors mandate denitrogenation (i.e., administration of 100% oxygen) before laryngoscopy and intubation in pregnant patients.

Mucosal vascular engorgement results in edema of the respiratory tract, including the oral and nasal pharynx, larynx, and trachea. Laryngeal edema may alter voice tone and/or quality.[123] Exacerbation of these changes may occur in patients with upper respiratory tract infections or preeclampsia. These changes make airway instrumentation more difficult and hazardous than in nonpregnant patients. Placement of a nasal airway may precipitate significant hemorrhage. Unfortunately, vasoconstrictor agents (e.g., cocaine, phenylephrine) may be absorbed systemically and cause uterine vasoconstriction and decreased uteroplacental perfusion. For oral tracheal intubation, the likelihood of edema in the false cords mandates use of a smaller endotracheal tube than in a similar-sized nonpregnant woman. A 6.5 mm cuffed endotracheal tube represents a prudent choice for intubation of most pregnant women.

Of healthy pregnant women, 60% to 70% have mild, intermittent dyspnea. The cause is not clear but may be related to alteration of chest wall proprioceptors and/or progesterone-related hyperventilation.[123] Diaphragm elevation may result in increased lung markings, mimicking mild congestive heart failure, on the chest radiographs of healthy pregnant women.

Central Nervous System Changes

A pregnant patient requires less local anesthetic to produce a given level of spinal or epidural anesthesia than does a similarly-sized nonpregnant patient. Earlier, it was believed that the decreased local anesthetic requirement of pregnancy was due to increased intraabdominal pressure, which caused epidural venous engorgement and decreased volume of the epidural and subarachnoid spaces. But Fagraeus et al. observed that during the first trimester (before significant uterine enlargement), epidural anesthesia spread similarly to that administered at term.[46] **Acid-base changes in cerebral spinal fluid and/or the hormonal changes of pregnancy may cause increased sensitivity to local anesthetics.**[41,46]

Pregnancy decreases the requirement for inhalation agents by as much as 40%.[99] **The mechanism is unclear. A concentration of an inhalation agent that would not produce loss of consciousness in a nonpregnant patient may render a pregnant patient unconscious, subjecting her to risk of airway loss and/or aspiration of gastric contents.**

Renal Changes

Renal blood flow and glomerular filtration rate (GFR) increase 50% to 60% during normal pregnancy. These changes begin early in the first trimester. Creatinine clearance increases, and blood urea nitrogen (BUN) and creatinine concentrations decrease. For example, a "normal" BUN concentration of 15 mg/dl, a serum creatinine concentration of 1.0 mg/dl, and a creatinine clearance of 100 ml/min suggest abnormal renal function in a pregnant woman who is near term. Glucosuria may occur in healthy pregnant women, because tubular reabsorption of glucose may not parallel the increased GFR. Glucosuria does not necessarily reflect carbohydrate intolerance. Similarly, modest proteinuria (less than 300 mg/24 hr) commonly occurs in the absence of a renal pathologic condition.

Maternal progesterone, a smooth muscle relaxant, causes dilatation of renal calyces, pelves, and ureters. After mid-pregnancy the enlarged uterus compresses the ureters at the pelvic brim, exacerbating ureteral dilatation. Urinary stasis then predisposes the pregnant woman to bacteriuria and pyelonephritis. Occasionally renal failure occurs solely as a result of ureteral obstruction by the gravid uterus.

Gastrointestinal Changes

The enlarged gravid uterus displaces the stomach cephalad. This changes the angle of the gastroesophageal junction and decreases the competence of the gastroesophageal sphincter. Not only does this facilitate the occurrence of gastric reflux and heartburn in as many as 70% of pregnant women, but it also places pregnant women at risk for regurgitation and aspiration of gastric contents during general anesthesia or any other loss of consciousness (e.g., generalized tonic-clonic seizure). Similarly, the enlarged uterus displaces the pylorus upward and backward, resulting in delayed gastric emptying.

Elevated concentrations of progesterone tend to delay gastric emptying during pregnancy. Opioid analgetics, often given to alleviate pain during labor, significantly delay gastric emptying.[97]

Hepatic Changes

There is little or no change in hepatic blood flow during normal pregnancy. In the absence of a hepatic pathologic condition, the healthy pregnant woman may have slight elevations of serum aspartate aminotransferase, lactic dehydrogenase, alkaline phosphatase, and/or cholesterol. Colloid oncotic pressure decreases as a result of decreased total protein and decreased albumin-globulin ratio. Colloid oncotic pressure decreases further after delivery, regardless of method of delivery or anesthesia.[39] The patient with preeclampsia may develop pulmonary edema with only a modest increase in pulmonary capillary wedge pressure.

Plasma cholinesterase activity decreases during pregnancy and immediately postpartum.[18,112] The decrease in cholinesterase activity usually is not sufficient to result in prolonged paralysis after a single dose of succinylcholine.[18]

Coagulation Factor Changes

There is no consistent change in platelet count or function during normal pregnancy, yet pregnancy produces a hypercoagulable state. All coagulation factors except XI and XIII increase. Fibrinolytic activity decreases during the third trimester as a result of decreased plasminogen activator concentration. These changes, combined with rapid contraction of the uterus after placental separation, help protect the gravid woman from major hemorrhage. Unfortunately, hypercoagulability also predisposes to thromboembolic disease. The parturient is at greatest risk for deep venous thrombosis and pulmonary embolism just after delivery.

Endocrine Changes

Mean blood glucose concentrations remain within the normal range although individual glucose concentrations may be somewhat lower than those before pregnancy. Increased release of insulin offsets the diabetogenic activity of human placental lactogen and steroid hormones.

The thyroid gland enlarges 50% to 70% during pregnancy. Concentrations of thyroid-binding globulin and total thyroxine increase, but concentrations of free thyroxine and triiodothyronine do not change.

Reproductive Tract Changes

The uterus weighs 50 to 70 g in the nonpregnant woman but weighs 1000 to 1200 g at term. Total uterine blood flow increases from 50 ml/min in the nonpregnant woman to 700 ml/min at term, representing approximately 10% of cardiac output. Approximately 80% of the gravid uterine blood flow perfuses the intervillous space; most of the remainder perfuses the enlarged myometrium.

The uterine vasculature seems to be maximally dilated in healthy pregnant women; therefore uterine blood flow decreases parallel with maternal arterial pressure. There is little or no autoregulation of uterine blood flow during pregnancy. Any factor that decreases venous return and cardiac output (e.g., aortocaval compression, positive-pressure ventilation) will decrease uterine blood flow. Uterine contractions also decrease uterine blood flow. No known drugs specifically and directly increase uterine blood flow. Drugs used to treat preterm labor may improve uteroplacental perfusion in some cases, not by directly increasing uterine blood flow but by decreasing or eliminating uterine contractions.

Alpha-adrenergic agonists are potent uterine vasoconstrictors and markedly decrease uterine blood flow. In contrast, ephedrine—a mixed alpha- and beta-agonist—seems to protect uterine blood flow and is the vasopressor of choice in most cases of hypotension in obstetric practice. The conventional wisdom is that ephedrine's beta-agonist activity helps maintain cardiac output and uterine blood flow. Recent data suggest that ephedrine exerts a protective effect on uterine blood flow independent of beta-agonist activity.[26,29] The protective effect may result in part from ephedrine's ability to produce greater venoconstriction than arterial constriction.[74,106] Recently it has been contended that small doses of alpha-adrenergic agonists (e.g., phenylephrine), administered in doses just sufficient to correct hypotension, may be safely administered in situations where administration of a beta-agonist is undesirable.[91,105]

SURGERY DURING PREGNANCY

Approximately 1% to 2% of all pregnant women require anesthesia for surgery unrelated to delivery.[114] The anesthesiologist must consider the physiologic changes of pregnancy and should also consider all possible fetal effects of the maternal disease process. Protection of the mother is paramount, but other goals of anesthetic management include maintenance of uterine blood flow and fetal oxygenation, avoidance of teratogenic drugs, and prevention of preterm labor.

Maternal Considerations

Earlier we discussed factors that place pregnant patients at an increased risk for a "full stomach" and aspiration of gastric contents during general anesthesia. It is not clear when these factors become clinically important during pregnancy. Maternal concentrations of progesterone increase early during pregnancy, but the uterus does not enlarge significantly until mid-pregnancy. Wyner and Cohen compared gastric pH and volume during general anesthesia in 20 nonpregnant women vs. 62 women undergoing elective abortion at a mean ($\pm$ SEM) gestational age of 15 ($\pm$ 3) weeks. Mean gastric volume was identical in the two groups, and gastric pH was actually lower (i.e., worse) in the nonpregnant group although the mean pH was less than 2.5 in both groups. Approximately half of the patients in each group were considered "at risk" for aspiration. The authors concluded that pregnancy of less than 20 weeks' gestation did not increase gastric volume or acidity compared with nonpregnant women undergoing gynecologic surgery. This study did not consider any potential effect of progesterone on the gastroesophageal sphincter.[133] At present, there is no consensus on whether one should take extra precautions to protect the airway during early pregnancy, but it seems prudent to take such precautions after the first trimester.

Anesthesia and Outcome of Pregnancy
Teratogenesis

Perhaps the greatest concern of the patient is whether anesthetics might increase the risk of congenital anomalies. Presently, no data exist to base a contention that modern anesthetic agents or techniques are teratogenic in humans.

Animal studies. Prolonged exposure of pregnant rats to high concentrations of volatile agents has produced an increase of fetal anomalies and wastage. Unfortunately physiologic abnormalities such as hypoventilation and hypothermia occurred during these experiments and may have caused adverse reproductive outcomes.[34] Mazze et al. observed an increased incidence of cleft palate in mice exposed to isoflurane, but that species is especially susceptible to that anomaly.[87] The latter has not been observed after similar anesthetic exposure in rats.[85]

There has been concern that administration of nitrous oxide during pregnancy may increase the risk of fetal anomalies. Nitrous oxide inactivates maternal and fetal methionine synthetase.[5] Inhibition of methionine synthetase decreases production of endogenous folinic acid, which is necessary for conversion of uridine to the DNA building block thymidine. Impaired DNA synthesis and inhibition of cell division might be theoretically possible. Administration of nitrous oxide to pregnant rats did increase the incidence of fetal anomalies and/or resorption.[73,85] In one study, a control group of animals that received xenon (an agent with anesthetic potency similar to that of nitrous oxide) did not experience adverse fetal outcome.[73] This suggests that nitrous oxide toxicity might be prevented by pretreatment with folinic acid

because the latter bypasses the biochemical defect created by nitrous oxide–induced inhibition of methionine synthetase. Subsequent studies observed that both halothane and isoflurane, but not folinic acid, decreased the likelihood of fetal anomalies and resorption.[48,84] Fujinaga et al. concluded that these results "cast doubt on the methionine synthetase inhibition theory" of nitrous oxide teratogenicity.[48] Mazze et al. suggested that there was "no basis for administering folinic acid to pregnant women anesthetized with this drug [nitrous oxide]."[84]

Human studies. Shnider and Webster evaluated the medical records of 9073 women who delivered infants between July 1959 and August 1964.[114] Of those women, 147 (1.6%) had surgery during pregnancy. There was no increased incidence of congenital anomalies in the surgical group, but the authors noted that most of these patients received anesthetics during the second or third trimester, after organogenesis. Brodsky et al. mailed questionnaires to 287 women who had surgery during pregnancy. Among these women, 187 had surgery during the first trimester. There was no significant increase in the number of congenital anomalies in the infants born to women who had surgery during pregnancy, compared with a suitable control group of pregnant women who didn't have surgery.[19]

Duncan et al. used health insurance records to evaluate fetal risks of anesthesia among all pregnant women in Manitoba between 1971 and 1978. Each of 2565 women who underwent surgery during pregnancy was paired by maternal age and area of residence with a pregnant woman who did not undergo surgery. Again, there was no significant difference betwee the two groups in the incidence of congenital anomalies.[44]

Mazze and Kallen recently obtained data from three Swedish health care registries to evaluate the risk of adverse reproductive outcomes after anesthesia and surgery during pregnancies between 1973 and 1981. They identified 5405 women who underwent surgery during pregnancy. Of these, 42% underwent surgery during the first trimester. Among these women, 65% received general anesthesia, and nitrous oxide was given in over 98% of those cases for a total of 1433 nitrous oxide administrations during the first trimester. The authors observed no increased incidence of congenital anomalies among women who underwent surgery during pregnancy. They specifically noted no increased incidence of congenital anomalies among women who underwent surgery during the first trimester. Administration of general anesthesia was not associated with an increase in any adverse outcome.[86]

No human study suggests that the administration of anesthetics during surgery on pregnant patients

increases the risk of fetal anomalies. However, these retrospective studies are insufficient to allow one to state categorically that anesthetics are not teratogenic. It is possible that exposure to anesthetic "X" for 6 hours at exactly 28 days' gestation might increase the incidence of anomaly "Y" from 2/1000 to 4/1000. No epidemiologic study could allow for the exclusion of all such possibilities. When discussing the risks of anesthetics with a pregnant patient scheduled for surgery, one should remind the patient that a 3% baseline incidence of fetal anomalies exists among all pregnant women, but there is no clinical evidence that administration of anesthetics increases this risk.

Spontaneous abortion and preterm labor

There is perhaps greater reason to be concerned that anesthesia and surgery during pregnancy might increase the risk of fetal wastage and/or preterm labor. Shnider and Webster noted that preterm delivery occurred in 8.8% of women who underwent surgery during pregnancy although they did not report the incidence of preterm delivery among nonsurgical control patients. Perinatal mortality incidence was 7.5% among surgical patients, compared with only 2.0% in nonsurgical patients. The authors suggested that "premature labor and delivery following operation was due mainly to the patient's surgical disease rather than to either the surgical or anesthetic technique per se."[114]

Brodsky et al. noted that women who underwent surgery during either the first or second trimester had an increased incidence of spontaneous abortion when compared with nonsurgical control patients.[19] Duncan et al. observed no increase in spontaneous abortion incidence among all women who underwent surgery during pregnancy. When they limited their analysis to those women who received general anesthetics for surgery during pregnancy, they observed a significant increase in spontaneous abortion (estimated risk ratio = 1.58) when compared with matched controls. They found the increased risk was greatest among those women having obstetric or gynecologic surgical procedures (estimated risk ratio = 2.0).[44] Unfortunately, there were too few obstetric or gynecologic procedures performed under alternate anesthetic techniques to evaluate the effect of any particular surgical procedure alone. Cohen criticized by noting that the group receiving general anesthetics had undergone more complex surgical procedures.[35] In reply, Duncan noted that there had been significantly increased risk of spontaneous abortion among women undergoing operations at other sites but only when performed with general anesthetics.[43]

Mazze and Kallen observed a twofold increase in incidence of very low- and low-birthweight infants among women who underwent surgery during pregnancy. The reduced birthweight was secondary both to prematurity and to intrauterine growth retardation. In addition, there was an increase in infants born alive but who died within 7 days of delivery. Most deaths occurred in infants of very low birthweight. These adverse outcomes did not seem associated with a specific type of anesthetic.[86]

Anesthesiologist's Approach to the Patient

Elective surgery should be avoided during pregnancy. If surgery should become necessary, it is prudent to delay the procedure until the end of the first trimester, if possible.

Regardless of the surgical procedure or anesthetic technique, aortocaval compression should be avoided after 18 to 20 weeks' gestation; supplemental oxygen should be given to the mother, and maternal blood pressure should be maintained near preanesthetic measurements. If hypotension should occur, a mixed agonist such as ephedrine remains the drug of choice in most cases.

The anesthesiologist and surgeon should consult with the obstetrician before surgery. Beginning at 18 to 20 weeks' gestation, one should monitor the electronic fetal heart rate before, during, and immediately after anesthesia. This may be difficult, if not impossible, to accomplish during abdominal surgery. It is often helpful for an obstetrician or obstetric nurse to be present during surgery to interpret changes in the fetal heart rate tracing. When the mother receives a general anesthetic, the fetus does also, and a decreased beat-to-beat variability of the fetal heart rate will occur.[16,78]

Other changes (e.g., decelerations, bradycardia, persistent tachycardia) may signal fetal compromise, and one should take steps to improve uteroplacental perfusion and fetal oxygenation. These might include exaggeration of left uterine displacement, administration of a higher inspired concentration of oxygen, adjustment of maternal ventilation, augmentation of maternal circulating blood volume, and/or pharmacologic treatment of hypotension. After surgery, one should continue to monitor fetal heart rate, so one should monitor uterine activity with an external tocodynamometer. Residual anesthetic and analgetic drugs may blunt perception of uterine contractions. If preterm labor should occur, the obstetrician might begin pharmacologic tocolytic therapy.

Choice of anesthetic technique

At least three arguments favor regional anesthesia. First, Duncan et al. noted an increased likelihood of spontaneous abortion after administration of general but not regional or local anesthesia.[44] Second, local

anesthetic agents are not teratogenic in either animals or humans. Third, successful regional anesthesia avoids manipulation of the airway and the risk of aspiration. Some argue that spinal anesthesia is preferable to epidural anesthesia. Others favor continuous epidural anesthesia because of its slower onset and greater flexibility. One would also expect a smaller risk of spinal headache with epidural anesthesia than with spinal anesthesia.

Choice of anesthetic agents

If an anticholinergic agent is given before surgery, one should remember that glycopyrrolate, unlike atropine, does not cross the placenta. If general anesthesia is necessary, there are no data that mandate any particular choice of agents. One anesthetic agent that should be avoided is high-dose ketamine, which increases uterine tone. Otherwise it seems reasonable to use agents that have a "track record" in pregnant patients. It is probably not wise to use new agents or techniques in pregnant patients until those agents and techniques have undergone rigorous scrutiny elsewhere. Administration of a potent halogenated agent seems wise in most cases, especially if one anticipates uterine manipulation during surgery. The halogenated agents relax uterine smooth muscle; thus administration of a halogenated agent might prevent preterm labor. In addition, halogenated agents allow administration of higher oxygen concentrations.

It seems unncessary to avoid nitrous oxide altogether. Avoidance of nitrous oxide might prompt administration of a high concentration of a potent halogenated agent. Prolonged fetal exposure to a high concentration (e.g., 2 MAC) of a potent halogenated agent can result in fetal myocardial depression and acidosis.[17] If one anticipates administration of nitrous oxide for a prolonged procedure, some would advocate administration of folinic acid to the mother. But folinic acid does not exert a protective effect in an animal model,[48,84] and this practice is not standard. Finally, one should avoid maternal hyperventilation (which may decrease uteroplacental perfusion) unless there is a specific indication (e.g., increased intracranial pressure).

On occasion it may be necessary to deviate from these principles. One might need to perform deliberate hypotension during clipping of an intracranial aneurysm. Fortunately most fetuses are remarkably resilient. There have been successful uses of deliberate hypotension,[42,94] **hypothermia,**[57] **and/or cardiopulmonary bypass,**[14,36] **followed by maintenance of pregnancy and delivery of a healthy infant. When one encounters such a challenging case, it is useful to remember that what is best for the mother is probably best for the fetus.**

PRETERM LABOR AND DELIVERY

Preterm delivery remains the leading cause of perinatal morbidity and mortality in the United States. Approximately 7% to 8% of all infants born in the United States are delivered preterm.[51] **Indeed, two thirds of infant deaths occur among infants weighing less than 2500 g at birth.**

An infant is preterm when delivered between 20 and 37 weeks after the first day of the last menstrual period (i.e., at least 3 weeks before the expected date of term delivery). Heretofore, any infant weighing less than 2500 g at delivery was considered preterm. Some of these neonates actually are small-for-gestational age (SGA) and are not preterm. An infant of unknown gestational age who weighs less than 2500 g at birth is considered a low-birthweight infant, and an infant who weighs less than 1500 g at birth is considered a very low-birthweight infant.

Box 28-1 lists factors associated with preterm labor and delivery. These associations do not necessarily reflect cause-and-effect relationships. In most cases, the etiologic factor is unclear. Not all preterm births result from preterm labor. As many as 25% of all preterm deliveries are performed electively. The obstetrician may elect to perform preterm delivery for maternal or fetal indications (e.g., severe preeclampsia, chronic intrauterine fetal stress). Unfortunately some infants are delivered electively before term because of inappropriate assessment of gestational age. Preterm elective repeat cesarean section remains an occasional cause of neonatal respiratory distress syndrome.

Diagnosing Preterm Labor

Diagnosing preterm labor is not always easy. Advanced preterm labor is obvious, but early symptoms of preterm labor may be subtle. Conversely, not all symptomatic women are in true labor. Gonik and Creasy suggested the following criteria for the diagnosis of preterm labor: (1) gestational age of 20 to 37 weeks, (2) documented uterine contractions, and (3) documented change in cervix, cervical effacement of 80%, or cervical dilation of 2 cm.[51] Castle and Turnbull suggested that the use of real-time ultrasonography might improve sensitivity and specificity of the diagnosis of preterm labor. They noted that if fetal breathing movements were present during ultrasonographic examination, preterm parturients were probably not in true labor.[22]

Obstetric Management

The initial assessment and therapy of preterm labor includes maternal bedrest, hydration, and fetal surveillance, including electronic fetal heart rate monitoring. Contractions will often cease with bedrest and hydration alone. In the remaining patients, the obstetrician must decide whether to begin tocolytic therapy. Obstetricians typically reserve tocolytic therapy for those patients with a gestational age of less than 34 weeks and no evidence of fetal distress. Most U.S. obstetricians have abandoned the use of ethanol for tocolysis. Tocolytic agents used in modern obstetric practice include (1) beta-adrenergic agents, (2) magnesium sulfate, (3) prostaglandin synthetase inhibitors, and (4) calcium-entry blocking agents.

Beta-adrenergic agents

Beta-adrenergic agents (e.g., ritodrine, terbutaline) represent the most common drugs used for tocolytic therapy in the United States and Europe. In fact, ritodrine is the only drug specifically approved by the U.S. Food and Drug Administration for tocolysis. Although these agents are relatively selective for the $beta_2$ receptor (which includes uterine smooth muscle), $beta_1$ stimulation does occur and results in increased maternal heart rate and systolic arterial pressure, decreased diastolic arterial pressure, and unchanged or decreased mean arterial pressure. Other side effects include hyperglycemia and hypokalemia. Hypokalemia does not result from increased urinary excretion of potassium; rather, it occurs as a result of insulin-mediated passage of potassium and glucose from the extracellular to the intracellular space.

ECG changes suggestive of ischemia may occur during beta-adrenergic therapy. Fortunately, true myocardial ischemia seems rare during beta-adrenergic tocolytic therapy. Hendricks et al. concluded that these changes typically represent "a physiologic expression of ritodrine-induced tachycardia or hypokalemia."[60] They questioned the validity of the use of electrocardiograms of asymptomatic patients as a sole criterion for discontinuation of beta-adrenergic therapy. At The University of Iowa Hospitals and Clinics, we do not obtain electrocardiograms or serial potassium measurements in asymptomatic, healthy patients receiving beta-adrenergic tocolytic therapy.

Pulmonary edema represents an infrequent but serious complication of beta-adrenergic tocolytic therapy. It typically occurs 24 to 48 hours after the start of therapy. The cause of this complication is unclear. Fluid overload might occur in some patients as a result of inappropriate hydration before and during tocolytic therapy and/or as a result of fluid retention secondary to beta-adrenergic receptor stimulation. Beta-receptor stimulation increases release of antidiuretic hormone and also increases renal tubular reabsorption of sodium.[7,71,110] There have been cases of pulmonary edema in preterm parturients who have not received beta-adrenergic agents but have received other tocolytic agents (e.g., magnesium sulfate). Thus some have suggested that pulmonary edema is not a direct effect of beta-adrenergic tocolytic therapy. Benedetti suggested that unrecognized infection may result in pulmonary capillary injury in preterm parturients.[8] Recently Hatjis and Swain observed a strong association between pulmonary edema and maternal infection in patients given tocolytic therapy for preterm labor.[55]

Thus it seems reasonable to monitor hemoglobin oxygen saturation in patients who are receiving parenteral beta-adrenergic tocolytic therapy. One may notice a decrease in oxygen saturation before other symptoms of pulmonary edema become apparent. Should pulmonary edema occur, one should immediately discontinue the beta-adrenergic agent and administer supplemental oxygen. Most patients will respond to simple fluid restriction. Pisani and Rosenow recently reviewed 58 cases of pulmonary edema associated with tocolytic therapy. Only four patients required intubation and mechanical ventilation.[101]

Magnesium sulfate

Magnesium sulfate ($MgSO_4$) has emerged as a popular alternative to beta-adrenergic therapy. Bolus administration of $MgSO_4$ typically results in only transient decreases in systemic vascular resistance and mean arterial pressure. Randomized studies of patients who received either beta-adrenergic therapy or $MgSO_4$ have consistently noted fewer cardiovascular side effects in patients who received $MgSO_4$. Thus many clinicians consider $MgSO_4$ to be the tocolytic agent of choice in patients at risk for hemorrhage. Recently, we observed that $MgSO_4$, but not ritodrine, worsened maternal hypotension during hemorrhage in gravid ewes.[28] We speculated that Mg^{++} attenuated the compensatory cardiovascular response to hemorrhage in that study. We also speculated that ritodrine's inotropic and chronotropic activity helped maintain maternal cardiac output and mean arterial pressure during hemorrhage.[28]

Prostaglandin synthetase inhibitor

Prostaglandin synthetase inhibitors (e.g., indomethacin) seem attractive for tocolytic therapy. Prostaglandins are a major hormonal stimulus of uterine contractions, and prostaglandin synthetase inhibitors significantly decrease the prostaglandin concentration. Indomethacin has received the most extensive evaluation. Unlike aspirin, which permanently inactivates cyclooxygenase, indomethacin causes reversible inhibition of the enzyme and thereby causes transient impairment of platelet function. Indomethacin may be administered either orally or rectally, is effective, and has few maternal side effects. Unfortunately, there has been widespread concern regarding potential adverse fetal effects of exposure to indomethacin *in utero*. Specifically, there has been concern that indomethacin might cause antenatal closure of the ductus arteriosus, persistent fetal circulation after birth, and/or neonatal bleeding disorders. Niebyl and Witter suggested that adverse

neonatal effects are unlikely if indomethacin is used in short courses, is restricted to patients who are at less than 34 weeks' gestation, and is stopped at an appropriate interval before delivery.[96] Moise et al. performed serial fetal echocardiography in pregnant women who received indomethacin for treatment of preterm labor. Detection of ductal constriction in 7 of 14 fetuses led to discontinuation of indomethacin. The authors concluded that indomethacin causes transient constriction of the ductus arteriosus in some fetuses, even after short-term maternal use.[90]

Calcium-entry blocking agents

Calcium-entry blocking agents appear to be potent tocolytic agents, with perhaps less severe cardiovascular side effects than the beta-adrenergic agents. Unfortunately, initial enthusiasm for these agents has been tempered by reports of decreased uteroplacental blood flow, fetal hypoxia, and fetal acidosis in laboratory animals. These effects may occur with some but not all calcium-entry blocking agents. Further studies are needed before there is widespread use of these agents for tocolysis in pregnant women.

Anesthesiologist's Approach to the Patient

There are at least three situations when obstetric patients require anesthesia during or after tocolytic therapy.[23] First, tocolytic therapy is not always successful, so preterm delivery occurs. Parturients may desire epidural anesthesia for analgesia during labor and vaginal delivery. Some physicians consider regional anesthesia medically indicated in such cases because epidural or spinal anesthesia may inhibit inappropriate maternal expulsive efforts and facilitate an atraumatic, controlled delivery. Operative delivery mandates administration of anesthesia. Malloy et al. recently reported that 44% of all very low-birthweight infants delivered in Missouri between 1980 and 1984 were delivered by cesarean section.[80]

Second, some obstetricians advocate administration of a tocolytic agent before and during performance of cervical cerclage, an operation performed to prevent preterm delivery. Third, some obstetricians advocate administration of a tocolytic agent for treatment of acute fetal distress.[65,100] The goal is to improve uteroplacental perfusion by relaxing the uterus and thereby facilitate fetal resuscitation *in utero*. Although this may allow obstetricians to avoid operative delivery in some patients, the remaining women will require emergency induction of anesthesia for cesarean section.

Specific anesthetic requirements for vaginal delivery of the preterm infant include the following: (1) inhibition of inappropriate maternal expulsive efforts before complete cervical dilation, especially with the breech presentation; (2) avoidance of precipitous de-

livery, which causes rapid decompression of the fetal head and increased risk of intracranial hemorrhage; and (3) provision of a relaxed maternal pelvic floor and perineum to facilitate smooth, controlled delivery of the vulnerable, preterm fetal head.

Unfortunately, appropriately timing the administration of regional anesthetics is more difficult with women in preterm labor than in term labor. The preterm parturient often has a prolonged latent phase of labor. She may be hospitalized for days or weeks while receiving tocolytic therapy. When tocolysis fails, the patient typically is in advanced labor and delivery may be imminent. After a few strong contractions, she may have cervical dilatation of 5 cm. Full cervical dilation is sufficient to allow retraction of the cervix over the fetal head. In the preterm parturient, 7 cm may constitute full cervical dilation, rather than 10 cm as at term. The obstetrician may ask the anesthesiologist to provide epidural anesthetics immediately.

Considerations after beta-adrenergic tocolytic therapy

The half-lives of ritodrine and terbutaline are prolonged in pregnant women. Kuhnert et al. observed that the distribution phase and equilibrium phase half-lives for ritodrine in pregnant women are 32 ± 20 minutes and 17 ± 10 hours, respectively.[72] The cardiovascular effects of these agents also persist after discontinuation. There are sparse data on the effects of anesthesia shortly after administration of a beta-adrenergic tocolytic agent. Shin and Kim retrospectively observed that maternal hypotension occurred in two of three women who received epidural anesthesia within 30 minutes of discontinuation of ritodrine, compared with one of eight women for whom there was a delay of more than 30 minutes ($p = .15$).[111] Abouleish contended that regional anesthetics should not be administered unless the beta-adrenergic agent has been discontinued for at least 2 hours before cesarean section.[2]

Women with failed tocolysis typically require emergency induction of anesthesia. A proscription against regional anesthesia deprives the parturient of enjoying the emotional experience associated with childbirth and subjects her to the risks of general anesthesia (i.e., failure to intubate the trachea and/or aspiration of gastric contents).

Recently we observed that ritodrine did not worsen maternal hypotension during epidural lidocaine anesthesia in gravid ewes.[27] The inotropic and chronotropic activity of ritodrine seemed to preserve cardiac output and uterine blood flow during epidural lidocaine anesthesia. As with all animal studies, one should use caution before extrapolating these results to humans. Nonetheless, our study suggests that admonitions against use of epidural anesthesia in patients who have recently received a beta-adrenergic

agent may not be valid. We believe that careful induction of epidural anesthesia may be safely performed in patients who have recently received beta-adrenergic therapy, provided that tachycardia is not severe. A delay of 15 minutes often results in sufficient slowing of maternal heart rate to allow one to proceed with epidural anesthesia.

One should probably avoid vigorous hydration before administering an epidural anesthetic in these patients. A large bolus of crystalloid may precipitate pulmonary edema. One should first give a modest bolus of crystalloid (e.g., 500 ml of Ringer's lactate) and then slowly establish epidural anesthesia. One can then add crystalloid to maintain normal maternal blood pressure.

If general anesthesia is required after administration of a beta-adrenergic agent, one should avoid agents that will exacerbate maternal tachycardia (e.g., atropine, glycopyrrolate, pancuronium). It also seems appropriate to avoid halothane, which sensitizes the myocardium to catecholamine-induced dysrhythmias more than do enflurane or isoflurane. Some anesthesiologists administer an intravenous lidocaine bolus during rapid-sequence induction of anesthesia to reduce the likelihood of maternal arrhythmias during laryngoscopy and intubation. Finally, residual maternal tachycardia from the beta-adrenergic agent complicates assessment of hydration and depth of anesthesia.

Considerations after magnesium sulfate ($MgSO_4$) therapy

Magnesium alters neuromuscular function as follows: it (1) attenuates acetylcholine release at the neuromuscular junction, (2) reduces end-plate sensitivity to acetylcholine, and (3) decreases muscle membrane excitability. Accordingly, magnesium potentiates activity of both depolarizing and nondepolarizing muscle relaxants. One should not administer a "defasciculating" dose of nondepolarizing muscle relaxant before administration of succinylcholine in patients who have recently received $MgSO_4$. Rather, one should give an intubating dose of muscle relaxant (e.g., 1 mg/kg of succinylcholine) and then use a nerve stimulator to monitor neuromuscular function before giving additional muscle relaxant.

Should there be a delay between discontinuation of $MgSO_4$ and induction of regional anesthesia? Suresh and Lawson stated that $MgSO_4$ "should be discontinued prior to initiation of lumbar epidural analgesia because magnesium can increase the likelihood of hypotension through its generalized vasodilating properties."[120] On the other hand, epidural anesthesia is commonly given safely to preeclamptic women who continue to receive $MgSO_4$ during anesthesia and surgery. One cannot assume that normotensive preterm parturients given MgSO$_4$ for tocolysis will respond to regional anesthesia in the same manner as preeclamptic parturients. Recently we observed that MgSO$_4$ decreased maternal blood pressure but not uterine blood flow or fetal oxygenation during epidural lidocaine anesthesia in gravid ewes.[124] If applicable to humans, hypermagnesemia may interfere with maintenance of blood pressure and increase the likelihood of modest hypotension during regional anesthesia in normotensive pregnant women. In our judgment, it is not necessary that one withhold epidural anesthetics from patients who have recently received MgSO$_4$ for tocolysis. But in most cases, the slower onset of epidural anesthesia seems preferable to the faster onset of spinal anesthesia.

Considerations after prostaglandin synthetase inhibitor therapy

Indomethacin reversibly inhibits cyclooxygenase; it thereby produces a transient abnormality in platelet function. Some anesthesiologists measure the bleeding time before administering regional anesthesia in patients who have recently received a prostaglandin synthetase inhibitor to treat preterm labor. Williams et al. reported one case of cervical epidural hematoma after steroid injection into the cervical epidural space of a man who had been taking indomethacin. This complication occurred after the seventh epidural steroid injection over 2 years.[132] However, epidural hematoma is a rare complication in obstetric patients.

In some circumstances, it may be impossible to measure bleeding time with sufficient speed to guide management. Further, the predictive value of the bleeding time is unclear. In these cases, the anesthesiologist should assess all risks and benefits of regional anesthesia vs. alternatives. In the absence of other risk factors for abnormal bleeding and/or coagulation, we will administer regional anesthesia, without first measuring bleeding time, in selected patients who have received indomethacin.

PREECLAMPSIA

Preeclampsia is a hypertensive disorder unique to pregnancy. It complicates 5% to 10% of all pregnancies and is associated with 20% of maternal deaths in the United States. Cerebral hemorrhage and/or edema are the most frequent causes of death. Preeclampsia is also a major cause of intrauterine growth retardation and perinatal morbidity and mortality.

Traditionally the diagnosis of preeclampsia has required the presence of (1) hypertension and (2) proteinuria (at least 300 mg/24 hr) or pathologic edema. Unfortunately, most healthy pregnant women

---

BOX 28-2
HYPERTENSIVE DISORDERS OF PREGNANCY

Pregnancy-induced hypertension
Preeclampsia
  Mild
  Severe
Eclampsia

Chronic hypertension preceding pregnancy

Chronic hypertension with superimposed pregnancy-induced hypertension
Superimposed preeclampsia
Superimposed eclampsia

From American College of Obstetricians and Gynecologists: Management of preeclampsia, ACOG Technical Bulletin #91, Washington, D.C., 1986.

---

experience dependent edema. There are no standardized methods for identifying pathologic edema diagnostic of preeclampsia. Sibai recently proposed that edema not be used in the diagnosis of preeclampsia.[115]

Box 28-2 lists the classification of the hypertensive disorders of pregnancy, as suggested by the American College of Obstetricians and Gynecologists.[3] Preeclampsia is classified as either mild or severe. There is no classification for "moderate" preeclampsia. Preeclampsia is regarded as severe if one or more of the following are present[3]:

- Systolic blood pressure at least 160 mm Hg on two occasions at least 6 hours apart
- Diastolic blood pressure at least 110 mm Hg on two occasions at least 6 hours apart
- At least 5 g protein in a 24-hour urine collection
- Oliguria (less than 400 ml/24 hr)
- Cerebral or visual disturbances
- Cyanosis or pulmonary edema
- Epigastric or right upper quadrant pain
- Impaired liver function of unclear cause
- Thrombocytopenia or disseminated intravascular coagulation

Not all hypertensive pregnant women have preeclampsia. Preeclampsia is primarily a disease of nulliparous women and is not usually recurrent.[115] Among hypertensive preterm or parous women suspected of having preeclampsia, the likelihood of an incorrect diagnosis is high. Women with early-onset (i.e., before term) hypertension have a high likelihood of unrecognized, chronic renal disease.[64,115] The laboratory findings, clinical course, and perinatal outcome of early-onset preeclampsia are worse than those in women who develop preeclampsia after 34 weeks' gestation (i.e., the earlier the onset of preeclampsia, the sicker the patient).[115,117]

Although not all hypertensive pregnant women have preeclampsia, the diagnosis of preeclampsia may be inappropriately excluded in *normotensive* pregnant women with other signs of preeclampsia (e.g., coagulopathy, liver dysfunction, or thrombocytopenia). Weinstein identified a group of preeclamptic women with hemolysis, elevated liver enzymes, and low platelet count (i.e., HELLP syndrome).[129,130] Often this variant of severe preeclampsia is incorrectly given a nonobstetric diagnosis such as a hematologic or gastrointestinal disease. Regardless of the *initial* presentation, preeclampsia ultimately includes vasoconstriction, reduced uteroplacental blood flow, and hypertension.

Etiology and Pathophysiology

The cause of preeclampsia remains unknown. Past theories have suggested that preeclampsia results from (1) uteroplacental ischemia, (2) genetic predisposition, (3) a primary immunologic disorder, (4) humoral factors, and/or (5) environmental factors. No single theory adequately explains preeclampsia. There is evidence that preeclampsia is not primarily a hypertensive disorder, but a disease process related to endothelial cell injury.[108,127] Roberts et al. proposed that "poorly perfused placental tissue releases a factor into the systemic circulation that injures endothelial cells. The changes initiated by endothelial cell injury set in motion a dysfunctional cascade of coagulation, vasoconstriction, and intravascular fluid redistribution that results in the clinical syndrome of preeclampsia."[108]

Recently there has been emphasis on identifying successful prophylaxis of preeclampsia. Women who develop preeclampsia begin to lose the pregnancy-associated refractory response to angiotensin II as early as 18 weeks of gestation.[50] Preeclamptic women have an imbalance in placental production of prostacyclin (a vasodilator and inhibitor of platelet aggregation) and thromboxane (a vasoconstrictor and stimulator of platelet aggregation). In normal pregnancy, the placenta produces equal amounts of prostacyclin and thromboxane. In preeclamptic women, the placenta produces seven times more thromboxane than prostacyclin.[127] Prophylactic administration of a prostaglandin synthetase inhibitor (e.g., low-dose aspirin) may restore prostacyclin/thromboxane balance and reduce the incidence of preeclampsia,[126] but aspirin is not a treatment for the syndrome of preeclampsia, once it has developed.

Direct measurements of plasma volume have demonstrated decreases in preeclamptic women.[56] Hemoconcentration (e.g., increased hematocrit level)

occurs. Invasive and noninvasive monitoring of preeclamptic women have revealed heterogenous hemodynamic findings. Pulmonary capillary wedge pressure may be low, normal, or high. Potential reasons for heterogeneity include the following: (1) variation in patient selection and severity of disease, (2) variation in disease progression (e.g., early vs. late disease), and (3) variation in fluid and pharmacologic management before and during the hemodynamic measurements. Alternatively, preeclampsia may not be a single disease entity. Weiner stated: "It may well be that, rather than a single disease with a singular cause, preeclampsia is a clinical syndrome having multiple causes, each activating a common pathway culminating in endothelial damage, vasospasm, and hypertension."[128]

Obstetric Management

Most obstetricians in the United States now agree on the following method of seizure prophylaxis and the definitive treatment of preeclampsia.

Seizure prophylaxis

Magnesium sulfate (MgSO$_4$) remains the cornerstone of seizure prophylaxis in the United States. MgSO$_4$ is not an antihypertensive agent, and there remains debate as to whether it is even an anticonvulsant. Bolus infusion of MgSO$_4$ (4 g IV over 15 min) has a transient hypotensive effect that does not continue during infusion.[37] Obstetricians and obstetric nurses monitor deep tendon reflexes in patients receiving MgSO$_4$ because the reflexes are lost when the magnesium concentration reaches approximately 10 mEq/L. This is below the concentration needed to cause the worst side effects, namely respiratory paralysis (15 mEq/L), sinoatrial and atrioventricular block (15 mEq/L), and cardiac arrest (25 mEq/L).[54] Magnesium is excreted by the kidneys and must be given cautiously when renal function is impaired.

Delivery

Delivery is the definitive treatment of preeclampsia, but in some cases of early-onset preeclampsia, the obstetrician may attempt to delay delivery to allow development of fetal lung maturity. There is no agreement about the utility and safety of delayed delivery in women in whom preeclampsia is diagnosed between 28 and 36 weeks' gestation. Management of second trimester preeclampsia is even more problematic. Sibai et al. retrospectively observed that conservative management of such cases was not associated with improved perinatal outcome. Delayed delivery was also associated with a very high rate of maternal morbidity.[117]

Although delivery may represent definitive treatment of preeclampsia, the disease does not abruptly cease. Some patients remain severely ill after delivery, and pulmonary edema is most likely to develop postpartum as a result of delayed intravascular mobilization of extravascular fluid, unaccompanied by spontaneous diuresis.[11,116]

Cardiovascular Assessment and Management

Current controversies in cardiovascular assessment and management include the following: What are the indications for invasive hemodynamic monitoring? What are the roles of blood volume expansion? Should oliguria be treated? What is the appropriate treatment of severe hypertension?

Invasive hemodynamic monitoring

Proponents of aggressive use of invasive hemodynamic monitoring in patients with severe preeclampsia give the following arguments. First, oliguria does not always reflect volume depletion.[33] Urinary diagnostic indices are not useful indicators of volume status in patients with severe preeclampsia.[75] Clark et al. studied nine patients with severe preeclampsia complicated by oliguria (i.e., less than 30 ml/hr for 3 hours) who failed to respond to a modest fluid challenge (e.g., 300 to 500 ml of Ringer's lactate over 20 minutes).[33] They identified three hemodynamic subsets: (1) patients with low pulmonary capillary wedge pressures, modest elevations of systemic vascular resistance, and hyperdynamic ventricular function treated with volume expansion, (2) a single patient with markedly elevated systemic vascular resistance and decreased cardiac output given hydralazine for afterload reduction, and (3) a final group of patients who appeared to be hypertensive primarily due to increased cardiac output. The latter group had high cardiac outputs, normal or only slightly increased systemic vascular resistance, and normal or increased pulmonary capillary wedge pressures, yet remained oliguric. The authors concluded that these patients had selective renal arteriospasm disproportionate to systemic vasoconstriction. They were treated with afterload reduction with hydralazine or preload reduction with nitroglycerin.

A second argument for invasive hemodynamic monitoring is that pulmonary edema of preeclampsia may be cardiogenic or noncardiogenic (i.e., decreased colloid osmotic pressure with or without increased pulmonary capillary permeability).[32,59,119] Colloid osmotic pressure is often low and typically declines further after delivery.[9,39] Therefore small increases in pulmonary capillary wedge pressure may result in pulmonary edema. The third argument is that there is a poor correlation between central venous pressure and pulmonary capillary wedge pressure in women with severe preeclampsia.[10,38,119]

Opponents of aggressive invasive monitoring counter with the following arguments. First, there is little need to treat oliguria per se in preeclamptic patients because antepartum oliguria is rarely followed by postpartum renal failure in preeclamptic women. Second, a management protocol that includes fluid restriction and early delivery and restricts antihypertensive therapy to hydralazine for treatment of diastolic blood pressure that is at least 110 mm Hg results in a low incidence of pulmonary edema.[102] Third, if central venous pressure is less than 6 mm Hg, the pulmonary capillary wedge pressure is unlikely to be markedly elevated.[125] Fourth, most labor and delivery units are not staffed and equipped to safely use invasive hemodynamic monitoring. Most critical care units are not prepared to care for a pregnant woman and her fetus and are often some distance from the labor and delivery unit. (In some hospitals, critical care nurses are transferred to the labor and delivery unit to facilitate safe use of invasive monitoring.) Fifth, preeclamptic women are most likely to develop pulmonary edema postpartum.[11,116] Sibai et al. reviewed 37 cases of pulmonary edema associated with preeclampsia-eclampsia. Of the 37 patients, 26 had postpartum pulmonary edema, and the onset was greater than 48 hours postpartum in 16 of those patients.[116] Because the incidence of pulmonary artery catheter–associated complications increases in proportion to duration of catheterization, the catheter may be removed before or during the period of greatest risk for pulmonary edema.[25,47] Thus some have advocated noninvasive monitoring while providing antepartum care on the labor and delivery unit and then transfer to the critical care unit for invasive hemodynamic monitoring after delivery.

Masaki and Greenspoon retrospectively reviewed 1 year's experience with pulmonary artery catheterization in patients with pregnancy-induced hypertension (PIH) at Los Angeles County Hospital.[83] Among these patients, pulmonary artery catheterization was limited to patients with one of the following two criteria: (1) oliguria unresponsive to fluid challenge of 500 to 1500 ml and/or (2) clinically severe pulmonary edema. During the study, 16,383 deliveries were performed at the hospital, but only seven patients met these criteria for pulmonary artery catheterization. Thus the rate of catheterization for patients with pregnancy-induced hypertension was 1 in 2340 obstetric patients. Among the patients who did not receive pulmonary artery catheterization, there were no cases of renal failure, cardiac failure, or death that might have been prevented by pulmonary artery catheterization. The authors concluded that "the lack of serious sequelae in noncatheterized patients with PIH suggests that more frequent use of the PA catheter would be of questionable benefit in the management of PIH."[83]

Blood volume expansion

Proponents of blood volume expansion argue that blood volume expansion in preeclamptic women may cause vasodilation and decreased maternal arterial pressure.[49,67] Second, if one can improve renal perfusion, uteroplacental perfusion may also improve. Third, hydration before either vasodilator therapy or administration of epidural anesthesia prevents abrupt hypotension.[40] Opponents of blood volume expansion note that it does not consistently decrease mean arterial pressure,[40,53] improve uteroplacental perfusion,[6] or decrease likelihood of fetal distress during labor.[70] Second, administration of large volumes of crystalloid and/or colloid may predispose the patient to pulmonary and/or cerebral edema postpartum.[11,12]

Treatment of severe hypertension

Obstetricians usually reserve antihypertensive therapy for patients with systolic blood pressure of at least 160 mm Hg or diastolic pressures of at least 110 mm Hg. They fear that more aggressive treatment of hypertension may cause decreased uteroplacental perfusion. Hydralazine remains the mainstay of intrapartum antihypertensive therapy. It decreases blood pressure but increases uterine blood flow during phenylephrine-induced hypertension in gravid ewes.[107] Hydralazine has an established safety record in pregnant patients. Disadvantages include delayed onset, reflex tachycardia, and prolonged duration of action. Although safe in most patients, it occasionally precipitates abrupt, profound hypotension. It is unlikely that hydralazine would decrease blood pressure in a preeclamptic patient who is hypertensive because of increased cardiac output.[32]

There is no consensus on appropriate alternatives to hydralazine. Diuretics further reduce intravascular volume, thereby further decreasing uteroplacental perfusion, and are inappropriate antepartum. Diuretics may be necessary in postpartum patients who do not undergo spontaneous diuresis, especially those who were given antepartum volume expansion. Most obstetricians avoid diazoxide, which causes sodium and water retention and hyperglycemia, and inhibits uterine contractions. The ganglionic blocker trimethaphan is still used occasionally and is unlikely to precipitate abrupt hypotension. Recently there has been enthusiasm for use of labetalol.[79,103] Incremental injection of labetalol is unlikely to precipitate abrupt hypotension and does not necessarily require invasive hemodynamic monitoring. The decrease in blood pressure is not accompanied by reflex tachycardia, which occurs with hydralazine. Disadvantages of labetalol include significant interpatient dosage variability,[79] as well as prolonged duration. The effects of labetalol on the fetus and neonate must be further evaluated to help clarify its role in the treatment of severe hypertension in pregnancy.

The use of sodium nitroprusside and nitroglycerin remains controversial. Naulty et al. observed cyanide toxicity in fetal lambs after maternal administration of nitroprusside—namely, 25 μg/kg/min—which was sufficient to decrease maternal mean arterial pressure by 20% for 1 hour.[93] This is at least three times greater than the maximal short-term recommended human dose. Risk of fetal cyanide toxicity with smaller doses of nitroprusside in humans is undetermined, but short-term infusions have been given without toxicity.[118] In patients with severe hypertension and low pulmonary capillary wedge pressure, either nitroprusside or nitroglycerin may precipitate sudden, severe hypotension. Cotton et al. evaluated the cardiovascular effects of nitroglycerin, both with and without volume expansion, in six patients with severe preeclampsia.[40] Nitroglycerin alone significantly reduced the cardiac index and oxygen delivery. Two patients experienced abrupt, profound hypotension accompanied by fetal heart rate abnormalities. Blood volume expansion resulted in the nitroglycerin being no longer able to lower arterial pressure, as would be expected after volume expansion plus a venodilator. The cardiac index and oxygen delivery were maintained. Kirshon et al. concluded: "The benefit of volume expansion in pregnancy-induced hypertension appears to be the prevention of sudden and profound drops in blood pressure with antihypertensive therapy."[70] Clearly neither nitroprusside nor nitroglycerin should be given without invasive hemodynamic monitoring.

In summary, invasive hemodynamic monitoring seems indicated in patients with severe preeclampsia plus pulmonary edema. Otherwise, it seems reasonable to reserve invasive monitoring for patients with severe hypertension unresponsive to conventional antihypertensive therapy (e.g., hydralazine) and for *selected* patients who will receive epidural anesthesia. Volume expansion does not seem indicated in preeclamptic patients with oliguria alone because there is little evidence that oliguria in this setting requires treatment. Careful blood volume expansion should be performed if the patient will receive vasodilators, including epidural anesthesia.

Anesthesiologist's Approach to the Patient

In a review of hypertension in pregnancy, Lindheimer and Katz concluded: "Epidural block should be avoided, since in preeclampsia it is associated with sudden falls of blood pressure and on occasion with vascular collapse."[77] Undoubtedly this scenario did occur 3 decades ago when spinal anesthetics were given to preeclamptic women with unrecognized, uncorrected hypovolemia. Norris et al. recently observed profound hypotension in two of five mildly preeclamptic women who received spinal anesthesia for nonemergent cesarean section.[98] With appropriate hydration and slow induction of anesthesia, epidural anesthesia is currently the preferred technique in most centers.

Graham and Goldstein and Newsome et al. demonstrated stability of maternal cardiac output after administration of a epidural anesthesia in patients with severe preeclampsia.[52,95] Epidural anesthesia provides excellent analgesia during labor and allows the patient to remain awake and alert during vaginal or cesarean delivery. Epidural anesthesia has at least three specific advantages in preeclamptic women. First, it reduces circulating concentrations of catecholamines in laboring women, facilitating control of blood pressure and improving intervillous blood flow[1,67,113]; second, it allows better control of systemic and pulmonary arterial pressures during cesarean section than does general anesthesia[61]; and third, epidural anesthesia does not require laryngoscopy and intubation, which may be hazardous and/or difficult because of severe pharyngolaryngeal edema.[58]

Assessment of platelet function in preeclamptic patients is controversial. Patients with severe preeclampsia are at increased risk for coagulopathy. If the platelet count is greater than 100,000, it is unlikely that indices of coagulation are abnormal, but patients with preeclampsia may have abnormal platelet function despite a normal platelet count.[69] Platelet dysfunction in preeclampsia seems related to the severity of the disease (i.e., only women with severe preeclampsia seem at risk for platelet dysfunction and prolonged bleeding times).[63] We usually obtain a bleeding time before performing epidural anesthesia in a patient with severe preeclampsia. On the other hand, we are aware that the predictive value of the bleeding time is unclear. Further, we know of only one case (unpublished) of epidural hematoma after the administration of epidural anesthesia in a patient with preeclampsia.

Another unresolved question is whether there should be assessment of platelet function in a patient who has received low-dose aspirin during pregnancy. Benigni et al. noted that daily administration of 60 mg of aspirin to women at risk for preeclampsia caused a small but significant prolongation of the bleeding time (i.e., 6.2 ± 1.8 minutes in the aspirin-treated group vs. 4.7 ± 1.2 minutes in the control group).[13] Our approach to this question is similar to that noted in the earlier discussion of anesthetic management of patients who have received indomethacin for tocolysis.

FETAL STRESS AND DISTRESS
Etiology

It is useful to distinguish between chronic fetal stress and acute fetal distress.

Chronic fetal stress

First, chronic fetal stress may occur with inadequate maternal nutrition and/or oxygenation. The former may occur in a patient with alcohol or drug addiction, and the latter may occur in a patient with asthma or a right-to-left shunt. Second, inadequate placental oxygen delivery may result in chronic fetal stress. Examples include patients with anemia, nicotine abuse, or vascular disease secondary to chronic hypertension or diabetes. Third, there may be inadequate oxygen transfer across the placenta, as might occur with placenta previa or partial separation of the placenta. Fourth, chronic fetal stress may be due to inadequate fetal circulation, as might occur with fetal tachydysrhythmia or hemolytic disease secondary to Rh sensitization. Fifth, anomalous fetuses often show signs of chronic stress. These fetuses have an increased incidence of heart rate abnormalities.

Acute fetal distress

Acute fetal distress occurs as a result of one of three basic causes: (1) uteroplacental dysfunction, (2) umbilical cord compression, and/or (3) uterine hypertonus.

Uteroplacental dysfunction. Uterine contractions decrease uteroplacental blood flow. When superimposed on chronic uteroplacental insufficiency (e.g., such as may occur with diabetes or postdatism), labor may result in acute fetal distress. Maternal hypotension (as may occur during administration of spinal or epidural anesthesia) can cause acute fetal distress despite a normal uteroplacental unit.

Umbilical cord compression. Umbilical cord compression may occur before labor as a result of oligohydramnios (i.e., decreased volume of amniotic fluid). Mann recently suggested that undetected antenatal umbilical cord compression may be a cause of "unexplained brain damage."[81] Accordingly, obstetricians today pay careful attention to assessment of amniotic fluid volume. Frank prolapse of the umbilical cord (as might occur with a footling breech presentation) may also result in cord compression. Umbilical cord compression also occurs during the second stage of labor and results in variable fetal heart rate decelerations.

Uterine hypertonus. Dehydration may cause inappropriate uterine activity. Abruption of the placenta also may cause a tetanic uterus. Most often, uterine hypertonus occurs as a result of hyperstimulation with parenteral oxytocin.

Obstetric Management
Chronic fetal stress

An important goal of obstetric management is to detect and treat fetal stress before development of frank distress. Examples of treatment include the following: (1) bedrest in the left lateral decubitus position to improve uteroplacental perfusion, (2) maternal administration of supplemental oxygen to improve fetal oxygenation, (3) maternal or fetal administration of an antidysrhythmic agent, to try to convert a fetal tachydysrhythmia to normal sinus rhythm, (4) intrauterine transfusion of blood to a fetus that is anemic due to Rh sensitization, and (5) maternal administration of a glucocorticoid (e.g., betamethasone, dexamethasone), to try to accelerate fetal lung maturity.

If the fetal condition can possibly be improved and if the fetus is preterm, then a delay in delivery may be sought; however, frequent reassessments of fetal condition are required. If the fetal condition cannot be improved and/or the fetus is term, delivery should be effected, either by induction of labor or by performance of elective cesarean section.

Acute fetal distress

In situations of acute fetal distress, it remains advisable to attempt resuscitation of the fetus in utero. Resuscitation in utero has several advantages. First, it allows anesthesiology and operating room personnel time to prepare. Second, one may be able to avoid performance of emergency cesarean section. Third, it may result in the delivery of a resuscitated rather than a depressed newborn. And fourth, it may allow use of regional rather than general anesthesia.

To attempt resuscitation in utero, first one must ensure proper positioning of the mother. Regrettably some caregivers still allow parturients to remain supine during labor, which can cause aortocaval compression. With the mother in the lateral decubitus position, the compression is rapidly relieved, and uteroplacental perfusion and fetal condition often improve. This position may also relieve umbilical cord compression. Second, parenteral oxytocin should be discontinued. Third, supplemental oxygen should be administered to the mother. Fourth, one should ensure maintenance of normal maternal blood pressure. Relief of aortocaval compression may be sufficient to restore maternal blood pressure. If hypotension persists, a bolus of non-dextrose–containing balanced salt solution (e.g., Ringer's lactate) can be given. Bolus administration of a dextrose-containing solution may cause maternal-fetal hyperglycemia and hyperinsulinemia, which can later result in neonatal hypoglycemia. In some cases, administration of ephedrine is indicated. This mixed alpha- and beta-agonist is the vasopressor of choice for most hypotension in obstetric practice.

In cases of acute fetal distress secondary to uterine hypertonus, the obstetrician may give a bolus of a beta-adrenergic tocolytic agent (e.g., terbutaline). The goal is to relax the uterus and thereby allow improved uteroplacental perfusion. Indeed, there is evidence

that this technique may improve fetal acid-base status and may even obviate emergency delivery.[65,100] If this technique is unsuccessful, the anesthesiologist may be asked to give anesthesia to a patient with severe tachycardia due to recent administration of a beta-adrenergic agent.

Intrauterine infusion of normal saline (i.e., saline amnioinfusion) may relieve umbilical cord compression and eliminate variable decelerations of the fetal heart rate.[88,89,92] The procedure involves infusion of 200 to 1000 ml of normal saline into the uterine cavity through the intrauterine pressure catheter. This can be accomplished while transferring the patient to the operating room and preparing for cesarean section, should the amnioinfusion fail. Recently Wenstrom and Parsons suggested a second reason for performing amnioinfusion.[131] Specifically, they suggested that saline amnioinfusion be considered for thick meconium-staining of the amniotic fluid. In such cases, saline amnioinfusion should dilute the meconium and perhaps reduce the adverse consequences of meconium aspiration, should that occur.

Unfortunately, attempts at resuscitation in utero are not uniformly successful. With ongoing fetal distress, emergency delivery is necessary. If the cervix is fully dilated and the obstetrician does not anticipate a difficult application and delivery, he/she may opt for instrumental vaginal delivery. Otherwise, cesarean section must be performed.

Anesthesiologist's Approach to the Patient

Every parturient is a potential candidate for emergency administration of anesthesia. Ideally an anesthesia care provider should evaluate the parturient after admission to the labor and delivery unit. If evaluation has not occured, the anesthesia care provider may be required to provide emergency anesthesia to a patient who has not undergone any preanesthetic evaluation. In such cases, degree of obstetric urgency should affect the extent of the preanesthetic evaluation. Regardless of the extent of the emergency, the anesthesiologist must obtain some history and physical examination. One should not proceed with rapid-sequence induction of general anesthesia unless one is satisfied with airway assessment and is confident that intubation can be accomplished.

How does one choose an anesthetic technique in situations of fetal stress or distress? In situations of chronic fetal stress, either a regional or general anesthetic can be administered safely in most patients. In contrast, dire distress (e.g., prolonged and fixed bradycardia, placental abruption, uterine rupture) almost always mandates administration of general anesthesia. Many cases of fetal distress are intermediate between chronic stress and dire distress.

In these cases regional anesthesia is not necessarily contraindicated.[82,104] The following represents one approach to these cases[24]:

1. If a partial level of epidural anesthesia already exists and there is hemodynamic stability, extension of epidural anesthesia is appropriate for either instrumental vaginal delivery or cesarean section. We give a bolus of Ringer's lactate and inject epidural 3% 2-chloroprocaine in 5-ml increments while the urethral catheter is inserted and the abdomen is prepared and draped. Often there will be satisfactory anesthesia when the surgeon is ready to make the skin incision. If not, the ongoing fetal heart rate pattern will dictate whether a delay is acceptable. Surgery should not be delayed in the presence of ongoing, severe fetal distress. In cases of partial but incomplete epidural anesthesia, the obstetrician can supplement with local infiltration of a dilute solution of local anesthetic. In such cases, one might use 1% 2-chloroprocaine or 0.5% lidocaine.

2. Use of spinal anesthesia in the presence of acute fetal distress remains controversial. Spinal anesthesia is associated with a more rapid onset of sympathetic block than is epidural anesthesia. Although spinal hypotension occurs less frequently in women in labor than in those pregnant women who are not, risk of hypotension remains important.[31] Some anesthesiologists have had good results with spinal anesthesia during fetal distress.[82] Before using spinal anesthesia in such circumstances, these questions should be asked: (1) Could fetal distress be due to concealed abruption with attendant hypovolemia? (2) Can a successful block be achieved quickly, without delaying surgery? (3) Can hypotension be avoided?

3. After the patient is transferred to the delivery room, the fetal heart rate abnormality may resolve. In those cases one may now consider administering spinal or epidural anesthesia. We cannot overemphasize the importance of continuing to monitor fetal heart rate after transfer to the operating room. This should be accomplished with a fetal scalp electrode, which will allow monitoring of fetal heart rate during and after induction of anesthesia, until immediately before delivery. Fetal heart rate monitoring may facilitate administration of regional anesthesia because it may encourage the obstetrician and anesthesiologist to wait for satisfactory regional anesthesia. Fetal heart rate monitoring may also guide management in cases of failed intubation.

4. In the absence of satisfactory regional anesthesia and in the presence of ongoing, acute fetal distress, induction of general anesthesia is indicated for cesarean section. The anesthesiologist should *not* indiscriminately perform rapid-sequence induction of general anesthesia. A history and/or suspicion of difficult intubation should prompt either awake intubation or regional anesthesia, despite presence of fetal distress. It is possible to perform local infiltration with a dilute solution of a local anesthetic and deliver the baby with local anesthesia as the primary anesthetic technique. After delivery, the anesthesiologist can secure the airway by awake intubation to allow the obstetrician to complete surgery during general anesthesia. This may sound horrific, but it is preferable to ill-advised rapid-sequence induction with subsequent loss of airway. One must not endanger the mother in an effort to deliver a distressed fetus.

Anesthesiologists should remain sensitive to the emotional needs of the mother and father. Cases of fetal distress result in significant parental concern. Often the anesthesiologist qualifies as the best individual to reassure and comfort distressed parents. All members of the obstetric team should remember that chaos need not accompany urgency in these cases.

Finally, every hospital should develop a strict policy on the presence of the husband or support person in such cases. In our hospital, we permit the husband to remain with the patient when a regional anesthetic is used. If general anesthesia is required, the husband is asked to leave the operating room. Once the patient is stable, he may return to watch the delivery of the infant, but he again leaves the operating room when the pediatrician departs with the infant.

KEY POINTS

- Unlike other operations where the patient is primarily concerned with himself/herself, the pregnant patient is usually primarily concerned with her baby's welfare.

- The anesthesiologist should be able to detail the pregnancy-induced cardiovascular and respiratory changes.

- The central nervous system effects of pregnancy include a markedly reduced local anesthetic requirement when those agents are given intrathecally or epidurally.
- The anesthesiologist must clearly understand that pregnant patients are at increased risk for aspiration of gastric contents.
- Alpha-adrenergic agonists are potent uterine vasoconstrictors, and they markedly decrease uterine blood flow. Ephedrine, a mixed alpha- and beta-agonist, seems to protect uterine blood flow and is therefore the vasopressor of choice in most cases of hypotension in obstetric patients.
- No human studies suggest that the administration of an anesthetic during surgery increases risk of fetal anomalies. On the other hand, there is evidence that anesthesia and surgery during pregnancy might increase risk of fetal wastage and/or preterm labor. Therefore elective surgery should be avoided during pregnancy or, if not possible, at least delayed beyond the first trimester.
- Fetal monitoring should be attempted during surgery on the pregnant patient.
- Regional anesthesia may well be the preferred technique for performance of surgery on pregnant patients.
- Preterm delivery remains the leading cause of perinatal morbidity and mortality in the United States. Preterm labor is often treated with beta-adrenergic tocolytic therapy, and these agents interact with anesthetics. These interactions must be carefully understood by the anesthesiologist.
- Magnesium sulfate is also often used for treatment of preterm labor. It potentiates both depolarizing and non-depolarizing muscle relaxants.
- Preeclampsia, which traditionally includes hypertension and proteinuria, is another condition with which the anesthesiologist should be quite familiar.
- Magnesium sulfate remains the cornerstone of seizure prophylaxis in preeclampsia.
- There is considerable controversy about the use of invasive monitoring in preeclamptic patients.
- Hydralazine remains the mainstay of intrapartum antihypertensive therapy for severe preeclampsia. Recently labetalol has emerged as an attractive alternative.
- Epidural anesthesia is the preferred anesthetic technique in most patient's with preeclampsia.
- In the situation of acute fetal distress, resuscitation in utero should be attempted with proper positioning, oxygen, discontinuance of oxytocin, and maintenance of maternal blood pressure.
- Every parturient is a potential candidate for the emergency administration of anesthesia.

KEY REFERENCES

American College of Obstetricians and Gynecologists: Management of preeclampsia, *ACOG Technical Bulletin #91,* Washington, DC, 1986.

Chestnut DH: Fetal distress. In James FM, Dewan DL, and Wheeler AS, eds: *Obstetric anesthesia: the complicated patient,* ed 2, Philadelphia, 1988, FA Davis.

Chestnut DH: Anesthesia for preterm labor and delivery. In Hood DD, ed: *Problems in anesthesia: anesthesia in obstetrics and gynecology,* Philadelphia, 1989, JB Lippincott.

Duncan PG, Pope WD, Cohen MM et al: Fetal risk of anesthesia and surgery during pregnancy, *Anesthesiology* 64:790, 1986.

Marx GF, Luykx WM, and Cohen S: Fetal-neonatal status following caesarean section for fetal distress, *Br J Anaesth* 56:1009, 1984.

Mazze RI, Kallen B: Reproductive outcome after anesthesia and operation during pregnancy: a registry study of 5405 cases, *Am J Obstet Gynecol* 161:1178, 1989.

REFERENCES

1. Abboud T, Artal R, Sarkis F et al: Sympathoadrenal activity: maternal, fetal, and neonatal responses after epidural anesthesia in the preeclamptic patient, *Am J Obstet Gynecol* 144:915, 1982.
2. Abouleish E: Preterm labor. In Datta SJ, Ostheimer GW, eds: *Common problems in obstetric anesthesia,* Chicago, 1987, Year Book.
3. American College of Obstetricians and Gynecologists: Management of preeclampsia, *ACOG Technical Bulletin #91,* Washington, DC, 1986.
4. Archer GW, Marx GF: Arterial oxygen tension during apnoea in parturient women, *Br J Anaesth* 46:358, 1974.
5. Baden JM, Serra M, and Mazze RI: Inhibition of fetal methionine synthase by nitrous oxide, *Br J Anaesth* 56:523, 1984.
6. Belfort M, Kirshon B, Akovic K et al: *Umbilical and uterine artery impedance following volume expansion and verapamil therapy in severe preeclampsia* (abstract), Houston, Texas, 1990, Proceedings of the Annual Meeting of the Society of Perinatal Obstetricians.
7. Bellow-Reuss E: Effect of catecholamines on fluid reabsorption by the isolated proximal convoluted tubule, *Am J Physiol* 238:F347, 1980.
8. Benedetti TJ: Life-threatening complications of betamimetic therapy for preterm labor inhibition, *Clin Perinatol* 13:843, 1986.
9. Benedetti TJ, Carlson RW: Studies of colloid osmotic pressure in pregnancy-induced hypertension, *Am J Obstet Gynecol* 135:308, 1979.
10. Benedetti TJ, Cotton DB, Read JC et al: Hemodynamic observations in severe preeclampsia with a flow-directed pulmonary artery catheter, *Am J Obstet Gynecol* 136:465, 1980.
11. Benedetti TJ, Kates R, and Williams V: Hemodynamic observations in severe preeclampsia complicated by pulmonary edema, *Am J Obstet Gynecol* 152:330, 1985.
12. Benedetti TJ, Quilligan EJ: Cerebral edema in severe pregnancy-induced hypertension, *Am J Obstet Gynecol* 137:860, 1980.
13. Benigni A, Gregorini G, Frusca T et al: Effect of low-dose aspirin on fetal and maternal generation of thromboxane by platelets in women at risk for pregnancy-induced hypertension, *N Engl J Med* 321:357, 1989.
14. Bernal JM, Miralles PJ: Cardiac surgery with cardiopulmonary bypass during pregnancy, *Obstet Gynecol Survey* 41:1, 1986.
15. Bevan DR, Holdcroft A, Loh L et al: Closing volume and pregnancy, *Br Med J* 1:13, 1974.
16. Biehl DR: Foetal monitoring during surgery unrelated to pregnancy, *Can Anaesth Soc J* 32:455, 1985.
17. Biehl DR, Yarnell R, Wade JG et al: The uptake of isoflurane by the foetal lamb *in utero:* effect on regional blood flow, *Can Anaesth Soc J* 30:581, 1983.
18. Blitt CD, Petty WC, Alberternst EE et al: Correlation of plasma cholinesterase activity and duration of action of succinylcholine during pregnancy, *Anesth Analg* 56:78, 1977.
19. Brodsky JB, Cohen EN, Brown BW Jr et al: Surgery during pregnancy and fetal outcome, *Am J Obstet Gynecol* 138:1165, 1980.
20. Capeless EL, Clapp JF: Cardiovascular changes in early phase of pregnancy, *Am J Obstet Gynecol* 161;1449, 1989.
21. Caritis SN, Edelstone DI, and Mueller-Heubach E: Pharmacologic inhibition of preterm labor, *Am J Obstet Gynecol* 133:557, 1979.
22. Castle BM, Turnbull AC: The presence or absence of fetal breathing movements predicts the outcome of preterm labour, *Lancet* 2:472, 1983.
23. Chestnut DH: Anesthesia for preterm labor and delivery. In Hood DD, ed: *Problems in anesthesia: anesthesia in obstetrics and gynecology,* Philadelphia, 1989, JB Lippincott.
24. Chestnut DH: Fetal distress. In James FM, Dewan DL, and Wheeler AS, eds: *Obstetric anesthesia: the complicated patient,* ed 2, Philadelphia, 1988, FA Davis.
25. Chestnut DH, Lumb PD, Jelovsek F et al: Nonbacterial thrombotic endocarditis associated with severe preeclampsia and pulmonary artery catheterization, *J Reprod Med* 30:497, 1985.
26. Chestnut DH, Ostman LG, Weiner CP et al: The effect of vasopressor agents upon uterine artery blood flow velocity in the gravid guinea pig subjected to ritodrine infusion, *Anesthesiology* 68:363, 1988.
27. Chestnut DH, Pollack KL, Thompson CS et al: Does ritodrine worsen maternal hypotension during epidural anesthesia in gravid ewes? *Anesthesiology* 72:315, 1990.
28. Chestnut DH, Thompson CS, McLaughlin GL et al: Does the intravenous infusion of ritodrine or magnesium sulfate alter the hemodynamic response to hemorrhage in gravid ewes? *Am J Obstet Gynecol* 159:1467, 1988.
29. Chestnut DH, Weiner CP, Wang JP et al: The effect of ephedrine upon uterine artery blood flow velocity in the gravid guinea pig subjected to terbutaline infusion and acute hemorrhage, *Anesthesiology* 66:508, 1987.
30. Clapp JF: Maternal heart rate in pregnancy, *Am J Obstet Gynecol* 152:659, 1985.
31. Clark RB, Thompson DS, and Thompson CH: Prevention of spinal hypotension associated with cesarean section, *Anesthesiology* 45:670, 1976.
32. Clark SL, Cotton DB: Clinical indications for pulmonary artery catheterization in the patient with severe preeclampsia, *Am J Obstet Gynecol* 158:453, 1988.
33. Clark SL, Greenspoon JS, Aldahl D et al: Severe preeclampsia with persistent oliguria: management of hemodynamic subsets, *Am J Obstet Gynecol* 154:490, 1986.
34. Cohen SE: Non-obstetric surgery during pregnancy. In *Annual Refresher Course Lectures,* American Society of Anesthesiologists, 142:1, 1988.
35. Cohen SE: Risk of abortion following general anesthesia for surgery during pregnancy: anesthetic or surgical procedure? (letter), *Anesthesiology* 65:706, 1986.
36. Conroy JM, Bailey MK, Hollon MF et al: Anesthesia for open heart surgery in the pregnant patient, *South Med J* 82:492, 1989.
37. Cotton DB, Gonik B, and Dorman KF: Cardiovascular alterations in severe pregnancy-induced hypertension: acute effects of intravenous magnesium sulfate, *Am J Obstet Gynecol* 148:162, 1984.
38. Cotton DB, Gonik B, Dorman K et al: Cardiovascular alterations in severe pregnancy-induced hypertension: relationship of central venous pressure to pulmonary capillary wedge pressure, *Am J Obstet Gynecol* 151:762, 1985.
39. Cotton DB, Gonik B, Spillman T et al: Intrapartum to postpartum changes in colloid osmotic pressure, *Am J Obstet Gynecol* 149:174, 1984.
40. Cotton DB, Longmire S, Jones MM et al: Cardiovascular alterations in severe pregnancy-induced hypertension: effects of intravenous nitroglycerin coupled with blood volume expansion, *Am J Obstet Gynecol* 154:1053, 1986.
41. Datta S, Lambert DH, Gregus J et al: Differential sensitivities of mammalian nerve fibers during pregnancy, *Anesth Analg* 62:1070, 1983.
42. Donchin Y, Amirav B, Sahar A et al: Sodium nitroprusside for aneurysm surgery in pregnancy, *Br J Anaesth* 50:849, 1978.
43. Duncan PG: Risk of abortion following general anesthesia for surgery during pregnancy: anesthetic or surgical procedure? (letter), *Anesthesiology* 65:706, 1986.
44. Duncan PG, Pope WD, Cohen MM et al: Fetal risk of anesthesia and surgery during pregnancy, *Anesthesiology* 64:790, 1986.
45. Enein M, Zina AA, Kassem M et al: Echocardiography of the pericardium in pregnancy, *Obstet Gynecol* 69:851, 1987.
46. Fagraeus L, Urban B, and Bromage P: Spread of epidural analgesia in early pregnancy, *Anesthesiology* 58:184, 1983.
47. Ford SE, Manley PN: Indwelling cardiac catheters, *Arch Pathol Lab Med* 106:314, 1982.
48. Fujinaga M, Baden JM, Yhap EO et al: Reproductive and teratogenic effects of nitrous oxide, isoflurane, and their combination in Sprague-Dawley rats, *Anesthesiology* 67:960, 1987.

49. Gallery EDM, Delprado W, and Gyory AZ: Antihypertensive effect of plasma volume expansion in pregnancy-associated hypertension, *Aust N Z J Med* 11:20, 1981.

50. Gant NF, Daley GL, Chand S et al: A study of angiotensin II pressor response throughout primigravid pregnancy, *J Clin Invest* 52:2682, 1973.

51. Gonik B, Creasy RK: Preterm labor: its diagnosis and management, *Am J Obstet Gynecol* 154:3, 1986.

52. Graham C, Goldstein A: Epidural analgesia and cardiac output in severe preeclamptics, *Anaesthesia* 35:709, 1980.

53. Groenendijk R, Trimbos JBMJ, and Wallenburg HCS: Hemodynamic measurements in preeclampsia: preliminary observations, *Am J Obstet Gynecol* 150:232, 1984.

54. Gutsche BB, Cheek TG: Anesthetic considerations in preeclampsia-eclampsia. In Shnider SM, Levinson G, eds: *Anesthesia for obstetrics,* ed 2, Baltimore, 1987, Williams & Wilkins.

55. Hatjis CG, Swain M: Systemic tocolysis for premature labor is associated with an increased incidence of pulmonary edema in the presence of maternal infection, *Am J Obstet Gynecol* 159:723, 1988.

56. Hays PM, Cruikshank DP, and Dunn LJ: Plasma volume determination in normal and preeclamptic pregnancies, *Am J Obstet Gynecol* 151:958, 1985.

57. Hehre FW: Hypothermia for operations during pregnancy, *Anesth Analg* 44:424, 1965.

58. Heller PJ, Scheider EP, and Marx GP: Pharyngolaryngeal edema as a presenting symptom in preeclampsia, *Obstet Gynecol* 62:523, 1983.

59. Henderson DW, Vilos GA, Milne KJ et al: The role of Swan-Ganz catheterization in severe pregnancy-induced hypertension, *Am J Obstet Gynecol* 148:570, 1984.

60. Hendricks SK, Keroes J, and Katz M: Electrocardiographic changes associated with ritodrine-induced maternal tachycardia and hypokalemia, *Am J Obstet Gynecol* 154:921, 1986.

61. Hodgkinson R, Husain FJ, and Hayashi RH: Systemic and pulmonary blood pressure during caesarean section in parturients with gestational hypertension, *Can Anaesth Soc J* 27:389, 1980.

62. Howard BK, Goodson JH, and Mengert WF: Supine hypotension syndrome in late pregnancy, *Obstet Gynecol* 1:371, 1953.

63. Huff DL, Thurnau GR: Platelet dysfunction in preeclampsia (abstract), Las Vegas, 1988, Proceedings of the 1988 Annual Meeting of the Society of Perinatal Obstetricians.

64. Ihle BU, Long P, and Oats J: Early onset pre-eclampsia: recognition of underlying renal disease, *Brit Med J* 294:79, 1987.

65. Ingemarsson I, Arulkumaran S, and Ratnam SS: Single injection of terbutaline in term labor. I. Effect on fetal pH in cases with prolonged bradycardia, *Am J Obstet Gynecol* 153:859, 1985.

66. Jouppila P, Jouppila R, Hollmén A et al: Lumbar epidural analgesia to improve intervillous blood flow during labor in severe preeclampsia, *Obstet Gynecol* 59:158, 1982.

67. Joyce TH, Loon M: Pre-eclampsia: effect of albumin 25% infusion (abstract), *Anesthesiology* 55:A313, 1981.

68. Kambam JR, Handte RE, Brown WU et al: Effect of normal and preeclamptic pregnancies on the oxyhemoglobin dissociation curve, *Anesthesiology* 65:426, 1986.

69. Kelton JG, Hunter DJS, and Neame PB: A platelet function defect in preeclampsia, *Obstet Gynecol* 65:107, 1985.

70. Kirshon B, Moise KJ Jr, Cotton DB et al: Role of volume expansion in severe pre-eclampsia, *Surg Gynecol Obstet* 167:367, 1988.

71. Kleinman C, Nuwayhid B, Rudelstorfer R et al: Circulatory and renal effects of β-adrenergic-receptor stimulation in pregnant sheep, *Am J Obstet Gynecol* 149:865, 1984.

72. Kuhnert BR, Gross TL, Kuhnert PM et al: Ritodrine pharmacokinetics, *Clin Pharmacol Ther* 40:656, 1986.

73. Lane GA, Nahrwld ML, Tait AR et al: Anesthetics as teratogens: nitrous oxide is fetotoxic, xenon is not, *Science* 210:899, 1980.

74. Lawson NW, Wallfisch HK: Cardiovascular pharmacology: a new look at the "pressors." In Stoelting RK, Barash PG, and Gallagher TJ, eds: *Advances in anesthesia,* Chicago, 1986, Year Book Medical Publishers.

75. Lee W, Gonik B, and Cotton DB: Urinary diagnostic indices in preeclampsia-associated oliguria: correlation with invasive hemodynamic monitoring, *Am J Obstet Gynecol* 156:100, 1987.

76. Lees MM, Taylor SH, Scott DB et al: A study of cardiac output at rest throughout pregnancy, *J Obstet Gynaecol Br Commonw* 74:319, 1967.

77. Lindheimer MD, Katz AI: Current concepts: hypertension in pregnancy, *N Engl J Med* 313:675, 1985.

78. Liu PL, Warren TM, Ostheimer GW et al: Foetal monitoring in parturients undergoing surgery unrelated to pregnancy, *Can Anaesth Soc J* 32:525, 1985.

79. Mabie WC, Gonzalez AR, Sibai BM et al: A comparative trial of labetalol and hydralazine in the acute management of severe hypertension complicating pregnancy, *Obstet Gynecol* 70:328, 1987.

80. Malloy MH, Rhoads GG, Schramm W et al: Increasing cesarean section rates in very low-birth weight infants, *JAMA* 262:1475, 1989.

81. Mann LI: Pregnancy events and brain damage, *Am J Obstet Gynecol* 155:6, 1986.

82. Marx GF, Luykx WM, and Cohen S: Fetal-neonatal status following caesarean section for fetal distress, *Br J Anaesth* 56:1009, 1984.

83. Masaki DI, Greenspoon JS: Selective criteria for the identification of patients requiring peri-partum pulmonary artery catheterization for the management of pregnancy-induced hypertension (abstract), New Orleans, 1989, *Proceedings of the Annual Meeting of the Society of Perinatal Obstetricians.*

84. Mazze RI, Fujinaga M, and Baden JM: Halothane prevents nitrous oxide teratogenicity in Sprague-Dawley rats; folinic acid does not, *Teratology* 38:121, 1988.

85. Mazze RI, Fujinaga M, and Rice SA: Reproductive and teratogenic effects of nitrous oxide, halothane, isoflurane, and enflurane in Sprague-Dawley rats, *Anesthesiology* 64:339, 1986.

86. Mazze RI, Kallen B: Reproductive outcome after anesthesia and operation during pregnancy: a registry study of 5405 cases, *Am J Obstet Gynecol* 161:1178, 1989.

87. Mazze RI, Wilson AI, Rice SA et al: Fetal development in mice exposed to isoflurane, *Teratology* 32:339, 1985.

88. Miyazaki FS, Nevarez F: Saline amnioinfusion for relief of repetitive variable decelerations: a prospective randomized study, *Am J Obstet Gynecol* 153:301, 1985.

89. Miyazaki FS, Taylor NA: Saline amnioinfusion for relief of variable or prolonged decelerations: a preliminary report, *Am J Obstet Gynecol* 146:670, 1983.

90. Moise KJ, Huhta JC, Sharif DS et al: Indomethacin in the treatment of premature labor: effects on the fetal ductus arteriosus, *N Engl J Med* 319:327, 1988.

91. Moran DH, Perillo M, Bader AM et al: Phenylephrine in treating maternal hypotension secondary to spinal anesthesia (abstract), *Anesthesiology* 71:A856, 1989.

92. Nageotte MP, Freeman RK, Garite TJ et al: Prophylactic intrapartum amnioinfusion in patients with preterm premature rupture of membranes, *Am J Obstet Gynecol* 153:557, 1985.

93. Naulty J, Cefalo RC, and Lewis PE: Fetal toxicity of nitroprusside in the pregnant ewe, *Am J Obstet Gynecol* 139:708, 1981.

94. Newman B, Lam AM: Induced hypotension for clipping of a cerebral aneurysm during pregnancy: a case report and brief review, *Anesth Analg* 65:675, 1986.

95. Newsome LR, Bramwell RS, and Curling PE: Severe preeclampsia: hemodynamic effects of lumbar epidural anesthesia, *Anesth Analg* 65:31, 1986.

96. Niebyl JR, Witter FR: Neonatal outcome after indomethacin treatment for preterm labor, *Am J Obstet Gynecol* 155:747, 1986.

97. Nimmo WS, Wilson J, and Prescott LF: Narcotic analgesics and delayed gastric emptying in labour, *Lancet* 1:890, 1975.

98. Norris MC, Leighton BL, and DeSimone CA: Spinal anesthesia and preeclampsia (abstract), Seattle, 1989, *Proceedings of the Annual Meeting of the Society for Obstetric Anesthesia and Perinatology.*

99. Palahniuk RJ, Shnider SM, and Eger EI: Pregnancy decreases the requirements for inhaled anesthetic agents, *Anesthesiology* 41:82, 1974.

100. Patriarco MS, Viechnicki BM, Hutchin-

son TA et al: A study on intrauterine fetal resuscitation with terbutaline, *Am J Obstet Gynecol* 157:384, 1987.

101. Pisani RJ, Rosenow EC: Pulmonary edema associated with tocolytic therapy, *Ann Intern Med* 110:714, 1989.

102. Pritchard JA, Cunningham FG, and Pritchard SA: The Parkland Memorial Hospital protocol for treatment of eclampsia: evaluation of 245 cases, *Am J Obstet Gynecol* 148:951, 1984.

103. Ramanathan J, Sibai BM, Mabie WC et al: The use of labetalol for attenuation of the hypertensive response to endotracheal intubation in preeclampsia, *Am J Obstet Gynecol* 159:650, 1988.

104. Ramanathan J, Ricca DM, Sibai BM et al: Epidural versus general anesthesia in fetal distress with various abnormal fetal heart rate patterns, *Anesth Analg* 67:S180, 1988.

105. Ramanathan S, Grant GJ: Vasopressor therapy for hypotension due to epidural anesthesia for cesarean section, *Acta Anaesthesiol Scand* 32:559, 1988.

106. Ramanathan S, Grant G, and Turndorf H: Cardiac preload changes with ephedrine therapy for hypotension in obstetrical patients (abstract), *Anesth Analg* 65:S125, 1986.

107. Ring G, Krames E, Shnider SM et al: Comparison of nitroprusside and hydralazine in hypertensive pregnant ewes, *Obstet Gynecol* 50:598, 1977.

108. Roberts JM, Taylor RN, Musci TJ et al: Preeclampsia: an endothelial cell disorder, *Am J Obstet Gynecol* 161:1200, 1989.

109. Russell IF, Chambers WA: Closing volume in normal pregnancy, *Br J Anaesth* 53:1043, 1981.

110. Schrier RW, Liberman R, and Ufferman RC: Mechanism of antidiuretic effect of beta-adrenergic stimulation, *J Clin Invest* 51:97, 1972.

111. Shin YK, Kim YD: Anesthetic considerations in patients receiving ritodrine therapy for preterm labor (abstract), *Anesth Analg* 65(suppl):140, 1986.

112. Shnider SM: Serum cholinesterase activity during pregnancy, labor and puerperium, *Anesthesiology* 26:335, 1965.

113. Shnider SM, Abboud TK, Artal R et al: Maternal catecholamines decrease during labor after lumbar epidural anesthesia, *Am J Obstet Gynecol* 147:13, 1983.

114. Shnider SM, Webster GM: Maternal and fetal hazards of surgery during pregnancy, *Am J Obstet Gynecol* 92:891, 1965.

115. Sibai BM: Pitfalls in diagnosis and management of preeclampsia, *Am J Obstet Gynecol* 159:1, 1988.

116. Sibai BM, Mabie BC, Harvey CJ et al: Pulmonary edema in severe preeclampsia-eclampsia: analysis of thirty-seven consecutive cases, *Am J Obstet Gynecol* 156;1174, 1987.

117. Sibai BM, Taslimi M, Abdella TN et al: Maternal and perinatal outcome of conservative management of severe preeclampsia in midtrimester, *Am J Obstet Gynecol* 152:32, 1985.

118. Stempel JE, O'Grady JP, Morton MJ et al: Use of sodium nitroprusside in complications of gestational hypertension, *Obstet Gynecol* 60:533, 1982.

119. Strauss RG, Keefer JR, Burke T et al: Hemodynamic monitoring of cardiogenic pulmonary edema complicating toxemia of pregnancy, *Obstet Gynecol* 55:170, 1980.

120. Suresh MS, Lawson NW: Anesthesia for parturients with toxemia of pregnancy. In Datta SJ, Ostheimer GW, eds: *Common problems in obstetric anesthesia,* Chicago, 1987, Year Book Medical Publishers.

121. Ueland K, Hansen JM: Maternal cardiovascular dynamics. III. Labor and delivery under local and caudal analgesia, *Am J Obstet Gynecol* 103:8, 1969.

122. Ueland K, Novy MJ, Peterson EN et al: Maternal cardiovascular dynamics. IV. The influence of gestational age on the maternal cardiovascular response to posture and exercise, *Am J Obstet Gynecol* 104:856, 1969.

123. Varner MW: Physiologic changes in normal pregnancy, *Iowa Perinatal Letter* 6:1, 1985.

124. Vincent RD, Chestnut DH, Sipes SL et al: Magnesium sulfate decreases maternal blood pressure but not uterine blood flow during epidural anesthesia in gravid ewes, *Anesthesiology* 74:77, 1991.

125. Wallenburg HCS: Hemodynamics in hypertensive pregnancy. In Rubin PC, ed: *Handbook of hypertension,* New York, 1988, Elsevier.

126. Wallenburg HCS, Dekker GA, Makovitz JW et al: Low dose aspirin prevents pregnancy induced hypertension and preeclampsia in angiotensin sensitive primigravida, *Lancet* 1:1, 1986.

127. Walsh SW: Preeclampsia: an imbalance in placental prostacyclin and thromboxane production, *Am J Obstet Gynecol* 152:335, 1985.

128. Weiner CP: The role of serotonin in the genesis of hypertension in preeclampsia, *Am J Obstet Gynecol* 156:885, 1987.

129. Weinstein L: Preeclampsia/eclampsia with hemolysis, elevated liver enzymes, and thrombocytopenia, *Obstet Gynecol* 66:657, 1985.

130. Weinstein L: Syndrome of hemolysis, elevated liver enzymes, and low platelet count: a severe consequence of hypertension in pregnancy, *Am J Obstet Gynecol* 142:159, 1982.

131. Wenstrom KD, Parsons MT: The prevention of meconium aspiration in labor using amnioinfusion, *Obstet Gynecol* 73:647, 1989.

132. Williows KN, Jadcowshi A, and Enous PJD: Epidural haematoma requiring surgical decompression following repeated cervical epidermal steroid injections for chronic pain, *Pain* 42:197, 1990.

133. Wyner J, Cohen SE: Gastric volume in early pregnancy: effect of metoclopramide, *Anesthesiology* 57:209, 1982.

CHAPTER 29

Evaluation of the Obese Patient

DOUGLAS S. SNYDER

LINDA S. HUMPHREY

Obesity affects 25 to 45% of the American adult population[111] and is generally believed to increase the risks of anesthesia and surgery. The precise degree of risk is not known, but obese patients often develop significant impairments of their cardiovascular, pulmonary, and gastrointestinal/metabolic systems. Medical conditions statistically associated with obesity include hypertension, diabetes mellitus, coronary artery disease, cancer, cholelithiasis, and sudden death.[83] Complex psychosocial issues may also contribute to management difficulties. This chapter reviews the multiple factors that may contribute to perioperative risk and explores management implications.

DEFINITION

A definition of obesity requires standardization; this has proved difficult and elusive. The insurance industry was among the first to define obesity, eager to identify subsets of the population likely to submit early claims. Height and weight tables (desirable weight for height, Table 29-1)[99,100] may be skewed to one subset of the population (e.g., white, middle-class males seeking insurability).[16,89] Relative mortality would be underestimated with this approach by including more favorable risk individuals.[16,46] This possibility is supported by a longitudinal Veterans Administration study which found a higher early mortality among the obese population than that cited by the insurance industry[46] (Fig. 29-1). If individuals are covered by more than one policy, sampling error is a potential problem.[16]

Nevertheless, "ideal" weight for height tables are standard in the insurance industry and suggest that mortality is lowest in individuals within a certain weight for a given height.[99,100] **According to the height-weight tables of the insurance industry, "overweight" individuals weigh less than 20% above predicted ideal body weight, whereas "obese" individuals weigh more than 20% above ideal body weight. Morbid obesity is defined as body weight two times the predicted ideal body weight or greater than 100 pounds above ideal body weight.**[17,24]

Accurate measurement of body fat has been fraught with difficulty. Although not proved, body fat is generally considered to be a more important concern than body mass. The simplest method is to measure fat "directly" using special calipers to determine skinfold thickness at specific body sites. This technique is limited by its relative imprecision, variability among investigators, and sampling of only subcutaneous fat. The more complex method of measuring body

Table 29-1 1983 Metropolitan height and weight tables for men and women according to frame, ages 25-59				
Height (in shoes)*		Weight in pounds (in indoor clothing)†		
Feet	Inches	Small frame	Medium frame	Large frame
Men				
5	2	128-134	131-141	138-150
5	3	130-136	133-143	140-153
5	4	132-138	135-145	142-156
5	5	134-140	137-148	144-160
5	6	136-142	139-151	146-164
5	7	138-145	142-154	149-168
5	8	140-148	145-157	152-172
5	9	142-151	148-160	155-176
5	10	144-154	151-163	158-180
5	11	146-157	154-166	161-184
6	0	149-160	157-170	164-188
6	1	152-164	160-174	168-192
6	2	155-168	164-178	172-197
6	3	158-172	167-182	176-202
6	4	162-176	171-187	181-207
Women				
4	10	102-111	109-121	118-131
4	11	103-113	111-123	120-134
5	0	104-115	113-126	122-137
5	1	106-118	115-129	125-140
5	2	108-121	118-132	128-143
5	3	111-124	121-135	131-147
5	4	114-127	124-138	135-151
5	5	117-130	127-141	137-155
5	6	120-133	130-144	140-159
5	7	123-136	133-147	143-163
5	8	126-139	136-150	146-167
5	9	129-142	139-153	149-170
5	10	132-145	142-156	152-173
5	11	135-148	145-159	155-176
6	0	138-151	148-162	158-179

*Shoes with 1-inch heels.
†Indoor clothing weighing 5 pounds for men and 3 pounds for women.
Data from *Build Study, 1979,* Society of Actuaries and Association of Life Insurance Medical Directors of America, 1980. Copyright 1983 Metropolitan Life Insurance Company.

density requires total immersion in water with exhalation to residual volume. Obviously this technique is impractical for routine use. Indices based on height and weight have been developed to eliminate the contribution of height to weight.[15,82,89,98,124] These include the weight-to-height ratio (W/H), the ponderal index (either $^3\sqrt{W}/H$ or $H/^3\sqrt{W}$) and the Quetelet's index or body mass index (BMI), W/H^2.[44,82,89,98,124] Densi-

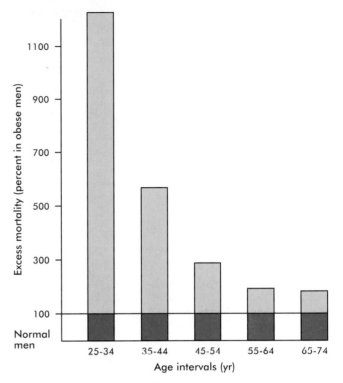

Fig. 29-1. Excessive mortality among morbidly obese men, computed by decade, compared with overall mortality for American men. (From Drenick EJ, Bale GS, Seltzer F et al: Excessive mortality and causes of death in morbidly obese men, *JAMA* 243:443, 1980.)

tometry has been found to best correlate with BMI.[15,82] The ponderal index overestimates obesity among short people and underestimates obesity among tall people, whereas the weight-to-height ratio has the opposite result. BMI has been adopted as the most useful index for evaluating obesity.* A BMI (kg/ m²) less than 25 is considered normal, greater than 30 obese, and between 25 and 30 overweight but at minimal risk of morbidity or mortality.[19,24,124] A BMI greater than 40 kg/m² reflects morbid obesity.[19]

PHYSIOLOGIC CHANGES ASSOCIATED WITH OBESITY
Pulmonary System

Hypoxemia commonly accompanies obesity. This can be attributed to (1) increased minute ventilation at rest to meet metabolic demands of the increased tissue mass, (2) increased work and energy cost of breathing, and (3) changes in lung volumes that result in closure of small airways and ventilation/perfusion ($\dot{V}/\dot{Q}$) mismatch during normal breathing.

---

* References 19, 24, 44, 81, 100, 124.

The basal metabolic rate of the obese individual is normal.[24] Efforts to discover a metabolic defect with an etiologic role in obesity have been unsuccessful.[44,89] The large mass of adipose tissue is metabolically active and oxygen consumption and carbon dioxide production are linearly increased with increasing weight.[4] As a result minute ventilation is increased at rest; with exercise or fever, the increase in metabolic demand will further stress an already stressed system. In a study of oxygen consumption at various levels of ventilation, 18 of 25 obese subjects increased oxygen consumption with increasing ventilation considerably more than nonobese control subjects.[80] The discrepancy became progressively greater at the higher ventilatory levels (Fig. 29-2). There was a tendency for the patient with the highest cost of increased ventilation to have the lowest resting Pao_2s and the highest $Paco_2$s. Both airway resistance and lung compliance were normal in two patients with the highest cost of ventilation and $Paco_2$. Considering that hypoventilation might represent an adaptive mechanism, hypoxemia and hypercapnia may be tolerated to spare an inordinate energy expenditure that would be required to normalize ventilation. Superimposed pulmonary disease could so greatly increase the metabolic cost of breathing that decompensation could result.

Efficiency of the respiratory muscles in the obese patient is reported to be well below normal.[56] In a study comparing five obese patients with dyspnea on exertion to seven normal controls, mechanical work (estimated from the area under the transpulmonary pressure–volume curve) was above normal in two of the obese patients and normal in the other three. However, energy expended to perform the work was greatly increased and percent efficiency (work performed/total energy expended for breathing) was reduced. As workload increased, energy expenditure increased in excess of the amount of work done on the lungs, presumed to be secondary to work moving extrapulmonary structures. Cherniak and Guenter found the work of breathing was not significantly different for normal and for obese subjects, despite differences in elastic resistance of the chest wall.[30] Banding the chest wall in normal subjects to simulate the reduced compliance of the obese patient produced similar inefficiency, implying that abnormally low lung volumes, as well as reduced chest wall compliance, may alter respiratory muscle efficiency. In a contrast-

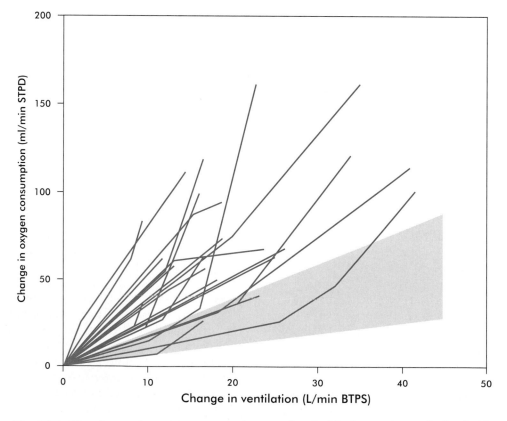

Fig. 29-2. The changes in oxygen consumption associated with changes in ventilation in 25 obese subjects. The stippled area represents the range found in normal subjects. (From Kaufman BJ et al: Hypoventilation in obesity, *J Clin Invest* 38:500, 1959.)

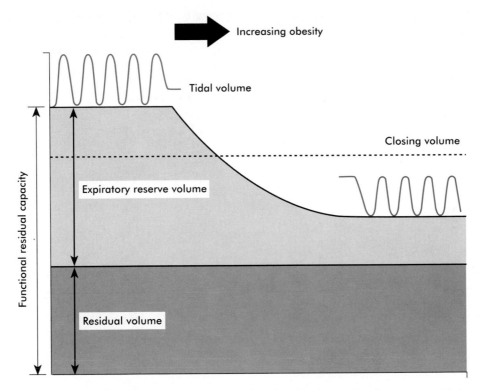

Fig. 29-3. The progressive decrement in functional residual capacity that occurs with increasing weight results in tidal ventilation occurring at or below closing volume. (From Fox GS: Anaesthesia for intestinal short circuiting in the morbidly obese with reference to the pathophysiology of gross obesity, *Can Anaesth Soc J* 22:307, 1975.)

ing report, Sharp et al. found that mechanical work in obese subjects averaged 1.3 times normal while that of patients with obesity-hypoventilation syndrome averaged 2.9 times normal.[116]

Reduced resting lung volumes in the obese patient also contribute to hypoxemia. Functional residual capacity (FRC), vital capacity, and total lung capacity (TLC) are all reduced as a result of lower respiratory compliance.[17,24,66,112,124] **The reduction in FRC is due primarily to a lower expiratory reserve volume (ERV); residual volume (RV) is unchanged (Fig. 29-3). This adversely influences the relationship between FRC and closing capacity (CC), the lung volume at which small airways begin to close. Since CC is unchanged in obesity, reduced FRC can result in lung volumes below CC in the course of normal tidal ventilation.**[66] **As perfusion of nonventilated distal alveoli continues, $\dot{V}/\dot{Q}$ mismatch and venous admixture develop.**[36,41-43,113,124] Such $\dot{V}/\dot{Q}$ mismatch has been documented by Barrera et al.[8] and Holley et al.[69] The distribution of ventilation to various lung regions in the obese patient does not differ significantly from normal unless ERV is drastically reduced, but overperfusion of underventilated areas or perfusion of completely unventilated areas occurs. Premature air-

way closure is most likely to occur in dependent regions[35] that are better perfused, as in normal weight individuals.[69] The supine position further aggravates the lung volume changes (Fig. 29-4). The supine position reduces FRC in normal individuals[36,42,43] since abdominal pressure increases more rapidly per centimeter of tissue height than thoracic pressure, causing the diaphragm to shift cephalad.[57] It is presumed that this effect is exaggerated in the obese, resulting in a further reduction in FRC, closure of more small airways, and increased work of breathing. Paul et al. found a clinically significant increase in both intrapulmonary shunting and oxygen consumption as a group of obese patients changed from sitting to supine positions.[104] General anesthesia is also known to decrease FRC.[41,42,66,86] Thus a supine, anesthetized obese patient is at significant risk of developing hypoxemia.[24,66]

Several studies examine the effects of weight loss on pulmonary function in the obese. Thirty-seven obese patients who achieved an average weight loss of 52 kg (Fig. 29-5) significantly increased their ERV.[132] Mean Pao_2 increased from 83 to 87 (p = .053) in the eleven patients evaluated. The increase in Pao_2 and the decrease in alveolar–arterial oxygen tension difference ($P(A-a)o_2$) correlated with the

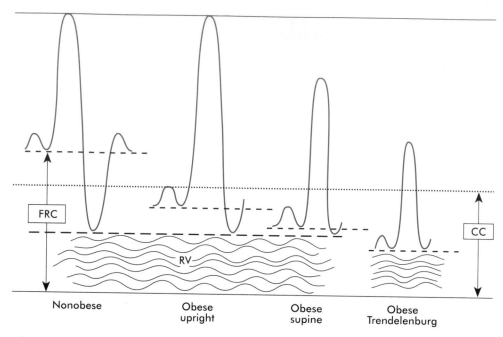

Fig. 29-4. Effect of position change on lung volumes in obese subjects. Further decline in functional residual capacity *(FRC)* worsens the relationship between FRC and closing volume or capacity *(CC)*. *RV,* residual volume. (From Vaughan RW: Pulmonary and cardiovascular derangements in the obese patient. In Brown BR et al, eds: Anesthesia and the obese patient. In *Contemporary anesthesia practice,* vol 5, Philadelphia, 1982, FA Davis.)

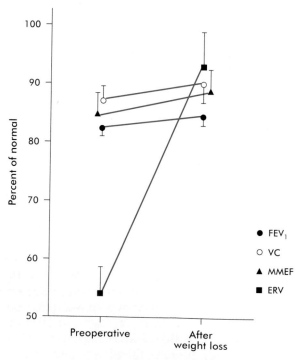

Fig. 29-5. Pulmonary function tests (PFTs) measured in 37 obese patients before and after weight loss averaging 52 kg. *FEV$_1$,* forced expiratory volume in 1 second; *VC,* vital capacity; *MMEF,* maximum mid-expiratory flow rate; *ERV,* expiratory reserve volume. (From Vaughan RW, Cork RC, and Hollander D: The effect of massive weight loss on arterial oxygenation and pulmonary function tests, *Anesthesiology* 54:325, 1981.)

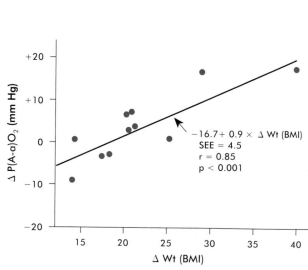

Fig. 29-6. Change in alveolar-to-arterial oxygen tension difference *(P(A-a)o$_2$)* as a function of weight loss, expressed in units of body mass index *(BMI)*. A change in BMI of >20 results in improved oxygenation. (From Vaughan RW, Cork RC, and Hollander D: The effect of massive weight loss on arterial oxygenation and pulmonary function tests, *Anesthesiology* 54:325, 1981.)

increase in ERV (Fig. 29-6). Sugerman and Fairman suggest that oxygenation improves even more significantly following weight loss in patients with obesity-hypoventilation syndrome.[120]

Cardiovascular System

Longitudinal studies of large populations have clarified the relationship between obesity and cardiovascular disease. After a 12-year follow-up, the Framingham Study, which originated in 1948, reported an association between angina pectoris and initial weight for both sexes and between sudden death and initial weight in men.[77] However, after controlling for elevated blood pressure and cholesterol (both frequently associated with obesity), these relationships held true for men only. The association of obesity with either elevated blood pressure or cholesterol, or both, resulted in potentiation of risk beyond that observed for either factor alone or in combination, independent of obesity. Interestingly, no association between obesity and myocardial infarction was demonstrated. **After 26 years of study, the Framingham population again showed obesity to be an important predictor of cardiovascular disease, particularly in individuals younger than 50 years of age.[71] Risk of coronary artery disease, myocardial infarction, and sudden death was increased among the obese of both sexes. Risk of congestive heart failure increased in men but in women was greater only in the heaviest subgroup. The risk of atherothrombotic stroke was increased primarily in women.** The effect of obesity on risk was demonstrated independently of other risk factors although only a small percentage of the obese individuals were free of these other factors.

Several other investigators accounted for the risk of cardiovascular disease among the obese solely on the basis of coexisting risk factors. Keys et al. suggested that obese individuals are often older, having gained weight with age, and thus were more likely to suffer from "ill health."[81,82] Mann summarized these findings in 1974 noting that the contribution of obesity to coronary heart disease is either small or nonexistent in the absence of other risk factors.[89] Differing results from the Framingham Study may be due to different levels of obesity between populations or to different lengths of follow-up.[71] Bray suggested that the issue of obesity as an independent risk factor may be irrelevant; for a particular obese patient the risk of cardiovascular disease is enhanced regardless of mechanism.[19]

Although the association of obesity and hypertension is well established, there is no proved cause and effect relationship.[89,96] Of course, an appropriately sized blood pressure cuff must be used to avoid artifactual elevation of the measurement.[19,26,90] **In the Framingham study, obese individuals were found to**

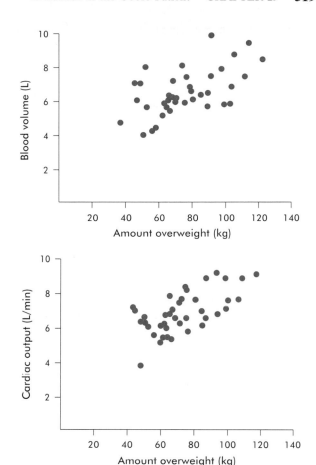

Fig. 29-7. Relationships between excessive weight, blood volume, and cardiac output in 40 obese subjects. (From Alexander JK: The cardiomyopathy of obesity, *Prog Cardiovasc Dis* 27:325, 1985.)

have an incidence of hypertension 10 times greater than the norm. The pathophysiology contributing to the development of hypertension is not completely understood. Blood volume has been noted to increase as weight increases above ideal body weight* (Fig. 29-7), suggesting a hydraulic basis for blood pressure elevation. Systemic vascular resistance (SVR) in morbidly obese patients has been reported to be normal.[2,4,39] The expanded blood volume in the obese patient causes an increased cardiac output with a lower calculated SVR for the same level of arterial blood pressure.[95,96] Therefore hypertension and obesity could coexist with a normal SVR.[96] The expanded blood volume is distributed between the peripheral and central circulations as in the nonobese person; both right and left ventricles are distended at end-diastole, which causes the observed increase in stroke volume.[95,112,124] This accounts for the increased cardiac output and the consistent increase in left ventricular stroke work.[3,39,96] As one would expect, a larger body

---

* References 4, 5, 6, 72, 96, 111, 124.

mass requires a higher total body oxygen consumption; hence cardiac output must be increased to meet the demand.* Organ blood flow does not change appreciably with increasing weight. The additional cardiac output is primarily perfusing adipose tissue.[4,5,17,111,124] For morbidly obese patients, blood volume and cardiac output are twice the values predicted for ideal body weight.[3,4,6,17] However, cardiac output normalized for body surface area is generally normal[4] or slightly below normal.[96]

What are the consequences of such altered physiology? **The chronically elevated preload causes both dilatation and hypertrophy of the left ventricle, so-called eccentric hypertrophy**[96] **(Fig. 29-8). Workload increases correspondingly and both systolic performance and compliance suffer. Elevated left ventricular end-diastolic volume and reduced compliance cause abnormally high left ventricular end-diastolic pressures (LVEDP) and pulmonary artery occlusion pressures (PAOP).** SVR might increase over time in the presence of chronically elevated cardiac output and blood volume. The high preload with obesity cou-

* References 5, 17, 19, 39, 95, 96, 111, 124.

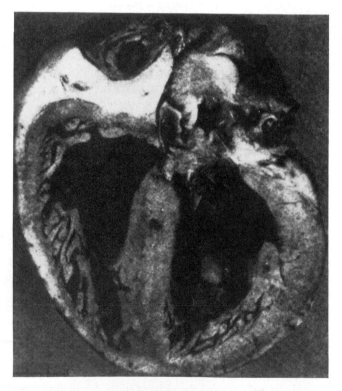

Fig. 29-8. Gross appearance of the heart at postmortem examination of an obese man dying of cardiac failure at age 42 (body weight 225 kg). Biventricular hypertrophy with chamber dilatation is demonstrated. (From Alexander JK: The cardiomyopathy of obesity, *Prog Cardiovasc Dis* 27:325, 1985.)

pled with a high SVR can lead to early left ventricular dysfunction and congestive heart failure[95] (Fig. 29-9). Alexander has proposed that grossly obese patients with congestive signs and symptoms may be subdivided into two categories.[4] The first group consists of those patients in whom the hypertrophic response has been sufficient to normalize wall stress; left ventricular systolic function is maintained and congestive symptoms develop because of the inappropriately elevated central blood volume and altered left ventricular compliance. In the second group are patients with dilated left ventricular chambers, "inadequate" hypertrophy, and chronically elevated wall stress. These patients are predisposed to depressed systolic function and myocardial decompensation with pulmonary congestion developing as a consequence.

Pulmonary hypertension, either at rest or during exercise, is also a common finding.[4,39] Most of the 40 obese patients studied by Alexander et al. had pulmonary hypertension accompanied by elevated PAOP, suggesting high LVEDP as the source of the pulmonary hypertension.[3,5] On the other hand, patients with obesity-hypoventilation syndrome often suffer from both right- and left-sided heart failure.[3,4,112] The right-sided signs and symptoms, presumably due to hypoxia-induced pulmonary hypertension, are often the predominant clinical problem.

The highly significant association between obesity and sudden death led Messerli et al. to investigate the incidence of dysrhythmias in obese subjects.[97] **Holter monitoring of 15 obese hypertensive patients without other cardiac disease revealed an incidence of premature ventricular contractions 10 times higher than control patients.** A second group of **obese subjects with eccentric left ventricular hypertrophy (n = 14) had 30 times more ventricular ectopy, including asymptomatic runs of trigeminy, quadrigeminy, and ventricular tachycardia.** Left ventricular mass and end-systolic wall stress were elevated in all obese subjects but were maximally increased in those with eccentric hypertrophy. **Although ventricular ectopy has not been proved to cause sudden death, the findings were considered ominous.**

Significant changes in cardiovascular parameters with postural changes were reported by Paul et al.[104] Both PAOP and cardiac output increased significantly as the supine position was assumed by a group of obese subjects. Oxygen consumption was significantly increased in the supine position because of the increased work of breathing and may have contributed to the elevated cardiac output. Paul et al.[104] believe that the ability of the heart to respond to increased preload by increasing cardiac output minimized the elevation in both left heart and pulmonary artery pressure. Pulmonary congestion or edema might be expected in individuals unable to tolerate the

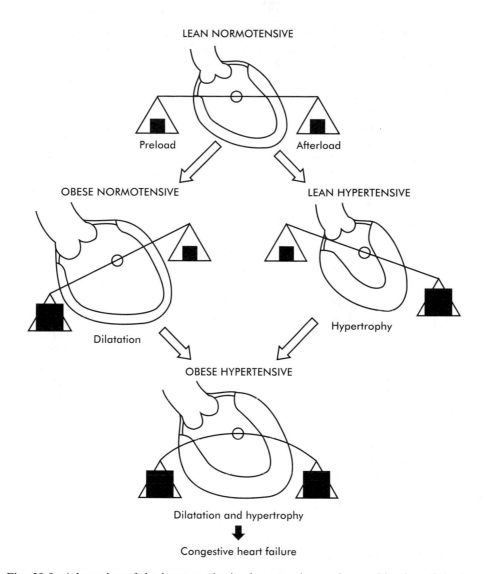

Fig. 29-9. Adaptation of the heart to obesity, hypertension, and a combination of the two. Although hypertension produces concentric hypertrophy only, obesity plus hypertension produces hypertrophy and dilatation (eccentric hypertrophy), associated with a high incidence of congestive heart failure. (From Messerli FH: Cardiovascular effects of obesity and hypertension, *Lancet* 1:1165, 1982.)

higher venous return and further elevated central blood volume.

How does weight loss affect hypertension that is associated with obesity? Because there is little support that obesity causes hypertension, weight loss would presumably be unlikely to improve hypertension.[89] Nevertheless, many studies have found that weight reduction in the obese person is commonly associated with a decrease in arterial blood pressure.[4,19,44,96,111]

Gastrointestinal-Metabolic System

Obesity influences gastrointestinal and metabolic physiology. Gastric volume and acidity are increased in the fasting state. Hepatic function is altered; drug metabolism may be affected both qualitatively and quantitatively. Diabetes mellitus is commonly associated with obesity, the severity of the diabetes being dependent on the duration and degree of obesity.[44,45] This section reviews the implications of these findings.

Not unlike the term parturient with increased abdominal girth, the obese patient is also at particular risk for aspiration with anesthesia.[133] Vaughan et al. compared 56 healthy obese patients with a similar number of nonobese controls.[133] Of the obese patients, 86% had a gastric fluid volume exceeding 25 ml (mean 42.3 ml), the theoretic volume above which risk from aspiration increases, and 88% had a gastric pH below 2.5 (mean 1.7), below which risk of pulmonary damage would increase following aspiration. **Of obese patients, 75% had both a high gastric volume and acidity and were therefore considered to be at high risk.** Vaughan et al. speculated that gastric emptying is delayed by the increased abdominal mass that causes antral distention, gastrin release, and a decrease in pH with parietal cell secretion. Others have confirmed finding high volume and low pH of gastric contents in the fasting obese patient,[85,88,137] but gastric emptying time was normal.[31,85] The mechanism is not entirely clear. This risk of aspiration is also potentially increased by other factors, including an increased incidence of hiatal hernia and increased intraabdominal pressure. Increased intraabdominal pressure has been shown to cause stress reflux of gastric contents into the esophagus.[40]

Pharmacologic intervention appears to reduce the number of patients at risk for aspiration. H₂ antagonists such as cimetidine and ranitidine effectively modify gastric pH. In the morbidly obese patient, cimetidine given orally in two 300 mg doses or intravenously (300 to 600 mg) at least 60 minutes before surgery increases pH but does not consistently decrease gastric volume.[85,137] Cimetidine has been

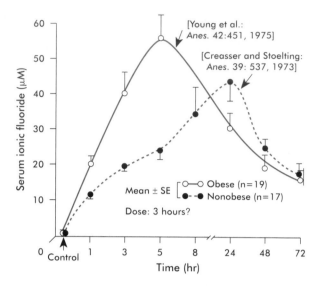

Fig. 29-10. Serum ionic fluoride concentration with time following approximately 3 hours of methoxyflurane anesthesia in obese (n = 19) and nonobese (n = 17) patients from two nonconcurrent studies. (From Vaughan RW: Biochemical and biotransformation alterations in obesity. In Brown BR et al, eds: Anesthesia and the obese patient. In *Contemporary anesthesia practice,* vol 5, Philadelphia, 1982, FA Davis.)

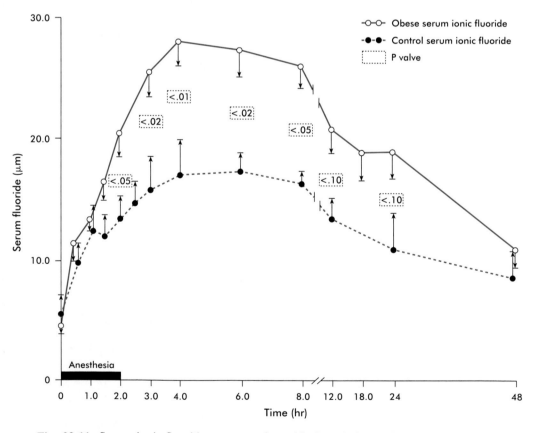

Fig. 29-11. Serum ionic fluoride concentration with time during and following 2 hours of enflurane anesthesia in obese (n = 24) and nonobese (n = 7) patients. (From Bentley JB, Vaughan RW, Miller MS et al: Serum inorganic fluoride levels in obese patients during and after enflurane anesthesia, *Anesth Analg* 58:409, 1979.)

found, however, to reduce hepatic blood flow and inhibit microsomal enzyme activity.[85] Intravenous administration of cimetidine has also been associated with bradycardia and asystole. Ranitidine is a newer H_2 blocker and appears to have fewer side effects than cimetidine. In one study, 150 to 300 mg of ranitidine given orally the night before and again the morning of surgery resulted in an increase in the pH in all 40 morbidly obese patients; the gastric volume was also somewhat decreased.[88] Addition of metoclopramide 10 to 20 mg orally on the morning of surgery decreased gastric volumes to less than 25 ml in all patients. **The administration of ranitidine and metoclopramide together appears to optimize pharmacologic prophylaxis against aspiration.**

Drug metabolism largely depends on liver function that is often abnormal in the obese patient.[24,128] For example, biotransformation of methoxyflurane in the obese patient is significantly higher[139] (Fig. 29-10). Unexpectedly high levels of free fluoride ion (F^-) after 4 MAC-hours of enflurane have been reported (a peak value of 52 μM and a mean of 22 μM overall).[34] Even with an enflurane anesthetic of less than 2 MAC-hours (Fig. 29-11), a more rapid rate of rise, increased peak concentration, and more prolonged elevation of F^- was found in the obese group (n = 24) than in the seven nonobese control patients.[12] Although clinical nephrotoxicity was not seen after this brief anesthetic exposure, the research-

ers speculated that prolonged exposure to enflurane might result in concentrations of F^- associated with subclinical renal dysfunction (30 μM)[34,91] or even frank nephrotoxicity (90 μM).[48,92] Isoflurane administration, however, is not associated with clinically significant F^- concentrations in the obese[119] (Fig. 29-12). One study using halothane found an increase in F^- concentration to 10.4 μM in the obese group, although other studies reported no change in F^- concentration in nonobese subjects.[91] This has been attributed to reductive metabolism of halothane[9,12] (Fig. 29-13). Bentley et al. speculated that obese individuals might be at increased risk for this type of injury, similar to reductive metabolism of halothane observed in animals with hepatic injuries. Although reductive metabolism is no longer considered to be a primary factor in "halothane hepatitis," 38% of obese patients in one large series developed unexplained jaundice following administration of halothane. Serum concentrations of bromide ion in the obese patient following halothane anesthesia were approximately double those measured in the nonobese but did not achieve sedative levels.[10] It is possible that protracted exposure to halothane could generate sedative levels of bromide ion. The concentration of bromide ion was found to peak in the obese patient on the third postoperative day, suggesting a theoretic cause for any prolonged sedation.

The mechanism of enhanced biotransformation of volatile anesthetics by the obese patient is not well understood. Increased hepatic uptake of lipid-soluble anesthetics resulting from higher than normal hepatic lipid could cause enhanced exposure of microsomal enzymes to the anesthetic. As an alternative, increased uptake of the agent into adipose tissue could

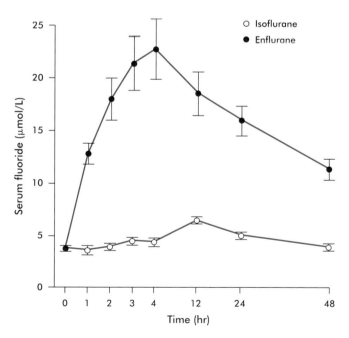

Fig. 29-12. Serum ionic fluoride concentration with time after enflurane (●, n = 5) and isoflurane (○, n = 5) anesthesia in obese patients. (From Strube PJ, Hulands GH, and Halsey MJ: Serum fluoride levels in morbidly obese patients: enflurane compared with isoflurane anaesthesia, *Anaesthesia* 42:685, 1987.)

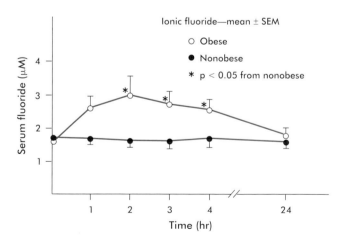

Fig. 29-13. Serum ionic fluoride concentration with time after halothane anesthesia in obese (n = 17) and nonobese (n = 8) patients. (From Bentley JB et al: Halothane biotransformation in obese and nonobese patients, *Anesthesiology* 57:94, 1982.)

cause subsequent prolonged delivery of the drug to the liver.[13,139] Other speculative mechanisms include increased splanchnic blood flow with a greater fraction of cardiac output and volatile agent delivered to the liver[13,139] and also higher than normal levels of cytochrome P-450 enzymes.[101,128] In the case of enflurane, a decreased blood–gas partition coefficient has been found in the obese, which results in more rapid uptake of anesthetic.[18,101] Lower affinity of enflurane for blood might result in greater tissue-blood partitioning, increasing the volume of distribution for enflurane.[101]

Morphologic and biochemical abnormalities of the liver have been associated with obesity.[24,128] Fatty infiltration occurs in the majority of massively obese individuals; other histopathologic changes include inflammation, focal necrosis, and cirrhosis. There is no recognized causal relationship between fatty infiltration and cirrhosis.[128] One study reported mortality from cirrhosis among obese men to be 250% of expected although this is disputed by others.[46] Hepatic enzymes may be slightly elevated in the obese, possibly due to the disruption of hepatocytes and/or obstruction of canaliculi by extravasated lipid.[88,128] Pathologic changes can also occur secondarily from cholelithiasis, which is commonly associated with obesity.[124]

Excess adipose tissue can also affect the serum half-life of fixed agents. Serum concentration and half-life are affected by two pharmacokinetic parameters, volume of distribution and clearance. If an agent is lipid-soluble, its steady-state volume of distribution will be larger in an obese person, the serum concentration resulting from a given dose will be lower, and the terminal elimination half-life will be greater (assuming the same clearance). Midazolam, a commonly used benzodiazepine for control of anxiety, is a perfect example. The elimination half-life of midazolam, which is highly lipophilic, is markedly longer in obese subjects than in normal weight controls (8.4 vs. 2.7 hours).[65] This occurs because there is a significantly greater volume of distribution; clearance is unchanged. Although midazolam is generally considered to be a short-acting sedative, it has the potential to produce prolonged sedation in obese patients, particularly because higher loading doses (based on body weight) are required to achieve adequate serum concentrations. In contrast, fentanyl, a lipophilic narcotic, has been found to have similar pharmacokinetic parameters in obese and nonobese subjects and should be administered on the basis of lean body weight.[10] This result is surprising because a larger volume of distribution in the obese would be anticipated for such a lipid-soluble agent. On the other hand, alfentanil, a newer synthetic narcotic, has a longer termi-

nal elimination half-life in the obese as a result of decreased clearance.[12] **The unpredictability of these pharmacokinetics highlights the need for careful drug studies in obese patients. In the absence of such studies, it is critical that data obtained in lean individuals not be assumed to apply to the obese.**

Drug studies in the obese are limited but do include digoxin, thiopental, theophylline, and the neuromuscular blockers. Digoxin half-life is unchanged following weight reduction, suggesting that its dosage should be calculated on the basis of lean body weight.[51] The commonly used induction agent thiopental, like midazolam, has a larger volume of distribution in the obese patient and repeated doses can lead to accumulation and prolonged somnolence.[76] In contrast, theophylline loading doses are best based on total body weight because the volume of distribution is similar in obese and normal weight subjects.[59] Because theophylline clearance is similar in obese and normal individuals, maintenance doses should be given on the basis of ideal body weight (a prolonged $T_{\frac{1}{2}}$ in the obese subjects was attributed to an enlarged volume of distribution and suggests less frequent dosing may be required). Despite its low fat solubility, requirements for pancuronium, a nondepolarizing neuromuscular blocker, are significantly increased in the obese patient.[122] However, once a correction is made for body surface area, the same dosage may be used in obese and nonobese patients. Tsueda et al. postulated that the additional requirement is accounted for by the increased extracellular fluid space into which the drug is distributed[122] although this explanation has been questioned.[52] Recovery of twitch response with vecuronium (0.1 mg/kg) was longer in obese than nonobese patients (82 ± 30 min vs. 50 ± 9 min, respectively, for time to 75% recovery).[136] There was no difference in recovery of twitch responses with atracurium (0.5 mg/kg). The authors attributed the prolonged duration of action of vecuronium in the obese patient to impaired hepatic clearance and/or a dose effect. The absence of prolongation of atracurium was presumed to be because of its lack of dependence on organ elimination. Pseudocholinesterase activity increases linearly with increasing weight; this factor, coupled with the larger extracellular fluid compartment, means that a larger dose of succinylcholine is required in the obese individual.[14] Dosage on the basis of total body weight results in appropriate twitch depression and a recovery time equivalent to that seen in nonobese patients dosed on a similar mg/kg schedule. Since adequate relaxation can be critical to both surgical exposure and wound closure in the obese, monitoring of neuromuscular function is recommended. Excessive subcutaneous adipose tissue can overlie peripheral nerves. Vaughan has recommended the use of needle electrodes for neuromuscular junction monitoring in obese patients.[24]

Renal System

There has been some concern that obese individuals are at increased risk for renal impairment. Proteinuria, the most frequently cited abnormality, has been reported to occur in greater than 40% of obese patients.[107] More recent studies suggest the incidence is far lower.[64,79] Mechanisms of glomerular injury are poorly understood, but an increase in glomerular filtration (by approximately 40%) in obesity is well documented[21] and may be an important contributing factor.[20] In remnant kidney models (prepared by surgical reduction in renal mass), compensatory increases in glomerular filtration are associated with development of focal segmental glomerular sclerosis, marked proteinuria, and declining renal function.[70] A study of 17 massively obese patients with marked proteinuria without clinically apparent systemic disease did find an increased relative incidence of focal glomerulosclerosis and occult diabetic nephropathy.[78] All of the patients had a normal serum albumin despite urinary protein excretion that was comparable to control, nonobese subjects. The finding of lesions typical for a diabetic nephropathy was unexpected; although some of the patients had mild glucose intolerance, none required insulin or had diabetic retinopathy. It may be that renal disease in the morbidly obese person differs from that seen in normal weight individuals and multiple factors (e.g., increased pressure or flow, glucose intolerance) may contribute to histopathologic changes. However, Kasiske and Napier reported that among 46 autopsied, massively obese patients there was no significant difference in the percentage of global glomerular sclerosis from normal weight controls.[79] This finding is consistent with clinical observations of Drenick et al. in which renal disease did not contribute to mortality in a 7.5 year follow-up of 200 morbidly obese men.[46] Further study is required to clarify any association between obesity and kidney disease.

OBESITY-HYPOVENTILATION SYNDROME

Morbidly obese individuals who represent about 5% to 7% of the obese population[44] may be subdivided into those with simple obesity and those with obesity-hypoventilation syndrome (OHS) or "Pickwickian" syndrome.[24,112,124] This latter group may constitute approximately 5% of the morbidly obese population[24,45] and is distinguished by the presence of carbon dioxide retention due to alveolar hypoventilation.[28,118] The term "Pickwickian" was coined by Burwell to describe an obese, somnolent patient reminiscent of Dickens' "Joe, the Fat Boy" from *The Posthumous*

Papers of the Pickwick Club.[28] Although the syndrome is not directly correlated with weight, all of its sufferers are massively obese and may improve greatly with even minor weight loss. **The cardinal sign of hypercapnia is not a feature of simple obesity. Associated characteristics include severe hypoxemia, somnolence, periodic breathing, pulmonary hypertension, biventricular enlargement (particularly the right ventricle), dependent edema, polycythemia, rales, and pulmonary edema.[28,45,111]**

Total pulmonary compliance is decreased by 20% in simple obesity, but it is reduced to 60% in OHS.[112,116] The work of breathing is dramatically elevated, approximating three times the normal level, as opposed to 0 to 30% above normal in the obese.[112,116] Oxygen cost of breathing is high, respiratory muscle efficiency is reduced, and weakness of inspiratory muscles has been identified. Rochester and Enson envisioned a vicious cycle of transient hypercapnia with an inadequate ventilatory response and worsening hypoxia, leading to pulmonary hypertension and transudation of fluid into the lung.[112] Lung compliance is thereby reduced, work of breathing is further increased, and deterioration in ventilation/perfusion matching occurs. In some patients pulmonary hypertension may be worsened by left ventricular dysfunction, but in general a drop in pressure across the pulmonary circuit (i.e., between pulmonary artery diastolic pressure and LVEDP or PAOP) is noted. If untreated, the result of this cycle is extreme hypoxemia and cyanosis, hypercapnia, pulmonary edema, and cor pulmonale. The characteristic somnolence is ascribed to intermittent nocturnal upper airway obstruction leading to apnea, followed by arousal and resumption of respiration. Daytime somnolence then results from sleep deprivation.[84,134]

The cause of hypercapnia in OHS is not completely understood. It has long been assumed that central responses are diminished in association with mechanical chest wall abnormalities. Although the majority of morbidly obese subjects remain eucapnic, a subset of individuals represents a spectrum between eucapnia/acute hypercapnia with sleep and chronic waking hypercapnia. Standard pulmonary function tests in the eucapnic, morbidly obese typically show a restrictive ventilatory defect, with decreased TLC, FRC, and total thoracic compliance and no associated airway obstruction. Respiratory rate is increased without a significant reduction in tidal volume. The increase in frequency reflects a significant reduction in T_E, the expiratory time/breath.[27] Thus T_I/T_E, the inspiratory time to expiratory time ratio, is greater in obese subjects. Because T_I is not altered, Burki and Baker speculated that termination of inspiration is unchanged in eucapnic obesity and that the T_E is possibly due to the decreased chest wall compliance or even active contractions of expiratory muscles.[27] Inspiratory neuromuscular drive/breath is also significantly increased (mouth occlusion pressure, $P_{0.1}$, the mouth pressure developed 0.1 sec after the start of inspiratory effort against a total occlusion at FRC, and the dp/dt_{max}, the maximal rate of increase of this pressure in the first 0.2 seconds), but this finding is difficult to interpret with the increased mechanical hindrance. Obese subjects were found to have an increased sensitivity to hypoxic stimulation exhibiting a greater ventilatory and mouth occlusion pressure response although resting values for $\dot{V}_E$, V_T, frequency, $P_{0.1}$, and dp/dt_{max} were also higher at baseline. No significant differences were observed in sensitivity to carbon dioxide; however, an inappropriately low central respiratory output for a given CO_2 stimulus was reported ($\dot{V}_E$ to $Paco_2$). This finding suggests that morbidly obese subjects could be at some risk in responding to a rise in $Paco_2$, possibly counteracted by increased sensitivity to hypoxia. Attenuation of hypoxic responsiveness could lead to the development of the OHS. The researchers concluded that the observed increase in resting inspiratory neuromuscular drive may not fully compensate for increased mechanical hindrance and that eucapnia is achieved by an alteration in central breath timing.

Emirgil and Sobol studied the effect of weight reduction (62 to 150 pounds) of four obese subjects (at least 50% above ideal body weight) on pulmonary function and respiratory center sensitivity.[49] The observed increase in FRC/TLC was due solely to an increase in ERV. The ventilatory response to carbon dioxide decreased after weight loss, which was interpreted by the researchers as a reduction in oxygen cost of breathing rather than a less sensitive respiratory center. **Obesity itself was not found to decrease respiratory center sensitivity to CO_2. Therefore hypercapnia in the obese subject suggests the presence of intrinsic disease of the respiratory center or the ventilatory system.**

Rapoport et al. performed a very interesting study in eight patients with OHS to discern the contribution of periodic upper airway obstruction.[108] The same laboratory had previously demonstrated no differences in obese patients with obstructive sleep apnea (OSA) and chronic hypercapnia and those with OSA and eucapnia with respect to the number and duration of apneas, degree of obesity, or severity of hypersomnolence.[60] After instituting tracheostomy (seven patients) or nasal CPAP (one patient), the patients fell into two separate groups: four of eight (including one with nasal CPAP) became eucapnic within 2 weeks, the others remained hypercapnic (despite a similar degree of improvement in sleep apnea symptoms). There were no differences regarding anatomic dead space, ventilatory chemore-

sponsiveness (all patients were in a low range of CO_2 responsiveness before therapy), residual apneas, or changes in pulmonary function. The researchers concluded that at least two different mechanisms are important for chronic hypercapnia to exist in the morbidly obese patient with OHS: (1) an unfavorable balance between normal ventilation during time awake and hypoventilation during periods with apnea (demonstrated by those that normalized CO_2 after therapy), and (2) sustained hypoventilation present even when fully awake, the true "Pickwickian" syndrome (demonstrated by those who failed to normalize CO_2 after therapy). Investigation of OHS is hampered by the inherent difficulty in assessing CO_2 responsivity. It would appear that these patients do represent a spectrum of disease, in part due to ventilatory control abnormalities, which assume great importance in perioperative management.

Clearly, patients with OHS present an extremely high anesthetic and surgical risk. Simply assuming the supine position can prove fatal for these patients. A history of sleeping in the sitting position should be taken very seriously.[121] Since even relatively minor weight loss can improve the physiologic state of these patients significantly,[28,112] weight loss should be strongly encouraged before elective surgery. When this is not possible or the surgery is urgent, aggressive cardiopulmonary management, including early endotracheal intubation, has been recommended.[102]

PERIOPERATIVE MANAGEMENT
Preoperative Evaluation

In addition to the usual preoperative assessment, our attention should focus on the issues unique to the obese patient. For example, the cardiorespiratory status requires a more thorough evaluation than would normally be warranted by age. The patient's tolerance for both activity and change in position should be carefully noted. Chest radiography, ECG, serum electrolyte panel (including glucose), and possibly liver function tests should be obtained preoperatively in addition to the usual urinalysis and hematologic assessment. An arterial blood gas measurement will help identify patients with OHS and establish a baseline level of oxygenation.[112] Results of pulmonary function tests of massively obese, otherwise healthy subjects (> 153% predicted body weight) generally fell within 95% confidence limits for predicted values; therefore, the researchers concluded that any abnormalities encountered were probably due to intrinsic lung disease rather than obesity (but excluded "extreme" obesity).[110] Spirometry has not been useful in predicting postoperative pulmonary complications in young to middle-aged morbidly obese patients lacking other risk factors.[37] Pulmonary function tests are advisable in older individuals and those with concurrent pulmonary disease, OHS, or a significant smoking history.

The utility of preoperative medication must be carefully evaluated. Many obese individuals have a tenuous respiratory status that narrows the safety margin for sedation.[17] Some experts recommend avoidance of narcotics; others eliminate sedative premedication entirely.[7,24] Small doses of oral benzodiazepines are generally well tolerated. Prolonged respiratory depression from long-acting agents such as lorazepam or scopolamine may delay weaning and extubation postoperatively. The "intramuscular" route of injection is not recommended because it may deposit medication into adipose tissue, making uptake and distribution unpredictable.[7,24,32] There is some evidence that diazepam is more predictable if given orally to the obese patient, but intramuscular diazepam is notoriously variable in action regardless of the patient's weight. As noted, these patients require protection against aspiration that includes the appropriately timed administration of an H_2 antagonist and metoclopramide.[88]

The current emphasis on cost containment is forcing older and sicker patients to undergo more complicated surgery as outpatients. Careful consideration must be taken regarding the appropriateness of outpatient surgery for such patients. Whereas federal government requirements for outpatient surgery were developed with regard to the complexity of the surgical procedure, little or no attention was paid to concurrent disease or potential anesthetic difficulties. Thus ASA III and IV patients are now occasionally managed without hospital admission. Several experts have questioned the wisdom of handling the morbidly obese patient in this fashion. Apfelbaum and Conahan have suggested that the likelihood of cardiopulmonary pathology and the potential for intraoperative problems make the morbidly obese, as well as some moderately obese individuals, unsuitable candidates for ambulatory surgery.[7] They have proposed that active morbidly obese persons (an unusual combination) who are highly motivated can be considered for surgery as outpatients.

Intraoperative Management

Even the most stalwart anesthesiologist may momentarily hesitate when faced with the responsibility of caring for the morbidly obese patient. These patients are technically demanding, and imprudent management could have serious consequences. Despite perceived advantages of regional (vs. general) anesthesia, technical difficulties, patient tolerance (e.g., issues as simple as positioning for a block or lying supine for the duration of the procedure), and airway control requirements (especially under emergency conditions) often limit regional anesthesia's use as an individual modality. Regardless of anesthetic technique, the obvious major concerns are to maintain oxygenation and ventilation and to avoid hemodynamic embarrassment in this vulnerable population.

The technical difficulties begin with transport of the patient to the operating room and transfer to the operating room table. The table width is often inadequate to accommodate both the patient's body and the upper extremities comfortably. In extreme cases two tables pushed together may be required.[17] This adaptation is not a perfect solution, however. Hand controls may interfere with close approximation of the tables and necessitate reversing the position of one of the tables. If repositioning is required, the anesthesiologist may forfeit the ability to adjust table position readily (Trendelenburg, height, tilt, etc.), which would interfere with optimal control. If the patient's arms must be tucked, careful padding of the ulnar nerves is important, with or without the addition of a metal "sled" to protect the limbs (Fig. 29-14). If

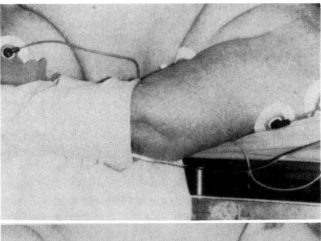

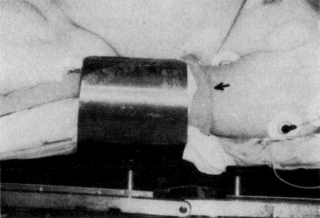

Fig. 29-14. A, Demonstration of the difficulty in safely positioning an obese patient's arms by the side. The potential for ulnar nerve injury is great when the elbow dangles off the mattress in this fashion. **B,** Use of a foam pad *(arrow)* and metal slide protects the extremity from harm.

the arms remain extended on arm boards, extreme abduction to accommodate the operating team must be avoided.

Establishing vascular access is the next hurdle, a procedure that is occasionally so difficult that venous cut-down is required.[17,24,29] Arterial, central venous, and pulmonary artery catheters are similarly difficult to place since landmarks and arterial pulses can be obscured by subcutaneous fat.

Blood pressure measurements will be artifactually elevated if a cuff too small for the arm is used.[19,89,90] This can be avoided by using cuffs with bladders that encircle a minimum of 75% of the upper arm circumference or, preferably, the entire arm.[24,89] A thigh cuff may be required in this circumstance. Because an excessively large cuff may artifactually lower blood pressure, some experts have suggested that 50% of arm circumference is the ideal bladder size. Others believe that width rather than length of the cuff is the key feature.[26] Even with the appropriate size cuff, Korotkoff sounds can be difficult to hear. Because of these problems and the fact that measurement of arterial blood gases might be required during surgery, the use of intraarterial pressure monitoring is recommended.

Airway management is notoriously difficult in the morbidly obese individual and may account for a significant percentage of perioperative morbidity.[50] Mask ventilation can be complicated by inadequate mask fit, airway obstruction by soft tissue, and laryngospasm. In addition, the stomach can become inflated with air as a result of the high pressures required for controlled or assisted mask ventilation, increasing the risk of regurgitation.[53] Endotracheal intubation may be difficult,[25] yet must be accomplished expediently to ensure protection of the airway from aspiration of gastric contents. A "rapid sequence" induction with cricoid pressure has been recommended[7] and has heretofore been our practice. The frequent horror stories of obese patients who prove to be neither intubatable nor ventilatable have encouraged a more conservative approach. Tracheostomy can also be technically difficult.[62] A "rapid sequence" induction might be more appropriate for the moderately obese and has been recommended when it is "certain" the patient can be intubated. (Numerous lawsuits raise the question of whether this is ever the case). The alternative is awake intubation, with or without fiberoptic visualization, which in experienced hands need not be traumatic. After the airway is secured and anesthesia is induced, placement of a gastric tube to evacuate the stomach is generally recommended to minimize risk of aspiration.

The obese patient's reduced FRC results in rapid desaturation in the absence of ventilation.[25] Jense

et al. evaluated the safe duration of apnea in humans after full preoxygenation, which was defined as the time arterial saturation remained $\geq 90\%$.[74] Normal, obese, and morbidly obese patients were found to desaturate after 6.1, 4.1, and 2.7 minutes respectively, demonstrating the widely held clinical impression that obese patients are at increased risk of developing hypoxemia when apneic. Goldberg et al. compared two methods of preoxygenation in morbidly obese patients: administering 100% oxygen with normal ventilation for 3 minutes vs. 100% oxygen with four vital capacity breaths within 30 seconds.[63] Patients were not allowed to remain apneic until desaturation to 90% occurred, but rather were ventilated after intubation and arterial blood gas sampling. Similar increases in Pao_2 were observed (~ 400 mm Hg) in both groups, whereas, $Paco_2$ was mildly but significantly increased in the group breathing 100% oxygen for 3 minutes. Because hypoventilation did not occur in the group taking four vital capacity breaths, the researchers suggest that this approach may be preferable. Regardless of preoxygenation technique, it is important to recognize that obese patients may have a remarkably limited tolerance for apnea. This should influence the approach to airway management.

Chronic physiologic abnormalities in obese patients can deteriorate during surgery. Unexplained deaths occurring intraoperatively and immediately postoperatively are reported in older literature. As recently as 1972 the mortality rate following abdominal operations in the obese was said to be 2.5 times that of the nonobese.[106] Part of this morbidity and mortality rate may be attributable to the tenuous cardiopulmonary status of the obese patient.

Obese patients may frequently develop intraoperative respiratory problems. The diminished FRC of these patients is reduced in the supine position and further reduced with the induction of general anesthesia.[24,42,66] Subsequent tidal ventilation occurs at a lung volume that can be below the closing capacity throughout its cycle, resulting in progressive hypoxemia.[24,41,43] Adequate oxygenation is not guaranteed with an FIO_2 of 0.4 of less.[126] Additional decrements in FRC occur with 15-degree head down positioning (Trendelenburg) or placement of an abdominal pack beneath the diaphragm. In the latter instance, a Pao_2 less than 65 mm Hg has been reported in all patients receiving an FIO_2 of 0.4.[126]

Several strategies can offset the reduction in FRC. Positive end-expiratory pressure (PEEP) is a standard therapy that is designed to expand the FRC primarily by increasing alveolar volume and alveolar recruitment. Santesson found improved Pao_2 and decreased $P(A-a)o_2$ in a group of extremely obese patients receiving 10 to 15 cm H_2O PEEP.[115] Unfortunately, cardiac output fell progressively with increasing

PEEP and oxygen delivery was thereby reduced despite improved O_2 content (Fig. 29-15). Salem et al. found improved PaO_2 and decreased $P(A-a)O_2$ after PEEP was discontinued[114] (Fig. 29-16). Although there was disagreement regarding the mechanism, both groups of researchers found PEEP detrimental to oxygen delivery in the obese. For any critical situation, benefits of PEEP therapy should be documented by evaluating its effects on oxygen delivery. Alternatively, large tidal volumes can be delivered by mechanical ventilation to prevent airway closure and atelectasis.[24] This recommendation, however, conflicts with data supporting the calculation of tidal volumes on the basis of ideal body weight to avoid hyperventilation.[58] High intrathoracic pressure can also increase pulmonary vascular resistance and right heart afterload. Another unique approach to increase

the FRC involves hydraulic suspension of the abdominal panniculus, thereby relieving the high transdiaphragmatic pressure[102,138] (Fig. 29-17). This maneuver is reportedly successful for increasing arterial oxygen tension.

Given that a normal weight individual could be expected to develop hypoxemia undergoing a lateral thoracotomy with one-lung anesthesia, the morbidly obese individual in the same circumstance would be cause for greater concern. Data on 22 morbidly obese patients undergoing transthoracic gastric stapling revealed marked shunting during collapse of the nondependent lung but adequate oxygenation in all patients.[23,103] This result may be due in part to the decrease in abdominal pressure resulting from lateral displacement of the panniculus. Patients undergoing thoracic procedures did not differ postoperatively from those undergoing upper abdominal procedures. The researchers did not address the problem of

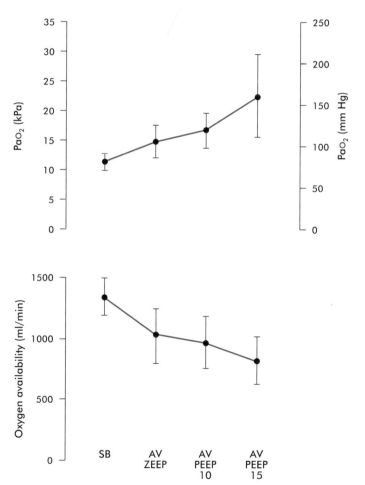

Fig. 29-15. Arterial oxygen tension (PaO_2) and oxygen availability during spontaneous breathing *(SB)* and artificial ventilation *(AV)* with zero end-expiratory pressure *(ZEEP)* and positive end-expiratory pressure *(PEEP)* of 10 and 15 cm H_2O. (From Santesson J: Oxygen transport and venous admixture in the extremely obese. Influence of anaesthesia and artificial ventilation with and without positive end-expiratory pressure, *Acta Anaesthesiol Scand* 20:387, 1976.)

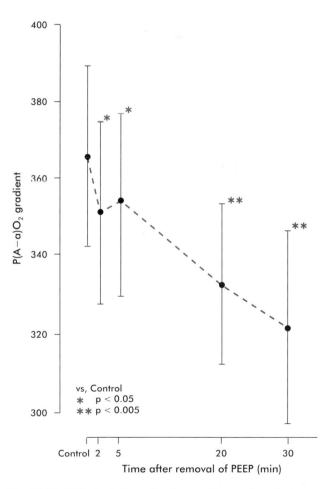

Fig. 29-16. Effect of discontinuing positive end-expiratory pressure *(PEEP)* on alveolar-to-arterial oxygen tension *(P[A-a]O_2)* gradient. (From Salem MR, Dalal FY, Zygmunt MP et al: Does PEEP improve intraoperative arterial oxygenation in grossly obese patients? *Anesthesiology* 48:280, 1978.)

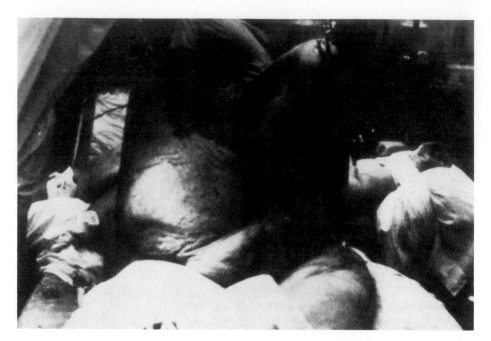

Fig. 29-17. Mechanical suspension of the abdominal panniculus in a morbidly obese patient. Marked improvement in arterial oxygen tension resulted. (From Wyner J, Brodsky JB, and Merrell RC: Massive obesity and arterial oxygenation, *Anesth Analg* 60:691, 1981.)

positioning a double lumen tube in a massively obese individual while protecting the airway against aspiration.

Morbidly obese individuals were reported to have abnormal hemodynamic responses to anesthesia and surgery.[1] Throughout the course of gastric stapling procedures, filling pressures were elevated above preoperative values, as well as values observed in nonobese patients undergoing abdominal surgery. Cardiac index and right ventricular stroke work were significantly lower than those obtained in nonobese patients, while left ventricular stroke work was reduced by 40% (not significant). Left ventricular stroke work remained depressed postoperatively.

General anesthesia in obese patients has broad support as the preferred technique. The primary advantage of general anesthesia is the assurance of adequate oxygenation and ventilation while protecting the airway. A high regional anesthetic could theoretically impair accessory respiratory muscle function in a patient who required all available ventilatory capability. On the other hand, there are several undesirable features of general anesthesia in this population. High concentrations of volatile anesthetic might be required since the obligate high FIO_2 restricts N_2O administration. As noted earlier, increased metabolism of these agents is a concern. Hemodynamic instability and dysrhythmias have been reported during induction of general anesthesia in the obese.[54] Recovery from general anesthesia by mor-

bidly obese individuals was assessed by Cork et al.[33] Despite theoretic concerns based on lipid solubility and biotransformation of volatile anesthetics, neither delayed awakening nor excessive recovery room stay was found. In addition, there was no difference in recovery time among patients receiving halothane, enflurane, or fentanyl anesthesia. However, fentanyl doses were low (average 2.6 μg/kg), and thiopental was the only other intravenous agent. The effect of increased doses or other agents on awakening is unknown.

In the obese patient the optimal timing for extubation should be carefully considered. In several series few of these patients were ventilated postoperatively.[94,109,123] A decision to transport the intubated patient to the recovery room or intensive care unit need not alter a plan for early extubation. As with any difficult intubation, extubation should occur only when the patient is judged alert and able to protect the airway; the patient should demonstrate full reversal of neuromuscular blockade, as well as sufficient inspiratory force and vital capacity. Obese patients extubated in the operating room should receive oxygen during transport regardless of distance because hypoxia can develop extremely rapidly. The head of the bed should be elevated as soon as possible or, alternatively, the patient can be placed in the lateral position.

Many of the problems associated with general anesthesia can be avoided with a carefully administered regional anesthetic. The patient remains awake and can protect the airway. At least one group has data to suggest that arterial blood gases are not compromised by even a high spinal anesthetic.[105] Complete relaxation of abdominal musculature is provided, which otherwise might be accomplished only with deep general anesthesia and/or large doses of neuromuscular blockers. Metabolism of volatile or fixed agents is not a concern. Postoperative pain relief can be provided, avoiding the respiratory depressant effects of systemic narcotics.[22] Undoubtedly the biggest drawback to regional anesthesia is its technical difficulty. Vertebral spines and iliac crests may not be palpable. One ingenious solution to this problem is the placement of two 26-gauge needles to mark the spinous processes above and below the desired interspace.[87] Standard spinal and epidural needles may or may not be sufficiently long. Specially designed equipment may decrease the problem of holding the hub indented far enough into the skin to permit administration of an agent or passage of an epidural catheter.[25,54] Another problem is that anesthetic levels during spinal or epidural anesthesia can be unpredictable.[29,47,93,105] Levels may be higher than expected[93] and can creep up slowly over at least 30 minutes.[29,67] This fact might explain the sudden deaths reported during spinal anesthesia.[29] The sitting position maintained for 5 minutes after administration of an epidural block limited the spread of anesthesia in a group of 250 obese parturients.[68] Epidural anesthesia might be preferable to spinal anesthesia since anesthetic levels are somewhat more titratable[87] although continuous spinal anesthesia has a few proponents.[29,73] Precipitous hypotension can follow sympathetic blockade in the obese.[29,54]

The combination of epidural and general anesthesia has been used by several groups. The use of lumbar epidural combined with general anesthesia was reported by Fox.[54] Sixteen patients undergoing intestinal bypass surgery received epidural lidocaine combined with a balanced (nitrous-narcotic) general anesthetic. None of the patients required postoperative mechanical ventilation, and postoperative narcotics were avoided. The suggestion was made that respiratory status was improved by the absence of abdominal "splinting" although subsequent data in 110 patients from the same group revealed no difference in blood gas tensions between patients receiving epidural analgesia and those receiving narcotics postoperatively.[55] Pneumonia was slightly less common in the epidural group (2.9% vs. 5.0% in the narcotic group). Gelman et al. compared thoracic epidural combined with general anesthesia (N_2O/O_2) and "balanced" anesthesia (N_2O/O_2/fentanyl and/or enflurane) in morbidly obese patients undergoing gastric bypass surgery.[61] Patients receiving epidural anesthesia continued to be treated with epidural

bupivacaine postoperatively for pain relief, whereas patients receiving balanced anesthesia were treated with morphine sulfate intravenously. The epidural space could not be identified in 5 of the first 12 patients, and subsequent epidurals were performed under fluoroscopic control. Although Gelman's study demonstrated no particular intraoperative advantage to epidural anesthesia, all patients in this group were extubated at the end of the surgical procedure, whereas 12 of 17 of the patients in the balanced anesthesia group were too sedated to permit immediate extubation. Postoperative epidural analgesia provided more predictable pain relief, causing significantly less sympathetically mediated hemodynamic responses. With adequate pain relief, restoration of vital capacity did not differ between the groups. In a similar study (although not prospective or randomized), Buckley et al. found a greater number of postoperative pulmonary complications in patients receiving general anesthesia than in those receiving epidural plus general anesthesia although the operative procedures were significantly shorter in the latter group.[25]

Postoperative Management

Because obese patients are at significant risk for postoperative hypoxemia,[123] adequacy of oxygenation (and ventilation) is a primary concern in the postoperative period. Room air PaO_2 remains depressed for up to 4 days. Hypoxemia is worse after surgery is performed through a vertical abdominal incision.[125,131] A semirecumbent position is recommended postoperatively to minimize deterioration in oxygenation associated with the supine position (Fig. 29-18).[127,129]

Because the pulmonary status of the obese patient is potentially compromised, particular attention should be directed to postoperative pain management. Narcotics are still the mainstay of therapy, administered intravenously, intramuscularly, or epidurally.[22,109] A randomized, double-blind study by Rawal et al. compared intramuscular with epidural morphine for patients undergoing elective gastroplasty for weight reduction.[109] Patients receiving epidural morphine were more likely to sit, stand, or walk unassisted during the first postoperative 24 hours than those patients receiving morphine intramuscularly. Pulmonary complications were less common in the epidural group, and these patients had significantly shorter hospital stays. These investigators provide the most compelling evidence supporting the superiority of a regional anesthetic technique in the obese, at least for postoperative management.

The surgical treatment of obese patients with obstructive sleep apnea (OSA) provides the opportunity to assess postoperative experience in a subset of patients with serious physiologic derangements. In a retrospective review of 135 patients, Esclamado et al.

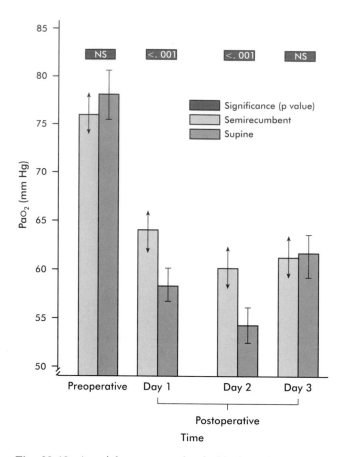

Fig. 29-18. Arterial oxygen tension in 22 obese female subjects in the semirecumbent and supine positions preoperatively and on days 1 through 3 postoperatively. On postoperative days 1 and 2 a significant effect on PaO_2 resulted from changing to the supine position. (From Vaughan RW, Wise L: Postoperative arterial blood gas measurement in obese patients: effect of position on gas exchange, *Ann Surg* 182:705, 1975.)

found a 13% incidence of perioperative complications (7 failed intubations, 7 with airway obstruction postextubation, 3 postoperative hemorrhages, 1 postoperative dysrhythmia).[50] Despite an acknowledged limited predictive value, the researchers suggest that an apnea index ≥ 70 (apneas plus hypopneas/hr), a minimum O_2 saturation $< 80\%$, and a "difficult" airway are indicators for perioperative airway risk. They also reported that patients who had received a significantly higher dose of narcotic intraoperatively (dose/kg body weight or dose/length of procedure) were at greater risk of developing an extubation complication. Although ill-defined, this information does target potential contributory factors to perioperative problems. Johnson and Sanders, responding to the unexpected death of a patient at home 36 hours after uvulopalatopharyngoplasty (UPPP), evaluated three obese patients prospectively undergoing UPPP

using polysomnography.[75] There was no difference in the mean duration of postoperative apneas on the second postoperative night, but the nadir SaO_2 during apnea in one patient was markedly lower (reported as 15% by ear oximetry, a methodology generally inaccurate below 60%). This result was associated with the longest apneic period of 189 seconds. Upper airway functions during sleep appear to be unchanged immediately following UPPP, and patients are reported to be at increased risk for ventricular dysrhythmia if oxygen saturation declines below 60% to 70%.[117] The researchers speculated that patients who preoperatively had awake hypercapnia and hypoxemia with significant sleep-associated hemoglobin desaturation may be at greatest risk for postoperative complications and that careful monitoring after surgery is indicated. The recommended duration for postoperative monitoring is not addressed, but one can infer a minimum of 48 hours. It is also important to recognize that UPPP fails to significantly influence OSA in approximately 50% of patients.

Although all postsurgical patients are at increased risk of thrombophlebitis, obese patients may be especially prone to develop this complication.[53] Early ambulation is therefore desirable. Investigators whose patients ambulate sooner after a particular technique often suggest that this represents a significant advantage to the technique. For example, Fox found that continuous epidural analgesia permitted the patients to perform "vigorous leg exercises," which he believed to be important in the prevention of deep venous thrombosis.[55] Nevertheless, the percentage of patients having pulmonary embolism was greater in the group who received epidural analgesia than in the group who received narcotics (5.7% vs. 2.5%). In addition, Rawal et al. were unable to document a difference in the incidence of thrombophlebitis with epidural anesthesia using a radioisotope technique.[109] Postoperative pain control should be adequate to permit early transfer of the patient to a bedside chair and subsequent ambulation. There is little question that prolonged bed rest increases the risk of thrombophlebitis.

SUMMARY

Obesity is a common condition that is frequently associated with multisystem disease and occurs in patients who are apt to require surgery. The anesthesiologist should appreciate that these patients may have a significantly altered physiology and present major technical and intellectual challenges. A carefully focused preoperative evaluation should guide the development of a perioperative plan to ensure a safe and uneventful course.

KEY POINTS

- Obesity has been statistically associated with a large number of chronic diseases and significant derangements in baseline physiology. These factors make the obese patient a high-risk consumer of anesthetic and surgical services.

- It has been known for many years that obesity is typically accompanied by hypoxemia. Several mechanisms underlie this hypoxemia: (1) increased work and energy cost of breathing, (2) higher minute ventilation at rest to handle the metabolic needs of the increased tissue mass, and (3) changes in lung volumes that result in closure of small airways and $\dot{V}/\dot{Q}$ mismatch during normal breathing.

- The relationship between obesity and cardiovascular disease has been elucidated through longitudinal studies of large populations. Follow-up of the Framingham population at 26 years showed obesity to be an important predictor of cardiovascular disease, particularly in individuals younger than 50 years of age. Risk of coronary artery disease, myocardial infarction, and sudden death was higher among obese persons of both sexes.

- The association of hypertension with obesity is well-known although cause and effect have not been established. Regardless of the level of blood pressure, increasing blood volume has been noted as weight increases above ideal. Excess body mass increases total body oxygen consumption, and hence cardiac output must be increased to meet the demand. Chronically elevated preload results in dilatation and hypertrophy of the left ventricle. Workload increases correspondingly and both systolic performance and compliance suffer. Consequently pulmonary hypertension is a common finding.

- The association between obesity and sudden death led investigators to conduct Holter monitoring of obese patients. They found an increase in premature ventricular contractions from 10 to 30 times control patients, including runs of ventricular tachycardia in patients with left ventricular hypertrophy.

- The gastrointestinal physiology of the obese differs from normal in two primary respects: (1) high gastric volume and low pH in the fasting state and (2) abnormalities of hepatic function. The obese are at risk for aspiration during the induction of anesthesia; the combination of metoclopramide and ranitidine appears to provide the best protection against aspiration. Biotransformation of volatile anesthetic agents is both qualitatively and quantitatively different in obese and nonobese subjects.

- Alterations in drug metabolism are common in obese patients. The unpredictability of pharmacokinetics in obese persons highlights the need for careful studies. In the absence of such studies, it is critical that data obtained in lean individuals not be assumed to apply to the obese individual.

- Patients suffering from obesity-hypoventilation syndrome (OHS) constitute approximately 5% of the morbidly obese population. The cardinal sign of OHS is hypercapnia; other characteristics include severe hypoxemia, somnolence, periodic breathing, pulmonary hypertension, enlargement of both ventricles but particularly the right, dependent edema, polycythemia, rales, and pulmonary edema. Patients with OHS represent an extremely high anesthetic and surgical risk. Simply assuming the supine position can prove fatal.

- In addition to the usual preoperative evaluation certain issues unique to the obese patient must be addressed: (1) the cardiorespiratory status requires a more thorough evaluation than would normally be warranted by age, and (2) pulmonary function tests are advisable in older individuals and those with concurrent pulmonary disease, OHS, or a significant smoking history.

- The tenuous respiratory status of many obese individuals makes excessive sedation hazardous.

KEY REFERENCES

Agarwal N, Shibutani K, San Filippo A et al: Hemodynamic and respiratory changes in surgery of the morbidly obese, *Surgery* 92:226, 1982.

Alexander JK: The cardiomyopathy of obesity, *Prog Cardiovasc Dis* 27:325, 1985.

Brown BR et al, eds: Anesthesia and the obese patient. In *Contemporary anesthesia practice*, vol 5, Philadelphia, 1982, FA Davis.

Fox GS, Whalley DG, and Bevan DR: Anaesthesia for the morbidly obese. Experience with 110 patients, *Br J Anaesth* 53:811, 1981.

Manchikanti L et al: Effect of preanesthetic ranitidine

and metoclopramide on gastric contents in morbidly obese patients, *Anesth Analg* 65:195, 1986.

Rawal N, Sjöstrand U, Christoffersson E et al: Comparison of intramuscular and epidural morphine for postoperative analgesia in the grossly

obese: influence on postoperative ambulation and pulmonary function, *Anesth Analg* 63:583, 1984.

Ray CS, Sue DY, Bray G et al: Effects of obesity on respiratory function, *Am Rev Respir Dis* 128:501, 1983.

REFERENCES

1. Agarwal N, Shibutani K, San Filippo A et al: Hemodynamic and respiratory changes in surgery of the morbidly obese, *Surgery* 92:226, 1982.
2. Alexander JK: Chronic heart disease due to obesity, *J Chron Dis* 18:895, 1965.
3. Alexander JK: Obesity and cardiac performance, *Am J Cardiol* 14:860, 1964.
4. Alexander JK: The cardiomyopathy of obesity, *Prog Cardiovasc Dis* 27:325, 1985.
5. Alexander JK, Dennis EW: Circulatory dynamics in extreme obesity, *Circulation* 20:662, 1959.
6. Alexander JK, Dennis EW, Smith WG et al: Blood volume, cardiac output, and distribution of systemic blood flow in extreme obesity, *Cardiovasc Res Cent Bull* 1:39, 1962-1963.
7. Apfelbaum JL, Conahan TJ: An approach to the management of a patient with morbid obesity scheduled for outpatient surgery, *Soc Ambul Anesth News* 1:3, 1986.
8. Barrera F, Reidenberg MM, Winters WL et al: Ventilation-perfusion relationships in the obese patient, *J Appl Physiol* 26:420, 1969.
9. Bentley JB, Borel JD, Vaughan RW et al: Weight, pseudo-cholinesterase activity, and succinylcholine requirement, *Anesthesiology* 57:48, 1982.
10. Bentley JB, Vaughan RW, Cork RC et al: Does evidence of reductive halothane biotransformation correlate with hepatic binding of metabolites in obese patients? *Anesth Analg* 60:548, 1981.
11. Bentley JB, Vaughan RW, Gandolfi A et al: Halothane biotransformation in obese and nonobese patients, *Anesthesiology* 57:94, 1982.
12. Bentley JB, Vaughan RW, Miller MS et al: Serum inorganic fluoride levels in obese patients during and after enflurane anesthesia, *Anesth Analg* 58:409, 1979.
13. Bentley JB et al: Fentanyl pharmacokinetics in obese and nonobese patients, *Anesthesiology* 55:A177, 1981.
14. Bentley JB et al: Obesity and alfentanil pharmacokinetics, *Anesth Analg* 62:245, 1983.
15. Billewicz WZ, Kemsley WF, Thomson AM et al: Indices of adiposity, *Br J Prev Soc Med* 16:183, 1962.
16. Blackburn H, Parlin RW: Antecedents of disease. Insurance mortality experience, *Ann N Y Acad Sci* 134:965, 1966.
17. Blass NH: Morbid obesity and other nutritional disorders. In Katz J et al, eds: *Anesthesia and uncommon diseases,* Philadelphia, 1981, WB Saunders.

18. Borel JD, Bentley JB, Vaughan RW et al: Enflurane blood-gas solubility: influence of weight and hemoglobin, *Anesth Analg* 61:1006, 1982.
19. Bray GA: Obesity and the heart, *Mod Concepts Cardiovasc Dis* 56:67, 1987.
20. Brenner BM: Hemodynamically mediated glomerular injury and the progressive nature of kidney disease, *Kidney Int* 23:647, 1983.
21. Brochner-Mortensen J et al: Renal function and body composition before and after intestinal bypass operation in obese patients, *Scand J Clin Lab Invest* 40:695, 1980.
22. Brodsky JB, Wyner J, Ehrenwerth J et al: One-lung anesthesia in morbidly obese patients, *Anesthesiology* 57:132, 1982.
23. Brodsky JB, et al: Epidural morphine following abdominoplasty, *Plast Reconstr Surg* 78:125, 1986.
24. Brown BR et al, eds: Anesthesia and the obese patient. In *Contemporary anesthesia practice*, vol 5, Philadelphia, 1982, FA Davis.
25. Buckley FP, Robinson NB, Simonowitz DA et al: Anaesthesia in the morbidly obese: a comparison of anaesthetic and analgesic regimens for upper abdominal surgery, *Anaesthesia* 38:840, 1983.
26. Burch GE, Shewey L: Sphygmomanometric cuff size and blood pressure recordings, *JAMA* 225:1215, 1973.
27. Burki NK, Baker RW: Ventilatory regulation in eucapnic morbid obesity, *Am Rev Respir Dis* 129:538, 1984.
28. Burwell CS, Robin ED, Whaley RD: Extreme obesity associated with alveolar hypoventilation–a Pickwickian syndrome, *Am J Med* 21:811, 1956.
29. Catenacci AJ, Anderson JD, and Boersma D: Anesthetic hazards of obesity, *JAMA* 175:657, 1961.
30. Cherniack KM, Guenter CA: The efficiency of the respiratory muscles in obesity, *Can J Biochem Physiol* 39:1215, 1961.
31. Christian PE, Datz FL, and Moore JG: Gastric emptying studies in the morbidly obese before and after gastroplasty, *J Nucl Med* 27:1686, 1986.
32. Cockshott WP, Thompson GT, Howlett LJ et al: Intramuscular or intralipomatous injections? *N Engl J Med* 307:356, 1982.
33. Cork RC, Vaughan RW, and Bentley JB: General anesthesia for morbidly obese patients–an examination of postoperative outcomes, *Anesthesiology* 54:310, 1981.
34. Cousins MJ, Greenstein LR, Hitt BA et al: Metabolism and renal effects of

enflurane in man, *Anesthesiology* 44:44, 1976.
35. Couture J et al: Airway closure in normal, obese, and anesthetized supine subjects, *Fed Proc* 29:269A, 1970.
36. Craig DB, Wahba WM, Don HF et al: "Closing volume" and its relationship to gas exchange in seated and supine positions, *J Appl Physiol* 31:717, 1971.
37. Crapo RO, Kelly TM, Elliot CG et al: Spirometry as a preoperative screening test in morbidly obese patients, *Surgery* 99:763, 1986.
38. Creasser CW, Stoelting RK: Serum inorganic fluoride concentrations during and after halothane, fluroxene, and methoxyflurane anesthesia in man, *Anesthesiology* 39:537, 1973.
39. de Divitiis O, Fazio S, Petitto M et al: Obesity and cardiac function, *Circulation* 64:477, 1981.
40. Dodds WJ, Dent J, Hogan WJ et al: Mechanisms of gastroesophageal reflux in patients with reflux esophagitis, *N Engl J Med* 307:1547, 1982.
41. Don HF, Craig DB, Wahba WM et al: The measurement of gas trapped in the lungs at functional residual capacity and the effects of posture, *Anesthesiology* 35:582, 1971.
42. Don HF, Wahba WM, and Craig DB: Airway closure, gas trapping, and the functional residual capacity during anesthesia, *Anesthesiology* 36:533, 1972.
43. Don HF, Wahba WM, Cuadrado L et al: The effects of anesthesia and 100 percent oxygen on the functional residual capacity of the lungs, *Anesthesiology* 32:521, 1970.
44. Drenick EJ: Definition and health consequences of morbid obesity, *Surg Clin North Am* 59:963, 1979.
45. Drenick EJ: Risk of obesity and surgical indications, *Int J Obes* 5:387, 1980.
46. Drenick EJ, Bale GS, Seltzer F et al: Excessive mortality and causes of death in morbidly obese men, *JAMA* 243:443, 1980.
47. Edelist G: Extreme obesity, *Anesthesiology* 29:846, 1968.
48. Eichhorn JH, Hedley-Whyte J et al: Renal failure following enflurane anesthesia, *Anesthesiology* 45:557, 1976.
49. Emirgil C, Sobol BJ: The effects of weight reduction on pulmonary function and the sensitivity of the respiratory center in obesity, *Am Rev Respir Dis* 108:831, 1973.
50. Esclamado RM, Glenn MG, McCulloch TM et al: Perioperative complications and risk factors in the surgical treatment of obstructive sleep apnea syndrome, *Laryngoscope* 99:1125, 1989.

51. Ewy GA, Groves BM, Ball MF et al: Digoxin metabolism in obesity, *Circulation* 44:810, 1971.
52. Feingold A: Pancuronium requirements of the morbidly obese, *Anesthesiology* 50:269, 1979.
53. Fisher A, Waterhouse TD, and Adams AP: Obesity: its relation to anaesthesia, *Anaesthesia* 30:633, 1975.
54. Fox GS: Anaesthesia for intestinal short circuiting in the morbidly obese with reference to the pathophysiology of gross obesity, *Can Anaesth Soc J* 22:307, 1975.
55. Fox GS, Whalley DG, and Bevan DR: Anaesthesia for the morbidly obese. Experience with 110 patients, *Br J Anaesth* 53:811, 1981.
56. Fritts HW et al: The efficiency of ventilation during voluntary hyperpnea: studies in normal subjects and in dyspneic patients with either chronic pulmonary emphysema or obesity, *J Clin Invest* 38:1339, 1959.
57. Froese AB, Bryan AC: Effects of anesthesia and paralysis on diaphragmatic mechanics in man, *Anesthesiology* 41:242, 1974.
58. Furgerson CL et al: Ventilator settings to mitigate hypocarbia in the obese patient, *Anesth Analg* 64:S53, 1986.
59. Gal P, Jusko WJ, Yurchak AM et al: Theophylline disposition in obesity, *Clin Pharmacol Ther* 23:438, 1978.
60. Garay SM, Rapoport D, Sorkin B et al: Regulation of ventilation in the obstructive sleep apnea syndrome, *Am Rev Respir Dis* 124:451, 1981.
61. Gelman S, Laws HL, Potzick J et al: Thoracic epidural vs. balanced anesthesia in morbid obesity: an intraoperative and postoperative hemodynamic study, *Anesth Analg* 59:902, 1980.
62. Ghorayeb BY: Tracheotomy in the morbidly obese patient, *Arch Otolaryngol Head Neck Surg* 113:556, 1987.
63. Goldberg ME, Norris MC, Larijani GE et al: Preoxygenation in the morbidly obese: a comparison of two techniques, *Anesth Analg* 68:520, 1989.
64. Goldszer R et al: Renal findings in obese humans, *Kidney Int* 25:165, 1984.
65. Greenblatt DJ, Abernethy DR, Locniskar A et al: Effect of age, gender, and obesity on midazolam kinetics, *Anesthesiology* 61:27, 1984.
66. Hedenstierna G, Santesson J, and Norlander O: Airway closure and distribution of inspired gas in the extremely obese, breathing spontaneously and during anesthesia with intermittent positive pressure ventilation, *Acta Anaesthesiol Scand* 20:334, 1976.
67. Hodgkinson R, Husain FJ: Obesity and the cephalad spread of analgesia following epidural administration of bupivacaine for cesarean section, *Anesth Analg* 59:89, 1980.
68. Hodgkinson R, Husain FJ: Obesity, gravity, and spread of epidural anesthesia, *Anesth Analg* 60:421, 1981.
69. Holley HS, Milic-Emili J, Becklake MR et al: Regional distribution of pulmonary ventilation and perfusion in obesity, *J Clin Invest* 46:475, 1967.

70. Hostetter TH et al: Hyperfiltration in remnant nephrons: a potentially adverse response to renal ablation, *Am J Physiol* 241:F85, 1981.
71. Hubert HB, Feinleib M, McNamera PM et al: Obesity as an independent risk factor for cardiovascular disease: a 26-year follow-up of participants in the Framingham Heart Study, *Circulation* 67:968, 1983.
72. Huff RL, Feller DD: Relation of circulating red cell volume to body density and obesity, *J Clin Invest* 35:1, 1956.
73. Jacobs LL, Berger HC, and Fierro FE: Obesity and continuous spinal anesthesia: a case report, *Anesth Analg* 42:547, 1963.
74. Jense HG, Dubin SA, Silverstein PI et al: Effect of obesity on safe duration of apnea in anesthetized humans, *Anesth Analg* 72:89, 1991.
75. Johnson JT, Sanders MH: Breathing during sleep immediately after uvulopalatopharyngoplasty, *Laryngoscope* 96:1236, 1986.
76. Jung D, Mayersohn M, Perrier D et al: Thiopental disposition in lean and obese patients undergoing surgery, *Anesthesiology* 56:269, 1982.
77. Kannel WB, LeBauer EJ, Dawber TR et al: Relation of body weight to development of coronary heart disease, *Circulation* 35:734, 1967.
78. Kasiske BL, Crosson JT: Renal disease in patients with massive obesity, *Arch Intern Med* 146:1105, 1986.
79. Kasiske BL, Napier J: Glomerular sclerosis in patients with massive obesity, *Am J Nephrol* 5:45, 1985.
80. Kaufman BJ et al: Hypoventilation in obesity, *J Clin Invest* 38:500, 1959.
81. Keys A, Aravanis C, Blackburn H et al: Coronary heart disease: overweight and obesity as risk factors, *Ann Intern Med* 77:15, 1972.
82. Keys A, Fidanza F, Karvonen MJ et al: Indices of relative weight and obesity, *J Chron Dis* 25:329, 1972.
83. Kral JG: Morbid obesity and related health risks, *Ann Intern Med* 103(6 pt 2):1043, 1985.
84. Kryger M, Quesney LF, Holder D et al: The sleep deprivation syndrome of the obese patient. A problem of periodic nocturnal upper airway obstruction, *Am J Med* 56:531, 1974.
85. Lam AM, Grace DM, Penny FJ et al: Prophylactic intravenous cimetidine reduces the risk of acid aspiration in morbidly obese patients, *Anesthesiology* 65:684, 1986.
86. Laws AK: Effects of induction of anaesthesia and muscle paralysis on functional residual capacity of the lungs, *Can Anaesthetist Soc J* 15:325, 1968.
87. Maitra AM et al: Continuous epidural analgesia for cesarean section in a patient with morbid obesity, *Anesth Analg* 58:348, 1979.
88. Manchikanti L et al: Effect of preanesthetic ranitidine and metoclopramide on gastric contents in morbidly obese patients, *Anesth Analg* 65:195, 1986.
89. Mann GV: The influence of obesity on health, *N Engl J Med* 291:(I)178, (II)226, 1974.

90. Maxwell MH, Waks AU, Schroth PC et al: Error in blood pressure measurement due to incorrect cuff size in obese patients, *Lancet* 2:33, 1982.
91. Mazze RI, Calverley RK, Smith NT et al: Inorganic fluoride nephrotoxicity: prolonged enflurane and halothane anesthesia in volunteers, *Anesthesiology* 46:265, 1977.
92. Mazze RI, Trudell JR, and Cousins MJ: Methoxyflurane metabolism and renal dysfunction: clinical correlation in man, *Anesthesiology* 35:247, 1971.
93. McCulloch WJD, Littlewood DG: Influence of obesity on spinal analgesia with isobaric 0.5% bupivacaine, *Br J Anaesth* 58:610, 1986.
94. McKenzie R et al: Anesthesia for jejunoileal shunt: review of 88 cases, *Anesth Analg* 54:65, 1975.
95. Messerli FH: Cardiopathy of obesity—a not-so victorian disease, *N Engl J Med* 314:378, 1986.
96. Messerli FH: Cardiovascular effects of obesity and hypertension, *Lancet* 1:1165, 1982.
97. Messerli FH, Nunez BD, Ventura HO et al: Overweight and sudden death. Increased ventricular ectopy in cardiopathy of obesity, *Arch Intern Med* 147:1725, 1987.
98. Metropolitan Life Insurance Co.: Measurement of overweight, *Statistical Bulletin* 65:20, 1984.
99. Metropolitan Life Insurance Co.: New weight standards for men and women, *Statistical Bulletin* 40:1, 1959.
100. Metropolitan Life Insurance Co.: 1983 Metropolitan height and weight tables, *Statistical Bulletin* 64:1, 1983.
101. Miller MS, Gandolfi AJ, Vaughan RW et al: Disposition of enflurane in obese patients, *J Pharmacol Exp Ther* 215:292, 1980.
102. Neuman GG, Baldwin CC, Petrini AJ et al: Perioperative management of a 430 kilogram (946 pound) patient with pickwickian syndrome, *Anesth Analg* 65:985, 1986.
103. Oakes DD, Cohn RB, Brodsky JB et al: Lateral thoracotomy and one-lung anesthesia in patients with morbid obesity, *Ann Thorac Surg* 34:572, 1982.
104. Paul DR, Hoyt JL, and Boutros AR: Cardiovascular and respiratory changes in response to change of posture in the very obese, *Anesthesiology* 45:73, 1976.
105. Pitkanen MT: Body mass and spread of spinal anesthesia with bupivacaine, *Anesth Analg* 66:127, 1987.
106. Postlethwait RW, Johnson WD: Complications following surgery for duodenal ulcer in obese patients, *Arch Surg* 105:438, 1972.
107. Preble WE: Obesity: observations on one thousand cases, *Boston M & S Journal* 188:617, 1923.
108. Rapoport DM, Garay SM, Epstein H et al: Hypercapnia in the obstructive sleep apnea syndrome, *Chest* 89:627, 1986.
109. Rawal N, Sjöstrand U, Christoffersson E et al: Comparison of intramuscular and epidural morphine for postoperative analgesia in the grossly obese: influence on

postoperative ambulation and pulmonary function, *Anesth Analg* 63:583, 1984.

110. Ray CS, Sue DY, Bray G et al: Effects of obesity on respiratory function, *Am Rev Respir Dis* 128:501, 1983.

111. Reisin E, Frohlich FD: Obesity: cardiovascular and respiratory pathophysiological alterations, *Arch Intern Med* 141:431, 1981.

112. Rochester DF, Enson Y: Current concepts in the pathogenesis of the obesity-hypoventilation syndrome, *Am J Med* 57:402, 1974.

113. Said SI: Abnormalities of pulmonary gas exchange in obesity, *Ann Intern Med* 53:1121, 1960.

114. Salem MR, Dalal FY, Zygmunt MP et al: Does PEEP improve intraoperative arterial oxygenation in grossly obese patients? *Anesthesiology* 48:280, 1978.

115. Santesson J: Oxygen transport and venous admixture in the extremely obese. Influence of anaesthesia and artificial ventilation with and without positive end-expiratory pressure, *Acta Anaesthesiol Scand* 20:387, 1976.

116. Sharp JT, Henry JP, Sweaney SK et al: The total work of breathing in normal and obese men, *J Clin Invest* 43:728, 1964.

117. Shepard JW et al: Relationship of ventricular ectopy to oxyhemoglobin desaturation in patients with obstructive sleep apnea, *Chest* 88:335, 1985.

118. Sieker HO et al: A cardipulmonary syndrome associated with extreme obesity, *J Clin Invest* 34:916, 1955.

119. Strube PJ, Hulands GH, and Halsey MJ: Serum fluoride levels in morbidly obese patients: enflurane compared with iso-flurane anaesthesia, *Anaesthesia* 42:685, 1987.

120. Sugerman HJ, Fairman RP: Massive weight loss will improve arterial oxygenation in selected patients, *Anesthesiology* 55:604, 1981.

121. Tsueda K, Debrand M, Zeok SS et al: Obesity supine death syndrome: reports of two morbidly obese patients, *Anesth Analg* 58:345, 1979.

122. Tsueda K, Warren JE, McCafferty LA et al: Pancuronium bromide requirement during anesthesia for the morbidly obese, *Anesthesiology* 48:438, 1978.

123. Vaughan RW: Anesthetic considerations in jejunoileal small bowel bypass for morbid obesity, *Anesth Analg* 53:421, 1974.

124. Vaughan RW, Conahan TJ: Cardiopulmonary consequences of morbid obesity, *Life Sci* 26:2119, 1980.

125. Vaughan RW, Wise L: Choice of abdominal operative incision in the obese patient: a study using blood gas measurements, *Ann Surg* 181:829, 1975.

126. Vaughan RW, Wise L: Intraoperative arterial oxygenation in obese patients, *Ann Surg* 184:35, 1976.

127. Vaughan RW, Wise L: Postoperative arterial blood gas measurement in obese patients: effect of position on gas exchange, *Ann Surg* 182:705, 1975.

128. Vaughan RW, Bauer S, and Wise L: Effect of position (semirecumbent versus supine) on postoperative oxygenation in markedly obese subjects, *Anesth Analg* 55:37, 1976.

129. Vaughan RW, Bauer S, and Wise L: Volume and pH of gastric juice in obese patients, *Anesthesiology* 43:686, 1975.

130. Vaughan RW, Cork RC, and Hollander D: The effect of massive weight loss on arterial oxygenation and pulmonary function tests, *Anesthesiology* 54:325, 1981.

131. Vaughan RW, Engelhardt RC, and Wise L: Postoperative alveolar-arterial oxygen tension difference: its relation to the operative incision in obese patients, *Anesth Analg* 54:433, 1975.

132. Vaughan RW, Engelhardt RC, and Wise L: Postoperative hypoxemia in obese patients, *Ann Surg* 180:877, 1974.

133. Vaughan RW, Gandolfi AJ, and Bentley JB: Biochemical considerations of morbid obesity, *Life Sci* 26:2215, 1980.

134. Walsh RE, Michaelson ED, Harkleroad LE et al: Upper airway obstruction in obese patients with sleep disturbances and somnolence, *Ann Intern Med* 76:185, 1972.

135. Walton B, Simpson BR, Stranin L et al: Unexplained hepatitis following halothane, *Br Med J* 1:1171, 1976.

136. Weinstein JA, Matteo RS, Ornstein E et al: Pharmacodynamics of vecuronium and atracurium in the obese surgical patient, *Anesth Analg* 67:1149, 1988.

137. Wilson SL et al: Effects of atropine, glycopyrrolate, and cimetidine on gastric secretions in morbidly obese patients, *Anesth Analg* 60:37, 1981.

138. Wyner J, Brodsky JB, and Merrell RC: Massive obesity and arterial oxygenation, *Anesth Analg* 60:691, 1981.

139. Young SR, Stoelting RK, Peterson C et al: Anesthetic biotransformation and renal function in obese patients during and after methoxyflurane or halothane anesthesia, *Anesthesiology* 42:451, 1975.

CHAPTER 30

Evaluation of the Patient With Alcoholism and Other Drug Dependencies

CHARLES BEATTIE

LYNETTE MARK

ANNIE UMBRICHT-SCHNEITER

Substance abuse is a major public health problem in the United States. The increasing complexities of patient presentation to medical care necessitate a multidisciplinary approach to medical evaluation and management. The anesthesiologist should be knowledgeable regarding issues related to prevalence, detection, medical management, perioperative treatment, and strategies for rehabilitation of the substance abuse patient, thereby contributing to comprehensive health care. Continued vigilance for unrecognized and undiagnosed substance abuse is important because behaviors associated with such abuse are a threat not only to the patient but also to the anesthesiologist and other members of the health care team. The risk of accidental transmission of infections such as viral hepatitis and the human immunodeficiency virus (HIV) has reached such major proportions that universal precautions have become necessary to protect the clinician and coworkers. Equally important, and because of the easy accessibility to substances with high abuse liability, anesthesiologists should be alerted to their own increased risk of impairment, as well as that of their colleagues.[43,100]

Patients recovering from drug and alcohol addiction are in remission from a debilitating chronic illness. Although they are most frequently happy, healthy, and productive members of the community, they often seek medical attention because of related morbidities and unrelated conditions. These patients require and deserve an appropriate response to their special needs by physicians and other health care professionals. It is hoped that the material in this chapter will contribute to that goal, pending formal specific directives from the field of addiction medicine.

ANESTHESIA FOR PATIENTS IN ACTIVE CHEMICAL DEPENDENCY

The scope of the problem represented by individuals abusing psychoactive substances and the impact of addictive diseases on the community can be better appreciated by consideration of the following facts:

- Alcoholism is the third leading cause of death and disability in the United States. Conservative estimates suggest that between 10 and 15 million Americans have the disease. This high prevalence and the association of alcoholism with trauma and with gastrointestinal hemorrhage make alcoholics frequent surgical patients.[110]
- Fetal alcohol syndrome (FAS) is one of the top three known causes of birth defects with accompanying mental retardation and hyperactivity—and the only preventable cause among those three. In early 1990, the Centers for Disease Control (CDC) estimated that more than 8000 infants are born each year with FAS.[106] The overall perinatal mortality is 17%, compared with 2% in the nonalcoholic population.[18]
- Estimates of the total number of heroin users in the United States range from 1 to 3 million.[108] The overall perinatal morbidity and mortality rate in infants born to mothers who abuse narcotics is significantly increased,[15] manifested by low birth weight, neurologic and mental disorders, as well as the neonatal withdrawal syndrome.[53]
- An estimated 10 million Americans are regular cocaine users and another 5 million have tried the drug.[26]
- It has been estimated that between 13,600 and 22,600 U.S. physicians are or will become alcoholics.[11]
- The Medical Association of Georgia Impaired Physician Program evaluated 1225 physicians *nationally* between July 1975 and September 1987 for diagnosis and treatment of impairment. More than 90% of the physicians treated had been chemically dependent[111]; 11% of these were anesthesiologists.[22,32] By contrast, fewer than 4.0% of all U.S. physicians are anesthesiologists.[94,117]

As patients who abuse various substances present to the medical community for care, there is increasing recognition of a need for specialty training in addiction medicine. Most physicians do not receive formal training in this field during medical school or residency[2] and thus lack knowledge and confidence for detection and constructive management of substance abuse in their patients. McDougal[73] addresses this problem as follows:

> As a professional community, we do poorly. Again and again, addicts tell of visiting emergency rooms, grossly under the influence of drugs, without a word or an action about the cause [of their medical problem]. Office-based practitioners will prescribe narcotics, sedatives, and antidepressants to persons who should be asked if they have or ever had drug difficulty. Teaching hospitals are not better; the majority of urban university hospital ward patients may be alcoholics or heroin addicts, each being skillfully and enthusiastically treated for the complications of the disease that brought them to the hospital. You will look long and hard to find a problem list with addiction as *the* diagnosis, or even *a* diagnosis. The primary, underlying disease is invisible, like the proverbial clothes of the emperor. Addiction is not diagnosed, treated, or staged; the need or fitness for recovery programs postdischarge are usually not part of discharge planning or prescribing.[73]

As the medical community acknowledges the magnitude of the problems associated with these patients, anecdotal experiences are being replaced by more systematic research in attempts to optimize medical care. In the last decade, a large medical institution developed a multidisciplinary, comprehensive, and integrated educational approach to issues of alcohol and other substance abuse.[77] As part of this process, all new admissions to the adult inpatient services of this academic hospital were surveyed with a questionnaire that included screening instruments (CAGE and an abbreviated version of the MAST) (Boxes 30-1 and 30-2)[13,25,34,77,125] to detect alcohol abuse. Results indicate that screen-positive alcohol abuse (defined as two or more positive answers on the CAGE or a score of five or more on the short MAST) is found in approximately 25% of the patients (for both medical and surgical admission). Detection rates by the house staff and faculty

---

BOX 30-1
CAGE ALCOHOLISM SCREENING TEST

Have you ever felt you should **C**ut down on your drinking?
Have people **A**nnoyed you by criticizing your drinking?
Have you ever felt bad or **G**uilty about your drinking?
Have you ever had a drink, as an **E**ye-opener, in the morning?

From Bush B et al: Screening for alcohol abuse using the CAGE questionnaire, *Am J Med* 82:231, 1987.

physicians caring for those patients who were admitted to medical and surgical wards were between 25% and 50%, and the rate was greater than 50% in psychiatry. If they did recognize an alcohol abuse problem, physicians intervened in only 50% to 75% of the cases. Based on their findings, Moore et al.[77] recommended that:

- Alcoholism-screening tests should be used with all patients as part of the physician's routine history-taking
- Alcohol abuse can affect all demographic and socioeconomic strata; physicians, however, tended to recognize it more often in the lower socioeconomic group
- A brief physician's intervention can be effective in motivating patients who abuse alcohol to change their behaviors or to seek appropriate treatment

The goals of this part of the chapter are to introduce issues of substance abuse and dependence, identify classes of abused substances, highlight associated medical problems (such as withdrawal syndromes), discuss strategies of perioperative management, and present options for postoperative analgesia and discharge planning. In the Appendix, we include the *1991 Resource and Referral Guide,* published by the National Council on Alcoholism and Drug Dependence, Inc.,[93] along with summary boxes for quick reference.

In the next part of the chapter, issues are presented relating to the perioperative management of persons who are in recovery from alcoholism or drug addiction and who are thus abstinent at the time of surgery but remain at risk for relapse. These individuals require special care to avoid exacerbation of their chemical dependency by injudicious use of psychoactive agents; however, they also need appropriate analgesia to minimize the stress of surgery, which can itself contribute to relapse.

Definitions, Mechanisms, and Consequences of Addiction

To understand the phenomenon of addiction it is useful to understand the mechanisms of drug self-administration and the abuse liability of the different drugs that are self-administered (for a nonmedical purpose). Drug self-administration is the rule rather than the exception in modern society; most of us consume caffeine, with an average daily U.S. ingestion of 320 mg.[33] Also an estimated 90% of the U.S. adult population drinks alcohol, and 30% smoke nicotine-containing tobacco.

The abuse liability of a drug is a function of the environment, the characteristics of the drug in question, and the population using it.[113]

A. Environment: For a subject to use a drug, he/she must first be exposed to it; then the drug must remain available for continued use; finally, the expectation(s) of the subject or of the observer will influence the subjective effect of the drug (e.g., peer pressure).

B. Four characteristics of a drug influence its rate of self-administration:

1. Its ability to cause a desired subjective effect, that is, to act as a *positive reinforcer.*
2. A *short latency* between administration and onset of action, in the order of seconds to

---

BOX 30-2
BRIEF MICHIGAN ALCOHOLISM SCREENING TEST (MAST)

Questions	Check One	
1. Do you feel you are a normal drinker?	Yes (0)	No (2)
2. Do friends or relatives think you are a normal drinker?	Yes (0)	No (2)
3. Have you ever attended a meeting of Alcoholics Anonymous (AA)?	Yes (5)	No (0)
4. Have you ever lost friends or girlfriends or boyfriends because of drinking?	Yes (2)	No (0)
5. Have you ever gotten into trouble at work because of drinking?	Yes (2)	No (0)
6. Have you ever neglected your obligations, your family, or your work for 2 or more days in a row because you were drinking?	Yes (2)	No (0)
7. Have you ever had delirium tremens or severe shaking, heard voices, or seen things that were not there after heavy drinking?	Yes (2)	No (0)
8. Have you ever gone to anyone for help about your drinking?	Yes (5)	No (0)
9. Have you ever been in a hospital because of drinking?	Yes (5)	No (0)
10. Have you ever been arrested for drunk driving or driving after drinking?	Yes (2)	No (0)

Note: Alcoholism is indicated by a score of greater than 5. Test scores are determined by tallying values of answers, which are on a progressive scale of 0, 2, and 5.
From Yersin B et al: Accuracy of the Michigan Alcoholism Screening Test for screening of alcoholism in patients of a medical department, *Arch Intern Med* 149:2071, 1989.

BOX 30-3
DIAGNOSTIC CRITERIA FOR PSYCHOACTIVE SUBSTANCE USE DISORDERS

Diagnostic criteria for psychoactive substance dependence

A. At least three of the following:
1. Substance often taken in larger amounts or over a longer period than the person intended
2. Persistent desire or one or more unsuccessful efforts to reduce or control substance use
3. A great deal of time spent in activities necessary to obtain the substance (e.g., theft), taking the substance (e.g., chain smoking), or recovering from its effects
4. Frequent intoxication or withdrawal symptoms when person is expected to fulfill major role obligations at work, school, or home (e.g., does not go to work because "hung over," goes to school or work "high," intoxicated while caring for children), or when substance use is physically hazardous (e.g., driving when intoxicated)
5. Important social, occupational, or recreational activities given up or reduced because of substance use
6. Continued substance use despite knowledge of having a persistent or recurrent social, psychologic, or physical problem that is caused or exacerbated by the use of the substance (e.g., continued heroin use despite family arguments about it, cocaine-induced depression, or an ulcer worsened by drinking)

7. Marked tolerance or the need for markedly increased amounts of the substance (i.e., at least a 50% increase) to achieve intoxication or desired effect or markedly diminished effect with continued use of the same amount

Note: The following items may not apply to cannabis, hallucinogens, or phencyclidine (PCP) abuse:

8. Characteristic withdrawal symptoms (see specific withdrawal syndromes under Psychoactive Substance–Induced Organic Mental Disorders)
9. Substance often taken to relieve or avoid withdrawal symptoms

B. Some symptoms of the disturbance have persisted for at least 1 month or have occurred repeatedly over a long period of time

Diagnostic criteria for psychoactive susbtance abuse

A. A maladaptive pattern of psychoactive substance use indicated by at least one of the following:
1. Continued use despite knowledge of having a persistent or recurrent social, occupational, psychologic, or phsyical problem that is caused or exacerbated by use of the psychoactive substance
2. Recurrent use in situations in which use is physically hazardous (e.g., driving while intoxicated)

B. Some symptoms of the disturbance have persisted for at least 1 month or have occurred repeatedly over a longer period of time

C. Never met the criteria for psychoactive substance dependence for this substance

Modified from Spitzer RL, Williams JB, eds: *Diagnostic and statistical manual of mental disorders: DSM-III-R*, ed 3, Washington, DC, 1987, American Psychiatric Association.

---

minutes (importance of the memory-linking stimulus to effect); for instance, phenobarbital has a low abuse potential compared to thiopental.
3. Drug *concentration* (e.g., alcoholics, in testing conditions, will self-administer alcohol in higher doses when it is in the form of liquor vs. beer).
4. **Ratio** between the desired subjective effect and the medical therapeutic efficacy: drugs with a high ratio have a low abuse potential.

C. Population: Different individuals show different drug preferences; there seem to be ethnic, racial, and inherited differences in the vulnerability of an individual to become chemically dependent[21]; the corollary is that the abuse liability of a drug is a function of the population tested (e.g., normal volunteers vs. drug abusers).

Drug dependence is a medical disorder that has been recognized as such by the American Medical Association (AMA)[6] and the American College of Physicians (ACP).[5]

Psychoactive substance use disorders constitute a diagnostic entity classified in the *Diagnostic and Statistical Manual of Mental Disorders,* 3rd edition, revised (DSM-III-R).[101] **Psychoactive substance dependence** (Box 30-3) is characterized by a progressive loss of control over the quantity of substance consumed, a narrowing of the range of activities around substance using, the onset of tolerance (i.e., the need for larger quantities of the drug to obtain the same effect), and with continued use, the development of drug-specific withdrawal syndromes. **Psychoactive substance abuse** (Box 30-3) is described as a maladaptive pattern of substance use that has not met the criteria for dependence but is continued despite recurrent social, occupational, psychologic, or physical problems, or in situations when use is physically hazardous (driving while intoxicated). The essential feature of both dependence and abuse is the conception that the person has impaired control of use of a substance(s) and experiences a compulsion to use despite adverse consequences. The clinical course may vary as a function of the substance used or the susceptibility of the individual to the toxic effect(s) of the drug so that patients may come for medical attention under different circumstances. For example, a young adolescent may present to the emergency room with an acute psychotic episode after ingesting phencyclidine for the first time (pathologic intoxication), or a surgical patient may develop opioid withdrawal symptoms after elective surgery although neither spouse nor colleagues may notice any cognitive impairment (they may state, however, that the patient had missed work more frequently recently, that he/she avoided social contacts, and that he/she seemed irritable).

The degree of **tolerance** for the toxic effects of a drug does not increase in parallel with the degree of tolerance for the desired euphoric effect, so that the risk of a toxic reaction increases as the dose is increased.[124] Tolerance is explained through pharmacologic (e.g., increased elimination), neurophysiologic (e.g., decreased number of postsynaptic receptors), and behavioral mechanisms (stimulus-conditioned compensatory response). The last factor may explain sudden decrease in tolerance when the drug is administered in an environment that is unusual to the subject (e.g., hospital).

The **spectrum** of intensity of the dependence syndrome ranges from mild to severe. The patient may be in partial or full remission although he/she can never be considered cured since the risk of relapse remains a potential threat (see later discussion).

Eleven classes of psychoactive drugs are commonly taken nonmedically: alcohol; sedatives, hypnotics, and anxiolytics; amphetamines and other sympathomimetics; cocaine; opioids; hallucinogens; phencyclidine and other arylcyclohexylamines; cannabis; inhalants; caffeine; and nicotine. All of these substances are open to abuse and dependence except for nicotine (for which no abuse syndrome is described but which leads to dependence in the majority of its users) and caffeine (although recent research indicates that

withdrawal symptoms occur when daily consumption of caffeine is abruptly interrupted). This caffeine dependence syndrome has been associated with postoperative headaches and other complaints.[45]

The Appendix at the end of this chapter lists, by class of substance, the symptoms and signs associated with intoxication, tolerance and dependence, and withdrawal along with suggestions for their management. Specific implications for anesthesia are included.

In a patient who is physically dependent on a psychoactive drug (mainly alcohol, sedative/hypnotic, or opioid), a reduction or abrupt discontinuation of drug use may precipitate a **withdrawal syndrome,** the nature of which varies depending on the drug (see the Appendix). Hospitalization for trauma or other acute medical or surgical illness, by causing an interruption in the patient's lifestyle, may initiate the syndrome. In the case of opioid dependence, the patient's anxiety, triggered by the justified fear that the health care team may decide not to treat withdrawal, will exacerbate the syndrome, making him/her less able to cope with pain and other stressful stimuli. In fact, few physicians realize that opioid withdrawal is associated with hyperalgesia (although animal studies have clearly demonstrated this phenomenon).[121] Such a situation sets the stage for conflicts, promotes patient noncompliance, and further complicates clinical management.

In the case of alcohol dependence, the onset of withdrawal can be acute or delayed up to 10 days after the last ingestion of alcohol. In the case of sedatives, the onset can be delayed even further, depending on the half-life of the drug. For opioid dependence, withdrawal typically occurs within 48 hours of the last drug administration.

The emergence of physiologic and psychologic symptoms of withdrawal in the perioperative period may be both confusing and dangerous. The following should be considered:

- **Intermittent or recurrent withdrawal:** The syndrome is recognized and the intervention initiated; however, the process is interrupted by repeated surgical procedures and use of anesthetic polypharmacy.
- **Complicated withdrawal:** The syndrome is recognized, but the intervention is limited by the cardiovascular or neurologic instability of the patient under concurrent surgical or medical stress. In the case of alcohol withdrawal, the instability of the patient may preclude the necessary sedation that optimal withdrawal management would imply.
- **Perioperative transition:** From intoxication to withdrawal, such as during a lengthy surgical procedure on a patient with multiple trauma, the

syndrome may express itself through diametrically opposed cardiovascular responses. Pharmacologic treatment of the first state may exaggerate the second; a narcotic overdose complicated by trauma with unknown blood loss and hypotension may require use of vasopressors. The situation may change abruptly with onset of withdrawal, confusing the estimation of volume of electrolyte solution needed to truly stabilize the patient.

The same patient may progress through more than one of the previous stages at different times during hospitalization. It should be noted that underdiagnosis as well as overdiagnosis of withdrawal can lead to patient mismanagement.

- **Unrecognized withdrawal:** A medical intervention is initiated on the basis of a presumed medical condition, with similar signs and symptoms that mislead the clinician as to the real cause. Such diagnostic error may worsen the patient's condition (e.g., an unrecognized opioid-dependent patient under anesthesia develops acute tachycardia, hypertension, and acidosis, and is treated with dantrolene for presumed malignant hyperthermia).
- **Unrecognized medical event, interpreted as withdrawal:** An intervention is initiated, with success, to stabilize a patient with presumed alcohol withdrawal during general anesthesia, thus leaving undiagnosed the true medical condition (e.g., tachycardia and hypertension caused by pheochromocytoma). Indeed, use of beta-blocking agents or clonidine may be appropriate in both situations although the pheochromocytoma remains undiagnosed.

The following principles are suggested to minimize undesirable consequences of withdrawal during the perioperative period. A thorough preanesthetic assessment of the pattern of psychoactive substance use is essential for good patient management and is reviewed in the next section. In addition, the following should be stressed:

- The withdrawal syndrome should be part of the differential diagnosis (but not the sole diagnosis considered) of any complication occurring during the perioperative period.
- Narcotic analgetics should not be withdrawn during the immediate postoperative period, but, on the contrary, should be administered as required (often in larger doses and for shorter intervals than for a nonchemically dependent patient). If an open, respectful physician-patient relationship is developed in the preanesthetic evaluation, it is less likely that the patient will engage in what is commonly called "drug-seeking

behavior." Two mechanisms explain the patient's requirement for increased analgetic doses: tolerance and the hyperalgesia of opioid withdrawal (related to dysfunction of the endogenous opioid system, which will be reviewed later in the chapter). Although hyperalgesia has not been clearly demonstrated during alcohol withdrawal, the associated anxiety decreases the tolerance threshold to nociceptive stimuli. Moreover, pharmacologic and psychologic tolerance can clearly be observed across different classes of psychoactive drugs.

- Pharmacologic management of the withdrawal syndrome should be directed at the prevention of serious complications (seizure, hyperthermia, hypertension with wound hemorrhage, injury to self and others), the relief of subjective symptoms including anxiety, and the attenuation of detrimental stresses both endogenous (fever of sepsis) and exogenous (noisy environment, bright lights). Therapy includes the use of specific pharmacologic agents (as indicated in the Appendix) as well as rehydration, electrolyte replacement, and nutritional supplementation, including thiamine and other vitamins.
- After successful withdrawal management and clinical stabilization, it is the clinician's duty to confront the patient with the consequences of his/her substance use pattern, emphasizing that he/she seems to have lost control over the compulsion to use, despite his/her otherwise sound judgment, so as to attenuate detrimental guilt (which may externalize itself in the form of aggressive, defiant behavior). The patient's responsibility is not in having a disease, but in developing the appropriate support system to achieve abstinence, or perhaps, in the case of opioid dependence, rehabilitation in the setting of a methadone treatment program.
- If available, early consultation with an addiction specialist may circumvent impending disasters, accelerate recovery, and facilitate discharge planning by organizing treatment of the substance use disorder. A resource guide to aid this process can be found in the Appendix at the end of this chapter.

Preanesthetic Evaluation

The anesthesiologist becomes involved in the medical management of substance-abusing or dependent patients in a variety of clinical situations. The purpose of this section is to highlight the comorbid conditions associated with acute or chronic use of psychoactive drugs; the Appendix provides a short overview by specific substance class with potential implications for the conduct of anesthesia. The anesthesiologist should consider these, as well as the presence of any known concurrent illnesses, when evaluating patients for surgery.

The following principles should be applied to the preanesthetic evaluation:

- All patients should be screened for alcohol and substance abuse preoperatively. Boxes 30-1 and 30-2 show two examples of alcohol-abuse screening instruments that are short, reliable, and widely used.[13,25,34,125] When indicated (traumatic injuries, uncooperative patient, etc.), blood alcohol level and a toxicity screen (blood and urine) should be obtained because the results aid in the assessment of the degree of tolerance, the risk for subsequent withdrawal, and the specific symptoms and signs that may be expected. Such objective information is useful later in the patient's clinical course to confront a possible denial of an alcohol or drug problem.

- A nonjudgmental, compassionate, but assertive approach to the alcohol or drug problem lays the groundwork for a fruitful therapeutic relationship and decreases the patient's anxiety (and thus the intensity of a potential withdrawal syndrome). At this stage, if the patient's state of consciousness allows, the clinician should ask about previous episodes of withdrawal and clearly state that, if such a complication threatens to occur, it will be addressed and promptly treated. This may encourage the patient to share past experiences and will guide the clinician in his/her choice of therapeutic intervention. Patients usually remember clinicians who show respect for them, and this will be beneficial in later clinical management. Moreover, when clinical signs are confusing, verbal information (or other forms of patient communication, if intubation is necessary) may clarify the situation.

- Once a good rapport has been established, and the patient is confident that his/her alcohol or drug dependence will be part of comprehensive clinical management, the clinician should assess the extent of the problem. Inquiries about each class of drugs should be made because polysubstance abuse is the rule. The majority of alcoholics are heavy smokers, and a significant proportion have used benzodiazepines to treat their alcohol-related anxiety or insomnia. The CAGE questions can be used to detect loss of control in the use of any type of drug.

Although the previous assessment may seem cumbersome to conduct for every preanesthetic evaluation, the high prevalence of undetected alcohol and substance abuse in hospitalized patients must be recognized. If negative, this assessment will take only a few minutes; if positive, it will potentially save invaluable time and resources in the perioperative period, in addition to providing the opportunity for intervention and recovery.

Complications

There are a number of complications associated with intravenous drug abuse and its associated lifestyle that are not substance specific. Although many of these (e.g., endocarditis) are well known to anesthesiologists, especially in large urban hospital settings, other, less extensively studied complications (pulmonary fibrosis) may be of clinical relevance as well.

Infections are the major complications of intravenous drug use.[49,50] Systemic infections include viral hepatitis (A, B, delta, and C), HIV, syphilis, bacterial sepsis, and tuberculosis. A history of hepatitis has been found in 50% of addicts screened, with one third having repeat episodes. Hepatitis B surface antigen screening is positive in 2.2% of addicts—four times the incidence in the general population.[38] In 1981, acquired immunodeficiency syndrome (AIDS) was first reported in drug abusers in the United States. By 1989, between 5% and 20% of intravenous drug abusers in the United States were infected with HIV and accounted for 75% of all heterosexually transmitted cases of AIDS.[123] Preoperative HIV testing is suggested by some, but the issue is controversial. Many states require informed patient consent, which may not be possible at the time of initial patient presentation. Even before the onset of AIDS, it was recognized that chemically dependent persons had multifactorial impairments of the immune response.[78] Chronic alcoholics are prone to pneumococcal pneumonia, dental decay, and aspiration pneumonia, often complicated by lung abscesses. Intravenous drug abusers are even more likely than other patients with AIDS to be exposed to opportunistic infections, which tend to have a more rapidly fatal course. Tuberculosis is again reaching epidemic proportions in this population, as a result of worsened living conditions (crowded shelters for the homeless) and the AIDS epidemic. This has special importance for anesthesia because tuberculosis can be contracted by other patients through insufficiently decontaminated ventilators or by the anesthesiologist through inhalation of infected air droplets (when suctioning a patient's airway without the anesthesiologist wearing a protective mask).

Localized infections include abscesses at the injection sites, involvement of inner organs with endocarditis (usually of the tricuspid valve) and lung abscesses possibly followed by metastatic abscesses to the left heart or the brain (with progressive or sudden change in mental status), and kidney abscesses (with recurrent, unexplained urinary tract infections and urosepsis).

The injection of unknown contaminants, used to "cut drugs," into the bloodstream is responsible for other complications of intravenous drug use. Talc or other inert substances lodge in the pulmonary capillaries and cause an inflammatory reaction that, over time, can result in pulmonary fibrosis and restrictive lung disease. Administration of quinidine/quinine in a patient deficient in glucose-6-phosphate dehydrogenase may cause hemolysis. Repeat injection of highly antigenic, contaminated solutions stimulates the immune system chronically, resulting in an increase in circulating globulins and hyperproteinemia. False-positive serologic test results are common in intravenous drug users.

Liver function tests (LFTs) are frequently abnormal secondary to hepatitis, HIV, and/or toxicity from fillers used to cut pure drugs.[36,61] Hepatic dysfunction associated with alcohol abuse usually takes 10 to 15 years to develop; however, cirrhosis with permanent and/or reversible changes can occur in the liver following one or more acute episodes.[85] Narcotic addicts have been reported in one series to have an 83% incidence of abnormal, clinically asymptomatic LFTs with increases of alanine aminotransferase, asparate aminotransferase, and alkaline phosphatase.[38] Possible explanations include malnutrition and chronic reaction to talc and other contaminants of abused drugs, concurrent infection with hepatitis B or C virus, and chronic alcohol abuse. This chronic toxic reaction may explain the prevalence of cirrhosis in young addicts (with significantly earlier onset than in abusers of alcohol only).[21]

Special attention should be directed to electrocardiographic abnormalities, including atrial and ventricular disturbances, prolonged QTc interval, evidence of previous myocardial infarction (cocaine), left ventricular hypertrophy or, as indicators of pulmonary hypertension, right ventricular hypertrophy, right atrial enlargement, and biphasic T waves. Transthoracic or transesophageal echocardiograms are invaluable techniques to view valvular pathologic conditions, investigate sources of embolic events, and assess cardiac function. Right-sided endocarditis and complications of septic emboli are reemerging as major problems with drug abusers. Issues of prophylactic antibiotic coverage or cardiac surgery may need to be addressed.[85]

Chest radiographs may show evidence of pneumothorax (after intrajugular or supraclavicular drug injection), interstitial infiltrate, scarring, abscesses, cardiac enlargement, and hilar lymphadenopathy. Pulmonary function tests are particularly useful to assess both obstructive and restrictive lung disease; both are prevalent in this population.

Toxicologic assays may be useful in both acute and elective circumstances. In patients with acute intoxication who exhibit clinical signs and symptoms characteristic of various psychoactive substances, blood and urine tests are a necessity. Most results for both urine and blood screens are available within the hour. In urgent or trauma situations, blood and urine samples are obtained by the trauma team preoperatively or by the anesthesiologist perioperatively. Because most psychoactive substances can be detected in the urine for up to 48 hours or longer, toxicology screens can be obtained on patients seen in the preadmission testing center for elective surgery to corroborate the presence of psychoactive substances. In addition, certain drug metabolites may be present in chronic abusers for longer time periods (greater than 48 hours). If a patient presents with symptoms of confusion that may indicate a withdrawal syndrome, a positive urine test result may aid in the diagnosis and facilitate appropriate therapy. Specific blood levels of psychoactive substances may be useful in determining drug tolerance (i.e., high blood levels without clinical evidence of toxicity may indicate chronic use of that substance or a cross-tolerant substance).

Complete blood counts may reveal suppression of erythropoiesis, leukopoiesis, and thrombopoiesis, reflecting a direct substance effect (e.g., ethanol),[109] or a secondary effect due to poor nutrition or an infectious process. A 25% incidence of chronic anemia was reported in one series of methadone maintenance patients.[26]

Serum electrolyte test results may reflect primary renal pathologic conditions or secondary effects from poor health and nutrition, intravenous dehydration, and trauma with resultant myoglobinemia from tissue necrosis and subsequent obstruction of renal tubules leading to failure. In addition, Na^+/K^+ disturbances may reflect initial diuresis (decreased levels of antidiuretic hormone) followed by antidiuretic effects of alcohol. Rhabdomyolysis has been reported in heroin addicts, probably secondary to unknown components in adulterated heroin, and is diagnosed by dark urine with myoglobin and free hemoglobin present.[38] Rhabdomyolysis has also been described as a reperfusion injury in cocaine users.

Premedication

Simple rules to premedicate for anesthesia should be followed to meet the physiologic and psychologic needs of patients who abuse various substances. The most important principle is to avoid withdrawal perioperatively; detoxification should never be done at the time of surgery. Such a procedure is not only counterproductive but dangerous. The premedication should provide sufficient sedation and anxiolysis while accounting for increased tolerance to most sedatives and narcotics. Caution is required in recording patients' self-reports of the daily dose of "street drug" used since they may be misinformed themselves; drugs are "cut" several times by dealers to increase profit, and the consumer usually gets a variable portion of the "dose" bought.

Alcohol-dependent patients should be premedicated with a long-acting cross-tolerant drug such as benzodiazepine (diazepam, chlordiazepoxide) or a barbiturate (phenobarbital). An adequate premedication will attenuate the patient's anxiety and thus the intensity of a potential withdrawal.

Opioid-dependent patients who are actively using drugs should receive enough narcotics to manage both pain and withdrawal. The patient's daily dose should be considered a physiologic baseline to which normal premedication is added. As stressed earlier, if good communication has been established, the patient can be a reliable indicator in relating the subjective effect. A dose of 20 mg of methadone (IM) can effectively stabilize a patient before the induction of anesthesia and may attenuate symptoms of withdrawal postoperatively.

Opioid-dependent patients enrolled in a methadone program should receive their usual oral daily dose before surgery. Physicians should not rely on the patient's information regarding the daily dose but should call the program for this information. This also allows the program to note the patient's hospitalization, so that the client will not be terminated from the program because of unexplained "no-show."

There is little information regarding special premedication for **other drug dependencies.** Neuroleptics and benzodiazepines may be indicated to treat psychotic states and agitation, cocaine-induced paranoia, and other thought disorders. Anxiolytics with little or no reinforcing properties, such as buspirone,[62] hydroxyzine, and halazepam[46] (benzodiazepine with slow onset of action), can provide the necessary sedation, without attracting the patient to a new substance (see section on analgesia, alternative treatments).

Premedication of the chemically dependent patient in remission merits special attention and is addressed in a later section of this chapter.

Anesthetic Techniques

General pharmacologic considerations should be remembered when planning anesthesia for patients who abuse various substances. Altered and variable pharmacokinetics influence the type of anesthetic agents used, as well as the doses. Drug interactions can lead to increased or decreased elimination and decreased or increased toxicity.[23] For example, alcohol can acutely protect the liver against enflurane toxicity, but chronic alcohol ingestion may, through enzyme induction (microsomal P450IIE1), cause significant elevation of transaminase.[114] A chronically damaged liver with borderline function can be precipitated into failure through the added stress of a surgical illness or the toxicity of some anesthetic agents. Substances with high lipid solubility (e.g., PCP) accumulate in the fat tissues and are released unpredictably into the circulation, with consequent fluctuation in mental states over a period of time of several days to weeks. Chronic use of nicotine accelerates the elimination of certain drugs (aminophylline) and slows the metabolism of others. Acute smoking cessation during hospitalization may unpredictably reverse these trends.

No single choice of anesthetic technique addresses all the issues that surround patients who abuse substances. Relevant features include severity of presentation and associated illnesses, surgical requirements, and ability of the anesthesiologist.[28] The Appendix lists perioperative considerations of specific psychoactive drugs and anesthetic interactions. Choice of agents or technique is often dictated by contraindications or limitations.

Limitations of regional techniques include patient cooperation, presence of coagulopathy, infection at site of placement, intravascular dehydration, true allergy to an anesthetic/narcotic or inability to metabolize a drug, neuropathy, potentially unprotected airway, technical difficulty, and/or site of surgical procedure. Depending on the patient and experience of the anesthesiologist, any or all of these limitations may apply. In addition, the anesthesiologist faces an increased risk of infection with every invasive procedure performed on such patients.

Limitations of general anesthesia include use of polypharmacy, which may result in untoward drug interactions; decreased ability by the patient to metabolize and excrete certain classes of anesthetics with increased potential for toxicity from such agents; masking of potential withdrawal signs with anesthetics and nonanesthetic agents that ultimately may increase the severity of the withdrawal syndrome; and potential for profound dysrhythmogenic and depressant effects of general anesthetics on the cardiovascular system.

Specific limitations of general anesthetic agents must be individualized to the degree of organ dysfunction of the patient. Patients with enzyme induction may increase the metabolism of inhalational agents, resulting in toxicity. Isoflurane is theoretically the agent of choice in patients with less than 1% liver metabolism but may be limited by dose-dependent cardiovascular effects. Actions of nondepolarizing neuromuscular blocking agents may be increased secondary to decreased K^+ or Mg^{++} or may be decreased as a result of altered protein binding or decreased cholinesterase activity at the motor end plate. Actions of succinylcholine may be increased secondary to diminished plasma cholinesterase production. Atracurium, with partial Hoffman elimination, may be the agent of choice. Clinical literature concerning requirements of anesthetics in chronic alcoholics is confusing. Does enzyme induction result in increased metabolism of anesthetic agents with subsequent increased toxicity, or rather does increased tolerance lead to increased requirements?[110] The anesthetic requirements of chronic alcoholics for induction of anesthesia with thiopental were investigated using an electroencephalographic (EEG) measure of thiopental's central nervous system drug effect and pharmacodynamic modeling to relate thiopental serum concentrations to drug effect. The investigation reported no differences in thiopental pharmacokinetic and pharmacodynamic parameters or dose requirements, according to EEGs, between alcoholics and nonalcoholics. Swerdlow et al.[110] suggested reconsideration of a priori increases in barbiturate induction doses in these patients. To date, there is no definitive study of minimum alveolar concentration (MAC) and alcoholism. Clinical experience affirms the broad spectrum of individual responses.[11]

The use of combined regional/general techniques intraoperatively with uninterrupted transition to postoperative pain management may be ideal for these patients. There are few literature reports to guide the anesthesiologist.

General considerations for the operative management of these patients include difficulties assessing preoperative intravascular states and assessing ongoing fluid losses in the face of ascites and sympathomimetic effects of abused drugs. Electrolyte imbalances and problems in maintaining body temperature may predispose the patient to life-threatening dysrhythmias.

Postoperative Pain and Other Considerations

A noxious neural stimulus is not passively received but is filtered, even at the first sensory synapse, by complex modulatory systems.[119] Endorphins are endogenous substances with analgetic properties similar to exogenous opioids such as morphine and seem to function as neuromodulators rather than classical neurotransmitters[76]; other and less understood nonopioid pain-modulating systems also exist, such as in environmentally produced analgesia, which is only partially antagonized by the opioid antagonist naloxone.[39] The Pavlovian classical paradigm demonstrates that the production of analgesia can be conditioned, and this type of analgesia can be completely reversed by use of naloxone.[119] Use of naloxone can decrease

the pain threshold of volunteers with naturally high pain thresholds but will not influence volunteers with low pain thresholds.[86] Use of naloxone also increases the intensity of pain in subjects already experiencing pain, whereas the increase in pain threshold produced by acupuncture, but not by hypnosis, can be entirely reversed by administration of naloxone.[119] Thus the experience of pain is modulated by the endogenous system of analgesia located in the spinal cord and the periaqueducal gray matter in the brainstem. This system, in turn, is a function of the individual's affective state (anxiety, depression), previous conditioning (cultural influences), and the environment in which nociception occurs (quiet or noisy room, friendly or hostile caregivers).[55] Consequently, pain is enhanced during withdrawal (such as naloxone-precipitated hyperalgesia),[10,121] fear,[96] depression, and after a previous negative experience in a hospitalized setting. Moreover, it has been shown that chronic administration of morphine decreases the endogenous production of endorphins.[40] Reports in the medical literature have often impugned patients with chemical dependencies for their "neurotic, even psychotic, nervous behavior, lowered tolerance to pain,"[57] and nagging "drug-seeking behavior." However, when considering the aforementioned scientific information, **patients who are opioid dependent should rather be treated on the model of patients who are corticoid dependent, with exogenously induced adrenal insufficiency, who need extra corticosteroid when faced with the stress of surgery.** Indeed, withdrawing adequate postoperative opioid analgesia from a dependent patient induces the behavioral components of endogenous opioid deficiency. This section of the chapter attempts to provide clinicians with some strategies to provide adequate analgesia to patients who are chemically dependent, with the understanding that:

Attempting to change drug habits in the face of acute illness is dangerous. Proper treatment is rational therapy for the illness with full realization of the disease associated with the drug abuse. An organized plan of approach is more important than choices in therapeutic agents.[85]

For the patient actively using mu agonists, use of opioids such as methadone, morphine sulfate, or a combination of both is indicated for the first 3 to 4 days after surgery. Methadone's duration of action for analgesia is only about 5 hours, so that accumulation is likely to occur during adequate pain control. If morphine alone is used, it should be administered at frequent and fixed intervals (e.g., every 2 to 3 hours) and at higher doses than for a nontolerant patient. Patient-controlled analgesia (PCA) may be indicated. Using methadone to stabilize the patient's opioid system (10 to 20 mg IM, or 20 to 40 mg orally, once a day) and then adding morphine at the usual analgetic dose may be the most appealing option because it clearly addresses the two problems separately. If this option is chosen, the short-acting opioid can be discontinued after the acute postoperative period and the opioid dependence can then be addressed, if possible with consultation with a specialist in addiction medicine. Several alternate therapeutic algorithms are possible depending on the patient's status and are discussed following:

- For a patient desiring referral to a methadone program on discharge (and such arrangements can be made), the individual should continue to use the methadone dose that suppresses withdrawal objectively and subjectively without causing drowsiness, and discharge should be coordinated with the methadone program. Some programs give priority admissions for patients with positive HIV serologies.

- For patients not interested in methadone treatment, who would rather be detoxified, three options are offered. The first is to taper the methadone use, decreasing the dose by 10% every third day. This can be done with the adjunct of a clonidine transdermal patch.[72,77] In the second option, a rapid detoxification protocol can be obtained by administering increasing doses of naltrexone with decreasing doses of clonidine.[17] A third approach is to begin use of buprenorphine, a partial mu agonist/antagonist with high receptor affinity that provides good analgesia and is associated with a very mild withdrawal syndrome.[87] Its use, however, cannot be mixed with other mu agonists, and it should be administered at least 12 hours after the last short-acting opioid, or 24 hours following the last methadone dose. A brief review of the pharmacology of buprenorphine is included in the Appendix.

- If the patient is already enrolled in a methadone treatment program, the usual daily dose is given (also on the day of surgery; see discussion of premedication), and short-acting opioids are added for treatment of analgesia at the same dose as for a usual patient, for 3 to 4 days. Patient care should be coordinated with the patient's methadone program; the methadone program must know when to prepare the patient's dose on the first day after discharge, and some programs can provide basic primary care, including administration of daily medications (antibiotics, AZT, Antabuse) or even dressing changes.

- If the patient is in remission from opioid dependence, systemic mu agonists should be used with caution, because the mu receptors are thought to

be responsible for inducing dependence.[1,20] Spinal analgesia may be preferred for these patients. because the opioid receptors located in the spinal cord are both kappa[48,122] and mu and euphoria caused by rostral spread to the midbrain is unlikely. In this population, effective systemic analgesia can be obtained safely by use of kappa agonist/mu antagonist agents such as dezocine[83] or nalbuphine[24] or even the new nonsteroidal antiinflammatory drug (NSAID) ketorolac[14,68] (see the section on patients in recovery).

Postoperative pain management in patients addicted to alcohol and other nonopioid substances follows similar considerations. Adequate analgesia is essential to prevent agitation and anxiety, both of which can precipitate or worsen an impending withdrawal syndrome. The best analgesia, requiring less medication, is obtained when withdrawal states and anxiety are prevented.[96] A combination of pharmacologic, behavioral, and physical approaches results in optimal patient care, minimizing the incidence of metabolic complications, and hopefully preparing the patient for further drug treatment and rehabilitation.

Analgesia is provided with adequate narcotics in the early postoperative period. Table 30-1 lists equi-analgetic doses of a variety of commonly used opioids for the treatment of moderate-to-severe pain. The narcotic dose should be individualized for each patient daily; pharmacologic cross-tolerance with other central nervous system depressants, like alcohol, explains the possible requirement for higher doses of narcotics. Conversely, liver failure (which can be unsuspected in patients with normal transaminase levels) necessitates a decrease in narcotic requirement. The stress of surgery and various pharmacologic interactions may alter the narcotic requirement over time. Use of PCA circumvents these problems, and in cooperative patients is an excellent alternative. Moreover, it gives the patient a sense of control over his/her fate, which often has been long lost in the addiction process.

Although use of mu agonists is not contraindicated in alcohol- or other drug-dependent patients who are actively using substances, because of an increased vulnerability to cross-addiction in this population, it may be preferable to use partial angonists/antagonists such as dezocine, butorphanol, nalbuphine, or pentazocine, with consideration that these agents have a ceiling effect for analgesia (and respiratory depression) and that high-dose usage (equivalent to more than 90 mg of pentazocine) can induce hallucinations. Dezocine seems to have a higher ceiling for analgesia than other drugs of this class. Because of their kappa agonist actions, use of these drugs is unlikely to cause dependence or withdrawal syndrome after abrupt

Table 30-1 Equianalgetic drug chart*

Analgetic	IM route (mg)†	Oral route (mg)†	Comments‡
Morphine	10	60	IM and oral doses of morphine have durations of action of 4-6 hours; oral dose for sustained-release tablets and rectal suppositories is 3-6 times the IM dose; the lower oral dose is suggested by several clinicians; it may be appropriate for some patients, especially elderly patients with chronic cancer pain; however, practice is on anecdotal evidence, not experimental research
Buprenorphine (Buprenex)	0.4 (0.3)		Narcotic agonist-antagonist that may precipitate withdrawal in patients very physically dependent on narcotics; dose for the sublingual form (not available in the United States) is 0.8 mg; compared with morphine, it is longer acting and more likely to produce nausea and vomiting; respiratory depression is rare but serious because it is not readily reversed by administration of naloxone; not available in Canada
Butorphanol (Stadol)	2		Narcotic agonist-antagonist that may produce withdrawal in patients physically dependent on narcotics; may also produce psychomimetic effects such as hallucinations; not available in Canada
Codeine	130	200	Relatively more toxic in high doses than morphine, causing more nausea and vomiting and considerable constipation; oral dose is about 1½ times the IM dose
Fentanyl (Sublimaze)	0.05		Most common use is for anesthesia, given IV; onset of action when given IM is about 15 minutes, and duration of action is about 90 min; analgetic effect is not significantly increased by use of droperidol; has been used as a substitute for high-dose IV morphine in terminally ill patients when use of morphine causes excitation; used IV in neonates and for brief procedures
Hydromorphone (Dilaudid)	1.5	7.5	Somewhat shorter acting than morphine; also available as rectal suppository and in high-potency injectable form (10 mg/ml); the oral dose is 5 times the IM dose
Levorphanol (Levo-Dromoran)	2	4	Longer acting than morphine when given in repeated, regular doses; useful alternative to oral methadone; careful titration required because drug accumulates; both dose and interval must be adjusted; onset of action with oral dose occurs within 1½ hours; initial oral dose is twice the injectable dose; the SQ route is recommended over the IM route
Meperidine (Demerol)	75	300	Shorter acting (2-4 hours) than morphine; watch for toxic effects on CNS caused by accumulation of the active metabolite normeperidine, which produces neuroexcitability; use with caution in patients with renal disease; because of the CNS risks, 300 mg oral is not recommended; since normeperidine has a long half-life (15 hours or longer), decreasing the dose in patients exhibiting a toxic reaction may increase CNS excitability, causing seizures; effects of normeperidine are increased (not reversed) by use of naloxone; oral dose is 4 times the IM dose
Methadone (Dolophine)	10	20	Longer acting than morphine when given in repeated, regular doses; careful titration required because drug accumulates; both dose and interval must be adjusted; analgetic effect may increase with repeated doses; onset with oral dose within 1 hour; initial oral dose is twice the IM dose
Methotrimeprazine (Levoprome)	20		Phenothiazine (nonnarcotic) drug; duration of action is 4-5 hours; common adverse effect is hypotension; not recommended for ambulatory patients
Nalbuphine (Nubain)	10 (20)		Narcotic agonist-antagonist that may produce withdrawal in patients physically dependent on narcotics; longer acting and less likely to cause hypotension than morphine; in doses 10 mg/70 kg, no additional respiratory depression is caused so patient may be started on a high dose

*The equianalgetic doses in this chart are based primarily on recommendation of the American Pain Society and Analgesic Study Section, Sloan-Kettering Institute for Cancer Research, New York, based on double-blind analgetic research. Values in parentheses refer to differences of opinion among clinicians.
†Approximate doses for moderate-to-severe pain.
‡All IM and oral doses in this chart are considered equivalent to 10 mg IM morphine in analgetic effect.
From McCaffery M, Beebe A: *Pain: clinical manual for nursing practice,* St Louis, 1989, Mosby–Year Book.

Table 30-1   Equianalgetic drug chart*—cont'd

Analgetic	IM route (mg)†	Oral route (mg)†	Comments‡
Opium (Pantopon) (Opium tincture)	20 (13.3)	6 ml	Infrequently used; pantopon is the injectable form; opium tincture, the oral form; pantopon, 20 mg, equals 10 mg IV morphine or 15 mg IM morphine; opium tincture contains 1% morphine; that, is 0.6 ml equals 6 mg oral morphine; therefore 6 ml equals 60 mg oral morphine
Oxycodone		30	Has faster onset and higher peak effect than most oral narcotics; duration of action up to 6 hours; in one study of postoperative pain, a preparation similar to the old formulation of Percodan (containing oxycodone, aspirin, phenacetin, and caffeine) was more effective and caused fewer adverse reactions than 90 mg of oral codeine or 75 mg oral pentazocine and was almost equivalent to 12.5 mg IM morphine; the oral dose is 1 or 2 times the IM dose
Oxymorphone (Numorphan)	1.5		Also available as rectal suppository; 10 mg given rectally equals 10 mg IM morphine; up to 1.5 mg IM now recommended as equal to 10 mg IM morphine
Pentazocine (Talwin)	60	180	Narcotic agonist-antagonist that may produce withdrawal in patients who are physically dependent on narcotics; could produce psychomimetic effects; the oral dose is 3 times the IM dose
Propoxyphene		500	One recognized use is for mild-to-moderate pain unrelieved by non-narcotics; never give as much as 500 mg orally; only low oral doses (65-130 mg) are recommended; the IM form is not available in the United States

discontinuation; however, they can induce withdrawal if administered shortly after a mu agonist.

Other analgetic techniques with low abuse potential include spinal and epidural opioid analgesia,[48,122] but higher doses will be required in opioid-tolerant patients. The new NSAID ketorolac achieves good postoperative analgesia in nondependent patients. Although theoretically attractive, its utility in chemically dependent patients who are actively using substances has not been fully evaluated. Known side effects could add to the gastrointestinal toxicity of chronic alcohol abuse although concurrent use of sucralfate may protect the gastric mucosa and circumvent this effect.[14,112]

Chronic alcoholics and cocaine users and possibly other drug users have a high prevalence of chemically induced anxiety disorders and depression that worsens in the early phase of abstinence.[92] These symptoms can be quite debilitating and lower the patient's tolerance to aversive stimuli, such as pain, frequently encountered in the course of hospitalization. It is appropriate to mention alternative pharmacologic strategies to address these symptoms.

Benzodiazepines have a role in the treatment of withdrawal syndromes; in the brain, alcohol dependence is accompanied by a decrease in gamma-aminobutyric acid (GABA), a neurotransmitter controlling the influx of chloride ions into the neurons,

thus acting as an inhibitor of neuronal discharge. After abrupt cessation of ingestion of alcohol, which is a central nervous system depressant, there is a sudden decrease in neuronal transmembrane potential and thus a propensity to hyperexcitability and seizures. Benzodiazepines (and barbiturates) attach to independent receptors at the same chloride-ion–gate channels to increase the affinity of GABA for its receptors and thereby act as specific antiwithdrawal agents and anticonvulsants. Beyond the detoxification period, however, in this patient population the most current prescribed benzodiazepines (diazepam, alprazolam, lorazepam) have a high abuse potential because of their short onset of action and positive reinforcing properties. Benzodiazepines with longer onset of action, such as halazepam, may have a role for the longer-term treatment of anxiety in the postoperative period.[46]

Alternative agents are buspirone[44] or antihistamines such as hydroxyzine. Buspirone also increases the affinity of GABA for its receptor through an unknown mechanism.[33] It has little, if any, abuse potential (recreational benzodiazepine users dislike its effect) although it has equivalent antianxiety efficacy to diazepam or clorazepate. It does not produce impairment in psychologic performances nor sedation as with benzodiazepines.[29,62]

Antidepressants are usually not necessary in the

treatment of depression that accompanies chemical dependence because most of its symptomatology improves dramatically[107] with continued abstinence. However, in some cases (prolonged hospitalization, presence of an affective illness antedating the chemical dependence syndrome) the use of antidepressants hastens recovery and decreases the need for chronic analgetic agents.[112]

Anticonvulsants, such as phenytoin and carbamazepine, also have a use in pain treatment by decreasing the frequency of neuronal discharge.[74]

Nonpharmacologic interventions can also decrease the analgetic requirement postoperatively.[65] Transcutaneous electrical nerve stimulator (TENS) units can be placed close to the surgical wound in the operating room. Biofeedback and relaxation techniques can be useful in a cooperating patient and are better taught preoperatively. They can be started at any time, however, since they may be a welcome distraction to a patient obsessed by pain.

When treating patients who abuse substances, it is essential for health care providers to function as a cohesive team. Clear contracts with spelled-out behavioral incentives (punitive sanctions such as restriction to one's room for any in-hospital drug use or abusive behavior), reinforced by regular, randomized urine toxicity testing (including alcohol) may save many patients from being discharged against medical advice, spare the energy of the health care team, and ultimately allow for better patient management. Discharge planning should include alcohol and drug treatment rehabilitation. The anesthesiologist is ideally positioned to lead the team effort regarding these issues, as he/she becomes progressively more involved in the preoperative assessment (through preoperative consultation) and postoperative care. The Appendix includes a resource guide that presents a broad range of private and public agencies for information referral of patients and/or their families for alcohol and drug rehabilitation programs.

ANESTHESIA FOR PATIENTS IN RECOVERY FROM CHEMICAL DEPENDENCY

Even as drug and alcohol abuse continues to escalate in the United States, with the devastating effects on social and physical health, so also has grown the population of persons successfully treated for the disease of addiction. Such individuals presenting for surgery may benefit from modification of standard procedures by surgeons, anesthesiologists, and nurses. Patients with a previous history of chemical dependency, who are abstinent at the time of surgery, have special concerns regarding adequacy of pain relief in the perioperative period and exacerbation of their chemical dependency (relapse). These concerns are in addition to the common anxieties shared with nondependent surgical patients, including loss of control, body disfigurement, mortality, outcome of the procedure, and prognosis.

No widely disseminated publication has addressed in detail the perioperative treatment of formerly addicted persons, currently in recovery, although the issue is under active consideration by a committee of the American Society of Addiction Medicine.[7] Although there is a paucity of published investigative material, clearly an extensive body of clinical experience must exist among practitioners across the nation. The information and opinions presented in this section were obtained largely from interviews with surgeons, anesthesiologists, addictionists* and other specialists, professionals, and laymen with personal experience. These sources are acknowledged where appropriate.

Scope of the Problem

The National Council on Alcoholism and Drug Dependency[82] estimates the number of alcoholics in the general population to be approximately 10 million. Alcoholics Anonymous (AA) estimates its American membership at slightly more than 1 million (1991).[4] Thus it may be roughly calculated that one in 10 alcoholics is in remission at any time. Approximations may be obtained for drugs other than alcohol, although they are probably less accurate. Narcotics Anonymous (NA) World Services believes their membership is about 400,000.[80] Estimates of the total number of drug addicts vary widely, depending on specific definitions and the inclusion of "softer" substances such as marijuana. The National Clearing House for Alcohol and Drug Information claims that about 13,000,000 Americans have used an illicit drug in the last month.[81]

About 100,000 persons are under treatment for their opioid addictions with chronic methadone therapy (methadone maintenance).[63] Although controversy exists within the field of addictionology regarding the classification of these individuals as "recovered," from the patient's perspective exactly the same perioperative concerns need to be addressed.[51]

Finally, the previous estimates leave uncounted those persons formerly addicted to mood-altering substances who have managed to become abstinent through means other than the 12-step (AA, NA, etc.) anonymous programs. Vaillant reports that only two fifths of alcoholics in his study group who were

---

* *Addictionist* is the appellation officially adopted by the Nomenclature Committee of the American Society of Addiction Medicine to identify physicians with formal training in the diagnosis and treatment of alcoholism and other chemical dependencies.[7]

"securely abstinent" at the time of interview identified themselves as members of AA.[116] If this ratio is accurate and broadly applicable to the chemically dependent population, there are possibly 3 million formerly addicted/currently abstinent persons in the United States. What is the expected number of encounters between patients formerly addicted and anesthesiologists?

Based on a prospective study using established screening instruments, Moore et al. found that one in four patients admitted for surgery at a major, urban, academic hospital had overt or occult evidence of alcoholism.[77] Clearly, this astounding figure reflects the serious short- and long-term health consequences of alcohol use and its common coaddictions (i.e., tobacco). From the previously mentioned estimates, anesthesiologists at that institution should expect to encounter between 800 and 1600 formerly addicted/currently abstinent persons/year (based on 20,000 surgeries). The need for special consideration that these patients represent requires some understanding of the psychology of addiction and recovery.

Chemical Dependency: Recovery and Relapse

The predominant approach to rehabilitation adopted by treatment facilities and 12-step programs or "fellowships" views addiction within the model of a medical disease, and it is recognized as such by both the American Medical Association[6] and the American College of Physicians.[5] Thus chemical dependency is thought to have an etiology, a clinical course, and a treatment.[67]

The disease of chemical dependency affects all socioeconomic classes. Stereotypes of appearance or behavior of either actively addicted or formerly addicted persons frequently are inaccurate. Accomplished, successful professionals (including physicians, administrators, businessmen, etc.) may be chemically dependent at the time of surgery, although this fact goes unreported and unrecognized. On the other hand, thousands of disadvantaged, derelict, and criminal alcoholics and addicts have recovered from their disease to become responsible, productive, and honest citizens. For those unfortunate individuals who do not receive treatment or who do not respond to treatment, chemical dependency is frequently a chronic, debilitating, progressive disease that leads to insanity, incarceration, or death. The reversals of this disorder, which do occur, are regarded by many as a modern marvel, and relapse would be viewed as reprehensible if promoted by an iatrogenic process. Such a danger may arise in the perioperative management of the recovering addict or alcoholic. Virtually all successful rehabilitation programs have advocated rigorous abstinence from serious mood-altering substances as a touchstone of recovery.[3] Exposure to sedatives and opioids can trigger "addictive thinking" and cause a return to drug use in susceptible individuals, unless the potential for this eventually is recognized and appropriate precautions are taken.

Relapse may be viewed simply as an acute exacerbation of a chronic illness, previously in remission. Its cause, manifestations, and prognoses are complex and varied. Recovered addicts will have suffered many problems in their personal and professional lives. Estrangement from parents, spouse and children, loss of jobs, indebtedness, legal difficulties, and health disorders may be experienced during the years of chemical dependency and to varying degrees into the recovery period. Stress and discouragement inhibit rehabilitation, and therefore relapse in early recovery is common. These episodes can be exceedingly disruptive to the patient's social structure and may destroy residual support systems, leading to discontinuance of treatment, overdose, or suicide. On the other hand, many persons with stable, secure, abstinent lives – that is those successfully treated for the disease of chemical dependency – have experienced relapse in the early days of their recovery. Therefore, whereas its avoidance is a desirable goal worthy of heightened awareness and special procedures, by no means is relapse an inevitable tragedy.

Why are recovered persons susceptible to relapse? The psychodynamics and neurochemical mechanisms of chemical dependency are under active study by many groups throughout the world.[52] Alteration of neurotransmitter (or receptor) activity in discrete midbrain structures associated with pleasure has been suggested as the common pathway of addiction caused by drugs from several classes. Whether this change is reversible is unclear. Meanwhile, epidemiologic studies have shown a hereditary influence for at least some significant portion of alcohol and amphetamine addictions. Thus susceptibility to relapse in former addicts could have a neurochemical basis.

From a psychologic perspective, the experience of the 12-step fellowships as originally formulated (in 1935) by Alcoholics Anonymous[3] merits consideration. The rehabilitation process is separable into several phases. Recovery is preceded by detoxification, but it is only after physical dependence has abated that the real process of healing may begin. Recovering persons learn to largely remodel their reactions to life events, both positive and negative. Their values change. Over time, in recovery, the outlook and behavior of dependent persons is transformed to be indistinguishable from individuals never addicted. Some attain a "state of self-respecting independence, of personal growth, and self-realization."[37] Recovered addicts occasionally may be noted for their exceptional degree of tolerance, reliability, integrity, and wit. Nevertheless, it is assumed, and well substantiated by numerous experiences, that **the potential for return to old attitudes and behavior resides, at some level, within the recovering person even after many years.** An extraordinarily high proportion of persons who relapse after a successful period of abstinence report moods of irritability and discontent that presage their return to drug or alcohol use by weeks or months. The zest for living and effective performance that many alcoholics and addicts in recovery manifest is thought to be contingent on the maintenance of a healthy psychologic and spiritual condition.[3] This, in turn, is accomplished by practicing the principles of their program. Some individuals diminish their active participation in recovery programs with the passage of time. These persons, although abstinent, may be more vulnerable to the stress encountered and more readily seduced by incidental drug-induced euphoria in the perioperative period.

It seems likely that the risk of relapse in the perioperative period is merely reflective of the overall risk of relapse, both being inversely proportional to the quality of the person's recovery program. Assessment of the *quality* and hence, it is proposed, the *stability* of a patient's recovery clearly is subjective, but there is some interest in quantifying this characteristic with psychologic questionnaires (the "Purpose of Life" Index).[56,66] If this instrument proves reliable, then preoperative assessment of relapse risk might be placed on a firmer foundation.

Regardless of the quality or the duration of a patient's recovery at the time of surgery, it is possible for that individual to **intensify** the practices of his/her program in preparation for the stressful period ahead.[16] Recovering persons commonly draw on the resources of their fellowship (phone calls, visits from other members) during particularly difficult times. This feature of the recovered person's support system (along with strengthened family relationships) constitutes a powerful defense against relapse and it will be exploited in the management strategies to be presented.

Fear of Pain

Fear of pain after major surgery is almost universal and thus is considered normal. Patients in recovery from chemical dependency have these fears exaggerated partially because they are concerned with rekindling the addictive process and partially because they believe their pain may be undertreated. Several publications have addressed the inadequacy of common analgetic regimens in the general surgery population.[8,71,102] Two additional considerations create a serious dilemma for the recovered addict—they may exhibit an elevated analgetic requirement, and well-meaning but misinformed health caregivers may withhold narcotics, either from a humanitarian perspective (not wanting to trigger relapse) or because of a moralistic attitude that interprets requests for pain medication as "drug-seeking" behavior. The dilemma for the patient clearly becomes the dilemma for the treating professional.

Variabilities in human individual pain threshold, intensity of noxious stimuli, and efficacy of inhibition at the receptor level are extremely broad, even for the same surgical procedure (or chronic condition).[59,88,115] Whereas clinicians repeatedly encounter examples of this fact, few manage to alter their prescribing practice and adjust doses appropriately to ensure adequate pain relief for all patients.[69,75] Conversely, respiratory depression and suppression of protective airway reflexes are always of concern in the immediate postoperative period and, clearly, aggressive pain management, if accomplished with narcotics, must be balanced with heightened vigilance.

Although it is a common perception that persons with active addictions require larger doses of analgesics and sedatives (probably true, but not universal), the needs of recovered addicts are unappreciated. Anecdotal information suggests that some formerly addicted, currently abstinent persons may fall predominantly into the category of individuals requiring **higher** doses of analgetic drugs.[27,41,103] This has not been formally investigated in humans, and the assumption must be treated with caution, but the possibility should be considered when interpreting intraoperative drug requirements and postoperative requests for analgetics.

The reluctance by health professionals to adequately treat acute pain in the general population has been noted, analyzed, and decried.* Indeed, some consider the apparent inhumanity of inadequate pain relief to be a crisis of major proportions.[69,75] The patient in recovery may be exposed to added hazard in this regard. Several instances of relapse to drug use have occurred in abstinent individuals after major surgery when analgetic administration was deliberately restricted.[27] The purported "cause" for return to addictive behavior in these persons was a psychologic reaction to the prolonged suffering that was experienced, although this was, of course, superimposed on other issues of health and well-being.

Effective Treatment Strategies

Several elements of a medical treatment conundrum have been identified regarding anesthesia and analgesia in recovering patients: the desirability of adequate pain relief, the possibility of increased analgetic requirements, the appropriate fear of relapse, and the widespread ignorance of health care professionals

---

*References 8, 59, 69, 71, 88, 102, 115.

regarding these issues. Although literature reports offer little guidance regarding resolution of this problem, the Medical Care in Recovery Committee of the American Society of Addiction Medicine (ASAM) has issued a public policy statement that is quoted verbatim in Box 30-4.

This policy statement is broadly applicable to the medical treatment of recovering persons but it does not explicitly address the perioperative period. The overall tenor of these recommendations seems to highlight the risk of relapse rather than promoting the

---

BOX 30-4
AMERICAN SOCIETY OF ADDICTION MEDICINE PUBLIC POLICY STATEMENT: MEDICAL CARE IN RECOVERY

Background

Alcoholism and other dependencies (addictive disorders) are primary, chronic, and often progressive diseases that affect almost every aspect of health. The medical, surgical, and psychiatric treatment of a recovering chemically dependent patient may have a profound effect on the patient's risk of relapse. Any potentially addicting drug which alters mood may be hazardous to recovery even if the patient has not previously been dependent upon that substance.

Policy recommendations

The American Society of Addiction Medicine recommends that:

For comprehensive medical care, all disease states, including addictive diseases, either active or in remission, must be taken into account in treatment planning.

Abstinence from all potentially addicting, mood-altering drugs is the goal for patients in recovery from addiction. However, such drugs occasionally may be a necessary adjunct in the management of a given patient for a specific condition. Judicious prescribing and close monitoring are necessary to minimize the risk of relapse into active addiction.

When potentially addicting drugs are medically necessary, their dosages should be determined by the therapeutic requirements, bearing in mind variations in individual tolerance.

Physicians are encouraged to seek consultation with a physician knowledgeable in addiction medicine, when treating a patient with a history of alcoholism or other addictive disease.

Adopted by American Society of Addiction Medicine Board of Directors 9/25/89.

---

adequacy of pain relief. The ASAM statement does provide for the possibility of opioid administration (not specifically identified), but its emphasis on the hazards of mood-altering substances could be misinterpreted. The majority of persons closest to the issue, including formerly addicted persons who have recently undergone major surgery and recovery-knowledgeable surgeons, nurses, and addictionists, report that **conventional attitudes are more likely to result in inadequate perioperative pain relief rather than excessive opioid administration.**[*] Their collective experience may be summarized as follows:

- Recovered addicts/alcoholics should receive adequate analgesia appropriate to their perception of the severity of the noxious stimulus
- Special nerve blocks, nonopioid analgetics, and other alternate modalities should be considered first when feasible
- Treatment may involve opioids and still be accomplished with minimal risk of relapse, provided certain precautions are observed

The remainder of this chapter is devoted to an elaboration and expansion of these statements toward the comprehensive perioperative management of recovering persons.

Specific aspects of anesthetic management that must be addressed include preoperative evaluation, preoperative medication, intraoperative regional techniques, general anesthesia, postoperative narcotics, PCA, other special regional techniques, and newer nonnarcotic pharmacologic therapy.

Preoperative issues

The preoperative medical evaluation of recovering persons should include a search for the stigmata of chronic drug ingestion, which may linger for months or years. Nicotine abuse remains especially common in these patients even though they have favorably modified most other destructive personal habits. This is a testimony to nicotine's addictive potency.

Two pharmacologic agents that have implications for the perioperative period, **disulfiram and naltrexone,** are occasionally used as drug-deterrent adjuncts to therapy in the early months of recovery. Disulfiram (Antabuse), taken orally once a day, inhibits alcohol metabolism, causing a buildup of acetaldehyde. The drug is prescribed for several months after detoxification in primary alcoholics while an effective recovery program is established. After ingestion of even small amounts of alcohol the patient experiences flushing, choking, nausea, tachycardia, and hypotension. All alcohol-containing medications, including skin preparation solutions, should be avoided. Some

---

*References 27, 41, 54, 84, 91, 103.

patients taking Antabuse have elevated hepatic aminotransferase levels. Naltrexone is an oral medication that demonstrates pure opioid antagonist action. Although opioid ingestion does not cause unpleasant symptoms, the threshold to induce euphoria is greatly elevated. The drug is prescribed as part of a multifaceted approach to recovery from opioid addiction. Patients taking naltrexone at the time of surgery will have markedly elevated opioid requirements if opioids are chosen for pain relief. Both naltrexone and disulfram may be continued up to the day of surgery if deemed desirable by those supervising the patient's recovery. In-hospital continuance of naltrexone is probably not advisable since opioid antagonism is counterproductive.

Patients receiving chronic methadone therapy should have their regular daily dose ascertained, then administered as a baseline, with further opioids given to ameliorate pain as required[51,63] (see earlier discussion).

A desirable objective in the modulation of preoperative anxiety is to treat effectively without producing a conscious euphoria that could stimulate dormant mood/thinking/behavior cycles.[69] Relaxation techniques and soothing music with personal earphones have been used in lieu of preoperative medication.[66] The latter should either be avoided or else given in sufficient doses to induce hypnosis, thereby avoiding the euphoric state.[69] Other anxiolytics with minimal abuse potential include buspirone and hydroxizine[29] (see earlier discussion).

Intraoperative management

Intraoperative anesthesia may be performed with a broad range of agents and techniques, although the advantages of regional anesthesia in this patient population are manifest and therefore the method is indicated whenever feasible and commensurate with the expertise of the practitioner. The art and science of regional anesthesia continues to advance. Virtually all forms of surgery can be performed using a regional technique as a supplement to general anesthesia or as the sole modality. Skills and experience, however, vary widely and the complete spectrum of neural blocks may not be available everywhere. In addition, various relative and absolute contraindications to regional techniques exist and the failure rate is not insignificant. Fortunately, other options are viable. General anesthesia in all its variations may be used safely, provided postoperative planning has been complete as discussed in the next section. Even the use of opioids, as part of a rational, balanced anesthetic, need not be feared. The most difficult issues of perioperative management begin at the termination of surgery.

Postoperative care

Problems of the postoperative period may be divided into the time immediately after surgery, the in-hospital convalescence, and the discharge medications. Obviously, if continuous regional anesthesia has been used intraoperatively, this may be continued. Some practicioners believe that the benefits of regional techniques are so significant (and the dangers of narcotics so serious) that postoperative pain management should virtually always involve neural blockade.[69] Continuous spinals, lumbar and thoracic epidurals, and even continuous plexus and axillary infusions may be used. In this scheme the effort to avoid narcotics includes prolongation of hospital care until pain has abated sufficiently to allow discharge without medication.[69] The latter maneuver, while helpful, may not be supported by third-party payors.

The extraordinarily conservative approach just described is not validated by the majority of practitioners.[16,27,54,84,103] Although some abstinent persons could require strict adherence to the no-narcotic rule, at least those large numbers of former addicts and alcoholics recovering within the 12-step fellowships have resources that may be used to broaden the range of safe and acceptable analgetic methods. The first step is to assess the extent and adequacy of the patient's recovery program. Sharing the details of one's thinking and feeling state with others in their fellowship is standard behavior for active participants in AA, NA, etc. An important individual in this process is the patient's "sponsor." The patient should be encouraged to escalate his/her contact with this person as the time of surgery approaches.[16,27,54,84] In the majority of cases it will be helpful for the sponsor or surrogate to be introduced to the surgeon and anesthesiologist. A relationship between these caregivers could help resolve questions that may arise regarding analgetic requirements in the postoperative period. Keys to success include an addiction/recovery-knowledgeable physician who orders pain medication in response to the patient's level of discomfort and active participation by individuals important in the patient's recovery program (fellowship members, sponsor, spouse, counselor). Both of these elements should be present. The second provision means that the patient's level of comfort and use of narcotics (including cumulative dosages) should be discussed daily by the patient, the treating health professional, and the recovery contact person. These procedures have been successfully used for some time by several practitioners.*

Intravenous PCA with opioids has been used routinely in recovering persons after major sur-

---

* References 16, 27, 54, 60, 84, 103.

gery[54,103-105] — the matter, however, is controversial. The use of PCA has been questioned on theoretic grounds (harmful psychodynamics of self-administration),[69,70] but clinical experience has shown the method to be safe and effective, at least in recovering alcoholics, when used in the context of program intensification and daily discussions as described. Well-designed clinical studies may not be ethical and clinicians may have to rely on anecdotal reports of successful and unsuccessful cases. Neural axis narcotics have advantages over as-needed parenteral or IV PCA modalities, since there is probably less alteration of mood (euphoria) with spinal or epidural dosing. Recent developments in opioid receptor classification suggest that spinal cord analgesia is modulated by both kappa and mu subtypes, but rostral spread to midbrain structures may be minimal.

Nothing in the previous recommendations should imply that narcotics are not capable of initiating relapse — only that clinical practice has shown that opioid analgesia may be used, and used effectively, with appropriate attention to detail. Whether patients formerly addicted to different classes of mood-altering substances have different relapse risks or would benefit from selected treatment regimens are topics of current discussion.[60,66,91] Although it seems reasonable that primary opioid abusers would be at greatest danger with perioperative narcotic administration, the nature of the abused substance may or may not prove to be overriding compared to the quality of the individual's sobriety. In any case the proportion of "polydrug" multiple-substance addicts is growing and clear distinctions are frequently not possible.

Alternate therapies have emerged that show promise for use in recovering patients. Ketorolac, a parenteral NSAID, has analgetic potencies comparable to morphine with the following intramuscular equivalence: 30 to 90 mg ketorolac = 6 to 12 mg morphine.[12] There is increasing evidence that suggests that ketorolac is effective in treating moderate-to-severe pain with an adverse effect rate similar to morphine (although different in nature) and without, of course, addiction potential. Somnolence and gastric upset are reported in some patients. Ketorolac has been used successfully in recovering patients after surgery.[27]

Kappa agonist/partial antagonist opioids (nalbuphine, dezocine, butorphanol, pentazocine) present a low (but finite) abuse potential while providing good analgesia.[83] These agents may be preferred, perhaps as adjuncts to ketorolac.

The alpha$_2$-receptor agonist, clonidine, or subsequently developed congeners may prove useful for both recovering addicts and active addicts as well as never-addicted persons in the perioperative period. In addition to its salubrious effects on the withdrawal syndrome mentioned earlier, clonidine has been identified as (1) an anxiolytic, (2) a sedative, (3) synergistic with anesthetic agents, and (4) analgetic, especially in the epidural space.[72] Further developments with this class of drugs and clear indications for their use in the amelioration of perioperative stress will be closely monitored by clinicians.

If a patient continues to require analgetic medications after discharge from the hospital, which occurs more frequently in these times of "managed care" and shortened hospitalizations, a new and potentially hazardous period ensues.

Unsupervised and unrestricted access to opioid-containing drugs personally possessed by the patient is extremely unwise, regardless of the primarily abused substance, even for persons with a strong recovery program and years of stable sobriety. These medications should be dispensed, if possible, by the patient's spouse, significant other, sponsor, or other knowledgeable person.[60,84] The appropriate individual to accept this responsibility must be chosen with due regard to any emotional conflicts that may exist between him/her and the patient. The doses, refills, and continued need for opioid analgetics should be openly discussed by the relevant parties on a daily basis. Provided these precautions are taken and procedures followed, adequate pain relief may be assured with effective safeguards against relapse.[54,84] Oral NSAIDs should be used when possible. TENS has been used with intermittent success[66] in recovering patients for incisional pain.

Clinical mistakes

The following anecdotes exemplify errors of omission and commission by treating physicians and their patients in recovery that have led to identified episodes of relapse (or near-miss)[19,60,90]:

- Postoperative narcotics were administered in the hospital to a primary IV opioid abuser only 6 months into recovery, with no special "program intensification." The patient developed drug ideation in the hospital and returned to drug use immediately after discharge.
- Hypnotics and anxiolytics were prescribed for "nerves" after major abdominal surgery for neoplasm in a recovering, chemically dependent person. There was no program intensification. The patient soon relapsed to alcohol use, his primary drug of choice.
- Tylenol with codeine tablets were given to a 50-year-old physician after oral surgery; the medication was to be taken home. The patient was in stable recovery from alcoholism for 10

years. The patient experienced euphoria and drug ideation after the fourth tablet and immediately destroyed the remaining drug.

■ An alcoholic patient with more than 10 years of sobriety developed chronic back pain and was given unsupervised narcotics and diazepam. Although abstinent for many years, she did not actively participate in a 12-step fellowship or otherwise have an alternate support system. The patient relapsed and died of alcohol-related illness within the year.

These vignettes are quite representative of known cases of relapse. In each example, serious mistakes were made in patient management. Informal surveys (ongoing) have failed to reveal a relapse incident related to perioperative medications when the suggested treatment strategies have been used.

Specifically omitted from consideration in this chapter are discussions regarding the treatment of chronic pain conditions and/or analgesia for the terminally ill. Management of chronic pain in recovering persons is extraordinarily complex.[30,89] Unfortunately, such patients are often interminably poised on a narrow edge between psychic distress and somatic pain.[120] Their care requires management by a specialist in addiction medicine. Similarly, the recovering person who develops severe pain in the setting of a terminal illness needs support and treatment by individuals sensitive to the range of spiritual, psychologic, and physical issues involved.

SUMMARY

Patients in recovery from the disease of chemical dependency represent a special group with perioperative needs that are paradoxic. Both under-treatment and over-treatment with mood-altering analgetics or sedatives is inappropriate and probably dangerous. Pending definitive studies, concerned professionals must rely on cumulative clinical experience. Hopefully, the material in this chapter will provide reassurance and guidance to both patient and clinician until such information is forthcoming.

ACKNOWLEDGMENT

The authors recognize Stephen A. Derrer, M.D., who participated in the original planning of this project, and Marigail Wynne, M.D., who provided encouragement and suggestions. We also thank the several members of the fellowships of Alcoholics Anonymous and Narcotics Anonymous who shared their experiences with us.

KEY POINTS

■ Patients in recovery from alcohol and other drug addictions should have adequate analgesia in the perioperative period. Physicians and nurses should neither unnecessarily promote nor unreasonably restrict analgetics.

■ Patients who are in recovery through 12-step fellowships should intensify their program preoperatively and arrange for visits and discussion of feeling state and cumulative drug dosing in the postoperative period with their sponsor or other fellowship contact.

■ Optimal care is achieved by a trusting, cooperative relationship among a recovery-knowledgeable physician, the patient, and his/her support person.

■ The risk of relapse to drug use is real but manageable. This risk may be less for patients in an active, stable, recovery program.

■ Regional or regional-supplemented general anesthesia may be preferred if the technique can be performed with alacrity and maintained with vigilance. If possible, continuous infusions should extend into the postoperative period.

■ Nonopioid analgetics, especially ketorolac, should be considered first-line therapy.

■ Abstinent patients may have elevated requirements for analgesia even many years after the discontinuation of mood-altering substances.

■ Narcotics (opioids) may be safely and effectively used, provided they are administered by a recovery-knowledgeable practitioner and patients continue intensified contact through a 12-step fellowship.

■ Patient-controlled analgesia (PCA) has been used successfully while the patient is monitored closely with support from intensified contact with a 12-step fellowship. Primary opioid addicts, as compared to primary alcoholics, may or may not be at higher risk with this modality.

■ Epidural and spinal narcotics, managed by an acute pain service, may have the highest margin of safety of the opioid therapies.

■ Discharge medications must be supervised by 12-step program contacts and the treating physician. Unsupervised access to narcotic analgetics may place the patient at high risk for relapse.

■ The services of an addictionist or pain specialist are helpful in difficult cases, especially those involving chronic pain and the terminally ill.

KEY REFERENCES

American College of Physicians Health and Public Policy Committee: Chemical dependence, *Ann Intern Med* 102:405, 1985.

Bruce DL: Alcoholism and anesthesia, *Anesth Analg* 62:84, 1983.

Gevirtz C: The intravenous drug abuse patient. In Frost EA, ed: *Pre-anesthetic assessment,* Boston, 1988, Birkhauser.

Holloway M: Treatment for addiction, *Sci Am* 263(2): 94, 1991.

Melzak R: The tragedy of needless pain, *Sci Am* 262:2, 1990.

Stuart G, Sundeen S: Substance abuse. In Stuart G, Sundeen S, eds: *Principles and practice of psychiatric nursing,* St Louis, 1986, CV Mosby.

REFERENCES

1. Aceto M et al: Effect of β-funaltrexamine (β-FNA) on morphine dependence in rats and monkeys, *Eur J Pharmacol* 123:387, 1986.
2. Adler GR, Potts FE, Kirby RR et al: Narcotics control in anesthesia training, *JAMA* 253:3133, 1985.
3. Alcoholics Anonymous: *The Big Book,* ed 3, New York, 1976, World Services.
4. Alcoholics Anonymous World Services, General Office, 468 Park Ave, South, New York, NY 10016.
5. American College of Physicians Health and Public Policy Committee: Chemical dependence, *Ann Intern Med* 102:405, 1985.
6. American Medical Association, Council on Mental Health: Medical school education on the abuse of alcohol and other psychotropic drugs, *JAMA* 219:1746, 1972.
7. American Society of Addiction Medicine, 5235 Wisconsin Ave, NW, Washington, DC 20015.
8. Angell M: The quality of mercy, *N Engl J Med* 306:98, 1982.
9. Antelman SM: Amitriptyline provides long-lasting immunization against sudden cardiac death from cocaine, *Eur J Pharmacol* 69:119, 1981.
10. Bederson J, Field H, and Barbaro N: Hyperalgesia during naloxone-precipitated withdrawal from morphine is associated with increased on-cell activity in the rostral ventromedial medulla, *Somatosen Motor Res* (7)2:185, 1990.
11. Bruce DL: Alcoholism and anesthesia, *Anesth Analg* 62:84, 1983.
12. Buckley MMT, Brogden RN: Ketorolac—a review, *Drugs* 39:86, 1990.
13. Bush B et al: Screening for alcohol abuse using the CAGE questionnaire, *Am J Med* 82:231, 1987.
14. Caldwell JR et al: Sucralfate treatment of nonsteroidal anti-inflammatory drug-induced gastrointestinal symptoms and mucosal damage, *Am J Med* 83(suppl B):74, 1987.
15. Campaigning for healthy babies,: *The New York Times Magazine,* p 4a, April 7, 1991.
16. Chambers J, Addictionist, Kensington, Md, personal communication, April 1991.
17. Charney D, Riordan C, Kleber H et al: Clonidine and naltrexone. A safe, effective, and rapid treatment of abrupt withdrawal methadone therapy, *Gen Psychiatry* 39:1327, 1982.
18. Clarren SK: The diagnosis and treatment of fetal alcohol syndrome, *Comp Ther* 8:41, 1982.
19. Davis J, Director, Resource Group Counseling and Education Center, Baltimore, Md, personal communication, April 1991.
20. DeLander GE, Porthoghese PS, and Takemori AE: Role of spinal mu opioid receptors in the development of morphine tolerance and dependence, *J Pharmacol Exp Ther* 231(1):91, 1984.
21. Drug Abuse Warning Network: 1982 annual data, National Institute on Drug Abuse, Rockville, Md, 1982, National Institutes of Health.
22. Editorial, *Anesthesia* 25:163, 1970.
23. Elliott HW: Effects of street drugs on anesthesia, *Int J Clin Pharmacol* 12:134, 1975.
24. Errick JK, Heel RC: Nalbuphine. A preliminary review of its pharmacological properties and therapeutic efficacy, *Drugs* 26:191, 1983.
25. Ewing J: Detecting alcoholism. The CAGE questionnaire, *JAMA* 252(14): 1905, 1984.
26. Fabiani CA: From coca chewing to cocaine smoking, *Resident Staff Physician* 37:101, 1991.
27. Farley W, Medical Director, Perspectives Health Program, Hampton, Va, personal communication, April 1991.
28. Farley WJ, Talbott GD, eds: Anesthesiology and addiction, *Anesth Analg* 62:465, 1983.
29. Feighner J, Merideth C, and Hendrickson G: A double-blind comparison of buspirone and diazepam in outpatients with generalized anxiety disorder, *J Clin Psychiatry* 43(12):102, 1982.
30. Filshie J: The non-drug treatment of neuralgic and neuropathic pain of malignancy, *Cancer Surv* 7(1):161, 1988.
31. Fultz J, Senay E: Guidelines for the management of hospitalized narcotic addicts, *Ann Intern Med* 82(6):815, 1975.
32. Gallegos KV, Browne CH, Veit FW et al: Addiction in anesthesiologists: drug access and patterns of substance abuse, *QRB* 116, April, 1988.
33. Garattini S, Caccia S, and Mennini T: Notes on buspirone's mechanisms of action, *J Clin Psychiatry* 43(12):19, 1982.
34. Garzotto N et al: Validation of a screening questionnaire for alcoholism (MAST) in an Italian sample, *Compr Psychiatry* 29(3):323, 1988.
35. Gawin F, Ellinwood E: Cocaine and other stimulants. Actions, abuse, and treatment, *N Engl J Med* 318(18):1173, 1988.
36. Gelb AM, Mildvan D, and Stenger RJ: The spectrum and causes of liver disease in narcotic addicts, *Am J Gastroenterol* 67:314, 1977.
37. Gerard DL, Saenger G, and Wile R: The abstinent alcoholic, *Arch Gen Psychiatry* 6:83, 1962.
38. Gevirtz C: The intravenous drug abuse patient. In Frost EA, ed: *Pre-anesthetic assessment,* Boston, 1988, Birkhauser.
39. Gianoulakis C, Drouin JN, Seidah NG et al: Effect of chronic morphine treatment on beta-endorphin biosynthesis by the rat neurointermediate lobe, *Eur J Pharmacol* 72:313, 1981.
40. Gold M, Pottash A, Sweeney D et al: Opiate withdrawal using clonidine. A safe, effective, and rapid non-opiate treatment, *JAMA* 243(4):343, 1980.
41. Goodwin G, Division Medical Officer, US Postal Service, Baltimore, Md, personal communication, April 1991.
42. Gorelick DA, Wilkins JN: Special aspects of human alcohol withdrawal. In Galanter M, ed: *Recent development in alcoholism,* vol 4, New York, 1986, Plenum Publishing.
43. Gravenstein JS, Kory WP, and Marks RG: Drug abuse by anesthesia personnel, *Anesth Analg* 62:467, 1983.

44. Griffith J et al: Investigation of the abuse liability of busiprone in alcohol-dependent patients, *Am J Med* 80(suppl 3B):30, 1986.
45. Griffiths R et al: Low-dose caffeine physical dependence in humans, *J Pharmacol Exp Ther* 255(3):1123, 1990.
46. Griffiths R, Wolb B: Relative abuse liability of different benzodiazepines in drug abusers, *J Clin Psychopharmacol* 10(4):237, 1990.
47. Guiffrida JG, Bizzarri DV, Saure AC et al: Anesthetic management of drug abusers, *Anesth Analg* 49(2):272, 1970.
48. Gustaffson L, Wiesenfeld-Hallin Z: Spinal opioid analgesia. A critical update, *Drugs* 35:597, 1988.
49. Haverkos H: Infectious diseases and drug abuse: prevention and treatment in the drug abuse treatment system. In *European Symposium on AIDS and Drug Abuse: Providing Care for HIV-infected Drug Users*, Vienna, Austria, August 1990, World Health Organization, Geneva, (draft).
50. Haverkos H, Lange W: Serious infections other than human immunodeficiency virus among intravenous drug abusers, *J Infect Dis* 161:894, 1990.
51. Hayes MG, Medical Director, Man Alive Research, Inc., Baltimore, Md, personal communication, May 1991.
52. Holloway M: Treatment for addiction, *Sci Am* 263(2):94, 1991.
53. Horowitz J: Anesthetic implications of substance abuse in the parturient, *J Am Assoc Nurse Anesthetist* 56:510, 1988.
54. Hyde G, Professor of Surgery, University of Kentucky Medical Center, Lexington, Ky, personal communication, May 1991.
55. Hymans S, Cassem N: Pain, *Sci Am*, 1990.
56. Jacobson GR, Rigger DP, and Mueller L: Purpose in life and personal values among adult alcoholics, *J Clin Psychol* 33:314, 1977.
57. Jage J: Anaesthesie und analgesie bei opiatabhängigen, *Anaesthetist* 37:470, 1988.
58. Johnson R et al: Use of buprenorphine in the treatment of opiate addiction. I. Physiologic and behavioral effects during a rapid dose induction, *Clin Pharmacol Ther* 46:335, 1989.
59. Kaiko RF, Wallenstein SL, and Rogers AG: Sources of variation of analgesic responses in cancer patients with chronic pain receiving morphine, *Pain* 15:191, 1983.
60. Kent R, Medical Director, Oakview Treatment Center, Baltimore, Md, personal communication, May 1991.
61. Klatskin G: Alcohol and its relation to liver damage, *Gastroenterology* 41:443, 1961.
62. Lader M: Psychological effects of busiprone, *J Clin Psychiatry* 43(12):62, 1982.
63. Lane R, Executive Director of Man Alive Research, Inc., Baltimore, Md, personal communication, April 1990.
64. Lange W et al: Safety and side-effects of buprenorphine in the clinical manage-

ment of heroin addiction, *Drug and Alcohol Depend* 26:19, 1990.
65. Lau MP: Acupuncture and addiction: an overview, addictive disease, *Int J* 2(3):449, 1976.
66. Lawton MJ, Associated Professor and Director of Alcohol and Drug Education/Rehabilitation Program, Department of Rehabilitation Counseling, Virginia Commonwealth University, Richmond, Va, personal communication, June 1991.
67. Lewis DC: Comparison of alcoholism and other radical diseases, *Psychiatr Ann* 21:256, 1991.
68. Litvak K, McEvoy G: Ketorolac, an injectable non-narcotic analgesic, *Clin Pharm* 9:921, 1990.
69. Mangieri EA, Addictionist, Northport, Ala, personal communication, May 1991.
70. Mangieri EA: *Anesthesiol News,* March 1991 [letter].
71. Marks RM, Sachar EJ: Undertreatment of medical inpatients with narcotic analgesics, *Ann Intern Med* 78:173, 1973.
72. Maze M, Tranquilli W: Alpha$_2$- adrenoreceptor agonists: defining the role in clinical anesthesia, *Anesthesiology* 74:581, 1991.
73. McDougal DH: The role of the "non-addictionist" in the treatment and referral of addicts. In Physician Rehabilitation Committee: *Straight Forward,* Baltimore, April, 1991, Medical and Chirurgical Faculty of Maryland.
74. McQuay H: Pharmacologic treatment of neuralgic and neuropathic pain, *Cancer Surv* 7(1):141, 1988.
75. Melzak R: The tragedy of needless pain, *Sci Am* 262:2, 1990.
76. Millan M: Multiple opioid systems and pain, *Pain* 27:303, 1986.
77. Moore RD, Bone LR, Geller G et al: Prevalence, detection, and treatment of alcoholism in hospitalized patients, *JAMA* 261:403, 1989.
78. Moss AR: AIDS and intravenous drug use: the real heterosexual epidemic, *Br Med J* 294:389, 1987.
79. Nahas G: A calcium-channel blocker as antidote to the cardiac effects of cocaine intoxication, *N Engl J Med* 313:519, 1986.
80. Narcotics Anonymous World Services, personal communication, May 1990.
81. National Clearing House for Alcohol and Drug Information (NCADI), personal communication, May 1991.
82. National Council on Alcoholism and Drug Dependence, personal communication.
83. O'Brian J, Benfield P: Dezocine—a preliminary review of its pharmacodynamic and pharmacokinetic properties and therapeutic efficacy, *Drugs* 38(2):226, 1989.
84. Ohliger P, Laguna Miguel, Calif, personal communication, June 1991.
85. Orkin LR, Chen CH: Addiction, alcoholism, and anesthesia, *South Med J* 70:1172, 1977.
86. Osborne NN: Naloxone alters pain perception and somatosensory evoked potentials in normal subjects, *Nature* 270:620, 1977.

87. Parran TV Jr, Adelman CL, and Jasinski DR: Buprenorphine detoxification of medically unstable narcotic dependent patients: a case series, *Substance Abuse* 11(4):197, 1990.
88. Perry SW: Irrational attitudes toward addicts and narcotics, *Bull NY Acad Med* 61:706, 1985.
89. Portnoy RK: Chronic opioid therapy in non-malignant pain, *J Pain Symptom Managmnt* 5:546, 1990.
90. Quinn J, Director, Quinn Center, Inc. Baltimore, Md, personal communication, April 1991.
91. Radcliffe TB, Physician in Charge, Chemical Dependency Recovery Program, Kaiser Hospital, Fontana, Calif, personal communication, May 1991.
92. Regier D et al: Comorbidity of mental disorders with alcohol and other drug abuse. Results from the Epidemiologic Catchment Area (ECA) study, *JAMA* 264:2511, 1990.
93. *Resource and referral guide (1991): data source:* New York, 1991, National Council on Alcoholism and Drug Dependence.
94. Roback G et al: *Physician characteristics and distribution in the U.S.,* Chicago, 1986, American Medical Association.
95. Schweizer E et al: Carbamazepine treatment in patients discontinuing long-term benzodiazepine therapy, *Arch Gen Psychiatry* 48:448, 1991.
96. Scott LE, Clum GA, and Peoples JB: Preoperative predictors of postoperative pain, *Pain* 15:283, 1983.
97. Segal IS, Jarvis DJ, Duncan SR et al: Clinical efficacy of oral-transdermal clonidine combinations during the perioperative period, *Anesthesiology* 74:220, 1991.
98. Seller E, Naranjo C: New strategies for the treatment of alcohol withdrawal, *Psych Pharmacol Bull* 22(1):88, 1986.
99. Seller E, Naranjo C, Harrison M et al: Diazepam loading: simplified treatment of alcohol withdrawal, *Clin Pharmacol Ther* 34(6):822, 1983.
100. Spiegelman WG, Saunders L, and Mazze RI: Addiction and anesthesiology, *Anesthesiology* 60:335, 1984.
101. Spitzer RL, Williams JB, eds: *Diagnostic and statistical manual of mental disorders: DSM-III-R,* ed 3, Washington, DC, 1987, American Psychiatric Association.
102. Sriwatanakul K, Weiss FFA, and Alloza JL: Analysis of narcotic analgesic usage in the treatment of postoperative pain, *JAMA* 250:926, 1983.
103. Stacey BR, Pain Evaluation and Treatment Institute, University of Pittsburgh, Pittsburgh, Pa, personal communication, April 1991.
104. Stacey BR, Brody MD: *Anesthesiology News,* March 1991 (letter).
105. Stacey BR, Brody MC, and Burke DF: Patients with substance abuse history can effectively use PCA, *Anesthesiology* 73:A759, 1990.
106. *Straight Forward,* Baltimore, April, 1991, Medical and Chirurgical Faculty of Maryland.

107. Strain E, Stitzer M, and Gigelow G: Early treatment time course of depressive symptoms in opiate addicts, *J Nerv Ment Dis* 179(4):215, 1991.

108. Stuart G, Sundeen S: Substance abuse. In Stuart G, Sundeen S, eds: *Principles and practice of psychiatric nursing,* St Louis, 1986, CV Mosby.

109. Sullivan LW, Hervert V: Suppression of hematopoiesis by ethanol, *J Clin Invest* 43:2048, 1964.

110. Swerdlow BN, Holley FO, Maitre PO et al: Chronic alcohol intake does not change thiopental anesthetic requirement, pharmacokinetics, or pharmacodynamics, *Anesthesiology* 72:455, 1990.

111. Talbott GD: Elements of the impaired physicians program, *J Med Assoc Ga* 73:749, 1984.

112. Tarnaski A et al: Efficacy of sucralfate and cimetidine in protection of the human gastric mucosa against alcohol injury, *Am J Med* 83(suppl B):31, 1987.

113. Teshy B: Abuse liability of drugs in humans, Research Monograph 92, Rockville, Md, 1989, National Institute on Drug Abuse.

114. Tsutsumi R et al: Interaction of ethanol and enflurane metabolism and toxicity: role of P45011E1, *Alcohol Clin Exp Res* 14(2):174, 1990.

115. Tucker C: Acute pain and substance abuse in surgical patients, *J Neurosci Nurs* 22(6):339, 1990.

116. Vaillant GE: *The national history of alcoholism,* Cambridge, Mass, 1983, Harvard University Press.

117. Ward CF, Ward GS, and Saidman LJ: Drug abuse in anesthesia training programs: a survey: 1970 through 1980, *JAMA* 250:P922, 1983.

118. Wartenberg A et al: Use of the Revised Clinical Institute Withdrawal Assessment – Alcohol in an inpatient psychiatric unit: effects on treatment of alcohol withdrawal syndrome, *Substance Abuse* 12(1):36, 1991.

119. Watkins L, Mayer D: Organization of endogenous opiate and nonopiate pain control systems, *Science* 216:1185, 1982.

120. Weingarten MA: Chronic opioid therapy in patients with a remote history of substance abuse, *J Pain Symptom Managmnt* 6:2, 1991.

121. Wilcox RE, Mikula JA, and Levitt RA: Periaqueductal gray naloxone microinjections in morphine-dependent rats: hyperalgesia without "classical" withdrawal, *Neuropharmacology* 18:639, 1979.

122. Wood PL, Rackham A, and Richard J: Spinal analgesia: comparison of the mu agonist morphine and kappa agonist ethyldetazocine, *Life Sci* 28:2119, 1981.

123. Wood PR, Soni N: Anaesthesia and substance abuse, *Anaesthesia* 44:672, 1989.

124. Wright C, Bigelow GE, Stitzer ML et al: Acute physical dependence in humans: repeated naloxone-precipitated withdrawal after a single dose of methadone, *Drug Alcohol Depend* 27:139, 1991.

125. Yersin B et al: Accuracy of the Michigan Alcoholism Screening Test for screening of alcoholism in patients of a medical department, *Arch Intern Med* 149:2071, 1989.

APPENDIX

FEATURES OF PSYCHOACTIVE SUBSTANCES
Ethyl Alcohol

Ethyl alcohol

Characteristics of intoxication: (1) *Acute:* biphasic reaction with disinhibition, agitation followed by progressive CNS depression. Myocardial and respiratory depression. Electrolyte abnormalities. (2) *Chronic:* hepatic damage (enzymatic induction followed by insufficiency), gastrointestinal toxicity, pancreatitis; marrow suppression: anemia, leukopenia, thrombocytopenia; neurotoxicity: seizure, Wernicke's and Korsakoff's syndromes, dementia, polyneuropathy; malnutrition: protein and vitamin deficiencies.

Tolerance and dependence: Narrowing of the "therapeutic" index: tolerance to lethal dose remains constant in spite of tolerance to euphoric effect. Induction of the hepatic microsomal enzymatic system as well as similar depressant effect on the brain explains cross-tolerance to barbiturates, sedative, and hypnotics.

Characteristics of withdrawal: Neuronal hyperexcitability (seizure, delirium); hyperadrenergic state; *potentially fatal.*

Physiologic responses of withdrawal: Tachycardia, hypertension, dysrhythmias, cardiac failure; hyperpyrexia; agitation, hyperreflexia, tremors, hallucinations, sensory disturbances, delirium, seizures.

Assessment of withdrawal: Clinical Institute Withdrawal Assessment—Alcohol revised (CIWA-Ar), a short 10-item objective scale scoring withdrawal severity, simplifying communication and treatment (see opposite page).

Pharmacologic interventions for treatment of withdrawal[42] (see examples): (1) *Benzodiazepines:* enhance the affinity of GABA for its receptor, favoring influx of chloride in the neuron and hyperpolarization: allay anxiety, increase seizure threshold, prevent delirium. (2) *Antipsychotics:* (risk: lower seizure threshold). (3) *Beta-blockers:* adjunct to (1) to reduce hyperadrenergic state. (4) *Alpha-adrenoreceptor agonists*[72] (clonidine): adjunct to (1) to reduce hyperadrenergic state, anxiety, and provide sedation.[97] (5) *Alcohol infusion:* (does not protect against seizure, promotes further electrolyte disorders, toxic to many organ tissues including the brain) controversial.

Anesthetic implications: Withdrawal may present pre-, intra-, or postoperatively. (1) *Acute:* additive with anesthetics; lower doses required. Intoxicated, disoriented patients may be traumatized or injure others. Specific considerations: CNS pathology reflecting alterations in ICP, full stomach, aspiration, intravascular volume status masked by sympathomimetic HR, BP effects. (2) *Chronic effects:* cross-tolerance with anesthetics. Controversial literature for increased/normal dose requirements. Specific considerations (in addition to (1)): altered liver function may result in toxicity to agents undergoing hepatic metabolism. Inhalantional agents favor nitrous oxide, isoflurane; muscle relaxants—potential for prolonged blockage with succinylcholine secondary to ↓ plasma cholinesterase; nondepolarizing agents ↑ length secondary to ↑ acetylcholine. Atracurium may be choice with Hoffman elimination. Regional techniques may be limited by coagulopathy, ↓ metabolism with ↑ toxicity of local anesthetics, peripheral neuropathy, noncooperation, infection, or sepsis, profound intravascular dehydration.

Modified from Elliot HW: Effect of street drugs on anesthesia, *Int J Clin Pharmacol* 12:134, 1975; Horowitz J: Anesthetic implications of substance abuse in the parturient, *J Am Assoc Nurse Anesthetist* 56:510, 1988; Spitzer RL, Williams JB, eds: *Diagnostic and statistical manual of mental disorders: DSM-III-R,* ed 3, Washington, DC, 1987, American Psychiatric Association; and other sources cited in the text.

FEATURES OF PSYCHOACTIVE SUBSTANCES
Ethyl Alcohol

Special considerations

Anesthetic implications for the alcoholic parturient:
(1) *Presentation:* during first two trimesters, increased incidence of spontaneous abortion; at delivery, increased incidence of abruptio placentae, antepartum bleeding, and anemia; occurence of withdrawal syndrome. (2) *Regional anesthetic technique limitations* as discussed previously; general anesthetic limitations compounded by "physiological changes of pregnancy."

Anesthetic implications for the infant born to alcholic parturient: (1) *In utero consequences*: fetal alcohol syndrome (FAS) with CNS dysfunction, growth deficiency, possible renal, hepatic, and cardiac abnormalities, and facial characteristics. (2) *At delivery:* increased incidence of meconium staining, lower APGAR scores, and occurrence of withdrawal; potential for difficult airway (FAS).

CIWA-Ar[118] *Scale:* Items 1 to 9 are scored on a scale of 1 to 7; item 10 is scored on a scale of 1 to 4.
1. Nausea/vomiting:
   0 = no nausea, vomiting to
   7 = constant nausea, dry heaves/vomiting
2. Tremor (arms extended, fingers spread apart):
   0 = no tremor to
   7 = severe, even at rest
3. Sweats:
   0 = no sweats to
   7 = drenching sweats
4. Anxiety:
   0 = no anxiety to
   7 = state of panic delirium
5. Agitation:
   0 = normal activity to
   7 = in constant movement, thrashing about
6. Tactile disturbances:
   0 = none
   3-4 = increased sensitivity to touch
   7 = frightening, intense tactile hallucinations
7. Auditory disturbances:
   0 = none
   3-4 = increased sensitivity to noise
   7 = frightening, intense auditory hallucinations
8. Visual disturbances:
   0 = none
   3-4 = photophobia
   7 = intense visual hallucinations
9. Headache:
   0 = none to
   7 = worst headache ever
10. Orientation:
   0 = can do serial threes to
   4 = disoriented to time, person, and date.

Scoring: A score of 10 or above should prompt pharmacologic intervention.

Examples of Alcohol Withdrawal Protocols
Diazepam Loading Protocol[98,99]

Diazepam 20 mg orally, reevaluate with CIWA-Ar after 30-60 minutes.
CIWA-Ar above 10: give additional 20 mg diazepam orally, reevaluate after 2 hours.
Repeat one more time if CIWA-A above 10.
Reevaluate every 24 hours.

Theoretically, no further medication needed. Practically, patient may be more comfortable with one or two dose(s) of diazepam (10-20 mg) on day 2.

Advantage: Once withdrawal is controlled the drug tapers itself. In case of liver failure, the taper will be slower; consider cutting the dose in half to avoid oversedation.

Disadvantage: Small risk of oversedation in case of liver failure, however, less so than when cumulative doses are used.
(Delirium: IV diazepam 5 mg bolus, repeat every 5 minutes until good control is obtained. Then 10-20 mg diazepam orally every 4 hours for 24 hours. Maintain good hydration.)

Oxazepam Taper Protocol

Oxazepam: 60-90 mg every 2-4 hours x 24-48 hours
Oxazepam: 60 mg every 6 hours x 24 hours
Oxazepam: 30 mg every 6 hours x 24 hours
Oxazepam: 15 mg every 6 hours x 24 hours
Oxazepam: 15 mg every 6 hours x 12 hours

Advantage: Oxazepam is eliminated by the kidneys; no risk of oversedation with concurrent liver failure.

Disadvantage: Complicated protocol; potential for intermittent withdrawal between doses.

FEATURES OF PSYCHOACTIVE SUBSTANCES
Cocaine, Amphetamines, Barbiturates, Carbamates, Benzodiazepines, and Sedative-Hypnotics

---

Cocaine and amphetamines

Characteristics of intoxication[35]: CNS stimulation, hypervigilance, anxiety, agitation, psychosis (paranoia); tachycardia, hypertension, acute ischemic tissue damage (stroke, myocardial, intestinal infarction, etc.) or reperfusion injury (rhabdomyolysis).

Tolerance and dependence: Limited tolerance; marked psychic tolerance (cocaine mimics instinctual drives); unclear physical dependence, rather abstinence syndrome with behavioral symptoms.

Characteristics of withdrawal: Hypersomnia, hyperphagia, anhedonia, fluctuating depression, anxiety, agitation.

Physiologic response of withdrawal: None reported.

Pharmacologic interventions for treatment of toxicity and abstinence: (1) *Cocaine-associated dysrhythmias:* beta-blockers. (2) *Cocaine-associated sudden cardiac arrest:* amitriptyline (10 mg/kg),[9] calcium channel blockers.[79] (3) *Abstinence syndrome:* combination therapy including bromocriptine, amantadine, antidepressants, amino acids, flupenthixol, decanate, carbamazepine, buprenorphine.[26]

Anesthetic implications: Sympathomimetic effects may make assessment of intravascular volume/blood loss and depth of anesthesia difficult. Distinctions between drug toxicity and onset of withdrawal are difficult; differential diagnosis of sympathomimetic state must include ischemia, anesthetic drug interaction, malignant hyperthermia, thyroid storm, pheochromocytoma, etc.

Special considerations

Anesthetic implications for the cocaine/amphetamine abuse parturient: (1) *Presentation:* increased vasoconstriction in placenta with decreased fetal blood flow; during first two trimesters, increased incidence of spontaneous abortion; during third trimester, increased premature labor, abruptio placentae. (2) *Anesthetic techniques:* guided by acute or chronic use and implications to cardiovascular response as outlined previously.

Anesthetic implications for the infant born to parturient: (1) *In utero consequences:* hypoxia, increased incidence of cryptorchism and hydroenphrosis, case reports of cerebral infarcts. (2) *At delivery:* increased impairment of homeostatic control, potential for withdrawal.

Barbiturates, carbamates, benzodiazepines, sedative-hypnotics

Characteristics of intoxication: Biphasic reaction with disinhibition, agitation followed by progressive CNS depression and coma. Except for benzodiazepines, potentially fatal respiratory and cardiovascular depression.

Tolerance and dependence: Limited tolerance to lethal effects but marked tolerance to sedation.

Characteristics of withdrawal: Neuronal hyperexcitability (seizure, delirium); hyperadrenergic state; potentially fatal.

Physiologic response of withdrawal: Hypertension with orthostatic hypotension, tachycardia; hyperpyrexia; anxiety, irritability, weakness, insomnia, headache, tremors, delirium, seizures.

Pharmacologic interventions for treatment of withdrawal: (1) If severe, or symptoms not tolerated because of old age, substitute with cross-tolerant long-acting agent (e.g., phenobarbital) with slow gradual taper (several weeks). (2) Clonidine, as useful agent to (1). (3) Carbamazepine.[95]

Anesthetic implications: (1) *Acute:* additive with anesthetics, lower doses required. (2) *Chronic:* cross-tolerance to anesthetics, higher doses required.

Modified from Elliot HW: Effect of street drugs on anesthesia, *Int J Clin Pharmacol* 12:134, 1975; Horowitz J: Anesthetic implications of substance abuse in the parturient, *J Am Assoc Nurse Anesthetist* 56:510, 1988; Spitzer RL, Williams JB, eds: *Diagnostic and statistical manual of mental disorders: DSM-III-R,* ed 3, Washington, DC, 1987, American Psychiatric Association; and other sources cited in the text.

FEATURES OF PSYCHOACTIVE SUBSTANCES
Cannabis, Hallucinogens, Inhalants, and Volatile Solvents

Cannabis

Characteristics of intoxication: Anxiety, panic attacks, hallucinations, fear of "going crazy." Conjunctival injection, sympathetic discharge.

Tolerance and dependence: Psychic dependence possible. No physical dependence.

Characteristics of withdrawal: None reported.

Physiologic response of withdrawal: None reported.

Pharmacologic interventions for treatment of withdrawal: None reported.

Anesthetic implications: *With acute use:* ↑ levels of circulating catechols with ↑ anesthetic requirements.[123] Epinephrine-induced dysrhythmias occur at much lower dosages. *With chronic use:* patients will develop depletion of catecholamines, which may decrease their anesthetic needs. Choice of technique may be influenced by physiologic effects of cannabis: (1) cardiovascular: variable, includes direct depressant effect, tachydysrhythmia, bradydysrhythmia, orthostatic hypotension; (2) respiratory: variable, includes bronchodilation, respiratory depression, pulmonary edema, bronchorrhea; (3) anticholinergic effect: potentiation of nondepolarizing neuromuscular blocking agents; (4) depression of thermoregulating mechanism: regional techniques may be limited by psychologic state.

Special considerations

Anesthetic implications for the cannabis abuse parturient: (1) *Presentation:* increased use in first trimester related to antiemetic effects; at delivery: increased incidence of protracted and arrested labor. (2) *Anesthetic techniques:* choice influenced as above.

Anesthetic implications for the infant born to the parturient: (1) *In utero:* occurrence of fetal alcohol syndrome–like characteristics. (2) *At delivery:* altered response to visual stimuli, high-pitched cry, FAS-like facial abnormalities may result in difficult airway.

Hallucinogens, LSD, Psilocybin, Mescaline

Characteristics of intoxication: Anxiety, panic attacks, hallucinations, fear of "going crazy."

Tolerance and dependence: Rapid onset of tolerance (tachyphylaxis); no physical dependence.

Characteristics of withdrawal: None reported.

Physiologic response of withdrawal: None reported.

Pharmacologic interventions for treatment of withdrawal: Not applicable.

Anesthetic implications: No cross-tolerance to anesthetics. A "trip" may be stopped by sedatives or phenothiazines. Possible metabolic effects in chronic users may prolong succinylcholine neuromuscular block and delay metabolism of ester type local anesthetics, histamine, and serotonin; may potentiate narcotics, analgetics, and sympathomimetic drugs. Rarely precipitates postoperative psychosis.

Inhalants, Volatile Solvents

Characteristics of intoxication: Similar to gaseous anesthetics; photophobia, eye irritation, diplopia, tinnitus, sneezing, rhinorrhea, cough, nausea, vomiting, diarrhea, anorexia, chest pain, dysrhythmia, myalgia.

Tolerance and dependence: Rapid onset of tolerance; no physical dependence.

Characteristics of withdrawal: None reported.

Physiologic response of withdrawal: None reported.

Pharmacologic interventions for treatment of withdrawal: Not applicable.

Anesthetic implications: Problems of dealing with intoxicated patient. Possible hepatic, renal, bone marrow, and other organ pathology from halogenated and impure chemicals.

Modified from Elliot HW: Effect of street drugs on anesthesia, *Int J Clin Pharmacol* 12:134, 1975; Horowitz J: Anesthetic implications of substance abuse in the parturient, *J Am Assoc Nurse Anesthetist* 56:510, 1988; Spitzer RL, Williams JB, eds: *Diagnostic and statistical manual of mental disorders: DSM-II-R,* ed 3, Washington, DC, 1987, American Psychiatric Association; and other sources cited in the text.

Narcotics: heroin, morphine, etc.

Characteristics of intoxication and overdose: Euphoria, lethargy, miosis, constipation, coma, slow respiration, hypotension, pinpoint pupils with overdose (except meperidine).

Tolerance and dependence: Marked tolerance and dependence to mu agonists; mu receptors appear to be responsible for the induction of tolerance.[11] Partial agonist/antagonists have low dependence potential.

Characteristics of withdrawal: Yawning, lacrimation, rhinorrhea, diarrhea, dehydration, fever, sweating, gooseflesh (cold turkey).

Physiologic response of withdrawal: (1) Cardiovascular: tachycardia, hypertension. (2) Respiratory: tachypnea, rhinorrhea, lacrimation. (3) Thermogenic: sweating, gooseflesh, hyperpyrexia. (4) Neurologic: dilated pupils, drug craving, [91] fixed position. NOTE: Withdrawal responses are similar for morphine, heroin, and methadone and distinguished by delayed onset with methadone (12 hours vs. 6) peak (day 6 vs. 72 hours) and completion (day 14 vs. 7).

Pharmacologic interventions for treatment of withdrawal: (1) Methadone; (2) buprenorphine; (3) clonidine and anticholinergic agents. (See management strategies.)

Anesthetic implications: Strategies for inpatient management of opioid dependence:
A. The patient is on methadone treatment:
Continue same daily dose. Beware of drug interactions (phenytoin, rifampin) that decrease the half-life of methadone and cause withdrawal in the second half of the night. Contact the program to clarify the dose, and coordinate drug treatment and medical treatment. Contact is essential so that the patient is not discharged definitively from the program while in the hospital. The Methadone Program needs to be informed of discharge date, to medicate the patient on the following day.
B. The patient is self-administering short-acting opioids:
Stabilize the patient perioperatively (e.g., 10-20 mg methadone IM), additional analgesia with short-acting mu agonist opioids. After medical/surgical stabilization of the patient, and if the patient cannot be admitted to a Methadone Program on discharge, start detoxification.
C. Detoxification protocols.
Buprenorphine: A safe alternative for detoxification of medically unstable patients. Buprenorphine is a partial mu agonist, with high affinity for the opiate receptors; duration of action independent of serum half-life. Buprenorphine produces little

physical dependence as the withdrawal symptoms are much milder and more tolerable than those associated with methadone withdrawal.[58, 64] Provides analgesia; ceiling effect to respiratory depression and analgesia. Buprenorphine precipitates withdrawal when administered directly after a mu agonist. Once administered, it blocks the effect of mu agonists (naltrexone-like effect). Buprenorphine 0.3-0.9 mg SQ or IM every 3-4 hours during 72 hours, then halve the dose for 72 hours, and discontinue. If needed, use clonidine transdermal patch to attenuate any withdrawal.[87]

Methadone taper: Causes discomfort, protracted withdrawal. Reduce dose by 10% every third day. Add clonidine transdermal patch, as above. Methadone taper can be accelerated with concurrent use of naltrexone.[17]

Clonidine taper[40]: Only treats the cardiovascular response, not the subjective symptoms. Clonidine 0.2-0.3 mg orally x 1; 0.01 mg orally every 4 hours x 5; 0.1 mg orally every 6 hours x 4; 0.1 mg orally every 8 hours x 3. Add dicyclomine 10 mg orally every 6 hours as needed for abdominal cramps.

Special considerations

Anesthetic implications for narcotic-abusing parturient: (1) *Presentation:* increased incidence of pregnancy-induced hypertension. Manifestations of withdrawal start approximately 4-6 hours after last dose, reach greatest intensity at 72 hours, and are gone within 10 days. Treatment as above. Consultation recommended. (2) *Anesthetic techniques:* In addition to risk related to pregnancy, several case reports reveal severe hypotension during general anesthesia administered within 2-6 hours of patient's last dose. Intraoperative administration of morphine or dose of patient's preferred drug abated symptoms.[114] Regional anesthesia, given as early as possible, is recommended.

Anesthetic implications for the infant born to the narcotic-abusing parturient: (1) *In utero:* intrauterine growth retardation, chromosomal damage, decreased mental and neurologic ability. (2) *At delivery:* increased incidence of breech presentation; tendency to respiratory depression and hypoxic episodes, problems with interactive behavior and homeostatic control; overall, higher morbidity/mortality rate. [NOTE: similar effects with parturients/infants on methadone]. *Neonatal narcotic withdrawal:* may appear within 12-14 hours with maternal narcotic abuse; within 1-7 days with maternal methadone therapy. Symptoms may persist for up to 4 months and include: autonomic hyperirritability, tachypnea, high-pitched cry. Treatment includes: phenobarbital, paregoric, chlorpromazine, methadone, diazepam. Clonidine 3-4 µg/kg/day has been reported effective without toxicity.

For sources see p. 563.

1991 RESOURCE AND REFERRAL GUIDE

■ADULT CHILDREN OF ALCOHOLICS
Central Service Board
PO Box 3216
Torrance, Ca 90505
(213) 534-1815

■ADVOCACY INSTITUTE
1730 Rhode Island Ave., NW
Ste. 600
Washington, DC 20036
(202) 659-8475

■AL-ANON FAMILY GROUP HEADQUARTERS
PO Box 862, Madison Square Station
New York, NY 10018
(212) 302-7240

■ALATEEN
Same as above

■ALCOHOL AND DRUG PROBLEMS ASSOCIATION OF NORTH AMERICA
1400 Eye St. NW, Ste. 1275
Washington, DC 20005
(202) 289-6755

■ALCOHOL RESEARCH GROUP LIBRARY
1816 Scenic Ave.
Berkeley, CA 94709
(415) 642-5208

■ALCOHOLICS ANONYMOUS (AA)
General Service Board
PO Box 459
Grand Central Station
New York, NY 10163
(212) 686-1100

■AMERICAN BAR ASSOCIATION'S SPECIAL COMMITTEE ON DRUG CRISIS
1800 M St., NW
Washington, DC 20036
(202) 331-2279

■AMERICAN COUNCIL ON ALCOHOL PROBLEMS
3426 Bridgeland Dr.
Bridgeton, MO 63044
(314) 739-5944

■AMERICAN COUNCIL FOR DRUG EDUCATION
204 Monroe St., Ste. 110
Rockville, MD 20854
(301) 294-0600

■AMERICAN SOCIETY OF ADDICTION MEDICINE
5225 Wisconsin Ave., NW,
Ste. 409
Washington, DC 20015
(202) 244-8948

■ASSOCIATION OF HALFWAY HOUSE ALCOHOLISM PROGRAMS OF NORTH AMERICA
786 E. Seventh St.
St. Paul, MN 55106
(612) 771-0933

■CENTER FOR ALCOHOL AND ADDICTION STUDIES
Box G, Brown University
Providence, RI 02912
(401) 863-1109

■CENTER FOR SCIENCE IN THE PUBLIC INTEREST (CSPI)
1875 Connecticut Ave., NW
Washington, DC 20009
(202) 332-9110

■CHILDREN OF ALCOHOLICS FOUNDATION, INC.
555 Madison Ave., 4th Fl.
New York, NY 10166
(212) 754-0656

■COALITION ON ADVERTISING AND FAMILY EDUCATION
c/o CSPI

■COCAINE ANONYMOUS
6125 Washington Blvd.
Ste 202
Culver City, CA 90232
(213) 839-1141

■CO-DEPENDENTS ANONYMOUS
PO Box 5508
Glendale, AZ 85312-5508

■EMPLOYEE ASSISTANCE PROFESSIONALS ASSOCIATION
4601 N. Fairfax Dr.
Ste. 1001
Arlington, VA 22203
(703) 522-6272

■ENTERTAINMENT INDUSTRIES COUNCIL
4444 Riverside Dr., Ste. 203
Burbank, CA 91505
(818) 841-9933

■FAMILIES IN ACTION
National Drug Information Center
2296 Henderson Mill Rd
Ste. 204
Atlanta, GA 30345
(404) 934-6364

■BETTY FORD FOUNDATION
39000 Bob Hope Dr.
Rancho Mirage, CA 92270
(619) 340-3911

■HAZELDEN FOUNDATION
Box 11
Center City, MN 55012
(800) 328-9000

■INTERNATIONAL COUNCIL ON ALCOHOL AND ADDICTION
Case postale 189
Avenue Tribunall-Federal 1
1001 Lausanne, Switzerland
021 20 98 65/66

■JEWISH ALCOHOLICS, CHEMICALLY DEPENDENT PERSONS AND SIGNIFICANT OTHERS
197 E. Broadway
New York, NY 10002
(212) 473-4747

■INSTITUTE ON BLACK CHEMICAL ABUSE
2614 Nicollet Ave.
Minneapolis, MN 55408
(612) 871-7878

■THE JOHNSON INSTITUTE
7151 Metro Blvd., Ste. 250
Minneapolis, MN 55439
(612) 944-0511

■LEGAL ACTION CENTER
153 Waverly Pl.
New York, NY 10014
(212) 243-1313

■MULTI-CULTURAL TRAINING RESOURCE CENTER
1540 Market St., Ste. 320
San Francisco, CA 94102
(415) 861-2142

■MULTI-MEDIA CENTER
(formerly CORK INSTITUTE)
720 Westview Dr., SW
Atlanta, GA 30310-1495
(404) 752-1530

■NARCOTICS ANONYMOUS
World Service Office
PO Box 9999
Van Nuys, CA 91409
(818) 780-3951

■NATIONAL ASSOCIATION FOR CHILDREN OF ALCOHOLICS (NACoA)
31582 Coast Hwy., Ste. B
South Laguna, CA 92677-3044
(714) 499-3889

■NATIONAL ASSOCIATON FOR PERINATAL ADDICTION RESEARCH AND EDUCATION
11 E. Hubbard St., Ste. 200
Chicago, IL 60611
(312) 329-2512

■NATIONAL ASSOCIATION OF ADDICTION TREATMENT PROVIDERS (NAATP)
25201 Paseo De Alicia
Ste. 100
Laguna Hills, CA 92653
(714) 837-3038

■NATIONAL ASSOCIATION OF ALCOHOLISM AND DRUG ABUSE COUNSELORS (NAADC)
3717 Columbia Pike, Ste. 642
Arlington, VA 22204
(730) 920-4644

■NATIONAL ASSOCIATION OF STATE ALCOHOL AND DRUG ABUSE DIRECTORS (NASADAD)
444 N. Capital St., NW
Ste. 642
Washington, DC 20001
(202) 783-6868

■NATIONAL CATHOLIC COUNCIL ON ALCOHOLISM AND RELATED DRUG PROBLEMS
1200 Varnum St., NE
Washington, DC 20017-2796
(202) 832-3811

■NATIONAL CLEARINGHOUSE FOR ALCOHOL AND DRUG INFORMATION (NCADI)
PO Box 2345
Rockville, Md 20852
(800) 729-6686

■NATIONAL COALITION TO PREVENT IMPAIRED DRIVING
c/o Advocacy Institute

■NATIONAL COUNCIL ON ALCOHOLISM AND DRUG DEPENDENCE
12 W. 21st St., 8th Fl.
New York, NY 10010
(212) 206-6770

■NATIONAL HIGHWAY TRAFFIC SAFETY ADMINISTRATION
400 7th St., SW
Washington, DC 20590
(202) 366-0123

■NATIONAL HISPANIC FAMILY AGAINST DRUG ABUSE
151 K St., Ste. 1029
Washington, DC 20005
(202) 732-7227

■NATIONAL INSTITUTE ON ALCOHOL ABUSE AND ALCOHOLISM (NIAAA)
Parklawn Bldg., Rm. 16-105
5600 Fishers Ln.
Rockville, MD 20857
(301) 443-3885

■NATIONAL NURSES SOCIETY ON ADDICTIONS
5700 Old Orchard Rd.
Skokie, IL 60077
(708) 966-5010

■NATIONAL SAFETY COUNCIL
444 North Michigan Ave.
Chicago, IL 60611
(312) 527-4800

■NATIONAL SELF-HELP CLEARINGHOUSE
33 W. 43rd St., Rm. 620
New York, NY 10036
(212) 642-2944

■OFFICE FOR SUBSTANCE ABUSE PREVENTION (OSAP)
Alcohol, Drug Abuse and Mental Health Adminstration,
Rockwall II
5600 Fishers Ln.
Rockville, MD 20857
(301) 443-0373

■PARENTS RESOURCE INSTITUTE FOR DRUG EDUCATION (PRIDE)
The Hurt Bldg., Ste. 210
50 Hurt Plaza
Atlanta, GA 30303
(800) 241-7946

■REMOVE INTOXICATED DRIVERS (RID)
PO Box 520
Schenectady, NY 12301
(518) 372-0034

■RESEARCH SOCIETY ON ALCOHOLISM
Box 1203, State University of New York
Health Science Center at Brooklyn
450 Clarkson Ave.
Brooklyn, NY 11203
(718) 270-2911

■RUTGERS UNIVERSITY CENTER OF ALCOHOL STUDIES
Smithers Hall, Busch Campus
Piscataway, NJ 08855-0969
(201) 932-4442

■THE CHRISTOPHER D. SMITHERS FOUNDATION
PO Box 67
Mill Neck, NY 11765
(516) 676-0067

■STEPPING STONES FOUNDATION
PO Box 452
Bedford Hill, NY 10507
(914) 232-4822

■SUBSTANCE ABUSE LIBRARIANS AND INFORMATION SPECIALISTS (SALIS)
Alcoholism and Drug Abuse Institute Library
3937 15th Ave., NE, NL-15
Seattle, WA 98105
(206) 543-0937

■SUZANNE SOMERS INSTITUTE
340 South Farrell Dr.
Ste. A203
Palm Springs, CA 92262
(619) 325-0110

■THERAPEUTIC COMMUNITIES OF AMERICA
1250 24 St., NW, Ste. 875
Washington, DC 20037
(202) 466-0511

■WOMEN FOR SOBRIETY
PO Box 618
Quakertown, PA 18951
(215) 536-8026

From *Resource and Referral Guide (1991) Data Source,* New York, 1991, National Council on Alcoholism and Drug Dependence.

CHAPTER 31

Evaluation of the Psychiatric Patient

STEPHEN A. DERRER

MARK A. HELFAER

For most anesthesiologists, providing care to a psychiatric patient requires skills not readily acquired from caring for patients with other disorders. During the preoperative interview the clinician often may have difficulty establishing rapport with the patient and gathering reliable, believable information. The adequacy of "informed consent" may be uncertain more often in caring for a psychiatric patient. Many psychiatric patients are receiving drugs that may have significant effects on the central nervous system (CNS), cardiovascular system, and other organ systems. These drugs also may interact with agents used during the perioperative period. Finally, many psychiatric patients under an anesthesiologist's care are being referred for electroconvulsive therapy (ECT), a procedure that carries many specific concerns.

PREOPERATIVE INTERVIEW

Preoperatively, an anesthesiologist is accustomed to interviewing patients who have voluntarily sought medical care. These patients are motivated to supply the clinician with any information necessary to promote safe, effective anesthesia and a positive outcome from the procedure. Although some psychiatric patients are so motivated, many others are not. The anesthesiologist may be confronted with a patient lacking insight into his/her problem and using denial and resistance. The patient may be delusional or, more often, depressed and totally uncommunicative. The patient may provide misinformation or no information at all. **Therefore the anesthesiologist should be prepared to rely more on the physical examination and a review of the patient's records for data. Also, the anesthesiologist should use the interview as an opportunity to develop a physician-patient relationship.**

The anesthesiologist/interviewer should provide understanding as well as reassurance to the patient.[56,80] This is often made more difficult by the interviewer's frequent frustration when dealing with a depressed individual. The anesthesiologist should probably avoid direct discussion of the patient's psychiatric history with the patient during the preoperative interview.[68] **If issues in the pyschiatric history are of specific concern to the anesthesiologist, they should be addressed to the patient's psychiatrist whenever possible.**

The clinician should remember that many serious medical illnesses may mimic psychiatric disease[40,53] (Box 31-1). Patients with thyroid disease,[35,52,80]

BOX 31-1
MEDICAL PROBLEMS THAT CAN MIMIC PSYCHIATRIC DISORDERS

Endocrine abnormalities

Hypothyroidism
Cushing's syndrome

Neurologic diseases

Seizure disorders (particularly temporal lobe
  epilepsy)
Demyelinating disease
Head trauma
Brain tumors
Encephalitis

Alcohol and drug abuse

Toxic and metabolic disorders

Heavy metal poisoning
Vitamin B_{12} or folate deficiency
Anticholinergic poisoning
Drug-induced toxicity

Collagen vascular disorders

---

especially hypothyroidism (Fig. 31-1); seizure disorders[7,41,66]; and chemical dependency often have psychiatric manifestations of their disease. Less common disturbances that can mimic psychiatric disorders include Cushing's syndrome,[8,20,51] encephalitis[64] and other neurologic disorders,[2,23,75] collagen vascular disease,[12] heavy metal toxicity,[6,19,57] and various meta-bolic disorders.[28,72] **Many drugs,**[65] including anti-cholinergics,[14] cimetidine,[1] reserpine,[37] digoxin,[38] monoamine oxidase (MAO) inhibitors,[73] indometha-cin,[17] and phencyclidine,[67] **can produce or mimic chronic psychiatric disorders.** Also, the psychiatric patient is susceptible to all the medical problems en-countered in the general population. Diabetes, for example, may occur more often among depressive persons than the general population.[81] Similarly, cer-tain specific personality types appear to be more sus-ceptible to coronary artery disease and its associated morbidity and mortality.[9,32] **The clinician thus must be alert to possible previously undiagnosed disorders while performing the preoperative evaluation.**

INFORMED CONSENT

Obtaining informed consent is an important compo-nent of an anesthesiologist's preoperative interview. For most surgical patients, the clinician describes the plan and risks involved and answers questions from a patient who is alert and communicative and demon-strates some understanding of the procedure, indica-tions, and risks. The psychiatric patient more often has blunted verbal and facial responses, which the clinician may regard as feedback indicating that the patient understands and agrees to the clinician's proposal. **Although the clinician should always at-tempt to have the patient demonstrate understanding of the proposed procedure, the lack of such a demonstration should not be equated with either a lack of informed consent or a lack of competency to provide consent.**[70] If the anesthesiologist leaves the interview uncertain of the adequacy of the consent,

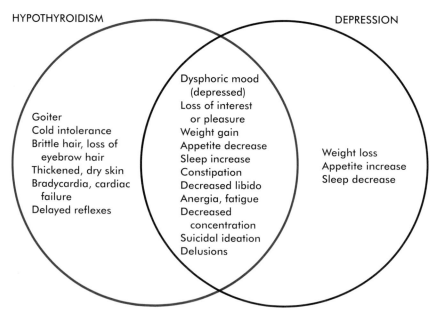

Fig. 31-1. Signs and symptoms of hypothyroidism and depression. (From Extein I, Gold MS: *Medical mimics of psychiatric disorders,* Washington, DC, 1986, American Psychiat-ric Press.)

he/she should consult the patient's chart or the referring psychiatrist or surgeon to determine who consented to the procedure. If that individual is not the patient, the consent for anesthetic care should be sought from the same source. **The anesthesiologist should not hesitate to discuss legitimate concerns regarding the adequacy of consent with the referring physician.** A further discussion of informed consent can be found in Chapter 101.

ANESTHETIC INTERACTIONS WITH PSYCHOTROPIC MEDICATION

Psychiatric practice, as with anesthetic practice, involves the use of a wide variety of powerful pharmacologic agents unfamiliar to specialists in most other specialties. These drugs have prominent effects on the CNS and cardiovascular systems that often affect the patient's responses to surgical stress and agents used in anesthesia. An understanding of psychotropic medications, their side effects, and their interactions with anesthetics is useful in the preoperative assessment of the psychiatric patient. A review of some of the important drug interactions is found in Table 31-1.

Major Tranquilizers

The major tranquilizers include members of several chemical classes: phenothiazines, butyrophenones, and thioxanthenes. Among the specific agents are chlorpromazine, promazine, triflupromazine, fluphenazine, trifluoperazine, haloperidol, and thiothixene. Although some individual differences exist among these agents in their effects on various receptors, **all possess antidopaminergic, anticholinergic, and antiadrenergic properties.** Pronounced hypotension during anesthesia has been attributed to these agents.[34]

Because the phenothiazines are selective alpha-adrenergic blockers, antihypertensive agents that have mixed alpha and beta agonist actions, such as **epinephrine, ephedrine, and mephentermine, may demonstrate reduced effectiveness or may even worsen hypotension.** This is caused by the relative enhancement of beta-adrenergic-induced vasodilation during alpha-adrenergic blockage, so-called epinephrine reversal.[79] The alpha-blockade produced by the major tranquilizers blunts reflex-mediated vasoconstriction in response to hypovolemia or drug-induced cardiac depression. This contributes to the observed incidence of intraoperative hypotension seen in patients treated with this class of drugs.

The anticholinergic effects of the major tranquilizers can increase the tendency toward undesirable side effects of anticholinergics typically used intraoperatively. Foreseeable problems include fever, adynamic ileus, tachycardia, urinary retention, and confusion. Clearly, anticholinergics should be given in judicious doses for patients receiving major tranquilizers. The severity of some side effects may be further reduced or eliminated by using a quaternary anticholinergic compound (e.g., glycopyrrolate) when an anticholinergic drug is indicated.

Besides their autonomic effects, the major tranquilizers can be potent sedatives and as such are capable of enhancing the CNS depressant effects of anesthetics and narcotics. Several members of this class, notably chlorpromazine, promazine, and promethazine, are sometimes used to enhance narcotic-induced analgesia and sedation. **The possibility of exaggerated CNS depression must be considered when planning an anesthetic for patients receiving these drugs to avoid prolonged postoperative somnolence.**[21]

A small minority of patients who take neuroleptics may develop *neuroleptic malignant syndrome,* characterized by muscle rigidity, tachycardia, and fever. These symptoms bear a strong resemblance to the signs of *malignant hyperthermia,* and the syndrome is treated with dantrolene (and bromocriptine). Since an association may exist between the two disease processes,[18] the anesthesiologist should avoid agents

Table 31-1   Interactions of psychotropic drugs with intraoperative agents

Psychotropic agent	Intraoperative agent	Interaction	References
Tricyclic antidepressants	Halothane, pancuronium	Tachydysrhythmias	24, 74
	Sympathomimetics	Hypertension	10, 44, 74
	Anticholinergics	Exaggerated anticholinergic responses	26, 63
Monoamine oxidase inhibitors	Meperidine	Hypertension, hyperpyrexia, seizures	25, 62, 78
	Sympathomimetics	Hypertension	48, 69
Phenothiazines	Enflurane, isoflurane	Hypotension	34
Lithium	Barbiturates	Prolonged somnolence	49, 58
	Nondepolarizing relaxants	Prolonged blockade	42
	Depolarizing relaxants	Prolonged blockade	4, 60

that trigger malignant hyperthermia (especially succinylcholine and halothane) in patients with neuroleptic malignant syndrome.

With a sound understanding of the interactions between the major tranquilizers and specific anesthetic agents, the anesthesiologist can safely prepare for elective surgery with the appropriate precautions.

Tricyclic Antidepressants

Tricyclic antidepressant agents are currently the mainstay in pharmacologic treatment of depression. Frequently used members of this class include amitriptyline, imipramine, nortriptyline, and doxepin. **Each of these drugs blocks the presynaptic reuptake of catecholamines and thereby increases central adrenergic tone.**[5] The resulting increase in concentration of catecholamines in the synaptic spaces enhances postsynaptic receptor stimulation, which is likely the mechanism of the tricyclic antidepressants' therapeutic effects. Tricyclic antidepressants increase circulating catecholamine levels.[44] These agents also have a quinidine-like effect on the heart and can slow atrioventricular conduction.[77,82]

The tricyclics have been shown to cause many adverse drug interactions with several classes of agents typically used intraoperatively (see Table 31-1). **The use of halothane-pancuronium anesthesia during treatment with tricyclic antidepressants has lead to reports of complications from serious dysrhythmias.**[24] Apparently, the catecholamine release caused by pancuronium is enhanced by the action of tricyclics. This exaggerated catecholamine release can then trigger serious dysrhythmias in the halothane-sensitized myocardium.

Chronic therapy with tricyclic antidepressants similarly produces an exaggerated response to sympathomimetics. When sympathomimetics are used, even in the doses administered as vasoconstrictors with local anesthetics, dangerous levels of hypertension as well as tachycardia and dysrhythmias are possible. **Pressors thus should be used cautiously.** Treatment should be available to deal with possible adverse consequences.

Because of the occasional seriousness of these interactions, some have recommended withdrawal of tricyclics for 2 weeks before elective surgery.[47] This is probably unnecessary, and it is generally desirable to continue any long-term medical regimen beneficial to the patient. The clinician must be aware of the nature and possible seriousness of drug interactions involving tricyclics when planning an anesthetic for patients receiving these drugs (see Table 31-1).

Monoamine Oxidase Inhibitors

The MAO inhibitors increase the availability of catecholamines in the CNS by blocking their break- down by the enzyme monoamine oxidase. MAO inhibitors have a therapeutic effect in the treatment of depression, although their use has largely been supplanted by the tricyclics. Several MAO inhibitors—phenelzine, pargyline, isocarboxazid, and tranylcypromine—are still sometimes used in patients with refractory depression.

The combination of MAO inhibitors and either sympathomimetics or meperidine has resulted in numerous reports of profound reactions, including hyperpyrexia, hypertension, and seizures.[16,29] The response to sympathomimetics is mediated by the large quantities of catecholamine available for release, a result of the inhibiting effect of MAO inhibitors on catecholamine breakdown. The mechanism for the response to meperidine is poorly understood. This phenomenon has caused debate as to whether MAO inhibitors should be withdrawn preoperatively.[20] Because narcotics other than meperidine do not seem to trigger a dramatic reaction,[22] most patients can probably be managed safely with proper monitoring. Avoiding the surgical delay may decrease patient suffering that can occur following withdrawal. By avoiding agents that would trigger these interactions, the MAO inhibitors can be safely continued up to and through the perioperative period.

Lithium

Lithium salts are frequently used for patients with manic-depressive illness and appear particularly effective in limiting the manic phases of this disorder. **Lithium has a rather narrow toxic/therapeutic ratio and probably exerts both its toxic and its therapeutic effects via an effect on sodium channels.** Lithium can produce both cardiac conduction abnormalities and T-wave changes of uncertain clinical significance.[13] **The effect of lithium on sodium channels causes a general depression of excitable tissues, such as cardiac and nervous tissue.**

Concentrations of lithium above the therapeutic range (0.5 to 1.5 mEq/L) can produce obvious confusion and somnolence. Even in the absence of clinical symptoms of global depression, **lithium can prolong barbiturate-induced sleep time, postoperative unconsciousness, and recovery time.**[49,58] **Lithium can also enhance the neuromuscular blockade produced by succinylcholine**[43] **or pancuronium.**[11] Interestingly, however, lithium is reported to have no effect on the blockade produced by gallamine or d-tubocurarine.[42]

Although chronic lithium use probably represents some additional risk during elective surgery, the risk is apparently not great in the absence of overt toxicity. The risks of proceeding with elective surgery in a patient receiving lithium must be balanced against the risks to the patient's well-being imposed by withdrawing effective therapy. **In proceeding, the clinician must be aware of the effects of lithium on such diffuse areas as cardiac conduction, neuromuscular function, and global cerebral function.**

Other Psychotropic Medications

Reserpine is no longer used to any appreciable extent in psychiatric practice. It is still used occasionally as an antihypertensive agent and sympatholytic. Reserpine depletes catecholamine stores. The effects of sympathomimetic agents on patients receiving reserpine can be quite abnormal. The action of direct-acting sympathomimetics may be enhanced because of receptor hypersensitivity, whereas the action of indirect-acting agents is substantially blunted because of the diminished quantity of catecholamines available for release from presynaptic storage.[3]

Fluoxetine (Prozac) has become the most frequently prescribed antidepressant. It is a bicyclic that inhibits the reuptake of serotonin and lacks the anticholinergic and alpha-adrenergic blocking properties of the tricyclic antidepressants. Life-threatening interactions with MAO inhibitors have been reported. Less severe reactions have been reported with the concomitant use of lithium, haloperidol, tryptophan, and carbamazepine. These reactions have been neurologic or behavioral effects.[61] Fluoxetine may increase the toxicity of tricyclics by inhibiting their metabolism. The drug is also strongly bound to plasma proteins and therefore may displace protein-bound drugs such as digoxin or warfarin. Although no interactons between fluoxetine and anesthetics have been reported, the clinician should use antiemetics such as droperidol and prochlorperazine with caution.

Trazodone is an antidepressant agent unrelated to the tricyclics that inhibits serotonin reuptake. Although its use has been popularized because of its favorable side effects profile, exacerbation of serious dysrhythmias in patients with mitral valve prolapse has been reported with trazadone use.[46] Overall, however, trazadone compares favorably with the tricyclic antidepressants and MAO inhibitors.

Maprotiline (Ludiomil) is a tetracycline antidepressant agent. As yet, experience with perioperative problems is limited with this class of drugs. However, their clinical pharmacology is similar to that of the tricyclics, and tetracyclic antidepressants should be considered to have the same potential for adverse drug interactions.

PREOPERATIVE EVALUATION FOR ELECTROCONVULSIVE THERAPY

ECT is a useful and effective, although sometimes controversial, treatment for depression. It is also occasionally used to treat acute schizophrenia, particularly if the patient has a refractory affective component. This treatment modality was developed during the 1930s based on the observation that psychiatric symptoms in a schizophrenic patient were somewhat alleviated by a seizure. Various pharmacologically induced seizure regimens, including insulin-induced hypoglycemia, were used before the standardization of electrical induction as the epileptogenic stimulus of choice. The later development of ECT was hampered by some degree of abuse and adverse publicity, culminating in legal restriction in some jurisdictions. The technique survived and currently has renewed popularity because it is an effective and relatively safe modality, comparing favorably to drugs in the treatment of depression.[71]

The mechanism of the antidepressant effect of ECT is unknown. Its effectiveness, however, is *not* related to the production of cerebral hypoxia or memory disturbances or to general cerebral or sympathetic stimulation. A seizure must be produced by the electrical stimulus for the treatment to be effective, and seizures less than 25 seconds in duration are of little benefit.

The safety and acceptability of ECT are greatly enhanced by the use of muscle relaxants and anesthetics.[76] For the anesthesiologist, ECT presents several interesting challenges. **The treatment itself produces profound but short-lived changes in the cardiovascular system, particularly cerebral blood flow and metabolism.** Finally, although the procedure is brief and noninvasive, potential complications are possible in many areas of concern to the anesthesiologist, including the airway, the musculoskeletal system, and drug interactions involving the anesthetic agents. Drug interactions are discussed in the previous section; the other areas of specific concern in ECT are considered here.

Physiologic Effects

ECT produces an immediate and profound autonomic activation (Box 31-2).[33] **This is often apparent as an immediate bradycardia, followed shortly by tachycardia and hypertension.** Other electrocardiographic (ECG) changes, such as repolarization abnormalities, atrioventricular dissociation, and ventricular and supraventricular ectopy, are possible.[39] The patient often salivates profusely.[45,54] Plasma catecholamine levels are also increased,[50] which can lead to an episode of tachycardia and hypertension of greater duration than the initial autonomically mediated event.

The seizure activity produced by ECT is accompanied by the expected increases in cerebral metabolism, cerebral blood flow, and intracranial pressure.[15,22,55] ECT is also accompanied by increases in intraocular[27] and intragastric[59] pressures. ECT appears to have an aggravating effect on diabetes,[30,31,36]

BOX 31-2
PHYSIOLOGIC EFFECTS OF
ELECTROCONVULSIVE THERAPY (ECT)

Cardiovascular effects
   Immediate: parasympathetic stimulation
      Bradycardia
      Hypotension
   Late (after 1 minute): sympathetic stimulation
      Tachycardia
      Hypertension
      Dysrhythmias
      ↑ Myocardial oxygen consumption
Cerebral effects
   ↑ Cerebral oxygen consumption
   ↑ Cerebral blood flow
   ↑ Intracranial pressure
↑ Intraocular pressure
↑ Intragastric pressure

From Gaines GY, Rees I: Electroconvulsive therapy and anesthetic considerations, *Anesth Analg* 65:1345, 1986.

---

probably because of the increases in plasma cortisol, glucagon, and catecholamine levels.[50]

Preanesthetic Workup

The laboratory evaluation in preparation for ECT of a reasonably healthy patient need not be extensive. **Because of the magnitude of the cardiomuscular impact of the treatment, an ECG is mandatory.** Although others have recommended batteries of routine tests, including blood count, urinalysis, chest radiograph, blood chemistries, and thyroid function tests,[59] performance of these or other tests should be dictated by the patient history, physical examination, and medical regimen and need not be performed routinely.

With advances in the understanding of disease processes, drug interactions, monitoring, and airway management, the list of conditions contraindicating ECT has diminished. ECT should never be undertaken lightly, but it should be regarded as an important and worthwhile therapy that the anesthesiologist should accommodate whenever possible. A patient with serious pulmonary or neuromuscular disease should be managed with the same considerations used during urgent surgical procedures. A patient with advanced cardiac disease, for example, may require invasive hemodynamic monitoring, including pulmonary artery catheterization. Once the patient's response to ECT and response to drugs used to modify the hemodynamic response to ECT have been quantified, subsequent treatments can often be performed with routine monitoring.

CONCLUSION

The psychiatric patient often presents unique challenges to the anesthesiologist, specifically in the areas of interpersonal communication, drug interactions, and preparation for ECT and its implications. With a detailed understanding of the potential problems and their mechanism, these patients can be handled safely in almost all situations.

KEY POINTS

- Preoperative assessment of the psychiatric patient may be based more on the physical examination and review of the patient's record than on the interview results.

- Many serious medical illnesses can mimic psychiatric disease, as can many drug effects. Among these diseases are thyroid disorders, seizure disorders, Cushing's syndrome, encephalitis, collagen vascular disease, heavy metal toxicity, and chemical dependency. Drugs that produce psychiatric symptoms include anticholinergics, cimetidine, reserpine, digoxin, monoamine oxidase (MAO) inhibitors, indomethacin, and phencyclidine.

- Sympathomimetics may have reduced effectiveness or may even cause hypotension when used with phenothiazines.

- The use of halothane-pancuronium anesthesia during treatment with tricyclics can lead to complications resulting from serious dysrhythmias.

- Chronic therapy with tricyclics may produce an exaggerated response to sympathomimetics.

- When MAO inhibitors are combined with either sympathomimetics or meperidine, profound reactions can result, including hyperpyrexia, hypertension, and seizures.

- Lithium produces effects on cardiac conduction, neuromuscular function, and global cerebral function, prolonging barbiturate-induced sleep time, postoperative unconsciousness, and recovery time.

■ Elective surgery can be safely performed with appropriate precautions when psychotropic medicines are being concomitantly administered.

■ Electroconvulsive therapy (ECT) produces an immediate and profound autonomic activation (immediate bradycardia, followed shortly by tachycardia and hypertension).

KEY REFERENCES

Selvin BL: Electroconvulsive therapy—1987, *Anesthesiology* 67:367, 1987.

Viegas OJ: Psychiatric illness. In Stoelting RK, Deerdorf SF, eds: *Anesthesia and co-existing disease*, New York, 1983, Churchill-Livingstone.

REFERENCES

1. Adler LE, Sadja L, and Wilets G: Cimetidine toxicity manifested as paranoia and hallucinations, *Am J Psychiatry* 137:1112, 1980.
2. Alarcon RD, Thweatt RW: A case of subdural hematoma mimicking severe depression with conversion-like symptoms, *Am J Psychiatry* 140:1360, 1983.
3. Alper MH, Flacke W, and Krager O: Pharmacology of reserpine and its implications for anesthesia, *Anesthesiology* 24:524, 1963.
4. Amidsen A: Lithium and drug interactions, *Drugs* 24:133, 1982.
5. Anderson BO: Long term prognosis in geriatric surgery: 2-17 year follow-up of 7922 patients, *J Am Geriatr Soc* 20:255, 1972.
6. Baker EL, Feldman RG, White RF et al: The role of occupational lead exposure in the genesis of psychiatric and behavioral disturbances, *Acta Psychiatr Scand* 67:38, 1983.
7. Bear D, Levin K, Blumer D et al: Interictal behavior in hospitalized temporal lobe epileptics: relationship to idiopathic psychiatric syndromes, *J Neurol Neurosurg Psychiatry* 45:481, 1982.
8. Becker L, Gold P, and Chrousos G: Analogies between Cushing's disease and depression: a case report, *Gen Hosp Psychiatry* 5:89, 1983.
9. Blumenthal JA, Williams RB Jr, Kong Y et al: Type A behavior pattern and coronary atherosclerosis, *Circulation* 58:634, 1978.
10. Boakes AJ, Laurence DR, Teoh PC et al: Interactions between sympathomimetic amines and antidepressant agents in man, *Br Med J* 1:311, 1973.
11. Borden H, Clarke M, and Katz H: The use of pancuronium bromide in patients receiving lithium carbonate, *Can Anaesth Soc J* 21:79, 1974.
12. Borson S: Behçet's disease as a psychiatric disorder: a case report, *Am J Psychiatry* 139:1348, 1982.
13. Brady HD, Gargan JH: Lithium and the heart: unanswered questions, *Chest* 93:166, 1988.
14. Brizer DA, Manning DW: Delirium induced by poisoning with anticholinergic agents, *Am J Psychiatry* 138:1343, 1982.
15. Brodersen P, Paulson OB, Bolwig TG et al: Cerebral hyperemia in electrically induced epileptic seizures, *Arch Neurol* 28:334, 1973.
16. Brownlee G, Williams GW: Potentiation of amphetamine and pethidine by monoamine oxidase inhibitors, *Lancet* 1:699, 1963.
17. Carney MWP: Paranoid psychosis with indomethacin, *Br Med J* 2:994, 1977.
18. Caroft SN, Rosenberg H, Fletcher JE et al: Malignant hyperthermia susceptibility in neuroleptic malignant syndrome, *Anesthesiology* 67:20, 1987.
19. Chandra SV: Psychiatric illness due to manganese poisoning, *Acta Psychiatr Scand* 67:49, 1983.
20. Cohen SI: Cushing's syndrome: a psychiatric study of 29 patients, *Br J Psychiatry* 136:120, 1980.
21. Dobkins AB: Potentiation of thiopental anesthesia by derivatives and analogues of phenothiazine, *Anesthesiology* 21:292, 1960.
22. Dressler DM, Folk J: The treatment of depression with ECT in the presence of a brain tumor, *Am J Psychiatry* 132:1320, 1975.
23. Dubin WR, Weiss KJ, and Zeccardi JA: Organic brain syndrome: a psychiatric imposter, *JAMA* 249:60, 1983.
24. Edwards RP, Miller RD, Roizen MF et al: Cardiac responses to imipramine and pancuronium during anesthesia with halothane and enflurane, *Anesthesiology* 50:421, 1979.
25. El-Ganzouri AR, Ivankovich AD, Braverman B et al: Monoamine oxidase inhibitors: should they be discontinued preoperatively? *Anesth Analg* 64:592, 1985.
26. El-Jousef MK et al: Reversal of antiparkinsonian drug toxicity by physostigmine: a controlled study, *Am J Psychiatry* 130:141, 1973.
27. Eptein HM, Fagman W, Bruce DL et al: Intraocular pressure changes during anesthesia for electroshock therapy, *Anesth Analg* 54:479, 1975.
28. Evans DL, Edelson GA, and Golden RN: Organic psychoses without anemia or spinal cord symptoms in patients with vitamin B_{12} deficiency, *Am J Psychiatry* 140:218, 1983.
29. Evans-Prosser CDG: The use of pethidine and morphine in the presence of monoamine oxidase inhibitors, *Br J Anaesth* 40:279, 1968.
30. Fakhri O, Fadhli A, and Rawi R: Effect of electroconvulsive therapy on diabetes mellitus, *Lancet* 2:775, 1980.
31. Finestone DH, Weiner RD: Effects of ECT on diabetes mellitus, *Acta Psychiatr Scand* 70:321, 1984.
32. Friedman M, Byers SO, Diamant J et al: Plasma catecholamine response of coronary artery–prone subjects (type A) to a specific challenge, *Metabolism* 24:205, 1975.
33. Gaines GY, Rees I: Electroconvulsive therapy and anesthetic considerations, *Anesth Analg* 65:1345, 1986.
34. Gold MI: Profound hypotension associated with preoperative use of phenothiazines, *Anesth Analg* 53:844, 1974.
35. Goldman V: Local anaesthetics containing vasoconstrictor, *Br Med J* 1:175, 1971.
36. Goldney R, Thomas A, and Phillips P: Depression, electroconvulsive therapy and diabetes mellitus, *Aust N Z J Psychiatry* 17:289, 1983.
37. Goodwin FK, Bunney WE: Depressions following reserpine: a reevaluation, *Semin Psychiatry* 3:435, 1971.
38. Gorelick DA, Kussin SZ, and Kahn I: Single case study: paranoid delusions and auditory hallucinations associated with digoxin intoxication, *J Nerv Ment Dis* 166:817, 1978.
39. Gould L, Gopalaswamy C, Chandy F et al: Electroconvulsive therapy–induced ECG changes simulating a myocardial infarction, *Arch Intern Med* 143:1786, 1983.
40. Hall RCW et al: Physical illness presenting as psychiatric disease, *Arch Gen Psychiatry* 35:1315, 1978.
41. Hara T, Hoshi A, Takase M et al: Factors related to psychiatric episodes in epileptics, *Folia Psychiatr Neurol Jpn* 34:329, 1980.
42. Hill GE, Wong KC: Lithium carbonate and neuromuscular blocking agents, *Anesthesiology* 46:122, 1977.
43. Hill GE, Wong KC, and Hodges MR: Potentiation of succinylcholine neuromuscular blockade by lithium carbonate, *Anesthesiology* 44:439, 1976.

44. Hollister LE: During therapy: tricyclic antidepressants, *N Engl J Med* 299:1106, 1161, 1978.

45. Hurwitz TD: Electroconvulsive therapy: a review, *Compr Psychiatry* 15:303, 1974.

46. Janowsky D, Curtis G, Zisook S et al: Ventricular arrhythmias possibly aggravated by trazadone, *Am J Psychiatry* 140:796, 1983.

47. Janowsky EC, Risch SC, and Janowsky DS: Psychotropic agents. In Smith NT, Miller RD, and Corbasco AN, eds: *Drug interactions in anesthesia,* Philadelphia, 1981, Lea & Febiger.

48. Jenkins LC, Graves HB: Potential hazards of psychoactive drugs in association with anesthesia, *Can Anaesth Soc J* 12:121, 1965.

49. Jephcott G, Kerry RJ: Lithium: an anesthetic risk, *Br J Anaesth* 46:389, 1974.

50. Jones RM, Knight PR: Cardiovascular and hormonal responses to ECT, *Anesthesia* 36:795, 1981.

51. Kelly WF, Checkley SA, Bender DA et al: Cushing's syndrome and depression: a prospective study of 26 patients, *Br J Psychiatry* 142:16, 1983.

52. Klein I, Levey GS: Unusual manifestations of hypothyroidism, *Arch Intern Med* 144:123, 1984.

53. Koranyi EK: Morbidity and rate of undiagnosed physical illness in a psychiatric clinic population, *Arch Gen Psychiatry* 36:414, 1979.

54. London SW, Glass DD: Prevention of electroconvulsive therapy–induced dysrhythmias with atropine and propranolol, *Anesthesiology* 62:819, 1985.

55. Lorett-Doust JW, Raschka LB: Enduring effects of modified ECT on cerebral circulation in man, *Psychiatr Clin North Am* 8:293, 1975.

56. MacKinnon RA, Michels R: General principles of the interview. In *The psychiatric interview in clinical practice,* Philadelphia, 1971, WB Saunders.

57. Maghazaji HI: Psychiatric aspects of methyl mercury poisoning, *J Neurol Neurosurg Psychiatry* 37:954, 1974.

58. Mannisto PT, Saarnivarra L: Effect of lithium and rubidium on the sleeping time caused by various intravenous anesthetics in the mouse, *Br J Anaesth* 48:185, 1976.

59. Marks RJ: Electroconvulsive therapy: physiologic and anaesthetic considerations, *Can Anaesth Soc J* 31:541, 1984.

60. Martin BA, Kramer PM: Clinical significance of the interaction between lithium and a neuromuscular blocker, *Am J Psychiatry* 139:1326, 1982.

61. *Med Let* 32:83, 1990.

62. Michaels I et al: Anesthesia for cardiac surgery in patients receiving monoamine oxidase inhibitors, *Anesth Analg* 63:1041, 1984.

63. Milner G, Hills N: Adynamic ileus and nortriptyline, *Br Med J* 1:1421, 1966.

64. Oommen AJ, Johnson PC, and Ray CG: Herpes simplex type II virus encephalitis presenting as psychosis, *Am J Med* 73:445, 1982.

65. Paykel ES, Fleminger R, and Watson JP: Psychiatric side effects of antihypertensive drugs other than reserpine, *J Clin Pharmacol* 2:14, 1982.

66. Perez MM, Trimble MR: Epileptic psychosis—diagnostic comparison with process schizophrenia, *Br J Psychiatry* 137:245, 1980.

67. Rappolt RT, Gay GR, and Farris RD: Emergency management of acute phencyclidine intoxication, *J Am Coll Emerg Physicians* 8:68, 1979.

68. Rich CL, Smith NT: Anaesthesia for electroconvulsive therapy: a psychiatric viewpoint, *Can Anaesth Soc J* 28:153, 1981.

69. Schwartz AJ, Woollman H: Anesthetic considerations for patients on chronic drug therapy: L-dopa, monoamine oxidase inhibitors, tricyclic antidepressants, and propranolol, *Anesthesiology* 44:98, 1976.

70. Schwartz HI, Blank K: Shifting competency during hospitalization: a model for informed consent decisions, *Hosp Community Psychiatry* 37:1256, 1986.

71. Selvin BL: Electroconvulsive therapy—1987, *Anesthesiology* 67:367, 1987.

72. Shalmlam R: An overview of folic acid deficiency and psychiatric illness. In Botz MI, Reynolds EH, eds: *Folic acid in neurology, psychiatry and internal medicine,* New York, 1979, Raven Press.

73. Sheehy LM, Maxmen JS: Phenelzine induced psychosis, *Am J Psychiatry* 135:1422, 1978.

74. Spies CK, Smith CM, and Marge M: Halothane-epinephrine arrhythmias and adrenergic responsiveness after chronic imipramine administration in dogs, *Anesth Analg* 63:825, 1984.

75. Strauss I, Keshner M: Mental symptoms in cases of tumor of the frontal lobe, *Arch Neurol Psychiatry* 33:986, 1935.

76. Valentine M, Keddie KM, and Dunne D: A comparison of techniques in electroconvulsive therapy, *Br J Psychiatry* 114:989, 1968.

77. Veith RC, Raskind MA, Caldwell JH et al: Cardiovascular effects of tricyclic antidepressants in depressed patients with chronic heart disease, *N Engl J Med* 306:954, 1982.

78. Viegas OJ: Psychiatric illness. In Stoelting RK, Deerdorf SF, eds: *Anesthesia and co-existing disease,* New York, 1983, Churchill-Livingstone.

79. Weiner N: Drugs that inhibit adrenergic nerves and block adrenergic receptors. In Goodman AG et al, eds: *The pharmacologic basis of therapeutics,* ed 7, New York, 1985, Macmillan.

80. Whitehorn JC: Guide to interviewing and clinical personality study, *Arch Neurol Psychiatry* 52:197, 1944.

81. Wilkinson DG: Psychiatric aspects of diabetes mellitus, *Br J Psychiatry* 138:1, 1981.

82. Williams RB, Sherter C: Cardiac complications of tricyclic antidepressant therapy, *Ann Intern Med* 74:395, 1971.

CHAPTER 32

Evaluation of the Burn Patient

WILLIAM R. FURMAN
KENT S. PEARSON

Burn injury is a specific form of trauma in which the largest organ in the body, the skin, is damaged. **Major burns cause subtotal destruction of the skin and mucous membranes and are associated with severe metabolic, cardiovascular, and respiratory disorders.** Burn patients require many lifesaving, function-preserving, and appearance-saving surgical procedures during their hospital stay. **Many such operations cannot be delayed until the underlying systemic disorders are corrected. Much of the metabolic, cardiovascular, and respiratory dysfunction associated with burn injury is perpetuated by the burn wound and thus cannot be fully corrected until the burn wound has been excised and grafted.**

These factors make it necessary and proper to anesthetize critically ill burn patients many times during their course of treatment and likewise make it impossible to completely reverse their underlying ailments before surgery. One useful way to deal with the discomfort inherent in this need to provide anesthesia to metabolically imbalanced patients is to view their transfer to the operating room as merely another aspect of their intensive care. In this respect, the anesthesiologist's responsibility is to continue (and modify as needed) metabolic, cardiovascular, and respiratory support during transport to the operating room, during surgery, and return transport to the burn unit. To effectively perform that role, it is necessary to understand the biology of burn injury, the direct and indirect metabolic, hemodynamic, and pulmonary consequences of burns, and the logistic problems these consequences impose. These factors are considered in the preoperative visit.

BIOLOGY AND CONSEQUENCES OF BURN INJURY

Burns may be directly caused by heat or by the heat energy generated by chemicals, electricity, or ionizing radiation. This energy directly injures the skin and may also affect mucous membranes. Chemical mediators and vasoactive substances are released after burn injury, and many of the metabolic, cardiovascular, and pulmonary abnormalities that subsequently develop may be attributable to the effects of these mediators.

Characterization of Burns

Burns are classified according to their severity, the energy source, and the presence of associated inhalational injury. The severity of a burn is related to its depth and extent. The depth of skin destruction is characterized as **first-, second-** or **third-degree,** based on whether there is superficial, partial-thickness, or full-thickness destruction of the skin and its appendages. The term **fourth-degree** is sometimes used to identify burns that injure structures beneath the skin, such as muscle and fascia. The extent of the burn is the percentage of the total body surface area (TBSA) that is affected, usually estimated by use of the Lund and Browder chart[38,44] (Fig. 32-1).

ADMISSION BURN EVALUATION SHEET

Date of Admission: ______________________ Weight: ______________________

AREA	PERCENT OF BURN					SEVERITY OF BURN		TOTAL PERCENT
	0-1 Year	1-4 Years	5-9 Years	10-15 Years	ADULT	2°	3°	
Head	19	17	13	10	7			
Neck	2	2	2	2	2			
Ant. Trunk	13	17	13	13	13			
Post. Trunk	13	13	13	13	13			
R. Buttock	2½	2½	2½	2½	2½			
L. Buttock	2½	2½	2½	2½	2½			
Genitalia	1	1	1	1	1			
R.U. Arm	4	4	4	4	4			
L.U. Arm	4	4	4	4	4			
R.L. Arm	3	3	3	3	3			
L.L. Arm	3	3	3	3	3			
R. Hand	2½	2½	2½	2½	2½			
L. Hand	2½	2½	2½	2½	2½			
R. Thigh	5½	6½	8½	8½	9½			
L. Thigh	5½	6½	8½	8½	9½			
R. Leg	5	5	5½	6	7			
L. Leg	5	5	5½	6	7			
R. Foot	3½	3½	3½	3½	3½			
L. Foot	3½	3½	3½	3½	3½			
				Total				

Code: Blue areas indicate 2°
Red areas indicate 3°

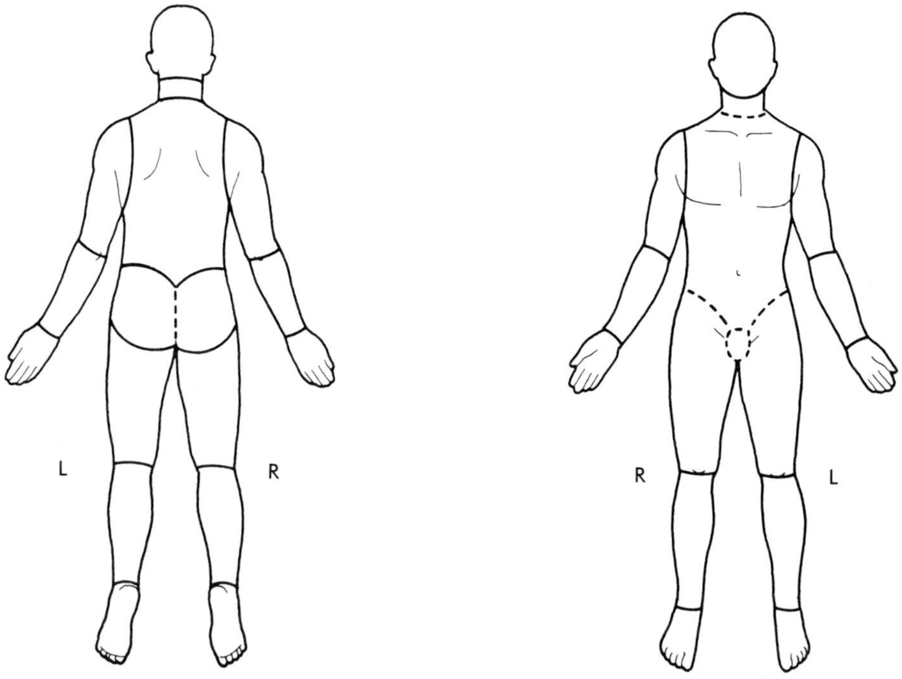

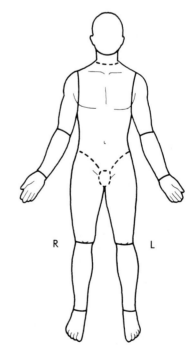

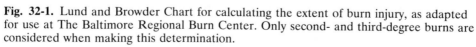

Fig. 32-1. Lund and Browder Chart for calculating the extent of burn injury, as adapted for use at The Baltimore Regional Burn Center. Only second- and third-degree burns are considered when making this determination.

In terms of prognosis, it is helpful to make a single distinction between first- or superficial second-degree burns and deep second- or third-degree burns because the latter do not heal spontaneously or do so with poor cosmetic and functional result. Superficial partial-thickness burns involve only the epidermis and outer dermis, resulting in only minor physiologic changes. The burned areas appear blistered, with pink or red epidermis below the blister (Table 32-1). The burned skin is very painful because of exposed nerve endings. Deep partial-thickness burns extend further into the dermis but spare portions of the epidermal skin appendages (hair follicles, nerve endings, sweat glands, and sebaceous glands). These burns appear white but are soft and elastic to touch. Full-thickness burns spare no epithelial remnants in the wound and appear hard, dry, and white or tan-colored. Pain is usually absent in areas of full-thickness burns because the nerve endings have been destroyed.

Deep second- and third-degree burns require surgical debridement and coverage, whereas more superficial burns generally do not. **Mortality from thermal injury is related to the area involved by deep second- or third-degree burns.** Other factors associated with mortality are age, **the presence of inhalational injury,**[27,28,51] and the presence of a burn caused by high-tension (more than 1000 V) electrical shock.[33] The decision to refer a patient to a regional burn center after resuscitation and stabilization is usually based on the determination that the burn is *major*. In adults, major burns are usually considered to be those involving 20% or more of the TBSA in deep partial-thickness or full-thickness burns (5% to 10% TBSA in infants and children) as well as those complicated by smoke inhalation or large facial, hand, or perineal burns. High-tension electrical burns are also considered major.

Direct Effects of Burn Injury
Injury to the skin

Mediator release. **Thermal injury to skin and its microvasculature incites an inflammatory response consisting of activation of leukocytes and release of biologic response mediators (BRMs).**[42] In general terms, this response consists of the cellular processes that localize injury, combat infection, and promote healing of the wound. Local blood flow increases and white blood cells (WBC) migrate into the affected area. Complement is activated, and prostaglandins (PG), interleukins, platelet-aggregating factor, interferons, colony-stimulating factors, and other WBC-derived polypeptides (cytokines) are released into the wound and the bloodstream.[7,19,20]

Patients with burn wounds typically present with three concentric zones of injury. The *central zone of coagulation* contains necrotic tissue and thrombosed

Table 32-1 Classification of burn depth	
Burn type	**Characteristics**
First degree	Only epidermis damaged
	Painful erythema
	Minimal local edema
	Spontaneous healing in 48-72 hours
Superficial second degree (superficial partial-thickeness)	Outer layers of dermis destroyed
	Vesicles formed
	Erythema, blanching with pressure
Deep second degree (deep partial-thickness)	Only deepest dermal appendages not damaged
	Skin pale, blistered, edematous
Third degree (full-thickness)	All of epidermis and dermis destroyed
	Burned area is anesthetic, dry, and charred or white

blood vessels and is nonviable. The *outer zone of hyperemia* is viable, but develops a significant increase in capillary permeability and tissue edema. The clinical course of the *intermediate zone of stasis* evolves over the first 48 hours after the burn injury; this zone may survive or suffer tissue death, depending on the type of burning medium and the duration of exposure.[8] The occlusion of blood vessels, increases in capillary permeability, and vasodilation that occur in these three zones are believed to be mediated by locally released BRMs. These BRMs also have profound systemic effects, which contribute to alterations in metabolism, hemodynamics, and pulmonary function.

Local edema. **Edema formation and resultant loss of plasma volume are the primary reasons why burn victims require copious fluid resuscitation** (see Chapter 86). An immediate increase in microvascular permeability to large molecular weight proteins occurs in the burn wound.[15,25] Although this is partly related to the thermal insult, histamine, prostaglandins (PGE_2 and prostacyclin), serotonin, and oxygen-free radicals are known to be released into the wound,[42] and are probably also involved.

Direct injury to the respiratory system

Inhalational injury comprises carbon monoxide (CO) poisoning, upper airway swelling and obstruction, and damage to the lower respiratory tract (Box 32-1). Each of these can lead to respiratory failure and the requirement for early endotracheal intubation. **Inha-**

lational injury is a serious complication of burn exposure because when present, on the average, it increases mortality rates by 40%.[28]

Carbon monoxide poisoning. Carbon monoxide poisoning occurs at the scene of the injury and exerts its adverse effects in the first few hours. Carbon monoxide causes tissue hypoxia, despite a high Po_2, because it binds to hemoglobin 200 times more readily than oxygen, thus reducing the oxygen-carrying capacity of the blood. The reduction in oxygen-carrying capacity leads to a decrease in oxygen delivery, which is compounded by the fact that carbon monoxide also increases the stability of the oxyhemoglobin molecule and thus impedes release of oxygen to the tissues.[18,32]

Carbon monoxide poisoning should be suspected in victims of closed-space fires (buildings and automobiles). Clinical signs and symptoms of hypoxia may be present: headache, shortness of breath, nausea, angina pectoris, tachypnea, and mental status changes; however, the patient will not have cyanosis. **Standard (two-wavelength) pulse oximetry does not distinguish between the oxyhemoglobin and the carboxyhemoglobin molecules.** Newer three-wavelength devices capable of such distinction are being developed.[3]

The diagnosis of carbon monoxide poisoning is made by measuring the carboxyhemoglobin level, expressed as a percent saturation of hemoglobin in arterial blood. Saturations in excess of 15% are usually toxic, and those exceeding 50% are almost always lethal. The treatment is removal from the source of carbon monoxide and administration of 100% oxygen. Use of 100% oxygen displaces carbon monoxide from the hemoglobin molecule by reducing the half-life for dissociation of carbon monoxide from hemoglobin from 5 hours (breathing room air) to 45 to 60 minutes. Hyperbaric oxygen therapy has been recommended as a treatment for carbon monoxide poisoning because it can further reduce this half-life to 23 minutes. Hyperbaric oxygen therapy is not available in all burn centers and is controversial because outcome studies have not consistently shown it to be beneficial.[21,39] Even with appropriate treatment and despite apparent initial recovery from the acute effects of carbon monoxide poisoning, delayed neurologic symptoms may develop after several weeks. This is more common in elderly patients and in those with especially high initial carbon monoxide levels.[11]

Upper airway injury. **Inhaled flames, toxic chemicals, and hot air can injure the upper airway and lower respiratory tract.**[35] Inhalational injury is common in victims of structural fires (buildings and vehicles). **Life-threatening swelling of the tissues of the upper airway,** defined as those structures above the true vocal cords, occurs in 20% to 30% of patients with inhalational injury.[14,22] In these patients, the direct injury is initially manifested as erythema, blistering, and necrosis of the epithelium. After a latent period of 4 to 48 hours, however, significant edema of the epiglottis and laryngeal structures develops.[5,40]

The diagnosis of evolving airway obstruction is best made by examination of the upper airway. The clinical signs of facial burns, sooty oral or nasal secretions, hoarseness, and a swollen, erythematous tongue are suggestive but not diagnostic.[24,45] **When clinical suspicion is high, a fiberoptic nasopharyngoscopy or direct laryngoscopy is required.**[30,36] **If upper airway damage is confirmed, the safest course is to secure the airway for at least 72 hours with an endotracheal tube.**[32] Although it is easier to diagnose this problem than to exclude it, pulmonary flow-volume loops that are consistently normal or mildly abnormal and do not worsen when repeated at frequent intervals (every 2 to 3 hours) correlate well with the absence of physiologically significant obstruction.[23]

If only minimal damage is observed, reexamination at frequent intervals is an alternative to immediate intubation of the airway; however, this approach incurs an increased risk of failure or complications. The implication of the delay inherent in reexamination is that the intubation may be performed under more difficult conditions after the swelling has become more severe and the anatomic structures less easily recognizable.

Lower respiratory tract injury. **Direct thermal injury to the lower respiratory tract is rare, except when live steam or burning gases are inhaled, because the thermal energy of hot air is dissipated in the upper airway.**[14,35,48] However, the tracheobronchial tree and lungs are not protected from exposure to noxious chemicals and particulates contained in smoke. Respiratory failure related to chemically mediated pulmonary insufficiency may develop as early as 3 hours after smoke inhalation. Pulmonary edema, associated with an increase in pulmonary transvascular fluid flux, and bronchopneumonic infections may follow.

Smoke exposure unassociated with burns can cause noncardiogenic pulmonary edema, usually within the first 2 to 5 days after the burn injury. Initially, mucociliary clearance and pulmonary surfactant activity are impaired, and histamine, kinins, and other

BRMs are released within the lungs. Abnormalities of gas exchange develop because of bronchospasm, local atelectasis, and pulmonary edema. After several hours, depending on the chemicals contained in the smoke, pseudomembranous tracheobronchitis may develop and hyaline membrane formation, fibrin deposition, intraalveolar hemorrhage, and pulmonary edema follow. Surface burns, especially if greater than 25% TBSA, can be synergistic with smoke in producing pulmonary injury.[46]

Special aspects of electrical injury

The passage of electrical current through the body generates heat in proportion to the square of the current flow (amperage). High-tension (>1000 V) exposures are particularly dangerous because the amperage is proportional to the voltage, making the heat produced proportional to the voltage squared. The majority of the heat production occurs in tissues with the highest electrical resistance. Almost all internal tissues (except bone) offer very low resistance, but skin resistance is relatively high.[41] As a result, considerable heat is produced in the body at points of entrance and exit of electric current, causing extensive damage to the skin and underlying blood vessels, muscles, and nerves.[9,41] Ignition of clothing and subsequent flame burns also often occur during electrical injury.

Significant deep tissue destruction, disproportionate to the amount of surface burn, is common after high-tension injury. For this reason, extremely aggressive fluid resuscitation is recommended (7 ml/kg/percent TBSA burned) during the first day of therapy.[41] Compartment syndromes frequently develop in these patients, and they require fasciotomies or amputations because of the tissue destruction that occurs in the limbs.[29,33]

Two important visceral sequelae of electrical injury are myocardial damage and renal failure. Myocardial damage appears more likely to occur in larger burns caused by high-tension exposure when the electricity actually passes through the heart. A major risk factor is a vertical pathway of current flow (entrance and exit wounds on opposite sides of the pubic symphysis).[10] Skeletal muscle damage is associated with hypermyoglobinemia, myoglobinuria, and renal failure. Although it is not proved that heme pigments are causative of renal dysfunction, measures to alkalinize and increase the volume of the urine continue to be recommended as the treatment of choice for pigmenturia after electrical injury.

Systemic Effects of Burn Injury
Metabolic effects

Hypermetabolism, usually beginning at the end of the first week after burn injury, is a prominent feature of burn injury with the degree of increase in metabolic rate directly related to burn size. Oxygen consumption is elevated to as much as 2.5 times predicted baseline levels, and heat production, body temperature, and protein catabolism also increase.[2] Increased levels of catecholamines, cortisol, glucagon, and growth hormone are all seen after burn injury. Collectively, they stimulate gluconeogenesis, and, despite elevated insulin levels, glucose transport into tissues is impaired, often leading to hyperglycemia.[6,49]

Hypermetabolism and hyperthermia are common after burn injury. Circulating catecholamines appear to play a role in mediating the inherent temperature elevation seen in burn patients and their preference for a warmer environment.[50] The disruption of the skin in burned areas constitutes a breakdown in the normal barriers to evaporative heat and fluid loss. Excessive heat loss can lead to shivering, which further increases oxygen consumption. **As a consequence of hypermetabolism, there is a dramatic increase in caloric requirements; more than 4000 kcal may be required daily to prevent protein catabolism.** At the time of the preoperative visit, the anesthesiologist should consider continuing the patient's enteric feedings as long as possible to minimize the length of the starvation interval.

Edema forms in both burned and nonburned tissue after burn injury[16] and is probably multifactorial in origin. Hypoproteinemia typically develops during the first week, when large volumes of intravenous fluid are being administered. In addition, the biologic response mediators that promote local edema at the burn site are also released into the bloodstream. There is speculation that they may also act systemically to increase vascular permeability and fluid flux in nonburned areas.[42] Plasma protein levels are typically depressed after burn injury, and remain depressed for a prolonged period.

Cardiovascular effects

Death from burn shock is now quite rare as a result of the widespread appreciation among health care providers that burn victims require between 2 and 4 ml/kg of fluid in the first 24 hours for each 1% TBSA burned. Several effective formulas (see Chapter 86) for preventing burn shock have been developed; all involve administration of large quantities of crystalloid fluids. **The use of colloids remains controversial.**

Edema formation after burn injury proceeds for approximately 24 to 36 hours, with most edema developing during the first 6 hours.[16] Large quantities of exogenously administered fluids and solutes are required during the first 2 days to maintain the plasma volume and cardiac preload. Spontaneous resorption of fluid begins thereafter, and fluid requirements decrease.

Cardiac output declines in the first 24 hours, often before the decrease in filling pressures. Circulating myocardial depressant factors have been implicated as the reason for this decrease in myocardial contractility, which may be mediated by oxygen-derived free radicals. These factors have yet to be identified, however.[17] Cardiac output usually increases toward normal after the first 24 hours, and later exceeds normal during the hypermetabolic phase if coronary artery disease does not limit myocardial oxygen supply.

Pulmonary effects

Pulmonary complications of burns may be temporally divided into early, delayed, and late events. The early complications occur in the first 24 to 48 hours and include carbon monoxide exposure, upper airway swelling, and noncardiogenic pulmonary edema. The adult respiratory distress syndrome (ARDS) usually develops at an intermediate time, within 2 to 5 days, and is a principal cause of death in hospitalized burn patients.[1,12] Important late complications are pneumonia, with and without atelectasis, and pulmonary emboli.

ARDS can develop after surface burns unassociated with inhalational injury. A primary defect in pulmonary vascular permeability may be causative; however, the exact mechanism remains unknown.[26] The complement cascade, cytokines, oxygen-derived free radicals, and eicosanoids (products of white blood cells) have all been implicated and may interact in a multifactorial manner. In addition, endotoxemia may also be involved in activating leukocytes and causing them to aggregate in the lung.[46]

Burn patients who survive into the second week are especially susceptible to pneumonia and atelectasis, even in the absence of inhalational injury. Their immune systems are suppressed in direct proportion to the magnitude of the burn injury.[37] Patients are often immobilized during treatment and commonly have bacteremia. Development of pulmonary emboli is another potential pulmonary complication that occurs after burn injury in up to 30% of patients.[13] Risk factors for this complication may include immobilization and hypercoagulability. The latter is evidenced by thrombocytosis and elevated levels of factors V and VII.[46]

PREOPERATIVE CONCERNS FOR BURN PATIENTS

Surgery may be needed for burn patients at any time during their hospital stay. The most frequently performed surgical procedures involve wound debridement and coverage. In some centers, excision and grafting are begun as early as the first 24 hours

---

> **BOX 32-2**
> **MAJOR PREOPERATIVE CONSIDERATIONS IN BURN WOUND DEBRIDEMENT AND GRAFTING PROCEDURES**
>
> Altered muscle relaxant pharmacology
> Potential for massive blood loss
> Anticipated position of the patient during surgery
> Airway management
> Ventilatory management
> Monitoring
> Intravascular access
> Safe transport to and from the operating room

---

after injury. Other procedures required in the course of recovery from burn injury include escharotomies, fasciotomies, tracheostomies, fracture repairs, and exploratory procedures related to blunt trauma associated with the burn.

During the acute phase, patients generally are metabolically compromised with hemodynamic and pulmonary dysfunction, yet the surgical procedure is necessary and may not be delayed in expectation of recovery. In cases of wound debridement and grafting, the surgery is viewed as the treatment. The role of the anesthesiologist in such cases is to understand the degree of physiologic compromise that exists and can be expected to complicate anesthetic care and to be prepared to meet the challenges imposed by it. Burn patients' unique care needs include their altered muscle relaxant pharmacologic state, potentially massive transfusion requirements, difficulties encountered in positioning the patient for surgery, airway management, ventilatory management (each discussed in detail in Chapter 86), difficulties encountered in monitoring and intravascular access, and the details of safe transport to and from the operating room (Box 32-2).

Monitoring and Intravascular Access

During the preoperative visit, the means of monitoring blood pressure, ECG, and oxygen saturation should be planned, especially if there are burns of the extremities and chest. Blood pressure cuffs can be applied on any nonburned arm or leg, but, when all four limbs are involved, use of a percutaneous arterial catheter is usually required. Arterial lines are often inserted for monitoring the initial fluid resuscitation and maintained for use during surgical procedures. A nonburned site of insertion is preferred; radial and femoral arteries are most commonly used. Use of an axillary artery is an alternative.

Standard ECG electrode placements are difficult when the chest and arms have been burned. The electrodes will not adhere to moist surfaces. To minimize the risks of contamination, an effort is usually made to avoid applying electrodes to burned or debrided dermis. Nonstandard lead arrangements result and make interpretation of the nature of dysrhythmias and the shape of the QRS complex more difficult. In near-total burns, it is impossible to monitor the ECG and avoid placing electrodes in burned areas. Skin staples may be applied over the chest or arms and "alligator" clips used to achieve electrical contact. If the arms are not part of the operative field, a gauze wrap may be used to hold electrodes in place on the arms. Topical antibacterial ointments are good electrical conductors.

Pulse oximeters have become an important part of intraoperative monitoring during anesthesia, especially for burn patients who frequently suffer respiratory disease. Unfortunately, burns of the extremities and face often make it impossible to obtain a signal from an oximeter probe and preclude the use of this valuable technology in situations when it could be most useful. More frequent measurements of arterial blood gases are sometimes necessary because of this.

Other standard monitoring modalities are generally unaffected by burn injury, and difficulties with their application are not usually anticipated. Capnometry, auscultation of heart tones and breath sounds, and urine output and body temperature measurements can and should be used as for other surgical procedures.

Ventilator management if the patient's airway is already intubated

The plan for intraoperative management of the patient who is already being treated for respiratory failure begins with a survey of the current ventilator settings (rate, tidal volume, inspired oxygen percentage, and level of positive end-expiratory pressure, if any). Oxygen consumption and carbon dioxide production are increased after thermal injury in proportion to the burn size, and inhalational injury impairs oxygenation and increases the dead space/tidal volume ratio.[43] For these reasons, burn patients usually require an elevated minute volume. An adult patient with a large burn may need more than 20 L/min. In larger patients, minute volumes greater than 30 L/min, which exceeds the capability of some standard anesthesia machine ventilators, may be required.

At the time of the preoperative visit, an estimate is usually made regarding the patient's postoperative ventilatory support needs. **The decision to wean from mechanical support and extubate a burn patient is based on the same principles as in any intensive care setting. Weaning is not attempted in the presence of cardiovascular instability, hypothermia, significant metabolic derangement, sepsis, or signs of worsening pulmonary function.** Extubation is delayed until the patient is alert enough to protect the upper airway from obstruction or aspiration of secretions.

An extensive debridement and grafting procedure in a patient with a major burn may be considered a variable significant enough to warrant postoperative ventilatory support for several hours. This ensures the adequacy of oxygenation and ventilation during a period of potential risk for hypoxia or hypoventilation. Another situation when a patient with airway mechanics suitable for extubation might require continued postoperative intubation is when grafts have been applied to the patient's back and the postoperative plan calls for the patient to remain prone after surgery. Reintubation in the event of decompensation would require turning the patient supine and would compromise the grafts.

Safe Transport to and from the Operating Room

Transportation to and from the operating room can be extremely hazardous for patients who have hemodynamic instability or respiratory failure. Measures must be taken to ensure the safety of the critically ill patient in hallways, corridors, and other areas where help may be unavailable. In some institutions, transfer necessitates the use of an elevator, a situation that completely isolates the transport team for some period of time. The transport team therefore must be able to provide emergency medical care in isolation and be prepared to perform reintubation and advanced cardiac life support.

At least two anesthesia personnel are usually required to manage the airway, observe the monitors,

---

BOX 32-3
CONSIDERATIONS WITH RESPECT TO TRANSPORT OF CRITICALLY ILL BURN PATIENTS TO THE OPERATING ROOM

Monitoring

Vital signs
Oxygen saturation

Oxygen delivery to lungs

High-flow system
Ability to provide high inspiratory pressures
Ability to provide PEEP
Sufficient volume of oxygen to withstand high flows
and unexpected delays
Successful trial of oxygen delivery system before
departure from Burn Unit

and administer medications. In preparation for transport, consideration should be given to how pulse, blood pressure, and oxygen saturation monitoring will be established and how ventilatory support is to be continued during this difficult interval (Box 32-3). If the patient is combative, the use of sedatives and muscle relaxants should also be contemplated.

Monitoring and ventilatory support. Consideration should be given to the use of continuous displays of ECG, arterial pressure, and arterial oxygen saturation (Sao_2) by using portable battery-powered instruments during transport. Special attention must be given to the means by which oxygenation and ventilation will be accomplished during transport because of the severe nature of pulmonary dysfunction that occurs in patients with surface burns complicated by inalational injury. It is often necessary to use a system capable of delivering high flows of 100% oxygen, positive end-expiratory pressure (PEEP), and very high inspiratory pressures for an extended period of time.

An anesthesia gas delivery apparatus, such as the Mapleson D system, is a good choice because it avoids many of the problems encountered in the standard manual resuscitators. Most standard bag-valve systems cannot provide 100% oxygen unless high flow rates are used and a reservoir component is added to the system, and most cannot provide PEEP. One oxygen tank may be inadequate for transfer of a burn patient to the operating room because it is not uncommon for a burn patient to require as much as 30 L/min of fresh gas flow to support ventilation. To provide such a high flow, two tanks may be yoked together because the standard regulators are limited at 15 to 20 L/min. In addition, a standard E cylinder of oxygen contains only 620 L when filled (20 minutes at 30 L/min).

For patients with severe pulmonary disease, it is advisable to perform a 5-minute trial of oxygenation and ventilation in the intensive care unit with the breathing system that will be used during transport. If there is any doubt about the adequacy of the portable breathing system at that point, arterial blood gases can be obtained for confirmation. Occasionally, the degree of pulmonary dysfunction is so great that respiratory function simply cannot be supported during transfer to the operating room and surgery remains impossible until clinical improvement occurs.

At times, the patient is so combative that effective ventilation and oxygenation are impeded, and safe transfer to the operating room can only be accomplished if sedatives and muscle relaxants are administered. Use of benzodiazepines is safe in these patients if amnesia is desired; however, if muscle paralysis is required, as discussed in Chapter 86, only nondepolarizing muscle relaxants should be used.

RECONSTRUCTIVE PROCEDURES

For months to years after the burn wounds have been successfully grafted, there follows a reconstructive phase during which repeated surgical procedures are performed to remove or reduce scar tissue and so improve both functional and cosmetic outcomes. In general, these patients can be treated as most other plastic surgery patients although the safety of using succinylcholine during the first 1 to 2 years after the burn injury remains controversial.[34]

For this patient group, the most important ongoing anesthetic problems relate to the physical effects of scar contractures and the psychologic effects of repeated hospitalizations (especially in burn-injured children). Intubation of the trachea continues to be difficult in patients with scar contractures of the face and neck until these scars have been released.

SUMMARY

The management of burn patients challenges the anesthesiologist's ability to successfully treat patients with advanced physiologic and pharmacologic disorders. The preoperative evaluation and intraoperative care are arduous; however, it is most rewarding to participate in the progressive recovery of victims of such severe injuries.

KEY POINTS

- Major burns cause subtotal destruction of the skin and mucous membranes and are associated with severe metabolic, cardiovascular, and respiratory disorders.

- Burn patients require many life-saving, function-preserving, and appearance-saving surgical procedures during their hospital stay. Many of these procedures cannot be delayed long enough to allow correction of the underlying systemic disorders.

- Much of the metabolic, cardiovascular, and respiratory dysfunction associated with burn injury is perpetuated by the burn wound and thus cannot be fully corrected until the burn wound has been excised and grafted.

- Burns are classified according to their severity, the energy source, and the presence of associated inhalational injury.

- In terms of prognosis, it is helpful to make a single distinction between *first-degree or superficial second-degree burns* and *deep second-degree or third-degree burns* because the latter do not heal spontaneously or do so with poor cosmetic and functional result.

- Mortality from thermal injury is related to the area involved by deep second- or third-degree burns and the presence of inhalational injury.

- Thermal injury to skin and its microvasculature incites an inflammatory response consisting of activation of leukocytes and release of biologic response mediators.

- Edema formation and resultant loss of plasma volume are the chief reasons that burn victims require copious fluid resuscitation.

- Inhalational injury is an extremely important complication of burn exposure because when present, on the average, it increases mortality rates by 40%.

- Carbon monoxide (CO) poisoning should be suspected in any victim of a closed-space fire (buildings and automobiles).

- Standard pulse oximetry does not distinguish between the oxyhemoglobin and the carboxyhemoglobin molecules.

- The diagnosis of CO poisoning is made by measuring the carboxyhemoglobin level, expressed as a percent saturation of hemoglobin in arterial blood.

- Inhaled flames, toxic chemicals, and hot air can produce life-threatening swelling of the tissues of the upper airway.

- The presence of evolving airway obstruction may be suggested by the clinical signs of facial burns, sooty oral or nasal secretions, hoarseness, and a swollen, erythematous tongue, but the diagnosis is best made by fiberoptic or direct layrngoscopic examination of the upper airway.

- If upper airway damage is confirmed, the safest course is to secure the airway for at least 72 hours with an endotracheal tube.

- Direct thermal injury to the lower respiratory tract is rare, except when live steam or burning gases are inhaled, because the thermal energy of hot air is dissipated in the upper airway.

- Hypermetabolism, usually beginning at the end of the first week after the burn injury, is a prominent feature of burn injury with the degree of increase in metabolic rate directly related to burn size.

- As a consequence of hypermetabolism, there is a dramatic increase in caloric requirements; more than 4000 kcal may be required daily to prevent protein catabolism.

- Death from burn shock is now quite rare as a result of widespread appreciation among health care providers that burn victims require between 2 and 4 ml/kg of fluid in the first 24 hours *for each 1% TBSA burned.* The use of colloids remains controversial.

- ARDS can develop after surface burns unassociated with inhalational injury.

- Burn patients who survive into the second week are especially susceptible to pneumonia and atelectasis even in the absence of inhalational injury.

- During the preoperative visit, the means of monitoring blood pressure, ECG, and oxygen saturation should be planned, especially if there are burns of the extremities and chest.

- During mechanical ventilation, burn patients usually require an elevated minute volume because oxygen consumption and carbon dioxide production are increased after thermal injury in proportion to the burn size and because inhalational injury impairs oxygenation and increases the dead space/tidal volume ratio.

- After surgery, the decision to wean from mechanical support and extubate a burn patient is based on the same principles as in any intensive care setting: in the presence of cardiovascular instability, hypothermia, significant metabolic derangement, sepsis, or signs of worsening pulmonary function, weaning is not attempted.

- Transportation to and from the operating room can be extremely hazardous for patients who have hemodynamic instability or respiratory failure.

KEY REFERENCES

Demling RH, Kramer G, and Harmes B: Role of thermal injury-induced hypoproteinemia on fluid flux and protein permeability in burned and non-burned tissue, *Surgery* 95:136, 1984.

Fong Y, Moldawer LL, Shires GT et al: The biologic characteristics of cytokines and their implication in surgical injury, *Surg Gynecol Obstet* 170:363, 1990.

Haponik EF, Meyers DA, Munster AM et al: Acute upper airway injury in burn patients: serial changes on flow-volume curves and nasopharyngoscopy, *Am Rev Respir Dis* 135:360, 1987.

Wilmore DW, Long JM, Mason AD Jr et al: Catecholamines: mediator of the hypermetabolic response to thermal injury, *Ann Surg* 180:653, 1974.

Wilmore D, Mason AD, Johnson DW et al: Effect of ambient temperature on heat production and heat loss in burn patients, *J Appl Physiol* 38:593, 1975.

REFERENCES

1. Achauer BM, Allyn PA, Furnas DW et al: Pulmonary complications of burns: the major threat to the burn patient, *Ann Surg* 177:311, 1973.
2. Aulick LH, Hander EH, Wilmore DW et al: The relative significance of thermal and metabolic demands on burn hypermetabolism, *J Trauma* 19:559, 1979.
3. Barker SJ, Tremper KK, Hufstedler S et al: The effects of carbon monoxide inhalation on noninvasive oxygen monitoring, *Anesth Analg* 65:S12, 1986.
4. Bartlett RH: Types of respiratory injury, *J Trauma* 19:918, 1979.
5. Beal DD, Conner GH: Respiratory tract injury: a guide to management following thermal and smoke injury, *Laryngoscope* 80:25, 1970.
6. Bessey PQ, Watters JM, Aoki TT et al: Combined hormonal infusion simulates the metabolic response to injury, *Ann Surg* 200:264, 1984.
7. Border J: Hypothesis: sepsis, multiple systems organ failure, and the macrophage, *Arch Surg* 123:285, 1988.
8. Boykin JV, Eriksson E, and Pittman RN: In vivo microcirculation of scald burn and the progression of postburn dermal ischemia, *Plast Reconstr Surg* 66:191, 1980.
9. Burke JF, Quinby WC Jr, Bondoc C et al: Patterns of high tension electrical injury in children and adolescents and their management, *Am J Surg* 133:492, 1977.
10. Chandra NC, Siu CO, and Munster AM: Clinical predictors of myocardial damage after high voltage electrical injury, *Crit Care Med* 18:293, 1990.
11. Choi IS: Delayed neurologic sequelae in carbon monoxide intoxication, *Arch Neurol* 40:433, 1983.
12. Clark WR, Monaventura M, and Myers W: Smoke inhalation and airway management at a regional burn unit: 1974-1983, *J Burn Care Rehabil* 10:52, 1989.
13. Coleman JB, Chang FC: Pulmonary embolism: an unrecognized event in severely burned patients, *Am J Surg* 130:697, 1975.
14. Crapo RO: Smoke-inhalation injuries, *JAMA* 246:1694, 1981.
15. Demling RH, Will JA, Belzer FO et al: Effect of major thermal injury on the pulmonary microcirculation, *Surgery* 83:746, 1978.
16. Demling RH, Kramer G, and Harmes B: Role of thermal injury-induced hypoproteinemia on fluid flux and protein permeability in burned and nonburned tissue, *Surgery* 95:136, 1984.
17. Demling RH: Pathophysiological changes after cutaneous burns and approach to initial resuscitation. In Martyn JAJ, ed: *Acute management of the burned patient,* Philadelphia, 1990, WB Saunders.
18. Dreisbach RH: *Handbook of poisoning: diagnosis and treatment,* Los Altos, Calif, 1974, Lange Medical.
19. Faist E, Mewes A, Strasser T et al: Alteration of monocyte function following major injury, *Arch Surg* 123:287, 1988.
20. Fong Y, Moldawer LL, Shires GT et al: The biologic characteristics of cytokines and their implication in surgical injury, *Surg Gynecol Obstet* 170:363, 1990.
21. Grube BJ, Marvin JA, and Heimbach DM: Therpeutic hyperbaric oxygen: help or hindrance in burn patients with carbon monoxide poisoning? *J Burn Care Rehabil* 28:110, 1980.
22. Haponik EF, Munster AM, Wise RA et al: Upper airway function in burn patients: correlation of flow-volume curves and nasopharyngoscopy, *Am Rev Respir Dis* 129:251, 1984.
23. Haponik EF, Meyers DA, Munster AM et al: Acute upper airway injury in burn patients: serial changes of flow-volume curves and nasopharyngoscopy, *Am Rev Respir Dis* 135:360, 1987.
24. Haponik EF: Clinical and functional assessment. In Haponik EF, Munster AM, eds: *Respiratory injury: smoke inhalation and burns,* New York, 1990, McGraw-Hill.
25. Harms BA, Bodai BI, Kramer GC et al: Microvascular fluid and protein flux in pulmonary and systemic circulations after thermal injury, *Microvasc Res* 23:77, 1982.
26. Head JM: Inhalation injury in burns, *Am J Surg* 139:508, 1980.
27. Heimbach DM: Smoke inhalation: current concept. In Wachtel TL, Kahn V, and Frank HA, eds: *Current topics in burn care,* Rockville, Md, 1983, Aspen Systems.
28. Herndon DN, Thompson PB, Linares HA et al: Postgraduate course: respiratory injury, part I, *J Burn Care Rehabil* 7:184, 1986.
29. Holliman CJ, Saffle JR, Kravitz M et al: Early surgical decompression in the management of electric injuries, *Am J Surg* 144:733, 1982.
30. Hunt JL, Agee RN, and Pruitt BA: Fiberoptic bronchoscopy in acute inhalational injury, *J Trauma* 15:641, 1975.
31. Reference deleted in proofs.
32. Lamb JD: Anaesthetic considerations for major thermal injury, *Can Anaesth Soc J* 32:84, 1985.
33. Luce EA, Gottlieb SE: "True" high-tension electric injuries, *Ann Plast Surg* 12:321, 1984.
34. Marytn JA, Goldhill DR, and Goudsouzian NG: Clinical pharamcology of muscle relaxants in burned patients, *J Clin Pharmacol* 26:680, 1986.
35. Moritz AR, Henriques FC, and McLean R: The effects of inhaled heat on the air passages and lungs, *Am J Pathol* 21:311, 1945.
36. Moylan JA, Adib K, and Birnbaum M: Fiberoptic bronchoscopy following thermal injury, *Surg Gynecol Obstet* 140:541, 1975.
37. Munster AM, Eurenius K, Katz RM et al: Cell-mediated immunity after thermal injury, *Ann Surg* 177:139, 1973.
38. Munster AM: Burn wound. In Cameron JL, ed: *Current surgical therapy,* St Louis, 1986, CV Mosby.
39. Norkol DM, Kirkpatrick JN: Treatment of acute carbon monoxide poisoning with hyperbaric oxygen: a review of 115 cases, *Ann Emerg Med* 14:1168, 1985.

40. Reed GF, Camp HL: Upper airway problems in severely burned patients, *Ann Otol Rhinol Laryngol* 78:741, 1969.
41. Remensnyder JP: Acute electrical injuries. In Martyn JAJ, ed: *Acute management of the burned patient,* Philadelphia, 1990, WB Saunders.
42. Riley-Paull KL, Munster AM: The role of cytokines in thermal injury, *Crit Care Rep* 2:4, 1990.
43. Robinson NB, Hudson LD, Robertson HT et al: Ventilation and perfusion alterations after smoke inhalation injury, *Surgery* 90:352, 1981.

44. Robson MC, Kucan JO: The burn wound. In Wachtel TL, Kahn V, and Frank HA, eds: *Current topics in burn care,* Rockville, Md, 1983, Aspen Systems.
45. Sendak MJ, Furman WR: Anesthetic aspects. In Haponik EF, Munster AM, eds: *Respiratory injury: smoke inhalation and burns,* New York, 1990, McGraw-Hill.
46. Strongin J, Hales CA: Pulmonary disorders in the burn patient. In Martyn JAJ, ed: *Acute management of the burned patient,* Philadelphia, 1990, WB Saunders.
47. Reference deleted in proofs.

48. Trunkey DD: Inhalation injury, *Surg Clin North Am* 58:1133, 1978.
49. Wilmore DW, Long JM, Mason AD Jr et al: Catecholamines: mediator of the hypermetabolic response to thermal injury, *Ann Surg* 180:653, 1974.
50. Wilmore DW, Mason AD Jr, Johnson DW et al: Effect of ambient temperature on heat production and heat loss in burn patients, *J Appl Physiol* 38:593, 1975.
51. Zikria BA, Weston GC, Chodoff M et al: Smoke and carbon monoxide poisoning in fire victims, *J Trauma* 12:641, 1972.

CHAPTER 33

Evaluation of the Patient with Dermatologic Problems

NEIL T. SAKIMA

Providing anesthesia for patients with skin diseases involves understanding the disease process, including its mucous membrane and systemic manifestations, and avoiding exacerbation of the patient's condition while performing the maneuvers necessary to deliver the anesthetic. This chapter reviews important general medical concerns in patients with skin disease and then studies specific skin diseases and their anesthetic considerations.

GENERAL CONSIDERATIONS IN SKIN DISEASE

Risk of Skin Trauma

Friction, pressure, and needle punctures may induce or exacerbate skin lesions. Friction from bed sheets when the patient is moved from the stretcher to the operating room table may be avoided by lifting the patient, or by having the patient lift himself or herself to the operating room table without sliding. **Pressure points such as the elbows, heels, and occiput should be carefully padded.** Padding should also be placed on the operating room table to protect the patient's torso. Skin under the blood pressure cuff should be lubricated to minimize potential injury from friction. Lubricated gauze or padding can further minimize possible pressure injury. Use of a hydrocortisone-containing ointment or cream as a lubricant has been advocated but is not of proven benefit. **A stethoscope placed under the blood pressure cuff to listen for Korotkoff sounds may cause trauma and should be avoided.** Oscillometry or palpation of a distal pulse are preferred techniques to measure blood pressure. Some authors recommend not measuring blood pressure at all because of the risk of inducing new bullae.[19] However, other authors have found careful wrapping of the arm under the blood pressure cuff with moist gauze to be safe.[31] **Needle punctures from intravenous catheter insertion or intramuscular/subcutaneous injections should be kept to a minimum.**

Tape and adhesives should be used only when necessary and their use should be kept to a minimum. A precordial stethoscope may be placed on the patient's chest without adhesive. Electrocardiogram electrodes with the adhesive outer ring removed may be placed gel side up under the patient. The endotracheal tube may be secured by gauze tied to the endotracheal tube and wrapped around the patient's neck. Alternatively, the anesthesiologist or an assistant may manually hold the endotracheal tube in place during surgery without securing it to the patient's skin. The eyes should be protected with ophthalmic ointment and should not be taped shut.

Airway Management

Visualization of the laryngeal structures may be hindered by the patient's inability to open the mouth because of perioral scarring (epidermolysis bullosa dystrophica (EBD), scleroderma, Behçet's disease) or temporomandibular joint dysfunction (scleroderma). Edema, bullae, secretions, and/or bleeding in the oropharynx and nasopharynx may not only make visualization of the laryngeal structures difficult, but also place the patient at significant risk for airway obstruction (EBD, pemphigus). **Involvement of the larynx and trachea may also occur (junctional epidermolysis bullosa, cicatricial pemphigoid, Stevens-Johnson's syndrome).**[21]

Trauma during laryngoscopy and intubation should be kept to a minimum because of tissue friability and the risk of inducing new lesions (EBD, pemphigus). The laryngoscope blade should be well lubricated and a MacIntosh blade should be used to minimize trauma to the posterior surface of the epiglottis. **A smaller than usual, well-lubricated endotracheal tube should be used to minimize trauma to the larynx and trachea.** The endotracheal tube may also be warmed to soften it. Care should be taken not to overinflate the endotracheal tube cuff. Suctioning of the airway should be performed with a minimum of mucosal contact. Use of oropharyngeal and nasopharyngeal airways, nasal or esophageal temperature probes, nasogastric tubes, and esophageal stethoscopes should be avoided, if possible. **If bleeding from the oropharynx is encountered, epinephrine-soaked sponges (1:200,000 solution) have been reported to control bleeding with only mild tachycardia and hypertension when 40 ml were used in a man weighing 77 kg.**[41] Before the endotracheal tube is removed, the upper airway must be carefully reassessed.

If a mask is used, the patient's face should be protected by lubricant-soaked cotton or gauze sponges to minimize friction and pressure injury.

Because of the risks involved with airway instrumentation, techniques that use spontaneous respiration with ketamine anesthesia have proved popular in patients with significant mucosal involvement.[4,19,32,34,55]

Vascular Access

Intravenous access may be difficult to obtain in patients with generalized skin disease. **If possible, an uninvolved area of skin should be used for venous access.** Sterile technique minimizes the risk of infection. **Antiseptic should be poured or placed on the skin without rubbing.** The catheter may be sutured in place or secured with a gauze wrap. If a peripheral vein cannot be cannulated, central venous access may be required.

Heat Regulation

The skin plays a major role in regulation of body temperature. **Heat loss by evaporation is normally controlled by regulation of sweat production. However, in denuded skin, increased insensible fluid losses occur because of breakdown of the barrier function of the skin.** Increased heat loss may also occur because of increased blood flow to diseased skin.[17]

Evaporative heat loss may be minimized by keeping as much of the patient's body covered as possible. Increasing the operating room temperature and use of a warming blanket, humidifier, and warmed intravenous and irrigation fluids may be helpful in maintaining body temperature.

Conversely, **if a patient cannot perspire because of a skin disorder, hyperthermia may result.** Evaporative heat loss can be enhanced by keeping the skin moist and maintaining air circulation over the skin. A cooling blanket may be used to enhance conductive heat loss. Ice packs may be applied to the patient's axillae and groin in more extreme circumstances. Decreasing ambient air temperature and keeping the patient uncovered will maximize convective and radiant heat loss.

Temperature measurement may be problematic in patients with diffuse mucosal disease. Use of esophageal, rectal, or nasal thermometers may be ill advised because of the risk of trauma to mucosal tissues. Use of axillary thermometers is a possible alternative.

Risk of Infection

Lack of integrity of the skin and/or mucous membranes predisposes patients to infection. In addition, the underlying disease process and treatment (i.e., steroids or other immunosuppressive drugs) may place patients at increased risk of infection. Any monitoring device or material that contacts denuded skin should be clean. Patients should be treated with appropriate antibiotic regimens and care must be taken to prevent the spread of infection to other patients. Disposable equipment should be used when possible. Contaminated equipment should be thoroughly cleaned, gloves must be worn by all health care providers, and handwashing should be thorough. Contaminated outer garments should be removed when health care workers leave the operating room.

Corticosteroid Therapy

Many patients with skin disorders may be taking systemic corticosteroids. Because of the risk of suppression of the hypothalamic-pituitary-adrenal (HPA) axis, corticosteroid therapy needs to be continued and possibly increased during the perioperative period. **Intensive therapy with topical steroids may also cause temporary suppression of the HPA axis,[37] and systemic corticosteroid coverage is indicated in these patients.** Although HPA axis suppression may resolve in several days after topical steroid therapy is discontinued,[37] suppression of normal adrenal responses may persist for as long as 9 months to 1 year after systemic therapy.[43] Therefore Roizen recommends glucocorticoid supplementation for any patients who have received steroids within the previous year.[43]

Kehlet[30] and Symreng et al.[50] advocate low-dose corticosteroid therapy with a bolus of 25 mg of hydrocortisone at induction of anesthesia followed by a constant infusion of 100 mg over 24 hours. The mean cortisol levels obtained with this regimen are higher than nonsteroid-treated, normal controls for the first 2 hours and are similar thereafter. Alternatively, high-dose therapy with 300 to 400 mg of hydrocortisone given in divided doses may be used.[39]

Cardiovascular Status

Cardiovascular disease may occur in association with many skin diseases. Myocarditis or pericarditis may be associated with the collagen vascular disorders, Stevens-Johnson's syndrome, mucocutaneous lymph node syndrome, and Behçet's disease.[11,27] Dysrhythmias and conduction disturbances have occurred in patients with Stevens-Johnson's syndrome, scleroderma, dermatomyositis, and mucocutaneous lymph node syndrome.[9,27] Heart failure may occur secondary to myocardial fibrosis in scleroderma. High-output heart failure may occur because of increased blood flow to diseased skin.[46] Hypertension related to renal dysfunction may be seen in patients with EBD. Unexplained hypertension in the setting of neurofibromatosis may be related to pheochromocytoma.

An electrocardiogram should be obtained for any patient with systemic cardiovascular manifestations of skin disease who is suspected of having dysrhythmias or conduction defects. An echocardiogram may be used to assess myocardial function if heart failure is suspected. Serum urea nitrogen and creatinine levels may be used to screen for renal dysfunction. **Hypertension in the setting of neurofibromatosis should prompt a search for pheochromocytoma.**

Pulmonary Status

The pulmonary system has mucous membranes and is at risk in any skin disease that involves the mucous membranes. Restrictive lung disease secondary to pulmonary fibrosis and kyphoscoliosis may occur in patients with scleroderma and neurofibromatosis, respectively. Pneumonitis may occur in cases of dermatomyositis.[45] Pneumothorax may occur in patients with Stevens-Johnson's syndrome, secondary to blebs in the visceral pleura.[11]

Chest radiographs should be obtained in any patient suspected of having pulmonary disease. Pulmonary function tests and arterial blood gas tests are recommended in patients who are suspected of having significant pulmonary compromise.

Gastrointestinal and Nutritional Status

The gastrointestinal mucosa has the same embryologic origin as the skin and may be affected by the same pathologic processes that affect the skin. Oral lesions, as may be seen in EBD, pemphigus, and Stevens-Johnson's syndrome, can interfere with adequate nutrition. Anemia may result from nutritional deficiencies or ulceration in the gastrointestinal tract, leading to bleeding. Decreased clotting factors from hepatic disease or malabsorption of fat-soluble vitamins may lead to a bleeding diathesis, as in mast cell disease.[47] Hypoalbuminemia from hepatic dysfunction or malnutrition may alter protein binding and affect the response to a given dose of medication.

Preoperative nutritional support may be appropriate in malnourished patients. The metabolic and hematologic evaluation of patients with significant gastrointestinal and nutritional deficiencies should be determined by the clinical history and physical examination.

ANESTHETIC CONSIDERATIONS IN SPECIFIC SKIN DISEASES
Epidermolysis Bullosa Dystrophica

Epidermolysis bullosa constitutes a group of rare genetic disorders characterized by formation of blisters at sites of minor physical injury (Table 33-1). It may be divided into scarring (dystrophic) and nonscarring forms. Epidermolysis bullosa dystrophica (EBD) is a scarring form and is further divided into forms with dominant and recessive inheritance. The dominant form is usually mild and the mucous membranes are only occasionally involved. The recessive form is more severe and is characterized by extensive bulla formation with scarring of the skin as well as the mucosa of the lips, tongue, oropharynx, and esophagus, particularly after friction. **Rarely, laryngeal stenosis may occur.[42,52] Severe microstomia with limited mouth opening may result from scarring of the commissures of the lips.** Poor dentition from dysplastic teeth and the patient's inability to maintain adequate oral hygiene is common. Dysphagia may

Table 33-1 Epidermolysis bullosa

Disease	Cutaneous manifestations	Systemic manifestations	Anesthetic considerations
Intraepidermal			
Epidermolysis bullosa (EB) simplex, generalized (Koebner)	Characterized by bullae formation in areas of repeated trauma; oral mucosa may be involved in EB herpetiformis; healing occurs without scarring; lesions usually appear in the first year of life, but may occur at any age; autosomal dominant inheritance		
EB simplex, localized (Weber-Cockayne)			
EB herpetiformis (Downing-Meara)			
EB simplex (Ogna)			
EB simplex with mottled pigmentation			Friction, pressure, needle punctures, and tape may exacerbate skin lesions and should be kept to a minimum; manipulation of the airway and other mucosal membranes should be avoided, if possible; perioral scarring in EBD may make direct laryngoscopy difficult; heat, fluid, and electrolyte losses may occur from denuded skin; porphyria should be ruled out before barbiturates are used in patients with EBD; general and regional anesthetic techniques have been used successfully in these patients; subcutaneous infiltration of local anesthetics should be avoided because of the risk of skin sloughing
Junctional (intralamina lucida)			
EB atrophicans generalisata gravis (EB letalis, Herlitz's disease)	EB letalis is characterized by generalized bullae with little or no healing; severe disease may be fatal within a few months; all mucosal membranes may be involved; cicatricial junctional EB notable for scarring that may produce syndactyly, contractures, and stenosis of the anterior nares; autosomal recessive inheritance	Respiratory distress from laryngeal and bronchial lesions, sepsis, pyloric atresia, anemia, and growth retardation may be seen in EB letalis	
EB atrophicans generalisata mitis			
EB atrophicans localisata			
EB atrophicans inversa			
EB progressiva			
Generalized atrophic benign EB			
Cicatricial junctional EB			
Dermolytic or dystrophic (sublamina densa)			

Dominant forms:
  Dystrophic EB (EBD), hyperplastic variant (Cockayne-Touraine)
  Dystrophic EB, albopapuloid variant (Pasini)
Recessive forms:
  Generalized (gravis or mitis)
  Localized
  Inverse
	All forms characterized by bullae that heal with scarring; EBD with dominant inheritance is usually mild with relative sparing of mucous membranes; EBD with recessive inheritance is marked by generalized bullae with significant mucosal involvement; there is an increased risk of skin carcinoma in both forms	Esophageal stricture, poor nutrition, growth retardation, iron deficiency anemia, chronic infections with amyloidosis, meningitis and seizures, poststreptococcal glomerulonephritis, hypertension related to renal disease, contractures, and possible association with porphyria	

BOX 33-1
DRUGS THAT MAY EXACERBATE PORPHYRIA

Hypnotics

Althesin
Barbiturates
Benzodiazepines:
   Chlordiazepoxide
   Clonazepam
   Diazepam
   Flurazepam
   Oxazepam
Chlormethazanone
Glutethimide
Meprobamate
Methyprylon
Sulphonal
Trional

Inhalational agents

Enflurane
Halothane
Methoxyflurane

Narcotics

Fentanyl
Pentazocine

Anticonvulsants

Carbamazepine
Ethosuximide
Mephenytoin
Methsuximide
Phensuximide
Phenytoin
Primidone
Trimethadione
Valproate

Antihypertensives

Clonidine
Furosemide
Hydralazine
Methyldopa
Pargyline
Phenoxybenzamine
Spironolactone

Antimicrobials

Chloramphenicol
Chloroquine
Griseofulvin
Novobiocin
Pyrazinamide
Rifampin
Sulfonamides

Analgetics

Amidopyrine
Aminopyrine
Antipyrine
Dichloralphenazone
Diclofenac
Phenylbutazone

Other agents

Dapsone
Diethylpropion
Dramamine
Ergot preparations
Ethchlorvynol
Ethyl alcohol
Hormones
   Estrogens
   Progesterones
Hyoscine-N-butylbromide
Imipramine
Nikethamide
Pyrazinamide
Sedormid
Sulfonylureas
   Chlorpropamide
   Tolbutamide
Theophylline

Bickers DR, Pathak MA: The porphyrias. In Fitzpatrick TB et al, eds: *Dermatology in general medicine,* New York, 1987, McGraw-Hill; Meyer UA: Porphyrias. In Isselbacher KJ et al, eds: *Harrison's principles of internal medicine,* ed 9, New York, 1980, McGraw-Hill; and Wood AJ, Oates JA: Adverse reactions to drugs. In Braunwald E et al, eds: *Harrison's principles of internal medicine,* ed 11, New York, 1987, McGraw-Hill.

---

result from esophageal webbing and stricture secondary to trauma to the membranes of the esophagus. Iron deficiency anemia may occur because of poor nutritional intake. Chronic infections of the skin may lead to chronic debilitation, amyloidosis, meningitis and seizures, and poststreptococcal glomerulonephritis. Hypertension related to renal problems is common. Foot and hand lesions may heal with fusion and flexion contractures of the digits.[4] There is an association between EBD and porphyria,[35] and some authors recommend screening all patients with EBD for porphyria.[22] Some patients with presumed epidermolysis bullosa dystrophica involving only the skin may have porphyria cutanea tarda (PCT). Bickers and Pathak state that drugs associated with induction of attacks of acute intermittent porphyria, variegate porphyria, and hereditary coproporphyria (Box 33-1) do not appear to cause exacerbations of PCT, although ethyl alcohol and estrogenic hormones can induce PCT in susceptible individuals.[3] However, it would be prudent to use drugs that are safe in any patient with porphyria[36] (Box 33-2).

Anesthetic considerations in patients with EBD include avoidance of trauma to the skin (see "Risk of Skin Trauma" section for specific recommendations). **Although oropharyngeal bulla formation and hemorrhage have been widely reported, laryngeal and tracheal complications related to airway instrumentation are uncommon.**[2] James and Wark reported a series of 131 patients with EBD who were intubated and had no postoperative laryngeal bulla formation.[24] It has been suggested that because the mucosa of the

---

BOX 33-2
DRUGS CONSIDERED SAFE IN PATIENTS
WITH ACUTE INTERMITTENT PORPHYRIA,
VARIEGATE PORPHYRIA, AND HEREDITARY
COPROPORPHYRIA

Analgetics

Salicylates
Morphine and related compounds

Antibiotics

Penicillins

Psychoactive drugs

Phenothiazines

Antihistamines

Diphenhydramine

Antihypertensives

Guanethidine
Propranolol
Reserpine

Miscellaneous

Atropine
Neostigmine
Propanidid
Procaine
Succinylcholine
Ether
Nitrous oxide

From Meyer UA: Porphyrias. In Isselbacher KJ et al, eds: *Harrison's principles of internal medicine*, ed 9, New York, 1980, McGraw-Hill.

---

larynx and trachea is primarily pseudostratified ciliated columnar epithelium as opposed to the stratified squamous epithelium of the lips, tongue, oropharynx, and epiglottis, the former structures are less susceptible to bulla formation.[2] Therefore **tracheal intubation may be a less damaging procedure than placement of oral or nasal airways.** However, laryngoscopy may be difficult in patients with EBD and there is significant risk for oropharyngeal trauma from laryngoscopy.[24,53] In contrast, all mucosal surfaces are affected in junctional epidermolysis bullosa, a nonscarring form of epidermolysis bullosa, and tracheal lesions may occur spontaneously or in response to trauma related to endotracheal intubation.[21]

Ketamine, alone or in combination with a benzodiazepine, has been used in many patients with EBD.[4,19,32,34] Use of ketamine has the advantage of maintaining airway reflexes in a spontaneously breathing patient while providing analgesia and am-

nesia for the surgical procedure. Emergence delirium is controlled by concurrent use of the benzodiazepine. Excessive salivation may be controlled with atropine or glycopyrrolate. Although ketamine is effective in blocking somatic pain, it is not as effective in blocking visceral pain.

Regional anesthesia has been used successfully in patients with EBD. Broster, Placek, and Eggers described use of an epidural anesthetic in a pregnant patient for whom the epidural catheter was secured with sutures and gauze wrapped around the patient's abdomen during labor.[7] The patient subsequently had a cesarean section under epidural anesthesia without sequelae. Successful subarachnoid and axillary blocks have also been reported without sequelae.[28,31,48] Subcutaneous infiltration of local anesthetic should be avoided because of the risk of skin sloughing.[47] Needle punctures should not be performed through involved or infected skin.

Inhalational anesthesia has been used with success in cases of EBD. If appropriate precautions are taken, the risk of traumatic bulla formation is small whether the airway is managed by mask or intubation.[24]

Pemphigus and Pemphigoid

Pemphigus refers to a group of entities characterized by loss of adhesion between epidermal cells (acantholysis) (Table 33-2). It is associated with the presence of circulating autoantibodies to an intercellular epidermal antigen. Pemphigus vulgaris has been associated with use of penicillamine, captopril, penicillin, rifampin, and thiopronine. There may also be an association with myasthenia gravis and thymoma. Pemphigus vulgaris may involve all skin surfaces and mucous membranes, including the oropharynx and nasopharynx, esophagus, anus, penis, vagina, and conjunctiva.

Pemphigoid is characterized by subepidermal bullae without acantholysis (see Table 33-2). Immunoglobulin G antibody to basement membrane is present. Pemphigoid has been associated with use of furosemide, penicillamine, and clonidine. Mucosal lesions are usually small and not significant. The larynx is usually not involved except in the rare variant, cicatricial pemphigoid, which involves primarily mucosal surfaces and may cause web adhesions of the vocal cords.[13,18]

Treatment regimens for pemphigus include use of corticosteroids, immunosuppressive agents (methotrexate, azathioprine, and cyclophosphamide), gold therapy, and adrenocorticotropic hormone.[27] The treatment of pemphigoid is the same as for pemphigus except that the disease is more responsive to corticosteroid therapy, and immunosuppressive therapy should be required only occasionally.[1]

There is a paucity of reports on the anesthetic

Table 33-2   Pemphigus and pemphigoid

Disease	Cutaneous manifestations	Systemic manifestations	Anesthetic considerations
Pemphigus			
Pemphigus vulgaris Pemphigus vegetans (Neumann type, Hallopeau type)	Affects the suprabasilar layer of the skin; may begin as localized bullous disease before becoming generalized; oropharyngeal and nasopharyngeal lesions occur in nearly all patients; pemphigus vegetans is a variant characterized by bullae that form fungoid or papillomatous vegetations; onset usually between 40 and 60 years		
Pemphigus folicaeus Brazilian pemphigus Pemphigus erythematosus (Senear-Usher)	Affects the subcorneal layer of the skin; milder than pemphigus vulgaris and usually spares the mouth; onset usually 40 to 50 years but may occur as early as 3 years; Brazilian pemphigus is a variant endemic in areas of Brazil and occurs more commonly in children and young adults; pemphigus erythematosus has some characteristics of discoid lupus		Friction, pressure, needle punctures, and tape may exacerbate skin lesions and should be kept to a minimum; manipulation of the airway and other mucosal membranes should be avoided, if possible; heat, fluid, and electrolyte losses may occur from denuded skin; corticosteroids are commonly used to treat these disorders and replacement or increased doses may be required during the perioperative period; general and regional anesthetic techniques have been used successfully in these patients; subcutaneous infiltration of local anesthetics should be avoided because of the risk of skin sloughing
Benign familial chronic pemphigus	Affects the suprabasilar layer of the skin; mild disease that rarely involves the mouth; incompletely penetrant autosomal dominant inheritance		
Pemphigoid			
Bullous pemphigoid Pemphigoid gestationis (herpes gestationis)	Subepidermal bullae without acantholysis; mucosal lesions usually minor; pemphigoid gestationis is a variant that usually occurs in the second trimester and resolves within 3 months of delivery		
Cicatricial pemphigoid	Mucous membrane vesicles that heal with scarring; may present with web adhesions of the vocal cords; onset late in life	Esophageal stricture, deafness from middle ear involvement, blindness from conjunctival involvement	

management of patients with pemphigus and pemphigoid. It is generally thought that the anesthetic considerations are similar to those described for patients with EBD. **Use of intravenous ketamine infusion combined with a benzodiazepine in a spontaneously breathing patient has been advocated to minimize airway manipulations.**[55] **Epidural and continuous spinal anesthesia has been used successfully in patients with buccal pemphigus**[25] **and bullous pemphigoid,**[40] respectively. Because these patients are commonly receiving steroid therapy, replacement or stress doses of steroids may be required (see the "Corticosteroid Therapy" section for specific recommendations).

Erythema Multiforme and Related Disorders

Erythema multiforme (EM) is a reaction pattern in the skin and mucous membranes that manifests as maculopapular or bullous lesions (see Table 33-3). It is hypothesized that foreign antigens are sequestered in the epidermis and are an immune stimulus for cytotoxic responses that damage epidermal cells.[1] Onset can occur at any age, but the disease is most commonly seen in patients between 10 and 30 years of age. It has been associated with infections (Box 33-3),

vaccinations, drugs (Box 33-4), collagen vascular disease, allergic skin contactants,[16] malignancy, radiation therapy, and hormonal changes associated with pregnancy and menstruation.[1,23,27,57] Treatment involves avoidance, removal, or treatment of the possible causes of EM. In early cases, administration of systemic corticosteroids may arrest progression and lead to a more rapid recovery.[1]

Stevens-Johnson's syndrome was historically thought to be a severe form of EM, but many experts now believe that it represents a separate entity. It is characterized by widespread bulla formation and has a mortality rate of 3% to 18%.[1,11] Mucous membranes of the entire body may be involved. Ulcers may occur in the nasopharynx, oropharynx, larynx, trachea, and bronchi. Bullae of visceral pleura have resulted in pleural effusions and bronchiolar-alveolar-pleural fistulas with bilateral pneumothoraces and subcutaneous emphysema.[6] Pneumonitis may occur with clinical features similar to those of atypical pneumonia.[49] Acute atrial fibrillation has been reported and acute myocarditis has been found at autopsy. Löffler's syndrome with eosinophilia may also occur. Ulceration of the esophagus and colon has caused perforation and fatal gastrointestinal hemorrhage. Anemia

Table 33-3   Erythema multiforme and related disorders

Disease	Cutaneous manifestations	Systemic manifestations	Anesthetic considerations
Erythema multiforme (EM) and Stevens-Johnson's syndrome	Lesions in EM are maculopapular with variegated tints and iris lesions; Stevens-Johnson's syndrome is more severe with widespread bulla formation; all mucous membranes and pleura may be involved, including the upper and lower airways; most commonly seen in patients between 10 and 30 years	Pleural effusions, bronchopleural fistulas, pneumothoraces, pneumonitis, myocarditis and atrial fibrillation, gastrointestinal hemorrhage and anemia, poor nutrition, and nephritis	Friction, pressure, needle punctures, and tape may exacerbate skin lesions and should be kept to a minimum; manipulation of the airway is particularly hazardous because of involvement of subglottic structures; positive pressure ventilation may cause tension pneumothorax and should be avoided if possible; heat, fluid, and electrolyte losses may occur from denuded skin; there are no ideal anesthetic techniques; intravenous ketamine anesthesia with spontaneous respirations has been used with success
Toxic epidermal necrolysis (TEN) Staphylococcal scalded skin syndrome (SSSS)	Characterized by toxin-induced epidermal cleavage in the granular layer of the skin, most commonly seen in young children		
TEN from other causes	Characterized by basal cell disintegration with generalized bulla formation and desquamation; mucous membranes commonly involved		

BOX 33-3
INFECTIONS ASSOCIATED WITH
ERYTHEMA MULTIFORME

Bacterial	Viral
Diphtheria	Herpesvirus
Erysipeloid	Viral upper respiratory
Glanders	infection
	Asian flu
Yersinia infections	Lymphogranuloma
Mycoplasma	venereum
pneumonia	Infectious mononu-
Psittacosis	cleosis
Tuberculosis	Measles
Tularemia	Milkers' nodules
Lepromatous leprosy	Mumps
Typhoid fever	Smallpox vaccination
	Coxsackie viruses
Mycotic	Echoviruses
Coccidioidomycosis	Poliomyelitis
Histoplasmosis	

Protozoan

Malaria
Trichomoniasis

From Arnold HL Jr, Odom RB, and James WD: *Andrews' diseases of the skin,* Philadelphia, 1990, WB Saunders.

BOX 33-4
DRUGS ASSOCIATED WITH ERYTHEMA
MULTIFORME, STEVENS-JOHNSON'S
SYNDROME, OR TOXIC EPIDERMAL
NECROLYSIS

Allopurinol	Mercurials
Aminopyrine	Mithramycin
Antipyrine	Nalidixic acid
Arsenic	Penicillamine
Barbiturates	Penicillins
Bromides	Phenylbutazone
Chlorpropamide	Phenolphthalein
Codeine	Phenytoin
Dapsone	Procaine
Digitalis	Salicylates
Ethosuximide	Sulfonamides
Gold salts	Sulfones
Hexametaphosphate	Tetracyclines
Hydralazine	Thiazides
Iodides	Tolbutamide

From Arnold HL Jr, Odom RB, and James WD: *Andrews' diseases of the skin,* Philadelphia, 1990, WB Saunders; and Wood AJ, Oates JA: Adverse reactions to drugs. In Braunwald E et al, eds: *Harrison's principles of internal medicine,* ed 11, New York, 1987, McGraw-Hill.

---

secondary to bleeding, infection, and poor nutrition is common. Nephritis may cause acute renal failure. Seizures, coma, arthritis, myositis, urethritis, balanitis, vulvovaginitis, conjunctivitis, and corneal ulceration may also occur. In fatal cases, sepsis is the usual cause of death. Steroids and antihistamines have been used to treat Stevens-Johnson's syndrome with inconsistent results.[11] Antibiotics for infectious complications and nutritional support are given as indicated.

Toxic epidermal necrolysis (TEN) is a severe disease and is separated into two forms: one associated with staphylococcal toxins (staphylococcal scalded skin syndrome [SSSS]/Ritter's syndrome), and another associated with other infections and drugs (Lyell's disease). The SSSS is seen mainly in young children with staphylococcal infection of phage type 71. The epidermal cleavage is in the malpighian or granular layer and is caused by an exotoxin produced by the bacteria. Treatment is with antibiotics. In TEN from other causes, epidermal cleavage occurs just above or at the basal layer as a result of basal cell disintegration. Because the full thickness of the epidermis is separated in TEN, the serum loss is greater and the prognosis is more guarded than in SSSS. Unlike the SSSS, the mucous membranes are

often involved and associated membranoproliferative glomerulonephritis has been noted.

General precautions should be taken to avoid skin trauma. (See "Risk of Skin Trauma" section.) **Bladder catheterization should be avoided, if possible, because of the risk of urethritis.** Special care should be taken to protect the eyes because of the risk of conjunctivitis and corneal ulceration. Replacement or stress doses of corticosteroids may be required if patients are receiving steroid therapy (see "Corticosteroid Therapy" section).

There are no ideal anesthetics for use in the Stevens-Johnson's syndrome and TEN. **Manipulation and trauma of the airway should be avoided, if possible. Endotracheal intubation is particularly hazardous in this group of patients. Trauma to the laryngeal and tracheal mucosa by the endotracheal tube may cause abrasion and bleeding in ulcerated areas or cause bulla formation with severe compromise of the airway after extubation.** There is a risk of tension pneumothorax with positive pressure ventilation because of the occurrence of pleural blebs and pneumothorax. Regional anesthetics may be considered depending on the condition of the overlying skin and the presence of systemic infection. However, the meninges are epithelial surfaces and death from meningoencephalitis in Stevens-Johnson's syndrome has been reported.[5] **Infiltration of local anesthetics may be used if appropriate for the surgical procedure.** Ketamine as the sole anesthetic agent has been used with success in spontaneously breathing patients.[11]

Scleroderma

Scleroderma may be either localized to the skin (morphea and linear scleroderma) or may present as a generalized disorder of connective tissue (progressive systemic sclerosis (PSS) and CREST syndrome) (see Table 33-4). PSS is characterized by thickening and fibrosis of the skin with widespread systemic involvement. Raynaud's phenomenon involving the extremities is present in more than 95% of cases. There is also evidence that there is cold-induced vasospasm in the circulation of the heart, lungs, and kidneys, suggesting that internal organ "Raynaud equivalents" may play a role in the visceral abnormalities of scleroderma. Skin involvement usually begins on the fingers and hands and may progress to involve the face, arms, legs, and trunk. Scleroderma occurs most commonly between

Table 33-4 Scleroderma			
Disease	Cutaneous manifestations	Systemic manifestations	Anesthetic considerations
Generalized			
Progressive systemic sclerosis (PSS)	Thickening and fibrosis of the skin with Raynaud's phenomenon, occurs most commonly between 35 and 55 years	Interstitial pneumonitis, pulmonary fibrosis, pulmonary hypertension, interstitial myocardial fibrosis with heart failure or conduction defects, renal dysfunction associated with malignant hypertension, muscularis atrophy, and fibrosis of the gastrointestinal tract with esophageal dysmotility and reflux esophagitis, myositis, and arthritis	Mouth opening may be limited by thickening of the skin of the face and temporomandibular joint dysfunction; oral and nasal telangiectasias associated with the CREST syndrome may bleed if traumatized during instrumentation of the airway; prophylaxis with antacids, anticholinergics, H_2 blockers, and/or metoclopramide with awake or rapid sequence intubation may be indicated in patients with esophageal involvement because of the increased risk of reflux and aspiration; the patient should be kept warm to avoid Raynaud's phenomenon; arterial cannulation should be avoided because of the risk of vasospasm; chronic corticosteroid use may require replacement or increased doses during the perioperative period. Prolonged anesthesia after local anesthetic administration has been reported
Childhood PSS	Raynaud's phenomenon less frequent than in adult form	Cardiac involvement more common and renal involvement less common than in adult form	
CREST syndrome	Subcutaneous calcinosis, esophageal dysmotility, sclerodactyly, and telangiectasia	Variant of scleroderma with less risk of involvement of the heart, kidneys, muscles, and joints, but with increased risk of pulmonary hypertension in the absence of significant pulmonary interstitial fibrosis	
Localized			
Morphea Localized Guttate Generalized Profunda (pansclerotic morphea of childhood) Linear	Nonelastic, rigid macules or plaques with hypopigmentation or hyperpigmentation	Morphea profunda may present not only with sclerosis of the dermis, but also of the panniculus, fascia, muscle, and bone	

BOX 33-5
SYNDROMES ASSOCIATED WITH
PROGRESSIVE SYSTEMIC SCLEROSIS

Hashimoto's thyroiditis
Sjögren's syndrome
Dermatomyositis
Congenital hypogammaglobulinemia
Myasthenia gravis
Mycosis fungoides
Muscular dystrophy
Urticaria pigmentosa
Hyperthyroidism
Alopecia
Vitiligo
Pretibial myxedema
Melanoderma

From Arnold HL Jr, Odom RB, and James WD: *Andrews' diseases of the skin,* Philadelphia, 1990, WB Saunders.

BOX 33-6
SYNDROMES ASSOCIATED WITH
SCLERODERMATOUS SKIN CHANGES

Porphyria cutanea tarda
Primary systemic amyloidosis
Sjögren's syndrome
Werner's syndrome
POEMS syndrome
Carcinoid syndrome
Phenylketonuria
Progeria
Ataxia telangiectasia
Hurler's syndrome
Congenital poikiloderma
Exposure to:
  Pentazocine
  Bleomycin
  Silica
  Epoxy resins
  Hydrocarbons
  Chlorethylene
  Vinyl chloride

From Arnold HL Jr, Odom RB, and James WD: *Andrews' diseases of the skin,* Philadelphia, 1990, WB Saunders.

---

the ages of 35 and 55, but may occur at any age. The childhood form of PSS is notable for an increased risk of cardiac involvement. PSS may be associated with many other diseases (Box 33-5), and sclerodermatous skin changes may be present in other disease processes or toxic exposures (Box 33-6).

The CREST syndrome (subcutaneous *c*alcinosis, *R*aynaud's phenomenon, *e*sophageal dysmotility, *s*clerodactyly, and *t*elangiectasia) is a variant of scleroderma (see Table 33-5) and has a relatively benign course with substantially lower risk of involvement of muscles, joints, heart, and kidneys.[20] However, **these patients are at increased risk of progressive pulmonary hypertension in the absence of significant pulmonary interstitial fibrosis.**

Anesthetic considerations include limited airway access because of the patient's inability to open the mouth as a result of thickening of the skin of the face and dysfunction of the temporomandibular joint.[56] These patients are at increased risk of aspiration because of gastroesophageal reflux and intestinal dysmotility. Prophylaxis with antacids, anticholinergics, H_2-blockers, and/or metoclopramide with awake intubation or rapid sequence induction may decrease the risk of aspiration. Oral and nasal telangiectasias associated with the CREST syndrome may bleed if traumatized during instrumentation.[51] Cold-induced vasospasm has been implicated in the pathogenesis of the disease in multiple organs and must be avoided. Arterial cannulation in patients with Raynaud's phenomenon should be avoided, if possible, because of the risk of vasospasm. Intravenous administration of methohexital into a dorsal hand

vein has been reported to provoke a transient, painful, cyanotic reaction in the fingers similar to Raynaud's phenomenon.[12] **If pulmonary hypertension or impaired cardiac function is suspected, pulmonary artery catheterization may be indicated, especially in the presence of impaired renal function and possible large intravascular volume shifts.**[58] Peripheral venous access may be difficult to establish because of thickening of the skin. These patients may also be receiving chronic steroid therapy and require additional steroids during the perioperative period. (See "Corticosteroid Therapy" section.)

Regional anesthesia has the advantage of producing peripheral vasodilation and therefore decreasing the risk of Raynaud's phenomenon. **However, prolonged anesthesia after local anesthetic administration subcutaneously, epidurally, and with axillary and digital nerve block has been reported.**[14,33,51]

Mast Cell Disease

Mast cell disease is a group of entities in which excessive numbers of mast cells infiltrate various organs, including the skin (Table 33-6). The classic mast cell infiltrate appears as a reddish-brown pigmented macule, as in urticaria pigmentosa, that develops urticaria with a surrounding erythematous flare from histamine release when stroked (Darier's

Table 33-5 Clinical manifestations of scleroderma and CREST syndrome

Manifestations	Incidence	
	Scleroderma (systemic sclerosis)	CREST syndrome
Interstitial pulmonary fibrosis	75%	Rare
Pulmonary hypertension	Rare	10%
Myocardial involvement	15% to 50%	5%
Renal involvement	25%	Rare
Esophageal dysmotility	90%	90%
Tendon friction rubs	60%	<1%
Arthritis	40%	20%
Myositis	20%	<5%

Modified from Harris ED: Systemic sclerosis. In Wyngaarden JB, Smith LH, eds: *Cecil textbook of medicine,* Philadelphia, 1985, WB Saunders.

sign). Half the cases of mast cell disease have their onset before 6 months of age, with another fourth occurring before puberty. Systemic effects such as flushing, pruritus, hypotension, and shock, or local edema sufficient to produce vesicles and bullae may also occur with histamine release induced by mechanical manipulation, psychologic stress, temperature change, alcohol, vomiting, exercise, or pharmacologic agents (Box 33-7).[10,44,47] Skin involvement occurs most commonly in children, with clearing in half the patients and improvement in almost all before adult life.

Urticaria pigmentosa without systemic involvement accounts for 90% of persons affected with mast cell disease. When urticaria pigmentosa has its onset in adulthood, or when there is diffuse skin involvement, extracutaneous organ involvement must be suspected. Any tissue where mast cells are found can be affected. **Clotting factors may be reduced because of the combined effects of hepatic fibrosis and malabsorption of fat-soluble vitamins secondary to intestinal lesions.[47] Perioperative hemorrhagic diathesis related to heparin release from mast cells is a potential concern, although it is uncommon.** Protamine sulfate

Table 33-6 Mast cell disease

Disease	Cutaneous manifestations	Systemic manifestations	Anesthetic considerations
Childhood types			
Solitary mastocytoma	Reddish-brown macule that forms a wheal when stroked (urticaria pigmentosa)	Hypotension, pruritus, and flushing from histamine release, hepatic fibrosis, intestinal malabsorption, ulcers and gastrointestinal bleeding, osteoporosis, bone marrow infiltration, anemia, leukopenia, thrombocytopenia, and bleeding diathesis from nutritional deficiency and heparin release from mast cells	Avoid maneuvers that may cause degranulation, such as physical trauma, emotional stress, and drugs that release histamine; succinylcholine and meperidine produce minimal histamine release and have been used with success; antihistamines (H₁ and H₂ blockers) and antiserotonin agents may be useful in treating symptoms of histamine release; nifedipine may raise the threshold for mast cell degranulation; perioperative heparin release causing hemorrhagic diathesis has been successfully treated with protamine sulfate
Diffuse cutaneous mastocytosis	Same lesion as above but with widespread distribution		
Pseudoxanthomatous mastocytosis (Xanthelasmoidea)	Rare variant with pale yellow nodular lesions that develop erythema but no urticaria with rubbing		
Adult types			
Erythrodermic mastocytosis	Diffuse cutaneous disease		
Systemic mastocytosis	Same as above with systemic involvement		
Familial urticaria pigmentosa	A familial form of mastocytosis characterized by giant mast cell granules with autosomal dominant transmission and incomplete penetrance		

BOX 33-7
DRUGS ASSOCIATED WITH
HISTAMINE RELEASE

Opiates

Morphine
Meperidine (slight)

Anticholinergics

Atropine
Scopolamine

Muscle relaxants

Tubocurarine
Metocurine (slight)
Atracurium (slight)
Succinylcholine (slight)

Barbiturates

Thiopental
Thiamylal

Miscellaneous drugs

Dextran
Aspirin
Polymyxin
Guinine
Thiamine
Papaverine

---

has been used successfully in the treatment of bleeding in such patients.[10] Increased circulating histamine may lead to increased gastric acid secretion with ulcer formation and gastrointestinal bleeding.[10] Osteoporosis from bone involvement may occur. Mast cell infiltrates may occur in the bone marrow and mast cell leukemia may rarely develop. Anemia, leukopenia, and thrombocytopenia may occur. Mast cell infiltrates may also occur in the spleen and lymph nodes. There may be an increased incidence of non-mast cell leukemias and lymphomas associated with mast cell disease.

Therapy involves avoidance of maneuvers that lead to mast cell degranulation. Chronic administration of antihistamines (both H_1-blockers and H_2-blockers) and the antiserotonin drugs such as cyproheptadine are useful in relieving symptoms related to mastocytosis.[1] However, use of antihistamines does not prevent degranulation and release of histamine from the mast cells.[10] Use of nifedipine may improve symptoms by raising the threshold for degranulation in mast cells.[15] **Anesthetic agents that release histamine should be avoided.**

Inhalation anesthetics do not cause degranulation and may be used safely. Pancuronium, vecuronium, fentanyl, sufentanil, and alfentanil do not release histamine and should also be safe. Succinylcholine and meperidine produce minimal histamine release and have been used with success.**[10,44]

Neurofibromatosis

Neurofibromatosis (von Recklinghausen's disease) represents overgrowth of Schwann cells and endoneurium. It occurs in one of 3000 births and has a prevalence of 0.04%. Half the cases are sporadic, presumably representing a new mutation, but once expressed the disease is transmitted as a mendelian dominant characteristic. Neurofibromatosis presents as smooth, flesh-colored papules on the skin in association with café-au-lait spots (Table 33-7). Diffuse interstitial lung disease occurs in 7% of patients.[8] Mental deficiency, dementia, and epilepsy may be associated with brain involvement. Acoustic neuromas may lead to deafness. Gliomas of the optic nerve present with exophthalmia and decreased visual acuity. There may be nodules of the iris and hamartomas of the retina. Neuromas of spinal nerves may cause paralysis. Mesenteric and colonic neurofibroma may cause obstruction or result in bleeding. Cystic lesions in bone may produce scoliosis, kyphoscoliosis, lordosis, pseudoarthrosis, spina bifida, dislocations, and atraumatic fractures.[1] Ten percent to 15% of cases of pheochromocytoma are associated with neurofibromatosis.[27] Other endocrine disorders such as acromegaly, cretinism, hyperparathyroidism, myxedema, or precocious puberty may be present.[1]

Anesthetic management of these patients involves a careful physical examination to search for extracutaneous manifestations of the disease. In particular, a careful neurologic examination should be performed. Use of general anesthesia may be preferred over regional anesthetic techniques if involvement of the axial or peripheral nervous systems is suspected in the area considered for anesthetic blockade. **Unexplained hypertension should raise the possibility of pheochromocytoma.**

Mucocutaneous Lymph Node Disease

Mucocutaneous lymph node syndrome (Kawasaki's disease) is a disease of unclear origin characterized by fever of more than 5 days, conjunctival infection, mouth lesions, desquamation of the fingers and toes, an erythematous rash, and lymph node enlargement. Gingivitis, rhinitis, proteinuria, pyuria, diarrhea, aseptic meningitis, arthralgias, photophobia, anemia, leukocytosis, thrombocytosis, and mild icterus with elevated transaminase levels may also be seen. Coronary aneurysms or ectasia occur in 15% to 25% of patients.[38] In patients with angiographically documented coronary aneurysms, 50% have persistent abnormalities 5 to 18 months after the acute stage

Table 33-7 Miscellaneous skin disorders

Disease	Cutaneous manifestations	Systemic manifestations	Anesthetic considerations
Neurofibromatosis	Smooth, flesh-colored papules in association with café-au-lait spots; autosomal dominant inheritance	Interstitial lung disease, mental deficiency, seizures, paralysis secondary to spinal nerve neuromas, cranial nerve lesions, cystic bone lesions, kyphoscoliosis, lordosis, bowel obstruction and bleeding secondary to mesenteric and colonic neurofibromas, associated with pheochromocytoma and other endocrine abnormalities	Suspect pheochromocytoma in the presence of unexplained hypertension
Mucocutaneous lymph node disease	Desquamation of fingers and toes, erythematous rash, and oral lesions	Myocarditis, pericarditis, coronary artery lesions, proteinuria, diarrhea, mild icterus with elevated transaminases, aseptic meningitis, arthralgias, and anemia	Cardiac involvement is a prominent manifestation of this disease and must be considered when planning the patient's perioperative care
Dermatomyositis	Erythematous and sometimes edematous rash; heliotrope rash on upper eyelids and face are highly suggestive of the diagnosis	Aspiration, interstitial pneumonitis, pneumonia, asymptomatic electrocardiographic abnormalities, congestive heart failure, heart block, dysphagia, symmetric proximal muscle weakness, arthritis, and coexistent malignancy	Pulmonary status and ability to protect the airway must be carefully assessed; there is anecdotal evidence that these patients are more sensitive to nondepolarizing muscle relaxants
Behçet's disease	Oral and genital erosions, inflammatory ocular disease, erythema nodosum-like lesions, hyperirritable skin, and pustular skin lesions	Gastrointestinal ulcers, hemiplegia, paraplegia, cerebellar dysfunction, psychologic dysfunction, and arterial or venous occlusion	Trauma to the skin and mucosa, membranes should be minimized; oral lesions may make intubation difficult

of illness.[29] Echocardiography is also an effective means of documenting coronary artery aneurysms.[29] **Sudden death, presumably as a result of cardiac involvement, has been reported in 1% to 2% of patients.**[1] Other cardiac manifestations include angina, ECG changes (prolonged PR or QT intervals, Q waves, ST elevation, or flat T waves), myocarditis, pericarditis, pericardial effusion, and mitral regurgitation.[29]

Kawasaki's disease is treated with aspirin. High doses (100 mg/kg/day) are used during the acute phase of the illness and are decreased as the patient improves (3 to 5 mg/kg/day). If doses are not decreased, salicylate toxicity may result from improved absorption from the gastrointestinal tract. Steroid use has not been shown to be effective and may increase the risk of myocardial infarction.[1] Use of high-dose intravenous gamma globulin may decrease the incidence of coronary artery abnormalities.[38]

Anesthetic consideration must be given to possible cardiac manifestations during both the active and recuperative phases of the disease.

Dermatomyositis

Dermatomyositis is a category of polymyositis with skin involvement. The typical rash is erythematous, sometimes edematous, and occurs on the forehead, neck, shoulders, trunk, and arms. A heliotrope rash on the upper eyelids and face is highly suggestive of the diagnosis of dermatomyositis. Other criteria for the diagnosis of polymyositis are symmetric proximal muscle weakness, elevation of muscle enzyme activities in serum, typical electromyographic abnormalities, and a positive result from muscle biopsy. Arthralgias occur in about one fourth of patients with dermatomyositis, but true arthritis is usually mild. Dysphagia may occur related to weakness of the striated musculature of the posterior pharynx, and pneumonia as a result of aspiration is a major cause of morbidity and mortality in these patients. Interstitial pneumonitis occurs in 5% to 10% of patients. Asymptomatic electrocardiographic abnormalities are common, but congestive heart failure or heart block is uncommon. There is also an incidence of coexistent malignancy in 15% of patients with dermatomyositis. Treatment is with bed rest and administration of corticosteroids.

Anesthetic considerations include careful assessment of the patient's pulmonary status, including the ability to protect the airway. **There is only anecdotal evidence that these patients may be more sensitive to the nondepolarizing muscle relaxants, but caution is still advised in titrating the dose of nondepolarizing muscle relaxants in such patients.**[26]

Behçet's Disease

Behçet's disease is an inflammatory disorder of unknown origin that affects small blood vessels, particularly venules, and is characterized primarily by oral and genital erosions with inflammatory ocular disease. Scarring in the mouth is unusual but may cause difficulties at intubation.[54] Cutaneous lesions, such as erythema nodosum–like eruptions, superficial thrombophlebitis, pustular skin lesions, and hyperirritability of the skin occur in approximately 80% to 85% of patients. Behçet's disease is also associated with arthritis of the knees, ankles, elbow, and wrists. Gastrointestinal lesions include erosions or superficial ulcers in the terminal ileum or colon. Central nervous system manifestations include hemiplegia, paraplegia, cerebellar dysfunction, and psychologic dysfunction. Arterial or venous vascular occlusion may occur. The onset is usually in the third or fourth decade. Sterile pustules may occur after intradermal injection of normal saline solution or a mere needle puncture.

Corticosteroids may be used to palliate inflammation. Immunosuppressive therapy with azathioprine and cyclophosphamide is used to reduce the need for corticosteroids. Use of chlorambucil has been reported to prevent blindness in patients with posterior retinal involvement. Administration of colchicine is sometimes effective in treating the mucocutaneous and cutaneous lesions. A trial of sulfasalazine may be useful in patients with gastrointestinal manifestations.

Anesthetic considerations include careful airway management and avoidance of skin trauma. Patients receiving steroids will require appropriate steroid replacement therapy (see section on corticosteroid therapy). Preoperative assessment for extracutaneous manifestations, especially of the neurologic system, should be performed.

SUMMARY

Patients with skin disease present multiple challenges in their anesthetic management. Care must be taken to avoid further injury to diseased skin regardless of its specific cause. Maneuvers that are ordinarily assumed as safe, such as moving the patient from a stretcher to the operating room table, may cause frictional injury to friable skin. Adhesives normally used to secure monitoring devices, intravascular catheters, and endotracheal tubes may be injurious to skin, and alternatives may be required.

The normal barrier function of the skin may be impaired, leading to increased risk of infection. Increased losses of fluids, electrolytes, and heat may occur through diseased skin and must be treated appropriately.

Airway management may be complicated by perioral and mucosal involvement. Perioral scarring may limit mouth opening and mucosal bullae, bleeding, swelling, and secretions may make laryngoscopy difficult. In certain cases, endotracheal intubation is relatively contraindicated because of the risk of traumatic injury to the tracheal mucosa. Even mask ventilation may pose the risk of pressure injury to the skin.

Many systemic disorders may present as diseases of the skin. It is important to appreciate these associations and to fully evaluate the patient to assess potential involvement of other organ systems. Anesthetic management must consider the systemic as well as the dermatologic manifestations of skin diseases.

KEY POINTS

- In general when providing anesthesia for patients with dermatologic conditions, it is important to avoid maneuvers that exacerbate the condition.

- Friction, pressure, and needle punctures may induce or exacerbate skin lesions.

- Pressure points should be carefully padded.

- Visualization of the laryngeal structures may be hindered by the patient's inability to open the mouth because of the perioral scarring.

- Involvement of the larynx and trachea may also occur.

- Trauma during laryngoscopy and intubation should be minimized because of tissue friability and the risk of inducing new lesions.

- Heat regulation may be difficult in patients with dermatologic conditions.

- Patients may become hypothermic or hyperthermic depending on their condition.

- Lack of integrity of the skin predisposes patients to infection. In addition, the underlying disease process and treatment may place the patient at increased risk of infection.

- Intensive therapy with topical steroids may cause temporary suppression of the HPA axis, and systemic corticosteroid coverage is indicated in these patients.

- Cardiovascular disease may occur in association with many skin diseases.

- The pulmonary system has mucous membranes and is at risk in any skin disease that involves the mucous membranes.

- The gastrointestinal mucosa has the same embryologic origin as the skin and may be affected by the same pathologic processes that affect the skin.

KEY REFERENCES

Fox RH, Shuster S, Williams R et al: Cardiovascular, metabolic and thermoregulatory disturbances in patients with erythrodermic skin diseases, *Br Med J* 1:619, 1965.

James I, Wark HI: Airway management during anesthesia in patients with epidermolysis bullosa dystrophica, *Anesthesiology* 56:323, 1982.

Kelly RE, Kolf HD, Rothaus KO et al: Brachial plexus anesthesia in eight patients with recessive dystrophica epidermolysis bullosa, *Anesth Analg* 66:1318, 1987.

Prasad KK, Chen L: Anesthetic management of a patient with bullous pemphigoid, *Anesth Analg* 69:537, 1989.

Smith GB, Shribman AJ: Anesthesia and severe skin disease, *Anaesthesia* 39:443, 1984.

REFERENCES

1. Arnold HL Jr, Odom RB, and James WD: *Andrews' diseases of the skin,* Philadelphia, 1990, WB Saunders.
2. Berryhill RE, Benumof JL, Saidman LJ et al: Anesthetic management of emergency cesarean section in a patient with epidermolysis bullosa dystrophica polydysplastica, *Anesth Analg* 57:281, 1978.
3. Bickers DR, Pathak MA: The porphyrias. In Fitzpatrick TB et al, eds: *Dermatology in general medicine,* New York, 1987, McGraw-Hill.
4. Block MS, Gross BD: Epidermolysis bullosa dystrophica recessive: oral surgery and anesthetic considerations, *J Oral Maxillofac Surg* 40:753, 1982.
5. Boe J, Dalgaard JB, and Scott D: Mucocutaneous-ocular syndrome with intestinal involvement, *Am J Med* 25:857, 1958.

6. Broadbent RV: Stevens-Johnson disease presenting with pneumothorax, *Rocky Mountain Med J* 64:69, 1967.
7. Broster T, Placek R, and Eggers GW Jr: Epidermolysis bullosa: anesthetic management for cesarean section, *Anesth Analg* 66:341, 1987.
8. Burkhalter JL, Morano JU, McCay MB et al: Diffuse interstitial lung disease in neurofibromatosis, *South Med J* 79:944, 1986.
9. Clements PJ, Furst DE, Cabeen W et al: The relationship of arrhythmias and conduction disturbances to other manifestations of cardiopulmonary disease in progressive systemic sclerosis (PSS), *Am J Med* 71:38, 1981.
10. Coleman MA, Liberthson RR, Crone RK et al: General anesthesia in a child with urticaria pigmentosa, *Anesth Analg* 59:704, 1980.

11. Cucchiara RF, Dawson B: Anesthesia in Stevens-Johnson syndrome: report of a case, *Anesthesiology* 35:357, 1971.
12. Davidson-Lamb RW, Finlayson MC: Scleroderma, *Anaesthesia* 32:893, 1977.
13. Drenger B, Zibenbaum M, Reifen E et al: Severe upper airway obstruction and difficult intubation in cicatricial pemphigoid, *Anaesthesia* 41:1029, 1986.
14. Eisele JH, Reitan JA: Scleroderma, Raynaud's phenomenon, and local anesthetics, *Anesthesiology* 34:386, 1971.
15. Fairley JA, Pentland AP, and Voorhees JJ: Urticaria pigmentosa responsive to nifedipine, *J Am Acad Dermatol* 11:740, 1984.
16. Fisher AA: Erythema multiforme-like eruptions to contactants, *Cutis* 38:101, 1986.

17. Fox RH, Shuster S, Williams R et al: Cardiovascular, metabolic, and thermoregulatory disturbances in patients with erythrodermic skin diseases, *Br Med J* 1:619, 1965.

18. Hallenborg C, Rowe LD, Gamsu G et al: Severe upper airway obstruction caused by bullous pemphigoid: diagnostic usefulness of the flow-volume curve, *Otolaryngol Head Neck Surg* 90:20, 1982.

19. Hamann RA, Cohen PJ: Anesthetic management of a patient with epidermolysis bullosa dystrophica. *Anesthesiology* 34:389, 1971.

20. Harris ED: Systemic sclerosis. In Wyngaarden JB, Smith LH, eds: *Cecil textbook of medicine*, Philadelphia, 1985, WB Saunders.

21. Holzman RS, Worthen HM, and Johnson KL: Anaesthesia for children with junctional epidermolysis bullosa (letalis), *Can J Anaesth* 34:395, 1987.

22. Hubbert CH, Adams JG: Anesthetic management of patients with epidermolysis bullosa, *South Med J* 70:1375, 1977.

23. Huff JC: Acyclovir for recurrent erythema multiforme due to herpes simplex, *J Am Acad Dermatol* 18:197, 1988.

24. James I, Wark H: Airway management during anesthesia in patients with epidermolysis bullosa dystrophica, *Anesthesiology* 56:323, 1982.

25. Jeyaram C, Torda TA: Anesthetic management of cholecystectomy in a patient with buccal pemphigus, *Anesthesiology* 40:600, 1974.

26. Johns RA, Finholt DA, and Stirt JA: Anaesthetic management of a child with dermatomyositis, *Can Anaesth Soc J* 33:71, 1986.

27. Johnson M: Skin diseases. In Wyngaarden JB, Smith LH, eds: *Cecil textbook of medicine*, Philadelphia, 1985, WB Saunders.

28. Kaplan R, Strauch B: Regional anesthesia in a child with epidermolysis bullosa, *Anesthesiology* 67:262, 1987.

29. Kato H, Ichinose E, Yoshioka F, et al: Fate of coronary aneurysms in Kawasaki disease: serial coronary angiography and long-term follow-up study, *Am J Cardiol* 49:1758, 1982.

30. Kehlet H: A rational approach to dosage and preparation of parenteral glucocorticoid substitution therapy during surgical procedures, *Acta Anaesthesiol Scand* 19:260, 1975.

31. Kelly RE, Koff HD, Rothaus KO et al: Brachial plexus anesthesia in eight patients with recessive dystrophic epidermolysis bullosa, *Anesth Analg* 66:1318, 1987.

32. Lee C, Nagel EL: Anesthetic management of a patient with recessive epidermolysis bullosa dystrophica, *Anesthesiology* 43:122, 1975.

33. Lewis GB: Prolonged regional analgesia in scleroderma, *Can Anaesth Soc J* 21:495, 1974.

34. LoVerme SR, Oropollo AT: Ketamine anesthesia in dermolytic bullous dermatosis (epidermolysis bullosa), *Anesth Analg* 56:398, 1977.

35. Marshall BE: A comment on epidermolysis bullosa and its anaesthetic management for dental operations, *Br J Anaesth* 35:724, 1963.

36. Meyer UA: Porphyrias. In Isselbacher KJ et al, eds: *Harrison's principles of internal medicine*, ed 9, New York, 1980, McGraw-Hill.

37. Munro DD: The effect of percutaneously absorbed steroids on hypothalamic-pituitary-adrenal function after intensive use in in-patients, *Br J Dermatol* 94(suppl 12):67, 1976.

38. Newburger JW, Takahashi M, Burns JC et al: The treatment of Kawasaki syndrome with intravenous gamma globulin, *N Engl J Med* 315:341, 1986.

39. Plumpton FS, Besser GM, and Cole PV: Corticosteroid treatment and surgery, *Anaesthesia* 24:12, 1969.

40. Prasad KK, Chen L: Anesthetic management of a patient with bullous pemphigoid, *Anesth Analg* 69:537, 1989.

41. Pratilas V, Biezunski A: Epidermolysis bullosa manifested and treated during anesthesia, *Anesthesiology* 43:581, 1975.

42. Ramadass T, Thangavelu TA: Epidermolysis bullosa and its E.N.T. manifestations, *J Laryngol Otol* 92:441, 1978.

43. Roizen MF: Anesthetic implications of concurrent diseases. In Miller RD, ed: *Anesthesia*, New York, 1986, Churchill-Livingstone.

44. Rosenbaum KJ, Strobel GE: Anesthetic considerations in mastocytosis, *Anesthesiology* 38:398, 1973.

45. Schwarz MI, Matthay RA, Sahn SA et al: Interstitial lung disease in polymyositis and dermatomyositis: analysis of six cases and review of the literature, *Medicine* 55:89, 1976.

46. Shuster S: High-output cardiac failure from skin disease, *Lancet* 1:1338, 1963.

47. Smith GB, Shribman AJ: Anaesthesia and severe skin disease, *Anaesthesia* 39:443, 1984.

48. Spielman FJ, Mann ES: Subarachnoid and epidural anaesthesia for patients with epidermolysis bullosa, *Can J Anaesth Soc J* 31:549, 1984.

49. Stanyon JH, Warner WP: Mucosal respiratory syndrome, *Can Med Assoc J* 53:427, 1945.

50. Symreng T, Karlberg BE, Kagedal B et al: Physiological cortisol substitution of long-term steroid treated patients undergoing major surgery, *Br J Anaesth* 53:949, 1981.

51. Thompson J, Conklin KA: Anesthetic management of a pregnant patient with scleroderma, *Anesthesiology* 59:69, 1983.

52. Thompson JW: Epidermolysis bullosa dystrophica of the larynx and trachea. Acute airway obstruction, *Otolaryngol Head Neck Surg* 89:428, 1980.

53. Tomilson AA: Recessive dystrophic epidermolysis bullosa: the anaesthetic management of a case for major surgery, *Anaesthesia* 38:485, 1983.

54. Turner ME: Anaesthetic difficulties associated with Behçet's syndrome, *Br J Anaesth* 44:100, 1972.

55. Vatashsky E, Aronson HB: Pemphigus vulgaris: anaesthesia in the traumatised patient, *Anaesthesia* 37:1195, 1982.

56. Weisman RA, Calcaterra TC: Head and neck manifestations of scleroderma, *Ann Otol Rhinol Laryngol* 87:332, 1978.

57. Wood AJ, Oates JA: Adverse reactions to drugs. In Braunwald E et al, eds: *Harrison's principles of internal medicine*, ed 11, New York, 1987, McGraw-Hill.

58. Younker D, Harrison B: Scleroderma and pregnancy, *Br J Anaesth* 57:1136, 1985.

CHAPTER 34

Evaluation of the Trauma Patient

JOHN K. STENE, Jr.
CHRISTOPHER M. GRANDE
(JOHN) S.T. SUM PING

The well-trained trauma anesthesiologist/critical care specialist (TA/CCS) plays a multipart role in the care of a trauma patient, particularly in preoperative essentials such as securing the airway and providing adequate ventilation, appropriate intravenous fluid management, and indicated sedation, analgesia, and anesthesia. The anesthetic care of a trauma patient differs from that of an elective or nontraumatic surgical patient. The trauma patient's acute condition and need for immediate, lifesaving intervention requires concurrent (rather than the more traditional sequential) examination, diagnosis, and treatment, often according to preexisting protocols rather than formal diagnoses.[24,98] For this reason, and to preclude

trying to anesthetically manage an unfamiliar trauma patient in the operating room, the TA/CCS must be present and involved with the trauma patient's admission and initial survey (Box 34-1).[100]

This early involvement affords several advantages. First, since trauma care mandates making maximal use of every minute of the "golden hour," the TA/CCS who is present on admission does not need to duplicate efforts at defining the patient's condition and so avoids undue delay in instituting appropriate therapy. Second, early involvement ensures the delivery of a properly prepared patient to the operating room, along with the equipment to monitor the patient during transport. Third, the TA/CCS can control most patients' airways via endotracheal intubation, thereby reducing the incidence of emergency tracheostomies. For the patient who requires tracheostomy (e.g., one with facial trauma), a secure airway has already been provided. In addition, the TA/CCS is qualified to perform an emergency cricothyroidotomy.

Thus the trauma patient benefits from the TA/CCS's early involvement in his/her care. This same involvement also facilitates the TA/CCS's responsibility for providing adequate, appropriate, and individualized preoperative analgetic and anesthetic care.[41,43]* Because trauma patients often require sur-

---

* In 1988 concerned individuals formed the International Trauma Anesthesia and Critical Care Society (ITACCS) to recognize and further these mutual benefits to patients and practitioners. Currently, with more than 300 members, ITACCS is both an overseeing agency and a professional society dedicated to the advancement of scientific, educational, social, and political issues related to anesthesia subspecialists who spend a significant amount of time with trauma patients. These objectives are critical to the overall goal of increasing sophistication for trauma management systems. As the trauma surgeon's abilities expand, the trauma anesthesiologist must be able to cope with these new demands. ITACCS is responsible for appreciating these demands and devising means to meet them.

BOX 34-1
RESUSCITATION PROTOCOLS—
PRIMARY SURVEY

I. Scan: 2- to 15-second overview for obvious injuries.
II. Obtain patient's history from emergency medical services personnel.
III. Ask patient to describe injuries, if able.
IV. Ascertain the "ABCDEs":
   A. Airway: patent?
      1. Look for chest wall movements, retraction, nasal flaring.
      2. Listen for breath sounds: stridor, stertorous respirations.
      3. Feel for air movement.
   B. Breathing: any obstruction? (Patient may require intubation.)
      1. Determine presence or absence of adequate spontaneous ventilation.
      2. Inspect thoracic cage for symmetric chest movement (open pneumothorax, sucking chest wound).
      3. Check for flail segments.
      4. Auscultate for bilateral air movement.
      5. Provide mechanical ventilatory assistance for ventilatory failure.
   C. Circulation: adequate perfusion?
      1. Check peripheral pulses, capillary refill, arterial blood pressure.
      2. Obtain electrocardiogram.
      3. Grade shock by vital signs.
      4. Correct circulatory shock: start intravenous lines and obtain blood sample for cross-match and laboratory analysis.
   D. Disability: neurologic injury?
      1. Evaluate central function:
         a. A—*a*lert
         b. V—responds to *v*ocal stimuli
         c. P—responds to *p*ainful stimuli
         d. U—*u*nresponsive
      2. Evaluate pupil size, responsiveness to light.
      3. Determine motor function, reflexes in all four extremities.
      4. Use Glasgow Coma Scale.
   E. Expose patient for complete examination.
V. Remember: treat problem when identified; do not wait for completion of primary survey.

Modified from Stene JK, Grande CM, Bernhard WN et al: Overview of perioperative anesthetic management of the trauma patient: thoracoabdominal and orthopaedic injuries. In Stene JK, Grande CM, eds: *Trauma anesthesia*, Baltimore, 1991, Williams & Wilkins.

gery with varying degrees of urgency—immediately, urgently, and even electively—and at any time, the TA/CCS must be prepared to provide appropriate interpretation at all hours. The TA/CCS must have a proper understanding of trauma patients' special problems to minimize mortality and morbidity from traumatic illness. Certification as an instructor or provider for the Advanced Trauma Life Support (ATLS) course, developed by the Committee on Trauma of the American College of Surgeons,[24] is an important method of preparing the TA/CCS for managing trauma patients.

DEMOGRAPHICS OF TRAUMA

Trauma has become a national health concern over the past decade and is the leading cause of death and disability in the young, productive portion of the U.S. population. Trauma is now the third leading cause of death at any age, after heart disease and cancer. Every year 175,000 persons die from trauma in the United States, and this number continues to increase rapidly, in contrast to decreasing mortality from heart disease, cancer, and cerebrovascular accident (CVA, stroke).[107-109] Direct cost of trauma care represents 7% of all health care expenditure.[71] One third of all hospital admissions, or 19 million hospital days, result from trauma.[15] This represents more hospital days than all heart disease patients require and four times the number hospitalized cancer patients require.[109]

Mortality from trauma is age related. Although more trauma patients are in the younger generation, the elderly are likely to suffer most. The elderly account for almost 33% of health care trauma resources and are five times more likely to die of an equivalent injury than younger people.[60] If elderly trauma patients survive, they often face a major decrement in the quality of life.[75]

Trauma deaths occur in a trimodal pattern.[109] Fifty percent of deaths occur within 1 hour of injury. Intermediate deaths occur within a few hours of injury and constitute 30% of deaths. Late deaths occur from 2 to 6 weeks after injury and account for 20% of all trauma deaths (see Fig. 85-1).

PREHOSPITAL CARE

Today, paramedical personnel are usually well trained in the performance of advanced life support. This improved care has reportedly led to reduced mortality in San Diego County, Calif., during 1980 to 1982.[56] Controversy surrounds how much to extend relatively time-consuming advanced life support care to the trauma scene. Proponents of "scoop and run" believe that trauma patients should not be stabilized at the scene but simply transported, since decreased time for patients to reach definitive medical care has been correlated with increased survival.[14] Others have suggested that cardiopulmonary resuscitation (CPR) with endotracheal intubation, vigorous fluid administration, and rapid transport can be effective in critically ill trauma patients.[26] Clearly, benefit from resuscitation at the trauma scene must depend on the individual trauma patient's condition. These types of decisions should be made by physicians with experience in managing trauma, such as the involvement of the TA/CCS in prehospital care in Europe.[41]

INITIAL ASSESSMENT

The TA/CCS's assessment of the trauma patient begins by communication with emergency medical services (EMS) personnel following notification of the patient's impending arrival. The patient's Trauma Score (TS) (Table 34-1) is quickly calculated from EMS information because it correlates with survival rate.[20] A TS of 12 or less is associated with a decreased chance of survival (Table 34-2).

Equipped with background information on the patients' condition, the TA/CCS is better prepared to

---

Table 34-1   Trauma score

Parameter	Measurement	Score	Total
A. Respiratory rate	10-24/min	4	
	25-35/min	3	
	>35/min	2	
	<10/min	1	
	0/min	0	A. _____
B. Respiratory effort	Normal	1	
	Shallow or retractive (use of accessory muscles)	0	B. _____
C. Systolic blood pressure	> 90 mm Hg	4	
	70-90 mm Hg	3	
	50-69 mm Hg	2	
	< 50 mm Hg	1	
	0 mm Hg	0	C. _____
D. Capillary refill	Normal	2	
	Delayed (>2 seconds)	1	
	None	0	D. _____
E. Glasgow Coma Scale (GCS)			
1. Eye opening			
Spontaneous	___ 4	(14-15)* 5	
To voice	___ 3	(11-13) 4	
To pain	___ 2	(8-10) 3	
None	___ 1	(5-7) 2	
		(3-4) 1	E. _____
2. Verbal response			
Oriented	___ 5		
Confused	___ 4		
Inappropriate words	___ 3		
Incomprehensible words	___ 2		
None	___ 1		
3. Motor response			
Obeys commands	___ 6		
Purposeful movements (pain)	___ 5		
Withdraw (pain)	___ 4		
Flexion (pain)	___ 3		
Extension (pain)	___ 2		
None	___ 1	Trauma Score	
Total GCS points (1 + 2 + 3) _____		(Total points A + B + C + D + E)	

*Numbers in parentheses refer to the total GCS points from the last entry in the left-hand column.
From Champion HR, Sacco WJ, Carnazzo AJ et al: Trauma score, *Crit Care Med* 9:672, 1981.

Table 34-2   Survival rate from Trauma Score

Trauma Score	Survival (%)
16	99
13	93
10	60
7	15
4	2
1	0

organize immediate care on the trauma patient's arrival. **When the patient arrives, an assessment of the airway, breathing, circulation, and neurologic status (ABCN) can be done in under 1 minute.** While this is being done, other trauma team members can establish venous access and place the appropriate monitors (e.g., blood pressure, electrocardiogram [ECG], pulse oximeter). A trauma patient who is conscious, moving all extremities, and normotensive without respiratory embarrassment, tachycardia, or neck pain is likely to be in stable condition, and adequate time is available for a more thorough assessment. If the patient does not take a deep breath on command, the TA/CCS begins ventilation of the lungs with a bag and mask. The TA/CCS then prepares to intubate the trachea to secure the airway.

Airway Management

Airway management can be complex in trauma patients because of potential cervical spine, maxillofacial, upper airway, and lower respiratory tract injuries, as well as the frequent occurrence of a full stomach. The extent of these injuries is usually unknown, and insufficient time may be available to investigate their extent and severity before committing to one of several options to achieve airway management.

The ability to speak virtually guarantees a patent airway and confirms the patient's ability to breathe. If adequate respirations are present, the TA/CCS has time to analyze available options and develop a treatment plan. While the TA/CCS is formulating the plan, the following steps are instituted: (1) a baseline measurement of arterial blood gases (ABGs), (2) administration of supplemental oxygen (O_2) supplied by face mask, (3) exposure of a lateral cervical spine radiograph to check for a possible cervical spine fracture, and (4) placement of a gastric tube. If the patient is unable to speak, the TA/CCS must rule out acute airway obstruction. Even if the patient is unconscious but shows adequate tidal respiratory gas exchange, time exists to formulate a plan for airway

management. The TA/CCS must act emergently to secure a patent airway if the patient is unconscious and not breathing. The TA/CCS must protect spinal cord neurologic function during all maneuvers to secure a patent airway. If damage has been ruled out by radiographs or a computed tomographic (CT) scan, the TA/CCS can work with assurance that iatrogenic spinal cord injury is unlikely.

Airway control options

The unconscious patient may obstruct the airway from the tongue falling back against the posterior pharynx (soft tissue obstruction) or from a foreign body stuck in the pharynx or upper respiratory tract. Several maneuvers, such as chin lift, neck lift, or jaw thrust, may be employed to relieve the soft tissue obstruction. These maneuvers involve a significant amount of head and neck movement and are usually inappropriate for a trauma patient who has a suspected cervical spine fracture unless no alternative exists. Establishment of an airway may be aided by using an artificial nasopharyngeal or oropharyngeal airway, but the TA/CCS must consider accompanying risks, including agitation, retching, coughing, vomiting, and bleeding. All these may contribute to complications such as elevated intracranial pressure (ICP) or pulmonary aspiration of gastric contents.

Inability to obtain or maintain a patent airway by these maneuvers may indicate foreign body obstruction. Exploration with a finger or a Yankauer suction catheter may clear the airway. If not immediately successful, the pharynx and larynx must be visualized to identify the foreign body and facilitate its removal. **Laryngoscopy should be done with the precautions described later whenever cervical spine injury is suspected.** Cervical spinal injury must be suspected if the lateral radiograph shows a reaction or if the patient received blunt injury consistent with head and neck injury.

Nasal intubation

Some anesthesiologists consider "blind" nasal intubation to be the method of choice in a patient with restricted neck movement, but this technique is not without important complications,[39] as described following.

- **Patients with cervical spine injuries also may have head injury accompanied by basilar skull fracture with disruption of the cribriform plate of the ethmoid bone deep inside the nose. Nasal intubation is contraindicated because the endotracheal tube may traverse the fractured cribriform plate and disrupt the brain substance. Furthermore, the nasal tube increases the risk of spreading bacterial infection from sinusitis to the meninges in a basilar skull fracture.**

- Nasal intubation is not easy to perform in confused and combative patients, who may thrash about and worsen cervical spine injury.
- Inadequate topical anesthesia or nerve block may allow retching and vomiting when the endotracheal tube is manipulated into the pharynx and larynx. This may result in a significant increase in ICP or cause laryngospasm, bronchospasm, and aspiration pneumonia.

Although blind nasal intubation undoubtedly has a place in airway management of patients with cervical spine injuries, other techniques should be considered.

Oral intubation

The major concern with oral intubation in a patient with cervical spine injury is that obligatory movement of the head and neck during laryngoscopy for an anesthetized paralyzed patient may cause further cervical cord injury. Fiberoptic intubation with the patient awake following bilateral superior laryngeal nerve blocks plus appropriate topical anesthesia is an option but may be difficult. Awake intubation may be dangerous in a confused patient because further damage to the cervical spine may occur with sudden, inappropriate movements. **Stabilization of suspected cervical spine injury during direct laryngoscopy can** be obtained with *manual in-line axial traction* (**MIAT**) (Fig. 34-1), a technique accepted by the American College of Surgeons as part of the ATLS protocol for emergency intubation.[24,98] Most trauma patients are now routinely transported from the field with a cervical collar to stabilize the cervical spine. Before oral intubation is attempted, the anterior portion of the cervical collar is removed and MIAT applied by a specialist in the management of cervical spine injury. This procedure also provides access to the anterior neck should a surgical airway be needed.

Because most trauma patients should be considered to have full stomachs, many anesthesiologists recommend cricoid pressure[87] until the trachea is intubated. Properly applied cricoid pressure requires a force of 44 newtons (N) ($kg \cdot m/s^{-2}$) to prevent regurgitation of gastric contents;[118] the concern is that too great a force on an unstable cervical spine fracture may cause further cervical cord injury. Cricoid pressure should only be used after the TA/CCS has considered the risks of further cervical spine injury vs. aspiration pneumonia. Failure of oral intubation with MIAT for the trauma patient with cervical spine injury after induction of anesthesia and paralysis usually requires establishment of an emergency surgical airway.

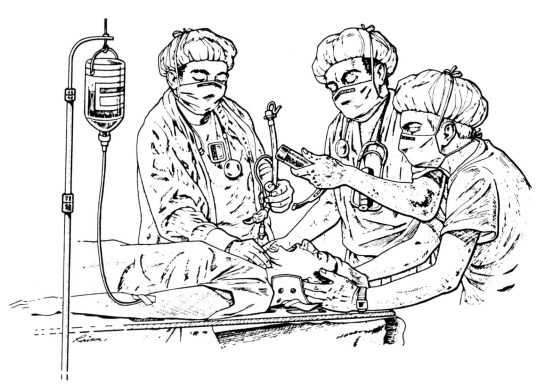

Fig. 34-1. Manual in-line axial traction (MIAT), also known as manual cervical spine immobilization/stabilization. (From Stene JK: Anesthesia for the critically ill trauma patient. In Siegel J, ed: *Trauma, emergency surgery and critical care,* New York, 1987, Churchill-Livingstone.)

Surgical options

If nasal or oral intubation is technically difficult and is not successful after a reasonable number of attempts, some type of "surgical airway" must be obtained. The number of attempts considered reasonable depends on the specific conditions of each trauma patient and the skill and experience of the anesthesiologist. O_2 jet insufflation can be provided with a 14-gauge catheter through the cricothyroid membrane or the anterior tracheal wall, attached directly to the gas outlet of the anesthetic machine. This setup can then be used similarly to a Sanders Injector by intermittently pressing on the O_2 flush to provide an O_2 flow at 50 psi pressure.[84,96] The Venturi effect created entrains air, which, together with the O_2 flow, produces inflation of the lungs. Complications of this technique usually result from pulmonary barotrauma to the lung or obstruction to gas outflow through the larynx.[93] Such O_2 insufflation is only a temporary alternative until a more permanent cricothyroidotomy or tracheostomy is performed.

Cricothyroidotomy, followed by the insertion of a 5 to 6 mm endotracheal tube through the surgical opening, is preferred to a more formal tracheostomy for the patient in an emergency situation because it is less time-consuming, easier to perform, and more likely to result in a dependable airway. Cricothyroidotomy may later be converted to a tracheostomy under more controlled conditions.[30] The prepackaged cricothyroidotomy "kits" available today (e.g., Weiss Airway, NuTrach, Abelson Airway) have all the necessary equipment in a box and may save time and confusion during resuscitation. However, the user must become familiar with a particular kit before the emergency to avoid misuse.

Some trauma patients arrive in the hospital already intubated. The TA/CCS must personally check proper positioning of the endotracheal tube. The esophageal obturator airway (EOA) and esophageal gastric tube airway (EGTA) are still being used in the field by EMS technicians and paramedics in some communities, although the safety and efficacy of these devices are in question.[7,31,85] Once inserted, the EGTA/EOA must not be removed until the airway has been protected by a cuffed endotracheal tube and the stomach suctioned. A new emergency airway product, the pharyngeotracheal lumen airway (see Fig. 84-3), is currently undergoing extensive evaluation. Although initial reports about its effectiveness appear promising,[9,74] it is too early to comment on its dependability.

Resuscitation

Thirty percent of trauma patients die during the initial hour following a traumatic injury. The cause of these early deaths is hemorrhage or central nervous system (CNS) laceration.[107] During this hour, proper assessment and appropriate management of volume status are critical to outcome. Clinically, this can be a challenging task, especially in an unresponsive, multiply traumatized patient.

Intravascular volume is estimated with palpation of a peripheral pulse, measurement of arterial blood pressure (Table 34-3), observation of general skin condition, and assessment of mental status. The acutely volume-depleted trauma patient will have cool, moist, pallid, or cyanotic skin, especially at the extremities, and a depressed level of consciousness. A major goal in resuscitating these patients is to replete intravascular volume to maximize tissue O_2 delivery. **Cardiac output and perfusion of the vital organs are more important determinants of outcome than arterial blood pressure. Vasopressor agents therefore must be used sparingly, if at all, and only with the intention of temporarily gaining a little time until hypovolemia can be corrected.**

As volume status is being assessed, other trauma

Table 34-3   American College of Surgeons classes of acute hemorrhage

Parameter	Class I	II	III	IV
Blood loss (ml)	750	1000-1250	1500-1800	2000-2500
Blood loss (% of blood loss in 70 kg patient)	15	20-25	30-35	40-50
Pulse rate (normal: 72 beats/min)	>72-84	>100	>120	>140
Blood pressure (normal: 120/80)	118/82	110/80	70-90/50-60	<50 systolic
Pulse pressure (mm Hg)	36	30	20-30	10-20
Respiratory rate	14-20	20-30	30-40	>35
Urine output (normal: 40-50 ml/hr)	30-35	25-30	5-15	Negligible
CNS-mental status	Slightly anxious	Mildly anxious	Anxious/confused	Confused/lethargic

Courtesy the American College of Surgeons.

team members are evaluating and managing the airway, obtaining blood for laboratory studies (typing and cross-matching, complete blood count [CBC] with platelet count, electrolytes, glucose, blood urea nitrogen [BUN], toxicology screen), and establishing intravascular access for fluid replacement. If necessary, open surgical cannulation of a peripheral vein should be performed without hesitation. The choice of either the saphenous vein or the antecubital vein for a cutdown is controversial.[69,90] The disadvantages of using the lower-limb venous system are as follows:

- The veins may be smaller or occluded from chronic venous disease.
- The MAST may interfere with the cutdown and reduce the rate of fluid infusion at that site.
- The patient may have intrapelvic or abdominal bleeding, which may render such fluid replacement ineffective or even deleterious.

The problems with a cutdown at the antecubital fossa are that it is technically more difficult and that resuscitation of intravascular volume may not be effective with unsuspected bleeding from the superior vena cava, in a similar fashion to intraabdominal bleeding. When a cutdown is necessary, it is preferable to establish venous access rapidly with the saphenous vein first and then proceed to the veins of the upper limbs, if indicated. Literature review indicates approximately a 5% rate of catheter-related sepsis.[63] In most patients the catheter initially becomes colonized by the patient's own cutaneous flora invading the insertion site. Thus careful aseptic placement is important, even during resuscitation and induction of general anesthesia. A new subcutaneous, silver-impregnated cuff has been reported to reduce the incidence of catheter-related bacteremia fourfold,[63] but this can be placed later and should not be considered until the patient's condition is stabilized.

Rapid resuscitation of the trauma patient is best accomplished with large-gauge, short intravenous (IV) catheters.[68] Other considerations include length and size of the infusion set and flow resistance of fluid warmers when rapid infusion is needed. Using wide-bore urology irrigation tubing can more than double the flow rate.[68] A recently introduced fluid warmer that has large-bore tubing (Level One Technology, Marshfield, Mass.) can rapidly warm and infuse a large volume of fluid (500 ml/min for blood), which should meet the needs of most trauma patients. In major centers that have extensive trauma teams, overtransfusion and fluid resuscitation can now be done if careful monitoring is not already being conducted.

Initial resuscitation is begun with a balanced salt solution while blood samples are sent to the laboratory and blood bank. A longstanding controversy exists about whether colloid or crystalloid solutions should be used for resuscitation. The data available at present are confusing and conflicting.[33,35,78,81] Different study designs, difficulties in measuring small changes in pulmonary function, and different patient populations may account for opposite conclusions having been reached in previous studies. During hemorrhage, the interstitial space, as well as the intravascular compartment, are diminished with the compensatory increase in reabsorption of fluid into the capillaries (Starling equilibrium of capillary exchange). To replenish the intravascular and interstitial compartment rapidly and efficiently, both colloid and crystalloid should be given (see Chapter 85). Although no data exist on the "correct" combination of colloid and crystalloid, one reasonable approach is to start with a 1:1 ratio until the patient's condition is more stable.

The patient who has severe blood loss and is in shock (classes III and IV of acute hemorrhage [see Table 34-3]) requires blood administration. Available options are type O negative low-titer, type-specific, typed and screened, or typed and cross-matched blood. The initial choice depends on the degree of hemodynamic instability. Type O negative red blood cells (RBCs) have no major antigens and can be given reasonably safely to patients of any blood type; the accompanying serum may contain antibodies to A and B antigens. Even packed RBCs may have a significant amount of serum present, but the risk of a major hemolytic transfusion reaction remains low. Unfortunately, only 8% of the population has O negative blood, and blood bank reserves on O negative, low-antibody-titer blood are usually very low. For this reason, O positive RBCs are frequently used. This is a reasonable approach in males but may be a problem in females of childbearing age who are Rh negative.

If 50% to 75% of the patient's blood volume has been replaced with type O blood, one probably should continue to administer type O blood. Otherwise, risk of a major cross-match reaction increases since the patient may have received enough anti-A or anti-B antibodies to precipitate intravascular hemolysis if A, B, or AB units are subsequently given. If temporizing measures can gain the 5 minutes necessary to obtain type-specific blood, it is preferable to use it instead of type O.[36] If time permits, the patient's blood should be typed and screened blood should be available. When blood is typed and screened, the patient's blood group is identified, and the serum is screened for major blood group antibodies. A full cross-match generally requires about 45 minutes and involves mixing donor cells with recipient serum to rule out any antigen-antibody reactions.

Fluid resuscitation of the patient is continued until improved perfusion and restoration of organ function occur or until vital organ monitoring indicates that cardiac failure is incipient. In the awake patient, mental status usually improves as hypovolemic shock resolves. Other manifestations of improved cardiac output include increased pulse pressure, decreased heart rate, increased urine output, resolution of lactic acidosis, and brisk capillary refill. Direct arterial pressure monitoring may allow detection of intravascular volume deficits early. Degree of systolic pressure variation with each mechanical breath correlates positively with the amount of hemorrhage. Trends in cardiac filling pressure (central venous pressure [CVP] or pulmonary capillary wedge pressure [PCWP]), rather than absolute numbers, is also helpful in fluid management.

Mechanism of Injury

The anesthesiologist caring for the trauma patient should have at least a basic understanding of the mechanisms of injury to facilitate diagnosis and treatment and guard against "pitfalls." The patient's past medical history and details of the trauma incident are both important in trying to establish the extent and consequences of the injury.[38,41]

Injuries can be classified into penetrating, blunt, or a combination of both. Penetrating trauma can range as a spectrum of disease that extends from the frequently ignored minor pinprick to the devastating results caused by high-powered firearms. The extent of damage caused is influenced by three factors:

- Character of the wounding instrument (e.g., knife's degree of sharpness and shape)
- Instrument's velocity at time of impact
- Characteristics of the tissue through which instrument passes

A detailed explanation how those three factors interact to produce the final injury is beyond the scope of this chapter.

Blunt trauma is the result of an abrupt change of either linear or rotary velocity, as experienced in high-speed crashes or falls from significant heights. Newton's first law (an object in motion tends to remain in motion until affected by an outside force) can explain most injuries incurred by blunt trauma. The force, which acts to stop the object, is directly proportional to the square of the change in velocity and the mass of the object; that is, the faster and heavier an object, the more extensive is the injury when the object comes to a complete stop. This force is a form of gravity and is known as g force. The magnitude of g force generated by a particular motor vehicle accident (MVA) can be estimated using the following formula[67]:

$$g = \frac{mph^2}{30 \times \text{Stopping distance (feet)}}$$

As the human body decelerates, the organs continue forward at the original velocity. Under such conditions the body and its organs assume "apparent weights" that vary with initial velocity. The organs, as they move forward, may be torn from their attachments through rotary and shearing forces, with disruption of connective tissue, blood vessels, and nerves.

Changes in velocity of less than 12 mph are rarely associated with significant injuries. Changes in velocity greater than 20 mph usually cause severe injuries, depending on the circumstances. When velocity change exceeds 30 mph, the trauma patient is likely to have severe injury.[106] The trauma patient's extent of injury might indicate the speed of impact and change in velocity for an MVA.

TYPES OF INJURY
Head Injuries

Brain damage resulting from an injury to the head is a common cause of mortality and morbidity. **In a trauma patient with brain injury, one must minimize and prevent further insults to the already damaged brain.** With early institution of ventilation, restoration of cerebral perfusion, and reduction of an elevated ICP, the outcome is more favorable.[21] In a conscious patient, presence and extent of brain injury can be assessed with a thorough neurologic examination. CT scanning is necessary for the unconscious patient as soon as his/her general condition is stabilized. One must diagnose the cause of coma in a trauma patient because delay in evaluating intracranial hemorrhage may have devastating effects. Mortality was found to be 30% in patients undergoing surgery for an acute subdural hematoma within 4 hours of injury vs. 90% in those who had surgery after 4 hours.[86]

Thoracic Injuries

Thoracic injuries are directly responsible for more than 25% of trauma death and contribute significantly in at least another 25%.[13] The primary site of injury in patients with penetrating injury is usually obvious. Often the extent of injury appears superficially minor, but the patient may have massive bleeding from the lung, cardiac injuries (usually with tamponade), large vessel damage (aorta, vena cava, pulmonary, subclavian and innominate arteries and veins), and chest wall vessels (intercostal or internal mammary arteries). Blunt trauma presents an even greater diagnostic dilemma because external injury may not be apparent.

In every patient with thoracic trauma, penetrating or blunt, one must investigate for any major injury to the lung/chest wall/diaphragm, the cardiovascular system, or both. In blunt trauma, rib fractures are the most common injuries, followed in order by hemothorax, pneumothorax, and flail chest. The first and second ribs are difficult to fracture, and patients who have fractures of these two ribs are likely to have significant thoracic or thoracic outlet vascular injuries.[115] Patients with severe thoracic injuries should have serial chest radiographs (every 6 to 12 hours for 24 to 48 hours) to exclude a pneumothorax or hemothorax, which may develop more than 6 to 24 hours after the initial injury. A small pneumothorax or hemothorax does not require immediate intervention if the patient is in stable condition. These injuries must be observed closely, and thoracostomy tubes should be inserted if one suspects that they are enlarging in size. Thoracostomy tubes (26 to 32 French for a pneumothorax, 30 to 40 French for a hemothorax or hemopneumothorax) should be placed in the fourth or fifth interspace in the midaxillary line and directed posteriorly and toward the pulmonary apex to reduce the possibility of damaging a high-lying diaphragm.

The frequency and extent of lung contusions are usually proportional to the severity of thoracic injuries. Chest radiographic changes in lung contusion tend to lag 24 to 48 hours behind the patient's condition and laboratory changes, and the extent of lung injury is usually greater than suspected radiologically. The ABGs tend to deteriorate progressively over the initial 48 to 72 hours as increasing water moves into the area of parenchymal lung injury. Treatment primarily involves maintenance of adequate ventilation of the lung and good tissue oxygenation. If spontaneous ventilation is inadequate, mechanical support with synchronized intermittent mandatory ventilation (SIMV) provides better ventilation/perfusion matching, better hemodynamics, and quicker weaning than does controlled ventilation. Contusions usually begin to resolve in 2 to 5 days if other pulmonary complications are not superimposed.[116] **Urgent surgery (e.g., fracture reductions) should not necessarily be postponed because of pulmonary contusions.**

Injuries to bronchi result from the g forces shearing the more mobile distal bronchi from relatively fixed proximal structures during rapid deceleration. One should always suspect this injury when a massive subcutaneous or mediastinal emphysema or a persistent pneumothorax with a continuing large air leak is found. Most of these injuries occur within 2 cm of the carina and are diagnosed by bronchoscopy. Bronchial injuries should be repaired surgically; otherwise they will result in repeated pulmonary infections, severe bronchial stenosis, or severe mediastinitis.

The most common cardiac injuries from trauma are contusion, tamponade, and rupture. Trauma patients with cardiac rupture are normally dead on arrival. Cardiac tamponade usually results from a penetrating injury. If tamponade is the problem, Beck's triad (distended neck veins, decreased blood pressure, depressed heart tones) may be present, as well as signs such as tachycardia, paradoxic pulse, and a narrowed pulse pressure. If the patient is hypotensive, immediate treatment should consist of fluids, inotropic support, and open surgical drainage.

The incidence of cardiac contusion after severe blunt chest trauma varies from 20% to 76%.[27] Diagnosing myocardial contusion[104] may be problematic. Most often it is diagnosed on the basis of abnormal ECG (ST-T wave abnormalities, bundle branch block, dysrhythmias) and creatine kinase isoenzymes (CK-MB) changes. Further tests, including 2-D echocardiography, radionuclide angiography, and coronary angiography, are done in selected patients. Patients with cardiac contusions are normally monitored in the intensive care unit for 2 to 3 days for early detection and treatment of complications, especially dysrhythmias and congestive heart failure. Whether patients with cardiac contusion should have their urgent surgery delayed is controversial. Every such patient should be assessed individually, with special consideration for the urgency of surgery and hemodynamic instability.

Traumatic rupture of the aorta occurs infrequently, but mortality is very high. From 80% to 90% of patients die within a few minutes of their injuries. Of those who survive for 1 hour, 90% die within 10 weeks.[76] The most common site of injury is just distal to the left subclavian artery,[76] followed by the innominate or left subclavian artery at the thoracic inlet. Aortic injuries are easily missed since about one third of patients have little or no external evidence of chest trauma. Definitive diagnostic tools include an arch aortogram or a contrast-enhanced CT scan. Surgical repair of the aortic injuries can be done with or without cardiopulmonary bypass, depending on the extent of the damage.

Abdominal Injuries

With penetrating injuries to the abdomen, the decision to perform surgery is usually clear soon after admission. In patients with blunt trauma, intraabdominal injuries can be difficult to diagnose, and clinical manifestations of serious injuries may be delayed for hours or days. The most common injuries are splenic rupture and laceration of the liver, which result in significant bleeding. Bowel injuries, with perforations from direct trauma or ischemia caused by mesenteric damage, can occur with blunt or penetrating injuries. When it is difficult to determine clinically or by abdominal radiographs whether intraperitoneal bleeding or contamination are present, diagnostic peritoneal lavage (DPL) is most useful.[8,82] In equivocal cases, a CT scan with contrast should help in the decision regarding laparotomy.[16]

Injuries to the urinary tract can be difficult to diagnose. Urethral injury should be suspected with blunt trauma to the pelvis or perineum, particularly if blood is seen at the urethral meatus or hematoma in the perineum. A Foley catheter should generally not be inserted until a definite diagnosis is obtained with a urethrogram.

Patients with urethral injuries should have a suprapubic cystostomy. Injuries higher up the urinary tract can be assessed with a cystogram and IV pyelogram if hematuria continues after bladder catheterization.

Injuries to the major vessels in the abdomen occur infrequently and are related primarily to gunshot and stab wounds.[17] They are diagnosed if one has a high index of suspicion regarding patients with penetrating injuries who have deteriorating vital signs; positive peritoneal lavage and laparotomy should be instituted. If the abdominal aorta is involved, mortality is reported to be 50%.[17]

Musculoskeletal Injuries

In the patient with acute trauma, one must evaluate the extent of the musculoskeletal injuries to assess the amount of hemorrhage, both apparent and occult. Visual inspection for asymmetry, palpation of distal pulses, feeling for skin distension or tightness, and location of pain is necessary when looking for fractures. In comatose patients, areas of abnormal range of motion or crepitation may be the only objective evidence of a fracture. Obvious fractures should be splinted early, and dislocations with neurovascular impairment should be reduced as soon as possible. One must remember that pain from fractures is occasionally referred to more distal portions of the extremity, and therefore radiographs must be obtained of all areas that might have a fracture.

ANESTHETIC MANAGEMENT
Preoperative Assessment and Preparation for Anesthesia
Preanesthetic diagnosis and management
Optimal resuscitation of the critically injured trauma patient depends on concurrent diagnosis and treatment. To accomplish this goal, the TA/CCS must work with the surgical team, following the protocols delineated by ATLS guidelines.

Step 1: initial assessment. The first step is to rapidly assess for cardiac arrest, the need for CPR, and the baseline neurologic status (using a combination of the Glasgow Coma Scale and quick evaluation of extremity motor strength). This is followed by intervention to secure the airway and provide artificial ventilation as indicated. Through all maneuvers and diagnostic procedures, the TA/CCS must pay particular attention to avoiding manipulations of the cervical spine until cervical spine injury can be ruled out.[98]

Step 2: history. As the second step, after or concurrently with ensuring appropriate initial intervention, the TA/CCS continues the preanesthetic diagnosis by obtaining details of patient and incident history from the patient, family members, primary care physician, prehospital personnel, and witnesses at the scene.

PATIENT DETAILS. The TA/CCS can care for a trauma patient better if the TA/CCS can obtain information about the patient's past medical history and condition at the scene. If the patient is comatose and other sources of information are not available, knowledge of the diseases and conditions typical of general populations corresponding to the patient's age and state of health will help the anesthesiologist prepare for possible complications.[70,80] Ideally the TA/CCS should gather the following information:

- Allergies or preexisting medical conditions and diseases such as cirrhosis of the liver, which is known to increase the mortality of trauma patients, or diabetes, which can complicate anesthesia because of the chronic use of insulin[70,80]
- Previous surgical procedures, which might indicate a potential for developing malignant hyperthermia,[18] a known contributor to trauma mortality
- Other untoward reactions to previous anesthetics and any history of drug or alcohol abuse or ingestion, which is often a "chronic" condition among trauma patients[61,94]

Much can be learned about the patient's injuries from information about the type and magnitude of the trauma involved (i.e., mechanism of injury).[25,38] Knowledge of the mechanism (in essence, the "etiology" of the "disease") involved can (1) assist in the diagnosis of the complete zone of injury and associated injuries, (2) help as a written prediction of the patient's physiologic response, (3) indicate intervention priorities, and (4) help avoid complications, such as an expanded pneumothorax or pneumocephalus secondary to the inappropriate use of nitrous oxide (N_2O). For example, a patient with a femoral fracture and maxillofacial trauma from an MVA may have a cribriform plate fracture and an occult pneumocephalus that could become a tension pneumocephalus with the use of N_2O.

Step 3: physical examination. The necessary physical examination and laboratory testing must follow the airway, breathing, circulation, and neurologic priorities as outlined by any life-support management protocol system (e.g., advanced cardiac life support, advanced burn life support, ATLS). Trauma patients frequently require simultaneous anesthesia, fluid resuscitation, and initiation of surgery.

AIRWAY AND BREATHING. The upper airway of the nonintubated patient should be examined to determine the potential for intubation difficulties and airway obstruction. The examination should include tongue size, tonsilar pillars, teeth, and presence of direct injuries.[66] The extensive techniques of airway management for the trauma patient were discussed earlier.[42]

CIRCULATION. The clinician should evaluate the circulatory system for hemorrhagic shock and blood loss and the chest for signs of pneumothorax, myocardial contusion, and pericardial tamponade. Hypotension mandates rapid replacement of the automatically assumed major fluid loss, unless spinal shock (no hemorrhagic loss) has been demonstrated.

NEUROLOGIC SYSTEMS. The brief neurologic examination includes assessment of the patient's level of consciousness, Glasgow Coma Scale score, pupil size and reactivity, and extremity motor function.

LABORATORY ANALYSES. Initial analyses include chest and cervical spine radiographs; hemoglobin and hematocrit measurements; determination of serum glucose, BUN, creatinine, electrolytes, and ABGs; and an ECG.

EVALUATION. Several rating systems exist besides the Trauma Score (TS) with which to evaluate a trauma patient. Some systems share certain characteristics and some are unique, but all are designed to quantify the extent of a trauma patient's injuries in terms of severity, risk of complications, and prognosis. All have advantages and disadvantages, strengths and weaknesses. The Physical Status designation of the American Society of Anesthesiologists can aid in predicting mortality from blunt trauma, but does not detect small differences in severely injured patients.[57,110] The TS and Injury Severity Score (ISS) use physiologic and anatomic bases to evaluate prospectively the seriousness of a patient's injuries. The TA/CCS uses the scores from these rating systems in conjunction with the patient's core body temperature on admission (which negatively correlates with ISS) to confirm his/her preoperative analysis of the patient's injury severity.

Step 4: treatment. In the immediate preoperative period the TA/CCS primarily focuses on management of the patient's respiratory, circulatory, and central nervous systems. The first concern may involve interventions that are lifesaving, life sustaining, or adjunctive therapy for shock and head injuries.[83] **If treatment for hemorrhagic shock (inadequate microcirculatory blood flow and suboptimal cellular O_2 delivery and utilization) is not begun within the first 60 minutes after surgery, the "golden hour," no subsequent intervention will avert the inevitable fatal result. Therefore treatment of hemorrhagic shock must begin on admission and continue throughout the**

perioperative period. It must be aggressive, must control traumatic hemorrhage, must deliver appropriate fluid replacement, and must ensure adequate perfusion of the brain with oxygenated blood. Such measures are performed while the cervical spine is protected against injury or possible aggravation of an existing injury.[101]

Monitoring

Concurrently with the patient's evaluation and resuscitation, the TA/CCS must consult with the surgeon about the type of surgical interventions (indicated by the patient's injuries and his/her overall condition). In this way appropriate preparations for monitoring and anesthetic/pharmacologic support during the procedures can be made, including precautions for any

---

Table 34-4 Basic monitoring

Parameter	Specific need
Personnel	Trained anesthesia provider continuously with patient
Oxygenation	Pulse oximeter O_2 analyzer on anesthesia machine or ventilator to monitor O_2 supply Mass spectrometer or similar device to monitor inspired and expired O_2 concentrations (optional)
Ventilation	Tidal volume and respiratory rate monitored by observation of breathing bag, respirometer, or ascultation of breath sounds Impedance pneumograph CO_2: inspired and expired gas monitored using capnograph with waveform display Airway pressure monitor to signify disconnection from mechanical ventilation
Circulation	Electrocardiograph: to monitor pulse rate and cardiac rhythm Arterial blood pressure (noninvasive): arm or leg cuff (oscillometric, Doppler, Korotkoff sounds) or digital (Finipress) Capillary perfusion: inspection of capillary refill or pulse oximeter
Temperature	Core temperature monitored by thermistor in esophagus, rectum, bladder, or tympanic membrane

From Stene JK, Grande CM, Bernhard WN et al: Overview of perioperative anesthetic management of the trauma patient: thoracoabdominal and orthopaedic injuries. In Stene JK, Grande CM, eds: *Trauma anesthesia*, Baltimore, 1991, Williams & Wilkins.

Table 34-5   Advanced monitoring

Parameter	Specific need
Depth of anesthesia	Mass spectrometer or anesthesia gas analyzer to monitor end-tidal anesthetic concentrations Blood concentrations of fixed drugs Electroencephalogram and sensory-evoked potentials
Oxygenation	Arterial blood gases (in combination with "oxygenation" equipment)
Circulation	Arterial catheter for continuous intraarterial pressure monitoring Central venous catheter for continuous right atrial/superior vena cava pressure monitoring Pulmonary artery catheter for monitoring central venous pressure, pulmonary artery pressure, and wedge/left atrial pressure Cardiac output: monitored by thermal dilution using a pulmonary artery catheter, by transthoracic electrical impedance, or by Doppler probe to detect pulsatile volume changes in aorta Indwelling urinary catheter (to monitor urinary output as function of adequate perfusion status) Transesophageal echocardiography
Ventilation	Mass spectrometer to monitor CO_2 waveform O_2 consumption, CO_2 production at the airway (indirect calorimeter)

From Stene JK, Grande CM, Bernhard WN et al: Overview of perioperative anesthetic management of the trauma patient: thoracoabdominal and orthopaedic injuries. In Stene JK, Grande CM, eds: *Trauma anesthesia*, Baltimore, 1991, Williams & Wilkins.

potential complications.[41] Part of the preparation involves ensuring that the patient has at least two large-bore IV catheters in place and selecting basic (Table 34-4) or advanced (Table 34-5) monitoring.

Basic noninvasive techniques

Noninstrumented monitoring. Although modern medical science has developed a sophisticated armamentarium of electronic and computerized monitoring devices, the basics of good monitoring practice must not be forgotten or ignored: the attentive presence of a well-trained anesthesiologist who incorporates the "gold standard" of look, listen, and feel with extensive physiologic, anatomic, and pharmacologic knowledge.[10,49] The basic techniques become

even more important when sophisticated resources are unavailable, such as at the site of a battlefield, a disaster, a primitive medical facility, or an accident (motor vehicle, industrial, nuclear).[10,29,40]

The "look, listen, and feel" technique involves the following steps: (1) observing the patient's eyes (for tearing, pupil size, pupil motion) and skin and nails (for color, capillary refill responses to pressure), (2) listening for irregular or absent breath sounds, and (3) feeling for the pulse (approximate systolic blood pressure), skin temperature and moisture, and muscle tone. For example, shock is associated with tachycardia, diaphoresis, weak and thready pulse, and tachypnea.

Instrumentation. Modern technology can enhance the anesthesiologist's evaluation and monitoring of a trauma patient. In particular, computers can be used to store data from monitors and to calculate ongoing parameters and ratios between those parameters as a guide to interventions.[97,102]

CARDIOVASCULAR SYSTEM. Monitoring can begin with basic auscultation of heart sounds with a precordial or esophageal stethoscope (see also following section on combination monitors).

Blood pressure (BP) can be monitored in a variety of ways. An inflatable sphygmomanometer around an extremity can indicate arterial BP, and needle oscillations of an aneroid pressure manometer during cuff deflation will measure systolic BP. Auscultating Korotkoff sounds distal to the cuff will provide more accurate measurements of systolic and diastolic BP. Other monitoring devices include electronic oscillometers and Doppler probes (that can also detect cardiac air emboli); these devices are accurate, create reproducible results, and reliably free the anesthesiologist for other tasks.[5,34]

Circulatory system function monitoring involves the ECG (at least a limb lead and a precordial lead), which can indicate ischemia in a patient with coronary artery disease and can generate an impedance pneumogram[3] (see later discussion), and the pulse oximeter to monitor heart rate and arterial oxyhemoglobin saturation.[5,88,119] The presence of a pulse or high O_2 saturation level on the pulse oximeter indicates adequate blood volume and perfusion; a low saturation level indicates ventilation or perfusion impairment.

RESPIRATORY SYSTEM. The basic techniques include monitoring rate and depth of respiration with a precordial or esophageal stethoscope and a respirometer; many of the latter digitally display respiratory frequency, tidal volume, and minute ventilation. Ventilators often have alarms to indicate low- or high-delivered volume levels.

Pulmonary gas exchange, as an indicator of ventilation and perfusion levels, can be analyzed by a capnometer (respiratory rate, CO_2 concentration),[44] mass spectrometer (inspiratory and expiratory gases, halogenated anesthetic agents), or colorimetric semiquantitative devices (breath-by-breath end-tidal CO_2).[37,103] Impedance pneumography indicates relative tidal changes in thoracic gas volume.[102]

COMBINATION MONITORS. Body temperatures, both skin and core, can indicate a variety of system "malfunctions" in the trauma patient. Thermistors are often connected to and used with other monitoring devices (esophageal stethoscope, Foley urinary catheter, pulmonary artery catheter) so that the TA/CCS has a range of temperature readings displayed on equipment monitors. Liquid crystal display patches applied to the forehead supply skin temperature readings; readings from thermistors in the rectum, bladder, esophagus, or tympanic membrane most closely approximate body core temperature.[52]

Cardiopulmonary function monitoring includes finger plethysmographs, transesophageal echocardiographs, impedance plethysmographs (changes in thoracic blood volume during cardiac cycle), transcutaneous O_2 and CO_2 sensor readings, and two-beamed, pulse-Doppler suprasternal probes (cardiac output).*

NEUROMUSCULAR SYSTEM. Percutaneous nerve stimulation should be as routine as temperature monitoring. Neuromuscular transmission and degree of muscle relaxant–induced neuromuscular receptor blockade can be assessed, monitoring the inversely proportional muscular activity produced by transcutaneous motor nerve stimulation.[1,89]

Minimally invasive techniques

The increased risk of morbidity (e.g., hematoma, undetected hemorrhage from intraarterial catheters) to a trauma patient from even minimally invasive monitoring techniques is usually outweighed by the risk of less adequate monitoring from noninvasive techniques. Because noninvasive alternatives can supply acceptable alternatives for "routine" monitoring (e.g., frequent BP readings), a medical indication must exist to use any invasive monitoring device. For example, extremely low BP associated with traumatic shock may not be accurately measured by indirect, noninvasive techniques.

Devices. Most lifesaving protocols mandate the insertion of an indwelling urinary catheter (Foley) to monitor urine output in a trauma patient.[24] Although it can increase the risk of a urinary infection by providing an entrance route for bacteria, that risk is outweighed by the benefits it provides: it decreases risk of urinary infection from nonvoiding and permits monitoring of organ perfusion and effectiveness of fluid resuscitation. Even the presence of blood at the

---

* References 6, 50, 73, 95, 111, 117.

meatus, an indication of possible direct trauma to the urethra and normally an absolute contraindication to catheter insertion, may be judged less of a risk than not using a urinary catheter for trauma patients with specific injuries.

Esophageal monitoring devices include a thermistor-containing stethoscope, esophageal ECG lead, Doppler probe to measure cardiac output,[111] ultrasound probe for echocardiography, and esophageal balloon to monitor distal esophageal muscle tone as an indicator of depth of anesthesia. The risks of invasive esophageal monitoring can be minimized by avoiding the use of these devices in patients with esophageal disease.

Neurologic monitoring devices in this category include the electroencephalogram (EEG).[4] Electrodes placed into the skin of the scalp[46] record visual-evoked, auditory-evoked, and somatosensory-evoked potentials[115] and thus monitor CNS function during neurosurgical anesthesia as well as that in patients with CNS trauma that cannot be managed surgically or with impaired cerebral perfusion. Changes in the recordings could indicate changes in blood flow to the spinal cord,[54] in ICP, or in brainstem CNS function.[46,120]

Laboratory analyses. Laboratory analyses (Box 34-2) form an important part of trauma patient monitoring and must begin with baseline readings on admission.

Respiratory analyses begin with ABGs (cardiorespiratory function). The initial sample, optimally taken while the patient spontaneously breathes room air, supplies a known fraction of inspired oxygen (FIO_2) for evaluating arterial oxygen tension (PaO_2) as an index of gas exchange; readings can thereafter be taken while the patient breathes O_2.

Invasive techniques

Because of the complications inherent in invasive monitoring, in the TA/CCS's clinical judgment a sufficient medical indication must exist to justify placing the already compromised patient at additional risk. The anesthesiologist must document the conditions prompting such monitoring and be prepared to defend his/her decision based on knowledge of the devices, the complications, the procedures, and the risk/benefit ratio.

Despite the drawbacks, there are some benefits. Aggressive hemodynamic monitoring has been shown to reduce mortality and reinfarction rate in surgical patients with a history of myocardial infarction;[79] a trauma patient with a similar history appears to derive equal benefit from similar hemodynamic monitoring. Hemodynamic monitoring can also indicate whether or not tissue oxygenation is adequate, based on continuous measurement of hemoglobin saturation of

---

BOX 34-2
LABORATORY ANALYSES

Pulmonary function

Frequent arterial blood gases
Occasional mixed venous blood gasses and
pulmonary shunt determination

Hematologic function

Hematocrit/hemoglobin concentration
White blood cell count
Platelet count
Prothrombin time
Partial thromboplastin time
Fibrinogen concentration
Blood type and cross-match

Chemistry laboratory

Serum electrolyte concentration (sodium, potas-
sium, chloride)
Carbon dioxide content (bicarbonate)
Blood urea nitrogen concentration (serum)
Creatinine concentration (serum and urinary)
Glucose concentration
Toxicology for prescribed/illicit agents (serum,
urine)
Ionized calcium concentration
Phosphorus concentration
Magnesium concentration
Sodium concentration (urine)
Osmolarity (serum, urine)

From Stene JK, Grande CM, Bernhard WN et al: Overview of
perioperative anesthetic management of the trauma patient:
thoracoabdominal and orthopaedic injuries. In Stene JK,
Grande CM, eds: *Trauma anesthesia*, Baltimore, 1991, Williams
& Wilkins.

---

mixed venous blood with O_2. This is a valuable tool for the trauma patient whose tissue oxygenation level has decreased from normal to low as sepsis develops.[91]

Pharmacology

The trauma patient with an isolated injury may benefit from the use of regional anesthesia, but general anesthesia is usually more appropriate for the severely injured patient[28,41,98] **for several reasons:**

- **General anesthesia provides for easier accommodation of or attention to hemodynamic and resuscitative changes.**[19,77,98,99]
- **It allows the TA/CCS to use a balanced combination of pharmacologic agents to provide the four components of anesthesia — sleep, amnesia, analgesia, and muscle relaxation — to optimize the patient's physiologic stability.**[19,23,45,72,99]

- **It facilitates "customizing" the choice of pharmacologic agents to fit the individual patient's condition and injuries, ensuring a safe procedure and avoiding the aggravation of any existing shock state.**[19,45,72,99]
- **It does not require an awake patient to endure the discomforts of long surgeries.**
- **It permits procedures on more than one site, a frequent necessity for the multiply traumatized patient.**

General anesthesia can be safely administered to a multiply injured patient by using the following:

- Agents that minimize cardiovascular depression and intracranial hypertension
- Small, titrated IV doses to achieve the desired anesthetic effect without hypotension (Reduced blood volume probably concentrates the delivered dose at the active site in the brain and reduces hepatic blood flow.)[51,114]
- A combination of drugs for a balanced anesthesia technique to promote ventilation/perfusion relationships that optimize gas exchange[2,32]
- Normal doses of muscle relaxants to facilitate emergency tracheal intubation through rapid paralysis

Because hypnosis or amnesia is secondary in importance to maintaining cardiovascular homeostasis and adequate cerebral perfusion in the trauma patient, the TA/CCS must be cognizant of drug effects and the conditions for which they would be contraindicated (Table 34-6). He/she should also ensure that all anesthesia machines can deliver O_2 in combination with air or other gases. Air/O_2 mixtures can decrease FIO_2, and heliox mixtures (up to 80% helium, 20% O_2) can reduce the viscosity of gas, enabling patients with extreme airway obstruction to generate spontaneous ventilation until surgical removal of the obstruction. Heliox is rarely required for the trauma patient, but air/O_2 mixtures are used routinely for this patient population because N_2O is frequently contraindicated.

State-of-the-art agents

To date, analyses of the effect of various anesthetic agents on the outcome of shock, both in experimental animal models[11,62,92,105,113] and in clinical trauma patient management,* have failed to identify one "best" anesthetic. However, effective lactate clearance forms a common ground for correlated interpretation.† Preservation of visceral blood flow to the liver and kidneys (to maintain lactate clearance) appears to be a very important factor in anesthetic interaction with circulatory shock.

---

* References 6, 22, 47, 53, 59, 61, 65.
† References 11, 62, 65, 105, 112, 113.

Table 34-6 Contraindications for specific drugs

Drug type	Contraindications
Hypnotics	Shock: a relative contraindication; all hypnotics should be carefully titrated to effect (sleep) to avoid aggravating hypotension Closed head injury: ketamine potently increases intracranial pressure
Inhalationals	Closed air space (pneumothorax, pneumocephalus, bowel distension): N_2O accumulates and places air space under tension Air embolism: N_2O (see above) Head injury: all agents increase cerebral blood volume and intracranial pressure; however, these effects can be counteracted by deliberate hyperventilation and administration of moderate concentrations Malignant hyperthermia: halothane, enflurane, and isoflurane can cause this Myocardial depression: N_2O aggravates this
Muscle relaxants	Shock: all histamine-releasing muscle relaxants (e.g., curare) aggravate shock Malignant hyperthermia: succinylcholine can cause this Burns: 48 hours after injury, succinylcholine exaggerates $[K^+]$ increase Spinal cord injury: 48 hours to 6 months after injury; succinylcholine exaggerates $[K^+]$ increases
Opioids	Shock: relative contraindication; use caution and titrate to effect to avoid aggravating hypotension

From Stene JK, Grande CM, Bernhard WN et al: Overview of perioperative anesthetic management of the trauma patient: thoracoabdominal and orthopaedic injuries. In Stene JK, Grande CM, eds: *Trauma anesthesia*, Baltimore, 1991, Williams & Wilkins.

Table 34-7 Usefulness of anesthetic agents for emergency and follow-up trauma surgery*

	Emergency		Follow-up
Agent	**ER**	**OR**	**OR**
Hypnotics			
Thiopental	4	4	4
Ketamine	3	3	2
Etomidate	2	1	3
Midazolam†	2/4	3	3
Propofol	1	1	4
Inhalation anesthetics			
Enflurane	0	2	3
Halothane	0	2	2
Isoflurane	0	4	4
Nitrous oxide	1	0	1
Muscle relaxants			
Pancuronium	2	2	2
Succinylcholine	2	2	3
Vecuronium	4	4	4
Atracurium	1	1	4
Opioids			
Alfentanil	1	2	4
Fentanyl	2	3	4
Morphine	1	1	2
Nalbuphine	3	2	2
Sufentanil	3	4	4

ER, Emergency room; *OR*, operating room.
*Drugs are graded on a scale of 0 to 4: *0*, not useful; *1*, minimally useful; *2*, somewhat useful; *3*, useful; *4*, very useful.
†Midazolam during emergency, unstable trauma is somewhat useful as a hypnotic induction agent; however, as an amnestic agent, at this point in management, it is very useful. During intraoperative management, midazolam becomes less useful, since the stablized trauma patient is now able to better tolerate introduction of a potent inhalant.
From Stene JK, Grande CM, Bernhard WN et al: Overview of perioperative anesthetic management of the trauma patient: thoracoabdominal and orthopaedic injuries. In Stene JK, Grande CM, eds: *Trauma anesthesia*, Baltimore, 1991, Williams & Wilkins.

beta-adrenergic (not alpha-adrenergic) stimulation.[55]

Studies have shown that trauma patients with preexisting cirrhosis of the liver have a higher mortality as a group because of poor hepatic perfusion and lactate clearance. As hemorrhagic shock decreases O_2 delivery to the muscles, they produce more lactic acid, which is transported to the liver and kidney for clearance by gluconeogenesis and conversion to pyruvate for fuel-energy metabolism.[48,58] This metabolic clearance of lactate requires adequate hepatic intracellular O_2, which, if impaired by anesthesia, will reduce lactate clearance. The decreased lactate clearance rate results in the development of lactic acidosis (greater than 5 mmol/L; arterial pH [pHa] less than 7.25), which exerts a negative inotropic effect on the heart already compromised by the shock state, leading

In the experimental studies, cyclopropane and fluroxene have been associated with high shock-induced mortality, increased catecholamine and lactate concentrations (lactic acidosis), and central lobular hepatic necrosis.[62] However, ketamine, another sympathomimetic anesthetic, is not associated with these results, perhaps because it enhances

to the irreversible heart failure seen in "terminal" shock.[12,58,101] Experimental studies have shown that anesthetics that reduce splanchnic blood flow to maintain systemic BP result in high mortality, a fact that validates the clinical observation that cirrhosis of the liver is the most fatal of all preexisting diseases or conditions for a trauma patient.[70] Therefore anesthetics used for any trauma patient should not impair visceral blood flow or hepatorenal lactate clearance. Table 34-7 lists useful pharmacologic agents for the trauma patient, both in the acute and in the "reoperative" (or follow-up) phases.

SUMMARY

We have discussed subjects germane to the preoperative anesthetic management (e.g., monitoring, pharmacology) of any surgical patient in the light of trauma care. In addition, we have examined issues we believe to be unique to the practice of trauma anesthesia. As opposed to conventional anesthesiology practice, these issues include a greater familiarity with topics such as history taking (e.g., patient details, studies of the cause-and-effect relationship of mechanisms and patterns of injury) and more intense involvement with initial physical assessment of and therapeutic interventions for the trauma patient at the earliest opportunity. This early involvement, which benefits both the patient and the anesthesiologist, may begin in the field, the emergency room, or (least desirably) in the operating room.

All trauma patients are not in the "urgent/emergent" category. A significant percentage of trauma patients are seen again in the operating suite either as inpatients or as ambulating patients returning to the trauma center for follow-up procedures. This proportion of "chronic" trauma patients is projected to increase as initial field and early intrahospital care continues to improve and to reduce mortality from trauma. Thus anesthesiologists' participation in the management of the patient's morbidity must inevitably increase as trauma assumes an increasingly large part of anesthesia practice.

KEY POINTS

- The anesthesiologist must be a part of the trauma team and participate in the emergency department trauma resuscitation and diagnosis.
- Airway management is frequently best achieved with oral intubation assisted with muscle relaxants.

- Anesthetic drugs are chosen to minimize circulatory compromise and maintain hepatic lactate clearance.
- Early aggressive therapy followed by less aggressive care when no longer needed is far better than continually responding to a patient's deterioration with increasingly aggressive care.

KEY REFERENCES

Baskett PJF: The trauma anesthesia/critical care specialist in the field, *Crit Care Clin* 6:13, 1990.

Bavister PH, Longnecker DE: Influence of anesthetic agents on the survival of rats following acute ischemia of the bowel, *Br J Anaesth* 51:921, 1979.

Border JR, Lewis FR, Aprahamian C et al: Prehospital trauma care: stabilize or scoop and run? *J Trauma* 23:708, 1983 (panel discussion).

Brown DL: Anesthetic agents in trauma surgery: are there differences? *Int Anesthesiol Clin* 25(1):75, 1987.

Gervin AS, Fischer RP: Resuscitation of trauma patient with type-specific uncrossmatched blood, *J Trauma* 24:327, 1984.

Grande CM: Mechanisms and patterns of injury: the key to anticipation in trauma management, *Crit Care Clin* 6:25, 1990.

Grande CM, Stene JK and Barton CR: The trauma anesthesiologist, *Md Med J* 37:531, 1988.

Halford FJ: A critique of intravenous anesthesia in war surgery, *Anesthesiology* 4:67, 1943.

Jowitt MD, Knight RJ: Anaesthesia during the Falklands campaign, *Anaesthesia* 38:776, 1983.

Longnecker DE, Sturggill BC: Influence of anesthetic agent on survival following hemorrhage, *Anesthesiology* 45:516, 1976.

McIntyre JWR: The difficult tracheal intubation, *Can J Anaesth* 34:204, 1987.

Morris JA, MacKenzie EJ, and Edelstein SL: The effect of pre-existing conditions on mortality in trauma patients, *JAMA* 263:1942, 1990.

Oreskovich MR et al: Geriatric trauma: injury patterns and outcome, *J Trauma* 24:565, 1984.

Peters RM: Fluid resuscitation and oxygen exchange

in hypovolemia. In Siegel JH, ed: *Trauma: emergency surgery and critical care,* New York, 1987, Churchill-Livingstone.

Sellick BA: Cricoid pressure to control regurgitation of stomach contents during induction of anaesthesia, *Lancet* 2:404, 1961.

Spoerel WE, Narayanan PS, and Singh NP: Transtracheal ventilation, *Br J Anaesth* 43:932, 1971.

Stene JK, Grande CM: Trauma anesthesia: past, present and future. In Stene JK, Grande CM, eds: *Trauma anesthesia,* Baltimore, 1991, Williams & Wilkins.

Trunkey DD: Trauma, *Sci Am* 249(2):28, 1983.

Wraight WJ, Chamney AR, and Howells TH: The determination of an effective cricoid pressure, *Anaesthesia* 38:461, 1983.

REFERENCES

1. Ali HH, Miller RD: Monitoring of neuromuscular function. In Miller RD, ed: *Anesthesia,* ed 2, New York, 1986, Churchill-Livingstone.
2. Anjow-Lindskog E, Broman L, Broman M et al: Effects of intravenous anesthesia on VA/Q distributions, *Anesthesiology* 62:485, 1985.
3. Anonymous: Apnea monitoring by impedance pneumography, *Health Devices* 16:80, 1987.
4. Anonymous: EEG monitors, *Health Devices* 15:71, 1986.
5. Anonymous: Pulse oximeter, *Health Devices* 18:185, 1989.
6. Anonymous: The question of intravenous anesthesia in war surgery, *Anesthesiology* 4:74, 1943.
7. Auerbach PS, Geehr EC: Inadequate oxygenation and ventilation using the esophageal gastric tube airway in the pre-hospital setting, *JAMA* 250:3067, 1983.
8. Bagwell CS, Ferguson WW: Blunt abdominal trauma: exploratory laparotomy or peritoneal lavage? *Am J Surg* 140:368, 1980.
9. Bartlett RL, Martin SD, Perina D et al: The pharyngotracheal lumen airway: an assessment of airway control in the setting of upper airway hemorrhage, *Ann Emerg Med* 16:145, 1987.
10. Baskett PJF: The trauma anesthesia/critical care specialist in the field, *Crit Care Clin* 6:13, 1990.
11. Bavister PH, Longnecker DE: Influence of anesthetic agents on the survival of rats following acute ischemia of the bowel, *Br J Anaesth* 51:921, 1979.
12. Bersin RM, Arieff AI: Recent advances in therapy of lactic acidosis, *Intensive Care World* 4:128, 1987.
13. Blair E, Topuzlu C, and Deane RS: Major blunt chest trauma, *Curr Probl Surg* 2:64, 1969.
14. Border JR, Lewis FR, Aprahamian C et al: Pre-hospital trauma care: stabilize or scoop and run? *J Trauma* 23:708, 1983 (panel discussion).
15. Boyd DR, Cowley RA: Comprehensive regional trauma/emergency medical services (EMS) delivery systems: the United States experience, *World J Surg* 7:149, 1983.
16. Bressler MJ: Computed tomography of the abdomen, *Ann Emerg Med* 15:280, 1986.
17. Brinton M et al: Acute abdominal aortic injuries, *J Trauma* 22:660, 1986.
18. Britt BA: Malignant hyperthermia, *Can Anaesth Soc J* 32:666, 1985.
19. Brown DL: Anesthetic agents in trauma surgery: are there differences? *Int Anesthesiol Clin* 25(1):75, 1987.
20. Champion HR, Sacco WJ, Carnazzo AJ et al: Trauma Score, *Crit Care Med* 9:672, 1981.
21. Changaris DG, McGraw CP, and Richardson JD: Correlation of cerebral perfusion pressure on mortality and long-term recovery, *J Trauma* 26:670, 1986.
22. Chasapakis G, Kekis N, Sakkalis C et al: Use of ketamine and pancuronium in patients with hemorrhagic shock, *Anesth Analg* 52:282, 1973.
23. Clarke RSJ, Carson IW: Anaesthesia for trauma and shock. In Nunn JF, Utting JE, and Brown BR, eds: *General anaesthesia,* ed 5, London, 1989, Butterworth.
24. Committee on Trauma: *The Advanced Trauma Life Support Program: instructor's manual,* Chicago, 1989, American College of Surgeons.
25. Committee on Trauma Research: *Injury in America: a continuing public health problem,* Washington DC, 1985, National Academy Press.
26. Copass MK, Oreskovich MR, Bladergroen MR et al: Pre-hospital cardiopulmonary resuscitation of the critically-injured patient, *Am J Surg* 148:20, 1984.
27. Demuth WE, Baue AE, and Odum JA: Contusions of the heart, *J Trauma* 7:443, 1967.
28. Desai SM, Bernhard WN, and McAlary B: Regional anesthesia: management considerations in the trauma patient, *Crit Care Clin* 6:85, 1990.
29. Donchin Y, Wiener M, Grande CM et al: Military medicine: trauma anesthesia and critical care on the battlefield, *Crit Care Clin* 6:185, 1990.
30. Donegan JH: Cardiopulmonary resuscitation. In Miller RD, ed: *Anesthesia,* ed 2, New York, 1986, Churchill-Livingstone.
31. Donen N, Tweed WA, Dashfsky S et al: The esophageal obsturator airway: an appraisal, *Can Anaesth Soc J* 30:194, 1983.
32. Eger EI II: *Anesthesia uptake and action,* Baltimore, 1974, Williams & Wilkins.
33. Falk JL, Rackow ER, and Weil MH: Colloid and crystalloid fluid resuscitation. In Shoemaker WC, Ayres S, Grenvik A et al, eds. *Textbook of critical care,* Philadelphia, 1989, WB Saunders.
34. Finnie KJC, Watts DG, and Armstrong PW: Biases in the measurement of arterial pressure, *Crit Care Med* 12:965, 1984.
35. Gallagher JD, Moore RA, Kerns D et al: Effects of colloid or crystalloid administration on pulmonary extravascular water in the postoperative period after coronary artery bypass grafting, *Anesth Analg* 64:753, 1985.
36. Gervin AS, Fischer RP: Resuscitation of trauma patient with type-specific uncrossmatched blood, *J Trauma* 24:327, 1984.
37. Goldberg JS, Rawle PR, Zehnder JL et al: Colorimetric end-tidal carbon dioxide monitoring for tracheal intubation, *Anesth Analg* 70:191, 1990.
38. Grande CM: Mechanisms and patterns of injury: the key to anticipation in trauma management, *Crit Care Clin* 6:25, 1990.
39. Grande CM, Barton CR, and Stene JK: Appropriate techniques for airway management of emergency patients with suspected spinal cord injury, *Anesth Analg* 67:714, 1988.
40. Grande CM, Baskett PJF, Donchin Y et al: Trauma anesthesia for disasters: anything, anytime, anywhere, *Crit Care Clin* 7(1), 1991.
41. Grande CM, Stene JK and Barton CR: The trauma anesthesiologist, *Md Med J* 37:531, 1988.
42. Grande CM, Stene JK, and Bernhard WN: Airway management: considerations in the trauma patient, *Crit Care Clin* 6:37, 1990.
43. Grande CM, Stene JK, Bernhard WN: Trauma anesthesia and critical care: the concept and rationale for a new subspecialty, *Crit Care Clin* 6:1, 1990.
44. Gravenstein JS, Paulus DA, and Hayes TS: *Capnography in clinical practice,* Boston, 1989, Butterworth.

45. Graves CL: Management of general anesthesia during hemorrhage, *Int Anesthesiol Clin* 12(1):1, 1974.

46. Grundy BL: Intraoperative monitoring of sensory evoked potentials, *Anesthesiology* 58:72, 1983.

47. Halford FJ: A critique of intravenous anesthesia in war surgery, *Anesthesiology* 4:67, 1943.

48. Haljamae H: Lactate metabolism, *Intensive Care World* 4:1181, 1987.

49. House of Delegates: *Standards for basic intra-operative monitoring*, Chicago, 1990, American Society of Anesthesiologist Directory of Members.

50. Huch R, Lubbers DW, and Huch LA: The transcutaneous measurement of oxygen and carbon dioxide tensions for the determination of arterial blood-gas values with control of local perfusion and peripheral perfusion pressure. In Payne JP, Hill DW, eds: *Oxygen measurement in biology and medicine*, London, 1975, Butterworth.

51. Hug CC Jr: Pharmacokinetics of drugs administered intravenously, *Anesth Analg* 57:704, 1978.

52. Imrie MM, Hall GM: Body temperature and anaesthesia, *Br J Anaesth* 64:346, 1990.

53. Jowitt MD, Knight RJ: Anaesthesia during the Falklands campaign, *Anaesthesia* 38:776, 1983.

54. Judson J, Cant BR, and Shaw NA: Early prediction of outcome from cerebral trauma by somatosensory-evoked potentials, *Crit Care Med* 18:363, 1990.

55. Kaukinen S: Effects of antihypertensive medication on the cardiovascular response to ketamine in rats, *Acta Anesthesiol Scand* 22:437, 1978.

56. Klauber MR, Marshall LF, Toole BM et al: Cause of decline in head injury mortality rate in San Diego County, California, *J Neurosurg* 62:528, 1985.

57. Koch JP, McClelland BA, Wortzman D et al: Is the ASA physical status clarification adequate in predicting mortality in blunt trauma? *Anesthesiology* 67: A482, 1987.

58. Kruse JA: Blood lactate and oxygen transport, *Intensive Care World* 4:120, 1987.

59. Kuznetsova OIU, Marusanov VE, Biderman FM et al: Anesteziia ketalarom na dogospital nom etape u postradaushikh/s/tiazheloi travmoi c raumaticheskim shokom (Ketalar anesthesia in the first-aid stage with the victims of severe injury and traumatic shock), *Vestnik Khirurgii Imenirt I Grekova* 132(7):88, 1984.

60. Lauer AR: Age and sex in relation to accidents, *Traffic Safety Res Rev* 3:21, 1959.

61. Lenz G, Stehle R: Anesthesia under field conditions: a review of 945 cases, *Acta Anaesthesiol Scand* 28:351, 1984.

62. Longnecker DE, Sturggill BC: Influence of anesthetic agent on survival following hemorrhage, *Anesthesiology* 45:516, 1976.

63. Maki DG, Cobb L, Garman JK et al: An attachable silver impregnated cuff for prevention of infection with central venous catheters: a prospective randomized multicenter trial, *Am J Med* 85:307, 1988.

64. Marzuk PM, Tardiff K, Leon AC et al: Prevalence of recent cocaine use among motor vehicle fatalities in New York City, *JAMA* 263:250, 1990.

65. McGown RGL: A technique of anaesthesia in haemorrhagic shock, *Anaesthesia* 30:616, 1975.

66. McIntyre JWR: The difficult tracheal intubation, *Can J Anaesth* 34:204, 1987.

67. McSwain NE: Mechanisms of injuries in blunt trauma. In McSwain NE, Kertein MD, eds: *Evaluation and management of trauma*, Norwalk, Conn, 1987, Appleton-Century-Crofts.

68. Millihan JS, Cain TL, and Hansbrough J: Rapid volume replacement for hypovolemic shock: a comparison of techniques and equipment, *J Trauma* 26:428, 1984.

69. Moore EE: Resuscitation and evaluation of the injured patient. In Zuidema GD, Rutherford RB, and Ballinger WF, eds: *The management of trauma*, ed 4, Philadelphia, 1985, WB Saunders.

70. Morris JA, MacKenzie EJ, and Edelstein SL: The effect of pre-existing conditions on mortality in trauma patients, *JAMA* 263:1942, 1990.

71. Munoz E: Economic cost of trauma, United States, 1982, *J Trauma* 24:237, 1986.

72. Nicholls BJ, Cullen BF: Anesthesia for trauma, *J Clin Anesth* 1:115, 1988.

73. Niclou R, Teague SM, and Lee R: Clinical evaluation of a diameter sensing Doppler cardiac output meter, *Crit Care Med* 18:428, 1990.

74. Niemann JJ, Rosborough JP, Myers R et al: The pharyngeotracheal lumen airway: preliminary investigation of a new adjunct, *Ann Emerg Med* 13:591, 1984.

75. Oreskovich MR et al: Geriatric trauma: injury patterns and outcome, *J Trauma* 24:565, 1984.

76. Parmley LF, Manion WC, and Mattingly TW: Non-penetrating traumatic injury to the heart, *Circulation* 18:371, 1958.

77. Peters RM: Fluid resuscitation and oxygen exchange in hypovolemia. In Siegel JH, ed: *Trauma: emergency surgery and critical care*, New York, 1987, Churchill-Livingstone.

78. Rachow EC, Falk JL, Fein IA et al: Fluid resuscitation in circulatory shock: a comparison of the cardiorespiratory effects of albumin, hetastarch, and saline solutions in patients with hypovolemic and septic shock, *Crit Care Med* 11:839, 1983.

79. Rao TLK, Jacobs JK, and El-Etr AA: Reinfarction following anesthesia in patients with myocardial infarction, *Anesthesiology* 59:449, 1983.

80. Rembert FC: State of health at time of injury. In Giesecke AH, ed: *Anesthesia for the surgery of trauma*, Philadelphia, 1976, FA Davis.

81. Rodman GH, Kirby RR: Post-traumatic respiratory failure: role of fluid therapy. In Brown BR, ed: *Contemporary anesthetic practice: fluid and blood therapy*, Philadelphia, 1983, FA Davis.

82. Root HD, Hauser CW, McKinley CK et al: Diagnostic peritoneal lavage, *Surgery* 57:633, 1965.

83. Safar P, Bircher NG: *Cardiopulmonary cerebral resuscitation*, ed 3, London, 1988, WB Saunders.

84. Sanders RD: Two ventilating attachments for bronchoscopes, *Del Med J* 39:170, 1967.

85. Schofferman J, Oill P, and Lewis AJ: The esophageal obturator airway: a clinical evaluation, *Chest* 69:67, 1976.

86. Seelig JM, Becker DP, Miller JD et al: Traumatic acute subdural hematoma, *N Engl J Med* 304:1511, 1981.

87. Sellick BA: Cricoid pressure to control regurgitation of stomach contents during induction of anaesthesia, *Lancet* 2:404, 1961.

88. Severinghaus JW, Naifeh KH: Accuracy of response of six pulse oximeters to profound hypoxia, *Anesthesiology* 67:551, 1987.

89. Sharpe MD, Lam AM, Nicholas JF et al: Correlation between integrated evoked EMG and respiratory function following atracurium administration in unanesthetized humans, *Can J Anaesth* 37:307, 1990.

90. Shires T: Initial care of the injured patient, *J Trauma* 10:940, 1970.

91. Siegel JH, Vary TC: Sepsis, abnormal metabolic control, and the multiple organ syndrome. In Siegel JH, ed: *Trauma: emergency surgery and critical care*, New York, 1987, Churchill-Livingstone.

92. Smith DP, Fabian LW, and Carnes MA: Comparative evaluation of fluothane and cyclopropane anesthesia during hemorrhage hypovolcmia: changing concepts in the management of anesthesia, *Anesth Analg* 40:137, 1961.

93. Smith RB, Shaer WB, and Pfaeffle H: Percutaneous transtracheal ventilation for anesthesia and resuscitation: a review and report of complications, *Can Anaesth Soc J* 22:607, 1975.

94. Soderstrom CA, DuPriest RW Jr, Benner C et al: Alcohol and roadway trauma: problems of diagnosis and management, *Am Surg* 45:129, 1979.

95. Spinale FG, Smith AC, and Crawford FA: Relationship of bioimpedence to thermodilution and echocardiographic measurements of cardiac function, *Crit Care Med* 18:414, 1990.

96. Spoerel WE, Narayanan PS, and Singh NP: Transtracheal ventilation, *Br J Anaesth* 43:932, 1971.

97. Sramek BB: The impact on diagnosis and therapy of computerized integration, processing and display of noninvasive hemodynamic and cardiodynamic parameters, *Intensive Care World* 6:205, 1989.

98. Stene JK: Anesthesia for the critically ill trauma patient. In Siegel JH, ed: *Trauma: emergency surgery and critical care*, New York, 1987, Churchill-Livingstone.

99. Stene JK, Grande CM: General anesthesia: management considerations

in the trauma patient, *Crit Care Clin* 6:73, 1990.

100. Stene JK, Grande CM: Trauma anesthesia: past, present and future. In Stene JK, Grande CM, eds: *Trauma anesthesia,* Baltimore, 1991, Williams & Wilkins.

101. Stene JK, Grande CM, and Giesecke AH: Resuscitation of traumatic shock. In Stene JK, Grande CM, eds: *Trauma anesthesia,* Baltimore, 1991, Williams & Wilkins.

102. Stene JK, Long JF: Hemodynamic monitoring with use of a bedside computer terminal, *CVP* 10(1):66, 1982.

103. Sum-Ping ST, Mehta MP, and Anderton JM: A comparative study of methods of detection of esophageal intubation, *Anesth Analg* 69:627, 1989.

104. Tenzer ML: The spectrum of myocardial contusion: a review, *J Trauma* 25:620, 1985.

105. Theye RA, Perry LB, and Brzica SM Jr: Influence of anesthetic agent on response to hemorrhagic hypotension, *Anesthesiology* 40:32, 1974.

106. Trunkey DD: Force in blunt trauma. In Trunkey DD, Lewis FR: *Current therapy of trauma,* ed 2, Toronto, 1986, BC Becker.

107. Trunkey DD: The nature of things that go bang in the night, *Surgery* 92:123, 1982.

108. Trunkey DD: Shock trauma, *Can J Surg* 27:479, 1984.

109. Trunkey DD: Trauma, *Sci Am* 249(2):28, 1983.

110. Trunkey DD, Siegel J, Baker SP et al: Panel: current status of trauma severity, *J Trauma* 23:185, 1983.

111. Urbanowicz JH, Shaaban MJ, Cohen NH et al: Comparison of transesophageal echocardiographic and scintigraphic estimates of left ventricular end-diastolic volume index and ejection fraction in patients following coronary artery bypass grafting, *Anesthesiology* 72:607, 1990.

112. Weiskopf RB, Bogetz MS, Roizen MF et al: Cardiovascular effects of the volatile anesthetics during hypovolemia, *Anesthesiology* 61:A51, 1984.

113. Weiskopf RB, Townsley MI, Riordan KK et al: Comparison of cardiopulmonary responses to graded hemorrhage during enflurane, halothane, isoflurane, and ketamine anesthesia, *Anesth Analg* 60:481, 1981.

114. Wilkinson GR: Pharmacokinetics in disease states modifying body perfusion. In Benet LZ, ed: *The effects of disease states on drug pharmacokinetics,* Washington DC, 1976, American Pharmaceutical Association.

115. Wilson JM, Thomas AN, Goodman PC et al: Severe chest trauma: morbidity implication of first and second rib fracture in 120 patients, *Arch Surg* 113:846, 1978.

116. Wiot JF: The radiologic manifestations of blunt chest trauma, *JAMA* 231:500, 1975.

117. Wong DH, Mahutte CK: Two-beam pulsed Doppler cardiac output measurement: reproducibility and agreement with thermodilution, *Crit Care Med* 18:433, 1990.

118. Wraight WJ, Chamney AR, and Howells TH: The determination of an effective cricoid pressure, *Anaesthesia* 38:461, 1983.

119. Yelderman M, New NJ: Evaluation of pulse oximetry, *Anesthesiology* 59:349, 1983.

120. York D, Legan M, Benner S et al: Further studies with a noninvasive method of intracranial pressure estimation, *Neurosurgery* 14:456, 1984.

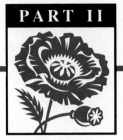

PART II

ANESTHETIC CARE

CHAPTER 35

Anesthesia Risk

ALAN F. ROSS
JOHN H. TINKER

What are the risks of anesthesia? Patients frequently ask this question and anesthesiologists provide examples to answer it. Minor risks may include nausea or vomiting, sore throat, chipped teeth, etc., whereas major risks might involve perioperative myocardial infarction. The patient is reassured that major risks, such as myocardial infarction, are only a problem in patients with known heart disease, and, in fact, much research and progress has been accomplished in that area. Yet the true thrust of the question remains unanswered. Consider these remarks by Thomas Dry in 1952:

Through the years patients having heart disease who have had to undergo operation have been the cause of considerable apprehension. This is understandable since patients with normal hearts have died unexpectedly on the table during procedures as minor as tonsillectomy.[58]

The fearfulness of this subject often allows both anesthesiologist and patient to be satisfied with more superficial explanations of risk. For example, an extensive survey of patients' concerns regarding anesthesia omitted direct questions about death to avoid undue patient anxiety.[185] **It is easier to accept that one is just "going to sleep," rather than consider that the anesthetized state, which allows surgical trespass into the deepest recesses of the body, is achieved only by pharmacologically overwhelming the human body's most tenacious defenses.**

Our specialty has clearly had difficulty facing this issue. Studies of anesthesia risk have existed for more than 30 years, yet only recently has the subject received major attention.[13,16-18,71,72,200] Early investigators, such as Ruth,[175] MacIntosh,[135] and Edwards et al.,[68] recommended formal anesthesia study commissions to openly and frankly discuss cases of adverse outcomes, but this was before the massive increase in medical malpractice lawsuits.[21] The recent British confidential inquiry into perioperative deaths required evocation of "crown privilege" to prevent individual legal representatives from using the data.[12] Another problem has been an assumption that some increase in mortality is inevitable as physicians more aggressively contest disease. Ament noted in 1960: "It is obvious that by rarely refusing any patient the benefits of surgery, we may expose ourselves to a higher mortality rate."[2]

Cases of anesthetic death are rare, amid millions of successful and uncomplicated administrations. This has contributed to the mistaken assumption by clinicians that "it can't happen to me." After collection and analysis of these rare events, it is clear that

anesthetic death may occur at any time despite years of safe practice.[20, 221]

The resurgence in concern for anesthetic risk is encouraging. **The American Society of Anesthesiologists (ASA) has become a leader in establishment of medical practice standards. The Anesthesia Patient** Safety Foundation has provided risk reduction educational programs. Quality assurance programs have been mandated by the Joint Commission on Accreditation of Hospitals Organizations (JCAHO) to monitor outcomes, attempt to analyze problems, and address solutions.

Despite these developments, the task confronted is major.[75] In the United States alone approximately 24 million operations are performed annually.[211] If the risk of death due to anesthesia is estimated at 1/10,000,[134] then there may be 2400 deaths each year primarily related to anesthesia. In addition, major anesthesia-related morbidity causes great suffering and drains health care dollars for long-term supportive care. Unlike numerous modifiable health risks, such as cigarette smoking and obesity, patients cannot voluntarily reduce their personal risk from anesthesia. The responsibility of anesthesia risk reduction rests squarely on the shoulders of those who practice our specialty. The challenges ahead include the necessity to follow thousands of cases to collect even a handful of events for analysis. Litigation is likely to jeopardize release of available information. Technology and equipment to reduce risk may need to be applied to thousands of patients to save even one life, and, even then, the events are rarely crystal clear. Perspective is provided by the comments of Beecher and Todd from their 1954 landmark study of anesthetic mortality:

Data are presented to show that death from anesthesia is of sufficient magnitude to constitute a public health problem. Anesthesia kills several times as many citizens each year out of the total population of the country as does poliomyelitis [even in 1954]. Consideration of the millions of dollars rightly spent in attacking poliomyelitis and the next to nothing, comparatively, spent in anesthesia research makes clear an urgent need.[9]

Today, polio has been silenced. The call for anesthesia risk reduction has only recently been sounded.[75,115-117,119,122]

PROBLEMS IN THE STUDY OF ANESTHESIA RISK

A major difficulty in the study of anesthesia risk is to separate anesthetic factors from those related to surgery or patient disease. In a 1988 study, Cohen, Duncan, and Tate concluded after studying 100,000 anesthetics that surgical risk factors and patient diseases were much more important predictors of 7-day mortality than were anesthesia factors.[28] This is not surprising. The overall mortality rate was 71.4/10,000 anesthetics, yet primary anesthesia mortality is elsewhere estimated to be less than 1/10,000. Their study asks the question: "Does anesthesia contribute to operative mortality?" Although the answer must be "yes" to some extent, the influences of surgery and patient disease prevent accurate assessment of the anesthesia contribution. An example of such confounding influences is the large number of studies that have failed to demonstrate that any particular anesthetic technique for coronary artery bypass surgery results in fewer postoperative myocardial infarctions.[138,166,188,194,207]

In 1956, Edwards et al. attempted to distinguish among the various factors involved in mortality by using peer review committees.[68] As might be expected, even the experts disagreed and the cause of death[68] — anesthetic, surgical, or patient disease — was often decided by vote. In 1983, Lunn, Hunter, and Scott attempted to assess the role of anesthesia in mortality in the United Kingdom.[133] Importantly, questionnaires were sent to both the anesthetists and the surgeon. Not surprisingly, the assessments differed significantly. Recent attempts to separate various causes of adverse outcome have used multivariate statistical analysis, which can help unravel these components.

A major goal of anesthesia risk studies is to identify common patterns that occur in cases of adverse outcome.[47] However, if mortality due to anesthesia occurs at a rate of less than 1/10,000, then the population studied must be enormous.[12] Several strategies have been used. Retrospective analysis allows access to sufficiently large data bases, but must rely on potentially incomplete past records, which reflect changing practice standards over time. Keenan and Boyan used this method to identify factors associated in anesthesia-related intraoperative cardiac arrest.[120] Another retrospective strategy is to study cases of adverse outcome that have been the subject of lawsuits that either resulted in settlements or judgments. Such studies are called "closed claims" studies. Caplan et al. used this approach to identify a potential problem with unexpected arrest during spinal anesthesia and to gain original insight into possible mechanisms.[17] Utting (1979) analyzed cases from the British Medical Defense Union to determine anesthetic contributory factors.[213] These methods have generated useful information, although not every case of adverse anesthetic outcome is subjected to legal action. Caplan et al.[16] used closed claims data to analyze cases of respiratory adverse outcomes and postoperative peripheral nerve dysfunction. Keats editorialized that the most useful function of closed claims is in recognition of patterns that contribute to adverse outcomes.[118]

A prospective approach to study of anesthetic risk

must take place over many years and/or involve multiple institutions. The Confidential Enquiry into Perioperative Death (CEPOD) in 1987, headed by JN Lunn of Britain, accessed nearly half a million cases over a 1-year period, but required participation of three large regions of the United Kingdom.[12] **Problems encountered in such a massive study included incomplete participation by all physicians and regional variations in reporting. In fact, the authors reported that "pockets of resistance to CEPOD" occurred in each region. Some hospitals returned a majority of the questionnaires, whereas elsewhere fewer than 20% were completed.[13]**

A different strategy was used by Cooper et al. in 1978 to cope with the logistic problems of risk study.[35] Rather than study outcome events, Cooper et al. assessed "critical incidents,"[77] defined as occurrences that led or could have led to an undesirable outcome.[32-35] This definition led to inclusion of events that had no or only transient effects on the patients. This study generated useful information regarding factors that contributed to "critical incidents," but did not further define actual risks of permanent negative outcome. It is a landmark focus on the *process* by which we conduct our business.

EARLY STUDIES: BEFORE 1980

Before the founding of the American Medical Association in 1846, ether had been used clinically by Crawford W. Long and demonstrated publicly by Morton. In 1848, shortly after the introduction of chloroform, the first recognized anesthetic death, namely that of Hannah Greener, was reported.[190] In the months and years that followed other deaths occurred. Expert commissions, researchers, and clinicians professed widely divergent views as to causes. Laboratory scientists provided evidence that chloroform overdosage caused death in animals as a result of respiratory depression before cardiac failure. Clinicians held that cardiac toxicity was the primary mechanism. Still others assessed that the resuscitation attempts; e.g., forced sips of brandy, rather than the chloroform, caused asphyxiation. **John Snow (1858) carefully analyzed 50 clinical cases of death during chloroform anesthesia. His clinical observations provided the first formal investigation of anesthetic mortality.[190]** In contrast to early deaths that occurred in relatively healthy patients during minor surgeries, subsequent cases often involved patients with significant preoperative diseases during more extensive surgery. How to distinguish anesthetic variables from other factors contributing to operative mortality was then and still remains a major challenge. Contributions of early studies included development of study methods plus estimation of overall risk incidence (Table 35-1).

In 1944, Gillespie emphasized the importance of precise definitions of anesthetic mortality and stressed the need of record keeping.[86] By this time, the ability to provide support for respiration was a recognized skill of the anesthesiologist. In contrast, he stated "when circulation fails, little can be done." In the seven case descriptions provided, evidence for airway difficulty, overdose, and lack of monitoring was present. The practice of telephoning a blood donor *after* major hemorrhage from a vascular tumor has occurred would today be considered inadequate preparation.

In Philadelphia in 1935, Ruth helped establish the first anesthesia study commission to analyze deaths

Table 35-1   Estimates of the incidence of mortality related to anesthesia before 1980

Investigator(s)	Year	Number of anesthetics	Primary cause	Primary and associated cause
Beecher & Todd[9]	1954	599,548	1 : 2680	1 : 1560
Dornette & Orth[54]	1956	63,105	1 : 2427	1 : 1343
Schapira, Keyes, and Hurwitt[179]	1960	22,177	1 : 1232	1 : 821
Phillips et al.[163]	1960	–	1 : 7692	1 : 2500
Dripps, Lamont, and Eckenhoff[57]	1961	33,224	1 : 852	1 : 415
Clifton and Hotton[22]	1963	205,640	1 : 6048	1 : 3955
Memery[146]	1965	114,866	1 : 3145	1 : 1082
Gebbie[83]	1966	129,336	–	1 : 6158
Minuck[148]	1967	121,786	1 : 6766	1 : 3291
Harrison[100]	1968	177,928	–	1 : 3068
Marx, Matteo, and Orkin[144]	1973	34,145	–	1 : 1265
Bodlander[11]	1975	211,130	1 : 14,075	1 : 1703
Harrison[101]	1978	240,483	–	1 : 4537
Hovi-Viander[108]	1980	338,934	1 : 5059	1 : 1412

From Ross AF, Tinker JH: Anesthesia risk. In Miller RD, ed: *Anesthesia.* ed 3, New York, 1990, Churchill-Livingstone.

related to anesthesia.[175] The voluntary submission of cases was deemed inadequate because many fatalities were not reported. Years later the commission's practice of determining cause of death by majority vote would also be deemed inadequate. Still, Ruth's report in the 1945 study revealed the state of anesthesia practice in the early years.

... when anesthetic difficulties are encountered, intracardiac injections of epinephrine, often in overdose, are too popular and the simple, indicated corrective measures ignored.... the more dramatic needles, analeptics, and stimulants too often have a wider application than the indicated patent airway and simple, quiet inflations of the lungs with pure oxygen.[175]

In 1948, Sir Robert MacIntosh voiced his strong opinion that many anesthetic-related deaths were preventable and that improved education was the best means to avoid unnecessary mortality.[135] **His report discouraged the widespread practice of attributing anesthetic deaths to meaningless conditions, such as "status thymicolymphaticus" and thereby condemning others to repeat the actual mistakes. Instead, MacIntosh emphasized that understanding real mechanisms, such as airway obstruction, intravenous injections of local anesthetic, and overdoses of drugs such as pentothal, could lead to improvement in practice.** A particular statement is noteworthy:

The anesthetist's skill lies in getting good results with safe doses. The inexperienced man whose technique is at fault relies on massive doses and even tends to increase these until confronted with an emergency.[135]

Even today a report stating that "the patient required flush dopamine to maintain blood pressure" signals that MacIntosh's insight is still applicable.

In 1951, Ehrenhaft, Eastwood, and Morris reported the benefits of artificial circulatory support for intraoperative cardiac arrest.[70] Before 1948, therapy had consisted of intravenous or intracardiac medications and artificial ventilation, yet none of the 11 patients survived. After 1948, direct (open) manual cardiac compression was instituted with 25% survival. The authors emphasized the importance of a patent airway and advocated use of intravenous procaine to reduce cardiac irritability plus electric shock to reverse ventricular fibrillation. West in 1954 also added to the early knowledge of intraoperative cardiac arrest.[220]

Beecher and Todd in 1954 published a landmark study of anesthetic death in 10 institutions.[9] They analyzed a variety of factors including technique (e.g., spinal vs. general), agent, patient age, anesthetist, and equipment used for 599,548 anesthetics. Anesthesia was deemed the primary factor contributing to mortality in 1/2680 anesthetics. The study was best

known for its condemnation of "curare drugs" that were associated with markedly increased mortality rates. Bias against "curare drugs" may have prevented appreciation that supported ventilation was essential with these agents. Instead, curare agents were deemed "inherently toxic" drugs that caused circulatory failure even when artificial respiration of "a generally effective type" was used.

An important development was that of Jude, Kouwenhoven, and Knickerbocker in 1961.[111] They reported the successful application of closed chest external cardiac massage (Table 35-2). Particularly interesting was the report that cardiac function was restored in all 31 patients who experienced cardiac arrest while in the operating room or recovery room. This group included seven arrests during induction of anesthesia and 15 during surgery. In contrast, a group of 24 patients with acute myocardial infarction had only a 42% success rate in restoring cardiac function. Factors contributing to the good results in the surgical population probably included younger age, more rapid institution of resuscitation, and absence of severe coronary disease. Ventricular fibrillation was present more often in acute myocardial infarctions, whereas asystole was seen in most operative arrests. It is likely that some of the intraoperative arrests in their study represented vagal bradycardia with hypotension, which may account for the high success with closed chest massage. Nonetheless, it is also likely that these events could have resulted in adverse outcomes had resuscitation not been attempted.

A major contribution in 1956 was that of Edwards et al. who developed a classification scheme by which cases of operative mortality caused by anesthesia could be separated from factors such as surgery and patient disease.[68] The system included categories for cases in which the cause of death could not be ascertained. Prior studies, notably that of Beecher

---

Table 35-2 Cardiac arrests treated with external cardiac massage

Circulatory condition	Patients in operating and recovery rooms (n = 31)	Patients with myocardial infarction (n = 24)
Asystole	86%	12%
Ventricular fibrillation	14%	88%
Proof of arrest	28%	96%
Cardiac action restored	100%	42%

From Jude JR, Kouwenhoven WB, and Knickerbocker GG: Cardiac arrest: report of application of external cardiac message on 118 patients, *JAMA* 178:1063, 1961.

and Todd, had deemed that when no cause of death could be determined, the case constituted a "presumptive anesthesia death."[9] After assessing 1000 cases of operative mortality, Edwards et al. concluded that departures from accepted practice occurred in cases where anesthesia had contributed to death.[68]

Dripps in 1957 emphasized the hazards of the immediate postoperative period.[56] In 1960, Collins recognized the benefit of work/rest cycles to maintain alertness.[30] In 1960, Phillips et al. emphasized the need for routine postanesthetic recovery rooms.[163] Further Clifton and Hotton in 1963 reported the dangers of gastric aspiration, respiratory obstruction, and thiopentone overdose,[22] and Harrison in 1968 reported improvement in anesthetic risk claimed as a result of advances in patient monitoring, recovery room use, and supervision in training programs.[100]

Before the 1980s, reports of anesthetic risk came from the United Kingdom, United States, Australia, South Africa, Finland, and Vancouver.* The reported incidence of primary anesthetic mortality ranged from a high of 1/852 reported by Dripps, Lamont, and Eckenhoff in 1961,[57] to a low of 1/14,075 reported by Bodlander in 1975 from Sydney, Australia.[11] Bodlander noted that the contribution of anesthesia to operative mortality had decreased from 21% in the prior decade to 3.7% at the time of his report. Despite apparent progress, traditional causes of anesthetic deaths, namely respiratory obstruction, gastric contents aspiration, and cardiovascular collapse remained.[11] Bodlander's data, compared to earlier data from the same institution published by Clifton and Hotton,[22] raise questions (Table 35-3). Although deaths due solely to anesthesia were a smaller proportion of overall operative mortality in Bodlander's data, the total operative mortality had increased 2.5 times. Further, there were more cases in Bodlander's series in which anesthesia contributed to mortality than in Clifton and Hotton's series. When both primary and contributory causes of mortality were considered, there was actually a higher incidence in Bodlander's data. One must wonder if any real reduction in risk had occurred, or whether the numbers merely represent different counting techniques.

In 1979, Keats critically renewed prior anesthesia risk studies and concluded that in fact "precious little" was actually known about the role of anesthesia in operative mortality.[115] Widespread bias toward identification of errors rather than mechanisms of toxicity made prior estimates of anesthetic mortality unacceptable. Of note are the editorial remarks of Hamilton also in 1979, who disagreed and contended that errors in management were major factors in

---

* References 10, 11, 51, 100, 108, 135, 209, 212, 220.

Table 35-3   Deaths associated with anesthesia at Royal Prince Alfred Hospital, Sydney, Australia

	Clifton and Hotton[22] 1952-1962	Bodlander[11] 1963-1972
Total anesthetics	205,640	211,130
Total operative mortality	162	408
Deaths due solely to anesthesia	34 (20.9)*	15 (3.7%)*
When anesthesia partly contributed to death	18 (11.2)*	109 (26.7%)*
Total anesthetic risk	52/205,640 = 1/3955	124/211,130 = 1/1702

*Figures in parentheses denote the percentage of total operative mortality for each category.

anesthetic risk.[99] Actually, the early studies had established that both errors (respiratory insufficiency, gastric aspiration, and overdose) and drug toxicity (chloroform, curare, ether, cyclopropane) were important factors.

STUDIES DURING THE 1980s
United Kingdom

Sponsored by the Nuffield Provincial Hospitals Trust, ongoing efforts in the United Kingdom have made major contributions to the study of anesthetic risk. The most recent and extensive study is the Confidential Enquiry into Perioperative Deaths (CEPOD).[12,66,192] **Prior to CEPOD, the same group, namely Lunn, Mushin, and colleagues at Cardiff, established important groundwork—an anonymous and confidential system to report deaths** occurring within 6 days of surgery from five regions in England, Wales, and Scotland.[133,134] Reports were analyzed by two assessors, and differences in opinion were decided by arbitration. The overall 6-day operative mortality was 6/1000 (.6%). The rate at which anesthesia was partly or totally causative of mortality was 1 to 2 per 10,000 cases. The rate at which anesthesia was totally causative was 0.8 to 0.9 per 10,000. In addition, the study provided information regarding the various anesthesia practice standards in the United Kingdom. Extrapolations by the authors suggested that nearly 300,000 patients were not seen preoperatively by their anesthetist, 468,000 did not have blood pressure recorded intraoperatively, 534,000 cases did not have the anesthesia machine tested by the anesthetist beforehand, and in 1,290,000 cases, interoperative monitoring did not include ECG.[134] This extrapolation may have been invalid because the study identified only 62% of the perioperative deaths known by the government to have occurred. Detailed reports were requested only when the anesthetist or surgeon considered that anesthesia had in some way contributed to the death. Thus only one of 16 deaths was analyzed in detail. These early results were published in 1982, followed by a second report in 1983, which illustrated the importance of multiple opinions in outcome assessment.[133,134] The asesssors agreed with the anesthetist only in one third of the cases, the surgeon only in one third, and *neither* in one fifth.[133]

The Confidential Enquiry into Perioperative Deaths (CEPOD)[12] was based in methodology on earlier works by Lunn et al.,[132] Lunn, Hunter, and Scott,[133] and Lunn and Mushin.[134] The CEPOD study, however, included both the Association of Surgeons of Great Britain and Ireland, and the Association of Anesthetists of Great Britain and Ireland.[12] **Both surgical and anesthetic causes of perioperative death were assessed. Voluntary anonymous reports of perioperative death were submitted by anesthetists and surgeons, facilitated by "crown privilege" government support of total confidentiality.**

The Secretary of State is satisfied that the disclosure of documents about individual cases prepared for the Enquiry into Perioperative Deaths would be against the public interest and would undermine the whole basis of a confidential study. Therefore, the data/information sent to the confidential Enquiry into perioperative deaths is protected from subpoena . . .[12]

Included for study were deaths that occurred within 30 days of surgery in three regions of the United Kingdom over a 12-month period. Overall, there were approximately 500,000 operations with a crude mortality rate of 0.7% to 0.8%.

Specific conclusions were reached from the CE-POD study regarding patient mortality and medical practices (Table 35-4). Most mortality occurred in patients over age 75 years and was considered unavoidable because of the patients' preoperative diseases. Many anesthetists and surgeons did not conduct regular morbidity and mortality audits, and joint meetings between the two groups were rare. There were examples of surgeons operating for conditions for which they were not trained, and deaths in which junior surgeons or anesthetists did not seek senior advice before, during, or after the operation. Preoperative preparation was sometimes inadequate because of "undue haste to operate." There were cases in which moribund or terminally ill patients underwent surgery that would not have improved their condition.[12]

Specific findings for anesthetic practice were also noted. Patients were seen preoperatively in more than 80% of the cases, but postoperatively in less than 50%. More than 90% of patients had preoperative hemoglobin, electrolytes, and blood urea nitrogen determinations, and more than 80% had a preoperative chest radiograph and electrocardiogram. The older age of the CEPOD patients may have contributed to the relatively high use of preoperative laboratory studies. Intraoperative monitoring of CE-POD patients was deemed inadequate by the anesthetist assessors in over 20% cases. For example, muscle relaxants were used in more than 50% of cases, but a nerve stimulator was used in only 14%[12] (Table 35-5).

In light of the prominent role of ventilation in anesthetic risk, the low use of ventricular alarms is surprising. Particularly striking is the use of inspired oxygen analyzers in only 16.2% of cases. Apparently even the assessors thought that monitoring of inspired

---

Table 35-4   Leading factors contributing to deaths in CEPOD study

Anesthesia-related	Surgical-related
Failure to apply knowledge	Inappropriate preoperative management
Poor standard of practice	Inappropriate operation
Failure of organizations	Inappropriate level of surgeon

Buck N, Devlin HB, and Lunn JL: *Report of a Confidential Enquiry into Perioperative Deaths*, Nuffield Provincial Hospitals Trust, London, 1987, The King's Fund Publishing House.

Table 35-5   Use of intraoperative monitoring in CEPOD study

Monitor	% Used
Electrocardiogram	97%
Indirect blood pressure	90%
Manual pulse	66%
Ventilator alarm	39%
Stethoscope	28%
Exhaled carbon dioxide	19%
Inspired oxygen	16%
Nerve stimulator	14%
Core temperature	7%

Buck N, Devlin HB, and Lunn JL: *Report of a Confidential Enquiry into Perioperative Deaths*, Nuffield Provincial Hospitals Trust, London, 1987, The King's Fund Publishing House.

oxygen was less important "provided that rotameters were known to be functional." Anesthesia was judged to have contributed in some way to perioperative death in 410 cases but was assessed to be totally responsible for death in only three cases. **Thus anesthesia was contributory to seven deaths per 10,000 operations, but was totally responsible for only 1 death per 185,000 operations**[12] **(Table 35-6). These data are quite different from those reported by Lunn and Mushin in 1982,**[134] **and the reported risk is much lower.** One explanation is that improvement occurred over that time. Another is that numerous deaths were classified as "anesthesia contributory" rather than "totally causative" in the CEPOD study. Among the so-called "misadventures" during anesthesia were nine cases of aspiration of vomit and 18 cases of cardiac arrest.[13] Perhaps the true incidence of anesthetic risk lies between these numbers. Although it is tempting to quote the lower incidence, verification is needed.

Another significant aspect of the CEPOD study was assessment of surgical factors contributing to mortality. These data were evaluated by surgical assessors and represent a different medical perspective. An important note is that the data represent only patients who died; thus extrapolation to all surgery is problematic. The most common operations and most common clinical causes of death are listed in Tables 35-7 and 35-8.

It might be assumed that the relatively high incidence of orthopedic deaths was simply a reflection of the elderly patients who comprised the CEPOD population. The assessors concluded that these deaths occurred in elderly females with fractures of the femur neck and were inversely related to seniority of operating surgeon and preoperative preparation. The operating surgeon was a consultant (most senior) in only 19% of orthopedic cases, compared to the overall CEPOD sample in which a consultant was the operating surgeon in 47% of the operations. In comparison to general surgery cases, fewer physicians examined orthopedic cases preoperatively and fewer preoperative tests were ordered. Other specific findings included inadequate preoperative fluid and transfusion resuscitation in cases of incarcerated hernia and peptic ulcer. Some important similarities between surgical and anesthetic characteristics of CEPOD cases are evident. The seniority of physician was dependent on when the surgery was performed. Senior anesthetists and surgeons were more likely to be present during day cases, and junior physicians were more likely present at night (Table 35-9).

Table 35-6   Variation in incidence of anesthesia risk in United Kingdom studies

Role of anesthesia in perioperative mortality	Lunn and Mushin[134] (1982)	CEPOD[12] (1987)
Contributory only	1-2/10,000	7/10,000
Total cause	.8-.9/10,000	.054/10,000*

*This is equivalent to the 1/185,000 figure.

Table 35-7   CEPOD—the five most common operations

Operation	% Total
Laparotomy	21.9%
Dynamic hip screw	10.8%
Hemiarthroplasty	4.8%
Hemicolectomy	4.8%
Aortic aneurysm repair	4.6%

Buck N, Devlin HB, and Lunn JL: *Report of a Confidential Enquiry into Perioperative Deaths*, Nuffield Provincial Hospitals Trust, London, 1987, The King's Fund Publishing House.

Table 35-8   CEPOD—the five most common clinical causes of death

Causes of death	% Total
Bronchopneumonia	13.5%
Congestive heart failure	10.8%
Myocardial infarction	8.4%
Pulmonary embolism	7.8%
Respiratory failure	6.5%

Buck N, Devlin HB, and Lunn JL: *Report of a Confidential Enquiry into Perioperative Deaths*, Nuffield Provincial Hospitals Trust, London, 1987, The King's Fund Publishing House.

Table 35-9   Grade of CEPOD physician according to hour of operation

Grade	Anesthetist		Surgeon	
	Day*	Night†	Day	Night
Consultant	50%	25%	45%	34%
Others	50%	75%	55%	66%

*Day represents Monday through Friday, 9 AM to 7 PM.
†Night represents Monday through Friday, 7 PM to 9 AM, and Saturday and Sunday.
‡Indicates senior physician.
Buck N, Devlin HB, and Lunn JL: *Report of a Confidential Enquiry into Perioperative Deaths*, Nuffield Provincial Hospitals Trust, London, 1987, The King's Fund Publishing House.

Both anesthetists and surgeon assessors concluded that avoidable elements were present in about 20% of cases. Contributing factors for both anesthetists and surgeons tended to be failures to act appropriately with existing knowledge rather than knowledge deficiency, equipment malfunction, or fatigue. The issue of fatigue depends on definition of excessive duty. The CEPOD report states:

The graph shows little evidence of excessive duty hours. The great majority of operating surgeons being on duty for less than 24 hours prior to undertaking the surgical intervention reported. A further group was on duty for up to 36 hours, but there are few examples of surgeons being on duty for excessive hours of duty longer than this.[12]

The French Survey

In 1977, the French Ministry of Health directed that a study of anesthetic complications in France be undertaken.[102,202] A prospective survey of 460 public and private institutions from 1978 to 1982 identified 198,103 anesthetic cases, which composed a "representative sample" (one thirteenth) of France's total anesthetic practice, estimated to be approximately 2.5 million cases per year. Major complications occurred in 268 cases, which resulted in death within 24 hours in 67 cases or persistent coma in 16 cases. Death or persistent coma was considered in some way related to anesthesia in 1/2387 cases and totally related to anesthesia in 1/7924. Thus the mortality totally attributable to anesthesia is similar to the 1/10,000 figure identified by early United Kingdom studies. Other findings by the French survey confirmed that major complications were more frequent in older age groups, emergency operations, poor preoperative ASA physical status class, and patients with multiple associated diseases. The causes of anesthetic mortality reveal important and unique findings of the French survey[202] (Table 35-10).

Most striking are the adverse outcomes associated with postoperative respiratory depression. The authors indicate that almost all of these patients had received narcotics and muscle relaxants during anesthesia, *which had not been reversed*. A contributing factor was infrequent use of recovery rooms in France, which resulted in half of all study patients being returned directly to the ward after anesthesia. Confirmation is indicated by the fact that although most complications (58%) occurred during the operation, most deaths occurred during the postoperative period[202] (Table 35-11).

A second unique finding was the high incidence of "anaphylactoid shock" reported as a complication. The authors contended that evidence for overdose was absent in the anaphylactoid shock cases, and instead incriminated use of Althesin and succinylcholine. It should be noted that a category for drug overdose was not included as a cause of complication.[202]

The French survey did have potential advantages because of its prospective nature, rather than studying perioperative deaths, as in the United Kingdom studies. First was the ability to assess the incidence of nonfatal complications. Second, the total number of anesthetics was known rather than estimated. Third, a potentially more complete reporting of deaths was possible than in the voluntary system used in the United Kingdom studies. Refusal to participate was also noted as a problem in the French survey. An important disadvantage of the French survey was limitation of occurrence of death to 24 hours, a much more restrictive period than in the United Kingdom study.[12] In fact, the CEPOD study determined that when a period of 30 days after surgery was considered, only 50% of perioperative deaths occurred during the first week.[13] Thus patients with respiratory failure, myocardial infarction, and congestive heart failure who died after 24 hours would have been missed by the French survey.

Table 35-10 Causes of death or coma totally attributable to anesthesia in French survey

Problem	Number of complications	Number of deaths	Number of comas
Equipment failure	5	1	1
Intubation complication	16	1	1
Aspiration gastric contents	27	4	2
Postoperative respiratory depression	28	7	5
Anaphylactoid shock	31	1	1
Cardiac arrest	17	1	—

From Tiret L, Desmonts JM, Hatton F et al: Complications associated with anaesthesia—a prospective survey in France, *Can Anaesth Soc J* 33:336, 1986.

Table 35-11 Timing of complications and mortality occurrence in French survey

	During operation	Postoperative
Number of complications (n = 268)	156 (58%)	112 (42%)
Number of deaths (n = 67)	25 (37%)	42 (62%)

From Tiret L, Desmonts JM, Hatton F et al: Complications associated with anaesthesia—a prospective survey in France, *Can Anaesth Soc J* 33:336, 1986.

New South Wales, Australia

In New South Wales, Australia, a committee representing anesthesia, surgery, obstetrics, and general practice, formed in 1960, has investigated deaths related to anesthesia since that time.[103,104] Deaths are identified by coroners' reports, and questionnaires are voluntarily returned. The guarantee of confidentiality required legislation, but has generated a response rate greater than 90%. The reports are classified and those deemed associated with anesthesia are assessed for errors. The findings of this committee were most recently reported by Holland in 1987, and include analysis of anesthetic errors, changes in anesthesia personnel, and an overall reduction of the risk of anesthesia.[104] The occurrence of errors in anesthesia-associated deaths has decreased over time although 90% of cases were still deemed associated with error. **Although some errors, such as hypoxic gas mixture, have diminished in frequency, the top five errors of the 1960s—overdose, wrong choice of anesthetic, inadequate preparation, inadequate crisis management, and inadequate postoperative management—were still the leading errors of the 1980s.** Despite an overall reduction in anesthetic-related deaths, mortality in good and fair-risk patients continues to be a significant proportion the recent period's total[104] (Table 35-12).

Holland's ongoing committee assessment did demonstrate an overall reduction in anesthesia-related mortality. The incidence of anesthesia-related deaths was 1/5,500 in 1960, 1/10,250 in 1970, and 1/26,000 in 1984. Holland estimates that it was five times safer to undergo anesthesia (in Australia) in 1987 than it was in 1960.[104] Improvement is the result of reduction of errors and is attributed to elimination of nonspecialists from the anesthesia work force. Holland also attributes improvement to the influence of the Faculty of Anesthetists in its settings of standards, training, and credentialing requirements for fellowship.

In the Australian report, identification of deaths is facilitated by law, which requires that any patient who dies "whilst under, as a result of, or within 24 hours of an anaesthetic" be reported to the coroner. As in the French survey, the time limitation may have caused late deaths to be missed. Also, it is not clear whether adverse neurologic outcomes were counted. Finally, the denominator of total anesthetics administered was estimated. The proportions of this total for different personnel, such as specialists, registrars, nonspecialists, may be imprecise. Nonetheless, Holland is to be congratulated for his perserverance in providing the most longitudinal anesthesia risk studies in anesthesiology literature.[103,104]

United States Studies

The legal system in the United States has probably been responsible for the absence of any large-scale study of anesthesia risk in this country, compared to such accomplishments in the United Kingdom. An organized collection and assessment of such material by a national panel would greatly aid understanding of the problem. Instead, cases with adverse outcomes are argued for years by lawyers and insurance companies. It is unlikely that this adversarial system determines true mechanisms that caused adverse outcomes. This system, which, in essence is an inspection of sorts *after* the fact, contributes little to the prevention of similar problems. **Ironically, this resembles the observations of MacIntosh in 1948: "Similar accidents occurred at neighboring towns which might well have been avoided had the anaesthetist had available to him the details of the other mishaps."**[135]

Keenan and Boyan studied intraoperative cardiac arrest over a 15-year period at the Medical College of Virginia.[120] From 163,240 administered anesthetics, 449 cases of cardiac arrest were identified, 27 of which were judged solely attributable to anesthesia (1.7 arrests per 10,000 anesthetics). Subsequent death occurred in half these cases, for a mortality of approximately 1/10,000 anesthetics. Mechanisms leading to cardiac arrests were judged to be failure to ventilate in 45% of the cases and anesthetic overdose in 55%. Half the ventilatory arrests (7 of 12) and half the overdose arrests (8 of 15) resulted in death. Thus, despite the presence of trained personnel, resuscitation drugs, equipment, and monitors, the outcome of a witnessed cardiac arrest was death in roughly half the cases. The poor outcome may indicate the need to improve resuscitation skills or that cardiac arrest is a late sign of a progressive deterioration that has irreversibly damaged less robust essential organs. The arrests were deemed avoidable in three fourths of the cases.[120]

If cardiac arrest is a late sign, an early indicator of impending arrest would be extremely desirable. **Per-**

Table 35-12 Number of cases and proportion of anesthetic-related mortality in good- and fair-risk patients over time		
	1960-1969 (n = 335)	**1970-1980** (n = 239)	**1983-1985** (n = 50)
Good risk	65 (19%)*	42 (18%)	9 (18%)
Fair risk	80 (24%)	72 (30%)	14 (28%)

*Thus from 1960 to 1969, a total of 65 anesthetic-related deaths occurred in good-risk patients and represent 19% of the total of anesthetic-related deaths for that period.
From Holland R: Anaesthetic mortality in New South Wales, *Br J Anaesth* 59:834, 1987.

haps the single most important contribution of Keenan and Boyan was that such a sign—progressive bradycardia—was noted to precede cardiac arrest in 26 of the 27 cases. Unfortunately, the significance of this sign was not appreciated, as evidenced by atropine therapy rather than use of 100% oxygen. Keenan and Boyan concluded that adminstration of atropine did "little but waste time."[120] An unanswered question is whether early therapy of bradycardia with 100% oxygen would have altered the outcome. Another question is whether today's use of capnography and pulse oximetry has decreased the incidence of ventilatory failure cardiac arrests.[200] Also of interest is whether use of isoflurane,[170] with its more favorable toxic therapeutic ratio, has decreased the incidence of overdose cardiac arrests, compared to Keenan and Boyan's data, which were obtained from cases that used halothane and enflurane.[120]

Other findings of Keenan and Boyan include the facts that intraoperative cardiac arrest was more frequent in the following cases: emergency rather than elective surgery, ASA III and IV classes rather than ASA I and II classes, and children under age 12 compared to adults. These results would be expected because sicker patients have less reserve, but it is also possible that errors are more frequent or less easily detected in complicated cases. It should be noted that the incidence of overall anesthetic mortality is likely to be underestimated by the data of Keenan and Boyan, because patients may die as a result of aspiration of gastric contents, preoperative myocardial infarction, hypoxic brain damage, etc. without suffering an *intraoperative* cardiac arrest, which was the only complication studied. The distinctiveness of intraoperative cardiac arrest, however, offers a useful marker for study and comparison.[120]

Another study of cardiac arrest was that of Caplan et al. in 1988, who reviewed 14 closed legal claims cases of unexpected cardiac arrests in healthy patients who had received competently administered spinal anesthetics.[17] Several common patterns were noted. First, in patients who had been sedated, cyanosis was noted before the arrest, suggesting that unappreciated respiratory insufficiency had been present. Second, potent inotropic/vasoconstrictor agents were administered either late or in insufficient doses when cardiac arrest occurred (again, with the admonition regarding the likelihood that atropine was a time-waster).[120] It was speculated that in the presence of spinal anesthetic–induced vasodilation, the limited blood flow generated from cardiopulmonary resuscitation might be diverted away from the brain and heart. This explanation was advanced as a possible reason that, despite successful cardiac resuscitation, only four of the 14 patients regained con-

Table 35-13   Closed claims negative outcomes considered preventable by additional monitors

Complication	Preventable	Nonpreventable
Death	241 (57.1%)	158 (37.4%)
Brain damage	83 (58.4%)	51 (35.9%)
Nerve damage	1	164 (92.1%)

From Tinker JH, Dull DL, Caplan RA et al: Role of monitoring devices in prevention of anesthetic mishaps: a closed claims analysis, *Anesthesiology* 71:541, 1989.

sciousness and only one returned to normal activities. This outcome was much worse than out-of-hospital resuscitations from cardiac arrest.[128]

The landmark study by Caplan et al. illustrates the important contribution available from studies of rare events.[17] Their findings were applauded as demonstrating that a careful search for mechanisms of toxicity could explain the occurrence of anesthetic risk.[115,118] The exhaustive search for management errors by the American Society of Anesthesiologists Closed Claims Study was responsible for grouping these cases together, facilitating these discoveries.

The second report from the ASA Closed Claim Study was that of Tinker et al. in 1989, who assessed the potential role of monitoring devices in the prevention of anesthetic mishaps[200] **(Table 35-13). Review of 1097 anesthetic-related closed malpractice claims, by claims reviewers who were all experienced practicing anesthesiologists, determined that 31.5% of the negative outcomes could have been prevented by the use of additional monitors, primarily pulse oximetry and capnography, regardless of whether such monitors existed at the time of the incident.** Importantly, the preventable injuries were significantly more severe in terms of degree of injury and cost of settlement than were injuries judged nonpreventable by additional monitoring. These results applied to adverse outcomes from regional as well as general anesthesia. Thus, considering the adverse outcomes of death and brain damage, additional monitoring would have prevented the negative outcome in approximately 58% of the cases in which major incidents occurred. These conclusions assume that the additional monitors would have been in use, functioning continuously and correctly, and correctly interpreted at the time of the accident. This is a challenging expectation for any piece of equipment, particularly high-technology devices subjected to daily use and artifact vulnerability. **The conclusions assume that output from the monitoring device would have been "assimilated, interpreted and acted upon cor-**

Table 35-14 Clinical signs noted in records of closed claims cases

Sign	Number of preventable cases	Number nonpreventable cases
Bradycardia	182	50
Asystole	170	81
Hypotension	157	75
Cyanosis	142	29

Note: A total of 346 cases were judged preventable by additional monitoring while 751 cases were judged nonpreventable.
From Tinker JH, Dull DL, Caplan RA et al: Role of monitoring devices in prevention of anesthetic mishaps: a closed claims analysis, *Anesthesiology* 71:541, 1989.

Table 35-15 Monitors potentially efficacious in preventing injuries or deaths

Additional monitors	Number cases (%) n = 346
Pulse oximetry alone	138 (40%)
Capnography alone	8 (2%)
Both pulse oximetry and capnography	176 (51%)

From Tinker JH, Dull DL, Caplan RA et al: Role of monitoring devices in prevention of anesthetic mishaps: a closed claims analysis, *Anesthesiology* 71:541, 1989.

Table 35-16 Distribution of adverse respiratory events

Event	Number of cases	Percent of 522 respiratory claims
Inadequate ventilation	196	38%
Esophageal intubation	94	18%
Difficult tracheal intubation	87	17%
Inadequate FIO_2	11	2%

From Caplan RA, Posner K, Ward RJ et al: Adverse respiratory events in anesthesia: a closed claims analysis, *Anesthesiology* 72:828, 1990.

rectly." Pertinent to this issue was the finding that in almost 90% of the preventable cases (305 of 346 cases), at least one clinical sign, and in some cases several clinical signs, of abnormality had been present from existing monitors (Table 35-14). Pulse oximetry and capnography together were determined to be the most useful additional monitors.[200]

Similar to the findings of Keehan and Boyan,[120] despite warnings, adverse events still occurred. It is arguable whether pulse oximetry and capnography provide a more clear warning of respiratory problems than signs such as bradycardia. Fully half of the preventable outcomes were judged, arbitrarily, to require *both* pulse oximetry *and* capnography to establish preventability. In other words, despite providing a clear signal of systemic oxygen saturation, pulse oximetry alone would have established preventability of only 40% of the cases. Despite providing a clear indication of exhaled carbon dioxide and inspired oxygen, capnography alone would have established preventability in only 2% of the cases. This result was obtained because of an arbitrary decision by the Closed Claims Committee, namely that in cases of unrecognized esophageal intubation, *both* pulse oximetry *and* capnometry would be deemed capable of preventing the complication when used together (Table 35-15).

There is also the assumption that the correct therapy would be timely and of sufficient magnitude to convert all negative outcomes to positive ones. The possibility that some cases of death would be converted to brain damage only was not mentioned. The potential role of monitoring in prevention of anesthetic mishaps, thus, represents a *best case* scenario, when everything works. The question remains why 37% of deaths and 36% of brain damage outcomes were considered not preventable by additional monitors.

The third Closed Claims Report, again by Caplan et al., specifically concerned adverse respiratory events[16] (Table 35-16). The outcomes represented the single largest class of injury in the Closed Claims Study and were responsible for death or brain damage in 85% of the cases. Inadequate ventilation, esophageal intubation, and difficult intubation accounted for three fourths of all adverse respiratory events. Notable for their small contributions were: equipment failures, such as breathing circuit disconnection and misconnection and inadequate inspired oxygen concentrations. In general, cases of inadequate ventilation and esophageal intubation were more likely to be judged as substandard care, preventable by better monitoring, resultant in death or brain damage, and associated with larger ultimate settlements or judgments than were cases of difficult intubation. A mechanism of injury was not distinguishable for cases of inadequate ventilation. This perhaps represented an indictment of traditional clinical signs, such as reservoir bag motion, breath sounds, and chest excursion, to assure adequate ventilation. Several important points regarding esophageal intubation centered on ability to detect the problem promptly. The authors emphasized the unreliability of breath sound auscultation, which was associated with misdiagnosis in 48% of these problem cases. **Hemodynamic indicators, such as bradycardia, asystole, and hypotension, were present in 84% of esophageal intubation cases but seem to have been perceived as independent threats to life rather than symptoms of esophageal intubation.** Cyanosis was noted in less than half of the cases, representing the known limited sensitivity of the human eye for this condition plus the latter's dependence on sufficient hemoglobin, plus difficulty in detection in Black patients. Finally, the authors speculate that adequate preoxygenation may have contributed to misdiagnosis by providing an appearance of normalcy for some time after intubation and thus falsely supporting the misdiagnosis by breath sound auscultation.[16]

A fourth report from the closed claims data is that of Kroll et al. in 1990, who addressed the issue of perioperative peripheral nerve injury.[123] Such cases comprised 15% of all the closed claims reviewed, and were dominated by ulnar, brachial plexus, and lumbosacral nerve root injury. Mechanisms of this troubling risk of anesthesia were not forthcoming from this study. The fifth closed claims report is that of Chadwick et al. in 1991,[18] which examines obstetric anesthesia closed claims (see the section on obstetric risks).

RISK INDICES

Early studies of operative risk identified certain patient characteristics that appeared to increase the likelihood of adverse outcome. The strongest overall predictor was the presence of a recent myocardial infarction, which markedly increased the risk of perioperative myocardial infarction.* Although today a patient's cardiovascular profile may include angiographic delineation of disease or be modified by prior coronary bypass surgery, the presence of a recent myocardial infarction remains a significant risk factor.† **In the late 1970s, a variety of characteristics were included to form preoperative checklists that might facilitate prediction of postoperative adverse outcomes.** The well-known Cardiac Risk Index (CRI) was published by Goldman et al. in 1977.[90] Several points must be remembered. The concept of a classification scheme was not new because the ASA Physical Status had been in use since 1961.[57,176,214] Neither were the individual risk factors discovered by Goldman et al. Instead, Goldman et al. organized the material into a scheme that could be easily applied for preoperative assessment. Unfortunately, the scheme did not withstand subsequent prospective evaluation of its predictive value. Other risk indices have also

been proposed. Cooperman et al.[37] in 1978, Detsky et al.[49] in 1986, and most recently, Shah et al.[184] in 1990 have published various risk indices to predict cardiac events. Tiret et al. in 1988 proposed a risk factor index that utilized the following: ASA physical status, age, complexity of operation, and urgency of surgery to predict postoperative outcomes.[203]

A critical requirement of the various proposed indices is that their predictive ability should be subsequently independently verified. Only the Goldman et al. CRI has been evaluated and the results are mixed. In 1984 Zeldin prospectively applied the CRI to 1140 surgical patients, and found that high-risk patients experienced only half the predicted rates of cardiac complications.[223] Some bias may have been introduced because Zeldin was the primary surgeon for all the patients studied. Domaingue, Davies, and Cronin[53] (1982) and Jeffrey et al.[109] (1983) prospectively applied the CRI to patients undergoing vascular surgery. Detsky et al. applied CRI to patients for whom preoperative cardiac consultation had been requested.[49] All found a significantly worse cardiac complication rate than predicted by the Goldman index. Gerson et al.[84] (1985) and Mangano et al.[139] (1990) also failed to demonstrate the predictive capacity of the CRI. Charlson et al.[19] (1987) noted that the various results obtained by these risk index studies were significantly influenced by differences in study population, surveillance methods, and outcome criteria (Table 35-17). **In this respect, it is significant that the only validation study that enrolled patients in a manner similar to Goldman was the study by Waters et al. in 1981.[219] They found the CRI no more predictive of postoperative cardiac events than the ASA Physical Status Classification scheme.**

In addition to combination indices, some investigators have studied the utility of single preoperative characteristics in predicting outcome. Goldman and Caldera (1979) did not find that preoperative hypertension increased the incidence of postoperative myocardial infarction.[89] The presence of diabetes was noted by MacKenzie and Charlson to increase perioperative complications.[136] The inability to perform a specified amount of exercise was correlated by Gerson et al. with an increased incidence of cardiac and pulmonary complications.[84] One problem in such studies is that a population selected for one characteristic, e.g., hypertension, includes patients with other dissimilar problems. Thus, among the patients with hypertension studied by Charlson et al., patients with cardiomegaly had a greater risk for complications than those without cardiomegaly.[19]

Another approach has been to collect data on all perioperative patient characteristics to determine which correlated with adverse outcomes.[76] Fowkes et al. (1982) used this method to analyze 108,878

---

* References 4, 69, 80, 88, 90, 178, 194, 197, 199, 206.
† References 41, 78, 112, 121, 137, 180.

Table 35-17   Effect of various eligibility criteria on population selection

Author	Goldman et al.[90]	Jeffrey et al.[109]	Detsky et al.[49]	Gerson et al.[84]
Patient eligibility	All ward patients	Abdominal aneurysm surgery	Suspected cardiac disease	Elderly abdominal or thoracic surgery
Percent of prospective population enrolled	100%	13%	60%	38%

From Charlson ME, Ales KA, Simon R et al: Why predictive indexes perform less well in validation studies, *Arch Intern Med* 147:2155, 1987.

anesthetics administered in Cardiff.[79] Characteristics that increased risk of operative mortality included cardiac failure, impaired renal function, ischemic heart disease, diabetes, chronic lower respiratory tract infection, obesity, and emergency operation. Cohen, Duncan, and Tate (1988) also used an extensive data collection system and a multiple logistic model to ascertain individual predictive risk factors.[28] Factors associated with increased mortality included age, male gender, physical status class, major surgery, emergency operation, and intraoperative complications. Duration of anesthesia and experience of the anesthesiologist did not correlate with increased mortality. Questions are raised by the finding that narcotic techniques and those using one or two anesthetic drugs rather than multiple agents were associated with increased mortality, whereas inhalation techniques were not. In addition, patients who were monitored with four or more monitors had five times the mortality of patients who had either none or only one monitor. Although the explanation may be that sicker patients had multiple monitors and received narcotics, it might be contended that this represents inherent "toxicity" of monitors or narcotic agents. The conclusion of Cohen et al. that patients and surgical risk factors were more important than anesthesia factors in predicting surgical mortality illustrates an important point of all risk index–type studies.[28] When high-risk patients are studied, mortality related to anesthesia is often obscured by overwhelming influences of other factors.

More than three decades before the various cardiac risk indices were popularized, the concept of preoperative classification of physical status had been developed and implemented by anesthesiologists. The original scheme was developed by a committee of the ASA and was intended to provide a common terminology and a means to facilitate collection of statistical data. Saklad (1941) reported that label of "operative risk" was purposely avoided because it included variables such as proposed operation and skill of the surgeon.[176] Instead, the classification was

restricted to preoperative characteristics and was called the physical state of the patient. The original scheme contained six classes, which included provision for emergency surgery. A seventh class was subsequently added for moribund patients. In their 1961 report of the role of anesthesia in surgical mortality, Dripps, Lamont, and Eckenhoff modified the ASA system, which they called a physical status (PS) rating.[57] These modifications were subsequently adopted by the ASA in 1962 and are the system in use today. Keats, however, asserted that credit for the scheme rightly belongs to its innovators, Saklad, Rovenstine, and Taylor.[114] Indeed, Dripps violated the original intentions of avoiding surgical variables by describing Class I as: "normal healthy patient for elective operation."[57] Worse was the demeaning 1977 contention by Goldman et al. that called the scheme the "Dripps-American Surgical Association" classification.[90] Although some may assert that these were minor editorial mistakes, it should be noted that Eagle et al. perpetuated the error in 1987 and 1989.[60,61]

Because the ASA Physical Status classification uses general descriptions rather than specific disease states, the reproducibility of these subjective classifications was addressed by Owens in 1978.[161] Ten hypothetical patients were classified by 255 anesthesiologists. Six of the cases were classified consistently by most of the respondents, whereas four cases elicited divergent responses. The problematic cases included cases with variables of advanced age, recent bleeding, obesity, and old myocardial infarction. **Despite this, the PS classification has facilitated assessment and communication for 30 years. Its widespread application today in essentially its original form is testimony to its usefulness.** An inevitable question was whether the preoperative PS classification was predictive of outcome. Indeed, class 5 included expected outcome, namely death, in its definition. Goldstein and Keats (1970) deemed the ASA physical status "not a sensitive predictor of anesthetic mortality" because the combined data of six prior studies demonstrated that 41% of anesthetic-

Table 35-18   Relationship of total operative mortality to preoperative physical status

Physical status class	Vacanti et al. Operative mortality[214]	Marx et al. Operative mortality[144]
1	1 : 1179	1 : 1665
2	1 : 371	1 : 212
3	1 : 55	1 : 23
4	1 : 13	1 : 4
5	1 : 11	1 : 2

Table 35-19   Relationship of anesthetic mortality to preoperative physical status

Physical status class	Dripps et al. Anesthetic mortality[57]	Marx et al. Anesthetic mortality[144]
1	0	1/9160*
2	1/1013	1/10609*
3	1/151	1/347
4	1/22	1/134
5	1/11	1/64

*Note that for Physical Status Classes 1 and 2, the data from Marx, Matteo, and Orkin demonstrate an anesthetic risk of 1:10,000.

related deaths occurred in ASA Class I or II patients.[91] It should be noted that the majority of cases for the combined data came from the early reports of Beecher and Todd[9] (1954) and Edwards et al.[68] (1956), and was the basis for the direct association between physical status and anesthetic mortality found by Dripps[57] in 1961. Preoperative physical status might be expected to reflect a patient's ability to withstand the stress of surgery. If so, then preoperative physical status might correlate with overall operative mortality. Vacanti, Van Houten, and Hill[214] (1970) and Marx, Matteo, and Orkin[144] (1973) demonstrated such a relationship, despite significant differences in their patient populations (Table 35-18).

Another hypothesis is that the sicker patients with less physiologic reserve would be less able to withstand an error, overdose, or critical incident from the anesthetic. If so, the preoperative physical status might be expected to also correlate with mortality resulting from anesthesia. Such an association was found by Dripps in 1961[57] and can be calculated from the data of Marx, Matteo, and Orkin[144] in 1973 (Table 35-19).

Other examples of the correlation of preoperative physical status with outcome include the data of Waters et al., who found the physical status to be as predictive as the Goldman CRI for postoperative adverse cardiac events.[219] Keenan and Boyan (1985) determined that intraoperative cardiac arrests related to anesthesia were more frequent in class III and IV than class I and II patients.[120] In addition, when cardiac arrest occurred in class III and IV patients, it carried a 60% mortality, whereas only a 30% mortality in class I and II patients, which demonstrates the usefulness of the physical status classification.

AGENT VS. ANESTHESIOLOGIST, TOXICITY VS. ERRORS

One opinion is that anesthetic agents themselves are inherently toxic and that despite appropriate admin-

istration, untoward effects, either singly or in combination, can result in mortality. This view was first championed by Keats (1979), who criticized earlier studies of anesthetic risk because of their biased assumptions that errors were the only explanation for anesthetic mortality.[115] Keats provided this example of Sir Robert MacIntosh's views of anesthetic risk in 1948:

As I hold that there should be no deaths due to anesthetics, I am very uneasy as to how far we are justified in testing new drugs when the correct administration of those already available to us will give excellent operating conditions to the surgeon at negligible risk to the patient.[135]

Another example is the protocol used to classify postoperative deaths by the Baltimore Anesthesia Study Committee 1960.[93] If the anesthetic was thought to contribute to the death, the choices were limited for classification. Which phase of the anesthetic management of such case was principally at fault? The choices were (1) preoperative preparation and medication, (2) error in selection of agent or method, (3) improper management of the anesthetic, (4) improper resuscitation, and (5) postoperative medication or management.

Keats was concerned that preoccupation with such classification of errors might preclude discoveries about inherent toxicity of the agents themselves and/or in combination.[115] Before the recognition of malignant hyperthermia, deaths caused by this disease had likely been attributed to errors in airway management because of accompanying hypercarbia. Before understanding of hyperkalemia associated with succinylcholine use in burn patients, such a death could be classified as improper resuscitation. In each case, error classification would *end the analysis,* despite the fact that knowledge of the mechanism of death had not been advanced. Instead of the "error bias," Keats recommended a thorough search for true causality of adverse reactions.[115] The recent ASA closed claims analysis of spinal anesthesia by Caplan et al. has substantiated this perspective. These authors analyzed 14 cases of cardiac arrest that occurred in healthy patients despite an appropriately managed spinal anesthetic.[17] Common patterns were noted and a hypothesis for a new mechanism of toxicity was proposed, which can now be tested experimentally and chemically.

The opposing view is that most cases of anesthetic mortality occur not from drug toxicity, but from errors in management. Hamilton's 1979 editorial view about Keats' argument notes that historically adverse outcomes attributed to patients' conditions or drug toxicity also failed to advance knowledge of anesthetic risk.[99] Thus explanations for death such as "status lymphaticus" prevented the assessment of correctable anesthetic management problems. In fact, in 1948 MacIntosh visited Royal Air Force hospitals and found that anesthetic accidents were occurring commonly, yet efforts were being made to suppress that information. This policy, he stated, "is all very bad for the nation because many of these deaths might have been avoided if the anesthetist had known from the tragic experiences of others of the dangers to which he was exposing his patient."[135]

It should be noted that the recent work by Caplan et al. (1988) concerning spinal anesthesia resulted from insurance company closed malpractice claims cases.[17] It was the exhaustive search for management errors by the practicing anesthesiologists of the ASA Professional Liability Committee that grouped these cases and facilitated elucidation of a possible mechanism. Further, the recent emphasis on error prevention with pulse oximetry plus capnography holds promise for real reductions in anesthetic mortality.[20,200] Despite Keats' warning that emphasis on management errors has contributed to the malpractice problem, the specialty's efforts to reduce errors have resulted in reductions in malpractice insurance.

Risk according to agent used

A discussion of "what is the safest anesthetic" was reported in the *Journal of the American Medical Association* in 1887. Ether vs. chloroform was compared and benefits of inhalers rather than the outmoded towel-cone were emphasized. The report included a timeless quotation: "All anesthetics are dangerous, and become more so when administered in unknown quantities and in an unsafe manner."

Among the characteristics of ether is its dose-related depression of respiration. This feature prevented uptake of high concentrations that caused circulatory depression, and thus was a safety feature. Overwhelming concern about flammability led to its abandonment, along with cyclopropane, ethylene, and fluroxene. Senior readers of this chapter may mourn

the passage of some or all of these agents. Some have called cyclopropane the "champagne of anesthesia." This chapter's senior author (JHT) has used all of these except ethylene and strongly disagrees. Today's agents are much better.

Most, if not all, anesthetic agents have been questioned with regard to relative safety. The process often begins with clinical reports of untoward reactions and proceeds to clinical trials or laboratory research to establish whether claims of toxicity have merit. This process has identified the nephrotoxicity of methoxyflurane[40] and succinylcholine toxicity in trauma patients, burn patients,[205] and those with neuromuscular disease.[36] The multi-institutional National Halothane Study evaluated claims of hepatic necrosis.[64,196] This massive research determined that halothane use was associated with hepatic necrosis but the incidence was extremely rare. However, studies with large numbers of patients do not guarantee conclusions that will stand the test of time. **Beecher and Todd (1954) reported a large multihospital survey of more than 500,000 patients.[9] Those who had received "curare agents" had a six times worse operative mortality.** Because these adverse outcomes occurred for both experienced and unexperienced physicians, and often in "good risk" patients, the authors concluded that these drugs possessed "inherent toxicity." The authors' bias toward toxicity is illustrated by their contention that curare agents precipitated circulatory failure in cases when artificial respiration "of a generally effective type" was employed. Further illustration of bias is the contributory role assigned to curare:

Even if the assumption was correct, for example, that an air embolus was the immediate cause of death, it is conceivable that a patient's circulatory system might have been so weakened by the 'curare' that he succumbed when he otherwise would not.[9]

The issue of curare's inherent toxicity was not settled until the report by Dripps, Lamont, and Eckenhoff (1961) that 6000 patients had received a "curare" muscle agent and not one had died.[57] In retrospect, perhaps firm conviction about inherent toxicity prevented attention to management errors. The dangers of "toxicity" bias are also illustrated by the report that preoperative propranolol contributed to adverse outcomes in a small series of cardiac surgical patients.[216] The bias against propranolol was so widespread in the medical community that many physicians changed their practices on the basis of this small report without corroborating research. Many cases of angina, dysrhythmia, and myocardial infarction were precipitated by unwarranted preoperative discontinuation of propranolol.[147]

A recent claim of anesthetic toxicity is the reported

causative association of isoflurane to "coronary steal" in 1983.[167] Like propranolol, this purported toxicity of isoflurane was reported in a small group of patients (n = 27) who underwent coronary artery bypass surgery. The facts are that the ECG changes were not dramatic, other reasons such as decreased blood pressure could account for the observations, and the critical measurement of coronary sinus flow is known to have important inaccuracies. The authors concluded that isoflurane was a "powerful" coronary vasodilator responsible for the ischemic changes by a coronary steal mechanism. Rather than widespread confirmation of these findings by clinicians, support for "coronary steal" toxicity was forthcoming only from complex nonclinically relevant animal preparations. Clinical reports appeared to instead indicate that isoflurane was not inherently more toxic than other agents/techniques. Substantial toxicity bias continued to be injected by the editorial comments of Becker (1987) who concluded that isoflurane could be "dangerous."[7] It is unknown how many physicians changed their practices on the basis of this editorial.

The issue of editorial views by nonanesthesiologists deserves comment. Consider a report in the *Wall Street Journal* that a drug commonly used by anesthesiologists to control hypertension had resulted in nine cases of cyanide poisoning.[141] Although nitroprusside's pharmacology and toxicity[201] had been reviewed years earlier, to nonphysicians, such a drug must appear frightening and one to be avoided. Similarly, a cardiologist who has little or no experience with general anesthetics and is given such adverse data may be expected to form a negative opinion, especially if it seems to confirm his own previously reported animal model. The key point is that the terms "dangerous" and "safe" are *comparative* terms, never absolutes unless complete avoidance can be accomplished. Patients still need some kind of anesthesia. Thus safety or toxicity *must* be assessed in light of available alternatives.

The question of whether general or regional anesthesia is safer continues to be argued. In 1961 Dripps, Lamont, and Eckenhoff reported that death related to anesthesia occurred less frequently when regional rather than general anesthesia was used.[57] A recent review by Scott and Kehlet (1988) found that only two of 12 mortality studies of patients undergoing hip surgery demonstrated significant benefit of regional over general anesthesia.[182] Yeager et al. demonstrated that epidural anesthesia plus light general anesthesia with postoperative epidural analgesia had fewer complications than general anesthesia.[222] A different perspective was provided by Olsson and Hallen, who assessed 115 cases of anesthetic-related cardiac arrest, of whom nine died.[158] Although spinal and epidural anesthetics accounted for only 10 cases of cardiac arrest, five of these patients died. The authors indicated that this high mortality occurred when spinal or epidural anesthesia was administered to patients with poor physical status, including hypovolemia. This explanation correlates with the assessment by Caplan et al. that cardiopulmonary resuscitation may be difficult in patients who have received a spinal anesthetic because of vasodilation from sympathetic blockade.[17]

Does choice of hospital influence patient risk?

This emotionally and politically charged question is applicable to all fields of medicine. There are many published examples of outcome variation between institutions. Hotchkiss (1960) reported that mortality from patent ductus arteriosus repair was significantly worse in nonteaching centers than in university centers, which had higher caseloads.[107] Easton and Sherman (1977) reported that the combined stroke plus mortality rate for carotid endarterectomy in two community hospitals was 21%, nearly tenfold worse than previously published results.[62] The Coronary Artery Surgery Study demonstrated regional mortality variations. The National Halothane Study demonstrated a 24-fold variation in postoperative mortality among the 34 participating institutions despite attempts at standardization for patients and surgery.[155] Six institutions had mortality rates under 1%, whereas 10 institutions had rates higher than 3%. The most recent and most controversial published institutional variation is the public report of hosptial-specific death rates for U.S. Medicare patients.[110] The first report was released in 1986 and has been followed by yearly updates. Despite the unpopularity and dubious clinical or statistical validity of such reports, they do have impact.[95] For example, the American Heart Association Stroke Council had called for voluntary restrictions on carotid endarterectomy.[8] A recent major multi-institutional trial indicating efficacy (once again) for the operation is likely to increase the number of operations performed and rekindle the issue of institutional variability.[157] It is inevitable that the future will bring more disclosures of medical outcomes.

Does the risk of anesthesia depend on who administers the anesthetic?

This question is also explosive. Its answer depends in part on how data are collected and interpreted. For example, Slogoff and Keats (1985) published data indicating that the patients of one anesthesiologist, #7, had significantly more perioperative myocardial infarctions after anesthesia for coronary bypass surgery than did patients of other anesthesiologists.[187]

They stated:

We believe the varying rates of ischemia during anesthesia among anesthesiologists reflect their varying skills in managing patients for CABG operations and may represent an objective measure for assessing clinical skills.[187]

Despite this contention, review of the data suggests that other anesthesiologists had similar frequencies of ischemia. Although anesthesiologist #7 had more episodes of hypertension and tachycardia, that person's incidence of intraoperative hypotension was less than any other anesthesiologist. These findings conflict with studies of noncardiac surgery that have implicated intraoperative hypotension, but not tachycardia or hypertension, as predictors of postoperative infarction. Our interpretation of the data of Slogoff and Keats cannot discern why more infarctions occurred for #7. It is somewhat surprising that editorial comments concluded that the study represented "an hypothesis confirmed."[129] We are not so sure. This is an important issue because quality assurance activities can be used to try to improve patient care or be subverted to deny recredentialing. **Whatever indicators are chosen, they must represent deviation from recognized standards of care rather than arbitrary definitions of "acceptable" clinical parameters (Table 35-20).**

Different conclusions concerning the role of the individual anesthesiologist were reached by Cohen, Duncan, and Tate (1988) in their study of operative mortality for 100,000 cases in a tertiary care center in Manitoba.[28] The experience of the anesthesiologist was not found to be related to operative mortality. All anesthesiologists were board certified with at least 1 or 2 years of further training. Only two levels of experience were assessed, determined by whether the anesthesiologist had performed more than 600 procedures/year for 8 years. Both groups were thus likely to be composed of relatively experienced

persons. Unaddressed questions included comparisons among different hospitals, subspecializations in anesthesia, board certified vs. general practitioner anesthesiologists, or physician anesthesiologists vs. nonphysician anesthetists.[28]

The issue of non-anesthesiologist anesthesia providers is also a controversial subject. Holland (1987) reported that a 25-year survey of anesthetic mortality in New South Wales, Australia, demonstrated that nonspecialist general practitioners and resident medical officers not training in anesthesia contributed least to mortality, especially in recent years, largely because their participation in the anesthesia work force had declined[104] (Table 35-21).

A unique aspect of the Confidential Enquiry into Perioperative Death (CEPOD) report was that approximately 175 cases were reported in which patient death had occurred after a surgeon had administered the anesthetic.[12] **Anesthetics involved sedation for endoscopy, regional techniques, and local anesthesias. The authors concluded that (1) patients were frequently not weighed before surgery; (2) the maximum safe dose was often not known; (3) intraoperative monitoring was frequently ignored; and (4) records of anesthetic agent and dose administered were not always kept.**[12] An earlier report by Grimes and Cates in 1976 also illustrates the potential danger of the administration of anesthetics by non-anesthesia personnel.[98] Three deaths from paracervical block for first-trimester abortions were reported, and the authors concluded that administration of the appropriate dose of local anesthetic was the single most important factor. Despite this, in each case, cardiopulmonary arrest occurred after convulsion. Thus, arguably, the most important factor might have been lack of resuscitation skills. Despite the potential dangers, the authors recommended: ". . . If tremor, twitching or convulsions occur, the patient should be treated with intravenous diazepam or a rapid-acting

Table 35-20 Variation in postoperative infarction rates among anesthesiologists			
Anesthesiologist	Arrival ischemia	During anesthesia ischemia	Postoperative infarction
1	19%	29%	2.9%
4	22%	38%	5.1%
7	20%	45%	12.5%
8	26%	32%	1.9%

From Slogoff S, Keats AS: Does perioperative myocardial ischemia lead to postoperative myocardial infarction? *Anesthesiology* 62:107, 1985.

Table 35-21 Cases of anesthetic mortality for good-risk patients according to grade of anesthetist			
	1960 to 1969	1970 to 1980	1983 to 1985
Specialists	8	19	7
Registrars	6	2	—
Nonspecialists	45	18	1
Resident	6	1	—

From Holland R: Anaesthetic mortality in New South Wales, *Br J Anaesth* 59:834, 1987.

Table 35-22 Incidence of anesthesia deaths/10,000 anesthetics in North Carolina

Provider	Rate/10,000
Surgeon/dentist	.87
CRNA	.48
Anesthesiologist	.41
Anesthesiologist and CRNA	.36

From Bechtoldt AA: Committee on anesthesia study of anesthesia-related deaths: 1969-1976, *NC Med J* 42:253, 1981.

Table 35-23 Percentage of nonfatal complications for 112,271 anesthetics

Complication occurrence	1975 to 1978	1979 to 1983
Intraoperative	7.6%	10.6%
Recovery room	3.1%	5.9%
Postoperative: major	0.4%	0.45%
minor	8.9%	9.4%
Total in patients seen	25.5%	31.6%
Total for all patients	14.0%	17.8%

From Cohen MM, Duncan PG, Pope WDB et al: A survey of 112,000 anaesthetics at one teaching hospital (1975-83), *Can Anaesth Soc J* 33:22, 1986.

barbiturate.... If convulsions persist, intubation should be instituted with the aid of succinylcholine ..."[98]

A second consideration of obstetrician-administered anesthesia is that two patients may simultaneously be at risk. Chadwick et al. described a case of saddleblock anesthetic wherein bradycardia of the fetus occurred at the same time as respiratory distress of the mother.[18] Finally, a report by Bechtoldt of North Carolina's Committee on Anesthesia Study compared rates of anesthesia mortality among various providers[6] (Table 35-22). Surgeons or dentists had the highest rate, whereas CRNAs working with anesthesiologists had the lowest rate. All groups had rates lower than the commonly accepted 1/10,000.

These raw statistics are perhaps misleading because there is no correction for severity of illness. For example, Bechtoldt reported that anesthetic deaths occurred most often in patients aged 71 to 80 years, with intraabdominal operations, and in physical status class 3 patients.[6] Were these cases equally distributed among surgeon/dentists, CRNAs, and anesthesiologists? The type of anesthesia reported included general, regional, local infiltration, and intravenous sedation. Were these cases equally distributed? Thus Bechtoldt's data, like other risk studies, were unlikely to have accurately compared different types of anesthesia providers.

NONFATAL ANESTHESIA RISKS

Nonfatal complications are an important aspect of risk.[169] This is a diverse category, including adverse reactions, such as halothane-associated hepatic necrosis[196] and malignant hyperthermia,[92] as well as complications, such as postintubation granuloma of the larynx.[191] Fortunately, major nonfatal adverse events, like anesthetic mortality, occur rarely. In contrast, minor complications, such as nausea and vomiting, are noted with considerable frequency.[27] For a particular patient, even minor adverse events

may constitute an important source of discomfort and dissatisfaction.

A major contribution to understanding the incidence of nonfatal anesthetic complications was provided by investigators at the University of Manitoba at Winnipeg. Burnham and Craig (1980) reported the organization of a postanesthetic follow-up service.[14] Cohen et al. (1986) reported the results of this study, which surveyed 112,721 anesthetics administered over 9 years[27] (Table 35-23). Overall, 17.8% of cases were determined to have some anesthetic-related complication. The frequency of complications appeared to increase rather than decrease over time. The high rate is partly a function of definition. Arrhythmias constituted the most common intraoperative complication, and use of intraoperative electrocardiography increased over time. Nausea, vomiting, and sore throat were the most frequent postoperative complications. **Only the incidence of complications was reported, not their impact or outcome. For example, intraoperative cardiac arrest was noted to occur at a rate of seven arrests/10,000 anesthetics. It is likely that this complication resulted in substantial morbidity and mortality, whereas the complication of intraoperative arrhythmia had negligible impact despite its frequency of 356 arrhythmias/10,000 anesthetics.[27]**

Another question raised by the Winnipeg data concerns the total number of complications. The rates are higher for patients who were actually seen by the postoperative nurse because it was assumed that patients who were discharged had no complications. This suggests that the incidence of minor complications is probably higher than the reported 17.8%.

A subsequent report by Duncan and Cohen (1987), using the same data base, determined which factors correlated with the occurrence of complicatons.[59] As expected, there was an increased incidence of postoperative respiratory complications in patients with preoperative respiratory disease. Unexpectedly, there was a markedly higher incidence of intraoperative cardiac arrest in patients with preoperative renal disease. Still other findings were controversial, such as an increase in postoperative complications in patients who received spinal or pure narcotic techniques vs. inhalation anesthetics. Perhaps the most provocative finding was that greater experience of the anesthesiologist correlated with reduced risk of postoperative complications. In a later report concerning operative morality, Cohen, Duncan, and Tate (1988) found that the experience of the anesthesiologist was not a factor.[28]

The Winnipeg investigators also investigated nonfatal complications of obstetric anesthesia. Ong et al. (1987) reported that during the years 1975 to 1983, more than 30,000 infants were delivered at Winnipeg Womens Hospital.[159] Epidural anesthesia for vaginal deliveries and cesarean sections increased, whereas use of general anesthetics decreased. The primary complications noted during anesthesia were hypotension and unintended dural puncture. Delayed complications included back pain, headache, and sore throat. The frequency of most complications decreased over the study time period, except headache, which remained relatively constant. The impact of these complications is not addressed by the report. Of particular interest are the infrequent complications, including aspiration, convulsions, and postoperative neurologic symptoms.[159]

In contrast to large-scale studies of all anesthetic complications are reports that concentrate on a single type of complication. **One such recent report by Kroll et al. (1990) concerned perioperative peripheral nerve injury.**[123] **Using data from the ASA Closed Claims study, the authors noted that 15% of all closed claims studied involved nerve injury.** Ulnar, brachial plexus, and lumbosacral nerve root injury predominated. Although the mechanism of injury was rarely discernible, some patterns were noted. The ulnar nerve was most frequently affected and accounted for one third of the claims. A 3:1 male preponderance was noted for ulnar injuries. General anesthesia was the technique most often used. In contrast, brachial plexus and lumbosacral nerve root injury–related claims were more commonly filed by females. Brachial plexus injury occurred with both general and regional techniques, and was associated with use of shoulder braces, prone position, arm suspension, techniques, etc. Lumbosacral nerve root injuries were most often associated with pain or paresthesia accompanying a regional anesthetic technique. Reviewers judged that care was more often satisfactory in nerve injury cases than in other claims, such as adverse respiratory events.[123]

Another specific anesthetic complication involves

Table 35-24   Distribution of 1223 dental injuries

Type of injury	Percent cases
Dislodgement of loose or mobile teeth	47%
Chip or fracture of natural tooth	39%
Damage to dental prosthesis	12%

From Lockhart PB, Feldbau EV, Gabel RS et al: Dental complications during and after tracheal intubation, *J Am Dent Assoc* 112:480, 1986.

dental damage.[23] Lockhart et al. (1986) surveyed 133 anesthesia training programs and found 1223 dental injuries occurring in 1,135,212 cases in which tracheal intubation was used, for an incidence of 1 injury/1000 cases[127] (Table 35-24).

In addition, Lockhart et al. retrospectively reviewed 5 years of dental consultations for one teaching hospital and found 32 cases of dental trauma associated with general anesthesia. Oroendotracheal intubation accounted for 75% of the cases, whereas 25% occurred during extubation or in the recovery room. **Recovery room episodes were often related to biting on oropharyngeal airways or "bite blocks." The upper left central incisor was affected most often and accounted for half of the injuries. More than half of all incidents occurred during difficult or emergency intubations.** The authors suggest that some form of "tooth protector" could have prevented most of the incidents.[127]

ANESTHETIC RISK IN SPECIAL PATIENT GROUPS
Obstetrics

Maternal mortality has been reported for many years, often as the number of maternal deaths per number of births* (Table 35-25). Variation in the methods of calculation makes direct comparison of rates problematic.

Overall, maternal mortality is similar to the 1/10,000 rate estimated for overall risk of anesthesia. Hospitals with delivery rates of 1000/year might not suffer a maternal death for several years. **Because *anesthetic-related* maternal death represents a small percentage of maternal deaths in a particular hospital, anesthetic-related maternal deaths are quite unusual.** In fact, Endler et al. (1988) determined that from 1972 through 1984, anesthetic-related maternal deaths occurred at a rate of 1 to 4 per year for the entire state of Michigan.[74] The exact role of anesthesia in maternal mortality is difficult to assess because

---

* References 42, 97, 143, 150, 152, 172, 209, 210.

Table 35-25 Recent reports of maternal mortality rates and the proportion related to anesthesia complications

Comparison issues	Kaunitz et al.[113] 1974-1978	Endler et al.[74] 1972-1984	Rochat et al.[171] 1980-1985	Confidential Enquiry 1982-1984[210]
Region(s) studied	50 U.S. states	Michigan	19 areas of U.S.	England and Wales
Maternal deaths per 100,000 live births	15.3	12.8	14.1	8.6
Anesthetic deaths per 100,000 live births	0.6	0.82	0.98	1.1
Percent anesthetic deaths of total maternal deaths	4.0%	6.9%	7.0%	13.0%

the number of live births does not equal the number of anesthetics administered. Gibbs et al. (1986), in a national survey of nearly 1200 hospitals, determined that epidural block, spinal block, or general anesthesia was used in only one of four vaginal deliveries.[85] Although cesarean section almost always requires one of these techniques, it represents less than one fourth of all deliveries. The problem can be illustrated by the following studies. Both Kaunitz et al.[113] (study period 1974 to 1978) and Rochat et al.[171] (study period 1980 to 1985) identified anesthetic complications as sixth on the list of causes of maternal deaths, considerably lower than embolic diseases and hypertensive diseases. **However, Rochat et al. noted that between the two periods, all direct causes of maternal mortality decreased except anesthesia and cerebrovascular accident.[171] This could imply that anesthesia progress has not kept pace with other medical advancements. Alternatively, because all rates are based on numbers of live births, the finding may simply represent increased use of anesthesia in childbirth.** Another issue is the time frame used for definition of maternal death. Some reports include deaths occurring within 1 year of the end of pregnancy, whereas the National Center for Health Statistics defines only death occurring up to 42 days after the end of pregnancy as maternal. Rochat et al. noted that this limited definition would have excluded 10% of anesthetic-related maternal deaths.

Despite these problems, reports of mortality rates can illustrate important issues. Kaunitz et al. (1985) surveyed maternal mortality throughout the United States. Anesthesia mortality was more frequent in women over age 30 and in nonwhites.[113] Hospital size and geographic region of the country did not demonstrate trends in anesthetic mortality. Endler et al. (1988) noted 15 cases of primary anesthetic maternal death in the state of Michigan over the years 1972 to 1984.[74] Failure to secure a patent airway was the predominant cause of death. Emergency procedure, obesity, and hypertension of pregnancy were often present. The incidence of anesthetic death was

Table 35-26 Types of injuries in obstetric anesthesia closed claims

Type of injury	claims regional anesthesia* (n = 124)	of claims general anesthesia (n = 62)
Maternal death	15	26
Newborn brain damage	23	15
Newborn death	8	6
Maternal brain damage	9	5
Headache	23	0
Pain during anesthesia	16	0
Maternal nerve damage	12	4
Emotional distress	9	3
Back pain	9	0

*Numbers of claims are indicated, not percentage.
From Chadwick JS, Posner K, Caplan RA et al: A comparison of obstetric and nonobstetric anesthesia malpractice claims, *Anesthesiology* 74:242, 1991.

markedly higher in blacks than whites, suggesting the difficulty of detection of cyanosis. Rochat et al. (1988) surveyed 19 regions of the United States and found that anesthesia-related maternal deaths were more frequent in mothers over age 30 and in nonwhites.[171] The Confidential Enquiry into Maternal Deaths in England and Wales has regularly assessed maternal death rates since 1952. The 1979-1981 report noted 82 direct anesthetic maternal deaths and seven in which anesthesia was contributory.[210] Aspiration of gastric contents and difficulty with intubation were leading factors. Postoperative respiratory failure related to use of narcotics and long-acting muscle relaxants also contributed.

Another perspective on anesthetic causes of maternal mortality is provided by the ASA Committee on Professional Liability. In 1991, Chadwick et al. reported a review of closed malpractice claims for 190 obstetric cases representing 127 cases of cesarean section and 63 of vaginal delivery[18] (Table 35-26).

Maternal death and newborn brain damage were the most frequent injuries in obstetric closed claims. Some injuries and events seemed related to the type of anesthetic technique. For example, claims involving maternal death and respiratory system events were more prevalent in cases involving general anesthesia, whereas claims for convulsions, headache, pain during anesthesia, and backache were more common in cases involving regional anesthesia (Table 35-27). Other authors have also commented on maternal complications of regional anesthesia.[43,142] Some injuries were related to factors other than anesthetic technique. For example, 17 of the 38 cases of newborn brain injury could be attributed to anesthesia, 14 could be attributed to obstetric or congenital problems, and 5 to difficulty with newborn resuscitation.

The most complete reporting of maternal mortality related to anesthesia comes from the United Kingdom via the Report on Confidential Enquiries into Maternal Deaths in England and Wales (CEMD).[210] The most recent report covers the years 1982 to 1984 and represents the eleventh such triennial evaluation.[210] Maternal mortality has decreased by half every 10 years. The CEMD reports between 1970-1972 and 1982-1984 have demonstrated that anesthetic maternal deaths have also decreased (Table 35-28).

The magnitude of the decrease in anesthetic deaths is even greater because the number of anesthetics administered increased over time. This point is illustrated by the data concerning cesarean sections, where it is likely that anesthesia was used. Thus overall maternal mortality has decreased by half over the last 10 years, but maternal mortality related to anesthesia for cesarean section may have fallen by 75%. Despite this progress, authors of the CEMD report point out that anesthesia continues to be an important cause of direct maternal deaths, remaining the third most common cause of maternal death, following pulmonary embolism and hypertensive diseases of pregnancy. These anesthetic maternal deaths were all considered to represent cases of substandard care.[210]

In the 1982-1984 CEMD report, 18 direct anesthetic maternal deaths and one anesthesia contributory death occurred.[210] Three fourths of the deaths occurred in emergency cases. The largest category,

---

Table 35-27 Nature of damaging event in obstetric anesthesia closed claims compared to non-obstetric closed claims

Category	Percent of nonobstetric claims (n = 1351)	Percent of obstetric claims with regional anesthesia (n = 124)	Percent of obstetric claims with general anesthesia* (n = 62)
Respiratory	35%	11%	53%
Convulsion	1%	15%	2%
Equipment	4%	6%	6%
Wrong drug	3%	2%	10%
Cardiovascular	7%	3%	2%

*Numbers indicate the percentage of claims within the column. The total number of claims for each column is in parentheses.
From Chadwick JS, Posner K, Caplan RA et al: A comparison of obstetric and nonobstetric anesthesia malpractice claims, *Anesthesiology* 74:242, 1991.

Table 35-28 Anesthesia related direct maternal deaths from CEMD* reports (1970-1989)

	1970-1972	1973-1975	1976-1978	1979-1981	1982-1984
Direct anesthesia deaths	37	27	27	22	18
Anesthesia deaths as percentage of direct maternal deaths	10.8	11.9	12.4	12.4	13.0
Estimated number cesarean sections in NHS hospitals	103,310	101,410	120,570	167,020	185,820
Anesthetic deaths in National Health Service cesarean sections	22	17	18	19	8
Calculated anesthetic deaths per 10,000 anesthetics for cesarean section	2.13	1.67	1.49	1.14	0.43

*Confidential Enquiries into Maternal Deaths.
From Turnbull A, Tindall VR, Beard RW et al: *Report on Confidential Enquiries into Maternal Deaths in England and Wales 1982-1984*, London, 1989, Her Majesty's Stationery Office. Data for anesthesia deaths on p. 97 and data for cesarean sections on p. 87.

difficulty with endotracheal intubation, accounted for 10 deaths. Aspiration of stomach contents accounted for seven deaths. Inadequately reversed neuromuscular blockade accounted for two postoperative ward deaths. It was considered that inexperienced junior anesthetists were left to care for complicated patients. Lack of cooperation and discussion between anesthesia and obstetrics services contributed to deaths that could have been prevented. Other notable findings included aspiration deaths in patients who had received particulate antacids, hemorrhage death from attempted tracheostomy, total spinal blockade with epidural "top up" dose, and hypoxemia from an outmoded ventilator.[210]

The conclusions of the CEMD report of 1982-1984 included an overview of the 33 years during which the data have been kept. This overview concluded that maternity patients had not been provided with the same standard of anesthesia care that was available to surgical patients. In each of the last five triennial reports, anesthetic deaths were characterized by a high incidence of avoidable factors or substandard care. Raising the standard of obstetric anesthetic care to that of other surgery was deemed a major goal.[210]

Pertinent to this subject is the survey by Gibbs et al. of obstetric anesthesia in the United States and the reason that anesthesiologists were not more involved.[85] In almost 1200 surveyed hospitals, anesthesiologists, including residents, were available exclusively for labor and delivery cases in only 21% of hospitals. Labor and delivery coverage by dedicated anesthesiologists at night and on weekends was available in only 15% of hospitals. The more common arrangement was that anesthesiologists covered labor and delivery in addition to other commitments. **The most striking deficiencies were noted in hospitals with fewer than 500 deliveries per year. In smaller U.S. hospitals, 55% of general anesthetics were provided by a CRNA directed by an obstetrician. Newborn resuscitation was often performed by "other" personnel, who were not anesthesiologists, obstetricians, pediatricians, or CRNAs. Epidural anesthesia for cesarean section is performed by the obstetrician in 20% of cases. Yet hospitals with fewer than 500 deliveries/ year accounted for 54% of the hospitals that provided obstetric care in 1985.** Leading responses by anesthesiologists for the reason for lack of involvement included (1) lack of predictability of labor and delivery, making difficult scheduling, (2) high risk of malpractice claims, (3) dictation of anesthesia type and timing by obstetricians, and (4) less financial remuneration than general operating room anesthetics.[85] The significance of these findings is underscored by cesarean section rates in the United States. The cesarean section rate rose from 5.5% in 1970 to 24.4%

in 1987, which has prompted concern and strategies for reduction.[193]

Pediatrics

Two concepts emerge from the study of anesthetic risk in pediatric surgery. First, the pediatric age group, particularly infants less than 1 year of age, appears to be at increased risk for anesthetic complications. The second is that anesthetic risk for pediatric patients is reduced in centers where specialized pediatric anesthesia is available. Many reports emphasize the pediatric respiratory system.[5,50,126,168,174]

Many reports have demonstrated increased anesthetic risk in pediatric patients.* In Beecher and Todd's 1954 multi-institutional study, a "disproportionate number" of anesthetic deaths were noted to have occurred in patients under age 10.[9] Anesthetic deaths were three to five times more frequent in this age group than in the second or third decade age groups. Similarly, the analysis by Edwards et al. (1956) of "1000 anesthetic deaths" suggested an increased mortality in patients under age 10 years.[68] Graff et al. (1964) reported the findings of the Baltimore Anesthesia Study Committee, which specifically concerned pediatric anesthetic mortality.[93] Anesthetic-associated deaths accounted for about one of six perioperative deaths, a percentage that applied to adults as well as children. In infants less than 1 month old, deaths ascribed to anesthesia accounted for one of four perioperative deaths. A disturbing finding was that over half the pediatric anesthesia deaths occurred in good-risk patients. When factors contributing to mortality were assessed, over 80% involved the respiratory system (Table 35-29). A relatively minor role was played by cardiac dysrhythmia, despite widespread attention on this "complication."[93]

Comparison among these reports is prevented by the lack of a denominator indicating total number of anesthetics. Qualitative comparisons can be made between institutions that specialize in pediatrics vs. those that do not. Graff et al. (1964) studied pediatric anesthetic mortality over 11 years in Baltimore. They listed tonsillectomy as the operative procedure most frequently associated with anesthetic deaths. In contrast, Ament (1960) reported 10 years of data from the Buffalo Children's Hospital, which included 23,186 adenotonsillectomies with only one death.[2] Similarly, Davies (1964) reported that only one primary anesthetic death occurred during 21,500 cases of tonsillectomy and/or adenoidectomy at the University of London.[44] These results suggest that expertise in pediatric airway management is an important factor.

---

* References 9, 26, 65, 68, 93, 204.

Table 35-29 Factors contributing to pediatric anesthetic mortality from the Baltimore Anesthesia Study Committee			
Respiratory (n = 48)		**Cardiovascular (n = 9)**	
Airway obstruction	15	Hypovolemia	6
Aspiration	15	Myocardial depression	2
Central nervous system depression	10	Dysrhythmia	1
Lung disease	5		
Neuromuscular depression	3		

From Graff TD, Phillips OC, Benson DW et al: Baltimore Anesthesia Study Committee: factors in pediatric anesthesia mortality, *Anesth Analg* 43:407, 1964.

Table 35-30 Incidence of operative pediatric cardiac arrest related to anesthesia		
	Rackow, Salanitre, and Green[165] (1961)	**Tiret et al.[204] (1988)**
Infants	14/10,000	19/10,000
Children	4.3/10,000	2.1/10,000
Adults	3.8/10,000*	7/10,000

*Data of Rackow H et al. for adults includes cardiac arrests that were related to anesthesia and to unknown causes.

A different approach to pediatric anesthetic risk involves assessment of incidence of intraoperative cardiac arrest. Reports by Rackow, Salanitre, and Green[165] (1961), Salem et al.[177] (1975), Keenan and Boyan[120] (1985), and Tiret et al.[204] (1988) indicated that the pediatric patient, particularly the infant, is at increased risk. Rackow, Salanitre, and Green studied the incidence of pediatric cardiac arrest related to anesthesia over a 10-year period at Columbia.[165] Infants younger than 1 year of age constituted only 12.5% of the pediatric surgical population, but suffered nearly 30% of the cardiac arrests. In children aged 1 to 13 years, the incidence of cardiac arrest related to anesthesia was not significantly different from the rate in adults (older than 13 years). The outcome of cardiac arrests in all children was poor, with complete recovery occurring in only 16% and death in 68%. In contrast, adults suffering operative cardiac arrest had a 50% complete recovery rate. Salem et al. (1975) described 73 instances collected from seven institutions over 12 years in which anesthesia contributed to cardiac arrest.[177] No "denominator" was available, so the incidence was unknown. Twenty cardiac arrests related to hypovolemia were reported. Seven of these occurred in patients with preoperative anemia who received halothane; most had just been intubated and positive pressure ventilation initiated. No deaths occurred. Thirteen cardiac arrests occurred as a result of intraoperative blood loss that was underestimated or inadequately replaced. This illustrates that the pediatric patient may be remarkably resilient, but margin for error is limited. Respiratory problems in the immediate postoperative period accounted for many of the respiratory cardiac arrests and deaths. Keenan and Boyan noted that the incidence of cardiac arrest related to anesthesia in patients under age 12 was three times higher than that of older patients.[120]

The most recent study of pediatric anesthetic risk is that of Tiret et al. (1988).[204] A prospective study of major anesthetic complications in pediatric patients in 440 French hospitals was conducted between 1978 and 1982. A total of 27 major anesthetic complications occurred during 40,240 administered anesthetics, which included 12 cases of cardiac arrest but only one death. The major findings involved differences between infants younger than 1 year of age and children aged 1 to 13 years. The incidence of major complications and cardiac arrests were significantly higher for infants than children. The major causes of complications in infants occurred during the maintenance period and involved the respiratory system, such as airway problems and aspiration. In contrast, in older children complications were divided equally between respiratory and cardiovascular causes, and were most frequent during induction and recovery.[204]

This incidence of anesthetic death was quite low—1 death per 40,000 administered anesthetics. Nearly all patients who had cardiac arrests apparently recovered without major sequelae. Both findings are at variance with other studies of anesthetic risk. Table 35-30 compares the incidences of cardiac arrest reported by Rackow, Salanitre, and Green[165] in 1961 and Tiret et al.[204] in 1988.

Despite improved outcomes reported by Tiret et al., some questions remain. Remarkable is a comparison of the pediatric data of Tiret et al. in 1988, with data prospectively obtained for adults during the same period in France, also by Tiret et al.[202] (1986). The total incidence of complications and cardiac arrests was higher in infants than adults, but infant anesthetic mortality was zero, whereas anesthetic-related death and coma occurred in adults at a rate of 1/2387 anesthetics. In adults, half the cases of death and coma attributable to anesthesia were related to postoperative respiratory depression. Such postoperative respiratory depression was not mentioned as a complication in infants and accounted for only two of 18 complications in older children. Narcotic-based anesthetics likely played a major role in adults, whereas inhalation techniques predominated in pediatrics. Of interest is that the *only* pediatric death occurred in a 13-year-old patient who received nitrous oxide, succinylcholine, narcotic, and neuroleptic agents for wrist fracture repair. Death was related to postoperative respiratory depression on the ward.

The most recent report concerning pediatric morbidity and mortality is that of Cohen, Cameron, and Duncan, who assessed 29,220 anesthetics administered over a 6-year period at Winnipeg Children's Hospital.[26] Major complications, such as cardiac arrest and death, were reported as well as events such as vomiting, arrhythmia, sore throat, etc. Neonates were found to have the highest incidence of adverse events, including cardiac arrest and death although no distinction was made regarding anesthesia or surgery as the cause. Neonates were more likely to have undergone major cardiac or vascular surgery, whereas older children mostly underwent otolaryngologic or orthopedic procedures. With these qualifications, the data of Cohen, Cameron, and Duncan support the findings of Rackow, Salanitre, and Green[165] and Tiret et al.[204] that cardiac arrest is more frequent in infants than older children. Intraoperative and postoperative complications in neonates and infants were dominated by respiratory problems, blood pressure problems, and temperature problems. It is noteworthy that intraoperative temperature monitoring was performed in less than half the cases in the overall study. Complications in children aged 1 to 5 years were mostly related to respiratory problems although recovery room vomiting was significant. In children older than age 5, postoperative vomiting was the major complication.[26] Other investigators using pulse oximetry have demonstrated that the postoperative period is also a risk for hypoxemia.[39,151]

Elderly

Whether the elderly are at increased risk from anesthesia is not well defined.[24,106,149] Some studies have identified that older age correlates with increased operative mortality. Denny and Denson (1972) reported on 272 patients over age 90.[46] Overall mortality was 29%; two thirds of the operations were orthopedic, mostly hip fractures. The worst outcomes were in patients who had surgery for bowel obstruction (63% mortality), preoperative pulmonary disease (63% mortality), and preoperative congestive heart failure (50% mortality). Goldman et al. (1977) identified advanced age as a factor contributing to

poor operative outcome.[90] None of these reports distinguishes mortality related to anesthesia.

Anesthetic risk studies do not provide clarification. For example, Beecher and Todd (1954) commented that anesthetic deaths appeared more frequently in the elderly.[9] Data from Edwards et al. (1956) also suggested this trend, but neither study had an accurate denominator of the number of anesthetics administered to the elderly.[68] Marx, Matteo, and Otkin (1973) assessed 27 cases of primary anesthetic death. Nearly half occurred in patients over age 65, but most were also in preoperative ASA classes IV and V.[144] Cohen, Duncan, and Tate (1988) contended that advanced age was an important factor in operative mortality but did not correlate age with anesthetic factors.[28] Similarly, Djokovic and Hedley-Whyte (1979) reported on 500 surgical patients over age 80. The overall mortality was 6.2%, and marked differences were noted between different ASA classifications; fewer than 1% of ASA class II patients died, whereas 25% of ASA class IV patients died.[52]

Many reviews have concerned potential problems of aging,[29,48,96,217] such as atherosclerosis,[153,218] reduced left ventricular function during exercise,[164] alterations in respiratory reserve,[124,154] impaired temperature regulation, and reduced glomerular filtration. Nonetheless, Edmunds et al. demonstrated that many patients over age 80 years can successfully undergo open heart surgery for coronary artery disease or valve replacement.[67]

Evidence that the elderly may be at increased risk for anesthetic problems is offered by Tiret et al. in the prospective French survey. They identified markedly increased frequency of major anesthetic complications in patients over age 45, with a peak at age 75.[202] Whether these complications actually resulted in adverse outcomes or recovery is not clear. In contrast, Keenan and Boyan failed to demonstrate a predilection of anesthetic-related cardiac arrests in the elderly.[120] Possible explanations include that elderly patients were recognized to be at increased risk and thus were better monitored, more lightly anesthetized, more often admitted to the intensive care unit, or assigned to more experienced anesthetists.

The most extensive recent survey of anesthetic and surgical mortality, the Confidential Enquiry into Perioperative Deaths, noted that 79% of reported deaths occurred in patients over age 65, remarkable because patients over age 65 years accounted for only 22% of the surgical population.[12] Despite the predominance of elderly patient deaths, the CEPOD study did *not* conclude that anesthetic-associated deaths were more likely in the elderly. This may have reflected a bias that operative deaths in younger patients were more likely considered to represent anesthetic complications.

Despite lack of clear evidence that the elderly are at increased anesthesia risk, several studies suggest potential problems.[181] Del Guercio and Cohn (1980) assessed 148 patients over age 65.[45] Patients having good cardiopulmonary function had good outcomes, whereas those assessed as having poor function suffered high perioperative mortality. Before the assessment by Del Guercio and Cohn, all of the patients had been evaluated as "cleared for surgery" by an internist.[45] Gerson et al. (1985) found that inability to perform a specific amount of bicycle exercise correlated well with adverse postoperative outcomes.[84] A second problem identified by Kronenberg and Drage (1973) is that ventilatory and heart rate responses to hypoxemia and hypercapnia are attenuated by aging.[124] Thus it might be anticipated that the elderly would be more susceptible to respiratory insufficiency and that the anesthesiologist may be less able to detect such a condition by vital sign changes. Murphy et al. (1989) reported that cardiopulmonary resuscitation may be difficult in elderly patients.[156] It is possible that perioperative cardiac arrests in the elderly are related to underlying cardiac disease rather than the circumstances associated with anesthesia.

STRATEGIES FOR RISK REDUCTION
National Risk Reduction Strategies

Major large-scale efforts by the ASA and its Anesthesia Patient Safety Foundation have been undertaken to try to reduce anesthesia risk. **The 1980s brought two major developments (Table 35-31). The ASA adopted formal statements of practice standards. Coincidentally, techniques of pulse oximetry**[25,31,145] **and capnography were popularized.**[63] There was debate regarding possible drawbacks of such standards, including medicolegal problems, potential distraction by additional alarms and monitors, and less vigilance as a result of assuming that added monitors will catch abnormalities. However, like prior monitors, such as the ECG and oxygen analyzer, pulse oximetry and capnography have rapidly been assimilated into practice. **The standards and monitors have been widely embraced and applied by anesthesiologists, largely because risk reduction is a universal goal.**[21,94,189]

Implementation of standards and oximetry/capnography monitoring holds promise of reduction of anesthetic risk. It is critical that any risk reduction be understood. ASA standards and oximetry/capnography are separate and distinct entities, despite their common concerns for oxygenation, ventilation, and circulation. Specifically, oximetry and capnography are not (yet) mandated by ASA standards (1991) although they are strongly encouraged. A provocative

Table 35-31   ASA standards for basic intraoperative monitoring*

Standard I	Qualified anesthesia personnel shall be present in the room throughout the conduct of all general anesthetics, regional anesthetics, and monitored anesthesia care
Standard II	During all anesthetics, the patient's oxygenation, ventilation, circulation, and temperature shall be continually evaluated

*Approved by House of Delegates, Oct. 21, 1986.

report by Eichhorn (1989) is pertinent to both these issues and is reviewed in some detail.[71] Readers are also referred to the editorial review by Orkin.[160]

Eichhorn examined major intraoperative anesthetic accidents and deaths in healthy patients in nine component Harvard-affiliated hospitals before and after adoption of the Harvard minimal monitoring standards.[72,105] Detailed descriptions of the eleven cases considered were provided.[71] Eichhorn concluded that adoption of practice standards in July 1985 had a positive impact in terms of risk reduction. Specifically, a 3.22-fold decrease in the incidence of accidents was observed. The decrease in accidents could have been the result of requirements explicitly stated in the standards or the use of specific oximetry/capnography monitors. Is the assumption valid that standards or new monitors would have prevented adverse outcomes noted in the *earlier* period?

Assessment of the cases in the Eichhorn report suggests that issues quite separate from monitoring standards may have been key factors.[71] Eight of the eleven cases were assessed to represent inadequate supervision of residents or CRNAs. Problems with equipment included: copper kettle that administered liquid isoflurane, positive end-expiratory pressure (PEEP) ball valve that obstructed breathing circuit, and an anesthesia machine that had a left-sided oxygen flowmeter. Whether monitoring standards would have prevented these poor outcomes is debatable. In at least two cases airway obstruction was clearly recognized but could not be alleviated. In four other cases respiration was apparently monitored by "bag motion," "rising and falling" of chest, or observation of spontaneous breathing. In one case attempts to repair the ECG monitor, a mandated standard, actually distracted the anesthesiologist from the patient.

The argument that oximetry and capnography would have prevented the adverse outcomes is stronger but not overwhelming. Neither capnography nor oximetry would have prevented liquid isoflurane administration (one case) or overdose of dextran 40 (another case). Nor would the cases of *recognized* airway obstruction have been relieved by the monitors. Finally, in two cases additional discoveries would have been necessary to avoid adverse outcome. In one, the left-sided oxygen flowmeter would need to be understood, and in the other, the site of airway obstruction at the PEEP valve would require discovery. Overall, at least three cases and possibly an additional two cases, could not have been prevented by standards or oximetry/capnography. If these nonpreventable accidents have simply not yet occurred since the standards and monitoring advances, it is premature to conclude that any risk reduction has taken place. Another validity problem with Eichhorn's assertion is that practice *before* the standards should *not* have included these activities. **Most practitioners followed mandated procedures *long before* they were so required.**

Strategies for the Individual Anesthesiologist

The larger scale efforts to adopt practice standards and monitoring techniques provide a framework to reduce risk of anesthesia, but reduction of risk can only be accomplished at the practitioner level. Although adherence to practice standards, utilization of monitors, and maintenance of vigilance are important, our roles must be enlarged to include risk education of patients, anesthesia trainees, and other hospital physicians.

The anesthesiologist must assess risks for each patient to determine an anesthetic plan that best assures safety. Conflicting goals often require prioritization. For example, the Risk Management Foundation determined that the most frequent anesthesia-related claim from 1976 to 1983 involved dental damage. In an effort to avoid dental damage, some authors have recommended use of succinylcholine rather than nondepolarizing drugs for intubation, avoidance of bite blocks at any time, and use of nasal airway.[15] Clokie, Metcalf, and Holland (1989) stated: "Vulnerable dentition may force the anaesthetist to consider the use of fiberoptic bronchoscopy, lighted stylets or the complete avoidance of tracheal intubation."[23] These recommendations may not be in the patient's best interest, although they are in the best interest of dentition. A case description by Endler et al. (1988) is pertinent. An obese pregnant patient underwent emergency cesarean section with general anesthesia by mask *because* of poor dentition. The mask airway may have prevented dental damage, but the patient died as a result of massive pulmonary aspiration of gastric contents.[74]

Quality assurance programs may facilitate im-

provement in anesthesia risk, *provided* such programs are applied appropriately. A recent report by Gold et al. (1989) stated that the most common reasons for unanticipated admission to the hospital after ambulatory surgery included pain and vomiting, whereas postoperative somnolence was substantially less frequent.[87] Is it reasonable for an individual anesthesiologist to increase the amount of administered narcotic and antiemetic drugs in an effort to meet a quality assurance (QA) committee's standard? Instead of simply assessing the frequency of admissions, quality assurance must also judge the appropriateness. Teplick et al. (1983) determined that the incidence of serious, unpredictable problems justified overnight intensive care unit admission for *all* vascular surgery patients.[198]

The individual anesthesiologist is in a key position to recognize patterns of patient risk and to develop strategies for risk reduction. Recognition that fatigue may affect physician performance should encourage scheduling of appropriate rest cycles.[162] Recognition of rapid arterial desaturation in pregnancy has emphasized adequate preoxygenation.[3] Other examples of risk reduction strategies include difficult intubation drills[38,183,208] and simulation of risk situations.[81,82]

A second role of the anesthesiologist is to educate trainees regarding the incidence and circumstances of anesthesia risk.[1] Cheney contended that in the typical scenario of esophageal intubation, the patient has a deceptively normal appearance with good skin color as a result of preoxygenation and thoracic "breath sounds." When crisis occurred, it appeared to be a life-threatening cardiac condition instead of a respiratory problem.[20] Training programs must emphasize scenarios of crisis management to facilitate appropriate therapy. When time is limited and disorder impending, thoughtful consideration of options is nearly impossible. In CPR training, the practice of drills facilitates emergency management. Are cardiac arrest drills conducted in your OR? The studies by Gaba et al. to develop anesthesia simulators hold promise.[81,82] Yet electronic equipment and mannequins are not essential for sources of anesthetic risk to be discussed early and often. Practical experience is also available. Patients with correctly placed nasogastric tubes might provide opportunity for simulation of "breath sounds over the stomach." Unfortunately, some anesthesiologists learn this sound amid the frightening confusion of an intraoperative cardiac arrest. Many such teaching opportunities are probably available. The first step is that training programs establish that risk education occupy a priority position.

A specific area for education may be in anesthesia apparatus checkout.[55] One study found that 190 meeting attendees who examined anesthesia machines with prearranged problems detected an average of only 2.2 of five faults.[13] Professional background did not influence results although persons with 10 or more years experience scored better than those with less experience. Recently, March and Crowley (1991) found that use of the FDA Anesthesia Apparatus Checkout Recommendations did not substantially improve the ability of 188 anesthesiologists to detect prearranged machine faults compared to their own checkout methods.[140] With either method the rate of detection was about one of four faults detected. Anesthesiologists in residency training detected more faults than those who primarily practiced direct patient care. Maintenance of equipment is another key issue.[33] Kumar, Hintze, and Jacob (1988) demonstrated that objective review of equipment function can enhance patient safety.[125]

The third goal of education is directed at other physicians and the hospital itself. If other physicians understand the nature of anesthetic risk, they will be supportive of practices that assure safety. The necessity of this cooperation is most clear when it is lacking. For example, a 1991 obstetric editorial by Elkington explored the question of what constitutes a rational safe policy regarding oral intake for the women in labor.[73] Traditionally, standards have restricted oral intake, a policy that Simkin (1986) found as a cause of dissatisfaction in 27% of new mothers.[186] Elkington also reviewed several studies of maternal mortality and noted that anesthetic causes of death, particularly aspiration, are infrequent. Elkington reached a conclusion *that is the antithesis of at least half a century of anesthetic risk studies:*

One can only conclude that these policies are the result of tradition rather than thoughtful decision. These policies may persist on the basis of anecdotal experience, institutional inertia to change policies begun in the 1940s, compromise with anesthesia department policy to ensure adequate coverage, exaggerated notions of risk, or fears of litigation.[73]

Included in Elkington's recommendations is the use of regional anesthesia "whenever possible as well as liberal use of supplemental techniques for inadequate blocks (e.g., low-dose ketamine or fentanyl, 30% to 40% nitrous oxide)." Although this commentary is disturbing, its publication in the prestigious *Obstetrics and Gynecology* journal, without an opposing point of view, suggests that neither patients nor their obstetricians appreciate the risks of anesthesia. **Ironically, these misperceptions may have arisen because of years of efforts by anesthesiologists that have made anesthesia relatively safe. Thus a major task for the anesthesiologist is make the risks of anesthesia clear to others.** It may necessitate the establishment of

practice guidelines. Finally, some degree of "reeducation" is necessary to undo some of the misconceptions that have evolved. **Euphemistic expressions applied to anesthetic practices should be abandoned in favor of terms that convey meaningful reality. The first term that should be abandoned is "muscle relaxant," a name that suggests a soothing, quieting effect. Why not call the drugs "paralysis agents," a name that appropriately describes their action and conveys the sense that these drugs must be used with appropriate caution?**

SUMMARY

The 1980s brought important developments to the subject of anesthetic risk. New mechanisms of injury have been identified and new strategies for risk reduction implemented. These portend progress, but some expectations may fall short.[119] This summary primarily addresses problems yet to be resolved.

One example is the multi-institutional study of anesthetic agents that was anticipated to provide new insight into the risk of anesthesia.[195] Instead, the study focused on such a small number of patients that the incidence of major adverse outcomes was too rare to draw conclusions. Another example is a large new study of pediatric anesthetic complications.[26] This study noted mortality but failed to distinguish which deaths occurred as a result of anesthesia versus surgery, particularly important because cases of cardiovascular surgery were included in the data. As a result, these two major studies focused on issues, such as blood pressure and heart rate, rather than major adverse outcomes. One reason may be that too many patients are needed to adequately study rare events. It may be that the adversarial medicolegal environment of the United States and Canada has precluded study of major adverse outcomes until the case has been financially settled, such as in the closed claims studies (which are often *years,* sometimes *decades* after the events in question). **We must instead salute the British, especially Lunn and his colleagues at Cardiff, who recognized that improvement in patient safety is a higher priority than individual lawsuits, and thus have provided the world's most comprehensive understanding of mortality and morbidity in general surgery.**[130-134,215]

A second major issue involves our assessment of progress. Anesthesia risk studies have been plagued for years by problems in counting deaths, estimating denominators, and speculating mechanisms. The 1980s brought two new strategies—practice standards and oximetry/capnography—but it is critically important to assess the impact of these developments. Unfortunately, the same counting problems and speculations appear to threaten accurate assessment

Table 35-32 Incidence of anesthetic mortality from three sources		
Lunn and Mushin[134]	CEPOD[12]	Harvard[71]
1/10,000	1/185,000	1/200,000

of change. In our opinion, the data supplied by Eichhorn[71] do *not* support that Harvard standards for *minimal* monitoring are responsible for reduction in intraoperative accidents. Evidence that oximetry/capnography decreased the intraoperative accident rate is better but not overwhelming. However, most disturbing is the assessment of overall anesthetic mortality at the Harvard hospitals. Using the Harvard insurance data from 1976 through 1988, Eichhorn notes that five deaths occurred in 1,001,000 anesthetics administered to healthy patients (Table 35-32). On this basis, Eichhorn suggests that the mortality from anesthesia is closer to that noted by CEPOD data than the "popularly cited (but old)" anesthetic mortality estimate of 1/10,000. The cases described by Eichhorn appear to be the same old types of accidents noted by Lunn et al. Why are Eichhorn's estimates so much better? The most likely explanation is that not all the deaths were counted. Specifically, only cases occurring in ASA I or II patients were counted. Only intraoperative accidents were counted, specifically excluding postoperative or transportation events. Thus no cases of postoperative respiratory insufficiency related to narcotics or muscle relaxants are mentioned. Also notably absent are deaths that resulted from intraoperative aspiration of gastric contents. It would be expected that some such events must have occurred over the 12½-year period in over 1 million anesthetics. Eichhorn clearly stated these exclusions. Yet it is also fair to say that such data cannot be directly compared to those of other studies that did not use such exclusions. **The result is that an improvement in anesthetic risk may be perceived when, in fact, no change of such magnitude may have occurred at all.** Some may contend that risk improvement must have occurred because malpractice insurance companies have actually lowered premiums for anesthesiologists. Malpractice insurance rates actually began to decrease before implemented standards and safety monitoring. Why might monitors and standards be so important for an insurance carrier? One reason is that cases of hypoventilation are a common cause of malpractice claims. Deaths from respiratory causes have occurred as a result of aspiration and difficulty with intubation, as well as esophageal intubation or airway disconnections. However, deaths due to a *known* problem, such as failed intubation that received immediate even though ineffective therapy, often result in smaller settlements than deaths that occurred because of errors that were unnoticed and untreated.[20] Oximetry and capnography should at least establish that a problem exists and give the anesthesiologist an opportunity to administer correct therapy. It may be expected that *even if no change occurs in outcome,* malpractice premiums will drop because unnoticed and untreated problems will at least be noticed and treatment attempted. Perhaps the most accurate conclusion is that many more cases must be accumulated before an accurate assessment can be made. Where does the individual anesthesiologist stand? We believe that standards and oximetry/capnography will reduce anesthetic accidents somewhat. Adverse outcomes related to difficult intubation, aspiration, and overdose may be unaffected. The best approach is to redirect education efforts as to the nature of anesthetic accidents, strategic planning for crisis management, and protocols for prevention. **Anesthetic deaths are rare events. It is possible that an anesthesiologist is as likely to encounter an out-of-hospital cardiopulmonary resusitation as an intraoperative anesthetic crisis. Most anesthesiologists routinely practice and renew skills to deal with the rare event of out-of-hospital CPR. We ought to similarly practice and teach approaches for anesthetic crises. Monitors and standards will help, but only if decisions are made correctly.**

KEY POINTS

■ Numerous recent studies, none from the United States, have suggested that the risk of death from anesthesia may be between 1 in 10,000 and 1 in 200,000. Based on this range, we really don't know very much about the exact risk of death from anesthesia. In the United States, in particular, because of legal considerations, we know nothing about the actual risk of dying from anesthesia per se.

- Another way to look at anesthesia risk is to study "critical incidents." The studies of Cooper et al. are important in this regard.
- The Beecher and Todd study published in 1954 on deaths associated with anesthesia and surgery is important for its assessment of risk as well as the illustration of bias against curare drugs.
- The Confidential Enquiry into Perioperative Death (CEPOD) study should be considered the most definitive work that exists to date on the subject of anesthesia risk. It is the most recent of many accomplishments of Dr. Lunn et al. whose work has set the standard for our current understanding of the risk of anesthesia.
- The French survey of 1977 established the real need for postanesthetic recovery room facilities.
- The New South Wales Studies of Holland et al., taken longitudinally over more than 30 years, present convincing evidence that increasing educational levels of practitioners contributed to dramatic reduction in anesthesia deaths.
- The study by Keenan and Boyan is a landmark study of intraoperative cardiac arrest. Progressive bradycardia was noted to precede cardiac arrest in over 95% of cases.
- Another landmark study is that of Caplan whose 14 cases of unexpected cardiac arrest during spinal anesthesia confirmed that the study of rare events can yield new understanding of mechanisms. Other studies emanating from the American Society of Anesthesiologists' Closed Claims Study concern respiratory events, monitoring issues, peripheral nerve damage, and obstetric cases.
- The ASA physical status system is a fairly useful predictor of patient outcome.
- This chapter places in perspective the importance of understanding the value and the dangers of single case reports regarding side effects, toxicity, or other adverse outcomes. Examined are effects from drugs like curare, nitroprusside and cyanide toxicity, isoflurane and coronary steal, and propranolol.
- A report by Bechtoldt about anesthetic deaths in North Carolina purports to be a study about provider-associated risk. This study has so many flaws as to be unusable. The issue of anesthesia risk as a function of who provides anesthesia care is a topic that cries out for legitimate study.
- The survey of Gibbs et al. of obstetric anesthesia in the United States is one of the rare studies in which U.S. outcome data are summarized. Out of 1200 hospitals surveyed, however, physician anesthesiologists, including residents, were available exclusively for labor and delivery in only 21% of hospitals. At night and on weekends, this coverage by dedicated anesthesiologists, including residents, dropped to only 15%.
- Studies of pediatric anesthesia risk clearly indicate that special care is necessary.
- It is not known whether establishment by a national organization of "standards" for anesthesia practice or "practice guidelines" will, in fact, lower anesthesia risk. There are contentions to this effect, but these studies have their problems.
- It is correct, however, that both ASA standards and new monitoring techniques have been rapidly assimilated by anesthesiologists primarily because anesthesia risk reduction is a universal goal.

SUGGESTED READINGS

Brown EM: Quality assurance in anesthesiology — the problem-oriented audit, *Anesth Analg* 63:611, 1984.

Cheney FW, Posner K, Caplan RA et al: Standard of care and anesthesiology liability, *JAMA* 261:1599, 1989.

Cote CJ, Rolf N, Liu LMP et al: A single-blind study of combined pulse oximetry and capnography in children, *Anesthesiology* 74:980, 1991.

Editorial: What is the safest anesthetic? *JAMA* 8:520, 1887.

Gravenstein JS, Holzer JF, eds: *Safety and cost containment in anesthesia,* Stoneham, Mass, 1988, Butterworths.

Kraft H: More on standards, monitoring, and outcome, *Anesthesiology* 71(3):472, 1989.

Rosenblatt RA, Hurst A: An analysis of closed obstetric malpractice claims, *Obstet Gynecol* 74:710, 1989.

Turnbull A, Tindall VR, Beard RW et al: *Report on Confidential Enquires into Maternal Deaths in England and Wales 1982-1984,* London, 1989, Her Majesty's Stationery Office.

Whitcher C, Ream AK, Parsons D et al: Anesthetic mishaps and the cost of monitoring: a proposed standard for monitoring equipment, *J Clin Monit* 4:5, 1988.

KEY REFERENCES

Beecher HK, Todd DP: A study of the deaths associated with anesthesia and surgery, *Ann Surg* 140:2, 1954.

Buck N, Devlin HB, and Lunn JL: *The Report of a Confidential Enquiry into Perioperative Deaths,* Nuffield Provincial Hospitals Trust, London, 1987, The Kings Fund Publishing House.

Caplan RA, Posner K, Ward RJ et al: Adverse respiratory events in anesthesia: a closed claims analysis, *Anesthesiology* 72:828, 1990.

Caplan RA, Ward RJ, Posner K et al: Unexpected cardiac arrest during spinal anesthesia. A closed claims analysis of predisposing factors, *Anesthesiology* 68:5, 1988.

Chadwick HS, Posner K, Caplan RA et al: A comparison of obstetric and nonobstetric anesthesia malpractice claims, *Anesthesiology* 74:242, 1991.

Cooper JB, Long CD, Newbower RS et al: Critical incidents associated with intraopertaive exchanges on anesthesia personnel, *Anesthesiology* 56:456, 1982.

Cooper JB, Newbower RS, and Kitz RJ: An analysis of major errors and equipment failures in anesthesia management: considerations for prevention and detection, *Anesthesiology* 60:34, 1984.

Cooper JB, Newbower RS, Long CD et al: Preventable anesthesia mishaps: a study of human factors, *Anesthesiology* 49:399, 1978.

Eichhorn JH: Prevention of intraoperative anesthesia accidents and related severe injury through safety monitoring, *Anesthesiology* 70:572, 1989.

Eichhorn JH, Cooper JB, Cullen DJ et al: Standards for patient monitoring during anesthesia at Harvard Medical School, *JAMA* 256:1017, 1986.

Gibbs CP, Krischer J, Peckham BM et al: Obstetric anesthesia: a national survey, *Anesthesiology* 65:298, 1986.

Hamilton WK: Unexpected deaths during anesthesia: wherein lies the cause? *Anesthesiology* 50:381, 1979.

Holland R: Anaesthetic mortality in New South Wales, *Br J Anaesth* 59:834, 1987.

Keats AS: What do we know about anesthetic mortality? *Anesthesiology* 50:387, 1979.

Keats AS: Anesthesia mortality—a new mechanism, *Anestheisology* 68:2, 1988.

Keats AS: Anesthesia mortality in perspective, *Anesth Analg* 71:113, 1990.

Keats AS: The closed claims study, *Anesthesiology* 73(2):199, 1990 (editorial).

REFERENCES

1. Allnut MF: Human-factors in accidents, *Br J Anaesth* 59:856, 1987.
2. Ament R: Classification of operating room mortality; review of cases in a pediatric medical center during the 10-year period, 1949-1958, *Anesth Analg* 39:158, 1960.
3. Archer GW, Marx GF: Arterial oxygen tension during apnea in parturient women, *Br J Anaesth* 46:358, 1974.
4. Arkins R, Smessaert AA, and Hicks RG: Mortality and morbidity in surgical patients with coronary artery disease, *JAMA* 190:485, 1964.
5. Badgwell JM, McLeod ME, and Friedberg J: Airway obstruction in infants and children, *Can Anaesth Soc J* 34:90, 1987.
6. Bechtoldt AA: Committee on anesthesia study of anesthesia-related deaths: 1969-1976, *NC Med J* 42:253, 1981.
7. Becker LC: Is isoflurane dangerous for the patient with coronary artery disease? *Anesthesiology* 66:259, 1987.
8. Beebe HG, Clagett P, DeWeese JA et al: Assessing risk associated with carotid endarterectomy, *Circulation* 79: 472, 1989.
9. Beecher HK, Todd DP: A study of the deaths associated with anesthesia and surgery, *Ann Surg* 140:2, 1954.

10. Boba A, Landmesser CM: Total cardio-respiratory collapse (cardiac arrest): contributory and causative errors of omission and commission for which anesthesiologists must assume responsibility, *NY State J Med* 61:2928, 1961.
11. Bodlander FMS: Deaths associated with anaesthesia, *Br J Anaesth* 47:36, 1975.
12. Buck N, Devlin HB, and Lunn JL: *The Report of a Confidential Enquiry into Perioperative Deaths,* Nuffield Provincial Hospitals Trust, London, 1987, The Kings Fund Publishing House.
13. Buffington CW, Ramanathan S, and Turndorf H: Detection of anesthesia machine faults, *Anesth Analg* 63:79, 1984.
14. Burnham M, Craig DB: A post-anaesthetic follow-up program, *Can Anaesth Soc J* 27(2):164, 1980.
15. Burton JF, Baker AB: Dental damage during anesthesia and surgery, *Anaesth Intens Care* 15:262, 1987.
16. Caplan RA, Posner K, Ward RJ et al: Adverse respiratory events in anesthesia: a closed claims analysis, *Anesthesiology* 72:828, 1990.
17. Caplan RA, Ward RJ, Posner K et al: Unexpected cardiac arrest during spinal anesthesia. A closed claims analysis of

predisposing factors, *Anesthesiology* 68:5, 1988.
18. Chadwick HS, Posner K, Caplan RA et al: A comparison of obstetric and nonobstetric anesthesia malpractice claims, *Anesthesiology* 74:242, 1991.
19. Charlson ME, Ales KA, Simon R et al: Why predictive indexes perform less well in validation studies, *Arch Intern Med* 147:2155, 1987.
20. Cheney FW: Anesthesia: potential risks and causes of incidents. In Gravenstein JS, Holzer JF, eds: *Safety and cost containment in anesthesia,* Stoneham, Mass, 1988, Butterworths.
21. Cheney FW: Anaesthesia and the law: the North American experience, *Br J Anaesth* 59:891, 1987.
22. Clifton BS, Hotton WIT: Deaths associated with anaesthesia, *Br J Anaesth* 35:250, 1963.
23. Clokie C, Metcalf I, and Holland: Dental trauma in anaesthesia, *Can J Anaesth* 36(6):675, 1989.
24. Cogbill CL: Operation in the aged, *Arch Surg* 94:202, 1967.
25. Cohen DE, Downes JJ, and Raphaely RC: What difference does pulse oximetry make? *Anesthesiology* 68:181, 1988.
26. Cohen MM, Cameron CB, and Duncan

PG: Pediatric anesthesia morbidity and mortality in the perioperative period, *Anesth Analg* 70:160, 1990.

27. Cohen MM, Duncan PG, Pope WDB et al: A survey of 112,000 anaesthetics at one teaching hospital (1975-83), *Can Anaesth Soc J* 33:22, 1986.

28. Cohen MM, Duncan PG, and Tate RB: Does anaesthesia contribute to operative mortality? *JAMA* 260:2859, 1988.

29. Cole WH: Medical differences between the young and the aged, *J Am Geriatr Soc* 18:589, 1970.

30. Collins VJ: Fatalities in anesthesia and surgery: fundamental considerations, *JAMA* 172:549, 1960.

31. Cooper JB, Cullen DJ, Nemeskal R et al: Effects of information feedback and pulse oximetry on the incidence of anesthesia complications, *Anesthesiology* 67:686, 1987.

32. Cooper JB, Long CD, and Newbower RS: Human error in anesthesia management. In Grundy BL, Gravenstein JS, eds: *Quality of care in anesthesia,* Springfield, Ill, 1982, Charles C Thomas.

33. Cooper JB, Long CD, Newbower RS et al: Critical incidents associated with intraopertaive exchanges on anesthesia personnel, *Anesthesiology* 56:456, 1982.

34. Cooper JB, Newbower RS, and Kitz RJ: An analysis of major errors and equipment failures in anesthesia management: considerations for prevention and detection, *Anesthesiology* 60:34, 1984.

35. Cooper JB, Newbower RS, Long CD et al: Preventable anesthesia mishaps: a study of human factors, *Anesthesiology* 49:399, 1978.

36. Cooperman   LH: Succinylcholine-induced hyperkalemia in neuromuscular disease, *JAMA* 213:1867, 1970.

37. Cooperman M, Pflug B, Martin EW et al: Cardiovascular risk factors in patients with peripheral vascular disease, *Surgery* 84:505, 1978.

38. Cormach RS, Lehane J: Difficult tracheal intubation in obstetrics, *Anaesthesia* 39:1105, 1984.

39. Cote CJ, Goldstein EA, Cote MA et al: A single-blind study of pulse oximetry in children, *Anesthesiology* 68:184, 1988.

40. Crandell WB, Pappas SG, and MacDonald A: Nephrotoxicity associated with methoxyflurane anesthesia, *Anesthesiology* 27:591, 1966.

41. Crawford ES, Morris GC, and Howell JF: Operative risk in patients with previous coronary artery bypass, *Ann Thorac Surg* 26:215, 1978.

42. Crawford JS: Some maternal complications of epidural analgesia for labour, *Anaesthesia* 40:1219, 1985.

43. Crawford JS: The anesthetists's contribution to maternal mortality, *Br J Anaesth* 42:70, 1970.

44. Davies DD: Anaesthetic mortality in tonsillectomy and adenoidectomy, *Br J Anaesth* 36:110, 1964.

45. Del Guercio LRM, Cohn JD: Monitoring operative risk in the elderly, *JAMA* 243:1350, 1980.

46. Denny JL, Denson JS: Risk of surgery in patients over 90, *Geriatrics* 27:115, Jan 1972.

47. Derrington MC, Smith G: A review of studies of anaesthetic risk, morbidity and mortality, *Br J Anaesth* 59:815, 1987.

48. Desmeules H, Fourneir L, and Tremblay PR: Systematic changes in the elderly patient and their anaesthetic implications, *Can Anaesth Soc J* 32:184, 1985.

49. Detsky AS, Abrams HB, Forbath N et al: Cardiac assessment for patients undergoing noncardiac surgery, a multifactorial clinical risk index, *Arch Intern Med* 146:2131, 1986.

50. Dierdorf SF, Krishna G: Anesthetic management of neonatal surgical emergencies, *Anesth Analg* 60:204, 1981.

51. Dinnick DP: Deaths associated with anesthesia, *Anaesthesia* 19:536, 1964.

52. Djokovic JL, Hedley-Whyte J: Prediction of outcome of surgery and anesthesia in patients over 80, *JAMA* 242:2301, 1979.

53. Domaingue CM, Davies JM, and Cronin KD: Cardiovascular risk factors in patients for vasuclar surgery, *Anaesth Intensive Care* 10:324, 1982.

54. Dornette WHL, Orth OS: Death in the operating room, *Anesth Analg* 35:545, 1956.

55. Dorsch JA, Dorsch SE: *Understanding anesthesia equipment, construction, care and complications,* ed 2, Baltimore, MD, 1984, Williams & Wilkins.

56. Dripps RD: Hazards of immediate postoperative period, *JAMA* 165:795, 1957.

57. Dripps RD, Lamont A, and Eckenhoff JE: The role of anesthesia in surgical mortality, *JAMA* 178:261, 1961.

58. Dry TJ: The surgical risk of patients with heart disease, *Surg Gynecol Obstet* 120, July 1952.

59. Duncan PG, Cohen MM: Postoperative complications: factors of significance to anaesthetic practice, *Can J Anaesth* 34(1):2, 1987.

60. Eagle KA, Coley CM, Newell JB et al: Combining clinical and thallium data optimizes preoperative assessment of cardiac risk before major vascular surgery, *Ann Intern Med* 110:859, 1989.

61. Eagle KA, Singer DE, Brewster DC et al: Dipyridamole-thallium scanning in patients undergoing vascular surgery, *JAMA* 257:2185, 1987.

62. Easton JD, Sherman DG: Stroke and mortality rate in carotid endarterectomy: 228 consecutive operations, *Stroke* 8:565, 1977.

63. ECRI Technology Assessment: deaths during general anesthesia, *J Health Care Technol* 1:155, 1985.

64. Editorial: The national halothane study, *JAMA* 197:811, 1966.

65. Editorial: Complications of anaesthsia in infants and children. *Lancet* 2:1466, 1988.

66. Editorial: NCEPOD (National confidential enquiry into perioperative deaths), *Lancet* 2:1320, 1988.

67. Edmunds LH, Stephenson LW, Edie RN et al: Open-heart surgery in octogenarians, *N Engl J Med* 319:131, 1988.

68. Edwards G, Morton HJV, Pask EA et al: Deaths associated with anaesthesia: a report on 1,000 cases, *Anaesthesia* 11:194, 1956.

69. Eerola M, Eerola R, Kaukinen S et al: Risk factors in surgical patients with verified preoperative myocardial infarction, *Acta Anaesthesiol Scand* 24:219, 1980.

70. Ehrenhaft JL, Eastwood DW, and Morris LE: Analysis of twenty-seven cases of acute arrest, *J Thorac Surg* 22:592, 1951.

71. Eichhorn JH: Prevention of intraoperative anesthesia accidents and related severe injury through safety monitoring, *Anesthesiology* 70:572, 1989.

72. Eichhorn JH, Cooper JB, Cullen DJ et al: Standards for patient monitoring during anesthesia at Harvard Medical School, *JAMA* 256:1017, 1986.

73. Elkington KW: At the water's edge: where obstetrics and anesthesia meet, *Obstet Gynecol* 77:304, 1991.

74. Endler GC, Mariona FG, Sokol RJ et al: Anesthesia-related maternal mortality in Michigan, 1972-1984, *Am J Obstet Gynecol* 159:187, 1988.

75. Epstein RM: Morbidity and mortality from anesthesia: a continuing problem, *Anesthesiology* 49:388, 1978.

76. Farrow SC, Fowkes FGR, Lunn JN et al: Epidemiology in anaesthesia II: factors affecting mortailty in hospital, *Br J Anaesth* 54:811, 1982.

77. Flanagan JC: The critical incident technique, *Psychol Bull* 51:327, 1954.

78. Foster EO, Davis KB, Carpenter JA et al: Risk of noncardiac operation in patients with defined coronary disease: The Coronary Artery Surgery study (CASS) Registry Experience, *Ann Thorac Surg* 41:42, 1986.

79. Fowkes FGR, Lunn JN, Farrow SC et al: Epidemiology in anaesthesia, III: mortality risk in patients with coexisting physical disease, *Br J Anaesth* 54:819, 1982.

80. Fraser JG, Ramachandran PR, and Davis HS: Anesthesia and recent myocardial infarction, *JAMA* 199:318, 1967.

81. Gaba DM, De Anda A: A comprehensive anesthesia simulation environment: recreating the operating room for research and training, *Anesthesiology* 69:387, 1988.

82. Gaba DM, Maxwell M, and DeAnda A: Anesthetic mishaps: breaking the chain of accident evolution, *Anesthesiology* 66:670, 1987.

83. Gebbie D: Anaesthesia and death, *Can Anaesth Soc J* 13:390, 1966.

84. Gerson MC, Hurst JM, Hertzberg VS et al: Cardiac prognosis in noncardiac geriatric surgery, *Ann Intern Med* 103:832, 1985.

85. Gibbs CP, Krischer J, Peckham BM et al: Obstetric anesthesia: a national survey, *Anesthesiology* 65:298, 1986.

86. Gillespie DM: Death during anesthesia, *Br J Anaesth* 19:1, 1944.

87. Gold BS, Kitz DS, Lecky JH et al: Unanticipated admission to the hospital following ambulatory surgery, *JAMA* 262:3008, 1989.

88. Goldman L: Cardiac risks and compli-

cations of noncardiac surgery, *Ann Intern Med* 98:504, 1983.

89. Goldman L, Caldera DL: Risks of general anesthesia and elective operation in the hypertensive patient, *Anesthesiology* 50:285, 1979.

90. Goldman L, Caldera DL, Nussbaum SR et al: Multifactorial index on cardiac risk in noncardiac surgical procedures, *N Engl J Med* 297:845, 1977.

91. Goldstein A, Keats AS: The risk of anesthesia, *Anesthesiology* 33:130, 1970.

92. Gordon RA, Britt BA, and Kalow W, eds: *International symposium on malignant hyperthermia*, Springfiled, Ill, 1973, Charles C Thomas.

93. Graff TD, Phillips OC, Benson DW et al: Baltimore Anesthesia Study Committee: factors in pediatric anesthesia mortality, *Anesth Analg* 43:407, 1964.

94. Gravenstein JS, Holzer JF, eds: *Safety and cost containment in anesthesia*, Stoneham, Mass, 1988, Butterworths.

95. Green J, Wintfeld N, Sharkey P et al: The importance of severity of illness in assessing hospital mortality, *JAMA* 263:241, 1990.

96. Greenburg AG, Saik RP, and Pridham D: Influence of age on mortality of colon surgery, *Am J Surg* 150:65, 1985.

97. Greiss FC, Anderson SG: Elimination of maternal deaths from anesthesia, *Obstet Gynecol* 29:677, 1967.

98. Grimes DA, Cates W: Deaths from paracervical anesthesia used for first trimester abortion 1972-1975, *N Engl J Med* 295:1397, 1976.

99. Hamilton WK: Unexpected deaths during anesthesia: wherein lies the cause? *Anesthesiology* 50:381, 1979.

100. Harrison GG: Anaesthetic contributory death—its incidence and causes, *S Afr Med J* Part I, 42:514, 1968; Part II, 42:544, 1968.

101. Harrison GG: Death attributable to anesthesia: a 10 year survey (1967-1976), *Br J Anaesth* 50:1041, 1978.

102. Hatton F, Tiret L, Vourc'h G et al: Morbidity and mortality associated with anaesthesia—French Survey: preliminary results. In Vickers MD, Lunn JN, eds: *Mortality in anaesthesia*, Berlin, 1983, Springer-Verlag.

103. Holland R: Special committee investigating deaths under anaesthesia: report on 745 classified cases, *Med J Aust* 1:573, 1970.

104. Holland R: Anaesthetic mortality in New South Wales, *Br J Anaesth* 59:834, 1987.

105. Hornbein TJ: The settting of standards of care, *JAMA* 256:1040, 1986.

106. Hosking MP, Warner MA, Lobdell CM et al: Outcomes of surgery in patients 90 years of age and older, *JAMA* 261:1909, 1989.

107. Hotchkiss WS: Patent ductus arteriosus and the occasional cardiac surgeon, *JAMA* 173:244, 1960.

108. Hovi-Viander M: Death associated with anaesthesia in Finland, *Br J Anaesth* 52:483, 1980.

109. Jeffrey CC, Kunsman J, Cullen DJ et al: A prospective evaluation of cardiac risk index, *Anesthesiology* 58:462, 1983.

110. Jones L: HCFA releases hospital mortality studies, *American Medical News*, Jan 12, 1990.

111. Jude JR, Kouwenhoven WB, and Knickerbocker GG: Cardiac arrest: report of application of external cardiac massage on 118 patients, *JAMA* 178:85, 1961.

112. Kannel WB, McGee D, and Gordon T: A general cardiovascular risk profile: the Framingham study, *Am J Cardiol* 38:46, 1976.

113. Kaunitz AM, Hughes JM, Grimes DA et al: Causes of maternal mortality in the United States, *Obstet Gynecol* 65:605, 1985.

114. Keats AS: The ASA classification of physical status—a recapitulation, *Anesthesiology* 49:233, 1978.

115. Keats AS: What do we know about anesthetic mortality? *Anesthesiology* 50:387, 1979.

116. Keats AS: Anesthesia mortality—a new mechanism, *Anestheisology* 68:2, 1988.

117. Keats AS: Anesthesia mortality in perspective, *Anesth Analg* 71:113, 1990.

118. Keats AS: The closed claims study, *Anesthesiology* 73(2):199, 1990 (editorial).

119. Keats AS, Siker ES: International symposium on preventable anesthetic morbidity and mortality, Boston, Massachusetts, Oct 8-19, 1984, *Anesthesia* 63:349, 1985.

120. Keenan RL, Boyan CP: Cardiac arrest due to anesthesia: a study of incidence and causes, *JAMA* 253:2373, 1985.

121. Kennedy JW, Kaiser GC, Fisher LD et al: Clinical and angiographic predictors of operative mortality from the collaborative study in coronary artery surgery (CASS), *Circulation* 63:793, 1981.

122. Klaucke DN, Rericki DA, and Brown RA: *Investigation of mortality and severe morbidity associated with anesthesia: pilot study final report*, American Association of Anesthesiologists and Centers for Disease Control, Atlanta, Ga, Dec 1, 1988.

123. Kroll DA, Caplan RA, Posner K et al: Nerve injury associated with anesthesia, *Anesthesiology* 73:202, 1990.

124. Kronenberg RS, Drage GW: Attenuation of the ventilatory and heart rate responses to hypoxia and hypocapnia with aging in normal man, *J Clin Invest* 52:1812, 1973.

125. Kumar V, Hintze MS, and Jacob AM: A random survey of anesthesia machines and ancillary monitors in 45 hospitals, *Anesth Analg* 67:644, 1988.

126. Kurth CD, Spitzer AR, Broennle AM et al: Postoperative apnea in preterm infants, *Anesthesiology* 66:483, 1987.

127. Lockhart PB, Feldbau EV, Gabel RS et al: Dental complications during and after tracheal intubation, *J Am Dent Assoc* 112:480, 1986.

128. Longstreth WT, Inui TS, Cobb LA et al: Neurologic recovery after out-of-hospital cardiac arrest, *Ann Intern Med* 98(part I):588, 1983.

129. Lowenstein E: Perianesthetic ischemic episodes cause myocardial infarction in humans—a hypothesis confirmed, *Anesthesiology* 62:103, 1985.

130. Lunn JN: Anaesthetist, lawyers, and the public, *Anaesthesia* 44:1, 1989.

131. Lunn JN, Devlin HB: Lessons from the confidential enquiry into perioperative deaths in three NHS regions, *Lancet* 2:1384, 1987.

132. Lunn JN, Farrow SC, Fowkes FGR et al: Epidemiology in anaesthesia I: anaesthetic practice over 20 years, *Br J Anaesth* 54:803, 1982.

133. Lunn JN, Hunter AR, and Scott DB: Anaesthesia related surgical mortality, *Anaesthesia* 38:1090, 1983.

134. Lunn JN, Mushin WW: *Mortality associated with anaesthesia*, Nuffield Provincial Hospitals Trust, London, 1982, The Kings Fund Publishing House.

135. MacIntosh RR: Deaths under anaesthetics, *Br J Anaesth* 21:107, 1948.

136. MacKenzie CR, Charlson ME: Assessment of perioperative risk in the patient with diabetes mellitus, *Surg Gynecol Obstet* 167:293, 1988.

137. Mahar LJ, Steen PA, Tinker JH et al: Perioperative myocardial infarction in patients with coronary artery disease with and without aorto-coronary artery bypass grafts, *J Thorac Cardiovasc Surg* 76:533, 1978.

138. Mangano DT: Anesthetics, coronary artery disease, and outcome: unresolved controversies, *Anesthesiology* 70:175, 1989.

139. Mangano DT, Browner WS, Hollenberger M et al: Association of perioperative myocardial ischemia with cardiac morbidity and mortality in men undergoing noncardiac surgery, *N Engl J Med* 323:1781, 1990.

140. March MG, Crowley JJ: An evaluation of anesthesiologists' present checkout methods and the validity of the FDA checklist, *Anesthesiology* 75:724, 1991.

141. Marcus AD: Suits spur FDA probe of blood pressure drug's label, *Wall Street Journal* p B-11, Feb 14, 1990.

142. Marx GR: Maternal complications of regional analgesia, *Reg Anaesth* 6:104, 1981.

143. Marx GF: Comment, *Obstet Anesth Digest* 110, Sept 1985.

144. Marx GH, Matteo CV, and Orkin LR: Computer analysis of post-anesthetic deaths, *Anesthesiology* 39:54, 1973.

145. McKay WPS, Noble WH: Critical accidents detected by pulse oximetry during anesthesia, *Can J Anaesth* 35:265, 1988.

146. Memery HN: Anesthesia mortality in private practice, *JAMA* 194:127, 1965.

147. Miller RR, Olson HG, Amsterdam EA et al: Propranolol withdrawal rebound phenomenon, *N Engl J Med* 293:416, 1975.

148. Minuck M: Death in the operating room, *Can Anaesth Soc J* 14:197, 1967.

149. Mohr DN: Estimation of surgical risk in the elderly: a correlative view, *Am Geriatr Soc* 31:99, 1983.

150. Moir DD: Maternal mortality and anaesthesia, *Br J Anaesth* 52:1, 1980.

151. Montoyama EK, Glazener CH: Hypoxemia after general anesthesia in children, *Anesth Analg* 65:267, 1986.

152. Morgan M: Anaesthetic contribution to maternal mortality, *Br J Anaesth* 59:842, 1987.

153. Morley JE, Reese SS: Clinical implications of the aging heart, *Am J Med* 86:77, 1989.

154. Morrison JN, Richardson J, Dunn L et al: Respiratory muscle performance in normal elderly subjects and patients with COPD, *Chest* 95:90, 1989.

155. Moses LE, Mosteller F: Institutional differences in postoperative death rates; commentary on some findings of the National Halothane Study, *JAMA* 203: 150, 1968.

156. Murphy DJ, Murray AM, Robinson BE et al: Outcomes of cardiopulmonary resuscitation in the elderly, *Ann Intern Med* 111:199, 1989.

157. North American Symptomatic Carotid Endarterectomy Trial collaborators: Beneficial effects of carotid endarterectomy in symptomatic patients with high grade carotid stenoses, *N Engl J Med* 325:445, 1991.

158. Olsson GL, Hallen B: Cardiac arrest during anaesthesia. A computer-aided study in 250,543 anaesthetics, *Acta Anaesthesiol Scand* 32:653, 1988.

159. Ong B, Cohen M, Cumming M et al: Obstetrical anaesthesia at Winnipeg Women's Hospital 1975-1983: anaesthetic techniques and complications, *Can J Anaesth* 34(3):294, 1987.

160. Orkin FK: Practice standards: the Midas touch or the emperor's new clothes? *Anesthesiology* 70(4):567, 1989.

161. Owens WD: ASA physical status classifications: a study of consistency of ratings, *Anesthesiology* 49:239, 1978.

162. Parker JBR: The effects of fatigue on physician performance—an underestimated cause of physician impairment and increased patient risk, *Can J Anaesth* 34(5):489, 1987.

163. Phillips OC, Frazier TM, Graff TD et al: The Baltimore Anesthesia Study Committee. A review of 1,024 postoperative deaths, *JAMA* 174:2015, 1960.

164. Port S, Cobb FR, Coleman E et al: Effect of age on the response of the left ventricular ejection fraction to exercise, *N Engl J Med* 303:1133, 1980.

165. Rackow H, Salanitre E, and Green LT: Frequency of cardiac arrest associated with anesthesia in infants and children, *Pediatrics* 28:697, 1961.

166. Rao TL, Jacobs KH, and El-Etr AA: Reinfarction following anesthesia in patients with myocardial infarction, *Anesthesiology* 59:499, 1983.

167. Reiz S, Balfors E, Sorensen MB et al: Isoflurane—a powerful coronary vasodilator in patients with coronary artery disease, *Anesthesiology* 59:91, 1983.

168. Richardson MA, Colton RT: Anatomic abnormalities of the pediatric airway, *Pediatr Clin North Am* 31:821, 1984.

169. Riding JE: Minor complications of general anaesthesia, *Br J Anaesth* 49:91, 1975.

170. Roberts SL, Gilbert M, and Tinker JH: Isoflurane has a greater margin of safety than halothane in swine with and without major surgery or critical coronary stenosis, *Anesth Analg* 66:485, 1987.

171. Rochat RW, Koonin LM, Atrash HK, et al: Maternal mortality in the United States: report from the Maternal Mortality Collaborative, *Obstet Gynecol* 72: 91, 1988.

172. Rosen M: Deaths associated with anesthesia for obstetrics, *Anaesthesia* 36:145, 1981 (editorial).

173. Ross AF, Tinker JH: Anesthesia risk. In Miller RD, ed: *Anesthesia*, ed 3, New York, 1990, Churchill-Livingstone.

174. Roy WL, Lerman J: Laryngospasm in paediatric anaesthesia, *Can J Anaesth* 35:93, 1988.

175. Ruth HS: Anesthesia study commissions, *JAMA* 127:514, 1945.

176. Saklad M: Grading of patients for surgical procedures, *Anesthesia* 2:281, 1941.

177. Salem MR, Bennett EJ, Schweiss JF et al: Cardiac arrest related to anesthesia; contributing factors in infants and children, *JAMA* 233:238, 1975.

178. Sapala JA, Ponka JL, and Duverrow WSC: Operative and nonoperative risks in the cardiac patient, *J Am Geriatr Soc* 23:529, 1978.

179. Schapira M, Keyes ER, and Hurwitt ES: An analysis of deaths in the operating room and within 24 hours of surgery, *Anesth Analg* 39:149, 1960.

180. Scher KS, Tice DA: Operative risk in patients with previous coronary artery bypass, *Arch Surg* 111:807, 1976.

181. Scott DL: Anaesthetic experiences in 1,300 major geriatric operations, *Br J Anaesth* 33:354, 1961.

182. Scott NB, Kehlet H: Regional anesthesia and surgical morbidity, *Br J Surg* 75:299, 1988.

183. Sellick BA: Cricoid pressure to control regurgitation of stomach contents during induction of anesthesia, *Lancet* 2:404, 1961.

184. Shah KB, Kleinman BS, Rao TLK et al: Angina and other risk factors in patients with cardiac diseases undergoing noncardiac operations, *Anesth Analg* 70:240, 1990.

185. Shevde K, Panagopoulos G: A survey of 800 patients' knowledge, attitudes, and concerns regarding anesthesia, *Anesth Analg* 73:190, 1991.

186. Simkin P: Stress, pain and catecholamines in labor. Part 2. Stress associated with childbearing events: a pilot survey of new mothers, *Birth* 13:234, 1986.

187. Slogoff S, Keats AS: Does perioperative myocardial ischemia lead to postoperative myocardial infarction? *Anesthesiology* 62:107, 1985.

188. Slogoff S, Keats AS: Randomized trial of primary anesthetic agents on outcome of coronary artery bypass operation, *Anesthesiology* 70:179, 1989.

189. Smith G, Norman J: Complications and medico-legal aspects of anaesthesia, *Br J Anaesth* 59:813, 1987.

190. Snow J: *On chloroform and other anesthetics,* London, 1858, John Churchill.

191. Snow JC, Harano M, and Balogh K: Post intubation granuloma of the larnyx, *Anesth Analg* 45:425, 1966.

192. Spence AA: The lessons of CEPOD, *Br J Anaesth* 60:753, 1988.

193. Stafford RS: Alternative strategies for controlling rising cesarean section rates, *JAMA* 263:683, 1990.

194. Steen PA, Tinker JH, and Tarhan S: Myocardial reinfarction after anesthesia and surgery, *JAMA* 239:2566, 1978.

195. Strunin L, Forrest JB, Lunn JN et al: Panel summary: toward excellence in anesthesia, *Can J Anaesth* 35:278, 1988.

196. Subcommittee on the National Halothane Study of the Committee on Anesthesia, National Academy of Sciences—National Research Council: Summary of the National Halothane Study; possible association between halothane anesthesia and postoperative hepatic necrosis, *JAMA* 197:775, 1966.

197. Tarhan S, Moffitt EA, Taylor WF et al: Myocardial infarction after general anesthesia, *JAMA* 220:1451, 1972.

198. Teplick R, Caldera DL, Gilbert JP et al: Benefit of elective intensive care admission after certain operations, *Anesth Analg* 62:572, 1983.

199. Tinker JH: Perioperative myocardial infarction, *Semin Anesth* 1:253, 1982.

200. Tinker JH, Dull DL, Caplan RA et al: Role of monitoring devices in prevention of anesthetic mishaps: a closed claims analysis, *Anesthesiology* 71:541, 1989.

201. Tinker JH, Michenfelder J: Sodium nitroprusside: pharmacology, toxicity, and therapuetics, *Anesthesiology* 45:340, 1976.

202. Tiret L, Desmonts JM, Hatton F et al: Complications associated with anaesthesia—a prospective survey in France, *Can Anaesth Soc J* 33:336, 1986.

203. Tiret L, Hatton F, Desmonts JM et al: Prediction of outcome of anaesthesia in patients over 40 years: a multifactorial risk index, *Stat Med* 7:947, 1988.

204. Tiret L, Nivoche Y, Hatton F et al: Complications related to anaesthesia in infants and children, *Br J Anaesth* 61:263, 1988.

205. Tolmie JD, Joyce TH, and Mitchell GD: Succinylcholine danger in the burned patient, *Anesthesiology* 28:467, 1967.

206. Topkins MJ, Artusio JF: Myocardial infarction and surgery, *Anesth Analg* 43:716, 1964.

207. Tuman KJ, McCarthy RJ, and Spiess BD: Does choice of anesthetic agent significantly affect outcome after coronary artery surgery? *Anesthesiology* 70: 189, 1989.

208. Tunstall ME: Failed intubation drill, *Anaesthesia* 31:856, 1976.

209. Turnbull KW, Farcourt-Smith PF, and Banting GC: Death within 48 hours of anesthesia at the Vancouver General Hospital, *Can Anaesth Soc J* 27:159, 1980.

210. Turnbull A, Tindall VR, Beard RW et al: *Report on Confidential Enquiries into Maternal Deaths in England and Wales 1982-1984,* London, 1989, Her Majesty's Stationery Office.

211. US Bureau of Census: *Vital and health statistics of the United States,* 1988 ed, 1987, Washington, DC, US Government Printing Office.

212. Utting JE: Pitfalls in anaesthetic practice, *Br J Anaesth* 59:877, 1987.

213. Utting JE, Gray TC, and Shelley FC: Human misadventure in anesthesia, *Can Anaesth Soc J* 26:472, 1979.

214. Vacanti CJ, Van Houten RJ, and Hill RC: A statistical analysis of the relationship of physical status to postoperative mortality in 68,388 cases, *Anesth Analg* 49:564, 1970.

215. Vickers MD, Lunn JN: *Mortality in an-aesthesia,* Berlin, 1983, Springer-Verlag.

216. Viljoen JF, Estafanous G, and Kellner GA: Propranolol and cardiac surgery, *J Thorac Cardiovasc Surg* 64:826, 1972.

217. Wahba WM: Influence of aging on lung function—clinical significance of charges from age twenty, *Anesth Analg* 62:764, 1983.

218. Waller BF, Roberts WC: Cardiovascular disease in the very elderly: analysis of 40 necropsy patients aged 90 years and over, *Am J Cardiol* 51:40, 1983.

219. Waters J, Wilkinson C, Golmon M et al: Evaluation of cardiac risk in noncardiac surgical patients, *Anesthesiology* 55:A343, 1981.

220. West JP: Cardiac arrest during anesthesia and surgery, *Ann Surg* 140:623, 1954.

221. Wylie WD: "There but for the grace of God . . ." *Ann R Coll Surg Engl* 56:171, 1975.

222. Yeager MP, Glass DD, Neff RK et al: Epidural anesthesia and analgesia in high risk surgical patients, *Anesthesiology* 66:729, 1987.

223. Zeldin RA: Assessing cardiac risk in patients who undergo noncardiac surgical procedures, *Can J Surg* 27:402, 1984.

CHAPTER 36

Critical Incidents in Anesthesia

HUGH L. FLANAGAN

History
  Critical incidents in the 19th century
  Development of critical incident technique
Detection of Critical Incidents
Prevention of Critical Incidents

HISTORY

Critical incident technique (CIT) was applied to the study of anesthesia mishaps by Cooper et al. in 1975.[12] They defined a critical incident as[11]:

... A human error or equipment failure that could have led (if not discovered or corrected in time) or did lead to an undesirable outcome, ranging from increased length of hospital stay to death.

Although this technique was not described until the 20th century, early anesthesiologists reported anesthesia-related incidents that would meet Cooper's critical incident criteria even today. **Anesthesiologists of the 19th century developed the rudiments of critical incident analysis, peer review, and patient safety activities.** Public outcry ensued after early anesthesia accidents. Adverse outcomes were frequently reported in the medical journals for peer review.[45,48] The Boston Society for Improvement of Medical Care investigated anesthesia safety in the mid-19th century. After reviewing the world literature of deaths related to ether anesthesia ($n = 41$), the committee concluded[28]:

Sulphuric ether is safer than any other anesthetic and this conviction is gradually gaining ground.

The advantages of chloroform are exclusively those of convenience. Its dangers are not averted by its admixture with sulphuric ether in any proportions. The combinations of these two agents cannot be too strongly denounced as a treacherous and dangerous compound. Chloric ether, being a solution of chloroform in alcohol needs the same condemnation.

Critical Incidents in the 19th Century

The safety of ether anesthesia was unknown when first publicly demonstrated by Charles Morton on Oct. 16, 1846. Anesthesia safety was subsequently addressed by Snow's treatise on the inhalation of ether published in 1847.[47] He described 75 cases of successful ether anesthesia at two hospitals in London. There were no deaths during induction of anesthesia or the operation itself in this series. He reported five deaths in the postoperative period. The hospital course and autopsies of those patients indicate that the majority died of sepsis ("erysipelas") in that prelisterian era. Anesthetic mortality was therefore less than 1.3%. However, the surgical mortality of limb amputation was 23%. This no doubt made the anesthesia risk seem trivial when compared to the benefits.

The first anesthetic death from chloroform was reported in 1848 by Snow.[48] Hanna Greener, 15 years old, died suddenly during the excision of a toenail while she was receiving chloroform general anesthesia.[34,42] This event raised concern about the safety of chloroform, particularly since the patient had previously had a toenail excised while receiving ether anesthesia without incident. In addition, death would not have been anticipated if the surgery had been performed without anesthesia. Controversy ensued for many years regarding the safety of ether vs. chloroform.

659

Nineteenth-century equipment failures were also reported. Josiah Flagg's textbook of anesthesia published in 1851 included chapters on the production and use of ether and chloroform. He described an occurrence when a patient suffered awareness and extreme pain during a dental extraction with ether. Afterward, Flagg was perplexed by the lack of ether odor on the breath of his patient. He stated "I then examined the mouth-piece of my inhaler, and discovered that the inner valve had stuck in such a manner as to preclude the possibility of the passage of its vapour!"[20] This represents an early critical incident related to equipment failure.

The early anesthesiologists recognized that an obstructed airway was a critical incident that could lead to asphyxia and cardiac arrest. Primitive appliances were developed to assist in opening the mouth (Fig. 36-1) and retracting the tongue (Fig. 36-2) when the airway was obstructed.[39, 43] Apnea or hypoventilation was considered an "anesthesia accident." Recommended treatment ranged from slapping the chest vigorously with a wet towel, to artificial respiration[43] (Fig. 36-3) or transcutaneous "galvanic stimulation" (pacing) of the phrenic nerves in the neck.[33]

Conditions for advances in anesthesia safety were not favorable in the mid- to late 19th century. **Patient monitoring was subjective, accomplished by the unaided human senses. Anesthesia records were not seriously considered until advocated by Cushing in 1895.**[2] Few physiologic data were available following an intraoperative death. Measurement of blood pressure by sphygmomanometry[18] and electrocardiographic[19] monitoring of the heart would not occur

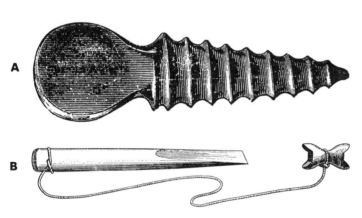

Fig. 36-1. Oral screw (**A**), and wooden wedge with mouth gag (**B**), used to separate clenched teeth during airway obstruction in patients under general anesthesia. (From Patton J: *Anaesthesia and anaesthetics,* Chicago, 1903, Cleveland Press, and Robinson H, ed: *Anaesthetics and their administration,* ed 2, London, 1920, Henry Frowde, Hodder & Stoughton.)

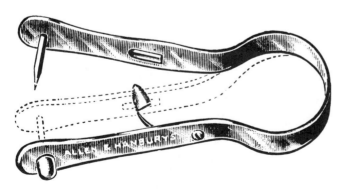

Fig. 36-2. Instrument used to grasp (pierce) the tongue and pull it anteriorly to relieve airway obstruction in patients under general anesthesia. (From Robinson H: *Anaesthetics and their administration,* ed 2, London, 1920, Henry Frowde, Hodder & Stoughton.)

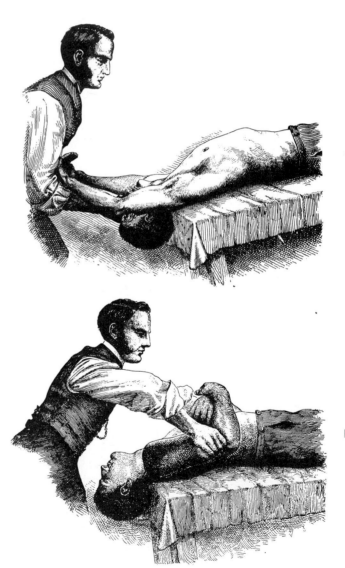

Fig. 36-3. Treatment of an anesthesia accident (apnea) by Silvester's method of artificial respiration. **A,** Inspiration. **B,** Expiration. (From Robinson H, ed: *Anaesthetics and their administration,* ed 2, London, 1920, Henry Frowde, Hodder & Stoughton.)

until the 20th century. Autopsies, primitive by today's standards, usually failed to determine the cause of death during anesthesia.

Lyman's textbook, published in 1881, prophetically included chapters on anesthesia accidents and medicolegal problems.[33] Sykes' review of the first 100 years of anesthesia included a list of lethal critical incidents in a chapter entitled "Thirty-seven Little Things Which Have Caused Death"[51] (Box 36-1).

As the numbers of anesthetics administered grew, early investigators published morbidity and mortality studies. Comparison of the different studies was confounded by many variables. **Figures for death caused solely by anesthesia ranged from 1/2000 for chloroform anesthesia[51] in the late 19th century to 1/10,000 in the mid-20th century.**[9] Approximately 20 million anesthetics are administered annually in the

United States. The latter mortality rate predicts 2000 preventable anesthesia deaths *each year*. **In the last decade a study in the United Kingdom has revised this mortality figure to 1/185,000.**[5] In 1988 the Centers for Disease Control (CDC) pilot study of anesthesia morbidity and mortality surveyed approximately 8000 anesthetics conducted in five hospitals over a 3-month interval.[31] The reviewers identified six adverse outcomes in which anesthesia was contributory (6.25/10,000) and one adverse outcome totally related to anesthesia (1.25/10,000). The CDC figures understate the extent of safety problems because they do not quantify critical incidents in which the patient escaped injury or an adverse outcome.

Development of Critical Incident Technique

Lack of data and inability to assess the degree to which human behavior contributed to an anesthetic catastrophe hampered the early anesthesiologist's attempts to improve patient safety. The U.S. military experienced similar problems in assessing the performance of men and machines in the 20th century during World War II.

Critical incident technique (CIT) was refined by Flanagan[22] from a process described in the late 19th century by Sir Francis Galton. Flanagan found CIT to be[21]:

. . . very effective in obtaining information from individuals concerning their own errors, from subordinates concerning errors of their superiors, from superiors, with respect to their subordinates, and also from participants with respect to coparticipants.[22]

The CIT procedure is divided into three parts (Box 36-2). The procedures used in the CIT developed by Flanagan are outlined in Boxes 36-3 to 36-5. **CIT is used to identify human behaviors that are critical in achieving *or* preventing a planned outcome.** Current CIT evolved from studies in the Aviation Psychology Program of the United States Army Forces in World War II in 1941. The Air Force used CIT to develop

---

BOX 36-1
COLLECTION OF LETHAL CRITICAL INCIDENTS (1873-1961)

Faulty Junker apparatus delivers excessive chloroform vapour (1873)
Phosgene gas liberated from exhaled chloroform by gaslight
Incorrect assembly of tubing in Junker inhaler delivers liquid chloroform to the patient
Tilted reservoir delivers liquid chloroform
Excessive chloroform vapour dose from safety inhaler
Correctly assembled Junker inhaler delivers excessive chloroform dose
"Chloroform" explosion (ether seeped by faulty valve)
Esophageal intubation
Endotracheal tube cuff explosion
CO_2 cylinder swap for oxygen
N_2O cylinder swap for oxygen
Trilene-generated poisonous trichloroacetylene in the presence of soda lime
Drug swap (1.0% percaine instead of 0.1% procaine)
Spinal meningitis (infected equipment)
Air embolism (gas pressurized–inverted glass bottle for blood transfusion)
Air embolism (entrainment from leaky IV tubing)
Air embolism (motorized transfusion pump with faulty one-way valve, permitting air entrainment)
Air embolism (hole in vein from suture ligature for transfusion cannula)
Air embolism while vein open during difficult cannulation for transfusion

From Sykes SW: *Essays on the first hundred years of anesthesia,* Edinburgh, 1961, E & S Livingstone.

BOX 36-2
OUTLINE OF CRITICAL INCIDENT PROCEDURE

Objectively gather certain important facts concerning behavior in defined situations
Classify the critical incidents
Develop inferences regarding practical procedures for improving performances

From Flanagan JC: The critical incident technique, *Psychol Bull* 51:327, 1954.

BOX 36-3
CRITICAL INCIDENT ANALYSIS PROCEDURES

Establish the general aim(s) of the activity
Establish plans and specifications (specification of observers, groups to be observed, and observations to be made [see Box 36-4])
Collect the data
Analyze the data
Interpret and report

From Flanagan JC: The critical incident technique, *Psychol Bull* 51:327, 1954.

BOX 36-4
SPECIFICATIONS REGARDING OBSERVATIONS

Persons to make the observations

Knowledge concerning the activity
  Relation to those observed
  Training requirements

Groups to be observed

General description
  Location
  Persons
  Times
  Conditions

Behaviors to be observed

General type of activity
  Specific behaviors
  Criteria of relevance to general aim
  Criteria of importance to general aim (critical points)

From Flanagan JC: The critical incident technique, *Psychol Bull* 51:327, 1954.

---

procedures for the selection of aircrews. Miller used CIT to study the reasons that pilot instructors and check pilots used to eliminate candidates from flight school.[36] These comments, in addition to a number of specific observations of particular behaviors, became a tool for a research program on selecting pilots. In 1944 the Army Air Forces used this technique to help characterize combat leadership qualities (positive and negative). Combat veterans were asked to recount incidents when they observed pivotal behavior that was especially helpful or inadequate in accomplishing the assigned mission. This study helped define the "critical requirements" of combat leadership.[55]

Critical incident technique consists of a set of procedures (Box 36-3) for collecting direct observations of human behavior in a way that facilitates the solving of practical problems in human behavior. Williamson notes that[11, 57]:

The CI approach does not require death or injury ("substantive negative outcome")[11] to identify errors. Rather it utilizes not just the small 'visible tip of mortality' of the metaphorical 'iceberg of clinical anaesthesia mistakes'[27] but also samples the relatively large and to date mostly untapped 'submerged body' of errors that do not cause patient harm.[11,57]

In the late 1960s the National Transportation Safety Board sought to augment data collection for critical incident analysis and proposed installation of automated data recorders (the "black box") on all large commercial jetliners. The pilots' union fought this proposal vigorously because they feared faulty data collection and unwarranted disciplinary actions. Finally, a Federal Aeronautics and Aviation directive mandated the installation of automated flight data recorders on large commercial jet aircraft.[37,53] However, the automated data recorders were placed on these aircraft with the proviso that data could only be examined in the event of a crash or a serious in-flight emergency. The data could not be used as a basis for

---

BOX 36-5
OUTLINE FOR AN INTERVIEW TO ESTABLISH GENERAL AIM FOR AN ACTIVITY

Introductory statement: We are making a study of (specific activity). We believe that you are particularly well-qualified to tell us about (specific activity).
Request for general aim: What would you say is the primary purpose of (specific activity)?
Request for summary: In a few words, how would you summarize the general aim of (specific activity)?

From Flanagan JC: The critical incident technique, *Psychol Bull* 51:327, 1954.

---

disciplinary actions or auditing performance.[53] A similar controversy has developed over the proposed use of automated chart recorders in anesthesia machines.[25]

Williamson posed a definition of an anesthesia-related critical incident[56] (Box 36-6). He points out several advantages of CIT studies over mortality studies (Box 36-7).

BOX 36-6
DEFINITION OF AN ANESTHESIA-RELATED CRITICAL INCIDENT

It is an error by a member of the anesthesia team or an equipment failure

It occurs while the patient is under the care of the anesthesia team

It is reported by someone either involved in or who witnessed directly the entire incident

It was clearly preventable

From Williamson J: Critical incident reporting in anesthesia, *Anaesth Intens Care* 16:100, 1988.

Table 36-1 Category and incidence of anesthesia-related injuries

Complication	Results	
Airway problems	Deaths	Brain damage
Difficult intubation	4	2
Esophageal intubation	4	2
Bronchospasm	6	
Obstruction	1	
Inadequate ventilation	14	2
Other	1	1
Subtotal	30	7
Total in 11-year study	49	8

Modified from Solazzi RW, Ward RJ: Analysis of anesthetic mishaps, *Int Anesthesiol Clinic* 22(2):43, 1984.

BOX 36-7
ADVANTAGES OF CIT STUDIES IN ANESTHESIA

Substantive negative outcome not required

Validity unaffected by advances in anesthesia

All aspects of anesthesia practice monitored

Focus is on prevention

Evaluation is done of new corrective strategies

From Williamson J: Critical incident reporting in anesthesia, *Anaesth Intens Care* 16:100, 1988.

DETECTION OF CRITICAL INCIDENTS

Early investigators searched for large databases as a resource in characterizing anesthesia mishaps and patient injuries. These efforts included reviews of open and closed claims recorded by medical liability insurers. Critical incidents culled from these sources were biased in that they were retrospective and had actually resulted in patient injury and litigation. Denominators were not available. Rates of injury could not be assessed or compared. In the mid-1970s several investigations studied the causes of anesthesia-related injury. It was hoped that this information would help in the development of strategies to improve quality of care. During this time there was an increase in the number, severity, and size of malpractice settlements. Concerned insurers cooperated with investigators by opening their files for analysis. As a result of accelerating losses, many insurers stopped issuing medical liability insurance policies altogether. This precipitated a crisis in many locales where insurance became unavailable or prohibitively expensive.

Investigators found it difficult to study patient injuries that led to insurance payouts. A national registry of patient injuries or malpractice claims did not exist. The terms of many settlements were not public information. During this malpractice crisis the National Association of Insurance Commissioners (NAIC) conducted a 3½-year closed claim study[50] between July 1975 and December 1978. Insurers that had written $1 million or more in medical malpractice premiums in any year since 1970 were included in the study. Anesthesia injuries accounted for only 4.6% of all paid claims but a disproportionate 8.7% of all dollars indemnified. The NAIC study determined that human error occurred in 69% of the incidents. Solazzi and Ward reviewed 11 years of malpractice claims in Washington state from 1971 to 1982.[49] **The authors found that 61% of the anesthesia-related deaths and 88% of the incidents of anesthesia-related brain damage were caused by embarrassment of the respiratory system** (Table 36-1).

The theme of respiratory embarrassment as a major contributor to patient injury was reinforced in a contemporaneous European study. Green and Taylor reviewed cases presented to the Medical Protection Society in the United Kingdom for the 5 years between January 1977 and December 1982.[26] In this review, 54% of the 71 anesthesia-related mishaps that led to death or neurologic damage were caused by impairment of the respiratory system (Table 36-2).

A retrospective review of intraoperative cardiac arrests by Keenan and Boyan determined that critical incidents grouped in the category of inadequate pulmonary ventilation caused almost 50% of the avoidable arrests.[30] Unrecognized esophageal intubation occurred in 30% of the cardiac arrests due to inadequate ventilation. Caplan et al. reviewed claims involving adverse respiratory events from 20 U.S.

Table 36-2 Primary causes of mishaps during anesthesia leading to death or neurologic damage

Difficulty	No. of cases
Respiratory obstruction	14
In recovery room (5)	
In operating theater (9)	
Intubation difficulties	10
Esophageal intubation	6
Respirator failures	8
Disconnections (3)	
Transpositions (3)	
Electrical failure (1)	
Unspecified (1)	
Subtotal	38
Other	33
Total cases of brain damage or neurologic damage	71

Modified from Green RA, Taylor TH: An anaylsis of anesthesia medical liability claims in the United Kingdom, 1977-82, *Int Anesthesiol Clin* 22(2):78, 1984.

insurance carriers between 1975 and 1985.[6] Death or brain damage occurred in 85% of the cases. Pulse oximetry and capnography were not widely used during the interval of this study. **The three most common causes of respiratory events leading to claims were inadequate ventilation, unrecognized esophageal intubation, and airway obstruction.** They noted with alarm that in 48% of these cases, auscultation of the chest failed to detect an esophageal intubation.

Governmental agencies attempted to quantify anesthesia injuries on a comprehensive prospective basis. This effort represented an advance over the previous sporadic retrospective studies. Federal and state regulatory agencies attempted to reduce patient injuries and improve quality of care through legislative initiatives. The Commonwealth of Massachusetts has defined two categories of incidents (Box 36-8) that must be reported to the Massachusetts Board of Registration and Discipline in Medicine with the names of the health care providers included. On a federal level, the National Practitioner Data Bank (NPDB) was formed to help assess the frequency and severity of medical injuries and relate them to individual practitioners.[35] Currently, state medical boards and hospital credentialing committees must query the NPDB for the claims history of physicians applying for clinical privileges. They thought that restriction of privileges of selected practitioners would reduce the frequency of patient injuries. This approach will not be successful if the cause of the patient's injury was related to the *process* or *system of*

BOX 36-8
REPORTABLE MAJOR INCIDENTS DEFINED BY MASSACHUSETTS BOARD OF REGISTRATION AND DISCIPLINE IN MEDICINE

Category one incidents
1. Maternal deaths that are related to delivery.
2. Fetal deaths as defined by Massachusetts General Law (MGL) c. 111, s. 202 means death prior to the complete expulsion or extraction from its mother of a fetus, irrespective of the duration of pregnancy, as indicated by the fact that after such expulsion or extraction the fetus does not breathe or show any other evidence of life such as beating of the heart, pulsation of the umbilical cord, or definite movement of voluntary muscles.
"Fetal death" does not include an abortion as definied in MGL c. 112, s. 12K.
3. Chronic vegetative state resulting from medical intervention.
4. Death in the course of or resulting from ambulatory surgical care.

Category two incidents
1. Major or permanent impairments of bodily functions or deaths that are not ordinarily expected as foreseeable results of the patient's condition or of appropriately selected and administered treatment.

From Commonwealth of Massachusetts Regulation: 243 CMR 3:08a2, a and b.

---

health care rather than the practitioner's management.

In a more comprehensive approach, the Joint Commission on Accreditation of Healthcare Organizations (JCAHO)[1] recommended monitoring of occurrence screens that were thought to be potentially indicative of substandard care (Box 36-9). This more broad-based screening will help quantify many near-injury cases as well as incidents leading to litigation.

Comparison of hospital death rates has also been advocated by some for assessment of quality of care.[29] Based on computerized billing data, the Department of Health and Human Services reported results of a study that calculated the death rates for 17 diagnostic categories in every hospital that treated Medicare patients. A predicted death rate was calculated that included 95% of all hospitals. Hospitals with death rates two standard deviations above the mean mortality rate were identified. This study was heavily critized because of a large number of uncontrolled variables. The Health Care Financing Administration

---

BOX 36-9
ANESTHESIA CARE INDICATORS

---

1. Patients diagnosed with a CNS complication occurring during procedures involving anesthesia administration or within 2 postprocedure days of its conclusion, subcategorized by ASA-PS class, patient age, and CNS vs. non-CNS related procedures.
2. Patients developing a peripheral neurologic deficit during procedures involving anesthesia administration within 2 postprocedure days of its conclusion.
3. Patients with an acute myocardial infarction during procedures involving anesthesia administration or within 2 postprocedure days of its conclusion, subcategorized by ASA-PS class, patient age, and cardiac vs. noncardiac procedures.
4. Patients with a cardiac arrest during procedures involving anesthesia administration or within 24 postprocedure hours of its conclusion, excluding patients with required intraoperative cardiac arrest, subcategorized by ASA-PS class, patient age, and cardiac vs. noncardiac procedures.
5. Patients with an unplanned respiratory arrest during procedures involving anesthesia administration or within 24 postprocedure hours of its conclusion.
6. Death of patients during procedures involving anesthesia administration, or within 48 postprocedure hours of its conclusion, sub-categorized by ASA-PS class and patient age.
7. Unplanned admission of patients to the hospital within 1 postprocedure day after outpatient procedures involving anesthesia administration.
8. Unplanned admission of patients to an intensive care unit within 1 postprocedure day of procedures involving anesthesia administration.
9. Patients with a discharge diagnosis of fulminant pulmonary edema developed during procedures involving anesthesia administration or within 1 postprocedure day of its conclusion.
10. Patients diagnosed with aspiration pneumonitis occurring during procedures involving anesthesia administration or within 2 postprocedure days of its conclusion.
11. Patients developing a postural headache within 4 postprocedure days after procedures involving spinal or epidural anesthesia administration.
12. Patients experiencing a dental injury during procedures involving anesthesia care.
13. Patients experiencing an ocular injury during procedures involving anesthesia care.

From the Joint Commission on Accreditation of Healthcare Organizations: *Accreditation manual for hospitals*, Oakbrook Terrace, Ill, 1990, The Commission.

Table 36-3   Ten most frequent critical incidents

Critical incident description	Percent of total critical incidents
Breathing circuit disconnection	8
Inadvertent gas flow change	6
Syringe swap	5
Gas supply problem	4
Intravenous apparatus disconnection	3
Laryngoscope malfunction	3
Premature extubation	3
Breathing circuit connection error	3
Hypovolemia	3
Tracheal airway device position changes	2

From Cooper JB, Newbower RS, Long CD et al: Preventable anesthesia mishaps, *Anesthesiology* 49:399, 1978.

study did not determine if hospitals with high mortality rates admitted unusually ill patients or provided substandard care. This approach did not account for comorbidities or consider that effective therapy may have been intentionally withheld. "Do Not Resuscitate" orders may have been written for patients with coexisting terminal illness because of quality of life issues or family concerns. This study did not identify specific errors leading to avoidable deaths. Harrison notes that "counting the dead is a crude method for gauging the quality of anesthesia."[27]

The CIT provides an opportunity to identify human behaviors that could have a positive or negative impact on patient safety. Cooper et al. used a modified CIT to retrospectively study preventable anesthesia mishaps in an urban teaching institution.[10] They recorded 359 events that met their critical incident definition. **Human error was a factor in 82% of the incidents; equipment failure accounted for another 14%.** Approximately half of the errors described were "near misses"—they had no effect or only a transient effect on the patient. The 10 most common incidents account for 39% of the total cases (Table 36-3). They identified 44 categories of "associated factors" that were thought to facilitate the occurrence of a negative critical incident (Table 36-4). In a follow-up study, Cooper, Newbower, and Kitz found that more than 90% of substantive negative outcomes were the result of human errors[11] (Table 36-5). A prospective component to their study produced similar event frequencies compared to earlier retrospective studies. They listed the distribution of the most frequent incidents (Table 36-6).

A prospective study from the Netherlands identified 148 episodes of "faults, accidents or near accidents" during the administration of 113,074 anesthetics. The incidence of cardiac arrest was 1/3362.

Table 36-4 Most common factors associated with critical incidents

Associated factors	Percent of total
Inadequate experience	16
Inadequate familiarity with equipment/device	9
Poor communication	6
Haste	5
Inattention/carelessness	5
Fatigue	5
Excessive dependency on other personnel	5
Failure to perform a normal check	5
Training or experience—other factors	5
Supervisor not present enough	4
Environment or colleagues—other factors	4
Visual field restricted	4
Mental or physical—other factors	4
Inadequate familiarity with surgical procedure	3
Distraction	3
Poor labeling of controls, drugs, etc.	2
Supervision—other factors	2
Other	13

Modified from Cooper JB, Newbower RS, Long CD et al: Preventable anesthesia mishaps, *Anesthesiology* 49:399, 1978.

Table 36-5 Distribution of human error and disconnection incidents according to the nature of the activity or system involved

Event	Percent of total
Drug administration	24
Anesthesia machine use	22
Airway management	16
Breathing circuit/ventilation	11
Fluid and electrolyte management	5
IV apparatus	6
Monitoring device	4
Other	12

Modified from Cooper JB, Newbower RS, and Kitz RJ: An analysis of major errors and equipment failures in anesthesia management: consideration for prevention and detection, *Anesthesiology* 60:34, 1984.

Table 36-6 Distribution of frequent critical incidents

Incident description	Number of incidents
Breathing circuit disconnection during mechanical ventilation	57
Syringe swap	50
Gas flow control technical error	41
Loss of gas supply	32
Intravenous line disconnection	24
Vaporizer off unintentionally	22
Drug ampule swap	21
Drug overdose (syringe, judgmental)	20
Drug overdose (vaporizer, technical)	20
Breathing circuit leak	19
Unintentional extubation	18
Misplaced tracheal tube	18
Breathing circuit misconnection	18
Inadequate fluid replacement	15
Premature extubation	15
Ventilator malfunction	15
Misuse of blood pressure monitor	15
Other	87
Total incidents	507

Modified from Cooper JB, Newbower RS, and Kirz RJ: An analysis of major consideration for prevention and detection, *Anesthesiology*, 60:34, 1984.

Thirteen of the cardiac arrests were anesthesia related (1/7500). Almost half of the patients with anesthesia-related cardiac arrests could not be resuscitated; 62% had a fatal outcome. The mortality rate after preventable cardiac arrest was higher (100%) in ASA IV-V patients compared to ASA I-III patients (47%).[9] In the latter group, preventable causes were identified in 47% of the cases. Drug administration error was the most common cause of preventable cardiac arrest.

Currie monitored the frequency of critical incidents prospectively during an 18-month period in two teaching hospitals in Sydney, Australia.[14] A preprinted form was completed if a critical incident occurred. Mishaps were defined as errors in judgment, errors in technique, equipment failure, and failure to check equipment. A total of 167 incidents were identified and reviewed in the 23,713 anesthetics administered during this period. The compliance rate was not known. Ventilatory impairment related to human error occurred in 61% of these incidents.

Recovery room impact events (RRIEs) were studied by Cooper et al.[10] RRIEs included a number of critical incidents and adverse events that were not necessarily life threatening in themselves. The authors reported intraoperative rates of hypotension and hypoxemia of 5.4% and 0.34%, respectively. In a single-blind study, Cote et al. demonstrated that oximetry diagnosed hypoxemia before signs and symptoms of hypoxia were apparent in pediatric surgical patients.[13] The rate of serious hypoxia ($Sao_2 < 85\%$ for longer than 30 seconds) was less in the group of patients monitored by oximetry ($Sao_2 < 85\%$) in ambulatory patients. In a study of ambulatory surgery patients, Raemer noted that anesthesiologists failed to detect any incidents of mild hypoxia, whereas only 29% of the episodes of severe hypoxia were detected without the aid of oximetry. Preventability was not assessed. The high rate of hypoxia (10%) in this healthy adult outpatient population is disturbing.[41]

The previously mentioned studies detected a higher rate of hypoxia than Cooper's RRIE study that depended on voluntary reporting of hypoxic incidents. This suggests that automated chart recorders may provide a more accurate assessment of the frequency, severity, and duration of intraoperative hypoxia.

Critical incidents also occur outside the operating room during transport between critical care areas or in the postanesthesia care unit. Monitoring in these areas is less intense. Critical incidents may not be detected as quickly. A pulse oximetry study conducted with recovery room patients by Morris et al. indicated that hypoxia developed in 14% of ambulatory patients ($Sao_2 < 90\%$) after undergoing minor gynecologic surgery.[38] The rate of hypoxia increased with time, rising from 2% on admission to the postanesthesia care unit to 9% on discharge.

The ASA closed claims study found that 7.1% of closed claims arose from incidents that developed in the recovery room.[59] Respiratory incidents occurred in 58% of these patients, and the cardiovascular system was involved in 11% of cases. In addition, the proportion of serious outcomes was higher compared to events occurring in the operating room. Of these patients, 78% died or suffered brain damage. Reviewers thought that pulse oximetry would have prevented the complications in 39% of the cases.

Smith, Fleming, and Ceraianu found that patients being transported between critical care areas for elective and emergency procedures had mishap rates in excess of 40%.[46] Braman et al. reported a significant incidence of acidosis related to hypoventilation and cardiac dysrhythmias during transport of critically ill patients.[4]

PREVENTION OF CRITICAL INCIDENTS

Cooper, Newbower, and Kitz listed a number of factors associated with critical incidents (Table 36-7).[11] These factors deal exclusively with the performance of the anesthesia practitioner and the equipment used to induce and maintain anesthesia. The scope of this analysis may be too limited to discover all the opportunities for improving quality of care. The fact that anesthesiologists are consumers as well as providers of services should also be considered. Laffel and Blumenthal suggest a broader approach to the analysis of adverse outcomes.[32] They note that variation in outcome may not be solely determined by the

Table 36-7   Potential strategies for prevention or detection of 70 incidents with substantive negative outcome

Strategies	Number of incidents
Additional training	38
Improved supervision/second opinion	20
Specific protocol development	7
Equipment or apparatus inspection	8
More complete preoperative assessment	8
Equipment/human factor improvements	18
Additional monitoring instrumentation	18
Other specific organizational improvements	21
Improved communication	8
Improved personnel selection procedures	5

Modified from Cooper JB, Newbower RS, and Kitz RJ: An analysis of major errors and equipment failures in anesthesia management, *Anesthesiology* 60:34, 1984.

practitioner and his equipment: "Quality experts suggest that processes, not individuals should be the objects of quality improvement."[32] The quality of anesthesia care rendered also depends on the data supplied by medical consultants, medical records, clinical laboratories, and diagnostic services within and outside the hospital. The cause of variation in quality or outcome (e.g. hypoxic brain damage) is frequently assigned to the attending anesthesiologist through malpractice litigation. However, it is possible that this low-frequency outcome would be equally likely with another practitioner. If this is true, then withdrawing the medical license of the involved practitioner may not be effective in reducing the frequency of hypoxic brain damage. Laffel and Blumenthal[32] and Berwick[3] think that setting arbitrary intervention thresholds for occurrence screens (e.g., <2% rate of intraoperative hypoxia) may not optimize patient care. Such goals promote tolerance of a finite rate of critical incidents. Consequently, practitioners do not search for the profound knowledge that will result in breakthroughs capable of eliminating the adverse event altogether.

After a review of malpractice data supplied by their insurer, the Risk Management Committee of the Harvard Medical School Anesthesia departments rejected the "bad apple" approach to prevention. The committee thought standards of care would promote patient safety by ensuring early warning of critical incidents. The committee reviewed the mechanisms of injury in all anesthesia-related claims or incidents provided by their medical liability insurer. In 1985 the committee proposed standards of anesthesia care that might prevent the injuries noted in the claims review. The Harvard Risk Management Committee proposed methods for continuous monitoring of ventilation and circulation.[16] The committee chose to change the *process* of care instead of sanctioning individual practitioners.

Regulatory agencies appear to be pursuing the "bad apple" approach. State licensing boards have been under pressure to identify and discipline physicians who provide substandard care. The Massachusetts Board of Registration and Discipline in Medicine has published its own mandatory occurrence screens (see Box 36-8). Positive screens must be reported to the Board by Institutional Patient Care Assessment Committees, which are also mandated by law. Information thus reported is used by the medical board when processing applications for medical license renewals. The federal government has established a National Practitioner Data Bank (NPDB) to receive claims data from the nation's malpractice insurers.[35] Medical boards and hospitals are required to query this data bank to ensure that credentialing materials are complete and accurate when evaluating physicians who request medical privileges. Licensing boards and credentialing committees presumably will not grant privileges to practitioners who fail to meet the reviewing body's standard of care. Removing the "bad apples" sanctions a portion of the providers whose activities have resulted in patient injuries.

The efficacy of this approach is unknown. A follow-up study by Eichhorn after the clinical adoption of the Harvard Anesthesia Standards demonstrated a 3.22-fold reduction in preventable accidents in ASA 1 and 2 patients.[16, 17] In the 3 years following the introduction of the Harvard Standards, only one injury occurred (one month after the standards were introduced). This represented a 71% reduction in injuries. Although the difference is not statistically significant, Eichhorn thought the standards played a key role in providing early warning of unsafe conditions. Whether they were causal is debatable. Eichhorn noted that coincident factors, such as the availability of oximetry, heightened awareness, and increased knowledge of factors leading to anesthesia mishaps, may have been responsible for this change.

Several alternative efforts have been proposed to reduce patient injuries and near-injuries while improving quality of care. The JCAHO has mandated continuous monitoring and evaluation of anesthesia care. Anesthesia departments must select a number of indicators that define a measurable dimension of the quality and appropriateness of an important aspect of patient care (e.g., tracheal reintubation). Criteria are then developed that define an expected level of performance (e.g., tracheal reintubation is necessary for no more than 1% of patients undergoing anesthesia). Clinical privileges are renewed periodically on the basis of individual competence as determined by the above monitoring processes.

Practice guidelines have been advocated to reduce the frequency of critical incidents and patient injuries. The concept of guidelines for medical care is receiving growing interest at the local and national level.[58] Practice guidelines offer several advantages, although some physicians undoubtedly will object to interference with their practice of medicine. Advocates believe guidelines will be effective in reducing inappropriate care, controlling unwarranted geographic variations in practice, and making more effective use of the shrinking health care dollar. At the national level, the federal government has created a new U.S. Public Health Service agency with the responsibility for practice guidelines.[58] Guidelines address the human error element contributing to patient injury. A smaller fraction of injuries is related to equipment failure. Such efforts are being made continuously. Equipment manufacturers have responded to safety concerns by modifying their equipment. Dorsch and Dorsch outline many anesthesia equipment design criteria that represent a direct response to specific incident(s) of patient injuries.[15] The FDA regulates the safety of anesthesia equipment through the medical device amendment of the Federal Food, Drug, and Cosmetic Act. Under section 501(k) manufacturers must notify the FDA 90 days before marketing a new device or substantially modifying an existing device to allow time for FDA review. Manufacturers are also required to notify the FDA of complaints or problems involving medical devices.[54]

Cooper suggested 10 preventive strategies for the 70 human error incidents with substantive negative outcomes.[11] Three of these strategies were mandated by the Harvard Standards for anesthesia monitoring—protocol, monitors, and inspection. Cooper studied the impact of education by feedback of critical incident data collected during a study of adverse incidents. He failed to demonstrate an overall change in RRIEs, but noted a significant reduction in hypotensive and hypovolemic RRIE after the introduction of oximetry.[12] A causal relationship was not established. The use of pulse oximetry during anesthesia care has been associated with fewer major hypoxic events.[13] Tinker et al. thought that oximetry and capnography were most helpful in reducing critical incidents.[52] Cheney analyzed 100 claims in the ASA closed claims study in which oximetry was in use at the time of the incident and noted that reviewers were able to rule out preexisting hypoxia in seven circulatory-related occurrences (a convenient hypothesis frequently used by the plaintiff's attorney.)[8]

The review by Pedersen and Johansen of serious anesthesia morbidity suggests that high-risk patients are more likely than healthy patients to be affected by errors and suffer substantially negative outcomes.[40]

After the wide-scale introduction of pulse oximetry in Massachusetts, Zeitlin estimated a 13-fold reduction in anesthetic deaths based on a closed claim study.[59] Since the Joint Underwriters Association promoted the use of oximetry and capnography through malpractice premium discounts, there has been only one anesthesia-related hypoxic injury.[7] Gaba et al. have proposed a schema to break the chain of accident evolution[24] (Box 36-10).

Efforts in anesthesia education have moved toward the use of simulators to provide learning opportunities for resident and staff anesthesiologists. This allows simulation of a wide range of serious "intraoperative" critical incidents free of patient risk.[23,44] Simulators show promise in the development and testing of strategies and protocols designed to prevent patient injury from critical incidents.

BOX 36-10
STRATEGIES FOR RECOVERING FROM ANESTHESIA INCIDENTS

Detect one or more manifestations of the incident in progress

Verify the manifestations and reject false alarms

Recognize that manifestations represent an actual or potential threat

Assure continued maintenance of life-sustaining functions

Implement "generic" diagnostic or corrective strategies to provide failure compensation and allow continuation of surgery if possible

Achieve specific diagnosis and therapy of the underlying causes

Provide follow-up of recovery to ensure adequate correction or compensation

From Gaba DM, Maxwell M, and DeAnda A: Anesthetic mishaps: breaking the chain of accident evolution, *Anesthesiology* 66(5):670, 1987.

KEY POINTS

- Critical incidents occur in all phases of anesthesia care, including the operating room, postanesthesia care unit, transport of patients between critical care areas, and pain management.

- The philosophy of continuous quality improvement must be adopted to seek the profound knowledge necessary for breakthroughs in patient safety.

- Solutions must involve thoughtful analysis of the process of care, including the consumer-provider relationships of the supporting health care workers as well as the anesthesiologists and their equipment.

- Preventive strategies must ensure the prompt recognition of infrequent sentinel events that herald swift and potentially catastrophic critical incidents.

- Anesthesiologists must be educated to promptly use effective therapies to ensure recovery from critical incidents.

KEY REFERENCES

Berwick DM: Continuous improvement as an ideal in health care, *N Engl J Med* 320(1):53, 1989.

Cooper JB, Newbower RS, and Kitz RJ: An analysis of major errors and equipment failures in anesthesia management: consideration for prevention and detection, *Anesthesiology* 60:34, 1984.

Keenan RL, Boyan CP: Cardiac arrest due to anesthesia, *JAMA* 253(16):2373, 1985.

Solazzi RW, Ward RJ: Analysis of anesthetic mishaps, *Int Anesthesiol Clin* 22(2):43, 1984.

REFERENCES

1. *Accreditation manual for hospitals,* Joint Commission on Accreditation of Healthcare Organizations, Oakbrook Terrace, Ill, 1990.

2. Beecher HK: The first anesthesia records, *Surg Gynecol Obstet* 71:689, 1940.

3. Berwick DM: Continuous improvement as an ideal in health care, *N Engl J Med* 320(1):53, 1989.

4. Braman SS, Dunn SM, Amico CA et al: Complications of intrahospital transport in critically ill patients, *Ann Intern Med* 107(4):469, 1987.

5. Buck N, Devlin HB, and Lunn JN: *The report of a confidential enquiry into perioperative deaths,* London, 1987, Nuffield Provincial Hospitals Trust and The King's Fund.

6. Caplan RA, Posner KL, Ward RJ et al: Adverse respiratory events in anesthesia: a closed claims analysis, *Anesthesiology* 72(5):828, 1990.

7. Cass WA, Director of Risk Management, Joint Underwriters of Massachusetts: Personal communication, Oct 29, 1990.

8. Cheney FW: The ASA closed claims study after the pulse oximeter: a preliminary look, *Am Soc Anesthesiol Newslet* 54(2):10, 1990.

9. Chopra V, Bocvill JG, and Spierdijk J: Accidents, near accidents and complications during anaesthesia, *Anaesthesia* 45:3, 1990.

10. Cooper JB, Cullen DJ, Nemeskal R et al: Effects of information feedback and pulse oximetry on the incidence of anesthetic complications, *Anesthesiology* 67:686, 1987.

11. Cooper JB, Newbower RS, and Kitz RJ: An analysis of major errors and equipment failures in anesthesia management: consideration for prevention and detection, *Anesthesiology* 60:34, 1984.

12. Cooper JB, Newbower RS, Long CD et al: Preventable anesthesia mishaps, *Anesthesiology* 49:399, 1978.

13. Cote CJ, Goldstein EA, Cote MA et al: A single-blind study of pulse oximetry in children, *Anesthesiology* 68:184, 1988.

14. Currie M: A prospective survey of anaesthetic critical events in a teaching hospital, *Anesth Intens Care* 17:403, 1989.

15. Dorsch JA, Dorsch SE: *Understanding anesthesia equipment,* Baltimore, 1984, Williams & Wilkins.

16. Eichhorn JH: Prevention of intraoperative accidents and related severe injury through safety monitoring, *Anesthesiology* 70:572, 1989.

17. Eichhorn JH, Cooper JB, Cullen DJ et al: Standard for patient monitoring during anesthesia at Harvard Medical School, *JAMA* 256:1017, 1986.

18. Faulconer A, Keys T: *Foundations in anesthesiology,* Springfield, Ill, 1965, Charles C Thomas, p. 822.

19. Faulconer A, Keys T: *Foundations in anesthesiology,* Springfield, Ill, 1965, Charles C Thomas, p.1043.

20. Flagg JFB: *Ether and chloroform: their employment in surgery, dentistry, midwifery, therapeutics, etc,* Philadelphia, 1851, Lindsay & Blakston.

21. Flanagan JC: The aviation psychology program in the Army Air Forces, *Army Air Force Aviation Psychology Program Research Report No 1,* Washington, DC, 1947, US Government Printing Office.

22. Flanagan JC: The critical incident technique, *Psychol Bull* 51:327, 1954.

23. Gaba DM, DeAnda A: The response of anesthesia trainees to simulated critical incidents, *Anesth Analg* 68:444, 1989.

24. Gaba DM, Maxwell M, and DeAnda A: Anesthetic mishaps: breaking the chain of accident evolution, *Anesthesiology* 66(5): 670, 1987.

25. Gibbs RF: The present and future medicolegal importance of record keeping in anesthesia and intensive care: the case for automation, *J Clin Monit* 5(4):251, 1989.

26. Green RA, Taylor TH: An analysis of anesthesia medical liability claims in the United Kingdom, 1977-1982, *Int Anesthesiol Clin* 22(2):78, 1984.

27. Harrison GG: Anesthetic accidents, *Clin Anesthesiol* 1:415, 1983.

28. Hodges RM et al: Report of a committee of the Boston Society for Medical Improvement on "The alleged dangers which accompany the inhalation of the vapor of sulphuric ether," Boston, 1861, David Clapp.

29. Jencks SF, Daley J, Draper D et al: Interpreting hospital mortality data, *JAMA* 260:3611, 1988.

30. Keenan RL, Boyan CP: Cardiac arrest due to anesthesia, *JAMA* 253(16):2373, 1985.

31. Klaucke DN, Revicki DA, and Brown RE: *Investigation of mortality and severe morbidity associated with anesthesia: a pilot study,* Washington, DC, 1988, Battelle Human Affairs Research Centers.

32. Laffel G, Blumenthal D: The case for using industrial quality management science in health care organizations, *JAMA* 262(20):2869, 1989.

33. Lyman HM: *Artificial anesthesia and anaesthetics,* New York, 1881, William Wood.

34. Meggison TN: *Lond Med Gaz* 6:254, 1848 (letter).

35. Milazzo VL: The national practitioner data bank (NPDB) in summary, *Natl Med Leg J* 1(2):10, 1990.

36. Miller NE: Psychological research on pilot training, *Army Air Force Aviation Psychology Program Research Report No 8,* Washington, DC, 1947, US Government Printing Office.

37. Montgomery M: Chief, engineering services division bureau of technology, National Transportation Safety Board, Washington, DC: Personal communication, 1990.

38. Morris RW, Bushman A, Warren DL, et al: The prevalence of hypoxemia detected by pulse oximetry during recovery from anesthesia, *J Clin Monit* 4:16, 1988.

39. Patton J: *Anaesthesia and anaesthetics,* Chicago, 1903, Cleveland Press.

40. Pedersen T, Johansen SH: Serious morbidity attributable to anesthesia, consideration for prevention, *Anaesthesia* 44: 504, 1989.

41. Raemer DB, Warren DL, Morris R, et al: Hypoxemia during ambulatory gynecologic surgery as evaluated by the pulse oximeter, *J Clin Monit* 3:244, 1987.

42. Report of inquest, *Lond Med Gaz* 6:250, 1848.

43. Robinson H, ed: *Anaesthetics and their administration,* ed 2, London, 1920, Henry Frowde, Hodder & Stoughton.

44. Schwid HA, O'Donnell D: The anesthesia simulator-recorder: a device to train and evaluate anesthesiologists' response to critical incidents, *Anesthesiology* 72(1): 191, 1990.

45. Simpson JY: The alleged cases of death from chloroform, *Lancet* 1:175, 1848.

46. Smith I, Fleming S, and Ceraianu A: Mishaps during transport from the intensive care unit, *Crit Care Med* 18(3):278, 1990.

47. Snow J: *On the inhalation of the vapor of ether,* London, 1847, John Churchill.

48. Snow J: Remarks on the fatal cases of the inhalation of chloroform, *Lond Med Gaz,* p. 277, 1848.

49. Solazzi RW, Ward RJ: Analysis of anesthetic mishaps, *Int Anesthesiol Clin* 22(2): 43, 1984.

50. Sowka MP: *Malpractice claims—final compilation,* Brookfield, Wis, 1980, National Association of Insurance Commissioners.

51. Sykes SW: *Essays on the first hundred years of anaesthesia,* Edinburgh, 1961, E & S Livingstone.

52. Tinker JH, Dull DL, Caplan RA et al: Role of monitoring devices in prevention of anesthetic mishaps: a closed claims analysis, *Anesthesiology* 71:541, 1989.

53. Title 14 Aeronautics and Space, chp 1, Federal Aviation Agency, (Reg Doc No 3008; Amendments 4b-15,40-48.41-13,42-12, 91-4, 514-73). Installation of cockpit voice recorders in large airplanes used by an air or commercial operator, *Fed Reg* 8401, 1964.

54. Veale JR: Role of the FDA in regulating the safety of anesthesia equipment, *Med Instrum* 19(3):127, 1985.

55. Wickert F: Psychological research on problems of redistribution, *Army Air Force Aviation Psychology Program Research Report No 14,* Washington, DC, 1947, US Government Printing Office.

56. Williamson JA: Critical incident reporting in anesthesia, *Anaesth Intens Care* 16:101, 1988.

57. Williamson JA, Webb RK, and Pryor GL: Anaesthesia safety and the 'critical incident technique,' *Aust Clin Rev* 5:57, 1985.

58. Woolf S: Practice guidelines: a new reality in medicine, *Arch Intern Med* 50:1811, 1990.

59. Zeitlin GL: Possible decrease in mortality associated with anesthesia, a comparison of two time periods in Massachusetts, USA, *Anaesthesia* 44:432, 1989.

60. Zeitlin GL: Recovery room mishaps in the ASA closed claims study, *Am Soc Anesthesiol Newslet* 53(7):28, 1989.

CHAPTER 37

Cardiopulmonary Resuscitation

CHARLES L. SCHLEIEN
MARK C. ROGERS

The field of cardiopulmonary resuscitation (CPR) has existed in its modern form since the original descriptions of closed-chest CPR in 1960 by Kouwenhoven et al.[173] Clearly though, many CPR procedures, such as artificial ventilation, epinephrine, defibrillation, and even emergency intravenous access, including intraosseous injections, are based historically on scientific experiments done many years before Kouwenhoven. CPR was once thought to be a miracle cure for patients suffering from cardiac arrest, but it is clear now that without certain underlying preexisting conditions of the patient, CPR does not work terribly well. **Many outcome studies have shown that the**

survival rate following CPR is well below 50%, and in many cases even below 15%. Because of this poor survival rate, there are many who claim that CPR is ineffective. What many forget, though, is that without the use of basic CPR, survival following a cardiac arrest is rare. Today many patients continue to lead highly functioning lives following a cardiac arrest as a result of the efficacy of CPR. Controversies abound regarding principles of the basic physiology of blood flow during CPR and indications for many of the drugs used in advanced life support. These controversies will be discussed in this chapter.

BASIC LIFE SUPPORT
Techniques

The use of basic life support techniques is intended to externally support the circulation and ventilation of a patient who has suffered either a respiratory or a cardiorespiratory arrest. **From a physiologic standpoint, the objective of performing CPR is to provide oxygen to the vital organs, the heart, and the brain until normal circulation is restored.** The algorithms for basic CPR are shown in the box. **As usual, the ABCs of CPR should always be followed—airway, breathing, and circulation (Box 37-1) (Fig. 37-1).**

Cricothyroidotomy

This technique, first described in 1956 by Jacoby et al., was designed to deliver oxygen to the patient without particular concern for adequate ventilation.[145] Use of the Venturi principle for oxygen delivery[279] with jet ventilation for intraoperative bronchoscopy was first utilized in 1967. **Spoerel et al., using wall oxygen (50 psi), demonstrated a gas flow of 500 ml/sec producing**

671

BOX 37-1
BASIC CPR

Airway

Assess
Call for help
Position
Open airway
   Head tilt/chin lift
   Jaw thrust

Breathing

Determine breathlessness
Perform breathing
   Two breaths (1-1.5 seconds each)
Cricoid pressure

Circulation	Adult	Child	Infant
Determine pulselessness	Carotid artery	Carotid artery	Brachial artery
Activate EMS system			
Chest compressions			
Placement	Two hands	One hand	Two fingers or encircling method
Depth of compression	1.5-2 in	1-1.5 in	0.5-1 in
Rate/min	80-100	80-100	100

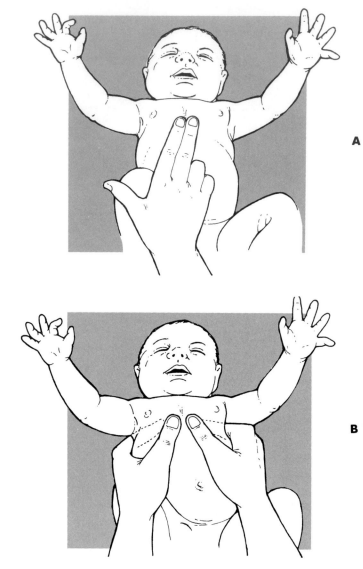

Fig. 37-1. **A,** Two-finger method of external chest compression in infants. Rescuer places two fingers on sternum, one fingerbreadth below line intersecting nipples and compresses ½ to 1 inch at a rate of 100 compressions/minute. Ventilation is not shown for the sake of clarity. **B,** Encircling method of external chest compression in infants. Rescuer places thumbs over sternum one fingerbreadth below line intersecting nipples and clasps hands behind infant's back. (From Schleien CL: Recent advances in pediatric CPR, *Anesthesiology Report* 1:6, 1988.)

adequate blood gas values in normally compliant lungs.[298] In 1972 Jacobs described the first use of emergency cricothyroidotomy, delivering oxygen via a ventilator through a 14-gauge catheter in arrested patients.[144] It has also been used in arrested pediatric patients.[296] When percutaneous transtracheal jet ventilation was compared with high frequency ventilation and intermittent positive pressure ventilation (IPPV), oxygenation was adequate.[311] **One hundred percent oxygen allowed adequate oxygenation *without* providing adequate ventilation.**[228]

Advantages often cited for the use of the cricothyroidotomy include its ease of placement in adult patients, the capability of continuing cardiac massage during placement of a tracheal catheter, and the ability to suction the pharynx if needed. In addition, the use of jet ventilation in this manner has been able to dislodge a foreign body in the trachea by increasing intrapulmonary pressure.[267]

Emergency cricothyroidotomy is the last access to the airway for an anesthesiologist who is faced with a patient in whom he/she is unable to intubate the trachea. Inability to intubate the trachea could be due to any of a number of anatomic deformities, including oropharyngeal edema secondary to a burn, allergy, infection, a foreign body causing obstruction, trauma to the face or larynx causing distortion or obstruction, or cervical spine injury impeding adequate positioning (Box 37-2).

Performing a cricothyroidotomy is simple and necessitates equipment that is readily available to the

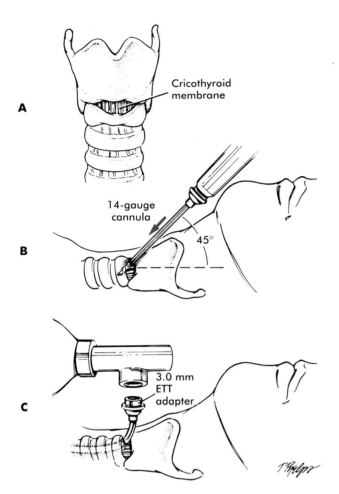

A

Cricothyroid membrane

B

14-gauge cannula

45°

C

3.0 mm ETT adapter

Fig. 37-2. Cricothyroidotomy. **A,** Anatomic view. **B,** Insertion of 14-gauge IV cannula. **C,** Bag attached to 3.0 endotracheal tube (ETT) adaptor connected to IV cannula. (From Yaster M: Airway management. In Nichols DG, Yaster M, Lappe DG et al, eds: *Johns Hopkins Hospital Golden Hour: the handbook of advanced pediatric life support,* St Louis, 1991, Mosby–Year Book.)

---

anesthesiologist. **A 16-gauge angiocath (18-gauge in smaller children) is passed through the cricothyroid membrane, located between the inferior edge of the thyroid cartilage and the upper edge of the cricoid cartilage.** The larynx is stabilized with the fingers while palpating the cricothyroid membrane. The angiocath is placed at a caudad angle in the midline of the neck into the trachea to avoid injury to the larynx. This is done while aspirating gently on an attached syringe to determine when the trachea is successfully entered (Fig. 37-2). Once air is aspirated, the plastic catheter is advanced into the trachea. The connector from a 3.0 endotracheal tube fits snugly onto the angiocath. As an alternative, the barrel of a 3-ml syringe will also fit into the angiocath, which can then be attached to a 7.0 endotracheal tube connector. This setup allows attachment of an Ambu-bag or other source of oxygen. It is prudent to have this

---

BOX 37-2
CAUSES OF A DIFFICULT AIRWAY

Edema of oropharynx
Burn
Allergy
Infection

Foreign body obstruction

Trauma
Face
Larynx
Trachea

Tumor
Oral cavity
Pharynx
Larynx

Cervical spine injury

Anatomic abnormality
Anterior placement of larynx
Congenital anomaly

BOX 37-3
CONNECTORS TO ANGIOCATH
FOR CRICOTHYROIDOTOMY

Angiocath → 3.0 endotracheal tube connector → Ambu-bag
Angiocath → 3 ml syringe → 7.0 endotracheal tube connector → Ambu-bag

---

BOX 37-4
COMPLICATIONS OF CRICOTHYROIDOTOMY

Difficult anatomy
Trauma
Obesity

Subcutaneous or mediastinal emphysema

Traumatized
Vascular structures
Nerves
Airway

Infection

False passage

Fistula formation

Laryngeal edema

attachment available on an arrest crash cart or an anesthesia cart for ready use[284] (Box 37-3). Complications secondary to cricothyroidotomy are listed in Box 37-4.

ADVANCED CPR
Vascular Access and Fluid Administration During CPR

One of the essential aspects of CPR is the early establishment of an intravenous line for the administration of fluids and medications. **If an intravenous line cannot be established rapidly because of technical difficulties, one of the other alternatives — endotracheal, intraosseous, or intracardiac injection — can be used.**

Intravenous access

During CPR, if a central venous line is in place, as is often the case in the operating room, it should be used to administer fluids and medications. If there is no preexisting line, a large peripheral vein such as the antecubital vein should be used. Attempts to use either the jugular or subclavian vein frequently interfere with bag-mask ventilation during CPR. Once the patient's trachea is intubated, central venous cannulation is much easier. Possible approaches to circulation via the venous system include the internal and external jugular veins, subclavian vein, femoral vein, saphenous vein via cutdown, or peripheral sites such as the antecubital or axillary veins (Figs. 37-3 to 37-6).

There may be a significant delay in the circulation time of drugs administered from a peripheral site during CPR.[130,179] Peak drug levels may be reduced when peripheral sites are used compared with central sites of drug administration, although in a canine study levels were equal.[15,91,179]

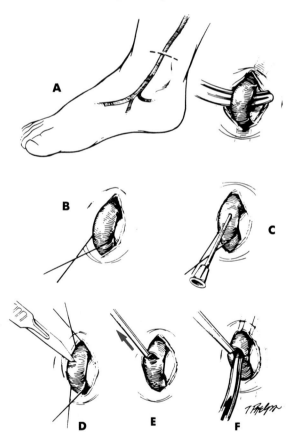

Fig. 37-3. Saphenous vein cutdown. **A,** Transverse incision 1 cm medial to the medial malleolus. Blunt dissection with hemostat. **B,** Control of vein with ligature. **C,** Direct puncture with IV catheter or **D,** proximal and distal control with ligature and incision with No. 11 scalpel blade. **E,** Insertion of right angle vein guide. **F,** Insertion of Silastic catheter underneath vein guide. (From Schleien CL: Cardiopulmonary resuscitation. In Nichols DG, Yaster M, Lappe DG et al, eds: *Johns Hopkins Hospital Golden Hour: the handbook of advanced pediatric life support,* St Louis, 1991, Mosby–Year Book.)

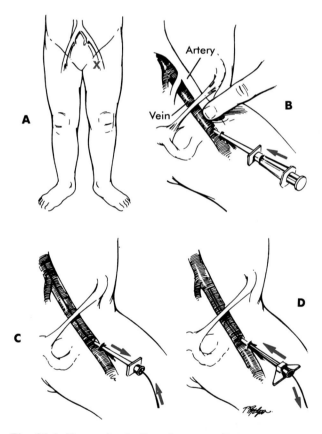

Fig. 37-4. Femoral vein line placement (Seldinger technique). **A,** Femoral vein midway between anterosuperior iliac crest and symphysis pubis. **B,** Insertion of needle into femoral vein just medial to femoral arterial pulse. **C,** Insertion of guide wire through needle in the vein. Needle removed once guide wire in place. **D,** Infusion catheter advanced over guide wire into vein. Guide wire removed after catheter in place. (From Schleien CL: Cardiopulmonary resuscitation. In Nichols DG, Yaster M, Lappe DG et al, eds: *Johns Hopkins Hospital Golden Hour: the handbook of advanced pediatric life support,* St Louis, 1991, Mosby–Year Book.)

Endotracheal administration

During CPR the rapid establishment of an intravenous line can be difficult. This is especially true in obese patients or in infants and small children. The endotracheal route can be used in these settings. **The drugs that can be given through the endotracheal tube include lidocaine, atropine, naloxone, and epinephrine (LANE) (Box 37-5).**

The use of the endotracheal route for ionized medications such as sodium bicarbonate or calcium chloride is not recommended. The rate of absorption and physiologic effects of lidocaine, epinephrine, and atropine administered via the endotracheal route compares favorably with the intravenous route in most studies.[138,265,266] The peak level of drugs such as epinephrine or lidocaine administered via the endotracheal route may be less compared with the intraosseous route of administration. There is inconsistency in obtaining therapeutic levels of lidocaine when administered to humans by this route during CPR.[208] Roberts et al. found the peak drug concentration of epinephrine to be one tenth following endotracheal administration compared with intravenous administration in anesthetized dogs. In a canine arrest model, the endotracheal epinephrine dose producing 50% resuscitation success was 130 μg/kg.[253] Thus the effective dose of epinephrine by the endotracheal route may be much larger than presently recommended.

The volume and the diluent in which the medications are administered may play an important role in the success of this technique. When large volumes of fluid are utilized, pulmonary surfactant may be

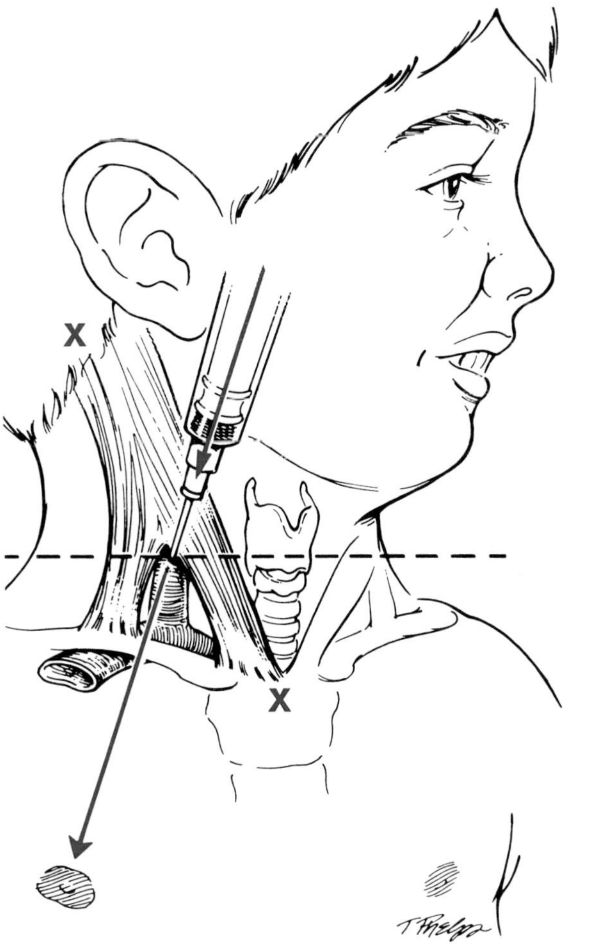

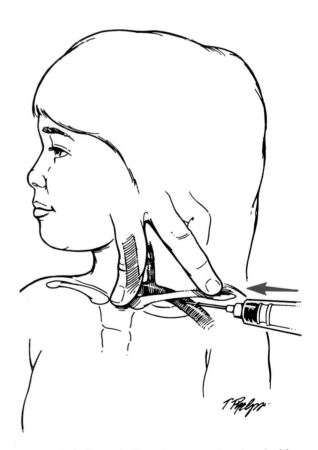

Fig. 37-5. Internal jugular vein line placement. Head turned to the opposite side and needle puncture at the apex of the triangle formed by the heads of the sternocleidomastoid muscle (midway between the sternal notch and the mastoid process). Needle aimed at the ipsilateral nipple. (From Schleien CL: Cardiopulmonary resuscitation. In Nichols DG, Yaster M, Lappe DG et al, eds: *Johns Hopkins Hospital Golden Hour: the handbook of advanced pediatric life support,* St Louis, 1991, Mosby–Year Book.)

Fig. 37-6. Subclavian vein line placement. Landmarks identified by placing operator's thumb in the sternal notch and index finger at the junction of the clavicle and first rib. Needle puncture 1 cm lateral and 1 cm inferior to clavicle-rib junction aiming for the sternal notch. Seldinger technique used for line placement. (From Schleien CL: Cardiopulmonary resuscitation. In Nichols DG, Yaster M, Lappe DG, et al, eds: *Johns Hopkins Hospital Golden Hour: the handbook of advanced pediatric life support,* St Louis, 1991, Mosby–Year Book.)

BOX 37-5
ENDOTRACHEAL ADMINISTRATION
OF DRUGS

Lidocaine	*Do not administer*
Atropine	Bicarbonate
Naloxone	Calcium
Epinephrine	

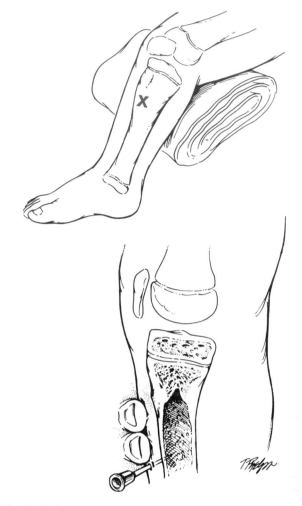

Fig. 37-7. Intraosseous needle placement. Insert needle at the level of tibial tubercle on the medial portion of the tibia. The needle is aimed caudally and laterally. (From Schleien CL: Cardiopulmonary resuscitation. In Nichols DG, Yaster M, Lappe DG, et al, eds: *Johns Hopkins Hospital Golden Hour: the handbook of advanced pediatric life support,* St Louis, 1991, Mosby–Year Book.)

altered or destroyed, resulting in atelectasis. **The total volume of fluid delivered into the trachea should not exceed 10 ml in the adult or 5 ml in the infant.**[109] **The use of normal saline may have the least detrimental effects on lung mechanics**[109] **and may be important for the absorption of medication from the bronchial tree.**[256] Absorption into the systemic circulation may be enhanced by deep intrapulmonary administration.[252] This is performed by passing a Swan-Ganz catheter to a wedged position deep into the bronchial tree.

The risk associated with the route of administration is the formation of an intrapulmonary depot of drug that may prolong its effect. This could result in postresuscitation hypertension or the recurrence of fibrillation after normal circulation is restored. **We still lack a clear understanding of the optimal dose of endotracheal epinephrine, but its use in larger doses than presently recommended, diluted in saline and given deeply into the bronchial tree, is probably warranted.**

Intraosseous administration

The intraosseous route of fluid and medication administration, described originally in 1934,[152] has regained popularity recently in the CPR literature. **All medications used during CPR and fluids, including whole blood, have been given by the intraosseous route.** This technique should be considered a temporary measure during emergencies when other vascular sites are not available.

The technique of placing an intraosseous line is straightforward. A standard 16-gauge or 18-gauge needle, spinal needle with stylet, or bone marrow needle is inserted into the anterior surface of the tibia, 1 to 3 cm below the tibial tuberosity. The needle is directed to a 90 degree angle to the medial surface of the bone or slightly inferior to avoid the epiphyseal plate. The infusion is successful if the needle is in the marrow cavity as evidenced by the needle standing upright without support. It will lose the upright position if it has slipped into the subcutaneous tissue. In addition, there is a loss of resistance after the needle passes through the bony cortex of the tibia. Bone marrow can be aspirated into a syringe connected to the needle. Free flow of the drug or fluid infusion without significant subcutaneous infiltration also should be demonstrated[19] (Fig. 37-7).

In 1944 Meola reported 326 successful intraosseous infusions with only one complication. Heinild et al. reported the results of 984 infusions in which five children developed osteomyelitis without any other complications. Orlowski et al. revealed a high rate of occurrence of fat and bone marrow embolism following the administration of both fluids and medications by this route. Despite these findings, there were no significant alterations in Pa_{O_2} or intrapulmonary shunt.[234] Large amounts of isotonic fluid have been successfully administered to reverse hemorrhagic shock in a rabbit model.[219] Blood pH was raised equally by the administration of sodium bicarbonate through a central intravenous or intraosseous line.[297] The hemodynamic response, time of onset, and time to peak effect were similar when comparing epinephrine administration by these two routes.[8]

Types of fluids

Fluid management during CPR remains an ubiquitous part of the resuscitation process. **As in other types of shock, colloid does not appear to offer any advantage over crystalloid in respect to outcome. Following head injury and hemorrhagic shock, there may be an advantage in using a hypertonic solution instead of an isotonic crystalloid solution.** This benefit may be related to a combination of volume expansion,[225,294] enhanced cardiac performance,[*] vasodilation of systemic arterioles,[†] or decreased intracranial pressure and cerebral edema following head injury and hemorrhagic shock.[‡] The relationship that fluid management has to the resuscitation sequence is unknown.

Volume loading increases arterial blood pressure, carotid blood flow, and cardiac output during CPR.[74,126,337] Despite this, perfusion pressures to the heart and brain are decreased when volume loading occurs on the venous side of the circulation.[74,320,337] Thus there may be an advantage to volume loading on the arterial side of the circulation.

Monitoring During CPR

Assessment of the patient during CPR is similar to other clinical situations; the major points are listed in Box 37-6. A basic clinical examination and adherence to basic principles including inspection, palpation, and auscultation of the patient are performed. The chest is carefully observed for adequacy of chest expansion with artificial ventilation and for equal and normal breath sounds. In addition, the depth of compression and the position of the rescuer's hands in performing chest compressions should be reevaluated constantly. Palpation is essential in establishing pulselessness, in assessing the adequacy of blood flow during chest compressions, and in locating landmarks. **Simply palpating the peripheral pulses may not allow an accurate assessment of blood flow during CPR. This is due to the intense vasoconstriction that occurs with the use of epinephrine or other alpha-adrenergic agonist drugs.**

The amount of blood flow or function of any of the vital organs is not adequately assessed by the clinical examination. The use of an indwelling arterial catheter, when available, is an invaluable monitor in

---

* References 225, 240, 269, 322, 330, 349, 350.
† References 99, 100, 127, 200, 225, 229, 255, 300.
‡ References 118-120, 247-249, 319, 321, 352.

> **BOX 37-6**
> **ASSESSMENT OF PATIENT DURING CPR**
>
> **Inspection**
> Chest rise
> Depth of compression
> Position of rescuer's hands
>
> **Palpation**
> Establish pulselessness
> Assess peripheral pulses
> Locate landmarks
>
> **Auscultation**
> Breath sounds
> Heart sounds
>
> **Monitoring**
> ECG
> Arterial line
> Central venous line
> Pulse oximeter
> Transcutaneous O_2 monitoring
> End-tidal CO_2
> Temperature
> EEG
> Evoked potentials

assessing the arterial blood pressure. **The diastolic pressure is particularly important in assessing CPR because it is the critical pressure for determining coronary perfusion.** In addition, an arterial line allows for determination of arterial blood gases, as well as measuring pH, oxygenation, and ventilation. This line could be placed in the radial artery by percutaneous placement or cutdown. In addition, the femoral artery is easily accessible by the Seldinger technique. The degree of oxygen delivery can also be determined by transcutaneous monitoring of P_{O_2} or by pulse oximetry. Pulse oximetry can be used during CPR to determine not only the oxygen saturation but also the adequacy of pulsatile flow at the site of placement.[226,339]

The assessment of vital organ function has not been performed classically during CPR. Cardiac function or adequacy of coronary blood flow is typically assessed with the use of an electrocardiogram. This allows for an assessment of the cardiac rhythm and the presence of ischemia once a life-sustaining rhythm is restored. Direct measurement of cardiac output is feasible, but technically difficult because of the severity of the low-flow state.[67,293] **The use of end-tidal CO_2 monitoring as an indication of flow is a valuable adjunct during CPR.**[113,163,274,278,324] **End-tidal CO_2 has** been correlated with the coronary perfusion pressure,[274,278] the critical parameter for resuscitation of the heart. With epinephrine administration, the end-tidal CO_2 may not be an accurate indicator of blood flow, as it may cause increased pulmonary shunting.[203]

The neurologic examination, although routinely performed during CPR, should not be utilized as a predictor of outcome.[151] Use of the electroencephalogram has also been shown to be a poor predictor of survival during CPR.[218,220,356] Somatosensory-evoked potentials have been used as a monitor of adequacy of cerebral blood flow and function in an experimental animal model of CPR[104,285] and might be applied in humans in the neurosurgical operating room when available.

Temperature should be monitored routinely during CPR because it may vary widely during the resuscitation or at presentation to the hospital. Temperature may affect the success of resuscitation, the short-term neurologic status, and the eventual neurologic outcome. The possible use of hypothermia may be applied eventually to improve outcome from resuscitation.

Pharmacology
Adrenergic agonists

The use of adrenergic agonists during CPR was first described by Redding and Pearson in 1963, 3 years following the original description of closed-chest CPR.[258] These authors subsequently showed that earlier administration of epinephrine improved the success rate of CPR in a canine model of cardiac arrest.[258] They later showed that the increase in diastolic aortic pressure generated by the administration of adrenergic agonist drugs was responsible for the success of resuscitation.[236] They theorized that vasopressors such as epinephrine were of value because the drug increased peripheral vascular tone.

Yakaitis et al. investigated the relative importance of alpha-adrenergic and beta-adrenergic agonist actions during resuscitation.[355] Only 27% of dogs that received both alpha-adrenergic receptor antagonists and beta-adrenergic receptor agonists, such as isoproterenol, were resuscitated successfully. In contrast, all of the dogs that received alpha-adrenergic agonist drugs with beta-adrenergic antagonist drugs were resuscitated successfully. These data suggest that the alpha-adrenergic agonist receptor action of epinephrine is responsible for successful resuscitation.

More recent studies have reinforced this concept. Michael et al. demonstrated that the effects of epinephrine during CPR were mediated by the selective vasoconstriction of peripheral vessels except those supplying the brain and heart. During epinephrine infusion, higher aortic systolic and diastolic pressures were maintained as the effective downstream pressures for heart or brain (right atrial pressure or intracranial pressure, respectively), resulting in higher perfusion pressures to the heart and brain.[214] Despite the increase in aortic pressure, flow to other organs such as the kidneys and intestine decreased markedly.[168,214,288]

Coronary blood flow

As described above, the increase in aortic diastolic pressure during CPR is critical for maintaining coronary blood flow and success of resuscitation. In beating hearts, beta-adrenergic effects increase the contractile state of the myocardium. During CPR, these effects are thought to result in stimulation of spontaneous myocardial contractions and an increase in the intensity of ventricular fibrillation. In contrast, the inotropic effect of beta-adrenergic agonist drugs might actually be deleterious to the fibrillating heart by increasing intramyocardial wall pressure and hence the downstream pressure for coronary perfusion.[190] This would cause a decreased coronary perfusion pressure and lead to decreased subendocardial blood flow. In addition, beta-adrenergic stimulation might also increase the myocardial oxygen demand superimposed on the low coronary blood flow available during CPR. In normally beating hearts, subendocardial blood flow occurs almost entirely during diastole. Ventricular fibrillation has been shown to simulate a period of sustained contraction.[77] This leads to a higher intramyocardial wall pressure during fibrillation, producing a decrease in myocardial perfusion pressure and coronary blood flow. This combination of increased oxygen demand by the beta-agonist action and decreased oxygen supply by the decrease in coronary blood flow may cause further damage to an already ischemic heart.

Other adrenergic agonist drugs, some with pure alpha-adrenergic actions, have been used successfully during CPR. These drugs, such as phenylephrine and methoxamine, cause peripheral vasoconstriction during CPR, generating an increase in aortic diastolic pressure. Moreover, they may not cause an increase in oxygen demand of the heart because of the absence of beta-adrenergic stimulation. This would result in a more favorable oxygen demand-to-supply ratio in the ischemic heart (Box 37-7).

Successful resuscitation with alpha-adrenergic agonist medications has been shown clearly in animal studies.[236,258,285,355] These drugs maintain myocardial blood flow as well as epinephrine does during CPR.[355] Schleien et al. found that high aortic pressures can be sustained in a canine model of CPR with phenylephrine.[285] Moreover, the high level of myocardial perfusion pressure and coronary blood flow produced were

---

BOX 37-7
ALPHA-ADRENERGIC VS. BETA-ADRENERGIC
AGONIST EFFECTS

Alpha-adrenergic effects

Vasoconstrict peripheral vessels
Maintain aortic diastolic pressure
Improve coronary blood flow
No metabolic stimulatory effect

Beta-adrenergic effects

Vasodilate peripheral vessels
Decrease aortic diastolic pressure
Increase metabolic rate
Increase inotropic function
Increase intensity of ventricular fibrillation

---

equivalent in the phenylephrine and epinephrine animal groups. The use of either drug[285] resulted in a 75% success rate for resuscitation. There has been debate though regarding the relative merits of a pure alpha-adrenergic agonist vs. epinephrine for resuscitation.[32,35,137]

Cerebral blood flow

The generation of cerebral blood flow during CPR also appears to depend on the vasoconstriction of peripheral vessels.[170] **Cerebral blood flow, like coronary blood flow, is enhanced by the use of alpha-adrenergic agonists.** Epinephrine produces selective vasoconstriction of noncerebral peripheral vessels to other areas of the head and scalp (i.e., tongue, facial muscles, and skin) without causing cerebral vasoconstriction in adult[214,252] and infant models of CPR.[288] Phenylephrine has been found to be as effective in generating and sustaining cerebral blood flow as epinephrine in an adult canine model[285] and in an infant piglet model.[287] Cerebral oxygen uptake was maintained at prearrest levels in dogs in both an epinephrine and a phenylephrine drug group for 20 minutes of CPR, implying that cerebral blood flow was higher than is necessary to maintain adequate cerebral metabolism.[285] When epinephrine or phenylephrine was administered 9 minutes after fibrillation, one group of investigators failed to detect differences in neurological deficits 24 hours later.[29] Other investigators have found epinephrine to be beneficial in generating vital organ blood flow.[32,34,35] This may be due to the use of drug dosages that are not equally potent in generating vascular pressure and blood flow.

Cerebral oxygen uptake may be increased by central beta-adrenoceptors if sufficient amounts of

epinephrine cross the blood-brain barrier.[41,197] Additionally, epinephrine may vasoconstrict or vasodilate cerebral vessels, depending on the balance between alpha-adrenergic and beta-adrenergic effects.[353] When cerebral ischemia was brief, epinephrine and phenylephrine had similar effects on cerebral blood flow and metabolism. In this experiment, the blood-brain barrier most likely was not disrupted.[285] These drugs can cross the barrier if there is mechanical disruption or if the enzymatic barriers to vasopressors are overwhelmed in the presence of tissue hypoxia.[84,182] **During CPR the blood-brain barrier may be disrupted during the large fluctuation of cerebral venous and arterial pressures that is generated during chest compressions. The permeability of the barrier may also increase during the surge of arterial pressure that may occur in a maximally dilated vascular bed following resuscitation.**[9] An increase in cerebral oxygen demand when flow is limited could affect cerebral recovery adversely. Using a small amino acid, alpha-aminoisobutyric acid, as a marker of blood-brain barrier permeability in dogs, we recently showed no disruption of the barrier during CPR, immediately following resuscitation or 4 hours after resuscitation.[286] In young piglets, following 8 minutes of cardiac arrest, the blood-brain barrier was disrupted 4 hours after defibrillation[289] (Fig. 37-8).

Dosage

The most efficacious dose of epinephrine during CPR is still controversial. The dosage currently recommended by the American Heart Association is 10 μg/kg administered every 5 minutes.[5] **Increasing the usual and recommended dose of epinephrine by 20 to 200 times may have a beneficial effect on the generation of coronary and cerebral blood flow during closed-chest**[33] **or open-chest CPR.**[38] Koscove and Paradis reported on two patients who were resuscitated from ventricular fibrillation with high doses of epinephrine (5 mg) after failing conventional therapy.[171] In a recent study in humans, systolic and diastolic pressures were increased when 5 mg of epinephrine was administered.[106] Large doses of epinephrine failed, however, to improve the balance between myocardial oxygen supply and demand during CPR in dogs.[75] The use of constant infusions of larger doses may also be warranted.[285]

pH issues — sodium bicarbonate

Use of sodium bicarbonate during CPR is now one of the more controversial areas in the CPR literature. These controversies stem from a number of issues, including possible side effects of the drug such as hyperosmolality and hypernatremia, its unproved efficacy in increasing patient survival following cardiac arrest, the need for increased ventilation because

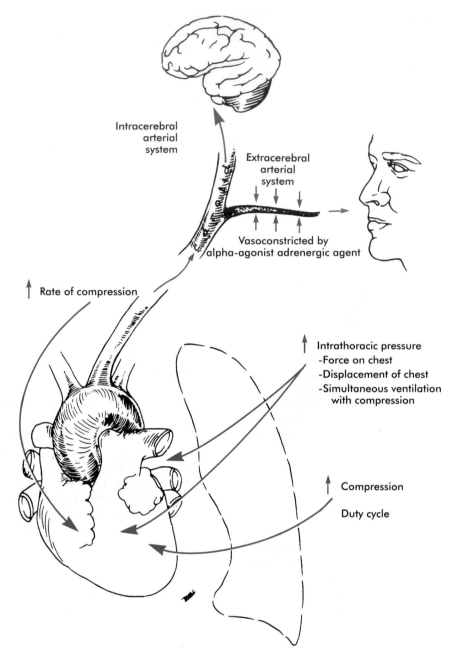

Fig. 37-8. Factors that increase blood flow from the heart are outlined. An increase in cerebral blood flow is also caused by vasoconstriction of extracerebral blood vessels that shunt blood to the intracerebral vessels. (From Schleien CL, Berkowitz ID, Traystman RJ et al: Controversial issues in cardiopulmonary resuscitation, *Anesthesiology* 71:136, 1989.)

of CO_2 production,[27] shift of the oxygen dissociation curve causing a decrease in the unloading of oxygen to tissues, and the creation of paradoxical intracellular acidosis by its dissociation into CO_2 (Box 37-8).

Sodium bicarbonate is indicated for significant metabolic acidosis occurring during cardiac arrest and CPR.[259] It has been shown to increase the success of resuscitation when accompanied by fluid loading in an experimental model.[277] The metabolic acidosis that

occurs during these periods may have widespread detrimental effects. Systemic acidosis depresses myocardial function by depressing spontaneous cardiac activity, diastolic depolarization, electrical threshold for ventricular fibrillation, the inotropic state of the myocardium, and cardiac responsiveness to catecholamines.[49,235,243] Peripheral vessels may also be affected by systemic acidosis, generally by causing a decrease in systemic vascular resistance. This may be par-

---

BOX 37-8
SIDE EFFECTS OF SODIUM BICARBONATE

Hyperosmolality
Hypernatremia
Hypercapnia
Decreased unloading of oxygen from hemoglobin
Paradoxical intracellular acidosis

---

ticularly catastrophic during CPR when peripheral vasoconstriction is the physiologic effect that is desired. **Moreover, the responsiveness of the peripheral circulation to both alpha-adrenergic and beta-adrenergic agonists is decreased with acidosis.**[183] This effect may be overcome by large doses of catecholamines[301,354] (Box 37-9).

Although the cardiovascular problems caused by acidosis during CPR may be severe, a number of possible offsetting problems due to sodium bicarbonate may preclude its use during CPR. **Sodium bicarbonate has not been shown to improve outcome from cardiac arrest in a randomized, controlled fashion.**[299] Guerci et al. did not find that bicarbonate had a more beneficial effect in defibrillating arrested dogs than saline,[115] although both groups had a high success rate of resuscitation. Graf et al. showed that bicarbonate may actually be deleterious from a hemodynamic standpoint in the treatment of lactic acidosis.[108] The mortality from acidosis induced in diabetic dogs was no different in a bicarbonate-treated group than in a control group. These models arguably may not be applicable to the clinical CPR situation. Following elevation of pH, there may be a leftward shift of the oxygen dissociation curve, causing oxygen to be bound more tightly to hemoglobin.

BOX 37-9
ADVERSE EFFECTS OF
ACIDOSIS DURING CPR

Decreased myocardial function

Depressed SA node
Depressed diastolic depolarization
Depressed threshold for ventricular fibrillation
Negative inotrope

Decreased catecholamine responsiveness

Heart
Peripheral vessels

Peripheral vasodilation

Theoretically this effect allows less oxygen to be available to tissues at a time when blood flow is already limited, further worsening the ischemic condition. The clinical relevance of this effect is undetermined. The incidence of hyperosmolality and hypernatremia by the administration of large doses of bicarbonate is documented.[5,206]

The paradoxical production of intracellular and central nervous system acidosis by bicarbonate might also be a contraindication to its use during CPR.[18] This occurs following the dissociation of bicarbonate, in the presence of carbonic anhydrase, to water and CO_2. CO_2 rapidly diffuses across cell membranes, faster than the egress of H^+ from cells. Thus there may be the generation of intracellular acidosis following bicarbonate administration.[291] This may have widespread consequences on central nervous system function[244] and the diaphragm.[153] This effect in the brain may not be clinically relevant. Sessler et al. demonstrated that administering bicarbonate to neonatal rabbits recovering from hypoxic lactic acidosis increased arterial pH without producing the phenomenon of paradoxical intracellular acidosis. If this effect is an important one, the use of noncarbon dioxide–generating buffers may be warranted.[22,164,291] Others argue that bicarbonate treatment is important and may be a temporizing measure that increases a potentially lethal pH until the underlying cause of acidosis is treated and adequate circulation is restored.[227]

An increase in central venous acidosis during CPR has been well documented in both animal[110] and human studies.[342] This occurs because of the large amount of CO_2 production associated with anaerobic metabolism during the low flow state of CPR. CO_2 is not eliminated despite hyperventilation because of inadequate pulmonary blood flow. Blood that reaches the lungs and subsequently enters the systemic arterial circulation may have a normal PCO_2 and thus a near-normal pH because of the relative hyperventilation during CPR. Despite this, most of the blood remains in the venous circulation and has a higher PCO_2, resulting in a lowered pH in the venous blood, seen mainly as a respiratory acidosis. This relationship between arterial and venous blood is witnessed any

---

BOX 37-10
INDICATIONS FOR USE
OF SODIUM BICARBONATE

Prior metabolic acidosis
Lengthy CPR
Hyperkalemia

time there is a marked decrease in cardiac output or an increase in cellular metabolism.[3] The clinical implications of an arterial-venous Pco_2 gradient are an increased level of Pco_2 in the coronary circulation leading to the appearance of myocardial acidosis, which may impair cellular function.[335]

In conclusion, the use of sodium bicarbonate for the treatment of acidosis during CPR remains controversial. The most critical step in treating lactic acidosis is the identification of the underlying cause. **The best treatment for a large arterial-venous gradient of pH and Pco_2 is improving cardiac output through the use of improved mechanical CPR and adrenergic agonists. Bicarbonate administration in the CPR setting may be warranted in patients who have had a long period of cardiac arrest or who have severe metabolic acidosis preceding their arrest in which the acidosis may have contributed to the cardiac arrest.** Thus bicarbonate is indicated when the CPR scenario is not going well after ventilation, chest compressions have been established, and 1 round of other medications has been administered (usually 10 minutes into the CPR sequence). In addition, bicarbonate is indicated when cardiac arrest is caused by hyperkalemia. **When bicarbonate is used, 1 mEq/kg should be given as the initial dose and no more than half this dose given every 10 minutes thereafter. If arterial blood gases have been obtained, the dose can be calculated as $0.3 \times$ base deficit $\times$ patient's weight (kg)** (Box 37-10).

Calcium salts

The use of calcium chloride during CPR is not in favor as it was as recently as 1985. This is primarily due to the finding that in the setting of cardiac arrest, calcium may prevent reflow of blood into ischemic areas of the brain and heart, which may ultimately worsen the prognosis. Cytoplasmic calcium accumulation appears to be the final common pathway of cell death.[157,347] Moreover, inhibition of calcium accumulation following an ischemic episode preserves myocardial function,[50] so that the use of calcium channel blocking agents may be more helpful than calcium in preventing or ameliorating damage during or following an ischemic event such as a cardiac arrest. Calcium channel blockers also raise the threshold of the ischemic heart to ventricular fibrillation.[261]

Calcium is essential in myocardial excitation-contraction coupling, in increasing contractility, and in enhancing ventricular automaticity during asystole.[110] These physiologic effects may make calcium useful in the setting of asystole and electromechanical dissociation.[159] Evidence for the successful use of calcium in these settings, however, is lacking.[69,304,305] Ionized hypocalcemia that leads to decreased ventricular performance, peripheral vasodilation, and blunt-

---

BOX 37-11
INDICATIONS FOR USE OF CALCIUM

Hypocalcemia
  Total
  Ionized
Calcium channel blocker overdose
Hyperkalemia
Hypermagnesemia

---

ing of the hemodynamic response to catecholamines[30,78,202,282,327] has been documented in patients suffering an out-of-hospital cardiac arrest.[328]

At present, the firm indications for calcium use during CPR is for patients suffering a cardiac arrest secondary to hypocalcemia, hyperkalemia, hypermagnesemia, or an overdose with a calcium channel blocking agent. Hypocalcemia is seen in patients with conditions leading to a decrease in total body calcium, such as hypoparathyroidism, renal failure, and pancreatitis. **More often, however, the condition is seen as a decrease in the circulating ionized calcium level associated with massive blood transfusion. This occurs most commonly in the operating room in patients undergoing major surgical procedures, following massive trauma, or during the course of orthotopic liver transplantation. It is also seen commonly in the emergency department following massive trauma.** Since calcium administration is at present not a first-line treatment during CPR, the anesthesiologist or other medical caretaker needs to consider hypocalcemia as the cause of the arrest and treat it appropriately when cardiac arrest occurs in the operating room. Recent reports document the occurrence of severe ionized hypocalcemia after out-of-hospital cardiac arrest.[328] Future recommendations will need to take these reports into account.

When calcium chloride is indicated during CPR (Box 37-11), **it is given in a dosage of 2 ml of a 10% solution in adults, and repeated as necessary. In children, the dose is 0.1 ml/kg of the 10% solution.** Two other calcium salts available for clinical use are calcium gluconate and calcium gluceptate. These drugs are equally effective in raising ionized calcium levels during CPR.[133] Calcium gluconate can be given in a dose of 100 mg/kg in adults and 100 to 120 mg/kg with a maximum dose of 2 g in the pediatric patient. Calcium gluceptate can be given in a dose of 5 ml to 7 ml. **Calcium solutions should be given by slow IV administration. When given rapidly to a beating heart, severe bradycardia or sustained contraction of the myocardium with ventricular standstill can occur.**

Atropine

Atropine is a parasympatholytic drug that works primarily by reducing cardiac vagal tone that causes an increase in the rate of discharge from the sinus node and improves conduction through the AV node.[72]

Atropine is indicated when bradycardia coexists with hypotension, ventricular ectopy, or symptoms associated with myocardial ischemia. The drug can also be used to treat second-degree and third-degree heart block, and slow idioventricular rates.[283] It may be effective in treating ventricular asystole.[37,222,306]

The recommended dose for bradycardia is 0.5 mg IV every 5 minutes to a total dose of 2.0 mg. When treating asystole, 1.0 mg IV is given and repeated in 5 minutes if asystole persists. The pediatric dose of atropine is 0.01 to 0.02 mg/kg with a minimum dose of 0.15 mg. A minimum dose is used because of the possibility of paradoxical bradycardia resulting from a central stimulatory effect on the medullary vagal nuclei.[172]

The side effects of atropine result from the resultant tachycardia after its administration. This tachycardia is especially dangerous in patients with acute myocardial ischemia or infarction because of the resultant increase in the myocardial oxygen requirement.[204,263] Ventricular fibrillation and tachycardia have been caused by the IV administration of atropine.[54,195,204]

Glucose

The use of glucose during CPR is controversial at this time because of the possible detrimental effects of hyperglycemia on the brain during ischemia. The association of hyperglycemia with aggravation of cerebral ischemic damage was initially reported by Meyers et al.[223] and confirmed subsequently by other investigators in animal models of both focal and global ischemia.[53,105,181,250] **These studies have demonstrated that when hyperglycemia is produced before a cerebral ischemic event, the neurologic outcome is worse than in normoglycemic animal controls.**

The pathophysiologic mechanism for neurologic damage is thought to be an increase in brain lactic acid levels. Lactic acid is produced during periods of anaerobic metabolism, which is increased during periods of hyperglycemia. The resultant acidosis aggravates neuronal injury.[176] There is evidence in humans that clinical outcome following an episode of cerebral ischemia is also worsened by hyperglycemia. Pulsinelli et al. found that patients with hyperglycemia had worsening of their neurologic outcome compared with patients who were normoglycemic after ischemic strokes.[251]

In the clinical context of cardiac arrest, a fluid containing glucose is frequently administered. In adults, a bolus of 50% glucose solution is often given to the unconscious patient to treat possible hypoglycemia as a cause of coma. However, hyperglycemia produced by the infusion of this high dose of glucose may worsen cerebral ischemic damage already produced by a cardiac arrest and subsequent reperfusion with low cerebral blood flow. D'Alecy et al.[61] demonstrated in a canine model of cardiac arrest and resuscitation that physiologic quantities of 5% dextrose solution administered before arrest worsened neurologic outcome following resuscitation. However, the clinical significance of this study is unclear because glucose infusion begins during, rather than before, cardiac resuscitation. In another study, Lundy et al. demonstrated that the administration of glucose during the commencement of ischemia and CPR also resulted in a higher mortality and worse neurologic outcome in dogs.[196] In addition, in that study, increased inotrope support was required to maintain blood pressure following resuscitation in those animals receiving glucose.

Even without glucose administration, Longstreth et al., in a retrospective study of neurologic outcome after out-of-hospital cardiac arrest, demonstrated worse neurologic recovery in patients who had a high blood glucose on admission. However, in a subsequent study, the authors suggested that the higher blood glucose level in those patients may have resulted from the prolonged and difficult resuscitation.[193] Because only a minimal amount of glucose, if any, was administered before admission to the hospital, they suggested that the rise of glucose level during CPR was due to the endogenous release of glucose.

With so much attention on the possibility of an adverse outcome due to hyperglycemia during CPR, hypoglycemia may now become more prevalent. **Hypoglycemia should be avoided, and its prompt treatment is critical. Patients prone to hypoglycemia, such as infants (who have low glycogen stores) or adults (those who are ill and have low glycogen stores or diabetics receiving insulin), should have serum glucose levels checked during CPR and treated if hypoglycemia does occur.**

In summary, the data are inconclusive regarding the effect of glucose levels on neurologic outcome following CPR. Laboratory studies have shown the adverse effect of hyperglycemia in animals suffering cerebral ischemia, when hyperglycemia preceded the period of cerebral ischemia. Thus, the effect of hyperglycemia, particularly when it is caused by the endogenous release of glucose secondary to high catecholamine levels present during a cardiac arrest and CPR, is unclear. **It is reasonable at this time to avoid the administration of supplemental glucose during CPR unless hypoglycemia is present.**

Oxygen

Even though thousands of articles refer to the various drug therapies and to new methods of CPR, few point out the need for oxygen. **Patients in cardiac arrest or low cardiac output states should receive 100% oxygen as soon as possible.** Oxygen will increase arterial oxygen tension and hemoglobin saturation if ventilation is supported, and continued tissue oxygenation when circulation is supported. During cardiac or pulmonary arrest the highest possible oxygen concentration (100%) should be administered to all patients regardless of the cause of the arrest.

Newer and experimental drug therapies

The field of brain resuscitation is one that has many positive claims but still only scant experimental data to support those claims. The number of pharmacologic and other therapeutic maneuvers to enhance cardiac or brain recovery following cardiac arrest or other ischemic events is varied. These therapies include the use of drugs such as calcium channel blockers, excitatory amino acid receptor blockers, oxygen radical scavengers, blockers of arachidonic acid metabolism, hypothermia, and others. The future for these therapies is unknown at this time. Whether any of these therapeutic modalities will play an essential role in the resuscitation process or will go the way of the barbiturates in primary brain protection is also unknown.

Defibrillation
Electric countershock

The three most common rhythm disturbances encountered during a cardiac arrest are ventricular fibrillation, electromechanical dissociation, and asystole. Ventricular fibrillation is the most common dysrhythmia in this setting and is caused by reentry impulse generation with multiple circuits with changing pattern. Many of the conditions encountered in the operating room — hypoxia, hypercapnia, ischemia, hypothermia, metabolic acidosis, and electrolyte disturbances — lower the threshold for ventricular fibrillation. Electric countershock is the treatment of choice for ventricular fibrillation and for ventricular tachycardia when a pulse is not present or the patient has signs reflecting a poor cardiac output.

The first successful use of electrical defibrillation occurred in 1775, when applied to a three-year-old child. In 1899, alternating current was used to defibrillate an open dog heart.[175] In fact, the electric utility companies funded much of the defibrillation research early in this century hoping to reverse the high number of electric shock fatalities in their workers.[174] In 1939 the Soviets, Furvich and Yuniev, described the first successful use of external electric countershock in dogs.[65] In 1947 Beck performed the first successful open-chest human defibrillation in an operating room.[16] Finally, in 1956, a full 4 years before external cardiac massage was described, the first successful external defibrillation was performed by Zoll.[357]

The technique of applying an electric countershock is a simple one. Most important, the appropriate personnel need to know where the defibrillator is located. In addition, it should be maintained to specifications. **An initial defibrillation of 200 joules is recommended in adult patients. The dose of the second shock is more controversial, therefore a dose of 200 to 300 joules is used. Should the first two shocks not be successful, a third shock of 360 joules is used. In children a dose of 2 joules/kg is used on the first defibrillatory attempt. If this is unsuccessful, a second shock of 4 joules/kg is used and repeated twice if needed.** If defibrillatory attempts are unsuccessful after three attempts, attention should be redirected to the oxygenation, acid-base status, and administration of CPR and drugs such as epinephrine. In addition, if defibrillation attempts fail, factors that may increase transthoracic impedance should be evaluated. These factors include pneumothorax, inadequate paddle–chest wall interface, inadequate paddle position, excessive distance between paddles, and inadequate paddle pressure on the chest.[5]

The placement of appropriate-sized paddles is important, particularly in the pediatric population. For adults 14-cm diameter paddles are used, for older children 8-cm paddles, and for infants 4.5-cm paddles. The largest paddle size appropriate for the patient is used so that the density of current flow is reduced, leading to less myocardial damage. The paddles are situated so that a majority of myocardium is included between them. **One paddle is placed to the right of the upper sternum below the clavicle, the other positioned just below and to the left of the left nipple. An alternative approach, particularly when appropriate-sized paddles are not available for infants or small children, is placement of one paddle anteriorly over the left precordium, with the other paddle on the back between the scapulae behind the heart. For patients with dextrocardia, the position should be reversed.** The interface between the paddle and the chest wall can be electrode cream, saline, soap, or gauze pads. The electrode cream produces lower impedance than the paste. The substance used should not form a complete circuit from one paddle to the other. This would cause the electric circuit to follow the path of least resistance and bypass the heart. Electric countershock, when properly administered, directs more than 2 amp through the heart. This current produces a sustained contraction in the normally beating heart. In the fibrillating heart it will terminate ventricular fibrillation by simultaneously depolarizing the entire myocardium. Following this massive depolarization, spontaneous cardiac contractions commence, assuming the metabolic milieu is normal.

Direct current (DC) shock is the sole method now used for defibrillation, because alternating current was found to be too hazardous to the patient and the operator. In addition, DC has the advantage of being portable. Most commonly a dampened sine wave is used to deliver energy, but a trapezoid waveform has also been used.[6] DC current is associated with hazards, including myocardial damage, inability to defibrillate, and the presence of postdefibrillation dysrhythmias.[59] In a majority of adult patients, 100 to 200 joules are successful when shocks are delivered with minimal delay. Very high voltages, 500 to 1000 joules, have been used,[314,315] but these do not appear to be necessary. Of adult patients 95%, including some weighing in excess of 100 kg, were successfully defibrillated with the use of 200 joules.[40] **In a prospective out-of-hospital study, survival was unrelated to the energy level used or the weight of the patient.**[341] These data have been reconfirmed in later studies.[70,98] There was no difference in heart weight or energy per gram of heart weight needed to defibrillate when postmortem examination was performed subsequently.[160]

With increasing levels of energy, there is an increase in myocardial damage[60,73] and in the incidence of postresuscitation dysrhythmias.[238] The increased incidence of dysrhythmias is thought to be associated with prolonged depolarization of the myocardial cell membrane.[7,149] In humans, dysrhythmia frequency and the degree of ST segment depression is greater with increased energy doses.[260] It has been argued that two low energy shocks cause more myocardial damage than one high energy shock, although this has not been substantiated.[2] In addition, transthoracic impedance declines with repeated shocks,[60,101] although this effect is only mild in humans.[161]

The time to defibrillation may be the most important aspect to successful resuscitation.[160,242] In one study, success of defibrillation was higher when the defibrillatory attempt occurred within 8 minutes of the cardiac arrest. In all of the unsuccessful attempts, the time following cardiac arrest to defibrillation averaged 17 minutes.[160] Acidosis and hypoxia have been correlated with decreased success of defibrillation[160]; mild to moderate hypothermia has not.[313] The concurrent use of antidysrhythmics such as lidocaine with electrical countershock may have its hazards. Lidocaine increases the energy required for ventricular defibrillation in dogs.[12,82] This effect appears to be enhanced by acidosis and reversed by alkalosis, effects consistent with the drug's sodium channel-blocking properties.[83] Another factor important for the success

of defibrillation is the simultaneous depolarization of a critical myocardial mass. Even though depolarization of every myocardial cell is not needed for successful defibrillation, placing the paddles appropriately is important to get the greatest mass of the heart between the paddles. The success of defibrillation may also depend on the cause of ventricular fibrillation. Patients who suffer an acute myocardial infarction with heart failure have a decreased success rate of defibrillation.[97]

Open-chest defibrillation can be used in the operating room when the thorax is already opened during surgery. When defibrillation is performed in this manner, 5 joules should be used on the first attempt. If unsuccessful, repeated doses can be used with energy levels up to 50 joules. Internal paddles are available: 6 cm diameter for adults, 4 cm for children, and 2 cm for infants. The handles should be insulated. The paddles are applied with saline-soaked pads. One electrode is placed behind the left ventricle and the other electrode over the right ventricle on the anterior surface of the heart.

Lidocaine

Lidocaine has many uses for the anesthesiologist. In the cardiac arrest setting it is frequently used following resuscitation for prophylaxis or treatment of ventricular ectopy or during unstable rhythms leading to cardiac arrest. Lidocaine is effective in terminating ventricular premature beats (VPBs) and ventricular tachycardia in humans in a number of settings, including intraoperative, preoperative, or postoperative cardiac surgery, following an acute myocardial infarction, and in patients with digitalis intoxication. It is also effective in preventing and treating ventricular dysrhythmias during cardiac catheterization. Lidocaine has not been found effective in the treatment of atrial or atrioventricular junctional dysrhythmias (Box 37-12).

Lidocaine is metabolized mainly in the liver by the microsomal enzyme system.[52] Its major degenerative pathway is by oxidative N-de-ethylation, followed by hydrolysis to 2-6 xylidine. Its minor degradative

---

BOX 37-12
INDICATIONS FOR USE OF LIDOCAINE

Frequent ventricular premature beats (> 6/min)
Coupled VPBS
Multiform VPBS
Ventricular tachycardia
Prophylaxis during cardiac catheterization
Prophylaxis following resuscitation

pathway is by hydroxylation of its aromatic nitrogen. Up to 10% of the drug is excreted unchanged in the urine. An acid urine increases its excretion.

From an electrophysiologic standpoint, lidocaine causes a decrease in automaticity by decreasing the slope of the normal phase 4 depolarization in Purkinje fibers.[24] Lidocaine also increases the threshold for ventricular fibrillation.[103] In addition, lidocaine can abolish dysrhythmias due to ventricular reentry. It has no effect on conduction times through the AV node or on intraventricular conduction time. The relevance of these effects to ischemic myocardium in vivo may be affected by changes in the microcirculation causing differences in local tissue levels of lidocaine.[52]

The toxic effects of lidocaine are mainly attributed to its central nervous system disturbances. These include seizures, psychosis, drowsiness, paresthesias, disorientation, muscle twitching, agitation, and respiratory arrest. Any time that lidocaine is given, drugs such as a benzodiazepine or short-acting barbiturate and airway equipment should be available to treat seizures. True allergic reactions to lidocaine are rare.

Cardiovascular side effects, although described, are unusual. In dogs, when lidocaine is given as a rapid IV bolus, there is a transient decrease of cardiac output, stroke work, blood pressure, and systemic vascular resistance, with a slight increase in heart rate.[10] In healthy adults, these hemodynamic changes do not occur.[147,290] In awake patients with cardiac disease, there was either no change or only a minimal decrease in ventricular function when lidocaine was given.[147,290] Thus in patients with cardiac disease, slow administration of lidocaine, 50 to 100 mg/min is advised[52] (Box 37-13).

Bretylium

Bretylium is used in suppressing serious ventricular dysrhythmias when other antidysrhythmics such as lidocaine have been unsuccessful.[167] Presently, it is indicated for the treatment of life-threatening ventricular dysrhythmias such as ventricular fibrillation and tachycardia resistant to treatment with adequate doses of first-line medications. Electrical cardioversion is the first line of treatment when ventricular tachycardia presents with hemodynamic compromise. The drug is not used to treat asymptomatic premature ventricular beats or atrial dysrhythmias. Bretylium compared favorably with lidocaine in treating out-of-hospital patients with ventricular fibrillation.[129]

Bretylium is a bromobenzyl quaternary ammonia compound unrelated to lidocaine. Its mean elimination half-life is 9.8 hours.[268] The drug is 80% excreted in the urine and remains unchanged over the first 24 hours. An additional 10% of the drug is excreted in the urine over the next 72 hours.[180]

The mechanism of action of bretylium lies in its adrenergic stimulatory properties and in its direct cardiac action. After intravenous administration, there is an initial release of norepinephrine with subsequent inhibition of release of norepinephrine.[201] There also appears to be a block of the reuptake mechanisms of norepinephrine and epinephrine into adrenergic nerve endings. This effect potentiates the action of these agonists on the adrenergic receptors. The importance of this adrenergic function of bretylium on its antidysrhythmic effect remains unknown.

The direct cardiac action of bretylium is not mediated by beta-adrenergic receptors.[25] Its actions persist despite pretreatment with reserpine or cardiac denervation. Bretylium increases the action potential duration of cardiac muscle and the effective refractory period of Purkinje and ventricular muscle fibers. Its major antidysrhythmic effect may lie in its ability to diminish the difference in action potential duration between normal and infarcted areas of the heart.[47] Bretylium also increases the electrical ventricular fibrillatory threshold in normal and infarcted hearts and appears to be more effective in doing so than lidocaine.[48] A combination of bretylium and lidocaine may cause a more rapid and prolonged antifibrillatory effect than either drug alone.[125] Bretylium has been noted to defibrillate the heart without electric countershock.[13]

The dosage of bretylium is 5 to 10 mg/kg body weight given by rapid intravenous bolus administration to treat ventricular fibrillation. If the drug can be given less urgently, 500 mg should be diluted to no less than 50 ml and given over 5 to 10 minutes. The patient should be closely monitored during its administration because of the frequency of blood pressure changes (see following). Its action in suppressing ventricular fibrillation is within minutes. When treating ventricular fibrillation, defibrillation should be administered first. If this maneuver is unsuccessful three times, epinephrine should be administered, followed by

---

BOX 37-13
TOXICITY OF LIDOCAINE

Central nervous system — common in dosage > 5 mg/kg
Allergy — rare
Cardiovascular — rare
  If seizures occur with use of lidocaine, administer:

Benzodiazepine:	Diazepam	0.1 mg/kg
	Midazolam	0.05 mg/kg
Barbiturate:	Thiopental	1-4 mg/kg
	Phenobarbital	5-15 mg/kg

another defibrillatory attempt. If that is unsuccessful, lidocaine should be given, followed by another defibrillatory attempt, which is followed by a dose of bretylium. This is followed by a defibrillatory attempt and then another dose of bretylium. If the dysrhythmia persists or recurs, additional drug can be given every 15 to 30 minutes, up to a total dose of 30 mg/kg.

Hemodynamic side effects are most common with the administration of bretylium. There is usually an initial increase in blood pressure due to the release of norepinephrine after an IV dose (if the patient is not in ventricular fibrillation). This could also result in a transient increase in the number of premature ventricular beats. Subsequently, a majority of patients exhibit a hypotensive response, which can be attenuated by placing the patient in the supine position.[167] This effect is due to its adrenergic-blocking actions. If this effect is severe, the patient should be supported with fluids and vasopressors. Patients may also exhibit extreme hypersensitivity to exogenous direct-acting catecholamines because of the impaired uptake of those drugs. When bretylium is rapidly infused, nausea and vomiting commonly occur. Parotid swelling and pain have been seen with oral use of the drug.[167]

Electromechanical Dissociation

Electromechanical dissociation (EMD) is defined as organized electrocardiographic activity without evidence of myocardial contractions. It may occur as either the primary dysrhythmia following cardiac arrest or an intervening rhythm associated with treatment for cardiac arrest. It is important to differentiate the two patterns of EMD. **It may be caused by a variety of noncardiac mechanisms including hypovolemia, pericardial tamponade, tension pneumothorax, or pulmonary embolism. In these cases, treatment is directed at the underlying disorder and usually results in a successful outcome.** Primary EMD may represent a failure of myocardial contractility caused by a depletion of intracellular energy stores.[332] In a large retrospective study of patients with EMD, age greater than 70 years, prearrest hypoxemia, and the presence of pulmonary disease or diabetes mellitus were associated with an increased risk of developing EMD[310] (Box 37-14).

Treatment of EMD has been, on the whole, very dissatisfying. Successful resuscitation rates are reported to approach zero.[143] In the previously cited study, 18% of 261 patients with cardiac arrest exhibited EMD either as the presenting rhythm or subsequent to defibrillation. Of these, only four patients survived EMD, although patients who presented with EMD had a higher mortality and a slower rate of cerebral recovery than patients presenting with other rhythms. Patients who developed EMD subse-

---

```
┌─────────────────────────────────────┐
│              BOX 37–14               │
│    CAUSES OF ELECTROMECHANICAL       │
│         DISSOCIATION (EMD)           │
├─────────────────────────────────────┤
│  Noncardiac (secondary)              │
│  Hypovolemia                         │
│  Pericardial tamponade               │
│  Tension pneumothorax                │
│  Pulmonary embolism                  │
│                                      │
│  Cardiac (primary)                   │
│  Failure of myocardial contractility │
└─────────────────────────────────────┘
```

quent to defibrillation had a better outcome than those patients presenting with EMD.[125] There does not appear to be an ECG-correlated finding in predicting outcome of EMD after prolonged ventricular fibrillation.[233]

Treatment of EMD has historically included the use of epinephrine or other catecholamines, calcium chloride, and atropine. Methoxamine, an alpha-agonist, has been used successfully in the treatment of EMD,[257] although a recent study showed no difference in human resuscitation comparing the use of epinephrine and methoxamine. In that study, only 1 patient out of 79 presenting with EMD survived to hospital discharge.[325] The use of calcium chloride alone does not appear to be warranted,[28] although improved resuscitation rates with calcium administration have been found if the QRS complex was more than or equal to 0.12 seconds[308] or there was ECG evidence of ischemia.[305] Glucagon had a favorable effect on dogs with EMD or asystole in restoring effective spontaneous circulation following unsuccessful CPR.[232]

Thus treatment of EMD should first be directed toward the noncardiac causes, such as hypovolemia or pneumothorax. When EMD presents as the primary dysrhythmia, the usual drug therapies during CPR should be utilized, although successful resuscitation in patients with this disorder is very limited. It is appropriate, though, to resuscitate patients with apparent EMD because of the inability, at times, to appreciate a pulse in low flow states following defibrillation. In these cases what is diagnosed as EMD may actually be a case of cardiogenic shock with weak pulses (Box 37-15).

Open-Chest CPR

The use of open-chest cardiac massage has been primarily replaced by closed-chest CPR since its inception in 1960.[173] From a physiologic standpoint open-chest CPR is superior to closed-chest CPR in

---

BOX 37-15
TREATMENT FOR
ELECTROMECHANICAL DISSOCIATION

Noncardiac
Check for secondary causes

Cardiac
Epinephrine
Calcium
Atropine
Glucagon

BOX 37-16
ALGORITHM FOR ASYSTOLE

Begin CPR
↓
IV access
↓
Epinephrine
↓
Atropine
↓
Sodium bicarbonate

---

generating vital organ blood flow. There continue to be a number of indications for its use.

The generation of cardiac output and vital organ blood flow is better with open-chest CPR compared with conventional CPR in animals[26,343] and humans.[68] When performed after 15 minutes of closed-chest CPR, open-chest CPR significantly improves coronary perfusion pressure and the rate of successful resuscitation.[276] By directly applying force to the heart in open-chest CPR, there is no elevation in intrathoracic pressure. Thus right atrial and intracranial pressure do not increase as in closed-chest CPR. This results in higher coronary and cerebral perfusion pressure.[275,285]

With evidence of superior blood pressure and blood flow with open-chest CPR, there are a number of indications for its use. Nevertheless, open-chest CPR is not a means of CPR that can be employed by lay people or by most physicians. The operating room is one situation that is more amenable to this technique. **The indications for its use in the operating room include cardiac arrest secondary to cardiac tamponade, cardiac arrest in the face of critical aortic stenosis or when associated with hypothermia, and cardiac arrest secondary to a ruptured aortic aneurysm when cardiopulmonary bypass facilities are immediately available.** Clearly, when cardiac arrest occurs during surgery in which the chest is already opened, open-chest CPR should be applied. **Other non-operating room indications for open-chest CPR include cardiac arrest secondary to penetrating chest injury or crushed chest injury, anatomic chest wall abnormalities that make closed-chest CPR impossible or ineffective, and failure of adequately applied closed-chest CPR.**[5] This last point remains controversial. When initiated earlier following failure of closed-chest CPR, open-chest CPR may improve resuscitation.[162,275]

Temporary Pacemaker Therapy

When emergency pacing is indicated, intravenous or transthoracic pacing can be initiated. Recently, exter-

nal noninvasive temporary pacemakers have been developed that greatly facilitate the use of temporary pacemaking. This system uses large, high impedance electrodes that allows relatively nonpainful stimuli without discomfort from skeletal muscle contraction.[358] **Temporary pacing is indicated for patients whose primary problem is impulse formation or conduction who have preserved myocardial function.** This is illustrated in patients with severe bradycardia or high-grade heart block who have a stroke volume sufficient to generate a palpable pulse. **At this time, no studies have shown temporary pacing to be effective for most cardiac arrest situations, so it is not recommended except for the specific situations outlined above.**[5,93]

Summary

Boxes 37-16 and 37-17 and Table 37-1 give summaries of advanced life support guidelines and procedures.

COMPLICATIONS

Since the original description of closed-chest CPR in 1960, a wide array of complications have been noted and published. Some of these have even occurred in the rescuer, including a Spigelian hernia sustained while training in a CPR course.[31]

Almost every organ system has suffered a complication. These complications include injuries to the neck, thorax, and abdomen, complications secondary to bone marrow and air emboli, those due to aspiration, others due to electrolyte problems, and complications secondary to equipment such as misplaced endotracheal tubes and esophageal obturator airways.

Complications involving the thoracic cavity make up the largest percentage of all complications during CPR. In a recent study, thoracic complications were observed in 42.7% of cases. A total of 31.6% had rib

```
┌─────────────────────────────────┐
│          BOX 37-17              │
│        ALGORITHM FOR            │
│     VENTRICULAR FIBRILLATION    │
├─────────────────────────────────┤
│                                 │
│  Begin CPR                      │
│      ↓                          │
│  Defibrillate 200 Joules        │
│      ↓                          │
│  Defibrillate 200 Joules        │
│      ↓                          │
│  Defibrillate 360 Joules        │
│      ↓                          │
│  Epinephrine 1 mg               │
│      ↓                          │
│  Defibrillate 360 Joules        │
│      ↓                          │
│  Lidocaine 1 mg/kg              │
│      ↓                          │
│  Defibrillate 360 Joules        │
│      ↓                          │
│  Bretylium 5 mg/kg              │
│      ↓                          │
│  Defibrillate 360 Joules        │
│      ↓                          │
│  Bretylium 5 mg/kg              │
│      ↓                          │
│  Defibrillate 360 Joules        │
│      ↓                          │
│  Bretylium or lidocaine         │
│                                 │
└─────────────────────────────────┘
```

fractures, 21.1% had sternal fractures, and 18.3% were reported to have anterior mediastinal hemorrhage. In that study, 20.4% of patients had an upper airway complication, 30.8% had abdominal visceral complications, and 13% had pulmonary complications not related to the chest wall.[177] The incidences of pulmonary edema, as illustrated above[177] and by others,[76] illustrate its frequency during CPR. Its cause is probably quite diverse and may include a number of factors (Box 37-18).

Electrolyte changes are frequently associated with CPR due to the large shifts of blood volume, severe swings in serum pH, and the administration of many drugs that increase the electrolyte load. Although hyperkalemia has been associated with CPR,[245] hypokalemia is the more common postresuscitation abnormality.[62,272,318] Hypokalemia may be caused by a rapid shift of potassium into the intracellular compartment by pH change or by epinephrine, or may be associated with the dysrythmia itself.[272]

Much has been written about the spread of infectious diseases including hepatitis B virus (HBV) and the AIDS virus (HIV).[142,264] Performance of mouth-to-mouth resuscitation or invasive procedures can result in exchange of blood between victim and rescuer if either has had breaks in the skin on or around the lips or in soft tissues of the oral cavity mucosa. Thus there is theoretic risk of HBV and HIV transmissions during mouth-to-mouth resuscitation. According to the position statement of the American Heart Association, the theoretic risk of infection is greater for salivary or aerosol transmissions of herpes simplex, *Neisseria meningitidis* infection, tuberculosis,

Table 37-1   Drug dosages during CPR

	Dosage	How supplied	Volume
Epinephrine	1 mg	1 : 10,000 solution	10 ml
	Pediatric: 10 μg/kg (repeat every 5 min)	1 : 1000 dilute to 1 : 10,000	0.1 ml/kg
Sodium bicarbonate	50 mEq	1 mEq/ml dilute with	50 ml
	Pediatric: 1 mEq/kg	saline 1 : 1 (infants)	1 ml/kg
	or		
	0.3 mEq × base deficit × wgt (kg)		
Atropine	0.5 mg every 5 min (up to 2 mg)	1 mg/ml	1 ml
	1 mg for asystole	0.1 mg/ml	10 ml
	Pediatric: 0.01-0.02 mg/kg (minimum dose-		
	0.15 mg)		
Calcium chloride	200 mg	100 mg/ml	0.1 ml/kg
	Pediatric: 10 mg/kg		
gluconate	100 mg/kg		
	Pediatric: 100-200 mg/kg (up to 2 g)		
gluceptate	5-7 ml		
Lidocaine	1 mg/kg followed by	1%, 2%, 4% solution	
	0.5 mg/kg every 8-10 min (up to 3 mg/kg)		
Bretylium	5 mg/kg (up to 30 mg/kg)		

Table 37-2 Complications during CPR

	Complications	References
Neck	Endotracheal tube placement in esophagus	224
	Esophageal tears—(especially with esophageal obturator airway)	117, 209, 215, 241, 281
	Trauma to hyoid bone	246
	Trauma to thyroid cartilage	246
Thorax	Rib fractures	134, 177, 224, 246
	Sternal fracture	177, 224, 246
	Hemopericardium	134, 177, 224, 246
	Ventricular contusion	224
	Cardiac laceration	348
	Cardiac rupture	14
	Pulmonary edema	76, 177, 224
Abdomen	Gastric distention	224
	Gastric laceration or rupture	4, 209, 333, 334
	Liver rupture	177, 185, 217, 224
	Splenic rupture	185
	Pneumoperitoneum	51
	Aspiration	224
Vascular	Fat emboli	329
	Bone marrow emboli	246, 329
	Disseminated intravascular coagulopathy (DIC)	211
	Thrombosis	128
Electrolytes	Hypokalemia	62, 272, 318
	Hyperkalemia	245
	Hypocalcemia	272
	Hypomagnesemia	272
Rescuer-associated	Infection (bacteria, TB, AIDS, hepatitis)	1, 131, 207
	Physical stress	191

and other respiratory infections. The transmission of HBV or HIV infection during mouth-to-mouth resuscitation has not been documented. However, to minimize the theoretic risks, mechanical ventilation or barrier devices should be accessible to all health care workers[264] (Table 37-2).

PHYSIOLOGY OF CPR
Mechanisms of Blood Flow
History

Beginning with Kouwenhoven's original description of closed-chest CPR, it was generally assumed that blood flow during closed-chest compression resulted from direct squeezing of the heart between the vertebral column and the sternum.[175] If the cardiac pump mechanism is responsible for generating blood flow during closed-chest CPR, the ventricles are compressed to a greater extent than the atria to generate an atrioventricular pressure gradient. This results in closure of the atrioventricular valves.

Ejection of blood from the ventricles is accompanied by a reduction in ventricular volume. During chest relaxation, atrial pressure increases above ventricular pressure, causing the opening of the atrioventricular valves and ventricular filling. This set of cardiac dynamics and flow events mimics the normal cardiac cycle and is definitely operable in open-chest CPR.

Several observations during CPR have been inconsistent with the cardiac pump mechanism of blood flow. Weale and Rothwell-Jackson noted that closed-chest CPR produced equivalent increases in arterial and right-atrial pressures.[340] Rudikoff et al. noted that closed-chest CPR failed to generate adequate blood pressure in patients with flail chest, a clinical circumstance that should permit direct cardiac compression more readily.[271] In those cases blood pressure could be generated when the chest was stabilized by external binding. In 1976 Criley made the dramatic observation that several patients who developed ventricular fibrillation during the course of cardiac catheterization could generate a cardiac output adequate to

---

BOX 37-18
CAUSES OF PULMONARY EDEMA
DURING CPR

Airway obstruction

Development of large negative intrathoracic
pressure

**Acute development of negative intrathoracic
pressure**

On resumption of spontaneous respiration

Aspiration

Overhydration

Increased hydrostatic pressure
Decreased plasma colloid osmotic pressure

Alpha-adrenergic agonists

Increased central blood volume

Leaky capillary syndrome

Due to hypoxic/ischemic injury

Left ventricular failure

Decreased lymph flow during CPR
Neurogenic pulmonary edema

---

preserve consciousness by repetitive coughing. This
was thought to be due to phasic elevation of intrathoracic pressure.[56] Cough CPR focused subsequent
research on whether direct cardiac compression or an
increase in intrathoracic pressure was responsible for
blood flow during CPR.[57]

Intrathoracic pump mechanism

Maneuvers that increase intrathoracic pressure during closed-chest CPR are shown to cause increases of
intrathoracic vascular pressures.[271] The increase of
intrathoracic pressure leads to an increase in carotid
blood flow, suggesting a different mechanism to
account for the forward blood flow during CPR. By
the thoracic pump mechanism, blood flow is thought
to be due solely to changes in intrathoracic pressure
without direct compression of the heart.[271,344] According to this model, closed-chest CPR produces a
generalized elevation of intrathoracic pressure transmitted equally to all chambers of the heart and
intrathoracic vascular structures. The gradient for
blood flow during closed-chest CPR is thought to be
due to a number of factors. The increase in intravascular pressure is transmitted from the intrathoracic to
the peripheral arteries. Because of competent venous
valves at the thoracic inlet, venous collapse at the

inlet, and a highly compliant peripheral venous
system, less pressure is transmitted to the extrathoracic veins compared with the arteries. Thus this
unequal transmission of vascular pressure provides
the gradient for extrathoracic blood flow.[271,344,345]
Implied in the thoracic pump mechanism is the
antegrade flow of blood through an open mitral valve
during chest compression. During relaxation, intrathoracic pressure falls below that of the extrathoracic venous pressure and blood returns to the lungs.
Thus the heart plays no active role as a blood pump
if the intrathoracic pump mechanism is accurate but
serves only as a passive conduit for blood flow.

A number of studies support the thoracic pump
mechanism. There is a close correlation between the
increase in intrapleural pressure and the change in
intrathoracic vascular pressures during closed-chest
CPR.[46,230] Others have demonstrated the existence of
a peripheral vascular gradient sufficient to satisfy the
thoracic pump theory in the form of a large pressure
gradient between the extrathoracic jugular veins and
the right atrium during chest compression in dogs and
humans.[230,271] Two-dimensional echocardiographic
studies during closed-chest CPR in both dogs[230] and
humans[262,346] have shown that the aortic and mitral
valve are open and that left ventricular dimensions are
reduced. In addition, it has been demonstrated
angiographically that there is a decrease in aortic
diameter during chest compression in dogs.[230] If direct
cardiac compression is responsible for ejection of
blood from the heart, an increase rather than a
reduction of aortic diameter would be expected. Thus
a number of findings are predicted by the thoracic
pump theory in which the heart is a conduit and not
a pump for blood flow.

Cardiac pump mechanism

The mechanism of blood flow during closed-chest
CPR remains controversial. When ventricular dimensions were measured, external chest compression has
been shown to produce changes in ventricular
shape.[199] In dogs undergoing high rate manual CPR,
the mitral valve has been shown to close rapidly at a
time when the left ventricle became deformed.[95] The
mitral valve has been shown to close early in CPR.[71]
Thus there remains evidence that the cardiac pump
mechanism may be important, depending on the
method of CPR administration.

Rate and duty cycle

**In 1986 the American Heart Association in the
Guidelines for CPR and Emergency Cardiac Care
increased the recommended rate of chest compressions from 60 to 100.**[5] This change represented a
compromise between advocates of the thoracic pump
mechanism and the direct cardiac compression mech-

anism.[5] Duty cycle is defined as the ratio, stated as a percent, of the duration of the compression phase to that of the entire compression-relaxation cycle. For example, at a rate of 30 compressions per minute, a 1 second compression equals a 50% duty cycle. If blood flow is generated by direct cardiac compression, the stroke volume is determined by the force of compression. Prolonging the compression (increasing the duty cycle) beyond the time necessary to achieve full ventricular ejection should have no further effect on stroke volume in this model. Increasing the rate of compressions increases cardiac output because a fixed blood volume is ejected with each cardiac compression. In contrast, if blood flow is produced by the thoracic pump, the mechanism of flow is analogous to a pressure pump. Blood must be ejected from the large capacitance thoracic vessels for systemic blood flow to occur. With the thoracic pump mechanism, flow is enhanced by increasing both the force of compression and the duty cycle, but is not affected by changes in compression rate over a wide range of rates.[46]

Mathematical models of the cardiovascular system have confirmed that blood flow is determined by the applied force and the compression duration with the thoracic pump mechanism.[23,123] It appears from the experimental animal data and more limited human data that both the thoracic pump and cardiac pump mechanisms can effectively generate blood flow during closed-chest CPR. Discrepancies among the results of various studies may be attributed to differences in CPR models and compression tech-niques. These differences may involve issues of chest compliance and geometry, maturity of different animal species, or chest compression techniques. For example, in an infant with a very compliant chest wall, either mechanism may come into play. Differences in techniques may include the magnitude of sternal displacement, compression force, momentum of chest compression, compression rate, and duty cycle (Fig. 37-9).

On the basis of their canine studies, Maier et al. recommended an increase in the chest compression rate to 120/min.[199] Proponents of the thoracic pump mechanism have suggested that more emphasis be placed on the duration of compression and a chest compression rate be chosen that can most readily achieve a duty cycle of 50%. At a rate of 60/min, a pause between chest compressions is required to achieve a 50% duty cycle. This is tiring and difficult for the rescuer to accomplish. At a faster rate of approximately 100/min, the resuscitator can more readily achieve a 50% duty cycle. Thus the change in the American Heart Association Guidelines for CPR satisfies those who recommend faster chest compres-sions[199] and those who recommend a longer duty cycle.[46]

Newer CPR Techniques
Simultaneous compression-ventilation CPR

A number of experimental techniques have been introduced over the past few years in an attempt to increase vital organ blood flow during CPR. The introduction of simultaneous ventilation-compression

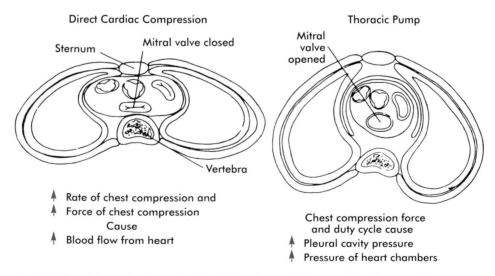

Fig. 37-9. Possible mechanisms for blood flow during CPR includes direct cardiac compression and the thoracic pump. With direct cardiac compression, an increase in chest compression rate causes an increase in blood flow by squeezing the heart between the vertebral column and sternum. With the thoracic pump mechanism, factors that increase pleural pressure cause an increase in pressure within the heart chambers and ultimately an increase in blood flow (From Schleien CL, Berkowitz ID, Traystman RJ et al: Contro-versial issues in cardiopulmonary resuscitation, *Anesthesiology* 71:136, 1989.)

CPR (SCV-CPR) was a logical development based on the thoracic pump mechanism of blood flow during CPR. Chandra et al. demonstrated that the simultaneous application of external chest compression and ventilation at high airway pressure (80 to 100 mm Hg) is a technique that increases intrathoracic pressure and vascular pressures compared with conventional CPR.[43] This technique generated higher aortic blood pressure, cardiac output, and carotid blood flow in both animal[45] and human[43] CPR studies than did conventional CPR techniques. Subsequent studies have confirmed these physiologic advantages in canine models of CPR.[169,194] However, in infant piglets[20] and small dogs,[273] SCV-CPR offers no advantage compared with conventional CPR techniques in raising intrathoracic pressure, systemic blood pressure, or vital organ perfusion. In these small animals, the high chest compliance and specific chest geometry may allow high intrathoracic pressure to be achieved by conventional CPR techniques.[63,64,288] Recently, 944 patients in an out-of-hospital setting were selected randomly to receive either SCV-CPR or conventional CPR. Survival to hospital admission and to discharge was superior in the conventional CPR group.[178] Coronary perfusion pressure was decreased in humans in another study.[312] The use of SCV-CPR would require more sophisticated mechanical equipment to be able to deliver very high airway pressure in an intubated patient. No study to date has shown an increased survival with the use of this technique.

Vest CPR

Vest CPR is a method of increasing intrathoracic pressure by phasically inflating a bladder around the chest, without significantly changing the dimensions of the chest.[122,124,194] There are two possible advantages of this technique compared with conventional CPR. The large increase in intrathoracic pressure occurs by a uniform, circumferential decrease in chest dimension rather than by the focal distortion of a small area of the chest. In addition, trauma to the abdominal viscera and to the chest wall may be obviated. With a vest inflation pressure of 280 mm Hg, cerebral blood flow was maintained at prearrest values while myocardial blood flow was reduced by 50%. No visceral trauma was produced in this group of animals.[194] Vest CPR lowered the coronary perfusion gradient despite increasing aortic systolic pressure in a human study.[312] Despite late application and severe acidosis, vest CPR augmented aortic pressure and coronary perfusion in humans in another study.[116] In the laboratory setting the technique has been applied to dogs to study brain bioenergetics and brain intracellular pH by nuclear magnetic resonance (NMR) spectroscopy.[90] Clinically, the use of vest CPR also depends on the use of sophisticated equipment, making it experimental at this time.

Abdominal compression

Limiting caudad movement of the diaphragm and the dissipation of the intrathoracic pressure that is generated may increase intrathoracic pressure.[231] These techniques, including abdominal binding or continuous abdominal pressure during conventional or SCV-CPR, have been shown to increase aortic pressure and carotid blood flow in both animal[231] and human[44] studies. In addition, these maneuvers may "autotransfuse" blood, resulting in an increase in central blood volume. However, despite the increase in aortic pressure, there is also an increase in right atrial pressure (used as the downstream pressure for coronary blood flow) that exceeds the increase in aortic diastolic pressure. This results in a decrease in coronary perfusion pressure.[292] Subsequent studies also have confirmed that abdominal binding in dogs fails to increase myocardial blood flow when compared with conventional CPR.[231] When applied during SCV-CPR, abdominal binding decreases the cerebral perfusion pressure. This occurs because of the transmission of intrathoracic pressure to the intracranial vault, resulting in increased intracranial pressure and lowered cerebral perfusion pressure.[114,169]

Military antishock trousers (MAST) used during conventional CPR produces the same vascular effects as continuous abdominal binding. Even though aortic pressure is increased, the effective downstream pressures for myocardial and cerebral perfusion are also increased, resulting in lower coronary and brain perfusion pressures respectively.[114,185] Clinical studies have also demonstrated that the use of the MAST suit during CPR does not increase the survival rate from cardiac arrest.[187,198]

The use of interposed abdominal counterpulsation (IAC-CPR) consists of the application of abdominal pressure either manually or by phasic inflation of a circumferential vest around the abdomen, during the relaxation phase of conventional CPR.[11] IAC-CPR increases venous return and compresses the abdominal aorta to produce retrograde aortic flow, closing the aortic valve and augmenting diastolic pressure. It may also act to sustain the increase of intrathoracic pressure, thus increasing the duty cycle.[168] In animal experiments, cardiac output and brain and coronary blood flow are substantially increased when compared with conventional CPR[85,336,338] but not in an infant model.[81] Human studies have also demonstrated an increase in aortic pressure and coronary perfusion pressure during IAC-CPR when compared with conventional CPR.[21,139,140] The frequency of complications, including laceration of abdominal viscera or esophageal regurgitation, is not increased with IAC-CPR.[21,205] However, there has not been improvement in long-term clinical outcome with the use of this technique.[21,139]

Cardiopulmonary bypass

The use of cardiopulmonary bypass (CPB) as a tool to increase survival and improve functional recovery has gained some popularity in the tertiary care clinical setting. In the canine model, CPB increased cardiovascular resuscitative ability in survival without neurologic deficit as compared to closed-chest CPR.[111,112] Clearly this technology may improve our survival but necessitates the use of a bypass team on call 24 hours a day in a very limited in-hospital setting.

OUTCOME

The use of CPR, as described in 1960, including the combination of mouth-to-mouth ventilation and closed-chest cardiac compressions, successfully oxygenates the blood and provides some circulation of blood.[173] The use of basic CPR in the 1990s is just one of the factors that contribute to the eventual outcome of the arrested patient, and is the factor that leads to successful resuscitation by the lay population. Other factors that dictate success in the in-hospital or sophisticated out-of-hospital scenarios include age, prior medical condition, and mechanism of cardiac arrest. Eisenberg et al. published a series of articles that confirmed that survival from cardiac arrest is determined by the interplay of many factors including age, sex, underlying severity of medical illness, presenting cardiac rhythm, and the time from arrest to the arrival of a resuscitation team.[86-89] The pharmacologic and physiologic advances that have evolved over the past 30 years have added much to the array of treatments available but have come under closer scrutiny lately as they relate to patient outcome. Clearly, the underlying factors that contribute to the cardiac arrest play a major role in the possible success of resuscitation.

With the development of basic CPR in the early 1960s, skilled resuscitation teams, both in and out of the hospital, were developed and lives were saved. Soon thereafter, reports of patients being successfully resuscitated by basic life support, defibrillation, and medications became common even as long as 5 hours after the commencement of CPR.[254]

A number of clinical studies have been published that studied out-of-hospital survival following CPR. **In King County, Washington, the survival rate for bystander-initiated CPR following a witnessed arrest was 32% compared with a survival rate of 3% for unwitnessed cardiac arrests without bystander CPR.**[58] The benefit of a witnessed arrest is that the bystander may notify the emergency system sooner and have nothing at all to do with the use of cardiac compression. The studies from Milwaukee demonstrate that, with the brief interval between the witnessed arrest and the arrival of emergency personnel, bystander

CPR contributes little to the success of resuscitation. It is the attempt at defibrillation that appears to be the critical element in the success of resuscitation when the arrest time is very short.[307,317]

The outcome following CPR in the hospital is not different from those studies of out-of-hospital arrests. Reviewing a heterogenous array of in-hospital studies, the resuscitation rate ranges from 13% to 52%. The long term survival rate for these patients from the same studies ranges from 5% to 27%. Much criticism has been made of the low rate of survival, but without the use of CPR these percentages would most likely be much lower.*

Predicting the survival of a patient resuscitated from a cardiac arrest may play an increasingly important role as medical resources shrink. Use of the Glasgow Coma Score during days 1 to 6 following resuscitation may be helpful in predicting outcome,[221] although another study showed that only the absence of spontaneous breathing on admission to the hospital following cardiac arrest was predictive of an unfavorable neurologic outcome. The use of CPR in patients at the extremes of ages has been reviewed as it relates to the prudent use of medical resources. Resuscitation of elderly patients in whom out-of-hospital arrest occurs was thought to be reasonable and appropriate by one group. Even though elderly patients were more likely than younger patients to die during hospitalization, the hospital stay of the elderly patient was not longer, the elderly did not have more residual neurologic impairments, and survival after hospital discharge was similar to that in younger patients.[323] Lack of survival was recently shown in the elderly following cardiac arrest.[152] Survival after CPR in infants less than 1500 g was found to be zero in 38 babies who received CPR in the first 3 days of life and was 36% in infants who received CPR after the third day of life. The authors thought that CPR may not be warranted in this population of patients. The study is flawed, however, in that many of the patients did not even receive chest compressions, infants who were successfully resuscitated in the delivery room were omitted from the study, and the interventions were generally very heterogenous and poorly defined.

The outcome of the patient who receives CPR in the operating room or other perioperative location will generally be balanced by two offsetting factors: the frequent severe underlying illness of the patient vs. the intense monitoring and rapid response that the arrested patient receives in those settings.

---

* References 17, 36, 39, 42, 55, 66, 79, 80, 92, 94, 96, 102, 107, 111, 121, 135, 136, 141, 146, 148, 150, 154-156, 158, 165, 166, 184, 186, 188, 189, 210, 213, 216, 237, 239, 270, 280, 295, 302, 303, 309, 316, 326, 331, 334, 351.

KEY POINTS

- The ABCs of CPR should always be followed — airway, breathing, and circulation.

- Performing a cricothyroidotomy is simple and requires equipment that is readily available to the anesthesiologist.

- If an intravenous line cannot be established rapidly because of technical difficulties, one of the other alternatives — endotracheal, intraosseous, or intracardiac injection — can be used.

- The drugs that can be given through the endotracheal tube include lidocaine, atropine, naloxone, and epinephrine (LANE).

- The use of end-tidal CO_2 monitoring as an indication of flow is a valuable adjunct during CPR. End-tidal CO_2 has been correlated with the coronary perfusion pressure, the critical parameter for resuscitation of the heart.

- Temperature may affect the success of resuscitation, the short-term neurologic status, and the eventual neurologic outcome.

- The most efficacious dose of epinephrine during CPR is still controversial. Increasing the usual and recommended dose of epinephrine by 20 to 200 times may have a beneficial effect on the generation of coronary and cerebral blood flow during closed-chest or open-chest CPR.

- Many outcome studies have shown that the survival rate following CPR is well below 50% and in many cases even below 15%.

- The use of the endotracheal route for ionized medications, such as sodium bicarbonate or calcium chloride, is not recommended.

- All medications used during CPR and fluids, including whole blood, should be given by the intraosseous route.

- Colloid does not appear to offer any advantage over crystalloid in respect to CPR outcome.

- The patient's diastolic pressure is particularly important in assessing CPR because it is the critical pressure for determining coronary perfusion.

- The alpha-adrenergic agonist receptor action of epinephrine is responsible for successful resuscitation.

- Sodium bicarbonate is indicated for significant metabolic acidosis occurring during cardiac arrest and CPR. In addition, bicarbonate is indicated when cardiac arrest is caused by hyperkalemia.

- The use of calcium chloride during CPR is not in favor. This is primarily because, in the setting of cardiac arrest, calcium may prevent reflow of blood into ischemic areas of the brain and heart, which may ultimately worsen the prognosis.

- Calcium, however, should be used during CPR for patients suffering a cardiac arrest secondary to hypocalcemia, hyperkalemia, hypermagnesemia, or an overdose with a calcium channel blocking agent.

- The use of glucose during CPR is controversial because of the possible detrimental effects of hyperglycemia on the brain during ischemia.

- The time to defibrillation may be the most important aspect in a successful resuscitation.

KEY REFERENCES

AHA standards and guidelines for cardiopulmonary resuscitation (CPR) and emergency cardiac care (ECC), *JAMA* 255(21):2905, 1986.

Brown CG, Werman HA, Davis EA et al: The effect of high-dose phenylephrine versus epinephrine on regional cerebral blood flow during CPR, *Ann Emerg Med* 16:743, 1987.

Criley JM, Blaufuss AJ, and Kissel GL: Cough-induced cardiac compression, *JAMA* 263:1246, 1976.

Dean JM, Koehler RC, Schleien CL et al: Age-related effects of compression rate and duration in cardiopulmonary resuscitation, *J Appl Physiol* 68:554, 1990.

Eisenberg MS, Bergner L, Hallstrom AP et al: Sudden cardiac death, *Sci Am* 254(5):37, 1986.

Feneley MP, Maier GW, Gaynor JW et al: Sequence of mitral valve motion and transmitral blood flow during manual cardiopulmonary resuscitation in dogs, *Circulation* 76:363, 1987.

Guerci AD, Shi AY, Levin H et al: Transmission of intrathoracic pressure to the intracranial space during cardiopulmonary resuscitation in dogs, *Circ Res* 56:20, 1985.

Koehler RC, Michael JR, Guerci AD et al: Beneficial effect of epinephrine infusion on cerebral and myocardial blood flows during CPR, *Ann Emerg Med* 14:744, 1985.

Longstreth WT Jr, Diehr P, Cobb LA et al: Neurologic outcome and blood glucose levels during out-of-hospital cardiopulmonary resuscitation, *Neurology* 36:1186, 1986.

Michael JR, Guerci AD, Koehler RC et al: Mechanisms by which epinephrine augments cerebral and myocardial perfusion during cardiopulmonary resuscitation in dogs, *Circulation* 69:822, 1984.

Rudikoff MT, Maughen WL, Effron M et al: Mechanisms of blood flow during cardiopulmonary resuscitation, *Circulation* 61:345, 1980.

Schleien CL, Koehler RC, Gervais H et al: Organ blood flow and somatosensory evoked potentials during and after cardiopulmonary resuscitation with epinephrine and phenyleprine, *Circulation* 79:1332, 1989.

Weil MH, Rackow EC, Trevino R et al: Differences in acid–base state between venous and arterial blood during cardiopulmonary resuscitation, *N Engl J Med* 315:153, 1986.

Yakaitis RW, Otto CW, and Blitt CD: Relative importance of alpha and beta adrenergic receptors during resuscitation, *Crit Care Med* 7:293, 1979.

REFERENCES

1. Achong MR: Infectious hazards of mouth-to-mouth resuscitation, *Am Heart J* 100:759, 1980.
2. Adgey AA, Patton JN, Campbell NP et al: Ventricular defibrillation: appropriate energy levels (editorial), *Circulation* 60:219, 1979.
3. Adrogue HJ, Rashad MN, Gorin AB et al: Assessing acid–base status in circulatory failure; differences between arterial and venous blood, *N Engl J Med* 320:1312, 1989.
4. Aguilar JC: Fatal gastric hemorrhage: a complication of cardiorespiratory resuscitation, *J Trauma* 21:573, 1981.
5. AHA standards and guidelines for cardiopulmonary resuscitation (CPR) and emergency cardiac care (ECC), *JAMA* 255(21):2905, 1986.
6. Anderson GJ, Suelzer J: The efficacy of trapezoidal wave forms for ventricular fibrillation, *Chest* 70:298, 1976.
7. Anderson GJ et al: Electro–physiological characterization of myocardial injury induced by defibrillation shocks, *Med Instr* 14:54, 1980 (abstract).
8. Andropoulos DB, Soifer SJ, and Schreiber MD: Plasma epinephrine concentrations after intraosseous and central venous injection during cardiopulmonary resuscitation in the lamb, *J Pediatr* 312, 1990.
9. Arai T, Watanabe T, Nagaro T et al: Blood–brain barrier impairment after cardiac resuscitation, *Crit Care Med* 9:444, 1981.
10. Austen WG, Moran JM: Cardiac and peripheral vascular effects of lidocaine and procainalol, *Am J Cardiol* 16:701, 1965.
11. Babbs CF, Tacker WA: Cardiopulmonary resuscitation with interposed abdominal compression, *Circulation* 74(suppl IV), 37, 1986.
12. Babbs CF, Yim GK, Whistler SJ et al: Elevation of ventricular defibrillation threshold in dogs by antiarrhythmic drugs, *Am Heart J* 98:345, 1979.
13. Bacaner MB: Bretylium tosylate for suppression of induced ventricular fibrillation, *Am J Cardiol* 17:528, 1966.
14. Baldwin JJ, Edwards JE: Rupture of right ventricle complicating closed chest cardiac massage, *Circulation* 53:562, 1976.
15. Barsan WG, Levy RC, and Weir H: Lidocaine levels during CPR: differences after peripheral venous, central venous, and intracardiac injections, *Ann Emerg Med* 10:73, 1981.
16. Beck CS, Pritchard WH, and Feil HS: Ventricular fibrillation of long duration abolished by electric shock, *JAMA* 135:985, 1947.
17. Bedell SE et al: Survival after cardiopulmonary resuscitation in the hospital, *N Engl J Med* 309:569, 1983.
18. Berenyi K, Wolk M, and Killip T: Cerebrospinal fluid acidosis complicating therapy of experimental cardiac arrest, *Circulation* 52:319, 1975.
19. Berg RA: Emergency infusion of catecholamines into bone marrow, *Am J Dis Child* 138:810, 1984.
20. Berkowitz ID, Chantarojanasiri T, Koehler RC et al: Blood flow during cardiopulmonary resuscitation with simultaneous compression and ventilation in infant pigs, *Pediatr Res* 26:558, 1989.
21. Berryman CR, Phillips GM: Interposed abdominal compression–CPR in human subjects, *Ann Emerg Med* 13:226, 1984.
22. Bersin RM, Arieff AL: Improved hemodynamic function during hypoxia with Carbicarb, a new agent for the management of acidosis, *Circulation* 77:227, 1988.
23. Beyar R et al: Computer studies of systemic and regional blood flow mechanisms during cardiopulmonary resuscitation, *Med Biol Eng Comput* 22:499, 1984.
24. Bigger JT Jr, Hoffman BF: Antiarrhythmic drugs. In Gilman AG, Goodman LS, Rall TW et al, eds: *The pharmacological basis of therapeutics*, New York, 1985, MacMillan Publishing.
25. Bigger JT Jr, Jaffe CC: The effect of bretylium tosylate on the electrophysiologic properties of ventricular muscle and Purkinje fibers, *Am J Cardiol* 27:82, 1971.
26. Bircher N, Safar P, and Stewart R: A comparison of standard, "MAST"-augmented, and open-chest CPR in dogs: a preliminary investigation, *Crit Care Med* 8:147, 1980.
27. Bishop RL, Weisfeldt ML: Sodium bicarbonate administration during cardiac arrest: effect on arterial pH, PCO_2, and osmolality, *JAMA* 235:506, 1976.
28. Blecic S, DeBacker D, Huynh CH et al: Calcium chloride in experimental electromechanical dissociation: a placebo-controlled trial in dogs, *Crit Care Med* 15(4):324, 1987.
29. Brillman JA, Sanders AB, Otto CW et al: Outcome of resuscitation from fibrillatory arrest using epinephrine and phenylephrine in dogs, *Crit Care Med* 13:912, 1985.
30. Bristow MR et al: Ionized calcium and the heart. Elucidation of in vivo concentration–response relationships in the open chest dog, *Circ Res* 41:565, 1977.
31. Brockman GF, Rodman GH: Acute Spigelian hernia, an unusual complication of cardiopulmonary resuscitation, *J Ky Med Assoc* 77:511, 1979.
32. Brown CG, Davis EA, and Werman RL: Methoxamine versus epinephrine on regional cerebral blood flow during cardiopulmonary resuscitation, *Crit Care Med* 15:682, 1987.
33. Brown CG, Werman HA, Davis EA et al: Comparative effects of graded doses of epinephrine on regional brain blood flow during CPR in a swine model, *Ann Emerg Med* 15:1138, 1986.
34. Brown CG, Birinyi F, Werman HA et al: The comparative effects of epinephrine versus phenylephrine on regional cerebral blood flow during cardiopulmonary resuscitation, *Resuscitation* 14:171, 1986.
35. Brown CG, Werman HA, Davis EA et al: The effect of high-dose phenylephrine versus epinephrine on regional cerebral blood flow during CPR, *Ann Emerg Med* 16:743, 1987.
36. Brown CS, Scott AA: Cardiopulmonary resuscitation: a review of 184 cases and some applications for future improvements, *Can Anaes Soc J* 17:565, 1970.
37. Brown DC, Lewis AJ, and Criley JM: Asystole and its treatment: the possible role of the parasympathetic nervous system in cardiac arrest, *JACEP* 8:11,448, 1979.
38. Brunette DD, Jameson SJ: Comparison of standard versus high-dose epinephrine in the resuscitation of cardiac arrest in dogs, *Ann Emerg Med* 19:8, 1990.
39. Camarata SJ et al: Cardiac arrest in the critically ill. I. A study of predisposing causes in 132 patients, *Circulation* 44:688, 1971.
40. Campbell NPS et al: Transthoracic ventricular defibrillation in adults, *Br Med J* 2:1379, 1977.
41. Carlsson C, Hägerdal M, Kaasik AE

et al: A catecholamine-mediated increase in cerebral oxygen uptake during immobilization stress in rats, *Brain Res* 119:223, 1977.

42. Castagna J, Weil MH, and Shubin H: Factors determining survival in patients with cardiac arrest, *Chest* 65:527, 1974.

43. Chandra N, Rudikoff M, and Weisfeldt ML: Simultaneous chest compression and ventilation at high airway pressure during cardiopulmonary resuscitation, *Lancet* 1:175, 1980.

44. Chandra N, Snyder LD, and Weisfeldt ML: Abdominal binding during cardiopulmonary resuscitation in man, *JAMA* 246:351, 1981.

45. Chandra N et al: Augmentation of carotid flow during cardiopulmonary resuscitation by ventilation at high airway pressure simultaneous with chest compression, *Am J Cardiol* 48:1053, 1981.

46. Chandra N et al: Contrasts between intrathoracic pressures during chest compression and cardiac massage, *Crit Care Med* 9:789, 1981.

47. Chatterjee K, Mandel WJ, Vyden JK et al: Cardiovascular effects of bretylium tosylate in acute myocardial infarction, *JAMA* 223:757, 1973.

48. Chow MSS, Kluger J, DiPersio DM et al: Antifibrillatory effects of lidocaine and bretylium immediately post cardiopulmonary resuscitation, *Am Heart J* 110:938, 1985.

49. Cingolani HE, Mattiazi AR, Blesa ES: Contractility in isolated mammalian heart muscle after acid–base changes, *Circ Res* 26:269, 1970.

50. Clark RE, Kristlieb IY, and Henry PD: Nifedipine: a myocardial protective agent, *Am J Cardiol* 44:825, 1979.

51. Clinch SL, Thompson JS, and Edney JA: Pneumoperitoneum after cardiopulmonary resuscitation: a therapeutic dilemma, *J Trauma* 23:428, 1983.

52. Collingsworth KA, Kalman SM, and Harrison DC: The clinical pharmacology of lidocaine as an antiarrhythmic drug, *Circulation* 50:1217, 1974.

53. Combs DJ, Reuland DS, Martin DB et al: Glycolytic inhibition by 2-deoxyglucose reduces hyperglycemic associated mortality and morbidity in the ischemic rat, *Stroke* 17:990, 1986.

54. Cooper MJ, Abinader EG: Atropine-induced ventricular fibrillation: case report and review of the literature, *Am Heart J* 97:225, 1979.

55. Coskey RL: Cardiopulmonary resuscitation impact on hospital mortality—a ten-year study, *West J Med* 129:511, 1978.

56. Criley JM, Blaufuss AJ, and Kissel GL: Cough-induced cardiac compression, *JAMA* 263:1246, 1976.

57. Criley JM, Ung S, and Niemann JT: What is the role of newer methods of cardiopulmonary resuscitation? *Cardiovasc Clin* 13:297, 1983.

58. Cummins RO, Eisenberg MS, Hallstrom AP et al: Survival of out-of-hospital cardiac arrest with early initiation of cardiopulmonary resuscitation, *Am J Emerg Med* 3:114, 1985.

59. Dahl CF et al: Myocardial necrosis from direct current countershock: effect of paddle electrode size and time interval between discharges, *Circulation* 50:956, 1974.

60. Dahl CF, Ewy GA, Ewy MD et al: Transthoracic impedance to direct current discharge: effect of repeated countershocks, *Med Instrum* 10:151, 1976.

61. D'Alecy LG, Lundy EF, Barton KS et al: Dextrose containing intravenous fluid repairs outcome and increases death after eight minutes of cardiac arrest and resuscitation in dogs, *Surgery* 100:505, 1986.

62. Daniell HW: Hypokalemia after resuscitation, *JAMA* 250:1025, 1983 (editorial).

63. Dean JM, Koehler RC, Schleien CL et al: Age-related changes in chest geometry during cardiopulmonary resuscitation, *J Appl Physiol* 62:2212, 1987.

64. Dean JM, Koehler RC, Schleien CL et al: Age-related effects of compression rate and duration in cardiopulmonary resuscitation, *J Appl Physiol* 68:554, 1990.

65. DeBard ML: The history of cardiopulmonary resuscitation, *Ann Emerg Med* 9:273, 1980.

66. DeBard ML: Cardiopulmonary resuscitation: analysis of six years' experience and review of the literature, *Ann Emerg Med* 10:408, 1981.

67. DelGuercio LRM, Coomaraswamy RP, and State S: Cardiac output and other hemodynamic variables during external cardiac massage in man, *N Engl J Med* 269:1398, 1963.

68. DelGuercio LRM, Felins NR, Cohn JD et al: Comparison of blood flow during external and internal cardiac massage in man, *Circ Suppl* 31:I171, 1965.

69. Dembo DH: Calcium in advanced life support, *Crit Care Med* 9:358, 1981.

70. DeSilva RA, Lown B: Energy requirement for defibrillation of a markedly overweight patient, *Circulation* 57:827, 1978.

71. Deshmukh HG, Weil MH et al: Echocardiographic observations during cardiopulmonary resuscitation: A preliminary report, *Crit Care Med* 13:904, 1985.

72. Dhingia R, Amat-y-Leon F, and Wyndham C: Electrophysiologic effects of atropine on human sinus node and atrium, *Am J Med* 38:492, 1976.

73. DiCola VC et al: Myocardial uptake of technetium-99m stannous pyrophosphate following direct current transthoracic countershock, *Circulation* 54:980, 1976.

74. Ditchey RV, Lindenfeld J: Potential adverse effects of volume loading on perfusion of vital organs during closed-chest resuscitation, *Circulation* 69:181, 1984.

75. Ditchey RV, Lindenfeld J: Failure of epinephrine to improve the balance between myocardial oxygen supply and demand during closed-chest resuscitation in dogs, *Circulation* 78:382, 1988.

76. Dohi S: Postcardiopulmonary resuscitation pulmonary edema, *Crit Care Med* 11:434, 1983.

77. Downey JM, Chagrasulis RW, and Hemphill V: Quantitative study of intramyocardial compression in the fibrillating heart, *Am J Physiol* 237:H191, 1979.

78. Drop LJ, Scheidegger D: Plasma ionized calcium concentration: important determinant of the hemodynamic response to calcium infusion, *J Thorac Cardiovasc Surg* 79:425, 1980.

79. Dupont B, Flensted-Jenson E, and Sandoe E: The long-term prognosis for patients resuscitated after cardiac arrest. A follow-up study, *Am Heart J* 78:444, 1969.

80. Dykema ML, Vasu CM: Cardiopulmonary resuscitation in a community hospital—a one year experience, *Mich Med* 72:469, 1973.

81. Eberle B, Schleien CL, Shaffner DH et al: Effects of three modes of abdominal compression on vital organ blood-flow in a piglet CPR model, *Anesthesiology* 73(A):300, 1990.

82. Echt DS, Cato EL, and Coxe DR: pH-dependent effects of lidocaine on defibrillation energy requirements in dogs, *Circulation* 80:1003, 1989.

83. Echt DS, Black JN, Barbey JT et al: Evaluation of antiarrhythmic drugs on defibrillation energy requirements in dogs: sodium channel block and action potential prolongation, *Circulation* 79:1106, 1989.

84. Edvinsson L, Hardebo JE, MacKenzie ET et al: Effect of exogenous noradrenaline on local cerebral blood flow after osmotic opening of the blood–brain barrier in the rat, *J Physiol (Lond)* 274:149, 1978.

85. Einagle V, Bertrand F, Wise RA et al: Interposed abdominal compressions and carotid blood flow during cardiopulmonary resuscitation: support for a thoracoabdominal unit, *Chest* 93:1206, 1988.

86. Eisenberg MS, Bergner L, and Hallstrom A: Paramedic programs and out-of-hospital cardiac arrest. I. Factors associated with successful resuscitation, *Am J Public Health* 69:30, 1979.

87. Eisenberg MS, Bergner L, Hallstrom A: Out-of-hospital cardiac arrest: improved survival with paramedic services, *Lancet* II:812, 1980.

88. Eisenberg MS, Copass MK, Hallstrom A et al: Management of out-of-hospital cardiac arrest: failure of basic emergency medical technician services, *JAMA* 243:1049, 1980.

89. Eisenberg MS, Bergner L, Hallstrom A et al: Sudden cardiac death, *Sci Am* 254:(5):37, 1986.

90. Eleff SM, Schleien CL, Koehler RC et al: Brain bioenergetics during cardiopulmonary resuscitation in dogs, *Anesthesiology* 76:77, 1990.

91. Emerman CL, Pinchak AC, Hancock D et al: Effect of injection site on circulation times during cardiac arrest, *Crit Care Med* 16:1138, 1988.

92. Fabricius-Bierre N, Astvad K, and Kiaerulff J: Cardiac arrest following acute myocardial infarction. A study of 285 cases from three medical depart-

ments using a joint acute admission section containing a coronary care unit, *Acta Med Scand* 195:261, 1974.

93. Falk FH et al: External noninvasive cardiac pacing in out-of-hospital cardiac arrest, *Crit Care Med* 11:779, 1983.

94. Farha GJ, Capehart RJ, and Barker PN: Cardiopulmonary resuscitation in a community hospital, *J Kans Med Soc* 72:406, 1972.

95. Feneley MP, Maier GW, Gaynor JW et al: Sequence of mitral valve motion and transmitral blood flow during manual cardiopulmonary resuscitation in dogs, *Circulation* 76:363, 1987.

96. Fusgen I, Summa JK: How much sense is there in an attempt to resuscitate an aged person?, *Gerontology* 24:37, 1978.

97. Gascho JA, Crampton RS, Cherwek ML et al: Determinants of ventricular defibrillation in adults, *Circulation* 60:231, 1979.

98. Gascho JA et al: Energy levels and patient weight in ventricular fibrillation, *JAMA* 242:1380, 1979.

99. Gazitua S et al: Effect of osmolarity on canine renal vascular resistance, *Am J Physiol* 217:302, 1969.

100. Gazitua S, Scott JB, Swindall B et al: Resistance responses to local changes in plasma osmolality in three vascular beds, *Am J Physiol* 220:384, 1971.

101. Geddes LA, Tacker WA, Cabler P et al: The decrease in transthoracic resistance during successive ventricular defibrillation trials, *Med Instrum* 9:179, 1975.

102. George AI Jr, Folk BP III, Crecelius PL et al: Prearrest morbidity and other correlates of survival after in-hospital cardiopulmonary arrest, *Am J Med* 87:28, 1989.

103. Gerstenblith G, Spear JF, and Moore EN: Quantitative study of the effect of lidocaine on the threshold for ventricular fibrillation in the dog, *Am J Cardiol* 30:242, 1972.

104. Gervais HW, Schleien CL, Koehler RC et al: Effect of adrenergic drugs on cerebral blood flow, metabolism, and evoked potentials after delayed cardiopulmonary resuscitation in immature swine, *Stroke* 22:447, 1991.

105. Ginsberg MD, Welsh FA, and Budd WW: Focal cerebral blood flow and glucose utilization, *Stroke* 1:347, 1980.

106. Gonzalez ER, Ornato JP, Garnett AR et al: Dose-dependent vasopressor response to epinephrine during CPR in human beings, *Ann Emerg Med* 18:920, 1989.

107. Grace WJ, Minogue WF: Resuscitation for cardiac arrest due to myocardial infarction, *Chest* 50:173, 1966.

108. Graf H, Leach W, and Arieff AI: Evidence for a detrimental effect of bicarbonate therapy in hypoxic lactic acidosis, *Science* 227:754, 1985.

109. Greenberg MI, Roberts JR, and Baskin SI: Use of endotracheally administered epinephrine in a pediatric patient, *Am J Dis Child* 135:767, 1981.

110. Greenblatt DJ, Gross PL, Bolognini V: Pharmacotherapy of cardiopulmonary arrest, *Am J Hosp Pharm* 33:579, 1976.

111. Greenfield I: Emergency red: a plan for hospital personnel in the treatment of cardiac and respiratory emergencies, *Minn Med* 47:745, 1964.

112. Grundler W, Weil MH, and Rackow EC: Arteriovenous carbon dioxide and pH gradients during cardiac arrest, *Circulation* 74:1071, 1986.

113. Gudipati CV, Weil MH, Bisera J et al: Expired carbon dioxide: a noninvasive monitor of cardiopulmonary resuscitation, *Circulation* 77:234, 1988.

114. Guerci AD, Shi AY, Levin H et al: Transmission of intrathoracic pressure to the intracranial space during cardiopulmonary resuscitation in dogs, *Circ Res* 56:20, 1985.

115. Guerci AD, Chandra N, Johnson E et al: Failure of sodium bicarbonate to improve resuscitation from ventricular fibrillation in dogs, *Circulation* 74:IV75, 1986.

116. Guerci AD et al: Vest CPR increases aortic pressure in humans, *Circulation* 80(4):II-496, 1989.

117. Guildner CW, Williams D, and Subitch T: Airway obstructed by foreign material: the Heimlich maneuver, *JACEP* 5:675, 1976.

118. Gunnar WP, Merlotti GJ, Barrett J et al: Resuscitation from hemorrhagic shock: alterations of the intracranial pressure after normal saline, 3% saline, and dextran-40, *Ann Surg* 204:686, 1986.

119. Gunnar WP et al: Elevated intracranial pressure and hemorrhagic shock: beneficial effects of hypertonic saline resuscitation in an experimental model, *Fed Proc* 46:805, 1987.

120. Gunnar W, Jonasson O, Merlotti G et al: Head injury and hemorrhagic shock: studies of the blood brain barrier and intracranial pressure after resuscitation with normal saline solution, 3% saline solution, and dextran-40, *Surgery* 103(4):398, 1988.

121. Hahn RG, Hutchinson JC, and Conte JE: Cardiopulmonary resuscitation in a university hospital. An analysis of the cost and survival, *West J Med* 131:344, 1979.

122. Halperin HR, Guerci AD, Chandra N et al: Vest inflation without simultaneous ventilation during cardiac arrest in dogs: improved survival from prolonged cardiopulmonary resuscitation, *Circulation* 74:1407, 1986.

123. Halperin HR, Tsitlik JE, Beyer R et al: Intrathoracic pressure fluctuations move blood during CPR: comparison of hemodynamic data with predictions from a mathematical model, *Ann Biomed Eng* 15:385, 1987.

124. Halperin HR, Tsitlik JE, Guerci AD et al: Determinants of blood flow to vital organs during cardiopulmonary resuscitation in dogs, *Circulation* 73:539, 1986.

125. Hanyok JJ, Chow MS, Kluger J et al: Antifibrillatory effects of high dose bretylium and a lidocaine–bretylium combination during cardiopulmonary resuscitation, *Crit Care Med* 16:691, 1988.

126. Harris LC, Kirimli B, and Safar P: Augmentation of artificial circulation during cardiopulmonary resuscitation, *Anesthesiology* 28:730, 1967.

127. Hauge A, Bo G: Blood hyperosmolality and pulmonary vascular resistance in the cat, *Circ Res* 28:371, 1971.

128. Hay E, Cohen H, Pasik S: Acute thrombosis of subclavian artery during CPR, *Ann Emerg Med* 16(4):447, 1987.

129. Haynes RE, Chinn TL, Copass MK et al: Comparison of bretylium tosylate and lidocaine in management of out of hospital ventricular fibrillation: a randomized clinical trial, *Am J Cardiol* 48:353, 1981.

130. Hedges JR et al: Central versus peripheral intravenous routes in cardiopulmonary resuscitation, *Am J Emerg Med* 2:385, 1984.

131. Heilman KM, Muschenheim C: Primary cutaneous tuberculosis resulting from mouth-to-mouth respiration, *N Engl J Med* 273:1035, 1965.

132. Heinild S, Sondergaard T, and Tudvad F: Bone marrow infusion in childhood: experiences from 1,000 infusions, *J Pediatr* 30:400, 1947.

133. Heining MPD, Band DM, and Linton RAF: Choice of calcium salt: a comparison of the effects of calcium chloride and gluconate on plasma ionised calcium, *Anaesthesia* 39:1079, 1984.

134. Himmelhoch SR, Dekker A, Gazzaniga AB et al: Closed-chest cardiac resuscitation, *N Engl J Med* 270:118, 1964.

135. Ho SK, Quattlebaum F: Cardiac resuscitation in a community hospital, *Minn Med* 50:1925, 1967.

136. Hollingsworth JH: The results of cardiopulmonary resuscitation. A 3-year university hospital experience, *Ann Intern Med* 71:459, 1969.

137. Holmes HR, Babbs CF, Voorhees WD et al: Influence of adrenergic drugs upon vital perfusion during CPR, *Crit Care Med* 8:137, 1980.

138. Hornchen U, Schuttler J, Stoeckel H et al: Endobronchial instillation of epinephrine during cardiopulmonary resuscitation, *Crit Care Med* 15:1037, 1987.

139. Howard M et al: Interposed abdominal compression CPR: its effects on coronary perfusion pressure—human subjects, *Ann Emerg Med* 13:989, 1984.

140. Howard M, Carrubba C, Foss F et al: Interposed abdominal compression-CPR: its effects on parameters of coronary perfusion in human subjects, *Ann Emerg Med* 16:253, 1987.

141. Hubbell RW, Okel BB: The value of a cardiac resuscitation program in a community hospital, *J Med Assoc Ga* 58:112, 1969.

142. Infection control guidelines for CPR providers, *JAMA* 262(19):2732, 1989.

143. Iseri L et al: Prehospital cardiac arrest after arrival of the paramedic unit, *JACEP* 6:530, 1977.

144. Jacobs HB: Emergency percutaneous transtracheal catheter and ventilator, *J Trauma* 12:50, 1972.

145. Jacoby JJ et al: Transtracheal resuscitation, *JAMA* 162:625, 1956.

146. Jeresaty RM, Godar TJ, and Liss JP: External cardiac resuscitation in a community hospital. A three-year experience, *Arch Intern Med* 124:588, 1969.

147. Jewitt DE, Kishow Y, and Thomas M:

Lidocaine in the management of arrhythmias after myocardial infarction, *Circulation* 37:965, 1968.

148. Johnson AL et al: Results of cardiac resuscitation in 552 patients, *Am J Cardiol* 20:831, 1967.

149. Jones JL, Lepeschkin E, Jones RE et al: Response of cultured myocardial cells to countershock-type electrical field stimulation, *Am J Physiol* 235:H214, 1978.

150. Jordan D, Lavin T, and Hamelberg W: Resuscitation experience within the hospital, *JAMA* 188:181, 1964.

151. Jorgensen EO, Malchow-Moller A: Cerebral prognostic signs during cardiopulmonary resuscitation, *Resuscitation* 6:217, 1979.

152. Josefson LM: A new method of treatment—intraossal injections, *Acta Medica Scand* 81:550, 1934.

153. Juan G, Calverley P, Talamo C et al: Effect of carbon dioxide on diaphragmatic function in human beings, *N Engl J Med* 310:874, 1984.

154. Jude JR, Kouwenhoven WB, and Knickerbocker GG: Cardiac arrest: report of application of external cardiac massage in 118 patients, *JAMA* 178:1063, 1961.

155. Jung MA, Selby A, Johnson JR et al: Value of a cardiac arrest team in a university hospital: results in a series of 100 patients, *Can Med Assoc J* 98:74, 1968.

156. Kaplan BM, Knott AP: Closed chest cardiac massage for circulatory arrest effectiveness in 100 consecutive cases, *Arch Intern Med* 114:5, 1964.

157. Katz AM, Reuter M: Cellular calcium and cardiac cell death, *Am J Cardiol* 44:188, 1979.

158. Kaunitz VH, Trivedi JM: Cardiopulmonary resuscitation in a community hospital, *NY State J Med* 72:2751, 1972.

159. Kay JH, Blalock A: The use of calcium chloride in the treatment of cardiac arrest in patients, *Surg Gynecol Obstet* 93:97, 1951.

160. Kerber RE, Sarnat W: Factors influencing the success of ventricular defibrillation in man, *Circulation* 60:226, 1979.

161. Kerber RE et al: Transthoracic resistance of human defibrillation: influence of body weight, chest size, serial shocks, paddle size and paddle contact pressure, *Circulation* 63:676, 1981.

162. Kern KB, Sanders AB, and Ewy GA: Open-chest cardiac massage after closed-chest compression in a canine model: when to intervene, *Resuscitation* 15:51, 1987.

163. Kern KB et al: Dynamic changes in expired end–tidal carbon dioxide as a prognostic guide during CPR in dogs, *Ann Emerg Med* 17:392, 1988.

164. Kindig NB, Sherrill DS, Shapiro JI et al: Extracorporeal bicarbonate space after bicarbonate or a bicarbonate–carbonate mixture in acidotic dogs, *J Appl Physiol* 67(6):2331, 1989.

165. Kirby BJ, McNicol MW: Results of cardiac resuscitation in one hundred patients: effects on acid–base status, *Postgrad Med J* 43:75, 1967.

166. Klassen GA, Broadhurst C, Peretz DI et al: Cardiac resuscitation in 126 medical patients using external cardiac massage, *Lancet* I:1290, 1963.

167. Koch-Weser J: Drug therapy—Bretylium, *N Engl J Med* 300:437, 1979.

168. Koehler RC, Michael JR: Cardiopulmonary resuscitation, brain blood flow, and neurologic recovery, *Crit Care Clin* 1:205, 1985.

169. Koehler RC, Chandra N, Guerci AD et al: Augmentation of cerebral perfusion by simultaneous chest compression and lung inflation with abdominal binding after cardiac arrest in dogs, *Circulation* 67:266, 1983.

170. Koehler RC, Michael JR, Guerci AD et al: Beneficial effect of epinephrine infusion on cerebral and myocardial blood flows during CPR, *Ann Emerg Med* 14:744, 1985.

171. Koscove EM, Paradis NA: Successful resuscitation from cardiac arrest using high-dose epinephrine therapy, *JAMA* 259:3031, 1988.

172. Kottmeier CA, Gravenstein JS: The parasympathomimetic activity of atropine and atropine methylbromide, *Anesthesiology* 29:1125, 1968.

173. Kouwenhoven WB, Jude JR, and Knickerbocker GG: Closed chest cardiac massage, *JAMA* 173:1064, 1960.

174. Kouwenhoven WB, Langworthy R: Cardiopulmonary resuscitation: an account of forty-five years of research, *Hopkins Med J* 132:186, 1973.

175. Kouwenhoven WB et al: Closed chest defibrillation of the heart, *Surgery* 42:550, 1957.

176. Kraig RP, Petito CK, Plum F et al: Hydrogen ions kill brain at concentrations reached in ischemia, *J Cereb Blood Flow Metab* 7:379, 1987.

177. Krischer JP, Fine EG, Davis JH et al: Complications of cardiac resuscitation, *Chest* 92(2):287, 1987.

178. Krischer JP, Fine EG, Weisfeldt ML et al: Comparison of prehospital conventional and simultaneous compression–ventilation cardiopulmonary resuscitation, *Crit Care Med* 17:1263, 1989.

179. Kuhn GH et al: Peripheral vs central circulation times during CPR: a pilot study, *Ann Emerg Med* 10:417, 1981.

180. Kuntzman R, Tsai I, and Chang R: Disposition of bretylium in man and rat: a sensitive chemical method for its estimation in plasma and urine, *Clin Pharmacol Ther* 11:829, 1970.

181. Lanier WL, Stangland KJ, Scheithauer BW et al: The effects of dextrose infusion and head position on neurologic outcome after complete cerebral ischemia in primates: examination of a model, *Anesthesiology* 66:39, 1987.

182. Lasbennes F, Sercombe R, and Seylaz J: Monoamine oxidase activity in brain microvessels determined using natural and artificial substances: relevance to the blood–brain barrier, *J Cereb Blood Flow Metab* 3:521, 1983.

183. Lathers CM, Tumer N, and Schoffstall JM: Plasma catecholamines, pH, and blood pressure during cardiac arrest in pigs, *Resuscitation* 18:59, 1989.

184. Lawrence RM, Haley EM, and Gillies AJ: Closed-chest cardiopulmonary resuscitation. Results and criteria for application, *NY State J Med* 64:2523, 1964.

185. Lee HR et al: MAST augmentation of external cardiac compression: role of changing intrapleural pressure, *Ann Emerg Med* 10:560, 1981.

186. Lemire JG, Johnson AL: Is cardiac resuscitation worthwhile? A decade of experience, *N Engl J Med* 286:970, 1972.

187. Lilja GP, Long RS, and Ruiz E: Augmentation of systolic blood pressure during external cardiac compression by use of the MAST suit, *Ann Emerg Med* 10:182, 1981.

188. Lillehei CW, Lavadia PG, DeWall RA et al: Four years experience with external cardiac resuscitation, *JAMA* 193:651, 1965.

189. Linko E et al: Resuscitation in cardiac arrest: an analysis of 100 successive medical cases, *Acta Med Scand* 182:611, 1967.

190. Livesay JJ, Follette DM, Fey KH et al: Optimizing myocardial supply/demand balance with alpha-adrenergic drugs during cardiopulmonary resuscitation, *J Thorac Cardiovasc Surg* 76:244, 1978.

191. Longergan JH, Youngberg JZ, and Kaplan JA: Cardiopulmonary resuscitation: physical stress on the rescuer, *Crit Care Med* 9:793, 1981.

192. Longstreth WT, Inui TS: High blood glucose level on hospital admission and poor neurological recovery after cardiac arrest, *Ann Neurol* 15:59, 1984.

193. Longstreth WT Jr, Diehr P, Cobb LA et al: Neurologic outcome and blood glucose levels during out-of-hospital cardiopulmonary resuscitation, *Neurology* 36:1186, 1986.

194. Luce JM, Ross BK, O'Quin RJ et al: Regional blood flow during cardiopulmonary resuscitation in dogs using simultaneous and nonsimultaneous compression and ventilation, *Circulation* 67:258, 1983.

195. Lunde P: Ventricular fibrillation after intravenous atropine for treatment for sinus bradycardia, *Acta Med Scand* 199:369, 1976.

196. Lundy EF et al: Infusion of five percent dextrose increases mortality and morbidity following six minutes of cardiac arrest in resuscitated dogs, *J Crit Care* 2:4, 1987.

197. MacKenzie ET, McCulloch J, O'Kean M et al: Cerebral circulation and norepinephrine: relevance of the blood–brain barrier, *Am J Physiol* 231:483, 1976.

198. Mahoney BD, Mirick MJ: Pneumatic trousers in refractory cardiopulmonary arrest, *Ann Emerg Med* 13:410, 1984.

199. Maier GW, Tyson GS Jr, Olsen CO et al: The physiology of external cardiac massage: high-impulse cardiopulmonary resuscitation, *Circulation* 70:86, 1984.

200. Maningas PA: Resuscitation with 7.5% NaCl in 6% dextran-70 during hemorrhagic shock in swine: effects on organ blood flow, *Crit Care Med* 15:1121, 1987.

201. Markis JE, Koch-Weser J: Characterizations and mechanisms of inotropic and chronotropic actions of bretylium tosylate, *J Pharmacol Exp Ther* 178:94, 1971.

202. Marquez J et al: Cardiovascular depres-

sion secondary to ionic hypocalcemia during hepatic transplantation in humans, *Anesthesiology* 65:457, 1986.

203. Martin GB, Gentile NT, Paradis NA et al: Effect of epinephrine on end–tidal carbon dioxide monitoring during CPR, *Ann Emerg Med* 19:396, 1990.

204. Massumi RA, Mason DT, Amsterdam EA et al: Ventricular fibrillation and tachycardia after intravenous atropine for treatment of bradycardias, *N Engl J Med* 287:336, 1972.

205. Mateer JR, Stueven HA, Thompson BM et al: Pre-hospital IAC–CPR versus standard CPR: paramedic resuscitation of cardiac arrests, *Am J Med* 3:143, 1985.

206. Mattar JA, Weil MH, Shubin H et al: Cardiac arrest in the critically ill: Hyperosmolal states following cardiac arrest, *Am J Med* 56:162, 1974.

207. McCormack AP, Damon SK, Eisenberg MS et al: Disagreeable physical characteristics affecting bystander CPR, *Ann Emerg Med* 18:283, 1989.

208. McDonald JL: Serum lidocaine levels during cardiopulmonary resuscitation after intravenous and endotracheal administration, *Crit Care Med* 13(11):914, 1985.

209. McGrath RB: Gastroesophageal lacerations: a fatal complication of closed-chest cardiopulmonary resuscitation, *Chest* 83:571, 1983.

210. McGrath RB: In-house cardiopulmonary resuscitation—after a quarter of a century, *Ann Emerg Med* 16:1365, 1987.

211. Mehta B et al: Disseminated intravascular coagulation following cardiac arrest: a study of 15 patients, *Am J Med Sci* 264:353, 1972.

212. Meola F: Bone marrow infusions as routine procedure in children, *J Pediatr* 25:13, 1944.

213. Messert B, Qualgieri CE: Cardiopulmonary resuscitation perspectives and problems, *Lancet* II:410, 1976.

214. Michael JR, Guerci AD, Koehler RC et al: Mechanisms by which epinephrine augments cerebral and myocardial perfusion during cardiopulmonary resuscitation in dogs, *Circulation* 69:822, 1984.

215. Michael TAD, Gordon AS: The esophageal obturator airway: a new device in emergency cardiopulmonary resuscitation, *Br J Med* 281:1531, 1980.

216. Minuck M, Perkins R: Long-term study of patients successfully resuscitated following cardiac arrest, *Can Med Assoc J* 100:1126, 1969.

217. Morgan RR: Laceration of the liver from closed-chest cardiac massage, *N Engl J Med* 265:82, 1961.

218. Morillo LE, Tulloch JW, Gumnit RJ et al: Compressed spectral array patterns following cardiopulmonary arrest. A preliminary report, *Arch Neurol* 40:287, 1983.

219. Morris RE, Schonfeld N, and Haftel AJ: Treatment of hemorrhagic shock with intraosseous administration of crystalloid fluid in the rabbit model, *Ann Emerg Med* 16:1321, 1987.

220. Moss J, Rockoff M: EEG monitoring during cardiac arrest and resuscitation, *JAMA* 244:2750, 1980.

221. Mullie A, Verstringe P, Buylaert W et al: Predictive value of glasgow coma score for awakening after out-of-hospital cardiac arrest, *Lancet:*Jan 23, 1988.

222. Myerburg RJ et al: Outcome of resuscitation from bradyarrhythmic or asystolic prehospital cardiac arrest, *J Am Coll Cardiol* 4:1118, 1984.

223. Myers R: Lactic acid accumulation as a cause of brain edema and cerebral necrosis resulting from oxygen deprivation. In Korbin R, Guilleminault C, eds: *Advances in perinatal neurology,* New York, 1979, Spectrum.

224. Nagel EL, Fine EG, Krischer JP et al: Complications of CPR, *Crit Care Med* 9:424, 1981.

225. Nakayama S, Sibley L, Gunther RA et al: Small-volume resuscitation with hypertonic saline (2,400 mOsm/liter) during hemorrhagic shock, *Circ Shock* 13:149, 1984.

226. Narang VPS: Utility of the pulse oximeter during cardiopulmonary resuscitation, *Anesthesiology* 65:239, 1986.

227. Narins RG, Cohen JJ: Bicarbonate therapy for organic acidosis: the case for its continued use, *Ann Intern Med* 106:615, 1987.

228. Neff CC, Pfister RC, and Van Sonnenberg E: Percutaneous transtracheal ventilation: experimental and practical aspects, *J Trauma* 23:84, 1983.

229. Nerlich M, Gunther R, and Demling RH: Resuscitation from hemorrhagic shock with hypertonic saline or lactated Ringer's (effect on the pulmonary and systemic microcirculations), *Circ Shock* 10:179, 1983.

230. Niemann JT et al: Pressure-synchronized cineangiography during experimental cardiopulmonary resuscitation, *Circulation* 64:985, 1981.

231. Niemann JT, Rosborough JP, Ung S et al: Hemodynamic effects of continuous abdominal binding during cardiac arrest and resuscitation, *Am J Cardiol* 53:269, 1984.

232. Niemann JT, Haynes KS, Garner D et al: Postcountershock pulseless rhythms: hemodynamic effects of glucagon in a canine model, *Crit Care Med* 15:554, 1987.

233. Niemann JT, Garner D, Pelikan PC et al: Predictive value of the ECG in determining cardiac resuscitation outcome in a canine model of postcountershock electromechanical dissociation after prolonged ventricular fibrillation, *Ann Emerg Med* 17:567, 1988.

234. Orlowski JP, Julius CJ, Petras RE et al: The safety of intraosseous infusions: risks of fat and bone marrow emboli to the lungs, *Ann Emerg Med* 18:1062, 1989.

235. Pannier JL, Leusen I: Contraction characteristics of papillary muscle during changes in acid–base composition of the bathing fluid, *Arch Int Physiol Biochim* 76:624, 1968.

236. Pearson JW, Redding JS: Influence of peripheral vascular tone on resuscitation, *Anesth Analg* 44:746, 1965.

237. Peatfield RC, Sillett RW, Taylor D et al: Survival after cardiac arrest in hospital, *Lancet* I:1223, 1977.

238. Peleska B: Cardiac arrhythmias following condenser discharges and their dependence upon strength of current and phase of cardiac cycle, *Circ Res* 13:21, 1963.

239. Peschin A, Coakley CS: A five year review of 734 cardiopulmonary arrests, *South Med J* 63:506, 1970.

240. Peters RM, Shackford SR, Hogan JS et al: Comparison of isotonic and hypertonic fluids in resuscitation from hypovolemic shock, *Surg Gynecol Obstet* 163:219, 1986.

241. Pilcher DB, DeMeules JE: Esophageal perforation following use of esophageal airway, *Chest* 69:377, 1976.

242. Pionkowski RS et al: Resuscitation time in ventricular fibrillation—a prognostic indicator, *Ann Emerg Med* 12:733, 1983.

243. Poole-Wilson PA, Langer GA: Effects of acidosis on mechanical function and Ca^{+2} exchange in rabbit myocardium, *Am J Physiol* 236:H525, 1979.

244. Posner JB, Plum F: Spinal-fluid pH and neurologic symptoms in systemic acidosis, *N Engl J Med* 277:605, 1967.

245. Powner DJ: Blood potassium measurements during CPR, *Chest* 69:371, 1981 (editorial).

246. Powner DJ, Holcombe PA, and Mello LA: Cardiopulmonary resuscitation-related injuries, *Crit Care Med* 12:54, 1984.

247. Prough DS, Johnson JC, Poole GV Jr et al: Effects on intracranial pressure of resuscitation from hemorrhagic shock with hypertonic saline versus lactated Ringer's solution, *Crit Care Med* 13:407, 1985.

248. Prough DS, Johnson JC, Stullken EH et al: Effects on cerebral hemodynamics of resuscitation from endotoxic shock with hypertonic saline versus lactated Ringer's solution, *Crit Care Med* 13:1040, 1985.

249. Prough DS, Johnson JC, Stump DA et al: Effects of hypertonic saline versus lactated Ringer's solution on cerebral oxygen transport during resuscitation from hemorrhagic shock, *J Neurosurg* 64:627, 1986.

250. Pulsinelli WA, Waldman S, Rawlinson D et al: Moderate hyperglycemia augments ischemic brain damage: a neuropathologic study in the rat, *Neurology* 32:1239, 1982.

251. Pulsinelli WA, Levy DE, Sigsbee B et al: Increased damage after ischemic stroke in patients with hyperglycemia with or without established diabetes mellitus, *Am J Med* 74:540, 1983.

252. Ralston SH, Voorhees WD, and Babbs CF: Intrapulmonary epinephrine during prolonged cardiopulmonary resuscitation: improved regional blood flow and resuscitation in dogs, *Ann Emerg Med* 13:79, 1984.

253. Ralston SH, Tacker WA, Showen L et al: Endotracheal versus intravenous epinephrine during electromechanical dissociation with CPR in dogs, *Ann Emerg Med* 14:1044, 1985.

254. Ramsay ID: Survival after imipramine poisoning, *Lancet* II:1308, 1967.

255. Read RC, Johnson JA, Vick JA et al:

Vascular effects of hypertonic solutions, *Circ Res* 8:538, 1960.

256. Redding JS, Asuncion JS, and Pearson JW: Effective routes of drug administration during cardiac arrest, *Anesth Analg* 46:253, 1967.

257. Redding JS, Haynes RR, and Thomas JD: Drug therapy in resuscitation from electromechanical dissociation, *Crit Care Med* 11:681, 1983.

258. Redding JS, Pearson JW: Evaluation for drugs for cardiac resuscitation, *Anesthesiology* 24:203, 1963.

259. Redding JS, Pearson JW: Resuscitation from ventricular fibrillation, *JAMA* 203:255, 1968.

260. Resnekov L: Present status of electroversion in the management of cardiac dysrhythmias, *Circulation* 47:1356, 1973.

261. Resnekov L: Calcium antagonist drugs—myocardial preservation and reduced vulnerability to ventricular fibrillation during CPR, *Crit Care Med* 9:360, 1981.

262. Rich S, Wix HL, and Shapiro EP: Clinical assessment of heart chamber size and valve motion during cardiopulmonary resuscitation by two-dimensional echocardiography, *Am Heart J* 102:368, 1981.

263. Richman S: Adverse effect of atropine during myocardial infarction: enhancement of ischemia following intravenously administered atropine, *JAMA* 228:1414, 1974.

264. Risk of infection during CPR training and rescue: supplemental guidelines, *JAMA* 262(19):2714, 1989.

265. Roberts J, Greenberg M, and Knaub M: Comparison of the pharmacologic effects of epinephrine administered by the intravenous and endotracheal routes, *JACEP* 7:260, 1978.

266. Roberts J, Greenberg M, and Knaub M: Blood levels following intravenous and endotracheal epinephrine administration, *JACEP* 8:53, 1979.

267. Rock JJ, Pfaeffle H, and Smith RB: High pressure jet insufflation used to prevent aspirations and its effect in the tracheal mucosal wall, *Crit Care Med* 4:135, 1976.

268. Romhilt DW, Bloodfield SS, and Lipicky RJ: Evaluation of bretylium tosylate for the treatment of premature ventricular contractions, *Circulation* 45:800, 1972.

269. Rowe GG, McKenna DH, Corliss RJ et al: Hemodynamic effects of hypertonic sodium chloride, *J Appl Physiol* 32:182, 1972.

270. Rozenbaum EA, Shenkman L: Predicting outcome of inhospital cardiopulmonary resuscitation, *Crit Care Med* 16:583, 1988.

271. Rudikoff MT, Maughen WL, Effron M et al: Mechanisms of blood flow during cardiopulmonary resuscitation, *Circulation* 61:345, 1980.

272. Salerno DM, Elsperger KJ, Helseth P et al: Serum potassium, calcium and magnesium after resuscitation from ventricular fibrillation: a canine study, *J Am Coll Cardiol* 10:178, 1987.

273. Sanders AB, Ewy GA, Alferness CA et al: Failure of one method of simultaneous chest compression, ventilation, and abdominal binding during CPR, *Crit Care Med* 10:509, 1982.

274. Sanders AB, Ewy GA, Bragg S et al: Expired Pco$_2$ as a prognostic indicator of successful resuscitation from cardiac arrest, *Ann Emerg Med* 14:948, 1985.

275. Sanders AB, Kern KB, Atlas M et al: Importance of the duration of inadequate coronary perfusion pressure on resuscitation from cardiac arrest, *J Am Coll Cardiol* 6:113, 1985.

276. Sanders AB, Kern KB, Ewy GA et al: Improved resuscitation from cardiac arrest with open-chest massage, *Ann Emerg Med* 13:672, 1984.

277. Sanders AB, Kern KB, Fonken S et al: The role of bicarbonate and fluid loading in improving resuscitation from prolonged cardiac arrest with rapid manual chest compression CPR, *Ann Emerg Med* 19:1, 1990.

278. Sanders AB, Kern KB, Otto CW et al: End–tidal carbon dioxide monitoring during cardiopulmonary resuscitation: a prognostic indicator for survival, *JAMA* 262:1347, 1989.

279. Sanders RD: Two ventilating attachments for bronchoscopes, *Del Med J* 39:170, 1967.

280. Saphir R: External cardiac massage prospective analysis of 123 cases and review of the literature, *Medicine* 47:73, 1968.

281. Sarr MG: Bilateral pneumothoraces after resuscitation with esophageal airway, *JAMA* 243:2154, 1980 (letter).

282. Scheidegger D, Drop LJ, and Laver MB: Interaction between vasoactive drugs and plasma ionized calcium, *Intensive Care Med* 3:200, 1977.

283. Scheinman MM, Thorburn D, and Abbott JA: Use of atropine in patients with acute myocardial infarction and sinus bradycardia, *Circulation* 52:627, 1975.

284. Schleien CL, Rogers MC: Cardiopulmonary resuscitation in infants and children. In Rogers MC, ed: *Textbook of pediatric intensive care*, Baltimore, 1987, Williams & Wilkins.

285. Schleien CL, Dean JM, Koehler RC et al: Effect of epinephrine on cerebral and myocardial perfusion in an infant animal preparation of cardiopulmonary resuscitation, *Circulation* 78:809, 1986.

286. Schleien CL, Koehler RC, Gervais H et al: Organ blood flow and somatosensory evoked potentials during and after cardiopulmonary resuscitation with epinephrine and phenylephrine, *Circulation* 79:1332, 1989.

287. Schleien CL, Koehler RC, Shaffner DH et al: Blood–brain barrier integrity during cardiopulmonary resuscitation in dogs, *Stroke* 21(8):1185, 1990.

288. Schleien CL et al: Effect of phenylephrine on cerebral and myocardial perfusion during cardiopulmonary resuscitation in infant piglets (abstract). *Anesthesiology* 65:A76, 1986.

289. Schleien CL, Koehler RC, Shaffner DH et al: Blood-brain barrier disruption after cardiopulmonary disruption in immature swine, *Stroke* 22:477, 1991.

290. Schunacher RR et al: Hemodynamic effects of lidocaine in patients with heart disease, *Am J Cardiol* 24:191, 1969.

291. Shapiro JI, Whalen M, Kucera R et al: Brain pH responses to sodium bicarbonate and Carbicarb during systemic acidosis, *Am J Physiol* 256:H1316, 1989.

292. Sharff JA, Pantley G, and Noel E: Effect of time on regional organ perfusion during two methods of cardiopulmonary resuscitation, *Ann Emerg Med* 13:649, 1984.

293. Silver DI, Murphy RJ, Babbs CF et al: Cardiac output during CPR: a comparison of two methods, *Crit Care Med* 9:419, 1981.

294. Smith GJ, Kramer GC, Perron P et al: A comparison of several hypertonic solutions for resuscitation of bled sheep, *J Surg Res* 39:517, 1985.

295. Smith HJ, Anthonisen NR: Results of cardiac resuscitation in 254 patients, *Lancet* I:1027, 1965.

296. Smith RB, Myers EN, and Sherman H: Transtracheal ventilation in paediatric patients, *Br J Anaesth* 46:313, 1974.

297. Spivey WH, Lathers CM, Malone DR et al: Comparison of intraosseous, central, and peripheral routes of sodium bicarbonate administration during CPR in pigs, *Ann Emerg Med* 14:1135, 1985.

298. Spoerel WE, Narayanan PS, and Singh NP: Transtracheal ventilation, *Br J Anaesth* 43:932, 1971.

299. Stacpoole PW: Lactic acidosis: the case against bicarbonate therapy, *Ann Intern Med* 105:276, 1986.

300. Stainsby WN, Barclay JK: Effect of infusions on osmotically active substances on muscle blood flow and systemic blood pressure, *Circ Res* 28(Suppl 1):I-33, 1971.

301. Steinhart CR, Permutt S, Gurtner GH et al: Beta-adrenergic activity and cardiovascular response to severe respiratory acidosis, *Am J Physiol* 244:H46, 1983.

302. Stemmler EJ: Cardiac resuscitation: a 1-year study of patients resuscitated within a university hospital, *Ann Intern Med* 63:613, 1965.

303. Stiles QR, Tucker BI, Meyer BW et al: Cardiopulmonary arrest: evaluation of an active resuscitation program, *Am J Surg* 122:282, 1971.

304. Stueven HA, Thompson B, Aprahamian C et al: Lack of effectiveness of calcium chloride in refractory asystole, *Ann Emerg Med* 14:630, 1985.

305. Stueven HA, Thompson B, Aprahamian C et al: The effectiveness of calcium chloride in refractory electromechanical dissociation, *Ann Emerg Med* 14:626, 1985.

306. Stueven HA, Tonsfeldt DJ, Thompson BM et al: Atropine in asystole: human studies, *Ann Emerg Med* 13:815, 1984.

307. Stueven H, Troiano P, Thompson B et al: Bystander/first responder CPR: ten years experience in a paramedic system, *Ann Emerg Med* 15:707, 1986.

308. Stueven H et al: Effectiveness of calcium chloride in refractory electromechanical dissociation, *Ann Emerg Med* 13:387, 1984.

309. Suljaga-Pechtel K, Goldberg E, Strickon P et al: Cardiopulmonary resuscitation in a hospitalized population: prospective study of factors associated with outcome, *Resuscitation* 12:77, 1984.

310. Sutton-Tyrrell K, Abramson NS, Safar P et al: Predictors of electromechanical dissociation during cardiac arrest, *Ann Emerg Med* 17:572, 1988.

311. Swartzman S, Wilson MA, Hoff BH et al: Percutaneous transtracheal jet ventilation for cardiopulmonary resuscitation: evaluation of a new jet ventilator, *Crit Care Med* 12:8, 1984.

312. Swenson RD, Weaver WD, Niskanen RA et al: Hemodynamics in humans during conventional and experimental methods of cardiopulmonary resuscitation, *Circulation* 78:630, 1988.

313. Tacker WA Jr, Babbs CF, Abendschein DR et al: Trans-chest defibrillation under conditions of hypothermia, *Crit Care Med* 9:390, 1981.

314. Tacker WA Jr, Ewy GA: Emergency defibrillation dose: recommendations and rationale, *Circulation* 60:223, 1979.

315. Tacker WA Jr et al: Energy dosage for human trans-chest electrical ventricular defibrillation, *N Engl J Med* 290:214, 1974.

316. Taffet GE, Teasdale TA, Luchi RJ et al: In-hospital cardiopulmonary resuscitation, *JAMA* 260:2069, 1988.

317. Thompson BM, Stueven HA, Mateer JR et al: Comparison of clinical CPR studies in Milwaukee and elsewhere in the United States, *Ann Emerg Med* 14:750, 1985.

318. Thompson RG, Cobb LA: Hypokalemia after resuscitation from out-of-hospital ventricular fibrillation, *JAMA* 248:2860, 1982.

319. Todd MM et al: The effects of acute isovolemic hemodilution on the brain: a comparison of crystalloid and colloid solutions, *Anesthesiology* 61:A122, 1984.

320. Tomaszemski CA, Meador SA: Theoretical effects of fluid infusions during cardiopulmonary resuscitation as demonstrated in a computer model circulation, *Resuscitation* 15:97, 1987.

321. Tommasino C, Moore S, and Todd MM: Cerebral effects of isovolemic hemodilution with crystalloid or colloid solutions, *Crit Care Med* 16:862, 1988.

322. Traverso LW, Bellamy RF, Hollenbach SJ et al: Hypertonic sodium chloride solutions: effect on hemodynamics and survival after hemorrhage in swine, *J Trauma* 27:32, 1987.

323. Tresch DD, Thakur RK, Hoffmann RG et al: Should the elderly be resuscitated following out-of-hospital cardiac arrest?, *Am J Med* 86:145, 1989.

324. Trevino RP, Bisera J, Weil MH et al: End–tidal CO2 as a guide to successful cardiopulmonary resuscitation: a preliminary report, *Crit Care Med* 13:910, 1985.

325. Turner LM, Parsons M, Luetkemeyer RC et al: A comparison of epinephrine and methoxamine for resuscitation from electromechanical dissociation in human beings, *Ann Emerg Med* 17:443, 1988.

326. Tweed WA, Bristow G, Donen N et al: Evaluation of hospital-based cardiac resuscitation, 1973-1977, *Can Med Assoc J* 122:301, 1980.

327. Urban P, Scheidegger D, Buchmann B et al: The hemodynamic effects of heparin and their relation to ionized calcium levels, *J Thorac Cardiovasc Surg* 91:303, 1986.

328. Urban P, Scheidegger D, Buchmann B et al: Cardiac arrest and blood ionized calcium levels, *Ann of Int Med* 109:110, 1988.

329. Vagn-Hansen PL: Complications following external cardiac massage with special emphasis on cerebral embolism, *Acta Pathol Microbiol Scand* (Sect A)79:505, 1971.

330. Velasco IT, Pontieri V, Rocha e Silva M Jr et al: Hyperosmotic NaCl and severe hemorrhagic shock, *Am J Physiol* 239:H664, 1980.

331. Vijay NK, Schoonmaker FW: Cardiopulmonary arrest and resuscitation, *Am Fam Physician* 12:85, 1975.

332. Vincent JL, Thijs L, Weil MH et al: Clinical and experimental studies on electromechanical dissociation, *Circulation* 64:18, 1981.

333. Visintine RE, Baick CH: Ruptured stomach after Heimlich maneuver, *JAMA* 234:415, 1975.

334. Volastro P, Sigmann P, and Oaks WW: Cardiac resuscitation in 512 hospitalized patients, *Pa Med* 73:45, 1970.

335. von Planta M, Weil MH, Gazmuri RJ et al: Myocardial acidosis associated with CO2 production during cardiac arrest and resuscitation, *Circulation* 80:684, 1989.

336. Voorhees WD, Babbs CF, and Niebauer MJ: Improved oxygen delivery during cardiopulmonary resuscitation with interposed abdominal compressions, *Ann Emerg Med* 12:128, 1983.

337. Voorhees WD, Ralston SH, Kougias C et al: Fluid loading with whole blood or Ringer's lactate during CPR in dogs, *Resuscitation* 15:113, 1987.

338. Voorhees WD, Ralston SH, and Babbs CF: Regional blood flow during cardiopulmonary resuscitation with abdominal counterpulsation in dogs, *Am J Emerg Med* 2:123, 1983.

339. Waxman K: Noninvasive monitoring in emergency resuscitation, *Ann Emerg Med* 15:1434, 1986.

340. Weale FE, Lond MS, and Rothwell-Jackson RL: The efficiency of cardiac massage, *Lancet* 1:990, 1962.

341. Weaver WD, Cobb LA, Copass MK et al: Ventricular defibrillation—a comparative trial using 175-J and 320-J shocks, *N Engl J Med* 307:1101, 1982.

342. Weil MH, Rackow EC, Trevino R et al: Differences in acid–base state between venous and arterial blood during cardiopulmonary resuscitation, *N Engl J Med* 315:153, 1986.

343. Weiser FM, Adler LN, and Kuhn LA: Hemodynamic effects of closed and open-chest cardiac resuscitation in normal dogs and those with acute myocardial infarction, *Am J Cardiol* 10:555,1962.

344. Weisfeldt ML, Chandra N: Physiology of cardiopulmonary resuscitation, *Annu Rev Med* 32:435, 1981.

345. Weisfeldt ML, Halperin HR: Cardiopulmonary resuscitation: beyond cardiac massage, *Circulation* 74:443, 1986.

346. Werner JA, Greene HL, Janko CL et al: Visualization of cardiac valve motion in man during external chest compression using two-dimensional echocardiography, *Circulation* 63:1417, 1981.

347. White BC, Winegar CD, Wilson RF et al: Possible role of calcium blockers in cerebral resuscitation: a review of the literature and synthesis for future studies, *Crit Care Med* 11:202, 1983.

348. Wild LM, Lajos TZ, Lee AB et al: Left ventricular laceration due to stented prosthesis, *Chest* 77:216, 1980.

349. Wildenthal K, Mierzwiak DS, and Mitchell JH: Acute effects of increased serum osmolality on left ventricular performance, *Am J Physiol* 216:898, 1969.

350. Wildenthal K, Skelton CL, and Coleman HN: Cardiac muscle mechanics in hyperosmotic solutions, *Am J Physiol* 217:302, 1969.

351. Wildsmith JAW, Dennyson WG, and Myers KW: Results of resuscitation following cardiac arrest. A review from a major teaching hospital, *Br J Anaesth* 44:716, 1972.

352. Wilson BJ et al: The effects of various hypertonic sodium salt solutions on cisternal pressure, *Surgery* 30:361, 1951.

353. Winquist RJ, Webb RC, and Bohr OF: Relaxation to transmural nerve stimulation and exogenously added norepinephrine in porcine vessels. A study utilizing cerebrovascular intrinsic tone, *Circ Res* 51:769, 1982.

354. Wood WB, Manley ES Jr, and Woodbury RA: The effects of CO2 induced respiratory acidosis on the depressor and pressor components of the dog's blood pressure response to epinephrine, *J Pharmacol Exp Ther* 139:238, 1963.

355. Yakaitis RW, Otto CW, and Blitt CD: Relative importance of alpha and beta adrenergic receptors during resuscitation, *Crit Care Med* 7:293, 1979.

356. Young WL, Ornstein E: Compressed spectral array EEG during cardiac arrest and resuscitation, *Anesthesiology* 62:535, 1985.

357. Zoll PM et al: Treatment of unexpected cardiac arrest by external electric stimulation of heart, *N Engl J Med* 254:727, 1956.

358. Zoll PM, Zoll RH, Falk RH et al: External noninvasive temporary cardiac pacing: clinical trials, *Circulation* 71:937, 1985.

CHAPTER 38

Positioning of Patients for Operation

LEROY D. VANDAM

Positioning of a patient refers to a body position or arrangement of the body members that is maintained by or imposed on a patient in the course of a particular diagnosis or treatment. In general, the posture of a patient is relevant during the course of a medical examination, during diagnostic radiology or endoscopy, and during anesthesia and surgery. **The purpose of positioning is to allow the procedure to be performed as simply as possible and to achieve the best possible results free of complications. In anesthesia, the importance of positioning is crucial under the following circumstances: tracheal intubation; regional procedures, particularly spinal and epidural blocks; invasive monitoring techniques; and intraoperative changing of a patient's position to improve respiration or circulation.** Moreover, positioning is important in specific situations, such as deliberate hypotension, which renders a relatively blood-free operative field to enhance delicate dissection. In addition to pharmacologic lowering of blood pressure, the patient should be properly positioned with the operative site uppermost to diminish venous congestion.

The emphasis in this chapter, however, is restricted to surgical procedures in which standard positions are used for various kinds of operations. The symbols useful in indicating positions on the anesthetic record are shown in Fig. 38-1.[8] Some eponymic designations for the more commonly used positions are listed in Table 38-1. Surgeons usually have their preferences, which should be allowed unless the patient is placed at higher risk for development of a complication. A surgical team must be cognizant of the surgeon's needs so that the operation can proceed expeditiously. **The fact that anesthetized patients are often placed in positions that they could not otherwise tolerate for long in the conscious state should not be overlooked. Moreover, during regional anesthesia with lack of sensation and loss of consciousness in general anesthesia, the patient cannot sense positionally induced changes and is thereby subject to a number of complications, both physiologic and pathologic.**

PREOPERATIVE CONSIDERATIONS

The position for surgery should be chosen based on preoperative history and physical examination. Has the patient had postural problems in the waking or anesthetized state? Arthritis with major joint dysfunc-

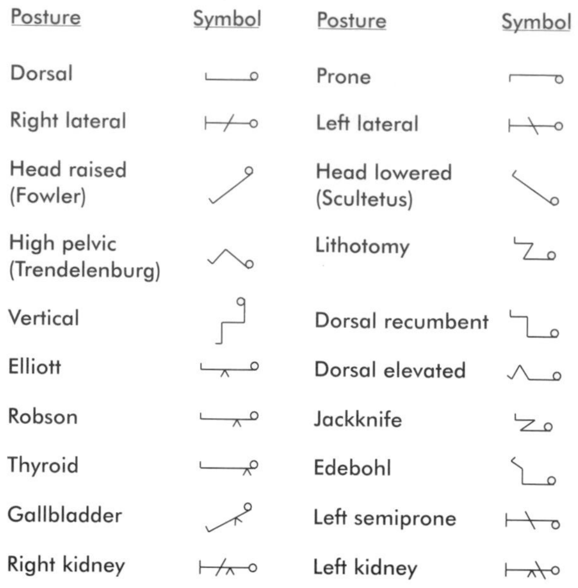

Fig. 38-1. Symbols for surgical positions. (From Miller AH: Surgical posture: with symbols for its record on the anesthetist's chart, *Anesthesiology* 1:247, 1940.)

tion causes problems in positioning the head and opening the mouth, not only for surgical access but also for tracheal intubation. A position can be tested beforehand (e.g., flexing of the hips and knees for lithotomy). Can the arms be comfortably abducted or pronated? Other physical conditions and ailments call for analysis and planning. Severe, generalized osteoporosis can predispose the patient to bone fracture even with the slightest trauma if the patient is not handled carefully. Morbid obesity poses many problems. Will it be feasible to move the anesthetized patient to the prone position without injury both to the patient and the operating room staff? There should always be adequate staff available for such activity because trauma to personnel is common, particularly back strain. Some anesthesiologists have attempted to mitigate the positioning problem in obese patients by intubating the trachea with topical anesthesia, then having the conscious patient move from the supine to the prone position on the operating table. General anesthesia is then induced with the airway assured.

Several diseases and physiologic conditions marked by autonomic nervous system insufficiency may cause arterial hypotension when the patient is made to assume any degree of the erect position, particularly when anesthetized. In this category are patients who are debilitated, bedridden, dehydrated, or with hemorrhage-induced hypovolemic conditions; diabetic or renal failure patients with peripheral neuropathy; and paraplegics or quadriplegics.[11] Before changing positions during anesthesia, the devel-

Table 38-1 Selected eponymic designations for surgical positioning

Position	Description
Bozeman's position 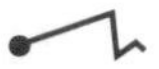	Patient rests on the knees and elbows and is supported by straps
Edebohl's position for vaginal operations 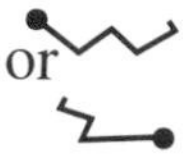	Patient lies on her back at the edge of the table, with hips and knees partly flexed; the feet are held up and apart by supports attached to the table
Fowler's position 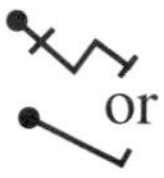	Dorsal position in which the knees and head and shoulders are elevated, thus forming a **V** with the pelvis at the apex, to ensure better dependent intraabdominal drainage
Robson's position (also known as Elliot's or Mayo's position) 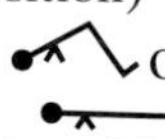	Position that enhances exposure for surgery on the biliary system in which a sandbag is placed posteriorly below the right costal margin
Sims' position 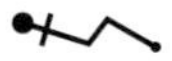	Lateral recumbent position for obstetric delivery, the woman lying on the left side with the under arm behind the back of the head, with thighs flexed, the upper one more than the lower
Trendelenburg position 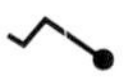	Patient lies supine with the knees bent and higher than the rest of the body; the legs extend over the edge of a supporting surface so that the knees form the apex of a right angle and the body forms an inverted **V** with the pelvis elevated over the head.

opment of hypotension can be minimized by blood volume replenishment, by wrapping the legs with elastic bandages, by the use of compression boots, or by use of a positive gravity suit. Choice of anesthesia is also relevant when peripheral vasodilation is to be expected. Thus for the erect positions vasodilation induced by histamine-releasing agents such as morphine or the use of spinal and epidural anesthesia with their accompanying sympathetic blockade may be avoided by choice of other agents.

PROTECTION OF MEDICAL DEVICES

Many surgical patients depend on life support systems for their immediate and long-term survival. Commonly used devices include intravenous lines, bladder catheters, and gastric tubes, which must be guarded during positioning. More important are the intravenous alimentation lines, arteriovenous shunts needed for hemodialysis, cardiac pacemakers, and insulin pumps. Similarly, maintenance of the neck in an extended, midline position when cervical fracture is suspected may entail the use of head tongs to maintain extension and its inclusion in the positioning schema.

Whenever the position of a patient is changed during anesthesia, attached apparatus must be reexamined both for intactness and correct placement. For example, a lawsuit was filed against an anesthesiologist because an insulin pump placed at a patient's side during general anesthesia allegedly led to pressure-paralysis of the radial nerve. This diabetic patient already had severe peripheral neuropathy, thus raising the possibility of antecedent neurologic disease, a problem well-known in relation to spinal anesthesia.

INJURY TO SOFT TISSUES AND SKELETON

Prolonged maintenance of any position on an operating table may induce pressure necrosis of the skin and underlying tissues. Injury most often occurs over bony prominences and is enhanced by the physical status of the patient and modifying physical circumstances. The paraplegic patient is particularly prone to development of pressure sores.[11] Other features such as debility, malnutrition with hypoalbuminemia, and fecal and urinary incontinence exaggerate the possibility of tissue ulceration, whereas vasoconstriction and hypothermia are additional risk factors.

Experimentally, it has been found that pressures greater than 70 mm Hg applied constantly over a period of 2 hours or longer can result in irreversible ischemia.[10] The injury may be graded as shown in Box 38-1. Such injuries can occur over the forehead and malar areas, the skin over the iliac crests, at bony prominences of arms and legs, and on the female breasts and scrotum in the male. During cardiopulmonary bypass operations with the patient supine, the occiput may sustain pressure injury of varying degree or simply subsequent development of alopecia.

The areas subject to pressure should be raised from time to time during surgery to prevent these kinds of injuries. Several kinds of mattresses are designed to avert pressure injury, such as the foam egg crate variety (also used to prevent nerve injury), water mattresses, and inflatable alternating pressure devices.

BOX 38-1
INJURY GRADING SYSTEM FOR PRESSURE INJURIES

Stage 1:   Blanching followed by nonblanching erythema
Stage 2:   Induration or edema with breakdown of the dermis
Stage 3:   Ulceration extending to subcutaneous tissues and still further to fascia, muscle, and bone

---

OCULAR INJURY

During anesthesia and particularly when the patient is in the prone decubitus, the orbital cavity and eye are at risk for injury. Because the consequences are grave and practically all such injuries are avoidable, anesthesiologists must constantly be alert to avoid them. Direct trauma from an improperly applied face mask plus excessive pressure may be equated with pressure on the eye with the patient in the prone or lateral position. Corneal abrasion may develop if the eyelids are not kept closed. In addition, periorbital edema, nerve palsies (supraocular and infraocular sensory nerves), and diminution in retinal artery blood flow with possible retinal infarction and blindness may occur with improper positioning.[2]

The cornea is easily abraded as a result of reduced lacrimation during general anesthesia. At the termination of general anesthesia, therefore, the eyes should be inspected for damage. After awakening, the patient may experience a foreign body sensation, with lacrimation and pain aggravated by lid closure and eye movement. Corneal abrasion can be detected under good illumination as an area of diminished light reflection. Ophthalmologic consultation should be sought not only for the patient's welfare but also for medicolegal reasons. Examination of the eye may involve use of a topical anesthetic that can delay corneal reepithelialization, instillation of fluorescein dye, and ophthalmoscopy. In treatment, a topical antibiotic, such as erythromycin, is instilled into the conjunctival sac, in addition to use of atropine to reduce the pain associated with ciliary spasm. The eye is securely patched with a sterile pad to reduce ocular movement and pain associated with blinking.

Corneal trauma is best prevented by taping the closed eyelids when pressure against the eye is anticipated. A plastic eye shield may be required when the eyes are out of view beneath surgical drapes or if the head is prone on a head rest. Sterile mineral oil, artificial tears, and methylcellulose have been used as benign lubricants for the conjunctival sac.

NERVE INJURY

Many reports have described the development of peripheral nerve injury during the course of anesthesia. **Nerves may be injured through stretch or by compression against bone or operating room equipment largely because protective muscle tone is lost during anesthesia and the patient cannot perceive pain and numbness.** Among the nerves commonly affected are the brachial plexus and its divisions, the ulnar and radial in the arm, and the common peroneal in the leg. Injury to branches of the facial and trigeminal nerve, to the long thoracic nerve, and to the obturator, femoral, sciatic, and lateral femoral cutaneous nerves in the thigh has been reported. It is worth noting that nerve injury and other kinds of trauma related to positioning cannot be detected by any current monitoring device. However, evoked potential recording can detect spinal cord ischemia as well as imminent intracranial nerve tract damage during craniotomy.

How molecular damage to nerves is produced by pressure or stretch has been studied by several researchers.[4,12] Based on their observations, the degree of injury can be graded with an eye to prognosis. In grade 1 injury (neuropraxis), a response to blunt force or compression, there is temporary dysfunction but only slight evidence of demyelinization without axonal degeneration. In 1929, Gasser and Erlanger found a gradient of susceptibility of nerve fibers to this kind of injury, ranging from the most susceptible group A, heavily melyinated motor fibers, through fibers of lesser diameter that subserve position and vibratory sense. In the wakeful state the effect of pressure is experienced as a motor paralysis that results from keeping the legs crossed for a time; the patient is unable to stand but sensation remains intact. This differential effect is also seen in the motor paralysis that follows excessive pressure created by using a pneumatic tourniquet.

In grade 2 injury (axonotmesis), destruction of axons occurs, including the myelin sheath but without injury to supporting matrix. Wallerian degeneration occurs distal to the injury site, although the connective tissue of the nerve is intact and endoneurium and Schwann's sheath are not disrupted. Thus the axon can regenerate, depending on proximity of the injury to the cell body, and function may be restored eventually. In this kind of neuronal injury it is not clear whether the cause relates to interruption of the endoneural blood supply or mere hypoxia.

In grade 3 injury (neurotmesis), the nerve may have been crushed, avulsed, or severed. Nerve fibers, connective tissue, and Schwann's sheath are completely disrupted, with loss of functional and anatomic continuity. Unless the damaged section of the nerve

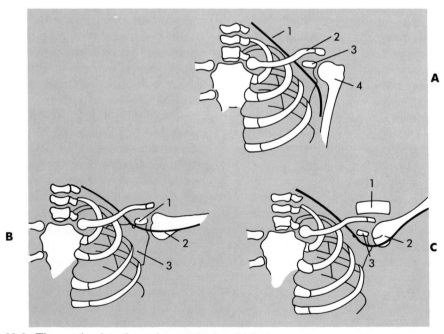

Fig. 38-2. The mechanics of traction on the brachial plexus. **A,** Arm at side: *1,* brachial plexus; *2,* clavicle; *3,* coracoid process of scapula; *4,* head of humerus. **B,** Arm at right angle: scapula *(3)* rotates and brachial plexus is stretched beneath coracoid process *(1)* and around head of humerus *(2)*. **C,** Arm hyperextended with shoulder brace *(1)* depressing scapula *(3)*. Brachial plexus stretched beneath coracoid process *(1)* and around head of humerus *(2)*. (From Dripps RD, Eckenhoff JE, and Vandam LD: *Introduction to anesthesia,* ed 7, Philaldephia, 1988, WB Saunders.)

can be excised and the surgically severed ends of the nerve are carefully approximated, little if any return of function can be anticipated. This is the type of injury wherein a painful neuroma develops as a result of disorganized regeneration of axons at a fibrous, endoneural scar.

Clinical Origin of Nerve Palsies

Because the brachial plexus and its peripheral branches are among the most frequently injured nerves, additional explanation may further clarify how the other nerves may be traumatized.

The nerves comprising the brachial plexus arise centrally at the transverse processes of the vertebrae and terminate peripherally at their points of entry to the arm (Fig. 38-2). Separation of these two points stretches the nerves, with resulting damage of the nature previously described. Flexion of the head in the opposite direction combined with downward displacement of the ipsilateral shoulder places additional tension on the nerves, while several fulcrums, such as the scalene muscles, the attachment of the pectoralis minor muscle to the coracoid process of the scapula, and the rounded head of the humerus, provide further possibilities for stretch. Hyperabduction, extension, and external rotation of the arm stretch the brachial plexus around these fulcrums. A supporting brace applied to the shoulder may not only act as a fulcrum but also compresses the brachial plexus against the first rib; a shoulder brace should not be used when the arm is extended on an arm rest. Rarely, the plexus may be pinched between the clavicle and first rib.

Ulnar and radial nerves are superficially placed and hence are easily compressed against bone or operating table and the common peroneal nerve against leg stirrups. Branches of the facial nerve may be injured by overenthusiastic attempts to elevate the jaw via pressure on the rami of the mandible or by tight application of a head strap to secure a face mask.

PHYSIOLOGIC RESPONSES TO CHANGE IN POSITION

The major physiologic effects of position changes relate to respiration and circulation. In the normal subject, measurements of circulation and respiration are usually made with the patient in the sitting position. However, a patient to be anesthetized is usually supine at the start, followed often during the anesthetized state by changes that involve varying degrees of erectness, as in head-down, prone, or lateral decubitus.

Systemic Circulation

When a recumbent subject assumes the erect position, as in getting out of bed, through a gravity effect the volume of blood in the venous system above and below the heart pools in the periphery and alters transmural venous pressures without directly affecting the driving force of the arterial circulation.[9] The degree of hydrostatic force can be calculated from the vertical distance between the right atrium and any point below. Thus above the atrium, the veins tend to empty while those below, in the abdomen and lower extremities, dilate. If, for example, the veins in the leg are 100 cm below the right atrium, the weight of the column of blood is about 77 mm Hg. The addition of another 10 mm Hg, representing dynamic venous pressure, results in a total rise in intravascular pressure of 87 mm Hg. This increase in hydrostatic pressure is transmitted to the capillaries where fluid exchange is negatively affected.

Severe hypotension, largely related to the decline in preload and a consequent decrease in cardiac output, results in the absence of the following compensatory mechanisms: reflex sympathetic vasoconstriction, changes in extravascular pressure and venous tone, pressure of the subcutaneous tissues in the legs related to venous engorgement, muscle contraction, and presence of valves in the veins, all of which oppose the hydrostatic effect. Venous constriction and increases in heart rate and cardiac output, the result of sympathetic activation, are the major adjustments that limit the decrease in systemic arterial pressure. This sympathetic response is mediated by a decrease in carotid sinus pressure via activation of pressor receptors.

It is not surprising that all studies on the effect of varying degrees of the upright position during anesthesia have shown a decrease in systemic arterial pressure, because of obtundation of sympathetic activation, the depressant effects on the heart, and the vasodilation produced both by inhalation and regional anesthesia. The situation is comparable to the passive head-up tilt in a conscious subject where fainting readily occurs.

In the 90-degree head-down position, a conscious individual may not be able to survive for more than several hours because of a rise in both arterial and venous pressures, plus the adverse effects on respiration discussed in the following sections. All of the other positions required for surgical procedures are variations on the erect or supine positions, including the prone and lateral decubitus, with corresponding circulatory changes.

Effects of position on the cerebral circulation

In the change from a supine to an erect position, as much as 300 to 800 ml of blood may pool in the extremities through gravity. Consequently, cerebral blood flow may decrease initially by as much as 80%, but restoration quickly occurs because of reflex vasoconstrictive action in the periphery and via

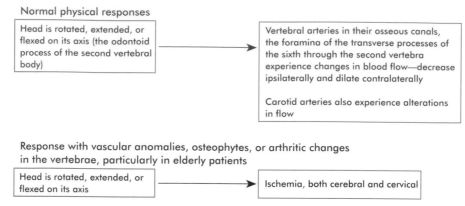

Normal physical responses

| Head is rotated, extended, or flexed on its axis (the odontoid process of the second vertebral body) | → | Vertebral arteries in their osseous canals, the foramina of the transverse processes of the sixth through the second vertebra experience changes in blood flow—decrease ipsilaterally and dilate contralaterally

Carotid arteries also experience alterations in flow |

Response with vascular anomalies, osteophytes, or arthritic changes in the vertebrae, particularly in elderly patients

| Head is rotated, extended, or flexed on its axis | ──────→ | Ischemia, both cerebral and cervical |

Fig. 38-3. Mechanism of cerebral ischemic development in relation to movement of the neck.

autoregulation of blood flow within the brain and spinal cord.[14] This is a normal response, but, in the presence of arteriosclerosis, or in elderly patients and in cases of antonomic nervous insufficiency, the compensation may be delayed or absent, with resulting cerebrovascular ischemia.

With regard to positioning, movements of the neck represent a possible source of ischemia, in relation to the cervical blood supply to the brain and spinal cord. Toole has pointed out that within the mobile isthmus between head and chest, the arteries and veins that supply the brain and spinal cord are constantly subject to mechanical stress[14]. Whenever the head is rotated, extended, or flexed on its axis (e.g., the odontoid process of the second vertebral body), the vertebral arteries located in the osseous foramina of the transverse processes of the sixth through the second vertebrae undergo changes in blood flow. For example, when the head is turned to one side, vertebral blood flow decreases ipsilaterally and increases on the contralateral side. Similar blood flow changes may also occur in the carotid arteries. These alterations in head position may cause cerebral and cervical ischemia, particularly in elderly patients in whom vascular anomalies, osteophytes, or arthritic changes may be present (Fig. 38-3).

Respiratory Alterations

The anesthetized subject lies at first in the supine, sleeping position, which is well tolerated by nearly every human being. Nevertheless, alterations in respiratory function related to a change from the erect to the supine position are not inconsiderable and, as in the case of the circulation, are further affected by the anesthetic technique.

The respiratory changes are primarily the result of alterations in the static behavior of the respiratory system, demonstrable by volume pressure relations, which are usually measured with the patient in a standard, sitting position. The subdivisions of the gas volumes of the lungs are well known (Fig. 38-4). Lung volumes vary with age, body size, and gender. As Agostini and Hyatt have described them, in the resting individual breathing can be defined as a volume variation initiated from a relaxed state at end-expiration, the functional residual capacity (FRC).[1] **In the supine position, as the abdomen and its contents resemble a container with a distensible wall, the diaphragm is thrust upward or distended by the weight of abdominal contents. Thus FRC is reduced relative to the erect position and is further compromised during general anesthesia. When the FRC declines below residual volume, the closing volume is approached (Fig. 38-5), and atelectasis and ventilation/perfusion abnormalities develop. These changes are ordinarily of little significance except in patients with respiratory compromise.** With use of higher than atmospheric inspiratory oxygen pressures, reliance on pulse oximetry and end-tidal carbon dioxide record-

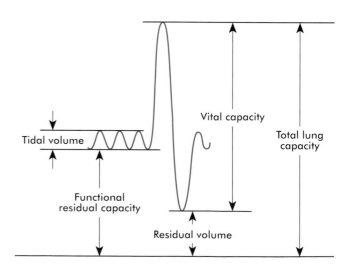

Fig. 38-4. Static lung volumes in humans.

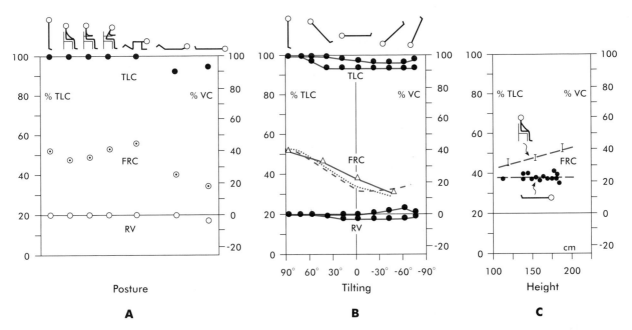

Fig. 38-5. Pulmonary subdivisions in various postures (**A**), during tilting (**B**), and as function of body height (**C**). In instances when residual volume *(RV)* was not determined, it was assumed to be 20% of total lung capacity *(TLC)* in upright posture. **A,** Standing (Mead J, unpublished observations); seated erect; seated erect, arms supported; seated leaning forward, arms supported; on hands and knees; prone; supine. **B,** During tilting; *triangles;* all remaining points (Mead J, unpublished observations). *Dotted* (supported at shoulders) and *broken lines* (supported by ankles) are average values for five subjects. Values of *TLC* and *RV* are for individual subjects. **C,** Seated; ranges are SE for groups of 10 subjects; *broken line* is fit by eye; supine. (From Agostoni E, Hyatt RE: Static behavior of the respiratory system. In Macklein PT, Mead J, eds: *Handbook of physiology: the respiratory system,* vol 3, part 1, ch 9, Bethesda, Md, 1986, American Physiological Society.)

ing, and use of mass spectrometry for analysis of respiratory and anesthetic gases, anesthesiologists may maintain respiratory exchange in a safe range. Variations in both the supine and erect positions affect lung volumes as already described for the supine position alone, and there are subtle influences on lung volume resulting from displacement of the heart and mediastinal contents.[6] In the lateral and prone positions, unless the chest wall is adequately supported, mechanical restriction of chest wall motion occurs. Finally, as initially demonstrated by Wade (Fig. 38-6), ventilation/perfusion relations follow a gravity-graded pattern with ventilation dominant and perfusion more pronounced in dependent regions.[15]

SURGICAL POSITIONS

Martin has edited an excellent, comprehensive monograph on this subject.[7] However, only the positional needs of the major specialties of surgery (from that monograph) are presented in this chapter. The information provided represents the opinions of practitio-

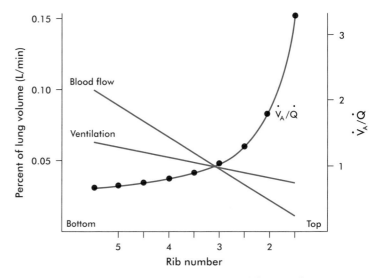

Fig. 38-6. Distribution of ventilation, blood flow, and ventilation/perfusion ratio up the normal upright lung. Straight lines have been drawn through the ventilation and blood flow data. Because blood flow decreases more rapidly than ventilation with distance up the lung, ventilation/perfusion ratios rise, slowly at first, then rapidly. (From Wade JB: *Ventilation, blood flow and gas exchange,* ed 3, London, 1977, Blackwell Scientific.)

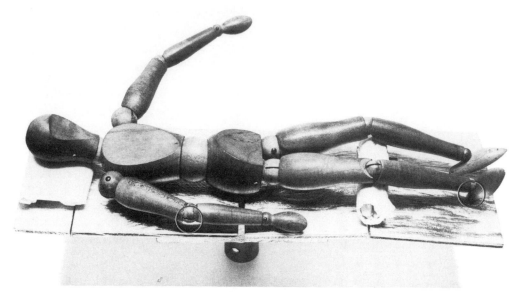

Fig. 38-7. Supine position. Table is level, head is slightly elevated on a pillow, knees slightly flexed on a pillow, right arm at the side-hand pronated, left arm (on a padded arm board) with moderate abduction, slightly dihedral. The elbows should be padded and the heels protected against pressure.

ners both in anesthesiology and in surgery, usually a combination of the two, and there is some repetition.

General Surgery

The positions required for general surgery are as follows:

- Supine
- Prone
- Right and left lateral decubitus
- Semisupine ("lawn chair" posture)
- Prone-jackknife
- Lithotomy

- "Kidney"
- Trendelenburg

The goal of these positions is **to improve operating conditions for the surgeon by facilitating exposure and providing a relatively bloodless field.**

Supine position

The **supine position** (Fig. 38-7) is the most commonly used with the least adverse physiologic effects, especially for the cardiovascular system, since there are essentially no pressure gradients above or below the heart. There is, however, V/Q mismatch and effects

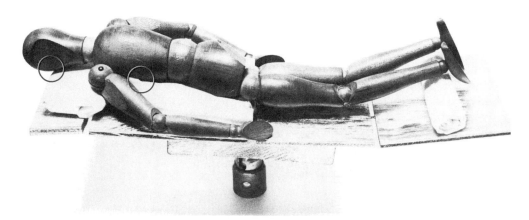

Fig. 38-8. Prone position. The table is positioned slightly head up, the patient's torso is elevated by bolsters, head in axial line, with arms at the sides (might be overhead). Elbows should be wrapped, knees flexed (padded), and ankles resting on a small blanket roll. In a modification of this position, the table might be flexed or the patient resting on a padded curved frame, to open the intervertebral spaces for disc surgery.

on FRC that arise from the "rolling up" of abdominal contents beneath the diaphragm, which impedes ventilation to the lower lung zones. Precautions for this position include brachial plexus and ulnar nerve protection if the arms are extended and avoidance of pressure on the heels during prolonged procedures.

Prone position

The **prone position** (Fig. 38-8), with the patient lying face down on an operating table, poses essentially the identical adverse physiologic effects as the supine decubitus position. Precautions include assurance that eyes, ears, nose, breasts, and male genitalia are not subject to excessive pressure. In a modification of the prone position, the patient may be placed on a curved frame or bolsters to elevate and flex the back, thereby opening the intervertebral spaces (as for spinal disc operations) and permitting the scapulae to slide laterally. The same precautions as with supine positioning are required to guard against excessive pressures. However, the hemodynamic effects are slightly more evident because the heart is at a higher level than both head and legs. If a frame or bolsters arc used, the legs should be wrapped with elastic bandages to prevent venous pooling, the knees should be flexed, and knees and feet padded. A frame of this generic kind permits the abdomen and its contents to hang freely, thus improving the position of the diaphragm and pulmonary ventilation. A final and essential precaution in relation to this position is that the components of the brachial plexus must not be stretched by hyperabduction or hyperextension of the arms.

Lateral decubitus

In the **right** or **left lateral decubitus** (Fig. 38-9), the patient rests on the side, with the dependent leg flexed and the nondependent leg extended, with a pillow placed between them. A so-called axillary roll is placed just caudal to the axilla so that the upper rib cage, not the contents of the axilla, rests on the roll. The dependent arm is usually extended at less than 90 degrees. The upper arm can be secured to the "ether screen," padded with gauze wrap, or placed in a special holder designed for the purpose. The dependent ear should be protected from pressure effects and the head propped on a firm pillow to prevent displacement from the central axis. Adverse physiologic effects of this position primarily result from compression of the dependent lung by downward shift of the mediastinal contents.

"Lawn chair" position

In the **"lawn chair" position** (Fig. 38-10), probably the most physiologically benign of all and used for operations on the neck (thyroid, parathyroid, radical neck dissection), adverse physiologic effects are mainly of a cardiovascular nature. Often an overzealous surgeon may rapidly crank up the upper end of the table shortly after induction of anesthesia, with a resulting decline in blood pressure. It is, therefore, advantageous to conduct anesthesia at a light depth until operation has begun.

Jackknife position

The **jackknife position,** a variant of the prone position, is used for rectal and perirectal procedures and

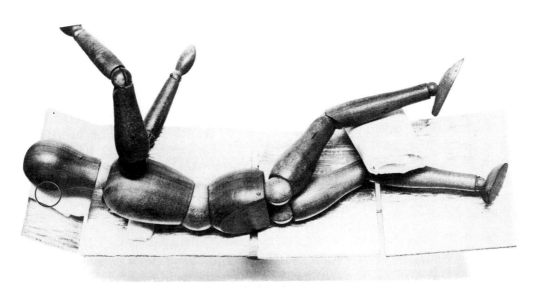

Fig. 38-9. Lateral decubitus, right or left position. The patient is positioned on the side, head on a pillow in the axial line, with axillary contents protected by an "axillary roll" beneath the upper rib cage. Arms are in a neutral position, the upper leg flexed with the lower leg slightly less flexed; the knees are separated by a pillow.

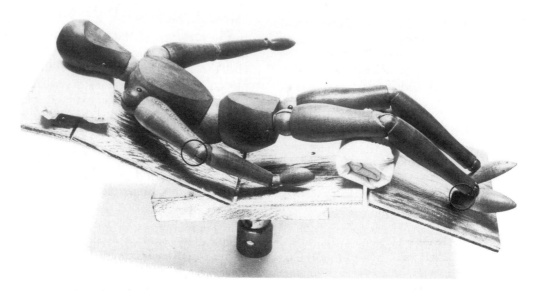

Fig. 38-10. "Lawn chair" position. The table is moderately flexed, with the upper body elevated, head in axial line (may be extended) resting on a pillow, knees are flexed resting on a pillow, the right arm at the side, left arm in safe abduction with hand pronated. Elbow joints and ankles should be padded.

pilonidal sinus excision. The body is flexed at the hips and the buttocks are uppermost since the operating table is tilted head-down. Use of spinal anesthesia may be preferable in this situation, thus avoiding airway problems. Because patients are anesthetized only below the waist, they can report any undue pressures in unanesthetized areas (face or upper extremity). During spinal anethesia in this position the legs are dependent, causing venous pooling, a decrease in cardiac output via reduction in preload, and a decline in blood pressure; therefore the legs should be wrapped before turning. Hypobaric or isobaric spinal anesthesia may be given with the patient in the lateral position; the patient is then immediately turned prone with frequent blood pressure recordings. When general anesthesia is required, the same precautions as noted for the prone position are used. The endotracheal tube is tied around the patient's neck instead of being taped at the mouth, where tape can be loosened by saliva.

Lithotomy position

The essential feature of the **lithotomy position** is that the hips are flexed, knees bent, and the legs suspended by stirrups. Otherwise the patient is supine, often with the table tilted down toward the head. The most important precaution is to ascertain that the peroneal nerve is not compressed between fibula and stirrups, or the leg inwardly rotated on the thigh, thereby stretching the common peroneal nerve around the head of the fibula. If the patient's hands are tucked in at the sides, precautions should be taken

to ensure that the fingers are not caught and crushed when the foot of the operating table is elevated at termination of operation. One advantage of the lithotomy position is that hemodynamics are preserved, with the legs elevated above heart level. However, if there has been major blood loss during the operation, hypotension can appear when the legs are removed from the stirrups, as a result of reperfusion and pooling of blood in the legs. Therefore the legs should be wrapped beforehand and slowly lowered to the horizontal.

Flexed lateral (kidney) position

In **the flexed lateral (kidney) position** (Fig. 38-11), the padding and precautions are similar to those for the lateral position alone. However, the nondependent arm need not be secured as in the lateral position because it is not in the path of the operation being performed at a lower level.

Trendelenburg position

Trendelenburg position (Fig. 38-12) is commonly used for pelvic surgery but actually has been modified from the original description because the surgeon merely wishes to have the head down so that the abdominal contents are out of the pelvis. Pressure of the viscera against the diaphragm plus the use of abdominal retractors markedly encroach on the FRC. Spinal or epidural anesthesia is often used for these operations. Cardiovascular stability is usually well maintained because venous return is improved. A common problem with the use of hyperbaric spinal

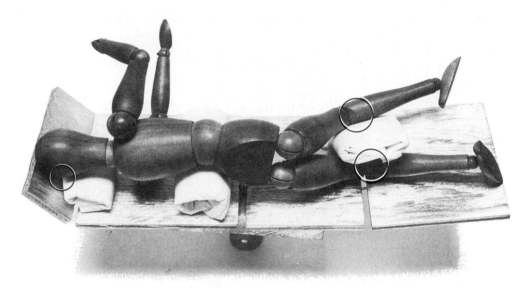

Fig. 38-11. Flexed lateral position. This is essentially the same as the lateral decubitus position, but the body is flexed at the thoracoabdominal junction by means of a "kidney rest" or a firm pillow. This maneuver separates the lower thoracic margin from the iliac crest, permitting access to the retroperitoneal area for kidney and adrenal operations or lumbar sympathectomy.

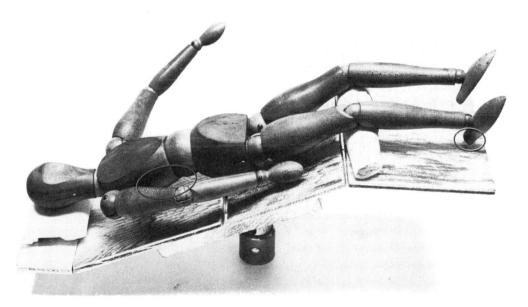

Fig. 38-12. Trendelenburg position. The original position as shown here entailed a marked head-down tilt of the table with knees flexed and legs elevated (held by an assistant). As a result, the abdominal contents were displaced from the pelvis for relatively blood-free operations on the pelvic structures. In current practice the Trendelenburg position consists mainly of a head-down tilt of the table with the patient otherwise supine.

anesthesia is the decision regarding when the patient can be safely placed in the head-down position without risking high levels of anesthesia.

Cardiac Surgery

For all patients undergoing cardiac surgery via a median sternotomy in which there is any possibility of using the saphenous veins for coronary bypass (this includes patients for valve replacement as well as those undergoing a scheduled coronary procedure), a standard frog-leg position is used (Fig 38-13). The patient lies supine and is positioned so that the vertex of the head extends only 1 or 2 inches onto the small head support. This is done so that the hand crank used

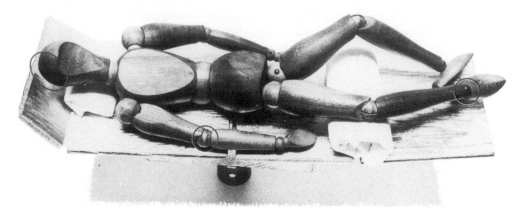

Fig. 38-13. Position for most types of cardiac surgery. As noted in the text, the legs are in the "frog" position to permit access to the groins; the vertex of the head does not quite extend to the edge of the head rest. Arms are at the sides but separated from the torso.

for raising and lowering the head or tilting the top of the table does not strike the surgeon at the knee. It is also important to have the "ether" screen tilted well toward the anesthesiologist so that the elbows of the operating surgeon (right- or left-handed) have clearance from the drapes and the operative field is directly in front of the surgeon rather than to the side. Resting on a soft pillow, the patient's legs are flexed at the knees and the soles of the feet approximated, which results in external rotation of the thighs for best access in harvesting saphenous veins from either thigh or lower leg, or the approach to femoral artery and vein. Care should be taken to pad the heels with soft plastic sponges. Use of blanket rolls or other dense props to elevate the legs should be avoided to minimize the possibility of sciatic nerve palsy. This virtually never occurs when a pillow is used, but some centers have reported this problem when using blanket rolls.

With the frog-leg position, the patient's arms are kept close to the body on each side, and, provided the arms rest on the mattress and are not allowed to press against the metal tabletop, elbow pads probably are not necessary, although a worthy precaution. A specially designed soft plastic sponge in a doughnut configuration is used to pad the back of the head. Some patients may emerge from anesthesia with a damaged area over the occiput, varying from 1 to 3 cm in diameter, ranging in severity from simple itching and scaling to full-thickness necrosis. There has been considerable effort to determine why such injuries occur, but with no success in reaching an explanation. Diminished perfusion or nonpulsatile blood flow may be contributory. Specifically, this lesion does not seem to be related to stray current from a cautery or any other type of electrical discharge. The problem does not seem to relate directly to pressure because lesions occur even with the use of the doughnut. Neverthe-

less, use of the doughnut seems to have reduced the incidence of injuries even though it does not eliminate them.

Some cardiac operations are performed through a right anterior thoracotomy; that position does require a blanket roll beneath the right side of the chest, posteriorly, with the right arm at the side (see lateral decubitus position). The elbow is bent so that the arm remains clear of the lateral wall of the chest. In this position, an attempt is made to flatten the pelvis so that the femoral vessels, especially on the left side, but if necessary also on the right, are readily exposed.

At times a left thoracotomy is required when placing the patient on bypass by way of the left femoral artery and vein at the groin. In this situation, a standard right lateral decubitus is appropriate, with the pelvis tilted backward to assist in exposure of the groin. Occasionally, this position is necessary in patients undergoing reoperation with grafting to the circumflex marginal arteries.

During the course of most cardiac operations the thorax is elevated approximately 30 degrees during cardiopulmonary bypass to provide a better view of the valves. In addition, this allows the iced saline solution, which is dripped onto the pericardium to produce topical hypothermia, to settle in the pericardial cavity. To assist in cooling for patients undergoing valvular surgery, the patient is generally tilted approximately 10 or 15 degrees to the left in order for the "toe" of the sabot-shaped pericardium to be in a dependent position. This also allows pooling of iced saline solution in the pericardial cavity, keeping the apex and left ventricular myocardium cold.

Vascular Surgery

Carotid endarterectomy calls for the supine, slightly sitting position (semi-Fowler's "lawn chair") (see Fig.

38-10); the neck is extended on a "dog" dish and rotated to the contralateral side. The angle of elevation, approximately 30 degrees, is favored to improve visibility and diminish venous bleeding. The surgeon favors placing himself/herself and the assistant on the operative side of the table with the ipsilateral arm at the patient's side, allowing the tracheal tube, ECG leads, and arterial line to be on the opposite side and fully available for the anesthesia team.

Thoracoabdominal aneurysm excision requires a lateral thoracotomy position with left side up and left arm across the chest, with the support of a kidney brace (similar to the left kidney position; see Fig. 38-11), plus support beneath the left hip so that the axis of the pelvis is less than 45 degrees from the horizontal. This position permits a thoracoabdominal incision, as well as access to the right groin if necessary. The table can be rolled back and forth to improve exposure at either end of the field. The patient's anatomic features are "unrolled" by this exposure in a manner compared to that of a frozen biscuit container. Some abdominal aortic aneurysms are managed via a similar position but with a retroperitoneal, nonthoracic incision.

Abdominal aortic aneurysmectomy or **aortic bypass** calls for a dorsal position with arms abducted. Head-down tilting is advantageous for proximal exposure of the aorta in a barrel-chested patient or for improved exposure of the pelvis.

Iliac artery surgery and **lumbar sympathectomy** are best done with the patient in a dorsal position with a support beneath the ipsilateral hip and intermittent rolling of the table. During infrainguinal bypass, a dorsal position with slightly less flexion and external rotation is convenient. Frequent rolling of the table from side to side helps in exposure. The prone position is optimal for repair of a **popliteal aneurysm.**

For **portacaval shunting,** a supine, dorsal position is used (see Fig. 38-8), with optional use of a roll or kidney bar beneath the right costal margin to improve exposure of the porta hepatis. In **vena caval interruption** the dorsal position is useful with the head down during venous manipulation to reduce the chance of air embolism.

Obstetrics

For vaginal delivery, the patient is placed in the lithotomy position. To avoid peripheral nerve injury, the ankles and knees should be cushioned to avoid pressure against the metal stirrups. To prevent backstrain, the hips and buttocks should be positioned without protruding over the table edge. When placed in stirrups or removed from stirrups, the legs should be flexed and elevated simultaneously to avoid strain on the back or groin.

In a **cesarean delivery,** the patient lies supine. However, the gravid uterus may obstruct the inferior vena cava, resulting in the "supine hypotensive syndrome." To prevent this, a semilateral tilt is maintained by placing a wedge beneath the right hip at an optimum tilt of 15 degrees. Crawford et al. reported less fetal acidosis and higher Apgar scores when left uterine displacement was maintained during cesarean delivery.[3] A clinically important observation regarding positioning of parturients during induction of spinal anesthesia is noteworthy. Sprague advised placing the patient in the right lateral position during induction of spinal anesthesia for cesarean delivery because subsequent placement in the left, semilateral decubitus with a wedge beneath the right hip may be associated with more even distribution of local anesthetic in the subarachnoid space.[13] This resulted in improved sensory anesthesia and a higher incidence of patient satisfaction.

Orthopedic Surgery

Surgical positions for foot and ankle, knee and hip, tibial osteotomy, femoral fracture, hand surgery and back surgery are discussed in the following paragraphs.

General precautions

A pillow is placed beneath the patient's head, with possible pillow support of lumbar lordosis, arms positioned (elbows padded) along the sides of the trunk, or abducted (not beyond 90 degrees) on padded arm boards with hands pronated. The patient should be observed for bony contact points at the occiput, sacrum, elbows, and heels. In general, the goal is to minimize the influence of gravity on the circulatory system with minimal perfusion gradient in mean arterial pressure from heart to periphery. In venous return, there should be a positive gradient from the periphery to the right atrium. Venous changes are most affected by cyclic respiratory variations in intrathoracic pressure. Easy access to the patient's face and airway is necessary. Respiratory V/Q relations are affected by cephalad migration of the abdominal contents and dorsal diaphragmatic curvature. Improved ventilation of the suffused lungs should be sought via assisted or controlled ventilation.

Possible adverse consequences are related to postural changes and include:

- **Hypotension with head-up tilt**
- **With head-down tilt, increase in cerebral venous and intracranial pressure as well as in myocardial oxygen consumption**
- **Worsened V/Q relations with head-down tilt as well as further problems with spontaneous or controlled ventilation**

Lateral decubitus

In the **lateral decubitus** (see Fig. 38-9), the patient is turned to one side with the trunk stabilized to prevent rolling, legs straight with pillows between them, or with the lower leg flexed 90 degrees at the hip and the knee bent to maintain the leg on the table. The lower leg is padded to prevent common peroneal nerve injury. A thoracic roll is placed caudal to the axilla to prevent compression of the shoulder and to relieve pressure on the neurovascular bundle as well as to ensure good blood flow to the lower hand. To prevent ventral circumduction of the shoulder, the lower shoulder is slightly dorsal. The head is supported to keep the cervical spine aligned with the thoracic spine. The arms are extended ventrally on a padded armboard (elbows padded) or with blanket supports between them, or the arms may be flexed at the elbows to prevent ventral rotation of the upper shoulder. The strap support to the table should not be placed over the thorax, which may impede ventilation, but rather should be located between the iliac crest and upper femur, or pelvic supports should be used.

Prone decubitus

In the **prone decubitus** (see Fig. 38-8), the patient's abdomen is kept free to prevent a rise in intraabdominal pressure and in the perivertebral plexus of veins. If the head is below the heart, venous congestion occurs. If the abdomen hangs free, decreases in FRC are less than in the supine position. The head and extremities may be lower than the spine. Ventral supports consist of parallel sheet rolls or a padded

---

> **BOX 38-2**
> **ESSENTIALS FOR THE SUPINE POSITION**
> (see also Fig. 38-7)
>
> Protect the ulnar nerves at the elbows
> Avoid brachial plexus stretch with the arms abducted
> Carefully position the head in the presence of cervical injury
> Wrap the legs or use compression boots

---

adjustable metal frame. The head is in the sagittal plane and supported on soft sponges to prevent pressure on the down side (eye and ear).

Neurosurgery

For patients undergoing neurosurgery, there are specific precautions to be taken depending on the position assumed (Fig. 38-14). These are outlined in Boxes 38-2 to 38-4.

SUMMARY

Proper positioning of patients intraoperatively is vital to facilitate the surgical procedure, to ensure cardiorespiratory stability, and to avoid trauma to the anesthetized patient. Although the supine position is used most often intraoperatively, this requires dili-

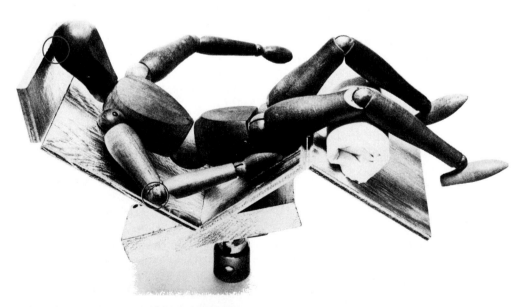

Fig. 38-14. Sitting position, used in neurosurgery for suboccipital exploration. The patient is in the sitting position, legs flexed, approximately at cardiac level. The head is flexed on a head rest (not shown in this illustration).

BOX 38-3
ESSENTIALS FOR THE PRONE POSITION
(see also Fig. 38-8)

Protect personnel from back strain while turning the patient

Place the patient's arms either at the sides or upward around the head

Avoid pressure on dependent eyes and ears

Avoid abdominal pressure and consequent rise in pressure in the perivertebral plexus of veins

Protect the tracheal tube by using tincture of balsam for the attachment and use a salivary drying agent

To detect possible changes in spinal neuronal conduction in the presence of spinal stenosis, use evoked potential monitoring

Watch for excessive extension or flexion of the cervical spine

Protect female breasts with sponge supports

Allow intravenous and arterial lines to travel over the patient during the turn to the prone position

Place all monitoring devices before turning the patient

BOX 38-4
ESSENTIALS FOR THE SITTING POSITION
(Fig. 38-14)*

To detect air embolism, use a Doppler device or echocardiography (end-expiratory carbon dioxide declines with embolism)

Be aware that peripheral vasodilation leads to a decrease in pulmonary artery wedge pressure, a decline in cardiac output, a reflex rise in pulse rate, and systemic vascular resistance while cerebral blood flow falls momentarily and then corrects

Protect the ulnar and peroneal nerves

Wrap the legs or use compression boots

Carefully flex the neck with the chin positioned a finger's breadth from the chest to prevent cervical vein obstruction

Do not use this position in patients with major cardiovascular disease because of induced sympathetic reflex hyperactivity

In the final position, place the patient's knees approximately at heart level

Use the head holder; an intravenous barbiturate should be given before placing the holder on the patient to avoid reflex sympathetic hyperactivity

*Rarely used now because of the possibility of cerebral air embolization.

---

gence on the part of the anesthesiologist to ensure that injury does not occur to the anesthetized patient, particularly with reference to positioning of upper and lower limbs. Patient position is most often dictated by the desire for maximum exposure of the operative field for the surgical team. However, the requirements for specific patient positions merely for surgical convenience should not jeopardize patient safety in terms of ensuring adequate respiratory and cardiovascular stability and avoidance of traumatic injury. The anesthesiologist should be familiar with the positioning requirements for various surgical procedures. Moreover, an understanding of the anatomic and physiologic alterations related to changes in patient positioning are essential to ensure intraoperative stability and prevent tissue injuries that may result in permanent impairment postoperatively.

KEY POINTS

■ The purpose of positioning is to allow the procedure to be performed as simply as possible and to achieve the best possible results free of complications. In anesthesia, the importance of positioning should not be underestimated: during tracheal intubation; regional procedures, particularly spinal and epidural blocks; invasive monitoring techniques; and intraoperative changing of a patient's position to improve respiration or circulation.

■ The fact that anesthetized patients are often placed in positions that they could not otherwise tolerate for long periods in the conscious state should not be overlooked. Moreover, during regional anesthesia with lack of sensation and loss of consciousness in general anesthesia, the patient cannot sense positionally induced changes and is thereby subject to a number of complications, both physiologic and pathologic.

■ The optimal patient position for surgery should be based on preoperative history and physical examination.

■ Prolonged maintenance of any position on an

operating table may induce pressure necrosis of the skin and underlying tissues. The injury most often occurs over bony prominences and is enhanced by the physical circumstances. Paraplegic patients are particularly prone to the development of pressure sores.

- During anesthesia and particularly in the prone decubitus, the orbital cavity and eye are at risk for injury. Because the consequences are grave and practically all such injuries are avoidable, anesthesiologists must be constantly alert to avoid them.

- The cornea is easily abraded as a result of reduced lacrimation during general anesthesia. At the termination of general anesthesia, therefore, the eyes should be inspected for damage.

- Nerves may be injured through stretch or by compression against bone or operating room equipment, largely because protective muscle tone is lost during anesthesia and the patient cannot perceive pain and numbness.

- In the supine position, because the abdomen and its contents behave like a container with a distensible wall, the diaphragm is thrust upward or distended by the weight of abdominal contents. Thus FRC is reduced relative to the erect position and is further compromised during general anesthesia. When the FRC declines below residual volume, the closing volume is approached, wherein atelectasis and ventilation/perfusion abnormalities develop. These changes are ordinarily of little significance except in patients with respiratory compromise.

- Possible adverse physiologic consequences related to postural changes include (1) hypotension with head-up tilt, (2) increase in cerebral venous and intracranial pressure as well as in myocardial oxygen consumption with head-down tilt, (3) worsened V/Q relations with head-down tilt as well as further problems with spontaneous or controlled ventilation.

KEY REFERENCES

Agostini, Hyatt RE: Static behavior of the respiratory system. In Macklein PT, Mead J, eds: *Handbook of physiology: the respiratory system,* vol 3, part 1, ch 9, Bethesda, Md, 1986, American Physiological Society.

Denny-Brown D, Doherty MM: Effects of transient stretch or compression of peripheral nerve, *Arch Neurol Psychiatr* 54:116, 1945.

Goode PS, Allman RM: The prevention and management of pressure ulcers, *Med Clin North Am* 73:1511, 1989.

Martin JT: *Positioning in anesthesia and surgery,* ed 2, Philadelphia, 1987, WB Saunders.

Miller AH: Surgical posture: with symbols for its record on the anesthetist's chart, *Anesthesiology* 1:241, 1940.

Toole JF: Effects of change of head, limb and body position on cephalic circulation, *N Engl J Med* 279:307, 1968.

REFERENCES

1. Agostini E, Hyatt RE: Static behavior of the respiratory system. In Macklein PT, Mead J, eds: *Handbook of physiology: the respiratory system,* vol 3, part 1, ch 9, Bethesda, Md, 1986, American Physiological Society.
2. Brooks GZ, Vandam LD: Ocular complications of anesthesia, *Weekly Anesthesiol Update* 3(13):1, 1979.
3. Crawford JS, Burton M, and Davies P: Time and lateral tilt at caesarian section, *Br J Anaesth* 44:477, 1972.
4. Denny-Brown D, Doherty MM: Effects of transient stretch or compression of peripheral nerve, *Arch Neurol Psychiatr* 54:116, 1945.
5. Goode PS, Allman RM: The prevention and management of pressure ulcers, *Med Clin North Am* 73:1511, 1989.
6. Kaneko K, Milic-Emili J, Dolovich MB et al: Regional distribution of ventilation and perfusion as a function of body position, *J Appl Physiol* 21:767, 1966.
7. Martin JT: *Positioning in anesthesia and surgery,* ed 2, Philadelphia, 1987, WB Saunders.
8. Miller AH: Surgical posture: with symbols for its record on the anesthetist's chart, *Anesthesiology* 1:241, 1940.
9. Milnor WR: Normal circulatory function. In Mountcastle VB, ed: *Medical physiology,* ch 40, ed 14, St Louis, 1980, CV Mosby.
10. National Pressure Ulcer Advisory Panel: *Decubitus* 2:24, 1989.
11. Rocco AG, Vandam LD: Problems in anesthesia for paraplegics, *Anesthesiology* 20:348, 1959.
12. Seldon HJ: Three types of nerve injury, *Brain* 66:237, 1943.
13. Sprague DH: Effects of position and uterine displacement on spinal anesthesia for cesarian section, *Anesthesiology* 44:164, 1976.
14. Toole JF: Effects of change of head, limb and body position on cephalic circulation, *N Engl J Med* 279:307, 1968.
15. Wade JB: Ventilation, blood flow and gas exchange, ed 3, London, 1977, Blackwell Scientific.

CHAPTER 39

Electricity, Electrical Safety, and Instrumentation in the Operating Room

ROBERT H. STIEFEL

The role of technology in medicine has steadily increased over the past few decades, and there is every indication that this will continue. Most of this technology has been in the form of new electronic equipment. Safety has sometimes been overlooked; at other times, specific aspects of safety (notably electrical safety) are overemphasized. This chapter describes the principles and practices of the safe use of medical equipment.

The safe use of modern medical technology depends first on an understanding of the operating principles of the technology. An understanding of electrical hazards is also necessary to operate electrical equipment safely. Such knowledge is based on an understanding of electricity and electronics. Therefore this chapter starts with a review of basic concepts of electricity and electronics. In the second section the hazards of medical equipment use are described and explained.

Standards and regulations for the use of medical equipment have been promulgated to avoid hazards to patients and personnel. The third section of this chapter describes the organizations that set standards, tells how and why they develop standards, and gives an overview of some of their more important standards. From this information, it becomes clear that the proper use of standards is to provide safe, and safe use of, medical technology.

All three of these sections provide the basis for development of an equipment safety program, as described in the final section. The need to understand and apply electrical engineering principles and practices, to analyze and avoid equipment hazards, and to apply equipment safety standards has spawned a new profession in health care. Known as clinical engineering, and practiced by biomedical engineers and technicians in hospitals, this field is described in the final section. This section concludes with a discussion of technology management—the term used to describe the involvement of clinicians, engineers, and administrators in planning and implementing the use of medical technology in the most effective manner.

An understanding and respect for the safe use of medical equipment is particularly important for anesthesiologists. Of the major disciplines of modern medicine, none depends more on technology for direct patient care and safety than does anesthesiology. Many of the devices used at the bedside for the diagnosis and treatment of patients were developed first for use in the operating room by anesthesiologists. Anesthesiologists use the widest variety of equipment, and routinely use it in the most precarious situations, of any of the medical disciplines.

ELECTRICITY

Current is the flow of electric charge, electrons being the most common charge carrier. The unit of measure of current is the ampere, or amp, abbreviated A. One ampere is the flow of one coulomb per second, and one coulomb is 6.2420×10^{18} units of electric charge. An electron has one unit of negative electric charge. The symbol for current is I; the symbol for charge (in coulombs) is Q.

Voltage, also called potential difference or electromotive force (EMF),* is the work (i.e., expenditure of energy) required to move electrons. It is also the difference in potential energy between two points due to differences in electrical charge, or the energy released when electrons move from higher to lower potential. The unit of measure of voltage is the volt, and the symbol for voltage is V (or sometimes E). One volt represents the amount of work to move one coulomb. The zero potential reference point is called ground or earth. Besides being a reference point, ground also plays a major role in electrical safety. Hazard currents can be safely drained by connection to ground, as will be discussed later.

A *conductor* is a material through which electrons move easily (e.g., copper) and an *insulator* is a material through which electrons move poorly (e.g., glass). A *semiconductor* is a material that is normally an insulator but acts like a conductor when certain conditions are met (e.g., silicon crystals with a particular impurity added).

---

* Electromotive force is not a force but an energy. The misnomer is a carryover from times when the distinction between force and energy was not clearly defined.

Direct Current

Direct current (DC) is unidirectional current and is constant in magnitude. Batteries provide a constant direct current. By convention, the direction of current is from the more positive to the more negative voltage (Fig. 39-1). This was based on a guess by Benjamin Franklin, when he needed to assign algebraic signs in equations describing electrical charges and forces. Unfortunately, his guess was incorrect. Electrons actually flow from negative to positive, opposite to the convention for current that was accepted before the discovery of electrons.

Resistance is the opposition to the flow of current. The unit of measure of resistance is the ohm, abbreviated Ω, and the symbol for resistance is R. A resistor is an electrical component designed to provide a specific value of resistance. Voltage, current, and resistance are related by Ohm's law, which states that voltage is directly proportional to current and to resistance (Fig. 39-2).

Power is work per unit time, or the rate at which electrical energy is used. Its unit of measure, the watt (abbreviated W), is equivalent to one joule per

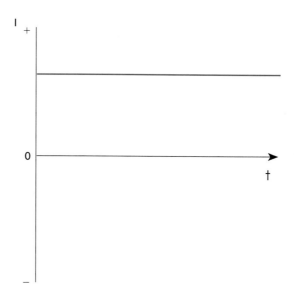

Fig. 39-1. Direct current.

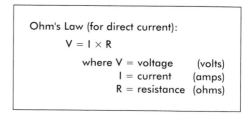

Fig. 39-2. Ohm's law for direct current.

second. The symbol for power is P, and it is calculated as $P = IV = I^2R$.

Alternating Current

Alternating current (AC) differs from direct current in that its polarity reverses periodically. As a result, its magnitude is constantly changing. A *cycle* is one complete wave pattern (from *O* to *A* in Fig. 39-3). A *period* is the time of one cycle. The average value of alternating current over one period is zero. *Frequency* (f) is the number of cycles per second (cps) and is the inverse of the period. The unit of measure is the hertz, abbreviated Hz. By definition, 1 Hz = 1 cps. There are 360 degrees in one cycle, and the *phase* is the number of degrees between two AC waveforms at the same time.

Common household voltage (that available at electrical receptacles in the home) and the voltage at most hospital receptacles is nominally 120 volts AC (VAC) and has a 60 Hz sinusoidal waveform (a period of 16.7 msec). The voltage given is the root-mean-square (RMS) value, which is 0.707 ($1\sqrt{2}$) of the peak value, or 0.354 of the peak-to-peak value of the voltage waveform (Fig. 39-4). The RMS value of AC voltage provides the same wattage as the same value of DC voltage. DC and AC currents are additive. Combinations of DC and AC currents can make virtually any desired waveform. Conversely, any electrical waveform can be described as a series of sine waves, each at a single frequency (this technique is called Fourier analysis).

AC adds a number of refinements (= complications) to the treatment of electricity. Resistance is no longer the only opposition to current. *Reactance* is the opposition to current that varies with frequency (resistance is constant). Together, resistance and reactance are called *impedance*. Impedance is still measured in ohms, but its symbol is Z. Reactance is also composed of two parts—*capacitive reactance* and *inductive reactance*. Reactance has the symbol X; capacitive reactance is X_C and inductive reactance is X_L. Impedance is calculated as

$$Z = R^2 + (X_L - X_C)^2$$

and Ohm's law becomes

$$V = I \times Z$$

A *capacitor* is an electrical component designed to provide a specific value of capacitance, the property of storing separated charges when a voltage is present between conductors. In construction, a capacitor is two conductive plates separated by an insulating material called a dielectric. The symbol for capacitance is C. Capacitance is measured in farads, abbreviated F. More often, values are given in microfarads (microfarads = μF, although mF is also used). Capacitance is related to current and voltage by the following formula:

$$I = C\,[dV/dt]$$

An *inductor* is an electrical component designed to provide a specific value of inductance, the property of a varying electric current to induce a voltage in a circuit. An inductor is a coil of wire, often around a metallic core. The symbol for inductance is L, and the unit of measure is the henry, abbreviated H. Inductance is related to current and voltage by the following formula:

$$V = L\,[dI/dt]$$

An important application of inductance is in transformers. A transformer is constructed by placing two coils close to each other. An AC source is applied to one coil, and a current is induced in the other. Voltage can be adjusted up or down by selecting the ratio of turns of wire in the two coils:

$$\frac{V_1}{V_2} = \frac{N_1}{N_2}$$

where N is the number of turns of wire (Fig. 39-5). In fact, AC is used for transmission from electrical generators because transformers can convert AC voltages but not DC voltages. Raising and lowering

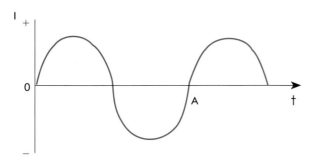

Fig. 39-3. Alternating current.

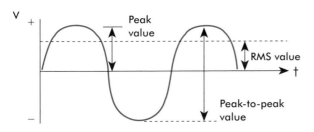

Fig. 39-4. Root-mean-square (RMS) voltage.

TRANSFORMER

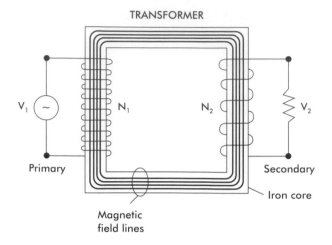

Fig. 39-5. Example of a transformer.

high voltages is practical only with transformers. High voltage is more efficiently transmitted over long distances. If current is cut in half, the voltage must be doubled to transmit the same power (recall that P = IV). However, this reduces the power loss in the transmission lines to one quarter (I^2R, where R is the resistance of the transmission line).

AC vs. DC

Sixty Hz was chosen for AC frequency for engineering reasons. Transformers work efficiently at 60 Hz. At higher frequencies, transmission losses increase. At lower frequencies, lights would flicker perceptibly. Unfortunately, 60 Hz also happens to be right in the middle of the range of frequencies to which muscles and nerves are most susceptible (see section on hazards of electricity).

An interesting historical note on the selection of alternating current over direct current involves William Kemmler, the first man legally electrocuted.[2]

In 1879, Thomas Edison invented the electric light. He then developed a DC distribution system, many of which were installed in the 1880s. George Westinghouse developed an AC distribution system late in the 1880s. Edison and Westinghouse waged an economic battle over whether AC or DC would become the standard for electrical distribution systems. The advantage of AC was that it could be transmitted at a high voltage over long distances, without the unacceptably high losses that both AC and DC suffer at low voltage, and then it could be dropped to a lower, safer voltage with a transformer for local distribution. Edison and others could show, however, that AC was more dangerous. In animal experiments, AC voltages of 200 volts were lethal, but DC was relatively safe at that level.

On June 4, 1888, Governor David Hill of New York

signed a law making electrocution the method of execution for capital crimes committed after January 1, 1889. Electrocution had been selected by a commission assigned the task of finding an effective, humane means of execution to replace hanging. In March 1889, an electrical engineer, Harold Brown, was contracted to provide execution systems for the Auburn, Sing Sing, and Clinton prisons. Brown had previously published on the dangers of AC and the comparative safety of DC. He naturally chose Westinghouse AC generators although he had to purchase them used because Westinghouse tried to prevent him from obtaining them at all (Westinghouse did not want his name associated with electrocution). The first system was installed in Auburn state prison in central New York State in June 1889.

Meanwhile, on March 29, 1889, in Buffalo, New York, William Kemmler killed his girlfriend after a drunken argument. On May 10 a jury found him guilty, and on May 14 he was sentenced to death by electrocution. Kemmler's attorney appealed on the grounds of cruel and unusual punishment. Hearings were conducted in New York City and Buffalo during July 1889. The defense attempted to prove that death by electric current was uncertain because people recovered after being struck by lightning. Brown testified on behalf of the State, describing his electrocution experiments on animals. Edison was also called by the State to testify. He opined that death by electrocution should be instantaneous. Kemmler's appeals were ultimately denied, and he was electrocuted on August 6, 1890.

Circuits

A *circuit* is any connection of electrical components. A *complete circuit* is one that starts and ends at the same point, and is required for current to flow (Fig. 39-6). A *series circuit* has two terminal components connected end to end, and the total current in the circuit passes through each component (i.e., the current is constant through a series circuit). A *parallel circuit* has two terminal components connected side by side. The current divides between the components, but the voltage drop across each component is the same (i.e., the voltage is constant across a parallel circuit) (Fig. 39-7).

Semiconductors

Electricity becomes more interesting and useful—as well as complicated—with semiconductors. Resistors, capacitors, and inductors are two-terminal, linear, and passive devices. In a linear device, a change in the input signal produces a proportional change in the output. A passive device is one with no built-in power source. A junction diode is the simplest semiconduc-

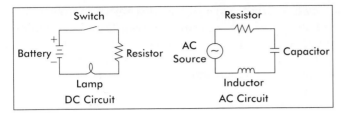

Fig. 39-6. Direct current (DC) circuit and an alternating current (AC) circuit.

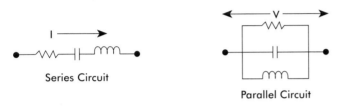

Fig. 39-7. Series and parallel circuits.

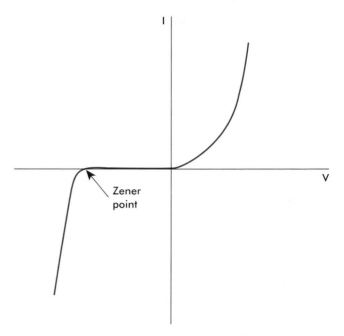

Fig. 39-9. Current vs. voltage in a zener diode.

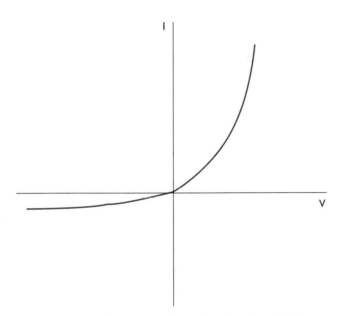

Fig. 39-8. Current vs. voltage in a junction diode.

tor. It is a two terminal, passive component, but it is nonlinear. It allows current in one direction and blocks current in the other (Fig. 39-8). This characteristic is used to convert AC to DC—*rectification.* A zener diode is a diode that can conduct in the reverse direction when a sufficiently large reverse voltage is applied (Fig. 39-9). This voltage is called the zener point, and a zener diode is used as a voltage regulator, which establishes a fixed voltage.

A transistor is a three-terminal, nonlinear, active device. Active means that the output can have more power than the input—*amplification.* The extra power comes from an external power supply. Characteristics

that are controlled by transistor circuits are input and output impedances, current and voltage gains, and phase and frequency responses. The most common transistor is the bipolar-junction-transistor. Its three terminals are called base, emitter, and collector. Depending on the polarity of these terminals, the transistor is npn or pnp (p is positive, n is negative). The field-effect-transistor (FET) is a newer device. Its three terminals are called gate, source, and drain. The gate is used to control the current between the source and the drain. The FET is unique because the gate draws almost no current from the signal source and has extremely high input impedance. Depending on polarity, a FET is either n-channel or p-channel. Depending on how the gate is constructed, a FET is either a junction (JFET) or metal-oxide-semiconductor (MOSFET) type. The symbols for resistors, capacitors, inductors, diodes, and transistors (as they appear in schematic drawings) are shown in Fig. 39-10.

Integrated circuits (IC) are single semiconductor "chips" into which have been etched numerous transistors and passive components. A single IC can be a complete amplifier, a chip capable of storing thousands of bytes of digital memory, a computer's microprocessor, or any of hundreds of different analog or digital circuits. ICs account for the miniaturization of instruments and computers, as well as for their phenomenal speed and versatility. Their reduced power requirements are another significant advantage.

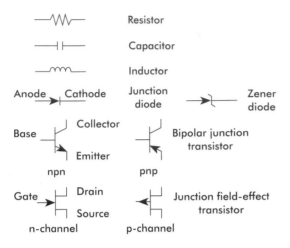

Resistor

Capacitor

Inductor

Anode — Cathode
Junction diode

Zener diode

Base — Collector / Emitter
npn

Bipolar junction transistor
pnp

Gate — Drain / Source
n-channel

Junction field-effect transistor
p-channel

Fig. 39-10. Electronic symbols.

Analog and Digital Circuits

Circuits that manipulate continuous waveform voltages are called *analog circuits.* Signals can have a wide range of magnitudes. Natural phenomena are typically analog. *Digital circuits* on the other hand, have only two discrete voltage values, called high and low (or 1 and 0). Analog data can be converted to digital, and vice versa, by A/D and D/A convertors. Data must be in digital form to be used by computers. Digital data also have greater immunity to electrical noise. Spurious voltages added to an analog signal will alter the signal's value. Digital low and high signals need only be within 1.5 V of their 0 to 5 V nominal values to be dependably interpreted.

Leakage Current

An unavoidable and undesirable side effect of electrical circuitry is leakage current. It is virtually impossible to contain all electrical energy within the wiring and components of electrical equipment. The primary source of leakage current is stray capacitance. Two conductors separated by insulation and air act like a capacitor, and alternating current is conducted between them. The electrical power cord usually has the greatest amount of stray capacitance because of the length and proximity of the wires. Interestingly, leakage current will flow in the ground wire of a power cord even when a device is not turned on, because AC voltage is applied as long as the power cord is plugged in.

There is also resistive leakage because insulation is less than perfect. Although resistive leakage current is a minor source, it does tend to increase as equipment ages. In addition to the degradation of insulation, there can be a buildup of dirt, dust, and moisture inside the equipment.

The ground wire in a three-wire power cord conducts leakage current from the chassis of equipment to ground. As we will see later, it also shunts fault currents (due to damaged insulation, wiring, or components) to ground. If a fault current is large enough, it will cause a fuse or circuit breaker to open, preventing shocks to patients or operators and further damage to equipment. If a ground wire is missing or broken, leakage current or fault current energizes the chassis until it finds an alternative path to ground. This alternative path can be a patient or an operator. This is one of the more important considerations in electrical hazards, which is the topic of the section on hazards of electricity.

Isolated Power

In a conventional power distribution system, three wires feed into a circuit breaker box. These three wires are called hot, neutral, and ground. (This discussion will be limited to 120 VAC systems.) The hot wire supplies current at 120 VAC, and the neutral wire provides the return path. The ground wire is for safety (i.e., for shock and fire protection from electrical faults). The circuit breaker box distributes power to branch circuits through individual circuit breakers. Each branch circuit feeds electrical receptacles, overhead lighting, and/or installed equipment (e.g., x-ray viewbox) (Fig. 39-11).

An isolated-power system is a more specialized type of power distribution system. An isolation transformer and a line-isolation monitor are installed directly in front of the circuit breaker box (Fig. 39-12). Neither of the output leads from the isolation transformer are connected to ground. The output leads are referred to as line 1 and line 2. Isolated power is sometimes called ungrounded, but it is important to realize that a ground wire is still used. In this context, ungrounded simply means that neither of the power lines is connected to ground. The line-isolation monitor (LIM) monitors the degree of isolation of the isolated-power system by measuring the amount of current that would flow to ground if either power line were connected directly to ground (total hazard current). If this current exceeds a preset limit, the monitor lights and sounds an alarm.

In a conventional power distribution system, a ground fault (a short circuit from the hot conductor to ground) allows a large current to flow until the circuit breaker opens (circuit breakers are typically rated at 15 or 20 A). **An ideal isolation transformer would not allow any current to flow from either power line to ground.** A direct fault from either power line to ground would merely convert the isolated-power system to a conventional power distribution system. A second fault, from the other power line to ground,

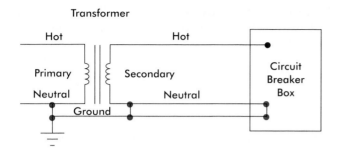

Fig. 39-11. Conventional power distribution system. Note the connections of neutral wires to ground terminals on both sides of the transformer and in the circuit breaker box.

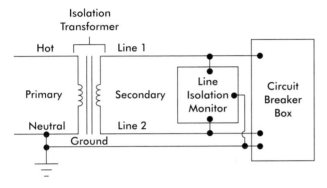

Fig. 39-12. Isolated-power system. Note that neither side of the secondary of the transformer is connected to ground terminals, either at the transformer or at the circuit breaker box.

would be required for a large current to flow to ground.

In reality, no isolation transformer is ideal. Capacitance between the transformer wiring creates a high-impedance path to ground. Additional high-impedance paths to ground exist within the line-isolation monitor and the power distribution wiring. Altogether, these allow up to 1.5 mA of leakage current. Each device connected to the system contributes its own inherent leakage current (generally less than 100 μA each). Because of this, the alarm point of the line-isolation monitor is usually set at 1.7 to 2.0 mA. This limits the shock and fire hazards due to ground faults. In 1978, the total hazard current limit was raised from 2 to 5 mA to reduce nuisance alarms. Isolated-power systems were originally employed in hospitals to eliminate sparks that could cause an explosion in the presence of flammable anesthetics. In the 1960s and early 1970s, when electrical safety first became a major concern, isolated-power systems were touted as panaceas for shock hazards. **The virtual elimination of flammable anesthetics and realistic, cost-effective electrical safety measures have minimized the use of isolated-power systems for shock and fire protection.**

The one remaining safety factor provided by isolated-power systems is branch circuit protection. In the event of a ground fault in a device connected to an isolated-power system, the LIM will activate both audible and visible alarms. These alert the operator to the fault and do no worse than converting the isolated-power system to conventional power (i.e., one power line is grounded). This allows the branch circuit to remain energized and equipment to continue operating. The circuit breaker does not open, because the only additional current that flows is limited to the previous value that the LIM was measuring. This benefit is also minimized by more realistic electrical safety measures applied to the design, construction, and maintenance of modern medical equipment.

Isolated-power systems were formerly required in anesthetizing locations and were strongly recommended in heavily instrumented areas (e.g., critical care units). They are, however, expensive—more than $2000 for the hardware, plus extra costs for installation. Since 1984 isolated-power systems have no longer been required in nonflammable anesthetizing locations, but they are still allowed and continue to be included in the design of most operating rooms.

Isolation Amplifiers

Amplifiers increase the magnitude of an electrical signal and/or modify the signal to filter out unwanted noise or other effects. As will be seen later, it is desirable to isolate electrial connections between instruments and patients from ground. To accomplish this, isolation amplifiers are used. They have the additional advantage of isolating the input connections from any AC-powered circuits. There are three basic design techniques employed by isolation amplifiers.

- Optical isolation amplifiers work by using light to transmit the signal. A light-emitting diode (LED) puts out light with intensity proportional to the strength of the signal. A photodiode then picks up the light signal and converts it back to an electrical signal.
- The transformer isolation amplifier uses a transformer to couple the input signal with the rest of the circuitry. To make the instrument usable down to DC levels, the input signal modulates a high-frequency carrier signal. After the transformer-coupling stage, the signal has to be demodulated before further processing.
- Capacitively coupled isolation amplifiers also need a high-frequency carrier signal to transmit the signal to be isolated across isolating capacitors. Again, the desired signal is subsequently removed via a demodulator circuit.

Interference

Electrical interference is any disturbance of the desired electrical signal. There are many possible sources of electrical interference, which may sometimes be hard to find or eliminate. The types of equipment most susceptible to electrical interference are physiologic monitors—equipment designed to detect generally low-level signals from a patient. Sources of interference include the following:

- Muscle artifact—muscle contractions produce electrical signals
- Broken input wires—open or intermittent circuits produce noisy signals
- Electrical power distribution system—electric and magnetic fields produced by power lines can produce interference
- Ground loops—current created when two devices are electrically grounded to points that are not at the same electrical potential, and are then connected to each other (e.g., through a patient); this current can subsequently interfere with the physiologic signal to be monitored
- Electromagnetic interference—transmitted signals picked up both by circuitry (especially patient lead wires) and by the patient, which act like antennas; common sources include such high-power, high-frequency equipment as electrosurgical units and x-ray machines

HAZARDS OF ELECTRICITY

The hazards of electricity for the human body can be divided into four main categories:

- Ventricular fibrillation
- Respiratory arrest
- Thermal burns
- Electrolytic burns

All of these are due to unwanted electric current flowing through the body. In addition, there can be hazards due to the electrical distribution system and connected equipment:

- Fire and explosion
- Electrical distribution system failure
- Electrical equipment failure

Finally, a very broad category can be added to the list of hazards—misuse.

Electrical Hazards to Patients

The human body is predominantly composed of conductive electrolyte solutions enclosed in a skin of high resistance. The skin's resistance varies depending on its condition. Dry, intact skin has a resistance in the neighborhood of one megohm (1 MΩ). Moisture (e.g., perspiration) reduces resistance to around 15 kilohms (15kΩ). Electrode paste reduces skin resistance to about 1000 ohms (1kΩ) by a combination of electrolytic action and mechanical abrasion. If the skin's resistance is breached by needles or catheters, resistance drops to a few hundred ohms.

Macroshock is the term used for current applied at the body's surface. *Microshock* describes current applied directly to the heart, and an electrically susceptible patient is one with a direct, conductive path to the heart (e.g., pacing catheter, fluid-delivery catheter). The effect of electricity on the human body varies depending on a number of factors. These include the magnitude, density, and frequency of the current; its path through the body; the weight of the subject; the duration of exposure; and the variability of response between subjects.

Fig. 39-13 shows the approximate threshold levels of different effects when a 60 Hz, 1-3 second duration current of different magnitudes is applied to the hands of a 70-kg man.[3,4,6,8] The threshold of perception is the minimum current that a subject can feel. As the current increases, the effect increases from a tingling sensation to pain. Further increases cause muscular contractions that prevent the subject from releasing his/her grasp—the let-go current. Just above the range of currents that prevent releasing the grip is the range that causes sustained contraction of the respiratory muscles. If the current is removed

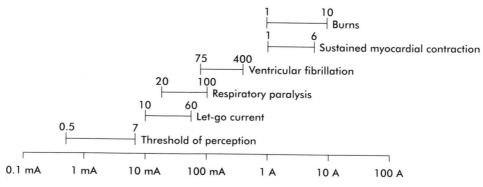

Fig. 39-13. Threshold ranges of different effects for 1- to 3-second application of 60 Hz current.

promptly, normal respiration resumes; if not, asphyxiation can result. Ventricular fibrillation occurs when a critical number of myocardial cells are excited by a current of sufficient magnitude. This condition is not reversed when the current is removed. However, if a current that causes sustained myocardial contraction is removed, normal cardiac activity resumes. This is a similar effect to defibrillation (the return of rhythmicity after an abrupt excitation and subsequent depolarization of a large portion of the myocardium). Skin burns occur at high currents due to heating of the high resistance of the skin (analogous to the heating of a high-resistance filament in a light bulb). High currents can cause muscle contractions so strong that tendons can tear away from bones. Nervous tissue, including the brain, ceases all activity when subjected to high currents. Of all these effects, ventricular fibrillation is the most dangerous to patients. For this reason, electrical safety in hospitals concentrates almost exclusively on preventing hazards that can cause ventricular fibrillation.

The path that the current takes through the body is important, because it is only the percentage of the total current that passes through the heart that has the potential for causing fibrillation.[6,8] For example, the two points of contact of the current source are on the same hand, there is little chance of fibrillation. A greater percentage of the current passes through the heart if it is applied between an arm and a leg rather than between both arms.

The longer the duration of the applied current, the less the magnitude of the current required to cause ventricular fibrillation.[4,5,8] There is a marked increase in the current required when the duration is reduced to less than 1 second. It can take 10 times as much current to cause fibrillation at 100 ms as it does at 1 s, but the current required at 5 second might be only about one half that required at 1 second.

The frequency of the applied current has an interesting effect on the susceptibility of the body.[4,13] The body is most susceptible to frequencies between 10 Hz and 1 kHz. The frequency at which the minimum current is required to induce fibrillation is in the 50 to 60 Hz range—the frequencies used for alternating current around the world. Below 10 Hz and above 1 kHz, the currents required to cause the same effects rise sharply. Studies of fibrillation thresholds have been conducted on dogs, pigs, sheep, and ponies. These have shown a direct relation between body weight and current, but the variability between subjects of the same weight is even greater.

There are two primary mechanisms for keeping equipment electrically safe: minimizing leakage current and grounding exposed conductive surfaces. Both are routinely tested as part of an electrical safety program, but there is no guarantee that either or both could not fail between equipment inspections.

Leakage current can increase because of degradation of insulation or because of a buildup of dust or other residue inside the instrument. Fault currents occur when something goes wrong—typically a short circuit to the device's chassis. If there is only a partial short, one in which the current that can flow to ground is limited, then the device continues to operate. This is likely when the fault is due to a failed component or a frayed wire, where only a few strands of wire might be touching the chassis. On the other hand, a direct short of the hot wire of the power cord to ground or neutral would cause the instrument's fuse or circuit breaker or the circuit breaker in the distribution system's branch circuit to open. The former is more likely, because the amperage rating of the instrument's fuse or breaker is much lower than the branch circuit's.

Grounding the chassis of an instrument shunts leakage current or fault current safely to earth ground and away from patients and personnel. Grounding can fail inside the instrument, the power cord, the electrical plug, or the electrical receptacle. As in the case of excessive leakage current or a partial short, if an instrument loses its ground connection, it will continue to operate.

There is no longer much likelihood that medical equipment with a two-wire power cord (i.e., ungrounded) will be in the patient's vicinity. However, it is possible for nonmedical equipment with a two-wire power cord to find its way to the bedside. The best example is entertainment equipment, such as a television, that can be brought in by visitors or supplied by well-meaning staff or volunteers.

Fig. 39-14 illustrates the protection normally provided by grounding. In the event of a fault to the chassis (1), the fault current is safely shunted to ground (arrowheads). If the ground continuity is broken at any point between the device and the circuit breaker box, the chassis of the device becomes electrically energized. Then if a patient contacts, or is connected to, the device (2) and a grounded surface (3), such as an electric hospital bed, then he/she becomes part of the circuit for the fault current (dashed line).

So far, this discussion of electrical hazards to patients has concentrated on macroshock—current applied to the surface of the body. **Electrically susceptible patients—those with a conductive path to the heart—are at risk for an additional hazard termed microschock.** When all of the hazard current passes through the heart, much lower levels can cause ventricular fibrillation. There is no unanimous agreement on the minimal level of microschock current that can cause ventricular fibrillation in humans, but 100 to

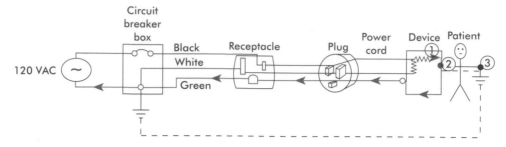

Fig. 39-14. Arrows indicate safe path for leakage or fault current. If ground continuity were broken, leakage or fault current would follow an alternate path, which includes the patient, indicated by the dashed line.

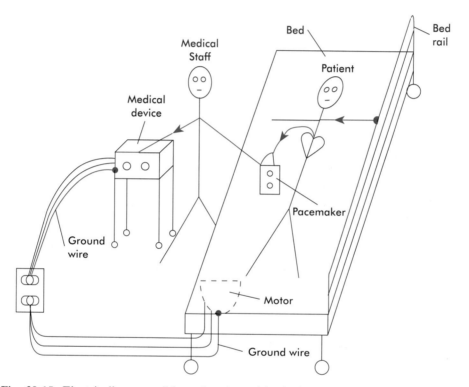

Fig. 39-15. Electrically susceptible patient is at risk of microshock if either the ground wire of the bed or the ground wire of the device is broken. (Arrows indicate current path through operator and patient.)

200 μA (microamps) is most commonly cited.[18-20,26,27] As little as 20 μA has caused fibrillation in a dog, using 60 Hz current, applied for 15 s through a 0.224 mm^2 contact area.[19]

Because the magnitude of the current that poses a microshock hazard is so small—roughly three orders of magnitude less than a macroshock hazard that can cause ventricular fibrillation—the problem of preventing it was originally more difficult. Temporary external pacemakers were AC-powered, and the catheters and connectors were not protected from casual contact. ECG monitors all had the right leg (RL) lead connected to chassis ground. Blood pressure transducers had metal cases that were also connected to ground. A variety of older equipment was still in use that had excessive leakage current and/or two-wire

power cords. There was a lack of appreciation for the importance of relatively small differences in electrical potential between grounds in the patient's environment. The importance of electrical safety programs was not acknowledged at all hospitals.

Very few accidental shocks or electrocutions in hospitals have ever been documented. Such incidents are rare; however, descriptions of hazards are accurate, because they have been found in hospitals. Although virtually all of these initial problems have been eliminated in modern hospitals, a brief review of the hazards is still worthwhile. It serves to reinforce the need for electrical safety programs, care in the design and selection of equipment, and the avoidance of practices that might be hazardous to electrically susceptible patients. Fig. 39-15 illustrates just one of

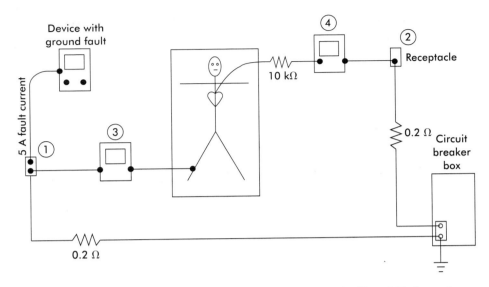

Fig. 39-16. A 5 A fault current raises the ground at receptacle *(1)* to 1 V above the ground at receptacle *(2)*. The patient is grounded via device *(3)* and has a fluid-filled cardiac catheter connected to device *(4)*. Up to 100 μA can flow through the patient's heart. (See text for analysis.)

many scenarios that would allow the leakage current of one device to flow through a patient's heart. If the ground wire of the bed were broken, the leakage current of the bed would flow through the bedrail, the patient's arm and heart, the pacing catheter, the nurse or doctor handling the catheter, and the grounded medical device. If the ground of the device were broken, the device's leakage current would follow the same path in the opposite direction.

Another, quite different scenario is presented in Fig. 39-16. In this figure, only the ground wiring of the power distribution system is drawn. There are two receptacles on separate branch circuits. A device with a ground fault, allowing a 5 A fault current, is connected to the receptacle *(1)*. Another device *(3)* grounds the patient via a RL connection (this might be an electrosurgical unit with a grounded return electrode). The patient also has a cardiac catheter with a relatively high resistance of 10 kΩ to ground. The resistance between the ground pins of each receptacle and the ground connection of the circuit breaker box is 0.2 Ω. The 5 A fault current through the 0.2 Ω ground resistance puts the ground of receptacle *(1)* at 1 V above the ground of receptacle *(2)*. This potential, across the 10 kΩ of the cardiac catheter (other resistances in the path, including the patient, are insignificant), allows 100 μA to flow through the patient's heart.

These types of events are now unlikely to occur, because reasonable, effective steps have been taken to prevent them. In particular, pacing catheters are protected from casual contact by the design of their connections and by precautions taken in their handling. Other catheters are typically effectively isolated

from ground. It is still possible that there can be broken ground wires or fault currents in equipment. However, they are less likely to occur, because of generally higher quality components and construction.

Thermal burns occur as a result of resistive heating of tissue. This type of heating is called joule heating. The amount of heat produced, in joules, is proportional to current, resistance, and time: $H = I^2RT$. The threshold current for causing burns depends on a number of factors. The smaller the contact area, the greater the current density and the greater the heating for a given current. From the equation for joule heating, it is clear that the longer the current is applied, the greater the heating. This is further affected by the ability of the tissue to dissipate heat. Well-vascularized tissue is able to carry away heat more effectively than poorly vascularized tissue. The higher the resistance of the tissue, the greater the heat production of a given current. Tissue resistance increases in this order: nerves, blood vessels, muscles, skin, tendons, fat, and bone. Although the joule heating of tissue is independent of frequency, the path that the current takes is not. This is because the impedance of different tissues varies at different frequencies. At DC and low AC frequencies, current distributes itself throughout the body. Skin tissue, however, exhibits a combination of high resistance and low capacitance. Therefore, at frequencies above 10 kHz, more current flows along the surface of the body (i.e., through the skin). This makes skin more susceptible to burns at radio-frequency currents from electrosurgical units, which operate from 500 kHz to 3 MHz.

DC causes burns at low potentials and currents due to electrolytic action. Saline in the body is converted to chlorine gas at the anode (positive) connection and sodium hydroxide and hydrogen at the cathode (negative) connection. Burns can occur at both connections but will be more severe at the cathode due to the caustic action of the sodium hydroxide.

Two points about electric shock hazards warrant emphasis. **The first is that leakage current is the significant hazard parameter, not voltage.** One reason for this is that it is current density that has the physiologic effect. The other reason is that the source impedance (the impedance "seen" when looking back into the leakage source) is usually much higher than the load (i.e., the patient). Thus there will be a relatively low current through the load, compared with the open circuit voltage (typically 120 VAC).

The second point is that there has historically been an overreaction to potential or theoretic electric shock hazards. This has, without a doubt, resulted in wasted resources. Time has been wasted hunting for escaping microamperes, and money has been wasted on multiple layers of redundant electrical safety hardware. There simply has not been enough of a real danger to justify these expenditures. Equipment and user performance problems, as will be described later, are more frequent and at least as serious. The overemphasis on electrical safety has detracted from attention to more important concerns, to the extent that some in-house equipment inspection programs only test safety and ignore performance measures.

Hazards of Electrical Distribution Systems and Equipment

Hazards with electrical distribution systems and equipment are generally more straightforward than the effects of electricity on patients. In spite of, or perhaps because of this, such hazards are more likely to occur. This section describes hazards associated with the use of electricity other than those which occur with the direct application of current to the body.

Historically, flammable anesthetics were the major explosion hazard. Now, nonflammable anesthetics are used almost exclusively, at least in the United States. **The risk of explosion in operating rooms has therefore been significantly reduced.** Other flammable liquids or aerosols may be used, however. These include some germicides and skin preparations. The use of such chemicals should be avoided. Finding a suitable substitute is probably easier than eliminating sources of ignition (e.g., electrical equipment, static electricity) or being sure to eliminate remnants of the liquid or its vapors.

Fire hazards are more difficult to avoid entirely than are explosion hazards. Fires can start under a much wider variety of circumstances. Electrical fires can start from the overheating of worn insulation, deteriorated components, excessive friction of moving parts, dirt or dust buildup on hot assemblies, and a variety of other possibilities. In the operating room the situation is exacerbated by the likelihood of increased oxygen or nitrous oxide concentrations, especially during head and neck surgery. Oxygen not only increases the intensity of a fire, but also reduces the temperature necessary for ignition. **New technologies can also introduce new fire hazards.** For example, lasers used for oropharyngeal procedures have ignited endotracheal tubes in patients' airways. The oxygen-enriched atmosphere produces a fearsome fire that is obviously life-threatening. Sloppy or thoughtless techniques are also a likely fire hazard (as well as being a surgical risk). Fires started by careless use of electrosurgical units continue to occur all too frequently.

Likewise, there are many ways that the electrical distribution system can fail. If there is a failure outside the hospital, the hospital should have an emergency alternate source of power. According to the National Fire Protection Association's standard, *Health Care Facilities* (NFPA 99),[17] hospitals must have an on-site generator, or generators, capable of powering what are defined as "essential electrical systems." This standard also has sections that provide detailed and specific requirements for wiring, distribution, circuit breakers, and grounding to reduce the potential for shocks, fires, and loss of power. This topic will be further discussed in the following section on standards. It should be obvious that, for the electrical system to be safe and dependable, it must be designed and installed properly. In addition, the electrical system must be inspected and tested periodically. This, too, will be described in detail in the section on standards of the National Fire Protection Association.

Many of the hazards attendant to the use of medical equipment have already been mentioned. Electric shock has been described in terms of its effects on the body, and it has been shown how a patient can be at risk for either macroshock or microshock. Operators can be equally at risk of macroshock—perhaps even more than patients—because they handle more equipment, more often, and under less controlled conditions. Operators have the additional hazard of a startle reaction to a shock that can lead to a secondary accident as they jerk or jump away. Defective equipment—in particular, improperly grounded equipment—poses a significant shock hazard.

Loss of power can immediately threaten a patient if equipment is sustaining his/her life. The best examples are undoubtedly heart-lung machines and ventilators. However, compressed gas can also be a power source. The loss of oxygen to an anesthesia machine or ventilator can be just as life-threatening as the loss of AC power. AC and compressed gas from a central source are fairly dependable and, at least with life support equipment, usually have some backup source. The same is not necessarily true for equipment that has a self-contained power source. External (temporary) pacemakers and portable ventilators are examples; the former depend on a battery and the latter on an oxygen cylinder. Equipment with a self-contained power source can be especially dangerous if power fails, because the patient might not be under direct observation by a clinician or might be in a location where adequate back-up support is not readily available (e.g., transport in an elevator).

A less common hazard is radio frequency (RF) interference. Some pieces of equipment generate RF signals that "escape" from their intended circuitry. The electrosurgical unit is the classic example. A powerful RF generator, such as an electrosurgical unit, can both conduct RF interference back through the power line and radiate it through the air, much like a radio transmitter. The former can be controlled by circuits called RF filters. The latter can be controlled by a combination of circuit design, physical layout, and shielding via the enclosure of subassemblies and the entire device. Devices can also be susceptible to RF interference. Devices with digital circuitry, including "micropocessor-controlled" devices, are particularly susceptible. Equipment that is susceptible to RF interference will also have RF filters built in to protect it. Unless properly designed, a characteristic of simple RF filters is to allow unacceptable leakage current to ground. Although modern medical equipment incorporates RF filters that do not have this flaw, older medical equipment (especially older physical therapy diathermy units) and many pieces of equipment not intended for medical applications have RF filters that cause high leakage current. An example of the latter is the personal computer. Often, an RF filter can be replaced with one designed for medical equipment. If not, a dedicated isolation transformer might have to be installed—a more expensive and cumbersome solution.

Fire and explosion hazards were described first, and separately, because they were a concern before the use of electrical equipment. These are still hazards that are not limited to electrical equipment. **Patients can also receive thermal injuries directly from equipment.** Sustained skin contact with a good thermal conductor at 42° to 44° C can burn the skin. As the temperature rises, the time required to burn falls rapidly. Hypo/hyperthermia machines, bloodwarmers, and infant radiant warmers are all devices intended to help maintain a patient's temperature. All of these should have safety (backup) thermostats but can overheat a patient if circuitry fails or if they are set improperly. The patient and the equipment should both be monitored. A malfunctioning heated humidifier in a ventilator circuit can burn a patient's airway or present a fire hazard. A patient can also be burned inadvertently by a laser or an electrosurgical unit. These are not theoretical hazards; they occur regularly in operating rooms as a result of even the slightest carelessness.

Moisture in equipment can reduce the insulating properties of wires, components, and printed circuit boards. This can easily lead to a malfunction, a shock hazard, or a fire. The most common cause of moisture getting into equipment is as a result of a container of liquid being placed "conveniently" on top and then being spilled or knocked over. Some equipment is built with holes or slots in the top to allow cooling. This is a poor design, usually compounded by having the top horizontal. It is much better to design equipment so that it does not need holes in the top and to have the top at any angle to prevent its use as a shelf.

Patients and staff can also suffer mechanical injury from equipment. A sharp corner or projection on a piece of equipment is almost a guarantee that someone will run into it. A top-heavy piece of equipment can fall onto a person as easily as onto the floor. A portable IV pole with small casters, a narrow wheel base, and two or three pumps clamped to the upper half is just waiting for a nudge. Overloaded or poorly installed shelves will eventually fail. Loose brackets or locking assemblies may lead to the collapse of a bed, operating room table, or wheelchair. What this should also point out is that, even if there is no human injury, the equipment will be damaged. This leads in turn to the damaged equipment not being available and a possibly expensive repair or early retirement.

Hazards of Misuse

Misuse of equipment is given many names that also indicate the breadth of this category: human or operator error, accidental activation, incorrect setting, confusing controls, misinterpreted displays, abuse, and so on. The types of hazards that can result from misuse are essentially the same as those previously described. It is all too easy, especially for a clinical engineer, to climb on a soapbox and preach about the sins of clinicians who do not have enough respect for medical equipment. It is much more useful to list steps to prevent misuse.

Anyone who operates medical equipment should read the operator's manual and understand the operating principles of the equipment, the function of all controls and displays, and any warnings. A copy of the manual should be available in a known, convenient location (with the equipment, if possible). An abbreviated instruction label on the instrument is often particularly useful. Operators should receive training; this might have to be repeated periodically, especially if they are only "occasional" users. New equipment should have undergone a careful selection process—ideally a comparative evaluation based on existing standards and an objective set of technical and clinical criteria. Trained technicians should periodically inspect and maintain the equipment. Malfunctioning or damaged equipment should be serviced promptly.

For the most critically important equipment, there should be plans or provisions for the eventuality of a failure. If there is sufficient justification, a backup unit is the best solution. There should be a long-range plan for how and when equipment should be considered for retirement and replacement. Criteria should include not only age and repair costs, but also functionality.

Above all is common sense. Psychologist Edward Titchener said, "Common sense is the very antipodes of science." This negative remark is obviously meant as sarcastic humor. More accurately, and more to the point, the physician Peter Latham said, "Common sense is, in medicine, the master workman."

STANDARDS

In a nation of rules, regulations, and recommendations, health care (including medical device manufacturers, hospitals, clinics, and other providers) is arguably the most regulated aspect of our society. The list of organizations that promulgate and/or enforce health care standards reads like a veritable alphabet soup of acronyms: FDA, NFPA, JCAHO, UL, ANSI, IEC, AAMI, ECRI, and so on. Their publications and pronouncements would overfill a good-sized bookcase. Keeping up-to-date and in compliance with their additions, editions, and updates can and does occupy the time of a significant number of health care employees. This section covers those organizations that have the most impact on the use of medical equipment. It describes the various groups, their standards, and the differences between their standards.

National Fire Protection Association (NFPA)
The NFPA is a nonprofit organization that produces scores of different fire safety–related codes and standards. Interestingly, none of them carry the force of law unless they are adopted by a state or local governing body. The two of most import to electrical safety in hospitals are the *National Electrical Code*[16] (NFPA 70), commonly known as the NEC, and *Health Care Facilities* (NFPA 99).[17] As with all NFPA

standards, these codes are under virtually constant review. Revisions appear, on the average, every 3 years. "Article 517" in the NEC pertains to electrical construction and installation in health care facilities. In its seven parts, it prescribes design, installation, and performance criteria of electrical distribution systems for general care, intensive care, and anesthetizing locations (including use of flammable and nonflammable anesthetics); electrical supplies for x-ray equipment; and low-voltage systems for communications, data, fire alarms, and so on. Two of the parts cover applications that are particularly unique to hospitals. **Emergency electrical power systems must provide continuous electrical service to specified areas of the hospital in the event of a disruption of normal electrical service. Isolated-power systems are required only in areas designated as hazardous anesthetizing locations (i.e., areas in which flammable anesthetics are used or stored).**

Health Care Facilities combines what used to be 12 separate standards. Its companion, *Health Care Facilities Handbook,*[12] provides guidance and commentary on the standard. This standard addresses fire, explosion, and electrical hazards in health care facilities. It covers performance, use, and maintenance of the physical facilities and equipment as they relate to hazards. Chapters 3 through 11 cover requirements categorized by systems or equipment (e.g., electrical, medical gas, and vacuum systems). Chapters 12 through 18 relate these requirements to different types of health care facilities (e.g., hospitals, medical and dental offices, and nursing homes). Chapter 12 is entitled "Hospital Requirements." Most of this chapter deals specifically with anesthetizing locations. **The requirements on anesthetizing locations are intended to protect against fire, explosion, shock, or mechanical injury hazards associated with the use of inhalation anesthetics.** Some very important changes have occurred in this section over the past few years. In particular, isolated power is no longer required "in facilities that have a written policy prohibiting the use of flammable inhalation anesthetizing agents." Although it is recognized that flammable anesthetics are probably not used in U.S. hospitals, the sections that pertain to flammable anesthetics have been retained. The rationale stated in the *Handbook* is that flammable anesthetics may be in use elsewhere in the world and that those areas may use NFPA standards for guidance in fire safety. In fact, over half of Chapter 12 deals with requirements that pertain only to flammable anesthetizing locations and therefore can be ignored by hospitals that do not use flammable anesthetics. Of importance to hospitals, Chapter 12 has several requirements that cover electrical and gas and vacuum systems and equipment. Chapter 12, like all of the chapters dealing with different types of facilities, refers to the earlier chapters on systems and equipment. Although this eliminates constant repetition of material, it requires constant leafing back and forth within the standard. This is exacerbated because, within the chapters on systems and equipment, there are further references to separate standards (e.g., the *National Electrical Code* and the *Life Safety Code*. The following discussion is limited to some of the more unique and important parts of the standard.

The electrical distribution system includes power to areas and functions for which there must be an alternate source of power in the event of disruption of the normal supply. The essential electrical system includes the alternate power sources, the distribution systems, and the areas and equipment that cannot safely be without power. The essential electrical system is divided into the emergency system and the equipment system. The emergency system must have power restored within 10 seconds. It includes the life safety branch, which provides power for lighting corridors and exits, alarm and communication systems, and lighting for the emergency generator and elevators. The emergency system also includes the critical branch for power to lighting, fixed equipment, and selected receptacles and power circuits in patient care areas. The equipment system includes service to primarily high-power (three-phase) equipment. Some equipment, such as central suction and compressed air, is to be automatically connected after a time delay to prevent overloading the generator. Other equipment—such as heating and ventilating systems, and elevators—can be connected either manually or automatically after a time delay. The alternate power source is to be tested under load at least once a month.

The electrical distribution system in patient care areas is to be tested according to criteria listed. Grounding voltage and impedance are to be tested in new construction before it is accepted and in existing construction whenever it has been altered (annual inspections are recommended). For new construction, the grounding voltage limit is 20 mV and the grounding impedance limit is 0.1 Ω. For existing construction, 500 mV is allowed in general care areas and 40 mV in critical care areas, although it is recommended that voltages over 20 mV be investigated. The impedance limit is 0.2 Ω. Receptacles are to be tested annually in general care areas and semiannually in critical care areas (unless longer intervals can be justified by performance history). Testing includes physical integrity, grounding, hot and neutral wiring polarity, and ground retention force (115 g).

Electrical equipment in hospitals includes both fixed and portable, patient care and non–patient care equipment. Of these, portable patient care equipment deserves the most attention. It is to be tested at least annually in general care areas and semiannually in critical care areas, unless the hospital can justify longer periods based on inspection history. Testing includes—and should be in the order of—physical inspection, grounding, and leakage current. Equipment should have an appropriate plug, power cord, and strain relief at the chassis. Ground resistance from chassis to ground pin should be less than 0.5 Ω, although double-insulated equipment is allowed to have a two-wire (ungrounded) power cord and plug. Ungrounded leakage current, with the unit on or off and with correct power line wiring polarity, is limited to 100 μA. Limits of 250 μA or 500 μA are allowed if specific, more stringent inspection criteria are employed to guarantee grounding integrity. Also, leakage current is measured as the RMS value from DC to 1 kHz. Leakage current limits increase to 10 mA proportional to frequency, for frequencies up to 100 kHz. If equipment is connected together such that one power cord supplies power to all pieces, leakage current is measured from the main power cord. Leakage current to ground of patients' leads is limited to 100 μA and 50 μA between leads for nonisolated input equipment, tested with power on, ground wire open and closed. The limits (to ground and between leads) for isolated input equipment are 10 μA with the ground closed and 50 μA with the ground open. In addition, isolated input equipment is tested with line voltage applied to each lead. Leakage current to ground is limited to 20 μA. Leakage current of non–patient care equipment used in patient care areas, such as housekeeping and maintenance items, is limited to 500 μA.

There are additional restrictions for equipment in anesthetizing locations. There is to be a storage device (e.g., cord wrap hooks) for the power cord of portable equipment to prevent damage during storage. Switches are not allowed in the power cord, except for splash-proof foot switches. Equipment is to be plugged into a fixed receptacle (i.e, not an extension cord). Allowable exceptions to this requirement are multiple-outlet strips permanently attached to a rack, table, or pedestal, and overhead (ceiling-drop) receptacles supplied by a flexible cord.

There are also some important administrative requirements. Only isolated input equipment is allowed to be connected to conductive catheters or pacemaker leads connected to a patient's heart. Equipment purchase orders are to require manuals that include operating, testing, and maintenance instructions. There is to be a scheduled inspection and preventive maintenance program. Electrical equipment for use with oxygen delivery equipment is to be listed for such use.

The hazards with centrally piped medical gas and vacuum systems include gases that intensify combustion (e.g., oxygen and nitrous oxide) being piped

throughout the hospital, gas cylinder storage, pipe leaks, cross-connection of gases, and poor performance or failure of the system. Most of these hazards can be avoided by proper design and installation of medical gas and vacuum systems. Almost all of the medical gas and vacuum requirements in NFPA 99 apply only to new installations, and all apply exclusively to centrally piped systems.

Alarms and pressure gauges must be located such that they are always under observation. In addition, there must be a local pressure alarm in critical care areas. Shutoff valves are to be installed at the main supply line and at each riser from the main supply line. Each branch must have a shutoff valve, followed by a pressure gauge, on the same floor that the branch serves. In critical care areas, this valve must be immediately outside each such area. In particular, each operating room must have shutoff valves for each gas outside the main door. Gas and vacuum outlets must be properly labelled and not allow connection of different gases. Either threaded or "quick-connect" (push-in) connectors are allowed, but threaded connections must comply with the Diameter-Index Safety System of the Compressed Gas Association.[17] There must be scheduled inspections and preventive maintenance. Alarms should be checked annually. Shutoff valves should be checked for external leaks, and outlets should be checked for leaks and flow. A new requirement is that hospitals must have a plan to respond to the failure of any medical gas system and the ability to implement it. While nonflammable waste anesthetic gases are allowed to be disposed of via the medical vacuum system, it is not recommended because of possible performance degradation.

Analogous to electrical hazards with electrical equipment, there are hazards associated with the gases used with medical gas equipment. In particular, care must be taken with oxygen and nitrous oxide, which are used with anesthesia equipment and (oxygen only) with respiratory therapy equipment. For example, after servicing components of the gas supply, it is necessary to test oxygen flowmeters and the oxygen flush valve to confirm that only oxygen is delivered. As with electrical equipment, gas equipment must have a scheduled inspection and preventive maintenance program.

Joint Commission on Accreditation of Healthcare Organizations (JCAHO)

JCAHO (formerly Joint Commission on Accreditation of Hospitals, or JCAH) is another private, nonprofit organization. It was formed in 1951 to improve the quality of health care to the public. JCAHO develops standards of quality in collaboration with health professionals and others. They publish and annually revise the *Accreditation Manual for Hospitals* (AMH).[10] Compliance with the requirements of the AMH is, in principle, voluntary. In practice, however, compliance is considered virtually mandatory. Medicare/Medicaid, many state health departments, and various other licensure organizations accept or require JCAHO accreditation as part of their own requirements.

The AMH has two dozen chapters, describing standards according to specialty, (e.g., diagnostic radiology, medical records, and nursing service). Of particular interest to anesthesiologists are the chapters on special care units and on surgical and anesthesia services. Of direct applicability to equipment safety is the chapter entitled "Plant, Technology, and Safety Management" (PTSM). Starting in 1985 the JCAHO initiated a process to convert the PTSM from a set of very specific standards to, in their words, "continuous quality improvement." Information gathered as a result of applying the PTSM standards is to be used to provide feedback on the performance of the institution and the results of changes made. This chapter has four sections, covering the management of safety, life safety, equipment, and utilities.

Hospitals are required to have a safety management program that includes accident reporting, training and education, and program evaluation. There must be a qualified safety officer responsible for the program and a safety committee that addresses safety management issues. Safety education is to be provided in orientation and continuing education. There must be hazardous materials and emergency preparedness programs.

The life safety management standard requires that hospitals comply with the current edition of the NFPA's *Life Safety Code,* NFPA 101. NFPA 101, and therefore this standard, addresses the fire safety of the building and staff education.

An equipment management program that identifies and controls hazards of medical and other electrical equipment is required. Equipment must be inventoried and receive scheduled inspections at least annually according to documented test procedures. Personnel who use or maintain equipment are to receive orientation and annual continuing education, unless there is documented evidence that no changes or hazards have occurred. Equipment problems are to be identified, evaluated, and remedied, and the actions evaluated.

The utility systems of a hospital include the following: electrical distribution and emergency power; elevators; heating, ventilating and air conditioning; plumbing; medical gases and vacuum; and data and communications. The utilities management program must reliably maintain these utilities and be prepared to handle any failures of such. As with the equipment management program, there must be an inventory, maintenance and training programs and proper handling of problems.

Food and Drug Administration (FDA)

Government regulation of medical devices is the responsibility of the FDA. Within the FDA, this falls to the Center for Devices and Radiological Health (CDRH).[24] The first federal law to protect the public from adulterated or misbranded food and drugs was The Food and Drugs Act, passed in 1906. In 1938 a new law—The Federal Food, Drug, and Cosmetic Act—established the FDA and expanded the authority to regulate food, drugs, and cosmetics. In 1976 the Medical Device Amendments established both the Bureau of Medical Devices and the Bureau of Radiological Health. (In 1982 the FDA combined these two bureaus into the CDRH.) The 1976 Amendments gave the FDA specific authority for the regulation of medical devices. Before this, the FDA's ability to regulate medical devices was severely hampered because they had to work within regulations intended for drugs. The 1976 Amendments differentiated medical devices from drugs by defining that the latter group works primarily through chemical action, whereas the former does not.

The 1976 Amendments also established a classification system for medical devices. Class I ("General Controls") devices require minimal regulation; they do not require performance standards or premarket approval. General controls require that manufacturers register annually with the FDA, follow published Good Manufacturing Practices (GMP) for establishing and documenting quality assurance practices, and comply with other labelling and documentation requirements of the Medical Device Amendments. Class II (" Performance Standards") devices must meet FDA-established standards that address safety and effectiveness. To date, however, the FDA has not adopted any standards for specific devices; the GMP is the only FDA device standard thus far. (Voluntary standards have been established by other organizations, and manufacturers almost invariably comply with them.) Examples of Class II devices include ventilators, monitors, and infant incubators. Class III ("Premarket Approval") devices must be demonstrated as safe and effective, typically via clinical testing. They include life support and implantable devices and devices that have a "potential unreasonable risk of illness or injury." Examples include implantable pacemakers, heart valves, and infant radiant warmers.

To market a new device, a manufacturer must submit a Premarket Notification, commonly called a "510(k)," referring to the section in the 1976 law. If the FDA determines that the new device is "substantially equivalent" to a device that was on the market before the enactment of the Medical Device Amendments (May 28, 1976), the device can be marketed. If not, the device is placed in Class III, unless the manufacturer successfully petitions the FDA for Class I or Class II classification. When a manufacturer or researcher wants to test a new device on human subjects, an Investigational Device Exemption (IDE) must be filed with the FDA. A major provision of the IDE is review by an institution's Institutional Review Board (IRB). The IRB ensures that patients' rights and safety are protected.

The 1976 Amendments established the Device Experience Network (DEN). The DEN collects data from voluntary reports of equipment problems by users (Problem Reporting Program [PRP]), Mandatory Device Reports (MDR) by manufacturers of equipment problems reported to them, and device recalls by manufacturers. The U.S. Pharmocopeia (USP, 1-800-638-6725) is under contract to the FDA to operate the PRP.

Congress became dissatisfied by the level of voluntary problem reporting by users. As a consequence, the Safe Medical Devices Act of 1990 (SMDA) was signed into law on November 28, 1990. **Effective November 28, 1991, users are required by law to report to manufacturers if a device contributed to a patient's or staff member's serious injury or illness.** If a device contributed to a death, the user must report to both the manufacturer and the FDA. Users include virtually all medical facilities except physicians' offices. Device is very broadly defined as an apparatus used to diagnose or treat a disease or function of the body. Reports must be submitted within 2 weeks of the time that the user became aware of the incident. A serious illness or injury is one that is life-threatening, results in permanent impairment, or requires immediate intervention to prevent permanent impairment. This law represents the first time that the FDA has directly regulated users of medical equipment. The user-reporting requirements of the SMDA are only 1 of the 18 parts of this law. The other sections all pertain to new or expanded regulations for manufacturers, including more authority for the FDA to require recalls of products.[21]

Underwriters Laboratories (UL)

The UL is an independent, nonprofit organization that develops safety standards. It tests materials, devices, and systems against these standards and "lists" (approves) products that meet the standards. **The UL is probably the most widely recognized safety testing organization in the country.** It was founded in 1894 as a result of fire insurance companies' (underwriters') concerns for the number of electrical fires occurring at the 1893 Columbian Exposition in

Chicago. Manufacturers seek UL listing to verify the safety of their products and, in many cases, to reduce their product liability insurance costs. In addition, some areas of the country *require* UL listing of products (e.g., Chicago, Oregon, and North Carolina).[23]

The UL standard for electrical medical equipment is UL 544, *Standard for Medical and Dental Equipment*.[22] Its various sections address construction, hazards to patients and users, electrical performance characteristics (including grounding impedance and leakage current), and labelling requirements. Grounding impedance is measured with a 6 V, 25 A, 60 Hz test current and is to be no more than 0.2 Ω from any exposed conductive surface to the ground pin of the power plug.

Leakage current is measured with the device in all combinations of power on and off, grounded and ungrounded (ground open), and power conductors (hot and neutral wires) connected normally and with reversed polarity. The AC values of leakage current are for leakage current frequencies up to 1 kHz. For frequencies up to 100 kHz, these AC values are multiplied by the frequency in kHz (e.g., 100 μA at 60 Hz becomes 10 mA at 100 kHz). This adjustment can be approximated by measuring leakage current through a test load (impedance) composed of a 1000 Ω resistor shunted by (i.e., in parallel with) a 0.15 μF capacitor and 10.2 Ω resistor in series (Fig. 39-17).

For patient care equipment, leakage current from chassis to ground cannot exceed 100 μA AC or 140 μA DC. This may be as high as 500 μA if the equipment incorporates a device that opens the power connection if ground continuity is lost. Leakage current from any patient connection to ground for nonisolated input equipment cannot exceed 50 μA AC or 70 μA DC. For isolated input equipment, these values are 10 μA AC and 14 μA DC. Isolated input connections are also tested by applying 120 V at 60 Hz between each lead and ground; the leakage current limit is 20 μA when measured at the patient end of a patient cable or 10 μA at the cable input connector. Non–patient care equipment leakage current from chassis to ground is limited to 500 μA AC and 700 μA DC.

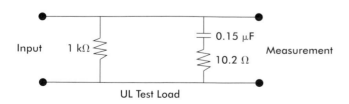

Fig. 39-17. Underwriters Laboratories (UL) test load.

Association for the Advancement of Medical Instrumentation (AAMI)

The AAMI is a private, nonprofit, professional membership organization. Members include engineers, technicians, physicians, nurses, and administrators. Membership categories include individual, institutional, and manufacturer. **One of the primary activities of AAMI is the writing of voluntary standards for medical devices. These standards are unique in that they cover more than safety; they also cover performance.** To date, the AAMI has published 19 standards and a number of "recommended practices" and "technical information reports." Their standards include *Electrosurgical Devices, Diagnostic Electrocardiographic Devices, Electronic or Automated Sphygmomanometers,* and *Cardiac Defibrillator Devices.*[1] Their standards are developed by a consensus process, in which manufacturers, users, researchers, consultants, and the FDA typically participate. All AAMI standards are submitted to the American National Standards Institute (see p. 737) for approval as a national standard. In addition, AAMI represents ANSI in the development of international standards for medical equipment with the IEC and ISO (see p. 737). It is the intention of the U.S. medical device standards writing organizations—including FDA, ANSI, and AAMI—to adopt IEC standards if at all possible, or to adapt them with minimal changes if not.

AAMI's electrical safety standard is ES1, *American National Standard, Safe Current Limits for Electromedical Apparatus.*[1] It specifies four classes of medical equipment: isolated patient connection, nonisolated patient connection, likely to contact patient (but no patient connection), and no-patient-contact. This standard does not include a specification for grounding impedance; it was not considered important enough. Leakage current is measured with every combination of power on and off, ground open and intact, and power line polarity normal and reversed. The leakage current limits are for frequencies from DC to 1 kHz. From 1 kHz to 100 kHz, the limit increases proportionately to the frequency (i.e., at 100 kHz, the limit is 100 times the 1 kHz limit). Above 100 kHz, the limit remains constant. This frequency response can be approximated with a test load. The AAMI test load was changed (it was originally similar to the load still used by UL) to resolve a problem when measuring high-frequency, low–source-impedance, leakage current (Fig. 39-18).

The chassis to ground leakage current limit is 100 μA for all four classes, except non-patient-contact equipment when the ground is open. Then 500 μA is allowed. Leakage current from any patient contact to ground cannot exceed 10 μA for isolated patient connection equipment and 50 μA for nonisolated patient connection equipment. With 120 V, 60 Hz applied to the input of isolated patient connection equipment, the leakage current limit is 10 μA; applied to the patient end of a patient cable, the limit is 20 μA. As the U.S. representative for IEC and ISO medical device standards, AAMI typically considers harmonizing U.S. and international versions of standards. However, AAMI has recently defeated an attempt, led by U.S. medical device manufacturers, to increase these leakage current limits to the IEC values (see Table 39-1).

American National Standards Institute (ANSI)

ANSI is a private, nonprofit organization that coordinates most other U.S. organizations that promulgate standards, including NFPA, AAMI, and ASTM. It administers voluntary consensus standards for virtually every type of product. These standards do not carry the force of law unless they are adopted and enforced by some other agency. ANSI is also the official U.S. representative to the IEC and ISO (see below). Within ANSI, the Medical Device Standards Board coordinates standards approved specifically for medical equipment.

ASTM (formerly American Society for Testing and Materials)

ASTM is also a private, nonprofit, organization that promulgates standards. It was founded in 1898 and currently has approximately 134 committees that write standards for materials, products, systems, and services. The F4 Committee writes standards for medical and surgical materials and devices, the F29 Committee for anesthesia and respiratory therapy equipment, and the F30 Committee for emergency medical devices. Of ASTM's 68 volumes of standards, Volume 13.01, *Medical Devices,* contains the ASTM standards for medical equipment, materials and supplies, and services. Examples include tracheal tubes, pediatric trauma facilities, and fixation pins and wires.

International Standards

International standards are assuming increasing importance because of the impending European Economic Community (EEC). A major provision of the EEC is the adoption of standards that will replace individual national standards of member countries. For any manufacturer to be able to market equipment in the EEC, it will have to comply with these standards. This is important to manufacturers because the EEC represent a very large market—second only to the United States.

The International Electrotechnical Commission (IEC) writes standards for electrical devices, and the International Organization for Standardization (ISO) writes standards for everything else. The IEC Technical Committee No. 62, which is responsible for standards on electrical equipment, publishes *IEC 601-1 Medical Electrical Equipment.* Part I, "The General Requirements for Safety," is the starting point for all IEC medical equipment standards. Part II requirements supplement (and amend as necessary) the general requirements to cover the characteristics of specific types of equipment. There are currently about 20 Part II requirements. Roughly one third of these standards cover x-ray and other ionizing radiation devices. They also have standards for such other devices as electrosurgical units, defibrillators, ventilators, and anesthesia machines. Like the AAMI standards, the IEC Particular Requirements cover safety and performance.

IEC 601-1 is much more difficult to read and use than any of the standards considered thus far. This seems particularly inappropriate because (1) this standard covers only the initial "general" requirements and (2) it is an "international" standard, intended for use by anyone and everyone. At the very least, an attempt should have been made to simplify the language. It also seems reasonable that the number and complexity of tests could be reduced without sacrificing safety.

There are dozens of definitions of terms in the section on "Terminology and Definitions." The majority of these defined terms seem redundant; other standards use descriptive terms that need no further definition. Some of the terms pertaining to electrical safety include the following:

Equipment classifications:
  - Class I—grounded
  - Class II—double-insulated
  - Within either class:
    Type B—defined by allowable level of leakage current
    Type BF—type B equipment with F-type patient connection
    Type CF—lower allowable leakage current than type B, with F-type patient connection
    F-type applied part—isolated patient connection

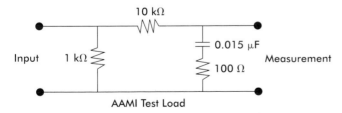

Fig. 39-18. Association for the Advancement of Medical Instrumentation (AAMI) test load.

Leakage currents:
- Earth—current in ground wire
- Enclosure—current from device enclosure to ground (i.e., measured through separate test lead)
- Patient—unintentional current from patient connection through patient to ground

Single-fault conditions:
- Loss of ground continuity
- Interruption of either power connection
- Voltage applied to an F-type applied part
- Voltage applied to signal or output connector
- And so forth

The upper limit on ground impedance between conductive surfaces of a device and the ground pin of its plug is 0.2 Ω. Leakage currents are measured under normal conditions and specified single-fault conditions with equipment on in all operating modes. The upper limits for leakage current pertain for frequencies up to 1 kHz. For frequencies between 1 kHz and 100 kHz, these values are multiplied by the frequency in kHz, to an upper limit of 10 mA. As with the UL and AAMI standards, a test load is suggested for measuring leakage current (Fig. 39-19).

The standard has a matrix of earth, enclosure, and patient leakage current limits vs. equipment types under normal and single-fault conditions. Earth leakage current (i.e., through the ground wire) is limited to 500 μA under normal conditions, 1 mA

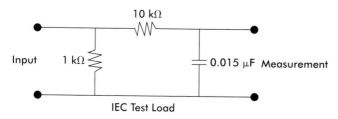

Fig. 39-19. International Electrotechnical Commission (IEC) test load.

under single-fault conditions, for equipment types B, BF, and CF. The enclosure leakage current (i.e., from exposed conductive surfaces) limit is 100 μA under normal conditions and 500 μA under single-fault conditions for all three equipment types. The patient leakage current (i.e., from patient connections) limit is 100 μA under normal conditions and 500 μA under single-fault conditions for equipment types B and BF. For type CF, these limits are 10 μA and 50 μA, respectively. With line voltage applied to an F-type applied part (i.e., isolated input patient connection), patient leakage current is limited to 50 μA for type CF equipment.

An interesting point about these leakage current limits is the difference between earth and enclosure leakage currents. If the impedance from the ground pin to the enclosure may not exceed 0.2 Ω, how can there be any difference in leakage current from these two locations? No other leakage current standard differentiates between leakage current through the ground wire and from the enclosure. The leakage current limits in the NFPA, UL, and AAMI standards are very similar, as are the equipment classification and test procedures. Not so with IEC 601-1; it has more classifications, more tests (only a few of which were described previously), and higher leakage current limits. Recently, an attempt to change the AAMI leakage current limits (the original and most widely recognized electrical standard in the United States; it is also the ANSI standard) to the same as the IEC values was defeated. The arguments in favor of changing were that this would create a world standard, would prevent possible retaliatory restriction of U.S.-made devices in countries where manufacturers designed to IEC 601-1 standards but did not meet AAMI ES1, and would allow all manufacturers to save costs by designing to less strict standards. A comparison of the grounding and leakage current specifications in AAMI, NFPA, UL, and IEC electrical safety standards for medical equipment appears in Table 39-1.

Table 39-1 Comparison of electrical safety standards, patient care equipment, ungrounded				
Specification	AAMI ES1	NFPA 99	UL 544	IEC 601-1
Ground impedance, plug to chassis	na	0.5 Ω	0.2 Ω	0.2 Ω
Leakage current, chassis to ground	100 μA	100 μA	100 μA AC 140 μA DC	500 μA
Leakage current, nonisolated patient connection	50 μA	100 μA	50 μA AC 70 μA DC	500 μA
Leakage current, isolated patient connection	10 μA	50 μA	10 μA AC 14 μA DC	50 μA
Leakage current, line voltage applied to isolated patient connection	20 μA	20 μA	20 μA	50 μA

ECRI (formerly Emergency Care Research Institute)

Since 1968, ECRI has been studying the safety and performance of medical equipment. **ECRI is a private, nonprofit organization that is the medical equipment analog of Consumers Union.** Their primary publication, *Health Devices,* publishes comparative evaluations of equipment and disposables and analysis and advice on technology and management issues relevant to health care. Although they do not publish standards per se, they do develop tests and performance criteria for the devices that they evaluate and for recommended inspection procedures. For years, their publication of these criteria and their direct involvement and interaction with organizations that promulgate standards have had a major impact on medical device standards.

SAFE USE OF EQUIPMENT
Hazards: A Reality Check

The hazards of medical equipment have been described in the previous sections of this chapter. These hazards all still exist, and new wrinkles on old types of problems continuously appear as new technologies are introduced. **However, the frequency of equipment-related hazards is reduced with understanding and experience. In addition, as more hospitals obtain the assistance of sophisticated clinical engineering departments, risk management and quality assurance functions improve. In fact, the current interest extends beyond risk management and quality control to quality improvement.**

The first reported instance of a fatal electric shock due to a medical device appeared in *Lancet,* April 16, 1960.[14] A patient died on the operating table when he was connected to a faulty cardiac monitor. Descriptions of electrical hazards in hospitals were published throughout the 1960s. Carl Walter, in 1970, claimed that 1200 patients were being electrocuted in U.S. hospitals per year.[25] This figure gained widespread notoriety when Ralph Nader repeated it in *Ladies Home Journal* in 1971.[15] This figure was never documented, however. Nevertheless, it led to a period of great, if often misplaced, activity that ultimately resulted in an understanding and appreciation of electrical safety. **The design and construction of modern medical equipment in combination with the practices employed in electrical safety programs have almost eliminated electrical shock incidents.** Although electrical safety concerns should not be ignored, perhaps their most important contribution is that now engineers and technicians have regular opportunities to test medical equipment. **The most important aspect of equipment inspections is performance testing.**

Fires and resulting burn injuries due to anesthetic gases have been eliminated because flammable anesthetic gases are no longer used in the United States. However, fires and burns still occur as a result of the use of electrosurgical units and lasers. Precautions are therefore still necessary. It is important to keep sources of fuel, oxidizing gas, and ignition separated. Most of the time, common sense and reasonable caution suffice to prevent fires. Additional precautions are necessary, in particular, for head and neck surgery. Basically, these precautions involve using nonflammable materials when possible, preventing the buildup of higher concentrations of oxidizing gases, and knowing where electrosurgical sparks or lasers are directed.

Burns also occur as a direct result of electrosurgical currents. Unintended burns may result from carelessness or improper technique with either the active or the return electrode. The active electrode should never be left on the patient when not in use. Inadvertent activation of the electrosurgical unit can cause a spark or current through layers of surgical drapes. Some electrosurgical units allow connection of more than one active electrode and may not always provide a means for selective activation. It becomes especially important that one active electrode not be lying on the patient when the other is activated, because current will be available from both. Burns at the site of the return electrode occur when there is inadequate electrical contact with the site, which may result if the electrode's conductive gel dries out. Gel can dry out in the package, if left open too long before application, or even during a particularly long surgical procedure. (Some return electrodes do not use electrode gel. They use either a conductive adhesive or capacitive coupling to the skin.) Another problem with elecrical contact occurs if not enough of the electrode is in contact with the skin. The entire surface must be firmly pressed to the skin. Bony areas should be avoided, because they make it difficult to maintain good contact. In addition, wrinkled electrodes, or "tenting" of the electrode over the skin, must be prevented. Poor electrical contact results in higher current densities, which can be sufficient to cause burns.

It is also possible to have burns occur at alternate sites. Contact with other conductive surfaces, such as ECG electrodes or the operating table, can cause the electrosurgical current to divide between return paths. This contact can be resistive or capacitive. At the frequencies used by electrosurgical units, capacitive coupling can occur with surfaces that would not appreciably conduct lower frequency currents. Two approaches are taken to avoid this. One is to always place the return electrode as close to the surgical site as possible. The other is, via the design of the electrosurgical unit, to ensure that all of the output current is returned to the electrosurgical unit through the return electrode. This can be accomplished by using an isolated output (analogous to isolated-power distribution systems) that does not allow current to return through alternate paths. Another technique is to compare the output current with the return current. If they are not the same, the electrosurgical unit deactivates the output and alarms (audible and visible).

It may be difficult to identify all contributing factors to a burn or burnlike injury. There are often multiple factors, any one of which by itself would not have caused an injury. Thermal burns can be due to direct contact or irradiant heat. Hyperthermia units can cause the former, and radiant warmers or high-intensity lights the latter. Ischemia due to pressure or surgery can exacerbate the problem, because circulating blood is an effective means for dissipating heat. Mechanical injuries can appear to be burns. Shearing forces—which result from changing the position of the operating table—can cause mechanical injury. Chemical burns can result from the application of some skin preparation agents (e.g., acetone, alcohol, iodine, or merthiolate). Injury is more likely if the agent is in constant contact with the skin and if heat or pressure is applied. Ethylene oxide, if not completely aerated from an anesthesia mask or hyperthermia blanket, may cause skin injury, especially if the skin is moist. Electrical burns can result from the unintended flow of electrical current. Not only electrosurgical units, but virtually any device that has an electrical output, can cause a burn if the current density is allowed to get too high. For example, muscle stimulators for testing the depth of anesthesia have caused burns when used with inappropriate electrodes.

Outright failure of medical equipment accounts for only a small percentage of patient injuries. Generally, a complete failure is obvious, and the real problem is the lack of availability of the device. **A more insidious problem occurs if the device is inaccurate.** This can lead to inappropriate treatment, either directly due to an incorrect output (e.g., defibrillator) or indirectly due to an inaccurate measurement (e.g., pressure monitor).

Although there are not many device-related patient injuries, more occur because of human error than device failure. This is probably because when a device fails an operator is likely to discover it. However, when the operator errs it may well go unnoticed. Operator error can take the form of misinterpretation, oversight, or misapplication. Any of these can be due, at least in part, to the design of equipment. Confusing or ambiguous controls and indicators increase the opportunities for mistakes. In addition, human error is likely to occur if operators do not receive adequate training or if a variety of models of

equipment are used interchangeably for the same applications.

Aspects of Equipment Safety

There are numerous aspects of equipment safety. Attention must be given to all of these aspects to provide the proper measure of safety. There are two broad categories to be considered: care of the equipment and care of the users.

Care of equipment requires conscientious application of engineering and management principles. Care of equipment also requires care of physical facilities; the former cannot work properly unless the latter also work properly. To provide this care, both clinical and plant engineering departments not only have to do their own jobs, they have to cooperate.

The clinical engineering department typically has responsibility for most electronic and pneumatic equipment that has a role in patient care. **The major functions of clinical engineering departments are inspections, repairs, and user assistance.** Every clinical engineering department should be providing these services. Biomedical equipment technicians are specially and specifically trained to provide these services. Appropriate education is either via a 2-year associates degree program or via special programs given by the armed services. Ongoing education, especially from manufacturers' service schools, maintains and updates their education.

Equipment inspections and preventive maintenance need to be done according to appropriate schedules and procedures. Developing the schedule depends on judgment and experience. Consideration is given to the likelihood of problems occurring, the seriousness of the consequences, and the manufacturer's specifications and recommendations. The procedures are developed from a combination of the manufacturer's procedures in the service manual, independently published standards and guidelines, and practical experience. Inspection procedures need to include safety (mechanical and electrical) and performance tests. In fact, the latter should be considered more important. Performance failures may or may not be more serious than are safety failures, but they are far more likely to occur. A successful inspection depends on two other things as well: appropriate test equipment and cooperative equipment users. The former is obvious; the latter too often is not. To locate equipment and ensure its availability, biomedical equipment technicians must have help from equipment users. Finally, the inspection program must be documented, including the schedule, procedures, and results.

To the uninitiated, medical equipment repair may seem to be an arcane art. Unfortunately, others seem to believe that repairs are trivial and may become unreasonably impatient when they are inconvenienced while waiting for equipment to be repaired. **The reality is that medical equipment repair is a technical skill that depends entirely on education and experience.** Necessary components of service work include service manuals, tools and test equipment, and repair parts. In addition, service schools and/or telephone technical support are often vital. Users can help in two important ways. The first is to take the time to explain the nature of the problem and a reasonable assessment of the priority of the equipment. The second is to give the time for the technician to concentrate on troubleshooting and repair. Documentation of repairs is important to the clinical engineering department to track trends with equipment and users. Such documentation should also be available to the users for their review.

User assistance implies that biomedical equipment technicians are themselves expert users. This is not unreasonable. By inclination, education, and experience, biomedical equipment technicians are uniquely qualified. By extension, technicians are often the most logical people to routinely use the most sophisticated medical equipment.

Other functions provided by more versatile clinical engineering departments include equipment evaluations, equipment-related incident investigations, in-service education, and design and fabrication of new or modified equipment. These are best left to engineers or experienced technicians with a demonstrated ability for these functions.

Plant engineering departments also provide inspections, preventive maintenance, and repairs. However, they typically do not provide user assistance to clinicians. The equipment for which they are responsible is predominantly nonmedical, but it is just as critical as is medical equipment to clinicians and patients. The medical equipment for which plant engineering departments are responsible usually includes patient beds, operating tables, operating room lights, nurse call systems, and such mechanical items as stretchers and wheelchairs.

Clinical engineering and plant engineering departments need to cooperate, particularly in areas in which their responsibilities overlap. Examples include the installation of equipment for patient monitoring, dialysis water treatment, and imaging, as well as other equipment that has unique installation or operational requirements.

Arguably the single most important facet of the safe and effective use of medical equipment is the end user. The end user is usually a nurse or a physician but may be an engineer, technician, or therapist. **The most vital component for their success is training.** The individual end user can be so skilled that he/she can even overcome shortcomings of particular equipment,

or so unskilled as to make hazardous the best of equipment. Training can and should be available from the manufacturer, both directly from its representatives and from its operators' manual, from the clinical engineering staff, and from other knowledgeable users. Users should understand the operating principles of the equipment, the operation of controls and indicators, and the applications for which the equipment is intended. They should observe the set-up and pre-use checks prescribed by the manufacturer. They have the right and the duty to insist that equipment is properly maintained and in proper working order. Finally, they must be observant and conscientious during the actual use of the equipment.

Another, occasionally overlooked, aspect of medical equipment use is cooperation with others in health care who are involved with the acquisition and use of medical technology. The institution's administration is responsible for planning, budgeting, and complying with myriad standards and regulations. They cannot be completely successful without the cooperation of clinicians. Support services, from housekeeping and nutrition departments to plant and clinical engineering departments, cannot successfully complete their responsibilities without cooperation from clinicians. All clinical areas have similar requirements. It is often just as important to share the availability of clinical equipment as it is to share clinical information to provide optimal patient care.

Technology Management

It is an oversimplification, but still useful, to categorize the approximately 30-year history of clinical engineering by decades. The 1960s were primarily concerned with electrical safety, the 1970s with performance assurance, and the 1980s with productivity and quality assurance. **The 1990s seem destined to be concerned with technology management, incorporating quality improvement.** The intention is for everyone involved in the acquisition and use of technology to cooperate to improve both this process and patient care within the constraints (primarily financial) imposed on health care.

Technology management is a complex subject, still in its infancy at least as far as its acceptance and application in health care institutions.[7] To bring a measure of order out of what is often a seemingly chaotic situation, technology management can be described as a five-step cycle (Fig. 39-20).

Appropriately enough, the first step is planning. New technology should be approached with equal measures of promise and caution. It takes time and objectivity to determine whether the new technology will actually improve health care, what the total cost will be, whether the cost is affordable, and whether the new technology fits properly with the mission and

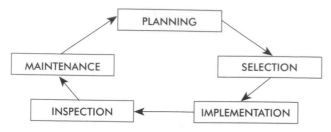

Fig. 39-20. Cycle of technology management.

other plans of the individual institution. Replacement of equipment is also involved in planning. Justification for replacement should include consideration of dependability and safety, operating and maintenance factors (including cost), and performance. Another consideration in planning is the quantity of equipment needed, both to satisfy peak demands and for backup. Related to this is the support for new equipment: trained users, installation requirements, supplies, and maintenance requirements.

If the decision is made to acquire new equipment, the second step is selection. Unless the technology is very new, there will probably be more than one source and/or more than one model or configuration. Technical and clinical criteria should be determined, based on available literature, the experience of other users, and the institution's unique needs. A comparative evaluation should be conducted. An engineer should test equipment samples to compare performance vs. the established criteria, any available standards, and the manufacturer's specifications. Acceptable equipment should then have a clinical trial that is long enough to expose the equipment to a representative sample of potential uses and users. Current users of each model at other institutions should be contacted for their reactions and opinions. Where possible, the institution should standardize on one model of a particular type of device, especially if users are likely to encounter different pieces of the same type of equipment. Finally, the institution should protect its negotiating position with vendors by not making its final decision (or at least letting it be known) until competitive bids are received and reviewed.

Implementation follows selection. The time to include all requirements and specifications to protect the investment is during order placement. Considerations for inclusion in the negotiation and ultimate order are operator and service training, warranty, supplies and accessories, price protection for future purchases, upgrades (especially software), and provision for maintenance, including parts and backups. This is also the time to consider installation requirements, such as special space or services, and who will perform the installation. Acceptance of, and payment for, the equipment should be contingent on a suc-

cessful initial inspection to be provided by personnel of the institution's choosing. **Before the new equipment is put into use, users must be trained. Ongoing training, both for new users and as reinforcement for others, should be available as needed.** The need for training simply cannot be overlooked or overemphasized.

Ongoing use of equipment requires an inspection program. As described previously, an inspection program should be done according to an established schedule, with procedures and test equipment that cover safety and performance aspects. Some equipment requires routine preventive maintenance (e.g., regular parts replacement or calibration). The inspection program must be properly documented, including the schedule, procedures, and results. Based on trends discovered as a result of analyzing inspection results, it might be appropriate to adjust the technology management program. If the equipment is not living up to expectations, it might be necessary to involve the manufacturer. If something were overlooked in the acquisition, the oversight should not only be corrected, but the selection and implementation processes might also be adjusted to prevent such occurrences in the future. As a result of trends, it might be necessary to increase the inspection frequency, or possibly to reduce it.

Ongoing use of equipment also requires maintenance. During the warranty period, a final decision can be made about whether service will be provided by the manufacturer, by an independent service organization, or by an in-house department. Then, before the warranty runs out, arrangements can be made so that there is no lapse in service. Again, documentation is necessary for — among other things — determining whether there are any trends in service problems that could be corrected. In addition, the service history of the equipment should be used to help decide on future purchases (e.g., buying more of the same device and repair or replacement choices). This, in turn, leads back to step one — planning.

Technology management is intended to combine and refine individual equipment programs, to make them work more efficiently, and to be directly involved in improving quality in general and patient care in particular (Box 39-1).

CONCLUSION

Medical technology is vital to modern health care. Its contributions to patient care and its rate of progress are awe-inspiring. The practice of anesthesiology depends largely on medical technology. In the operating room, the anesthesiologist is responsible for the patient. Equipment augments the anesthesiologist's ability to carry out this responsibility, but it certainly does not replace it. In fact, the anesthesiologist must know how to apply technology safely and effectively as part of this responsibility.

This chapter provides a background for both the principles and requirements of the safe use of medical equipment. Historically, scare tactics were used to convince clinicians to follow specific guidelines for the safe use of medical equipment. The better approach is to explain both the problems and the solutions, so that guidelines are understood and applied objectively. For example, medical device standards — when used as their originators intended — are generally a help and not a hindrance in providing safe and effective patient care.

This chapter has provided a review of basic electricity so that electrical hazards to patients can be explained. In response to such hazards, medical device standards have been developed. To apply these standards, electrical safety programs were instituted in hospitals. Experience with electrical safety programs showed the need for other safe practices in the application of technology. To acquire and implement new technology effectively, technology management programs are currently being developed.

Medical technology is indeed remarkable, but so are the people who use it safely and effectively. Two factors that may or may not be intuitively obvious are the following: (1) the safe and effective application of medical technology requires cooperation between clinical staff, support services, and administration, and (2) the justification for and application of medical technology is to improve the quality of patient care.

KEY POINTS

- Hazards to patients from medical equipment include fibrillation and burns, equipment failure, and misuse.
- Electrical safety concerns originating in the 1960s have led to the development of safety and performance standards, improved equipment designs, and in-house clinical engineering programs.
- Medical equipment standards are promulgated by a variety of national and international organizations. Both understanding and complying with them require clinical engineering expertise.

- Clinical engineering departments in hospitals help to ensure the safety and performance of medical equipment by providing evaluations, testing, maintenance, and training programs.
- The safe and effective use of medical equipment involves the cooperation of clinicans, administrators, support staff, and manufacturers. A clinical engineer is usually best able to orchestrate these efforts.
- A hospital-wide technology management program combines individual equipment programs and improves both efficiency and quality.

KEY REFERENCES

Dalziel CF: Reevaluation of lethal electric currents, *IEEE Transactions Industry Gen Appl* IGA-4(5): 467, 1968.

ECRI: Special report on technology management: preparing your hospital for 1990s, *Health Technol* 3:1, 1989.

Keil OR, Kitchin DJ, Gallagher L et al: The 1991 KIPS survey guide: hospital accreditation program. In Tomasik K, ed: *Plant technology and safety management series,* Oakbrook Terrace, Ill, 1990, Joint Commission on Accreditation of Healthcare Organizations.

Klein BR: *Health care facilities handbook,* ed 3, Quincy, Mass, 1990, National Fire Protection Association.

Starmer CF, Whalen RE: Current density and electrically induced ventricular fibrillation, *Med Instrument* 7(2):158, 1973.

REFERENCES

1. Association for the Advancement of Medical Instrumentation: AAMI standards and recommended practices, volume 1, *Biomedical equipment,* Arlington, Virginia, 1989, Association for the Advancement of Medical Instrumentation.
2. Bernstein T: A grand success, the first legal electrocution was fraught with controversy which flared between Edison and Westinghouse, *IEEE Spectrum* 54, February 1973.
3. Bruner JMR: Hazards of electrical apparatus, *Anesthesiology* 28(2):396, 1967.
4. Dalziel CF: Reevaluation of lethal electric currents, *IEEE Trans Industry Gen Appl* IGA-4(5):467, 1968.
5. Dalziel CF: Threshold 60-cycle fibrillating currents, *AIEE Trans (Power Apparatus and Systems)* 79:667, 1960.
6. Dalziel CF, Lee WR: Lethal electric current, *IEEE Spectrum* 6:44, 1969.
7. ECRI: Special report on technology management: preparing your hospital for the 1990s, *Health Technol* 3:1, 1989.
8. Geddes LA, Cabler P, Moore AG et al: Threshold 60-Hz current required for ventricular fibrillation in subjects of various body weights, *IEEE Trans Biomed Eng* 20:465, 1973.
9. International Electrotechnical Commission: *International standard, medical electrical equipment. Part 1. General requirements for safety,* ed 2, Genève, Suisse, 1988, Bureau Central de la Commission Electrotechnique International.
10. Joint Commission on Accreditation of Healthcare Organizations: *Accreditation manual for hospitals,* Oakbrook Terrace, Ill, 1991, The Commission.
11. Keil OR, Kitchin DJ, Gallagher L et al: The 1991 KIPS survey guide: hospital accreditation program. In Tomasik K, ed: *Plant technology and safety management series,* Oakbrook Terrace, Ill, 1990, Joint Commission on Accreditation of Healthcare Organizations.
12. Klein BR: *Health care facilities handbook,* ed 3, Quincy, Mass, 1990, National Fire Protection Association.
13. Kouwenhoven WB, Knickerbocker GG, Chestnut RW et al: A-C shocks of varying parameters affecting the heart, *AIEE Trans (Communication and Electronics)* 78:163, 1959.
14. Medicine and the law: fatal shock from a cardiac monitor, *Lancet* 1:872, 1960.
15. Nader R: Ralph Nader's most shocking exposé, *Ladies Home Journal* 98, March 1971.
16. National Fire Protection Association: *1990 edition of the national electrical code,* Quincy, Mass, 1989, The Association.
17. National Fire Protection Association: *Standard for health care facilities, 1990 edition,* Quincy, Mass, 1990, The Association.
18. Noordijk JA, Oey FTI, and Tebra W: Myocardial electrodes and the danger of ventricular fibrillation, *Lancet* 1:975, 1961.
19. Roy OZ, Scott JR, and Park GC: 60-Hz ventricular fibrillation and pump failure thresholds versus electrode area, *IEEE Trans Biomed Eng* 23(1):45, 1976.
20. Starmer CF, Whalen RE: Current density and electrically induced ventricular fibrillation, *Med Instrument* 7(2):158, 1973.
21. Stiefel RH: *The safe medical devices act of 1990: implications for health care personnel,* Arlington, Va, 1991, Association for the Advancement of Medical Instrumentation.
22. Underwriters Laboratories, Inc: *Standard for medical and dental equipment UL 544,* ed 2, Northbrook, Ill, 1991, The Laboratories.
23. Underwriters Laboratories, Inc: *Yesterday, today, tomorrow,* Northbrook, Ill, The Laboratories.
24. US Department of Health and Human Services: *The medical device amendments of 1976,* Public Health Service, Food and Drug Administration, Center for Devices and Radiological Health, Rockville, Md, 1984.
25. Walter CW: *Electric hazards in hospitals, proceedings of a workshop,* Washington, DC, 1970, National Academy of Sciences.
26. Watson AB, Wright JS, and Loughman J: Electrical thresholds for ventricular fibrillation in man, *Med J Aust* 1:1179, 1973.
27. Whalen RE, Starmer CF, and McIntosh HD: Electrical hazards associated with cardiac pacemaking, *Ann NY Acad Sci* 111:922, 1964.

CHAPTER 40

Standards for Patient Monitoring

JOHN H. EICHHORN

Anesthesia practice evolved significantly during the 1980s. Evidence that the overall outcome of anesthesia care improved is reflected by the fact that there were fewer anesthesia catastrophes that caused damage to patients at the end of the decade than at the beginning, and medical malpractice insurance premiums for anesthesiologists have been reduced, in many cases dramatically. However, careful epidemiologic studies have yet to "statistically prove" a decline in morbidity and mortality related to anesthesia care.

If the assumption that, in the aggregate, anesthesia care is safer now is accepted, developments during the 1980s contributed to this change. The most dramatic and visible factor is the concept of "safety monitoring" and the associated standards of care. **Monitoring standards cannot be the sole cause of reduced anesthesia accidents but rather are the tangible outward reflection of changes in attitudes and practices achieved by improvements in the following:**

- **The quality of people entering the anesthesiology profession**
- **Residency training**
- **Continuing education**
- **Research**
- **Anesthesia equipment**
- **Risk management initiatives**

Safety monitoring ("vigilance monitoring" or "accident-prevention monitoring") differs from physiologic monitoring with a pulmonary artery catheter or 2-D echo intended to allow fine-tuning of an anesthetic. Safety monitoring is designed to warn of "critical incidents," clinical developments that, if not corrected, would cause harm to the patient. In safety monitoring, both patient parameters and various features of the anesthetic delivery system are scrutinized. Classic safety monitors are the inspired oxygen concentration alarm and the breathing system disconnect warning device that alerts the anesthesiologist to breathing circuit leaks or disconnections. Pulse oximetry and capnography provide both safety information and physiologic data, as does the measurement of vital signs.

This chapter focuses on the principles of safety monitoring and how the study of past catastrophic anesthesia accidents led to recognized sets of monitoring standards for worldwide use. These safety monitoring standards specifically provide early warning signals of untoward developments during anesthesia so that the anesthesia provider(s) will have adequate time to correctly identify the problems and institute remedial action (such as reconnecting the breathing system tubing to the endotracheal tube), thereby preventing patient injury.[6]

Similar efforts to promulgate formal standards for physiologic monitoring are unlikely. Although physiologic monitoring may eventually be the subject of practice parameters, advisories, or "guidelines," adoption of formal standards would be difficult because of the wide variation in judgment and opinion in practice. Furthermore, the desirable endpoint of "good outcome" is much harder to define for physiologic parameters than for safety, for which the outcome is simply whether or not there is an untoward development that causes damage to the patient.

MAJOR ANESTHESIA ACCIDENTS

Monitoring standards in anesthesia practice are based on the belief that anesthesia accidents that cause death or major morbidity are not acceptable and must be reduced to an absolute minimum. By definition, the basis for eliminating such accidents must be an understanding of their type and nature.

Extensive, thoughtful discussion of major anesthesia accidents has occurred since Hannah Greener died while receiving chloroform anesthesia in 1848. Relatively recently, attention has been focused on the causes of mishaps, with comments such as, "Hypoxia from hypoventilation and low levels of inspired oxygen appeared to be the chief cause of cardiac arrest . . . ".[25] Attention turned to the role of medications in anesthesia-related mortality,[15] with the counterpoint of renewed emphasis on the role of human error in anesthesia catastrophes.[3,14,18] Increasingly in recent years, studies and reviews have revealed that relatively straightforward errors, often technical or mechanical, and the subsequent failure to recognize them until a very late stage in the evolution of the accident (most often at the time of a sudden, profound bradycardia) cause many such problems.*

The most common cause of anesthesia-related injury is failure of adequate ventilation, whether from an unrecognized esophageal intubation, a breathing system disconnection, kinked or dislodged endotracheal tube or breathing system tubing, incorrect ventilator settings, or simply inadequate spontaneous or assisted ventilation under anesthesia. This fact was recently reinforced by the American Association of Anesthesiologists (ASA) Closed Claims Study.[2] "Adverse respiratory events" represented the largest class of injuries, and 85% of these incidents led to death or brain damage. According to the study, 72% of the claims were considered preventable through better monitoring.

Other important problems involve incorrect fresh gas flows or deficiencies in the oxygen supply, but these are relatively less common. Overdose of anesthetic agent, either relative or absolute, has received attention and has elicited a debate as to whether untoward developments could be prevented through improved safety monitoring. It seems reasonable that scrupulous attention to vital signs and oxygenation should provide the best chance for early identification of this type of human error.

Even though the mechanism of injury is understood from retrospective studies, the actual number of major injuries related to anesthesia practice is not clear. Most insurance carriers are reluctant to share data to reveal information (even to academic investigators) that could be the subject of or relevant to medical malpractice lawsuits. The ASA closed claims study provides valuable information regarding mechanisms of accidents but still does not yield true accident rates because of the lack of a known complete numerator (all the major accidents in a given area for a given time) and an accurate denominator (the exact corresponding total number of anesthetics). Therefore estimates based on an amalgamation of multiple published and unpublished sources must be used. After higher earlier estimates,[10] a popular estimate in the early to mid-1980s was that among the 20 million patients anesthetized, possibly 2000 reasonably healthy patients (ASA class I or II) died from causes primarily attributable to anesthesia each year in the United States. How many of these were victims of outright accidents is less clear, but it is likely that the majority were. As early as 1986,[28] some improvement in these statistics was noted by insurance carriers. Any reduction in the rate of death or major morbidity related to anesthesia care is worthy of efforts to reduce it.

Historical Perspective

In 1984, the self-insurance medical malpractice carrier of Harvard Medical School expressed concern to the department heads of the nine component hospital anesthesia departments about the number of incidents and claims and associated indemnity that had arisen from anesthesia care since 1976. This led to appointment of a Risk Management Committee to investigate and suggest action. Review of the literature yielded the information previously listed, and review of all claims and incidents revealed that most cases involving major morbidity or death were judged preventable by this committee. Specifically, more meticulous monitoring would have given warnings early enough to allow the anesthesiologist to respond as appropriate to prevent the accident. Many cases, as expected, centered around failure of adequate ventilation, either spontaneous or mechanical.[7] However, review of the classic case outlined in Box 40-1 stimulated the formulation of the first committee decision: during all general anesthetics, oxygen monitors with lower limit alarms *must always* be used on all anesthesia machines.

For several reasons, the committee thought that the monitoring strategies and behaviors developed should be considered minimal safety monitoring, with the potential to help prevent catastrophic accidents. These were therefore expressed as formal standards of practice to be adopted by the consortium of hospitals and required of the staff.

---

* References 5, 9, 16, 17, 21, 22.

BOX 40-1
CLASSIC CASE REVIEWED BY RISK
MANAGEMENT COMMITTEE

A 27-year-old man with severe gastrointestinal bleeding was taken emergently to an angiographic suite for an attempt at arterial embolization. General anesthesia was needed, and, because there was no anesthesia machine in that suite, an old (1966) British machine was literally retrieved from a closet by a senior attending physician. Although all the operating room anesthesia machines then in use at that hospital had oxygen monitors, this old model did not. The attending physician was relieved by a resident who was unfamiliar with the British machine. At the end of the successful procedure, the room was still relatively dark. The resident intended to awaken the patient and turned the left gas flow knob off and the right one up (the correct procedure on a modern American machine). However, because of the configuration on the British machine, this action caused the delivery of 100% nitrous oxide. The quickly resulting cyanosis was masked by the dark room and a cardiac arrest resulted. Although resuscitated, the patient suffered hypoxic encephalopathy and was eventually allowed to expire.

BOX 40-2
FACTORS CONSIDERED IN
OPTIMIZING STANDARDS

Availability: For example, in 1984 use of capnography was uncommon and pulse oximeters were just beginning to gain acceptance
Cost
Simplicity of use
Distracting influence: For example, an unclear alarm message could delay rather than speed the needed response to an untoward development
Relative sensitivity: Offering few false-negatives
Relative specificity: Offering few false-positives
Predictability: Freedom from breakdown or aberrant output
Indicative of reasonable care[19]

---

cepted standards at the time of the untoward event.

Criteria for Monitoring Standards

No study offers "hard data" that statistically validate which monitoring modalities prevent anesthetic accidents. Furthermore, for ethical reasons, it is highly unlikely that prospective controlled trials of safety monitoring will be conducted. Therefore the committee relied on an intuitive approach, based on the experience of committee members and recognized authorities,* as well as on compromise among widely divergent opinions. If most accidents involve failure to ventilate the patient, then mandating the continuous monitoring of ventilation should alert the practitioner to ventilation problems in time to prevent injury. However, a balance was needed between what constituted too much monitoring and what represented too little. The factors considered in the effort to define the set of measurements and alarms are listed in Box 40-2. It should be noted that the last point, regarding reasonable care, refers to a doctrine of cost-to-benefit analysis applied to medical situations. It can be expressed as choosing to spend a relatively small amount of money (for example, on monitoring modalities) to potentially save a great deal of money (as in monetary settlements reached after anesthesia-caused injury or death). This is both reasonable and potentially a standard of care; the converse (spending a lot to save a little) is not reasonable.

Some other attributes of these standards deserve mention, such as:

- Standards must be realistic and attainable by the average practitioner

---

Among the goals set for the minimal monitoring standards were the following:

- **Reduction of patient injury arising from anesthesia accidents.** A secondary benefit from this goal should be a reduction in the number of malpractice claims, thus resulting in fewer and less expensive settlements and judgments, thereby creating the opportunity for eventual reductions in malpractice insurance premiums.
- **Application of collective experience toward the detection of very rare events.** Because the average anesthesiologist can expect to be involved in a catastrophic accident probably only once in an entire career, the individual will have difficulty developing a standard of care based on personal adverse experiences.
- **Provision of a means for objective evaluation.** If the standards are simple and clear, practitioners clearly either do or do not observe them. This allows the individual to assess his or her own practice as well as allowing supervisors to observe and quantify whether practice meets established criteria.
- **Codification of accepted practices.** This is seen as a significant aid to defense against malpractice claims when the practitioner can demonstrate documented adherence to published and ac-

---

* References 4, 12, 13, 23, 24, 27.

BOX 40-3
HARVARD MINIMAL MONITORING STANDARDS

These standards apply for any administration of anesthesia involving Department of Anaesthesia personnel and are specifically referable to preplanned anesthetics administered in designated anesthetizing locations (specific exclusion: administration of epidural analgesia for labor or pain management). In emergency circumstances in any location, immediate life support measures of whatever appropriate nature come first with attention turning to the measures described in these standards as soon as possible and practical. These are minimal standards that may be exceeded at any time based on the judgment of the involved anesthesia personnel. These standards encourage high-quality patient care, but observing them cannot guarantee any specific patient outcome. These standards are subject to revision from time to time, as warranted by the evolution of technology and practice.

Anesthesiologist's or nurse anesthetist's presence in operating room

For all anesthetics initiated by or involving a member of the department of anaesthesia, an attending or resident anesthesiologist or nurse anesthetist shall be present in the room throughout the conduct of all general anesthetics, regional anesthetics, and monitored intravenous anesthetics. An exception is made when there is a direct known hazard (e.g., radiation) to the anesthesiologist or nurse anesthetist, in which case some provision for monitoring the patient must be made.

Blood pressure and heart rate

Every patient receiving general anesthesia, regional anesthesia, or managed intravenous anesthesia shall have arterial blood pressure and heart rate measured at least every 5 minutes, where not clinically impractical.*

Electrocardiogram

Every patient shall have the electrocardiogram continuously displayed from the induction or institution of anesthesia until preparing to leave the anesthetizing location, where not clinically impractical.*

Continuous monitoring

During every administration of general anesthesia, the anesthetist shall employ methods of continuously monitoring the patient's ventilation and circulation. The methods shall include, for ventilation and circulation each, at least one of the following or the equivalent†:
For Ventilation—Palpation or observation of the reservoir breathing bag, auscultation of breath sounds, monitoring of respiratory gases such as end-tidal carbon dioxide, or monitoring of expiratory gas flow. Monitoring end-tidal carbon dioxide is an emerging standard and is strongly preferred.
For Circulation—Palpation of a pulse, auscultation of heart sounds, monitoring of a tracing of intraarterial pressure, pulse plethysmography/oximetry, or ultrasound peripheral pulse monitoring.
It is recognized that brief interruptions of the continuous monitoring may be unavoidable.

Breathing system disconnection monitoring

When ventilation is controlled by an automatic mechanical ventilator there shall be in continuous use a device that is capable of detecting disconnection of any component of the breathing system. The device must give an audible signal when its alarm threshold is exceeded. (It is recognized that there are certain rare or unusual circumstances in which such a device may fail to detect a disconnection.)

Oxygen analyzer

During every administration of general anesthesia using an anesthesia machine, the concentration of oxygen in the patient breathing system will be measured by a functioning oxygen analyzer with a low concentration limit alarm in use. This device must conform to the American National Standards Institute No. Z.79.10 standard.*

Ability to measure temperature

During every administration of general anesthesia, there shall be readily available a means to measure the patient's temperature.
Rationale—A means of temperature measurement must be available as a potential aid in the diagnosis and treatment of suspected or actual intraoperative hypothermia and malignant hyperthermia. The measurement/monitoring of temperature during *every* general anesthetic is not specifically mandated because of the potential risks of such monitoring and because of the likelihood of other physical signs giving earlier indication of the development of malignant hyperthermia.

*Under extenuating circumstances, the attending anesthesiologist may waive this requirement after so stating (including the reasons) in a note in the patient's chart.
†Equivalence is to be defined by the chief of the individual hospital department after submission to and review by the department heads, Department of Anaesthesia, Harvard Medical School, Boston.
From The Department of Anaesthesia, Harvard Medical School, adopted March 25, 1985; revised July 3, 1985.

- Standards should be technically achievable (not dependent on state-of-the-art high technology, which may not be available)
- Standards must be focused on behavior rather than on technology

This last point allowed individual variation in achieving the standard. For example, the original Harvard standards mandate continuous monitoring of ventilation. An amendable list of means to achieve this end is then given. Although capnography may have been the *best* available means, whether or not this was chosen was left to the individual anesthesiologist's evaluation. If auscultation of breath sounds via a precordial or esophageal stethoscope was used continuously to genuinely monitor ventilation, then the standard was being observed and the desired "early warning system" was functioning appropriately.

HARVARD STANDARDS

The minimal monitoring standards of the Harvard departments[8] were instituted in early 1985 and are reproduced in Box 40-3. The intent and reasoning are generally self-explanatory. The preamble and footnotes may seem cumbersome but they are as important as the standards themselves. These additional components reflect much thought in the standard-setting process. It was quickly realized that for every good idea or suggestion, an exception could be raised almost immediately. The standards are designed to acknowledge these exceptions and redirect the focus to the large majority of operative cases that are straightforward. The exclusion of epidural *analgesia* for labor (*not* delivery, which is equivalent to an operative case) or pain management resulted from two practical considerations. There had been no claims or incidents from this activity during the index period (or since), and it is not cost effective for an anesthesia caregiver to remain physically in the room with each patient during the entire duration of an epidural catheterization.

The standards specify, and it cannot be overemphasized, that these are *minimum* standards. It is expected and appropriate that these standards will routinely be exceeded. There was slight initial confusion that the standards might limit monitoring activity. This is not true—they prescribe care that is the *least* that must be provided in *all* cases.

The continuous monitoring of ventilation and circulation is the essence of the Harvard standards. To some, this may appear too lenient. The point is, however, that intermittent observations alone are insufficient. Achieving early warning of threatening situations rests on this concept. The standard allows for modifications, with approval, by a given department among the nine, but this has not happened. The

subsequent advent of the ASA standards is part of the reason, and various hospital departments have evolved de facto standards of care related to their particular circumstances. For example, all children receiving anesthesia have their temperatures monitored, but this has not been a formal written amendment to the published standards. The Harvard Risk Management Committee reevaluates these standards annually, always noting the emphasis on behavior and attitudes rather than on technology. However, as noted, the appearance and evolution of the ASA standards makes modification unlikely.

ASA MONITORING STANDARDS

Based on careful review of all available background material, the Ad Hoc Committee on Standards of Care of the ASA drafted standards for basic intraoperative monitoring in 1985 (Box 40-4). The concerns of this committee were to have a significant immediate impact in reducing intraoperative catastrophic events and to set standards for the profession rather than have arbitrary requirements forcefully imposed by other outside groups.

The caveats in the preamble of the ASA standards are broad, noting that some monitoring methods may be impractical in some cases and that even appropriate application of the methods may fail to detect untoward developments in rare or unusual cases (as in the Harvard standards' reference to the occasional failure of a breathing system low-pressure alarm to detect tubing disconnection). This reinforces both the extensive thought given in formulating this document and the desire for realistic rather than idealistic guidelines.

The ASA standards specifically mandate that oxygenation, ventilation, circulation, and temperature be continually (with a careful definition of the word "continually") evaluated. For each component section the objective of ensuring adequate patient status and anesthesia delivery system performance is stated. Then specific methods are outlined. There is strong emphasis on combining behavior with technology. Most significantly, there is a clear distinction between *qualitative* and *quantitative* evaluation, as well as an even clearer emphasis on the preference for the quantitative methods. In the original 1986 version, assessment of oxygenation by patient color was required, stating that this "may be adequate," but the quantitative monitoring modality, pulse oximetry, was "encouraged." Anesthesia practice in the United States in the late 1980s evolved to make intraoperative pulse oximetry a de facto standard of care. Accordingly, this was recognized by the ASA Standards of Care Committee. **In the amendment to the ASA Standards for Basic Intraoperative Monitoring effective in 1990, the standard was changed to mandate a**

BOX 40-4
AMERICAN SOCIETY OF ANESTHESIOLOGISTS
Standards for Basic Intraoperative Monitoring

These standards apply to all anesthesia care although, in emergency circumstances, appropriate life support measures take precedence. These standards may be exceeded at any time based on the judgment of the responsible anesthesiologist. They are intended to encourage high-quality patient care, but observing them cannot guarantee any specific patient outcome. They are subject to revision from time to time, as warranted by the evolution of technology and practice. This set of standards addresses only the issue of basic intraoperative monitoring, which is one component of anesthesia care. In certain rare or unusual circumstances, (1) some of these methods of monitoring may be clinically impractical, and (2) appropriate use of the described monitoring methods may fail to detect untoward clinical developments. Brief interruptions of continual† monitoring may be unavoidable. *Under extenuating circumstances, the responsible anesthesiologist may waive the requirements marked with an asterisk (*); it is recommended that when this is done, it should be so stated (including the reasons) in a note in the patient's medical record.* These standards are not intended for application to the care of the obstetric patient in labor or in the conduct of pain management.

Standard I

Qualified anesthesia personnel shall be present in the room throughout the conduct of all general anesthetics, regional anesthetics, and monitored anesthesia care.

Objective

Because of the rapid changes in patient status during anesthesia, qualified anesthesia personnel shall be continuously present to monitor the patient and provide anesthesia care. In the event there is a direct known hazard (e.g., radiation) to the anesthesia personnel that might require intermittent remote observation of the patient, some provision for monitoring the patient must be made. In the event that an emergency requires the temporary absence of the person primarily responsible for the anesthetic, the best judgment of the anesthesiologist will be exercised in comparing the emergency with the anesthetized patient's condition and in the selection of the person left responsible for the anesthetic during the temporary absence.

Standard II

During all anesthetics, the patient's oxygenation, ventilation, circulation, and temperature shall be continuously evaluated.

Oxygenation

Objective
To ensure adequate oxygen concentration in the inspired gas and the blood during all anesthetics.
Methods
1. Inspired gas: During every administraton of general anesthesia using an anesthesia machine, the concentration of oxygen in the patient breathing system shall be measured by an oxygen analyzer with a low oxygen concentration limit alarm in use.*
2. Blood oxygenation: During all anesthetics, a quantitative method of assessing oxygenation such as pulse oximetry shall be employed.* Adequate illumination and exposure of the patient is necessary to assess color.*

Ventilation

Objective
To ensure adequate ventilation of the patient during all anesthetics.
Methods
1. Every patient receiving general anesthesia shall have the adequacy of ventilation continually evaluated. While qualitative clinical signs such as chest excursion, observation of the reservoir breathing bag and auscultation of breath sounds may be adequate, quantitative monitoring of the CO_2 content and/or volume of expired gas is encouraged.

†Note that "continual" is defined as "repeated regularly and frequently in steady rapid succession," whereas "continuous" means "prolonged without any interruption at any time."
From The American Society of Anesthesiologists, adopted October 6, 1986; amended October 18, 1989; effective January 1, 1990.

BOX 40-4—cont'd
AMERICAN SOCIETY OF ANESTHESIOLOGISTS
Standards for Basic Intraoperative Monitoring

---

2. When an endotracheal tube is inserted, its correct positioning in the trachea must be verified. Clinical assessment is essential and end-tidal CO_2 analysis, in use from the time of endotracheal tube placement, is encouraged.

3. When ventilation is controlled by a mechanical ventilator, there shall be in continuous use a device that is capable of detecting disconnection of components of the breathing system. The device must give an audible signal when its alarm threshold is exceeded.

4. During regional anesthesia and monitored anesthesia care, the adequacy of ventilation shall be evaluated, at least, by continual observation of qualitative clinical signs.

Circulation

Objective
To ensure the adequacy of the patient's circulatory function during all anesthetics.
Methods
1. Every patient receiving anesthesia shall have the electrocardiogram continuously displayed from the beginning of anesthesia until preparing to leave the anesthetizing locaton.*
2. Every patient receiving anesthesia shall have arterial blood pressure and heart rate determined and evaluated at least every 5 minutes.*
3. Every patient receiving general anesthesia shall have, in addition to the above, circulatory function continually elevated by at least one of the following: palpation of a pulse, auscultation of heart sounds, monitoring of a tracing of intraarterial pressure, ultrasound peripheral pulse monitoring, or pulse plethysmography or oximetry.

Body temperature

Objective
To aid in the maintenance of appropriate body temperature during all anesthetics.
Methods
There shall be readily available a means to continuously measure the patient's temperature. When changes in body temperature are intended, anticipated, or suspected, the temperature shall be measured.

---

quantitative method of assessing oxygenation, transforming intraoperative pulse oximetry into a formal standard of care.

Similarly, ventilation must be continually evaluated. In the original version of the standards, qualitative methods were listed but with a stated preference for quantitative measurements (spirometry and capnography). Verification of correct endotracheal tube placement was also "encouraged." Although the use of capnography has become more prevalent during general anesthesia, still now its use is not as common as the use of pulse oximetry. However, an amendment to the ASA standards was proposed as a result of specific findings by the ASA closed claims study. This study revealed that unrecognized esophageal intubations and resultant patient injury continued to occur at an unacceptable rate, probably representing the type of anesthesia accident least impacted by the perceived general improvement in the safety of care. Accordingly, a proposal was adopted, to take effect in 1991, that the standard be amended to mandate the objective identification of expired carbon dioxide, via capnography, colorimetric indicator, or other technology, after placement of an endotracheal tube, to verify correct tube positioning in the trachea. This amendment will likely accelerate the implementation of capnography where it had not previously existed, and capnography will probably soon become a de facto standard of care, as pulse oximetry did before it was made a formal promulgated standard of care.

The arguments that oximetry and capnography should be mandatory intraoperative monitors were strengthened in a published analysis of preventability of the major anesthesia mishaps studied in the ASA closed claims study.[26] On the average, preventable accidents were significantly more severe than unpreventable occurrences. Importantly, 93% of the incidents judged to be preventable would have been prevented by applying a combination of pulse oximetry and capnography.

The ASA standards continued the concept that temperature measurement capability must be readily available during all anesthetic experiences, leaving

the practitioner some latitude to decide, for example, that temperature monitoring during brief noninvasive operative cases can safely be omitted. However, temperature measurement is mandated when changes in temperature are intended, anticipated, or suspected. This means, for instance, that temperature monitoring be established as the standard of care in cases involving lengthy, extensive intraabdominal or thoracic dissection because significant heat loss can be anticipated in these cases. In the late 1980s, those interested in the treatment of malignant hyperthermia repeatedly tried to make temperature monitoring mandatory during all uses of anesthetics. These proposals were not adopted because the temperature increase during this crisis is essentially always a comparatively late development and could not be relied on to provide the *initial* warning of an untoward development.

The ASA standards do include a critically important point directed at the recently increasing number of accidents involving inadequate ventilation by patients receiving intravenous sedation during regional anesthesia or monitored anesthesia care. At a minimum, continual observation of the adequacy of ventilation is required. Subsequent analysis from the ASA closed claims study intensified this concern by suggesting that unrecognized hypoventilation from sedation may contribute to sudden cardiac arrest during spinal anesthesia.[1]

OTHER COUNTRIES

Few, if any, countries other than the United States have the same emphasis on the term "standard of care." In the United States, this concept has profound medicolegal implications. Therefore the use of the term "standard" has been circumspect and reserved for the comparatively few circumstances when "the standard of care" was being established in a practical as well as a legal sense. In many other countries, documents concerning intraoperative monitoring are published with a wide variety of titles, including "guidelines," "recommendations," and "recommended practices," all of which are intended to establish the standard of care for anesthesia practitioners. Only some of these carry the same weight as the ASA standards in the United States.

Dutch anesthesiologists correctly point out that as early as 1978 the Netherlands Health Council formulated the first version of their monitoring standards, "Recommendations of the Health Council regarding monitoring requirements in the operating theater." The Dutch recommendations specify only what equipment must be available, not how it is to be used, which (while the implications are obvious) is left to the discretion of the individual practitioner. In the most recent version of this document, the following equipment was required: sphygomomanometer, ECG with recorder, pulse plethysmograph with recorder, pulse oximeter, spirometer, capnograph with recorder, and electric thermometer. In several European and some other countries, capnography was recognized and adopted as an essential safety monitor first, before pulse oximetry.

Most of the other relevant published documents from other countries appeared in the late 1980s, several closely following the two U.S. efforts chronicled earlier. In early 1987 "Guidelines to the practice of anaesthesia as recommended by the Canadian Anaesthetists' Society" was published. This document covers much more than monitoring. The opening of the monitoring section states, "The only indispensable monitor is the presence, at all times, of an appropriately trained and experienced physician. Mechanical and electronic monitors are, at best, aids to vigilance . . . ." The subsequent guidelines closely parallel the original Harvard standards.

The Faculty of Anaesthetists, Royal Australasian College of Surgeons "Policy statement — monitoring during anaesthesia" and the "Recommendations for standards of monitoring during anaesthesia and recovery" from the Association of Anaesthetists of Great Britain and Ireland both appeared in mid-1988. The U.K. document strongly recommended pulse oximetry and capnography and mentioned that a means to assess the degree of neuromuscular blockade must be readily available. Specific attention was directed to very brief anesthetics and to monitoring during transport. The Australian statement mandated pulse oximetry and stated that capnography must be available for those patients when it is clinically indicated. A significant component of the Australian standards is the attention given to the use of anesthetic assistants, with specific mandates that an assistant to the anaesthetist be present during induction and emergence and available if needed during the maintenance phase.

In late 1988 the Singapore Anaesthetic Society produced a comprehensive document, "Safety guidelines in anaesthesia," intended as a blueprint for countries of the Far East on all aspects of anesthetic care, with monitoring as only one section. Included, for example, were prescriptions for facilities and policies for administration of anesthesia for dentistry, radiographic imaging, and procedures performed in locations other than regular operating rooms. For regular intraoperative monitoring, capnography is called highly desirable and pulse oximetry is functionally mandated "where there is no financial restraint."

Similar types of monitoring standards documents have continued to appear. The recommendations from Finland include pulse oximetry and ECG during transfer of the patient, for example, to the recovery room. The German "Guidelines for quality assurance in anesthesiology" are similar to those from the Netherlands in only specifying what equipment must be available. However, a prior German regulation involving the requirement to identify failure of a mechanism providing medication led to the mandating of volatile anesthetic agent monitors on every anesthesia machine. In 1989 the French recommendations mandated pulse oximetry, recommended capnography, and emphasized that fresh gas "ratio protection" on modern anesthesia machines does not eliminate the requirement for an inspired oxygen concentration monitor. Several other countries, usually through their anesthesia professional societies but sometimes through their governments, have been or are in the process of formulating documents that will define standards of care for intraoperative monitoring.

SUMMARY

The concept of basic or minimal intraoperative monitoring can evoke various opinions.[11,20] **There can be no objection, however, to the goal of reducing major intraoperative anesthesia accidents. It seems intuitively reasonable that generating the earliest possible warning of an adverse development, such as a breathing system disconnection, will help prevent patient injury by allowing appropriate remedial intervention well before a patient is severely hypoxemic and the cyanosis and bradycardia are unmistakable. The intent of safety monitoring is to provide that warning. The focus must be on behavior and attitude, with technology playing only a supporting role. This approach to patient monitoring should prevail even though pulse oximetry is now mandatory in the United States and capnography probably soon will be.**

The cost-effectiveness of improved monitoring (behavior) and monitoring standards (technology) has not been determined precisely in rigid financial terms. However, monitoring standards and recommendations have been adopted locally, regionally, and nationally in several countries throughout the world. In each situation, the group that developed the standards considered the costs as well as the benefits of the proposed standards, and the recommended guidelines are noted more for their similarities than their differences. Cost-benefit ratios, or returns on investment, are difficult to calculate when dealing with rare occurrences that are likely to be devastating, if not fatal. The reasonable judgment of experts is probably more valuable than a quantitative calculation under these circumstances. In the United States,

the standards were adopted widely and promptly, indicating that the value of the investment in technology was apparent intuitively to both hospitals and practitioners.

Does safety monitoring affect anesthetic outcome? As noted, the ASA closed claims study analysis suggested that of the mishaps judged preventable, nearly all would have been prevented by a combination of pulse oximetry and capnography.[26] This supports the concept that continuous monitoring of oxygenation and ventilation should provide earlier warning of an untoward development; this, in turn, will facilitate the diagnosis and treatment of a developing problem in time to prevent patient injury. Furthermore, analysis of the Harvard data[16] reveals apparent reduction in the rates of major intraoperative anesthesia accidents and deaths after the implementation of the safety monitoring standards in 1985. The change is not statistically significant because of the difficulty of comparing very low rates. It is fully acknowledged that many positive developments in anesthesiology were occurring simultaneously, with the monitoring standards perhaps only the most visible.

As suggested earlier, the monitoring standards exemplify a set of changes in attitudes, behavior, and technology that led to safer anesthesia care. However, echoing earlier research, human errors are responsible for the majority of critical incidents, and such errors inevitably will continue to occur. Therefore the attitudes, behavior, and technology derived from the monitoring standards can reasonably be expected to cause these errors to be identified and corrected before the patient is damaged. These concepts have attracted the attention of the public and, by extension, public regulators. Several states in the United States have implemented or are proposing inclusion of specific monitoring practices into state health statutes or regulations, effectively giving them the force of law. In 1988, Massachusetts incorporated the ASA monitoring standards into state regulations. In 1989, both New York and New Jersey issued their own detailed regulations for intraoperative monitoring; both require pulse oximetry and capnography. Other states are contemplating similar action. Whether this strategy of government enforcement above and beyond the work of the profession and its societies will affect the rate of major anesthesia accidents remains to be seen.

The ASA standards for basic intraoperative monitoring have been widely publicized and distributed, including among medical malpractice plaintiff attorneys. It is certain that these standards will be cited as the established U.S. minimum standard of care for anesthesia safety monitoring. It can be hoped that these standards will be observed by anesthesia practitioners because of the desirable goals and reasonable nature of the standards. However, it must also be recognized that the potential medicolegal consequences of ignoring them are so great that this, too, will be an incentive for compliance. As noted, many medical malpractice insurance carriers, because of trends of fewer accidents and the prospect of still fewer in the future as a result of improvement in anesthesia care, best exemplified by the application of intraoperative monitoring standards, have lowered malpractice insurance premium rates for anesthesiologists. Eventually, even more clearly demonstrable decreases in the number and severity of major intraoperative anesthesia accidents and consequent patient injuries will validate all these efforts.

KEY POINTS

- The purpose of safety monitoring is to provide early warning of adverse developments, such as a breathing system disconnection.
- Safe anesthesia results in part from improved equipment; pulse oximetry is now mandatory in the United States and capnography is likely to become mandatory soon. However, technology should be regarded as secondary to forethought and a careful attitude.
- Monitoring standards and improvements in personnel, residency training, continuing education, research, anesthesia equipment, and risk management have all contributed to a reduction in anesthesia accidents.
- The most common cause of anesthesia-related injury is failure of adequate ventilation. It may result from an unrecognized esophageal intubation, a breathing system disconnection, a kinked or dislodged endotracheal tube or breathing system tubing, incorrect ventilator settings, or simply inadequate spontaneous or assisted ventilation under anesthesia.
- Monitoring standards generally define the minimum for safe practice; it is frequently appropriate to exceed these standards for high-quality care.
- The ASA Standards for Basic Intraoperative Monitoring (as amended in 1990) mandate a quantitative method of assessing oxygenation (i.e., pulse oximetry). They also suggest that temperature measurement capability must be readily available during use of all anesthetics, but need not necessarily be used during brief noninvasive cases.

KEY REFERENCES

Cooper JB, Newbower RS, Long CD et al: Preventable anesthesia mishaps: a study of human factors, *Anesthesiology* 49:399, 1978.

Eichhorn JH: Prevention of intraoperative anesthesia accidents and related severe injury through safety monitoring, *Anesthesiology* 70:572, 1989.

Eichhorn JH, Cooper JB, Cullen DJ et al: Standards for patient monitoring during anesthesia at Harvard Medical School, *JAMA* 256:1017, 1986.

Keats AS: What do we know about anesthetic mortality? *Anesthesiology* 50:387, 1979.

REFERENCES

1. Caplan RA, Ward RJ, Posner K et al: Unexpected cardiac arrest during spinal anesthesia: a closed claims analysis of predisposing factors, *Anesthesiology* 68:5, 1988.
2. Caplan RA, Posner KL, Ward RJ et al: Adverse respiratory events in anesthesia: a closed claim analysis, *Anesthesiology* 72:828, 1990.
3. Cooper JB, Newbower RS, Long CD et al: Preventable anesthesia mishaps: a study of human factors, *Anesthesiology* 49:399, 1978.
4. Duberman SM, Bendixen HH: Concepts of fail-safe in anesthesia practice, *Int Anesthesiol Clin* 22(2):149, 1984.
5. Craig J, Wilson ME: A survey of anesthetic misadventures, *Anesthesia* 36:933, 1981.
6. Eichhorn JH: Are there standards for intraoperative monitoring? In Stoelting RK, Barash PG, and Gallagher TJ, eds: *Advances in anesthesia*, vol 5, Chicago, 1988, Year Book Medical.
7. Eichhorn JH: Prevention of intraoperative anesthesia accidents and related severe injury through safety monitoring, *Anesthesiology* 70:572, 1989.
8. Eichhorn JH, Cooper JB, Cullen DJ et al: Standards for patient monitoring during anesthesia at Harvard Medical School, *JAMA* 256:1017, 1986.
9. Emergency Care Research Institute: Death during general anesthesia, *J Health Care Tech* 1:155, 1985.
10. Epstein RM: Morbidity and mortality from anesthesia: a continuing problem, *Anesthesiology* 49:388, 1978.

11. Gravenstein JS: Essential monitoring examined through different lenses, *J Clin Monit* 2:22, 1986.
12. Gravenstein JS, Paulus DA, eds: *Monitoring practice in clinical anesthesia,* Philadelphia, 1982, JB Lippincott.
13. Gravenstein JS, Newbower RS, Ream AK et al, eds: *An integrated approach to monitoring,* Stoneham, Mass, 1983, Butterworths.
14. Hamilton WK: Unexpected deaths during anesthesia: wherein lies the cause? *Anesthesiology* 50:381, 1979.
15. Keats AS: What do we know about anesthetic mortality? *Anesthesiology* 50: 387, 1979.
16. Keenan RL: Anesthesia disasters: incidence, causes and preventability, *Semin Anesth* 5:175, 1986.
17. Keenan RL, Boyan CP: Cardiac arrest due to anesthesia, *JAMA* 253:2373, 1985.

18. Newbower RS, Cooper JB, and Long CD: Failure analysis: the human element. In Gravenstein JS, Newbower RS, Ream AK et al, eds: *Essential noninvasive monitoring in anesthesia,* New York, 1980, Grune & Stratton.
19. Philip JH, Raemer DB: Selecting the optimal anesthesia monitoring assay, *Med Instrum* 3:122, 1985.
20. Pierce EC: Risk modification in anesthesiology. In Chapman-Cliburn G, ed: *Risk management and quality assurance: issues and interactions,* [A special publication of the Quality Review Bulletin], Chicago, 1986, Joint Commission on Accreditation of Hospitals.
21. Pierce EC, ed: Risk management in anesthesia, *Int Anesthesiol Clin* 27(3): 1989.
22. Pierce EC, Cooper JB, eds: Analysis of anesthetic mishaps, *Int Anesthesiol Clin* 22(2):1, 1984.

23. Saidman LJ, Smith NT, eds: *Monitoring in anesthesia,* ed 2, Stoneham, Mass, 1984, Butterworths.
24. Taylor G: What is minimal monitoring? In Gravenstein JS, Newbower RS, Ream AK et al, eds: *Essential noninvasive monitoring in anesthesia,* New York, 1980, Grune & Stratton.
25. Taylor G, Larson CP, and Prestwich R: Unexpected cardiac arrest during anesthesia and surgery, *JAMA* 236:2758, 1976.
26. Tinker JH, Dull DL, Caplan RA et al: Role of monitoring devices in prevention of anesthetic mishaps: a closed claim analysis, *Anesthesiology* 71:541, 1989.
27. Uhl RR: Monitoring: present concepts and future directions. In Gallagher TJ, ed: *Advances in anesthesia,* Chicago, 1984, Year Book Medical.
28. Wood M: Anesthesia claims decrease, *Anesthesia Patient Safety Foundation Newsletter* 1:21, 1986.

CHAPTER 41

Hemodynamic Monitoring

BRUCE D. SPIESS

Blood Pressure Monitoring
   Noninvasive methods
   Invasive methods
Central Venous Pressure Monitoring and
   Pulmonary Artery Catheter Monitoring
Noninvasive Determination of Cardiac Output
Summary

Hemodynamic monitoring is a vital part of the anesthesiologist's daily practice. Extensive understanding of the technology available and its function, limitations, applications, and complications is basic to modern practice of anesthesiology. Residents and young practitioners are often enamored of the "flashy technology" available, but the thrill of that electronic data gathering must be tempered by vigilant attention to patient care. Use of all the practitioner's senses forms the basis for hemodynamic monitoring. Palpation, inspection, and listening still are the cornerstones of data gathering. Not very long ago, a finger on the pulse was the only available hemodynamic monitor beyond a simple blood pressure cuff. Still, a great deal of information can be gathered from inspecting for peripheral perfusion, feeling the temperature of extremities, inspecting for cyanosis, and listening to esophageal breath and heart sounds. Indeed, if invasive and automated monitoring systems fail, those clinical skills are the only available data-gathering techniques that allow the clinician to ensure the patient a safe anesthetic. However, the skills just enumerated are highly individualized and the data gathered are subjective. There is no way to quantitate hemodynamic parameters measured by these techniques other than the heart rate. Therefore complex, mechanical, independent methods must be used if scientific, verifiable data are to be gathered.

The Latin *monere* means to warn or remind, and from it the word *monitor* is derived. The goal of all monitoring technology should be to give early warning to the practitioner so that patient care may be optimized. Included in that purpose is avoidance of preventable human errors or the early detection of such errors so that they may be corrected. Ultimately, application of monitoring technologies should improve patient care and therefore affect outcome.

The operating room and the crititical care unit are hostile environments for electronic technology. Under the best of circumstances, data acquisition may be impaired by interference. The clinician must be able to evaluate data generated by each individual technology. **Accuracy, reproducibility, specificity, sensitivity, and predictability are all features that affect usefulness of data delivered from any instrumentation.** Data that are reproducible but are not very accurate are of limited use or are potentially dangerous in the dynamic operating room situation. Invasiveness, rate and type of complications, ease of use, real-time vs. delayed data acquisition, and continuous vs. intermittent data input all affect the actual use of monitors. This chapter will outline available hemodynamic technologies and their use, application, and impact on patient care. The reader is cautioned to always be critical of these technologies, to be cognizant of those features that impact on their use, and to remember that any monitor is only as good as the human who ultimately decides patient care based on its output.

BLOOD PRESSURE MONITORING

For many patients, blood pressure monitoring, ECG, and pulse oximetry may provide adequate hemodynamic data for a routine anesthetic. Blood pressure within any portion of the vascular compartment represents the potential energy for perfusion contained within the bloodstream at that point and is therefore one of the most basic measurements of the cardiovascular system. Knowing the blood pressure is useful, but it can also be misleading. It is possible to have normal blood pressure or even quite elevated pressure and have a low cardiac output. In this case, systemic vascular resistance (SVR) would be elevated. Cardiac output can decrease to a level of severe organ hypoperfusion. Of course the opposite may also be true: a high cardiac output in a vasodilated patient, as seen in septic shock, may result in near-normal blood pressures. Therefore a normal blood pressure alone is an important hemodynamic finding but not one that proves normal hemodynamic function.

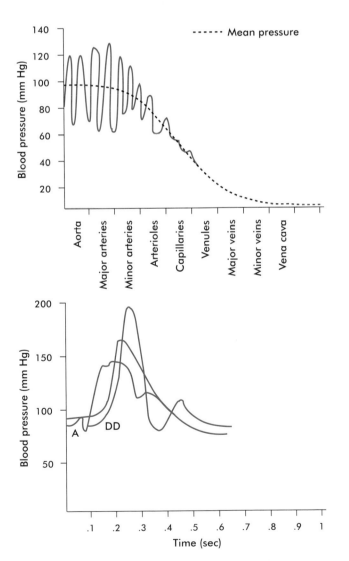

Fig. 41-1. Blood pressure as measured from different arterial and venous sites. Notice the different waveforms seen in the proximal (axillary artery) and progressively more distal (femoral and dorsalis pedis) arterial positions.

The pressure within either the arterial or venous circulation varies (Fig. 41-1), changing with both the cardiac and respiratory cycles. Therefore measurement of the blood pressure must be referenced to the site and measuring technique. Waveforms created by ejection of blood from the left ventricle are affected by the caliber of the vessels and any intercurrent obstructions. As blood flows down a tapered vessel, confinement of the pressure waveform occurs. Also, when a pressure wave meets a complete or partial obstruction, some of its energy is reflected. The subsequent pulse waves meeting that reflected wave are either partially enhanced or cancelled, depending on the wave's phasic overlap.

The speed of the advancing pressure wave with each cardiac cycle far exceeds the actual blood flow velocity.[39] In the aorta that speed may be 15 times faster than the flow of blood, whereas in an end-artery the pressure wave velocity may be as much as 100 times the speed of forward blood flow. The distensibility of the vascular tissue varies in many of the microenvironments of the arterial tree.[41] Therefore it is unreasonable to expect that blood pressures measured at different regions should be equal. With reasonable standardization of techniques and reproducibility of results, blood pressure can be a useful clinical tool.

Each method of measuring blood pressure has inherent inaccuracies, as well as artifacts, that actually change the derived reading. Therefore there is no easy way to know what the *true blood pressure* is. Not uncommonly, clinicians compare invasive and noninvasive blood pressures at the bedside and try to decide which technology to believe before treatment is instituted. Unfortunately, all too often the one chosen is the number that appears to be "the best" (i.e., a preconceived number closest to the physician's biases about the patient's condition). Understanding the limitations of the systems employed is necessary. When both invasive and noninvasive technologies are available and properly used, the site, system, and errors should be understood before deciding which to follow for treatment.

Noninvasive Methods

Noninvasive blood pressure measuring techniques use a cuff with an inflatable bladder applied to an extremity. The bladder inflation must be sufficient to occlude blood flow within the encaptured artery. Pressure must be transmitted from the cuff to the underlying tissues, therefore losing some energy in the process. Standards for size of blood pressure cuffs have been developed. If a cuff is too narrow for an extremity, higher pressures will be required to occlude the underlying artery. Artifactually elevated blood pressure readings result. The opposite is also true: a relatively wide cuff will yield a lower blood pressure reading.[55]

The bladder width ideally should be 40% of the circumference of the extremity to which it is applied. It does not matter whether pressure is determined from the upper arm, forearm, thigh, or calf; the rule still applies. The bladder length must be sufficient to encircle at least 60% of the extremity. Eighty percent is a better length and is used as the standard. There is no harm in actually having the bladder overlap as long as the blood pressure cuff can be secured. The standard size for each age group is shown in Table 41-1.

Normal systolic blood pressure is at its lowest level at birth or in the neonate (60 to 70 mm Hg), increasing in children ages 7 to 10 years (90 to 95 mm Hg). In adolescence, the normal level increases to 100 to 110 mm Hg and continues to increase throughout the aging process as the arterial tree stiffens. Hypotension and hypertension must always be qualified depending on the age group studied or the particular patient being monitored.

At the turn of the century Korotkoff noted that "short tones" may be auscultated distal to a Rivva-Rocci blood pressure cuff when its pressure was between systolic and diastolic pressure. Since his initial description, noises heard during auscultation of an artery as a blood pressure cuff is deflated have been referred to as Korotkoff sounds.[19] The physiologic basis for these sounds is the sudden reexpansion of the arterial walls distal to the cuff as a bolus or spurt of blood passes. Such a jet of blood apparently snaps the arterial walls and causes turbulent flow-producing sounds.[54]

If a clinician has excellent auscultatory skills, five different phases of sounds can be detected as the blood pressure cuff is deflated.[47,55] Phase I occurs after the pressure in the bladder drops such that a first tapping sound occurs. In phase II the tapping sounds give way to an actual bruit. Phase III is defined as the point where the sounds take on a more continuous nature, giving way to a muffled sound. Phase IV occurs when the muffling of the sounds becomes pervasive and the sound almost disappears. Phase V is the point at which the sounds actually do disappear. Systolic pressure corresponds closely to the sounds recorded at phase I. Diastolic pressure corresponds most closely to the end of phase IV or phase V. These phases, of course, are observer dependent. The skill of the practitioner using the stethoscope is important in determining accurate blood pressures. This may not be a problem in a normotensive individual, but in a patient who is hpotensive or in a noisy environment such as the recovery room, intensive care unit, or busy operating room, errors in measurement are sometimes large.[67]

Other methods of manual detection of blood pressure are possible besides listening for Korotkoff sounds. An oscillation method has been used but its limitations must be realized. If a manometer is attached to a standard cuff, oscillations will be seen near the systolic pressure. There is some argument whether the point of initial oscillation or the point of maximum oscillation should be used for determining systolic pressure. Maximum oscillation may be accurate within 30 mm Hg (not acceptable accuracy), and correlation of same with mean arterial pressure is perhaps better than with systolic pressure.[67]

Detection of the initial pulse wave transmitted to an artery distal to a blood pressure cuff may also be used to estimate systolic pressure. Fingertip palpation of the radial artery for the first transmitted pulsation can give a reasonable estimation of systolic blood pressure. Using this method for estimation of diastolic pressure is not reasonable. Pulse oximeters, fingertip plethysmographs, or other photoelectric pulse detectors can be mounted distal to the blood pressure cuff and used to detect the first initial pulse. Like the oscillation method these techniques can estimate systolic pressure, but they also seem to have a number of inaccuracies and therefore are not generally recommended for the operating rooms.

The use of automated blood pressure recording devices is so prevalent that the previous methods just described may now appear antiquated to the new resident in this specialty. An explosion of devices has occurred such that there are now scores of companies marketing noninvasive automated blood pressure

Table 41-1 Recommended blood pressure cuff standards

Arm circumference* at midpoint (cm)	Cuff type	Bladder dimensions	
		Width (cm)	Length (cm)
5-7.5	Newborn	3	5
7.5-13	Infant	5	8
13-20	Child	8	13
17-26	Small adult	11	17
24-32	Adult	13	24
32-42	Large adult	17	32
42-50†	Thigh adult	20	42

*Midpoint of the arm is halfway between acronion to olecranon.
†In persons of larger dimensions blood pressure may be measured in the leg or forearm.
From Kirkendall WM, Feinleib M, Freis ED et al: Recommendations for human blood pressure determination by sphygmomanometers: Subcommittee of the AHA Postgraduate Education Committee, *News from the American Heart Association* 1146A, 1981 (AHA reprint booklet 70-019-B).

systems. Every operating room and postanesthesia recovery station visited in the last few years has possessed such a device. It would seem to be a near requirement for anyone designing such facilities to include these machines, with sufficient backup units. Such devices offer the anesthesiologist a true time savings in the operating room. They free the practitioner for other necessary duties and also offer the advantage of automatic cycling. Therefore the patient is monitored at defined intervals and not just when the practitioner remembers to look at the blood pressure. Perhaps that automaticity coupled with some alerting system actually does enhance the vigilance of the anesthesia care team.

Automated machines that use an auscultatory technique have had problems with accuracy and will not be discussed.[44] Oscillometry devices are today's technology. The mechanism depends on sensing oscillations caused by arterial pulsation transmitted from the deflating blood pressure cuff. The amplitude of the oscillations has a relationship to systolic pressure (Fig. 41-2). An algorithm for estimation of systolic and diastolic pressures is constructed based on the point of maximum oscillation. The point of maximum oscillation closely approximates mean blood pressure. The individual algorithms used vary between manufacturers and are therefore proprietary information. For example, sometimes the definition of systolic pressure is the pressure at which the amplitude of the ascending oscillatory curve is 50% of the maximum oscillation.[34] Studies have shown that the actual correlation may vary between 45% and 57% of the maximum amplitude when the systolic blood pressure is between 100 and 195 mm Hg.[33] However, when hypotension occurs these relationships may not always be maintained.

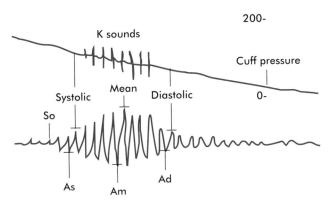

Fig. 41-2. Oscillometric measurement of blood pressure as compared to Korotkoff sounds. *So,* the initial point of cuff oscillation; *As,* auscultatory systolic pressure; *Am,* auscultatory mean blood pressure; *Ad* point at which diastolic blood pressure would be read by auscultation. (From Geddes LA: *Cardiovascular devices and their applications,* New York, 1984, John Wiley & Sons.)

Measurement of the mean pressure by this method also depends somewhat on the technique or algorithm developed by an individual manufacturer. Mean pressure may be physiologically defined by a number of different methods. To simply say that it is the arithmetic average of pressures is too simplistic. The most exact method of determining mean pressure from invasive monitoring is to integrate the area under the pressure-time curve and divide by the total time required for one cardiac cycle. Another method is to average all the measured pressures (oscillometrically) over one cardiac cycle—the Archimedes method. Or a geometric mean method may be defined wherein the pressure time curve is divided into two halves of equal area and the mean pressure is the point that defines the center of these two halves. These methods do *not* always produce the same numbers. Oscillometry techniques assume that the point of maximum oscillation amplitude corresponds to the approximate mean arterial pressure. Several clinical and theoretic studies have shown that this technique may, if anything, underestimate mean pressure. Sometimes error as great as 20% has been reported.[17,27,89] The reader should, by now, appreciate the complexity of measuring something as seemingly mundane as blood pressure.

The diastolic pressure measuring technique also varies from one automated equipment manufacturer to the next. They also use algorithms that examine relationships between the smallest detectable oscillations and the maximum oscillations.

The overall accuracy of these automated methods of detecting blood pressure is difficult to discern because every technique of measurement has inherent errors. One study of cardiac patients did examine mean blood pressure as measured by oscillometry vs. invasive techniques. Eighty-five percent of the readings by oscillometry were within 10 mm Hg of the corresponding measurements by an invasive method.[130] Bruner et al. disagreed, reporting a much less accurate correlation between oscillometric and direct measures.[17]

Another noninvasive automated technique has recently been introduced—photoplethysmography. Unlike the oscillometry methods that use arm or thigh cuffs, this method employs a small fingertip cuff. The external pressure exerted by this cuff is continuously maintained equal to that inside the digital artery such that the artery does not collapse. Blood flow to the finger is measured by infrared light transmission under the cuff, and a very rapidly reacting servo mechanism maintains the pressures throughout each cardiac cycle.[13,81,82] Heart rate and systolic, diastolic, and mean arterial pressures can be derived from such a system with a continuous readout. A calibration set-up procedure is required to find the maximum oscillation of pressure and calibrate mean arterial pressure from that. Once that has been set, an internal calibration must reset the system. This system is a continuous pulsatile monitor and may offer the advantage of working in a nonpulsatile environment such as cardiopulmonary bypass,[75] which, of course, is not the case for automated oscillometry.

A number of studies have compared the photoplethysmography technique with invasively gathered blood pressure data with satisfactory results.[59,109,123] There does appear to be some systematic error involved and at least one report has noted that this system reports lower systolic pressures than invasive systems.[123] They noted that error may be as much 13 mm Hg.[123] Two studies have compared this system to a routine automated oscillometry technique.[23,26] The oscillometry values for systolic pressures were consistently 7 mm Hg lower than those recorded by photoplethysmography. That difference may be explained by the fact that the oscillometry measurements were taken from the brachial artery, whereas the photoplethysmography measurements were taken from a more distal arterial system, the digital artery. Artifacts of pressure wave reflection and systolic augmentation do occur in such distal arteries.

Indeed, the authors note that when this new system is used continuously, its accuracy should be occasionally checked against routine automated oscillometry.[23,26,123] It is unclear where photoplethysmography will eventually fit into the armamentarium of blood pressure monitors. The technique so far has not been successfully applied to infants and neonates, and it should be more extensively tested in critically ill patients to establish its full applications.

Complications of the noninvasive blood pressure monitoring systems are seldom noted. If skinfolds or wrinkles are caught under the blood pressure cuff there is a potential for bruising or petechiae formation. Excessive cycling of an automated oscillometry system may cause peripheral ischemia. Cycling of older equipment may take up to 45 seconds to acquire blood pressure data. If a system cycles in a "STAT" mode every minute, a potential for tissue ischemia exists. The extremity could have the blood flow occluded 75% of the time. The photoplethysmography system needs to be widely tested, but there is concern about digital blood flow in states of shock. Unrecognized artifact is a real concern; patients have been treated based on aberrant numbers.

Invasive Methods

Although the previously mentioned techniques do have the advantage of being noninvasive, it should be obvious from the discussion that each has limitations. In 1949 Peterson et al. published their report of continuous recording of the brachial artery pressure of a human subject using a polyvinyl plastic catheter.[83] Development of hollow metal needles in the midnineteenth century had previously permitted measurement of arterial pressures during surgery using attached manometers. In 1934 Hamilton developed a brass membrane that could produce an optical tracing of blood pressure when attached to a needle and cannula.[40] In 1946 Lambert and Wood reported radial arterial cannulation and monitoring during human centrifugation experiments using the resistance wire strain gauge transducer, which is essentially unchanged today.[61] Peterson's technique reported in 1949 was the forerunner of today's routinely employed radial artery cannulation method.[83]

Today's invasive blood pressure monitoring systems use plastic or Teflon catheters, hollow, thick-walled tubing, electronic resistance wire strain gauge–based transducers, and oscillographic and/or hard copy monitors. These systems have inherent properties that affect measurement of blood pressure. Therefore something of the physics of the system and its component parts should be understood.

Cannula size depends on size of the artery (and patient) to be monitored. For routine radial artery cannulation a 20-gauge catheter is most widely employed although 18-gauge catheters have been used. The larger catheters may be more difficult to insert and occlude a greater portion of the arterial lumen. Smaller size catheters may be appropriate for the dorsalis pedis artery or for children (sizes 22 to 24). For femoral or axillary artery cannulation an 18-gauge, 12-cm catheter may be employed because smaller and shorter length catheters may kink or become dislodged from these larger arteries. Most catheters used are manufactured from Teflon because it is softer and less thrombogenic and offers an advantage for long-term placement.

Fluid-filled connecting tubing forms the mechanical link between the invasive cannula and the electronic transducer. The most ideal system, with the least distortion, would have the transducer directly connected to a metal needle. This is not desirable in the operating room or critical care setting. In contrast, the worst recording system might employ long distensible tubing with several stopcocks between the cannula and the transducer. Distensible tubing allows loss of kinetic energy and the stopcocks provide excellent places for trapping bubbles. The length of the connecting tubing should be limited to approximately 120 cm; however, a length of 60 cm is much better. The tubing should be thick walled with an internal lumenal diameter between 1.5 and 3 mm. The least number of stopcocks possible should be used in the line.[86]

All pressure-monitoring systems attempt to accurately convert the physical energy of pressure-induced

movements of a transducer diaphragm to electrical energy. The electrical signals can be calibrated proportional to changes in the inducing pressures. The fidelity with which the entire system performs is dependent on the transducer, its electrical components, and the previously mentioned parts (cannula, tubing, and stopcocks). The entire system behaves somewhat like a piston moving in a cylinder whose motion compresses a spring.[56] The components of a piston-spring system involve inertial forces (fluid movement in the catheter), elastic forces (the transducer diaphragm), and frictional forces (the viscosity of the fluid filling the tubing). If a mass attached to a spring is displaced from its equilibrium position, it creates a motion described as harmonic. That motion would create a sine wave if traced on a recording paper (Fig. 41-3). The number of oscillations/unit time are known as the frequency of the harmonic. In an ideal setting without frictional forces, if such a spring and mass system were set in motion, the harmonic frequency would proceed at the same rate for an infinite time. In the real world and in our monitoring system friction does occur. This is the interaction of the fluid with the catheter walls and resistance to movement of the diaphragm itself. That interaction is called *damping* and allows the decay of any natural oscillatory frequency back to baseline. The amount of damping of any system is important.

If there is no damping and the system oscillates indefinitely, it is called *undamped*. If there is just enough damping to prevent any oscillation then there is said to be critical damping. Overdamping occurs when the amount is beyond the critical level and when a mass is displaced from equilibrium, it returns to its equilibrium position in a nonoscillatory way. Obviously for any such "spring and piston" system

(monitoring transducer), there is an optimal degree of damping.

If an external force, such as a beating heart, produces its own oscillatory force and the frequency with which it drives the system corresponds to the undamped natural frequency of the system, then resonance occurs. Critically damped and overdamped systems cannot resonate, but they also cannot produce the most accurate pressure waveforms.

Hooke's law of the force on a spring is defined as:

$$F = kx$$

Where F = force (pressure is force/unit inside surface area), k = the spring constant, x = the position of a piston. Substituting pressure for the force, the equation can then be rewritten:

$$P = kx/A$$

or

$$x = (A/k)P$$

If x is the displacement of a piston or the movement of the transducer diaphragm, then the output voltage of the transducer can be made proportional to the pressure exerted on the transducer. The sensitivity of the transducer depends on how much movement is produced for each increment of pressure. Transducers sensitive to 1 to 2 mm Hg increment changes are adequate for use in clinical monitoring situations.

When a pressure waveform strikes the transducer, there is some inertial movement beyond the point of equilibrium to which the diaphragm would move if the same amount of pressure had been applied much more slowly. This excess is referred to as *overshoot*. In a very sensitive or compliant transducer, the amount of overshoot can be quite large and the diaphragm will oscillate with greater amplitude and slower frequency than in a tighter less sensitive diaphragm. The natural frequency of oscillation of the transducer system can be increased by decreasing the area of the membrane or by decreasing its compliance. If a transducer is tested with test waves, it should produce output that matches the input until the frequency of the input test wave is 0.2 times the natural frequency of the transducer system. That output is referred to as a "flat" frequency response curve. To avoid overshoot and undershoot, the transducer used should have a natural resonant frequency of five times or greater than the frequency pattern to be monitored. In a simplistic model of the human heart beating at a near maximum heart rate of 180 beats/minute (3 Hz), a transducer with a resonant frequency of at least 15 Hz is necessary.

Unfortunately, the biologic systems monitored do not produce simple sine waves of pulse by cardiac action. Arterial pulse waveforms are complex sum-

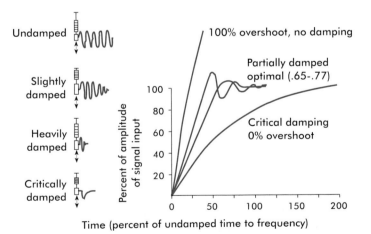

Fig. 41-3. Schematic representation of undamped to critically damped spring systems analogous to the transducers used in pressure monitoring systems.

mations of 6 to 10 harmonic sine waves superimposed (Fig. 41-4).[43] Therefore transducers should have resonant frequencies not at 15 Hz but at 10 times that level or at 150 Hz. Unfortunately, such a system is generally not practical, and other physical characteristics—namely damping—must be added to the system to overcome this problem.

Damping is added to keep the system from approaching its natural frequency and therefore "ringing." If it were undamped and allowed to be driven near its natural frequency, the transducer would destroy itself. All systems are damped by friction and the viscosity of the fluid filling the catheter. As discussed previously, the amount of damping must be optimal. Damping factors between 0.64 and 0.77 are thought to be optimal for blood pressure monitoring.

Another method of introducing damping is to have a bubble within the system. The bubble itself acts as a spring-loaded physical factor and therefore can reduce the natural frequency of the entire system. By so doing it may bring the entire transducer system out of conformity with the ideal system outlined previously. A small bubble can decrease the resonant frequency from 20 Hz to 8 to 10 Hz.[17] Indeed, such an occurrence would cause an overshoot of the systolic pressure and an underestimation of the diastolic pressure. One such artifactually produced experiment showed that changes of systolic pressure from 150 to 191 mm Hg and diastolic pressures from 50 to 47 mm Hg could be produced by varying the characteristics of the bubble.[104] The optimal system must provide adequate damping without decreasing the natural resonant frequency of the entire transducer system.

This can be accomplished with changes in fluid viscosity or addition of an impedance to fluid movement (catheter and tubing size).[1]

Movement of catheters within arteries and reflectance of pressure waves from end arteries introduce more artifact. It can be readily appreciated from the discussion of physical characteristics of transducers that artifact is a real influence on invasive monitoring.

Techniques for arterial catheter placement are numerous. Prepackaged arterial catheterization kits are also available. Some have cannulas with preplaced insertion wires. Successful placement of a radial artery catheter is like so many other techniques in medicine in that its successful practice is enhanced by experience and careful evaluation of anatomy before proceeding. Extension of the wrist will lift and elevate the radial artery so that it is more stabilized in the tissue planes (Fig. 41-5). Palpation of good pulsation is necessary. Palpation with two or three fingers gently to appreciate the pulse but not to occlude blood flow will outline the course of the artery. A gentle rolling of the fingertips medially and laterally will further outline the extent of arterial pulsation. Often the radial artery lies immediately adjacent to the flexor carpi radialis tendon, and, if its pulsation is not immediately obvious or if it is diffuse, the clinician should proceed medially until this landmark is found (Fig. 41-6). The skin in an awake patient should be adequately anesthetized with local anesthetic before insertion. The skin overlying the artery is quite sensitive, and the artery has a tendency to spasm so adequate dosages of anesthetic may help relieve this problem. The catheter-needle combination should be placed at a 30- to 45-degree angle to the skin in the long plane of the artery's course. Skin puncture with a slightly larger gauge needle has been contended to be helpful in preventing "burring" of the cannula itself when it passes through the dermis, but this has not ever been definitely proved. Any such imperfec-

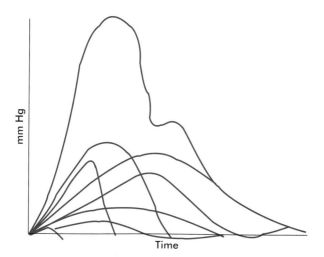

Fig. 41-4. Resultant final waveform recorded with invasive blood pressure measurements represents the summation of multiple harmonic waveforms present within the arterial tree. NOTE: This is a schematic demonstration and the pictured waveforms will not add up to the arterial waveform depicted.

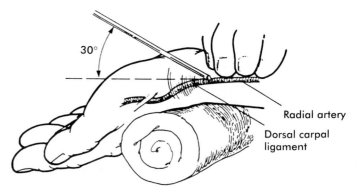

Fig. 41-5. Proper dorsiflexion of the wrist stabilizes the radial artery and eases cannulation.

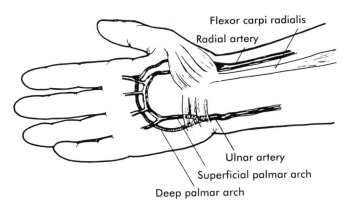

Fig. 41-6. Basic anatomic considerations of the radial and ulnar arteries. Note that the radial artery lies in very close proximity to the flexor carpi radialis tendon.

Labels: Flexor carpi radialis; Radial artery; Ulnar artery; Superficial palmar arch; Deep palmar arch

tion of the catheter will likely prevent it from advancing easily in the artery. The catheter/needle should always be filled with liquid (preferably heparinized saline) to allow the "flash" of arterial entrance to be instantly observed. The artery should be cannulated slowly and deliberately with continuous fingertip palpation of the arterial pulse. Once initial blood return is noticed, it is important to be sure that the cannula itself is in the arterial lumen before attempting to pass the catheter or the cannulation wire. Some practitioners prefer to use a transfixion (Seldinger) technique wherein the needle and cannula are passed through the entire artery and withdrawn until blood return is noted. If a guide wire is used and the catheter cannot be threaded, it is very important to not shear the guide wire by attempting to remove it forcibly against the needle. Failure of the catheter to advance is most often caused by not having the catheter's tip totally within the lumen of the artery.

The radial artery is often cannulated just proximal to the head of the radius or even more proximally. As it is followed more proximally it is more deeply imbedded in tissue and therefore often requires a more experienced "touch" to perceive its location and course. It can be a tortuous artery, particularly in elderly people with peripheral vascular disease, but it can also be cannulated between the proximal metacarpal bones in the anatomic snuffbox.[7,88]

It is possible to cannulate the ulnar artery. The ulnar and radial arteries represent end arteries of the brachial artery; together they feed the palmar arch. It is therefore *not* wise to attempt to cannulate one if the other has already been compromised.

The dorsalis pedis artery is an extension of the anterior tibial artery and can be palpated for cannulation over the dorsum of the foot as it courses superficial to the second or third metatarsals. It may

provide an alternative to the radial artery if that has already been cannulated or is thrombosed. My experience is that caution should be observed in using this artery in patients with diabetic circulatory problems as the potential for ulceration may be markedly enhanced.

The axillary artery is often quite easy to palpate, even in obese patients. One needs to remember the anatomic relationship of the brachial plexus and especially warn awake patients of possible paresthesias. This site is not widely used because catheters may become easily dislodged both intraoperatively and, particularly, postoperatively.

The femoral artery offers advantages and disadvantages. It is a large superficial artery and, therefore, should be relatively easy to cannulate. In patients with atherosclerotic disease that may not always be the case, and, even though initial arterial puncture is accomplished, a guide wire may become lodged in an atheroma. Often a flexible J wire can be passed. Caution must be used when cannulating the femoral artery to stay distal to the level of the inguinal ligament to avoid any chance of intraperitoneal passage of the cannula.

The assessment of adequacy of circulation before cannula insertion has been controversial. In the past, practitioners have used the Allen's test before cannulation of the radial artery to try to accomplish this goal. The Allen's test is performed by having a cooperative patient clench his/her fist to evacuate the blood of the hand while both the radial and ulnar arteries are occluded with the examiner's digital pressure. When the digital pressure is released from either the radial or the ulnar artery, refill should be seen in the hand within 5 to 7 seconds. The same procedure may be performed with release of the other artery to check its flow. Unfortunately, **complications of radial artery cannulation are *not* related to the adequacy or inadequacy of this test. Few practitioners today use it to make clinical decisions about whether or not to cannulate a radial artery. It is *not* of medicolegal importance either.**

In one study wherein radial artery cannulations took place despite an Allen's test showing inadequate collateralization, there was no evidence of ischemia in the 16 patients studied.[108] The incidence of congenitally or pathologically absent collaterals in the hand was 3% to 5% in one study and up to 10.4% in a group of older patients.[48,49] Ischemic damage to the hand or digits is extremely rare after radial artery cannulation and is probably not due to presence of patency of the other artery. Causes for ischemic damage include emboli, excessive trauma from long or large catheters, hypotension and shock states, prolonged use of high dosages of vasoconstrictors, presence of Raynaud's disease, and hypercoagulation due to hyperlipoproteinemia.* Reports of ischemic injury can be found in patients who had normal collateral blood flows by Allen's test.[4,18,69] Twenty-five percent to 50% of radial arteries are thrombosed by the time they are decannulated without major long-term sequelae because recanalization occurs in nearly all such vessels. Data from the surgical literature have shown that traumatic injury to the radial artery or even surgical ligation of it will not necessarily cause infarction or atrophy of distal tissues.[15,35,76,131] Therefore there is no reason to perform an Allen's test before radial artery cannulation.

There are some significant variations in recording of blood pressure from different cannulation sites in patients who are hypothermic or hypotensive or after cardiopulmonary bypass. Radial artery pressure after cardiopulmonary bypass may be quite different from that taken in a subclavian artery or femoral artery, by as much as 20% in some patients. For the majority of patients, that level of difference is not seen.[31,73,80,95,115] Some centers have gone to routine use of femoral arterial cannulas for their cardiopulmonary bypass cases because of these variations.

If disconnected, the 18-gauge size of femoral artery cannulas can lead to very rapid exsanguination with blood flows of up to 500 ml/min possible.[62] The femoral artery cannulation site is not at greater risk for infection than is a routine radial catheter.[118] Actually catheters placed at any site by cutdown have a higher incidence of infection than those placed percutaneously. In patients confined to bed (such as those in intensive care units) fecal microorganisms can be cultured from virtually any site. The thought that the femoral artery poses more infection risk is simply not true.

CENTRAL VENOUS PRESSURE MONITORING AND PULMONARY ARTERY CATHETER MONITORING

Invasive monitoring of the central circulation allows an estimate of cardiac preload. The placement of a catheter in the right atrium or very low superior vena cava yields a characteristic pressure waveform (Fig. 41-7). The supposition is that the mean central venous pressure (CVP) is reflective of right ventricular end-diastolic pressure. Those pressures should therefore be indicative of right ventricular filling. Unfortunately for this assumption, the right ventricle is a compliant cardiac chamber, and the relationship between changes in volume and changes in reflected pressure is not a straight line. The CVP does not always follow left ventricular filling, and at times it

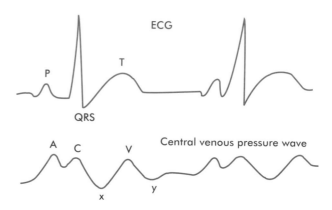

Fig. 41-7. Normal central venous pressure waveform compared to the ECG.

may trend in the opposite direction from pulmonary artery occlusion pressures.[99]

For either CVP or pulmonary artery (PA) monitoring, access to the central circulation must be gained. Anesthesiologists most often use the internal jugular vein as their approach. The basilic vein, external jugular, and subclavian approaches may be used in operating rooms, and it is wise for the anesthesiologist to be proficient at each of these techniques.

Cannulation of the internal jugular vein is a semi-blind technique but one that can be accomplished with a high degree of success if the anatomy involved is understood. There are at least three major approaches used, but the most common are the anterior and the median approaches. The internal jugular vein in the right side of the neck is most often cannulated because (1) it is convenient for right handed practitioners, (2) there is no thoracic duct on the right side, and (3), once cannulated, there is a relatively straight line for cannulation of the superior vena cava. The left internal jugular can be used, but caution should be used if attempting to cannulate it if attempts have already been made on the right side. Any time any such central venous access is attempted, the potential for a pneumothorax is always present. It is therefore important not to chance having a bilateral pneumothorax.

The internal jugular vein courses through the neck immediately deep to the body of the sternocleidomastoid muscle somewhat posterior and lateral to the carotid artery (Fig. 41-8). As it progresses caudally, it emerges from the body of the muscle to lie directly between the anterior and medial heads of that muscle. The anterior approach to cannulation is performed in the following manner. The pulsation of the carotid artery is appreciated with two fingers along the course. With those fingers defining its anatomy an explorer needle of small gauge is passed over the

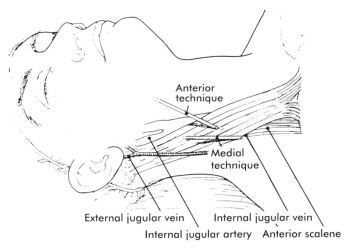

Fig. 41-8. Anterior and medial approaches to cannulation of the internal jugular vein. Note that the medial approach starts lower in the neck than does the anterior approach.

fingers under the body of the sternocleidomastoid muscle in the direction of the ipsilateral nipple. In most patients the internal jugular vein should be encountered within 2 to 4 cm. A syringe with constant negative pressure should be applied to the exploring needle so that a flash of blood will signify entrance into the vein. The jugular vein is easily compressed, especially if the venous pressure is not high. Most often cannulation should be attempted with the patient in the Trendelenburg position. Even then sometimes blood return may not be encountered until the needle is being withdrawn. If the carotid artery is encountered with the small-gauge seeking needle, trauma should be minimized. After the internal jugular vein has been located, a larger 18-gauge needle may be placed along the same path. Once this cannulation has been accomplished, it is wise to either transduce or attach a tubing to effect a manometer so that one can objectively assure that the carotid artery has not been accidently entered. Blood gases may also be obtained if there is doubt about whether the source of blood return is venous or arterial. The return of dark blood or the lack of pulsatile flow may not always be adequate indicators to assure that a carotid artery puncture is diagnosed.

Once the internal jugular vein is cannulated, a guide wire is passed followed by the final indwelling catheter. The type of catheter will vary from one practitioner to another and from one institution to another. Single or multiple lumen catheters are available for central venous pressure monitoring and infusions. If a pulmonary artery catheter is to be placed, a larger 8.5 French introducer should be placed.

The medial approach to the internal jugular vein is performed in the same manner as just described

except that the seeker needle and the eventual cannulation needle are introduced between the sternocleidomastoid and the anterior scalene muscle at the apex of the triangle that they form. The needle is again advanced toward the ipsilateral nipple until blood return is encountered.

Use of an exploring ("seeker") needle is controversial. Many believe it unnecessary and even potentially hindering to deliberately puncture the vein more than absolutely necessary because the resultant hematoma on removal immediately begins to compress the vein, making the actual cannulation more difficult.

Potential complications of internal jugular cannulation include the following: (1) failure to cannulate, (2) hematoma, (3) pneumothorax, (4) damage to brachial plexus, (5) carotid artery puncture, (6) hemothorax, (7) Horner's syndrome, and (8) chylothorax. Carotid artery puncture has been reported to occur in 2% of experienced attempts at performing the technique.[16] If a large bore introducer sheath is inadvertently placed into the carotid artery, it is recommended that neck exploration and repair be undertaken.[16] Local pressure will be helpful particularly if the needle puncture is small. Another alternative may be to prep the neck as part of the surgical site and be prepared to explore it should an expanding hematoma become apparent.[77]

Pneumothorax is a rare complication of internal jugular cannulation in experienced hands. There are no studies to show that one technique of insertion has any lower rate of complications than another. There is certainly a lower rate of pneumothorax with internal jugular cannulation vs. subclavian puncture.[45]

In patients with preexisting coagulopathy, it is important to carefully select the route of central line access. Basilic vein and external jugular routes allow the most easily accessible assessment for bleeding and the ability to tamponade or repair a bleeder. The internal jugular may be less preferable. Perhaps the least desirable approach is subclavian. If hemorrhage occurs into the pleura, it may go unnoticed until either hemodynamic compromise or lung compression becomes evident.

Air embolism is a potentially lethal consequence of central venous access. It is prudent to inspect intravenous lines for even small amounts of air before allowing them to be attached to the central line. During the process of cannulation, attention to technique is necessary to ensure that no air can gain entry through needles or cannulas as they are placed. Disconnections of the intravenous line from the central cannula, either in the Critical Care Unit or during transport, can cause air embolism or exsanguination. The PA catheter introducer contains a self-sealing rubber valve on its proximal end. Failure of this has been implicated as a source of air embolism. If the seal is defective or if a PA catheter has been in place for a prolonged period of time, the seal may leak.[22,125]

Catheter displacement or guide wire embolization are other potential problems that can occur. It is important to maintain control of these tools of cannulation so that they are *never* lost below the skin surface. The introducer wire should *never* be forcibly withdrawn through a needle because it is possible for it to shear off the wire end and embolize it to the right heart or pulmonary circulation.[9]

Once central venous access is secured, it may be used for monitoring or a PA catheter may be placed. Monitoring of pulmonary artery pressures is a method of following left ventricular function. Left ventricular preload is defined as the relative sarcomere stretch or length during end diastole, immediately before isovolumic contraction. This is also defined as LV end-diastolic wall stress, where stress is force/unit fiber cross-sectional area. Certainly in the clinical situation there is no way to measure such a microscopic parameter. Preload can also be approximated by thinking of it as left ventricular wall tension. Again that variable cannot be easily assessed. Left ventricular end-diastolic pressure (LVEDP) has some relationship to both of these true physiologic parameters, but LVEDP is often influenced by ventricular compliance and intraventricular volume. Therefore LVEDP is not always a direct indicator of left ventricular preload, but it has been accepted by clinicians as providing a reasonable estimate of that function. LVEDP should, under ideal circumstances, be reflected by left atrial pressure (again a very compliant heart chamber), which in turn should be reflected in pulmonary artery pressures (see Fig. 41-8).

The PA catheter was originally developed by Swan and Ganz to be flow-directed into the pulmonary artery to give information about patients with complicated myocardial infarctions.[117] In its present use today, the routine PA catheter is a triple lumen 7 French catheter with an imbedded thermistor wire (Fig. 41-9). A distal lumen opens beyond the balloon and is used for monitoring both pulmonary artery and pulmonary artery occlusion (pulmonary capillary wedge) pressures. A second monitoring lumen opens in the side of the catheter 25 cm behind the distal (PA) lumen. This allows continuous monitoring of the right atrial pressures. The third lumen allows balloon inflation so as to allow the catheter to be flow-directed.

The technique for flow-directing a PA catheter must be carried out under exacting sterile technique. Before insertion, the monitoring lumens should be flushed with heparinized saline and connected to proper transducers. The balloon should be checked for proper inflation and defects by inflating and

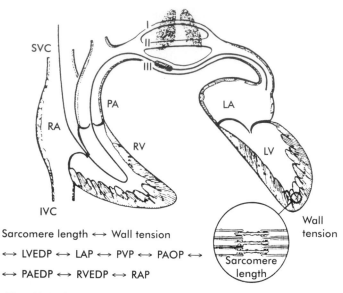

Sarcomere length ↔ Wall tension
↔ LVEDP ↔ LAP ↔ PVP ↔ PAOP ↔
↔ PAEDP ↔ RVEDP ↔ RAP

Fig. 41-9. Prediction of myocardial preload by pressure measurement supposes that pressure measured within various of the cardiac chambers or the pulmonary vasculature has a direct relationship to sarcomere length and wall tension. Such a supposition may be false in many circumstances.

holding with 1.5 ml of air. Care should be taken not to overinflate the balloon. The catheter has a natural curve placed during manufacture and that arc should be positioned so that on insertion the arc will point towards the right atrium, which, when viewed by the practitioner at the patient's head, will point down and left at the approximate 7 o'clock position. Once the catheter has been introduced into the indwelling 8.5 French sheath introducer, it should be advanced slowly to the 20-cm mark. At that point the balloon should be inflated with the full 1.5 ml of air, and inflation should be maintained. If any resistance to inflation is felt or if a sudden loss of the distal pressure wave is found, there may be a technical problem or the catheter may be lodged against either a vessel wall, valve, or the internal lumen of the introducer. The introducer is only 15 cm long, so that by passing the catheter to 20 cm it should be well beyond the end of the introducer and into the superior vena cava. After balloon inflation it is important to advance the catheter slowly and steadily to allow the normal blood flow to direct the PA catheter through the cardiac chambers. A characteristic change in pressure waveforms will be seen as the catheter traverses the right atrium, right ventricle, pulmonary valve, and eventually the pulmonary artery (Fig. 41-10). The catheter should be advanced until a pulmonary artery occlusion is completed, and the waveform changes to show the loss of the characteristic pulmonary artery trace. If a sudden resistance or a loss of the pressure tracing is noted, the catheter tip has become lodged against

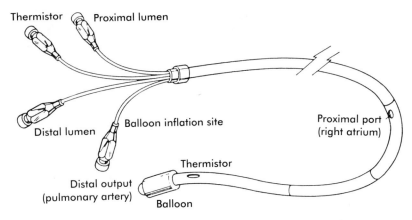

Fig. 41-10. Design of a routine pulmonary artery catheter.

an obstruction. The person placing the catheter must develop a feel for such obstructions and pull the catheter back after balloon deflation. Persistence or overzealous advancement can lead to some of the most feared iatrogenic complications of PA catheter placement.

Once in place, the PA catheter can generate very helpful data. With the catheter advanced to the position of balloon lodgement, a continuous fluid line is created between the catheter and the left atrium. Therefore this pulmonary artery occlusion pressure (PAOP, previously known as pulmonary capillary wedge pressure) is supposed to reflect left atrial pressure and therefore LVEDP. This relationship unfortunately occurs under normal physiologic conditions only and is affected by many internal and external forces.[28,122] Increases in pulmonary vascular resistance may change that special relationship. Diseases such as pulmonary embolism, acidosis, hypoxemia, and parenchymal pulmonary diseases, as well as catecholamine infusions, may affect the reflection of LVEDP in PAOP.[84,125] Tachycardia above a rate of 120 may introduce artifact into PAOP monitoring. Mitral incompetence, whether anatomic (e.g., rheumatic) or functional (e.g., loss of posterior papillary muscle function due to posterior left ventricular wall ischemia due in turn to circumflex inadequacy), can produce large waveforms (so-called V waves) in the PAOP wedge tracing.

When floated into position the PA catheter usually lodges in the right lower lobe of the pulmonary vascular tree. For accurate reflection of PAOP it must be placed in West's zone 3 of the lung. In West's classic descriptions of the pulmonary circulation, an upright individual possesses three zones of lung perfusion. In zone I the pressure in the alveolus (Palv) is greater than the arterial and venous pressures. Therefore little, if any, blood flow occurs. In zone II Palv is larger than PV but less than PA and therefore

the latter forms a resistance to flow. However, in zone III both PV and PA are greater than Palv and continuous flow of blood occurs. Therefore the PA catheter is only accurate in the zone III region of lung tissue. Most often it naturally flow-directs itself there anyway because that is where there is greatest blood flow. If a patient's position is changed, it is possible for the catheter to no longer be lying in zone III. Also, severe hypovolemia, pneumothorax, or excess positive end-expiratory pressure (PEEP) may convert a zone III region of the lung into a zone I or II physiology.

A routine chest radiograph may be helpful in diagnosing a PA catheter that has not gone to zone III. Also, if the following characteristics are found, one should suspect that the catheter is not appropriately placed: (1) the pulmonary artery end-diastolic pressure *cannot* be less than the PAOP and would be if blood would flow backward (which does not happen), (2) there is a totally flat PAOP trace, and (3) there is complete transfer of PEEP alveolar pressure to the PAOP.[8]

PEEP cannot only cause a change in the West zones of the lung but can also decrease cardiac venous return and change ventricular filling. Left ventricular compliance may change as well. The increase in pulmonary pressure may change the transmural pressure of the myocardial wall.[78] Usually a PEEP level below 10 mm Hg has little effect, and the normal relationship of PAOP to LVEDP appears to hold true.

Other factors that affect left ventricular compliance include valvular heart disease, hypertension, ischemia, and catecholamine therapy. Vasodilator therapy may increase ventricular compliance as well as decrease LVEDP. If compliance is held constant, there is a curvilinear relationship that relates LV volume to ventricular pressure. Heart function may be shifted from one curve to another depending on compliance. Routine PA catheter monitoring allows for "snapshot" measurements in time, but one may not know from the single data points on which pressure volume curve the heart is functioning. Shifts in cardiac compliance are dynamic. A sudden change in PAOP cannot always be inferred to be caused solely by changes in volume.

It is also possible for a significant diastolic pressure gradient to exist between the left atrium and ventricle. If mitral stenosis exists, the resistance to blood flow from the left atrium to the left ventricle is such that PAOP can be much higher than LVEDP. PAOP is not necessarily an accurate estimate of ventricular filling in this circumstance. Such a scenario may also occur with left atrial myxoma. With mitral regurgitation, a jet of retrograde ejected blood travels into the left atrium during systole and elevates diastolic left atrial pressure. A characteristic V wave may be seen on the PA tracing, and the practitioner must be careful during balloon inflation to interpret a subtle change of waveform as a PAOP tracing. Persistence in advancing the catheter in an attempt to obtain a "better looking" PAOP trace when mitral regurgitation is present may lead to disastrous consequences.

The complications of PA catheter use include those previously described for obtaining central venous access. During the attempt to float the catheter into position, ventricular and atrial dysrhythmias may occur, as well as heart block. Patients with preexisting bifascicular or even left bundle branch blocks may conceivably proceed to complete heart block.[77] Shah et al. reported one series of 6245 patients who had PA catheters inserted before surgery.[103] They noted PVCs in 3.1%, right bundle branch block in 0.048%, complete heart block in 0.016%, intrapulmonary hemorrhage in 0.064%, pulmonary infarcts in 0.064%, and death due to pulmonary artery rupture in 1 patient (0.016%). They concluded that this was a very low rate of complications and that the technique was therefore quite safe in experienced hands.[103] However, prevention of ventricular dysrhythmia with lidocaine during PA catheter placement does not appear to be effective.[97] Retraction of the catheter may relieve PVCs if encountered. If PVCs persist after catheter retraction, lidocaine may be useful. In any case, a PA catheter should *never* be placed without at least having lidocaine immediately available. If monitoring is deemed necessary and a preexisting heart block is present, a PA catheter equipped with pacing wires or a port for them may be used. Dysrhythmias may occur any time after the catheter has been placed. Patient movement or catheter displacement and coughing may all cause triggering of some dysrhythmia.[124]

Failure to get the catheter to pass through the heart may be due to a number of causes, including a low cardiac output syndrome, misdirection of the catheter

tip, balloon failure, and valvular obstruction. Catheters have the potential for coiling inside the right ventricle and can form loops. When such a looped catheter is retracted, it is possible to actually tie a knot in the catheter.[29,102] The PA catheter may dislodge or become entangled with pacemaker wires although this is rare. The presence of a well-established pacemaker is not generally considered a contraindication to passage of a PA catheter.

Upon removal, some of the same problems may arise as during passage of the catheter. It is possible to dislodge a clot that has formed on the catheter, resulting in a pulmonary embolus.[46] Catheters are now coated with heparin, and, although this decreases thrombosis formation, the potential for thrombosis cannot be eliminated. The PA catheter can also be inadvertently fixed with a suture during cardiac surgery, which will require surgical removal.[25] Valvular bacterial encrustations, endocarditis, and other infections have also been related to PA catheters.[14,38,65,79,85] Because of the potential for transmission of such infections, it is now recommended that catheters be changed every 3 to 4 days. It makes sense to find a new site for cannulation if there is the possibility of infection rather than to simply pass a sterile catheter through a possibly colonized central venous access. Catheter sheaths, iodophor ointments, and subcutaneous collagen barriers have been advocated to reduce risks of catheter infection. None can take the place of meticulous sterile technique and attention to detailed nursing care.

The most feared complication of PA catheter usage is rupture of the pulmonary artery and hemorrhage. Pulmonary hypertension, anticoagulation, excessive length of insertion (beyond 50 cm from the right internal jugular position), overinflation of the balloon, and hypothermia have been implicated as causes of pulmonary artery rupture.[5,24,94,103] Hemorrhage may be insignificant with faint blood-tinged sputum or blood noticed on suctioning the endotracheal tubing, or it can be so catastrophic as to cause massive hemoptysis and exsanguination. There is no best approach to care for these situations. PEEP has been applied with some help in resolving the hemorrhage.[113] Advancement of a single lumen endotracheal tube in an effort to isolate the lung usually fails because the bleeding is most often on the right side where the hastily passed tube is most likely also to lodge. A double lumen endotracheal tube may be placed to isolate the lungs but again that may prove quite difficult if bleeding is heavy. Supportive therapy is most often sufficient although angiography and surgical resection may eventually be required. A key point here is prevention. Just because balloon inflation to a proper wedge tracing initially required 1.5 ml of air does *not* mean it will require 1.5 ml again.

Catheters also tend to migrate distally into a smaller diameter pulmonary artery. The practitioner must *watch* the PA tracing continuously during *gradual* balloon inflation.

The pulmonary artery catheter allows more than just monitoring pressures in the PA, RA, and the wedge position. Other data that can be gathered include venous blood gases and even right atrial blood gases. With the thermistor present at the distal end of the catheter, thermodilution cardiac outputs can be determined. Cardiac output by the Fick equation is possible but quite cumbersome and not routinely performed. Dye dilution techniques historically have used an aliquot of indocyanine green dye injected peripherally. The dye concentration within the blood could be quantitated photometrically. The peripheral rate of rise of the dye was then used to calculate a cardiac output. Thermodilution has been shown to correlate well with these methods and is now the most widely used method of measuring this important physiologic function.[12,32,96,116] Thermodilution is essentially an indicator dilution technique similar to the indocyanine green method except that temperature change is used as the indicator. The basis for calculating cardiac output using temperature is the Stewart-Hamilton equation:

$$Q = \frac{V\,(Tb\text{-}Ti)K_1K_2}{Tb(t)dt}$$

Where Q = cardiac output, V = volume of injectate, Tb = blood temperature, Ti = injectate temperature, K_1 and K_2 = constants determined by catheter and electronic characteristics, and $Tb(t)dt$ = change in blood temperature over a given time.

Ten ml of cold crystalloid injectate is often used to determine cardiac outputs although room temperature injectate can also be employed. Smaller volumes may be used if fluid overload is a potential problem. The temperature of cold injectate should be below 24° C. If a colder injectate is used, a better signal to noise ratio is created and improved accuracy is expected. A cardiac output computer may be attached to the PA catheter to provide automated calculation of the cardiac output. Such a cardiac output computer has already been programmed with the Stewart-Hamilton equation. The constants in that equation are prescribed by the size, make, and type of catheter used. They vary because of luminal size and flow characteristics of individual catheters.[10] The computer should plot a curve of the temperature change measured by the thermistor. The area under that curve is inversely proportional to the cardiac output. If the curve is irregular, it may indicate that the thermistor has become lodged against the wall of the pulmonary artery or that other interference has been

detected such as electrocautery noise. The timing of the injection of the cold fluid is important. The respiratory cycle is associated with apparent changes in the cardiac output. Lung ventilation also can cause transients in blood temperature, which introduce error into the cardiac output measurements.[92,111] Most practitioners cease ventilating an anesthetized, paralyzed patient if possible during this measurement. Obviously this is not always desirable or possible.

Although thermodilution has become the most commonly employed method for obtaining cardiac output today, it is a very imprecise technique. Error even in experienced hands is approximately 10% to 20%.[60,63,101,117] Changes between individual measurements over time from the same patient and with the same computer must be greater than 22% before they can be said to be different.[117] In practice, thermodilution outputs should be taken in multiple groups (usually triplicate) and values that agree within 10% are selected for arithmetic averaging. That mean is then considered to represent cardiac output measurement at a particular time interval. It may be relevant here to remember the difference between *precision* and *accuracy*. *Precision* involves close agreement between repeated measures of a condition or value. *Accuracy* means that the measured value is in close agreement with the actual or true value. We need accuracy. We often settle for some degree of precision in the measurement.

With knowledge of pulmonary pressures, mixed venous and actual blood gases, right atrial pressures, and systemic blood pressures in conjunction with cardiac output, a number of useful hemodynamic calculations may be made. The derivations of the equations for these calculations can be seen in Table 41-2. It is incomplete to refer to cardiac output alone as a physiologic indicator of cardiac performance. A 5 L cardiac output may be hyperdynamic for a child or elderly 40-kg patient, or it may border on shock for a large male. Therefore it is important to consider such data in terms of *cardiac index*, which uses body surface area as a way to index actual output to body size. Vascular resistances may be calculated for both the systemic and the pulmonary circulation. Oxygen delivery and consumption may also be calculated. Left ventricular stroke work index may be used as a measure of cardiac workload. The rate pressure product (mean arterial pressure × heart rate) could be considered to be a gauge of cardiac risk for ischemia. Although it *is*, within limits, reasonably well correlated with myocardial O_2 demand, it is imprecise and can be misleading. A low heart rate and an elevated blood pressure may yield the same number as an elevated rate and a low blood pressure and both may have similar O_2 demand, but the slower rate allows better subendocardial supply. Applications

Table 41-2   Equations for common hemodynamic calculations

Hemodynamic parameters	Equation
Stroke volume	SV
Stroke volume index	SV/BSA (body surface area)
Cardiac output	CO = HR × SV
Cardiac index	= CO/BSA
Pulmonary artery pressure	= PA (systolic/diastolic/mean)
Pulmonary artery occlusion pressure	PAOP
Systemic vascular resistance	$\dfrac{\overline{MAP} - CVP}{CO} \times 80$
Pulmonary vascular resistance	$\dfrac{1.36\,(\overline{MAP} - PAOP)}{100} \times 51$
Left ventricular stroke work index	$\dfrac{1.36\,(\overline{PAP} - PAOP)}{100} \times 51$

and importance of the various permutations of hemodynamically derived data are elaborated on in pertinent chapters relating to subspecialty anesthesia in this text.

Mixed venous oxygen saturation ($S\overline{v}_{O_2}$) may be intermittently monitored by withdrawing blood gases from the distal port of the pulmonary artery catheter. The level of oxygen saturation in the pulmonary artery is affected by three major factors: (1) the initial blood arterial oxygen content, (2) total body oxygen consumption, and (3) cardiac output. Using $S\overline{v}_{O_2}$ as an indication of changes in cardiac output in anesthetized patients or patients in intensive care assumes, often incorrectly, that only one of these factors will change at once.[100] Pulmonary artery catheters with additional fiberoptic channels are now available. By passing higher energy down a fiberoptic channel and using a computer to examine the light absorbed and reflected from the pulmonary arterial blood, a continuous measurement of $S\overline{v}_{O_2}$ is possible.

$S\overline{v}_{O_2}$ measurement can be helpful in assessing the balance between peripheral metabolic oxygen demand and its supply. In critically ill patients, cardiac reserve will likely be extremely limited or nonexistent. If tissue oxygen demand increases or delivery decreases, a metabolic shift toward anaerobic metabolism may occur. $S\overline{v}_{O_2}$ monitoring has been advocated as an early warning monitor of changes in the oxygen supply/demand ratio.[52] Causes of decreased $S\overline{v}_{O_2}$

include hypoxemia, fever, hypermetabolic states, and decreased cardiac output. Sudden decreases in $S\overline{v}_{O_2}$ or downward trends have been shown to be predictive of major catastrophic events in critical care patients.[3,74] Increases in $S\overline{v}_{O_2}$ levels may signal increases in cardiac output or decreases in oxygen demand and vice versa. Clinical examples can be found in conditions of sepsis, cirrhosis, cyanide poisoning, liver transplantation or hypothermia or in cases of arterial venous fistulae formation.

Use of $S\overline{v}_{O_2}$ monitoring is still under evaluation. Its use with pulse oximetry to avoid multiple blood gas determinations when positive end-expiratory pressure therapy (PEEP) is being adjusted has been proposed.[91] The problem is that assumptions about changes in cardiac output based on changes or trends in $S\overline{v}_{O_2}$ are valid only if oxygen demand does not change. In the awakening, possibly shivering patient, in the septic patient, and even in the anesthetized, paralyzed patient who may be becoming hypothermic, these assumptions may be invalid.

New technologies have allowed further adaptation of the more standard pulmonary artery catheter design. A right ventricular catheter is now available for the assessment of right ventricular ejection fraction, RV preload, and RV end-systolic volume. Its ultimate use in the monitoring armamentarium is still to be determined. Addition of Doppler sound wave technology to the pulmonary artery catheter has allowed development of a continuous cardiac output catheter as well. These devices are in the very early stages of development.

NONINVASIVE DETERMINATION OF CARDIAC OUTPUT

Two-dimensional echocardiography is a new technique rapidly gaining popularity for intraoperative monitoring. It can provide a great deal of information about cardiac anatomy and physiology. Its use in detection of wall motion abnormalities has become widely publicized.* If abnormalities are found (hypokinetic or akinetic segments), inferences about cardiac function can be made. No routine quantitative data can as yet be gathered on cardiac output. Future work with computer-assisted measurements of the ventricular chamber size in end-diastole and end-systole may allow computations of cardiac output. The use of microbubble contrast injections may also be helpful.[129]

Doppler ultrasound is another recently applied technique that allows for the measurement of cardiac output. The theory behind this technology is based on

---

* References 2, 36, 42, 66, 110, 120, 127.

the classic Doppler equation:

$$FD = \frac{2fo}{C\ Vcos\theta}$$

where *FD* = change in frequency (Doppler shift), *fo* = frequency of sound transmitted, *C* = velocity of ultrasound in blood, *V* = velocity of moving blood (cardiac output if measured in the ascending aorta), and θ = the angle of the ultrasound waves to the blood flow being measured.

As ultrasound waves are reflected from a moving object (the bloodstream), the frequency of those waves is shifted. If the blood flow being measured is flowing toward the ultrasound beam, a positive Doppler shift or increase in frequency is noted. If blood is flowing away from the beam, then a negative or decrease in frequency is found. If the angle of the examining beam *(θ)* is great, then significant error in calculating flow velocity will be introduced. If the ultrasound beam is traveling in a parallel direction to the blood flow, then the angle becomes zero and no error is introduced. For clinical applications, the ultrasound beam must be directed at an angle of 20 degrees or less.[21] The flow velocity of blood in the aorta does not equal the cardiac output (CO). For that measurement (CO) the instantaneous cross-sectional area of the aorta must be entered simultaneously with the flow velocities. Both of these measurements change dramatically throughout the cardiac cycle. Some technologies in use today employ algorithms of the patient's sex, height, and weight to calculate aortic diameter. This may be a source of error, especially in patients who may not conform to normal anatomic descriptions, such as those with atherosclerotic aortic disease. More importantly, these technologies do not take instantaneous aortic diameter changes coupled with equally rapid flow velocity changes into account.

There are several applications of current Doppler cardiac output technologies that have been used by anesthesiologists. A suprasternal probe may be percutaneously angled toward the ascending aorta via the suprasternal notch. Also the Doppler probes have been mounted on esophageal stethoscopes or endotracheal tubes to measure descending and ascending aortic blood flow velocities, respectively. Once these probes have been placed and an adequate signal has been detected, continuous flow velocity monitoring is possible. Patient movement and surgical manipulation require repositioning of the Doppler probe. The flow velocities are reasonably accurate, but the process suffers greatly when assumptions about aortic diameter are "plugged in" to calculate "output."

Several recent studies have compared Doppler-derived cardiac output data with those by thermodilution and other technologies.[105,128] Closest agreement was found when esophageal Doppler probes were used in patients mechanically ventilated. Patients evaluated immediately following cardiopulmonary bypass and/or those not in sinus rhythm had considerably less agreement. The suprasternal notch probe also did not perform as well as the esophageal stethoscope–mounted probe.

It is not yet clear that such Doppler-derived cardiac output technology is reliable and clinically useful. Its place in the anesthesiologist's practice is not yet fully evaluated. Another basic problem yet to be answered is whether use of cardiac output monitoring alone without any measurements of preload, afterload, or contractility will prove useful. Unfortunately, Doppler monitoring provides only one parameter of the entire hemodynamic system.

Another relatively new technology that can provide noninvasive hemodynamic monitoring is thoracic bioimpedance.[10] Doppler ultrasound uses the frequency shift of sound waves to estimate cardiac output, whereas bioimpedance uses measured change of impedance to an electric current passed through the chest through a cardiac cycle to determine stroke volume. The chest can be modeled as a cylinder or cone partially filled with an electrolyte solution (blood). As the cardiac cycle progresses, the volume of electrolyte present within the chest changes and thus the impedance to electric current also changes. These changes produce a characteristic bioimpedance waveform that provides the measurements used in calculation of cardiac output (Fig. 41-11). There is considerable debate about the best equation for deriving cardiac output by bioimpedance. One of the original such expressions used by Bernstein is[11]:

$$SVbi = \frac{L^3 \times VETbi \times dZ/dtmax}{4.25 \times ZO}$$

where *SVbi* = the stroke volume, L^3 = the volume of electrically active tissue (calculated from nomograms), *VETbi* = ventricular ejection time as measured by bioimpedance, *dZ/dtmax* = the maximum rate of change of impedance, and *ZO* = static background impedance.

Today's commercially available bioimpedance hemodynamic monitoring systems use a 70 kHz, 2.5-mA current injected into the thoracic tissues. This current is thought to be biologically inactive. Four pairs of electrodes placed laterally on the chest and neck surround the thoracic cage and are used for injecting and sensing current (Fig. 41-12). Electrode placement and skin preparation are important for gathering accurate data. Once stroke volume is calculated, the computer derives cardiac output by multiplying it by the heart rate. The raw bioimpedance signal can be

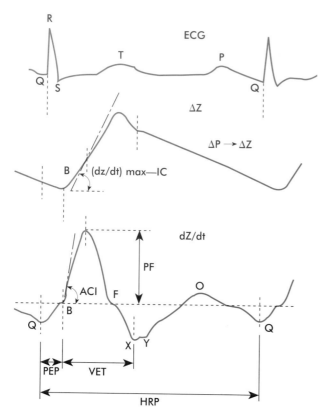

Fig. 41-11. Waveform changes as the pulmonary artery catheter traverses the right atrium, right ventricle, and pulmonary artery.

used to derive a number of other hemodynamic parameters as well. These include ejection fraction, systemic vascular resistance (assuming a constant CVP), end-diastolic volume index (preload), index of contractility, acceleration contraction index, and thoracic fluid index (Table 41-3).

The bioimpedance technology has been compared to thermodilution cardiac output in numerous studies.[10,11,51,112] Correlation coefficients between 0.68 and 0.93 have been reported. Because both are inexact tests of a physiologic function, use of correlation coefficient is probably not statistically appropriate for comparing these data. Other techniques such as regression analysis examination of bias and precision have shown that both bioimpedance and thermodilution are measuring the same physiologic events.[128] Cardiopulmonary bypass has been thought to affect measurement of bioimpedance cardiac output. Considerably more work is required before its use in these patients can be recommended.

In all new computer-driven monitoring technologies an evolutionary history of programming and software revision occurs. Development of thermodilution cardiac output computers went through such a process. Today's technology provides fewer errors, better detection of artifact, and more speed than that previously used. So it is with bioimpedance monitoring. The most recent software revisions have been tested during liver transplantation, a procedure with profound hemodynamic changes, and seem to be reliable.[112] There is little data that compare the

Table 41-3 Bioimpedance hemodynamic equations

Hemodynamic parameters	Normal subjects
Volume of electrically participating tissue (VEPT)	Calculated from algorithm
Stroke volume (SV) = VEPT × VET × IC	44 ml/min/m^{-2}
Stroke volume index (SI) = SV/BSA	
Cardiac output (CO) = SV × HR	
Cardiac index (CI) = CO/BSA	3.5 L/min/m^{-2}
Systolic time ratio (STR) = PEP/VET	
Ejection fraction (EF) = [0.84 − (0.64 × STR)] × 100 (%)	≥65%
End-diastolic volume (EDV) = 100 × SV/EF	
End-diastolic index (EDI) = EDV/BSA	45-100 ml^2
Systemic vascular resistance index (SVRI) = $\dfrac{\overline{MAP} - 6\ (constant)}{CI} \times 80$	
Index of contractility (IC) = (dz/dt)$_{max}$	0.045-0.075 (sec^{-1})
Peak flow index $\left(\dfrac{PF}{BSA}\right) = \dfrac{VEPT \times IC \times Constant}{BSA}$	270 ml/sec/m^{-2}
Thoracic fluid index (TFI)	
Acceleration contraction index (ACI)	0.9-1.6 sec^{-2}

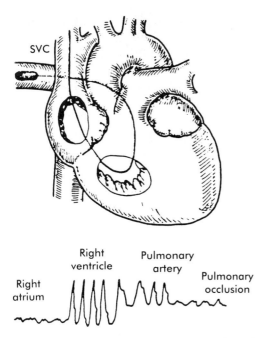

Fig. 41-12. Relationships of the ECG to chest impedance and its first derivative.

remainder of the bioimpedance-obtained hemodynamic functions with currently available monitoring. For example, bioimpedance ejection fraction and measures of preload have not been extensively tested in the operating room. These parameters, if proved reliable, would expand hemodynammic monitoring capabilities in that arena. The presently marketed technology can provide data either on a beat-to-beat basis or averaged over 16 beats. Concepts of an "index of contractility" or "acceleration contraction index" are foreign to most practitioners. The equations used to derive these parameters now appear complex, but there was a time when thermodilution was considered a complex new technology. Bioimpedance, particularly the possible monitoring of preload, afterload, and contractility, may be a promising technique for future use in operating rooms and intensive care situations. Coupled with a computer-driven data management system, the potential for nearly continuous hemodynamic monitoring with early warning and diagnosis assistance is on the horizon.

SUMMARY

Hemodynamic monitoring has changed drastically since the 1960s. Much of this change has been brought about by computer miniaturization development. Patient care has changed significantly because of these technologies. Critical care interventions are largely based on data gathered from invasive hemodynamic monitoring. It would seem that these ad-

vances have improved patient outcome significantly or at least are predictive of adverse outcomes.[68]

The ECG may identify ST-T wave changes indicative of cardiac ischemia, and perioperative identification of ischemia has been shown to be predictive of outcome events.[68,106,107] Monitoring changes in blood pressure, particularly hypotension, which can cause myocardial ischemia, and hypotension has been shown to affect perioperative outcome.[57,58,64,87] Efficacy of invasive hemodynamic monitoring, particularly the pulmonary artery catheter, has been less easily demonstrated.[90] Rao et al. demonstrated decreased myocardial infarctions in an outcome study, but their results were compared to previous reports, not concurrent controls.[90,114] Whether or not invasive monitoring played a role in the differences noted between these studies is still an issue. In patients undergoing cardiopulmonary bypass, one large study indicated that pulmonary artery catheters had no effect on patient outcome.[121] The problem may be that invasive monitoring technology may not be used by all practitioners in the same manner or to its full extent. A recent study indicated that a large segment of practitioners using PA catheters may not understand the technology well enough to use its information.[50] Further studies are needed to decide how invasive hemodynamic monitoring really impacts patient care and outcome.

Today the indications for the use of any monitoring technology, particularly invasive techniques, must be evaluated carefully for each patient. The future development and application of noninvasive complete hemodynamic systems is on the horizon now. As the computer world changes with each new technologic breakthrough, the accuracy and capability for hemodynamic monitoring systems should improve. Unfortunately, the application of that technology and its effect on outcome are difficult to prove. The patient population is changing, as are types of procedures performed. Clinicians use data from hemodynamic monitoring systems with varying opinions, therapies, and decision-making processes. There are few easy decisions with critically ill patients, and care based on hemodynamic monitoring leaves open much for interpretation. Although outcome as the ultimate determination of technology use is currently highly tainted, unfortunately outcome is so multifactorial that changes in one nontherapeutic technology, such as hemodynamic monitoring, cannot be easily sorted out from the dynamic changes affecting all of critical care and anesthesiology.

The future of hemodynamic monitoring will surely involve progressively more extensive use of computerization. Already computer-assisted diagnosis is available with bioimpedance technology. That type of assistance may be extended to other monitors as well.

Operating rooms and Critical Care Units of the future may see progressively less invasive monitoring in use. These technologic changes are exciting. The anesthesiologist must remain abreast of these changes because they will likely form a group of increasingly valuable tools for patient assessment.

KEY POINTS

- In hemodynamic monitoring, the anesthesiologist needs to understand the difference between accuracy, precision, reproducibility, specificity, sensitivity, and predictability.

- The speed of the advancing pressure wave with each cardiac cycle far exceeds the blood flow velocity. This is the reason blood pressure measurements in different regions are not equal. It is also one of the reasons why blood pressure is not necessarily reflective of blood flow.

- Automated oscillometry should be understood by the anesthesiologist in considerable detail, including potential errors and inaccuracies.

- The anesthesiologist should understand harmonic distortion, sometimes known as "fling," sometimes known as "poor frequency response," in invasive arterial blood pressure measuring systems and should become familiar with the term "damping" and how it is understood in arterial pressure monitoring systems.

- Complications of radial artery cannulation are not related to the adequacy or inadequacy of the Allen's test.

- A thorough understanding of the anatomy of the internal jugular vein region of the neck is essential if one is going to be successful with the semi-blind technique of pulmonary artery catheterization.

- Complications of pulmonary artery catheterization include ventricular and/or atrial dysrhythmias, heart block, intrapulmonary hemorrhage or infarct, and even death due to pulmonary artery rupture.

- Thermodilution cardiac outputs are very technique dependent and even then are fraught with accuracy and precision problems. Whether $S\bar{v}_{O_2}$ monitoring adds very much clinically to the monitoring armamentarium, when done continuously via a special pulmonary artery catheter, is quite controversial.

- Computer-driven sophisticated ECG monitoring techniques, including automated ST segment analysis, are proving quite useful in the detection of perioperative ischemia.

KEY REFERENCES

Barash PG, Nardi D, Hammond G et al: Catheter-induced pulmonary artery perforation, mechanisms, management, and modifications, *J Thorac Cardiovasc Surg* 82:5, 1981.

Bedford RF: Invasive blood pressure monitoring. In Blitt CD, ed: *Monitoring in anesthesia and critical care medicine,* New York, 1985, Churchill-Livingstone.

Carroll GC: Blood pressure monitoring. In Vender JS, ed: *Intensive care monitoring,* Philadelphia, 1988, WB Saunders.

Civetta JM, Gabel JC: Flow-directed pulmonary artery catheterization: indications and modifications in technique, *Ann Surg* 176:1193, 1979.

Clements FM, de Bruijn NP: Noninvasive cardiac monitoring. In Vender JS, ed: *Intensive care monitoring,* Philadelphia, 1988, WB Saunders.

Falicov RE, Resenkov L: Relationship of pulmonary artery end-diastolic pressure to left ventricular end-diastolic and mean filling pressures in patients with and without left ventricular dysfunction, *Circulation* 42:65, 1970.

Holland WW, Humerfelt S: Measurements of blood pressure: comparison of intra-arterial and cuff values, *Br Med J* 2:1241, 1964.

Kleinman B: Understanding natural frequency and damping and how they relate to the measurement of blood pressure, *J Clin Monit* 5:137, 1989.

Knight AA, Hollenberg M, London MJ et al: Perioperative myocardial ischemia: importance of the preoperative ischemic pattern, *Anesthesiology* 69: 232, 1988.

London MJ, Tuban JF, Wong MG et al: The "natural history" of segmental wall motion abnormalities in patients undergoing noncardiac surgery, *Anesthesiology* 73:644, 1990.

Mangano DT: Perioperative cardiac morbidity, *Anesthesiology* 72:153, 1990.

Mathew EB, Vender JS: Comparison of thermodilution cardiac output measured by different computers, *Crit Care Med* 15:989, 1987.

Mohr R, Lamee J, and Goor DA: Inaccuracy of radial artery pressure measurement after cardiac operations, *J Thorac Cardiovasc Surg* 94:286, 1987.

Murray IP: Complications of invasive monitoring, *Med Instrumentation* 15:85, 1981.

Prys-Roberts C: Invasive monitoring of the circulation. In Saidman L, Smith NT, eds: *Monitoring in anesthesia,* Boston, 1984, Butterworths.

Rao TK, Jacobs KH, and El-Etr AA: Reinfarction following anesthesia in patients with myocardial infarction, *Anesthesiology* 59:499, 1983.

Samaan HA: The hazards of radial artery pressure monitoring, *J Cardiovasc Surg* 12:342, 1971.

Siegel LC, Shafer SL, Martinez GM et al: Simultaneous measurement of cardiac output by thermodilution, esophageal Doppler and electrical impedance in anesthetized patients, *J Cardiothorac Anesthes* 2:590, 1988.

Slogoff S, Keats AS: Does perioperative myocardial ischemia lead to postoperative myocardial infarction? *Anesthesiology* 62:107, 1985.

Slogoff S, Keats AS: Further observations on perioperative myocardial ischemia, *Anesthesiology* 65:539, 1986.

Slogoft S, Keats AS, and Arlund C: On the safety of radial artery cannulation, *Anesthesiology* 59:42, 1983.

Swan HJC, Ganz W, Forrester JS et al: Catheterization of the heart in man with use of a flow-directed-balloon-tipped catheter, *N Engl J Med* 283:477, 1970.

Tuman KJ, McCarthy RJ, Spiess BD et al: Effect of pulmonary artery catheterization on outcome in patients undergoing coronary artery surgery, *Anesthesiology* 70:199, 1989.

Tuman KT: Pitfalls in interpretation of PA catheter data, *J Cardiothor Anesth* 3:625, 1989.

Van Egmond JV, Hasenbros M, and Crul JF: Invasive vs. non-invasive measurement of arterial pressure, *Br J Anaesth* 57:434, 1985.

Vender JS: Invasive cardiac monitoring. In Vender JS, ed: *Intensive care monitoring,* Philadelphia, 1988, WB Saunders.

Wong DH, Tremper KK, Stemmer EA et al: Noninvasive cardiac output: simultaneous comparison of two methods with thermodilution, *Anesthesiology* 72:784, 1990.

REFERENCES

1. Abrams JH, Olson ML, Marino JA et al: Use of a needle valve variable resistor to improve invasive blood pressure monitoring, *Crit Care Med* 12:978, 1984.
2. Aronson S, Bender EM, Feinstein SB et al: Contrast echocardiography: a method to visualize changes in regional myocardial perfusion in a dog model of CABG surgery, *Anesthesiology* 72:295, 1990.
3. Baele PL, McMichan JC, Marsh MB et al: Continuous monitoring of mixed venous oxygen saturation in critically ill patients, *Anesth Analg* 61:513, 1982.
4. Baker RJ, Chomprapaph B, and Nyhus LM: Severe ischemia of the hand following radial artery cannulation, *Surgery* 80:449, 1976.
5. Barash PG, Nardi D, Hammond G et al: Catheter-induced pulmonary artery perforation, mechanisms, management, and modifications, *J Thorac Cardiovasc Surg* 82:5, 1981.
6. Bartless RH, Munster AM: An improved technique for prolonged arterial cannulation, *N Engl J Med* 279:92, 1968.
7. Bedford RF: Invasive blood pressure monitoring. In Blitt CD, ed: *Monitoring in anesthesia and critical care medicine,* New York, 1985, Churchill-Livingstone.
8. Benumof JL, Saidman LJ, Arkin DB et al: Where pulmonary artery catheters go: intrathoracic distribution, *Anesthesiology* 46:336, 1977.
9. Bernhardt LC, Wegner GP, and Mendenhall JT: Intravenous catheter embolization to pulmonary artery, *Chest* 57:329, 1970.
10. Bernstein DP: Continuous noninvasive real-time monitoring of stroke volume and cardiac output by thoracic electrical bioimpedance, *Crit Care Med* 14:898, 1986.
11. Bernstein DP: A new stroke volume equation for thoracic electrical bioimpedance: theory and rationale, *Crit Care Med* 14:904, 1986.
12. Bilfinger TV, Lin CY, and Anagnostopoulos CE: In vitro determination of accuracy of cardiac output measurements by thermal dilution, *J Surg Res* 33:409, 1982.
13. Bochaner RD: Continuous, real-time, non-invasive monitor of blood pressure: Peñaz methodology applied to the finger, *J Clin Monit* 3:282, 1987.
14. Boscoe MJ, deLange S: Damage to the tricuspid valve with a Swan-Ganz catheter, *Br Med J* 283:346, 1981.
15. Boswick J: Injuries of the radial and ulnar arteries, *J Bone Joint Surg* 49(A):582, 1967.
16. Brown CQ: Inadvertent prolonged cannulation of the carotid artery, *Anesth Analg* 61:150, 1982.
17. Bruner JMR, Krenis LJ, Kunsman JM et al: Comparison of direct and indirect methods of measuring arterial blood pressure, part III, *Med Instrum* 15:182, 1981.
18. Cannon BW, Meshiew WT: Extremity amputation following radial artery cannulation in a patient with hyperlipoproteinemia type V, *Anesthesiology* 56:222, 1982.
19. Carroll GC: Blood pressure monitoring. In Vender JS, ed: *Intensive care monitoring,* Philadelphia, 1988, WB Saunders.
20. Civetta JM, Gabel JC: Flow-directed pulmonary artery catheterization: indications and modifications in technique, *Ann Surg* 176:1193, 1979.
21. Clements FM, de Bruijn NP: Noninvasive cardiac monitoring. In Vender JS, ed: *Intensive care monitoring,* Philadelphia, 1988, WB Saunders.
22. Doblar DD, Hinkle JC, Fay ML et al: Air embolism associated with pulmonary artery catheter introducer kit, *Anesthesiology* 56:307, 1982.
23. Dorlas JC, Nijboer JA, Butiju WT et al: Effects of peripheral vasoconstriction on the blood pressure in the finger, measured continuously by a new noninvasive method (the Finapres^R), *Anesthesiology* 62:342, 1985.
24. Eisenberg PR, Jaffe AS, and Schuster DP: Clinical evaluation compared to pulmonary artery catheterization in the hemodynamic assessment of critically ill patients, *Crit Care Med* 12:549, 1984.
25. Eliasen P, Vejlsted H: A mechanical complication with a balloon-tipped catheter during open heart surgery, *Scand J Thorac Cardiovasc Surg* 14:205, 1980.
26. Epstein RH, Kaplan S, Leighton BL etal: Evaluation of a continuous noninvasive blood pressure monitor in obstet-

ric patients undergoing spinal anesthesia, *J Clin Monit* 5:157, 1989.

27. Erlanger J: Studies in blood pressure estimation by indirect means, *Am J Physiol* 55:84, 1921.

28. Falicov RE, Resenkov L: Relationship of pulmonary artery end-diastolic pressure to left ventricular end-diastolic and mean filling pressures in patients with and without left ventricular dysfunction, *Circulation* 42:65, 1970.

29. Fibuch EE, Touhy GF: Intracardiac knotting of a flow-directed balloon-tipped catheter, *Anesth Analg* 59:217, 1980.

30. Forrester JS, Diamond G, McHugh TJ et al: Filling pressures in right and left sides of the heart in acute myocardial infarction. A reappraisal of central venous pressure monitoring, *N Engl J Med* 285:190, 1971.

31. Gallogher JD, Moore RA, McNicholas KW et al: Comparison of radial and femoral arterial blood pressures in children after cardiopulmonary bypass, *J Clin Monit* 1:168, 1985.

32. Ganz W, Donoso R, Marcus H et al: A new technique for measurement of cardiac output by thermodilution in man, *Am J Cardiol* 27:392, 1971.

33. Geddes LA: *The direct and indirect measurement of blood pressure*, Chicago, 1976, Year Book Medical Publishers, Inc.

34. Geddes LA: *Cardiovascular devices and their applications*, New York, 1984, John Wiley & Sons.

35. Gelberman RH, Nunley JA, Koman LA et al: The result of radial and ulnar arterial repair in the forearm, *J Bone Joint Surg* 64(A):383, 1982.

36. Gewertz BL, Krenser PC, Zarins CK et al: Transesophageal echocardiographic monitoring of myocardial ischemia during vascular surgery, *J Vasc Surg* 5:607, 1987.

37. Goodman EG, Howell AA: Further clinical studies in the auscultatory method of determining blood pressure, *Am J Med Sci* 142:334, 1911.

38. Greene JF, Fitzwater JE, and Clemmer TP: Septic endocarditis and indwelling pulmonary artery catheters, *JAMA* 233:891, 1975.

39. Guyton AC: *Textbook of medical physiology*, Philadelphia, 1976, WB Saunders.

40. Hamilton WF, Woodbury RA, and Harper HT: Optical tracing of human blood pressure, comparing critical and oscillographic criteria with the true blood pressure, *Am J Physiol* 113:59, 1936.

41. Hamilton WF, Woodbury RA, and Harper HT: Physiologic relationships between intrathoracic, intraspinal and arterial pressures, *JAMA* 107:854, 1936.

42. Hansen AM, Gangadharan V, Ramos RG et al: Sequence of mechanical, electrocardiographic and clinical effects of repeated coronary artery occlusion in human beings: echocardiographic observation during coronary angioplasty, *J Am Coll Cardiol* 5:193, 1985.

43. Hansen AT: Pressure measurement in the human organism, *Acta Physiol Scand* 19(Suppl):1, 1949.

44. Health devices: automatic sphygmomanometers. In Mosenkis R, ed: *Evaluation: sphygmomanometers, electronic, automatic [16-173]*, New York, 1986, Springer.

45. Herbst CA: Indication, management and complications of percutaneous subclavian catheters, *Arch Surg* 113:1421, 1978.

46. Hoar PF, Wilson RM, Mangano DT et al: Heparin bonding reduces thrombogenicity of pulmonary-artery catheters, *N Engl J Med* 305:993, 1981.

47. Holland WW, Humerfelt S: Measurements of blood pressure: comparison of intra-arterial and cuff values, *Br Med J* 2:1241, 1964.

48. Husum B, Palm T: Arterial dominance in the hand, *Br J Anaesth* 50:913, 1978.

49. Husum B, Palm T: Before cannulation of the radial artery: collateral arterial supply evaluated by strain-gauge plethysmography, *Acta Anaesthesiol Scand* 24:412, 1980.

50. Iberti TJ, Fischer EP, Leibowitz AB et al: Pulmonary artery catheter study group. A multicenter study of the physicians' knowledge of the pulmonary artery catheter, *JAMA* 264:2928, 1990.

51. Introna RPS, Pruett JK, Crumrine RC et al: Use of transthoracic bioimpedance to determine cardiac output in pediatric patients, *Crit Care Med* 16:1101, 1988.

52. Kandel G, Aberman A: Mixed venous oxygen saturation, its role in the assessment of the critically ill patient, *Arch Int Med* 143:1400, 1983.

53. Katz AM, Birnbaum M, Moylan J et al: Gangrene of the hand and forearm: a complication of radial artery cannulation, *Crit Care Med* 2:270, 1974.

54. King GE: Taking the blood pressure, *JAMA* 209:1902, 1969.

55. Kirkendall WM, Feinlab M, Freis ED et al: Recommendations for human blood pressure determination by sphygmomanometers. Subcommittee of the American Heart Association Postgraduate Education Committee, *News from the American Heart Association*, 1981, (AHA reprint booklet 70-019-B).

56. Kleinman B: Understanding natural frequency and damping and how they relate to the measurement of blood pressure, *J Clin Monit* 5:137, 1989.

57. Knight AA, Hollenberg M, London MJ et al: Perioperative myocardial ischemia: importance of the preoperative ischemic pattern, *Anesthesiology* 69:232, 1988.

58. Kotter G, Kotrly K, Kalbfleish J et al: Myocardial ischemia during cardiovascular surgery as detected by an ST segment trend monitoring system, *J Cardiothorac Anesth* 1:190, 1987.

59. Kurki T, Smith NT, Head N et al: Noninvasive continuous blood pressure measurement from the finger: optimal measurement conditions and factors affecting reliability, *J Clin Monit* 3:6, 1987.

60. LaMantia KR, O'Conner TO, and Barash PG: Comparing methods of measurement: an alternative approach, *Anesthesiology* 72:781, 1990.

61. Lambert EH, Wood EH: Direct determination of man's blood pressure on the human centrifuge during positive acceleration, *Fed Proc* 5:59, 1946.

62. Lantiegne KC, Civetta JM: A system for maintaining invasive pressure monitoring, *Heart Lung* 7:610, 1978.

63. Levett JM, Replogle RL: Thermodilution cardiac output: a critical analysis and review of the literature, *J Surg Res* 27:392, 1979.

64. Lickerman RW, Orkin FK, Jokes DR et al: Hemodynamic predictors of myocardial ischemia during halothane anesthesia for coronary artery revascularization, *Anesthesiology* 59:36, 1983.

65. Lindgren KM, McShane K, and Roberts WC: Acute rupture of the pulmonic valve by a balloon-tipped catheter producing a musical diastolic murmur, *Chest* 81:251, 1982.

66. London MJ, Tuban JF, Wong MG et al: The "natural history" of segmental wall motion abnormalities in patients undergoing noncardiac surgery, *Anesthesiology* 73:644, 1990.

67. Manck GW, Smith CR, Geddes LA et al: The meaning of the point of maximum in cuff pressure in the indirect measurement of blood pressure, *J Biomech Eng* 102:28, 1980.

68. Mangano DT: Perioperative cardiac morbidity, *Anesthesiology* 72:153, 1990.

69. Mangano DT, Hickey RF: Ischemic injury following uncomplicated radial catheterization, *Anesth Analg* 58:55, 1979.

70. Mathew EB, Vender JS: Comparison of thermodilution cardiac output measured by different computers, *Crit Care Med* 15:989, 1987.

71. Matthews JI, Gibbons RB: Embolization complicating radial artery puncture, *Ann Intern Med* 75:87, 1971.

72. Michaelson ED, Walsh RE: Osler's node — a complication of prolonged arterial cannulation, *N Engl J Med* 283:472, 1970.

73. Mohr R, Lamee J, and Goor DA: Inaccuracy of radial artery pressure measurement after cardiac operations, *J Thorac Cardiovasc Surg* 94:286, 1987.

74. Mohsinifar Z, Goldbach P, Tashkin DP et al: Relationship between O_2 delivery and O_2 consumption in the adult respiratory distress syndrome, *Chest* 84:267, 1983.

75. Molhoek GP, Wesseling KH, Settels JJM et al: Evaluation of the Peñaz servoplethysmomanometer for the continuous, noninvasive measurement of finger blood pressure, *Basic Res Cardiol* 79:598, 1984.

76. Morris GC Jr, Beall AC Jr, Roof WR et al: Surgical experience with 220 acute arterial injuries in civilian practice, *Am J Surg* 99:775, 1960.

77. Murray IP: Complications of invasive monitoring, *Med Instrumentation* 15:85, 1981.

78. O'Quin R, Marini JJ: Pulmonary artery occlusion pressure: clinical physiology, measurement, and interpretation, *Am Rev Respir Dis* 128:319, 1983.

79. O'Toole JD, Wurtzbacher JJ, Wearner NE et al: Pulmonary-valve injury and insufficiency during pulmonary-artery catheterization, *N Engl J Med* 301:1167, 1979.

80. Pauca AL, Meredith JW: Possibility of A-V shunting upon cardiopulmonary bypass discontinuation, *Anesthesiology* 67:91, 1987.

81. Peñaz J: Photoelectric measurement of blood pressure, volume and flow in the finger, *Digest 10th International Conference of Biological Engineering*, New York, 1973, Springer.

82. Peñaz J, Voigt A, and Teichmann W: Beitrag zur fortlaufenden indirekteu Blutduckmessung, *Zeitschr fur innere Med* 31:1030, 1976.

83. Peterson LH, Dripps RD, and Risman GC: A method for recording the arterial pressure pulse and blood pressure in man, *Am Heart J* 37:1, 1949.

84. Petty TL: Adult respiratory distress syndrome, *Semin Respir Med* 3:219, 1982.

85. Pinilla JC, Ross DF, Martin T et al: Study of the incidence of intravascular catheter injection and associated septicemia in critically ill patients, *Crit Care Med* 11:21, 1983.

86. Prys-Roberts C: Invasive monitoring of the circulation. In Saidman L, Smith NT, eds: *Monitoring in anesthesia,* Boston, 1984, Butterworths.

87. Prys-Roberts C, Meloche R, and Foex P: Studies of anesthesia in relation to hypertension. I. Cardiovascular responses to treated and untreated patients, *Br J Anaesth* 43:122, 1971.

88. Pyles ST, Scher KS, Vega ET et al: Cannulation of the dorsal radial artery: a new technique, *Anesth Analg* 61:876, 1982.

89. Ramscy M III: Noninvasive automatic determination of mean arterial pressure, *Med Biol Eng Comput* 17:1, 1979.

90. Rao TK, Jacobs KH, and El-Etr AA: Reinfarction following anesthesia in patients with myocardial infarction, *Anesthesiology* 59:499, 1983.

91. Räsänen J, Dours JB: Titration of continuous positive airway pressure by real-time dual oximetry, *Crit Care Med* 15:A395, 1987.

92. Riedringer MS, Shellock FG: Technical aspects of the thermodilution method for measuring cardiac output, *Heart Lung* 13:215, 1984.

93. Robard S: The significance of the intermediate Korotkoff sounds, *Circulation* 8:600, 1953.

94. Rosenbaum L, Rosenbaum SH, Ashkanazir T et al: Small amounts of hemophthisis as an early warning sign of pulmonary artery rupture by a pulmonary arterial catheter, *Crit Care Med* 9:319, 1981.

95. Rulf ENR, Mitchell MM, Prakash O et al: Measurement of arterial pressure after cardiopulmonary bypass with long radial artery catheters, *J Cardiothoracic Anesth* 4:19, 1990.

96. Runciman WB, Ilsley AH, and Roberts JG: An evaluation of thermodilution cardiac output measurements using the Swan-Ganz catheter, *Anaesth Inten Care* 9:208, 1981.

97. Salmenpera M, Peltola K, and Ronsenberg P: Does prophylactic lidocaine control cardiac arrhythmias associated with pulmonary artery catheterization? *Anesthesiology* 56:210, 1982.

98. Samaan HA: The hazards of radial artery pressure monitoring, *J Cardiovasc Surg* 12:342, 1971.

99. Samii K, Considles C, and Viars P: Central venous pressure and pulmonary wedge pressure, *Arch Surg* 111:1122, 1976.

100. Schueiss JF: Mixed venous hemoglobin saturation: theory and application, *Int Anesthesiol Clin* 25:113, 1987.

101. Schuster AH, Nauda NC: Doppler echocardiographic measurement of cardiac output: comparison with a non-golden standard, *Am J Cardiol* 53:257, 1984.

102. Schwartz KV, Garisa FG: Entanglement of Swan-Ganz catheter around an intracardiac structure, *JAMA* 237:113, 1987.

103. Shah KB, Rao TLK, Laughlin S et al: A review of pulmonary artery catheterization in 6245 patients, *Anesthesiology* 66:271, 1984.

104. Shinozaki T, Deana RS, and Mazuzau JE: The dynamic responses of liquid-filled catheter systems for direct measurement of blood pressure, *Anesthesiology* 53:498, 1980.

105. Siegel LC, Shafer SL, Martinez GM et al: Simultaneous measurement of cardiac output by thermodilution, esophageal Doppler and electrical impedance in anesthetized patients, *J Cardiothorac Anesthes* 2:590, 1988.

106. Slogoff S, Keats AS: Does perioperative myocardial ischemia lead to postoperative myocardial infarction? *Anesthesiology* 62:107, 1985.

107. Slogoff S, Keats AS: Further observations on perioperative myocardial ischemia, *Anesthesiology* 65:539, 1986.

108. Slogoff S, Keats AS, and Arlund C: On the safety of radial artery cannulation, *Anesthesiology* 59:42, 1983.

109. Smith JS, Cahalan MK, Benefiel DJ et al: Intraoperative detection of myocardial ischemia in high risk patients: electrocardiography versus two-dimensional transesophageal echocardiography, *Circulation* 72:1015, 1985.

110. Smith NT, Wesseling KH, and de Wit B: Evaluation of two prototype devices producing noninvasive, pulsatile calibrated blood pressure measurement from a finger, *J Clin Monit* 1:17, 1984.

111. Snyder JV, Powner DJ: Effects of mechanical ventilation on the measurement of cardiac output by thermodilution, *Crit Care Med* 10:677, 1982.

112. Spiess BD, Tuman KT: Bioimpedance hemodynamic monitoring compared to PA monitoring during liver transplantation, *J Surg Rev* (in press).

113. Sprung CL, Pozen RG, Rozanski JJ et al: Advanced ventricular arrhythmias during bedside pulmonary artery catheterization, *Am J Med* 72:203, 1982.

114. Steem PA, Tinker JH, and Tarhau S: Myocardial reinfarction after anesthesia and surgery, *JAMA* 239:2566, 1978.

115. Stern DH, Gerson JI, Allen FB et al: Can we trust the direct radial artery pressure immediately following cardiopulmonary bypass? *Anesthesiology* 62:557, 1985.

116. Stetz CW, Miller RG, Kelly GE et al: Reliability of the thermodilution method in the determination of cardiac output in clinical practice, *Am Rev Respir Dis* 126:1001, 1982.

117. Swan HJC, Ganz W, Forrester JS et al: Catheterization of the heart in man with use of a flow-directed-balloon-tipped catheter, *N Engl J Med* 283:477, 1970.

118. Thomas F, Burke JP, Parker J et al: The risk of infection related to radial versus femoral sites for arterial catheterization, *Crit Care Med* 11:807, 1983.

119. Thomson IR, Mutch WAC, and Culligan JD: Failure of intravenous nitroglycerin to prevent intraoperative myocardial ischemia during fentanyl-pancuronium anesthesia, *Anesthesiology* 61:385, 1984.

120. Topol EJ, Weis JL, Guzman PA et al: Immediate improvement of dysfunctional myocardial segments after coronary revascularization: detection of intraoperative transesophageal echocardiography, *J Am Coll Cardiol* 4:1123, 1984.

121. Tuman KJ, McCarthy RJ, Spiess BD et al: Effect of pulmonary artery catheterization on outcome in patients undergoing coronary artery surgery, *Anesthesiology* 70:199, 1989.

122. Tuman KT: Pitfalls in interpretation of PA catheter data, *J Cardiothor Anesth* 3:625, 1989.

123. Van Egmond JV, Hasenbros M, and Crul JF: Invasive vs. non-invasive measurement of arterial pressure, *Br J Anaesth* 57:434, 1985.

124. Vankydis PC, Cohen SI: Catheter-induced arrhythmias, *Am Heart J* 88:588, 1974.

125. Vender JS: Invasive cardiac monitoring. In Vender JS, ed: *Intensive care monitoring,* Philadelphia, 1988, WB Saunders.

126. West JB, Dollery CT, and Naimark A: Distribution of blood flow in isolated lung: relation to vascular and alveolar pressures, *J Applied Physiol* 19:713, 1964.

127. Wohlgelernter D, Cleman M, Highman HA et al: Regional myocardial dysfunction during coronary angioplasty: evaluation by two-dimensional echocardiography and 12-lead electrocardiography, *J Am Coll Cardiol* 7:1245, 1986.

128. Wong DH, Tremper KK, Stemmer EA et al: Noninvasive cardiac output: simultaneous comparison of two methods with thermodilution, *Anesthesiology* 72:784, 1990.

129. Wong DH, Tremper KK, Zaccari J et al: Acute cardiovascular response to passive leg raising, *Crit Care Med* 16:123, 1988.

130. Yelderman M, Rean AK: Indirect measurement of mean blood pressure in the anesthetized patient, *Anesthesiology* 50:253, 1979.

131. Zipperman HH: Acute arterial injuries in the Korean War, *Ann Surg* 139:1, 1954.

CHAPTER 42

Monitoring Respiratory Function

DANIEL B. RAEMER

Monitoring respiration during anesthesia is a critical responsibility of the clinician. Monitoring must be continuous, systematic, and vigilant. This requires a consistent approach to monitoring, as well as an understanding of respiratory physiology, the ventilatory system, and the associated instrumentation.

This chapter presents a systematic approach for evaluating respiration during anesthesia. Appropriate clinical monitoring of the respiratory pathway is described. The technology available to perform the monitoring tasks also is discussed.

RESPIRATORY PATHWAY

Cellular respiration requires the delivery of oxygen (O_2) and the removal of carbon dioxide (CO_2). In addition, cellular function requires delivery of substrate, removal of metabolic waste, and maintenance of homeostasis: pH, temperature, integrity, and absence of toxins. Although gas exchange is of primary importance during anesthesia, the clinician must consider all these requirements to evaluate respiration thoroughly.

Following the pathways for O_2 delivery and CO_2 elimination is a useful paradigm to monitor respiration systematically. Fig. 42-1 is a diagrammatic representation of the O_2 and CO_2 pathways demonstrating the critical points for monitoring. The five monitoring principles for consistently evaluating respiration are listed in Box 42-1.

MONITORING RESPIRATORY PATHWAY

Basic monitoring practice requires that the appropriate variables be measured continuously and that the information be conveyed to the clinician in a timely manner. Also, monitoring must not be unreasonably costly, and the patient should be at minimal, if any, risk.[69] Various aspects of monitoring respiratory function, including fraction of inspired oxygen (FIO_2), a disconnection monitor during mechanical ventilation, and "continuous monitoring of ventilation," are listed in the Minimum Monitoring Standards of the American Society of Anesthesiology (ASA).[2] A recent amendment requires the use of pulse oximetry, and respiratory CO_2 monitoring is encouraged.[3] Some medical malpractice insurance carriers have designated use of pulse oximeters and respiratory CO_2 monitors as a stipulation for coverage, whereas others have offered discounts for their purchase and use.[104]

Beyond the requirements set by standards, clinicians monitor variables that enable evaluation of the patient's clinical state at any given time.[69] For monitoring the respiratory system, this requires that the five principles listed in Box 42-1 be satisfied. Clinical circumstances dictate the most efficacious,

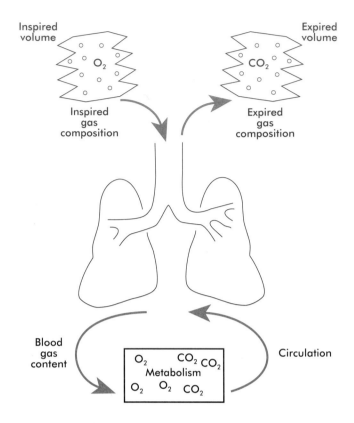

Fig. 42-1. Respiratory gas pathway.

safe, manageable, and economic monitoring array to accomplish this task.

Continuous measurement implies that the data are collected rapidly enough to determine changes in a variable. In an engineering sense, the data *must* be sampled twice as frequently and, in practice, *should* be sampled 3 to 10 times as frequently as the variable's most rapid changes to avoid missing information.[47] The implications for respiratory monitoring are that continuously changing variables (e.g., gas flow, expiratory gas composition) must be measured at least once per second. Variables that change each breath (e.g., tidal volume, breath-to-breath interval) must be measured every 1 or 2 seconds (or timed with each breath). Variables that change slowly (e.g., arterial CO_2 tension, pH) need to be measured only in 10-minute multiples or hours.

Conveying data to the clinician in a timely manner has several requirements. First, only data that contain information should be displayed. Some respiratory data are unchanging (e.g., set minute volume during mechanical ventilation, FIO_2) and only need to be displayed when changes occur. Similarly, data that are redundant with data already displayed contain no information. Second, data must be presented early to permit successful intervention. Acute changes in the respiratory system (e.g., failure of ventilation in a patient with 2 L of O_2 in functional residual capacity)

BOX 42-1
PRINCIPLES FOR CONSISTENT EVALUATION OF RESPIRATION

Knowing the composition of the inspiratory gas is important to evaluate whether adequate O_2 tension is available for the alveolar gas to oxygenate the blood. Also, determining the CO_2 tension of the inspired gas is valuable in assessing whether CO_2 can be eliminated from the blood efficiently.

Determining the tidal volume (V_T) delivered to the lung during inspiration is important to assess whether the airways are maintained open. Confirming that O_2 reaches the alveoli by the delivery of an adequate V_T is also important. Knowing the O_2 tension in this arterial blood is essential to infer that (a) the delivered O_2 has been distributed to the alveoli, (b) the alveolar membranes are functional, and (c) circulation to the alveoli has been removing O_2 from the alveolar gas. Determining the O_2 content in the arterial blood allows an appraisal of the adequacy of O_2 delivery to meet metabolic needs. Knowing the O_2 content in the venous blood relative to the arterial blood is important to conclude that O_2 has been extracted by the tissues. Determining the CO_2 tension of the arterial blood or alveolar gas is critical to confirm that CO_2 has been excreted in balance with metabolic CO_2 production.

Measuring the volume of expiratory gas is essential to assess whether the quantity of CO_2 being excreted is adequate to balance the CO_2 produced by metabolism.

---

requires detection and display before the 2 minutes when hypoxemia ensues. On the other hand, slow changes (e.g., slight hyperventilation) have less immediate consequences and do not require urgent notification of the clinician. Finally, the data must be accessible. As presented, monitored data sometimes contain artifacts, camouflage subtle and clinically significant changes, and can lead to paradoxic conclusions. In these situations the clinician must have access on demand to all collected data.

Safety in monitoring requires noninvasiveness whenever possible. The advent of the pulse oximeter and routine use of respiratory CO_2 analyzers are steps toward this goal. Use of more invasive technology (e.g., mixed venous saturation monitoring catheters) must be weighed carefully against its benefit.

Cost of respiratory monitoring must be balanced against benefits. The cost of respiratory function monitoring includes purchasing, operating, and maintaining equipment. Also, the indirect cost of failing to monitor for an event that leads to a poor patient outcome must be considered. On this basis, the cost of monitoring O_2 saturation in ambulatory gynecologic surgical patients has been justified.[76]

Composition of Inspired Gas

Clinically, the composition of the inspired gas can be monitored in three ways. First, the O_2 fraction or O_2 tension (Po_2) can be measured continuously with one of several analyzers. Second, the CO_2 can be monitored with a respiratory CO_2 analyzer. Third, the balance gases—nitrogen (N_2), nitrous oxide (N_2O), anesthetic agent, and helium—can be measured continuously with multigas analyzers.

A dedicated O_2 analyzer is always present in the breathing circuit. Usually, the sensor of this analyzer is located in the inspiratory portion of the breathing circuit to limit the exposure to troublesome water vapor.[13] Most analyzers are equipped with low-threshold and high-threshold alarms. The low O_2 alarm threshold is constrained above 18% to prevent a hypoxic inspired mixture from going undetected. Some multigas analyzers that sample gas from the breathing circuit near the patient's airway can measure inspiratory Po_2. In these analyzers the inspiratory Po_2 is distinguished from the expiratory Po_2 according to the timing of the respiratory CO_2 waveform.

O_2 analyzers typically display the FIO_2 on a digital (numeric) or analog (meter) display. Most O_2 analyzers actually measure Po_2, but are calibrated according to O_2 fraction (e.g., ambient, 20.9% and/or 100%) at ambient pressure. In the breathing circuit the total pressure during mechanical ventilation can be elevated. Thus these analyzers will read a higher fraction than expected. For example, an analyzer calibrated with 100% O_2 at ambient pressure will read an FIO_2 of 102% when ventilating with pure O_2 at an inspiratory pressure of 20 cm H_2O:

$$760 \text{ mm Hg} + (20 \text{ cm H}_2\text{O} \times 0.735 \text{ mm Hg/cm H}_2\text{O})/$$
$$760 \text{ mm Hg} = 101.9\%$$

The ASA guidelines for minimal monitoring require the use of an O_2 analyzer for all general anesthetic procedures.[2] In a modern anesthesia delivery system, when the O_2 analyzer reading is substantially different than expected, a technical problem is usually present. Since anesthesia machines that meet the ANSI Z-79.8 standard (sold after 1979) of the American National Standards Institute[56] have several mechanisms to prevent the delivery of hypoxic mixtures, the technical problem may be subtle. For example, the O_2 supply, either from a wall source or tank, may be contaminated with another gas.[94] Failure of the N_2O/O_2 proportioning device can lead to the delivery of a hypoxic mixture.[79] Also, under certain circumstances, disconnection of the fresh gas hose from the anesthesia machine can lead to a substantially lower inspiratory Po_2 than desired.[53]

The CO_2 tension (Pco_2) in the inspired gas should generally be near zero. An exception is when mechanical dead space is intentionally placed in the breathing circuit. Also, in some countries (e.g., United Kingdom) the addition of CO_2 gas to the breathing mixture or a bypass of the CO_2 absorber is frequently used to restore eucapnia at the end of surgery.[63] Common technical problems that cause elevated inspiratory Pco_2 include exhaustion of the CO_2 absorber, failure of one-way valves, and disconnection of the inspiratory side of the breathing circuit (spontaneous ventilation only).

A respiratory CO_2 analyzer can detect the presence of CO_2 in the inspired gas. Fig. 42-2 shows the trend of the Pco_2 when the CO_2 absorber has gradually failed. Fig. 42-3 demonstrates elevated inspiratory Pco_2 when excessive mechanical dead space is introduced in the breathing circuit. The unusual Pco_2 waveforms in Fig. 42-4 were produced when 500 ml/m of 5% CO_2 was added to the inspiratory side of a breathing circuit at the end of surgery in an attempt to restore eucapnia. Note the pulses of CO_2 in the inspired portion of the waveform that result from the 5% CO_2 gas accumulating on the inspired side of the circuit during the expiratory phase of ventilation.

Inspired Gas Volume

The delivery of gas to the patient must be monitored to ensure that (1) an adequate volume of gas can be delivered to the lung, (2) enough O_2 can be delivered to the arterial blood, and (3) an adequate expiratory volume can be achieved to eliminate CO_2. **Inspiratory gas volume must be adequate to meet five demands. First, inspired gas volume is necessary to expand the lung and prevent closure of airways (atelectasis) and shunting.[12]**

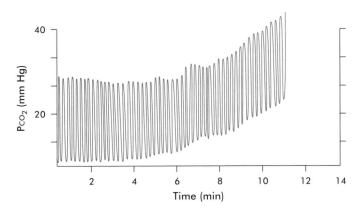

Fig. 42-2. Respiratory CO_2 analyzer waveform trend. Gradual increase in baseline CO_2 tension (Pco_2) results from failure of CO_2 absorber.

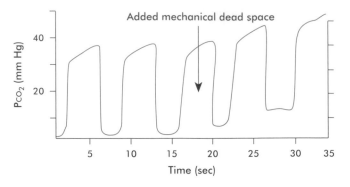

Fig. 42-3. Respiratory CO_2 analyzer waveforms demonstrating elevated inspiratory PCO_2 caused by mechanical dead space.

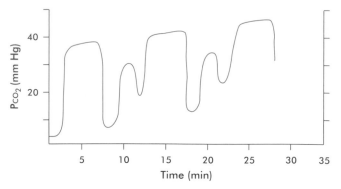

Fig. 42-4. Respiratory CO_2 analyzer waveforms demonstrating unusual PCO_2 changes caused by introduction of 5% CO_2 gas at 500 ml/min into inspiratory side of circle breathing circuit at the end of surgery in an attempt to rapidly restore eucapnia.

Second, an adequate volume of O_2 must be delivered to the alveolar space to meet the metabolic demands of the patient. The metabolic requirement for O_2 of an average male (weight, 70 kg) at rest is about 3.3 ml/kg/min.[62] During anesthesia and surgery, this value is modified primarily by muscle relaxants and, to a lesser extent, by temperature, stress, and other drugs. An estimate of 85% of basal oxygen consumption (2.8 ml/kg/min in a 70 kg male) has been suggested during uncomplicated anesthesia.

Third, excess inspired gas volume is necessary to fill the mechanical, anatomic, and alveolar dead space. The mechanical dead space of the breathing system includes all the breathing tubes in the circuit with two-way gas flow. In a circle breathing system the mechanical dead space is generally between the **Y** piece and the end of the tracheal tube. The anatomic dead space normally includes the pharynx, trachea, and major conducting airways and is about 170 ml. On one hand, when a patient is intubated, all the pharangeal and most tracheal volume is bypassed, thereby reducing the anatomic dead space to about 130 ml.[18] On the other hand, a face mask adds approximately 100 ml to anatomic dead space.[20] The alveolar dead space is equivalent to the portion of the total alveolar volume not exposed to pulmonary capillary blood. In normal awake adults, alveolar dead space is less than 10% of alveolar ventilation.[48] However, during anesthesia,[66] high FIO_2,[95] and positive pressure ventilation,[18] alveolar dead space may increase substantially. During anesthesia, total dead space may represent one third to two thirds of V_T, and it increases with age.[23]

Fourth, some of the gas volume delivered by a mechanical or manual ventilator during positive pressure ventilation must be provided to compensate for gas compression and breathing circuit distension. Typically, the loss of volume caused by compression

and circuit distension is about 150 ml.[30] With a peak inspired pressure (PIP) of 50 cm H_2O, an adult, rubber circle breathing circuit, including a heated humidifier, can have a compression and compliance volume of approximately 700 ml.[24]

Finally, the delivered inspired gas volume must be adequate to eliminate metabolic CO_2 during expiration. The inspired gas volume essentially determines the expired gas volume and is usually considered in that context clinically. Monitoring expired gas volume is discussed in a later section.

Inspired gas volume is not usually monitored directly but is typically evaluated in terms of a dependent variable: O_2 tension of arterial blood (PaO_2), O_2 saturation of arterial blood (SaO_2), PCO_2 of the expired gas, or CO_2 tension of arterial blood ($PaCO_2$). However, setting the mechanical ventilator, measuring the breathing circuit pressure, and monitoring the system for leaks, disconnections, and obstructions all indirectly monitor the adequacy of inspired gas volume.

Visually checking the ventilator settings is the first step in monitoring inspired gas volume. In most ventilators a calibrated accordion bellows is compressed with each inspiration. Observing that the bellows empties smoothly confirms that the set inspired gas volume is being delivered to the breathing circuit.

Monitoring breathing circuit pressures may also be used to indicate that the set inspired gas volume is being delivered. PIP depends on the resistance to flow of the breathing system and the compliance of the breathing system and thorax. PIP generally ranges from about 5 to 40 cm H_2O. Very low PIP indicates a very compliant breathing circuit, extremely compliant lungs, a significant leak in the system, or low inspiratory V_T. Very high PIP usually indicates that the respiratory system is extremely noncompliant, the resistance in the breathing circuit or airway is increased, or the inspiratory gas flow is high.

In addition to PIP, an airway plateau pressure can often be measured during an end-inspiratory pause. Measuring plateau pressure requires an end-inspiratory hold and depends on ventilator settings. Since inspiratory gas flow is zero, only the compliance of the breathing system and the lungs, not the resistance, contributes to the plateau pressure. An extremely low plateau pressure indicates that the V_T is not filling the system. An extremely high plateau pressure indicates the lung or breathing system is overfilled or stiff.

Breathing circuit leaks or obstructions are the most serious impediments to delivering an adequate inspired gas volume with intubated patients. Monitoring for faults in the breathing circuit must include one or more of the following: observing ventilation, auscultating breath sounds, measuring airway pressure, and measuring expiratory Pco_2.

Observing ventilation includes visualizing thoracic movements, abdominal movements, and, when the thorax is open, lung excursion. Observation also includes noting the appearance of condensation in the tracheal tube, the expansion and relaxation of the breathing circuit, sound and movement of the breathing bag or ventilator bellows, and the effect of the cycling intrathoracic pressure on cardiovascular variables (e.g., respiratory modulation of intraarterial, pulmonary artery, and central venous pressures and electrocardiogram [ECG]).

Breath sounds should be auscultated whenever a change in the airway status occurs. Preoperatively, this occurs after intubation, during a change in patient position, during changes in ventilation mode, and after resumption of ventilation following cardiopulmonary bypass. In the absence of other monitoring modalities such as respiratory Pco_2, continuous auscultation of breath sounds with a precordial or esophageal stethoscope is indicated.

Measuring airway pressure can detect many breathing circuit leaks, disconnections, and obstructions. As shown in Fig. 42-5, common points for breathing circuit disconnection include the tracheal tube adapter from the tracheal tube, the **Y** piece from the tracheal tube adapter, the corrugated breathing tube from the inspiratory and expiratory 15 mm adapters, and extubation. Also, Fig. 42-5 shows the common points for monitoring breathing circuit pressure. During positive pressure ventilation, PIP usually exceeds 15 cm H_2O and sometimes reaches 60 cm H_2O. The measured PIP achieved depends on several factors, including the breathing circuit compliance, airway resistance (primarily the tracheal tube adapter), the patient's compliance, the ventilator driving pressure, and the location of the measuring

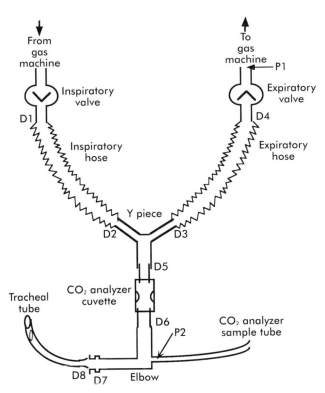

Fig. 42-5. Schematic of circle breathing system showing common points of disconnection: *D1*, inspiratory hose; *D2*, inspiratory Y piece; *D3*, expiratory Y piece; *D4*, expiratory hose; *D5*, common Y piece; *D6*, elbow; *D7*, tracheal tube adapter; *D8*, tracheal tube. Diagram shows two gas analyzer systems; mainstream CO_2 analyzer cuvette interposed between Y piece and elbow and sidestream CO_2 analyzer sample tube at elbow. Two common points *(P1, P2)* for measuring breathing circuit pressure are shown.

manometer.[30] Complete disconnections in the breathing circuit usually result in a loss of the positive pressure swings, and the pressure gauge usually shows greatly diminished peak pressures. Automatic disconnection detection systems are incorporated into most modern anesthesia machines that anticipate pressure changes above a threshold (e.g., 7.5 cm H_2O) at least once every 20 seconds. If no pressure fluctuation is observed, an alarm sounds.

Similarly, breathing circuit obstructions can occur at various points in the system. Fig. 42-6 shows the typical points for obstruction of the circuit with a tracheal tube, inspiratory valve, and expiratory valve. Sources of obstruction include foreign bodies,[81] mucous plugs, blood, or other patient-produced substances. Obstructions can also result from kinking of the expiratory tubing[54] or from mechanical faults[4,72] or manufacturing defects in the breathing circuit system.[6,34] Misplacement of one-way valves (e.g., positive end-expiratory pressure [PEEP] valves) can also result in circuit obstruction, and their use should be avoided.[7] Observed breathing circuit pressure

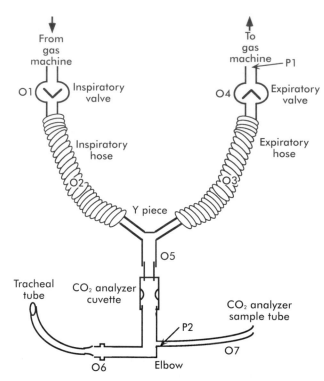

Fig. 42-6. Schematic of circle breathing system showing common points of obstruction: *O1,* inspiratory valve; *O2,* inspiratory hose; *O3,* expiratory hose; *O4,* expiratory valve; *O5,* common Y piece; *O6,* tracheal tube or adapter; *O7,* CO_2 analyzer sample tube. Diagram shows two gas analyzer systems; mainstream CO_2 analyzer cuvette interposed between Y piece and elbow and sidestream CO_2 analyzer sample tube at elbow. Two common points *(P1, P2)* for measuring breathing circuit pressure are shown.

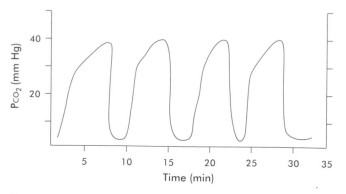

Fig. 42-7. Respiratory CO_2 analyzer waveforms demonstrating sloping upslope of P_{CO_2} during expiration. This usually results from partial airway obstruction, obstructive lung disease, or laryngospasm.

changes depend on the location of the pressure monitor tap, the location of the obstruction, and the mode of ventilation.

Automatic manometry systems that can detect breathing circuit obstruction are incorporated in many anesthesia machines. These systems detect high pressure in the breathing circuit (60 to 80 cm H_2O) or pressure that does not return to baseline within a predetermined interval (20 seconds). With a complete obstruction, some ventilators with adjustable inspiratory gas flow controls may not produce enough positive pressure to reach the alarm threshold of the high-pressure monitor.[11] Some systems have user-adjustable, high-pressure alarm thresholds to overcome this problem.

Monitoring respiratory CO_2 is an excellent method to detect breathing circuit problems. For example, complete obstruction or disconnection at most of the points shown in Figs. 42-5 or 42-6 during positive pressure ventilation of a paralyzed patient results in the absence of a CO_2 waveform. Partial disconnections may result in some ventilation and thus a CO_2 waveform, although it may look different than the

normal, rectangular-like waveshape. Partial obstruction of the expiratory valve (O4), expiratory hose (O3), the patient Y piece (O5), or the tracheal tube (O6) often results in CO_2 waveforms with sloping upstrokes (Fig. 42-7). Partial obstruction of the inspiratory valve or limb (D1 or D2) may or may not change the CO_2 waveform appreciably.

Tracheal tube misplacements such as esophageal intubation can also be detected via the CO_2 waveform.[58] In some cases a few pulses of CO_2 may result when ventilating the esophagus, but within the first three or four attempted breaths the CO_2 is absent.[49] Intubation of the right or left mainstem bronchus can sometimes be detected with CO_2 monitoring.[80] A sloping upstroke, similar to that seen with a partial expiratory obstruction, may be observed (Fig. 42-7).

Oxygen tension of the blood

The adequacy of oxygenation of the patient is best assessed in terms of the P_{O_2} or O_2 content in the blood. O_2 is present in the blood in two forms, bound to hemoglobin and dissolved in the plasma. The O_2 content is determined by the following equation:

$$O_2 \text{ content (g/dl)} = S_{O_2} \, (\%) \times Hb \, (g/dl) \times 1.34 \, (ml/g)$$
$$+ \, 0.003 \, (ml/dl/mm \, Hg) \times P_{O_2} \, (mm \, Hg)$$

where S_{O_2} is the percentage of hemoglobin (Hb) molecules saturated with O_2, and P_{O_2} is the O_2 tension. The value 1.34 is the molar O_2 capacity of Hb, and the value 0.003 is the solubility of O_2 in plasma. The typical O_2 content of arterial blood (Ca_{O_2}) of about 20 ml/dl is substantially greater than the O_2 content of the mixed venous blood (Cv_{O_2}) of 15 ml/dl because of O_2 extraction by the tissues. The ability of the Ca_{O_2} to provide for the metabolic demand depends on the distributional capability of the cardiovascular system. The following equation describes the relationship between the oxygen consumption

($\dot{V}O_2$), cardiac output ($\dot{Q}$), CaO_2, and CvO_2:

$$\dot{V}O_2 = \dot{Q} \times (CaO_2 - CvO_2)$$

Clinically, it is important to remember this relationship when assessing the adequacy of oxygenation. **For a given metabolic demand, inadequate oxygenation will result from a failure of one of three variables. First, circulation, as represented by $\dot{Q}$, may fail to meet distributional needs. Second, the arterial blood may not carry an adequate quantity of O_2, as reflected by low CaO_2. Finally, the tissues may be unable to extract O_2 because of a deficiency in the cellular metabolic apparatus, as reflected by a small CaO_2-CvO_2 difference.**

The first step in monitoring PO_2 of the blood is visual observation of the color of the patient's skin, lips, and blood. Observed cyanosis generally indicates severe hypoxemia, since it requires 5 g of deoxygenated Hb per deciliter of blood for cyanosis to be observable.[52] With a normal total hemoglobin (Hb_{TOT}) of 15 g/dl, this corresponds to an SaO_2 substantially less than 70%. In addition, observed or absent cyanosis is an unreliable monitor of oxygenation because of its subjectivity.[22]

The SO_2 is defined as 100 times the O_2 content divided by the O_2 capacity corrected for the dissolved O_2.[68] This corresponds to the fraction of oxyhemoglobin (HbO_2) to the total number of Hb molecules present in the blood. The remainder of the Hb may be functional or dysfunctional (i.e., incapable of carrying O_2). Dysfunctional species include carboxyhemoglobin (HbCO) and methemoglobin (Hb_{MET}).

Measuring SO_2 requires analysis of a blood sample in a co-oximeter analyzer. This type of analyzer generally measures and reports Hb, HbO_2, HbCO, Hb_{MET}, and Hb_{TOT} and the respective fractional saturations. Automatic blood gas analyzers often report SO_2, but this value is calculated from the measured PO_2, PCO_2, pH, and temperature using the HbO_2 dissociation relationship.[83] Dysfunctional hemoglobins and other factors that shift the HbO_2 dissociation curve (e.g., base excess, 2,3-diphosphoglycerate [2,3-DPG], citrate, phosphate, fetal Hb) are not always considered in the calculation.[42]

The SaO_2 can be estimated using a pulse oximeter measurement (SpO_2). Unlike SaO_2, the SpO_2 is a functional saturation defined as the HbO_2 relative to the total of oxyhemoglobin and deoxyhemoglobin. Since dysfunctional Hb species are not intended to be measured by the pulse oximeter, they are excluded from the Hb_{TOT} in the denominator of this relationship. Some manufacturers of the pulse oximeter have adjusted the displayed SpO_2 to account for the general population having approximately 2% HbCO in their blood.[102]

The SvO_2 may also be estimated using measure-

ment from a fiberoptic catheter spectrophotometer located in the right atrium or pulmonary artery. Similar to the pulse oximeter, these devices measure functional SO_2. These devices must be placed with a balloon flotation catheter. As such, they have the potential for complications, including embolism, knotting, dysrhythmias, infection, arterial perforation, and pneumothorax.[40] Also, these devices are expensive. Use of SvO_2 monitoring devices is generally indicated only when failure of O_2 extraction is suspected.

Measuring the PO_2 of a sample of arterial or venous blood is the most direct method to assess oxygenation of the blood. A small sample of blood must be collected anaerobically in a heparinized container for analysis. Syringe devices designed specifically for blood gas collection may contain a small quantity of freeze-dried heparin, thus preventing dilution of the sample.[38] The sample should be analyzed within 10 minutes or stored at 0° C for up to 30 minutes to avoid a decline in PO_2.[15] Automatic blood gas analyzers generally analyze the blood and report the results at 37° C. Correction of PO_2 to patient temperature can be accomplished mathematically.[5] It is arguable whether this correction is appropriate for clinical management.

The HbO_2 equilibrium relationship can be used to convert SO_2 to PO_2, and vice versa.[84,97] A rough estimate of PO_2 in mm Hg can be made from SO_2 in the range of 60% to 90% by subtracting 30 from the SO_2.

Complete assessment of the adequacy of oxygenation of the patient requires consideration of venous admixture. Drainage of the thebesian veins of the heart, bronchial veins, and intrapulmonary arteriovenous shunts cause mixed venous blood to enter directly into the arterial system without gas exchange. In addition, atelectasis, pneumothorax, pulmonary embolism, pulmonary edema, respiratory distress syndrome, and congenital heart disease can cause this venous admixture. Maldistribution of ventilation and perfusion in the lung, resulting in regional underventilation or overperfusion, can contribute to apparent venous admixture as well. The principal clinical observation resulting from shunting is a marked lowering of the PaO_2 and an increase in the difference between alveolar PO_2 (PAO_2) and PaO_2. The ratio of blood effectively bypassing gas exchange to the $\dot{Q}$ is termed the *shunt fraction* and is given by the equation:

$$\dot{Q}s/\dot{Q} = (PAO_2 - PaO_2)/(PAO_2 - PvO_2)$$

where $\dot{Q}$ is the shunted blood flow. The shunt fraction is difficult to measure because PvO_2 and PAO_2 must be determined. PvO_2 requires measurement of pulmonary artery blood via a balloon flotation catheter. PAO_2 cannot be measured directly but can be roughly estimated by:

$$PAO_2 = PIO_2 - (Paco_2/R)$$

where R is the respiratory exchange ratio ($\sim$ 0.8) and PIO_2 is inspiratory O_2 tension. The shunt fraction can also be approximated from measurement of the Pao_2 and the FIO_2. Fig. 42-8 is a diagram of the relationship between these variables showing bands of virtual shunt and assuming an Cao_2-Cvo_2 difference of 5 vol %. From Fig. 42-8 the virtual shunt can be approximated, and further changes in Pao_2 can be predicted as FIO_2 is changed by moving along the isoshunt bands.

Carbon dioxide tension of blood

The adequacy of minute ventilation appropriate to the patient's acid-base state is evaluated according to the Pco_2 in the arterial blood ($Paco_2$). $Paco_2$ in the normal range of 36 to 40 mm Hg is usually desirable. In some circumstances (e.g., elevated intracranial pressure), lower values of $Paco_2$ are sought. The alveolar ventilation required to achieve and maintain a desired $Paco_2$ can be estimated from the following equation:

$$V_A \text{ (L/m)} =$$
$$1.25 \text{ (mm Hg)} \times \dot{V}co_2 \text{ (ml/m)}/Paco_2 \text{ (mm Hg)}$$

where V_A is the required alveolar minute ventilation; 1.25 is a constant; $\dot{V}co_2$ is the predicted CO_2 production at standard temperature, pressure, dry (STPD); and $Paco_2$ is the desired $Paco_2$. The $\dot{V}co_2$

can be estimated from various tables and nomograms.[63] The minute volume necessary to achieve the required V_A must consider the mechanical, anatomic, and alveolar dead space. As discussed previously, during anesthesia and automatic ventilation at low tidal volumes (V_T), total dead space may represent one third to two thirds of V_T. Minute ventilation must therefore be increased to 1.5 to 3 times the required V_A to compensate for the dead space.

Considerations for sampling arterial blood to measure the $Paco_2$ are similar to those for Pao_2. **The end-tidal Pco_2 ($PETco_2$) monitored with a respiratory CO_2 analyzer can be used to estimate the $Paco_2$. The CO_2 in the pulmonary capillary blood, beginning with a Pco_2 about 6 mm Hg greater than arterial, reaches equilibrium with the alveolar gas. Theoretically, the gas at the end of an expiration is alveolar. Thus, in the healthy subject with little or no alveolar dead space, $PETco_2$ is an indirect measure of $Paco_2$. However, in anesthesia and intensive care settings, a difference between $Paco_2$ and $PETco_2$ is often observed.** This difference has been the subject of numerous investigations (selected studies are summarized in Table 42-1). Virtually all investigators have reported a difference. The observations differ somewhat among studies but average 3 to 4 mm Hg and can be as great as 18 mm Hg. Also, the variability of the difference between $Paco_2$ and $PETco_2$ among subjects is usually 3 to 4 mm Hg (1 standard deviation [SD]). Generally, this difference has been attributed to increased alveolar dead space caused by one of several conditions, including obstructive airway disease, surgery, mechanical ventilation, supine position, and various other clinical interventions and diseases. Clinically, it is important to recognize that $PETco_2$ underestimates $Paco_2$ by 3 to 4 mm Hg on average and not to rely on $PETco_2$ exclusively for managing ventilation.

$PETco_2$ measurements should be considered at body temperature and saturated with water vapor (BTPS). Some respiratory gas analyzers dry the sample and report the $PETco_2$ as measured. The reported values should be corrected for water vapor by applying the formula:

$$PETco_2 \text{ (BTPS)} \cong PETco_2 \text{ (dry)} \times (P_{BAR} - 47)/P_{BAR}$$

where P_{BAR} is the barometric pressure, and 47 is the saturated vapor pressure of water in mm Hg at 37° C.[85]

Expired Gas Volume

Monitoring expired volume ensures that the gas delivered to the patient has been successfully returned to the circuit and that the entire ventilation system is operational. As a reasonable estimator of alveolar ventilation, expired volume is often used to guide

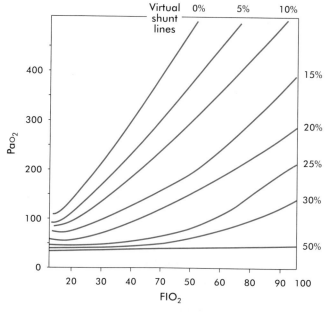

Fig. 42-8. Isoshunt diagram. Fraction of inspired O_2 is shown on the abscissa, and Pao_2 is shown on the ordinate. Bands of virtual shunt are shown from 0% to 50%. Hb of 10 to 14 g/dl, $Paco_2$ of 25 to 40 mm Hg, and (Cao_2 − Cvo_2) of 5 vol% are assumed. (Modified from Nunn JF: *Applied respiratory physiology,* London, 1977, Butterworths.)

Table 42-1   Selected differences between arterial and end-tidal CO_2 tension (P[a − ET]co_2) (1955 to present)

Author	Year	P (a − ET) co_2	Clinical setting*	Population†
Collier et al.[21]	1955	1.9 ± 2.4	Iron lung	41 patients, poliomyelitis
Nunn and Hill[66]	1960	4.5 ± 2.3	A/spon	12 patients, gynecologic surgery
		4.7 ± 2.3	A/IPPV	
Nunn[64]	1961	5.2 ± 1.5	A/IPPV	6 patients, thoracic surgery, prone
		10.5 ± 7.5	A/IPPV	6 patients, thoracic surgery, lateral
Askrog et al[8]	1964	5.9 ± 2.7	A/IPPV	7 patients, deliberate hypotension
Kowalski[46]	1966	2.0 ± 1.0	Awake	10 normal subjects
		7.0 ± 5.2	Awake	40 patients, COPD
		2.9 ± 3.2	Awake	12 patients, restrictive PD
Noe et al.[61]	1970	4.0 ± 3.5	Awake	10 normal subjects
		9.1 ± 3.3	Awake	15 patients, postoperative
Takki et al.[96]	1972	3.5 ± 2.5	A/IPPV	24 patients, 10 with COPD
Dahlgren and Symreng[26]	1974	2.3	A/IPPV	Neurosurgical patients
Poppius et al.[70]	1975	0.8	Awake	13 normal subjects
		3.8	Awake	13 patients, normal
		5.2	Awake	20 patients, restrictive PD
		7.5	Awake	17 patients, COPD
Dumpit and Brady[28]	1978			Arterialized capillary blood
		2.4	Awake	12 normal neonates
		8.2	Awake	7 restless neonates
		3.5	Awake	25 neonates recovered from RDS
		9.0	Awake	15 neonates, BPD
Prakash et al.[71]	1978	3.0	A/IPPV	29 infants, cardiac surgery
Luft et al.[51]	1979	6.7 ± 2.9	Awake	54 patients, PD
Fletcher[36]	1980	1.5 median	A/IPPV	87 patients, large V_T
		3.0 median	A/IPPV	86 patients, small V_T
Whitesell et al.[99]	1981	1.7 ± 3.5	A/IPPV	80 patients, general surgery
Raemer et al.[74]	1983	4.1 ± 2.6	A/IPPV	18 patients, major surgery
Epstein et al.[31]	1985	7.5 ± 4.5	IPPV	24 neonates, NICU
Bermudez and Lichtiger[14]	1987	4.6 ± 2.9	A/IPPV	25 patients, before cardiac bypass
		11.5 ± 3.5	A/IPPV	25 patients, after cardiac bypass
Fletcher[35]	1988	−0.3 ± 1.0	A/IPPV	13 children, normal circulation
		0.1 ± 1.4	A/IPPV	15 children, left-to-right shunts
		7.7 ± 4.9	A/IPPV	14 children, right-to-left shunts
		1.9 ± 2.6	A/IPPV	8 children, mixed shunts
Shankar et al.[91]	1989	0.5 (0.1-1.2)	A/IPPV	16 women, pregnant

*A, Awake; *IPPV*, intermittent positive pressure ventilation; *spon*, spontaneous ventilation.
†*COPD*, Chronic obstructive pulmonary disease; *PD*, pulmonary disease; *RDS*, respiratory distress syndrome; *BPD*, bronchopulmonary disease; V_T, tidal volume; *NICU*, neonatal intensive care unit.

adjustment of the mechanical ventilator or of manual ventilation.

The contribution of the gas compressed and stored in the distension of the breathing circuit must be considered in the expired ventilation measurement. This quantity of gas is a function of the ventilator parameters, the airway apparatus resistance, and compliance of the breathing circuit and patient. As cited earlier, the volume contributed to each measured expired V_T by gas compression and circuit compliance is typically about 150 ml.[30]

RESPIRATORY MONITORING TECHNOLOGY

Many devices are available for monitoring the patient's respiratory function in the operating room and postoperative care unit. Technical developments during the last decade have provided many choices for monitoring each component of the respiratory pathway. Understanding the principles of measurement, the operation, and the limitations of these devices is important to enable the clinician to choose the appropriate monitoring array and to use it effectively.

Devices for monitoring gas composition include O_2,

respiratory CO_2, and multigas analyzers. Pressure, flow, and volume instruments include manometers and respiratory flowmeters. Devices for monitoring O_2 and CO_2 in the blood include oximeters and blood gas analyzers. Many other technologies are available to make these measurements and are used frequently for clinical research (e.g., pneumotachographs, transcutaneous gas monitors, indwelling blood gas analyzers). However, only devices in widespread clinical use for monitoring respiratory function during and immediately after anesthesia are discussed here.

Gas Composition
Oxygen analyzers

The fraction of inspired oxygen (FIO_2) or fraction of expired oxygen (FEO_2) from an anesthesia breathing circuit is monitored with an O_2 analyzer. **Three types of O_2 analyzers typically are used for monitoring: those based on a polarographic sensor, a fuel cell, or a paramagnetic sensor. In addition to these methods, multigas analyzers using mass spectroscopy and Raman spectroscopy measure O_2 and are sometimes used as O_2 monitors.**

The *polarogaphic O_2 sensor* (Fig. 42-9) consists of a noble metal electrode (usually platinum) and a reference electrode in an electrolyte bath. An electrical potential of -0.6 to -0.8 volt is impressed across the electrodes, thus "polarizing" them. The sensor is exposed to the breathing circuit via an O_2-permeable membrane (usually Teflon). O_2 molecules traverse the membrane at a rate proportional to their partial pressure in the breathing circuit. The sensor consumes the O_2 molecules according to the following two-step oxidation-reduction reaction:

$$O_2 + 2H_2O + 2e^- \rightarrow H_2O_2 + 2OH^-$$
$$H_2O_2 + 2e^- \rightarrow 2OH^-$$

For every molecule of O_2 reduced, four electrons (e^-) are supplied by the electrical circuit. Thus the current, having been determined by the availability of O_2 molecules, is directly proportional to the O_2 partial pressure (PO_2) in the breathing circuit. Measurement of the current and conversion to units of PO_2 or equivalent concentration can easily be accomplished electronically and the results displayed on a digital (numeric) or analog (needle) meter.

The *fuel cell,* or *galvanic cell,* is basically an O_2

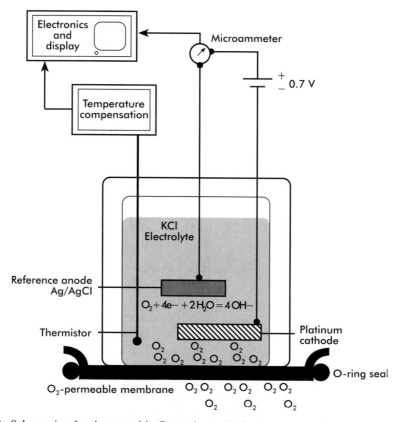

Fig. 42-9. Schematic of polarographic O_2 analyzer. O_2 in the gas sample permeates a Teflon or polyethylene membrane and enters a potassium chloride *(KCl)* electrolyte solution. When a potential of 0.7 volt from a battery is impressed across a platinum cathode and reference anode, current will flow through circuit in proportion to O_2 availability. Measured current is thus linearly related to PO_2 of gas sample. Temperature compensation is required for accurate measurement. *AgCl,* Silver chloride.

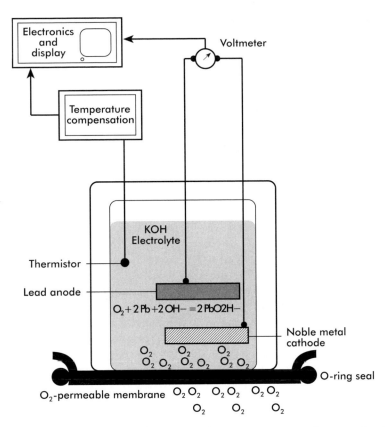

Fig. 42-10. Fuel cell O_2 analyzer. O_2 in gas sample permeates a membrane and enters a potassium hydroxide *(KOH)* electrolyte solution. A potential is established between a lead *(Pb)* anode and noble metal cathode as O_2 is supplied to anode. Measured voltage between electrodes is proportional to Po_2 of gas sample. Temperature compensation is required for accurate measurement.

battery consisting of a noble metal cathode and a lead (Pb) anode in a potassium hydroxide (KOH) electrolyte bath (Fig. 42-10). As with the polarographic electrode, an O_2-permeable membrane is exposed to the breathing circuit. O_2 is reduced at the cathode according to the following reaction:

$$O_2 + 2H_2O + 4e^- \rightarrow 4OH^-$$

The following reaction occurs at the anode:

$$2Pb + 6OH^- \rightarrow 2PbO_2H^- + 2H_2O + 4e^-$$

Thus a voltage develops that is proportional to the Po_2. No polarization potential is required. The galvanic sensor voltage can be measured and electronically scaled to units of Po_2 or equivalent concentration and displayed.

The *paramagnetic sensor* uses the strong, positive magnetic susceptibility of the gaseous O_2 molecule to measure the concentration in a breathing circuit. Because of two electrons in unpaired orbits, the O_2 molecule is attracted by a magnetic field. Modern paramagnetic O_2 sensors use this property by measuring a pressure differential between a stream of reference gas (air) and the measurement gas as the

streams are exposed to a changing magnetic field. An electromagnet is rapidly switched off and on, creating a changing magnetic field between its poles. The electromagnet is designed to have its poles in proximity, forming a narrow gap. The streams of measurement and reference gases are introduced to the gap between the magnet poles and then exit together. Assuming the measurement and reference gases have different Po_2, the pressure between the entrance and exit of the respective gas streams differs slightly because of the magnetic force on the O_2 molecules. A sensitive pressure transducer is used to convert this force to an electrical signal. The electrical signal can then be filtered appropriately and used to display the Po_2 or equivalent concentration.

All O_2 analyzers require periodic calibration. Since in all analyzers an electrical signal is produced proportional to Po_2, the constant of proportionality (gain) must be determined. Generally, the electrical signal in the presence of 0% O_2 is known to be near zero. Thus no offset correction is required. With the polarographic or fuel cell analyzer, the gain changes with time because of changes in electrolyte, electrode, and membrane. The gain of the paramagnetic sensor changes with temperature, humidity, and pneumatic factors. Calibration with a known gas, either room air (21% O_2) or 100% O_2, before each use is practical. Some oxygen analyzers perform their own periodic, computer-controlled, automatic calibration process.

The response time of O_2 analyzers differs. Polarographic and fuel cell analyzers respond to changes in Po_2 in the breathing circuit quite slowly because of their dependence on membrane diffusion. Response times are generally 20 to 30 seconds, prohibiting breath-by-breath measurements. Some analyzers use a single fuel cell to measure inspired and expired concentrations by directing the gas to the sensor with a valve. The valve is timed according to a CO_2 waveform to direct only inspired gas to the sensor for several sequential breaths. Then the valve is timed to direct only expired gas to the sensor for several breaths. Thus both inspired and expired concentrations are displayed, although averaged over several breaths. The paramagnetic analyzer, having no membrane, can respond on a breath-by-breath basis. Sampling from the breathing circuit Y piece, the paramagnetic O_2 analyzer can measure both inspired

and expired O_2 concentrations and display the real-time waveforms.

Respiratory gas analyzers

The infrared analyzer, photoacoustic spectrometer, Raman spectrometer, and mass spectrometer are the instruments typically used for respiratory CO_2 monitoring during anesthesia. The *infrared analyzer* is based on the relationship between light energy absorbed and the molar concentration of a gas, originally stated by Bouguer, rediscovered by Lambert, and finally refined by Beer.[43] The development of the first instrument for medical use has been attributed to Luft in 1943 in Germany.[93] Following World War II, Max Liston, an American engineer, obtained the patent for the detector Luft had developed. Liston developed the Model 16 CO_2 analyzer, a precursor to the LB-1 and LB-2 medical analyzers (Beckman Instruments Co.) typically used through the 1970s.

The *Raman spectrometer* is based on the elucidation of the phenomenon of spectral shift scattering by Raman and Krishnan in 1928.[77] This technology has

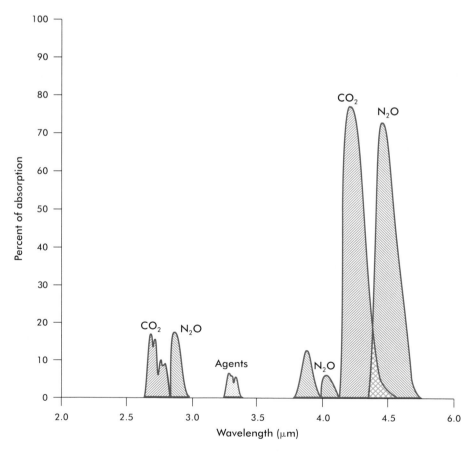

Fig. 42-11. Absorption bands of respiratory gases in infrared spectrum. CO_2 absorbs strongly at 4.25 μm center wavelength, N_2O absorbs strongly at 4.4 μm, and anesthetic agents have absorption bands of approximately 3.2 μm.

only recently been applied to medical gas analysis by Van Wagenen and associates.[98]

The first principles of *mass spectrometry* were presented by Thompson in 1912, and the first focusing instrument was developed 6 years later by Dempster.[27] The initial use of the mass spectrometer for respiratory measurements is credited to Fowler and Hugh-Jones in 1957.[37] Severinghaus and Ozanne[90] introduced the multiplexed mass spectrometer to the operating room and are generally recognized for developing this application.

Infrared analyzers. Infrared (IR) spectroscopy involves measuring energy absorbed from a narrow band of wavelengths of IR light passing through a gas sample. CO_2, N_2O, H_2O, and volatile anesthetic agents absorb IR energy when their atoms rotate or vibrate asymmetrically, resulting in a change in dipole moment. The nonpolar molecules argon (Ar), N_2, helium (He), xenon (Xe), and O_2 do not absorb IR energy. Since the number of molecules in the path of the IR energy determine the total absorption, IR analyzers measure *partial pressure* of a gas.

The respiratory and anesthetic gases exhibit absorption of IR radiation at unique bands in the spectrum (Fig. 42-11). CO_2 absorbs strongly between 4.2 and 4.4 micrometers (μm). N_2O absorbs strongly between 4.4 and 4.6 μm. Anesthetic agents have strong absorption bands at 3.1 and throughout the 9 to 12 μm regions. Because of the proximity of their absorption bands, some CO_2 analyzers are affected by high concentrations of N_2O.[88]

A separate phenomenon termed *collision broadening* may affect IR analyzer measurements. Molecular collisions cause a change in the dipole moment of the gas being analyzed. Thus the IR absorption band is broadened, and the apparent absorption at the measurement wavelength is altered.[60] In a typical IR CO_2 analyzer, 95% O_2 causes a 0.5% decline in the measured CO_2. N_2O causes a more substantial increase of about 0.1% CO_2 per 10% N_2O because of collision broadening. Some analyzers automatically compensate for the effect of collision broadening by measuring or estimating concentrations of interfering gases.

Fig. 42-12 shows a block diagram of an IR analyzer consisting of five components: light source, optical path, signal detector, signal processor, and gas sampler.

Light sources made of tungsten wires or ceramic resistive materials heated to 1500° to 4000° K emit energy over a broad wavelength range that includes the absorption spectrum of the respiratory gases.

Because energy output of IR light sources tends to drift, optical systems have been designed to stabilize the analyzers. Three common designs are distinguished by their use of single and dual IR beams and positive or negative filtering.[75]

In the *single-beam positive filter,* precision optical bandpass filters mounted on a spinning wheel (40 to 250 rpm) sequentially interrupt a single IR beam. The beam retains energy at a narrow band of wavelengths during each interruption. For each gas of interest, a pair of bandpass filters is selected at an absorption peak and at a reference wavelength where relatively little absorption occurs. The chopped IR beam then passes through a cuvette containing the sample gas. The ratio of IR beam intensity for each pair of filters is proportional to the partial pressure of the gas and is insensitive to changes in the intensity of the IR source.

Another single-beam positive filter design uses stationary optical filters instead of a spinning filter

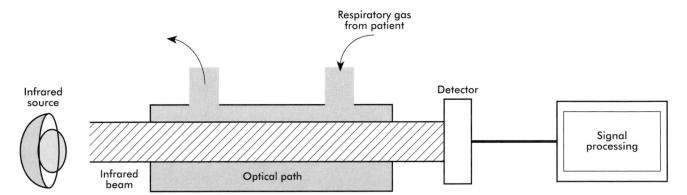

Fig. 42-12. Block diagram of infrared (IR) respiratory gas analyzer. An IR source emits a beam that passes through an optical path. Respiratory gas from patient is sampled and passes through optical path. An IR detector filters the beam and measures IR power absorbed by gas sample. Electrical signal from detector is processed to report gas composition in appropriate units of measure.

wheel. The pairs of filters are mounted close together within the circumference of the IR beam. A separate IR detector for each filter is used to measure the IR intensity. As before, the ratio of intensity at the absorption peak and reference wavelength is used to calculate the partial pressure of each gas in the sample.

In the *single-beam negative filter design,* the filters are usually gas-filled cells mounted in a spinning wheel. During each interruption the IR beam retains energy at all wavelengths except those absorbed by the gas. For each gas of interest, a cell with a high percentage of that gas and a cell with a nonabsorbing reference gas are used. The chopped IR beam then passes through a cuvette containing the sample gas. Similar to the positive filter design, the ratio of IR beam intensity for each pair of filter cells is proportional to the partial pressure of the gas and is insensitive to changes in the intensity of the IR source.

In the *dual-beam positive filter design,* the IR energy from the source is split into two parallel beams. One beam passes through the sample gas and the other through a reference gas. A spinning blade passes through the beams and sequentially interrupts one, the other, and both. The two beams are optically focused to a single point, where a bandpass optical filter selected at the absorption peak of the gas of interest is mounted over a single detector. As before, the intensity ratio of the sample and reference beams is proportional to the partial pressure of the gas.

For measuring CO_2, N_2O, and sometimes anesthetic agents, a radiation-sensitive solid-state material, lead selenide, is frequently used as a detector. Lead selenide is quite temperature sensitive and thus is usually thermostatically cooled or temperature compensated.[43]

Anesthetic agents and occasionally CO_2 and N_2O are sometimes measured with another detector type, the *Luft cell.* This detector uses a chamber filled with gas that expands as IR radiation enters the chamber and is absorbed. A flexible wall of the chamber acts as a diaphragm that moves as the gas expands, and a microphone converts the motion to an electrical signal.[50]

The signal processor converts the measured electrical currents to display the partial pressure of the gas. First, the ratios of detector currents at various points in the spinning wheel's progress (or from multiple detectors) are computed. Next, electronic scaling and filtering are applied. Finally, according to a table that contains the point-by-point conversion from electrical voltage to gas partial pressure, linearization is accomplished by a microprocessor. Compensation for cross-sensitivity or interference between gases can be accomplished by the microprocessor following linearization.

One of two methods for obtaining the gas sample are used clinically: mainstream or sidestream. *Mainstream instruments* locate a cuvette directly in the patient's respiratory gas stream. An IR optical measurement device is fitted over the cuvette, which is heated to about 40° C to prevent condensation on its windows. Advantages of the mainstream monitors include convenience, no waste gas disposal, and no compensation needed for water vapor. Bulkiness, vibration, and fragility of the sensor are limitations of these monitors.

Sidestream instruments continuously withdraw 50 to 500 ml/min from the breathing circuit through narrow-gauge sample tubing to the optical system, where the measurement is made. Sidestream monitors are sometimes considered more versatile than the mainstream monitors because the sample tubing can be put out of the way. Sample tubing is less cumbersome in the breathing circuit. The disadvantages of sidestream instruments are slower speed response and the need to deal with liquid water and water vapor. Water vapor from the breathing circuit condenses on its way to the sample cuvette and can interfere with optical transmission. Nafion tubing, a semipermeable polymer that selectively allows water vapor to pass from its interior to the relatively dry exterior, is sometimes used to eliminate water vapor.[45] A water trap is usually interposed between the patient sample line and the analyzer to protect the optical system from liquid water and body fluids.[32]

Photoacoustic spectrometer. As shown in Fig. 42-13, the photoacoustic spectrometer is similar to the basic IR spectometer. IR energy is passed through optical filters that select narrow-wavelength bands corresponding to the absorption characteristics of the respiratory gases. Evenly spaced windows are located along circumferences of a rotating wheel. The optical components are located on the wheel along one of its radii. Thus a series of IR beams pulse on and off at particular frequencies according to the rotation rate of the wheel and the spacing of the windows. The gas flowing through the measurement cuvette is exposed to the pulsing IR beams. As each gas absorbs the pulsating IR energy in its absorption band, it expands and contracts at that frequency. The resulting sound waves are measured with a microphone. The partial pressure of each gas in the sample is then proportional to the amplitude of the measured sound.

The photoacoustic technique has the distinct advantage over other IR methods because a simple microphone detector can be used to measure all the IR-absorbing gases. However, this device is sensitive to interference from loud noises or vibration.

Raman spectrometer. Most of the energy scattered as light strikes gas molecules is absorbed and reemitted in the same direction and at the same wavelength

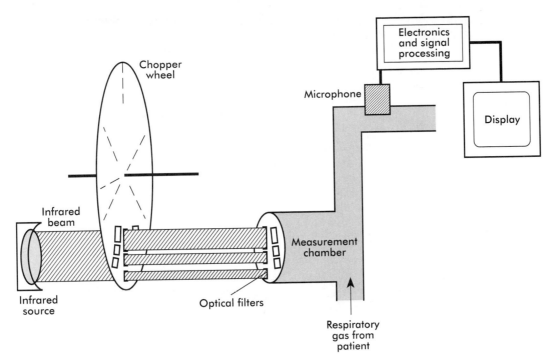

Fig. 42-13. Schematic diagram of photoacoustic spectrometer. An infrared (IR) source emits a beam that passes through a spinning "chopper wheel" having several rows of circumferential slots. Interrupted IR beams then pass through optical filters that select specific wavelengths of light chosen to be at absorption peaks of gases to be measured. Each interrupted IR light beam impinges on its respective gas in the measurement chamber, causing vibration of the gas as energy is absorbed and released from molecules. Vibration frequency of each gas depends on spacing of its slots on chopper wheel. A microphone converts gas vibration frequencies into electrical signals, which are converted to gas concentrations for display.

as the incoming beam (Rayleigh scattering). At room temperature, about 1 one-millionth of the energy is scattered at a longer wavelength, producing a so-called red-shifted spectrum. This Raman scattering can be used to measure the constituents of a gas mixture. Raman scattering is not limited to polar gas species as is IR spectroscopy. The gases CO_2, O_2, N_2, H_2O, N_2O, and anesthetic agents all exhibit Raman activity.

As shown in Fig. 42-14, the medical Raman spectrometer uses an ultraviolet laser to produce the incoming light beam. The measurement cuvette is located in the cavity of the laser so that the gas molecules are struck repeatedly by the beam. This results in enough Raman scattering to be collected and processed by the optical detection system. Photomultiplier tubes count the photons of scattered light at the characteristic, Raman-shifted wavelengths for each gas. Thus the Raman spectrometer measures the *partial pressures* of the gases in its measurement cuvette. Measurements are converted electronically to the desired units of measure and displayed on a screen.

Mass spectrometer. **A magnetic sector mass spec-**

trometer (Fig. 42-15) draws a minute fraction of the gas sampled from the breathing circuit into an evacuated measurement chamber. The gases are ionized by a stream of electrons. Fragments of predictable mass and charge are produced by the ionization process. An electrical field accelerates the ions through a constant magnetic field that deflects them according to their mass and charge. The heaviest ions have the longest trajectories. Strategically located metal dish collectors produce electrical currents as they receive the ions. An electronic system amplifies and scales these currents. The currents are summed in a circuit that ensures that the gas concentrations total 100%. Gases that are not measured, such as water vapor, are excluded by this process.

Unlike the magnetic sector mass spectrometer, the *quadrapole mass spectrometer* uses a varying magnetic field to establish the trajectory of the ions and a single dish to capture and measure them.

Clinical mass spectrometers are designed either to monitor a single patient continuously or to monitor several patients sequentially in different locations. Two types of systems share a single, centrally located

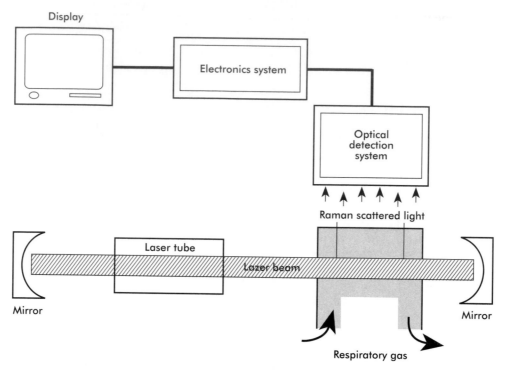

Fig. 42-14. Block diagram of Raman-scattering respiratory gas analyzer (Raman spectrometer). Laser tube generates monochromatic light that is contained within a cavity by mirrors. Respiratory gas from patient is sampled and passes through laser beam. Gas molecules scatter small amount of light at wavelengths different from those of incoming beam. Wavelength shift is characteristic of the gas species. The scattered light is detected, and gas composition is computed and displayed in appropriate units of measure.

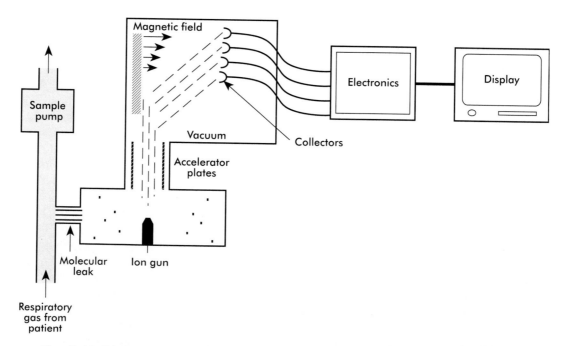

Fig. 42-15. Diagram of magnetic sector, respiratory mass spectrometer. Respiratory gas is sampled and passed by a molecular leak. Gas molecules enter a vacuum chamber, where they are ionized and electrically accelerated. A magnetic field deflects the ions. Mass and charge of ions determine their trajectory, where metal dish collectors are placed to detect them. Electrical currents produced by ions impacting collectors is processed, gas composition is computed, and results are displayed.

mass spectrometer. In one the gas is sampled from all locations through nylon tubing at a rate of about 250 ml/min. A rotary valve directs the gas samples, in turn, to the central mass spectrometer. The sampling locations may be up to 50 m from the central mass spectrometer.

In the second method the gas is continuously sampled from all patient locations at 90 ml/min to a waste line.[67] All the long sample tubing contains 20 seconds of inspired and expired gas. Solenoid valves sequentially switch each of the sample tubes to the inlet of the central mass spectrometer, where the gas is drawn into the evacuated inlet at twice the original sampling rate. The measurements are displayed at twice the speed to reproduce the proper timing of the waveforms. This method requires less time per patient location compared with direct sampling. The waveforms do not appear to be degraded when this technique is used.[67]

Pressure, Flow, and Volume
Manometers

Manometers for monitoring breathing circuit pressure are either analog gauges, solid-state transducers, or spring-loaded pressure switches.

An *analog dial gauge* usually is used to display the pressure in the breathing circuit at a location beyond the expiratory valve of the semiclosed circle system. The gauge itself is based on a Bourdon tube (Fig. 42-16), diaphram, or bellows. In the Bourdon tube design, an indicator needle mechanism is attached to the closed, free end of a curved piece of flattened, soft metal tubing. The open end of the tubing is in communication with the breathing circuit. Pressure in the circuit causes the tubing to become more circular, thus uncoiling the tubing and moving the indicator needle mechanism. A small adjustment screw is often used to align the indicator needle to the zero pressure mark when no pressure is applied. A high-quality Bourdon tube is accurate and reliable, requiring no mechanical stop at zero. Excessive pressures can bend the malleable tubing or indicator needle mechanism and ruin its operation.

Solid-state transducers are sometimes used to measure breathing circuit pressure because they permit an electronic display. The typical solid-state transducer is made from a crystal of the semiconductor silicon. A flexible diaphragm is etched into the crystal using integrated circuit techniques. A system of four resistive elements (Wheatstone's bridge) is produced in the diaphragm such that they predictably change value as the diaphram is deformed. During manufacture the resistances are trimmed with a laser, so no further calibration is required.

Pressure switches are often used to monitor breathing circuit pressures and are used in systems that

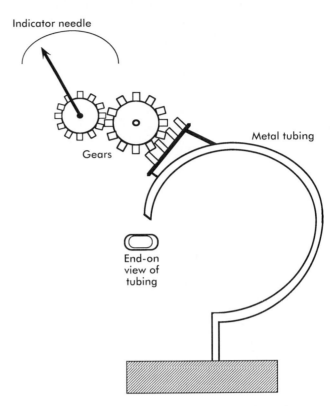

Fig. 42-16. Schematic representation of Bourdon tube pressure gauge. Gas pressure in oblong cross-sectional tubing causes slight straightening of coil. Tubing is attached to an indicator needle through mechanical linkage. Indicator needle is displayed in front of appropriately calibrated display.

detect excessive pressure, circuit integrity, and circuit obstruction. The pressure switch is designed such that the breathing circuit pressure is opposed by a linear spring or spring metal diaphragm (Fig. 42-17). In the diaphragm switch, when the pressure exceeds a threshold, the diaphragm is bent to a point where an electrical contact is made. The electrical contact is then used in an electronic circuit to detect breathing circuit pressure in excess of the specified value. An adjustment screw is sometimes provided to change the spring force and thus the threshold pressure value.

Flowmeters

Several types of respiratory flowmeters are used in anesthesia systems to monitor respiratory flow and volume. Generally, flowmeters are used to monitor V_T and minute volume. Occasionally, flowmeters capable of measuring instantaneous flow are used.

The *vane anemometer,* originally introduced into respiratory measurement by Wright,[101] is frequently used to measure V_T and minute ventilation. This device uses a rotating vane of low mass in the gas stream. Gas molecules colliding with the blades of the vane transfer their momentum in the direction of flow

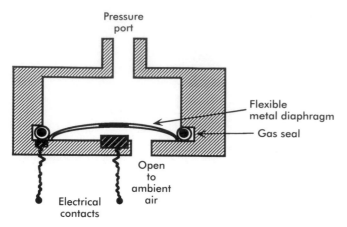

Fig. 42-17. Schematic cross section of pressure switch. Pressure of gas at pressure port forces metal diaphragm to make electrical contact when pressure exceeds a certain value. Some pressure switches have a spring and adjustment screw to allow calibration of switching pressure threshold.

and cause the vane to rotate. In the mechanical version the vane's rotation is connected to the dial via a gear mechanism resembling a watch. In an electronic implementation (Fig. 42-18), two pairs of light-emitting diodes (LEDs) and silicon photodetectors are used to measure the rate and direction of the vane rotation. The rotation rate is integrated electronically to determine the volume of gas passing the transducer over time.

Several physical factors limit the accuracy of the vane anemometer.[65] Since the principle of operation is momentum, the density of the gas affects the measurement. The gas flow is directed to the blades of the vane by tangential slots; thus the viscosity of the gas also influences the measurement. Furthermore, inertia and momentum of the vane are problematic. Accuracy is poor at low flows because of inertia and at high flows because of momentum. The accuracy of the Wright respirometer has been shown to be within 10% during anesthesia, whereas the modern electronic vane anemometer has not been evaluated.

A *sealed volumeter* (Fig. 42-19) is sometimes used to measure V_T and minute ventilation. This device

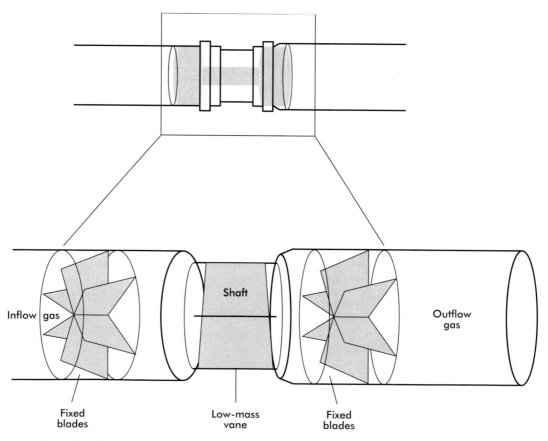

Fig. 42-18. Schematic drawing of electronic vane anemometer. Gas flow is directed by fixed vanes at inlet. Swirling gas causes a low-mass vane to spin. Light-emitting diodes (not shown) are positioned to detect rotations of the vane, which are converted into a flow measurement.

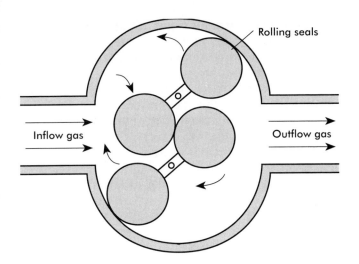

Fig. 42-19. Schematic drawing of sealed volumeter. Polystyrene rotating elements form a seal against interior of volumeter. Gas flow rotates elements, transferring fixed volumes from inlet to outlet. Measured volume is displayed on a gauge mechanically connected to rotating element shaft.

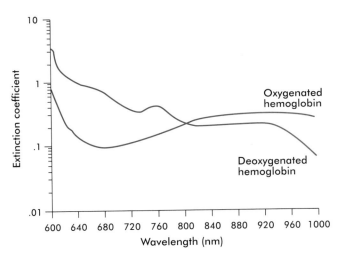

Fig. 42-20. Absorption spectra for oxygenated and deoxygenated hemoglobin.

consists of a pair of rotating elements in the gas flow path similar to a circular door at the entrance of an office building. A fixed volume of gas is passed across the transducer with each quarter rotation of the elements. A seal is formed between the polystyrene rotating elements and the interior wall of the tube.

The volumeter provides substantially more resistance to flow than the vane anemometer. The accuracy of the volumeter is affected by gas density and by inertia of the rotating elements. However, it is not influenced substantially by the flow pattern of the gas. The volumeter's accuracy has not been independently evaluated in an anesthesia setting.

A *pneumotachometer,* or *pneumotachograph,* is based on measurement of pressure across a resistive element in the flow path. The classic pneumotachometers, such as the Fleisch, use a series of parallel metal tubes or metal gauze mesh at the resistive element. The pressure measured across an appropriate element is essentially linear over a wide range of flow. The measurement is affected by gas viscosity and density.[41] Although highly accurate, the pneumotachometer is susceptible to fouling with moisture and mucus. Also, this device must be heated to prevent condensation from forming and must be calibrated frequently. Thus the pneumotachograph is not widely used in clinical anesthesia.

Oxygen in Blood
Oximeters

The oximeter is based on detecting the difference in absorption of particular wavelengths of light by oxygenated and reduced hemoglobin. The pulse oximeter uses this principle while employing the pulsatility of the arterial system to measure the saturation of arterial blood in vivo.

The modern pulse oximeter was conceived by Aoyagi in 1972, and the first instrument was produced in 1974 by the Minoruta Camera Co. in Japan.[87] Previously, oximeters had been developed that required some form of calibration, such as the exclusion of the venous blood from the earlobe.[86] Aoyagi's seminal idea was to use the pulsation of the optical transmission signal to discriminate between arterial blood saturation and background noise. The use of pulse oximetry with anesthesia in the United States was popularized by New and Lloyd in the early 1980s. They founded the Nellcor Corp. and developed a compact, convenient pulse oximeter specifically designed for use during anesthesia. By 1990, more than 27 companies marketed pulse oximeters for use during anesthesia, in the postanesthesia care unit (PACU), intensive care, and other health care specialties.

An oximeter for in vitro analysis uses multiwavelenth spectroscopy to perform its measurement. The absorption spectra for oxygenated (HbO_2) and deoxygenated hemoglobin (Hb) are shown in Fig. 42-20. Light in a particular wavelength band (e.g., 660 nm, a shade of red) is projected through a transparent cuvette, and the intensity of light transmitted is measured. When hemolyzed blood is placed in the cuvette, the amount of light transmitted is related to (1) the specific absorptions of Hb and HbO_2 at the particular wavelength band, (2) the total amount of Hb and HbO_2 in the light path, (3) the relative concentrations of Hb and HbO_2, and (4) the path length according to the Lambert-Beer law of absorption.[100]

Similarly, a second wavelength of light in another wavelength band (e.g., 940 nm, an infrared color just beyond the visible) can be simultaneously projected through the medium and the transmittance measured. By considering the ratio of the light transmitted at the two wavelengths, the dependence of the measurement on the total amount of Hb and HbO_2 and on the path length can be eliminated. Since the specific absorptions are known constants, the ratio of the transmitted light can be related to the proportion of HbO_2 to Hb.

In practice, laboratory oximeters use four to six wavelengths of light to measure other Hb species in the sample. Most oximeters can discriminate and measure Hb, HbO_2, HbCO, and Hb_{MET}.

To measure saturation of the arterial blood in vivo, the principle of pulse-added absorbance is used. Light in two wavelength bands is projected through tissue, such as a digit. The intensity of light transmitted is a function of the four variables previously listed. Also, the light transmitted is decreased by absorption by tissues other than blood. With each arterial pulsation, the amount of light transmitted is decreased by the quantity of Hb and HbO_2 in the new arterial blood that has entered the digit. Again, the ratio of light transmitted in each wavelength band and the ratio of the transmission at the peak and trough of the arterial pulsation are used to eliminate path length and total Hb and HbO_2 variables. Since the specific absorptions are known, only the relative concentrations of Hb and HbO_2 remain as variables.

An operation principle of the pulse oximeter is the Lambert-Beer law of absorption; in practice, however, light scattering causes a deviation from theory. Empiric calibration from human volunteer studies are generally used to compensate for this effect.

The pulse oximeter uses a pair of solid-state LEDs that efficiently emit narrow-wavelength bands of light. Usually, high-intensity LEDs with center wavelengths of 660 nm and 910 or 940 nm are used. The LEDs can transmit energy through a finger, nasal bridge, tongue, or ear lobe. The light is detected with a silicon photodiode.

The accuracy of the pulse oximeter has been the subject of many investigations. The agreement with a standard measurement, either an ex vivo oximeter or a calculated value from expired O_2 concentration, depends on the particular brand of pulse oximeter, the experimental method, and the range of values encountered. Generally, greater accuracy can be attained for SpO_2 greater than 70% because of the availability of data in this range. Extensive studies using healthy adult volunteers,[44,59,89,103] adult patients,[19,55] pediatric patients,[17,33] and neonates[29,57] have been performed using various manufacturers' models of pulse oximeters. These studies have shown, with some exceptions, that most devices agree with standard instruments within an average 2% and within 5% at a given value.

Various interferences with the accuracy of the pulse oximeter have been reported, including intravascular dye, fingernail polish, ambient light, electromagnetic radiation, and dysfunctional hemoglobins. Methylene blue, indocyanine green, and indigo carmine have been shown to interfere to some degree with the pulse oximeter, resulting in lower readings.[82,92] Coté et al.[25] demonstrated that various colors of nail polish caused artificially lower readings and recommended that polish always be removed from patients' fingers before application of a pulse oximeter sensor. Ambient light from a variety of sources, including common fluorescent light[39] and sunlight,[1] has been reported to cause artifactual readings from the pulse oximeter.

Electromagnetic interference from electrosurgical units (ESUs) is notorious for causing abberant readings from the pulse oximeter. Block and Detko[16] recommend placing the sensor as far as possible from the return plate, power cord, and cable of the ECU.

HbCO has been shown in animal experiments to interfere with pulse oximeters.[9,73] Since HbCO absorbs some light at each of the wavelengths used in the pulse oximeter, the magnitude of the artifact depends on the actual wavelength band used and the level of HbO_2 and Hb. An approximate correction equation follows:

$$SaO_2 = SpO_2 \times (1.0 - SaCO)$$

where $SaCO$ is the HbCO fraction. Hb_{MET} has a profound effect on the pulse oximeter and can increase or decrease the reading depending on the relative fractions of HbO_2 and Hb present.[10] Extremely high clinical levels of Hb_{MET} (greater than 40%) result in an SpO_2 reading around 85% regardless of the actual SaO_2. Fetal Hb has similar absorption characteristics to adult Hb, and the pulse oximeter readings are not appreciably affected.[78]

SUMMARY

Monitoring respiratory function during anesthesia requires a systematic approach for evaluating the patient's state. A five-step approach involves (1) knowing the composition of the inspired gas to evaluate the adequacy of O_2 and absence of CO_2 in the alveolar gas; (2) using V_T to assess opening of airways; (3) determining the PaO_2 to appraise the adequacy of O_2 delivery to meet metabolic needs; (4) knowing the $PaCO_2$ or $PACO_2$ to determine if CO_2 is being excreted in balance with metabolic production; and (5) measuring the expired gas volume to assess whether the quantity of CO_2 excreted is adequate.

Continuous respiratory monitoring is required

according to various standards. Timeliness of information display, noninvasiveness, and cost effectiveness are considerations in choosing the appropriate respiratory monitoring array.

Monitoring the inspired gas composition may be accomplished by measuring the P_{O_2}, P_{CO_2}, and balance gases with a variety of analyzers. Measuring P_{O_2} in the breathing circuit with an O_2 analyzer is required by standards. CO_2 should be near zero in the inspired gas unless mechanical dead space is intentionally placed in the common gas circuit or CO_2 is added to the inspired gas to restore eucapnia at the end of surgery. Otherwise, the presence of CO_2 usually indicates a technical problem with the breathing system.

Inspired gas volume must be adequate to expand the lung; deliver adequate O_2 to the alveolar gas; fill mechanical, anatomic, and alveolar dead space; compensate for gas compression and breathing circuit distension; and provide adequate volume for expiration of CO_2. Observing ventilation and measuring peak and plateau inspiratory pressures are useful in assessing the adequacy of inspired gas volume. Detecting breathing circuit leaks, disconnections, and obstructions is also critical. This can be accomplished by visualization, auscultation of breath sounds, measuring airway pressure, and monitoring respiratory CO_2.

The Pa_{O_2} or O_2 content of the blood determines the adequacy of the patient's oxygenation. Inadequate oxygenation can result from respiratory, circulatory, or metabolic failure. Observation of cyanosis is unreliable and a late indicator of inadequate oxygenation. Estimation of Sa_{O_2} by measuring Sp_{O_2} with a pulse oximeter is recommended. Measuring mixed venous Sa_{O_2} can be accomplished with a fiberoptic spectrophotometer, but the risk/benefit ratio of this monitor must be considered. Direct measurement of Pa_{O_2} from sampled blood is indicated to evaluate oxygenation fully. Consideration of venous admixture and its cause is important in the evaluation of oxygenation.

The Pa_{CO_2} must be evaluated to determine the adequacy of minute ventilation appropriate to the patient's acid-base state. Pa_{CO_2} can be estimated by measuring PET_{CO_2} with a respiratory CO_2 analyzer. The difference between Pa_{CO_2} and PET_{CO_2} resulting from alveolar dead space must be considered in this evaluation. Also, correction of PET_{CO_2} for water vapor is sometimes required, depending on the respiratory gas analyzer.

When monitoring the expired gas volume, one must consider the mode of ventilation as well as the contribution of gas compression and breathing circuit distension.

Various technologies are applied to monitoring respiratory function during anesthesia. Devices to monitor gas composition include O_2 analyzers based on polarography, fuel cells, and paramagnetism. Clinical analyzers for measuring CO_2, N_2O, and anesthetic agents based on infrared absorption are typically used. These include infrared spectrometers and photoacoustic spectrometers. Multigas analyzers that measure O_2, N_2O, N_2, anesthetic agents, and other gases are frequently used. These multigas analyzers include the Raman spectrometer and the mass spectrometer.

Pressure, flow, and volume of the breathing system are measured with a variety of devices. Manometers for pressure measurement include analog gauges, solid-state transducers, and pressure switches. Respiratory flowmeters and volume meters often used in anesthesia are mechanical and electronic vane anemometers, rolling seal volumeters, and, less frequently, pneumotachometers.

The pulse oximeter is based on measuring the pulse-added absorbance of two wavelengths of light shown through tissue. Although various minor interferences have been described, the accuracy and noninvasiveness of this device have made it an essential monitoring tool.

Using a systematic approach and the appropriate tools, the clinician can readily monitor the patient's respiratory function during anesthesia.

KEY POINTS

- Monitoring respiratory function during anesthesia requires a systematic approach for evaluating the patient's state. A five-step approach follows:
  1. Know the composition of the inspired gas to evaluate the adequacy of O_2 and absence of CO_2 in the alveolar gas.
  2. Determine V_T to assess opening of airways.
  3. Learn the Pa_{O_2} to appraise the adequacy of O_2 delivery to meet metabolic needs.

4. Know Pa_{CO_2} or PA_{CO_2} to determine if CO_2 is being excreted in balance with metabolic production.
  5. Measure the expired gas volume to assess whether the quantity of CO_2 excreted is adequate.

- Inspired gas volume must be adequate to expand the lung; deliver adequate O_2 to the alveolar gas; fill mechanical, anatomic, and alveolar dead space;

compensate for gas compression and breathing circuit distension; and provide adequate volume for expiration of CO_2.

- Observing ventilation and measuring peak and plateau inspiratory pressure are useful in assessing the adequacy of inspired gas volume.

- The Pao_2 or O_2 content of the blood determines the adequacy of a patient's oxygenation.

- Inadequate oxygenation can result from respiratory, circulatory, or metabolic failure. Observation of cyanosis is unreliable and a late indicator of inadequate oxygenation.

- Estimation of Sao_2 by measuring Spo_2 with a pulse oximeter is recommended to evaluate oxygenation.

- Oxygen is typically measured with one of two electrochemical devices, a polarographic sensor or a fuel cell or with a paramagnetic sensor, based on the physical properties of O_2

- Respiratory gas monitors based on several technol-

ogies are used to monitor CO_2 during anesthesia. The Raman spectrometer, infrared analyzer, and photoacoustic spectrometer are based on the optical properties of CO_2 gas. The mass spectrometer is based on molecular mass and charge.

- Pressure in an anesthesia breathing circuit is typically monitored using a mechanical analog dial gauge, an electronic solid state transducer, or an electromechanical pressure switch.

- Respiratory flow in an anesthesia system is most commonly measured using a vane anemometer that features a rotating low-mass vane in the gas stream or with a sealed volumeter that rotates a quarter turn in response to a fixed volume of gas.

- Oximeters and pulse oximeters are based on the differential absorption of light by HbO_2 and Hb. The pulse oximeter also depends on the change in light absorbance with the pulsatility of the arterial system.

KEY REFERENCES

Elliott WR, Topulos GP: The influence of the mechanics of anesthesia breathing circuits on respiratory monitoring, *Biomed Instrum Technol* 24:260, July 1990.

Linko K, Paloheimo M, and Tammisto T: Capnography for detection of accidental oesophageal intubation, *Acta Anaesthesiol Scand* 27:199, 1983.

Murray IP, Modell JH: Early detection of endotracheal tube accidents by monitoring carbon dioxide concentration in respiratory gas, *Anesthesiology* 59:344, 1983.

Nunn JF, Hill DW: Respiratory dead space and arterial to end-tidal CO_2 tension difference in anesthetized man, *J Appl Physiol* 15:383, 1960.

Philip JH, Raemer DB: Selecting the optimal anesthesia monitoring array, *Med Instrum* 19:122, 1985.

Raemer DB, Francis D, Philip JH et al: Variation in Pco_2 between arterial blood and peak expired gas during anesthesia, *Anesth Analg* 62:1065, 1983.

Severinghaus JW: Simple, accurate equations for human blood O_2 dissociation computations, *J Appl Physiol* 46:599, 1979.

Severinghaus JW, Ozanne G: Multioperating room monitoring with one mass spectrometer, *Acta Anaesthesiol Scand* 43:617, 1978.

Yelderman M, New W: Evaluation of pulse oximetry, *Anesthesiology* 59:349, 1983.

REFERENCES

1. Abbott MA: Monitoring oxygen saturation levels in the early recovery phase of general anesthesia. In Payne JF, Severinghaus JW, eds: *Pulse oximetry,* Dorchester, UK, 1986, Springer-Verlag.

2. American Society of Anesthesiologists: *Standards for basic intra-operative monitoring,* Las Vegas, 1986, House of Delegates, The Society.

3. American Society of Anesthesiologists: *Standards for basic intra-operative monitoring,* New Orleans, 1989, House of Delegates, The Society.

4. Anagnostou JM, Hults SL, and Moorthy SS: PEEP valve barotrauma, *Anesth Analg* 70:668, 1990.

5. Andritsch RF, Muravchick S, and Gold MI: Temperature correction of arterial blood gas parameters, *Anesthesiology* 55:311, 1981.

6. Arai T, Kuzume K: Endotracheal tube obstruction possibly due to structural fault (letter), *Anesthesiology* 59:480, 1983.

7. Arellano R, Ross D, and Lee K: Inappropriate attachment of PEEP valve causing total obstruction of ventilation bag, *Anesth Analg* 66:1049, 1987.

8. Askrog VF, Pender JW, and Eckenhoff JE: Changes in physiological dead space during deliberate hypotension, *Anesthesiology* 25:744, 1964.

9. Barker SJ, Tremper KK: The effect of carbon monoxide inhalation on pulse oximeter signal detection, *Anesthesiology* 67:599, 1987.

10. Barker SJ, Tremper KK, and Hyatt J: Effects of methemoglobinemia on pulse oximetry and mixed venous oximetery, *Anesthesiology* 70:112, 1989.

11. Bashein G, MacEvoy B: Anesthesia ventilators should have adjustable high-pressure alarms (letter), *Anesthesiology* 63:231, 1985.

12. Bendixen HH, Hedley-Whyte J, and Laver MB: Impaired oxygenation in surgical patients during general anesthesia with controlled ventilation, *N Engl J Med* 269:992, 1963.

13. Bengston JP, Sonander H, and Stenqvist O: Oxygen analyzers in anaesthesia: performance in a simulated clinical environment, *Acta Anaesthesiol Scand* 30:656, 1986.

14. Bermudez J, Lichtiger M: Increases in arterial to end-tidal CO_2 tension differences after cardiopulmonary bypass, *Anesth Analg* 66:690, 1987.

15. Biswas CK, Ramos JM, Agroyannis B et al: Blood gas analysis: effect of air bubbles in syringe and delay in estimation, *Br Med J* 284:923, 1982.

16. Block FE, Detko GJ: Minimizing interferences and false alarms from electrocautery in the Nellcor N-100 pulse oximeter, *J Clin Monit* 2:203, 1986.

17. Boxer RA, Gottesfeld I, Singh S et al: Noninvasive pulse oximetry in children with cyanotic congenital heart disease, *Crit Care Med* 15:1062, 1987.

18. Campbell EJM, Nunn JF, and Peckett BW: A comparison of artificial ventilation and spontaneous respiration with particular reference to ventilation-bloodflow relationships, *Br J Anaesth* 30:166, 1958.

19. Cecil WT, Thorpe KJ, Fibuch EE et al: A clinical evaluation of the Nellcor N-100 and the Ohmeda 3700 pulse oximeters, *J Clin Monit* 4:31, 1988.

20. Clarke AD: Potential deadspace in an anaesthetic mask and connectors, *Br J Anaesth* 30:176, 1958.

21. Collier CR, Affeldt JE, and Farr AF: Continuous rapid CO_2 analysis, *J Lab Clin Med* 45:526, 1955.

22. Comroe JH, Botlho S: The unreliability of cyanosis in the recognition of arterial anoxemia, *Am J Med Sci* 214:1, 1947.

23. Cooper EA: Physiological deadspace in passive ventilation: relationships with tidal volume, frequency, age, and minor upsets of respiratory health, *Anaesthesia* 22:199, 1967.

24. Coté CC, Petkau J, Ryan JF et al: Wasted ventilation measured in vitro with eight anesthetic circuits with and without inline humidification, *Anesthesiology* 59:442, 1983.

25. Coté CJ, Goldstein EA, Fuchsman WH et al: The effect of nail polish on pulse oximetry, *Anesth Analg* 67:683, 1988.

26. Dahlgren BE, Symreng T: Instant control of the alveolar pCO_2 in neurosurgical operations by the use of the Godart-Statham capnograph, *Opuscula Med* 19:271, 1974.

27. Davies NJH, Denison DM: Respiratory mass spectrometry. In Spence AA, ed: *Respiratory monitoring in intensive care,* Edinburgh, 1982, Churchill-Livingstone.

28. Dumpit FEM, Brady JP: A simple technique for measuring alveolar CO_2 in infants, *J Appl Physiol: Respir Environ Exerc Physiol* 45:648, 1978.

29. Duran M, Ramanathan R: Pulse oximetry for continuous oxygen monitoring in six newborn infants, *J Pediatr* 109:1052, 1986.

30. Elliott WR, Topulos GP: The influence of the mechanics of anesthesia breathing circuits on respiratory monitoring, *Biomed Instrum Technol* 24:260, July 1990.

31. Epstein MF, Cohen AR, Feldman HA, and Raemer DB: Estimation of $PaCO_2$ by two noninvasive methods in the critically ill newborn infant, *J Pediatr* 106:282, 1985.

32. Evaluation: carbon dioxide monitors, *ECRI Health Dev* 15:255, 1986.

33. Fait CD, Wetzel RC, Dean JM et al: Pulse oximetry in critically ill children, *J Clin Monit* 1:232, 1985.

34. Famewo CE: A not so apparent cause of intraluminal tracheal tube obstruction, *Anesthesiology* 58:593, 1983 (letter).

35. Fletcher R: Invasive and noninvasive measurement of the respiratory deadspace in anesthetized children with cardiac disease, *Anesth Analg* 67:442, 1988.

36. Fletcher R: *The single breath test for carbon dioxide,* thesis, 1980, University of Lund, Lund, Sweden.

37. Fowler KT, Hugh-Jones P: Mass spectrometry applied to clinical practice and research, *Br Med J* 1:1205, 1957.

38. Hamilton RD, Crockett AJ, and Alpers JH: Arterial blood gas analysis: potential errors due to the addition of heparin, *Anaesth Intensive Care* 6:251, 1978.

39. Hanowell L, Eisele JH, and Downs D: Ambient light affects pulse oximeters, *Anesthesiology* 67:864, 1987 (letter).

40. Hines R, Barash PG: Pulmonary artery catheterization. In Blitt CE, ed: *Monitoring in anesthesia and critical care medicine,* New York, 1990, Churchill-Livingstone.

41. Hobbes AFT: A comparison of methods of calibrating the pneumotachograph, *Br J Anaesth* 39:899, 1967.

42. Holbek CC: The radiometer ABL300 blood gas analyzer, *J Clin Monit* 5:4, 1989.

43. Hudson RD Jr: *Infrared system engineering,* New York, 1969, John Wiley & Sons.

44. Kagle DM, Alexander CM, Berko RS et al: Evaluation of the Ohmeda 3700 pulse oximeter: steady state and transient response characteristics, *Anesthesiology* 67:551, 1987.

45. Kertzman J: Paper 73425, 1973, Analytical Instrumentation Division, Instrument Society of America.

46. Kowalski JJ: Arterial to end-tidal CO_2 partial pressure gradient and the functional dead space in patients with obstructive or restrictive lung diseases, *Bull Phys Pathol Respir* 2:539, 1966.

47. Kuo BC: *Digital control systems,* New York, 1980, Holt, Rinehart & Winston.

48. Larson CP, Severinhaus JW: Postural variations in dead space and CO_2 gradients breathing air and O_2, *J Appl Physiol* 17:417-420, 1962.

49. Linko K, Paloheimo M, and Tammisto T: Capnography for detection of accidental oesophageal intubation, *Acta Anaesthesiol Scand* 27:199, 1983.

50. Luft K: Uber eine neue methods der registrierenden gasanalyse mit hilfe der absorbtion ultratoter strahlen ohne spektrale zerlegnung, *Z Techn Phys* 24:97, 1943.

51. Luft UC, Loeppky JA, and Mostyn EM: Mean alveolar gases and alveolar-arterial gradients in pulmonary patients, *J Appl Physiol: Respir Environ Exerc Physiol* 46:534, 1979.

52. Lundsgaard C, Van Slyke DD: Cyanosis, *Medicine* 2:1, 1923.

53. McGarrigle R, White S: Oxygen analyzers can detect disconnections, *Anesth Analg* 63:464, 1984 (letter).

54. McIntyre WR, Knopes KD, and Ossey KD: Anesthesia ventilators should have adjustable high-pressure alarms, *Anesthesiology* 63:231, 1985 (letter).

55. Mihm FG, Halperin DH: Noninvasive detection of profound arterial desaturations using pulse oximetry device, *Anesthesiology* 62:85, 1985.

56. Minimum performance and safety requirements for components and systems of continuous flow anesthesia machines for human use, ANSI Z-79.8, New York, 1979, American National Standards Institute.

57. Mok J, Pintar M, Benson L et al: Evaluation of noninvasive measurements of oxygenation in stable infants, *Crit Care Med* 14:960, 1986.

58. Murray IP, Modell JH. Early detection of endotracheal tube accidents by monitoring carbon dioxide concentration in respiratory gas, *Anesthesiology* 59:344, 1983.

59. Nickerson BG, Sakrison C, and Tremper KK: Bias and precision of pulse oximeters and arterial oximeters, *Chest* 93:515, 1988.

60. Nielsen JR, Thornton V, and Dalc EB: The absorption laws for gases in the infrared, *Rev Mod Phys* 16:307, 1944.

61. Noe FE, Alexander GD, and Brown EM: End-tidal and arterial gas tension levels in postanesthetic respiratory depression, *Anesth Analg* 49:637, 1970.

62. Nunn JF: *Applied respiratory physiology,* London, 1977, Butterworths.

63. Nunn JF: Carbon dioxide cylinders on anaesthetic apparatus, *Br J Anaesth* 65(2):155, 1990 (editorial).

64. Nunn JF: The distribution of inspired gas during thoracic surgery, *J Coll Surg* 28:223, 1961.

65. Nunn JF, Ezi-Ashi TI: The accuracy of the respirometer and ventigrator, *Br J Anaesth* 34:422, 1962.

66. Nunn JF, Hill DW: Respiratory dead space and arterial to end-tidal CO_2 tension differences in anesthetized man, *J Appl Physiol* 15:383, 1960.

67. Ozane GM, Young WG, Mazzei WJ et al: Multipatient anesthetic mass spectrometry: rapid analysis of data stored in long catheters, *Anesthesiology* 55:62-70, 1981.

68. Payne JP, Severinghaus JW, eds: *Pulse oximetry,* Berlin, 1986, Springer-Verlag.

69. Philip JH, Raemer DB: Selecting the optimal anesthesia monitoring array, *Med Instrum* 19:122, 1985.

70. Poppius H, Korhonen O, Viljanen AA et al: Arterial to end-tidal difference in respiratory disease, *Scand J Respir Dis* 56:254, 1975.

71. Prakash O, Jonson B, Bos E et al: Cardiorespiratory and metabolic effects of profound hypothermia, *Crit Care Med* 6:340, 1978.

72. Pyles ST, Berman LS, and Modell JH: Expiratory valve dysfunction in a semi-closed circle anesthesia circuit—verification by analysis of carbon dioxide waveform, *Anesth Analg* 63:537, 1984.

73. Raemer DB, Elliott WR, Topulos GP et al: The theoretical effect of carboxyhemoglobin on the pulse oximeter, *J Clin Monit* 5:246, 1989.

74. Raemer DB, Francis D, Philip JH et al: Variation in Pco₂ between arterial blood and peak expired gas during anesthesia, *Anesth Analg* 62:1065, 1983.

75. Raemer DB, Philip JH: Monitoring anesthetic and respiratory gases. In Blitt CD, ed: *Monitoring in anesthesia and critical care medicine,* New York, 1990, Churchill-Livingstone.

76. Raemer DB, Warren DL, Morris R et al: Hypoxemia during ambulatory gynecologic surgery as evaluated with the pulse oximeter, *J Clin Monit* 3:244, 1987.

77. Raman CV, Krishnan KS: The production of new radiations by light scattering. Part I, *Proc R Soc Lond* 122A:23, 1923.

78. Ramanathan R, Durand M, and Larrazabel C: Pulse oximetery in very low birth weight infants with acute and chronic lung disease, *Pediatrics* 79:612, 1987.

79. Richards C: Failure of a nitrous oxide–oxygen proportioning device, *Anesthesiology* 71:997, 1989 (letter).

80. Riley RH, Marcy JH: Unsuspected endobronchial intubation – detection by continuous mass spectrometry, *Anesthesiology* 63:203, 1985.

81. Sabo BA, Olinder PJ, and Smith RB: Obstruction of a breathing circuit, *Anesth Rav* 10:28, 1983.

82. Scheller MS, Unger RJ, and Kelner MJ: Effects of intravenously administered dyes on pulse oximetry readings, *Anesthesiology* 65:550, 1986.

83. Severinghaus JW: Blood gas calculator, *J Appl Physiol* 21:1108, 1966.

84. Severinghaus JW: Simple, accurate equations for human blood O₂ dissociation computations, *J Appl Physiol* 46:599, 1979.

85. Severinghaus JW: Water vapor calibration errors in some capnometers: respiratory conventions misunderstood by manufacturers? *Anesthesiology* 70:996, 1989.

86. Severinghaus JW, Astrup PB: History of blood gas analysis. VI. Oximetry, *J Clin Monit* 2:270, 1986.

87. Severinghaus JW, Honda Y: History of blood gas analysis. VII. Pulse oximetry, *J Clin Monit* 3:135, 1987.

88. Severinghaus JW, Larson CP, and Eger EI: Correction factors for infrared carbon dioxide pressure broadening by nitrogen, nitrous oxide, and cyclopropane, *Anesthesiology* 22:429, 1961.

89. Severinghaus JW, Naifeh KH: Accuracy of response of six pulse oximeters to profound hypoxia, *Anesthesiology* 67:551, 1987.

90. Severinghaus JW, Ozanne G: Multioperating room monitoring with one mass spectrometer, *Acta Anaesthesiol Scand* 43:617, 1978.

91. Shankar KB, Moseley M, Vemula V et al: Arterial to end-tidal carbon dioxide tension difference during anaesthesia in early pregnancy, *Can J Anaesth* 36:124, 1989.

92. Sidi A, Paulus DA, Rush W et al: Methylene blue and indocyanine green artifactually lower pulse oximetry readings of oxygen saturation: studies in dogs, *J Clin Monit* 3:249, 1987.

93. Smalhout B, Kalenda Z: *An atlas of capnography,* Netherlands, 1981, Kerckebosch-Zeist.

94. Sprague DH, Archer GW: Intraoperative hypoxia from an erroneously filled liquid oxygen reservoir, *Anesthesiology* 42:360, 1975 (letter).

95. Sykes MK, Finlay WEI: Deadspace during anaesthesia: effect of added oxygen, *Anaesthesiology* 26:22, 1971.

96. Takki S, Aromaa U, and Kauste A: The validity and usefulness of the end-tidal Pco₂ during anaesthesia, *Anal Clin Res* 4:278, 1972.

97. Tien YK, Gabel RA: Prediction of PO₂ from SO₂ using the standard oxygen hemoglobin equilibrium curve, *J Appl Physiol* 42:985, 1977.

98. Van Wagenen RA, Westenskow DR, Benner RE et al: Dedicated monitoring of anesthetic and respiratory gases by Raman scattering, *J Clin Monit* 2:215, 1986.

99. Whitesell R, Asiddao C, Gollman D et al: Relationship between arterial and peak expired carbon dioxide pressure during anesthesia and factors influencing the difference, *Anesth Analg* 60:508, 1981.

100. Wheeler L: Clinical laboratory instrumentation. In Webster JG, ed: *Medical instrumentation: application and design,* Boston, 1978, Houghton Mifflin.

101. Wright BM: A respiratory anemometer, *J Physiol (Lond)* 127:25P, 1955.

102. Wukitsch MW, Petterson MT, Tobler DR et al: Pulse oximetry: analysis of theory, technology, and practice, *J Clin Monit* 4:290, 1988.

103. Yelderman M, New W: Evaluation of pulse oximetry, *Anesthesiology* 59:349, 1983.

104. Zeitlin GL, Cass WA, and Gessner JS: Insurance incentives and the use of monitoring devices, *Anesthesiology* 69:441, 1988 (letter).

CHAPTER 43

Intraoperative Neurologic Monitoring

ROBERT W. McPHERSON

Neurologic assessment of patients during anesthesia differs from respiratory or cardiovascular monitoring under similar circumstances in several important ways. Injury to small areas of the nervous system may result in permanent disability. Other monitors are not available to confirm or refute changes in neurologic function, and equipment for neurologic monitoring is complex (computer based), expensive, and labor intensive. The brain has spontaneous electrical activity (electroencephalogram, EEG) and responds to stimuli applied to peripheral or cranial nerves (evoked potentials). Both EEG and evoked potentials (somatosensory-evoked potential, SSEP; brainstem auditory-evoked response, BAER; visual-evoked response, VER) may be monitored in the operating room to assess instantaneous function of parts of the nervous system.

Intraoperative monitoring differs from nonoperative monitoring of the same sensory modality in five important areas. First, monitoring is undertaken expectantly (indicated by disease or surgery rather than by symptoms). Second, most patients who may benefit from intraoperative monitoring have strong, easily obtainable waveforms. Third, for intraoperative monitoring to be successful, comparisons are made using the patient as his/her own control (i.e., pre-surgery; preevent such as aneurysm clip application) rather than using "normative values" to establish diagnosis (e.g., multiple sclerosis) or the degree of physiologic insult (e.g., head injury). Fourth, anesthesia and neuromuscular blocking agents change the patient's waveforms from those of the unanesthetized state but do not prevent rapid waveform generation and analysis. Finally, decisions concerning waveform changes must be made within minutes to prevent permanent neurologic injury.

Transient changes in brain electrical activity that are reversed spontaneously or by therapeutic interventions have presented difficulty in understanding what constitutes true positives and true negatives as well as false positives and false negatives for intraoperative monitoring. Changes or lack of changes in brain electrical activity that correlate with the presence or absence of postoperative neurologic changes are *true positives* or *true negatives*. Transient changes in electrical activity, responding to intraoperative events that are reversed by altering the clinical technique (e.g., elevation of systemic blood pressure, removal of spinal obstruction, removal of surgical retractor), are more difficult to evaluate. Strictly defined, those transient changes are *false positives,* since intraoperative waveform changes occur without changes in postoperative neurologic function when compared with preoperative function. Finally, there are *false negatives,* or changes in neurologic function without changes in monitored electrical activity. **Postoperative** neurologic changes following spinal surgery without intraoperative SSEP change may occur, and only modest changes in intraoperative SSEP waves may herald permanent neurologic changes.[27] Important in understanding false negatives is determining whether the monitor (EEG; sensory-evoked potential, SEP; BAER; VER) would be affected by the process that alters neurologic function. **Aggressive intraoperative monitoring of neurologic function does not guarantee prevention of neurologic injury, since not all parts of the brain are assessed using currently available monitoring.**

The neurologic system is particularly resistant to injury. Profound hypotension (mean arterial blood pressure of 12 to 25 mm Hg for 1 hour) leads to death in 40% of animals soon after hypotension caused by cardiac dysfunction or intestinal bleeding. In all survivors, EEG and SSEP waves that were severely depressed during hypotension recover with restoration of mean arterial blood pressure, and survivors have no apparent neurologic injury.[29]

In developing strategies for intraoperative monitoring, the following guidelines are helpful. The EEG reliably assesses only cortical function, although subcortical structures are involved in wave generation. The VER monitors functions of the retina, optic chiasm, optic radiations and occipital cortex. The SSEP assesses the neural axis from peripheral nerve through brainstem to cortex. The BAER assesses only brainstem function (waves occurring < 10 msec after stimuli), although long-latency cortical waves (> 20 msec after stimuli) can be assessed to evaluate cortical function. Finally, the motor-evoked potential (MEP) assesses functions of the motor cortex and descending tracts, with the peripheral response assessed by compound muscle action potential.

MONITORING TECHNIQUES

Electrical activity of the nervous system, both spontaneous and evoked, is measured by using a reference electrode system that records voltage changes over time at an active electrode compared with a reference electrode (electrically quiet). With both EEG and evoked potential monitoring, precise electrode placement is required. The international system of placement of 10 to 20 electrodes normalizes this placement for physiologic variability in skull shape and size and is used for electrode placement for both EEG and evoked-potential monitoring.

It is now presumed that EEG waves recorded from the surface of the brain are primarily caused by activity in postsynaptic and somatic membranes of cortical neuronal elements.[25] Excitatory and inhibitory postsynaptic potentials are involved in electrogenesis of EEG activities. According to Creutzfeld and Houchin, "the main elements which contribute to

the EEG are vertically oriented pyramidal cells."[25] In addition to neural phenomenon, glial cells may contribute to the electrogenesis of EEG waves.[137] The source of generation of characteristic EEG rhythms, such as posterior alpha rhythm (8 to 10 Hz), continues to be unclear; a thalamic origin has been suggested[1,43] but questioned by Lopes da Silva et al.[87,88] However, there is little doubt that the subcortical mechanism can influence the cortical EEG activity. Fig. 43-1 shows a schematic of simultaneous microelectrode recordings at several levels of the cortex. The electrical activity recorded by surface electrodes is the summation of groups of neuronal firing. Note that summation of multiple discrete discharges produces rhythmic waves recorded by surface electrodes.

Intraoperative monitoring has provided information concerning when intraoperative injury occurs and the success of interventions in reversing injury. Before widespread intraoperative monitoring, the timing and mechanism of injury were unclear. Successful monitoring requires a monitoring plan and philosophy that do not exclude any possible source of injury. For instance, surgical positioning may cause changes in brain electrical activity that suggest injury, but these changes are rapidly reversed by position change.[98]

ELECTROENCEPHALOGRAM

The EEG may be monitored to determine anesthetic level or to assess adequacy of brain oxygenation. Global or localized cerebral oxygen deprivation may occur intraoperatively, and the monitoring system should be capable of detecting either type of event. The EEG is evaluated for wave amplitude and frequency and patterns of brain waves with specific amplitude and frequency characteristics previously validated in normal individuals or under pathologic circumstances. **Intraoperative EEG monitoring requires recognition of several characteristic EEG patterns that occur normally or represent changes in the EEG caused by anesthetic agents or cerebral oxygen deprivation.** Characteristic rhythms are defined according to frequency, amplitude, and location.

Alpha rhythm has a frequency of 8 to 12 Hz and a variable amplitude less than 50 μV with rounded or sinusoidal waves. This rhythm is best seen when the patient's eyes are closed and he/she is relaxed. Alpha rhythm is blocked or attenuated by attention. Maximal alpha rhythm voltage is found over the occipital region. Beta rhythm (13 to 40 Hz) is found chiefly over the frontal and central regions, with amplitude less than 30 μV. Theta waves (4 to 7.5 Hz) have an amplitude of > 50 μV. Theta rhythm is usually found in infants and children but may persist up to 25 to 30 years of age. Delta waves (0.1 to 3.5 Hz, > 75 μV) occur during normal sleep. A small amount of theta rhythm is always found in a normal EEG. In the awake

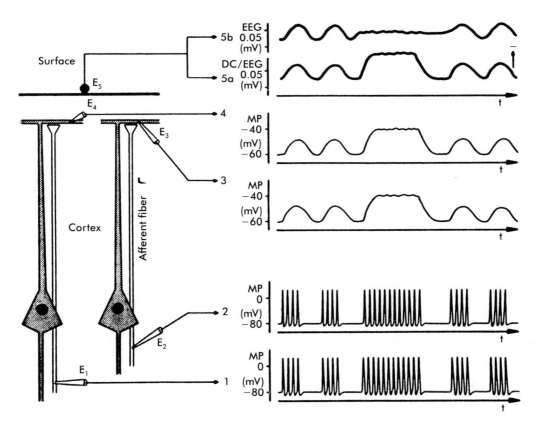

Fig. 43-1. Principles of wave generation. Excitatory synapses of two afferent fibers contact superficial dendritic arborization of two longitudinal neuronal elements. Afferent fiber activity is recorded by means of intracellular electrodes E_1 and E_2, and membrane potentials *(MP)* of dendritic elements are recorded by electrodes E_3 and E_4. Field potential at surface of neuronal structure *(cortex)* is led by electrode E_5. Synchronized groups of action potentials in afferent fibers (E_1, E_2) generate wavelike excitatory postsynaptic potentials (EPSPs) in dendritic areas (E_3, E_4) and corresponding field potentials in EEG and DC/EEG recording (E_5). Tonic activity in afferent fibers results in long-lasting EPSP with small fluctuations. During this period, EEG *(5b)* shows only a reduction in amplitude, whereas DC/EEG recording *(5a)* reflects depolarization of neuronal elements as well. (From Speckman EJ, Elger CE: Introduction to the neurophysiological basis of the EEG and DC potentials. In Niedermeyer E, Lopes da Silva F, eds: *Electroencephalography: basic principles, clinical application and related fields,* Baltimore, 1987, Urban & Schwarzenberg.)

individual the EEG consists of mainly beta activity with small amounts of delta and theta activity. If the individual is relaxed with eyes closed, alpha activity may be present.

Burst suppression is a dramatic EEG pattern in which short periods of electrocortical silence alternate with low-frequency, high-voltage activity. This pattern may be produced by high doses of barbiturates and etomidate, by high concentrations of isoflurane, and by hypothermia to the degree seen during cardiopulmonary bypass. This pattern may be seen as the brain is deprived of oxygen and during reoxygenation as the brain's metabolic status is repaired.

Intraoperative EEG monitoring requires data reduction to allow timely evaluation and therapeutic decisions. Data reduction must be accompanied by an extremely high validity of data processing. EEG monitoring in the operating room may be contaminated by rhythmic artifacts produced by pumps

and other machines that may be incorporated by computer-processed EEG. These artifacts may be presented as a normal EEG because of frequency or amplitude characteristics resembling brain waves. Thus all computer-processed EEGs should provide easy access to the unprocessed electrical signal for visual evaluation.

Multiple methods of computer EEG analysis are available,[86] all of which use analysis of amplitude, frequency, or both or some mathematic derivation of one or both to represent brain activity. Fast Fourier transformation (FFT) allows rapid evaluation of amplitude and latency and permits data to be displayed in a compressed spectral array (CSA) or density spectral array (DSA) (Fig. 43-2). The CSA is displayed in a pseudo-three-dimensional format in which large-amplitude segments may suppress information in earlier, lower-amplitude segments. DSA uses dot density to portray amplitude information, but

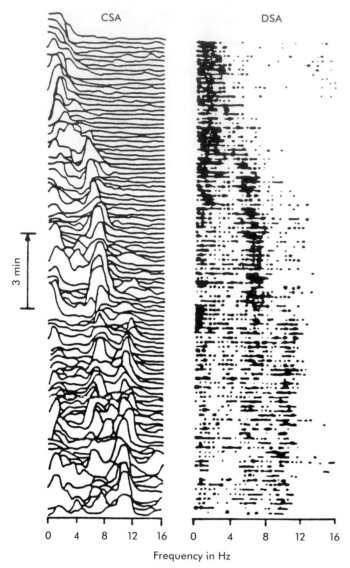

CSA   DSA

3 min

0   4   8   12   16   0   4   8   12   16

Frequency in Hz

Fig. 43-2. Compressed spectral array *(CSA)* and density spectral array *(DSA)* for same EEG data. (From Levy WJ, Shapiro HM, Maruchak G, et al: Automated EEG processing for intraoperative monitoring, *Anesthesiology* 53:223, 1980.)

the range of density is usually inadequate (varies from 1 to 10) to follow the range of EEG amplitude because EEG power ranges from 1 to 100. Another display method is band spectral analysis (BSA), in which power in bands (delta, theta, alpha, beta) is displayed.

Anesthetics

Thiopental causes a biphasic effect on the EEG, with an initial increase in fast activity (beta rhythm) and with slowing, burst suppression and electrocortical silence occurring with higher doses.[68] Etomidate causes a sustained theta activity with underlying fast activity that is similar to the effect caused by methohexital but with two to three times greater

efficacy.[48,149] With higher doses of etomidate, high-amplitude theta activity occurs and is followed by burst suppression.[148] Clonus associated with etomidate is not associated with EEG activity.[100] EEG frequency is inversely related to the serum etomidate concentration.[123]

Fentanyl causes a dose-dependent slowing of the EEG.[125] Other synthetic narcotics similar to fentanyl cause similar alterations in the EEG.[129] Narcotic-induced EEG changes lag behind serum narcotic concentration. The time lag during fentanyl infusion is about 6 minutes and may be caused by the large blood-brain partition coefficient for fentanyl. The steady-state serum concentration that causes one half of the maximal EEG slowing resulting from fentanyl is 6.9 ± 1.5 $\mu g/ml$.[124] Fig. 43-3 shows the typical dose-dependent EEG slowing with alfentanil and fentanyl. Note the similarity of waveform patterns as frequency decreases and wave amplitude increases.

Diazepam (Valium) (5 mg orally) reduces activity in the 4 to 7.5 Hz wave band and increases activity in the 13.5 to 26 Hz wave band.[5] In oral doses typically used for premedication, diazepam decreases alpha activity and increases beta activity, with the EEG effect reflecting blood levels.

Nitrous oxide produces fast activity (greater than 20 Hz) of the EEG in concentrations that produce unconsciousness in unpremedicated humans,[152] with activity predominantly in the frontal areas and a peak frequency of 34 Hz. Amplitude and quantity of increased activity increase with nitrous oxide concentration and return to control levels over 1 hour following discontinuation of nitrous oxide.

Halothane causes a progessive slowing of EEG frequency as concentration is increased[44] and does not appear to enhance epileptogenic activity.[99] EEG changes such as generalized slowing, a tendency toward posterior delta activity, and significant reduction in the frequency and amplitude of alpha rhythm may perist for 6 to 8 days following uncomplicated halothane anesthesia.[10]

Enflurane causes a dose-dependent loss of fast wave activity,[108] with periods of suppression occurring with high concentrations. **Enflurane may cause generalized seizures with characteristic tonic clonic activity and high-voltage EEG activity in humans,**[103] **even in concentrations less than necessary for satisfactory anesthesia.** Enflurane appears to encourage seizure activity in patients who have a prior history of seizures; an increased incidence accompanies hyperventilation.[81,104] **Animal studies have confirmed that hypocarbia lowers the seizure threshold during enflurane anesthesia.**[62] The complexity of enflurane's effects on brain electrical activity is demonstrated by a report of inhibition of seizure activity during enflurane anesthesia.[45] In this patient, addition of

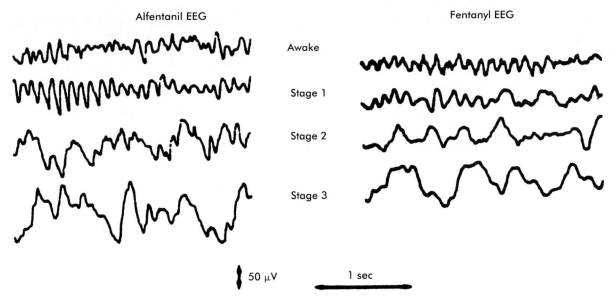

Fig. 43-3. Comparison of EEG effects of alfentanil and fentanyl. Note similarity of decrease in wave frequency and increase in amplitude. (From Scott JC, Ponganis KV, and Stanski DR: EEG quantitation of narcotic effect: the comparative pharmacodynamics of fentanyl and alfentanil, *Anesthesiology* 62:234, 1985.)

enflurane (40% MAC) to nitrous oxide anesthesia caused rapid (<5 min) disappearance of previously persistent seizure activity. Discontinuation of enflurane allowed return of seizure activity. EEG changes (increased amplitude and groups of high-frequency, high-voltage spikes in ventral posterolateral nucleus of thalamus, centromedian nucleus) persist for several days following enflurane administration in animals with long-term electrode placement[67] and may explain the postoperative seizure activity reported.[74]

Isoflurane initially produces a low-amplitude EEG with a frequency of 15 to 35 Hz. With loss of consciousness, 12 to 14 Hz activity is superimposed on 2 to 5 Hz, high-amplitude waves.[22] Anesthetic doses of isoflurane produce increasing periods of burst suppression, with complete electrocortical silence appearing at an end-inspiratory concentration of 2.5%.[38] Isoflurane is generally thought not to cause seizure activity and has been used successfully to treat status epilepticus.[72] However, seizure activity has been reported in a healthy patient during induction of anesthesia with isoflurane and nitrous oxide.[110] Some increase in amplitude and periodically recurring slowing have been observed in animals up to 24 hours following isoflurane administration.[67] Although isoflurane decreases EEG frequency and increases amplitude, it does not interfere with the diagnosis of intraoperative ischemia by EEG.[11]

Pathophysiology

The EEG is affected by oxygen deprivation to the brain (hypoxia or ischemia) or by the ability of the brain to use oxygen. In animals, respiration with 100% nitrogen causes a change in EEG from low-amplitude fast activity to high-amplitude slow activity associated with unconsciousness and lack of response to stimulation and complete flattening of the EEG within 40 seconds.[59] Cerebral utilization of oxygen and glucose diminish drastically when electrocortical silence occurs.[12]

Ernsting[39] reviewed the EEG changes of brief, profound hypoxia with a decrease in arterial oxygen tension (PaO_2) from 65 to 15 mm Hg over 1 to 2 seconds. With the onset of hypoxia, activity in the alpha band appears when the waves are present before onset of hypoxia. While the lack of oxygen is prolonged, electrical activity occurs with a lower frequency until the EEG is dominated by delta rhythm. In human volunteers, isocapnic hypoxia (O_2 saturation about 50%) decreases posterior alpha activity and causes the appearance of irregular slow waves with an amplitude of 50 μV over posterior and anterior head regions.[114] Metabolic encephalopathy causes a degree of slowing that parallels a depressed level of consciousness, with intermittent burst of rhythmic delta activity.[8] Hyperventilation (arterial carbon dioxide tension [$PaCO_2$], 18 to 19 mm Hg) causes slow waves not associated with changes in cerebral metabolic rates for oxygen or glucose[105] that may superficially resemble the EEG changes of hypoxia.

Zhongyuan et al. assessed acute and chronic hypoxia in human volunteers equivalent to about 8% inspired oxygen.[159] Acute hypoxia produces the

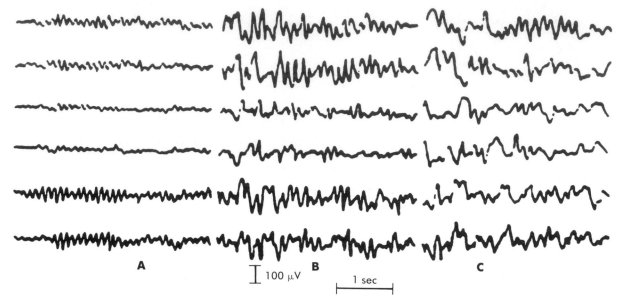

Fig. 43-4. Effect of acute hypoxia (PaO_2 about 55 mm Hg) on EEG in unanesthetized humans. **A,** EEG of normoxic subject. **B** and **C,** EEG during hypoxia in two subjects. (From Zhongyuan S, Deming Z, and Zhengzhong G: The influence of acute and chronic hypoxia on the electroencephalogram of human body, *Ann Physiol Anthropol* 6:111, 1987.)

abrupt onset of slow waves (3 to 7 Hz) with amplitude > 50 μV most obvious in frontal leads (Fig. 43-4). Less severe acute hypoxia causes an increase in alpha frequency and a decrease in alpha amplitude. Some subjects also have onset of theta waves (4 to 7 Hz). During acute hypoxia, EEG changes correlate with mental symptoms, and the EEG rapidly returns to normal with reoxygenation.

Carotid cross-clamping during carotid endarterectomy may produce global hemispheric ischemia in some patients. **EEG changes that may occur during carotid cross-clamping include a decrease in amplitude (including slow waves) or an increase in amplitude and decrease in frequency.** Unilateral changes are more frequent, but bilateral changes may occur with severely compromised, contralateral cerebral blood flow (> 90% stenosis). Blume and Sharbrough[4] concluded after reviewing several studies that moderate EEG changes from cross-clamping can be treated without temporary shunt insertion; however, severe changes with loss of all frequencies except for < 1 Hz activity probably require placement of a shunt. Severe EEG changes following carotid cross-clamping may be self-limited and may resolve before interventions such as temporary shunt placement can be accomplished.[113] The EEG most likely reflects essentially instantaneous adequacy of oxygen to the brain. The variability of EEG response and spontaneous resolution of these changes[113] undoubtedly represent a time-related return toward normal cerebral blood flow and oxygenation delivery via collateral channels following occlusion of a carotid artery.

Hypothermia decreases frequency of the EEG in patients undergoing hypothermic cardiopulmonary bypass (26° C). Approximately 76% of these patients demonstrate a linear relationship between power in higher frequencies (8 to 10 Hz) and temperature, and 25% demonstrate burst suppression.[85]

Anesthetic and other usual intraoperative physiologic changes (e.g., hypothermia) change the EEG from the awake state but allow diagnosis of both global and local ischemia. Computer-analyzed EEG is advantageous for intraoperative use because of data reduction. Monitoring should provide evaluation of multiple channels for each hemisphere and should provide access to the unprocessed waveform.

SENSORY-EVOKED POTENTIALS

Evoked potentials are computed averages of the brain's response to repetitive peripheral stimuli. These waves are small (1 to 2 μV) compared with the average EEG voltage (50 to 100 μV), and individual responses are usually hidden in the spontaneous EEG. Briefly stated, the averaging phenomenon reinforces electrical activity that occurs with the same time and polarity following each stimulation, whereas random electrical activity is eventually averaged to zero. The number of averages required to produce a stable waveform is inversely proportional to the amplitude of the wave. Fig. 43-5 shows the impact of increasing the number of averages on the development of characteristic waveforms for an upper extremity (median nerve) somatosensory-evoked potential (SSEP).

Waveforms are evaluated for latency (time after

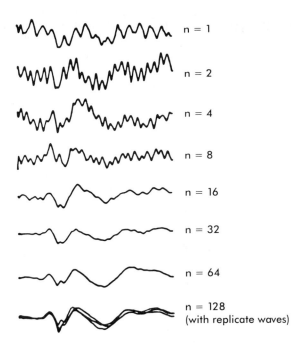

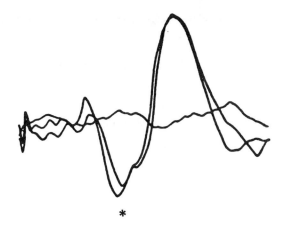

Fig. 43-6. Two visual-evoked responses generated with unanesthetized subject wearing goggles containing light-emitting diodes. Left eye was stimulated; active electrode over occipital region; reference electrode on forehead. Positive is down, and P100 (positive wave, 100 msec latency) is indicated by asterisk. Third trace without major deflections is average of EEG when retina was not stimulated.

Fig. 43-5. *Effect of number of stimuli on somatosensory-evoked potentials (SSEPs). Development of characteristic median nerve SSEP by averaging in anesthetized patient. Note that response is hidden in EEG (upper trace). With progressive number of stimuli, random noise is averaged out, leaving characteristic wave. Lowest trace shows several waves generated with 128 stimuli to demonstrate reproducible waves.*

stimulus) or size (amplitude) of characteristic waves. These data are provided by manually placing a cursor of the computer on the desired wave. Waveforms are designated for polarity, negative (N) or positive (P), plus nominal latency following stimulation for SSEP and visual-evoked response (VER). Brainstem auditory-evoked response (BAER) waves occurring within 10 msec of stimulation are designated in order of appearance by consecutive Roman numerals (I to VII), whereas later waves are designated similar to SSEP and VER waves by polarity and nominal latency. To evaluate monitoring technique properly, information about recording electrode sites, bandpass filter setting, stimulus rate, and stimulus intensity are required.

Brain electrical activity may be classified as near-field or far-field waves. *Near-field waves* are generated near the recording electrode, such as scalp-recorded SSEP waves. *Far-field waves* are recorded by electrodes distant from the neural generators. BAER waves are generated in the brainstem but recorded over the vertex of the skull; these are far-field waves.

Visual-Evoked Response

Stimulation of the retina produces an evoked response of the occipital cortex that is sensitive to changes in function of the visual apparatus caused by

tumors. Thus retina stimulation may be useful as a monitor in preventing injury during surgery near the optic chiasm. For intraoperative monitoring, the retina may be stimulated through closed eyelids. The patient wears goggles containing light-emitting diodes (LEDs), with recording electrodes over the occipital cortex (positions O_1 and O_2 according to 10 to 20 system). For electrophysiologic evaluation, flashes of white light or pattern-reversal stimulation presented on a screen have been used.

Characteristic waves of the VER are N70 (negative polarity, 70 msec latency) and P100 (positive polarity, 100 msec latency). Fig. 43-6 shows a VER generated using LED goggles in an unanesthetized subject. Duplicate waves are presented to show the reproducibility of the wave; included is a trace generated when the EEG was averaged in the absence of retinal stimulation. The wave frequently used for intraoperative monitoring is a positive wave (down position in Fig. 43-6) with a latency of about 100 msec (P100). More complex waves may be generated using either flashes of white light or pattern reversal with a television screen. These latter two methods of stimulation are difficult to use intraoperatively because of difficulty placing the stimulator such that a constant level of stimulation can be achieved throughout the monitoring period.

Since choice of stimulus type is not uniform, reported latency for waves vary from study to study. **Nominal latency of the wave appearing about 100 msec after stimulation are emphasized here, since that wave is generally the most resistant to anesthetic depression.** Although the waves reported are the same, nominal latencies reported may vary slightly because of technique (e.g., N65, N70 or P95, P100).

Table 43-1 Anesthetic effects on visual-evoked response (VER)

Drug	Amplitude	Latency (N70, P100)	Reference
Thiopental	Decrease	Increase	19
Etomidate (0.3 mg/kg)	No change	Increase	20
Fentanyl (60 μg/kg)	Decrease	No change	18
Diazepam (10 mg)	Decrease	No change	36
Nitrous oxide	Decrease	Variable	41
Halothane	Decrease	Increase	144
Enflurane	Decrease	Increase	16
Isoflurane	Decrease	Increase	17

Anesthetics

Intravenous anesthetic agents generally depress VER wave amplitude and increase latency. Table 43-1 summarizes effects of frequently used drugs on VER when administered individually. Less information is available concerning the effect of combinations of intravenous agents on the VER. Etomidate (0.3 mg/kg) alone does not change amplitude of P100 or N70 but slightly increases latencies of P60, N70, and P100 waves.[20] However, during fentanyl–nitrous oxide anesthesia, a similar dose of etomidate decreases the amplitude of P100, with an increase in P60 and N70 latency.

Anesthetic gases also generally depress amplitude and increase latency of the VER. The effect on both amplitude and latency is dose dependent. Nitrous oxide decreases the amplitude of the VER.[41] The N65 to P95 wave appears to be the most sensitive and is affected by as little as 10% nitrous oxide. The sensitivity of a pattern-reversal VER to nitrous oxide differs somewhat from a flash-evoked VER.[40] Halothane, enflurane, and isoflurane cause dose-dependent decreases in amplitude and increases in latency.[16,49,144] The inspired concentration of anesthetic agents that completely suppress the response varies; for example, isoflurane with a 1.2% end-tidal concentration completely abolishes the VER.[17]

Pathophysiology

Intraoperative waveform variability has shown that VER monitoring is of limited use during intracranial surgery. Cedzich et al. assessed a flash-evoked VER in 35 patients with tumors along the visual pathways (90% symptomatic).[13] Of the patients with perisellar lesions, 13 had a craniotomy and 12 had surgery via the transsphenoidal approach. During removal of the bone flap or during the transsphenoidal approach, the following were observed: a reversible loss of VER in 11 patients, a profound alteration of waveform in 8 patients, and a loss of single peaks in 15 patients. No correlation was found between intraoperative VER changes and postoperative changes in visual function. Thus instability of the waveforms is not simply a result of cranial bone flap removal.

Cedzich et al. found that an intraoperative flash-evoked VER is extremely variable and not useful for intraoperative monitoring because of difficulty obtaining reproducible peaks and amplitude changes.[14] They did find that patients with perisellar tumors had smaller wave amplitudes than patients with non-perisellar tumors who had similar surgery (craniotomies). The authors found complete intraoperative VER loss in 21 of 45 patients unassociated with postoperative neurologic changes.

The VER is altered by systemic effects such as increased intracranial pressure[153] and hypothermia.[115] In patients with hydrocephalus and head injury, an early VER wave (N70 recorded from an active vertex electrode) correlates with intracranial pressure.[153] An inverse relationship exists between temperature and VER amplitude and latency.[115]

Somatosensory-Evoked Potential

SSEPs are the response of the neural axis (from peripheral nerve to contralateral somatosensory cortex) to repetitive peripheral nerve stimulation. Function of the peripheral nerve, spinal cord (posterior columns) the brain (brainstem, medial leminscus, internal capsule, contralateral somatosensory cortex) can be assessed with this monitoring modality. The SSEP can be used for detection of localized injury to specific areas of the neural axis or as a nonspecific indicator of the adequacy of cerebral oxygen delivery by assessing cortically generated waves.

Powers et al. demonstrated that fibers in the ipsilateral dorsal column, ipsilateral dorsal spinocerebellar tract, and contralateral ventrolateral tracts carry SSEP responses to lower extremity stimulation.[111] A lesion of one half the dorsal column causes changes in the amplitude of both early and late scalp-recorded waves produced by stimulation ipsilateral to the side of the lesion, whereas a lesion of the dorsal spinocerebellar tract or ventrolateral tract causes changes only in later waves (>40 msec, amplitude decrease). Thus processes that produce major changes in the SSEP from lower extremity stimulation indicate injury to the posterior columns of the spinal cord.

Paired disk electrodes may be placed over the nerve (most often the median or posterior tibial nerve) for transcutaneous stimulation. Percutaneous 23-gauge needles can be placed near the nerve for stimulation. An advantage of needles for intraoperative use is constant stimulus location and intensity. Discomfort during SSEP stimulation may be reduced by minimizing current intensity and increasing the stimulus electrode surface area. The current required for adequate stimulation is less with subdermal needles placed near the nerve compared with surface electrodes and may decrease discomfort.

The signal-to-noise ratio affects the number of stimuli (averages) required to produce stable and reproducible waves. A large number of trials (> 1000) may be required to produce good waveforms in the awake patient because of muscle noise, whereas in the same patient under general anesthesia, a much smaller number of averages (128 to 256) may produce a stable waveform, which is different from the waveform with the patient awake. **Although anesthetics produce direct effects on the SSEP system, suppression of muscle artifacts by neuromuscular blocking agents and the ability to use a much higher stimulus intensity in the anesthetized patient allow rapid production of waves, which are reproducible but differ from those found in the awake patient.**

Fig. 43-7 shows variability in upper extremity SSEP in neurologically normal, unanesthetized subjects. It is unclear whether anesthetic depression differentially affects small or less complex waveforms. Fig. 43-8 demonstrates the effect of anesthetic induction as well as an increase in stimulus intensity in the

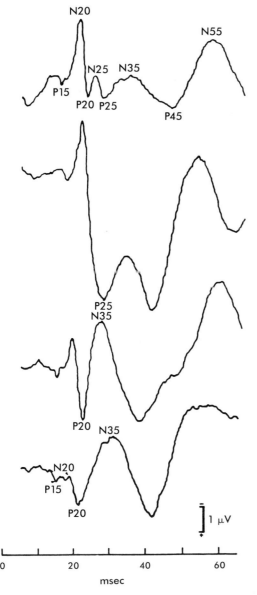

Fig. 43-7. Variability in morphology of upper extremity somatosensory-evoked potentials (SSEPs) in unanesthetized subjects using similar techniques. Normal latencies are provided. *N,* Negative; *P,* positive; numbers are milliseconds. (From Hume AL, Cant BR: Conduction time in central somatosensory pathway in man, *Electroencephalogr Clin Neurophysiol* 45:361, 1978.)

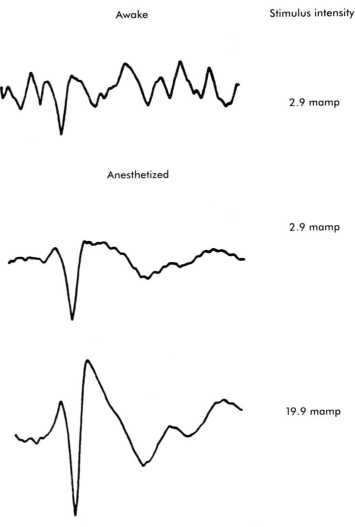

Fig. 43-8. Impact of anesthesia induction and increased stimulus intensity on median nerve SSEP. Anesthesia induction (thiopental plus fentanyl) plus pancuronium decreases muscle artifact. Increased stimulus intensity in anesthetized patient increases wave amplitude. Negative is up, and time is from 0 to 80 msec following stimulation.

anesthetized subject. The upper trace demonstrates some muscle artifact, which is completely suppressed by anesthetic induction with thiopental plus fentanyl and pancuronium for neuromuscular blockade. The lower trace demonstrates that increased stimulus intensity increases wave amplitude. The increased amplitude caused by a higher stimulus intensity may blunt anesthesia-related depression.

Optimizing the signal-to-noise ratio is particularly important in patients who have small waveforms resulting from disease, such as spinal cord stenosis or spinal cord compression from an extraaxial mass. With extremely small waves, generation of a reproducible lower extremity SSEP waveform may require 500 to 1000 stimuli delivered at 4 per second so that wave development time is 2 to 4 minutes. The level of electrical noise in the operating room is relatively high and usually cannot be greatly reduced. Generally the number of stimuli necessary to generate a good waveform is related to the signal-to-noise ratio in an exponential manner; thus a decrease in signal-to-noise ratio by one half requires a fourfold increase in the number of stimuli (and a fourfold increase in averaging time).

Fig. 43-9 shows a median nerve SSEP recorded from multiple levels in an unanesthetized patient and represents several important aspects of SSEP monitoring. Of particular importance is the ability to generate characteristic waves in unanesthetized pa-

tients in the electrically difficult operation room environment. Multiple traces are plotted to show waveform reproducibility. The ability to record signals at multiple levels of the neural axis is also demonstrated. In Fig. 43-9 an asterisk has been placed over the wave thought to originate near the monitoring electrode at each level. **The characteristic wave over the second cervical vertebra is N14 (negative, 14 msec latency) and over the brachial plexus is N9 (negative, 9 msec).** *Central conduction time* (CCT) is the delay from the second cervical vertebra to the cortex (i.e., N20 to N14). Simultaneous presentation of ascending locations allows rapid determination of the site of the signal's interruption. Attenuation of the scalp-recorded signal with maintenance of the signal over the upper spinal cord suggests a brainstem injury, whereas signal attenuation at the spinal cord level suggests peripheral nerve or brachial plexus injury.

Rapid localization injury sites using monitoring at ascending sites is shown in two patients with posterior fossa tumors in Fig. 43-10. Each pair of waves is simultaneously recorded from the scalp (upper trace) and the cervicomedullary junction (lower trace). In Fig. 43-10, *A*, surgical positioning of the patient resulted in rapid loss of waves at both locations, suggesting injury distal to the spinal cord. Proper positioning of the stimulated extremity caused rapid improvement of waves at both locations. In Fig. 43-10, *B*, surgical positioning of the patient produced loss of scalp-recorded waves with retention of waves recorded over the cervicomedullary junction, suggesting injury at the brainstem level. Repositioning of the head in the neutral position resulted in the return of scalp-recorded waves.

Several analysis methods for evoked potentials are available in addition to ensemble averaging. One method is the *moving window average* (MWA), which estimates by averaging within a window containing the *n* most recent sweeps, where *n* is some specific window length. The *exponentially weighted average* (EWA) estimates are obtained by weighted averaging of sweeps, with the weight of previous sweeps diminishing exponentially. Vaz et al. compared Fourier series modelling (*Fourier linear combined*, FLC) with MWA and EWA in a rapid change of evoked potential waveform (etomidate bolus). The algorithm outputs a fresh estimate after each sweep.[146] The authors showed that FLC follows transient evoked potential changes much faster than EWA or MWA.

Diagnostic criteria used to evaluate intraoperative waveform changes have been difficult to establish. Using conventional averaging techniques, latency changes of 7% to 15% and amplitude decreases of 45% to 50% occur without changes in postoperative neurologic function.[76,90,153] Use of the amplitude ratio of median nerve to posterior tibial nerve has been

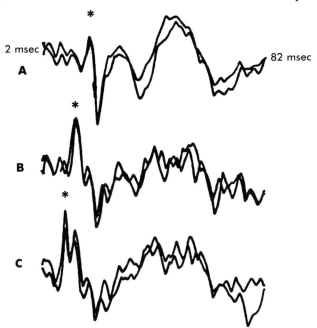

Fig. 43-9. Near-field recordings at ascending locations of neural axis following median nerve stimulation, referenced to forehead. **A,** Waves recorded over contralateral somatosensory cortex. **B,** Waves recorded over cervicomedullary junction (second cervical vertebra). **C,** Waves recorded over brachial plexus (Erb's point). In each trace an asterisk denotes near-field wave used for intraoperative monitoring.

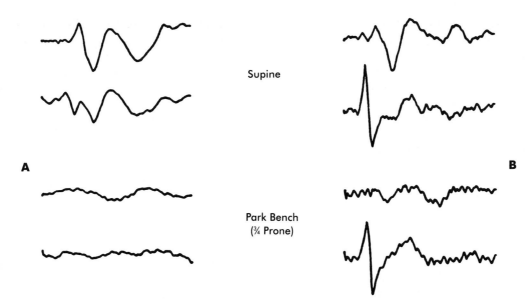

Supine

A

Park Bench
(¾ Prone)

B

Fig. 43-10. Position-related neurologic changes demonstrated by somatosensory-evoked potentials (SSEPs). Simultaneous recording over scalp (upper trace of each pair) and cervicomedullary junction (lower trace of each pair) in two patients. **A,** Patient had injury at level of brachial plexus. **B,** Return of patient's head to neutral position reversed waveform changes. (See text.)

suggested as a method to evaluate systemic effects on the posterior tibial waveform.

Two intraoperative monitoring techniques used frequently are stimulation of the median nerve for upper extremity monitoring and the posterior tibial nerve for lower extremity monitoring. Following stimulation of the median nerve, near-field waves can be recorded over the brachial plexus (Erb's point 2 cm superior to clavicular head of sternocleidomastoid muscle; N9), cervical spinal cord (N14), and somatosensory cortex (N20, P22). Stimulation of the posterior tibial nerve results in responses monitored over the popliteal fossa, lumbar spinal cord, and somatosensory cortex (P38, N49). Scalp-recorded waves following posterior tibial stimulation are frequently of the highest amplitude 1 to 2 cm lateral to the midline ipsilateral to the stimulation point because of paradoxic localization. Lesser et al. placed electrodes in the interhemispheric groove and found that maximal activity is recorded over the hemisphere contralateral to stimulation.[83] Paradoxic lateralization probably is related to a horizontal dipole located within the interhemispheric groove.

In unanesthetized subjects, stimulus frequencies of 1.6, 3.1, and 5.7 Hz do not change amplitudes or latencies.[26] In patients with spinal cord injury, amplitude following posterior tibial nerve stimulation is attenuated by a higher stimulus rate (>5.1 Hz), whereas good-quality waves could be obtained at a lower stimulus rate (1.1 or 2.1 Hz). Most patients (86%) who had a decrease in amplitude with an increase in stimulus rate had discrete sensory level

weakness, bilateral lower extremity weakness, or both. Only 28% of the patients whose SSEPs were not affected by an increased stimulus rate had similar neurologic impairment.[121] Fig. 43-11 shows the impact of a stimulus rate in a patient with abnormal spinal cord function. At the usual stimulus frequency used for intraoperative monitoring (4.1 Hz), a wave is not

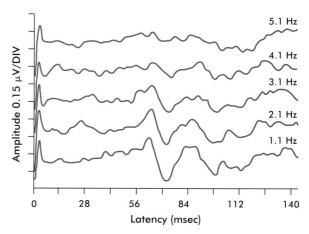

Fig. 43-11. Posterior tibial nerve SSEP attenuation caused by increasing stimulus rate in patients with spinal cord abnormalities. Note that at usual stimulus frequency for lower extremity monitoring (4.1 Hz), a very small wave is shown, whereas a lower stimulus frequency produces a wave robust enough to be used to detect intraoperative injury. (From Schubert A, Drummond JC, and Garfin SR: The influence of stimulus presentation rate on the cortical amplitude and latency of somatosensory-evoked potential recordings in patients with varying degrees of spinal cord injury, *Spine* 12:969, 1987.)

sufficiently distinctive to detect intraoperative injury. Reduction in stimulus rate allowed production of a wave sufficiently distinct to detect injury.

The spinal cord may be stimulated directly by percutaneous placement of flexible epidural electrodes. This electrode can be placed by fluoroscopic guidance and used to stimulate the spinal cord directly. This technique is useful during thoracic aneurysm surgery when aortic cross-clamping produces peripheral nerve ischemia. An epidural electrode can also be used to record large-amplitude waves that are relatively resistant to anesthetic depression.[54]

Cortical sensory-evoked potential recording can be used to localize the motor cortex because of its location next to the somatosensory cortex. The somatosensory cortex is identified by (1) approximately mirror-image waveforms recorded at electrode sites on opposite sides of the central sulcus (hand area) (i.e., P20 to N30 precentrally and N20 to P30 postcentrally), (2) a P25 to N35 wave of large amplitude in the postcentral gyrus near the central sulcus, and (3) regardless of component identification, maximal SSEP amplitude being recorded in the hand presentation area of the precentral and postcentral gyri.[151]

Anesthetics

Early components of the SSEP (< 40 msec for upper extremity nerve stimulation; < 80 msec for lower extremity nerve stimulation) are readily generated for intraoperative monitoring, and information about anesthetic effects on these waves is emphasized here. Table 43-2 summarizes effects of frequently used

drugs on SSEP when administered individually. Intravenous agents generally have only moderate effects on early parts of the waveforms and allow generation of waveforms adequate for rapid evaluation. **Barbiturates such as thiopental (5 mg/kg) cause moderate or no decrease in amplitude,**[32,73] **with a moderate increase in latency.** Diazepam depresses scalp recorded waves,[36] whereas the effect of midazolam is unclear with reports of no effect on amplitude with slight increase in latency[73] or 40% amplitude depression.[127] **Fentanyl has modest effects on early components of the SSEP waveform.** Amplitude is unchanged in doses of fentanyl up to 75 μg/kg,[28,95,107] but latency is increased.

A most surprising drug effect on SSEP waveform is the augmentation of amplitude (200% to 600%) caused by etomidate.[73,96] Waveform augmentation appears to be a cortical effect[96] and has been used clinically to augment abnormally small waves, thus allowing monitoring that otherwise would have not

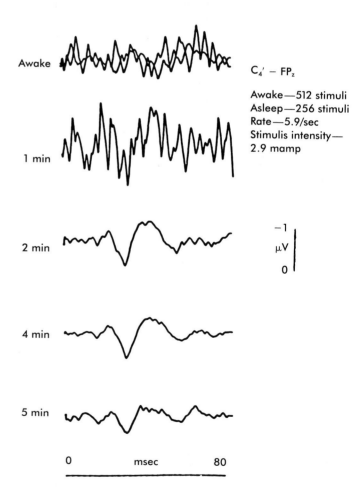

$C_{4}' - FP_z$

Awake—512 stimuli
Asleep—256 stimuli
Rate—5.9/sec
Stimulis intensity—2.9 mamp

Fig. 43-12. Augmentation of upper extremity SSEP by etomidate (0.4 mg/kg) in patient with severe cervical stenosis (complete spinal block at C4). In awake patient, SSEP waveform was not recognizable, whereas 2 minutes after induction of anesthesia with etomidate, a recognizable wave with increased latency was demonstrated.

Drug	Amplitude	Latency	Reference
Table 43-2	**Anesthetic effects on somatosensory-evoked potential (SSEP)**		
Thiopental	Small or no change	Increase	73
Etomidate	Increase	Increase	73, 96
Fentanyl	Moderate or no decrease	Moderate or no increase	28, 96, 107
Diazepam	Decrease	Increase	36
Midazolam	Decrease	Increase	127
Ketamine	Increase	Increase	122
Propofol	No change	Increase	118
Nitrous oxide	Decrease	No change	95, 109, 150
Halothane	Decrease	Increase	2, 106, 109
Enflurane	Decrease	Increase	126
Isoflurane	Decrease	Increase	22, 95

been possible.[128] Fig. 43-12 shows SSEP augmentation by etomidate. This was accomplished with a dose of etomidate routinely used for anesthesia induction. Ketamine (2 mg/kg) also increases SSEP amplitude, with the maximal increase occurring within 2 to 10 minutes.[122] Propofol (2.5 mg/kg) depresses deflections later than N20, increases N20 latency 8%, and increases CCT (N20 to N14 latency) 20%. N14 and N20 amplitudes are not affected by propofol.[118]

Volatile anesthetic gases and nitrous oxide depress the SSEP waveform, apparently in a dose-dependent manner.[106,109,126,150] With halothane, enflurane, and isoflurane, the amplitude is less and the latency greater with coadministration of nitrous oxide (60%). The effect of isoflurane on SSEP may occur within a few minutes.[6]

Enflurane decreases SSEP amplitude and increases latency in patients anesthetized with intravenous agents (fentanyl, thiopental).[95] Enflurane, 0.6% and 1.7%, under other circumstances may increase amplitude when compared with a control value.[23] Isoflurane decreases amplitude in a dose-dependent manner from 1.2 μV at 0.5 MAC (isoflurane plus nitrous oxide) to 0.3 μV at 1.5 MAC. Elimination of nitrous oxide increases amplitude by 100%.[150] Isoflurane decreases amplitude and increases latency in patients anesthetized with fentanyl and thiopental.[95] High concentrations of isoflurane (greater than 2%) completely suppress the scalp-recorded SSEP waves.[22]

Pathophysiology

Branston et al.[7] assessed the effects of ischemia on early components of SSEP in the brainstem thalamus and cerebral cortex and found that a cephalic-to-caudal decrease in cerebral blood flow (CBF) is required to maintain normal electrical activity. Initial changes in cortical SSEP waves occur at a mean arterial blood pressure (MABP) of 30 to 40 mm Hg, but thalamic and medical lemniscus flows are changed only at a lower MABP (<30 mm Hg). At MABP of 20 to 30 mm Hg, SSEP amplitudes in the cortex, thalamus, and medical lemniscus are 9%, 73%, and 91% of control values, respectively. In terms of blood flow, the threshold for SSEP change in the cortex is 15 to 20 ml/min/100 g; in the thalamus, 10 to 15 ml/min/100 g; and in the medial lemniscus, 10 ml/min/100 g.

During increased intracranial pressure SSEP latency does not increase until CBF falls >55% to 65%, corresponding to a 20% to 30% reduction in cerebral oxygen consumption ($CMRO_2$). CCT is prolonged when CBF falls below 15 to 20 ml/min/100 g and is associated with a decrease in $CMRO_2$ of 20% to 30%.[71]

Graf et al.[53] studied the effect of middle cerebral artery (MCA) occlusion on somatosensory response and found that ischemia is much more severe in the white matter pathways than in the somatosensory cortex. They concluded that SSEP loss in such circumstances is caused by white matter ischemia. Postischemic recovery of SSEP amplitude correlates with residual flow in both the ipsilateral MCA territory and the white matter during ischemia.[94] Animals that developed ischemic lesions of the cortex have more rapid loss and slower recovery of scalp-recorded SSEP than animals that did not subsequently develop lesions after reperfusion.[30]

Friedman et al. found during intracranial aneurysm ablation that from the time of dural opening until dural closure, prolonged CCT, decreased cortical amplitude, or disappearance of the SSEP wave was predictive of postoperative sensory or motor deficits, except when basilar artery surgery was involved.[42] Outcome of basilar artery surgery was not predicted by SSEP or BAER. The authors believed SSEP failed to correlate with outcome in basilar aneurysm surgery because the vascular distribution at risk (posterior cerebral arteries and basilar perforating vessels) does not reliably include either the BAER or the SSEP pathways. When they compared amplitude and latency values at dural opening to dural closure, they found a false positive incidence of only 2%. They found a 6% false negative incidence, but only 4% when basilar aneurysms were excluded.

Symon et al. assessed SSEP central conduction time (CCT; latency from cervical spinal cord to contralateral somatosensory cortex) in patients undergoing intracranial aneurysm ablation (34 procedures) and found that increases in CCT to 10 msec or disappearance of the scalp-recorded response was associated with postoperative neurologic deficits.[140]

Momma et al. assessed CCT during temporary clip application in 40 patients and found that 25% of patients had postoperative neurologic changes, although prompt recovery occurred in half these patients.[101] None of the patients whose CCT did not change intraoperatively had postoperative morbidity. In six patients, temporary arterial occlusion prolonged CCT up to 10 msec, and two of these patients had immediate postoperative neurologic deficit (one recovered). The scalp-recorded response became flat in 15 patients; seven of these had hemispheric deficits in the immediate postoperative period, and four recovered. Postoperative permanent deficit is unlikely if wave disappearance takes more than 3 to 4 minutes, and recovery is likely if N20 recovers within 20 minutes after reperfusion.[101]

Manninen et al. assessed SSEPs during temporary arterial occlusion during cerebral aneurysm surgery in 97 patients. SSEP changes during vessel occlusion were found in 24%, with 65% of these changes reversible with release of occlusion and 35% persisting.[92] In each case a persistent SSEP change predicted a postoperative neurologic deficit, whereas of the 15 patients with reversible changes, only five had postoperative deficits. Eighty percent of patients had no change in SSEP, and 14% had a new neurologic deficit postoperatively. Thus the false positive rate was 43%, and the false negative rate was 14%. If only persistent SSEP changes were considered as predictors of neurologic deficits, the false positive rate was 0%. **The SSEP was the better predictor of neurologic outcome in patients with temporary occlusion of the carotid system than of the vertebrobasilar system.** SSEP changes correctly predicted a neurologic deficit in only 38% of patients with vertebrobasilar artery aneurysms, compared with 75% of patients with MCA or carotid artery aneurysm.

Brinkman et al. compared intraoperative SSEP changes during carotid endarterectomy with postoperative neurophysiologic performance 7 days after surgery. They found that intraoperative loss of early waves in 4 of 14 patients was associated with worsening neurophysiologic performance, with two of these patients ultimately having a cerebrovascular accident (7 and 35 days after surgery). Patients who had amplitude decreases of 50% or more performed worse after surgery than those with less severe reduction of amplitude.[9]

Berenstein et al. studied SSEPs during spinal cord embolization of patients with arteriovenous malformation (AVM) under neuroleptanesthesia (droperidol, fentanyl). They found that the amplitude decreased coincident with opacification of the anterior spinal artery, with return of amplitude 2 to 4 minutes after catheter removal in all but one patient, who required 24 minutes for return of waves.[3] In three patients with an embolized AVM of the spinal cord, amplitude increased and SSEP changes were associated with immediate improvement of symptoms. The authors found in several patients that SSEP changes preceded motor weakness, which is different from findings in animal studies.

Dinner et al. assessed posterior tibial SSEPs in 220 patients (121 with scoliosis, 41 with neoplasm, 58 with other conditions).[27] Only three of seven patients who had worsening neurologic function after surgery had significant, persistent changes in intraoperative SSEPs (57% false negative). In an additional four patients, more than a 50% decrease in amplitude occurred without change in postoperative neurologic status (2% false positive).

Ginsburg et al. reported postoperative paraplegia with intraoperative preservation of SSEP in a patient with achondroplastic dwarfism.[49] The patient awoke paraplegic with preservation of cortical response to individual peroneal nerve stimulation and an absent pinprick response below the twelfth thoracic vertebra. Lesser et al.[84] described six patients who had postoperative deficits despite unchanged SSEPs. Zornow et al.[158] presented a case report of an autopsy-documented anterior spinal artery syndrome in which lower extremity SSEPs were retained.

Schmid et al. assessed SSEPs in 28 patients with symptomatic cervical radiculopathy.[119] They found that 68% of patients had false negative waveform changes on the side of symptoms and that 36% had false positive changes on the side contralateral to symptoms. Veilleux et al. reviewed median nerve SSEPs in patients undergoing surgery of the cervical spine who had baseline values available and who had no intradural process expanding or compressing the cervical cord.[147] In patients with preoperative evidence of spinal injury, intraoperative scalp-recorded waves could be lost without major changes in anesthesia or surgery. Intraoperative ulnar and tibial responses could be monitored in all patients in whom baseline studies could be obtained.

Hypothermia increases SSEP latency.[139,145] Latency change correlates with nasopharyngeal temperature. The impact of hypothermia on amplitude is less clear, with reports of no change[145] or decreased amplitude.[139] Latency of the initial waves is prolonged about 1.15 msec/° C, suggesting that a decrease in temperature of 2° to 3° C will increase latency about 3 msec,[145] an amount of change previously suggested to indicate neural injury. **Hyperthermia (42° C) suppresses SSEP amplitude.** The amplitude is only 15% of that at normothermia (37° C).[33]

Synek assessed median nerve SSEPs in the diagnosis of brachial plexus lesions in patients with injury, with cervical spondylopathic radioculopathies without myelopathy, and with brachial plexopathy and systemic cancer.[141] Median nerve SSEPs were normal in patients with injuries of the upper trunk and root avulsion confined to one or two root levels. Median nerve SSEPs were abnormal in multiple trunk lesions and multiple root avulsions. In patients with spondylopathic radiculopathies, median nerve SSEPs were normal in all but one patient.

Leandri et al. studied trigeminal nerve–evoked potentials in 23 patients with skull base tumors (perisellar or cerebellopontine angle).[78] They found altered waveforms in all patients with skull base tumors who had clinical signs in the trigeminal area and in 7 of 12 patients who did not have signs. Stimulation via two thin needles placed into the infraorbital foramen avoids activation of motor fibers and produces three negative waves within the first 3 msec after stimulation.[79] The first wave probably originates as the maxillary nerve joins the gasserian ganglion, where an extrinsic mass might compress the nerve. The second wave originates from the entry of the nerve into the pons, and the origin of the third wave is within the pons.

Intraoperative SSEP monitoring seems reliable for surgery involving the carotid artery system. SSEP monitoring is useful but less reliable in detecting injury in the vertebrobasilar system. Although initial clinical use involved monitoring during spinal surgery, neurologic injury may occur during surgery without waveform changes. The incidence of false positive changes (waveform change without alteration of neurologic function) appears to be increased in patients with compromised spinal cord function. Sophisticated waveform analysis currently under investigation may be more accurate in demonstrating waveform changes than the currently used technique of averaging.

Brainstem Auditory-Evoked Response

Auditory nerve stimulation produces both brainstem components and cortical components, although the latter have received only modest interest in intraoperative monitoring. **The BAER is the response of the auditory apparatus to stimulus of the auditory nerve and has been used extensively in patients at risk of brain injury during intracranial surgery and following head injury. Use of the BAER is widespread despite the extremely small amount of neural tissue involved and the resistance of BAER to oxygen deprivation compared with other neural monitors such as EEG or cortical SSEP waves.**[131]

The origin of the waves are wave I (auditory nerve), wave II (pontomedullary junction), wave III (caudal pons), wave IV (rostral pons), wave V (midbrain), and wave VI (thalamus). The BAER is generated by delivering pure tone clicks individually to each ear. Rarefaction clicks, condensation clicks, or alternation of rarefaction and condensation clicks may be used. Because of some crossover, the contralateral ear is masked with white noise. For intraoperative monitoring, small ear inserts that are easily secured work well. Technical difficulties may make intraoperative BAER interpretation difficult. Factors that decrease the effective stimulus intensity alter the waveform. Partial obstruction of the external auditory canal by cerumen or fluid will decrease the stimulus intensity, and increases in latency will occur that mimic neural injury.

Fig. 43-13 shows a BAER developed in the operating room using a small stimulator that can be secured for intraoperative monitoring. Several waves are superimposed to demonstrate constancy of the peaks. The characteristic peaks are labelled with Roman numerals. Interpeak latencies can be used to assess injury, and calculation of I to V interpeak latency assesses transmission from the eighth cranial nerve to the inferior colliculi.

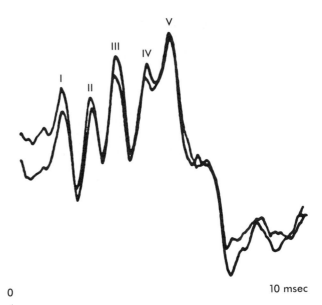

Fig. 43-13. Two separate brainstem auditory-evoked response (BAER) recordings performed in volunteer. Ear inserts were used for intraoperative click stimulation of left ear. Vertex was referenced to ipsilateral mastoid process. The rapid falloff following wave V is characteristic, and is used to localize wave V. Characteristic negative waves are indicated by Roman numerals.

BAER monitoring should be undertaken in all patients at risk, even if the primary disease causes hearing on the affected side to decrease below the functional level. Fig. 43-14 shows recordings from a patient with a large cerebellopontine angle tumor and greatly diminished hearing ipsilateral to the tumor. Unilateral BAER changes occurred with only a moderate degree of head turning and were reversed by returning the head to a neutral position.

In addition to brainstem response to auditory stimulation, longer latency responses occur. The P300 is a late auditory wave that appears to be an electrophysiologic correlate of complex processes such as directed attention, stimulus detection, sequential information processing, short-term memory, and decision making.[112] The P300 amplitude varies with stimulus probability (relative frequency, sequential structure), meaning (stimulus complexity, stimulus value), and information transmission (discrimination difficulty, allocation of attendance).[63] Middle-latency auditory responses (10 to 40 msec) are generated intracortically in neural elements of the primary auditory cortex.[70]

Anesthetics

BAER waves are particularly resistant to anesthetic agents, both intravenous and inhalational. Table 43-3 summarizes the effects of frequently used drugs on the BAER when used individually. Increasing levels of barbiturates and ketamine increase BAER inter-

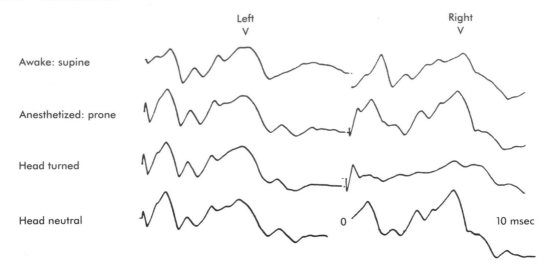

Fig. 43-14. Brainstem auditory-evoked responses (BAERs) in patient with cerebellopontine angle tumor. Left BAER recording is of normal latency, whereas right BAER recording has a wave V of increased latency because of large right cerebellopontine angle tumor. Mild head rotation caused a prolongation of wave V on right, which was reversed by placing patient's head in neutral position.

peak latency.[21,135] Propofol (2 mg/kg) with an infusion increases latency of the I, III, and V waves without change in amplitudes but completely suppresses middle-latency auditory waves.[15] Fentanyl in large doses does not alter the BAER.[116]

Houston et al.[60] found a linear decrease in BAER amplitude with an increase in nitrous oxide concentration (10% to 40%). They also found an increase in hearing threshold of sufficient magnitude to explain BAER changes caused by nitrous oxide. Nitrous oxide (33%) reduces the amplitude of long-latency auditory-evoked potentials without alteration in latency.[40,58] The effect of halothane in clinically useful concentrations on the BAER is unclear, with reports of no effect[35,117] and drug-induced increases in latency.[143] In one study the increase in wave V latency at a 1% end-expiratory concentration of halothane was slightly less than 1 msec. Slight increases in BAER latency occur in a dose-dependent manner during enflurane anesthesia.[34,143]

Table 43-3 Anesthetic effects on brainstem auditory-evoked response (BAER)

Drug	Latency	Reference
Thiopental	Increase	135
Fentanyl	No change	116
Propofol	Increase	15
Ketamine	Increase	21
Nitrous oxide	Increase	60
Halothane	Increase	117,142
Enflurane	Increase	34,142

Pathophysiology

In humans, hypercapnia (7.5 to 10% CO_2) does not change the BAER. In anesthetized cats, hypercapnia affects the BAER less than it affects the EEG. Hypercapnia increases latency slightly and is associated with a small decrease in amplitude. At $Paco_2$ of 90 mm Hg, the EEG is isoelectric but the BAER is essentially normal in experimental animals.[132]

Sohmer et al. found that the EEG became isoelectric at a cerebral perfusion pressure (CPP) of 24 mm Hg, whereas the BAER became isoelectric at 7 mm Hg. In most animals a stage of decreased CPP was reached in which wave I was preserved but brainstem waves were absent at about 14 mm Hg.[134] Sohmer et al.[133] assessed the BAER in cats during decreased CPP and found that at CPP of 26 mm Hg, the EEG and BAER rapidly decreased, with EEG changes occurring before significant BAER changes.[133] Goitein et al. assessed BAER in 25 children with reduced CPP and found that BAER became abnormal when CPP decreased to less than 30 mm Hg.[51]

Sohmer et al. compared the effect of severe hypoxia (Pao_2, 20 to 30 mm Hg) on the BAER, SSEP, and VER.[131] If MABP was maintained during severe hypoxia, no effect on SSEP or VER was seen, whereas the BAER and long-latency auditory-evoked potential waves were depressed. However, if MABP was allowed to decrease during hypoxia, all evoked potentials became severely depressed and isoelectric. **This suggests that BAER is altered early during hypoxia because of sensitivity of the cochlear microphonics to hypoxia rather than failure of brainstem conduction.**[130]

Kalmarchey et al. studied the BAER in patients during surgery for unilateral cerebellopontine angle

(CPA) tumors.[64] They found that BAER changes occur with lumbar drainage and tumor dissection in all patients, with bilateral latency prolongation in five of nine patients and an ipsilateral latency increase in six of nine patients. This suggests that the BAER is too sensitive for intraoperative monitoring. Patients with small CPA tumors may have a normal BAER at high stimulus intensity. At lower intensity, however, abnormal latency of wave V compared with the unaffected side may be demonstrated.[82,102]

Lam et al. reported BAER in three patients undergoing ablation of basilar artery aneurysm.[75] In two patients, ligation of the basilar artery and of a vertebral artery resulted in deterioration of the BAER and correlated with postoperative neurologic injury. In the third patient, transient postoperative neurologic changes correlated with intraoperative BAER changes.

An exponential increase in BAER latency occurs as temperature is decreased to 19° C in both primates[31] and rodents.[120] The increase in latency appears greater in the later waves.[136] Waves are easily identifiable at more frequently used levels of hypothermia (29° C) but are delayed by about 33%.[93] BAER latency is inversely related to temperature over the range of 36° to 42° C, with a decrease in amplitude as temperature increases.[52]

The BAER appears to be a sensitive monitor of the auditory apparatus in response to direct injury. **The BAER appears to be much less sensitive to diffuse insults such as hypoxia or intracranial hypertension than other modalities (e.g., EEG, SSEP).**

ELECTROMYOGRAPHY

Electromyography (EMG) is the response of the muscle to stimulation of the motor nerve. Facial nerve stimulation with EMG monitoring is frequently used to decrease the risk of facial nerve injury during surgery for CPA tumors. Since the response is generated by contraction of muscle, the use of neuromuscular blocking agents is somewhat restricted.

Kartush reviewed EMG and intraoperative facial nerve monitoring. He emphasized using a monopolar stimulator with an insulated tip, since cerebrospinal fluid can dispel the stimulus and lead to a false negative.[65] Typical stimulus parameters include a constant curve of 2 mamp at 5 cps for 200 μsec duration. EMG recording electrodes are placed in orbicularis oris and orbicularis oculi regions, with a ground electrode on the forehead. Anesthetic management, particularly the use of neuromuscular blocking agents, has been poorly studied. Clearly, the neuromuscular junction must be functional for an EMG response to occur when the nerve is stimulated.

The degree of neuromuscular blockade should be maintained at a light level until response of the respective muscles (orbicularis oris, orbicularis oculi) is verified. It is unclear if a nerve that has been stretched by a tumor or otherwise injured will respond to a normal level of stimulation.

MOTOR-EVOKED POTENTIALS

Limitation of SSEPs in monitoring the spinal cord has produced interest in directly monitoring the motor system with motor-evoked potentials (MEPs).

The motor cortex has been stimulated using transcranial electrical stimulation (E-MEP) and, more recently, magnetic stimulation (M-MEP). *Electrical stimulation* produces discomfort, is poorly tolerated in the awake subject, and has produced interest in magnetic stimulation of the motor cortex. Although less precise, *magnetic stimulation* offers the advantage of less discomfort and is well tolerated in the awake subject. Corticospinal response to direct stimulation of the motor cortex can be recorded from the lateral column of the spinal cord or from the spinal epidural space using percutaneous needles.[66] Monitoring of MEPs is difficult because of the efficiency of the central nervous system in conducting impulses via the spinal cord and peripheral nerves to muscle groups. These extremely small electrical impulses are difficult to record over the spinal cord or peripheral nerves. The muscle response to stimulation of the motor cortex is much larger than the neural response and therefore much easier to record.

Understanding the MEP is based primarily on potential responses of compound muscle action, despite both volatile anesthetic and neuromuscular blocking agents obtunding those responses. Latency is increased with magnetic generation compared with electrical generation of the MEP. Magnetic stimulation penetrates whole-body structures, including the skull, without creating large electrical fields at the surface; thus the patient feels little pain during stimulation of the cortex or peripheral nerves. Less stimulus artifact is produced with magnetic stimulation than with electrical stimulation. The stimulus artifact ceases when the magnetic stimulus terminates, whereas with electrical stimulation, artifact persists for a short time afterward.[24]

The M-MEP is produced by discharging an electromagnet near the skull over the motor cortex. Currently, both circular- and butterfly-shaped coils are being investigated for stimulation. Coil characteristic and orientation for stimulation are now under intensive investigation. The technique for the E-MEP is to place the anode 8 cm from midline, immediately posterior to the coronal suture, with the cathode placed at the bregma for hand area stimulation. For foot stimulation, the anode is placed at the bregma, and the cathode is placed 6 cm posterior in the midline. Electrical stimulation theoretically can cause seizures. Stimuli typically necessary to cause seizures are of greater duration than those required for MEP, and kindling is not produced at a stimulus rate less than three per second. Implanted metallic devices such as aneurysm clips pose increased risk with magnetic stimulation because of movement potential.

Anesthetics

Table 43-4 summarizes the effects of frequently used anesthetics on MEPs when administered individually.

In the monkey, Ghaly et al. studied the effect of incremental doses of ketamine on the M-MEP and found no depression (compared with basal ketamine anesthesia) at doses <20 mg/kg.[46] At higher doses, amplitude depression ranged from 14% to 45% with stimulation of the adductor pollicis brevis muscle and 57% to 82% with the adductor hallucis muscle. Latency increased 12% to 18%, and stimulus threshold also increased.

Nitrous oxide appears to depress both M-MEP and E-MEP. In humans, nitrous oxide during thiopental-fentanyl anesthesia depresses upper extremity response to 11% of baseline and lower extremity

Table 43-4 Anesthetic effects on motor-evoked potentials (MEPs)

Drug	Amplitude	Latency	Reference
Etomidate	No change	Increase	47
Fentanyl	No change?	No change?	155
Diazepam	Decrease	Increase	47
Ketamine	Decrease	Increase	46
Nitrous oxide	Decrease	Increase	46,156
Halothane	Decrease	Increase	57
Isoflurane (0.5%-1.5%)	Decrease	Increase	56

response to 7% of baseline in anterior tibial muscles. A similar depression is seen in human volunteers breathing 60% nitrous oxide.[155]

Loughman et al. studied halothane added to nitrous narcotic anesthesia using epidurally recorded E-MEP. They found that halothane did not alter amplitude or latency when compared with waves recorded during nitrous narcotic anesthesia.[89] Isoflurane (0.5% to 1.5%) increases latency and decreases

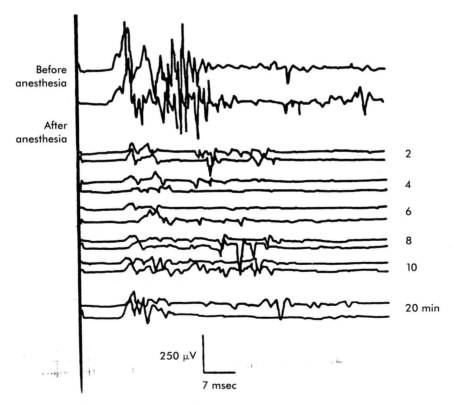

Fig. 43-15. Response of isoflurane on upper extremity magnetic motor-evoked potential (M-MEP). Two minutes after start of isoflurane, amplitude was decreased more than 75%. (From Haghighi SS, Green KD, Oro JJ et al: Depressive effect of isoflurane anesthesia on motor evoked potentials, *Neurosurgery* 26:993, 1990.)

amplitude of the E-MEP, with changes occurring within 2 minutes of anesthesia induction.[56]

Fig. 43-15 shows the effect of isoflurane on the compound motor action potential (cMAP) following electrical stimulation of the motor cortex. Isoflurane causes a rapid (within 2 minutes) and profound decrease in the amplitude of the cMAP. Although small compared with preanesthetic amplitudes, the amplitudes of these waves are much larger than scalp-recorded SSEP waves and thus should be easily monitored using conventional averaging technique. Haghighi et al.[57] compared volatile anesthetics with basal fentanyl-droperidol anesthesia on the E-MEP in rats and found a dose-dependent amplitude suppression, with halothane more depressant than isoflurane or enflurane.

Edmonds et al. assessed the response of bilateral anterior tibial muscles to M-MEP. They found that, preoperatively, 11 of 11 patients had recordable waves, whereas during nitrous narcotic anesthesia using a nondepolarizing muscle relaxant, only 9 of 11 had M-MEP waves. Anesthesia decreased amplitude from 523 to 163 μV.[37]

Pathophysiology

The proposed usefulness of the MEP is in those areas where monitoring of the SSEP has been found inadequate, especially when false negatives (injury without change in the SSEP) occur during spinal cord monitoring.[84] The E-MEP has been compared with the SSEP in patients with cortical and subcortical cerebrovascular accident (stroke) with varying degree of hemiparesis.[91] In patients with cortical infarcts, 55% had an abnormal MEP, and the remaining 45% had normal central motor conduction time. In three of five patients with subcortical infarct, both the MEP and the SSEP were absent. In all patients with subcortical infarct in which the MEP could be elicited, the SSEP could also be elicited. In two patients with cortical infarct, the MEP was absent but the SSEP was present; this was attributed to watershed infarcts. Subcortical infarcts prolonged central motor conduction time.

E-MEP has been assessed in animal studies of spinal cord ischemia using a thoracic aortic cross-clamping model.[77] Aortic cross-clamping produces a characteristic time-dependent and spinal level–de-pendent deterioration and loss of the MEP. Ischemic cord dysfunction, as evidenced by a change in the MEP, progressed from the distal to the proximal cord, with changes at L4 level occurring after 11 minutes and at T10 level after 17 minutes. In that study,[77] reperfusion resulted in MEP return, which progressed from proximal to distal. Although spinal cord blood flow was not assessed, this study suggests a significant time lag between events that limit blood flow to the spinal cord and changes in the transit of efferent impulses through the spinal cord. This time lag may be caused by the extremely small energy requirement for transmission of impulses via the spinal cord.

The E-MEP has been investigated in unanesthetized humans with space-occupying lesions of the brainstem or spinal cord using transcranial electrical stimulation and recording EMG from the contralateral thenar or anterior tibial muscle. Zenter and Rieder found a correct correlation between the MEP and the clinical motor status in 77% of thenar muscles and 84% of anterior tibial muscles, with 23% false positives in thenar recording and 16% in anterior tibial recording. There were no false negatives.[156]

The reliability of delivering stimuli to the motor cortex has led to clinical evaluation of E-MEP in patients at risk of injury during spinal surgery.[69,154] Zenter found that the E-MEP could be elicited in all 50 patients studied preoperatively. During neurolept-anesthesia, however, waves were absent in 12% of thenar muscles and 14% of anterior tibial muscles.[154] A 50% change in amplitude was used as a criterion for change. Zenter found that amplitude changes correlated with postoperative neurologic status in 81% of patients with stimulation of anterior tibial muscles (19% false negatives) and 76% with thenar muscles (24% false positives). In another clinical study,[69] 25% of patients had transient amplitude decreases of 50% that recovered completely and were associated with normal postoperative neurologic function. One patient had complete intraoperative loss of the MEP and awoke quadriplegic. Two patients had increased amplitude that was associated with improvement in motor function in the immediate postoperative period.

The MEP is very sensitive to anesthetics when the response is evaluated by recording the EMG response in a single twitch. Averaging the multiple responses may allow monitoring during volatile anesthesia.

KEY POINTS

- Postoperative neurologic changes following spinal surgery without intraoperative somatosensory-evoked potential (SSEP) change may occur, and only modest changes in intraoperative SSEP waves may herald permanent neurologic changes.

- Aggressive intraoperative monitoring of neurologic function does not guarantee prevention of neurologic injury, since not all parts of the brain are assessed using currently available monitoring.

- Intraoperative electroencephalographic (EEG) monitoring requires the recognition of several characteristic EEG patterns that occur normally or represent changes in the EEG caused by anesthetic agents or cerebral oxygen deprivation.

- Fentanyl causes a dose-dependent slowing of the EEG.

- Enflurane may cause generalized seizures with characteristic tonic-clonic activity and high-voltage EEG activity in humans, even in concentrations less than necessary for satisfactory anesthesia. Animal studies have confirmed that hypocapnia lowers the seizure threshold during enflurane anesthesia.

- EEG changes that may occur during carotid cross-clamping include a decrease in amplitude (including slow waves) or an increase in amplitude and a decrease in frequency.

- Hypothermia decreases the frequency of the EEG. Anesthetic and other usual intraoperative physiologic changes (e.g., hypothermia) alter the EEG from the awake state but allow diagnosis of both global and local ischemia.

- Evoked potentials are computed averages of the brain's response to repetitive peripheral stimuli.

- Nominal latency of the wave appearing about 100 msec after stimulation is important, since that wave is generally the most resistant to anesthetic depression.

- Intraoperative waveform variability has shown that visual-evoked response (VER) monitoring is of limited use during intracranial surgery.

- Although anesthetics produce direct effect on the SSEP system, suppression of muscle artifacts by neuromuscular blocking agents and the ability to use a much higher stimulus intensity in the anesthetized patient allow rapid production of waves, which are reproducible but differ from those found in the awake patient.

- The characteristic wave over the second cervical vertebra is N14 (negative, 14 msec latency) and over the brachial plexus is N9 (negative, 9 msec).

- The spinal cord may be stimulated directly by the percutaneous placement of flexible epidural electrodes.

- Barbiturates such as thiopental (5 mg/kg) cause moderate or no decrease in wave amplitude with a moderate increase in latency. Fentanyl has modest effects on early components of the SSEP waveform.

- A most surprising drug effect on SSEP waveform is the augmentation of amplitude (200% to 600%) caused by etomidate.

- Volatile anesthetic gases and nitrous oxide depress the SSEP waveform, apparently in a dose-dependent manner.

- During intracranial aneurysm ablation, the SSEP wave is predictive of postoperative sensory or motor deficits, except with basilar artery surgery.

- The SSEP is a better predictor of neurologic outcome in temporary occlusion of the carotid system than in the vertebrobasilar system.

- Hypothermia increases SSEP latency. Hyperthermia (42° C) suppresses SSEP amplitude.

- Intraoperative SSEP monitoring seems reliable for surgery involving the carotid artery system.

- The brainstem auditory-evoked response (BAER) is the response of the auditory apparatus to stimulus of the auditory nerve and has been used extensively in patients at risk of brain injury during intracranial surgery and following head injury.

- Resistance of the BAER to oxygen deprivation compares with other neural monitors, such as EEG or cortical SSEP waves.

- BAER waves are particularly resistant to anesthetic agents.

- The BAER is altered early during hypoxia because of sensitivity of the cochlear microphonics to hypoxia rather than failure of brainstem conduction.

- Increase in BAER latency occurs as temperature is decreased.

- BAER is much less sensitive to diffuse insults, such as hypoxia or intracranial hypertension, than other modalities (e.g., EEG, SSEP).

- The proposed usefulness of the motor-evoked response (MEP) is in those areas where monitoring of the SSEP has been found inadequate, especially when false negatives (injury without change in SSEP) occur during spinal cord monitoring.

- MEP is very sensitive to anesthetics.

KEY REFERENCES

Dong WK, Bledsoe SW, Eng DY et al: Profound arterial hypotension in dogs: brain electrical activity and organ integrity, *Anesthesiology* 58;61, 1983.

Lesser RP, Raudzens P, Luders H et al: Postoperative neurological deficits may occur despite unchanged intraoperative somatosensory evoked potentials, *Ann Neurol* 19:22, 1986.

Levy WJ, Shapiro HM, Maruchak G et al: Automated EEG processing for intraoperative monitoring: a comparison of techniques, *Anesthesiology* 53:223, 1980.

Manninen PH, Lam AM, and Nantau WE: Monitoring of somatosensory evoked potentials during temporary arterial occlusion in cerebral aneurysm surgery, *J Neurosurg Anesthesiol* 2:97, 1990.

Peterson DO, Drummond JC, and Todd MM: Effects of halothane, enflurane, isoflurane, and nitrous oxide on somatosensory evoked potentials in humans, *Anesthesiology* 65:35, 1986.

Scott JC, Ponganis KV, and Stanski DR: EEG quantitation of narcotic effect: the comparative pharmacodynamics of fentanyl and alfentanil, *Anesthesiology* 62:234, 1985.

Wolfe DE, Drummond JC: Differential effects of isoflurane/nitrous oxide on posterior tibial somatosensory evoked responses of cortical and subcortical origin, *Anesth Analg* 67:852, 1988.

Zentner J, Rieder G: Diagnostic significance of motor evoked potentials in space-occupying lesions of the brainstem and spinal cord, *Eur Arch Psychiatry Neurol Sci* 289:285, 1990.

REFERENCES

1. Andersen P, Andersson SA: Physiological mechanisms of the alpha waves. In Kellaway P, Petersen I, eds: *Clinical electroencephalography of children,* New York, 1968, Grune & Stratton.

2. Baines DB, Whittle IR, Chaseling RW et al: Effect of halothane on spinal somatosensory evoked potentials in sheep, *Br J Anaesth* 57:896, 1985.

3. Berenstein A, Young W, Ransohoff J et al: Somatosensory evoked potentials during spinal angiography and therapeutic transvascular embolization, *J Neurosurg* 60:777, 1984.

4. Blume WT, Sharbrough FW: EEG monitoring during carotid endarterectomy and open heart surgery. In Niedermeyer E, Lopes da Silva F, eds: *Electroencephalography: basic principles, clinical application and related fields,* ed 2, Baltimore, 1987, Urban & Schwarzenberg.

5. Bond A, Lader M, and Shrotriya R: Comparative effects of a repeated dose regimen of diazepam and busiprone on subjective ratings, psychological tests and the EEG, *Eur J Clin Pharmacol* 24:463, 1983.

6. Boston JR, Davis PJ, Brandon BW et al: Rate of change of somatosensory evoked potentials during isoflurane anesthesia in newborn piglets, *Anesth Analg* 70:275, 1990.

7. Branston NM, Ladds A, Symon L et al: Comparison of the effects of ischaemia on early components of the somatosensory evoked potential in brainstem, thalamus, and cerebral cortex, *J Cereb Blood Flow Metab* 4:68, 1984.

8. Brenner RP: The electroencephalogram in altered states of consciousness, *Neurol Clin* 3:615, 1985.

9. Brinkman SD, Braun P, Ganji S et al: Neuropsychological performance one week after carotid endarterectomy reflects intraoperative ischemia, *Stroke* 15:497, 1984.

10. Bruchiel KJ, Stockard JJ, Calverley RK et al: Electroencephalographic abnormalities following halothane anesthesia, *Anesth Analg* 57:244, 1978.

11. Campkin TV, Honigsberger L, and Smith IS: Isoflurane: effect on the encephalogram during carotid endarterectomy, *Anaesthesia* 40:188, 1985.

12. Cartheuser CF: Progressive hypoxia until brain electrical silence: a useful model for studying protective interventions, *Can J Physiol Pharmacol* 66:1398, 1988.

13. Cedzich C, Schramm J, and Fahbusch R: Are flash-evoked visual potentials useful for intraoperative monitoring of visual pathway function? *Neurosurgery* 21:709, 1987.

14. Cedzich C, Schramm J, Mengedoht CF et al: Factors that limit the use of flash visual evoked potentials for surgical monitoring, *Electroencephalogr Clin Neurophysiol* 71:142, 1988.

15. Chassard D, Joubaub A, Colson A et al: Auditory evoked potentials during propofol anaesthesia in man, *Br J Anaesth* 62:522, 1989.

16. Chi OZ, Field C: Effects of enflurane on visual evoked potentials in humans, *Br J Anaesth* 64:163, 1990.

17. Chi OZ, Field C: Effects of isoflurane on visual evoked potentials in humans, *Anesthesiology* 65:328, 1986.

18. Chi OZ, McCoy CL, and Field C: Effects of fentanyl anesthesia on visual evoked potentials in humans, *Anesthesiology* 67:827, 1987.

19. Chi OZ, Ryterband S, and Field C: Visual evoked potentials during thiopentone–fentanyl–nitrous oxide anaesthesia in humans, *Can J Anaesth* 36:637, 1989.

20. Chi OZ, Subramoni J, and Jasaitis D: Visual evoked potentials during etomidate administration in humans, *Can J Anaesth* 37:452, 1990.

21. Church MW, Gritzke R: Effects of ketamine anesthesia on the rat brainstem auditory evoked potential as a function of dose and stimulus intensity, *Electroencephalogr Clin Neurophysiol* 67:570, 1987.

22. Clark DL, Hosick EC, Adam N et al: Neural effects of isoflurane (Forane) in man, *Anesthesiology* 39:261, 1973.

23. Clark DL, Hosick EC, and Rosner BS: Neurophysiological effects of different anesthetics in unconscious man, *J Appl Physiol* 31:884, 1971.

24. Cracco RQ: Evaluation of conduction in central motor pathways: techniques, pathophysiology, and clinical interpretation, *Neurosurgery* 20:199, 1987.

25. Cruetzfeldt O, Houchin J: Neuronal basis of EEG waves. In Remond A, ed: *Handbook of electroencephalograpy and clinical neurophysiology,* Amsterdam, 1974, Elsevier.

26. Delberghe X, Mavroudakis N, Zegers-de-Beyl D et al: The effect of stimulus frequency on post- and pre-central short-latency somatosensory evoked po-

tentials (SEPs), *Electroencephalogr Clin Neurophysiol* 77:86, 1990.

27. Dinner DS, Luders H, Lesser RP et al: Intraoperative spinal somatosensory evoked potential monitoring, *J Neurosurg* 65:807, 1986.

28. Dolman J, Silvay G, Zappulla R et al: The effect of temperature, mean arterial pressure, and cardiopulmonary bypass flows on somatosensory evoked potential latency in man, *Thorac Cardiovasc Surg* 34:217, 1986.

29. Dong WK, Bledsoe SW, Eng DY et al: Profound arterial hypotension in dogs: brain electrical activity and organ integrity, *Anesthesiology* 58;61, 1983.

30. Dowman R, Boisvert DP, Gelb AW et al: Changes in the somatosensory evoked potential during and immediately following temporary middle cerebral artery occlusion predict somatosensory cortex ischemic lesions in monkeys, *J Clin Neurophysiol* 7:269, 1990.

31. Doyle WJ, Fria TJ: The effects of hypothermia on the latencies of the auditory brain-stem response (ABR) in the rhesus monkey, *Electroencephalogr Clin Neurophysiol* 60:258, 1985.

32. Drummond JC, Todd MM, and Hoi Sang U: The effect of high dose sodium pentothal in brainstem auditory and median nerve evoked response in humans, *Anesthesiology* 63:249, 1985.

33. Dubois M, Coppola R, and Buchsbaum MS: Somatosensory evoked potential during whole body hyperthermia in humans, *Electroencephalogr Clin Neurophysiol* 52:157, 1981.

34. Dubois MY, Sato S, and Chassy J: Effects of enflurane on brainstem auditory evoked response in human, *Anesth Analg* 61:898, 1982.

35. Duncan PG, Sanders RA, and McCullough DW: Preservation of auditory-evoked brainstem responses in anesthetized children, *Can Anaesth Soc J* 26:492, 1979.

36. Ebe M, Meier-Ewert KH, and Broughton R: Effects of intravenous diazepam (Valium) upon evoked potentials of photosensitive epileptic and normal subjects, *Electroencephalogr Clin Neurophysiol* 27:429, 1969.

37. Edmonds HL Jr, Paloheimo MP, Backman MH et al: Transcranial magnetic motor evoked potentials (tcMMEP) for functional monitoring of motor pathways during scoliosis surgery, *Spine* 14:683, 1989.

38. Eger EI II, Stevens WC, and Cromwell TH: The electroencephalogram in man anesthetized with Forane, *Anesthesiology* 35:504, 1971.

39. Ernsting J: The effects of hypoxia upon human performance and the electroencephalogram, *Int Anesth Clin* 4:245, 1966.

40. Fenwick P, Bushman J, Howard R et al: Contingent negative variation and evoked potential amplitude as a function of inspired nitrous oxide concentration, *Electroencephalogr Clin Neurophysiol* 47:473, 1979.

41. Fenwick P, Stone SA, and Bushman J: Changes in the pattern reversal visual evoked potential as a function of inspired nitrous oxide concentration, *Electroencephalogr Clin Neurophysiol* 57:178, 1984.

42. Friedman WA, Kaplan BL, Day AL et al: Evoked potential monitoring during aneurysm operation: observations after fifty cases, *Neurosurgery* 20:678, 1987.

43. Frost J: Physiological bases of normal EEG rhythms. In Remond A, ed: *Handbook of electroencephalography and clinical neurophysiology,* Amsterdam, 1976, Elsevier.

44. Gain EA, Paletz SG: An attempt to correlate the clinical signs of flurothane anaesthesia with the electroencephalographic levels, *Can Anaesth Soc J* 4:289, 1957.

45. Gallager TJ, Galindo A, and Richey ET: Inhibition of seizure activity during enflurane anesthesia, *Anesth Analg* 57:130, 1978.

46. Ghaly RF, Stone JL, Aldrete A et al: Effects of incremental ketamine hydrochloride doses on motor evoked potentials (MEPs) following transcranial magnetic stimulation: a primate study, *J Neurosurg Anesthesiol* 2:79, 1990.

47. Ghaly RF et al: The effect of etomidate on transcranial magnetic-induced motor evoked potentials in primates, *Anesthesiology* 73:3A, 1990.

48. Ghoneim MM, Yamada T: Etomidate: a clinical and electroencephalographic comparison with thiopental, *Anesth Analg* 56:479, 1977.

49. Ginsburg HH, Shetter AG, and Raudzens PA: Postoperative paraplegia with preserved intraoperative somatosensory evoked potentials, *J Neurosurg* 63:296, 1985.

50. Reference deleted in proofs.

51. Goitein KJ, Fainmesser P, and Sohmer H: Cerebral perfusion pressure and auditory brainstem responses in childhood CNS diseases, *Am J Dis Child* 137:777, 1983.

52. Gold S, Cahani M, Sohmer H et al: Effects of body temperature elevation on auditory nerve brain-stem evoked responses and EEGs in rats, *Electroencephalogr Clin Neurophysiol* 60:146, 1985.

53. Graf R, Kataoka K, Wakayama A et al: Functional impairment due to white matter ischemia after middle cerebral artery occlusion in cats, *Stroke* 21:923, 1990.

54. Grossi EA, Laschinger JC, Krieger KH et al: Epidural-evoked potentials: a more specific indicator of spinal cord ischemia, *J Surg Res* 44:224, 1988.

55. Reference deleted in proofs.

56. Haghighi SS, Green KD, Oro JJ et al: Depressive effect of isoflurane anesthesia on motor evoked potentials, *Neurosurgery* 26:993, 1990.

57. Haghighi SS, Madsen R, Green DG et al: Suppression of motor evoked potentials by inhalation anesthetics, *J Neurosurg Anesthesiol* 2:73, 1990.

58. Harkins SW, Benedetti C, Colpitts YH et al: Effects of nitrous oxide inhalation on brain potentials evoked by auditory and noxious dental stimulation, *Prog Neuropsychopharmacol Biol Psychiatry* 6:167, 1982.

59. Herin RA, Hall P, and Fitch JW: Nitrogen inhalation as a method of euthanasia in dogs, *Am J Vet Res* 39:989, 1978.

60. Houston HG, McClelland RJ, and Fenwick PBC: Effects of nitrous oxide on auditory cortical evoked potentials and subjective thresholds, *Br J Anaesth* 61:606, 1988.

61. Hume AL, Cant BR: Conduction time in central somatosensory pathway in man, *Electroencephalogr Clin Neurophysiol* 45:361, 1978.

62. Joas TA, Stevens WC, and Eger EI II: Electroencephalographic seizure activity in dogs during anesthesia, *Br J Anaesth* 43:739, 1971.

63. Johnson R Jr: A triarchic model of P300 amplitude, *Psychophysiology* 23:367, 1986.

64. Kalmarchey R, Avila A, and Symon L: The use of brainstem auditory evoked potentials during posterior fossa surgery as a monitor of brainstem function, *Acta Neurochir* 82:128, 1986.

65. Kartush JM: Electroneurography and intraoperative facial monitoring in contemporary neurotology, *Otolaryngol Head Neck Surg* 101:496, 1989.

66. Katayama Y, Tsubokawalt T, and Maejima S: Corticospinal direct response in humans: identification of the motor cortex during intracranial surgery under general anaesthesia, *J Neurol Neurosurg Psychiatry* 51:50, 1988.

67. Kavan EM, Julien RM, and Lucero JL: Persistent electroencephalographic alterations following administration of some volatile anaesthetics, *Br J Anaesth* 46:714, 1974.

68. Kiersey DK, Bickford RG, and Faulconer A: Electroencephalographic patterns produced by thiopental sodium during surgical operations: description and classification, *Br J Anaesth* 22:141, 1950.

69. Kitagawa H, Itoh T, Takano H et al: Motor evoked potential monitoring during upper cervical spine surgery, *Spine* 14:1078, 1989.

70. Knight RT, Brailowsky S: Auditory evoked potentials from the primary auditory cortex of the cat: topographic and pharmacological studies, *Electroencephalogr Clin Neurophysiol* 77:225, 1990.

71. Koehler RC, Backofen JE, McPherson RW et al: Cerebral blood flow and evoked potentials during Cushing response in sheep, *Am J Physiol* 256:H779, 1989.

72. Kofke AW, Snider MT, Young RS et al: Prolonged low flow isoflurane anesthesia for status epilepticus, *Anesthesiology* 62:653, 1985.

73. Koht A, Schutz W, Schmidt G et al: Effects of etomidate, midazolam, and thiopental on median nerve somatosensory evoked potentials and the additive effects of fentanyl and nitrous oxide, *Anesth Analg* 67:435, 1988.

74. Kruczer M, Albin MS, Wolf S et al:

Postoperative seizure activity following enflurane anesthesia, *Anesthesiology* 53: 175, 1980.

75. Lam AM, Keane JF, and Manninen PH: Monitoring of brainstem auditory evoked potentials during basilar artery occlusion in man, *Br J Anaesth* 57:924, 1985.

76. LaMont RL, Wasson SL, and Green MA: Spinal cord monitoring during spinal surgery using somatosensory evoked potentials, *J Pediatr Orthop* 3:31, 1983.

77. Laschinger JC, Owen J, Rosenbloom M et al: Direct noninvasive monitoring of spinal cord motor function during thoracic aortic occlusion: use of motor evoked potentials, *J Vasc Surg* 7:161, 1988.

78. Leandri M, Parodi CI, and Faval E: Early trigeminal evoked potentials in tumors of the base of the skull and trigeminal neuralgia, *Electroencephalogr Clin Neurophysiol* 71:114, 1988.

79. Leandri M, Parodi CI, and Faval E: Evoked potentials directly recorded from the trigeminal root in man, *Pain* 35:227, 1988.

80. Leandri M, Parodi CI, Zattoni J et al: Subcortical and cortical responses following infraorbital nerve stimulation in man, *Electroencephalogr Clin Neurophysiol* 66:253, 1987.

81. Lebowitz MH, Blitt CD, and Dillon JB: Enflurane induced CNS excitation: its relation to carbon dioxide tension, *Anesth Analg* 51:355, 1972.

82. Legatt AD, Pedley TA, Emerson RG et al: Normal brain-stem auditory evoked potentials with abnormal latency-intensity studies in patients with acoustic neuromas, *Arch Neurol* 45:1326, 1988.

83. Lesser RP, Luders H, Dinner DS et al: The source of paradoxical lateralization of cortical evoked potentials to posterior tibial nerve stimulation, *Neurology* 37:82, 1987.

84. Lesser RP, Raudzens P, Luders H et al: Postoperative neurological deficits may occur despite unchanged intraoperative somatosensory evoked potentials, *Ann Neurol* 19:22, 1986.

85. Levy WJ: Quantitative analysis of EEG changes during hypothermia, *Anesthesiology* 60:291, 1984.

86. Levy WJ, Shapiro HM, Maruchak G et al: Automated EEG processing for intraoperative monitoring: a comparison of techniques, *Anesthesiology* 53:223, 1980.

87. Lopes da Silva F: Dynamics of EEGs as signals of neuronal populations: models and theoretical considerations. In Niedermeyer E, Lopes da Silva F, eds: *Electroencephalography: basic principles, clinical application and related fields,* ed 2, Baltimore, 1987, Urban & Schwarzenberg.

88. Lopes da Silva F, van Lierop THMT, Schrijer CF et al: Organization of thalamic and cortical alpha rhythm: spectra and coherences, *Electroencephalogr Clin Neurophysiol* 35:627, 1973.

89. Loughman BA, Anderson SK, Hetreed MA et al: Effects of halothane on motor evoked potential recorded in the extradural space, *Br J Anaesth* 63:561, 1989.

90. Lubicky JP, Spadaro JA, Yuan HA et al: Variability of somatosensory cortical evoked potential monitoring during spinal surgery, *Spine* 14:790, 1989.

91. MacDonell RAL, Donnan GA, and Bladin PF: A comparison of somatosensory evoked and motor evoked potentials in stroke, *Ann Neurol* 25:68, 1989.

92. Manninen PH, Lam AM, and Nantau WE: Monitoring of somatosensory evoked potentials during temporary arterial occlusion in cerebral aneurysm surgery, *J Neurosurg Anesthesiol* 2:97, 1990.

93. Markland ON, Warren CH, Moorthy SS et al: Monitoring of multimodality evoked potentials during open heart surgery under hypothermia, *Electroencephalogr Clin Neurophysiol* 59:432, 1984.

94. Matsumiya N, Koehler RC, and Traystman RJ: Consistency of cerebral blood flow and evoked potential alterations with reversible focal ischemia in cats, *Stroke* 21:908, 1990.

95. McPherson RW, Mahla M, Johnson R et al: Effects of enflurane, isoflurane and nitrous oxide on somatosensory evoked potentials during fentanyl anesthesia, *Anesthesiology* 62:626, 1985.

96. McPherson RW, Sell B, and Traystman RJ: Effects of thiopental, fentanyl, and etomidate on upper extremity somatosensory evoked potentials in humans, *Anesthesiology* 65:584, 1986.

97. Reference deleted in proofs.

98. McPherson RW, Szymanski J, and Rogers MC: Somatosensory evoked potential changes in position-related brainstem ischemia, *Anesthesiology* 61:88, 1984.

99. Mecarelli O, DeFeo MR, Romanini L et al: EEG and clinical features in epileptic children during halothane anaesthesia, *Electroencephalogr Clin Neurophysiol* 52:486, 1981.

100. Meinck HM, Mohlenhof O, and Kettler D: Neurophysiological effects of etomidate, a new short-acting hypnotic, *Electroencephalogr Clin Neurophysiol* 50:515, 1980.

101. Momma F, Wang AD, and Symon L: Effects of temporary arterial occlusion on somatosensory evoked responses in aneurysm surgery, *Surg Neurol* 27:343, 1987.

102. Nataloni S, Gentili M, Pagni R et al: Prognostic value of brainstem auditory evoked potentials in pediatric patients with traumatic coma, *Resuscitation* 16: 127, 1988.

103. Niejadlik K, Galindo A: Electroencephalographic seizure activity during enflurane anesthesia, *Anesth Analg* 54:722, 1975.

104. Oshima E, Shingu K, and Mori K: EEG activity during halothane anaesthesia in man, *Br J Anaesth* 53:65, 1981.

105. Patel VM, Maulsby RL: How hyperventilation alters the electroencephalogram: a review of controversial viewpoints emphasizing neurophysiological mechanisms, *J Clin Neurophysiol* 4:101, 1987.

106. Pathak KS, Ammadio M, Kalamchi A et al: Effects of halothane, enflurane, and isoflurane on somatosensory evoked potentials during nitrous oxide anesthesia, *Anesthesiology* 66:753, 1987.

107. Pathak KS, Brown RH, Cascorbi HF et al: Effect of fentanyl and morphine on intraoperative somatosensory evoked potentials, *Anesth Analg* 63:833, 1984.

108. Persson A, Peterson E, and Wahlin A: EEG changes during general anesthesia with enflurane (Ethrane) in comparison with ether, *Acta Anaesth Scand* 22:339, 1978.

109. Peterson DO, Drummond JC, and Todd MM: Effects of halothane, enflurane, isoflurane, and nitrous oxide on somatosensory evoked potentials in humans, *Anesthesiology* 65:35, 1986.

110. Poulton TJ, Ellington RJ: Seizure associated with induction of anesthesia with isoflurane, *Anesthesiology* 61:471, 1984.

111. Powers SK, Bolger CA, and Edwards MS: Spinal cord pathways mediating somatosensory evoked potentials, *J Neurosurg* 57:472, 1982.

112. Pritchard WS: Psychophysiology of P300, *Psychol Bull* 89:506, 1981.

113. Rampil IJ, Correll JW, Rosenbaum SH et al: Computerized electroencephalogram monitoring and carotid artery shunting, *Neurosurgery* 13:276, 1983.

114. Rebuck AS, Davis C, Longmire D et al: Arterial oxygenation and carbon dioxide tensions in the production of hypoxic electroencephalographic changes in man, *Clin Sci Mol Med* 50:301, 1976.

115. Russ W, Kling D, Loesevitz A et al: Effect of hypothermia on visual evoked potentials (VEP) in humans, *Anesthesiology* 61:207, 1984.

116. Samra SK, Lilly DJ, Rush NL et al: Fentanyl anesthesia and human brainstem auditory evoked potentials, *Anesthesiology* 61:261, 1984.

117. Sanders RA, Duncan PG, and McCullough DW: Clinical experience with brainstem audiometry performed under general anesthesia, *J Otolaryngol* 8:24, 1979.

118. Scheepstra GL, de Lange JJ, Booij LH et al: Median nerve evoked potentials during propofol anaesthesia, *Br J Anaesth* 62:92, 1989.

119. Schmid UD, Hess CW, and Ludin HP: Somatosensory evoked potentials following nerve and segmental stimulation do not confirm cervical radiculopathy with sensory deficit, *J Neurol Neurosurg Psychiatry* 51:182, 1988.

120. Schorn V, Lennon V, and Bickford R: Temperature effects on the brainstem evoked responses (BAERs) of the rat, *Proc San Diego Biomed Symp* 16:313, 1977.

121. Schubert A, Drummond JC, and Garfin SR: The influence of stimulus presentation rate on the cortical amplitude and latency of intraoperative somatosensory-evoked potential recordings in patients with varying degrees of spinal cord injury, *Spine* 12:969, 1987.

122. Schubert A, Licina MG, and Lineberry PJ: The effect of ketamine on human somatosensory evoked potentials and its modification by nitrous oxide, *Anesthesiology* 72:33, 1990.

123. Schwilden H, Schuttler J, and Stoeckel H: Quantitation of the EEG and pharmacodynamic modelling of hypnotic drugs: etomidate as an example, *Eur J Anaesthesiol* 2:121, 1985.

124. Scott JC, Ponganis KV, and Stanski DR: EEG quantitation of narcotic effect: the comparative pharmacodynamics of fentanyl and alfentanil, *Anesthesiology* 62:234, 1985.

125. Sebel PS, Bovill JG, Wauquier A et al: Effects of high dose fentanyl on the electroencephalogram, *Anesthesiology* 55:293, 1981.

126. Sebel PS, Erwin CW, and Neville WK: Effects of halothane and enflurane on far and near field somatosensory evoked potentials, *Br J Anaesth* 59:1492, 1987.

127. Sloan TB, Fugina ML, and Toleikis JR: Effects of midazolam on median nerve somatosensory evoked potentials, *Br J Anaesth* 64:590, 1990.

128. Sloan TB, Ronai AK, Toleikis JR et al: Improvement of intraoperative somatosensory evoked potentials by etomidate, *Anesth Analg* 67:582, 1988.

129. Smith NT, DecSilver H, Sanford TJ et al: EEGs during high dose fentanyl, sufentanil or morphine-oxygen anesthesia, *Anesth Analg* 63:386, 1984.

130. Sohmer H, Freeman S, Gafni M et al: The depression of the auditory nerve brain-stem evoked response in hypoxemia—mechanism and site of effect, *Electroencephalogr Clin Neurophysiol* 64:334, 1986.

131. Sohmer H, Freeman S, and Malachi S: Multi-modality evoked potentials in hypoxemia, *Electroencephalogr Clin Neurophysiol* 64:328, 1986.

132. Sohmer H, Gafni M, and Chisin R: Auditory nerve–brain stem potentials in man and cat under hypoxic and hypercapnic conditions, *Electroencephalogr Clin Neurophysiol* 53:506, 1982.

133. Sohmer H, Gafni M, Goitein K et al: Auditory nerve brainstem evoked potentials in cats during manipulation of the cerebral perfusion pressure, *Electroencephalogr Clin Neurophysiol* 55:198, 1983.

134. Sohmer H, Gafni M, and Havatselet G: Persistence of auditory nerve response and absence of brain-stem response in severe cerebral ischaemia, *Electroencephalogr Clin Neurophysiol* 58:65, 1984.

135. Sohmer H, Goitein K: Auditory brainstem (ABP) and somatosensory evoked potentials (SEP) in an animal model of a synaptic lesion: elevated plasma barbiturate levels, *Electroencephalogr Clin Neurophysiol* 71:382, 1988.

136. Sohmer H, Gold S, Chani M et al: Effects of hypothermia on auditory brain-stem and somatosensory evoked responses: a model of a synaptic and axonal lesion, *Electroencephalogr Clin Neurophysiol* 74:50, 1989.

137. Somjen GG, Trachtenberg M: Neuroglia as generator of extracellular current. In Speckmann EJ, Caspters H, eds: *Origin of cerebral field potentials,* Stuttgart, 1979, Thieme.

138. Speckmann EJ, Elger CE: Introduction to the neurophysiological basis of the EEG and DC potentials. In Niedermeyer E, Lopes da Silva F, eds: *Electroencephalography: basic principles, clinical application and related fields,* ed 2, Baltimore, 1987, Urban & Schwarzenberg.

139. Stejskal L, Travnicek V, Sourek K et al: Somatosensory evoked potentials in deep hypothermia, *Appl Neurophysiol* 43:1, 1980.

140. Symon L, Wang AD, Costae Silva IE et al: Perioperative use of somatosensory evoked responses in aneurysm surgery, *J Neurosurg* 6:269, 1984.

141. Synek VM: Validity of median nerve somatosensory evoked potentials in the diagnosis of supraclavicular brachial plexus lesions, *Electroencephalogr Clin Neurophysiol* 65:27, 1986.

142. Thornton C, Catley DM, Jordan C et al: Enflurane anaesthesia causes graded changes in the brainstem and early cortical auditory evoked response in man, *Br J Anaesth* 55:479, 1983.

143. Thornton C, Heneghan CP, James MF et al: Effects of halothane or enflurane with controlled ventilation on auditory evoked potentials, *Br J Anaesth* 56:315, 1984.

144. Uhl RR, Squires KC, Bruce DL et al: Effect of halothane anesthesia on the human cortical visual evoked response, *Anesthesiology* 53:273, 1980.

145. Van-Rheineck-Leyssius AT, Kalkman CJ, and Bovil JG: Influence of moderate hypothermia on posterior tibial nerve, *Anesth Analg* 65:475, 1986.

146. Vaz CA, McPherson RW, and Thakor NV: Fourier series modeling of time-varying evoked potentials. III. Study of the human somatosensory evoked response to etomidate, *Electroencephalogr Clin Neurophysiol,* 80:108, 1991.

147. Veilleux M, Daube JR, and Cucchiara RF: Monitoring of cortical evoked potentials during surgical procedures, *Mayo Clin Proc* 62:256, 1987.

148. Waugier A: Profile of etomidate: a hypnotic, anticonvulsant and brain protective compound, *Anaesthesia* 38:26, 1983.

149. Waugier A, van-den-Broech WA, Verheyen JL et al: Electroencephalographic study of the short-acting hypnotics etomidate and methohexital in dogs, *Eur J Pharmacol* 47:367, 1978.

150. Wolfe DE, Drummond JC: Differential effects of isoflurane/nitrous oxide on posterior tibial somatosensory evoked responses of cortical and subcortical origin, *Anesth Analg* 67:852, 1988.

151. Wood CC, Spencer DD, Allison T et al: Localization of human sensorimotor cortex during surgery by cortical surface recording of somatosensory evoked potentials, *J Neurosurg* 68:99, 1988.

152. Yamamura T, Fukuda M, Takeya H et al: Fast oscillatory EEG activity induced by analgesic concentrations of nitrous oxide in man, *Anesth Analg* 60:283, 1981.

153. York DH, Chabot RJ, and Gaines RW: Response variability of somatosensory evoked potentials during scoliosis surgery, *Spine* 12:864, 1987.

154. Zentner J: Noninvasive motor evoked potential monitoring during neurosurgical operations on the spinal cord, *Neurosurgery* 24:709, 1989.

155. Zenter J, Kiss I, and Ebner A: Influence of anesthetics—nitrous oxide in particular—on electromyographic response evoked by transcranial electrical stimulation of the cortex, *Neurosurgery* 24:253, 1989.

156. Zentner J, Rieder G: Diagnostic significance of motor evoked potentials in space-occupying lesions of the brainstem and spinal cord, *Eur Arch Psychiatry Neurol Sci* 289:285, 1990.

157. Zhongyuan S, Deming Z, and Zhengzhong G: The influence of acute and chronic hypoxia on the electroencephalogram of human body, *Ann Physiol Anthropol* 6:111, 1987.

158. Zornow MH, Grafe MD, Tybor C et al: Preservation of evoked potentials in a case of anterior spinal artery syndrome, *Electroencephalogr Clin Neurophysiol* 77:137, 1990.

CHAPTER 44

Monitoring Neuromuscular Blockade

HASSAN H. ALI

The response to muscle relaxants is neither uniform nor predictable in the population at large. In addition, this response may be adversely modified by perioperative medication and/or disease states. These considerations have increased the awareness of many anesthesiologists for exploring ways to identify and monitor the response of individual patients to drugs that act on the neuromuscular junction. The most apparent goal is providing optimal surgical conditions (adequate surgical relaxation), while also ensuring timely restoration of neuromuscular function. This approach undoubtedly improves patient safety, increases efficiency and utilization of operating rooms, and prevents the backlog in the recovery room with the unnecessary burden on acute care personnel.

BASIC CONSIDERATIONS

The fundamental aspects of neuromuscular transmission and monitoring entail a brief overview of the clinical pharmacology of the neuromuscular junction as it pertains to the various patterns of neural stimulation and different measurement modalities.

Clinical Pharmacology of the Neuromuscular Junction

The neuromuscular junction (NMJ) is a synapse. The motor nerve loses its myelin sheath as it approaches the muscle and divides into many nerve filaments, each of which innervates a muscle fiber. The NMJ consists of two structures: the motor nerve terminal and the endplate region of the muscle membrane (Fig. 44-1). These two structures are separated by a gap, the synaptic cleft, which is continuous with the extracellular space. The nonmyelinated nerve terminal lies in a gutter on the surface of the muscle. The axoplasm is rich in mitochondria, endoplasmic reticulum, and synaptic vesicles. The complex molecules used in the synthesis of acetylcholine (Ach) (i.e., enzymes, transport protein, and new membrane for vesicles) are made in the cell body and transported through the axon to the nerve terminal.[38,44] The motor endplate is a chemosensitive, highly folded area of muscle membrane located opposite the motor nerve terminal. The surrounding sarcoplasm is also rich in mitochondria and calcium binding and storage sites. There are several specialized sites that interact with

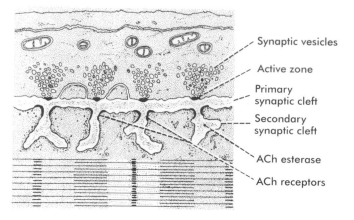

Synaptic vesicles

Active zone

Primary
synaptic cleft

Secondary
synaptic cleft

ACh esterase

ACh receptors

Fig. 44-1. Diagrammatic representation of the neuromuscular junction. Nerve terminal shows clusters of synaptic vesicles aggregated near the active zones. Synaptic gutter on the surface of the muscle membrane is comprised of the primary and secondary synaptic clefts that separate the nerve terminal membrane from the muscle membrane. Dense areas on the shoulders of the synaptic folds contain Ach receptors.

and modify the action of Ach. These are cholinergic receptors, the enzyme acetylcholinesterase, and Ach-sensitive area at the motor nerve terminals. For details, several excellent reviews are available.[10,18,42]

Synthesis, storage, and release of acetylcholine

Acetylcholine is synthesized within the motor nerve terminal[27] following acetylation of two simple molecules, choline and acetate, obtained from the environment of the nerve terminal. Choline is transported by a special system from the extracellular fluid to the axoplasm, and acetate is in the form of acetylcoenzyme A (acetyl CoA) from mitochondria. These two substrates with the enzyme choline acetyltransferase react to form Ach.[37] The newly formed Ach is transferred to and stored in synaptic vesicles. In the absence of stimulation, the endplate region of the muscle fiber displays spontaneous electrical activity in the form of discrete, randomly occurring miniature endplate potentials (mepp) on the order of 0.5 to 1.5 mV in amplitude. These resemble the much larger endplate potential (epp) evoked by the nerve impulse.[22] The mepp probably arises from the binding of a single quantum of Ach with the postjunctional membrane.[28] The normal epp is made up of statistical fusion of quantal components identical to the spontaneously occurring mepp. Depolarization opens specific calcium channels in the terminal axonal membrane and leads to an influx of Ca^{++}.[29] The latter then initiates the quantal release reaction. Katz has postulated that the quanta of Ach molecules are contained within synaptic vesicles that undergo frequent transient collisions with the axon membrane.[28] Cal-

cium ions cause attachment and local fusion between vesicular and axonal membranes followed by an all-or-none discharge of vesicular contents into the synaptic cleft. Numerous synaptic vesicles are gathered near the synaptic surface in several triangular formations. The apex of each triangle is close to a thickened area called the active zone (see Fig. 44-1). The active zone may be part of a system that orients and controls the site of release of Ach from synaptic vesicles. Each active zone lies opposite the opening of the junctional folds; the vesicles are opposite the shoulders of these folds where Ach receptors are highest in density. Acetylcholinesterase (AchE) is located in the basement membrane of the junctional folds and the depth of the secondary clefts. Molecules of Ach diffused from the receptors are hydrolyzed by AchE.

Repeated nerve stimulation requires the nerve ending to replenish its stores of releasable Ach, a process known as *mobilization.* The latter involves several steps to maintain the nerve ending capacity to release transmitter (i.e., choline transport, synthesis of acetyl-CoA, and the movement of vesicles to the release site). Failure of transmission during high-frequency stimulation has been attributed to the nerve's inability to mobilize Ach rapidly enough to replace that released,[9,19] that is, the output of Ach normally and spontaneously decreases as the stimulation frequency increases and continues. New techniques were developed to prevent muscle movement during nerve stimulation. This allowed the recording of epp and endplate current (epc) in the absence of curare-like drugs.[32] When this technique was used, there was relatively little epp or epc rundown during tetanic stimulation. However, in the presence of *d*-tubocurarine (dtc), there was a marked rundown or decrement in the epc amplitude. Therefore it seems clear that dtc actually causes the successive diminution of the epc in a train of responses.

Acetylcholine receptors

Acetylcholine receptors (AchR) are concentrated at the crests and shoulders of the junctional folds opposite the release sites of Ach. The use of the snake venom alpha-bungarotoxin (alpha-BUTX) facilitated the purification and biochemical analysis of AchR. The latter is a membrane protein that extends about 5.0 nm into the extracellular space and about 1.5 nm into the intracellular space.[41] The receptor protein has a molecular weight of about 250,000 daltons. It consists of five glycoprotein subunits. The two alpha-subunits are 40,000 daltons each; the others are 50,000, 60,000, and 65,000 daltons. The 40,000-dalton peptides carry the binding sites for both Ach and alpha-BUTX.[16,26] These five subunits are arranged in a ring that forms an ionophore or a channel for ions.[39]

When two Ach molecules bind to the two alpha-subunits, the channel opens. This allows sodium and calcium ions to flow into the cell while potassium exits. These ionic currents create the epp that triggers a muscle action potential (single fiber electromyogram [EMG]), and summation of these potentials leads to the compound action potential EMG. The muscle action potential spreads to the transverse tubules and activates the excitation-contraction coupling mechanism and muscle contraction[33] (mechanomyogram [MMG]).

Mechanism of evoked muscle fade

There is evidence that twitch depression and fade of tetanus are consequences of separate actions. Twitch depression may be explained in classic terms by blocking postjunctional cholinoceptor recognition sites. The mechanism underlying fade, however, is less obvious. **There appear to be two possible explanations:**

- **Relaxants act on certain receptors at the prejunctional membrane, blocking open sodium channels. This impairs mobilization of Ach from the mobilization store to the readily releasable store. Thus Ach output cannot keep pace with the demands of high-frequency stimulation.[42]**
- **High-frequency stimulation opens Ach receptor channels and causes the relaxant to exert an additional postjunctional channel block that** becomes more pronounced as the stimulus frequency increases.[18] **The prejunctional contribution to the phenomenon of fade is supported by the work of Bowman et al.[11] and Gibb and Marshall.[23]**

Types of Neuromuscular Blockade

The two main classes of muscle relaxants are listed in Box 44-1. It should be noted that with prolonged administration of a high dose of a depolarizing (phase I) relaxant, such as succinylcholine or decamethonium, or with interference with either metabolism or elimination, the block changes its characteristics as a result of the conformational change of Ach receptors. This process is referred to as passing from depolarizing to phase II block.

CLINICAL MONITORING OF NEUROMUSCULAR FUNCTION

The objectives of clinical monitoring are as follows:
- **Titration of individual dosage to achieve a desired effect**
- **Detection of abnormal sensitivity or possible decrease in clearance of a relaxant early in the course of the anesthetic**
- **Prediction of the optimal time of reversibility**
- **Accurate determination of adequate recovery as correlated with the clinical criteria of safe and optimal recovery**

Measurement of voluntary movements such as hand grip strength and head lift requires an awake and cooperative patient. However, tidal volume and inspiratory force can be measured in the unconscious patient, yet these measurements can be influenced by residual amounts of anesthetics and narcotics. Intraoperative monitoring of skeletal muscle relaxation that provides satisfactory surgical conditions, and ensures timely return of normal electromechanical function, can most reliably be achieved by stimulating an accessible peripheral motor nerve and feeling or recording the evoked response of the corresponding skeletal muscle or muscles.

The ulnar nerve–adductor pollicis brevis muscle provides the ideal human nerve-muscle preparation, which compares well with that of the experimental animal. The following briefly summarizes some of the possible nerve-muscle arrangements that may be available to the clinician.

Accessible Peripheral Motor Nerves
Ulnar nerve

The most accessible part of the ulnar nerve is behind the medial epicondyle of the humerus. At the wrist, the nerve lies superficially between the flexor carpi ulnaris tendon medially and the ulnar artery laterally

---

BOX 44-1
CHARACTERISTICS OF NEUROMUSCULAR BLOCKADE

Depolarizing (phase I) block

Muscle fasciculation preceding the onset of neuromuscular blockade
Sustained response to single-twitch stimuli
Sustained response to tetanic stimulation
Absence of posttetanic potentiation (PTP)
Lack of fade to train-of-four (TOF) stimulation
Block antagonized by nondepolarizing drugs
Block potentiated by anticholinesterases

Nondepolarizing (phase II) block

Appearance of tetanic fade and PTP
Absence of muscle fasciculation
TOF fade
Block antagonized by depolarizing drugs
Possible synergism between various groups of nondepolarizing relaxants
Block potentiates a nondepolarizing block
Partial or complete reversal with anticholinesterases

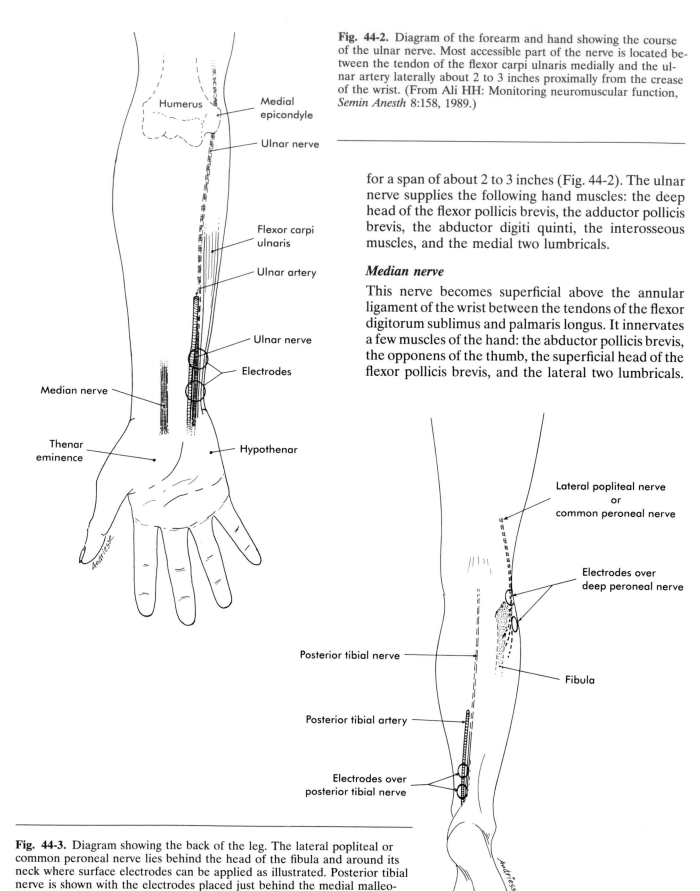

Fig. 44-2. Diagram of the forearm and hand showing the course of the ulnar nerve. Most accessible part of the nerve is located between the tendon of the flexor carpi ulnaris medially and the ulnar artery laterally about 2 to 3 inches proximally from the crease of the wrist. (From Ali HH: Monitoring neuromuscular function, *Semin Anesth* 8:158, 1989.)

for a span of about 2 to 3 inches (Fig. 44-2). The ulnar nerve supplies the following hand muscles: the deep head of the flexor pollicis brevis, the adductor pollicis brevis, the abductor digiti quinti, the interosseous muscles, and the medial two lumbricals.

Median nerve

This nerve becomes superficial above the annular ligament of the wrist between the tendons of the flexor digitorum sublimus and palmaris longus. It innervates a few muscles of the hand: the abductor pollicis brevis, the opponens of the thumb, the superficial head of the flexor pollicis brevis, and the lateral two lumbricals.

Fig. 44-3. Diagram showing the back of the leg. The lateral popliteal or common peroneal nerve lies behind the head of the fibula and around its neck where surface electrodes can be applied as illustrated. Posterior tibial nerve is shown with the electrodes placed just behind the medial malleolus of the tibia along the nerve. (From Ali HH: Monitoring neuromuscular function, *Semin Anesth* 8:158, 1989.)

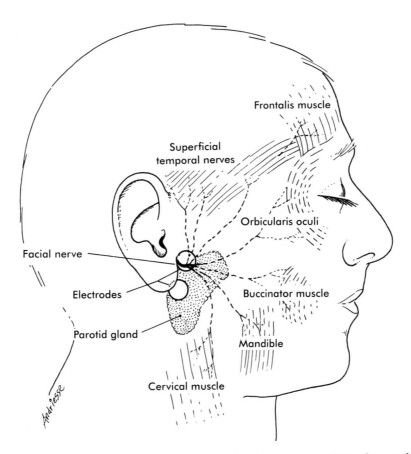

Fig. 44-4. Diagram shows the placement of the stimulating surface electrodes overlying the facial nerve just below the tragus of the ear. (From Ali HH: Monitoring neuromuscular function, *Semin Anesth* 8:158, 1989.)

The long flexors of the wrist and fingers are innervated by the ulnar and median nerves at and below the elbow.

Posterior tibial nerve

The nerve becomes superficial, covered by skin and fascia behind the medial malleolus of the tibia and posteromedial to the posterior tibial artery. Plantar flexion of the big toe can be assessed by stimulating the posterior tibial nerve at the above site (Fig. 44-3). The EMG response can be easily measured from some of the muscles of the sole of the foot: the flexor hallucis brevis, the abductor hallucis, and the adductor obliquus hallucis.

Lateral popliteal or peroneal nerve

This nerve runs behind the head of the fibula and around its neck. Its stimulation evokes dorsiflexion of the foot (see Fig. 44-3).

Facial nerve

The facial nerve emerges from the stylomastoid foramen and lies within the parotid gland as it branches to supply the various superficial facial muscles of expression (Fig. 44-4). These muscles, because of their superficial position, are vulnerable to direct stimulation by the overlying superficial electrodes. Stimulating the facial nerve close to the tragus of the ear as shown in Fig. 44-4 avoids to some extent direct stimulation of such muscles as the orbicularis oculi or the frontalis muscles. Caffrey, Warren, and Becker showed that when all four responses of the adductor pollicis brevis were abolished in response to train-of-four (TOF) ulnar nerve stimulation, the twitches of the orbicularis oculi muscle showed only minor fade to TOF stimulation.[13] This probably is the result of direct muscle stimulation, and may lead the observer to underestimate the degree of neuromuscular block and result in an unnecessary overdose with the nondepolarizing relaxant.

Methods of Assessment of Neuromuscular Function
Mechanical or contractile force measurement — mechanomyography

Muscle contraction can be assessed either isometrically, when the origin and insertion of the targeted muscle are fixed (i.e., the muscle is not allowed to shorten) or isotonically, when the origin of the muscle is fixed and the muscle is allowed to shorten during contraction.

Isometric measurement — tension devices

For isometric measurement, the muscle contraction can be quantified accurately by using a suitable tension device or force transducer. This requires immobilization of the muscle to be monitored with due regard to the preload tension, the capacity of the transducer, and positioning such that the direction of force is in line with the cantilever of the transducer (Fig. 44-5). **Adduction of the thumb in response to ulnar nerve stimulation is the most common human nerve-muscle preparation used in clinical research[3] (see Fig. 44-5). This preparation is used because the adductor pollicis brevis is conveniently located and is the only muscle supplied by the ulnar nerve to evoke thumb adduction.** Recording plantar flexion of the big toe in response to posterior tibial nerve stimulation or dorsiflexion of the foot in response to lateral popliteal

nerve stimulation can also be achieved with a special foot caliper. The measurement of the transduced response is more suited for clinical studies and is not practical for everyday clinical monitoring.

Isotonic contraction — accelerometry

For isotonic contraction, the range and acceleration of the motion of insertion of the muscle against a minimal or no load can be measured by **accelerometry.** Accelerometers have been used in the aerospace industry and to monitor other physiologic functions. The rationale for the concept of accelerometry as a measurement of force (isotonic contraction) comes from Newton's law, which states that $F = m \times a$ — force (F) equals mass (m) times acceleration (a). Assuming the mass is constant, the force then correlates with acceleration. The transducer used for measuring acceleration is either a piezoelectric ceramic wafer or a small aluminum rod with electrodes on both sides (e.g., a single-phase accelerometer transducer [Grass model SPA-1, Quincy, Mass.]).

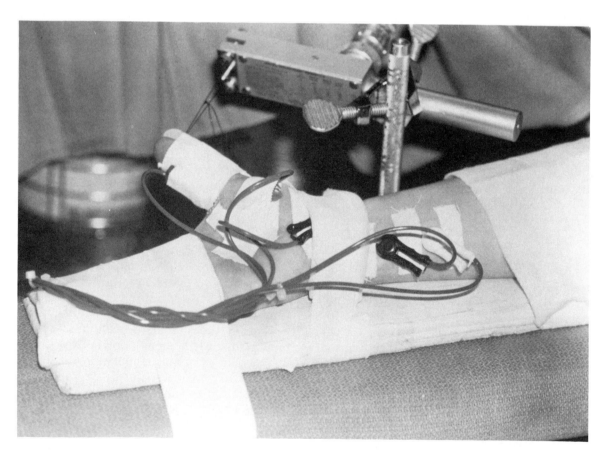

Fig. 44-5. Ulnar nerve–adductor pollicis assembly for simultaneous monitoring of transduced thumb adduction (isometric tension) and evoked integrated EMG of the adductor pollicis (thenar EMG). Note the transducer is aligned parallel to the fully abducted thumb with the direction of force in line with the cantilever of the transducer. Sensing EMG electrode is placed over the adductor pollicis, the reference electrode at the base of the thumb, and the ground electrode is placed at the crease of the wrist between the sensing and stimulating electrodes for EMG recording.

When the electrodes are exposed to a force, a voltage proportional to the acceleration is generated. This signal is amplified and can be measured. If the transducer is positioned, for example, on the thumb, so that the direction of force corresponds to the plane of acceleration, the voltage measured is proportional to the force of thumb adduction. Accelerometers do not need a preload, but a freely moving mass. It has been shown that there is a close relationship between TOF ratios measured by accelerometry of the thumb and evoked thumb adduction using a force transducer.[46] Accelerometers are easier to use than force transducers but more work must be done to evaluate the clinical relevance of these responses.

Tactile evaluation

Feeling the strength of a fully abducted thumb is a form of isometric measurement and is more reliable than feeling thumb adduction without a preload exerted on the muscle. Other muscles (the flexors or extensors) of the foot can be evaluated in a similar manner as the thumb.

Visual evaluation

The muscles usually used for observation of evoked contraction are hand, foot, and facial muscles. These are essentially isotonic contractions. This technique is at best unreliable and misleading.

Evoked electrical measurement — evoked electromyography

Evoked EMG is a more versatile method of measuring neuromuscular transmission because it can be obtained from muscles not accessible for tension measurement. The muscles commonly used for monitoring the EMG response are the adductor pollicis brevis (thenar EMG)[31] (see Fig. 44-2), the abductor digiti quinti (hypothenar EMG)[31] (see Fig. 44-2), or the first dorsal interosseous muscle of the hand.[6] These three muscles are innervated by the ulnar nerve. The facial muscles and the sole of the foot muscles, particularly in children, can likewise be used. Problems associated with transducer fixation, orientation, and overload are avoided when using evoked EMG.[24]

When the active sensing electrode (negative) is placed on the belly of the muscle, with the reference electrode (positive) on the point of insertion of this muscle and the ground electrode between the stimulating and sensing electrodes (see Fig. 44-5), a number of biphasic motor unit action potentials are recorded as a single summated compound action potential.[25] The potentials picked up by the sensing electrodes are usually small in amplitude. They are amplified to a level that can be easily studied. The main deflection of the compound action potential is usually displayed as an upright signal, although it is negative. The amplitude of the waveform or the area under the curve can be integrated and measured for assessment of neuromuscular transmission (Fig. 44-6). Until recently, routine evoked EMG monitoring in the operating room was not feasible because of the high cost and technical difficulties in recording high-speed events. The high-tech industry has provided small compact EMG monitoring equipment based on amplifying, filtering, rectifying, and integrating the area under the EMG waveform. This processing of the EMG signal made it possible to have a clinically useful tool in operating rooms and intensive care units. The

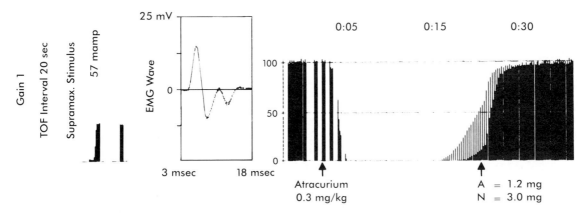

Fig. 44-6. Graphic printout of thenar EMG recording. From left to right, calibration response, compound action potential control waveform *(in the box),* and the integrated response. Atracurium 0.3 mg/kg was administered *(arrow),* and the paper speed was increased to show individual train-of-four (TOF) responses. At 20 minutes, reversal was achieved with atropine 1.2 mg and neostigmine 3.0 mg when the first response to TOF was approximately 55% of control and TOF ratio 25%. Note the fourth response of TOF *(dark shadow).* Time in minutes is represented on top of the tracing. (This recording was obtained from Datex® NMT 221 monitor, Helsinki, Finland.)

data are presented in both digital and graphic forms (see Fig. 44-6). It appears that EMG and tension measurements are comparable when measured from the same muscle.[1] It must be emphasized that EMG measurement reflects events at the neuromuscular junction. This can be demonstrated by the fact that use of dantrolene, a drug that essentially acts on the contractile mechanisms, does not depress EMG response when the MMG is significantly depressed.

Stimulators. The most desirable features in a peripheral nerve stimulator (PNS) (Box 44-2) are as follows:

- **Constant current output of sufficient amperage (up to 100 mamp) to ensure the delivery of a supramaximal stimulus; constant voltage output is not adequate because the current delivered will decrease with the increased resistance at the skin or electrode**

- **Generation of rectangular pulse of approximately 0.2 ms in duration to maintain the flow of current throughout the length of time that the stimulus is applied**
- **Battery operation with a battery level indicator**
- **Clearly marked negative (−) and positive (+) polarity**
- **Audible signal for each electrical pulse delivered**
- **Current meter indicator**
- **Capability of delivering a supramaximal stimulus via needle or surface electrodes at the standard frequencies (i.e., single stimulus, TOF, and tetanic stimulus at 50 Hz for 5 seconds)**

Electrodes. The following points should be remembered when electrodes are used:

- **Surface electrodes are preferred when possible**
- **Fresh, moist silver-silver chloride jelly disks of different sizes should be available**

BOX 44-2
CLINICAL APPLICATIONS OF A PERIPHERAL NERVE STIMULATOR (PNS)

Ideally, the anesthesiologist should be acquainted with the patient's baseline response after induction of anesthesia and before a relaxant is given to ensure that the electrodes are applied properly, the stimulator is functional, and the patient's response is normal. After succinylcholine is given, the physician waits until the twitch response becomes at least barely perceptible before laryngoscopy and tracheal intubation are attempted. Earlier attempts lead to bucking, coughing, and possibly traumatic intubation. If succinylcholine was administered earlier, no nondepolarizing relaxants should be given until recovery from the succinylcholine is demonstrated.

If succinylcholine infusion is planned for maintenance of surgical relaxation, the infusion should be titrated to a barely visible response. Intermittently the patient should be observed for early signs of phase II block development, which can be detected by the onset of fade to TOF stimulation. This fade may be seen at a total dose of 5 to 6 mg/kg succinylcholine if the maintenance anesthetic is enflurane, isoflurane, or halothane. The dose of succinylcholine needed to lead to phase II block during balanced nitrous oxide–opioid anesthesia is higher (10 to 12 mg/kg succinylcholine).[35,40]

If the succinylcholine infusion is discontinued because of the development of phase II block, tachyphylaxis, or prolonged surgery, relaxation can be maintained with a very small dose of a nondepolarizing agent (e.g., 3 mg *d*-tubocurarine, 0.5 to 1 mg pancuronium, 5.0 mg atracurium, or 0.5 to 1 mg vecuronium.) Each of these doses may ablate the twitch completely because nondepolarizing neuromuscular blockade is significantly potentiated by the preexisting phase II block.

Nondepolarizing relaxants may be given either as a bolus dose to facilitate tracheal intubation or titrated to about 95% twitch suppression (i.e., one response to TOF stimulation). Subsequent doses are usually indicated clinically when the single-twitch response recovers to approximately 25% twitch height or three responses to TOF stimulation. Variations exist from patient to patient, between lower abdominal and upper abdominal surgery, and with inhalation vs. balanced anesthesia. The supplemental doses for the long-acting relaxants *d*-tubocurarine, metocurine, and pancuronium are usually 3.0, 2.0, or 0.5 mg, respectively. For atracurium or vecuronium, the maintenance dose is about one fifth the intubating dose, or 100 μg/kg for atracurium and 20 μg/kg for vecuronium.

To monitor the continuous infusion of atracurium or vecuronium, the patient is usually allowed to recover to a TOF count of 1 (90% to 95% block). If an intubating dose was given earlier, the anesthesiologist may start with an infusion rate of approximately 10.0 μg/kg/min for atracurium or 2.0 μg/kg/min for vecuronium. The rate of infusion is adjusted up or down to maintain a TOF count of one or two responses. If the infusion of either drug follows an intubating dose of succinylcholine, a bolus of atracurium (0.2 mg/kg) or vecuronium (40 μg/kg) may be started as soon as evidence of recovery from succinylcholine is available. The infusion of either drug can follow the procedure previously outlined and be adjusted to a steady state of relaxation, which can be achieved within 10 to 15 minutes.

- **Skin overlying the nerve should be thoroughly cleaned, hairless, and dry**
- **Gentle pushing on the center of the pad ensures close skin contact with the electrode jelly**
- **Negative electrode should overlie the nerve to be stimulated. The positive electrode should be approximately 1 inch away, preferably along the course of the motor nerve**
- **Needle electrodes (e.g., 23-gauge stainless steel needles) should be used when surface electrodes are unlikely to deliver the needed supramaximal stimulus, for example, with thick or edematous skin or in obese patients**
- **Direct contact with the nerve or vascular injury should be avoided**
- **Needles must be kept apart without contact to avoid short circuiting**

PATTERNS OF NERVE STIMULATION

The muscle response to peripheral motor nerve stimulation depends on the pattern of the stimulus applied. Stimulus patterns include the following: single-twitch stimulus repeated at various frequen-cies, TOF, tetanic stimulation, posttetanic stimula-tion, and double-burst stimulation (DBS).

Single-Twitch Stimulus

The evoked response depends on the stimulus fre-quency. Changing the stimulus frequency from 0.1 Hz (one stimulus every 10 seconds) to 1.0 Hz (one stimulus every second) can significantly decrease the effective dose of a nondepolarizing relaxant needed to effect 95% twitch supression (ED_{95}). For example, the ED_{95} for *d*-tubocurarine decreases from 0.5 mg/kg to 0.16 mg/kg when the stimulus frequency is increased from 0.1 Hz to 1.0 Hz.[4] The onset time and the duration of the block also differ when the frequency is changed (Fig. 44-7). **The slow frequency of 0.1 to 0.15 Hz is more clinically relevant, since the degree of twitch suppression at these frequencies correlates with clinical relaxation.**[4] Use of the single-twitch stimulus requires the establishment of a control response before the administration of the relaxant (Fig. 44-8). Often the control or baseline twitch is either unavailable or forgotten. In clinical studies, when the baseline twitch is obtained, the percentage change from control response establishes the onset

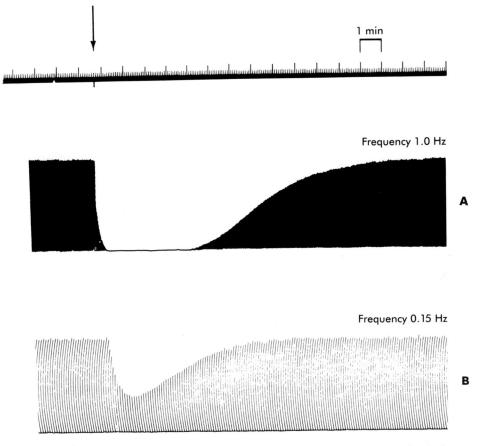

Fig. 44-7. Simultaneous recording of evoked thumb adduction to ulnar nerve stimulation in both right and left hands. **A,** At 1.0 Hz. **B,** At 0.15 Hz. Note the fast onset, deeper block, and delayed recovery during faster stimulation in **A.** (From Ali HH: Monitoring neuromuscular function, *Semin Anesth* 8:158, 1989.)

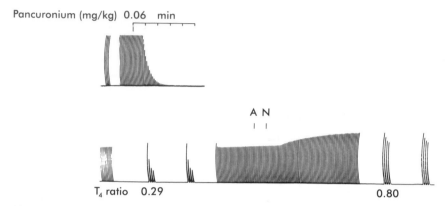

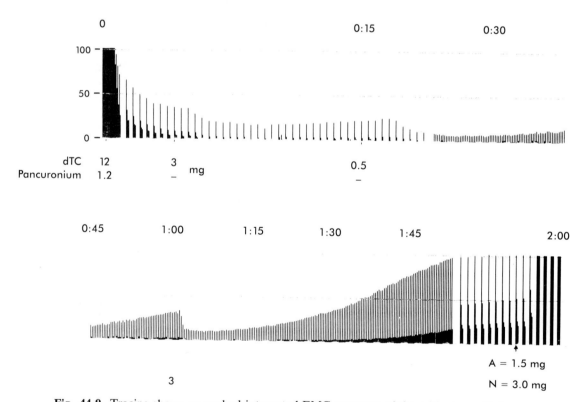

Fig. 44-8. Tracing shows evoked thumb adduction in response to ulnar nerve TOF and single-twitch (0.15 Hz) stimulation. *Upper panel:* TOF control response, single-twitch control twitch height. Use of pancuronium 0.06 mg/kg resulted in 99% block during N_2O-O_2 enflurane anesthesia. At 90 minutes, the single-twitch stimulus recovered to 70% of control with a TOF ratio of 0.29. Reversal with atropine *(A)* and neostigmine *(N)* resulted in complete recovery of the single twitch in 5 minutes, and, in 8 minutes, TOF ratio recovered to 0.8.

Fig. 44-9. Tracing shows an evoked integrated EMG response of the adductor pollicis during recovery from a combination of pancuronium and *d*-tubocurarine. Doses are in milligrams. Note at 1 hour and 52 minutes from the initial injection of the relaxant, the first twitch of TOF recovered completely to control height, yet TOF ratio was 0.15. Note the fourth response, which can be seen at faster paper speed *(dark shadow).* This residual fade was completely reversed within 2 minutes with atropine *(A)* 1.5 mg and neostigmine *(N)* 3.0 mg.

time, the potency of the relaxant, and the recovery to control height (duration).

The recovery rate or recovery index is defined as the time for the twitch to recover from 25% to 75% of control height. The recovery index is often used to compare different relaxants and identify the cumulative properties of the neuromuscular blocking drug. The return of the single twitch to control height does not necessarily mean complete restoration of neuromuscular transmission[8] (Fig. 44-9). In fact, there may be a substantial degree of residual curarization that varies with different relaxants.[5] Residual neuromuscular blockade can be more easily detected by one of the patterns of stimulation that follow.

Train-of-Four Stimulation

Train-of-four stimulation is essentially four stimuli applied at a frequency of 2 Hz for two seconds. Each train is repeated once every 10 to 12 seconds. Repeating TOF more frequently than 10 seconds conditions the first response of the train by the preceding TOF and leads to a falsely high TOF ratio. The TOF pattern can provide a quantitative estimate of the degree of nondepolarizing blockade without the need for a control response.[3] This provides a desirable clinical advantage over the single-twitch stimulus because it is not always feasible to establish a control response before the administration of a nondepolarizing relaxant. This is especially important when residual blockade is suspected in the perioperative period. The extent of fade determines the degree of neuromuscular blockade (NMB). It does not affect the course of recovery from nondepolarizing relaxants and causes less discomfort to the awake patient when compared to tetanic stimulation.

The ratio of the amplitude of the fourth to the first evoked response in the same train appears to provide

a convenient method for assessing neuromuscular function. The TOF proved to be a clinically useful stimulus pattern for detection and follow-up of the changing character of succinylcholine from phase I (depolarizing) to phase II NMB by virtue of the development of graded and progressive fade.[35,40] In addition, the response to TOF stimulation can be used clinically to determine the dose of a nondepolarizing relaxant required to produce a clinically relevant range of neuromuscular blockade (i.e., 75% to 95% twitch suppression) also termed *clinical relaxation,* without the need for transducing and recording the evoked response.[34] This is more reliably evaluated by feeling thumb adduction in response to ulnar nerve stimulation.

During titration of a nondepolarizing relaxant, the first response of TOF to decrease in amplitude is the fourth response (T_4). As more relaxant is given, the first response (T_1) becomes depressed and T_4 will be depressed more until a time when T_4 is eliminated at approximately 75% depression of T_1, when compared to the control response. The third and fourth responses (T_3 and T_4) are abolished at 80% block of T_1. In addition to the third and fourth responses, the second (T_2) response is ablated at about 90% suppression of T_1. This chronology may differ slightly among different relaxants, especially when doses are repeated. The disappearance of T_1 or all four responses indicates deep NMB. The recovery of these responses proceeds in the reverse order (i.e., T_1 response, followed by T_2, T_3 and the last to appear is T_4) when TOF ratio becomes measurable (Fig. 44-10). The time from peak effect of the relaxant (T_0 or T_1) to 25% recovery of T_1 (TOF count of 3) is generally termed **clinical duration** or **clinical relaxation** during nitrous oxide-oxygen-opioid anesthesia. At a TOF count of 3, abdominal relaxation generally becomes

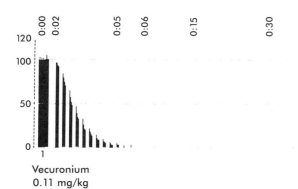

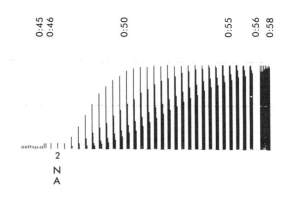

Fig. 44-10. Integrated evoked EMG to TOF stimulation shows the response to vecuronium 0.11 mg/kg. At 47 minutes the first response to TOF recovered spontaneously to 10% of control. Note during the onset there is minimal fade when compared to that during recovery. Neostigmine *(N)* 4.0 mg and atropine *(A)* 1.5 mg were administered. Note the development of T_2, T_3 and T_4, and the progressive increase in TOF ratio, which reached 0.8 after 11 minutes from reversal.

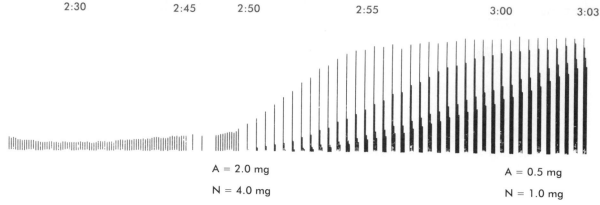

A = 2.0 mg

N = 4.0 mg

A = 0.5 mg

N = 1.0 mg

Fig. 44-11. This tracing contrasts with the recovery in Fig. 44-10. Note at 2 hours and 48 minutes after an intubation dose of a combination of pancuronium and *d*-tubocurarine and incremental doses of *d*-tubocurarine 3.0 mg alternating with pancuronium 0.5 mg, reversal was attempted with neostigmine (4.0 mg) and atropine (2.0 mg). At 12 minutes TOF ratio recovered to 0.5. Another dose of reversal as shown improved recovery of TOF ratio to 0.74.

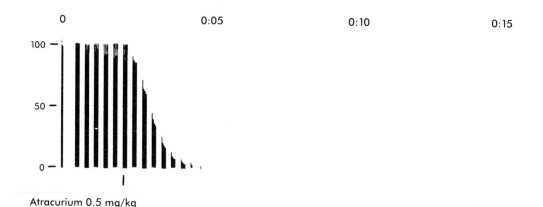

Atracurium 0.5 mg/kg

Fig. 44-12. Evoked integrated EMG showing the minimal fade during the onset of action of atracurium 0.5 mg/kg.

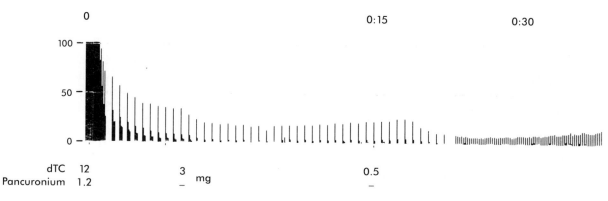

dTC   12

Pancuronium   1.2

3   mg

0.5

Fig. 44-13. Integrated evoked thenar EMG showing the onset of neuromuscular blockade after a combination of *d*-tubocurarine and pancuronium. Note the fade, which is more apparent than the fade after atracurium in Fig. 44-12. Doses of both relaxants are in milligrams.

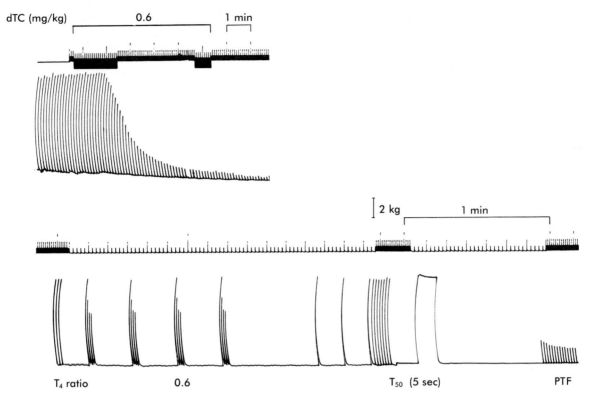

Fig. 44-14. Tracing shows evoked thumb adduction in response to single-twitch stimuli at 0.15 Hz and TOF. *Upper panel* shows the response to *d*-tubocurarine 0.6 mg/kg administered over 6 minutes. *Lower panel* shows the recovery of the single-twitch stimuli to control height, TOF ratio 0.6, and tetanic response at 50 Hz for 5 seconds with minimal fade, followed by minimal posttetanic facilitation *(PTF)*.

less satisfactory, signaling the need for a supplemental dose of the relaxant to maintain adequate surgical relaxation. This is especially important with relaxants, such as atracurium or vecuronium, because of their fast recovery. In the presence of potent inhalation anesthetics, lesser degrees of twitch depression are needed to provide satisfactory clinical relaxation. At the end of surgery spontaneous recovery of T_1 to 20% to 25% of control (TOF count of 2-3) allows rapid reversal of intermediate-acting relaxants. When long-acting drugs are used, the same degree of spontaneous recovery may require 10 to 12 minutes for adequate recovery after reversal (Fig. 44-11). During the onset of NMB, the degree of fade is less than that during recovery. The fade is also less during the onset of intermediate-acting relaxants than the fade following long-acting drugs (Figs. 44-12 and 44-13).

The ratio of the fourth to the first response correlates well with a simple clinical test commonly used for evaluating recovery from nondepolarizing NMB—head lift. With a TOF ratio about 0.6, patients were able to sustain head lift for ≥3.0 seconds.[6] In conscious unmedicated human volunteers, at a TOF ratio of 0.6 after incremental intravenous

d-tubocurarine administration, the vital capacity and inspiratory force differed significantly from control measurements. The lowest measurements, however, were well above the clinically acceptable limits for tracheal extubation.[7] A ratio greater than 0.75 was found to correlate with signs of adequate clinical recovery from nitrous oxide-oxygen-opioid balanced anesthesia.[2] This will be discussed in detail later. It should be emphasized that when the single-twitch stimulus at 0.15 Hz returns to control height, the TOF fade may still be significant (Fig. 44-14). This fade occurs more frequently with use of long-acting relaxants than with intermediate-acting drugs. The fade occurs more frequently with use of vecuronium than with atracurium at an equal degree of the recovery of the single-twitch stimulus or the first twitch of TOF[5] (Figs. 44-15 and 44-16). There are variable degrees of fade of TOF response even when mechanical tetanic response (50 Hz for 5 seconds) is fully sustained[8] (see Fig. 44-14).

It has been suggested that it is difficult to manually detect the fade during TOF stimulation when TOF ratio is 0.4 or greater. The method of detecting fade of thumb adduction is questionable. If the clinician

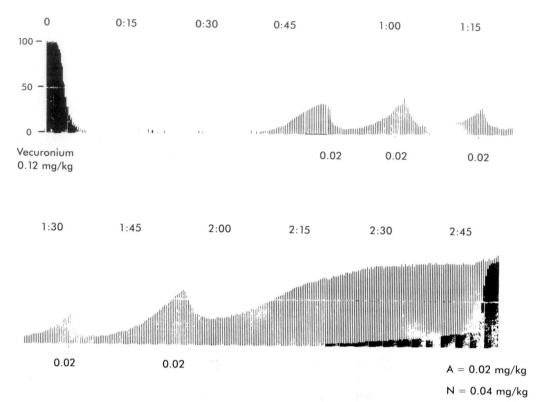

Fig. 44-15. Tracing of an evoked integrated thenar EMG. *Upper panel* shows the response to vecuronium 0.12 mg/kg followed by increments of 0.02 mg/kg every 15 minutes. *Lower panel* shows the response to another two similar increments followed by spontaneous recovery. Note appearance of the fourth response of TOF *(dark shadow)*. When T_1 recovered to control height, TOF ratio recovered to 0.15 and increased to 0.25 in 15 minutes. This residual blockade responded to reversal with atropine 20 μg/kg and neostigmine 40 μg/kg to a TOF ratio of 0.9 in 3 minutes.

observes thumb movement (visual assessment) or holds the thumb without exerting a preload tension on the adductor pollicis, this impression may be true. Conversely, if the thumb is fully abducted, subtle degrees of fade can be detected at a much higher TOF ratio (Ali HH, 1989, unpublished data). Engbaek, Ostergaard, and Viby-Mogensen[20] and Drenck et al.[17] studied another stimulation pattern called double-burst stimulation (DBS) in an attempt to increase the manual perception of fade.

Double-Burst Stimulation

This pattern of stimulation consists of two short bursts of three stimuli at a frequency of 50 Hz. The two bursts are separated by 750 ms. The response to each burst is perceived as a single strong response. During residual curarization, the response to the second burst of stimulation is conditioned by the first burst and appears smaller (fade).[20] The authors of this study believe that they can manually discern the degree of fade to DBS more than with TOF. They claim that with no manually detected fade of TOF response, there is only a 50% chance that TOF ratio is greater than 0.6.[17] They indicate that in the absence of fade to DBS, there is a 90% chance that TOF ratio measured

mechanically is about 0.6, and if there is a perceptible fade to DBS, there is a 75% chance that the true TOF ratio is less than 0.6.[18] The same authors were uncertain about the degree of manual or visual fade of tetanic response at 50 Hz for 5 seconds. It is known that DBS is more painful to patients recovering from anesthesia than TOF. Double-burst stimulation requires further clinical evaluation to ascertain its validity and clinical usefulness.

Tetanic Stimulation

The response to tetanic stimulation is well sustained over a certain range of frequencies (< 70 Hz)[43] in the absence of diseases of the neuromuscular junction, for example, myasthenia gravis, or absence of curare-like drugs. Higher-frequency stimulation increases the duration of the refractory period and it is possible that part of the fade seen is secondary to decreased ability of the muscle to respond rapidly rather than receptor blockade.[21] Moreover, fade has been observed after administration of neostigmine alone,[14] during the use of inhalation anesthetics,[15] and in the absence of neuromuscular blockade, at frequencies higher than 70 Hz.[8] **The tetanic frequency most commonly used to assess residual nondepolarizing neuromuscular**

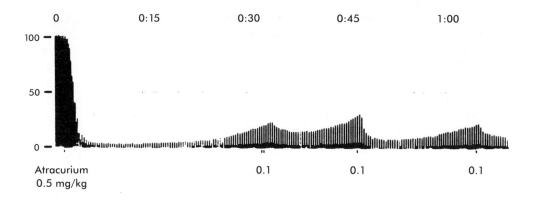

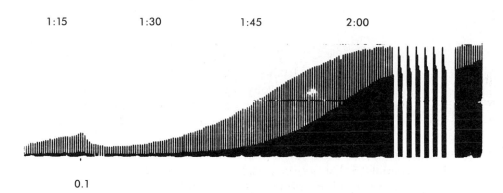

Fig. 44-16. This tracing is the same as Fig. 44-15 in response to atracurium 0.5 mg/kg and four increments of 0.1 mg/kg every 15 minutes. Note when T_1 spontaneously recovered to control height, TOF ratio was 0.74 and increased in the following 4 minutes to 0.85. No reversal was required because the patient met all criteria of adequate clinical recovery. (From Ali HH, Miller RD: Monitoring of neuromuscular function. In Miller RD, ed: *Anesthesia*, ed 2, vol 2, New York 1986, Churchill-Livingstone.)

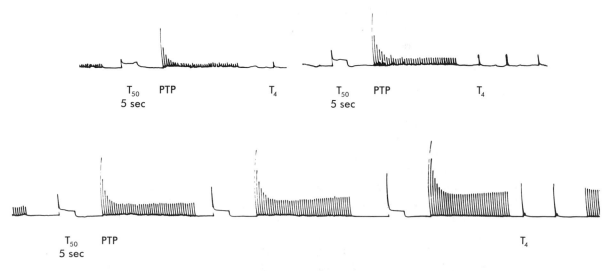

Fig. 44-17. *Upper* and *lower panels* show evoked thumb adduction in response to single-twitch stimulation at 0.1 Hz and repeated tetanic stimulation every 6 minutes at 50 Hz for 5 seconds. Note the tetanic fade, PTP (posttetanic potentiation), and the progressive recovery of the posttetanic single-twitch stimulation when compared with the pretetanic twitch height.

blockade is 50 Hz for 5 seconds, because the tension evoked by a 50 Hz tetanus compares with the tension developed during maximal voluntary effort.[36] Tetanic stimulation is painful to the awake patient. Furthermore, repeated tetanic stimulation leads to progressive recovery of the tetanized muscle (Fig. 44-17). This degree of tetanus-induced recovery does not reflect the systemic effects of the relaxant, for example, on the contralateral hand or the respiratory muscles. An occasional delivery of a 5-second tetanus at 50 Hz may be used when the response to single-twitch or TOF stimulus is absent. This is used to test for the presence of posttetanic potentiation (PTP). Tetanic stimulation at 50 Hz for 5 seconds can be applied at the end of the anesthetic, and before and after reversal of NMB to detect the presence or absence of tetanic fade.

Posttetanic Single-Twitch Stimulation

Posttetanic stimulation allows the detection of the presence or absence of PTP of the single-twitch stimulus at 0.1 Hz when delivered 3 to 5 seconds after the end of tetanic stimulation (see Fig. 44-17). During partial curarization, PTP can be explained by increased mobilization and enhanced synthesis of Ach during and after tetanic stimulation. The replenishment of the immediately available store of Ach leads to an increase in Ach release more than that before tetanic stimulation. Mechanical PTP can be demonstrated in the absence of neuromuscular blockade. This may be related to changes in the contractile response of the muscle induced by tetanic stimulation. This phenomenon does not appear during evoked EMG. Accordingly, the presence of evoked electromyographic PTP suggests residual curarization.[21]

Posttetanic Count and Profound Neuromuscular Blockade

Clinically, it is not desirable to ablate the response to single-twitch stimuli at 0.1 Hz or TOF, particularly when using long-acting relaxants. During most operative procedures, adequate surgical relaxation can be achieved by titrating the relaxant to 90% to 95% twitch suppression or one response to TOF. In exceptional conditions, deeper degrees of block may be needed or deep block may be produced by inadvertent overdose with complete ablation of the single-twitch, TOF, or even tetanic response. Some investigators[45] used repetitive tetanic stimulation at 50 Hz for 5 seconds every 6 to 10 minutes. After a pause of 3 seconds, single repeated twitch stimuli at 1.0 Hz follow the tetanic stimulus. The first appearance of a posttetanic response and the PTC can be evaluated. These authors found that a PTC of 1 indicates that the mean time to first detectable response to TOF stimulation is about 30 minutes during pancuronium-induced

NMB and 8 minutes after administration of atracurium or vecuronium. A PTC of 10 was found to coincide with appearance of the first twitch of TOF. I believe that intense NMB is not clinically indicated in most situations, as stated earlier, provided the patient is adequately anesthetized, because of the problems encountered in reversing this degree of block.

Repeated tetanic stimulation every 6 minutes leads to local muscle recovery and masking the real degree of NMB elsewhere in the body (see Fig. 44-17). An occasional application of a 5-second 50-Hz tetanus in the absence of any response to peripheral nerve stimulation is acceptable. This may reveal how soon spontaneous recovery will occur without distorting neuromuscular transmission at the site of stimulation.

REVERSAL OF NEUROMUSCULAR BLOCKADE

The ability to reverse a nondepolarizing NMB depends on the degree of spontaneous recovery before the administration of anticholinesterase drugs.[30] Some suggested guidelines follow:

- **In the absence of an evoked response to single-twitch stimulation at 0.1 Hz or TOF, do not attempt to reverse the block because antagonism will be difficult to achieve; on the contrary, recovery may be prolonged**
- **When there is only one response to TOF stimulation, adequate reversal may take as long as 30 minutes**
- **At a TOF count of two to three responses, recovery may take up to 10 to 12 minutes with long-acting relaxants and 4 to 5 minutes after intermediate-acting drugs**
- **When the fourth response to TOF stimulation appears, adequate recovery can be achieved within 5 minutes of reversal with neostigmine or 2 to 3 minutes after use of edrophonium**

These guidelines indicate the importance of monitoring neuromuscular function to determine the optimum time for administration of anticholinesterases and to predict adequate clinical recovery.

ASSESSMENT OF RECOVERY FROM NEUROMUSCULAR BLOCKADE
Recorded Response

Monitoring neuromuscular function during spontaneous recovery or after reversal of NMB provides a fairly reliable criterion of adequacy of clinical recovery. **When nondepolarizing relaxants are used, sustained tetanic response at 50 Hz for 5 seconds, absence of posttetanic potentiation, and absence of fade to TOF stimulation are the accepted criteria for adequate** recovery using evoked responses. A recorded TOF ratio of ≥ 0.75 is regarded by investigators as a reliable parameter indicating adequate recovery from nondepolarizing NMB. This ratio correlates with sustained head lift for 5 seconds, and adequate vital capacity and inspiratory force.[2,12]

When the single-twitch response at 0.1 Hz returns to control height, a substantial degree of fade of TOF may remain. Variable degrees of fade of TOF response may occur even when mechanical tetanic response at 50 Hz for 5 seconds is fully sustained.[8]

Without Recording Equipment

When recording equipment is not used, a nerve stimulator that is capable of delivering a TOF stimulus, tetanus at 50 Hz, or DBS is required.

If the thumb is held in full abduction (outstretched thumb) and there is no discernible difference between the fourth and the first responses to TOF stimulation, the TOF ratio is likely to be about 0.60 (Ali HH, 1989, unpublished data). Other workers[17] found that there is only a 50% chance that TOF ratio exceeds 0.60 with no manually detected fade to TOF stimulation. They recommended the use of DBS.

It should be emphasized that irrespective of the method used in assessing the adequacy of recovery from NMB, the clinician should use as many criteria as practical to ascertain the return of muscle strength to a level satisfactory enough to provide adequate pulmonary ventilation and protection of the upper airway. This assessment is discussed in Box 44-3.

With regard to varying sensitivity, eye and facial muscles should be observed. Drooping of the eyelids or ptosis and certain facial expressions similar to myasthenic or myopathic facies may indicate residual blockade. In addition, the intercostal muscles are more sensitive than the diaphragm. Because the diaphragm recovers earlier, there may be some incoordination of movement. For example, when the diaphragm contracts, the anterior chest wall muscles do not follow, which creates rocking respiratory movements.

The ability of certain groups of muscles to sustain a specific voluntary movement can be tested to assess the presence or absence of residual curarization. A nonsustained response is characterized by an initial strong contraction that becomes weaker when repeated rapidly. In particular, diplopia can be demonstrated in patients who may have recovered adequate respiratory function because of the exquisite sensitivity of eye muscles and failure to maintain sustained coordinated contraction. Sustained response of eye muscles can be tested by asking the patient to look to one side. The eye muscles initially pull the eyeball to that side, but the contraction immediately fades in the presence of residual curarization. Further trials lead to a nystagmus from repeated peak response and fade of tetanic contraction of the eye muscles. Jerky movements are related to a peak contraction followed by fade of voluntary activity. A failure to sustain muscle activity may be seen as head lift (for at least 5 seconds), hand grip, leg raising, opening the eyes widely, and protruding the tongue (Box 44-4).

Good signs of adequate recovery include effective swallowing (although in the absence of profuse oral secretions, repeated swallowing may indicate inadequate swallowing) and effective cough.

BOX 44-3
CLINICAL ASSESSMENT OF RESIDUAL NMB
WITHOUT A NERVE STIMULATOR

Assessment depends on two facts:
  Various muscles in the body have different
    sensitivities to muscle relaxants.
  Repetitive movement may reveal residual
    blockade by virtue of inability to sustain such
    movement.

BOX 44-4
CLINICAL CRITERIA OF
ADEQUATE RECOVERY

These clinical criteria depend on whether the patient is wide-awake, or is asleep or nonresponsive to commands.

Patient is awake:
Opens the eyes widely on command with no
    diplopia
Sustains protrusion of the tongue
Swallows effectively
Sustains a head lift for at least 5 seconds
Produces a sustained hand grip
Has an effective cough
Has an adequate vital capacity of at least
    15 ml/kg
Produces adequate inspiratory force of at least
    25 to 30 cm H_2O negative pressure

Patient is sleepy:
Has adequate tidal volume
Produces an inspiratory force of at least 25 to 30
    cm H_2O negative pressure
Has adequate evoked responses, including:
    Sustained tetanic response to 50 Hz for 5
        seconds
    TOF ratio > 0.75 or no discernible fade of
        the fully abducted thumb
    No fade to DBS

KEY POINTS

- The response to muscle relaxants is unpredictable in patients and more so in the presence of an array of drug and disease interaction.

- Monitoring neuromuscular blockade has gained wide acceptance by clinical anesthesiologist as providing adequate surgical relaxation and timely restoration of optimal neuromuscular function.

- In addition to the clinical criteria, monitoring neuromuscular function can be accomplished by measuring isometric contraction (tension—mechanomyography), isotonic contraction (accelerometry) or electrical activity (electromyography).

- Peripheral motor nerve stimulation can be in the form of repetitive single-twitch stimuli, train-of-four stimulation, tetanic stimulation, posttetanic stimulation (posttetanic count), and double-burst stimulation, for assessing both the depth of and recovery from neuromuscular blockade.

- Evoked train-of-four response appears to be a useful clinical tool for titrating relaxant requirement, determining the optimal time for administration of reversal drug, and predicting adequate clinial recovery without the need to establish a control response.

- The information generated from the evoked responses should be combined with other clinical criteria to formulate the final assessment for each patient's state of neuromuscular recovery from muscle relaxants.

- The technique involved in using a peripheral nerve stimulator (PNS) includes the following steps:

  1. Nerve stimulator should be tested and shown that it is capable of delivering a supramaximal stimulus.
  2. Anatomic landmarks should be checked and direct muscle stimulation avoided.
  3. Skin overlying the peripheral nerve to be stimulated should be prepared by adequately rubbing it with alcohol, allowing it to dry, and then applying the surface electrodes.
  4. Surface electrode disks must be moist.
  5. The negative electrode is applied over the accessible part of the motor nerve with the positive electrode about 1 inch away. The clinician should press on the center of the electrode to obtain good contact with the skin.
  6. For obese patients or those with thick or edematous skin, percutaneous needle electrodes may be indicated to ensure supramaximal stimulus.
  7. The patient should be kept warm, especially peripherally, where the neuromuscular response is being monitored, to avoid impaired nerve conduction or increased skin impedance.
  8. The response to ulnar nerve stimulation should be felt in the adduction of the outstretched thumb rather than in other finger movements.
  9. To monitor the facial muscles, the stimulating electrodes are applied just below the tragus of the ear and the movement of the orbicularis oculi or frontalis muscle (for example) is observed.
  10. The information from the evoked responses should be combined with other clinical criteria to formulate the final judgment of the patient's state of neuromuscular function.

KEY REFERENCES

Ali HH, Utting JE, and Gray TC: Quantitative assessment of residual antidepolarizing block (part I), *Br J Anaesth* 43:473, 1971.

Ali HH, Savarese JJ: Monitoring of neuromuscular function, *Anesthesiology* 45:216, 1976.

Ali HH, Savarese JJ, Lebowitz PW et al: Twitch, tetanus, and train-of-four as indices of recovery from nondepolarizing neuromuscular blockade, *Anesthesiology* 54:294, 1981.

Caffrey RR, Warren ML, and Becker KE: Neuromuscular blockade monitoring comparing the orbicularis oculi and adductor pollicis muscles, *Anesthesiology* 65:95, 1986.

REFERENCES

1. Ali HH, DeCesare R: Evoked EMG, integrated EMG (IEMG) and mechanical responses, *Anesthesiology* 71:A396, 1989.
2. Ali HH, Kitz RJ: Evaluation of recovery from nondepolarizing neuromuscular block, using a digital neuromuscular transmission analyser: preliminary report, *Anesth Analg* 52:740, 1973.
3. Ali HH, Savarese JJ: Monitoring of neuromuscular function, *Anesthesiology* 45: 216, 1976.
4. Ali HH, Savarese JJ: Stimulus frequency

and the dose response to *d*-tubocurarine in man, *Anesthesiology* 52:35, 1980.

5. Ali HH, Savarese JJ, and Basta SJ: Evaluation of cumulative properties of three new nondepolarizing neuromuscular blocking drugs BW A444U, atracurium and vecuronium, *Br J Anaesth* 55:107, 1983.

6. Ali HH, Utting JE, and Gray TC: Quantitative assessment of residual antidepolarizing block (part I), *Br J Anaesth* 43:473, 1971.

7. Ali HH, Wilson RS, Savarese JJ et al: The effect of tubocurarine on directly elicited train-of-four muscle response and respiratory measurements in humans, *Br J Anaesth* 47:570, 1975.

8. Ali HH, Savarese JJ, Lebowitz PW et al: Twitch, tetanus and train-of-four as indices of recovery from nondepolarizing neuromuscular blockade, *Anesthesiology* 54:294, 1981.

9. Birks RJ, McIntosh FC: Acetylcholine metabolism of a sympathetic ganglion, *Can J Biochem Physiol* 39:787, 1961.

10. Bowman WC: Prejunctional and postjunctional cholinoceptors at the neuromuscular junction, *Anesth Analg* 59:935, 1980.

11. Bowman WC, Gibb AJ, and Marshall IG: Prejunctional and postjunctional effects of vecuronium. In Agoston S, Bowman WC, Miller RD et al, eds: *Clinical experiences with Norcuron*[R], *Excerpta Medica, Current Clinical Practice Series 11*, 1983, Amsterdam.

12. Brand JB, Cullen DJ, Wilson NE et al: Spontaneous recovery from nondepolarizing neuromuscular blockade: correlation between clinical and evoked responses, *Anesth Analg* 56:55, 1977.

13. Caffrey RR, Warren ML, and Becker KE: Neuromuscular blockade monitoring comparing the orbicularis oculi and adductor pollicis muscles, *Anesthesiology* 65:95, 1986.

14. Chang CC, Chen SM, and Hong SJ: Reversal of the neostigmine-induced tetanic fade and endplate potential rundown with respect to the autoregulation of transmitter release, *Br J Pharmacol* 95:1255, 1988.

15. Cohen PJ, Heisterkamp CV, and Skovsted P: The effect of general anesthesia on the response to tetanic stimulus in man, *Br J Anaesth* 42:543, 1970.

16. Dolly JO: Biochemistry of acetylcholine receptors from skeletal muscle. In Tipton KF, ed: *International review of biochemical, physiological and pharmacological bio-*

chemistry 26:257, Baltimore, 1979, University Park Press.

17. Drenck NE, Ueda N, Olsen NV et al: Manual evaluation of residual curarization using double burst stimulation: a comparison with train-of-four, *Anesthesiology* 70:578, 1989.

18. Dreyer F: Acetylcholine receptor, *Br J Anaesth* 54:115, 1982.

19. Elmqvist D, Quastel DMJ: A quantitative study of end-plate potentials in isolated human muscle, *J Physiol (Lond)* 178:505, 1965.

20. Engbaek J, Ostergaard D, and Viby-Mogensen J: Double burst stimulation (DBS)—a new pattern of nerve stimulation to identify residual neuromuscular block, *Br J Anaesth* 62:274, 1989.

21. Epstein RA, Epstein RM: The electromyographic and the mechanical response of indirectly stimulated muscle in anesthetized man following curarization, *Anesthesiology* 38:212, 1973.

22. Fatt P, Katz B: Spontaneous subthreshold activity at motor endings, *J Physiol (Lond)* 117:109, 1952.

23. Gibb AJ, Marshall IG: Pre- and postjunctional effects of tubocurarine and trimetaphan involved in tetanic fade at the rat neuromuscular junction, *Br J Pharmacol* 78:86, 1983.

24. Gissen AJ: Standardized technique for transmission studies, *Anesthesiology* 39:567, 1973 (letter).

25. Grob D, Johns RL, and Harvey AM: Studies in neuromuscular function. I. Introduction and methods, *Johns Hopkins Hosp Bull* 99:115, 1956.

26. Heidmann T, Changeux JP: Structural and functional properties of the acetylcholine receptor protein in its purified and membrane-bound states, *Annu Rev Biochem* 47:371, 1978.

27. Hubbard JI: Mechanism of transmitter release, *Prog Biophys Mol Biol* 21:35, 1970.

28. Katz B: Quantal mechanism of neural transmitter release, *Science* 173:123, 1971.

29. Katz B, Miledi R: Further study of the role of calcium in synaptic transmission, *J Physiol (Lond)* 207:789, 1970.

30. Katz RL: Clinical neuromuscular pharmacology of pancuronium, *Anesthesiology* 34:550, 1971.

31. Katz RL: Electromyographic and mechanical effects of suxamethonium and tubocurarine on twitch, tetanic and post-tetanic responses, *Br J Anaesth* 45:849, 1973.

32. Kurihara T, Brooks JE: The mechanism of neuromuscular fatigue, *Arch Neurol* 32:168, 1975.

33. Landau EM: Function and structure of the Ach receptor at the muscle endplate, *Prog Neurobiol* 10:253, 1978.

34. Lee C: Train-of-four quantitation of competitive neuromuscular block, *Anesth Analg* 54:649, 1975.

35. Lee C, Katz RL: Dose relationships of phase II, tachyphylaxis and train-of-four fade in suxamethonium-induced dual neuromuscular block in man, *Br J Anaesth* 47:841, 1975.

36. Merton PA: Voluntary strength and fatigue, *J Physiol* 123:553, 1954.

37. Nachmansohn D, Machado AL: Formation of acetylcholine. New enzyme: "choline acetylase," *J Neurophysiol* 6:397, 1943.

38. Osborne MP: Role of vesicles with some observations on vertebrate sensory cells. In: Cottress GA, Usherwood PN, eds: *Synapses,* New York: 1977, Academic Press.

39. Raftery MA, Hunkapiller MW, Strader CD et al: Acetylcholine receptor: a complex of hemologous subunits, *Science* 208:1454, 1980.

40. Ramsey FM, Lebowitz PW, Savarese JJ et al: Clinical characteristics of long-term succinylcholine neuromuscular blockade during balanced anesthesia, *Anesth Analg* 59:110, 1980.

41. Ross MJ, Klymowski MW, Agard DA et al: Structural studies of a membrane-bound acetylcholine-receptor from *Torpedo californica, J Mol Biol* 116:635, 1977.

42. Standaert FG: Release of transmitter at the neuromuscular junction, *Br J Anaesth* 54:131, 1982.

43. Stanec A, Heyduk J, Stanec D et al: Tetanic fade and post-tetanic tension in the absence of neuromuscular block in anesthetized man, *Anesth Analg* 57:102, 1978.

44. Tucek S: *Acetylcholine synthesis in neurons,* New York, 1978, J Wiley & Sons.

45. Viby-Mogensen J, Howardy-Hansen P, Chraemer-Jorgensen B et al: Post-tetanic count (PTC). A new method of evaluating an intense nondepolarizing neuromuscular blockade, *Anesthesiology* 55:458, 1981.

46. Viby-Mogensen J, Jensen E, Werner M et al: Measurement of acceleration: a new method of monitoring neuromuscular function, *Acta Anaesthesiol Scand* 32:45, 1987.

CHAPTER 45

Monitoring of Hemostasis

DAVID J. MURRAY

Hemostatic Testing
 Preoperative screening
 Tests of the coagulation cascade
Monitoring in Special Circumstances
 Cardiopulmonary bypass
 Massive blood loss
 Disseminated intravascular coagulation
Intraoperative Blood Salvage
Coagulation Factor Replacement
Desmopressin, Aprotinin, and Antifibrinolysis

Normal hemostatic function can be interrupted by a variety of congenital and acquired diseases on an acute or chronic basis. Increased blood loss during surgery is a common finding in patients with hemostatic abnormalities, but multiple factors other than the hemostatic mechanism may be responsible for bleeding during surgery. When hemostatic abnormalities are the cause, clot formation will be absent and microvascular bleeding will be apparent. A bleeding patient who requires vascular volume resuscitation as well as correction of hemostatic abnormalities poses a serious therapeutic and diagnostic problem, particularly when a variety of coagulation tests and multiple blood components may be necessary to define the problem and correct the bleeding diathesis.

A simplistic method to assess excessive bleeding during surgery is to arbitrarily divide coagulation function into the four hemostatic problems that may lead to increased blood loss. These hemostatic problems may relate to (1) vascular factors, (2) platelet factors, (3) coagulation cascade abnormalities, and (4) clot retraction pathology.

Although all aspects of hemostatic function are interrelated, this arbitrary division of hemostatic steps is a useful clinical framework, particularly since each individual factor requires separate therapeutic intervention.

A normal hemostatic mechanism does not prevent blood loss that results from either large vessel disruption or when a large pressure gradient exists between the disrupted vasculature and the interstitium. In these situations, bleeding continues until intravascular pressure equals extravascular pressure. Frequently, increased bleeding during surgery is attributed to hemostatic disorders without considering the role of pressure gradients and major vessel disruption in contributing to blood loss. Bleeding from a ruptured intraabdominal aneurysm may cease when arterial pressure is decreased and extravasated blood increases intraabdominal pressure, but hemorrhage recurs when blood pressure is increased by volume resuscitation and intraabdominal pressure is decreased by laparotomy. Similarly, elevated venous pressure during surgery may also lead to an impression of increased blood loss secondary to a hemostatic disorder when hemostasis is normal. A patient in the prone position who has increased intraabdominal pressure from improper positioning experiences increased blood loss during laminectomy as a result of the distended venous plexus. A similar situation may occur during middle ear surgery if venous return from the head is obstructed from extensive lateral flexion of the neck. Although the initial approach to the bleeding patient requires an assessment of all the contributing factors currently, a problem with hemostasis during surgery is primarily a subjective impression of greater than normal blood loss in the absence of other causes of bleeding.

The severe bleeding reported in unprepared hemophiliac patients during minor surgery attests to the importance of the coagulation mechanism during surgery.[1] When hemostatic abnormalities are the causes of bleeding, bleeding from wound edges is unresponsive to electrocautery or suture ligature, bleeding may recur from a previously dry surgical field, and clot formation is absent.[11,62,65] Whereas severe abnormalities in hemostasis lead to profound blood loss, minor abnormalities in hemostasis may not significantly contribute to blood loss, and a method to monitor hemostasis is important.[1,51,62] Like most other organ systems, a considerable reserve of function exists for hemostasis, and increased bleeding during an operation does not occur until less than 30% of normal levels are present.[1,11,62] For a variety of coagulation factors, a clinically significant bleeding diathesis during surgery does not occur until coagulation factor levels are considerably less than 10% to 20% of normal.[1]

The approach to bleeding and coagulation function during the perioperative period must be based on the following: (1) an understanding of the normal response of the coagulation system to tissue injury (Table 45-1), (2) the changes from underlying disease drug therapy and blood volume replacement, (3) the requirements for surgical hemostasis, and (4) an appreciation of the effect of surgery and anesthesia on coagulation function. Monitoring all aspects of a complex coagulation system is difficult, particularly when the perioperative period creates dynamic changes in hemostatic function. An oversimplified approach to monitoring is to consider the integral relationship of vasculature, platelets, and coagulation

factors in the formation of a fibrin plug. If any one of these aspects is abnormal, persistent unrelenting clinical bleeding may occur during surgery.

HEMOSTATIC TESTING (Table 45-2)
Preoperative Screening

Preoperative laboratory assessment of hemostasis in the healthy patient with no bleeding history who requires minor surgery rarely, if ever, adds additional information that would help predict blood loss, alter an anesthetic or surgical plan, or contribute to medical care.[3,24,66,72] Screening coagulation tests such as the prothrombin time (PT) and partial thromboplastin time (PTT) are only infrequently abnormal in the absence of a history indicating coagulation dysfunction. In most circumstances, the presence of an unexpected abnormality in the PT and PTT does not appear to contribute to the care of the patient,[23,24] particularly if there are no signs and symptoms and the intended procedure is minor. In a retrospective review of unexpected abnormalities in 12 otherwise healthy patients with no history of bleeding abnormalities scheduled for minor surgery in my institution, the abnormal coagulation test results were not noted or followed in the postoperative period in five patients. All five patients had uneventful operations and perioperative recovery periods. In two patients, a repeat PT and PTT test was obtained in the postoperative period after an uneventful operation and recovery; the repeat tests were normal. In two patients a repeated set of preoperative PT and PTT tests were normal with uneventful operation. In two patients, the abnormality of the PTT delayed surgery. In one patient, the operation was undertaken later without further consultation evaluation. In the other patient, a hematologic consultation was obtained, and after extensive testing the abnormality was deemed clinically insignificant. Surgery in both patients was uneventful. In these healthy ASA physical status I

Table 45-1   Phases of hemostasis

Phases	Responses of coagulation system
Vascular (2-5 sec)	Contraction
	Loss of endothelial integrity with its antithrombin coating and capacity to release prostacyclin and fibrinolysin activator
	Attachment and activation of contact factors XII, prekallikrein
Platelet (3-10 sec)	Adhesion to damaged area
	Aggregation, coagulation factor activation, and release of Ca^{++}, thromboxane A_2, serotonin, ATP, ADP
Plasma (30-120 sec)	Activation intrinsic path XIIa-Xa-thrombin
	Fibrin clot formation, clot retraction
Repair (6-48 hr) (10-30 days)	Fibrinolysis
	Endothelial regeneration

Abbreviations: *ATP*, adenosine triphosphate; *ADP*, adenosine diphosphate.

Table 45-2   Normal values for coagulation tests

Coagulation tests	Values
Platelet count	150,000-350,000/mm³
Bleeding time	4-9 min
Activated partial thromboplastin time (aPTT)	25-37 sec
Activated coagulation time (ACT)	90-120 sec
Prothrombin time (PT)	10-15 sec
Thrombin time (TT)	15-19 sec
Fibrinogen level	150-350 mg/dl

patients, who had no history of bleeding problems and required minor surgery, even when an abnormal PT and PTT result was obtained, the tests did not appear to contribute to the perioperative care of the patients. If the detection of a laboratory abnormality in a healthy patient does not merit further evaluation or contribute to the patient's later medical care, then the screening test probably should be abandoned.

Although many patients do not require preoperative laboratory testing, many patients may potentially benefit from such testing. If hemostatic testing is judged to be indicated, the preoperative tests probably should include not only a PT and PTT but also fibrinogen levels. Obtaining a fibrinogen level is particularly helpful in management of acquired clotting disorders which are frequently associated with an imbalance between clot formation and dissolution, leading to fibrinogen consumption.[4,46,71,81]

A variety of obstetric diseases are associated with acute and chronic coagulation disorders that merit coagulation testing in the absence of symptoms.[9,13,55,63] The anticipated surgery may be an indication for obtaining a preoperative coagulation profile. Operative procedures associated with major blood loss, the use of cardiopulmonary bypass, and procedures involving systemic anticoagulation probably merit a preoperative coagulation profile, which frequently serves as a reference for later tests of coagulation.* Although the basis for obtaining PT and PTT tests may be too liberal at present, there are a variety of patients who do require preoperative hemostatic tests so that a rational plan for assessing hemostasis can be formulated in the perioperative period.

The availability of a variety of blood components to treat specific hemostatic abnormalities has grown as rapidly as the number of in vitro coagulation function tests. Thirty years ago patients with known bleeding disorders frequently had normal in vitro hemostatic tests.[47] In addition, the treatment for the patient suspected of having a hemostatic disorder was limited to fresh plasma or whole blood. Currently, the battery of tests required on donor blood before transfusion and the multiple roles for blood components in clinical medicine have essentially eliminated fresh whole blood as replacement for blood loss. The improved specificity and sensitivity of in vitro coagulation tests in the diagnosis of specific hemostatic abnormalities has markedly improved.[57,83] Similar to cardiovascular or respiratory monitoring, the monitoring of hemostasis requires a knowledge of the normal physiology of hemostasis, an understanding of coagulation pathology, the effects of anesthesia and surgery on hemostasis and an ability to interpret the

derived hemostatic monitoring information to formulate an effective plan of intervention.

The in vivo coagulation mechanism is not as clearly divided into platelet disorders, intrinsic or extrinsic coagulation disorders, or abnormalities related to fibrin deposition as suggested by the in vitro coagulation tests, but this arbitrary separation of coagulation function is helpful in diagnosis and therapy. A number of complex interrelationships among different elements of coagulation remain unanswered by this arbitrary separation. For example:

- How can a deficiency of part of the factor VIII complex in von Willebrand's disease lead to problems with platelet aggregation?
- Why do patients with severe deficiencies of certain coagulation factors with abnormal clotting test results experience minimal bleeding symptoms?
- Why do intrinsic coagulation factor disorders have severe clincial manifestations when the extrinsic coagulation cascade and common pathway of coagulation are intact?

Platelet count and bleeding time

Platelets play an integral role in all aspects of the hemostatic mechanism[86] (Box 45-1). The initial hemostatic plug formed at the site of vascular disruption is dependent on adequate platelet numbers and activity. The platelet plug is formed by the adhesion and aggregation of platelets. The coagulation mechanism activated by platelets leads to a fibrin meshwork at the site of the initial platelet plug. This integral platelet role explains why a decrease in platelet count increases surgical bleeding. An acute decline from normal levels to less than $50,000/mm^3$ leads to increased surgical bleeding.[43,54,59,60] Platelet transfusion is generally indicated to treat acute thrombocytopenia in the preoperative setting.[15,16,43] In a number of patients, chemotherapy for malignancies or autoimmune platelet disorders leads to the decreased production or increased destruction of platelets, and thrombocytopenia occurs more gradually.[15] Thrombocytopenia in this setting may not result in a bleeding tendency until platelet counts are considerably less than $50,000/mm.^3$ For this reason platelet counts of $50,000/mm^3$ in the perioperative period may be adequate in patients who have chronic thrombocytopenia.[15]

In addition to the important clinical relationship observed between decreased platelet count and increased bleeding during operation, the template or Ivy's bleeding time, a test of hemostatic plug formation, also progressively increases as the platelet count decreases.[29] The correlation among a decrease in platelet count, the increase in template bleeding time, and microvascular bleeding during operation sug-

---

* References 12, 50, 54, 60, 73, 75, 83.

**BOX 45-2
TESTS OF PLATELET FUNCTION**

Bleeding time (overall platelet function)
Response to ristocetin (platelet aggregation)
Aggregometer (platelet aggregation)
Rumpel-Leed (platelet adhesion)
Clot retraction

---

gests the bleeding time may be a convenient method to assess the impact of quantitative and qualitative platelet function abnormalities during the perioperative period. If a qualitative platelet abnormality markedly increases the template bleeding time, this may indicate that the abnormality requires correction with a homologous platelet transfusion.

Qualitative platelet abnormalities

A number of diseases and drugs may disturb platelet function in hemostasis. Although an in vitro abnormality in platelet function can often be demonstrated, a similar relationship between the qualitative abnormality and clinical bleeding during surgery may not follow.[48] In patients in whom qualitative platelet abnormalities are anticipated, a predictive test of in vivo platelet function is often helpful, particularly in deciding whether to proceed with elective operation. Similarly, the decisions about major regional anesthesia depend on measured coagulation function. The template bleeding time measures the time for a hemostatic plug to form after an incision of uniform depth and width.[29] The bleeding time is a relatively objective test of platelet function. When an experienced technician performs the test in a cooperative patient, the bleeding time is virtually the only platelet test available that assesses an easily understood and clinically relevant aspect of platelet function during the perioperative period. If increases in surgical blood loss parallel increases in bleeding time, then this would be an ideal test to determine whether significant platelet abnormalities exist in the perioperative period that require therapy. A large range of normal

bleeding times exist (4 to 9 minutes), and the relationship between increased bleeding time and increased blood loss is unfortunately not clearly demonstrated. Based on experience with other tests of coagulation, a bleeding time greater than 1.5 times a normal bleeding time (longer than 15 minutes) represents a clinically significant hemostatic abnormality.

The ability of platelets to aggregate, adhere to endothelium, and release chemotactic and vasoconstricting substances and initiate the coagulation cascade may be altered to varying degrees by disease or drugs. The best known of these interactions is the effect of acetylsalicyclic acid (ASA) and the nonsteroidal antiinflammatory drugs in disrupting thromboxane A_2 synthesis within the platelet.[86] In the case of ASA, inhibition of the cyclooxygenase enzyme systems prevents thromboxane synthesis from a precursor, arachidonic acid. Without thromboxane A_2, the ability of platelets to aggregate in response to Ca^{++} and vessel injury is decreased.[86] Although some studies suggest that surgical bleeding may be increased in the presence of ASA, an equivalent number suggest this in vitro abnormality may not increase blood loss during a major operation. When ASA is the causative agent, the platelet abnormality lasts the life of the platelet population (life span = 7 to 10 days), whereas with nonsteroidal antiinflammatory drugs the effect is more short lived.

Several platelet function tests are available (Box 45-2); the relationship between the qualitative platelet abnormalities detected by these tests and an increased bleeding tendency during an operative procedure is difficult to establish in clinical practice. Platelet aggregation and platelet roles in clot retraction can be tested and are used to identify qualitative platelet abnormalities caused by disease or drugs. Most drug effects on qualitative platelet function are reversible with discontinuation (e.g., dipyridamole and various analogs, calcium channel blockers, nonsteroidal antiinflammatory drugs) or occur only when large doses of drug (beta-lactam antibiotics on membrane glycoproteins) are administered. Although the effects of these drugs on hemostatic function represent an added threat to patients who already have coagulation problems (patients receiving either coumadin or heparin, or who have hemophilia or von Willebrand's disease), use of these drugs may not represent a bleeding threat to patients who otherwise have normal hemostatic function, particularly since the effects of most of these drugs on platelet function are transient and disappear shortly after discontinuation.

Tests of the Coagulation Cascade
PT and PTT

In the presence of hematologic abnormalities, whether a decline in hematocrit, platelet count, or coagulation factor level, the decision to transfuse blood components must be based on careful consideration of risk vs. benefit. Coagulation factors and platelet replacement based on laboratory assessment alone and not on clinical grounds must be considered a questionable practice.[14,15] Hemostatic monitoring must be used to determine which blood component to administer and may guide coagulation factor replacement.[11,62]

Two of the most commonly ordered in vitro tests of coagulation, the prothrombin time (PT) and activated partial thromboplastin time (aPTT), provide specific and sensitive coagulation cascade evaluation. **The PT provides sensitive information about the coagulation factor activity of the extrinsic coagulation system when a sample of blood is activated with a standardized clotting activator, such as tissue thromboplastin.**[6] **When a sample of blood is activated by using an incomplete thromboplastin activator, such as kaolin or silica, the aPTT is measured.**[83] **The aPTT provides relatively sensitive information about intrinsic coagulation factor levels.** The normal levels provided by laboratories for the PT and the aPTT include a range of two standard deviations from a sample of normal patients. These tests effectively exclude patients with significant coagulation factor deficits. With carefully controlled testing methods using newer reagents, the PT and aPTT increase above control values when coagulation factor activity in blood is less than 50% of normal levels.[57,83] The current specificity and sensitivity of the PT and aPTT might be contrasted with earlier testing methods when abnormalities were not observed until factor levels approached 10% to 15% of control levels, and often repeated tests on diluted serum were required to confirm that an abnormal hemostatic mechanism existed in patients with symptoms and signs that suggested a congenital or acquired deficiency of coagulation factors.[20,47] Despite an increased sensitivity of the PT and aPTT to actual levels of coagulation factors, clinicians must remember that a variety of reagents are used to conduct these tests and coagulation laboratories vary in their ability to detect coagulation factor deficiencies.[83] In general,

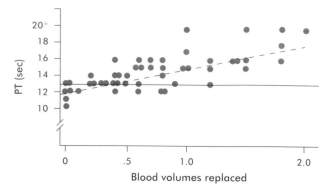

Fig. 45-1. Prothrombin time increases with progressive blood loss during packed red cell replacement in patients requiring major elective surgery. (From Murray DJ, Olson J, Strauss R et al: Coagulation changes during packed red cell replacement of major blood loss, *Anesthesiology* 69:839, 1988.)

the interpretation of a normal and abnormal aPTT test must be done in concert with an understanding of how sensitive the test is to actual coagulation factor levels and the clinical setting. For this reason, selecting an arbitrary upper limit without considering the sensitivity of the PT or aPTT and the hemostatic requirements for the operative procedure is similar to the arbitrary selection of a specific hematocrit to base red cell transfusion for all patients. The PT and aPTT tests also vary in their sensitivity to detect isolated deficiencies of individual coagulation factors of the extrinsic or intrinsic system, respectively. The PT is more sensitive to deficiencies of factor II and V than to VII and X. The aPTT is more sensitive to decreases in factors VIII and IX than to factors XI and XII (Figs. 45-1 and 45-2).

The question of what level of coagulation factor activity should be maintained during surgery is not clearly defined. The outcome of patients with isolated coagulation factor deficiencies as well as clinical studies of patients in whom coagulopathies developed during surgery suggest that a significant operative bleeding problem occurs when factor levels are less than 30% of normal.[1,11,62] **This information suggests that coagulation factor activity of 30% or more provides effective hemostasis during the perioperative period.** The primary laboratory tests used to assess the activity of coagulation factors, the PT and aPTT, are elevated above control levels when coagulation factor activity is less than 50% or 60% of normal levels.[57,83] Although the PT and aPTT tests are relatively sensitive in the detection of abnormalities of the extrinsic and intrinsic coagulation system, severe decreases in the conversion of prothrombin to thrombin or of fibrinogen to fibrin can also prolong the PT and aPTT. For this reason, decreases in fibrinogen levels also increase the PT and aPTT. When coagu-

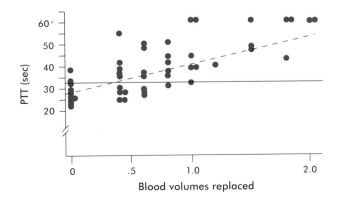

Fig. 45-2. Partial thromboplastin time increases in patients requiring major elective surgery. Replacement solutions are packed red cells and crystalloid. (From Murray DJ, Olson J, Strauss R et al: Coagulation changes during packed red cell replacement of major blood loss, *Anesthesiology* 69:839, 1988.)

lation factor activity approaches 30% of normal, the PT and aPTT generally are elevated to 150% of control values. The estimate of the relationship between the PT and aPTT and coagulation factor levels underlies the current recommendations that coagulation factor replacement should be withheld until PT and aPTT are greater than 1.5 times the control values.[11,15,62] **The transfusion of clotting factors (fresh frozen plasma) when diffuse microvascular bleeding occurs (bleeding from the puncture sites, recurrence of bleeding from operative sites) must be considered a *late indication* for the correction of coagulation factor deficits in patients during major surgery; but maintenance of in vitro tests of coagulation within a normal range with plasma components seems too liberal an indication for use of fresh frozen plasma based on a variety of clinical studies.**[11,60,62,65]

Measurement of coagulation factor levels

Do the PT and aPTT tests provide the clinician with enough specific and sensitive information about coagulation factor levels? With more specific forms of treatment for coagulation factor deficiencies available, more specific tests of coagulation factor levels might be a helpful guide to therapy. **If a test were available that could rapidly measure the level of a specific coagulation factor, the numerous interrelated processes that are involved in transforming an inactive coagulation factor to an active coagulation factor would not be tested. For this reason, laboratory tests that measure a desired end point, such as in vitro coagulation (the PT and aPTT), are currently the most appropriate approach for initial screening and monitoring of hemostatic therapy.** These tests have significant limitations in their use because a quality-controlled laboratory setting is required to reproduce

the results. In addition, the PT and aPTT test results can be abnormal when coagulation factor deficiencies not associated with abnormal surgical hemostasis exist (factor XII).

Fibrinogen. **The only quantitative coagulation factor level that is routinely available in clinical laboratories is the fibrinogen level.** The conversion of fibrinogen to fibrin in the formation of the hemostatic plug is the common final step to both the extrinsic and intrinsic coagulation systems. The steps from thrombin activation of fibrinogen to the final formation of the fibrin clot are important to understanding the action of heparin as well as disorders associated with clot lysis and disseminated intravascular coagulation. Thrombin acts on the fibrinogen molecule and a fibrin monomer is formed that in the presence of Ca^{++} and factor XIII is cross-linked with other fibrin monomers into the fibrin polymer. Heparin via antithrombin prevents thrombin activation of fibrinogen.[39,68,82] The local thrombolytic action of plasmin can degrade the fibrin meshwork. Excess plasmin, if not prevented by antiplasmin activity, acts on both fibrin and fibrinogen, leading to a variety of fibrinogen degradation products.

The synthesis of fibrinogen, like most other coagulation factors (except factor VIII), occurs in the liver and the volume of distribution is similar to many other coagulation factors (II, V, VII, IX, XI). A quantitative coagulation factor level can be a helpful guide to predicting levels of other coagulation factors. A normal fibrinogen level is between 150 to 350 mg/dl. The monitoring of a fibrinogen level during acute blood loss and replacement with whole blood or packed red cells can help define whether the problem is purely a dilutional decline or whether consumption of coagulation factors is also contributing to the decline. During packed red cell replacement, the decline in coagulation factors and fibrinogen levels generally decreases approximately 50% for each blood volume loss if dilution is the only factor contributing to the decrease (Fig. 45-3). When whole blood or modified whole blood is used for replacement because fibrinogen is stable during storage, a decline in fibrinogen levels based on dilution would not be anticipated.[50,54,59,60,62] If a consumptive coagulopathy or disseminated intravascular coagulation occurs, the fibrinogen level will decrease much faster than would be anticipated based on dilution with packed cell replacement.[62] The presence of a decreasing fibrinogen level during whole blood transfusion suggests a consumptive coagulation process that is activating and consuming fibrinogen.[59,60] Like the other coagulation factors, fibrinogen levels can decrease to 30% of normal levels before a coagulopathy develops. Fibrinogen levels of 75 to 100 mg/dl are associated with a clinical bleeding tendency.[11,62] Clin-

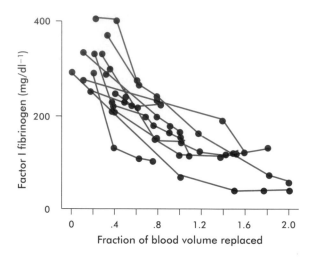

Fig. 45-3. Decreases in fibrinogen levels when packed red cells are used to replace blood loss during major elective surgery. (From Murray DJ, Olson J, Strauss R et al: Coagulation changes during packed red cell replacement of major blood loss, *Anesthesiology* 69:839, 1988.)

ical situations associated with consumption of coagulation factors can result in rapid changes in fibrinogen levels and are difficult to predict and monitor in clinical practice without assessments of fibrinogen levels.[11,54,62,65]

The fibrinogen level measures the level of the inactive precursor coagulation protein. This fibrinogen level does not assess the qualitative coagulation function of the protein.[46] Abnormal fibrinogen may be synthesized in severe liver disease, resulting in a dysfibrinogenemia and abnormal hemostasis. The hemostatic events that lead to the conversion of fibrinogen to fibrin in the final step in the coagulation cascade are also not assessed by a fibrinogen level determination. The fibrin clot formed may dissolve or may be prevented from final clot formation by circulating anticoagulants even though a normal fibrinogen level is present. Despite these limitations, the fibrinogen level may be of considerable value in predicting the level of other coagulation factors present and assessing the relative balance between dilution and consumption of coagulation factors when assessing hemostasis during major surgery.

A fibrinogen level between 150 and 350 mg/dl is normal; however, during pregnancy and in certain disease states, such as the recovery period after major trauma or burns, the physiologic response is an increase in fibrinogen levels, and the interpretation of a normal level in certain patients should be done in combination with an understanding of the changes associated with underlying conditions or disease.

Thrombin time. The thrombin time measures the duration between thrombin activation and the conversion of fibrinogen to fibrin formation. In the presence of normal fibrinogen levels, the test is sensitive to factors that might prevent or limit the conversion of fibrinogen to fibrin (i.e., abnormal fibrinogen, antithrombin effect of heparin or circulatory inhibitors, such as fibrinogen degradation products).[4,5] The thrombin time is prolonged with low fibrinogen levels, dysfibrinogenemia, use of heparin, and when fibrin degradation products interfere with fibrin polymerization. Additional variations of the thrombin time are available to define the specific problem preventing the conversion of fibrinogen to fibrin. Measuring a thrombin time in the presence of reptilase can help define whether the abnormality in thrombin time is related to heparin or other inhibitors of hemostases. Reptilase activates fibrinogen and produces a fibrin clot, because heparin does not inhibit this action of reptilase or fibrinogen; a normal reptilase time when combined with a prolonged thrombin time suggests a heparin effect.

Activated coagulation time. Similar to the other in vitro tests of coagulation, the activated coagulation time (ACT) (Box 45-3) is measured after whole blood is exposed to a specific activator of coagulation.[30] The time for in vitro clot formation (90 to 120 seconds) after whole blood is exposed to diatomaceous earth (celite) was defined as the ACT. Early in development, this test was found to be relatively insensitive to abnormalities in coagulation factor levels; but **the linear ACT increase with increasing doses of heparin provided a convenient method to monitor heparin's anticoagulant effect.**[72] The anticoagulation range required for cardiopulmonary bypass could be rapidly and predictably assessed with measurement of the ACT.[37,85,87] Unlike other in vitro coagulation tests that are profoundly abnormal in the presence of very low levels of circulatory heparin, the ACT increases in measurable increments from control levels with increasing heparin doses. Although the ACT test is simple, it lacks sensitivity to clotting abnormalities. When a normal activated coagulation time is obtained, serious clinical disorders of coagulation factors and platelets can be present. In addition, because small amounts of heparin can have profound effects on coagulation and produce little abnormality in the ACT, this test may not be an accurate method to ensure that no circulating heparin is present at the conclusion of cardiopulmonary bypass.[72]

Thromboelastogram (TEG). When multiple coagulation defects are possible, particularly after cardiopulmonary bypass and during liver transplantation,[42,77] an in vitro bedside coagulation test that separates various stages of clot formation including platelet activation, the formation of fibrin, and clot retraction would provide valuable information. At present, multiple coagulation tests are required to assess various steps of hemostasis. The thromboelastrogram assesses viscoelastic properties of whole blood and may be a useful perioperative screening test. Whole blood is placed in a heated rotating cuvette with a piston suspended, and, using an electronic amplification system, a tracing is recorded that helps define the viscoelastic properties of blood. The characteristic tracing can be quantified to provide information about initial platelet activation and fibrin formation as well as an index of clot retraction. The test may be less sensitive and specific than other in vitro coagulation tests, such as the PT, aPTT, platelet count, and fibrinogen levels, but may provide an overall assessment, which when normal, suggests that all elements involved in hemostasis are adequate for surgical hemostasis.

Whether enough information is available to use an abnormal TEG result to determine which component therapy should be administered is currently under investigation, primarily because of limited experience with interpretation and significance of an abnormal thromboelastogram tracing. When combined with other tests of coagulation, the TEG may provide relevant information about the adequacy of platelet function or the presence of clot lysis. At present, problems with platelet function and clot lysis frequently complicate cardiopulmonary bypass and liver transplantation and are difficult to evaluate rapidly in the operating room. This bedside test may help define that subset of patients who may benefit from platelet replacement despite adequate numbers of circulating platelets or in whom epsilon-aminocaproic acid might be indicated for the management of serious clot lysis.[41,42,77,84] More experience is required to define the role of this unique test in the perioperative setting. **At**

present, the test is a useful qualitative guide to *exclude* **significant coagulation disorders in the perioperative period,**[77] **but whether an abnormal TEG should be the basis to administer blood components requires further evaluation.**

MONITORING IN SPECIAL CIRCUMSTANCES
Cardiopulmonary Bypass

The dilution of vascular volume to prime the bypass circuit, contact activation of coagulation proteins and platelets from the surfaces of the artificial circulation, and the interface of blood with an oxygen exchanger (membrane or bubble oxygenator)[22] as well as the residual effects of heparin or heparin rebound may all contribute to development of a coagulopathy after cardiopulmonary bypass.[2,34,45,53] Although administering heparin prevents coagulation factor activation, heparin may also contribute to a qualitative and quantitative change in platelets during and after cardiopulmonary bypass.

Heparin

The rapid and profound activation of hemostasis associated with cardiopulmonary bypass was an early problem that limited the use of extracorporeal circuits. Heparin, which has multiple effects on coagulation, was an effective anticoagulant that prevented the activation of clotting when blood is exposed to the cardiopulmonary bypass circuit.[19,39] The optimal heparin dose and the subsequent monitoring of anticoagulation is based on the extent of the heparin effect to prevent macroscopic evidence of clot formation as well as microscopic activation of coagulation factors that can lead to an indolent activation of coagulation factors.[10,37,40,85,87] If anticoagulation is inadequate at any time during extracorporeal circulation, activation of coagulation factor occurs and the decrease in coagulation factors leads to bleeding problems during the perioperative period.

The initial dose of heparin required during cardiopulmonary bypass is based on pharmacokinetic principles of heparin distribution and metabolism.[10,40,85,87] Heparin is a strongly acidic drug that is bound to plasma protein and has a volume of distribution primarily limited to the plasma volume.[39] Factors that alter vascular volume are important in altering heparin dosage. The pharmacodynamic effect of heparin on anticoagulation is primarily the result of an interaction with antithrombin III that, when combined with heparin, prevents activation of thrombin. This interaction explains the occasional failure to achieve adequate anticoagulation in patients with decreased antithrombin III levels.[34,40,68]

The heparin concentration that results from an

intravenous dose is variable and depends on distribution and metabolism kinetics. In addition, the anticoagulant effect from a specific heparin level is also variable, depending on the sensitivity of a patient's coagulation system to heparin.[40] For this reason, heparin concentrations alone are not sufficient to indicate effective anticoagulation for cardiopulmonary bypass.

The activated clotting time (ACT) of whole blood,[30] **a simple bedside test, was adopted to monitor heparin anticoagulation during cardiopulmonary bypass.**[33] **More than a million patients who have undergone open heart procedures over the last two decades have had the adequacy of heparin anticoagulation measured with the ACT test. With a few modifications to improve the interpretation of the end point of the test (clot formation), the basic method is similar to its first description by Hattersley in 1966.**[30] **The linear increase in the ACT that occurs with increasing anticoagulant effect of heparin and the simplicity and rapid assessment of anticoagulation are distinct advantages of the ACT. The goal of anticoagulation during cardiopulmonary bypass is to provide enough anticoagulation to prevent activation of coagulation factors.**[87] **If an ACT of greater than 400 seconds is maintained during cardiopulmonary bypass, minimal evidence of coagulation factor activation is observed and fewer postoperative coagulation factor abnormalities are present.**[85,87] The normal ACT value ranges from 90 to 120 seconds. Although an individual dose response for heparin can be determined for each patient by using a smaller dose of heparin and checking the ACT,[11] this method is time consuming. The usual heparin requirements to achieve an ACT greater than 400 seconds is 3000 to 5000 IU/kg of body weight. At present, predicting the response of the ACT to this heparin dose is not possible, and effective coagulation must be checked before the initiation of cardiopulmonary bypass.

Alternative methods to predict heparin requirements or maintain heparin levels before or during cardiopulmonary bypass have not proved reliable. Additional doses of heparin may be required during cardiopulmonary bypass based on the response of the ACT, particularly since the half-life of heparin activity is 100 to 200 minutes. Although an initial ACT of greater than 400 seconds can easily be achieved, the dilution associated with the bypass circuit and the use of hypothermia during cardiopulmonary bypass alter heparin metabolism. In addition, hypothermia increases the ACT. Maintenance of adequate anticoagulation during hypothermic cardiopulmonary bypass is frequently more difficult to predict and requires continuous monitoring to assure adequate levels of anticoagulation.

Following the conclusion of cardiopulmonary bypass, heparin reversal with protamine is based on the reaction of protamine (a basic protein) with heparin (an acidic protein); reversal is based on a milligram of protamine for each 1000 IU of heparin. The use of the ACT as a method to initiate and maintain profound but measurable levels of anticoagulation during cardiopulmonary bypass is a valuable test, but the test by its nature is not sensitive to low levels of heparin or to decreases in platelet levels or coagulation factors. For this reason, the presence of a normal ACT may not be as good an indicator of complete heparin reversal as is the ACT level of greater than 400 seconds for the maintenance and initiation of cardiopulmonary bypass.

Alternative methods that assess the presence of heparin by testing the clotting time of blood in the presence of various titers of protamine (protamine titration) or a modified thrombin time are more sensitive to the presence of heparin and represent a more specific method to define whether the reversal of heparin is complete at the conclusion of cardiopulmonary bypass.

In view of the variability associated with heparin doses and the multiple effects of heparin on anticoagulation during cardiopulmonary bypass, a search for a more specific and predictable method to achieve anticoagulation as well as to monitor anticoagulation might result in an improvement in the hemostatic complications associated with cardiopulmonary bypass (Box 45-4). The most important modifications of systemic anticoagulation and monitoring of anticoagulation would be based on development of methods to more accurately predict, monitor, and prevent the

---

**BOX 45-4
METHODS TO IMPROVE ANTICOAGULATION DURING CARDIOPULMONARY BYPASS**

A drug or method that would predictably affect a single integral aspect of coagulation rather than have multiple anticoagulant effects

Anticoagulant effect unaltered by underlying disease or conditions

Distribution of anticoagulant drug more predictable

Metabolism of anticoagulant drug predictable and unaltered by hypothermia or underlying disease

Level of drug and anticoagulant effect that are integrally related and easily monitored

Reversal of drug possible with antagonist or technique that has no hemodynamic, hemostatic, or other sequelae

Method of monitoring that could reliably assess both the level of anticoagulant drug and the anticoagulant effect

irreversible coagulation problems associated with cardiopulmonary bypass.

Despite the titration of heparin according to the ACT and the use of protamine for reversal of heparin, multiple coagulation defects can occur after cardiopulmonary bypass. The hemostatic problems can lead to unrelenting bleeding in the perioperative period and represent a diagnostic challenge to the clinician. Various aspects of the bypass circuit contribute to the global problems that occur with coagulation after cardiopulmonary bypass. The decrease in platelet count associated with cardiopulmonary bypass is greater than anticipated with dilution alone and suggests a destruction or aggregation of platelets in the peripheral circulation.[34,79] In some patients use of heparin leads to thrombocytopenia. Large doses of heparin decrease platelet counts, and although a recovery in platelet level does not occur after the reversal of anticoagulation, significant abnormalities of platelet function persist, suggesting that many of the platelet abnormalities created by cardiopulmonary bypass are irreversible. In addition, additional abnormalities associated with major operative procedures can lead to increased bleeding in the perioperative period.

A list of potential causes of bleeding in the perioperative period includes:

- **Defects in vascular integrity (leaks in proximal or distal graft sites, sternal bleeding, bleeding aortotomy sites, etc.)**
- **Platelet abnormalities: quantitative decreases in platelet count; abnormal function of circulating platelets**
- **Coagulation factor abnormalities (residual heparin effect, coagulation factor deficiency related to dilution, consumption of coagulation factors due to microthrombi, and contact activation of factors during cardiopulmonary bypass)**
- **Contact activation of coagulation factors leads to activation of the fibrinolytic system; fibrin degradation products act as anticoagulants**

The identification and differentiation of medical from surgical causes of bleeding after cardiopulmonary bypass need to be formulated quickly, particularly since cardiac tamponade can result from excessive mediastinal bleeding. The differentation of a coagulopathy that requires blood component therapy or drug treatment, such as aminocaproic acid, from a vascular disruption requiring immediate surgical intervention is one of the key concerns in the care of the postoperative cardiopulmonary bypass patient. A viscoelastic bedside test of coagulation, the TEG, **is gaining acceptance as a test that may be helpful in differentiating problems related to coagulation function vs. surgical hemostasis.**[77] The frequency of false-positive and false-negative TEG tracings has not been addressed and this test currently must be considered an adjunct to coagulation monitoring methods in the operating room. Coagulation tests that provide rapid and relevant information about normal and abnormal surgical hemostasis would be an asset to the intraoperative management of many patients who have qualitative platelet abnormalities or problems with clot lysis after cardiopulmonary bypass surgery.

Massive Blood Loss
Blood replacement therapy

Vascular volume replacement, an adequate red cell mass, maintenance of acid-base balance, biochemical and thermal homeostases become of paramount importance during surgery associated with massive blood loss. One of the most serious consequences of massive blood loss is the development of a coagulopathy that contributes further to the exsanguination of the patient and often leads to a lethal operative outcome.[11,32,54,65]

A framework for assessing coagulation monitoring in massive blood loss might address these questions:

- **What is the relationship between coagulation factor loss and coagulation factor replaced (dilutional coagulopathy)? Are whole blood, undiluted whole blood, or packed cells used for replacement?**
- **Is a dilutional coagulopathy the only problem or is an ongoing consumptive coagulopathy also contributing to the problem? How is the diagnosis of these two problems separated by hemostatic testing?**
- **When and what blood components will be necessary to treat the coagulopathy?**

In situations when massive blood loss is anticipated, the preoperative coagulation assessment, whether normal or abnormal, provides a framework to base replacement of blood and hemostatic function. If the patient has multiple coagulopathies related to end-stage liver disease or has normal coagulation function, the dilutional hemostatic changes associated with blood replacement of massive blood loss alone are relatively simple to manage. The perioperative management of a patient experiencing massive blood loss associated not only with dilutional coagulopathy but with an ongoing disseminated coagulation problem is far more difficult to predict.

A shift to red cell components rather than whole blood over the last 20 years has required clinicians to reassess the role of dilutional changes in coagulation factors associated with major blood loss in the perioperative period. A rough guide to coagulation factor levels and platelets present in the circulation can be determined by an assessment of what coagulation factors are being lost during surgery and what

70 kg Man
Blood volume = 5000 ml

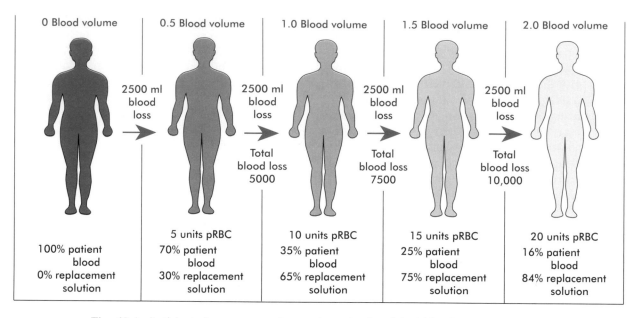

Fig. 45-4. Anticipated percentage changes in patient's original blood volume as replacement solutions are administered to replace blood loss.

solutions are being used to replace vascular volume and red cell losses (Fig. 45-4).[17,52,59,60,62] **Packed cells contain only a small amount of coagulation factor activity and no platelets, so replacement therapy with packed cells and crystalloid provides minimal hemostatic activity.** An estimate of platelet counts and coagulation factor levels might reasonably be based on these considerations.[18,62] These estimations of coagulation levels based on dilution alone tend to underestimate coagulation factor level because many coagulation factors and platelets are distributed to more than the vascular space and are also released into the circulation.[16,60,62] If disseminated coagulopathy is also present, coagulation factor estimates based on dilution may be overestimated. Activation of coagulation factors occurs when tissue thromboplastin is released into the circulation, when tissue trauma is severe,[32,54] or when shock has led to ischemic tissue injury.[28,74] These events lead to coagulation factor consumption and are particularly difficult to predict, monitor, and quantitate during a major operative procedure. When disseminated coagulopathy is present, the requirements for platelets and coagulation factors are much greater than estimates based on the dilutional formula. This is one of the primary reasons that prophylactic platelets or clotting components fail to restore hemostatic function and are not indicated in situations of dilutional or disseminated coagulopathy.[11,60,65,69,73]

Platelets[16,60,62] and factor VIII[11,62] have substantial circulatory reserve and if losses of these two coagulation determinants are based on dilution alone, the measured levels will frequently be greater than predicted based on dilution formula. For coagulation factors synthesized in the liver with volumes of distribution limited to the vascular space, the decline in coagulation factor activity more predictably follows dilution (fibrinogen, factors IX and V levels)[62] (see Fig. 45-3). If the replacement solution is packed red cells that contain minimal coagulation factor activity or platelets, then based on simple dilution after the loss of one blood volume, the percent of the original circulating volume (i.e., coagulation factor levels and platelets) would be 30% to 40%.

If whole blood or modified whole blood (platelets removed) is used for replacement, the activity of most coagulation factors will be maintained for at least the first 2 weeks of storage.[61] Factors V and VIII are labile in storage and decline to levels of 50% after 2 weeks of storage and slowly fall thereafter during storage. For the duration of whole blood storage, coagulation factors V and VIII activity is still adequate to provide effective surgical hemostasis. Platelets decline rapidly during the first 24 hours of whole blood storage, and the major dilutional problem during whole blood transfusion is thrombocytopenia. Based on dilution alone, platelet counts should be at least 30% of initial values after the replacement of an entire vascular volume with whole blood if dilution alone is responsible for coagulation. The declines in coagulation factor level would lead to abnormalities in the PT because this test is sensitive to factor V concentrations of less that 50% of normal.[51,57,62,83] Even with an increased PT, coagulation factor replacement in the form of FFP is not necessary until the PT and an aPTT are greater than 1.5 times control, a level that would be associated with coagulation factor levels of less than 30% of normal levels. It should be understood that dilutional changes can be predicted, but consumption of coagulation factors frequently occurs in situations of severe bleeding, and coagulation factor assessment may be difficult to predict based on dilutional formulas alone. In this setting, a fibrinogen level and platelet count are helpful because a decline greater than predicted on dilutional formulas alone would help confirm the presence of a disseminated coagulopathy.

In summary, when whole blood is used to replace blood loss, increased bleeding from thromocytopenia occurs before coagulation factor declines. If dilution alone is present, coagulation factor replacement is rarely necessary during whole blood replacement.[59] In the majority of patients who receive replacement packed red cells, a significant coagulopathy based on decreased platelet counts will also be observed before the need for coagulation factor replacement.[62] The dilutional decline in fibrinogen levels and factor V levels may lead to a coagulopathy requiring treatment when greater than one blood volume loss has occurred during packed red cell replacement.[62]

Autologous transfusion using blood scavenging techniques is an additional source of a dilutional decrease in coagulation factors and platelets. The use of the cell saver is an effective autologous method to decrease homologous red cell requirements, but red cell solutions are devoid of coagulation proteins as a result of the red cell washing to remove cellular debris. Failure to consider autologous replacement solutions will lead to a further dilutional decline in coagulation factors.

Disseminated consumption of coagulation factors and platelets as a result of shock, sepsis, or thromboplastin release into the circulation may occur in hypovolemic or septic shock, obstetric emergencies, or hemolytic transfusion reaction and lead to diffuse microvascular bleeding. Dramatic declines in platelet counts and fibrinogen levels may occur later after attention to the primary cause of the consumptive process. Correction of platelet counts and coagulation factor levels should be the focus of therapy, and blood components may be required. The use of fibrinolytic therapy or heparin is occasionally beneficial in this setting, provided attention has been directed to alleviating the primary problem that led to coagulation factor consumption.

Disseminated Intravascular Coagulation

Disseminated intravascular coagulation (DIC) is a poor descriptor for the spectrum of coagulation problems and variety of clinical conditions included within the definition of this syndrome.[9,13,25] The bleeding and hypocoagulable condition associated with the syndrome is the major manifestation rather than coagulation and thrombi in the microcirculation, as the term DIC implies.[55] A variable consumption of coagulation factors associated with circulatory anti-coagulants complicates treatment. At present, the best approach is to treat the primary disease process that has initiated DIC and support circulatory and hemostatic functions.

The physiology and pathology of clot formation have been elucidated by studies of patients with congenital and acquired coagulation disorders, but the spectrum of coagulation disorders associated with clot dissolution or clotting factor consumption is poorly understood (Box 45-5). Therapies directed at clot dissolution in acute myocardial infarction and acute pulmonary embolus with substances such as tissue plasminogen activators, streptokinase, and urokinase have been a major advance in acute thrombotic disorders. The serious bleeding complica-

---

BOX 45-5
CAUSES OF DISSEMINATED INTRAVASCULAR COAGULATION

Release of substances (tissue thromboplastin or cellular damage) leading to activation of coagulation

Acute
  Amniotic fluid embolism
  Abruptio placentae
  Tissue trauma (burns and tissue injury)
  Extracorporeal circulation
  Hemolytic transfusion reaction
  Near-drowning
Chronic
  Neoplasia
  Leukemia

Endothelial damage leading to coagulation factor activation

  Meningococcemia
  Viremia
  Hemolytic uremic syndrome
  Preeclampsia
  Transplant rejection
  Trauma and shock
  Dissecting aortic aneurysm
  Giant arteriovenous malformation
  Heat stroke
  Gram-negative sepsis

tions that may occur with thrombolytic therapy clearly indicate the importance of balance between clot formation and clot lysis and may enhance understanding of bleeding problems associated with extensive clot lysis.

Multiple clinical conditions can lead to an intravascular activation of the coagulation system that may be followed by clot lysis. Whether tissue thromboplastin activates clotting factors or activation of clot lysis consumes inactive circulatory coagulation factors, the result is a decline in coagulation factors and a syndrome known as DIC.

Almost all severe systemic disorders have been associated with a DIC syndrome that often occurs as a preterminal event, probably as a result of thromboplastin release from hypoxic, ischemic tissue beds.[7,28,78] A subset of conditions results in DIC when a large amount of thromboplastin-like substances are released into the circulation. The presence of endothelial cell damage is the basis for activation of coagulation that may lead to the syndrome of DIC. Amniotic fluid embolism, a hemolytic transfusion reaction, or abruptio placentae leads to activation of coagulation factors because of the release of thromboplastin into the circulation. A more chronic disseminated intravascular coagulation can occur (preeclampsia, sepsis, hemangioma) when vascular defects lead to the activation of coagulation factors and subsequent activation of clot dissolution. The coagulopathy has variable features depending on which aspect of coagulation is operative—excessive clot activation from thromboplastin or secondary clot lysis. The activation of coagulation factors in these conditions is followed by a profound decline in coagulation factor levels and activation of clot lysis. The presence of both coagulation factor activation and circulating anticoagulants makes the supportive care of patients with disorders a therapeutic dilemma. Often, not only is the replacement of deficient coagulation factors required, but methods to prevent activation of coagulation factors with the use of heparin. Alternatively, if the problem is believed to be excessive plasmin, the use of an inhibitor of plasminogen such as epsilon aminocaprioc acid (Amicar) may be considered. The delicate balance that is already disturbed in this syndrome makes therapy difficult. Without treatment and arrest of the underlying problem that caused DIC, this syndrome is frequently lethal.

Supportive therapy with coagulation factors, platelets, and occasionally an anticoagulant, heparin, or an agent that prevents clot lysis by an effect on plasminogen (epsilon aminocaproic acid) may be required while the underlying cause of DIC is treated. DIC is often observed as part of a terminal event and frequently signals irreversible multisystem organ failure. In such circumstances, often multiple factors have led to activation as well as consumption of coagulation factors.

INTRAOPERATIVE BLOOD SALVAGE

Scavenging blood loss at operative sites offers an effective method to decrease homologous transfusion.[8,26] Intraoperative scavenging may be a problem if (1) blood is contaminated by bowel contents or wound infection with bacterial organisms, (2) surgery for neoplasia creates a risk of intravenous tumor dissemination, (3) wound irritants (Betadine, neomycin) are aspirated into the suction device, or (4) damage of scavenged cells by excessive suctioning and the use of topical coagulants lead to hemolysis and cellular debris.

The simpler methods of scavenging include a self-contained collection and administration device that, when full, filters the blood and returns it to the patient. This method is primarily intended for postoperative use. The aspiration of citrated or heparinized blood collected from the surgical field, placed in a reservoir, and then processed and washed of debris from the cells using a cell saver device is more frequently used to create a red cell concentrate for reinfusion. **Blood loss must be anticipated to be at least 500 to 1000 ml to yield at least one processed red cell unit when automated cell scavenging systems are used.**[36,64,76,80]

The surgical procedure often dictates the degree of red cell processing required to prevent the reinfusion of free hemoglobin or cellular debris. In procedures in which systemic anticoagulation is used, such as cardiopulmonary bypass, or when rapid intermittent blood loss occurs (aneurysm repair), aspiration of tissue debris may be less problematic and wash cycles for scavenged red cells may not need to be extensive to provide a pure red cell concentrate.[58] In orthopedic procedures where blood loss is continuous throughout the procedure, tissue and bone debris and hemolyzed cells will be present in the collection device. Reinfused cellular debris may act as thromboplastin and initiate intravascular coagulation; for this reason wash cycles should be more extensive.[27,31]

The processed red cell concentrates, like packed red cells, contain minimal amounts of coagulation factors and may contribute to the dilutional coagulopathy of massive transfusion.

COAGULATION FACTOR REPLACEMENT

Plasma components with active coagulation factor activity include the following:
- Fresh frozen plasma
- Single donor plasma
- Cryoprecipitate

- Factor VIII concentrate
- Factor IX concentrate

Specific factor concentrations provide replacement for patients with isolated congenital or acquired coagulation factor deficiencies. The indication and effective dosages are outlined in Chapter 20. The goal of providing a specific coagulation factor has been realized for the congenital hemophilias. Cryoprecipitate, a fibrinogen- and factor VIII-rich preparation, provides replacement for von Willebrand factor and the rare patients with congenital fibrinogen or fibronectin deficits.

Coagulation factor replacement may be required in patients with acquired coagulation factor deficits, such as liver disease, DIC, dilutional coagulopathy of blood loss, or a coagulopathy after cardiopulmonary bypass. Multiple coagulation factor deficits may exist simultaneously, and the use of fresh frozen plasma is the most appropriate replacement. The coagulation factor replacement in one unit of fresh frozen plasma should increase coagulation factor levels by approximately 7% to 10% in a 70-kg male. If a reasonable goal of coagulation factor replacement is to achieve levels of 30%, a significant volume of fresh frozen plasma may be required when coagulation factors are indicated.

Although the routine prescription of fresh frozen plasma in patients with acquired coagulation deficits does not prevent microvascular bleeding, a subset of patients requires aggressive, ongoing replacement of coagulation factors to control microvascular bleeding from coagulopathy associated with massive transfusion,[11] DIC,[65] or after cardiopulmonary bypass. For patients in whom an ongoing coagulopathy develops, the maintenance of coagulation factor levels of 30% may require multiple units of fresh frozen plasma. It is difficult to identify these patients on a prospective basis. Coagulation monitoring needs to be frequent and timely results must be provided on which to base coagulation factor replacement.

Because fibrinogen or factor VIII problem alone rarely has led to a surgical coagulopathy, use of cryoprecipitate should not be an initial therapy in the acquired bleeding disorders found perioperatively.

DESMOPRESSIN, APROTININ, AND ANTIFIBRINOLYSIS

The role of pharmacologic agents in treating fibrinolysis (such as epsilon aminocaproic acid and tranexamic acid) is based on the concept that excessive plasmin leads to clot dissolution and circulating anticoagulants are contributory to or are primarily responsible for coagulation defects and abnormal bleeding.[2,35,36,45,56] Little information is available to support this concept, but a salutary effect in decreasing blood loss and in the therapy of severe coagulopathies has been reported during cardiopulmonary bypass and during the massive blood loss associated with liver transplant.[35,41,42,84] **The basis of this therapy is the inhibition of plasmin and the prevention of clot dissolution.**

Aprotinin may act as a plasmin inhibitor and perhaps prevent platelet membrane abnormalities believed to occur during cardiopulmonary bypass.[21,70,49] Desmopressin decreases bleeding time[44] and also is believed to prevent the qualitative platelet defect observed in patients during cardiopulmonary bypass and may be helpful in decreasing blood loss during spinal surgery.[44] The prospective use of desmopressin and aprotinin during cardiopulmonary bypass is under investigation. Preliminary reports with desmopressin appear promising. The major concerns relate to the shift of the coagulation balance from excessive clot dissolution to a situation that favors arterial and venous thrombosis. Improved understanding of the primary mechanism that alters the balance between clot formation and dissolution will help to establish fibrinolytic therapy as a more rational scientific basis approach rather than a "last-ditch" effort to treat a hemorrhaging patient. More recent investigations of desmopressin suggest a limited salutary effect, particularly in patients with uncomplicated cardiopulmonary bypass.[67]

KEY POINTS

- A simple and therefore useful way to describe perioperative bleeding is to divide it into causes related to vascular factors, platelet factors, coagulation cascade abnormalities, and clot retraction pathologic conditions.

- Current therapeutic nihilism toward any and all preoperative laboratory testing should be discarded with respect to many patients who are suspected of or are at risk for having possible bleeding disorders perioperatively.

- The prothrombin time (PT) and the activated partial thromboplastin time (aPTT) are currently the most appropriate approaches for individual screening and to monitor hemostatic therapy.
- The PT and aPTT become abnormal when coagulation factor activity decreases to 50% of normal levels.
- Some data suggest that coagulation factor activity of 30% or more provides reasonable hemostasis during the perioperative period, but the "ideal" activity levels are uncertain. Waiting to transfuse coagulation factors until there is microvascular bleeding is too late; but conversely, during major surgery, attempting to maintain all in vitro coagulation tests within laboratory normal limits is probably excessive.
- Understanding the usefulness of obtaining a bleeding time, for example, before use of epidural anesthesia in a patient with preeclampsia, is rapidly becoming a key test to assess platelet function.
- Monitoring fibrinogen levels is a helpful method in determining the contribution of coagulation factor

dilution and consumption to coagulopathy in the setting of massive blood loss.
- Other tests, such as the thrombin time and the activated coagulation time, have specific uses during various kinds of surgery (e.g., the use of the activated coagulation time during cardiopulmonary bypass).
- Although it has many problems, the ACT does seem to have a reasonable linear increase with increasing blood levels of heparin and does represent a convenient method to measure heparin's anticoagulation effect. The newer protamine titration methods have *not* been shown to be any more effective than the activated coagulation time in this particular regard.
- Bleeding following cardiopulmonary bypass surgery is frequently a multifactorial problem requiring rapid diagnosis and treatment.
- Thromboelastography will also (perhaps) be a useful test in the near future in cardiovascular procedures.

KEY REFERENCES

Bennett JS: Blood coagulation and coagulation tests, *Med Clin North Am* 68:557, 1984.

Bowie EJ, Owen CA: Clinical pathology of intravascular coagulation, *Bibl Hematolog* 49:217, 1983.

Ciavarella D, Reed RL, Counts RB et al: Clotting factor levels and the risk of diffuse microvascular bleeding in the massively transfused patient, *Br J Haematol* 67:365, 1987.

Colman RW, Marder VJ: Disseminated intravascular coagulation (DIC): pathogenesis, pathophysiology, and laboratory abnormalities. In Colman RW, Hirsh KJ, Marder J et al, eds: *Hemostasis and thrombosis: basic principles and clinical practice,* Philadelphia, 1982, JB Lippincott.

Consensus Conference: Fresh-frozen plasma, indications and risks, *JAMA* 253:551, 1985.

Consensus Conference: Platelet transfusion therapy, *JAMA* 257:1777, 1987.

Eisenberg JM, Clarke JR, and Sissman SA: Prothrombin and partial thromboplastin time as preoperative screening tests, *Arch Surg* 117:48-51, 1982.

Jobes DR, Schwartz AJ, Ellison N et al: Monitoring heparin anticoagulation and its neutralization, *Ann Thorac Surg* 31:161, 1981.

Mannucci PM, Federici AB, and Sirchia G: Hemostasis testing during massive blood replacement. A study of 172 cases, *Vox Sang* 42:113, 1982.

Murray DJ, Olson J, Strauss R et al: Coagulation changes during packed red cell replacement of major blood loss, *Anesthesiology* 69:839, 1988.

Rosenberg RD: Actions and interactions of antithrombin and heparin, *N Engl J Med* 292:146, 1975.

Weiss HJ: Platelet physiology and abnormalities of platelet function, *N Engl J Med* 293:531, 1975.

REFERENCES

1. Aggeler PM: Physiological basis for transfusion therapy in hemorrhagic disorders: a critical review, *Transfusion* 1:71, 1961.
2. Bachmann F, McKenna R, Cole ER et al: The hemostatic mechanism after open heart surgery. 1. Studies on plasma coagulation factors and fibrinolysis in 512 patients after extracorporeal circulation, *J Thorac Cardiovas Surg* 70:76, 1975.
3. Barentsky NG, Weinstein P: Partial thromboplastin time for screening, *Ann Intern Med* 91:498, 1979 (letter).
4. Bennett JS: Blood coagulation and coagulation tests, *Med Clin North Am* 68:557, 1984.
5. Bick RL, Bick MD, and Fekete LF: Antithrombin III patterns in disseminated intravascular coagulation, *Am J Clin Pathol* 73:577, 1980.
6. Biggs R, Douglas AS: The thromboplastin generation test, *J Clin Pathol* 6:23, 1953.

7. Blaisdell WF, Lim RC, and Stawne RF: Mechanism of pulmonary damage following hemorrhagic shock, *Surg Gynecol Obstet* 130:15, 1970.

8. Bovill DF, Moulton CW, Jackson WS et al: The efficacy of intraoperative autologous transfusion in major orthopedic surgery: a regression analysis, *Orthopedics* 9:1403, 1986.

9. Bowie EJ, Owen CA: Clinical pathology of intravascular coagulation, *Bibl Hematol* 49:217, 1983.

10. Bull BS, et al: Hemodensitometry—a new technique for the study of hemostasis in open heart surgery, *Ann Thorac Surg* 18:516, 1974.

11. Ciavarella D, Reed RL, Counts RB et al: Clotting factor levels and the risk of diffuse microvascular bleeding in the massively transfused patient, *Br J Haematol* 67:365, 1987.

12. Collins JA: Problems associated with the massive transfusion of stored blood, *Surgery* 75:274, 1974.

13. Colman RW, Marder VJ: Disseminated intravascular coagulation (DIC): pathogenesis, pathophysiology, and laboratory abnormalities. In Colman RW, Hirsh KJ, Marder J et al, eds: *Hemostasis and thrombosis: basic principles and clinical practice,* Philadelphia, 1982, JB Lippincott.

14. Consensus Conference: Fresh-frozen plasma, indications and risks, *JAMA* 253:551, 1985.

15. Consensus Conference: Platelet transfusion therapy, *JAMA* 257:1777, 1987.

16. Cote CJ, Liu LMP, Szyfelbeink SK et al: Changes in serial platelet counts following massive blood transfusion in pediatric patients, *Anesthesiology* 62:197, 1985.

17. Counts RB, Haisch C, Simon TL et al: Hemostasis in massively transfused trauma patients, *Ann Surg* 190:91, 1979.

18. Cullen JJ, Murray DJ, and Kealey GP: Changes in coagulation factors in patients with burns during acute blood loss, *J Burn Care Rehabil* 6:517, 1989.

19. Damus PS, Hicks M, and Rosenberg RD: Anticoagulant action of heparin, *Nature* 246:355, 1973.

20. Diamond LK, Porter FS: Inadequacy of routine bleeding and clotting times, *N Engl J Med* 259:1025, 1958.

21. Dietrich W, Barankay A, Dilthey G et al: Reduction of homologous blood requirement in cardiac surgery by intraoperative aprotinin application: clinical experience in 152 cardiac surgical patients, *J Thorac Cardiovasc Surg* 37:92, 1989.

22. Edmunds LH, Ellison N, Colman RW et al: Platelet function during cardiac operation: comparison of membrane and bubble oxygenators, *J Thorac Cardiovasc Surg* 83:805, 1982.

23. Eika C, Havie O, and Godal HC: The value of preoperative haemostatic screening, *Scand J Haematol* 21:349, 1978.

24. Eisenberg JM, Clarke JR, and Sissman SA: Prothrombin and partial thromboplastin time as preoperative screening tests, *Arch Surg* 117:48, 1982.

25. Fruchtman S, Aledort LM: Disseminated intravascular coagulation, *J Am Coll Cardiol* 8:159B, 1986.

26. Giordano GF, Goldman DS, Mammana RB et al: Intraoperative autotransfusion in cardiac operations: effect on intraoperative and postoperative transfusion requirements, *J Thorac Cardiovasc Surg* 96:382, 1988.

27. Griffith LD, Billman GF, Daily PO et al: Apparent coagulopathy caused by infusion of shed mediastinal blood and its prevention by washing of the infusate, *Ann Thorac Surg* 47:400, 1989.

28. Hardenway RM, Chun B, and Rutherford RB: Coagulation in shock in various species including man, *Acta Chir Scand* 130:157, 1965.

29. Harker LA, Slichter SJ: The bleeding time is a screening test for evaluation of platelet function, *N Engl J Med* 287:155, 1972.

30. Hattersley PG: Activated coagulation time of whole blood, *JAMA* 196:150, 1966.

31. Hauer JM: Controversies in autotransfusion, *Vox Sang* 46:8, 1984.

32. Hewson JR, Neame PB, Kumar N et al: Coagulopathy related to dilution and hypotension during massive transfusion, *Crit Care Med* 13:387, 1985.

33. Hill JD, Dontigny L, Leval M et al: A simple method of heparin management during prolonged extracorporeal circulation, *Ann Thorac Surg* 17:129, 1974.

34. Holloway DS, Summaria L, Sandesara J et al: Decreased platelet number and function and increased fibrinolysis contribute to postoperative bleeding in cardiopulmonary bypass patients, *Thromb Haemost* 59:62, 1988.

35. Horrow JC, Hlavacek J, Strong MD et al: Prophlylactic tranexamic acid decreases bleeding after cardiac operations, *J Thorac Cardiovasc Surg* 99:70, 1990.

36. Huddleston CB, Hammon JW, Wareing TH et al: Amelioration of the deleterious effects of platelets activated during cardiopulmonary bypass: comparison of a thromboxane synthetase inhibitor and a prostacyclin analogue, *J Thorac Cardiovasc Surg* 89:190, 1985.

37. Jaberi M, Bell WR, and Benson DW: Control of heparin therapy in open heart surgery, *J Thorac Cardiovasc Surg* 67:133, 1974.

38. Jacobs LM, Hsieh JW: A clinical review of autotransfusion and its role in trauma, *JAMA* 251:3283, 1984.

39. Jacques LV: Heparin: an old drug with a new paradigm, *Science* 206:528, 1979.

40. Jobes DR, Schwartz AJ, Ellison N et al: Monitoring heparin anticoagulation and its neutralization, *Ann Thorac Surg* 31:161, 1981.

41. Kang Y, Lewis JH, Navalgund A et al: Epsilon aminocaproic acid for treatment of fibrinolysis during liver transplantation, *Anesthesiology* 66:766, 1987.

42. Kang YG, Martin DJ, Marquez J et al: Intraoperative changes in blood coagulation and thromboelastograph monitoring in liver transplantation, *Anesth Analg* 64:888, 1985.

43. Kelton JG, Blajchman MA: Platelet transfusions, *Can Med Assoc J* 121:1353, 1979.

44. Kobrinsky NL, Gerrard JM, Watson CM et al: Shortening of the bleeding time by DDAVP in various disorders, *Lancet* 1:1145, 1984.

45. Kucuk O, Kwaan HC, Fredrickson J et al: Increased fibrinolysis in patients undergoing cardiopulmonary bypass opration, *Am J Hematol* 23:223, 1986.

46. Lamme B, Griffin JH: Formation of the fibrin clot: the balance of procoagulant and inhibitory factors, *Clin Haematol* 14:281, 1985.

47. Langdell RD, Wagner RH, and Brinkhoos KM: The partial thromboplastin time, *J Lab Clin Invest* 41:637, 1953.

48. Levine PH: Platelet function tests: predictive value, *N Engl J Med* 292:1346, 1973.

49. Longmore DB, Hoyle PM, Gregory A et al: Prostacyclin administration during cardiopulmonary bypass in man, *Lancet* 1:800, 1981.

50. Lucas CE, Ledgerwood AM, and Mammen EF: Altered coagulation protein content after albumin resuscitation, *Ann Surg* 196:198, 1982.

51. Lucas CE, Ledgerwood AM: Clinical significance of altered coagulation tests after massive transfusions for trauma, *Ann Surg* 47:125, 1981.

52. Lundsgaard-Hansen P: Component therapy of surgical hemorrhage: red cell concentrates, colloids and crystalloids, *Bibl Haematol* 46:147, 1980.

53. Mammen EF, Koets MH, Washington BC et al: Hemostasis changes during cardiopulmonary bypass surgery, *Semin Thromb Hemost* 11:281, 1985.

54. Mannucci PM, Federici AB, and Sirchia G: Hemostasis testing during massive blood replacement. A study of 172 cases, *Vox Sang* 42:113, 1982.

55. Mant MJ, King EE: Severe, acute disseminated intravascular coagulation, *Am J Med* 67:557, 1979.

56. Marengo-Rowe AJ, and Leveson JE: Fibrinolysis: a frequent cause of bleeding. In Ellison N, Jobes DR, eds: *Effective hemostasis in cardiac surgery,* Philadelphia: Saunders, 1988.

57. Marler RA, Baner RT, Endres-Broohm JL et al: Comparison of the sensitivity of commercial aPTT reagents in the detection of mild coagulopathies, *Am J Clin Pathol* 82:436, 1984.

58. McShane AJ, Power C, Jackson JF et al: Autotransfusion: quality of blood prepared with a red cell processing device, *Br J Anaesth* 59:1035, 1987.

59. Miller RD, Robbins TO, Tong MJ et al: Coagulation defects associated with massive blood transfusions, *Ann Surg* 174:794, 1971.

60. Miller RD: Complications of massive blood transfusions, *Anesthesiology* 39:82, 1973.

61. Moore GL, Peck CC, Sohmer PP et al: Some properties of blood stored in anticoagulant CPDA-1 solution. A brief summary, *Transfusion* 21:135, 1981.

62. Murray DJ, Olson J, Strauss R et al: Coagulation changes during packed red cell replacement of major blood loss, *Anesthesiology* 69:839, 1988.

63. Ockelford PS, Carter CJ: Disseminated intravascular coagulation: the application

and utility of diagnostic tests, *Semin Thromb Hemost* 8:198, 1982.

64. Popovsky MA, Devine PA: Intraoperative autologous transfusion, *Mayo Clin Proc* 60:125-134, 1985.

65. Reed RL, Ciaverella D, Heinback DM et al: Prophylactic platelet administration during massive transfusion, *Ann Surg* 203:40, 1986.

66. Robbins JA, Rose SD: Partial thromboplastin time as a screening test, *Ann Intern Med* 90:796, 1979.

67. Rocha E, Llorens R, Paramo JA et al: Does desmopressin acetate reduce blood loss after surgery in patients on cardiopulmonary bypass? *Circulation* 77:1319, 1988.

68. Rosenberg RD: Actions and interactions of antithrombin and heparin, *N Engl J Med* 292:146, 1975.

69. Roy RC, Stafford MA, Hudspeth AS et al: Failure of prophylaxis with fresh frozen plasma after cardiopulmonary bypass, *Anesthesiology* 69:254, 1988.

70. Royston D, Bidstrup BP, Taylor KM et al: Effect of aprotinin on need for blood transfusion after repeat open heart surgery, *Lancet* 2:1289, 1987.

71. Sakata Y, Yoshida N, and Matsoda M: Treatment of DIC with antithrombin III concentrations. *Bibl Hematol* 49:307, 1983.

72. Schriever HG, Epstein SE, and Mintz MD: Statistical correlation and heparin sensitivity of activated partial thromboplastin time, whole blood coagulation time, and automated coagulation time, *Am J Clin Pathol* 60:323, 1973.

73. Simon TL, Akl BF, and Murphy W: Controlled trial of routine administration of platelet concentrates in cardiopulmonary bypass surgery, *Ann Thorac Surg* 37:359, 1984.

74. Slichter SJ, Funk DD, Leandoer LE et al: Kinetic evaluation of hemostasis during surgery and wound healing, *Br J Haematol* 27:115, 1974.

75. Slichter SJ: Identification and management of defects in platelet hemostasis in massively transfused patients. In: Collings JA, Murawski K, and Shafer AW, eds: *Massive transfusion in surgery and trauma,* New York, 1982, Alan R. Liss.

76. Solomon MD, Rutledge MR, Kane LE et al: Cost comparison of intraoperative autologous versus homologous transfusion, *Transfusion* 28:379, 1988.

77. Spiess BD, Tuman KJ, McCarthy RJ et al: Thromboelastography as an indicator of postcardiopulmonary bypass coagulopathies, *J Clin Monit* 3:25, 1987.

78. String T, Robinson JA, and Blaisdell WF: Massive trauma, *Arch Surg* 102:406, 1971.

79. Tanaka T, Takao M, Yada I et al: Alterations in coagulations and fibrinolysis associated with cardiopulmonary bypass during open heart surgery, *J Cardiothorac Anes* 3:181, 1989.

80. Tawes RL, Scribner RG, Duval TB et al: The cell saver and autologous transfusion: an underutilized resource in vascular surgery, *Am J Surg* 152:105, 1986.

81. Thaler E, Lechner K: Antithrombin III deficiency and thromboembolism, *Clin Haematol* 10:369, 1981.

82. Thomas DP: Heparin, *Clin Haematol* 9:443, 1981.

83. Turi DS, Peerschke EI: Sensitivity of three activated partial thromboplastin time reagents to coagulation factor deficiencies, *Am J Clin Pathol* 85:43, 1986.

84. Vander Salm TJ, Ansell JE, Oike ON et al: The role of epsilon aminocaproic acid in reducing bleeding after cardiac operation: a double-blind randomized study, *J Thorac Cardiovasc Surg* 95:538, 1989.

85. Verska JJ: Control of heparinization by activated clotting time during bypass with improved postoperative hemostasis, *Ann Thorac Surg* 24:170, 1977.

86. Weiss HJ: Platelet physiology and abnormalities of platelet function, *N Engl J Med* 293:531, 1975.

87. Young JA, Kisker CT, and Doty DB: Adequate anticoagulation during cardiopulmonary bypass determined by activated clotting time and the appearance of fibrin monomer, *Ann Thorac Surg* 26:231, 1978.

CHAPTER 46

Monitoring and Management of Perioperative Fluid and Electrolyte Therapy

MICHAEL J. SENDAK

Perioperative fluid and electrolyte therapy is an integral component of a patient's anesthetic management and can play a critical role in surgical outcome. Most patients receiving anesthetic care are given some type of intravenous fluid therapy during a surgical procedure. Replacement of water, ions, protein, and/or red cells is necessary to overcome the pathophysiologic effects of surgery and to treat any underlying or associated medical disorders complicated by body fluid derangements. Depending on the particular patient and the planned surgical procedure, there can be a marked difference in the complexity of the fluid therapy needed for appropriate restoration of intravascular volume losses. A healthy patient undergoing a relatively brief and limited procedure (associated with minimal blood loss) might be given 1 or 2 L of crystalloid solution without much concern directed toward the patient's overall balance of fluids and electrolytes. This somewhat cavalier approach to fluid management is usually well tolerated by adult patients with normal renal, pulmonary, and cardiovascular function. Unfortunately, such a simplistic approach is not acceptable for infants and children or for adults undergoing extensive surgical procedures—with or without significant blood loss. Likewise, patients with major organ system dysfunction, intravascular volume disturbances, and/or electrolyte abnormalities require careful monitoring and replacement of fluids and electrolytes during the perioperative period.

Intravascular volume replacement should not be solely directed by memorized formulas, personal preference, or institutional bias. Fluid therapy must be individualized for each patient, with consideration of the functional status of most organ systems and based on accepted principles of basic science and physiology. Most diseases and many injuries, including operative trauma, impose a considerable impact on the physiology of body fluids and electrolytes. Thus the magnitude of the surgical procedure—as well as the patient's age, size, and preoperative physical status—all significantly influence fluid management. To adeptly manage all varieties of surgical patients and to maximize the quality of anesthetic care, the practicing anesthesiologist must recognize these many factors and (1) understand the volume and composition of normal body fluids; (2) anticipate, identify, and assess alterations of the compartmentalized fluid constituents; and (3) appropriately rectify abnormalities of these constituents in a timely manner.

This chapter is devoted to a review of normal fluid, electrolyte, and red blood cell physiology. In addition, frequently encountered perioperative disturbances of body water, ionic composition, protein concentration, and red cell mass are discussed. Finally, both theoretic and practical concerns about the correction of these abnormalities are addressed.

CRYSTALLOID THERAPY
Compartmentalization of Body Fluids

A prerequisite to understanding the rationale behind perioperative fluid management is a knowledge of the volume and composition of the various body fluid compartments. Through the use of radioactive isotope tracer techniques, these compartments have been relatively well defined.[183,184,329] For the most part, each compartment is physically separated from the others by a layer of functional semipermeable cell membranes, thereby allowing each compartment to be exquisitely dynamic. The range of normal values for the various fluid compartments is influenced by body habitus, age, weight, and gender, but within an individual patient (normal, steady state) the compartments are relatively stable in terms of size and composition.

Total body water

Water is the single most abundant compound in the body, constituting approximately 50% to 70% of body weight, and is the major solvent in which metabolism occurs. Total body water (TBW) refers to the amount of water in the body, expressed as a percentage of body weight. The average normal values (determined by the dilution technique; Table 46-1) for TBW are 60% and 50% in adult males and females, respectively, but there is a significant amount of normal variation ($\pm 15\%$) within each group.

As previously alluded to, the amount of TBW is a function of several variables, including lean body mass and age. Lean body mass is defined as the mass of functional tissues, consisting of bone, essential fat (i.e., structural lipid, which includes myelin, lecithin, cholesterol, and other lipids essential for body economy), and vital organs. Neutral or storage fat contains little water;[38,197,523] therefore TBW in a lean individual will be greater than in an obese person (e.g., perhaps

20% to 30% greater; Fig. 46-1). Lower values for TBW in adult females reflect a larger amount of subcutaneous adipose tissue and a smaller muscle mass, as compared with adult males.

The extremes of age are associated with the maximal and minimal values for TBW[182,473,523,693] (Table 46-2). Newborn infants have the highest proportion of their body weight represented by water (i.e., 75% to 80%). During the first several months after birth, body water is gradually lost so that by 1 year of age, TBW averages 65% and remains relatively constant throughout the remainder of infancy and childhood.[197] After adolescence, TBW declines steadily and significantly to a low of 52% and 46% in males and females, respectively.

Table 46-1 Total body water as percentage of body weight

Build	Total body water (% of body weight)	
	Male	Female
Thin	65	55
Average	60	50
Obese	55	45

From Scribner BH, ed: University of Washington teaching syllabus for the course on fluid and electrolyte balance, Seattle, 1969, University of Washington Press, and Rainey TG, English JF: Pharmacology of colloids and crystalloids. In Chernow B, ed: *The pharmacologic approach to the critically ill patient*, ed 2, Baltimore, 1988, Williams & Wilkins.

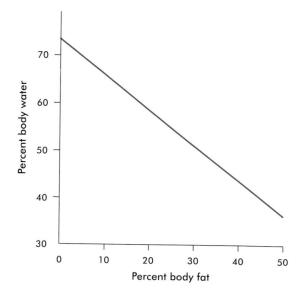

Fig. 46-1. Relationship between body fat and total body water in adults. (Modified from Behnke AR: Physiological studies pertaining to deep sea diving and aviation, especially in relation to the fat content and composition of the body, *Harvey Lect* 37:198, 1941-2.)

Table 46-2   Changes in total body water

Age	Male	Female
1 mo	76	76
1-12 mo	65	65
1-10 yr	62	62
10-16	59	57
17-39	61	50
40-49	55	47
>60	52	46

From Tonnesen AS: Crystalloids and colloids. In Miller RD, ed: *Anesthesia*, ed 3, New York, 1990, Churchill-Livingstone.

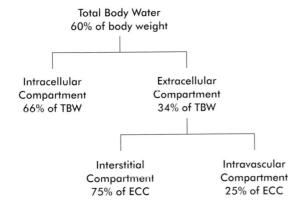

Fig. 46-2. Major body fluid compartments in a prototypic 70-kg adult male. (From Layon AJ, Kirby RR: Fluids and electrolytes in the critically ill. In Civetta JM, Taylor RW, and Kirby RR, eds: *Critical care,* New York, 1988, JB Lippincott.)

TBW exists in two major compartments: intracellular and extracellular fluid (Figs. 46-2 and 46-3). Fluid within the body's diverse cell population (i.e., intracellular water [ICW]) represents approximately 40% of body weight, with the largest proportion in the skeletal muscle mass[183,668] (Table 46-3). The total extracellular fluid volume constitutes approximately 20% of body weight and includes all body water external to the cells. This extracellular water (ECW), in turn, can be subdivided into several fluid compartments (Box 46-1). The blood plasma volume (intravascular compartment) composes—on the average—approximately 5% of body weight in the normal adult. The total functional extravascular ECW volume accounts for approximately 15% to 16% of body weight. For the purposes of this discussion the lymph fluid is considered extravascular, and it accounts for perhaps 2% of total body weight. The plasma volume, together with the rapid exchange component of interstitial fluid, is of the most practical importance in terms of perioperative fluid management. The remaining ECW subcompartments are relatively nonfunctional in that their equilibration time is so prolonged. The fluids within these subcompartments are diverse in terms of composition and range from simple transudates of plasma (e.g., "cavitary" fluids) to complex solutions formed by active transport mechanisms (e.g., transcellular fluids). These so-called nonfunctional components normally represent only a small percentage of the total ECW compartmental volume,[183,636] but in certain pathologic conditions the volume of these fluids can increase substantially. For example, the normal volume of all the transcellular water is roughly 15 ml/kg body weight

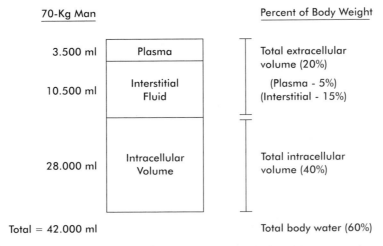

Fig. 46-3. Relative size of the major fluid compartments. (From Shires GT, Canizaro PC: Fluid, electrolyte, and nutritional management of the surgical patient. In Schwartz SI, ed: *Principles of surgery,* ed 2, New York, 1974, McGraw-Hill.)

Table 46-3 Contribution of body tissues to TBW*			
Tissue	% Body weight	% Water	Liters of water
Muscle	41.7	75.6	22.10
Skin	18.0	72.0	9.07
Skeleton	15.9	22.0	2.45
Adipose	±10.0	10.0	0.70
Blood	8.0	83.0	4.65
Liver	2.3	68.3	1.03
Brain	2.0	74.8	1.05
Intestine	1.8	74.5	0.94
Lung	0.7	79.0	0.39
Heart	0.5	79.2	0.28
Kidney	0.4	82.7	0.25
Spleen	0.2	75.8	0.10

*Approximate values for a lean 70-kg adult male.
From Skeleton H: The storage of water by various tissues of the body, *Arch Int Med* 40:140, 1927.

BOX 46-1
EXTRACELLULAR FLUID COMPARTMENTS

Intravascular

Plasma

Extravascular

Interstitial fluid and lymph
   Rapid exchange (with plasma) component
   Slow exchange (with plasma) component (e.g., cartilage, dense connective tissue)
Bone water (inaccessible)
"Cavitary" fluids (e.g., peritoneal, pericardial, pleural)
Transcellular fluids (e.g., salivary, hepatic, biliary, pancreatic, dermal, mucosal [respiratory, gastrointestinal], intraocular, intraluminal [gastrointestinal], intrathecal)

(1% to 2%); however, if there is intestinal obstruction, up to 20 L or more of transcellular fluid may accumulate within the lumen of the bowel.[640] Nevertheless, under normal conditions only a relatively small part of the ECW is liquid; most resides in a gel-like state loosely bound to the mucopolysaccharide connective tissue.

The previously noted alterations in TBW associated with differences in age and gender can be related to the influence of these variables on the size of the various functional fluid compartments. Table 46-4—using a practical ml/kg format—contrasts the volume of these compartments based on age and gender.

Table 46-4 Changes in fluid compartments on the basis of age and gender		
Compartment	Male (mg/kg)	Female (mg/kg)
ICW	450	400
ECW	200	150
Interstitial	165	120
Blood volume		
Neonate	80	80
Adult	60-70	55-65
Plasma volume	35-40	30-35
Red cell volume	25-30	20-25

ICW, intercellular water; *ECW*, extracellular water.
From Tonnesen AS: Crystalloids and colloids. In Miller RD, ed: *Anesthesia*, ed 3, New York, 1990, Churchill-Livingstone.

Ionic composition

In biologic systems, the physiologic and chemical activity of electrolytes depends on several variables, including (1) the number of particles present per unit volume (moles or millimoles per liter of solution), (2) the number of electric charges per unit volume (equivalents or milliequivalents per liter of solution), and (3) the number of osmotically active particles per unit volume (osmoles or milliosmoles per liter of solution). These variables can be measured or calculated and allow a physiologic comparison of the solutes present in a given solution. They are important for understanding and describing not only the composition of both body fluids and parenteral solutions, but also the complicated interactions between the various body fluid compartments. The following sections describe these variables, as well as other units of solute measurement, and address their clinical significance.

Electrical equivalence. The ionic composition of the body's various fluids is discussed in terms of chemical combining activity or chemical "equivalents." When the concentrations of different ions within each fluid compartment are so expressed, the sum of all positive ions (cations) exactly equals the sum of all negative ions (anions). Balance between cations and anions is mandatory, because all fluids or solutions within the body must be electrically neutral. Thus solute concentrations should be expressed consistently, with an understanding of the units used for measurement.

The atomic weight of an element is an arbitrarily selected number, with oxygen representing the relative standard of reference. The weight of one atom of oxygen has been chosen to be 16, and thus the atomic weight of all other elements is determined by their mass in relationship to that of oxygen (Table 46-5). The molecular weight of a compound can be determined by (1) knowing the chemical formula of the compound in question, and then (2) adding together the atomic weights of all the elements constituting that compound (Table 46-6).

A mole (M) of any substance is its molecular weight expressed in grams (i.e., gram-molecular weight) and contains 6.023×10^{23} molecules (Avogadro's number). Since most solutes in body fluids exist in relatively small concentrations, the term millimole (mM) is commonly used. A millimole of a substance is $\frac{1}{1000}$ of a mole or the substance's weight expressed in milligrams (see Table 46-6). In addition, 1 M of any gas (e.g., oxygen, carbon dioxide) under standard conditions occupies a constant volume of 22.4 L and 1 mM of gas occupies 22.4 ml. Regardless of whether a substance is ionized or nonionized, organic or inorganic, the terms mole and millimole are applicable.

Electrolytes combine with each other strictly in proportion to their ionic valences. Originally, oxygen was chosen as the standard of reference; 8 g of oxygen was arbitrarily designated as 1 equivalent.[541] This quantity of oxygen will combine with 1 g atomic weight of hydrogen. By convention, the chemical standard of reference for combining power is the electric charge (+) of 1 atomic weight (1 g) of hydrogen. Thus 1 equivalent (Eq) of an ion is that amount which can combine with 1 g of hydrogen and is therefore chemically equivalent to 1 g of hydrogen.

One Eq of hydrogen consists of 6.023×10^{23} particles, weighs 1 g, and carries a positive charge. This quantity of hydrogen ions neutralizes or balances 1 Eq of hydroxyl ions, which consists of 6.023×10^{23} particles, weighs 17 g, and carries a negative electric charge. The result of this neutralization is the formation of 1 M of water weighing 18 g. Such ions are termed univalent and balance each other in a 1:1 ratio. For all univalent ions, 1 Eq equals 1 M.

Certain ions (e.g., calcium, magnesium, sulfate) are divalent and carry either two positive charges (divalent cations) or two negative charges (divalent anions). These multivalent ions have greater chemical-combining power than do univalent ions. Because electrochemical neutrality must be maintained in all reactions, one divalent cation—such as calcium—will react with two univalent anions—such as chloride. In other words, 1 M of divalent cation (6.023×10^{23} particles) supplies 2 Eq and will combine with 2 M (1 Eq each) of univalent anion.

The ionic concentrations present in body fluids are relatively small and amount to fractions of an equivalent per liter. Therefore it is more convenient to express these concentrations in terms of milliequivalents (mEq) rather than equivalents. In the case of univalent ions, 1 mEq is equal to $\frac{1}{1000}$ of the gram-atomic weight (i.e., atomic weight expressed in

Table 46-5   Biologically important elements

Element	Symbol	Atomic weight*
Calcium	Ca	40
Chlorine	Cl	35
Hydrogen	H	1
Magnesium	Mg	24
Nitrogen	N	14
Oxygen	O	16
Phosphorus	P	31
Potassium	K	39
Sodium	Na	23
Sulfur	S	32

*Rounded off to the nearest whole number.

Table 46-6   Common ionized and nonionized substances

Substance	Formula	Atomic or molecular weight	Mole (M)	Millimole (mM)
Glucose	$C_6H_{12}O_6$	180	180 g	180 mg
Calcium chloride	$CaCl_2$	110	110 g	180 mg
Sulfate	SO_4^-	96	96 g	96 mg
Phosphate	HPO_4^-	96	96 g	96 mg
Sodium bicarbonate	$NaHCO_3$	84	84 g	84 mg
Potassium chloride	KCL	74	74 g	74 mg
Bicarbonate	HCO_{3-}	61	61 g	61 mg
Sodium chloride	NaCL	58	58 g	58 mg
Ammonium chloride	NH_4CL	53	53 g	53 mg
Calcium	Ca^{++}	40	40 g	40 mg
Sodium	Na^+	23	23 g	23 mg

Modified from Hays RM: Dynamics of body water and electrolytes. In Maxwell MH, Kleeman CR, eds: *Clinical disorders of fluid and electrolyte metabolism*, ed 2, New York, 1972, McGraw-Hill.

mg); is the same as 1 mM of the ion in question; and consists of 6.023×10^{20} particles. For divalent ions, 1 mEq consists of 3.012×10^{20} particles and weighs $\frac{1}{2000}$ of the gram-atomic weight. One mM of divalent ion equals two mEq. An equivalent (or milliequivalent) of any ion is its atomic weight expressed in grams (or milligrams) divided by the valence. It should be clear that electrolytes do not combine gram for gram or milligram for milligram; they combine equivalent for equivalent or milliequivalent for milliequivalent of opposite polarity. Therefore, in any given solution, the number of milliequivalents of cations is balanced by precisely the same number of milliequivalents of anions. An appreciation of this principle of electrochemical equivalence is paramount for understanding the ionic composition of body fluids and for administering crystalloid therapy appropriately.

Distribution of ions

The body's fluid compartments differ in concentrations of electrolytes, and the mean values listed in Table 46-7 are in no way absolute. There is a range (mean $\pm$ 2 SD) of accepted normal values for each ionic concentration. For instance, normal sodium concentrations are 138 to 146 mEq/L of plasma and chloride concentrations vary from 98 to 110 mEq/L. All other ions normally exhibit similar variations in concentration. In the extracellular compartment, the major cation is sodium, with the principal anions being chloride and bicarbonate. Sodium and chloride are free in solution, but appreciable fractions of calcium and magnesium are bound to protein. Of the total measured calcium, 35% to 45% is protein bound (pH dependent) with an additional 5% to 15% bound to anions such as phosphate and citrate to form nonionized components of calcium salts.[43] A measurement of ionized calcium is necessary for evaluation of the diffusible fraction of calcium. For plasma magnesium, approximately 30% is protein bound, 15% is complexed with anions, and 55% is in a free ionic form.[755]

The minor differences in ionic composition between plasma and interstitial fluid result from the differing compartmental protein concentrations.[722] Interstitial fluid represents an ultrafiltrate of plasma. A simple filtrate of plasma is free of all particulate matter (e.g., platelets, red and white blood cells), whereas an ultrafiltrate is, in addition, devoid of protein. In actuality, the interstitial fluid is not completely free of protein, but the total concentration is exceedingly low compared with either whole plasma or plasma water. The comparatively large and abundant plasma proteins display a net negative charge at a pH level of 7.4, and their diffusion across capillary endothelium is restricted. Thus, because of the greater plasma protein content (i.e., organic anions),

the total plasma concentration of cations is higher and the concentration of inorganic anions is slightly lower than in the interstitial fluid. Electroneutrality—by necessity—is maintained within each fluid compartment, but there is an important asymmetry of ion distribution between plasma and interstitial fluid. This asymmetry is an example of the Gibbs-Donnan rule, which describes the unequal distribution of *diffusible* ions on either side of the cell membranes bordering these fluid compartments.[197,296,541] Within each fluid compartment, the total cations must equal the total anions, but a greater number of diffusible ions reside in the compartment containing the organic anion. As a result, a slight osmotic pressure gradient is established, which can be effectively counterbalanced by capillary hydrostatic forces.

Because protein molecules are so abundant and widely distributed throughout the body and there are significant differences among the compartmental concentrations of protein (intracellular > plasma > interstitial), the Gibbs-Donnan principle is an important concept for understanding the distribution (i.e., concentration) of diffusible ions (see Table 46-7). When nondiffusible protein is excluded from a closed system, the product of the concentrations of any pair of diffusible cations and anions on one side of a membrane will equal the product of the same pair of ions on the other side. However, if a nondiffusible anion is present on only one side of a membrane or if unequal amounts of nondiffusible anion are present on either side of a membrane, then conditions are altered. For example, consider the closed system in Fig. 46-4 in which two equal volume compartments are separated by a rigid membrane that is permeable to sodium (Na^+) and chloride (Cl^-) ions but impermeable to protein (Pr^-) ions. Initially (starting condition), 5 Na^+ and 5 Pr^- ions are located on side *1* and 10 Na^+ and 10 Cl^- ions are located on side *2*. When an equilibrium condition is achieved (Fig. 46-4, *right*), there is an unequal distribution of both diffusible and nondiffusible ions. Nevertheless, electrical neutrality is maintained within each compartment and the products of the total concentrations of diffusible ions (i.e., Na^+ and Cl^-) are equal on either side of the membrane (the Gibbs-Donnan rule). Therefore at equilibrium conditions the following relationship exists:

$$Na_1^+ \times Cl_1^- = X \qquad \text{and} \qquad Na_2^+ \times Cl_2^- = X$$
$$9 \times 4 = 36 \qquad\qquad\qquad 6 \times 6 = 36$$

Despite the inequality of concentrations on either side of the membrane, there will be no further tendency toward equalization. If this system contains a variety of additional diffusible ions, all the cations and anions would distribute in a similar manner; the ratio of a specific ion's concentrations from both compartments will be the same as the ratio for any

Table 46-7   Electrolyte composition of body fluids (approximate)

Electrolyte	Plasma (mEq/L)	Plasma water (mEq/L)	Interstitial fluid (mEq/L)	Intracellular fluid (mEq/kg H_2O)
Cations				
Sodium	142	152	145	10
Potassium	4	4	4	156
Calcium	5	5	3	3
Magnesium	3	3	1	26
Total	154	164	153	195
Anions				
Chloride	103	109	114	2
Bicarbonate	27	29	30	10
Phosphate	2	2	2	108
Sulfate	1	1	1	20
Organic acids	5	6	5	
Protein	16	17	1	55
Total	154	164	153	195

Modified from Bergstrom J: Muscle electrolytes in man, *Scand J Clin Lab Invest* 14(suppl):68, 1962; Nanninga LB: Calculation of free magnesium, calcium, and potassium in muscle, *Biochem Biophys Acta* 54:338, 1961; Walser M: Extracellular fluid in individual tissues in relation to extracellular fluid in the body as a whole. In Bergner PE, Lushbaugh CC, eds: *Compartments, pools and spaces in medical physiology,* Washington, 1967; US Atomic Energy Commission Symposium 11.

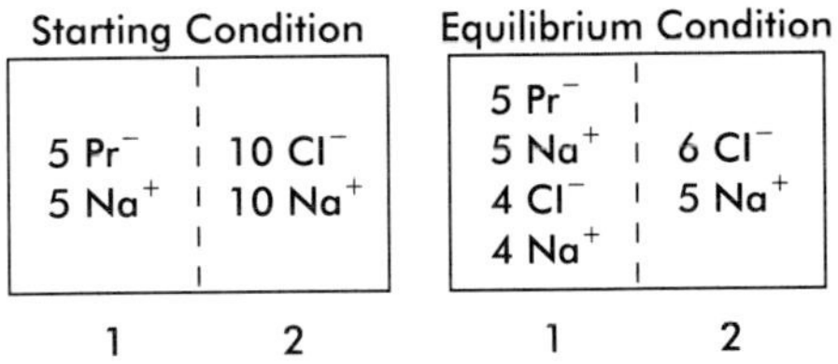

Fig. 46-4. Effect of nondiffusable protein anions on the distribution of diffusable cations and anions. (From Pitts RF: Volume and composition of the body fluids. In Pitts RF, ed: *Physiology of the kidney and body fluids,* ed 3, Chicago, 1974, Year Book Medical Publishers.)

other diffusible ion. For the example in Fig. 46-4, ionic distribution at equilibrium can be expressed as the following:

$$Na_1^+ \times Cl_1^- = Na_2^+ \times Cl_2^-$$

The equation can be rewritten as the following:

$$\frac{Na_1^+}{Na_2^+} = \frac{Cl_2^-}{Cl_1^-}$$

which would then yield these concentration ratios:

$$\frac{Na_1^+}{Na_2^+} = \frac{9}{6} = \frac{3}{2} \quad \text{and} \quad \frac{Cl_2^-}{Cl_1^-} = \frac{6}{4} = \frac{3}{2}$$

The ionic concentrations for plasma water differ from those of plasma due to the exclusion of solids—notably protein and lipids—which total approximately 7% (see Table 46-7). Plasma proteins

occupy a volume far out of proportion to the few milliequivalents of anion they represent. One L of plasma actually contains about 940 ml of water. The remaining volume is normally occupied, for the most part, by protein. Ions are generally dissolved in the aqueous phase of plasma, so that concentrations in plasma water exceed those in whole plasma by a factor of $1000\!/\!940$. Clinical laboratories usually report electrolyte values as the particular ionic concentration in a given volume of whole plasma or serum. These values, although not as accurate as plasma water values (mEq/L of plasma water), are nonetheless generally accepted. However, if the lipid or protein content of plasma is significantly elevated, there will be a corresponding decrease in the reported concentration of ions per liter of plasma. That is, the volume of water in the sample may be significantly less than the total volume; therefore the ionic concentrations will be underestimated. Under these circumstances, however, the number of ions per liter of plasma water will be unaffected.

The body's intracellular fluid is neither continuous nor homogenous. The many diverse cell types differ in terms of structure, water content (see Table 46-3), and chemical constitution.[48,475,492,770] In addition, the accurate measurement of intracellular ionic concentrations is exceedingly difficult. Skeletal muscle cells have provided the intracellular environment most thoroughly studied, and it is this intracellular composition represented by the mean values listed in Table 46-5. To assume that the ionic concentrations within a myocyte are the same as those within an erythrocyte, hepatocyte, or osteocyte not only is a gross oversimplification, but also is misleading. Nonetheless, there are specific intracellular ionic relationships that appear to be common to the majority of cells, and thus certain generalizations are allowed.

Within the intracellular compartment, potassium and magnesium are the predominant cations, whereas phosphate, sulfate, and protein are the most abundant anions. There is a marked difference between ICW and ECW in terms of ionic concentrations. The ratio of intracellular to extracellular potassium is almost 30:1. Likewise, sodium is portioned along a steep concentration gradient—albeit in the opposite direction. The total concentration of measured intracellular ions exceeds the concentrations within each of the extracellular compartments, which would seem to violate the concept of osmolar equilibrium (i.e., cells and extracellular fluid have equal osmolalities.)[425] This apparent discrepancy arises because the concentration of ions is expressed in milliequivalents (mEq) without regard to osmotic activity. It is likely that a portion of the intracellular ions are bound to protein and various other constituents, which results in osmotically inactive ions.[492] Hence equilibration of compartmental osmolalities occurs despite the differing ionic concentrations.

The preceding discussion highlighted several clinically important differences in compartmental ionic concentrations. An understanding of the origin of these differences is critical for a full appreciation of normal compartmental composition and the compositional changes associated with certain physiologic insults. The mechanisms responsible for the normal distribution of ions are highly complex and an area of intense research interest; many energy-dependent transport systems, carrier proteins and complexes, coenzymes, and cellular organelles are involved in this process. A detailed description of the intricate biophysical and chemical systems responsible for the normal ion concentrations within each fluid compartment is well beyond the scope of this chapter. Therefore the following discussion focuses on the major differences between intracellular and extracellular ion concentrations, providing a simplistic overview of the mechanisms involved.

As previously noted, normal cell membranes are impermeable to proteins and organic phosphate complexes and permeable to most other intracellular ions. Maintaining different ionic concentrations across cell membranes does not result primarily from the noted ionic impermeabilities, but rather from the active accumulation and extrusion of certain ions from within cells. Active, energy-dependent "ion pumps" (contained within cell membranes) generate the ionic concentration gradients observed among the various fluid compartments. Thus cells are effectively

rendered impermeable to ions by the function of these pumps. This effective impermeability exists despite the fact that radioactive isotope studies have demonstrated cell membranes to be permeable to a number of ions, including those which are arguably the most quantitatively and qualitatively important (e.g., sodium, potassium, and chloride). For example, the tendency for sodium ions to diffuse from extracellular fluid (high concentration) into cells (low concentration) is opposed by the active extrusion of sodium ions. Similarly, the tendency for potassium ions to diffuse along a concentration gradient from the intracellular fluid (high concentration) to the extracellular fluid (low concentration) is opposed by the active accumulation of potassium within the cells. It appears that the outward pumping of sodium is a process intimately linked to the inward pumping of potassium.[248,671]

The electrical polarization across cell membranes (negative inside, positive outside) also plays a role in maintaining normal ionic distribution. Large polyvalent protein and organic phosphate anions are confined intracellularly, due to their absolute membrane impermeability. Sodium is predominantly extracellular, because the function of the ion pumps results in effective membrane impermeability. In addition, it appears that cells are generally far more permeable to potassium than to sodium.[541] Thus positively charged potassium ions tend to diffuse down a concentration gradient and out of a cell. The result is an increasing negative charge within the cell that tends to counteract this diffusion. A state is established in which the outward diffusion of potassium (driven by the concentration gradient) is balanced by increasing cell negativity (loss of intracellular cations), thereby restraining further diffusion.

Membrane polarization is largely a function of the difference in potassium concentration on either side of the membrane. A crude quantitative description of the resulting potential difference can be derived through use of the simplified Nernst equation.* For most cells under normal conditions, the resting transmembrane potential difference is 60 to 90 mV. Abnormalities of ionic distribution can result in an altered potential difference and cellular dysfunction. Severe hypothermia, shock, anoxia, and various metabolic inhibitors each have the ability to inactivate ion pumps. With such occurrences, the characteristic differences between intracellular and extracellular concentrations tend to disappear as ions diffuse—unopposed—down their concentration gradients. Sodium and water tend to move intracellularly, whereas

---

*PD (in mV) $= -61 \times \log \dfrac{(K_i^+)}{(K_e^+)}$, where PD is the potential difference, K_i^+ is the intracellular concentration of potassium, and K_e^+ is the extracellular concentration of potassium.

potassium leaks out of cells with the potential for significant hyperkalemia.

Concentration. By convention, the concentrations of most parenteral solutions and the nonelectrolytes found in body fluids are expressed as percentages. Percent means "per hundred," and thus any concentration expressed as a percentage refers to units (usually weight in grams or milligrams per 100 ml of solution). For example, 0.9% saline solution (normal saline) represents 0.9 g sodium chloride/100 ml water and 5% glucose solution (D_5W) refers to 5 g dextrose/100 ml water (i.e., 50 g/L). In addition, laboratory measurements of glucose, albumin, total protein, urea, creatinine, cholesterol, and so on are expressed as milligrams percent (i.e., mg/100 ml of blood, serum, or plasma). A blood glucose concentration of 80 mg percent means 80 mg glucose/100 ml blood. Concentrations expressed as grams percent or milligrams percent will provide the weight of the electrolyte—or other substance—per unit volume but fail to allow a physiologic comparison of solutes present in the solution(s). Also, this method of expressing composition is temperature dependent; these concentrations may be inaccurate unless the temperature of the solution is accounted for at the time of administration or measurement.

A unit of measurement that is more physiologically appropriate, although seldom used clinically, is molal concentration, or molality (m). Molality is the concentration of a particular solute expressed as moles per 1000 g of solvent and is independent of temperature. A molal solution of saline will contain 58.5 g of sodium chloride dissolved in 1000 g of water. Alternatively, the molar concentration, or molarity (M), is the number of moles of solute per liter of solution (usually water) at a specified temperature. Because changes in temperature result in the expansion and contraction of liquids, the molar concentration of any solution varies with the temperature. As with other measurements of concentration for body fluids and parenteral solutions, the relatively small quantities of solute present are usually expressed as a thousandth of the particular unit. Thus for molal and molar concentrations the terms most commonly used are millimoles per kilogram (millimolal, [mm]) and millimoles per liter (millimolar [mM]). Of practical importance is the fact that molal and molar concentrations are often used interchangeably, because the difference between the two is negligible for the range of solute concentrations and temperature found within body fluids.

Distribution and movement of water

Because cell membranes are readily permeable to water molecules, there is a continual movement or exchange of water between the body's major fluid compartments (i.e., intracellular, interstitial, and intravascular). The major forces governing this water movement are hydrostatic and osmotic pressures. The following section reviews the origin of these pressures and discusses their impact on the flow and distribution of water among the fluid compartments.

Hydrostatic pressure. Hydrostatic pressure results from the weight of blood within the vasculature,[276] and the mechanical pressure generated by the heart.[597] In large arteries the normal mean pressure is approximately 95 mm Hg, but there is a gradual reduction in pressure along the arterial system as blood traverses more progressively distal vessels of diminishing caliber.[308] After reaching the capillary bed (the site of fluid exchange), the hydrostatic pressure is reduced to approximately 30 to 40 mm Hg and the effective net pressure is even less.[772] Nonetheless, the net hydrostatic pressure within the arterial end of the capillary is sufficient to transfer a small quantity of plasma water from the intravascular to the interstitial fluid compartment. Under normal conditions this process is reversed at the venous end of the capillary, where the filtered water is eventually returned to the intravascular compartment.

The preceding, relatively simplistic overview of hydrostatic water movement appears to be applicable to most capillary beds within the body. A notable exception does occur at the specialized capillary bed of the renal glomerulus.[221,420] Here, water moves out of the vascular space during the ultrafiltration of plasma, a process which occurs at a significantly greater net transcapillary pressure than is found in any other capillary bed. In addition, water movement back into the vascular space is incomplete, with some volume of the redistributed water ultimately excreted from the body as urine.

Thus, in most capillary beds, a relatively low hydrostatic pressure provides a force that results in the movement of water among fluid compartments. Excluding the glomeruli, the volume of water transferred as a consequence is relatively small. Quantitatively, a more important mechanism for the movement and redistribution of water is osmotic flow. Osmotic forces are responsible for a continual flux of water across cell membranes and among the vascular, interstitial, and cellular compartments.

When two aqueous solutions of unequal concentration are separated by a semipermeable membrane (i.e., permeable to water but not to solute), water will migrate from the more dilute to the more concentrated solution so as to equalize the concentrations of the two solutions.[197] Osmosis is the term used to describe this net flux of water. Osmotic pressure is the hydrostatic pressure that must be applied to the solution of greater concentration to prevent water movement across the membrane (Fig. 46-5).

Osmotic pressure. Osmotic pressure is one of the colligative properties of solutions: it is dependent on

ORIGIN OF OSMOTIC PRESSURE

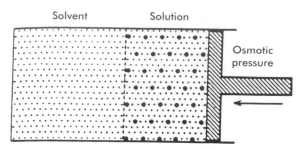

Solvent   Solution

Osmotic
pressure

Fig. 46-5. Origin of osmotic pressure. Pure solvent and solution (solvent + solute) separated by a semipermeated membrane. On the pure solvent side, molecules in a relatively unordered state strike the membrane with some passing through. On the solution side, the solvent is somewhat diluted by solute so that its concentration (i.e., activity, chemical potential, tendency to escape) is reduced. The result is fewer solvent molecules pass from solution to pure solvent than in the reverse direction. A net transfer of fluid (i.e., osmosis of solvent) occurs from pure solvent to solution. Osmotic pressure is the pressure that must be applied to the solution to increase the activity of solvent in solution to equal that of the pure solvent. (From Pitts RF: *The physiologic basis of diuretic therapy,* Springfield, Ill, 1959, Charles C Thomas.)

the *number* of osmotically active molecules in solution and not their molecular weight, electric charge, or valence number.[144,183] One gram-molecular weight (i.e., 1 mole) of a nondissociating compound (e.g., glucose, urea) consists of 6.023×10^{23} molecules and is termed 1 osmole (osmol, Osm). One Osm of a solute dissolved in 1 kg of water depresses the activity of the water by 22.4 atm. More applicable to biologic systems is the term milliosmole (mOsm), which is $\frac{1}{1000}$ of an osmole. For nondissociating compounds, 1 mM is equivalent to 1 mOsm. In turn, 1 mOsm of any solute dissolved in 1 kg of water will depress the activity of water by 17 mm Hg.

Ionized substances tend to dissociate in solution, thereby generating more osmotically active particles. For example, 1 gram-molecular weight of sodium chloride (NaCl)—consisting of 6.023×10^{23} molecules—dissociates into twice this number of ions in solution and exerts an osmotic effect of approximately 2 Osm.* One M of sodium sulfate (Na_2SO_4) results in 4 Eq (2 Na^+, SO_4^{--}) but dissociates so as to exert an osmotic effect approaching 3 Osm (Na, Na, SO_4).

OSMOLALITY AND OSMOLARITY. The concept of osmotic pressure is important for understanding normal body fluid homeostasis but clinically the term

---

* One M of sodium chloride in an extremely dilute solution will contribute 2 Osm. At physiologic concentrations, this dissociation is incomplete and actually results in only 1.85 Osm.[541]

is seldom used. Customarily, the osmotic concentration of a solution is expressed as the osmolarity or the osmolality (i.e., the sum of osmotically active molar concentrations of dissolved solutes). Osmolarity is the number of osmoles of solute *per liter* of solvent plus solute. A calculated osmolarity, usually expressed as mOsm/L of solution, can be found in nearly all parenteral solutions presently available. Osmolality, on the other hand, is the solute concentration *per kilogram* of solvent (water) and is theoretically more appropriate for a discussion of osmotic concentrations within body fluids. Osmolality is generally measured with a freezing point osmometer, although vapor pressure osmometers are available. Freezing point depression is another colligative property of solutions. Pure water freezes at 0° C, but a solution containing 1 Osm of solute per kg of water (i.e., 1 osmolal) freezes at −1.86° C. As solutions become more concentrated, the freezing point becomes lower and the freezing point depression becomes greater. When measured in this fashion, osmolality is usually expressed as mOsm/kg of water. Blood plasma normally freezes at −0.553° C, and therefore the osmolality is 0.553/1.86 = 0.297 (i.e., 297 mOsm/kg H_2O). The small differences between plasma osmolarity and osmolality are predominately due to protein and fat, which compose roughly 6% to 8% of the solutes in plasma.[640] The measurement of osmolality is unaffected by changes in plasma protein and fat (Table 46-8). Nonetheless, a freezing point osmometer depends on a physical change in the state of the original sample. Therefore inaccuracies may occur because of sample viscosity, particulate matter, or nonhomogeneity of the sample.[535] As with molal and molar concentrations, the difference between osmolarity and osmolality values is negligible when dealing with the small concentrations of solute present in body fluids.

Under normal conditions, all fluid compartments are essentially isoosmolar and there are no appreciable osmolar gradients except within the renal medulla.[370] The measured extracellular osmolality level is approximately 285 mOsm/kg H_2O (±10 mOsm/kg H_2O), and presumably the intracellular osmolality level is identical.[517] Since 1 mOsm/kg H_2O exerts an osmotic effect equivalent to 17 mm Hg, the osmotic pressure of most body fluids is roughly 300 × 17 = 5100 mm Hg. Quantitatively, osmotic pressures greatly exceed any hydrostatic pressure the body can achieve. The magnitude of these osmotic forces can be appreciated when one realizes that an osmotic pressure difference of only 6 mOsm/L, across a semipermeable membrane, can move as much water as the entire hydrostatic pressure generated by the heart.[308]

Recall that cell membranes are relatively impermeable to most solutes (e.g., sodium, glucose, man-

Table 46-8 The relationship between sodium, osmolality, and tonicity

Condition	Measured serum sodium	Measured serum osmolality	Tonicity
True hypotonicity	↓	↓	↓
Laboratory artifact	↓	Normal	Normal
Hyperlipemia			
Hyperproteinemia			
Increased ECF solute (nonsodium, impermeant)	↓	↑	↑
Glucose			
Mannitol			
Sorbitol			
Glycerol			
Increased ECF and ICF solute (nonsodium, permeant)	Normal	↑	Normal
Ethylene glycol			
Isopropyl alcohol			
Ethanol			
Methanol			
Urea			

Modified from Andreoli TE: Disorders of fluid volume, electrolyte and acid-base balance. In Wyngaarden JB, Smith LH, eds: *Cecil textbook of medicine*, ed 18, Philadelphia, 1988, WB Saunders.

nitol) but—on the other hand—are freely permeable to water, which will distribute according to osmotic gradients. The net result is that the osmolality of the intracellular and extracellular fluids equalize despite different compositions. In other words, the activity of water inside the cells (i.e., tendency to escape) will become the same as that within the surrounding fluid. The movement of water is governed by the compartmental concentrations of osmotically active substances (i.e., impermeant or semi-impermeant solute), predominantly electrolytes. Sodium, chloride, and bicarbonate account for 90% to 95% of the osmotic activity present in plasma and interstitial fluid.[541] Other ions and organic compounds (e.g., glucose, urea, amino acids) account for most of the remainder, with only a relatively small contribution provided by the large plasma proteins (see the section on colloid osmotic pressure). The major intracellular osmotic solutes are potassium, magnesium, phosphate, and protein.[238] Total body osmotic solute is portioned such that two thirds is contained within the intracellular fluid compartment and one third resides in the extracellular fluid compartment.[199] This localization of total body solute in turn explains the overall distribution of body water, as previously discussed (see Fig. 46-2).

In most situations, the concentrations of certain osmotically active substances can be combined to provide a remarkably accurate (within 10%) estimate of serum osmolality (S_{osm}) concentration:

$$S_{osm} \text{ (mOsm/kg H}_2\text{O)} = 2 \times [\text{Na}^+] + [\text{glucose}]/18 + [\text{BUN}]/2.8$$

where glucose and blood urea nitrogen (BUN) are expressed in mg/dl and Na^+ is the sodium concentration in mEq/l. Clinically, this formula has been found useful because (1) it is easy to recall and calculate, and (2) it provides valuable information for the diagnosis and management of fluid and electrolyte abnormalities. Additional information can be obtained when the calculated osmolality concentration is compared with the measured serum osmolality concentration.[678,794] The osmolal gradient or gap can be determined by subtracting the calculated osmolality value from the measured value and is normally less than 10 mOsm/kg H_2O.[238] This gradient is elevated in the presence of solutes (e.g., waste products, alcohol, and other drugs) that are unaccounted for and reside in the extracellular fluid compartment.

TONICITY. *Tonicity* is a term used to describe the relative osmolality of solutions. A solution is said to be isotonic when it is isosmotic (i.e., the same osmotic pressure) with the body fluids. For example, physiologic or "normal" saline is isotonic with respect to plasma. An isotonic solution added to either whole blood or packed red blood cells will neither increase nor decrease the size of the red blood cells, which function as tiny osmometers during acute changes in tonicity. In addition, an isotonic solution need not contain substances identical to those of a particular body fluid, because the osmolality of a solution is dependent on the *number* rather than the type of osmotically active particles present (see the section on hyponatremia). Therefore solutions of both 0.9% sodium chloride and 5% dextrose in water can be isotonic. Hypertonic solutions (e.g., 5% NaCl, 10%

mannitol) have a greater solute concentration and osmolarity than do body fluids and will cause cellular dehydration and shrinkage due to the outflow of water. Use of the term hypertonicity, therefore, implies intracellular volume depletion. On the other hand, hypotonic solutions (e.g., 0.45% NaCl) have fewer osmotically active particles per volume compared with the particular reference solution and tend to produce cellular swelling.

Although the terms tonicity and osmolality are frequently interchanged in clinical usage, an alteration (increase or decrease) in one of these factors does not always imply a similar change in the other. To maintain the intercompartmental osmolality, water distributes according to the amount of impermeant solute present in each fluid compartment. If tonicity is normal, there will be no shift in fluid between compartments. In hypertonic states the impermeant ECF solute concentration is increased, which results in a decreased ICF volume. High concentrations of permeant solute, such as urea, distribute evenly throughout TBW and therefore produce no lasting osmotic effect. Urea will not cause hypertonicity and ICF depletion but will cause hyperosmolality. With a molecular weight of 28, each 2.8 mg/dl increment in BUN concentration will raise the osmolality level by 1 mOsm/kg H_2O. The commonly employed methods for measuring the osmolality level—dependent on the colligative properties of solutions—are unable to differentiate permeant and impermeant solutes. Thus in certain situations, there can be an elevation of the measured serum osmolality level without an accompanying hypertonicity (see Table 46-8).[198,199,794] Hyperosmolality may exist with low, normal, or elevated tonicity.

Tonicity can also be thought of as the *effective osmolality* (E_{osm}) level. This latter term represents the concentration of those serum solutes which have the capacity to exert an osmotic force across semipermeable membranes and hence initiate water movement in and out of cells.[64,249,397,794] As noted previously, certain low–molecular-weight substances (e.g., urea, ethanol, methanol) rapidly penetrate cells according to their passive concentration gradients, thereby increasing both ECF and ICF solute. In general, these permeant substances fail to exert an effective osmotic force across cell membranes and have no lasting effect on net water movement. Effective osmolality concentration can be calculated from the following formula:

$$E_{osm} \text{ (mOsm/kg } H_2O) = 2 \times [Na^+] + [glucose]/18$$

where the urea term from the serum osmolality calculation has been omitted, since urea passes freely through cell membranes. The effective osmolality concentration is thus an estimate of tonicity, because it assumes that sodium and glucose are the only major

osmotically active solutes present. Tonicity can be calculated by summing the contribution of each impermeant solute in the ECF (i.e., 2 × sodium in mEq/L + glucose in mg/dl ÷ 18 + mannitol in mg/dl ÷ 18 + glycerol in mg/dl ÷ 9 + the contribution of all other impermeant solutes).[238] The obvious shortcoming of this calculation is that a knowledge of the concentration and osmotic effect of all ECF solutes is required. The presence of small permeant solutes can result in a disparity between the measured serum osmolality (accounting for all permeant and impermeant solutes) and the tonicity or effective osmolality (accounting for only the normally occurring, major osmotically active substances). If hyponatremia is superimposed on a condition associated with the presence of these permeant solutes (e.g., azotemia), the measured and calculated serum osmolality levels would fail to identify a true hypotonic state. In such a situation, calculation of the effective osmolality level would correctly reveal the hypotonicity (e.g., Na^+ = 125 mEq/L; glucose = 90; BUN = 140 mg/dl; S_{osm} = 305 mOsm/kg; and E_{osm} = 255 mOsm/kg). Using another approach, if the presence of a permeant solute is suspected, there is a high likelihood that the offending substance will be either urea or ethanol. An estimate of tonicity can be derived by subtracting the sum of (BUN mg/dl ÷ 18 + ETOH mg/dl ÷ 4.6) from the measured serum osmolality. Obviously, there are a number of potential pitfalls when using any of these methods for assessing tonicity, but in most clinical circumstances the formulas function satisfactorily.

Whenever fluid is added or removed from the body, osmotic forces rapidly and uniformly redistribute body water so as to eliminate all osmolar gradients and maintain isotonicity.[144] Fig. 46-6 schematically depicts the changes in volume and osmolality concentration of both the intracellular and extracellular fluid compartments resulting from the addition or loss of various fluids.

Unfortunately, the redistribution of body water cannot always compensate for pathologic or iatrogenic alterations of ionic and/or water content that may occur in a particular fluid compartment. When the serum osmolality level is less than 260 or greater than 325 mOsm/kg H_2O, neurologic abnormalities (e.g., confusion, obtundation, abnormal neuromuscular activity, or seizures) frequently occur.[22,369] The brain is particularly susceptible to volume shifts because of the delicate cerebral vasculature and because of the confinement of cerebral tissue within an enclosed rigid container. A reduced osmolality can occur with abnormal water retention (e.g., glucocorticoid deficiency, SIADH) or excessive loss of salt from either renal (e.g., diuretic overuse, primary adrenal insufficiency, nephropathy) or extrarenal

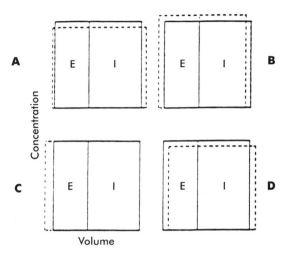

Fig. 46-6. Changes in volume and osmolal concentration of intracellular *(I)* and extracellular *(E)* fluids on addition of water to the body **(A)**, on addition of hypertonic salt solution **(B)**, on addition of isotonic salt solution **(C)**, and on loss of sodium chloride **(D)**. *Solid lines,* initial normal state. *Dashed lines,* final experimental state. Height of compartment represents osmolal concentration; width represents volume. (Original adaptation from Darrow DC, Yannet H: *Clin Invest* 14:266, 1935. In Pitts RF: Volume and composition of the body fluids. In *Physiology of the kidney and body fluids,* ed 3, Chicago, 1974, Year Book Medical Publishers.)

(e.g., gastrointestinal losses, burns) sources.[249] Although hypoosmolal states are frequently considered medical emergencies necessitating immediate intervention, the temporal aspects of therapy should be influenced by the duration and magnitude of the defect.[17,513] In addition, therapy will depend on the cause of the disturbance, as well as the ECF volume and the serum sodium concentration.[249,794] Management may be as simple as the restriction of water intake or as "complex" as the administration of hypertonic salt solutions (e.g., 3% or 5% NaCl).

Hyperosmolality may occur as the result of uremia, burns, dehydration, hyperglycemia, hyperalimentation, postobstructive uropathy, and numerous other conditions,[435,498] including the excessive use of bolus sodium bicarbonate (2000 mOsm/L) during cardiopulmonary resuscitation.[676] When hypertonicity develops rapidly, the body attempts compartmental osmolal equilibration primarily by water movement. If hypertonicity develops slowly (over days), certain cells (e.g., brain and red blood cells) can minimize osmotic losses by gaining solute.[794] The function of the cardiovascular and central nervous systems can become significantly compromised as the result of a rapidly occurring hyperosmolal state. Combined solute and water losses can produce hypotension or even shock; loss of CNS cellular volume results in traction on the cerebral vessels, which may lead to subcortical parenchymal hemorrhage, subarachnoid hemorrhage,

and/or venous thrombosis.[660,794] Hypertonicity resulting strictly from water loss is an unusual cause for a drop in systemic pressure (see the section on hypernatremia). In general, most patients with hypertonicity and water losses also have sodium deficits. Therefore treatment is aimed at replacing both water and salt deficits, matching intercurrent losses, and limiting any ongoing depletion. In contrast with low osmolal states and acute hyperosmolality, chronic hypertonicity should be corrected slowly and cautiously;[369,589] the compensatory generation of intracellular solute (i.e., idiogenic osmoles) within brain cells is a protective mechanism during the generation of the hypertonicity but becomes a predisposition for the development of cerebral edema as fluid replacement is undertaken.[322,546] Nevertheless, the expeditious initiation of treatment is warranted for any severe hyperosmolal condition, because a serum osmolality concentration of greater than 350 mOsm/kg H_2O for longer than 12 hours usually results in death.[435]

In summary, the plasma osmolality concentration is the main determinant of extracellular fluid volume; therefore disturbances in plasma osmolality are manifested chiefly as alterations in volume. Sodium ion alone accounts for 50% of the plasma osmotic pressure, and thus sodium and its anions are responsible for nearly all the extracellular fluid osmolality. For all practical purposes, control of the extracellular fluid compartment's osmolality concentration is synonymous with control of the sodium concentration.[498,794]

Alteration of Compartmental Constituents

Proper perioperative fluid management depends on an accurate evaluation of the patient's volume and electrolyte status. Historical information, appropriate laboratory data, and a physical examination provide the basis for this assessment. Together the subjective and objective information obtained can be used to diagnose a derangement of body fluids and also direct any therapeutic interventions that are indicated. If quantitative disturbances of red blood cells are excluded, then abnormalities of volume and/or electrolytes are—for all practical purposes—simply disorders of body water and/or solute. The analysis of such disorders is facilitated by categorizing them into *volume, concentration,* or *compositional* changes.[244,245,636] All of these categories are interrelated, and combined disturbances are quite common. Nonetheless, each category is a separate entity and will be addressed as such, unless otherwise noted.

Isolated changes in the *volume* of ECF result from the addition or removal of isotonic salt solutions. For example, acutely administering several liters of 0.9% NaCl or Ringer's solution results in expansion of the ECF compartment. In contrast, the relatively rapid loss of fluid from the small intestine results in diminished ECF. In such situations, there is an acute or subacute change in ECF volume with little or no change in ICF volume. The ICF volume remains stable as long as the osmolality concentration within the two compartments remains equilibrated.

The addition or loss of water, primarily involving the ECF compartment, alters the *concentration* of osmotically active particles. As previously discussed, sodium ion is quantitatively the single most important osmotically active substance within the ECF. The serum or plasma sodium concentration therefore generally reflects the tonicity of the compartmentalized body fluids. Thus abnormalities of sodium concentration usually indicate a redistribution of body water; water moves out of the ICF or ECF compartment (depending on the particular abnormality) until osmolal equilibrium is achieved.

An alteration of *composition* occurs when there is an imbalance in the ratio of certain substances suspended in body solutions. The concentration of most ions (excluding sodium) can be altered without inducing a significant change in the total number of osmotically active particles. This lack of change in osmolality concentration in no way implies that changes in composition are trivial. Relatively small changes in serum potassium, calcium, or magnesium have a negligible impact on the effective ECF osmotic pressure but may dramatically affect cellular or tissue performance.

Most of the preceding discussion has revolved around changes in ECF constituents. It is important to appreciate that there is an ongoing exchange of water and solute between the ICF and ECF compartments. As a consequence, there is rarely a significant alteration within one compartment that does not evoke some degree of compensatory response from the other compartment. Losses that involve a change in ECF concentration or composition are shared by the ICF. Even isotonic ECF losses have an impact on ICF volume, albeit a slow one. Nonetheless, in the operating room—where most fluid losses and gains occur rather quickly—changes in a patient's fluid status can be considered primarily as alterations in the ECF compartments.

Volume changes

Changes in volume occur frequently and require some investigation to obtain an accurate diagnosis. No readily available laboratory test can reliably identify acute volume changes, although a urine specimen (assuming normal renal function) that is significantly concentrated (e.g., 500 to 1400 mOsm/kg H_2O) with a high specific gravity and low sodium content (<20 mEq/L) can be helpful in identifying an ECF deficit.[164,337] In contrast, the diagnosis of long-standing

derangements in volume may be aided by certain laboratory tests. For example, with a prolonged ECF deficit, urea nitrogen (blood or serum) concentration rises gradually such that the ratio of urea nitrogen to serum creatinine is equal to or greater than 10:1.[615] Also, it is not unusual for a chronic ECF deficit to be associated with a "contraction" (metabolic) alkalosis.[351,371] However, the presence of a volume overload or deficit is best determined by the history and physical examination, including intake and output information, review of all medications, underlying medical/surgical conditions, changes in weight, and the presence of signs and symptoms compatible with either hypervolemia or hypovolemia. For an individual patient, these signs and symptoms depend not only on the relative or absolute quantity of ECF, but also on the rapidity of the change and the manifestations of any associated disease process(es). Thus changes in volume should be assessed at the bedside with little reliance on the clinical laboratory findings. Most importantly, this assessment must take place before the induction of anesthesia, because most of the available agents and techniques produce myocardial depression and/or vasodilation. Undertaking such an anesthetic administration in a patient with significant ECF depletion may lead to intractable circulatory collapse.[603,720]

Volume deficit. The single most common fluid disturbance in surgical patients is reduced ECF volume. Specifically, the reduction in the volume of plasma and the rapid exchange component of interstitial fluid are clinically most consequential. An important and highly dynamic relationship exists between the ECF volume and the subcompartmental intravascular volume. Most often, isotonic ECF losses either originate from or are quickly reflected in the intravascular volume. Such fluid losses contain water and electrolytes in approximately the same proportion as they exist in normal ECF. In surgical patients, an intensive preoperative work-up requiring restricted oral intake, purgatives, and enemas frequently results in a mild ECF deficit. More severe deficits may result from intractable vomiting, prolonged nasogastric suction, profuse diarrhea, fistulous drainage, severe diuresis, or hemorrhage.

The transfer of isotonic solution from a functional fluid compartment to a nonfunctional space is termed a *distributional* change.[244,245,636] For practical purposes, such changes can be considered a sub-type of ECF volume loss because of the following characteristics: (1) the fluid loss is isotonic, (2) both the interstitial fluid and the plasma volume contribute to the loss, and (3) the systemic manifestations of the loss are the same as those resulting from any other ECF deficit. As a result of surgical trauma, muscle injuries, burns, peritonitis, or ascites, functional body fluid is relo-

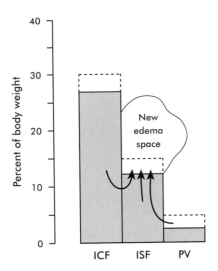

Fig. 46-7. Distributional fluid deficit. Contribution of various fluid compartments to the formation of acutely sequestered edema. *PV,* plasma volume; *ISF* and *ICF,* interstitial and intracellular fluids, respectively. *Dashed lines,* normal volume of each fluid compartment. (From Giesecke AH, Egbert LD: Perioperative fluid therapy—crystalloids. In Miller RD, ed: *Anesthesia,* ed 2, New York, 1986, Churchill-Livingstone.)

cated into an acutely formed sequestered edema space. This edema space is actually an appendage of the ISF compartment. The edema fluid has the same composition as the ISF and is derived from ICF, PV, and normal ISF (Fig. 46-7). Because it is unable to perform any of the physiologic duties of healthy ISF, this edema fluid is termed nonfunctional; it does not transport nutrients or metabolites and is unable to return to the vascular space in the event of sudden hemorrhage. It is difficult to gauge the size of the edema space, but after therapy that restores the normal ICF and ECF volumes, the patient will have gained weight equivalent to the volume of the sequestered fluid. When this transudation of fluid results from surgical trauma, it is often a major source of volume loss. Such "third spacing" of fluid does not cease immediately after termination of the surgical procedure. This fluid loss usually continues for 24 to 48 hours postoperatively.[635] An additional 24 to 72 hours is generally necessary to mobilize the sequestered fluid and eliminate it in the form of urine.

The search for an ECF deficit begins with subjective, historical information. Questions should be directed toward identification of any abnormal losses of blood, urine, feces, or perspiration. The presence of vomiting or diarrhea, as well as the use of diuretic medications, may be significant. The presence of thirst—a result of either hyperosmolality or hypovolemia—is also important. Estimates of urine volume and frequency are valuable, and the quantity

and composition of fluids administered or ingested should be ascertained.[731]

Objective evidence of ECF depletion usually confirms any suspicion raised by the historical data. In general, cardiovascular and central nervous system (CNS) signs predominate during the acute phase of ECF loss. Hypovolemia evokes reflex sympathetic stimulation, resulting in a sinus tachycardia. It usually requires a 15% to 30% loss of intravascular volume to elicit such a response while the patient is in the supine position.[731,762] A drop in arterial blood pressure can also be evidence for an ECF deficit, especially in infants because of their relatively fixed stroke volume.[222] In adults, the numerous compensatory mechanisms available make systemic pressure a less sensitive indicator of ECF loss;[79] usually a loss of intravascular volume of greater than 30% is necessary to elicit a decrease in arterial pressure.[682] The sensitivity of heart rate and blood pressure can be enhanced by evaluating the patient for orthostasis.[356,597]* With the upper body elevated at least 60 degrees, a persistent heart rate increase of >10 beats/min and a blood pressure decrease of >15% (compared with supine values) are indicative of moderately severe hypovolemia. Depending on the severity and duration of the hypotension, symptoms of impaired cerebral perfusion (i.e., dizziness, lightheadedness, syncope) may develop. Deficits of ECF volume tend to narrow the pulse pressure,[156,599] and filling pressures for both the right and left sides of the heart may become compromised.[730] Although there are multiple determinants of filling pressure, isolated hypovolemia produces a central venous pressure (CVP) of less than 7 mm Hg and a pulmonary artery occlusion pressure (PAOP) of less than 10 mm Hg. During mechanical ventilation, a fall in systolic pressure synchronized with inspiratory gas flow generally reflects hypovolemia.[544] In those patients requiring positive end-expiratory pressure (PEEP) support, a large difference in the PAOP as measured with and without PEEP is also suggestive of hypovolemia.

Moderate ECF deficits may produce sleepiness, apathy, anorexia, and diminished cognitive function. These CNS signs may progress with severe ECF deficits, resulting in hyporeflexia, stupor, or coma.[369]

Sympathetic stimulation produced by ECF volume loss results in cutaneous vasoconstriction. Patients exhibit cool, dry, pale skin with diminished capillary

---

* When a normal individual assumes an upright position, approximately 700 ml of venous blood is pooled in the lower extremities.[213,315] Mechanical factors (e.g., venous valves, leg muscle contraction) and reflex sympathetic activity (e.g., arteriolar and venous constriction, tachycardia) result in maintenance of venous return, stroke volume, and systemic arterial pressure.[140] Consequently, there is only a transient and mild decrease in systolic pressure (5 to 15 mm Hg), whereas diastolic pressure tends to increase and there is little or no change in mean arterial pressure.[356]

refill. As the deficit enlarges, skin turgor becomes poor, and tenting (lack of skin recoil after elevation) is evident. Dry mucous membranes are usually an early sign, with sunken eyes, longitudinal furrowing of the tongue, and collapsed veins occurring later, with more severe deficits.

Exact quantification of the ECF deficit is extremely difficult and probably unnecessary. The clinical findings with hypovolemia can be grouped so as to provide a rough estimate of the size of the deficit (Table 46-9). It is important to realize that the signs and symptoms related to a specific degree of volume loss may vary from patient to patient. The categorizations in Table 46-9 are by no means absolute; however, they can be clinically useful when initiating therapy.

Because pure ECF volume loss is an isotonic loss, the replacement fluid should always contain both water and salt. A polyionic balanced salt solution, such as lactated Ringer's, is preferable. For each estimated percentage of body weight lost as fluid, approximately 10 ml/kg of balanced salt solution will be needed for replenishment. Thus an average-sized adult with a moderate ECF loss (8% body weight) requires about 5.6 L of crystalloid. However, reliance on a formula or single clinical sign to determine the adequacy of therapy is totally inappropriate. Instead, restoration of normal CNS function and the stabilization of hemodynamic parameters should be used as therapeutic guidelines. Frequent clinical reevaluation is obligatory, and fluid replacement should be adjusted according to the patient's response.

Volume excess. In surgical patients, an excess of ECF occurs less frequently than a deficit but, nonetheless, reflects a fluid disturbance of significant importance. Most often volume excess is iatrogenic in origin, the result of excessive parenteral fluid administration. Also, specific varieties of cardiac, hepatic, and renal dysfunction may either initiate or contribute to the fluid retention. In addition, the rapid postoperative mobilization of isotonic fluid from a "third space" may result in expansion of the ECF volume despite appropriate intraoperative fluid management. Thus ECF volume excess does not necessarily imply congestive heart failure (CHF), which may be either the cause or the result of the hypervolemia. The history and physical examination are, again, the cornerstone for diagnosing ECF volume excess. A careful review of the patient's intake (oral and parenteral) and output is indicated, as well as a review of any alterations in body weight. Edema is frequently noted on physical examination and represents a significant increase in the interstitial compartment of the ECF volume.[37,277] Usually, edema is localized in dependent areas (i.e., lower extremities, presacral), but on occasion it can also be easily visualized in the scleral conjunctivae. In addition, an electrolyte and water diuresis[249] in the presence of excessive lacrimation and salivation, elevated arterial blood pressure, widened pulse pressure, relative bradycardia, bounding pulses, distended peripheral veins, and jugular venous distension* is highly suggestive of hypervolemia. On the other hand, when heart failure occurs in conjunction with hypervolemia, the clinical manifestations vary enormously and are determined by a multitude of factors. The signs and symptoms of heart failure are beyond the scope of this discussion but are thoroughly reviewed elsewhere.[80]

In most situations, therapy entails only the restriction of water and salt intake, because functioning kidneys allow a normalization of ECF volume. Intraoperative management may require the omission of maintenance fluids and the replacement of only that fluid volume which is "lost" during the procedure. Perioperative hormonal changes,[270,307,478,534,549] some anesthetic agents,[673] certain medications, and positive pressure ventilation[52,311,345] tend to limit renal output in surgical patients. For those patients with an ECF volume excess, an otherwise insignificant perioperative decrease in urine flow may have dire consequences. Therefore an occasional patient may require a small amount of potent diuretic, during or after surgery, so as to initiate or enhance the desired diuresis. However, diuretics generally should be reserved for situations where an ECF excess jeopardizes vital organ function (including the reparative

Table 46-9		Extracellular fluid deficits
Category	% Decrease in body weight	Clinical signs
Mild	3-5	Dry mucous membranes, oliguria
Moderate	6-10	Orthostatic hypotension, tachycardia, anorexia, apathy, poor skin turgor
Severe	11-15	Supine hypotension, stupor, sunken eyes, cool and dry skin, mild hypothermia
Catastrophic	>20	Coma, anuria, significant fall in core temperature, dicrotic pulse, pulsus paradoxus, circulatory collapse

---

* The height of the oscillating top of the distended proximal portion of the internal jugular vein reflects right atrial pressure. Quantitative evaluation of the jugular venous pulse should be initiated with the patient's upper body elevated 45 degrees. The upper limit of normal is 4 cm above the sternal angle, which corresponds to a central venous pressure of approximately 9 cm H_2O.[79]

processes involved in wound healing). When an enlarged ECF volume coexists with CHF, therapy depends on the severity, duration, and cause of the heart failure.[418,677] Regardless of the presence or absence of CHF, management of an expanded ECF volume should be directed by the patient's clinical condition and altered according to the observed responses.

Concentration changes

The second step in evaluating fluid and electrolyte balance is the consideration of concentration. Because the major component of body fluids is water (see the section on total body water), the addition or loss of compartmental water produces a change in solute concentration. The quantity of solute relative to the volume of water is thereby increased (concentrated) or reduced (diluted). Because water freely moves between fluid compartments, an initial isolated compartmental alteration in water volume is rapidly reflected in other compartments, resulting in osmolal equilibration. Concentration changes are therefore actually disorders of water balance. Most often, the initial aberration originates in the plasma. The plasma disturbance, in turn, evokes a response from the interstitial and intracellular compartments. Because sodium ion is relatively restricted from the intracellular space and is the predominant osmotically active substance in the ECF, changes in water volume are *generally* reflected by inverse changes in the serum sodium concentration and serum osmolality. On the other hand, primary alterations in the serum sodium content result in a redistribution of water, which in turn alters osmolality and compartmental solute concentrations. Sodium abnormalities uncomplicated by changes in water metabolism and distribution are uncommon; usually there are concurrent changes in both sodium and water.[640] Thus serum sodium levels are usually a key determinant of osmolality and a good indicator of concentration changes (i.e., water loss or gain). As a rule of thumb, similar and proportionate changes in serum sodium and chloride concentrations (e.g., a 10% reduction in both serum sodium and chloride concentrations) are usually due to changes in water volume.

The remainder of this section discusses concentration changes in terms of hyponatremic and hypernatremic syndromes, but a note of caution is in order. The use of serum sodium measurements alone as a basis for evaluation and therapy of concentration changes is a one-dimensional approach. In general, hyponatremia and hypernatremia reflect changes in TBW relative to total body sodium and do not reflect sodium balance alone. The sodium concentration and ECF volume may change in opposite directions (the so-called sodium paradox). Both reduced and elevated serum sodium concentrations may occur in the face of hypovolemia, hypervolemia, and normovolemia, and volume changes (isotonic fluid loss or gain) occur frequently without a change in serum sodium levels. Therefore a serum sodium concentration by itself fails to provide information about the patient's hydration or volume status; it merely reflects the ratio of total body water to salt.[64,575]

Sodium. The total body sodium concentration averages 60 mEq/kg of body weight in a healthy adult male[541] (i.e., 4200 mEq in a 70-kg man). Approximately 2000 to 2200 mEq is dissolved in the ECF. Another 1800 mEq resides within the skeletal system, which constitutes 15% to 16% of body weight.[49] Thus total body sodium is proportioned as follows: about 50% is extracellular, 40% is in bone, and 10% or less is intracellular.[197,541,731]

Body sodium is often discussed in terms of exchangeable and nonexchangeable moieties. Nonexchangeable sodium is that fraction adsorbed on hydroxyapatite crystals contained deep within the long bones of the skeleton.[575] It amounts to roughly 18 mEq/kg of the total body sodium concentration.[541] Clinically more important is the exchangeable sodium, which represents 42 mEq/kg of the total body sodium.[575,731,758,784] This exchangeable fraction includes all sodium within the extracellular and intracellular fluids and about half of the bone sodium. Exchangeable sodium is in diffusion equilibrium with plasma (serum) sodium and is reflected in the normal ECF concentration of sodium (i.e., 136 to 145 mEq/L). This exchangeable reservoir serves to mitigate concentration changes when sodium is either lost (e.g., sweat, diarrhea) or retained (e.g., cirrhosis, CHF). Accordingly, the concentration of sodium may provide little useful information about the total body sodium content.

The daily requirement for sodium (in adults) averages 1 to 2 mEq/kg/day, with the normal dietary intake ranging between 100 and 200 mEq/day. In contrast, preterm infants have large renal and intestinal sodium losses and require 4 to 5 mEq/kg/day during the initial postnatal period.[9,10] Sodium excretion (predominantly in urine) exactly balances intake in the healthy individual, because renal elimination can adequately compensate for intake ranging from 0.25 to 6 or more mEq/kg/day.[731] However, the turnover of sodium is relatively slow, requiring several days to excrete an ingested quantity of ion. The magnitude of the kidney's role in maintaining concentration can be appreciated when one realizes that 173 L of water and 24,000 mEq of sodium are filtered and resorbed by the kidney each day.[535] The kidney is able to regulate total body sodium through changes in the rates of glomerular filtration and tubular resorption.[674] These processes are modulated by several neurohumoral mechanisms, including the renin-angiotensin-aldosterone system, atrial natriuretic peptide, parathyroid hormone, antidiuretic hormone, and sympathetic stimulation. Both primary renal dysfunction and diseases affecting the neurohumoral regulatory systems may disrupt the kidney's ability to maintain sodium and water balance.

HYPONATREMIA. Hyponatremia exists when the serum (or plasma) sodium is less than 136 mEq/L. The measured value represents the ratio of sodium to volume in the serum (or plasma). Barring the existence of excess solute, hyponatremia implies hypo-osmolality of all body fluid compartments (i.e., TBW), but hyponatremia as an isolated finding does not imply anything about the patient's total body sodium content or volume status.[590] A low serum sodium concentration is significant because it can produce electrophysiologic disturbances. Effective depolarization of "excitable" cells and the subsequent generation of an action potential requires a proper ECF sodium concentration.[279] Neuronal and myocardial depolarization abnormalities can result in a wide range of CNS symptoms and dysrhythmias, respectively.

There are several ways to assess and classify hyponatremic states. A relatively simple method[249] for addressing clinical importance, cause, and management is to ask three pertinent questions: (1) Is the hyponatremia real or artifactual (pseudohyponatremia)? (2) Is the tonicity low, normal, or high? (Table 46-10), and (3) If the hyponatremia is real and associated with hypotonicity, what is the ECF volume status? The information gained can then be used to correctly diagnose and subsequently manage the hyponatremic state (Fig. 46-8).

Pseudohyponatremia is an example of isotonic hyponatremia and is characterized by low serum sodium and normal measured serum osmolality concentrations (see Table 46-8). The most common cause is hyperlipidemia, which may result (1) from an inborn error of lipoprotein metabolism, (2) secondary to a number of conditions, including diabetes mellitus, uremia, hypothyroidism, nephrotic syndrome, glucocorticoid excess, or alcohol abuse, or (3) as a side effect of oral contraceptives, beta-adrenergic blocking agents, or diuretics. Usually, the lipid concentration must be high enough to produce gross lactescence of the serum or plasma. Severe hyperproteinemia (e.g., Waldenström's macroglobulinemia, multiple myeloma) will also result in a low aqueous sodium concentration.[717] Typically, the serum or plasma is extremely viscid, attaining an almost gel-like state.[249]

Pseudohyponatremia exists when the laboratory provides a falsely low serum sodium estimate. Normally, a volume of plasma consists mostly (>90%) of water, but in the situations noted previously, there is a significant nonaqueous component. Because proteins have high molecular weights and lipids are hydrophobic, elevated protein and lipid concentrations displace water from a given volume of plasma and contribute little to the plasma osmolality concentration. With hyperproteinemia or hyperlipemia, these solids in plasma may increase from 7% to as much as 30%.[64,397] The sodium in solution will be diluted by the solid phase, which lacks sodium. Because the serum sodium concentration is normally reported as mEq/L of plasma, not mEq/L of plasma water, the measured concentration will be artificially low.[608] In other words, the serum sodium value is artifactually diminished because it is measured in a volume of plasma that contains a larger than normal percentage of nonaqueous solute. The recognition of pseudohyponatremia is important because no specific therapy for the low serum sodium concentration is warranted; true hyponatremia in this circumstance does not exist. The diagnosis can be confirmed by

Table 46-10	Categories of hyponatremia
Type	**Osmolality concentration (measured)**
Isotonic	Normal*
Hypertonic	Increased
Hypotonic	Decreased

*Approximate normal value for serum osmolality is 285 ± 10 mOsm/kg H₂O.

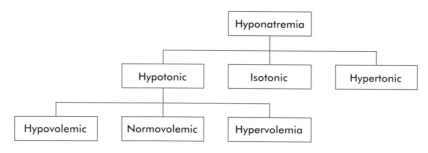

Fig. 46-8. Characterization of hyponatremic states.

obtaining a measurement of plasma water sodium or osmolality concentrations, which will reflect the activity of sodium in the aqueous phase.

Hypertonic hyponatremia arises when a diminished serum sodium concentration co-exists with an elevated serum osmolality (see Table 46-8). An increase in concentration of any osmotically active substance, which is confined predominately to the ECF (e.g., glucose, glycerol, mannitol), will result in water movement. Cellular dehydration occurs as water moves from the ICF to the ECF and the serum (plasma) sodium is diluted to a lower than normal value. The osmolar load usually evokes an osmotic diuresis, which produces a urinary loss of both sodium and free water (i.e., water free of solute). These losses, in turn, potentiate both the hypertonicity and the hyponatremia. The most frequent cause of this water and electrolyte disturbance is the occurrence of significant hyperglycemia in uncontrolled or poorly controlled diabetes mellitus. The measured serum sodium concentration falls approximately 1.6 mEq/L for each 100 mg/dl increment of blood glucose.[64,249] Any greater decrease in serum sodium concentration becomes a useful indicator of the degree of cellular dehydration. Another common cause of perioperative hypertonic hyponatremia is the overzealous use of intravenous mannitol.[30] Mannitol is often administered in an attempt to maintain or enhance renal performance (e.g., AAA repair with high aortic cross-clamp) and also used as an agent to minimize or diminish tissue edema (e.g., intracranial surgery).

When a patient's laboratory data reveal both hyponatremia and a normal or increased osmolality concentration, a state of hypertonic hyponatremia should be suspected. The presence or absence of hyperglycemia will be readily apparent from the results of routine blood work. If the impermeant ECF solute is one other than glucose, the osmolal gap will be significantly elevated. As noted previously, the measured osmolality concentration reflects the osmotic activity of all solutes present in the serum, whereas the calculated osmolality concentration accounts for the osmotic contribution of only sodium, glucose, and urea.[238] An osmolal gap of greater than 10 mOsm/kg provides clinically useful information, because it suggests the presence of another ECF solute. Management is directed toward restoration of the deficits in free water and volume and removal of the offending osmole. Significant hyperglycemia should be corrected with insulin therapy. The hyponatremia resulting from the elevated ECF solute concentration requires no specific therapy per se and will normalize as fluids are replaced and the offending solute is removed.

In most situations, hyponatremia develops with concurrent hypotonicity and a diminished serum osmolality concentration (see Table 46-8). This "true" hyponatremia is usually associated with an excess of body water. More importantly, the TBW will always be increased relative to the total body sodium.[92] Thus, despite the hyponatremia, the total body sodium content may be elevated, diminished, or unchanged as compared with normal.[64,244,397] In turn, total body sodium determines the ECF volume, and often these two terms are used interchangeably.[674] One important caveat does require mention: the ECF volume does not always parallel the effective intravascular volume or effective arterial plasma volume (e.g., the patient with severe congestive heart failure and accompanying hypotension and azotemia).[249] Nonetheless, it is clinically useful to classify the various hypotonic hyponatremic states on the basis of the associated ECF volume status: hyponatremia, hypernatremia, and normovolemia (see Fig. 46-8). Determination of the ECF volume status is a clinical judgment depending on the patient's history, physical examination, serial weights, medications, and laboratory data. Management of these perturbations in the amount of water and/or sodium will be directed by several factors, including the patient's (1) neurologic status,[16,19,29] (2) intravascular volume,[444] and (3) renal function.[7]

Hypovolemic hypotonic hyponatremia. For practical purposes, the potential causes of sodium depletion associated with a contracted ECF volume can be divided into two major categories: extrarenal and renal causes. Table 46-11 lists these underlying causes and summarizes the resultant urinary concentrations of sodium and chloride. These urine values are often helpful in establishing a correct diagnosis. As the body attempts to compensate for the underlying problem, volume and sodium regulatory systems are activated. The decreased ECF volume takes precedence over the diminished ECF tonicity (the so-called "law of circulating volume"). Volume depletion causes elevated antidiuretic hormone (ADH) levels, which will produce a retention of water in excess of sodium. With normal renal function, intact neuroendocrine responses, and a lack of diuretics, there is avid sodium and chloride retention by the kidneys along with reduced urine output. In general, a low urine sodium concentration (< 10 to 20 mEq/L) suggests that either the fluid and solute losses were extrarenal or the losses were originally renal in cause but have since subsided. An important exception may occur with metabolic alkalosis induced by the loss of gastric secretions. The elevated urine bicarbonate concentration may induce a significant urinary loss of sodium. Consequently, a diminished urine chloride concentration will provide the best evidence for contraction of the ECF volume in this situation.[249,371]

Another condition that may occur in the periop-

Table 46-11 Hypovolemic hypotonic hyponatremia

Cause	Urine sodium concentration (mEq/L)	Urine chloride concentration (mEq/L)
Extrarenal sodium losses		
Vomiting	<20	<20
With metabolic alkalosis	>20	<20
Diarrhea	<20	<20
Burns	<20	<20
"Third spacing"	<20	<20
Renal sodium losses		
Diuretics		
Continued use	>20	>20
After cessation	<20	<20
Primary adrenal insufficiency	>20	>20
Renal parenchymal disease	>20	>20

Modified from Goldberg M: Hyponatremia, *Med Clin North AM* 65:251, 1981.

Table 46-12 Hypervolemic hypotonic hyponatremia

Cause	Urine sodium concentration (mEq/L)	Urine chloride concentration (mEq/L)
Kidney disease		
Renal failure or severe insufficiency	>20	>20
Edematous states		
Cirrhosis of the liver	<20	<20
Congestive heart failure	<20	<20
Nephrotic syndrome	<20	<20
Severe hypoproteinemia	<20	<20

Modified from Humes HD, Narins RG, and Brenner BM: Disorders of water balance, *Hosp Pract* 3:133, 1979.

erative period is the loss of electrolyte-rich fluid (extrarenal source), which is then replaced with maintenance-type intravenous solutions (i.e., predominately free water). It is not uncommon to confront a patient suffering from a volume loss that is essentially isotonic, and yet the administered fluid therapy is hypotonic in nature. If the volume of this replacement therapy is inadequate, the signs and symptoms associated with hypovolemic hypotonic hyponatremia will develop.

The clinical manifestations associated with this form of hyponatremia are almost always due to the volume deficit. As one might expect, treatment is aimed at correcting the diminished ECF volume and generally involves the administration of isotonic sodium solutions. Parenteral fluids of this nature can replenish the ECF compartment and correct the impaired water excretion. Hypertonic salt solutions are rarely necessary, and fluid restriction or diuretics are inappropriate for this type of hyponatremia.

Hypervolemic hypotonic hyponatremia. This category of hyponatremia includes those conditions in which the total body sodium concentration is elevated, and there is a concomitant defect in the excretion of solute-free water. Water retention is proportionately greater than sodium retention, with the net result being an expanded ECF volume that is hypotonic. A dilutional hyponatremia is generated, and extensive edema formation is frequently observed.

The clinical disorders producing this particular variety of hyponatremia include renal failure, CHF, cirrhosis, and nephrotic syndrome (Table 46-12).

Patients with renal failure are frequently hyponatremic and volume expanded. As the functional nephron mass diminishes, the glomerular filtration rate (GFR) is reduced and there is limited excretion of both salt and free water.[85,376] If the total volume of both water intake (oral and parenteral) and production (endogenous) exceeds the volume of water excreted (insensible losses plus renal free water excretion), then water retention will occur with a decrease in serum sodium. In severe renal insufficiency or renal failure, the GFR may be 5% or less of the normal 180 L per day. Renal free water clearance is similarly reduced and may be significantly less than 1 L per day. Thus the intake of relatively small volumes of salt and/or water can easily overwhelm the remaining functional nephrons.

The second group of illnesses that may result in this type of hyponatremia are often categorized as the "edematous states." Patients with edema and underlying end stage nephrosis,[234] cirrhosis,[23,406,530] or CHF[326] tend to have markedly increased total body sodium concentrations and water. The increment in TBW is always proportionately greater in magnitude than the increase in the sodium concentration. An internal maldistribution of the ECF occurs, and most of the volume becomes redirected to the ISF compartment, the venous side of the circulation, and/or the intracorporeal fluid pools (e.g., pleural and ascitic fluid).[249] The plasma volume may be normal or even elevated, but the *effective* arterial plasma volume is reduced, and as a consequence, renal plasma flow and

GFR are diminished. The kidneys, baroreceptors, and hypothalamus respond as if there were true hypovolemia and sodium depletion. Renin, angiotensin, aldosterone, and ADH levels become elevated, a relative oliguria develops, and the urine sodium concentration drops to less than 10 to 20 mEq/L.[517] Patients afflicted with this pathophysiologic condition are often chronically hyponatremic but are usually not symptomatic from the hypotonicity unless they are rapidly administered a free water load.

As one might expect, therapeutic efforts should be aimed at stabilizing and then improving the primary cause of the edematous state. Further strategies for treatment should be based on the serum sodium concentration and the presence or absence of related clinical manifestations. In general, if the serum sodium concentration is between 120 and 130 mEq/L, rigid restriction of sodium and water intake is indicated. If the sodium concentration drops below 120 mEq/L and the stigmata of hypotonicity develop, more aggressive measures should be undertaken. As a result of the diminished effective arterial plasma volume, there is intense proximal tubular sodium resorption and minimal distal delivery of this ion. Conventional diuretic therapy is usually ineffective, because these agents work predominatcly on thc more distal sites of the nephron. On the other hand, diuretics such as zaroxolyn and acetazolamide have a theoretic advantage, because they inhibit a significant proportion of proximal tubular sodium rcsorption.[773] Often a combination of therapeutic agents is used in an attempt to increase the delivery of proximal tubular fluid to more distal sites where diuretics such as furosemide, bumetanide, spironolactone, and the thiazides can block salt and water reabsorption. Zaroxalyn and acetazolamide have also been used in this regard, as have aminophylline, dopamine, mannitol, and isooncotic plasma expanders. Regardless of the therapeutic option used, if the underlying condition is end-stage and irreversible, improvements in volume, tonicity, and/or sodium content are usually short lived.

Normovolemic hypotonic hyponatremia. There are several conditions where hyponatremia is associated with both a normal (or near-normal) total body sodium content and effective arterial plasma volume.[573] In most instances the diminished serum osmolality concentration results from excessive circulating ADH, which in turn produces a decrease in urine volume, a decrease in the serum sodium concentration, and a relative increase in urine osmolality concentration.[810] It is important to appreciate that the outpouring of ADH in this setting is unrelated to a volume deficit (either actual or effective). With an appropriate evaluation, an abnormality in the regulation of ADH secretion and/or

---

BOX 46-2
CONDITIONS ASSOCIATED WITH NORMOVOLEMIC HYPOTONIC HYPONATREMIA

Antidiuretic medications
Severe potassium depletion
Emotional stress
Psychogenic polydipsia
Severe hypothyroidism (myxedema)
Glucocorticoid deficiency
Reduced osmolal regulatory threshold
Parturition
Syndrome of inappropriate secretion of ADH (SIADH)

BOX 46-3
MEDICATIONS ASSOCIATED WITH HYPOTONIC HYPONATREMIA

Opiate derivates	Chlorpropamide
Clofibrate	Tolbutamide
Carbamazepine	Nonsteroidal antiinflam-
Cyclophosphamide	matory agents
Vincristine	Oxytocin
Vinblastine	Diuretics
Barbiturates	

---

sensitivity can usually be identified.[50,51] The causative pathophysiologic process or pharmacologic agent (Box 46-2) ultimately impairs renal water excretion. The hypotonicity thus generated is responsible for the observed clinical manifestations.

Numerous medications (other than diuretics) can impair water excretion and have been associated with normovolemic hyponatremia (Box 46-3). Most of these drugs can stimulate the release of ADH and/or potentiate the peripheral action of ADH (i.e., increased water permeability of the collecting ducts).[35,387,388,764] Conventional diuretics, especially those producing potassium depletion, may also generate hyponatremia;[395] the lowered sodium concentration is commonly attributed to a contraction of ECF volume, which in turn stimulates thirst and ADH secretion. An impaired urinary dilutional capacity with a relatively fixed minimal urinary osmolality concentration is a consequence of diuretic therapy.[64,773] Assuming there is limited variation in solute intake, hyponatremia then develops when water intake exceeds free water excretion. Diuretic-induced hypokalemia may produce a resetting of the "osmostat" such that clinically insignificant hypovolemia results in a substantial ADH response.[37,205] In addition, potassium depletion can lead to a shift of sodium ion into the ICF compartment, thereby exacerbating the hyponatremia.[205] Nonsteroidal anti-inflammatory agents can inhibit the synthesis of renal prostaglandins, which — in addition to their important vasoregulatory properties — also possess potent diuretic properties.[123] Thus a number of drugs are capable of creating a hyponatremic state that appears virtually identical to the syndrome of inappropriate secretion of ADH. One important difference between these two conditions is that the drug-induced syndrome rapidly dissipates with removal of the offending agent.

Psychogenic polydipsia is a rare cause of normovolemic hypotonic hyponatremia. It occurs in psychiatric patients, usually those taking one of the numerous phenothiazine medications. These drugs produce drying of the mucous membranes and thus stimulate thirst.[294] Generally, water intake must be extreme and associated with a decreased intake of salt and/or protein to generate symptomatic hyponatremia. A normal person can excrete 20 to 25 L of water per day (without developing hyponatremia or fluid retention), provided there is sufficient solute intake.[337] An important point to remember is that for any given urine osmolality concentration, water excretion is determined largely by solute intake and elimination.[64]

Both severe hypothyroidism (primary myxedema) and glucocorticoid deficiency increase water retention, probably through some degree of effective ECF volume contraction and compensatory ADH release.[408,672] In addition, cortisol has an important role in maintaining normal inhibitory control of ADH release.[7,36] Depending on the circumstance, physiologic doses of either thyroid extract (or the synthetic analog) or a glucocorticoid preparation will correct the hyponatremia and normalize the ADH levels.

Most cases of normovolemic hypotonic hyponatremia are iatrogenic in origin and arise from the administration of hypotonic fluids in the presence of a nonosmotic stimulus for ADH release. Emotional stress, anxiety, nausea, pain, and the administration of opiates are all common in surgical patients, and each condition promotes ADH release. The same conditions pertain to obstetric patients in whom the problem may be compounded by the administration of oxytocin, which simulates the physiologic actions of ADH.[766] Therefore fluid therapy and especially free water intake must be monitored carefully in these patients.

Certain patients with chronic debilitating disorders may suffer from a resetting of the "osmostat."[155] The level of serum osmolality or serum sodium that stimulates ADH release is reset downward to a lower value. These patients are relatively asymptomatic despite the existence of moderately severe hyponatremia. The serum sodium concentration typically ranges from 125 to 130 mEq/L, but the ADH response to water loading and hypertonicity is quantitatively normal. No specific therapy is indicated or necessary for this chronic hyponatremic state.

The syndrome of inappropriate secretion of ADH (SIADH) is a form of hypotonic hyponatremia caused by a sustained or intermittent release of ADH that is inappropriate for the physiologic conditions at hand (i.e., osmolality and ECF volume). Normally, a 3% or greater decrement in the serum sodium concentration produces a complete inhibition of ADH secretion and a urine osmolality concentration of 50 to 100 mOsm/kg. Despite the reduced serum osmolality and sodium concentrations, SIADH results in a natriuresis (> 20 mEq/L) and a urine osmolality concentration that is less than maximally dilute.[810]

The diagnosis of SIADH is largely one of exclusion, but the syndrome is often associated with a variety of central nervous system, neoplastic, and pulmonary disorders.[513] Some diseases result in ectopic production of an ADH-like substance, whereas others produce dysregulation of endogenous ADH secretion. A correct diagnosis requires the presence of normal renal, adrenal, and pituitary function.[35] The treatment of choice is usually water restriction. The acute form of the syndrome dissipates as the underlying illness (e.g., pneumonia) resolves. The more chronic form, however, is often associated with an incurable disease (e.g., unresectable cancer). In this situation, water restriction alone may be insufficient, and drugs such as lithium carbonate and demeclocycline (both capable of producing nephrogenic diabetes insipidus) have been used with some success.[50,71,666]

In all forms of hypotonic hyponatremia, the severity of the clinical manifestations depends on both the degree of hyponatremia and the rate of fall of sodium concentration.[22,136] Several days of progressive water retention and hypotonicity cause brain water to increase and nonspecific symptoms to develop. In general, at a serum sodium concentration of approximately 130 mEq/L, headache, restlessness, irritability, confusion, anorexia, muscle cramps, nausea, and vomiting may occur. An equivalent degree of hyponatremia that develops rapidly (< 24 hours) or a more pronounced reduction in serum sodium concentration (approximately 120 mEq/L) that arises gradually produces a greater increment in brain water; seizures, coma, papilledema, and a delayed relaxation phase of the deep tendon reflexes are often observed.[546] It is important to appreciate that even a relatively small excess water intake (oral or parenteral), in combination with a chronic but true hypotonic hyponatremic state, may result in acute water intoxication. The symptomatology is usually severe, the objective findings may be extreme (i.e., shock, widened QRS complexes, ST segment elevation, ventricular tachycardia, or fibrillation), and the overall mortality rate is approximately 50%.[19]

A serum sodium level of 120 mEq/L is often touted as the division between mild and severe reactions, but a note of caution is in order. Subacute (24 to 48 hours) and chronic hyponatremia evoke physiologic adaptations, and although the degree of serum sodium reduction generally parallels the clinical signs and symptoms, this relationship is not always consistent. Thus the decision to initiate therapy and the aggressiveness of the therapy should be individualized and based on the previously noted variables.[29] There have been reports of severe neurologic sequelae and even death after both slow and rapid correction of hyponatremia.[16,30,219,396,701,702] Nonetheless, most authors advocate prompt intervention when symptoms are severe or if the serum sodium concentration falls below 115 mEq/L.

Correction by 6 to 8 mEq/L/day is fast enough to allow a prompt and uncomplicated recovery and slow enough to remain below the limits of toxicity.[699]

The short-term goal is to achieve an acceptable level of the serum sodium level (i.e., a level associated with minimal symptoms), not a total correction of the sodium concentration.

Despite the premise that normovolemic hypotonic hyponatremia is associated with a normal ECF volume and total body sodium content, there is a disproportionate amount of water (i.e., relative deficit of sodium). A rough guide for rapidly correcting the hyponatremia can be obtained from calculating the sodium deficit:

$$Na^+_{deficit} = TBW \times (140 - \text{serum sodium concentration})$$

A reasonable approach is to administer half the deficit over the first 8 hours and, if symptoms resolve, the remaining half over the next 24 to 72 hours. A small volume of hypertonic saline solution (e.g., 3% or 5% sodium chloride, 513 mEq/L, and 856 mEq/L respectively) is most often recommended until seizures and/or coma resolve.[27,605,778] The simultaneous use of a loop diuretic prevents ECF volume overexpansion, enhances renal water excretion, and reduces urinary osmolality.[27] Also, it is crucial that urinary sodium and potassium losses be continuously replaced, and serum electrolyte and osmolality concentrations must be reassessed at frequent intervals.

For less severe cases of hyponatremia, normal (isotonic) saline can be administered in conjunction with a loop diuretic.[149,292] However, the use of normal saline (308 mOsm/L) alone may worsen the hyponatremia if the patient's urine osmolality is significantly greater than 308 mOsm/kg.[64]

There are two additional conditions occasionally associated with hyponatremia that are particular to surgical patients. Neither condition is a result of abnormal ADH secretion, and there is no consistent pattern of ECF volume. In the first condition, hyponatremia may result from the administration of hypotonic parenteral fluids (i.e., maintenance fluids) and the failure to appreciate the extent of endogenous water formation.[271,460,474,523] Endogenous water is generated from (1) oxidation, as nutrient fuels are used, and (2) mobilization, as cells undergo catabolism. Oxidation of 1 kg of fat generates approximately 1 L of solute free water. In addition, oxidation of 1 kg of lean body mass (73% to 82% water) mobilizes about 0.75 L of cellular water, and after a major operation it is possible to catabolize as much as 750 g of tissue daily. Therefore caloric intake must be adequate in the perioperative period; otherwise excessive endogenous water production may facilitate the development of hyponatremia.[151]

The second condition, one potentially resulting in postoperative or intraoperative hyponatremia, is the performance of transurethral surgery—in particular, transurethral prostatic resection (TURP). Surgical procedures of this nature require continuous irrigation of the operative field so as to improve visibility and distend the bladder or prostatic urethra. It is the systemic absorption of these irrigating solutions that can produce rapid and sometimes dramatic hyponatremia. The fluids used for intraoperative bladder irrigation must be nonelectrolytic to prevent dispersion of the high-frequency current from the resectoscope[432] and transparent to maintain visibility.[47] The solutions commonly employed include distilled water, glycine, mannitol, sorbitol, and a combination of the latter two, termed Cytal.* Because sterile water is so severely hypotonic (i.e., zero osmolarity) and because it has the potential for hemolyzing erythrocytes, its use has become limited mostly to the transurethral resection of bladder tumors. Sterile water in this situation produces osmotic lysis of tumor cells,[768] with a minimal risk of systemic hyponatremia so long as the procedure is relatively brief and the surgical trauma is not extensive. Most of the other so-called "isotonic" irrigating solutions are actually hypoosmolar, but when compared with water, their calculated osmolarity concentrations are much more acceptable (e.g., 1.2% glycine, 220 mOsm/L; 3% sorbitol, 165 mOsm/L). Intravascular absorption of these fluids does not generally cause a reduction in serum osmolality or hemolysis but can result in ECF volume expansion,

---

* References 218, 254, 423, 427, 616, 721.

CHF, interstitial edema, and/or unpredictably severe, dilutional hyponatremia.

During a TURP, systemic absorption of the irrigating solutions is influenced by the duration of exposure, the number and size of venous sinuses opened, extravasation of the fluid into tissues outside the bladder or prostatic capsule, and the hydrostatic pressure of the fluid.[1,83,206,511] In the past, numerous attempts have been made to quantitate the amount of fluid entrained. One study suggests estimating the average absorption at 10 to 30 ml per minute of operating time,[163] whereas other studies suggest indirectly measuring the fluid absorption by noting the immediate, postoperative weight gain.[427,721]

It is likely that all patients undergoing TURP absorb some quantity of irrigating fluid and thereby increase both their intravascular volume and pressure.[784] In addition, fluid absorption produces a dilution of the serum proteins with the net result within the intravascular compartment being an increase in hydrostatic pressure and a decrease in oncotic pressure. The severity and duration of these alterations are quite variable, but conditions do favor the movement of ECF volume from the intravascular compartment to the ISF compartment.[428] One reported case documents the movement of 1500 ml of fluid into the ISF compartment,[621] and for each 100 ml of redistributed fluid there is an associated relocation of 10 to 15 mEq of sodium ion. Thus the intravascular volume expansion may be relatively transient when compared with the duration of the hyponatremia and the excess ISF volume.

The early diagnosis of hyponatremia and/or volume overload during a transurethral procedure depends on frequently repeated assessments of the patient. This can be best accomplished with an anesthetic technique that neither alters the patient's sensorium nor significantly interferes with the compensatory cardiovascular mechanisms (e.g., a regional anesthetic).[342] The signs and symptoms of this rapid-onset hyponatremia are generally the same as those observed with acute water intoxication. However, acute hyponatremia with little or no decrease in the serum osmolality concentration is usually better tolerated in terms of symptoms and complications.[163] If clinical manifestations develop, the surgical procedure should be terminated as rapidly as possible and the corrective therapy (as previously outlined) should be initiated immediately.

HYPERNATREMIA. An elevated serum sodium concentration is a relatively uncommon, but nevertheless dangerous, abnormality with potentially dire consequences. Hypernatremia implies a relative free water deficit with a resultant increase in the solute concentrations within all body fluid compartments. Thus hypernatremia is associated with hypertonicity and hyperosmolality. When the serum osmolality level exceeds 295 to 300 mOsm/kg H_2O, ADH secretion is stimulated and the urine becomes severely concentrated (i.e., osmolality level greater than 800 to 1000 mOsm/kg H_2O).[538] The sensitive thirst response is activated in an attempt to stem cellular dehydration. Hypertonicity and hypernatremia rarely develop in the presence of an intact thirst mechanism and access to water, even if there is a complete absence of ADH and a total inability to concentrate the urine.[412,573] The imbalance between TBW and sodium that occurs in the hypernatremic states may develop from either water loss (i.e., pure water or hypotonic fluid) or salt gain. However, there must be some process or abnormality preventing water intake (oral and/or parenteral) for water loss to cause the hypernatremia.

The presence of hypernatremia per se implies nothing about total body sodium content. This distinction is crucial because it is the total body sodium, regardless of its serum concentration, that determines the net ECF volume. In turn, the relative size of the ECF volume may not necessarily correlate with the intravascular volume or the effective arterial plasma volume. With a pure water loss, the total body sodium content (and hence, the ECF volume) should remain normal. A combined sodium and water loss (i.e., water in excess of sodium) characterizes the removal of hypotonic fluids from the body and produces a diminished total body sodium content and hypovolemia. Conversely, an increment in total body sodium content will generally create a hypervolemic condition. This differentiation of the ECF volume status [50,794] is helpful in classifying the hypernatremic states (Fig. 46-9), but in actuality the categories are not as clearly distinct as has been implied. For any specific cause, a patient's ECF volume status depends on (1) the severity and duration of the disorder, (2) the actual composition of the fluid lost, (3) the total body sodium content, (4) the patient's baseline health status, (5) the presence of any underlying medical conditions, and (6) the quantity and composition of intake during the development of the hypernatremia. Nonetheless, this scheme for classifying the hypernatremic states is conceptually useful and applicable to the majority of clinical situations.

Hypotonic fluid loss. Probably the most common form of hypernatremia is that associated with the loss of hypotonic fluid (i.e., relatively greater water than sodium loss). The diminished ECF volume is usually associated with a reduced effective arterial plasma volume, and therefore the clinical manifestations mimic the findings in most other forms of hypovolemia (see the section on volume deficit). These losses can be grouped into two major categories: renal and extrarenal losses. The causes for a nonrenal loss of hypotonic fluid include excessive sweating (e.g., fever,

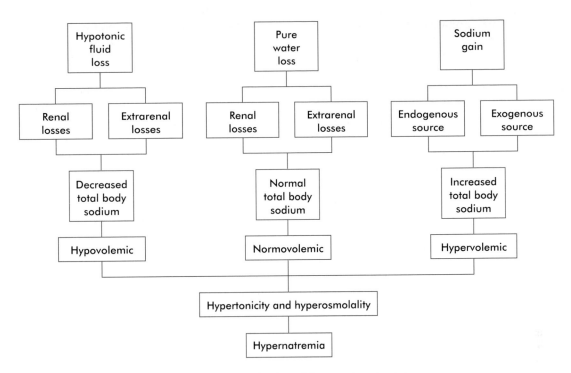

Fig. 46-9. Characterization of hypernatremic states.

strenuous exercise), heat stroke,[300,372] and diarrhea (especially in children).[384] However, there is significant variation exhibited in the fecal sodium loss resulting from diarrhea (e.g., 10 to 140 mEq/L).[656] The majority of gastrointestinal losses are isotonic and will not alter tonicity, the serum osmolality concentration, or the measured sodium concentration.

The renal causes of hypotonic fluid loss result in a solute diuresis, with the offending substance being either an electrolyte or a nonelectrolyte. As opposed to most other forms of total body sodium deficit, there will be an enhanced urine volume (i.e., polyuria) that is less than maximally concentrated because high urinary flows limit tubular reabsorption. The urine specific gravity will be approximately 1.01 and the osmolality level close to 300 mOsm/kg H_2O. In general, with an electrolyte diuresis the urine will contain a sodium salt, either chloride or bicarbonate.[665] The combined water and sodium chloride losses capable of producing hypernatremia may occur with chronic renal failure or insufficiency, salt-losing nephritides, Addison's disease, an isolated deficiency of aldosterone, or excessive use of conventional diuretics. Also, the limited ability to concentrate urine—often observed in elderly persons, preterm infants,[9,190] and those with hypoxic renal damage—results in a similar hypotonic fluid loss. The renal wasting of sodium bicarbonate (easily ruled out by a urine pH of less than 7.0) occurs with proximal renal tubular acidosis and Fanconi's syndrome.[495] The more common nonelectrolyte diuresis results from excess

solute such as glucose, fructose, mannitol, sorbitol, glycerol, urea, or amino acids.[198,241,249] These substances act as osmotic diuretics and produce a loss of solute, water, and sodium. This may occur unintentionally with high-protein diets,[794] inadequately diluted tube feedings,[233] or infant formulas,[207] and parenteral hyperalimentation, which can generate a nonketotic hyperosmolar state similar to severe diabetes.[18,90,442] Any substantial increase in protein intake can cause a urea-induced polyuria (1 g of protein contains 6 mM of urea), but exogenous intake is not the only means for creating this type of solute diuresis. The outpouring of urine after the relief of a urinary tract obstruction (i.e., postobstructive diuresis) is the result of normal endogenous urea production and continues until the previously accumulated urea is eliminated.

Regardless of the cause of the fluid loss, the mainstay of therapy is the administration of hypotonic crystalloid solutions. Fluids such as 0.45% normal saline can replace the water loss and gradually restore the total body sodium content. In certain situations, it may also be possible to remove a causative solute either directly (e.g., discontinuation of a parenteral hyperalimentation solution or a mannitol infusion) or indirectly (e.g., treating an underlying disorder such as Addison's disease).

Pure water loss. Total body sodium content and the relative size of the ECF volume usually remain normal with the isolated loss of solute-free water. Cell membranes are freely permeable to water, and, thus both the ICF and ECF compartments share the volume loss in proportion to their relative sizes.[198] However, the clinical manifestations (e.g., thirst, weakness, irritability, restlessness, seizures, and coma)[19,369] result from the diminished ICF volume. Two thirds of a pure water loss originates from the ICF compartment, and one third is contributed by the ECF compartment. Only one twelfth of the total water deficit is extracted from the intravascular fluids, because plasma volume constitutes only 25% of the ECF volume.[424] In addition, if oncotic pressure rises as a result of the water loss, this tends to limit any reduction in plasma volume.[286] As a consequence, the water loss must be massive in quantity (e.g., serum sodium concentration of greater than 170 mEq/L) to generate objective evidence of hypovolemia.

In general, the loss of pure water is characterized as being either renal or nonrenal in origin. The nonrenal causes produce an exaggeration of the normal, continuous insensible water losses that occur via the skin and lungs. Cutaneous evaporative losses may reach several liters per day in thyrotoxicosis or the subacute phase of a burn injury of significant magnitude. Pulmonary water loss increases with an elevated minute ventilation or ventilation with a dry (i.e., nonhumidified), inspired gas mixture, especially when accompanied by a high flow rate. Patients with endotracheal tubes or tracheostomies are more likely to suffer from the aforementioned pulmonary losses, and newborn infants are highly susceptible to all forms of increased insensible water loss[656] (Table 46-13).

The other major route of excess pure water loss is through the kidneys. This particular type of polyuric, euvolemic hypernatremia is seen with both neurogenic and nephrogenic diabetes insipidus. A diagnosis of diabetes insipidus (DI) implies an impaired renal concentrating mechanism that may result from either (1) a failure to synthesize, store, and/or secrete ADH or (2) an ineffectiveness of ADH at its target organ.[399,483,582] There are numerous causes for both forms of DI (Box 46-4), and distinction between the forms is crucial for administering the appropriate therapy.[68]

Neurogenic or central DI represents a defect in the formation or release of ADH due to the destruction of the supraoptic or paraventricular nuclei or from the interruption of the hypothalamic-hypophyseal tract above the median eminence.[573] In 30% to 50% of cases, no specific cause can be identified. Traumatic, neurogenic DI is usually triphasic in nature;[325] the initial polyuria caused by interrupted ADH secretion is followed by a phase of oliguria resulting from the sudden uncontrolled release of stored hormone that follows loss of cellular integrity. The last phase is again polyuric in nature and results from the depletion of stored ADH. Neurogenic DI may be associated with either a complete or partial absence of circulating ADH.[457]

Table 46-13 Factors associated with increased insensible water loss in neonates

Body system	Factors
Skin	Phototherapy, radiant warmers Decreased ambient humidity, gestational age Increased air currents, air temperature, motor activity, skin blood flow, core temperature
Lungs	Mouth breathing, increased minute ventilation, dry or cool inspired gases

Modified from Siker D: Pediatric fluids and electrolytes. In Gregory GA, ed: *Pediatric anesthesia*, ed 2, New York, 1989, Churchill-Livingstone.

BOX 46-4
CAUSES OF DIABETES INSIPIDUS

Neurogenic

Primary (idiopathic)
Secondary
  Trauma
  Hypoxia
  Neurosurgery
  Neoplasm: Primary of brain or pituitary; metastatic of lung or breast
  Granulomatous: Tuberculosis, sarcoid, eosinophilic granuloma, histiocytosis X
  Vascular: Aneurysm, thrombosis, Sheenan's syndrome
  Pituitary cysts
  CNS infections

Nephrogenic

Primary (familial)
Secondary
  Renal: Polycystic disease, medullary cystic disease, sickle cell disease, amyloidosis, pyelonephritis, radiation nephritis, posttransplantation, multiple myeloma, light chain nephropathy
  Drugs: Lithium, demeclocycline, amphotericin B, methoxyflurane, colchicine, vinblastine
  Electrolytes: Hypercalcemia, hypokalemia
  Dietary: Malnutrition, protein restriction, sodium restriction

Nephrogenic (ADH-resistant) DI is a disorder in which there is a lack of significant urinary concentration despite the presence of an adequate circulating ADH concentration. The collecting tubules may become unresponsive to ADH as a result of certain medications. There may be a loss of the normal medullary interstitial hypertonicity due to a lack of dietary protein (i.e., urea) or sodium chloride. Hypercalcemia[42] and hypokalemia both interfere with ADH binding to receptor sites. Primary or secondary renal disorders predominately affecting the intrarenal medulla and papilla (e.g., tubulointerstitial diseases) result in a hypotonic solute diuresis but are also included in this category, because of the presence of a poorly defined "uremic toxin" that antagonizes the effect of ADH.

The differentiation between neurogenic and nephrogenic DI is best accomplished by the fluid deprivation test,[50,457,809] which combines the stimuli of hyperosmolality, volume depletion, and exogenous ADH. Measurement of the resulting urine and serum osmolality levels should provide enough information to identify the form of DI responsible for the polyuria in about 80% of patients.[809] ADH levels can be used to confirm the diagnosis, but often there is a significant time lag (i.e., days to weeks) before the results are available.

The treatment of neurogenic DI should be carefully individualized. Mild forms of the syndrome may not require chronic therapy, whereas severe forms require hormone replacement and careful titration of water intake to avoid either dehydration or acute water intoxication. Replacement therapy is most often instituted with 1-desamino-8-D-arginine vasopressin (DDAVP) nasal spray. This synthetic analog of human ADH (arginine vasopressin) is minimally allergenic, possesses little pressor activity, and controls urine output for 12 to 24 hours after a single dose. Alternatively, vasopressin tannate in oil may be administered intramuscularly every 24 to 48 hours. Partial forms of neurogenic DI can often be controlled with chlorpropamide or clofibrate, which enhances the renal response to ADH or stimulates the central secretion of ADH, respectively.

For most forms of nephrogenic DI, removal of the causative agent (e.g., solute, drug) or correction of the underlying electrolyte abnormality (e.g., hypercalcemia, hypokalemia) is usually sufficient to rectify the disturbance. However, the DI associated with primary or secondary renal disorders is more difficult to control. Treatment is aimed at reducing the obligatory renal solute losses by restricting salt and protein intake. Thiazide diuretics, which decrease ECF volume and promote proximal tubular fluid reabsorption, have also been used with some success.

All forms of hypernatremia associated with a normal total body sodium content require water replacement. This may be administered either orally or parenterally, depending on the patient's condition and the severity of the abnormality. For those rare situations where hypotension accompanies water loss, isotonic fluids should be used to normalize the intravascular volume before initiating water replacement.

Salt gain. Excessive salt intake may be accidental, resulting from the ingestion of salt tablets or the improper preparation of infant formula (e.g., salt substituted for sugar). Just 1 g of table salt contains 34 mM of solute; therefore the consumption of large quantities of salt can readily produce sodium overload. In addition, the intake of seawater (approximately 1000 mOsm/kg H_2O) can generate a state of salt intoxication.[198]

Iatrogenic hypervolemic hypernatremia is perhaps the most common form of excess salt and usually results from the inappropriate use of sodium bicarbonate during cardiopulmonary resuscitation.[63,437] A less frequent cause is the incorrect use of 3% or 5% hypertonic sodium chloride during an attempt to rectify a hypotonic state. There is also the potential for inadvertent intravenous administration of 20% sodium chloride solution, which is intended for intraamniotic installation to induce a therapeutic abortion[613] (Table 46-14).

Disease states producing a mineralocorticoid excess (e.g., primary hyperaldosteronism [Conn's syndrome], Cushing's syndrome) may also cause sodium retention and hypernatremia. The use of hypertonic peritoneal dialysate in patients with chronic renal failure can produce severe hypotonic fluid losses with accompanying hypernatremia. However, the underlying renal dysfunction most often generates a state of sodium excess and expanded ECF volume; therefore this cause is included within the excess salt category.

An acute load of hypertonic salt produces intracellular fluid depletion (i.e., volume contraction) with a subsequent expansion of the ECF volume. Interstitial edema and CHF may develop. Thus the goal of therapy is to remove the excess sodium and replete the intracellular fluid volume. Diuretics are useful for establishing a salt loss, but agents that predominately disrupt the urinary-concentrating mechanisms (e.g., furosemide) may actually exacerbate the hypernatremia. Dialysis provides an alternative therapeutic modality if diuretics prove ineffective. Simultaneous water replacement is necessary to normalize the ICF volume.

Treatment. Because all three forms of hypernatremia require water (either alone, or in combination with sodium or a diuretic) to correct the abnormality, it becomes important to gauge the volume of water

Table 46-14 Hypertonic solutions

Solute	Concentration (% weight)	Calculated osmolarity concentration (mOsm/L)	Container size (ml)	Contents per container (mOsm)	Rise in osmolality concentration per container* (mOsm/kg H₂O)
Dextrose	10%	505	1000	505	12
	50%	2525	50	126	3
Mannitol	10%	549	500	275	6
	25%	1374	50	69	2
Sodium chloride	3%	1027	500	513	12
	5%	1711	500	856	20
	20%	6845	250	1711	40
Sodium bicarbonate	5%	1190	500	595	14
	8.4%	2000	50	100	2

*TBW assumed to be 42 L, and increment in osmolality $= \dfrac{\text{osmolal load}}{\text{TBW + volume of solution}}$.

Modified from Feig PU: Hypernatremia and hypertonic syndromes, *Med Clin North Am* 65:271, 1981.

required. With a pure water loss, the deficit can be estimated with the following equation:

$$\text{water deficit} = TBW \times \left(1 - \frac{140}{Na^+}\right)$$

where TBW is the calculated value for total body water as previously defined, and Na^+ is the current serum sodium concentration. In the case of an acute salt load, the relative water "deficit" can be approximated as follows:

$$\text{water "deficit"} = TBW \times \left(\frac{Na^+}{140} - 1\right)$$

where the "deficit" actually represents the volume of water necessary to dilute the elevated sodium concentration back to normal. The use of either equation requires a number of assumptions that, in turn, enhance the potential for inaccuracy.[198] Most importantly, the development or maintenance of hypernatremia usually involves the urinary loss of water and sodium during some phase of the abnormality. Use of these two equations therefore provides only a rough "guesstimate" as to the magnitude of the actual water deficit. Nevertheless, this can be a starting point from which to initiate therapy.

The potential for developing cerebral edema during therapy for chronic hypernatremic states has been previously discussed. The ideal rate of water replacement and normalization of the serum sodium concentration remain unknown. The recommendation most often quoted is for a maximal decline in the serum sodium concentration of 1 to 2 mEq/L/hr.[64,199,337,369,794] However, a recent review suggests that the rate of correction of chronic hypernatremia (>2 days) should not exceed 0.7 mEq/L/hr, whereas acute hypernatremia (<12 hours) may be corrected rapidly.[513] Equally important is the need for frequent clinical re-evaluation; any deterioration in neurologic function should prompt an immediate slowing of the corrective therapy.

Changes in composition

The final step in managing perioperative fluid and electrolyte therapy requires an evaluation of compartmental composition. An imbalance in the ratio of certain substances (specifically ions) suspended in the body fluids results in a compositional disturbance. The intravascular compartment is then scrutinized for the presence of abnormalities, and when a derangement is identified, certain assumptions can be made about the composition of the ISF and ICF compartments. Results of the history and physical examination may raise a clinical suspicion, but objective laboratory data are the usual means of discovering a perturbation in composition. These data are useful for assessing the severity of the problem and are also beneficial in determining the response to treatment. An alteration in composition may occur in conjunction with a volume and/or concentration disturbance, but it may also occur as an isolated entity. The compositional abnormalities of most importance, in terms of frequency and physiologic impact, include changes in acid-base balance and changes in the concentration of calcium, magnesium, potassium, or phosphorus.

Acid-base balance

ACID-BASE CHEMISTRY. In vivo acid-base reactions normally proceed in a rather restricted environment. The terminology used to describe these reactions—which occur at 37° C within the dilute, aqueous milieu of the body—is derived from the

Bröunsted-Lowry concept of acid-base chemistry. This approach defines an acid as a species having the capacity to donate or transfer a proton (i.e., H^+) to an acceptor and a base as a species having the capacity to accept or add a proton from a donor. The following example is representative of a simple acid-base reaction:

$$HA \longleftrightarrow H^+ + A^-$$

where *HA* is the H^+ donor (i.e., acid) and the anion, A^-, is the proton acceptor (i.e., base). Every acid-base reaction requires both a proton donor and proton acceptor, which, by convention, are designated a conjugate acid-base pair (HA and A^- in the above reaction).[145,328,402]

Each acid has a specific affinity for its proton that allows the acid to be characterized qualitatively in terms of its strength. Strong acids have a low proton affinity, readily give up hydrogen ions, and dissociate almost completely in aqueous solutions. In contrast, weak acids have a relatively high affinity for protons and dissociate only slightly in solution. For each acid-base reaction, there is an associated equilibrium constant, which is generally termed a dissociation constant and is denoted by K'. This dissociation constant is temperature dependent and reflects an acid's tendency to dissociate in solution. For the acid HA the following would be true:

$$K' = \frac{[H^+][A^-]}{[HA]}$$

where K' is the *apparent* dissociation constant (not the true, thermodynamic dissociation constant K) and the brackets indicate concentrations in moles/liter. The numeric value of K' is a measure of acid strength, because the value of K' is directly proportional to the strength of an acid. Since the K' values for the body's weak acids are so relatively small (e.g., at 25° C, 4.27×10^{-4} for H_2CO_3 and 4.8×10^{-13} for $HPO_4^=$), it is customary to indicate acid strength by means of the negative logarithm of K' and denote this value as pK' (e.g., at 25° C, the pK' values for H_2CO_3 and $HPO_4^=$ are 3.77 and 12.32, respectively).*Thus, as pK' values become smaller, the strength of the acid becomes greater.

Similar arguments can be made for compounds with basic properties; strong bases display nearly complete dissociation in solution, whereas weak bases do not. The equilibrium for an uncharged weak base (B) in aqueous solution would be formulated in the following manner:

$$B + H_2O \longleftrightarrow HB^+ + OH^-$$

---

* The logarithmic transformation of K':

$$pK' = \log_{10}\frac{1}{K'} = -\log_{10}K'$$

The equilibrium constant would be expressed as:

$$K' = \frac{[HB^+][OH^-]}{[B]}$$

Most textbooks of basic chemistry and biochemistry express this constant as K'_b to differentiate it from an acid constant K'_a. However, the important aspect of the Bröunsted-Lowry formalism is the tendency of protons to dissociate from a proton-donor species. Therefore both basic and acidic compounds are treated identically, and it is unnecessary to identify the dissociation constants as being specific for an acid or base (i.e., K'_a, K'_b).[402]

One of the simplest, yet most important, acid-base reactions is that which occurs in aqueous solution itself. Water is capable of functioning as both an acid and a base (i.e., it can donate and accept protons). A transfer of protons will occur when two water molecules react in an aqueous solution:

$$H_2O + H_2O \longleftrightarrow H_3O^+ + OH^-$$

Similarly, the dissociation of a single water molecule is an equilibrium process involving a conjugate acid-base pair:

$$H_2O \longleftrightarrow H^+ + OH^-$$

An equilibrium constant can be formulated in the usual manner:

$$K_{eq} = \frac{[H^+][OH^-]}{[H_2O]}$$

However, the concentration of water in an aqueous solution is very high, and for practical purposes, it is a constant (55.5 M). In other words, the minimal ionization of water (H^+ and OH^- concentrations of 1×10^{-7} M at 25° C) insignificantly alters its molar concentration. Therefore the equilibrium constant can be reformulated in a simplified form:

$$K_w = [H^+][OH^-]$$

where K_w is referred to as the ion product of water and has a value of 1.0×10^{-14} at 25° C. In an acidic solution, the H^+ is relatively large and the OH^- correspondingly small; in a basic solution, this relationship in concentration is reversed.

HYDROGEN ION CONCENTRATION AND pH. Within the body, the compartmental hydrogen ion concentrations are significantly less than one. For example, the normal concentration in the ECF is 40×10^{-6} mEq/L. Because these concentrations are rather cumbersome to report as milliequivalents per liter or moles per liter, the concept of pH was introduced; the previously discussed ion product of water is the basis for the pH scale. The measurement of pH provides a means for reporting the actual concentration of H^+ (and hence, OH^-) in solution with an acidity range between 1.0 M H^+ (pH 0) and 1×10^{-14} M H^+ (pH 14). By definition, pH is the negative logarithm (base 10) of the hydrogen ion concentration:

$$pH = \log \frac{1}{[H^+]} = -\log [H^+]$$

with the normal ECF pH being:

$$pH = -\log (40 \times 10^{-6} \text{ mEq/L}) = 7.4$$

In a healthy individual, there is little fluctuation in the hydrogen ion concentration as evidenced by the usual pH range of 7.38 to 7.42. However, the range of pH compatible with life is 6.8 to 7.8, representing a ten-fold difference in hydrogen ion concentration (160×10^{-6} to 16×10^{-6} mEq/L, respectively). The inverse relationship between pH and H^+ is evident from Table 46-15. It is important to note that when severe acidemia exists, a small change in the pH level reflects a large change in H^+. This occurs as a result of the logarithmic nature of the pH scale (Fig. 46-10).

BUFFERING AND EXCRETION OF ACIDS. Within the ECF the hydrogen ion concentration is normally quite stable (40 ± 5 nEq/L), despite the addition of a variable—but significant—daily acid load.[493] Although a number of potential pathologic alterations may cause an acid-base derangement, the daily acid load provides the greatest ongoing challenge to acid-base homeostasis in the normal individual. The body generates two types of acids: carbonic acid and metabolic acids. Carbonic acid (H_2CO_3, the so-called "volatile acid") is generated by the hydration of carbon dioxide (CO_2), which results from the oxida-

tive metabolism of carbohydrates and fat. Roughly 15,000 to 20,000 mEq of volatile acid may be excreted by the lungs (in the form of CO_2) each day.[460] A variety of metabolic or fixed acids are derived from either dietary intake (e.g., protein, organic acids) or cellular metabolism and result in 40 to 100 mEq of daily acid load. The majority of this H^+ is derived from the metabolism of sulfur-containing amino acids, which in turn generate sulfuric acid.[65] The nonvolatile acids (both organic and inorganic) are initially buffered, then may undergo further metabolism, and are ultimately excreted by the kidney. Together the renal and pulmonary systems provide a highly effective mechanism for eliminating parenterally administered, orally ingested, and endogenously produced acids, so long as organ function is not impaired and the buffer systems are not overwhelmed.

The massive production of H^+ and CO_2 results in a net surplus of acid that eventually enters the bloodstream. To minimize the likelihood of acidemia, the body uses several ICF and ECF buffer systems. In most instances, physiologic buffers are a mixture of weak acids (or bases) and their salts of strong bases (or acids). These conjugate acid-base pairs form a system that tends to resist (not prevent) changes in the pH level even when exposed to strong acids or bases.[296,402] Depending on the circumstances, the buffers will either donate or accept protons in an effort to stabilize the H^+. Most often, the body's buffer systems bind and carry free H^+. The portion of H^+ that is bound to such buffer systems cannot

Table 46-15 Relationship between pH and [H^+]	
pH	**[H^+] (nEq/L)***
0.0	$1,000 \times 10^6$
2.0	$1,000 \times 10^4$
4.0	$1,000 \times 10^2$
6.0	1,000
6.8	160
7.0	100
7.2	63
7.3	50
7.4	40
7.5	32
7.6	25
7.8	16
8.0	10
10.0	10×10^{-2}
12.0	10×10^{-4}
14.0	10×10^{-6}

*NOTE: One nanoequivalent (nEq) is equal to 1×10^{-9} Eq or 1×10^{-6} mEq.

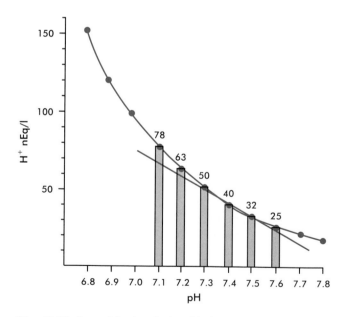

Fig. 46-10. Logarithmic relationship between H^+ ion concentration and pH. Notice the sharp increase in H^+ ion concentration as pH falls below 7.3. (From Geha DG: Blood gas monitoring. In Blitt CD, ed: *Monitoring in anesthesia and critical care medicine,* New York, 1985, Churchill-Livingstone.)

increase the acidity or lower the pH level of blood. The buffers effectively compensate for surges in acid intake or production and also facilitate the transport of acids to an appropriate site of excretion (i.e., kidney or lung). The extracellular buffers include the carbonic acid–bicarbonate, reduced and oxygenated hemoglobin, plasma protein or carbamino, and phosphate systems. In addition, there is a cellular contribution to ECF H^+ regulation via the membrane bound sodium pump, which exchanges Na^+ for K^+ and H^+.[640] Within the cytosol, proteins and phosphates are the major buffers, but the mechanisms of intracellular acid-base balance are poorly understood. In contrast, the workings of the carbonic acid–bicarbonate system (the predominant ECF buffer) have been intricately detailed, and it is this system which receives the most attention when dealing with clinical acid-base disorders.

From a purely chemical standpoint, the carbonic acid–bicarbonate buffer system appears relatively inefficient. However, when assessed biologically, the system is unique and highly efficient. One critical feature of this system is a reversible equilibrium involving hydrogen ion, carbonic acid, and carbon dioxide:

$$H^+ + HCO_3^- \longleftrightarrow H_2CO_3 \longleftrightarrow CO_2 + H_2O$$

Carbon dioxide and water are the major end products of aerobic metabolism. This CO_2 enters the intravascular compartment and is then transported in plasma or within red blood cells (RBCs). Most of the plasma CO_2 exists in three different forms: (1) bicarbonate (combined with certain cations), (2) carbonic acid (present in small amounts), and (3) protein bound (i.e., carbamino compounds).[297] In addition, a minimal quantity of dissolved CO_2 resides in the aqueous phase of plasma. Changes in the concentration of this CO_2 fraction are important, because they can shift (in either direction) the equilibrium of the above reaction. Most importantly, as this dissolved CO_2 transverses the body, it will interface and equilibrate (according to Henry's law) with gaseous CO_2. This CO_2 is then expelled through the lungs, and a potential source of H^+ is thereby eliminated.

The buffering capacity of whole blood greatly exceeds that of serum or plasma. Approximately 85% of the CO_2-carrying power of blood resides within RBCs and is provided by hemoglobin and phosphates.[297] However, most of the buffered CO_2 appears in the plasma as bicarbonate. In other words, the largest portion of the blood's buffering capacity is located intracellularly but is exerted in the plasma. The reason for this apparent inconsistency revolves around the presence of a specific RBC enzyme, carbonic anhydrase. Dissolved CO_2 freely permeates RBCs, and the carbonic anhydrase catalyzes its conversion to carbonic acid. A small amount of H_2CO_3 diffuses into the plasma, but most of this acid dissociates into H^+ and HCO_3^- (Fig. 46-11). The hydrogen ion is buffered by reduced hemoglobin. The

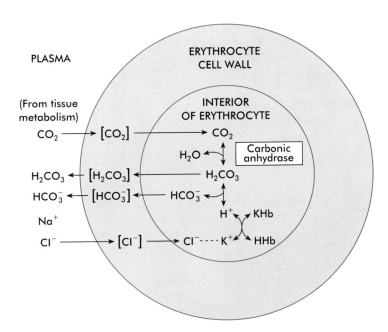

Fig. 46-11. Majority of the blood's buffer capacity resides within red blood cells, but most of the buffered CO_2 exists in plasma. The exchange of anions in the chloride shift maintains electroneutrality while allowing the plasma to carry additional CO_2 (as sodium bicarbonate). Within the red cell, hydrogen ion is buffered by hemoglobin (*Hb*). (From Harper HA: The chemistry of respiration. In Harper HA, ed: *Review of physiological chemistry,* Los Altos, Calif, 1973, Lange Medical Publications.)

bicarbonate is able to diffuse back into the plasma where it combines with sodium, and chloride ion moves from the plasma into the RBC to maintain electrical neutrality (the chloride shift). The net result is that dissolved CO_2 is replaced in the plasma by $NaHCO_3$, thereby allowing a greater CO_2-carrying capacity. In the pulmonary capillaries this entire process is reversed, because oxygen displaces H^+ from the hemoglobin molecule. H^+ and bicarbonate combine and eventually generate carbon dioxide and water. The carbon dioxide diffuses out of the blood, into the alveolar air sacs, and is eliminated by alveolar ventilation.

It should be apparent that carbonic acid is an exceptional compound, because it can behave as both an acid (i.e., H^+ donor) and a neutral gas (i.e., CO_2). The entire carbonic acid–bicarbonate system is uniquely suited for buffering because of its extensive distribution, the reversible equilibrium processes involving carbonic acid, and the presence of an enzyme catalyst. In addition, the quantity of available buffer can be adjusted as necessary through pulmonary excretion of carbon dioxide and renal excretion or reabsorption of bicarbonate (Fig. 46-12).

Ventilatory adjustments that affect CO_2 excretion (i.e., the rate and depth of respiration) are controlled by (1) central chemoreceptors in the medulla that are extremely sensitive to changes in the pH level (e.g., increased $Paco_2$ level) and (2) peripheral chemoreceptors (e.g., aortic arch, carotid body) that are responsive to changes in the Pao_2 level.[508] Renal regulation of acid-base balance occurs through several mechanisms. The kidneys are able to excrete bicarbonate when a positive base excess condition arises. They also excrete the daily load of metabolic acid (i.e., H^+), a process linked with the regeneration of bicarbonate and its subsequent diffusion into the bloodstream.[65,298,496,499] Both the proximal and the distal tubule cells of the nephron contain carbonic anhydrase, which facilitates this regeneration of

bicarbonate, and—in addition—allows the kidney to reclaim bicarbonate in the tubular filtrate. Distal tubular H^+ secretion occurs in conjunction with urinary buffers and results in the formation of titratable acid ($H^+ + HPO_4^{2-} \rightarrow H_2PO_4^-$) and ammonium ($H^+ + NH_3 \rightarrow NH_4^+$).[65,298,328,542] The mechanisms responsible for this renal H^+ secretion are valuable for conserving cations (predominately Na^+) and also fixed bases.

Although intracellular hemoglobin provides the largest portion of the blood's buffering capacity, acid-base disturbances are usually defined in terms of the predominant, plasma, conjugate acid-base pain (i.e., H_2CO_3 and HCO^-_3). The reasons for this include (1) the carbonic acid–bicarbonate system has a ubiquitous ECF distribution and all acid-base calculations assume that changes occur only in the ECF compartment, (2) an alteration in the carbonic acid–bicarbonate buffer system usually reflects a similar change in the nonbicarbonate buffers, and (3) the components of the carbonic acid–bicarbonate system can be easily quantified through calculation, estimation, or measurement. The Henderson-Hasselbach equation provides the usual means for describing the relationship between the pH level and the carbonic acid–bicarbonate system:

$$pH = pK' + \log \frac{[HCO_3^-]}{[H_2CO_3]}$$

Neutrality is regulated as the body attempts to maintain a 20:1 ratio of bicarbonate to carbonic acid. As long as this ratio is maintained, the ECF pH level will remain in the physiologic range. Alterations in the ratio (not the absolute concentrations) result in abnormalities of acid-base balance. An increased ratio (i.e., elevated pH level) results in alkalemia, and a decreased ratio (i.e., reduced pH level) produces acidemia.

To make the Henderson-Hasselbach equation less cumbersome and more clinically useful, certain manipulations can be made. Only a very small quantity of carbonic acid exists in the undissociated form. Therefore the equilibrium in the equation describing the hydration of carbon dioxide is normally far toward the side with dissolved CO_2.[237] Hence the concentration of dissolved CO_2 is substantially greater (approximately 1000 times), but directly proportional to, the concentration of H_2CO_3. In turn, dissolved CO_2 can be equated with $Paco_2$ by means of the Bunsen solubility coefficient for CO_2 in plasma[507]:

Dissolved CO_2 = (solubility coefficient) $\times$ $Paco_2$

Thus the activity of the carbonic acid–bicarbonate system can be expressed by a modified Henderson-Hasselbach equation:

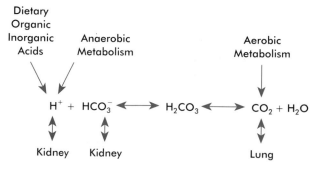

Fig. 46-12. Usual sources and routes of elimination for the acid and base components of the major ECF buffer system. (From Geha DG: Blood gas monitoring. In Blitt CD, ed: *Monitoring in anesthesia and critical care medicine,* New York, York, 1985, Churchill-Livingstone.)

$$pH = 6.1 + \log \frac{[HCO_3^-]}{0.03 \, Pa_{CO_2}}$$

where 6.1 is the apparent dissociation constant for carbonic acid at 37° C, and 0.03 is the solubility coefficient for carbon dioxide. All the components of this equation (i.e., pH, Pa_{CO_2} and $[HCO_3^-]$) are amenable to direct measurement, although determination of any two will permit calculation of the third component. Such is the case with an arterial blood gas sample where the Po_2, Pco_2 and pH levels are directly measured and CO_2 content (dissolved carbon dioxide, carbonic acid, and bicarbonate) or the bicarbonate concentration and base excess are calculated. A bicarbonate concentration by itself, regardless of the numeric value, will not provide a quantitative assessment of acid-base balance. It is the ratio of bicarbonate to carbonic acid or carbon dioxide that determines the pH level of the ECF. In clinical situations the pH, Pco_2, and either the CO_2 content or the bicarbonate concentration and base excess can be used to identify the type of abnormality (e.g., acidosis, alkalosis) and its origin (e.g., respiratory, metabolic, or mixed).

The ECF buffer systems (including hemoglobin) are important for limiting pH level changes that may result from respiratory and/or metabolic acid-base derangements. These systems all share in the buffering of a metabolic acid or alkali load. Hence the observed change in HCO_3^- concentration is less than the amount of acid or base added due to the involvement of the nonbicarbonate buffers.[328] In other words, measurements of the pH level and the HCO_3^- concentration will not directly account for hydrogen ions bound to or released from the buffer systems. Such measurements fail to reflect the total load of metabolic acid or alkali. As long as H^+ and OH^- remain bound to nonbicarbonate buffers, their impact on the pH level is negligible. When H^+ and OH^- interact with the carbonic acid–bicarbonate buffer system, the effect on both HCO_3^- concentration and pH level is minimized. As a result, only a very small portion of an excess acid-base load can be measured. A pH determination provides little direct information for quantitating the actual degree of acidosis or alkalosis.[328] In addition, the hydrogen ion concentration and pH level will not normalize until the entire acid or alkali load (carried by the buffer systems) is released and then neutralized.[328] Therefore, to quantitate the *total* metabolic acid-base load (a necessity for complete correction of the disturbance), a determination of base excess is usually necessary.

BASE EXCESS. The base excess (BE) provides a precise measure of the nonrespiratory component of an acid-base disturbance. It is a value that can be estimated through calculations,[653] derived from a nomogram,[652,654] or actually measured by titrating a blood sample. In clinical practice the BE is usually reported by the laboratory in conjunction with the results of a blood gas analysis. The measurement of BE involves the addition or removal of respiratory acid (i.e., Pco_2) so as to restore the pH level of the sample solution to normal (i.e., 7.4). Hence a correction is made for any respiratory-induced change in HCO_3^- concentration; the multibuffer system of the ECF is converted to a system that behaves similar to a simple HCO_3^- solution where the change in HCO_3^- concentration equals the amount of fixed acid added or removed from the blood.[328] Under these conditions the BE is then the difference between the patient's actual HCO_3^- concentration and the normal HCO_3^- concentration at a pH level of 7.4. Thus the BE may be either a positive or negative value, depending on relative surplus or deficiency of HCO_3^- in the patient's blood. The BE is normally reported in mEq/L; when multiplied by the volume of ECF, this value results in the quantity of acid or alkali required to correct the patient's metabolic abnormality.

CLINICAL CORRELATES OF ACID-BASE IMBALANCE. The clinical significance of a disruption in acid-base balance lies in its potential to produce an array of devastating effects. Most importantly, the concentration of hydrogen ions is a crucial determinant of proper enzyme activity throughout the body. Each enzymatic reaction has an optimal pH level at which the speed of the reaction is maximized.[202,401] Thus an alteration of the normal hydrogen ion concentration may increase the speed of some reactions and decrease the rate of others, thereby potentially creating metabolic chaos. These effects are always widespread, but a severe deterioration of organ performance is a relatively random and—for the most part—unpredictable occurrence.

Changes in the pH level will affect the degree of ionization for those molecules which normally exist in a partially ionized state. The protein-binding ability of certain ions (e.g., calcium) and drugs (e.g., thiopental) will be altered and may result in either an increase or decrease in the amount of "free" (i.e., active) ion or drug.[202] In addition, the actions of many drugs (e.g., epinephrine, digitalis, insulin) can be affected by pH changes in a manner unrelated to protein binding.

A temporary translocation of potassium between the ICF and ECF compartments occur with acidemia and alkalemia.[6] The normal transmembrane potential may be altered, and depending on the situation, electrocardiographic evidence of either hyperkalemia or hypokalemia may appear. In addition, pH-induced changes in 2,3-DPG metabolism can shift the oxyhemoglobin dissociation curve to the left (increased pH level) or to the right (decreased pH level).[41]

An acidosis (metabolic or respiratory) will have an impact on the performance of most organ systems, but

Table 46-16 Compensation in simple acid-base disturbances

Disturbance	Initial pH level	Initial alteration	Initial bicarbonate to carbonic acid ratio	Compensatory response	Compensated pH level
Respiratory acidosis	↓ ↓	↑ ↑ $Paco_2$	< 20:1	↑ HCO_3^-	↓
Metabolic acidosis	↓ ↓	↓ ↓ HCO_3^-	< 20:1	↓ $Paco_2$	↓
Respiratory alkalosis	↑ ↑	↓ ↓ $Paco_2$	> 20:1	↓ HCO_3^-	↑
Metabolic alkalosis	↑ ↑	↑ ↑ HCO_3^-	> 20:1	↑ $Paco_2$	↑

↑ = increased; ↓ = decreased; ↑ ↑ = greatly increased; ↓ ↓ = greatly decreased.
Modified from Shires GT, Canizaro PC: Fluid, electrolyte and nutritional management of the surgical patient. In Schwartz SI, ed: *Principles of surgery*, ed 2, New York, 1974, McGraw-Hill, and from Black RM: Metabolic acid-base disturbances. In Rippe JM, Irwin RS, Alpert JS et al, eds: *Intensive care medicine*, Boston, 1985, Little, Brown.

in the perioperative period the alterations in CNS, pulmonary, and cardiovascular function are of most concern. Acidemia produces a depression of cerebral processes, manifested by confusion and unresponsiveness that may culminate in unconsciousness.[548] Dilatation of the cerebral vasculature occurs as autoregulation is disrupted through direct and indirect mechanisms.[389,651] A metabolic acidosis initially stimulates respiration, producing an enhanced alveolar ventilation by enlarging the tidal volume (i.e., Kussmaul's respirations). However, a progressive decline in the pH level can impair the respiratory centers and produce apnea. Acidemia resulting from the administration or accumulation of carbon dioxide (e.g., intraperitoneal insufflation or inadequate ventilation, respectively) can produce an outpouring of catecholamines: heart rate, blood pressure, stroke volume, cardiac output, and both systemic and pulmonary vascular resistances will all increase despite a direct depressant effect of carbon dioxide (in high concentrations) on inotropic and chronotropic cardiac performance.[45] A more severe degree of acidemia will impair vasomotor function, which then leads to vascular dilatation and systemic hypotension. A profound reduction in the pH level can generate bradycardia and/or ventricular arrhythmias, including fibrillation.[242] As the pH level falls below 7.2, cardiac output decreases because contractility is compromised.[504,515,776] If the acidosis results in a pH level greater than 7.2, the diminished cardiac contractility may be partially blunted because the heart apparently develops an enhanced sensitivity to catecholamines.[463]

Alkalemia is often associated with marked cutaneous vasoconstriction and peripheral cyanosis.[202] Atrial and ventricular dysrhythmias may result from the associated hypokalemia. Acute hypocapnia increases cerebrovascular resistance and may produce cerebral hypoxia when combined with the shifting to the left of the oxygen-hemoglobin dissociation curve resulting from a respiratory alkalosis.[606,675,686] A rapid reduction

in the ionized fraction of calcium—the result of an acute respiratory-induced alkalemia—can produce Chvostek's and Trousseau's signs, muscle twitching, and seizure activity. Hypocapnia can also inhibit hypoxic pulmonary vasoconstriction[44,46] and incite bronchoconstriction, which may produce a decrease in pulmonary compliance and a mismatch of ventilation and perfusion. A substantial metabolic alkalosis may result in agitation, confusion, or lethargy, but the mechanism responsible for the CNS dysfunction is unclear because HCO_3^- does not readily diffuse across the blood-brain barrier.

SIMPLE ACID-BASE DISORDERS AND COMPENSATION. Simple acid-base disorders, both initially and primarily, alter either the arterial carbon dioxide tension or the serum bicarbonate concentration. Primary respiratory disturbances first affect the $Paco_2$ concentration, whereas primary metabolic disturbances initially change the HCO_3^- concentration. The primary disturbance will either increase or decrease the pH level, but this alteration is minimized by the major buffer systems in both the ICF and ECF. A secondary adaptation (often termed *compensation*) also occurs; the nonaffected component (i.e., $Paco_2$ or HCO_3^-) is adjusted so as to attenuate the severity of the pH change. These two homeostatic mechanisms attempt to maintain or reestablish the normal 20:1 ratio of HCO_3^- to H_2CO_3 (or $Paco_2$), since it is this ratio—not the individual values—that determines the pH level.

Primary respiratory disturbances evoke compensatory changes in the renal secretion, excretion, or resorption of acid or alkali[239] (Table 46-16). The compensation for primary metabolic disturbances occurs via alterations in alveolar ventilation. The temporal aspects of these compensatory processes differ markedly; respiratory compensation is maximized in approximately 12 hours, but renal compensation requires 1 to 3 days to reach its peak (Fig. 46-13). The magnitude of the particular adaptive

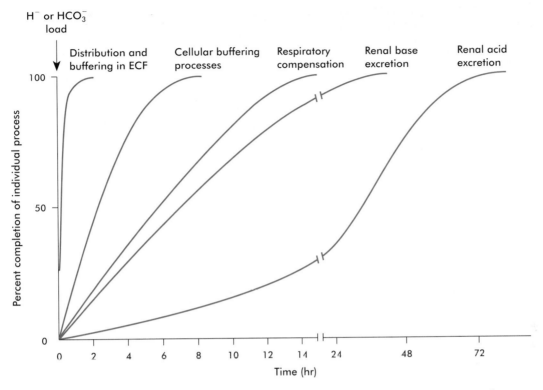

Fig. 46-13. Time course of the various compensatory mechanisms used in acid-base disturbances. (From Grogan MG, Rector FC, and Seldin DW: Acid-base disorders. In Brenner BM, Rector FC, eds: *The kidney,* ed 2, Philadelphia, 1981, WB Saunders.)

Table 46-17   Predicted compensatory responses in primary acid-base disturbances

Disturbance	Magnitude of primary alteration	Magnitude of compensatory response
Respiratory acidosis		
Acute	↑ $Paco_2$ 10 mm Hg	↑ HCO_3^- 1.0 mEq/L
Chronic	↑ $Paco_2$ 10 mm Hg	↑ HCO_3^- 3.5 mEq/L
Metabolic acidosis	↓ HCO_3^- 1.0 mEq/L	↓ $Paco_2$ 1.2 mm Hg
Respiratory alkalosis		
Acute	↓ $Paco_2$ 10 mm Hg	↓ HCO_3^- 2.0 mEq/L
Chronic	↓ $Paco_2$ 10 mm Hg	↓ HCO_3^- 5.0 mEq/L
Metabolic alkalosis	↑ HCO_3^- 1.0 mEq/L	↑ $Paco_2$ 0.7 mm Hg

↑ = increase, ↓ = decrease.
Modified from Rose BD, ed: *Clinical physiology of acid-base and electrolyte disorders*, ed 2, New York, 1984, McGraw-Hill.

response is fairly uniform and predictable[494] (Table 46-17), but the ultimate effect is limited in nature; compensation will redirect the pH level toward normal but will not completely correct the acidemia or alkalemia. During an evaluation of the measurable components of acid-base balance, knowledge of the expected compensatory response is important because an unanticipated response often indicates a mixed acid-base disturbance (e.g., the coexistence of two primary disorders such as a metabolic alkalosis

and a respiratory acidosis). In general, the most serious and life-threatening acid-base derangements are mixed disturbances in which the individual primary disorders each alter the pH level in the same direction (e.g., combined metabolic and respiratory acidoses). To appreciate the significance and potential impact of the mixed acid-base disturbances, a working knowledge of each primary disorder is required.

Respiratory acidosis. As long as intracellular processes are intact and there are sufficient quantities of oxygen and substrate, tissues will continuously produce carbon dioxide as a normal by-product of aerobic metabolism. Once generated, the carbon dioxide then is carried throughout the body in various forms that effectively minimize the impact of this volatile acid on the blood pH level. The plasma CO_2 content is a measure of this total quantity of circulating carbon dioxide and reflects the presence of carbon dioxide in the following forms and proportions: bicarbonate ion (94%), dissolved CO_2 (5%), carbonic acid (<1%), and carbamino CO_2 (negligible).[507] In addition, carbon dioxide diffuses into red blood cells (containing carbonic anhydrase), where a substantial amount exists as bicarbonate ion and also as carbamino CO_2 complexed with hemoglobin (Fig. 46-14). When carbon dioxide is added to capillary blood, approximately two thirds of it is transported in the plasma, but most of the buffering occurs within the red blood cells.[131] The mechanisms responsible for the transport and buffering of carbon dioxide represent a very dynamic system where bicarbonate, carbonic acid,

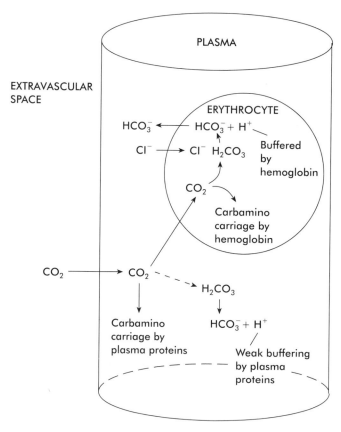

Fig. 46-14. Mechanisms for the transport and buffering of CO_2 in plasma and red blood cells. The largest portion of CO_2 diffuses into erythrocytes where it combines with hemoglobin or undergoes hydration to form carbonic acid—a process facilitated by carbonic anhydrase. (From Nunn JF: Carbon dioxide. In *Applied respiratory physiology,* ed 3, London, 1987, Butterworths.)

and carbamino CO_2 are in equilibrium with dissolved CO_2. In turn, the concentration of CO_2 in solution is determined by the partial pressure of CO_2 and its solubility coefficient.[312] The arterial carbon dioxide tension is normally maintained at 40 mm Hg through an intricate and efficient system that ultimately results in the pulmonary excretion of CO_2. Thus $Paco_2$ is a direct reflection of effective alveolar ventilation as denoted in the following relationship:

$$Paco_2{}^* = \frac{\dot{V}co_2}{\dot{V}A} \times K$$

where $\dot{V}co_2$ is the volume of CO_2 output per unit time, $\dot{V}A$ is the volume of alveolar ventilation per unit time, and K is a constant.[507,765] A normal $Paco_2$ value represents a steady state wherein the rates of CO_2 production and elimination are exactly balanced. Any disruption of this steady state that results in a $Paco_2$ level greater than 43 to 45 mm Hg creates a condition of respiratory acidosis.

In practice there are a number of potential causes for an increase in $Paco_2$ level (e.g., excessive CO_2 production, exogenous CO_2 administration, rebreathing endogenously produced CO_2, impairment of CO_2 diffusion, administration of carbonic anhydrase inhibitors, a large increase in the concentration of dissolved oxygen or the presence of a severe anemia). However, the development of a respiratory acidosis is almost always due to a defect in the pulmonary elimination of a normal CO_2 load. In other words, hypercapnia, the hallmark of respiratory acidosis, can be equated with hypoventilation.

With normal lungs, approximately two thirds of each breath reaches perfused alveoli and thus takes part in gas exchange (i.e., alveolar ventilation). The remaining one third of each breath does not participate in gas exchange and is termed physiologic dead space ventilation.[45] The relationship between alveolar ventilation and dead space[510] can be expressed as the following:

$$\dot{V}A = \text{respiratory rate} \times$$
$$(\text{tidal volume} - \text{physiologic dead space})$$

It follows that conditions associated with hypoventilation and respiratory acidosis (e.g., "central" respiratory depression, decreased compliance, increased airway resistance, and increased anatomic or alveolar

---

*By convention the alveolar and arterial Pco_2 values are assumed to be identical, because CO_2 freely permeates cell membranes and diffuses through aqueous solutions approximately 20 times faster than does O_2. The normal degree of shunting or scatter of ventilation/perfusion ratios results in an alveolar/arterial Pco_2 gradient of approximately 1 mm Hg. It is a rare circumstance (e.g., a severe and widespread diffusion defect) when this gradient exceeds 2 mm Hg. Thus, for practical purposes, there is no significant Pco_2 gradient between alveolar gas, pulmonary end-capillary blood, and arterial blood.[131,509,579]

dead space) have a detrimental impact on at least one of the determinants of alveolar ventilation. In the perioperative period there are a number of clinical conditions that can generate a respiratory acidosis, including upper airway obstruction, atelectasis, bronchospasm, pneumonia, saddle embolus, CHF, shock, abdominal distention, chest pain, flail chest, splinting of the diaphragm, and certain drugs (e.g., narcotics, volatile anesthetics, and neuromuscular blocking agents).

Three cardinal features of hypoventilation require emphasis. First, one must realize that hypoventilation is frequently caused by conditions that primarily alter the performance of organs or other structures outside the lungs; often the lungs are normal and are only indirectly affected by the primary process.[765] Second, despite the frequent presence of mild hypoxemia, severe oxygen desaturation usually does not develop with pure hypoventilation. For example, a doubling of the $Paco_2$ level that results in a substantial respiratory acidosis will decrease the alveolar partial pressure of oxygen to only approximately 60 mm Hg (Fig. 46-15). Third, the development of a significant respiratory acidosis is a relatively slow process. With a total respiratory arrest the rate of rise of the $Paco_2$ level is in the order of 3 to 6 mm Hg/min.[507] Therefore hypoventilatory states are associated with an even slower rate of $Paco_2$ increase.

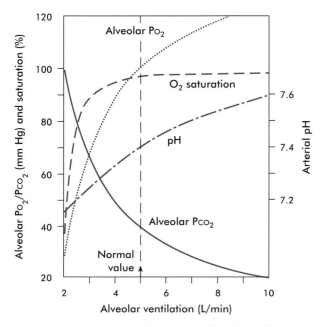

Fig. 46-15. Relationship between alveolar Pco_2, Po_2 and ventilation. During mild-to-mild moderate hypoventilation, a substantial rise in alveolar Pco_2 occurs in association with a relatively small reduction in arterial oxygen saturation. (From West JB: Gas exchange. In *Pulmonary pathophysiology,* ed 2, Baltimore, 1982, Williams & Wilkins.)

An increase in both the carbon dioxide tension and bicarbonate concentration and a decrease in the pH level are the primary findings in respiratory acidosis. The initial elevation in the $Paco_2$ level produces a rise in H^+ concentration, which—in turn—results in the compensatory generation of HCO_3^-. In acute respiratory acidosis, the H^+ is primarily buffered by hemoglobin. The intra-erythrocytic H^+ is derived from the dissociation of carbonic acid, which also results in the diffusion of HCO_3^- back into the blood. This adaptive response rapidly provides a limited quantity of HCO_3^-, because renal mechanisms do not participate in the compensation.[75,237] A serum HCO_3^- concentration of greater than 32 mEq/L or less than 24 mEq/L is indicative of a mixed acid-base disturbance.[75] In a simple but acute respiratory acidosis, the HCO_3^- concentration will increase 1.0 mEq/L for each 10 mm Hg increment in the $Paco_2$ level[494] (see Table 46-17). Treatment of the disorder is directed at restoring an adequate alveolar ventilation. Alkali therapy is rarely necessary, except perhaps in status asthmaticus where the acidosis blunts the effect of certain bronchodilator medications.[465,448]

A sustained respiratory acidosis may occur in individuals with chronic bronchitis, emphysema, bullous lung disease, congenital heart disease, extreme kyphoscoliosis, pickwickian syndrome, or Ondine's curse. In these chronic conditions there is renal compensation for the acidosis; the kidneys secrete H^+ and also regenerate and reabsorb HCO_3^-.[76,541] Hypochloremia develops, because a renal excretion of chloride is necessary to maintain electrical neutrality. When compared with acute respiratory acidosis, the chronic state produces a more efficient (but nevertheless, incomplete) compensation wherein the HCO_3^- concentration increases 3 to 4 mEq/L for each 10 mm Hg increase in the $Paco_2$ level.[76,239] In patients with normal renal function, a compensation of greater or lesser magnitude usually indicates a mixed disorder. No specific treatment is warranted in those with chronic respiratory acidosis. Occasionally an acute increase in CO_2 retention due to pneumonia, CHF, bronchospasm, or diminished hypoxic ventilatory drive (the result of oxygen administration) may become superimposed on the chronic disturbance. In this situation, therapy is aimed at correcting the acute process and alkalinizing salts are again not indicated.

Respiratory alkalosis. Hyperventilation is the sole cause of respiratory alkalosis. A supernormal minute ventilation may be spontaneous or iatrogenic in nature, but most commonly it is a secondary phenomena induced by either a drug or a disease process. Clinically, the acute state may result from fever, sepsis, salicylism, CHF, pneumonia, asthma, pulmonary emboli, damage to the CNS respiratory centers, or the hyperventilation syndrome associated with severe anxiety. An iatrogenic respiratory alkalosis (either intentional or inadvertent) may develop in the operating room or the intensive care unit as the result of mechanical ventilatory support. Pharmacologically-induced hyperventilation may result from the administration of doxapram during the immediate postanesthetic period, and chronic hyperventilation occurs in pregnancy, advanced hepatic insufficiency, restrictive lung disease, and acclimatization to high altitudes.[14]

The findings common to all forms of respiratory alkalosis are an elevation in the pH level and a reduction in both the $Paco_2$ and HCO_3^- concentrations. Acutely, protons shift from the ICF to the ECF so as to blunt the change in the pH level. For each 10 mm Hg fall in the $Paco_2$ concentration, the HCO_3^- concentration will decrease approximately 2 mEq/L. A severe, acute respiratory alkalosis may also produce significant changes in serum calcium and potassium concentrations. An enhanced binding of calcium to plasma proteins will reduce the ionized calcium concentration, with the potential for increased neuromuscular irritability, tetany, and seizures.[43] In addition, a fall in the $Paco_2$ level to less than 30 mm Hg results in a substantial intracellular translocation of potassium. The ensuing hypokalemia can produce cardiac dysrhythmias, including ventricular fibrillation. This latter problem can be potentiated by the coexistence of a metabolic alkalosis or the presence of digitalis. Therefore correction of any preexisting potassium deficit is essential. In general, therapy is directed at the underlying cause of the acute hyperventilatory state. If the respiratory alkalosis cannot be substantially reduced or ablated in a timely manner, then frequent evaluation of the serum calcium and potassium concentrations and/or continuous electrocardiographic monitoring should be performed.

In chronic hypocapnia, renal bicarbonate excretion provides the compensation for the diminished $Paco_2$ level. At least 24 to 48 hours are required for this adaptive mechanism to achieve its maximal function, but the end result is a near normal arterial pH level. For each 10 mm Hg decrease in the $Paco_2$ level, there is ultimately a reduction in HCO_3^- concentration of approximately 5 mEq/L. In most instances, it is unnecessary to treat a chronic respiratory alkalosis; if renal function remains normal, the elevation in the pH level will be minimal.

Metabolic acidosis. Metabolic acidosis results from a surplus of fixed acid (e.g., reduced excretion and/or increased production or intake) or a deficiency of bicarbonate (e.g., decreased regeneration or excessive loss). The relative abundance of H^+ results in low pH and HCO_3^- concentrations and a negative BE. This H^+ also stimulates medullary chemoreceptors;[204] a respiratory compensation occurs as alveolar hyperventilation develops and the $Paco_2$ concentration

subsequently falls. This adjustment in ventilation arises slowly and requires 12 to 24 hours to achieve a maximal response, because the H^+ cannot rapidly cross the blood-brain barrier.[204,537] Nevertheless, the magnitude of the compensatory response is predictable: a 1.2 mm Hg decrease in the $Paco_2$ concentration for each 1 mEq/L reduction in the HCO_3^- concentration. However, the $Paco_2$ level generally will not fall below 10 to 15 mm Hg,[98] even though the ventilatory response—for the most part—is proportional to the severity of the acidemia. In addition, this pulmonary adaptation is most effective during an acute acidosis because long-term reductions in the $Paco_2$ level may actually cause a decline in resorption of renal tubular bicarbonate.[122,422]

As a group, the metabolic acidoses exhibit tremendous variation in terms of severity. Regardless of initial pathophysiologic process, the degree of acidemia depends on the state of the body's buffer systems, the efficiency of the pulmonary compensatory mechanism, and the functional integrity of the kidneys. In certain situations the rate and duration of HCO_3^- loss or fixed acid production will also have an impact on the magnitude of the acidemia. In addition, the strength of the acid (i.e., pK') is important whenever there is an increased production or intake of fixed acid. The extent of the acidemia (as determined by the aforementioned factors), in conjunction with the cause of the acidosis, will then determine the quantitative and qualitative aspects of therapy.

Anion gap categorization of metabolic acidosis. A number of conditions may generate a metabolic acidosis in the perioperative period.[494] A convenient way to categorize these acidoses is by means of the corresponding anion gap. The anion gap represents the difference between unmeasured anions and cations within the serum or plasma. The basis for the determination of the anion gap is the principle of electroneutrality, which mandates that the total serum cations must exactly balance the total serum anions. Quantitatively, the most important ECF ions are sodium, chloride, and bicarbonate. All of the remaining ECF ions (excluding potassium) that are required for electroneutrality are neither measured nor reported with a routine electrolyte panel. Nevertheless, the following relationship exists:

$$[Cl^- + HCO_3^-] + \text{unmeasured anions} =$$
$$[Na^+] + \text{unmeasured cations}$$
$$\text{unmeasured anions} - \text{unmeasured cations} =$$
$$[Na^+] - [Cl^- + HCO_3^-]$$
$$\text{Anion gap} = [Na^+] - [Cl^- + H_2CO_3^-]$$

Thus the measured ionic concentrations used to calculate the anion gap actually reflect the concentrations of all the unmeasured ECF ions. Consequently, the anion gap represents the sum of the

Table 46-18   Components of the normal anion gap

Unmeasured anions (mEq/L)		Unmeasured cations (mEq/L)	
Protein	15	Calcium	5
Organic acids	5	Potassium	4.5
Phosphate	2	Magnesium	1.5
Sulfate	1		
Total	23	Total	11

Table 46-19   Causes of metabolic acidosis

Metabolic acidosis	Causes
Normal anion gap	
Loss of bicarbonate	Proximal renal tubular acidosis
	Primary hyperparathyroidism
	Carbonic anhydrase inhibitors
	Choelstyramine
	Dilutional acidosis
	Ureterosigmoidostomy
	Diarrheal states
	Biliary, pancreatic, and small bowel fistulas
Failure of bicarbonate regeneration	Distal renal tubular acidosis
	Hyporenin hypoladosteronism
	Diuretics: triamterene, spironolactone, amiloride
Administration of acid salts	Ammonium chloride
	Arginine hydrochloride
	Lysine hydrochloride
	Parenteral hyperalimentation
Increased anion gap	
Reduced excretion of inorganic acids	Renal failure
Accumulation of organic acids	Lactic acidosis
	Ketoacidosis: diabetic, alcoholic, starvation
	Ingestion: salicylate intoxication, paraldehyde intoxication, methanol intoxication, ethylene glycol intoxication

Modified from Andreoli TE: Disorders of fluid volume, electrolytes, and acid-base balance. In Wyngaarden JB, Smith LH, eds: *Cecil textbook of medicine*, Philadelphia, 1988, WB Saunders.

calcium, potassium, and magnesium concentrations subtracted from a larger total concentration of anions: sulfates and phosphates derived from tissue metabolism, ketoacids and lactic acid generated by the incomplete combustion of carbohydrates and fatty acids, and negatively charged proteins, predominantly albumin (Table 46-18). Under normal conditions the magnitude of the anion gap is approximately 10 to 12 mEq/L. In clinical situations where the ECF ionic concentrations are abnormal, the calculated anion gap may be elevated, reduced, or even normal; the actual value will be determined by the relative quantities of measured and unmeasured anions and cations.

The most important clinical use of the anion gap is in the differential diagnosis of a metabolic acidosis.[189] When such a condition exists, the anion gap will either increase or remain normal, depending on the cause of the acidosis (Table 46-19). Conversely, the finding of an increased anion gap is virtually synonymous with the presence of a metabolic acidosis.[227] In addition, the likelihood of an elevated anion gap representing a metabolic acidosis is enhanced as the magnitude of the gap increases:

- A normal anion gap (i.e., hyperchloremic) metabolic acidosis occurs whenever there is a significant net loss of bicarbonate. This may arise when (1) the kidneys fail to reabsorb or regenerate bicarbonate, (2) there are gastrointestinal losses of bicarbonate, or (3) the bicarbonate buffer system is overwhelmed by a net gain of acid (in the form of a chloride salt). Failure of the proximal tubule to resorb all the filtered bicarbonate may result from disease states (e.g., proximal renal tubular acidosis, Fanconi's syndrome, hyperparathyroidism), drugs (e.g., carbonic anhydrase inhibitors), or as a normal physiologic response to intravascular volume expansion (e.g., dilutional acidosis).[230] The secretions of the pancreas and small bowel are alkaline in nature; rapid transit of these secretions through the gastrointestinal tract[756] or external loss through a fistula prevents the

normal colonic reabsorption of bicarbonate. When significant quantities of chloride are presented to the colonic mucosa (e.g., urinary diverting procedures, cholestyramine), a chloride-bicarbonate exchange is activated that generates a gastrointestinal loss of alkali.[690] A failure of bicarbonate regeneration results from conditions (e.g., distal renal tubular acidosis) or drugs (e.g., amiloride) that disrupt the function of the distal nephron. A reduction in the serum bicarbonate concentration may also occur as hydrogen ions are generated by the metabolism of acidic chloride salts. A factor common to all these forms of metabolic acidosis is a normal anion gap; the decrease in serum bicarbonate concentration is totally offset by an increase in the serum chloride concentration.

- A high anion gap metabolic acidosis is similarly accompanied by a decrease in the serum bicarbonate concentration. The primary abnormality causes an accumulation of unmeasured anions and a corresponding decrease in the sum of the chloride and bicarbonate concentrations. These unmeasured anions will be acidic in nature and either organic or inorganic in composition. The most common clinical entities associated with this type of metabolic disturbance are uremic, lactic, and ketoacidosis.[226]

- Mild renal insufficiency results in decreased hydrogen ion secretion, ammonia synthesis, and bicarbonate resorption. Chloride then replaces bicarbonate in the serum, and a hyperchloremic metabolic acidosis is generated. However, when the normal glomerular filtration rate (GFR) is reduced by 70% to 80% (i.e., serum creatinine concentration of approximately 4 mg/100 ml), the kidneys are unable to excrete both H^+ and anions (principally, phosphates and sulfates).[189,771] The ensuing metabolic acidosis is usually associated with an anion gap in the range of 20 to 25 mEq/L. In uncomplicated uremia, the serum bicarbonate concentration rarely falls below 12 mEq/L and generally resides between 16 and 20 mEq/L.

- The accumulation of organic acids can lead to an acute and profound metabolic acidosis. This type of metabolic disturbance results from either an impairment of normal cellular respiration or an abnormality in the rates of lipolysis and glycolysis.[14] A relative decrease in tissue oxygenation (i.e., a diminished oxygen supply and demand ratio) or the presence of certain toxins and drugs can disrupt the processes of cellular respiration.[479] The ensuing reduction in aerobic, mitochondrial pyruvate metabolism leads to an accumulation of lactate.[421] Failure to oxidize and eliminate this strong organic acid ($pK' = 3.8$) may create a state of lactic acidosis,[383] where the pH level is often less than 7.1, the serum bicarbonate concentration is below 8 mEq/L, and the anion gap is frequently greater than 35 mEq/L.[189] The normal resting lactate concentration is approximately 1 mEq/L,[333] and concentrations greater than 5 mEq/L are generally considered diagnostic of the lactic acidosis syndrome.[341] Sustained lactic acidemia of this magnitude (as may occur with sepsis, dead bowel, cardiogenic or hemorrhagic shock) is often fatal,[466,529] al-

though rapid detection and intervention may occasionally improve this dismal prognosis. Lactic acidosis is probably the most common severe metabolic acidosis encountered in anesthetic practice.

- Ketoacidosis is also a metabolic disorder induced by organic acids and associated with a high anion gap. Most commonly, ketoacidosis occurs in conjunction with diabetes mellitus,[214] alcoholism,[289] or starvation.[521] The common pathogenic feature of these three disorders is an insulin deficiency that results in accelerated lipolysis with enhanced hepatic ketogenesis.[520] Acetoacetic acid and beta-hydroxybutyric acid will each reduce the bicarbonate concentration and increase the anion gap. In contrast, acetone (a ketone formed by the breakdown of acetoacetate) is not an acid and therefore will not contribute to the acidosis nor alter the anion gap.[711] Perioperatively, the quantitative evaluation of ketones is easily performed with Acetest tablets; however, this nitroprusside reactant is unable to detect the presence of beta-hydroxybutyric acid. This lack of reactivity precludes the use of Acetest tablets as the sole means for judging the efficacy of therapy. This is especially true of alcoholic ketoacidosis where frequently there is a disproportionate increase in the beta-hydroxybutyric acid to acetoacetic acid ratio.[289] This ratio will increase anytime a ketoacidosis coexists with diminished mitochondrial oxidation.[512] The resulting beta-hydroxybutyric acidosis maintains the lowered pH level and elevated anion gap despite an increasingly negative Acetest reaction. When evaluating and monitoring patients with ketoacidosis, one must appreciate that acetoacetic acid may spuriously elevate the serum creatinine concentration because of a colorimetric cross-reactivity between the chromogens.[65]

Therapy for metabolic acidosis. The ultimate goal of therapy for metabolic acidosis is restoration of the normal blood pH level and HCO_3^- concentration. The form of treatment should be determined by the acuteness, severity, and—most importantly—the underlying cause of the acidosis. Because metabolic acidosis is a manifestation of numerous syndromes and diseases, no one therapeutic regimen is appropriate for the many forms of this disorder. Whenever feasible, management should be primarily aimed toward correcting the process(es) that initiated the metabolic disturbance. Often, the acidemia per se requires no specific treatment unless the pH level is so profoundly low (e.g., less than 7.1) that it compromises cardiac contractility.[463,776] For example, diabetic ketoacidosis generally responds to fluid, electrolyte (e.g., phosphorus, potassium), and insulin replacement.[203,214,360,777] Alkali therapy is ordinarily unnecessary and may even make the situation worse.[57,327] Similarly, alcoholic and starvation ketoacidosis rarely require bicarbonate and usually resolve with the administration of saline and glucose.[289] The lactic acidosis resulting from generalized seizure activity may be moderately severe but is relatively short-lived once the convulsions subside[446,516] and does not require bicarbonate therapy. Type A lactic acidosis resolves when adequate tissue perfusion and oxygenation are restored.[466] Thus, depending on the clinical manifestations, the severity of the acidemia, and the expected rapidity of resolution, treatment of the acidosis with alkalinizing agents may not be necessary or indicated. However, when the process underlying the metabolic acidosis is complex, ongoing, unpredictable, and associated with a progressive decline in pH level, therapy specific for the acidemia is usually warranted.

The initial aim of treatment is to increase the ECF pH to a level that will alleviate or prevent the cardiovascular effects of severe acidemia so as to maintain hepatic metabolism and renal excretion of acid; a pH level of greater than 7.1 or 7.2 is generally desired. Sodium bicarbonate is most often the alkalinizing agent of choice, but the dose required is rather empirical.[65,328,512] The total extracellular base deficit can be estimated by multiplying BE × 0.2 × lean body weight in kilograms, but this calculation ignores ICF acid-base alterations. Alternatively, the difference between the desired and actual serum bicarbonate concentrations multiplied by the bicarbonate space can also provide an estimate of the necessary dose.* However, there are inaccuracies inherent in this estimate as well; the apparent volume of distribution may increase significantly (e.g., to 70% of body weight) in severe acidosis,[63,231] and the change in ventilation (i.e., $Paco_2$ concentration) after an acute increase in serum bicarbonate concentration cannot be accurately predicted. Therefore in clinical practice there is little need to calculate a bicarbonate dose. A reasonable approach — applicable to adults,

children, and infants — is to administer 1 mEq/kg of sodium bicarbonate (most often available in a concentration of 1 mEq/ml) and reevaluate the arterial pH level 20 minutes later.[108] Because the distribution of bicarbonate requires approximately 15 minutes, a pH level measured immediately after administration may overestimate the effectiveness of therapy.[65]

During the administration of sodium bicarbonate, it is both unnecessary and undesirable to totally to totally correct the ECF pH level; when the underlying cause of the metabolic acidosis is effectively treated, the excess acid will be metabolized and/or excreted. The use of sodium bicarbonate is thus merely a temporizing maneuver that allows time to identify and correct the pathophysiologic process(es) responsible for generating the metabolic acidosis. Sodium bicarbonate should always be administered cautiously, because there are certain hazards and limitations associated with its use. In patients with a sustained metabolic acidosis, rapid and significant increases in the pH level commonly produce an "overshoot alkalosis;" the plasma is alkalinized faster than the ISF of the brain due to the selective permeability of the blood-brain barrier.[464] The persistent CSF acidosis sustains the hyperventilatory response resulting in a blood pH level that is greater than normal.[537,548] In addition, bicarbonate administration can result in hypocalcemia, hypokalemia, hypernatremia, fluid overload, leftward shift of the oxyhemoglobin dissociation curve,[462] intracranial hemorrhage (in neonates),[660] tissue hypoxia, and enhanced production of organic acids.[21,217,497] Due to these potential side effects and complications, the role of bicarbonate therapy in metabolic acidosis is being reevaluated.[26,260,358,434] The current recommendation is for careful and judicious provision of relatively small amounts of sodium bicarbonate, because the dangers of inappropriate and overzealous use of this agent are well documented.[57]

The salts of organic acids are occasionally used as a bicarbonate substitute for the treatment of metabolic acidosis. These salts include citrate, lactate, and acetate. When metabolized, each milliequivalent of organic salt generates 1 mEq of HCO_3^- so that the dose of organic salt is identical to that of sodium bicarbonate. However, the effect on the pH level is delayed due to the required metabolism; if metabolism is impaired, there may be little or no impact on the ECF bicarbonate concentration. Consequently, the severity of the acidemia and the chosen mode of therapy will dictate the use of organic salts in metabolic acidosis. For example, peritoneal dialysis can be used as a means of treatment. Most of the commercial dialysates contain lactate (40 mEq/L), which undergoes hepatic metabolism and produces carbon dioxide, water, and eventually bicarbonate.

---

* The desired bicarbonate concentration can be calculated using the Henderson equation:

$$[H_+] = 24 \times \frac{Paco_2}{[HCO_3^-]}$$

where the H^+ at a pH level of 7.2 is 63 mEq/L (Table 46-15), the $Paco_2$ concentration is the patient's actual arterial carbon dioxide tension, and HCO_3^- is the concentration of bicarbonate necessary to achieve a pH level of 7.2 at the given Pco_2 value (i.e., the desired bicarbonate concentration). The dose of bicarbonate can then be derived as follows:

Bicarbonate dose (mEq/L) = ([HCO_3^-]$_{desired}$ − [HCO_3^-]$_{actual}$) × $VD_{HCO_3^-}$

where $VD_{HCO_3}^-$ is the volume of distribution for bicarbonate, which is theoretically 50% of lean body weight in kilograms.

Hemodialysis, on the other hand, most often uses acetate as a source of alkali because it is metabolized to bicarbonate, predominately by skeletal muscle.[65] Oral sodium citrate (e.g., Shohl's solution with a citrate concentration of 1 mEq/ml) is frequently used as a source of bicarbonate in the relatively small group of patients with renal failure who need ongoing alkali therapy. In general, these are patients with a serum bicarbonate concentration of less than 12 to 15 mEq/L who require 1 to 3 mEq/kg/day of bicarbonate substitute to balance the daily load of fixed acid. Certain intravenous crystalloid solutions also contain organic salts that can be metabolized to bicarbonate. However, the concentrations of the bicarbonate substitutes are so relatively low (e.g., 28 mEq/L of lactate in lactated Ringer's solution) that these solutions are inappropriate for the treatment of any significant metabolic acidosis.

Metabolic Alkalosis. Metabolic alkalosis occurs when there is a primary increase in the serum bicarbonate concentration. Metabolic alkalosis may occur in isolation when the pH level is elevated, or it may be superimposed on a respiratory or metabolic acidosis in association with a reduced ECF pH level. A sustained metabolic alkalosis requires two distinct physiologic derangements: there must be a condition that initially generates the alkalosis, and a second process is necessary to maintain the alkalosis.[387]

The *generation* of metabolic alkalosis occurs through a net gain of alkali, a loss of fixed acid, and/or a disproportionate loss of chloride compared with bicarbonate (Box 46-5). A gain of exogenous base is usually iatrogenic and results from the administration of sodium bicarbonate or a bicarbonate substitute. The loss of both hydrogen ion and chloride (produced by the parietal cells of the gastric mucosa) results from gastric suction or vomiting and is a common occurrence in surgical patients. Losses of hydrogen ion and chloride may also occur in the kidney. The terminal nephron is the site of two interrelated processes: bicarbonate regeneration and the sodium-potassium/hydrogen ion exchange. Situations that alter the normal pattern of distal exchange (e.g., mineralocorticoid excess, enhanced distal sodium delivery, respiratory acidosis, hypokalemia) can increase both renal acid excretion and bicarbonate regeneration.[354,409,545]

Once metabolic alkalosis is generated, an additional process is required for *maintenance* of the elevated serum bicarbonate concentration. In a normal individual, excess bicarbonate is rapidly excreted in the urine. Thus metabolic alkalosis can be sustained only if the kidneys fail to excrete the bicarbonate (e.g., increased proximal resorption or persistent distal regeneration). Increased bicarbonate resorption occurs with hypokalemia, decreased GFR, and — most importantly — volume depletion.[57] Since preser-

---

BOX 46-5
CONDITIONS GENERATING A METABOLIC ALKALOSIS

Net alkali gain
Sodium bicarbonate administration
Infusion of a bicarbonate substitute (acetate, lactate, citrate)
Milk-alkali syndrome

Gastrointestinal H^+ and Cl^- losses
Upper tract: gastric drainage, vomiting
Lower tract: villous adenoma, congenital chloridorrhea

Renal H^+ and Cl^- losses
Diuretics (thiazide and "loop")
Excess mineralocorticoid activity (primary hyperaldosteronism, Cushing's syndrome, Bartter's syndrome)
Post-hypercapnia
Nonresorbable anions (carbenicillin)
Severe potassium depletion

---

vation of the ECF volume takes precedence over pH homeostasis, hypovolemia causes the resorption sodium and bicarbonate despite the alkalemia. Contraction alkalosis is the term applied to this hypovolemic maintenance of a metabolic alkalosis.[14,106,230] Chloride depletion and its unavailability to accompany renal sodium resorption is also a result of intravascular volume contraction. In contrast, the continued distal regeneration of bicarbonate requires volume expansion as occurs with a mineralocorticoid excess where there is an increased distal sodium chloride delivery and often hypokalemia. In both situations, hypokalemia maintains the alkalosis, because the intracellular shift of hydrogen for potassium makes the hydrogen ion more readily available for distal tubular secretion.[95]

Characteristically, an increase in bicarbonate (i.e., a positive BE condition) is accompanied by a decrease in chloride because these are the two major ECF anions. In addition, most patients with metabolic acidosis will have some degree of hyperkalemia due to the mechanisms noted previously. The respiratory compensation elicited by the metabolic acidosis is quite variable and unpredictable; hospitalized patients with this disorder generally have superimposed illnesses that limit their ability to hypoventilate.[223] In an uncomplicated situation, there is a linear relationship in the rise of both the serum bicarbonate and the $Paco_2$ concentrations; each 1 mEq/L elevation in bicarbonate will increase the $Paco_2$ concentration by

Table 46-20 Urinary chloride in metabolic acidosis	
Chloride-responsive ($U_{cl}-$ < 10 mEq/L)	**Chloride-resistant** ($U_{cl}-$ > 20 mEq/L)
Gastrointestinal H^+ and Cl^- losses	Diuretic therapy
Post-diuretic therapy	Severe potassium depletion
Post-hypercapnia	Net alkali gain
Nonresorbable anions	Mineralocorticoid excess

$U_{cl}-$, urinary chloride concentration.
Modified from Narins RG, Krishna GG, Bressler L et al: The metabolic acidoses. In Maxwell MH, Kleeman CR, and Narins RG, eds: *Clinical disorders of fluid and electrolyte metabolism*, ed 4, New York, 1987, McGraw-Hill.

0.7 mm Hg until hypoxic ventilatory drive becomes an overriding factor (a $Paco_2$ concentration of approximately 55 to 60 mm Hg).[223,630] In addition to the aforementioned objective findings, the diagnosis and treatment of metabolic alkalosis are facilitated by measurement of the urinary chloride concentration (see below).

The first step in the management of metabolic alkalosis should be an evaluation for the cause of the disorder, as well as the mechanism responsible for its maintenance. It is important to appreciate that there may be a different cause for each of these two facets of the alkalosis and that definitive treatment requires correction of both processes. When combined with the patient's history and physical examination, the measurement of urinary chloride provides a convenient method for distinguishing certain types of metabolic alkalosis (Table 46-20). In turn, this chloride-dependent categorization has significant therapeutic implications. A low urinary chloride concentration (e.g., less than 10 mEq/L) often reflects a state of intravascular volume depletion. The therapy of choice is sodium chloride, which causes volume expansion and bicarbonate excretion. It is also prudent to administer potassium chloride, because this agent can correct the alkalosis as well as treat the frequently concomitant hypokalemia.[620] Moreover, the large bicarbonate diuresis that occurs during correction of the alkalosis can precipitate severe hypokalemia if this ion is not continually replaced. Potassium requirements of greater than 300 mEq per day are not unheard of. In patients with CHF or cirrhosis, the reduced urinary chloride may not reflect a loss of total body fluid; it may actually represent a reduced EABV despite an excess of total body water. Saline infusions are ill advised in these situations, and

therapy is best accomplished with a carbonic anhydrase inhibitor (e.g., acetazolamide), which impairs both renal sodium and bicarbonate resorption.

The elevation of the urinary chloride level (greater than 20 mEq/L) suggests volume expansion and diminished chloride resorption. Therefore chloride replenishment is unnecessary and ineffective. Measures that specifically address the underlying cause must be initiated (e.g., prevention of alkali intake; discontinuation of thiazide, loop diuretics, or potassium replacement). States of mineralocorticoid excess may require surgery, aldosterone antagonists, potassium-sparing diuretics, and/or sodium restriction to correct the metabolic alkalosis. In general, if the serum bicarbonate concentration is less than 30 to 32 mEq/L, therapy for the metabolic alkalosis is unnecessary. When treatment is required, a gradual correction of the alkalosis (as outlined previously) is usually acceptable. However, occasionally a more rapid and dramatic intervention is indicated. The severity of the alkalosis, the lack of renal function, and/or the presence of an excessive intravascular volume may necessitate the therapeutic usage of dilute hydrochloric acid. Acute correction of the alkalosis is possible with 0.05 to 0.2 normal HCl in distilled water.[4,778] The quantity of acid required can be determined as follows:

$$H^+ \text{ (mEq)} = ([HCO_3^-]_{actual} - [HCO_3^-]_{desired}) \times VD_{HCO3}-$$

where $VD_{HCO3}-$ is the theoretic volume of distribution for bicarbonate (i.e., $0.5 \times$ lean body weight in kilograms). Knowing the concentration of the available acid solution allows a determination of its H^+ content (e.g., 0.1 N HCl contains 100 mEq/L of H^+). The HCl solution should be slowly administered through a central venous catheter with the end-point of therapy being stabilization of the patient and not total correction of the alkalosis. However, the pH must be returned to an acceptable level in a relatively expeditious manner because extreme elevations of the pH level are associated with a high rate of mortality.[778]

Electrolyte imbalance. Perioperative electrolyte disturbances are relatively commonplace, and thus it is important for the practicing anesthesiologist to be adept at recognizing and managing these abnormalities. In most instances the first clue to an electrolyte imbalance is the presence of an abnormal serum electrolyte concentration. However, the serum level may or may not accurately reflect the total body content of the ion in question; for ions that are predominately intracellular, the serum concentrations are notoriously poor predictors of the total ion stores. Thus other methods must be employed to determine the approximate quantity of stored ion. An abnormal serum electrolyte concentration may reflect a true state of ion excess or depletion but, alternatively, may reflect a transcellular relocation of the ion or be factitious in nature. It is important to differentiate the states of ion excess and depletion from transient ion shifts and laboratory errors, because a therapeutic intervention in the latter two may have disastrous consequences. The following sections address this concern and review the presentation and management of the excess and depletion states associated with the cationic electrolytes calcium, magnesium, and potassium.

As a prelude to the following discussion, it is of practical importance for every clinician to be able to interchange electrolyte concentration units. For certain electrolytes (e.g., calcium and magnesium) the laboratory often provides measurements in terms of milligrams percent, milligrams per deciliter, or milligrams per 100 ml of serum. However, when one is dealing with intravenous solutions and electrolyte supplements, the ionic concentrations are usually expressed as milliequivalents per liter of solution. It is therefore crucial to possess the ability to equate these units of concentration. The following equation describes the relationship between mg/dl and mEq/L:

$$\frac{mg/100 \text{ ml}}{\text{atomic weight}} \times \text{valence} \times 10 = \frac{mEq}{\text{liter}}$$

where valence represents the number of electric charges associated with the element, ion, or compound. The utility of expressing electrolyte concentrations in milliequivalents per liter arises from the fact that electrolytes combine in terms of equivalents or milliequivalents. For example, an electrically neutral compound (e.g., sodium bicarbonate, potassium

---

chloride, and so on) has an equal number of both cationic and anionic milliequivalents. Also, each body fluid compartment has a total quantity of cationic milliequivalents that exactly balances the total number of anionic milliequivalents. Expressing electrolyte quantities in milligrams or millimoles will not reflect the chemical-combining power that is the basis of all electrolyte-containing parenteral solutions.

CALCIUM. Calcium is an essential inorganic element that plays a crucial role in many biologic functions (Box 46-6). It is the single most abundant electrolyte in the human body.[801] A normal adult contains between 1000 to 1400 g of calcium, of which 99% is located in bone, where it is the primary structural component. Approximately 1% of the total calcium pool resides in the soft tissues and the ECF compartment. However, soft-tissue intracellular calcium concentrations are roughly 1000-fold less than the ECF concentrations.[705] The portion of calcium that circulates in the blood exists in three forms: an ionized fraction (50%), a fraction bound to protein (mostly albumin), (40%), and a diffusible, nonionized fraction (10%) in which calcium is chelated with circulating anions (e.g., bicarbonate, phosphate, citrate).[798,801] It is generally (although not universally[655]) accepted that the ionized fraction is the portion of calcium that is physiologically active, and thus it is the concentration of this fraction that is closely regulated by parathyroid hormone, vitamin E, and calcitonin.[8,43,655] These substances alter the resorption of calcium from various target organs, including the skeletal system, the gastrointestinal tract, and the kidneys.

The average dietary intake of calcium is approximately 1000 mg per day.[397] Roughly 60% of the total calcium entering the gastrointestinal tract originates from ingested food, with the remainder derived from intestinal, biliary, and pancreatic secretions.[640] Under normal conditions, 30% to 70% of gastrointestinal calcium is resorbed in the small bowel.[705,801] In addition, the kidneys filter approximately 10 g of calcium each day and all but 1% to 2% is normally resorbed.[403] Thus, in a healthy adult, several hundred milligrams of calcium are excreted daily in the feces and urine, with a small amount also eliminated in sweat. Because of the formation of new bone, the daily calcium requirement for children (i.e., 20 mg/kg/day) is approximately twice as much as that for adults. In preterm infants the daily requirement may be as high as several hundred milligrams per kilogram because body reserves of calcium are exceedingly low.[656,750]

A measurement of total serum calcium (the analysis most often performed when a calcium level is requested) reflects the quantitative contribution of all three forms of circulating calcium. The normal value

---

BOX 46-6
CALCIUM-DEPENDENT PROCESSES

Muscle contraction
Neurotransmitter release
Cardiac pacemaker automaticity
Exocrine/endocrine secretion
Secretory vesicle exocytosis
Coagulation
Bone formation
Axonal flow
Enzyme activity
Cell motility
Cell division
Cell membrane integrity and function

Modified from Layon JA, Kirby RR: Fluids and electrolytes in the critically ill. In Civetta JM, Taylor RW, and Kirby RR, eds: *Critical care*, Philadelphia, 1988, JB Lippincott.

will vary depending on the particular laboratory but is generally in the range of 8.5 to 10.5 mg/dl (4.5 to 5.5 mEq/L, or 0.96 to 1.27 mmol/L). Because a considerable portion of the total serum calcium is bound to albumin, an "accurate" assessment of the total serum calcium concentration requires a simultaneous measurement of the serum albumin concentration. When a significant quantitative alteration occurs in the albumin concentration, a *corrected* total calcium concentration can be calculated; the adjustment necessary for the total serum calcium value is directly proportional (in either direction) to the magnitude of the albumin alteration. Specifically, for each 5 g/L increase or decrease in albumin concentration, 0.1 mmol/L should be added or subtracted (respectively) to the measured total calcium concentration.[487] In units that are more clinically useful, the *corrected* total serum calcium concentration can be derived by adjusting the calcium concentration by 0.8 mg/dl for each 1 g/dl change from the normal albumin concentration.[8,397] Hence the assessment of total serum calcium concentration is extremely limited unless there is a simultaneous evaluation of the serum protein concentrations.

A mathematically adjusted serum calcium concentration may be more representative of the total calcium concentration than a noncorrected value, but the calculated value may still not provide the information necessary to appropriately manage certain types of patients. In healthy individuals, there appears to be a linear correlation between total calcium concentration and the ionized fraction.[535] This relationship, however, may be unpredictably altered in many situations so that changes in the albumin and total calcium concentrations may actually mask hypercalcemia, hypocalcemia, and normocalcemia. For example, a normal total serum calcium concentration in a patient with hypoalbuminemia may reflect ionized hypercalcemia. Also, hyperproteinemia (e.g., prolonged tourniquet time during phlebotomy, non-synthetic colloid infusions) may elevate the total serum calcium concentration, resulting in a failure to identify a state of ionized hypocalcemia. Critically ill patients often have diminished albumin and total calcium levels, but the concentration of ionized calcium may be normal.[795,797,799,801] Most importantly, calcium binds to albumin with different affinities in different individuals, and presently there is no way to accurately predict this binding affinity.[797] Thus, in view of these pitfalls, it is essential to quantitatively assess the ionized portion of calcium in all moderately and severely ill patients;[391,801,806] a measured concentration of total calcium, a calculated ionized calcium concentration, or a *corrected* total calcium concentration will be unreliable in predicting the actual free ion concentration.

The ionized fraction of calcium is responsible for the majority of biologic activity, and thus hypercalcemia and hypocalcemia are most appropriately defined in terms of this fraction. If specifically requested, the ionized portion of calcium (i.e., the concentration of free calcium ions or the amount of elemental calcium) can be measured by most clinical laboratories. The normal values for this measurement usually range from 4 to 5 mg/dl (2.1 to 2.6 mEq/L, or 1.17 to 1.29 mmol/L) and are unaffected by the concentration of albumin or other proteins.[487] However, changes in the pH level will alter the ionized calcium concentration;[8,705] alkalemia increases the binding of calcium to protein, thereby reducing the ionized fraction. Acidemia, on the other hand, has the opposite effect and will enhance ionization. Thus alterations in pH level can evoke the signs and symptoms of hypocalcemia (increased pH level) or hypercalcemia (decreased pH level) despite a normal total serum calcium concentration.

Hypercalcemia. Hypercalcemia is associated with numerous conditions and disorders including hyperparathyroidism, immobilization, renal failure, adrenal insufficiency, pheochromocytoma, acromegaly, thyrotoxicosis, granulomatous diseases, and Paget's disease.[43,362] There are also a number of medications that have been implicated in the development of hypercalcemia[491] (Box 46-7). An abnormal elevation of the serum calcium concentration is usually caused by increased gastrointestinal absorption and/or bone resorption. In hospitalized patients, the single most common cause is a malignancy that results in excessive bone resorption.[211] This skeletal release of calcium may arise from either bony metastases or humoral substances generated by the tumor.[488,632,634,664,704]

Hypercalcemia is defined by a fasting, total serum calcium concentration of greater than 10.5 mg/dl (5.4 mEq/L or 5.25 mmol/L) or—more appropriately—by

---

BOX 46-7
DRUGS ASSOCIATED WITH HYPERCALCEMIA

Intravenous lipid emulsion
Vitamins D and A
Furosemide
Thiazides
Chlorthalidone
Lithium
Tamoxifen
Estrogens
Beta-adrenergic agonists

Modified from Nanji AA: Drug-induced electrolyte disorders, *Drug Intell Clin Pharm* 17:175, 1983.

an ionized calcium concentration in excess of 5.0 mg/dL (2.6 mEq/L or 1.29 mmol/L). A total serum calcium level below 12 mg/dl is usually not associated with symptoms. When the manifestations of hypercalcemia do occur, they tend to be independent of the cause. On the other hand, the chronicity and magnitude of the hypercalcemic state usually determine the clinical findings for a given patient. In addition, the presence of accompanying renal failure, cardiovascular impairment, electrolyte or acid-base disturbances, and the overall state of debilitation can alter the threshold for the signs and symptoms of hypercalcemia. The clinical manifestations may include nonspecific gastrointestinal complaints (e.g., nausea, vomiting, constipation, anorexia, pain), as well as arthralgias, weakness, bone pain, headache, lethargy, and confusion. Often there is an impaired renal concentrating mechanism, inappropriate polyuria, and progressive dehydration despite the presence of thirst and polydipsia. Cardiovascular effects include hypertension, dysrhythmias, increased systemic vascular resistance, and an increased sensitivity to digitalis preparations. The "classic" electrocardiographic finding is a shortened QT interval, but only a small percentage of patients develop this abnormality and the degree of QT shortening does not necessarily parallel the extent of calcium elevation.[188] Full-blown hypercalcemic crisis is a relatively rare occurrence but can result in prostration and shock. Persistence of this extreme state will result in death, with patients usually succumbing to renal failure, dysrhythmias, or CNS impairment.

In terms of specific anesthetic considerations, calcium availability plays an integral role in both CNS and neuromuscular function. It has been demonstrated that calcium ions facilitate the release of acetylcholine from the motor nerve terminal, enhance excitation-contraction coupling, and stabilize the postjunctional membrane.[430] In addition, calcium is partially or completely successful in antagonizing certain types of drug-induced neuromuscular blockade.[32,667,684] Nevertheless, there are no data available as to the effect of hypercalcemia on the development, duration, or resolution of a pharmacologically-induced neuromuscular blockade. However, there is some information available relative to CNS performance; it appears, at least in animal models, that hypercalcemia enhances the potency of inhalational anesthetics (i.e., decreases MAC).[200]

The critical level for total serum calcium appears to range from 16 to 20 mg/dl. If therapy is not initiated promptly and aggressively when such extreme concentrations exist, the symptoms may rapidly progress to death. A number of modalities are available to lower the serum calcium concentration, but the vigorousness of treatment will depend on the patient's symptoms and the absolute level of calcium. The mainstay of therapy is hydration, either with or without diuretics. Because the renal clearance of sodium and calcium are closely linked and most patients with hypercalcemia are dehydrated, normal saline (i.e., 0.9% sodium chloride) is usually the fluid of choice for volume loading. Alone, isotonic rehydration may decrease the serum calcium concentration,[614] but most commonly potent diuretics are also administered so as to obtain a vigorous sodium diuresis and enhance renal calcium excretion. For severe hypercalcemia, 2 to 3 L of normal saline should be given intravenously over 3 to 6 hours, along with *large* doses of furosemide (e.g., 40 to 100 mg IV every 2 to 4 hours). The goal is to obtain a urinary output of 3 to 5 ml/kg/hr, which should substantially lower the serum calcium concentration within 4 hours. Frequent evaluations of the patient's volume status are mandatory and can be facilitated by the use of invasive monitoring techniques. Electrolyte supplementation must be provided and the serum sodium, magnesium, phosphorus, and potassium concentrations checked often. In patients with renal or cardiac compromise, dialysis (hemodialysis or peritoneal dialysis) can be used, although improvements in the calcium concentration are usually short-lived.[706] Other alternative therapies include chelators (e.g., phosphates and EDTA), osteoclast inhibitors (e.g., mithramycin,[533,663] glucocorticoids,[528] calcitonin,[60] diphosphonates,[350,601] and calcium channel blockers. Verapamil has been used successfully to treat the cardiotoxic effects of life-threatening hypercalcemia.[803] However, use of this agent is merely a temporizing maneuver that is used in conjunction with the initiation of definitive therapy. The phosphates (e.g., potassium phosphate) are generally reserved for life-threatening situations because they are effective immediately (i.e., to bind and precipitate ionized calcium)[703] but often produce widespread metastatic calcification and occasionally renal failure or cardiac arrest.[8] Orally and rectally administered phosphates require several days for maximal effect but are safer than the intravenous preparations that are most efficacious several hours after the onset of administration. The intravenous phosphates should be given by continuous infusion at a dose of 20 to 30 mg of elemental phosphorus per kilogram of body weight over 12 to 16 hours. Phosphate therapy is contraindicated in patients with hyperphosphatemic hypercalcemia or any time the calcium-phosphorus product exceeds 60 to 70. In contrast, the osteoclast inhibitors are frequently used in less severe cases of hypercalcemia and require 1 to 3 days to attain peak effectiveness.

Hypocalcemia. Ionized hypocalcemia develops when there is inadequate compensation for ongoing calcium losses. In other words, the intake and/or skeletal mobilization of calcium are insufficient to offset the actual or functional loss of calcium from the intravascular fluid compartment. Ionized hypocalcemia (i.e., a measured value of less than 4 mg/dl) may result from any of four primary causes: (1) failure of parathyroid hormone secretion or action, (2) failure of vitamin D synthesis or action, (3) failure of bone to respond to parathyroid hormone and/or vitamin D, or (4) calcium chelation/precipitation.[797] Thus a number of conditions have the potential to generate hypocalcemia, including hypoparathyroidism (primary, secondary, or neonatal), hypermagnesemia, hyperphosphatemia, severe hypomagnesemia, burns, rhabdomyolysis, malabsorption, renal insufficiency, pancreatitis, hypothyroidism, sepsis and the fat embolism, hungry bone, and toxic shock syndromes.[43,714] In addition, a number of drugs can also produce hypocalcemia through the mechanisms previously noted (Box 46-8).[491]

Although hypocalcemia is an infrequent occurrence in healthy outpatients, it is a relatively common finding in ill, hospitalized patients due to insufficient

---

BOX 46-8
DRUGS ASSOCIATED WITH HYPOCALCEMIA

Albumin
Amnioglycosides
Amphotericin B
Calcitonin
*Cis*platinum
Citrate
Colchicine
Digitalis
Diphosphonates
EDTA
Estrogens
Ethylene glycol
Gallium nitrate
Glucorticoids
Glutethimide
Heparin
Loop diuretics
Magnesium
Mithramycin
Phenobarbital
Phenytoin
Phosphates
Propylthiouracil
Protamine
Radiocontrast dye
Sodium sulfate

Modified from Nanji AA: Drug-induced electrolyte disorders, *Drug Intell Clin Pharm* 17:175, 1983.

---

skeletal calcium mobilization. This is especially true of patients in both adult and pediatric intensive care units where the incidence of ionized hypocalcemia has been reported to range from 15% to 50%.[104,117,162,799] However, some of these patients (who would otherwise be hypocalcemic) may be protected from symptoms by the concurrent development of acidemia, which will raise the concentration of ionized calcium.

The hallmark of hypocalcemia is neuromuscular irritability, with symptoms ranging from paresthesias to tetany and seizures. In addition, hypocalcemia may augment the neuromuscular blockade caused by nondepolarizing muscle relaxants.[126,201] The cardiac consequences of hypocalcemia include bradycardia, heart block, cardiac arrest, and congestive failure.[132] The electrocardiogram may demonstrate prolongation of the QT and ST intervals but may also be completely normal despite severe hypocalcemia.[797] The diagnosis should also be considered in the presence of hypotension, which is refractory to fluids and pressor agents. Most of the patients who exhibit the manifestations of hypocalcemia (Box 46-9) have severe reductions in ionized calcium. Mild degrees of hypocalcemia (ionized calcium 3.2 mg/dl to 3.9 mg/dl), even in critically ill patients, usually do not evoke symptoms.

Acute symptomatic hypocalcemia is a medical emergency that warrants the intravenous administration of calcium.[796,799] Therapy should not be withheld, even if the cause of the hypocalcemia is unclear. In adults the recommended treatment is a 100-mg elemental calcium bolus (over 5 to 10 minutes), followed by a continuous infusion administered at a rate of 0.5 to 2 mg/kg/hr. Since a bolus dose of calcium will only increase the ionized calcium concentration for 1 to 2 hours, repeated boluses or an infusion is required. In general, the bolus/infusion regimen will normalize the ionized calcium concentration over 2 to 4 hours. However, the individual responses are variable and calcium levels should be frequently monitored; it is not uncommon that the maintenance rate for the elemental calcium infusion must be reduced (e.g., 0.3 to 0.5 mg/kg/hr).[797] In children and infants, the American Heart Association recommends the use of 5 to 7 mg/kg of elemental calcium (0.2 to 0.25 ml/kg of 10% calcium chloride solution) through an intravenous or intraosseous route.[577] This bolus dose may be repeated once in 10 minutes. This therapeutic guideline for pediatric patients specifically addresses pharmacologic intervention during advanced cardiac life support where the indicators for calcium administration have been limited to (1) suspected or documented hypocalcemia, (2) hyperkalemia, (3) hypermagnesemia, and (4) calcium channel blocker overdose. In neonates there is no evidence that calcium is useful during the acute phase

---

BOX 46-9
CLINICAL MANIFESTATIONS OF HYPOCALCEMIA

Neuromuscular

Paresthesias
Muscle weakness
Muscle spasm
Hyperactive reflexes
Chvostek's and Trousseau's signs
Tetany
Seizures

Cardiovascular

Bradycardia
Heart block
Cardiac arrest
Cardiac insufficiency
Hypotension
Insensitivity to digitalis and glucagon
T wave inversion
QT and ST interval prolongation

Respiratory

Laryngospasm
Bronchospasm
Apnea

Psychiatric

Irritability
Anxiety
Depression
Confusion
Dementia
Psychosis

Miscellaneous

Dry, scaly skin
Brittle nails and hair
Cataracts
Papilledema

Modified from Zaloga GP: Hypercalcemia in critically ill patients, *Crit Care Med* 20:251, 1992.

---

of cardiopulmonary resuscitation, and therefore it is generally not recommended. Neonatal tetany should be treated with elemental calcium in divided doses totalling about 2.4 mEq/kg daily.

There are three different calcium salt preparations that are readily available for intravenous administration (Table 46-21). Calcium chloride is the form most often recommended for use during cardiac resuscitation (when calcium is indicated) and during the rapid transfusion of large volumes of citrated blood. However, most clinicians consider calcium gluconate to be the salt of choice for the treatment of acute hypocalcemia. For many years, physicians have been taught that calcium chloride delivers ionized calcium directly to the intravascular fluid compartment, whereas calcium gluconate and calcium gluceptate (glucoheptonate) must first undergo hepatic metabolism.[577] Theoretically, the chloride salt should produce consistently higher and more predictable levels of ionized calcium when compared with the other calcium salts.[769] However, there is some evidence that equal elemental doses of the gluconate and chloride salts are equivalent in their ability to transiently increase the ionized calcium concentration.[134] Calcium chloride is very irritating to the peripheral vasculature and should be administered directly into the central venous circulation, if at all possible. In addition, the chloride salt is acidifying and theoretically should not be used when acidemia coincides with hypocalcemia. All parenteral calcium salts should be administered cautiously—if at all—to patients receiving cardiac glycosides, especially during cardiac resuscitation or during the treatment of hyperkalemia.

MAGNESIUM. Magnesium is the fourth most abundant cation within the body and is the second most prevalent intracellular cation next to potassium. The total body content of magnesium is approximately 25 to 30 g (~2000 mEq) in the average 70-kg adult. For infants, total body magnesium amounts to roughly 22 mEq/kg.[584] Within the body, magnesium is distributed such that 50% to 60% resides in the skeletal system and another 20% is located within muscle tissue.[559] The ICF to ECF concentration ratio is about 15:1. At

---

Table 46-21 Intravenous calcium preparations

	Concentration	Ampule/vial size	Total calcium	Elemental calcium/ml*
Calcium chloride	10%	10 ml	1 g	1.36 mEq; 27.2 mg
Calcium gluconate	10%	10 ml	1 g	0.45 mEq; 9 mg
Calcium gluceptate	22%	5 ml	1.1 g	0.9 mEq; 18 mg

*One mEq of elemental calcium is equivalent to 20 mg.

any one time, less than 1% of total body magnesium circulates within the intravascular fluid compartment, and thus serum levels do not reflect total body stores.[400] Depending on the particular laboratory, the normal total serum magnesium concentration ranges from 1.5 to 2.0 mEq/L. Similar to calcium, the circulating magnesium consists of three components: a chelated fraction (15%), a protein-bound fraction (30%), and an ionized, diffusible fraction (55%). It is this latter fraction which is physiologically active and therefore carefully regulated to maintain homeostasis. Presently, however, clinical laboratories are unable to measure an ionized magnesium concentration; the reported values actually reflect total circulating magnesium.[805]

Under normal conditions, magnesium balance is maintained by a dietary intake of 20 to 30 mEq/day.[559] The gastrointestinal tract absorbs 30% to 40% of this magnesium, with the remainder excreted in the feces.[262] Once absorbed, the circulating ionized magnesium is primarily regulated by the kidney; the majority of filtered magnesium is conserved through proximal tubular resorption.[137] There are, however, a number of situations where renal magnesium excretion can be enhanced: hypermagnesemia, hypercalcemia, hypophosphatemia, metabolic acidemia, ECF expansion, alcohol or protein intake, and the use of loop or osmotic diuretics.[714] In addition, renal resorption of calcium, sodium, and magnesium are all linked so that a primary renal loss of calcium or sodium generates a secondary magnesium loss.

Both parathyroid hormone (PTH) and vitamin D have regulatory influences on renal and gastrointestinal magnesium absorption. In turn, the ionized magnesium concentration influences PTH secretion (e.g., hypermagnesium and severe hypomagnesemia decrease secretion, whereas mild hypomagnesemia stimulates secretion).[119,400] Furthermore, the intercompartmental movement of magnesium ions is influenced by the pH level. Acidemia causes a net magnesium efflux from the ICF to the ECF, and alkalemia drives magnesium into cells. When all homeostatic mechanisms are intact, obligate magnesium losses (via feces, urine, sweat, and secretions) amount to roughly 0.3 mEq/kg/day.[800]

The importance of magnesium derives from its critical role in multiple cellular functions. This divalent ion is vital for the function of a number of enzyme systems, key for DNA transcription, and essential for the activity of many metabolic pathways including oxidative phosphorylation. Magnesium exerts a number of effects on the cardiovascular system and is also associated with neuromuscular contraction, protein synthesis, and thermoregulation. Therefore states of magnesium excess and depletion can have a profound and widespread impact on cellular performance.

Hypermagnesemia. Most often, hypermagnesemia is iatrogenic in origin and arises when magnesium-containing antacids, enemas, or total parenteral nutrition are administered to patients with renal insufficiency or failure.[595] The serum magnesium concentration tends to increase when the glomerular filtration rate falls below 15 ml/min.[81] Other less frequent causes of hypermagnesemia include Addison's disease, hypothyroidism, and lithium intoxication. Occasionally, a state of magnesium excess will develop in an eclamptic or preeclamptic parturient during continuous infusion magnesium sulfate therapy.[187,551]

Hypermagnesemia impairs neuromuscular function and can actually produce neuromuscular blockade.[187] There is a heightened sensitivity to both depolarizing and nondepolarizing muscle relaxants.[167,243] Magnesium also has direct cardiac as well as vascular effects. Excess magnesium may cause vasodilatation and hypotension,[802] and extremely high concentrations can result in cardiac arrest[352,524] and respiratory paralysis. The clinical manifestations of hypermagnesemia correlate fairly well with the total serum magnesium level (Table 46-22).

In acute situations (e.g., perioperatively), saline infusions and furosemide can be used to enhance renal magnesium excretion. The intravenous administration of calcium chloride or calcium gluconate can rapidly antagonize neuromuscular or cardiac toxicity;

Table 46-22   Clinical manifestations of hypermagnesemia

Effect	Total serum magnesium concentration (mg/dl)*	Total serum magnesium concentration (mEq/L)*
Normal	1.7-2.4	1.4-2.0
Diminished DTRs†	5-6	4-5
Anticonvulsant range	5-9	4-7
ECG changes§, bradycardia, hypotension	6-11	5-9
Somnolence	6-8	5-7
Loss of DTRs†	10-12	8-10
Respiratory compromise	10-12	8-10
Heart block	15	12
Respiratory arrest	18	15
Cardiac arrest	24	20

*With an atomic weight of 24.3 and a valence of two (+ +), a magnesium concentration of 1 mg/dl is equivalent to 0.8 mEq/L.
†Deep tendon reflexes.
‡Recommended serum levels during treatment of preeclampsia/eclampsia.
§Prolonged PR and ST intervals, widened QRS complexes, and/or elevated T waves.

however, the beneficial effect is usually transient. In patients with renal failure, peritoneal or hemodialysis can effectively remove excess magnesium.

Hypomagnesemia. In general, magnesium depletion results from excessive ion loss from either the gastrointestinal tract or the kidneys. Gut losses may be due to reduced mucosal surface area, increased intestinal secretions, and/or the formulation of insoluble magnesium soaps in the stool (the result of complexing with unabsorbed fat).[800] Therefore a number of diseases and conditions have the potential for generating hypomagnesemia. Normal colonic fluid contains 10 to 15 mEq/L of magnesium so that large amounts may be lost with diarrhea. The magnesium concentration of upper intestinal fluids is only 1 to 2 mEq/L; nevertheless, prolonged gastric suction/drainage can produce a state of depletion.[728] Renal losses of magnesium may become excessive as a result of hyperthyroidism, hyperaldosteronism, hypercalcemia, SIADH, diabetic ketoacidosis, infusions of calcium or sodium, the administration of certain drugs (Box 46-10), and intrinsic kidney disease.[804] Acute hypomagnesemia can also result from an internal redistribution as magnesium moves intracellularly after the administration of glucose or amino acids.[81]

Most patients with symptomatic hypomagnesemia also have low serum concentrations of calcium and/or potassium. It remains unclear whether magnesium depletion alone can cause symptoms.[366] Nevertheless, hypomagnesemia is characterized by neuronal irritability, and the neuromuscular manifestations are the same as those exhibited with hypocalcemia (see Box 46-9). The cardiovascular consequences include heart failure, vasospasm, hypertension, dysrhythmias, and

an increased sensitivity to digitalis and pressor agents.[94,127,340] Because of the risk of both perioperative dysrhythmias[229,380,381] and respiratory muscle dysfunction,[470] it has been recommended that magnesium deficiencies be partially or totally corrected before patients undergo anesthesia and surgery.[344]

Perioperative repletion of a magnesium deficit usually requires the administration of an intravenous supplement. The normal parenteral requirement for magnesium is roughly 12 to 30 mEq/day, assuming no unusual losses. A substantially greater amount is necessary to correct magnesium depletion. Despite an intracellular magnesium deficit and regardless of the process responsible for the deficit, much of the administered magnesium supplement is excreted in the urine. Therefore relatively large amounts of parenteral magnesium are required for several days to replenish intracellular stores.[344] Magnesium sulfate* is most often administered, but magnesium chloride is also available. When a bolus of magnesium sulfate is given intravenously, the onset of action is immediate and the duration of action is about 30 minutes. With an intramuscular injection, the onset of action occurs in approximately 1 hour and the effects last 3 to 4 hours.

In adults, mild degrees of magnesium deficiency can be treated with intramuscular magnesium sulfate (e.g., 1 g every 6 hr for four doses). In children with normal renal function, 1 mEq/kg/day of elemental magnesium can be added to the maintenance fluid solutions.[362] Overt and severe hypomagnesemia should always be treated with an intravenous magnesium supplement.[212,309] The deficit of magnesium is often 1 to 2 mEq/kg and requires a total dose of elemental magnesium in the range of 2 to 4 mEq/kg (given over several days). In adults, a 6 g loading dose of magnesium sulfate (slightly less than 600 mg of elemental magnesium) can be added to a liter of 5% dextrose in water and infused over 3 hours.[800,804] A continuous maintenance infusion of magnesium sulfate should then be administered for 4 to 7 days. This maintenance fluid should contain a total daily dose of 600 to 900 mg of elemental magnesium. In emergency situations the loading dose can be infused more rapidly, so long as continuous ECG monitoring is performed and the rate of administration does not exceed 15 mg of elemental magnesium per minute. For the duration of intravenous magnesium therapy,

---

BOX 46-10
DRUGS ASSOCIATED WITH HYPOMAGNESEMIA

Aminoglycosides*
Amphotericin B*
Calcium*
Carbenicillin*
Catecholamines
Cis-platinum*
Citrate
Digitalis*
Diuretics* (osmotic, loop, and thiazide)
Ethanol
Insulin
Purgatives/laxatives

*Inhibition of renal magnesium conservation.
Modified from Nanji AA: Drug-induced electrolyte disorders, *Drug Intell Clin Pharm* 17:175, 1983.

---

*Depending on the specific manufacturer, various concentrations of magnesium sulfate heptahydrate are available. Clinically, the 10% and 50% concentrations are frequently used and each gram of magnesium sulfate heptahydrate contains 8.1 mEq of magnesium. Thus each milliliter of the 10% magnesium sulfate heptahydrate solution (available in 20-ml and 50-ml vials) contains 0.8 mEq or 9.7 mg of elemental magnesium. Each milliliter of the 50% solution (available in 2-ml, 10-ml, and 20-ml vials) contains 4.1 mEq or 49.2 mg of elemental magnesium.

patients should be carefully monitored for evidence of magnesium toxicity. Frequent assessment of the total serum magnesium concentration is mandatory, as well as repeated evaluation of other pertinent variables (e.g., blood pressure, ECG, mental status, renal performance, and neuromuscular function). If signs or symptoms of hypermagnesemia develop, the infusion should be discontinued at least until the serum magnesium level normalizes.

POTASSIUM. Potassium is a key element for electrophysical cellular integrity. All cells have an electrical potential difference across their cell membranes.[279] The intracellular milieu carries a net negative charge relative to the fluid surrounding the cells. The membrane-dependent electrical potential is determined by the concentrations of various ions (predominately sodium, potassium, and chloride) in the ICF and ECF compartments. These ionic concentrations are a function of the selective permeability characteristics of the membrane and the presence of membrane-bound ionic transport pumps. The resulting membrane excitability allows cells (e.g., cardiac, neural, skeletal muscle, and so on) to perform specialized functions. Of all the ions responsible for generating cellular electrical properties, potassium is by far the most important. Thus when potassium homeostasis is altered, cellular function is disrupted and the manifestations of hypokalemia or hyperkalemia result.

The total body potassium concentration ranges from 50 to 55 mEq per kg of body weight or 3500 to 3850 mEq in a 70-kg person.[135,456,770] Of these body stores, 90% to 95% is exchangeable between the various fluid compartments.[748] Potassium is the most abundant intracellular cation, and approximately 98% of the total body potassium is located within the ICF compartment (i.e., only 60 to 70 mEq total in the ECF). Most of this intracellular potassium is contained in muscle cells at a concentration of approximately 150 mEq/L of water (see Table 46-7). However, the intracellular concentration of free (i.e., ionized) potassium may be considerably lower.[135] Because the normal potassium concentration in the fluid outside of the cells is 3.5 to 5.5 mEq/L, a huge concentration gradient exists between the ICF and ECF compartments. The primary mechanism for establishing and maintaining this concentration gradient is the sodium-potassium–activated ATPase "pump," which is located in the plasma membrane of all body cells. Therefore relatively small changes in the activity of this pump may have a significant impact on the plasma potassium concentration.

Normal dietary intake of potassium averages 1 to 1.5 mEq/kg body weight per day (i.e., roughly 50 to 100 mEq/day). Once absorbed, most of the potassium is rapidly sequestered within cells and is then gradually released and excreted.[56,685] Under normal conditions the apparent volume of distribution for a potassium load is approximately 60% to 70% of body weight (i.e., roughly the volume of TBW).[779] Of an acute load (oral or parenteral), 50% is excreted in the urine within 4 to 6 hours, but eventually the kidneys excrete 90% of the load and 10% is eliminated via the gastrointestinal tract.[685] Thus, under normal circumstances, potassium balance (intake vs. excretion) is predominately determined by the renal output (i.e., urinary loss) of potassium.

The kidneys can adjust urinary potassium excretion from less than 5 mEq/L to greater than 100 mEq/L.[397] Under normal conditions approximately 600 mEq of potassium is freely filtered through the glomeruli each day, and most of this potassium is then resorbed in the proximal tubules. However, it appears that the terminal nephron is the primary site of regulation for renal potassium excretion.[789,790] Potassium within these distal cells passively diffuses down concentration and electrochemical gradients into the tubular fluid. Thus secretion by the distal convoluted tubules and the collecting tubules is influenced by the intracellular potassium concentration, the rate of urinary flow, and the anionic charge of the urine. Also, conditions that increase distal sodium delivery will promote sodium resorption and potassium secretion.[58] This distal sodium for potassium exchange can be significantly augmented by aldosterone.[268] This hormone is a key regulator of renal potassium excretion, because it can dramatically alter the kidneys' capacity to eliminate this ion.

Disorders of potassium homeostasis are frequently discussed in terms of internal and external ion balance.[57,135] Internal potassium balance refers to the distribution of potassium between the ICF and ECF compartments, whereas external potassium balance represents the difference between potassium intake and excretion. Thus the external balance determines the quantity of total body potassium. Normally there is no net difference between potassium intake and excretion, and body stores of potassium are quantitatively stable. For a given individual, the magnitude of dietary potassium intake is relatively constant. The total potassium loss in sweat and feces is small, and thus renal excretion is the dominant factor governing external potassium balance. The internal distribution of potassium is directly affected by changes in acid-base balance, body fluid tonicity, and the secretion of insulin, catecholamines, and mineralocorticoids.[716] The influence of pH level alterations on potassium distribution is an aspect of internal balance that is appreciated by most clinicians. However, the generalization that changes in the pH and the serum potassium concentrations are invariably related in an inverse fashion and that the severity of these changes are proportional is an oversimplification. When the hydrogen ion concentration changes, the magnitude of the internal redistribution of potassium actually depends on the nature of the acid-base disturbance (e.g., acidemic, alkalemic, metabolic, or respiratory), the duration of the disturbance (e.g., acute, subacute, or chronic), and the cause of the disturbance (e.g., mineral acids, organic acids, and so on).[135,240]

Alterations of external potassium balance do not occur in isolation. When the external balance is altered, concomitant changes occur in the distribution of potassium between the ICF and ECF compartments that strongly influence the resulting serum potassium concentration. When there is a net total body loss or gain of potassium, the *proportional* change in serum potassium concentration is greater than the *proportional* change in total body potassium.[135,700] In other words, internal potassium balance is disrupted during fluctuations of external potassium balance and the serum concentration may provide misleading information. In addition, the serum value can be altered by variations in internal potassium balance that occur unrelated to changes in total body potassium (i.e., external potassium balance). Thus the serum potassium concentration (a function of both internal and external balance) is not reliable as an indicator of total body potassium stores during periods of altered potassium homeostasis. The electrocardiogram may be a more accurate indicator of potassium excess or depletion, because it can provide an electrophysiologic representation of overall potassium balance.[114,618] Nevertheless, in clinical practice, states of potassium imbalance are most often identified and then addressed (both diagnostically and therapeutically) in terms of the serum potassium concentration. Therefore the following sections conform to this approach and discuss disturbances of external and internal potassium balance as subgroups of hyperkalemia and hypokalemia.

Hyperkalemia. Hyperkalemia is generally defined as a serum potassium concentration of greater than 5.5 mEq/L. There are myriad conditions, diseases, and drugs that produce hyperkalemia by disrupting the normal external and/or internal potassium balance (Box 46-11). However, factitious hyperkalemia should always be considered in the differential diagnosis of an elevated potassium level, despite its rare occurrence. Lysis of the cellular elements of blood (e.g., erythrocytes, leukocytes, and platelets) may release significant quantities of potassium. The most common cause of factitious hyperkalemia is hemolysis occurring within a blood specimen. In vitro hemolysis that produces faintly visible xanthochromia will increase the serum potassium approximately 0.15 mEq/L.[397] This release of potassium from red blood cells, as well as the potassium release from ischemic muscle cells

---

BOX 46-11
CAUSES OF HYPERKALEMIA

Factitious
Hemolysis
Leukocytosis
Thrombocytosis

Altered internal potassium balance
Acidemia
Hypertonicity
Insulin deficiency
Hypoaldosteronism
Periodic paralysis
Malignant hyperthermia
Cell necrosis
  Rhabdomyolysis
  Hemolysis
  Burns
  Chemotherapy for certain leukemias/lymphomas
Drugs
  Succinylcholine
  Digitalis overdose
  Nonselective beta-blockers

Altered external potassium balance
Increased uptake
  Salt substitutes
  Replacement therapy
  Transfusions
  Antibiotics containing potassium salts
Decreased excretion
  Renal insufficiency/failure
  Post–renal transplantation
  Interstitial nephritis
  Hypoaldosteronism
  Diminished distal sodium delivery
  Drugs
    Heparin
    Betaconverting enzyme inhibitors
    NSAIDS
    Spironolactone
    Traimterene
    Amiloride

Modified from Solomon RJ, Katz JD: Disorders of potassium homeostasis. In Stoelting RK, ed: *Advances in anesthesia*, Chicago, 1986, Year Book Medical Publishers.

---

associated with a prolonged application of the phlebotomy tourniquet, will elevate both serum and plasma potassium concentrations.[135] Platelet counts in excess of $1,000,000/mm^3$ and white blood cell counts greater than $50,000/mm^3$ may also be associated with an increase in the potassium concentration. Such pseudohyperkalemia can be detected by measuring plasma, rather than serum potassium, concentration.

The plasma concentration is normally 0.3 to 0.5 mEq/L lower than the serum level, because the serum specimen allows in vitro clotting with associated cell lysis and intracellular potassium release.[685] A discrepancy of greater magnitude between the serum and plasma levels suggests a falsely elevated serum concentration that—if not correctly identified—may cause a great deal of unnecessary concern and even dangerous "therapeutic" interventions.

An abnormal potassium distribution can produce a significant (albeit transient) increase in the serum potassium concentration. A number of both well-defined and ill-defined mechanisms can generate the observed hyperkalemia. These transcellular shifts that alter the internal potassium balance are not uncommon to the perioperative period. Patients with severe diabetes,[250,505] burns, or acute metabolic acidosis[15,96] frequently require anesthesics and surgery and may exhibit this transcellular hyperkalemia. The use of nonselective beta-blockers, especially in patients with renal failure or insufficiency or diabetes mellitus, may also elevate the serum potassium concentration.[174,175,586,658,659] In addition, it is well documented that the depolarizing skeletal muscle relaxant succinylcholine can transiently elevate the serum potassium concentration by 0.3 to 0.5 mEq/L in normal subjects.[34,147,266] This potassium increase may be exaggerated in conditions where there is muscle membrane degeneration (e.g., trauma, burns, neuromuscular disorders) or neural denervation (e.g., cerebrovascular accidents, spinal cord injuries). It appears that when two or more conditions associated with altered internal potassium balance coexist (e.g., beta$_2$-blockade and succinylcholine), the hyperkalemic response is enhanced.[440]

A disruption of external potassium balance (e.g., increased intake or decreased excretion) can enlarge the total body stores of potassium and result in hyperkalemia. Increased potassium intake can elevate the serum potassium concentration; however, this is an unusual occurrence unless there is a concomitant reduction in potassium excretion. Impaired renal potassium elimination is by far the most common cause of hyperkalemia associated with a surplus of body potassium. Hyperkalemia is a prominent feature of the syndrome associated with acute renal failure. In contrast, many patients with chronic renal failure are able to maintain external potassium balance through enhanced gastrointestinal secretion and increased secretion by the remaining functional nephron mass.[155,657] Such patients are nevertheless prone to develop hyperkalemia with acute potassium loads, transcellular potassium shifts, and the ingestion of drugs that impair potassium secretion. In addition, hyperkalemia is a recurrent problem in patients with chronic renal disease who are oliguric (i.e., urinary output less than 1 L/day) or who have contracted diseases primarily affecting the renal medulla (i.e., the interstitial nephritides).[125,716]

Mineralocorticoids play an important role in modulating renal potassium secretion, and thus their absence or functional impairment may result in potassium retention and hyperkalemia. Generalized adrenal insufficiency (i.e., Addison's disease) is a relatively rare cause of hyperkalemia, but selective deficiencies of aldosterone are not uncommon. The syndrome of hyporeninemic hypoaldosteronism occurs with unusual frequency in patients with diabetes mellitus and is also associated with the use of certain nonsteroidal antiinflammatory drugs (NSAIDs), especially in patients with renal insufficiency.[120] Chronic administration of heparin (even the so-called "mini-dose" regimens) produces adrenal inhibition, diminished aldosterone secretion, and—occasionally—significant hyperkalemia.[145,514] The angiotensin-converting enzyme inhibitors reduce aldosterone secretion by preventing the conversion of angiotensin I to angiotensin II.[525] Hyperkalemia most often develops in the setting of renal insufficiency[723] or congestive heart failure.[433]

Hyperkalemia produces muscle weakness that can progress to flaccid quadriplegia. Initially, the weakness is most prominent in the lower extremities but then extends, involving the upper limbs (a so-called ascending "paralysis"). In postoperative patients, impaired respiratory muscle function may become significant when compounded by the respiratory depressant effects of residual inhalation and/or intravenous anesthetics. However, the most clinically important effect of hyperkalemia is its influence on the initiation and conduction of electrical impulses within the tissues of the heart.

The action potentials generated within cardiac cells result from sequential changes in membrane permeability for specific ions (Figs. 46-16 and 46-17). These permeability changes are due to the selective opening and closing of ion specific channels within the cell membranes.[277] In hyperkalemia the resting membrane potential is decreased toward the threshold potential (Fig. 46-18). With mild degrees of hyperkalemia (i.e., less than 6 to 7 mEq/L) there is increased automaticity as reflected by atrial and/or ventricular ectopy.[536] Hyperkalemia enhances rapid repolarization (phase 3), which causes shortening of the T-wave interval and peaking of the T wave,[713] especially in the chest leads. These symmetrically peaked T waves probably result from a merging of the normal U and T waves.[191] If the serum potassium concentration continues to rise, the inward movement of sodium (phase 0) and calcium (phase 2) will diminish; the PR interval becomes prolonged and eventually the P waves (atrial phase 0) will disap-

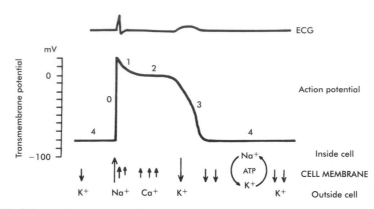

Fig. 46-16. Schematic representation of ventricular myocardial working cell action potential. *Arrows* indicate times of major ionic movement across cell membrane. (From Arrhythmias. In Jaffe AS: *Textbook of advanced cardiac life support,* Dallas, 1987, American Heart Association.)

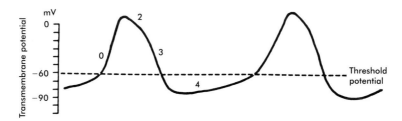

Fig. 46-17. Schematic representation of pacemaker cell action potential. (From Arrhythmias. In Jaffe AS: *Textbook of advanced cardiac life support,* Dallas, 1987, American Heart Association.)

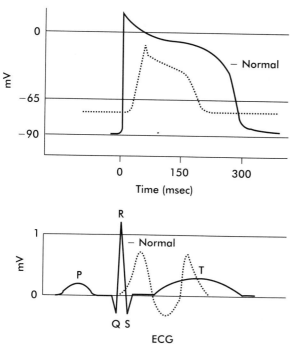

Fig. 46-18. Effect of severe hyperkalemia *(dotted line)* on actional potential and the ECG. (From Surawicz B: Relationship between electrocardiogram and electrolytes, *Am Heart J* 73:814, 1967.)

pear.[209,313] Within the ventricular muscle mass, both conduction velocity and the height of the action potential are reduced. The net result is a widened QRS complex and reduced contractility. If the hyperkalemia progresses (Fig. 46-19), the QRS complex will become smooth, wide, and sinusoidal as it merges with the T wave (serum potassium concentration of 10 to 12 mEq/L). If left untreated, the electrophysiologic manifestations of hyperkalemia will culminate in ventricular fibrillation or standstill.

Severe hyperkalemia (usually a serum concentration of greater than 7 mEq/L) requires prompt and appropriate management. Emergency treatment is aimed at quickly restoring normal transmembrane electrical potentials. With continuous ECG monitoring, 10 to 30 ml of 10% calcium gluconate can be administered over 3 to 5 minutes (a smaller quantity of calcium chloride may be substituted). The calcium will not change the ECF potassium concentration but will reduce both the threshold potential and the excitability of cell membranes. The duration of action is roughly 30 to 60 minutes; thus a second dose may be necessary. The calcium salt preparations must always be administered cautiously in patients receiving cardiac glycosides.

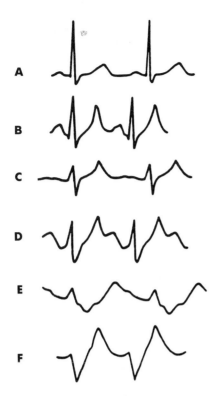

Fig. 46-19. Electrocardiographic changes of hyperkalemia. **A,** Normal tracing. **B** to **F,** Serial changes of elevated potassium levels. (From VanderArk CR, Ballantyne F III, and Reynolds EW Jr: Electrolytes and the electrocardiogram, *Cardiovasc Clin* 5(3):269, 1973.)

BOX 46-12
CAUSES OF HYPOKALEMIA

Altered internal potassium balance
  Alkalemia
  Insulin
  Beta$_2$-agonists
  Lithium overdose
  Anabolism
  Periodic paralysis

Altered external potassium balance
  Decreased intake
    Alcoholism
    Starvation
    Anorexia nervosa
  Increased renal excretion
    Primary and secondary hyperaldosteronism
    Hypomagnesemia
    Renal tubular acidosis
    Drugs
      Diuretics
      High-dose penicillin, carbenicillin, nafcillin, or ticarcillin
    Osmotic diuresis
    Myelomonocytic leukemia
  Increased gastrointestinal excretion
    Loss of gastric fluid
    Diarrhea

Emergency management also includes efforts to quickly increase the cellular uptake of potassium, thereby decreasing the ECF concentration. One to two ampules of 8.4% sodium bicarbonate can effectively lower the serum potassium level in 15 to 30 minutes.[217,397] Alkalinization must be undertaken cautiously in patients with hypocalcemia, because tetany may develop and patients with cardiac compromise may not be capable of handling the sodium load. A second method for shifting potassium intracellularly is the combined administration of glucose and insulin.[405] One unit of regular insulin is recommended for each 2 g of dextrose, with both agents given by intravenous bolus. For example, 1 ampule of D$_{50}$ (i.e., 50 ml of 50% dextrose) would be immediately followed by 12.5 units of regular insulin. A maintenance infusion containing 500 ml of 10% dextrose in water with 10 units of regular insulin may then be infused over 1 hour.[252] Again, this glucose and insulin therapy may require 15 to 30 minutes to achieve a maximal potassium translocation of 1 to 2 mEq/L. The effectiveness of these emergency measures can be best assessed by continuous ECG monitoring.

Strategies for reducing the total body potassium concentration should be undertaken simultaneously with acute management. If renal perfusion and function are adequate, loop diuretics (with or without zaroxalyn) should be used to obtain a kaliuresis. Orally or rectally administered calcium or sodium polystyrene sulfonate (e.g., Kayexalate), in combination with sorbitol, facilitates potassium excretion through a colonic exchange of calcium or sodium for potassium. These exchange resins are effective in approximately 60 minutes if given by enema or in 120 minutes if given by mouth.[397] Prolonged administration of diuretics and a high-salt diet are usually effective for treating hyporeninemic hypoaldosteronism, the most common form of chronic hyperkalemia.[512] Occasionally the synthetic mineralocorticoid fludrocortisone (Florinef) may also be required to stabilize external potassium balance. If these measures fail to control the hyperkalemia, then hemodialysis or peritoneal dialysis must be initiated to reduce total body potassium.

Hypokalemia. Hypokalemia is most often defined as a serum potassium concentration of less than 3.5 mEq/L. As with hyperkalemia, reduced potassium levels occur as a result of disrupted internal and/or external potassium balance (Box 46-12). A metabolic alkalemia may cause a transcellular potassium shift, but it is more likely that the associated hypokalemia is due to a depletion of total body potassium. Most chronic respiratory alkalemias have a minimal effect on the serum potassium concentration, but the acute respiratory alkalemia commonly associated with general anesthesia may decrease the serum potassium level by 0.5 mEq/L for each 10 mm Hg reduction in arterial carbon dioxide tension.[186] Stress-related catecholamine activity can produce a transient decrement in ECF potassium concentration.[481,710] Surgical stress may reduce the serum potassium concentration by 0.5 mEq/L.[290] The administration of exogenous catecholamines likewise may diminish the ECF potassium concentration via beta$_2$-receptor stimulation.[586] This effect has been demonstrated with epinephrine, isoproterenol, terbutaline, and ritodrine.[89,338,751] Thus hypokalemia of this nature may occur in critically ill patients requiring pharmacologic hemodynamic support and in pregnant patients with preterm labor who receive beta$_2$-receptor stimulants to suppress uterine activity. Acute hypothermia may also cause a redistribution hypokalemia that is reversible on rewarming.[689]

Hypokalemia resulting from altered external potassium balance usually implies a mechanism of increased renal or gastrointestinal excretion. An osmotic diuresis, regardless of the responsible solute (e.g., mannitol, urea, glucose), frequently lowers the total body potassium concentration. Similarly, the osmotic diureses associated with relief of a urinary obstruction and that occurring during recovery from acute tubular necrosis are both associated with hypokalemia. The common factor in the kaliuresis associated with each of these situations is an increased delivery of fluid and sodium to the terminal nephron. Diuretics that act proximal to the site of distal potassium secretion (e.g., furosemide, bumetanide, ethacrynic acid, acetazolamide, and possibly thiazides) also produce a kaliuresis of similar nature. In addition, large doses of certain antibiotics can increase fluid delivery to the terminal nephron (and thus increase potassium secretion) through the excretion of nonresorbable anions. There are a few primary and multiple secondary causes for hyperaldosteronism, including CHF, cirrhosis, and renovasculature hypertension. Many patients with these secondary disorders, however, may not develop hypokalemia unless treated with diuretics.

The potassium content of gastric fluid is normally less than 10 mEq/L. Direct gastric losses of potassium due to vomiting or suctioning are thus relatively small. However, the ongoing loss of gastric fluid creates hypovolemia, which in turn generates a state of secondary hyperaldosteronism. Also, the loss of gastric acid creates an alkalemia, and eventually the renal bicarbonate threshold is exceeded. The increased urinary bicarbonate enhances renal potassium secretion. Therefore the major source of potassium wasting associated with the loss of gastric fluid is actually renal rather than gastrointestinal.[64] In contrast, the lower gastrointestinal tract, which is normally responsible for only a small amount of potassium excretion, can dramatically increase its potassium loss with diarrhea. Stool water may contain from 29 to 147 mEq/L of potassium.[785] Thus large volumes of watery stool (e.g., laxative abuse, villous adenoma) may result in severe potassium depletion.

Because the degree of hypokalemia does not necessarily correlate with the total body potassium stores or the duration of the potassium deficit, it is difficult to predict the clinical manifestations for a given serum concentration. The signs and symptoms of hypokalemia result from the altered electrical forces across cell membranes. Potassium depletion causes the ratio of intracellular to extracellular potassium to increase, thereby reducing the resting potential (phase 4) and creating a state of hyperpolarization. When the action potential is initiated (phase 0), it is of super-normal magnitude. The time allotted for calcium entry (phase 2) is shortened, and repolarization (phase 3) is prolonged, leading to a greater relative refractory period. The diminished calcium entry may lead to malaise, myalgias, cramps, reduced exercise tolerance, and even paralysis. The altered permeability of the myocyte cell membrane results in an increased concentration of the creatine kinase MM isoenzyme. Severe hypokalemia (i.e., less than 2.5 mEq/L) may produce rhabdomyolysis.[59,373] Similar to hyperkalemia, potassium depletion may weaken the respiratory muscles, creating a need for postoperative mechanical ventilation. Hypokalemia may also appear to potentiate the effects of nondepolarizing skeletal muscle relaxants.

Smooth muscle function is also impaired; bladder dysfunction may produce urinary incontinence or retention, and ileus formation may result from the lack of peristalsis. The smooth muscle components of the peripheral vasculature are also affected. The pressor response to catecholamines is compromised, and orthostatic hypotension may develop.

Hypokalemia may alter the morphology of the heart's electrical activity as depicted on an ECG (Fig. 46-20). However, these morphologic changes are a relatively insensitive indicator of the severity of potassium depletion except in the face of extreme hypokalemia. The progression of ECG changes is classically described as follows: T-wave amplitude decreases, QT interval lengthens, U wave appears or becomes broader and taller, ST segment sags, and P-wave amplitude and QRS duration increase (Fig. 46-21). In contrast, cardiac dysrhythmias are a much

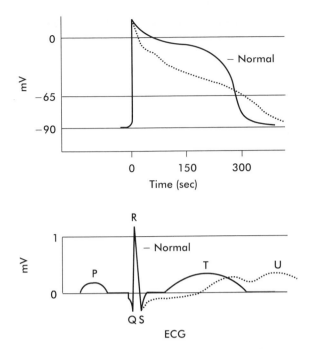

Fig. 46-20. Effect of severe hypokalemia *(dotted line)* on action potential and the ECG. (From Surawicz B: Relationship between electrocardiogram and electrolytes, *Am Heart J* 73:814, 1967.)

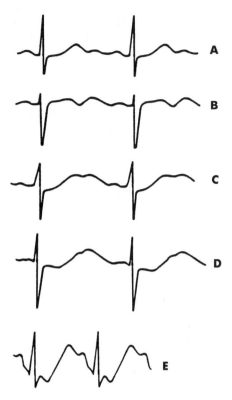

Fig. 46-21. Electrocardiographic changes of hypokalemia. **A,** Normal tracing with a typical U wave. **B** to **E,** Serial changes of hypopotassemia. (From VanderArk CR, Ballantyne F III, and Reynolds EW Jr: Electrolytes and the electrocardiogram, *Cardiovasc Cardiovascular Clin* 5[3]:269, 1973.)

more frequent and predictable occurrence. This vulnerability to rhythm disturbances results from the ability of hypokalemia to enhance intrinsic automaticity, sustain dysrhythmias, and alter conductivity. The most common dysrhythmias are atrial fibrillation and premature ventricular systoles, but supraventricular tachycardia, junctional tachycardia, and Mobitz type I second-degree atrioventricular block may also occur. Hypokalemia may induce digitalis intoxication and result in premature atrial and ventricular systoles, atrioventricular dissociation, paroxysmal atrial tachycardia with block, ventricular tachycardia (i.e., "torsades de pointes"), and ventricular fibrillation. It is important to note that most of the clinical data on the incidence and type of dysrhythmias associated with hypokalemia come from medical, not surgical, patients. These findings may or may not be applicable in the operating room.

Identifying significant hypokalemia, which creates an increased perioperative risk, is not an easy task.[299,320,445,784] This problem may be compounded if the decision to administer an anesthesic is based on a serum potassium concentration obtained in the immediate preoperative period. It appears that preanesthetic potassium levels may be consistently and significantly lower than those obtained 1 to 3 days preoperatively, due to the release of endogenous catecholamines.[320,361] The long-standing practice of withholding elective anesthetic services from patients with serum potassium levels of approximately 3.0 mEq/L or less finds little, if any, support within the clinical anesthesia literature. This practice may be based on the findings of in vitro experiments that have evaluated the effects of hypokalemia on cardiac cells.[305] On the other hand, there is some evidence that chronic hypokalemia in asymptomatic patients undergoing surgery and the administration of an anesthesic is not associated with an increased incidence of dysrhythmias.[753,754] Furthermore, hypokalemia combined with a halothane anesthesic and a catecholamine challenge does not increase the incidence of dysrhythmias, at least in one animal model.[390] It is likely that the duration of hypokalemia is an important factor in determining the threshold for perioperative dysrhythmias. Also, the presence or absence of additional factors that may potentiate the hypokalemia may be of equal or greater importance (e.g., release of endogenous catecholamines, administration of beta$_2$-agonists or diuretics, acute hyperventilation, underlying ischemic heart disease).

If therapy is required immediately before, during, or after surgery, intravenous potassium chloride is usually the agent of choice. The rate of replacement should be determined by the clinical manifestations;

however, the maximal recommended rate of infusion is 0.5 to 0.7 mEq/kg/hr.[153,685] This replacement infusion may be given in a concentration of 80 to 120 mEq per L of solution, and the patient should undergo continuous ECG monitoring. This is especially important in patients with insulin-dependent diabetes mellitus and those receiving nonselective beta-blockers, because these individuals are prone to develop hyperkalemia. The repletion of total body potassium stores requires approximately 200 mEq for each 1 mEq/L reduction in the serum potassium concentration. If hypomagnesemia coexists, magnesium repletion may be necessary to restore external potassium balance (i.e., total body stores) and normalize the serum concentration.[324,767]

Perioperative Fluids

The proper use of intravenous crystalloid solutions requires an understanding of the types of fluids available and the circumstances in which these fluids are indicated. The composition of body fluids and derangements of volume, concentration, and composition have previously been discussed. These concepts are extremely important and must be considered when planning perioperative fluid management. Changes in the volume, concentration, and/or composition of body fluids may occur at any time before, during, or after a surgical procedure. Therefore these parameters must be repeatedly assessed so as to provide the most appropriate fluid replacement. An accurate evaluation of a patient's preoperative fluid status and underlying disease process(es) combined with a knowledge of the proposed operation will allow the anesthesiologist to formulate a patient-specific plan for fluid therapy. This perioperative plan is basically composed of four components: (1) providing normal maintenance fluids, (2) correcting (partially or totally) any preexisting deficits, (3) replacing ongoing losses due to the surgical disease and its treatment, and (4) adjusting the type and quantity of fluids in accordance with the basal function of vital organ systems. A flexible approach to fluid management is key, because there is no precise, objective measure of the compartmental fluid volumes. In patients with complications or who have undergone extensive surgical procedures, it is relatively easy to underestimate or overestimate the required volume of replacement fluids. Quantitative errors of this type are important, because it is the fluid volume within the intravascular compartment (in conjunction with the rapid exchange component of the ISF) that is of most concern during the acute intraoperative period. A surplus or deficit of volume within the intravascular space may have dramatic consequences. Therefore, to prevent or correct a deterioration in clinical status, the plan for fluid therapy needs frequent reassess-

ment and—occasionally—acute intraoperative modification. From a simplistic but practical standpoint, perioperative fluid therapy is essentially an exercise in balancing the input and output of body water and electrolytes. A variety of intravenous solutions are available to achieve this end (Table 46-23). Depending on the circumstances, these fluids may be administered separately or in combination in an effort to maintain total body fluid homeostasis.

Basal energy requirements

The foundation of perioperative fluid management is the provision of maintenance fluids. There are a number of methods for calculating the basal fluid requirement, but the most commonly used scheme is based on energy metabolism (i.e., caloric expenditure).[323] The estimated or measured total body caloric expenditure per day can then be equated with the daily caloric requirement (i.e., a quantitative matching of caloric supply and demand) if basal conditions are to be maintained. It is assumed that the energy expended by an average hospitalized patient lies between the expenditures for an unstressed patient (i.e., basal metabolic requirement) and a stressed patient (i.e., active energy requirement). These expenditures appear to correlate with lean body weight and body surface area, although the relationship is nonlinear in nature (Fig. 46-22). Infants weighing less than 10 kg metabolize 100 kilocalories* per kilogram daily. This relatively large caloric requirement is necessitated by the rapid growth rate and proportionally large body surface area associated with infancy.[330] In children (i.e., 11 to 20 kg body weight) caloric requirements decrease to 50 kcal/kg/day; beyond 20 kg of body weight, metabolic requirements significantly decrease to 20 kcal/kg/day (Table 46-24).

Water is both consumed and produced by the processes involved in energy metabolism (i.e., gross energy changes associated with heat production, muscle activity, and the maintenance of vital functions). However, a substantially greater amount of water is required (1.15 to 1.2 ml/kcal) for these processes than is generated (0.15 to 0.2 ml/kcal) by them. The metabolism of 1 kcal is therefore associated with a net loss of approximately 1 ml of water (Table 46-25). Thus the basal metabolic requirement can be directly linked with the basal fluid requirement on a daily or even hourly basis.

---

* A kilogram-calorie or kilocalorie (kcal) is the amount of heat required (at a pressure of 1 atmosphere) to raise the temperature of a kilogram of water 1° (from 15° C to 16° C). In a resting state, all energy liberated from nutritional intake ultimately appears as heat. Therefore a heat unit was chosen as the most convenient means for measuring and expressing body energy metabolism. The kilocalorie or large calorie (i.e., Calorie or Cal., spelled with a capital C) is 1000 times greater in magnitude than the small calorie (i.e., calorie or cal.) used in physical measurements.[278]

Table 46-23 Commonly used perioperative crystalloid/sugar solutions

	Compounds (mg/100 ml)				Sugars g/100 ml	Electrolytes (mEq/L)				Other anions (mEq/L)	Osmolarity (calculated) mOsm/L	pH level
	Sodium chloride	Sodium lactate	Potassium chloride	Calcium chloride	Dextrose	Na	K	Ca	Cl	Lactate		
D_5W					5						252	4.5(3.5-6.5)
D_5W + 40 mEq/L KCl			300		5		40		40		333	4.5(3.5-6.5)
D_5 0.2% NaCl	200				5	34			34		321	4.0(3.5-6.5)
D_5 0.45% NaCl	450				5	77			77		406	4.0(3.5-6.5)
D_5 0.45% NaCl + 20 mEq/L KCl	450		150		5	77	20		97		447	4.5(3.5-6.5)
D_5 0.45% NaCl + 40 mEq/L KCl	450		300		5	77	40		117		487	4.5(3.5-6.5)
D_5LR	600	310	30	20	5	130	4	3	109	28	525	5.0(4.0-6.5)
LR	600	310	30	20		130	4	3	109	28	273	6.5(6.0-7.5)
RS	860		30	33		147.5	4	4.5	156		309	5.5(5.0-7.5)
0.45% NaCl	450					77			77		154	5.0(4.5-7.0)
0.9% NaCl	900					154			154		308	5.0(4.5-7.0)
4% NaCl	3000					513			513		1027	5.0(4.5-7.0)
D_{10}W					10						505	4.5(3.5-6.5)
D_{10} 0.9% NaCl	900				10	154			154		813	4.0(3.5-6.5)
D_{20}W					20						1010	4.5(3.5-6.5)

D_5W, 5% dextrose in water; $D_{10}W$, 10% dextrose in water; $D_{20}W$, 20% dextrose in water; LR, lactated Ringer's solution; RS, Ringer's solution.

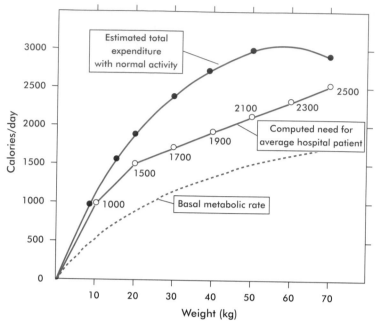

Fig. 46-22. Comparison of energy expenditures in basal and active states. Slope of the calculated curve is a function of three lines that correspond to body weights of 3-to-10 kg, 11-to-20 kg, and greater than 21 kg. (From Holliday MA, Segar WE: Maintenance need for water in parenteral fluid therapy, *Pediatrics* 19:823, 1957.)

Table 46-24	Basal metabolic requirements
Weight (kg)	**Calories needed (daily)**
0-10	1000 kcal/kg
11-20	1000 kcal + 50 kcal/kg for each kilogram over 10 kg
>20	1500 kcal + 20 kcal/kg for each kilogram over 20 kg

Table 46-25	Basal water requirement (ml/kcal)	
System		**Water (ml/kcal)**
Urine		0.73
Skin		0.30
Respiratory system		0.15
Metabolism		−0.15
Total		1.00

From Tonnesen AS: Crystalloids and colloids. In Miller RD, ed: *Anesthesia*, ed 3, New York, 1990, Churchill-Livingstone.

These guidelines for fluid and energy requirements were specifically derived for the average pediatric patient. There are a number of formulas and methods that estimate or measure adult caloric requirements more accurately. However, in an effort to simplify intraoperative fluid management, these guidelines are often applied to hospitalized adults, as well as children, infants, and neonates. This practice is acceptable during the acute, relatively short-term perioperative period but may not be appropriate in chronically ill or severely stressed patients (adult or pediatric). It is important to remember that these guidelines are merely an estimate of the net energy and fluid requirements and may need considerable adjustment when applied to a specific patient.

Energy metabolism is proportional to the body surface area rather than total body weight.[278] When the guidelines listed in Table 46-24 are used, lean body weight (expressed in kilograms) should be employed because it provides a better reflection of body surface area than does total body weight. In addition, there are a number of factors that influence the basal metabolic rate (Box 46-13). For example, fever can increase the basal energy requirement by roughly 10% for each 1° C elevation above normal, and general anesthetics may decrease energy requirements by about 10%. Thus large errors in the estimated fluid requirement may occur if such factors are not taken into account.

Maintenance fluids

As previously discussed, maintenance fluids can be based on basal energy requirements. These fluids should be continued throughout the perioperative period and supplemented by any replacements necessary for additional losses, deficits, and/or sequestration of body fluid.

Regardless of a patient's underlying state of health and the surgical disease or condition, there is a constant, unrelated loss of water and electrolytes from the body. These losses come about through several organ systems, including the skin, lungs, kidneys, and gastrointestinal tract. Maintenance fluids are provided to counterbalance these ongoing sensible and insensible losses. Insensible losses are so termed because they are not visible or readily measurable. They are mostly water losses occurring through the lungs (i.e., respiratory exchange) and evaporative

losses from the skin.[460,656] In a normal adult these losses total about 600 to 800 ml daily. Certain conditions or diseases can dramatically increase these insensible losses, which if not corrected will produce a concentration defect (i.e., a pure water deficit). Sensible losses are those which are visible and can be measured. Normally these losses occur only through feces and urine, but in the absence of diarrhea the fecal content of water and electrolytes is negligible. Thus, under normal conditions, sensible losses can be equated with urinary output. The daily volume of urine demonstrates substantial variation, from an obligatory minimum of 0.3 ml/kg/hr (i.e., 500 ml/day) to an "optimal" output of 1.0 ml/kg/hr or about 1700 ml/day in the average 70-kg patient. Appropriate maintenance fluid therapy will replace all sensible and insensible losses. These fluid losses are primarily water losses (i.e., minimal electrolyte content) and should be replaced with fluids of similar composition.

The quantitative daily water requirement can be estimated from the daily caloric need (see Table 46-24). Thus the water requirement is also a function of lean body weight. The "4-2-1 rule" puts this water requirement in a relatively simple form that is applicable for intraoperative use, because it provides the volume of water needed per hour (Table 46-26). As noted, this formula for water replacement is based on certain assumptions pertaining to the pediatric population; nevertheless, it has been applied successfully to adults in the operating room. The literature contains many other examples of formulas or guidelines for calculating maintenance fluid requirements. Most of these are based on patient weight or age and are derived from either energy expenditure studies or fluid balance studies (Table 46-27).

As alluded to, urine and insensible losses are composed primarily of water. However, even under normal circumstances small amounts of sodium, potassium, and chloride are also excreted. For surgical patients in a preoperative state of electrolyte homeostasis, a failure to provide these ions for a short period (e.g., during and immediately after surgery) is relatively inconsequential. However, if a patient is receiving only parenteral solutions for several days or

---

BOX 46-13
FACTORS INFLUENCING BASAL METABOLIC RATE (BMR)

Decreased BMR
  Starvation
  Hypothyroidism
  Addison's disease
  Obesity associated with hypothalamic or pituitary
    dysfunction
  General anesthetics

Increased BMR
  Skeletal muscle activity
  Ingestion of nutrients
  Caffeine
  Nicotine
  Fever
  Elevated ambient temperature
  Diabetes insipidus
  Leukemia
  Polycythemia
  Dyspnea associated with cardiac, pulmonary, or
    renal disease

Modified from Guyton AC: Energetics and metabolic rate. In *Textbook of medical physiology*, ed 8, Philadelphia, 1991, WB Saunders.

Table 46-26   Water replacement

Weight (kg)	Volume required
0-10	**4** ml/kg/hr
11-20	40 ml + **2** ml/kg/hr above 10 kg
>20	60 ml + **1** ml/kg/hr above 20 kg

Table 46-27   Maintenance fluids

Patient category	Volume required
Adult	1.5-2 ml/kg/hr
Child	2-4 ml/kg/hr
Infant	4-6 ml/kg/hr
Neonate	3 ml/kg/hr

weeks, these ions must be replaced or concentration and composition abnormalities will develop. Replacement is often based on the average daily requirement for these elements (e.g., sodium, 1 to 2 mEq/kg/day; chloride and potassium, 1 to 1.5 mEq/kg/day). A common practice is to include 1 mEq/kg/day (lean body weight) of each ion in the replacement solutions.

Glucose (in the form of dextrose) is frequently a component of maintenance solutions. As a caloric source, this carbohydrate can prevent ketosis; when administered in large enough quantities (e.g., 100 to 200 mg/kg/hr recommended, or 150 g/day minimal, in the average adult) it may spare nitrogen losses (i.e., protein catabolism).[171,278] In addition, the presence of dextrose significantly increases the osmolarity of intravenous solutions (see Table 46-23). Glucose has been routinely used in children to prevent hypoglycemia. Its use appears to be especially important when the patient has had NPO status for a prolonged period or has diminished glycogen stores.[261] Despite the recent concern that hyperglycemia may potentiate hypoxic brain damage,[648] there is insufficient clinical data to warrant the removal of dextrose from maintenance solutions. However, the use of 10% dextrose in water to prevent neonatal hypoglycemia must be carefully monitored, because hypervolemia and life-threatening hyperglycemia may develop.[538]

The solutions most often used as maintenance fluids include 5% dextrose in water (D_5W), 5% dextrose in 0.2% saline (D_5 .2% NaCl), and 5% dextrose in 0.45% saline (D_5 .45% NaCl) (Table 46-23). Small amounts of electrolytes can be added when indicated and the solution administered "piggyback" along with the replacement fluids.

Postoperatively, there are several factors that may necessitate a reduction in the rate of maintenance fluids. First, there are a number of hormonal changes associated with the stress of trauma and surgery.[84,640,787] After an operation, antidiuresis[271,736] and salt retention[141,306,474] frequently develop. During this period, many changes occur that can stimulate the nonosmotic release of ADH. Second, despite the fact that 5% dextrose in water is nearly isotonic at the time of administration, the carbohydrate is rapidly metabolized; the remaining free water then dilutes and expands the ICF and ECF compartments.[460] Third, there is increased endogenous water production. The use of nutrient fuels requires an oxidative process that generates water as a byproduct. Also, tissue catabolism mobilizes and releases intracellular water.[460,640] The increase in endogenous water production appears proportional to the extent of trauma and the nutritional status of the patient. Therefore the infusion rate of postoperative maintenance fluids may require a transient (24 to 72 hours) reduction of up to 30% to prevent hypervolemic, hypotonic hyponatremia.

Replacement fluids

The second component of perioperative fluid management is the administration of replacement fluids. These fluids are intended to replete preoperative deficits and replace both intraoperative and postoperative losses, including distributional deficits.

Preoperative deficits. In adults undergoing elective surgery, oral intake is usually restricted for at least 6 to 8 hours before the procedure. This period of restricted oral intake may be considerably longer when surgery is scheduled late in the day or may be shorter in infants and small children that are susceptible to dehydration. The resulting fluid deficit is primarily due to water losses and should be replaced with maintenance-type solutions. For an estimation of the deficit, the hourly maintenance fluid rate must first be calculated, as previously described. This hourly rate is then multiplied by the time of restricted intake, thus providing an estimate of the total deficit. In general, 50% of this deficit volume is replaced in the first hour of parenteral fluid therapy and 25% replaced in each of the ensuing 2 hours. The entire deficit will then be replaced in 3 hours and is easily accomplished by appropriately increasing the infusion rate of the maintenance fluids. During this repletion period, basal maintenance fluids must be continued. Hospitalized patients receiving intravenous fluids preoperatively may require little or none of this deficit replacement, depending on the infusion rate of the presurgical parenteral solutions.

Additional preoperative deficits may also occur. The most common and usually the most significant of these is a volume deficit (i.e., an isotonic reduction of the ECF volume), which may occur in isolation or in combination with a concentration or compositional disturbance. Clinically, these deficits are most easily categorized as originating from either internal or external fluid losses.

Internal losses are often categorized as distributional changes. These losses result from a relocation of ECF (i.e., both plasma and ISF), which creates an isotonic fluid loss and thus a volume deficit. In general, these losses fall into two categories: "cavitary" fluid losses and third-space fluid losses.* The cavitary losses (e.g., pleural, ascitic, and pericardial fluid) are simple transudates of plasma that often require a relatively prolonged period to accumulate in significant quantities. Therefore the impact on the

---

* For the purposes of this chapter, a third-space fluid loss is considered an isotonic fluid loss derived from the ICF, ISF, and PV. The resulting fluid pool is an appendage to the ISF and thus produces an increase in extracellular *tissue* fluid. In contrast, a "cavitary" fluid is considered a pathologic transudate of plasma that results in a fluid pool deposited in a preexisting body compartment, not in a tissue bed. However, other texts often consider the cavitary fluids as a component of the normal transcellular fluids. Depending on the reference source, the cavitary fluids may or may not be included as part of the third-space fluid losses.

Table 46-28   Electrolyte content of various body fluids

Source	24-hr volume (ml)	Sodium (mEq/L)	Potassium (mEq/L)	Chloride (mEq/L)	Bicarbonate (mEq/L)
Saliva	500-2000	2-10	20-30	8-18	30
Stomach	1000-2000	60-100	10-20	100-130	0
Pancreas	300-800	135-145	5-10	70-90	95-120
Bile	300-600	135-145	5-10	90-130	30-40
Small intestine	2000-4000	120-140	5-10	90-140	30-40
Ileum	100-2000	80-150	2-8	45-140	30
Colon		60	30	40	–

From Tonnesen AS: Crystalloids and colloids. In Miller RD, ed: *Anesthesia*, ed 3, New York, 1990, Churchill-Livingstone.

ECF volume is generally minor. A number of pathologic states affecting the lungs, abdominal viscera, and/or the peritoneal lining of the abdominal or pleural cavities may result in cavitary fluid losses. The third spacing of ECF has previously been discussed (see the section on volume deficit). In certain situations (e.g., obstructed, ischemic, or dead bowel), these losses may develop rather quickly and accumulate in significant quantities. The impact on the ECF volume may therefore be considerable. Both cavitary and third-space losses create a new ECF pool that is sequestered and essentially nonfunctional. However, the fluid lost in third spacing can probably be mobilized back into the functional fluid pool faster and easier than can fluid deposited in body cavities.

Internal blood losses will also diminish the ECF volume. Such losses may be significant with a retroperitoneal hematoma, leaking aneurysm or vascular anastomosis, pelvic or femoral fracture, or a splenic rupture. Depending on the acuteness of the hemorrhage, some degree of compensation or treatment may occur before the initial anesthetic evaluation. Thus the impact on the ECF volume may be blunted. In such cases a thorough clinical evaluation will be necessary to ascertain the full extent of the ECF loss. In addition, the hemoglobin concentration will not accurately reflect the true degree of blood loss until several hours or even days after the bleeding has subsided, depending on the patient's fluid intake. This will not be true if crystalloid or colloid fluid resuscitation has repleted the ECF volume. In this latter situation, the hemoglobin concentration will mirror any prior or ongoing blood loss.

Preoperative external fluid losses most often originate from the gastrointestinal tract and can produce a deficit of several liters. Vomiting, gastric suction, diarrhea, ostomy output, and overzealous bowel preps can produce such deficits. In addition, these losses may be hidden within the lumen of the intestine as occurs with a bowel obstruction or an ileus. A key component of these fluid losses is the excretion of transcellular fluids (Table 46-28). Thus the ECF volume deficit is frequently accompanied by concentration and composition disturbances.

External blood loss is also a frequent cause of preoperative isotonic volume depletion. Upper and lower gastrointestinal bleeding (i.e., hematemesis and melena), along with traumatic injuries, are the usual sources of this loss. However, more subtle external losses may also occur. Insensible losses may become excessive with hyperventilation, fever, sweating, denuded skin, burns, and the use of nonhumidified oxygen (via face mask) administered at high flow rates. Each of these conditions has the potential to create a hypovolemic concentration defect.

The first step in treating these preoperative deficits is to determine the extent of the problem. The assessment of ECF volume deficits is described elsewhere (see the section entitled "Volume Deficit"). Eventually, a measurement or "guesstimate" of the severity of the deficit must be made (see Table 46-9). Each 1% decrease in body weight will ultimately require approximately 10 ml/kg of isotonic fluid replenishment. Most of this fluid will not remain in the intravascular compartment; it will redistribute predominately to the ISF compartment where most of ECF deficit resides. The fluids used to replace pure volume losses should be nearly isotonic with respect to plasma and should also contain salt. In general, a polyvalent, balanced salt solution (e.g., mildly hypotonic, lactated Ringer's solution) is used, but normal saline (isotonic 0.9% NaCl) is certainly an acceptable alternative. Theoretically, both internal and external preoperative fluid deficits should undergo total correction before the administration of an anesthesic. However, an urgent need for surgery may preclude replacement of the entire deficit. Relatively small volume deficits (i.e., less than 20% of the blood volume) can often be replaced with an isotonic or balanced salt solution administered over a period of 15 minutes or less. Most patients will tolerate this degree of acute intravascular volume expansion.

Furthermore, 40% to 60% of the infused solution will redistribute to the ISF compartment within 15 to 30 minutes and 75% will redistribute by 1 hour. If the patient has a large deficit or there is little time before surgery, 25% to 50% of the replacement can be given over 1 hour with the remainder infused in a decremental fashion over several hours. Large deficits can also be replaced by a continuous infusion given over 8 to 24 hours, when time allows. These guidelines should be adjusted in accordance with the total quantity of fluid required, the patient's underlying state of health, and the presence of ongoing losses. Seriously ill patients or those requiring large replacement volumes may require central venous or pulmonary artery occlusion pressure monitoring. Coexisting concentration and composition abnormalities may be suggested by a thorough preanesthetic evaluation but are often confirmed by laboratory measurements. Deficits due to insensible losses should be replaced with hypotonic solutions, and electrolyte disorders should be corrected as outlined in previous sections of this chapter. Thus the goal of preoperative fluid therapy is to correct all concentration and composition disturbances and, most importantly, to attain a normal or slightly expanded functional ECF volume. Mild hypervolemia may help blunt the detrimental cardiovascular effects of both regional and general anesthesics, and will also provide some degree of hemodilution. This latter effect may prove beneficial in limiting the intraoperative decrement in red cell mass.

Intraoperative fluid losses. For organizational purposes, intraoperative fluid losses—similar to preoperative losses—can be categorized as either internal or external losses. The resulting deficits develop rather quickly and should be replaced in an immediate and ongoing fashion. Most of these losses are the result of isotonic reductions in the ECF and therefore should be corrected with a balanced salt solution or normal saline.

The most significant internal fluid loss during surgery is the distributional volume deficit frequently termed "third spacing" (see the section on volume deficit). This type of fluid loss occurs to some degree with every surgical procedure.[638] It appears that the volume of fluid sequestered is proportional to the amount of surgical trauma. Thus major orthopedic procedures, surgery within the chest cavity, bowel resections, and hysterectomies are some examples in which a significant quantity of third spacing occurs (i.e., perhaps 4% to 5% of body weight). The exact quantity of sequestered fluid is difficult to ascertain, and replacement of these third space losses is—at best—an approximation. Estimates for replacement with balanced salt solutions range from 0 to 67 ml/kg/hr of surgery.[639] This tremendous variation of

proposed infusion rates simply reinforces how difficult it is to objectively quantify these losses. In practice it appears that the required volume of replacement fluid is at the lower end of this spectrum. Initially, a somewhat subjective assessment must be made about the degree of surgical trauma. This assessment, in turn, will determine the initial infusion rate of the replacement solution: minimal trauma, 2 to 4 ml/kg/hr; moderate trauma, 4 to 6 ml/kg/hr; extensive trauma, 6 to 8 ml/kg/hr. It must be stressed that these infusion rates are estimates for initiating isotonic replacement. The rate will need to be adjusted in accordance with the patient's response. It is clear that this third spacing of fluid continues into the postoperative period, but it is unclear how this fluid loss varies (quantitatively) over time. In all probability, this third space has specific characteristics and limitations.[121,277] If this is, in fact, true, this appendage of the ISF compartment is not a limitless repository for ECF, and thus the distributional losses at the start and finish of surgery may not be equivalent. Therefore an argument could be made for gradually reducing the replacement infusion over the course of the surgical procedure.

External fluid losses during surgery are predominately due to insensible losses and blood loss. The insensible losses may increase with fever, an elevated ambient temperature, perspiration (e.g., a "lightly" anesthetized patient), hyperventilation, and high flow rates of nonhumidified gases. In addition, significant evaporative losses may occur when either the peritoneal or pleural surfaces are exposed to ambient conditions, a problem exacerbated by the high rate of air exchange in the operating room (e.g., 20 to 25 times per hour). As might be expected, these insensible losses may vary substantially and are difficult to quantify. Depending on the conditions, 1 to 4 ml/kg/hr of hypotonic fluid may appropriately replete this deficit.

Intraoperative blood loss is a relatively frequent occurrence, but it remains difficult to quantify. Even when all surgical losses have been identified and accounted for, the estimated blood loss (EBL) is usually less than the actual blood loss. If the blood volume is normalized and kept constant by the infusion of red cell free solutions (e.g., crystalloids or colloids), the intraoperative hemoglobin concentration will reflect the quantity of red blood cells lost. On the other hand, if the ECF volume repletion is inadequate or constantly changing, the hemoglobin concentration will not provide an accurate reflection of the true blood loss. Depending on the amount of blood lost, the preoperative hemoglobin concentration, and the patient's tolerance to a reduced red cell mass (i.e., tissue oxygen delivery), crystalloid solutions alone may be administered to maintain or normalize the blood volume. A volume of 2 to 4 ml of isotonic or balanced salt solution should be infused for each 1 ml of blood loss. The replacement fluid should be given concurrently with the blood loss at a rate that exactly balances the ongoing loss.

Often, hemorrhagic losses of less than 2 to 3 units are replaced with only normal saline or lactated Ringer's solution, whereas larger losses of blood may require the use of colloid solutions and/or transfusions. This is especially true when a rapid and overwhelming blood loss results in hemorrhagic shock. However, there are increasing reports of the successful treatment of hemorrhagic shock using asanguineous, hypertonic salt solutions. Animal studies employing a bolus infusion of hypertonic saline have revealed significant improvement (at least transiently) in mean arterial pressure, mean circulatory filling pressure, cardiac output, myocardial contractility, renal and cerebral blood flows, and acid-base balance.* In patients, hypertonic saline solutions appear to be an effective therapy for hypovolemic shock[103,152,321,634,793] and also the acute ECF deficits associated with thoracoabdominal aortic operations.[27,138,626,627] The infusion of hypertonic saline promptly expands the PV as water is osmotically extracted from erythrocytes, myocytes, and the vascular endothelium.[439] A single bolus of hypertonic saline may expand the PV by 24%,[793] but unless isotonic volume resuscitation is continued, the beneficial effects dissipate rather quickly. It appears that a critical factor in correcting hypovolemia is the amount of sodium administered and not simply the volume of fluid infused.[626,627] Thus volume resuscitation with hypertonic solutions significantly reduces the total quantity of both crystalloids and blood required to achieve hemodynamic stabilization.[626,627,793] This makes hypertonic saline an especially attractive therapeutic option when increased intracranial pressure and hypovolemia coexist.[552,553,555] Potential side effects of this therapy include hypernatremia, hyperchloremia, hyperosmolality, hypokalemia, and possibly acute hypotension (via decreased systemic vascular resistance) with extremely rapid administration.[364] Although transient concentration and composition disturbances do occur, the reported clinical trials have yet to identify a complication secondary to these abnormalities.[627,793] The solution most often used is 7.5% NaCl (2400 mOsm/L) with a dose of 4 ml/kg administered via bolus infusion. Despite the observed and theoretic benefits of this therapy,[625] the role of hypertonic solutions in perioperative fluid management has yet to be adequately defined. Therefore the

use of such fluids is controversial and is not presently an accepted standard of practice.[435]

Postoperative fluid losses. Both internal and external fluid losses continue into the postoperative period. Depending on the patient's preoperative status, intraoperative management, and surgical procedure, combinations of volume, concentration, and composition disturbances are not infrequent. As previously noted, sequestration or third spacing of ECF continues after surgery. The magnitude and duration of this fluid loss is poorly defined but most likely is influenced by the degree of surgical trauma and the intraoperative fluid management. In general, this edema fluid remains sequestered for 1 to 3 days and is then mobilized into the functional ECF compartment. Other potential sources of internal fluid loss include bleeding and the accumulation of fluid within body cavities. Deficits created by the external loss of body fluids may result from hemorrhage, enhanced insensible losses, or the loss of transcellular fluids (e.g., bile, pancreatic juices, CSF, and so on). Maintenance fluids should be continued postoperatively until the patient can tolerate an adequate degree of oral intake. Super-normal insensible losses can be easily replaced by appropriately increasing the infusion rate of the hypotonic maintenance fluids. Crystalloid replacement of all other postoperative fluid losses can be accomplished with a balanced salt solution and supplemental electrolytes, when indicated.

COLLOID THERAPY

In most patients the proper administration of crystalloid solutions will adequately replace perioperative fluid deficits and losses, thereby maintaining an acceptable level of vital organ perfusion. There are certain patients, however, that may require supplemental infusions of red blood cells or colloid solutions to attain this end. Patients with large blood or other fluid losses, patients in hypovolemic shock, and those patients designated "critically ill" (regardless of the cause) are often considered candidates for receiving blood products and/or colloid therapy. If the red cell mass is replaced appropriately (see the section entitled "Red Blood Cell Therapy"), two categories of fluid are then available for plasma volume expansion: crystalloids and colloids. Physiologic saline (e.g., 0.9% NaCl) and balanced salt solutions are often preferred, because they are relatively safe and inexpensive and do not directly alter hemostasis. However, when compared with a colloid solution, the crystalloid volume must be two to six times greater to achieve the same physiologic end points;[110] in addition, large quantities of crystalloid reduce the serum colloid osmotic (oncotic) pressure.[565,566] The clinical significance of these two findings remains question-

---

* References 398, 416, 490, 503, 554, 555, 585, 612, 733, 749.

able, and it is this uncertainty that is fundamental to the crystalloid vs. colloid controversy.

Under normal conditions the body possesses numerous mechanisms for regulating both the concentration of red cells and the composition of plasma. The red cell mass accounts for 45% of the blood volume, and the remaining 55% is plasma that contains water, solutes, electrolytes, and colloids. Free water, such as that contained in hypotonic solutions (e.g., D_5W), permeates all cell membranes and is distributed throughout total body water in accordance to osmotic gradients. Electrolytes are relatively impermeable to cell membranes but pass freely through vascular membranes. Thus crystalloid solutions (e.g., lactated Ringer's) equilibrate in the intravascular and ISF compartments and determine the total osmolality level that governs water movement between the ECF and ICF compartments. Colloids and colloid-containing fluids (e.g., 5% albumin) are predominately, but not totally, restricted to the intravascular compartment. Therefore the distinct difference between plasma and the ISF is the greater protein (colloid) concentration within the plasma. Although these proteins represent only a small fraction of the total number of dissolved particles in plasma, their size-related membrane impermeability creates an effective osmotic force—the colloid osmotic pressure (COP).[197,563] The capillary COP thus serves to retain plasma water in the intravascular fluid compartment.

The plasma COP is related to the *number* of protein particles per unit of solution. Albumin, with a molecular weight of 69,000 d, normally accounts for nearly two thirds of the plasma COP; it is the most oncotically active plasma protein and is responsible for a major portion of intravascular fluid retention.[563,564] The globulins within plasma have molecular weights that extend upward to 1,000,000 d but exert less of an oncotic effect, because the total number of these proteins is relatively small. These negatively charged proteins attract a large number of cations to maintain electroneutrality. The resulting unequal distribution of diffusible ions increases the number of osmotically active particles within plasma, which—in turn—increases the plasma COP. This example of the Gibbs-Donnan equilibrium results in a plasma COP that is about 50% greater than would be expected from the plasma proteins alone[195] (i.e., the serum or plasma protein concentration is an unreliable predictor of COP). On the other hand, red blood cells are suspended within plasma and are not a solute component of the plasma solution. These cellular elements do not exert an osmotic force, and thus the COP of blood and plasma are identical.[195]

The COP can be measured through samples of blood, serum, or plasma using a colloid osmometer

Table 46–29 Colloid osmotic pressure (COP)

Condition	Approximate plasma COP (mm Hg)
Normal adult, upright	25
Normal adult, supine	20
Critically ill adult	18-20

(i.e., oncometer).[761] This transducer–semipermeable membrane system measures the osmotic effects of molecules larger than 30,000 d and can provide a digitally displayed result in less than 1 minute.[563] The COP can be calculated, but the derived values are relatively inaccurate in critically ill patients (i.e., the patient group in whom the values would be most desired).[688] For the "average" patient in the intensive care unit, the measured plasma COP is in the range of 18 to 20 mm Hg[568,761] (Table 46-29).

The capillary circulation provides a means for the movement of water and solutes between the plasma and ISF. In an adult, the total filtering surface of the body's capillary membranes is on the order of 6300 m^2.[308] Quantitatively, the plasma COP is a rather weak force compared with the total osmotic pressure, but it nevertheless plays a vital role in the distribution of water between the intravascular and interstitial compartments. However, the plasma COP is only one of several forces that determine the fluid flux across a vascular membrane. The Starling equation describes the forces and principles that regulate the movement of fluid between the intravascular and ISF compartments:

$$Q_f = K_f [(P_c - P_t) - \sigma (\pi_c - \pi_t)]$$

where Q_f = net flow of fluid across the capillary membrane (i.e., filtration rate), K_f = fluid ultrafiltration coefficient, P_c = capillary hydrostatic pressure, P_t = interstitial (i.e., tissue) hydrostatic pressure, σ = Staverman reflection coefficient, π_c = capillary (i.e., plasma) COP, and π_t = interstitial COP.[691,692] The filtration coefficient is a function of the permeability and surface area of the capillary bed in question. The numeric value represents the net volume of fluid crossing the capillary membrane under a specific set of conditions. The reflection coefficient is a mathematic expression (ranging from 0 to 1) of the capillary membrane's permeability to a particular substance. Thus the reflection coefficient will vary with both the tissue bed and substance in question. If a substance is completely permeable to the capillary membrane, the reflection coefficient will be 0; if it is totally impermeable, the coefficient will be 1. For protein, the approximate reflection coefficients for liver, lung, and brain are 0.1, 0.7, and 0.99,

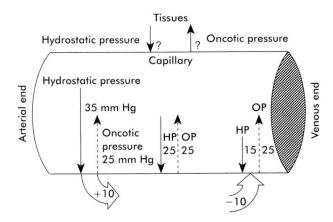

Fig. 46-23. Schematic representation of a normal capillary depicting the forces involved in the Starling equilibrium. At the arterial end, hydrostatic pressure exceeds oncotic pressure and there is a net efflux of capillary fluid. At the venous end, hydrostatic pressure is reduced and the oncotic pressure causes a net reabsorption of interstitial fluid. (From Maxwell MH: The nephrotic syndrome in adults, *Postgrad Med* 23:427, 1958.)

respectively.[780] The COP difference is of greatest magnitude in the brain, kidney, and systemic capillary beds ($\sigma = 0.9$). When a pulmonary insult creates a leaky capillary state, the protein-lung reflection coefficient may decrease to approximately 0.4.[86]

It should be apparent that the forces responsible for normal or abnormal fluid flux are the net colloid and hydrostatic pressures on either side of the capillary membrane. The capillary hydrostatic pressure is the driving force for fluid moving out of the intravascular compartment (Fig. 46-23). Because the interstitial hydrostatic pressure is usually negative or zero,[274,283,454] the plasma COP is the force primarily responsible for counterbalancing the capillary hydrostatic pressure. Any alteration of these forces that enhances filtration may induce changes that retard further transcapillary fluid loss (e.g., increased tissue hydrostatic pressure, increased plasma COP, and decreased tissue COP). In addition, the lymphatic system provides a means for returning filtered capillary water and protein back to the intravascular compartment.[719] The rate of lymphatic flow appears linked to filtration characteristics of the capillary wall and interstitium and the net flow of transcapillary fluid,[718] whether because of hypoproteinemia,[295,379] increased capillary hydrostatic pressure,[284] or enhanced membrane permeability.[581] When one or more of these conditions overwhelms the protective adaptations, the rate of interstitial fluid accumulation may surpass the rate of lymphatic drainage; edema will result, which—if present in the form of extravascular lung water—may have dire consequences for the patient.[569]

It is generally accepted that crystalloids are effec-

tive and appropriate for the initial management of ECF losses associated with hemorrhagic shock, major surgery, and/or trauma. After this acute resuscitation, there usually is a significant degree of hemodilution and a diminished plasma COP.[73,124,331,417,670] This reduction in plasma COP has been associated with the development of edema and transudates. It is often argued that continued fluid resuscitation should include colloid solutions in an attempt to minimize interstitial edema within vital organs (e.g., heart, brain, and lung).[413] In both patient* and animal studies,[291,382,610] colloid-containing resuscitation protocols have demonstrated the ability to either maintain or increase the plasma COP. A number of colloidal preparations have been used to achieve this COP stabilization. When compared with the normal electrolyte components of plasma, these solutions contain rather large natural or synthetic molecules that are relatively impermeable to the normal capillary membrane.

Albumin

Albumin is a natural blood colloid with a normal serum concentration of 3.5 to 5.0 g/dl in adults. Its molecular weight ranges from 65,000 d to 69,000 d. It is isoelectric at a pH level of 4.4 to 5.4, normally contains multiple negative charges at a pH level of 7.4, and is water soluble. Hepatocytes are responsible for albumin synthesis, with production regulated by perihepatic interstitial osmoreceptors and influenced by several circulating hormones.[195] The size (i.e., molecular weight) of this protein precludes glomerular filtration, and the half-life of circulating albumin is approximately 18 to 20 days.[53] Within the body, there are both intravascular and extravascular (i.e., interstitial) pools of albumin, which represent 40% and 60%, respectively, of the total body content (4 to 5 g/kg lean body weight).[53] Under normal conditions, only a small portion of the free or unbound albumin moves between the intravascular and ISF compartments. Approximately 6% to 11% of the circulating albumin pool undergoes degradation each day.[397,591] An abundance of hydrophilic amino acids creates a high affinity for water that allows each gram of albumin to bind a maximum of 18 ml of water.[314,562,609] As a result of this affinity for water and because albumin is the most abundant plasma protein, it accounts for roughly 70% to 80% of the plasma COP. In addition, the binding properties of albumin allow it to serve as a carrier protein for multiple substances, including certain drugs, hormones, enzymes, ions, dyes, amino and fatty acids, and intermediate metabolites (e.g., bilirubin).

---

* References 253, 419, 484, 550, 566, 637, 752.

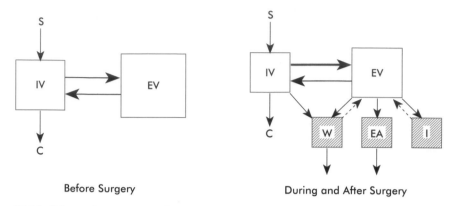

Before Surgery

During and After Surgery

Fig. 46-24. Schematic representation of the perioperative redistribution of albumin resulting from major abdominal surgery. *IV,* intravascular albumin, *EV,* extravascular albumin, *S,* synthesis, and *C,* catabolism. Albumin sequestration sites associated with surgery are denoted as *W,* wound, *EA,* extraabdominal, and *I,* intestinal. (From Hoye RC et al: Fluid volume and albumin kinetics occurring with major surgery, *JAMA* 222:1255, 1972.)

Major surgical procedures are associated with significant changes in albumin distribution.[331,506] It appears that the normal intravascular and interstitial pools of albumin are partially depleted, because this protein is sequestered in abnormal extracellular sites (Fig. 46-24). This sequestration creates new extracellular albumin reservoirs and is associated with a decrease in plasma COP, an increase in interstitial fluid, and a disproportionate reduction in plasma volume. The magnitude of the plasma volume deficit seems to parallel the extent of surgical trauma. However, the total decrement in ECF volume and plasma COP is partially offset by the prompt mobilization of normal extravascular albumin stores[438,669] and an acceleration in the rate of albumin synthesis.[195,592]

Parenteral albumin preparations are often used to normalize both plasma volume and COP. Albumin is commercially available in concentrations of 5% (250-ml and 500-ml vials) and 25% (50-ml and 100-ml vials). These solutions are derived from pooled human blood, serum, or plasma and have been pasteurized at 60° C for 10 hours. In addition, these preparations contain no clinically important antibodies and may be administered without regard to the recipient's blood group or Rh factor. The more frequently used 5% solution contains 50 mg of albumin per milliliter of physiologic salt solution, whereas the 25% solution contains an albumin concentration of 250 mg/ml. All commercial albumin products contain 130 to 160 mEq of sodium per liter of solution. *In vitro* analysis reveals that the 5% solution is isooncotic with respect to human plasma and that the more concentrated albumin preparation is five times more oncotically active than is an equivalent volume of normal plasma (Table 46-30).

Table 46-30 Colloid solutions

	Average molecular weight (daltons)	Approximate peak COP (mm Hg)
5% Albumin	69,000	20
25% Albumin	69,000	100
5% Plasma protein fraction	119,000	20
6% Hetastarch	450,000	30
10% Pentastarch	260,000	40
10% Dextran 40	40,000	70
6% Dextran 70	70,000	60

The response to an infusion of albumin is not simply a function of the solution's concentration or COP. In both human and animal studies, the volume expansion resulting from albumin therapy is inconsistent in nature; the magnitude and duration of the PV increase can not be accurately predicted. Nevertheless, it is clear that albumin solutions given during states of acute hypovolemia will rapidly produce some degree of plasma volume expansion and hemodilution that persist for many hours. On the other hand, if albumin is administered to normovolemic normoalbuminemic individuals, the excess water, sodium, and protein are lost from the vascular compartment within a few hours. In dehydrated patients, it appears that crystalloid solutions must be infused concurrently with albumin; otherwise, there is often little or no clinical improvement. However, after the administration of albumin in any patient, the amount of protein retained in the bloodstream and the associated increment in PV are not dependent on the concentration of the albumin solution. Rather, it is the total amount (i.e., grams) of infused albumin, the baseline plasma COP, and the preexisting PV deficit that are crucial in determining the clinical response.[393,562]

In general, solutions containing 5% albumin are used during the initial resuscitation of patients with hypovolemia. The more concentrated 25% solution is often reserved for patients in whom fluid and sodium intake must be minimized (e.g., infants, neonates, patients with cerebral edema, and patients with both edema and hypovolemia). In clinical practice, 25% albumin is often combined with a potent diuretic in an attempt to mobilize edema and/or ascitic fluid. It is assumed that such therapy will return the sequestered fluid to the intravascular compartment, where it will eventually undergo renal excretion. However, there is no scientific data supporting the efficacy of this combined therapeutic regimen that may be fraught with complications in fragile or critically ill patients.[397]

Albumin preparations are relatively nontoxic, and the safety of these solutions has been well demonstrated. Allergic reactions are usually mild (e.g., nausea, urticaria, fever, and chills) and occur at a rate of 0.5% to 1%. Albumin solutions do not appear to directly alter the coagulability of blood. Even when large quantities of albumin are infused during hypovolemic or septic shock, the incidence of bleeding and dysfunctional coagulation is the same as that associated with crystalloid resuscitation.[193,347] The major drawback to the use of commercial albumin preparations is the cost, which can be several times greater than that associated with the artificial macromolecular colloids.

Plasma Protein Fraction

Plasma protein fraction (PPF) is a 5% solution of selected proteins prepared from pooled human blood, serum, or plasma. It undergoes the same pasteurization process used for albumin and likewise can be administered without regard for the recipient's blood group or Rh factor. PPF is a mixture of proteins consisting mostly of albumin in an amount equal to or greater than 83% of the total protein composition. No more than 17% of the solution is composed of alpha and beta globulins, and gamma globulin accounts for less than 1%. PPF 5% solutions are approximately isooncotic with human plasma. These solutions also contain sodium (130 to 160 mEq/L), chloride ($\sim$90 mEq/L), and potassium (2 mEq/L maximum) but are devoid of the coagulation factors contained in fresh whole blood or fresh frozen plasma.

The pharmacologic properties of PPF are very similar to those previously described for albumin. PPF is used for plasma volume expansion in the treatment of certain types of shock and hypovolemia. Although PPF and 5% albumin are often viewed as interchange-

Table 46-31   Composition of fresh frozen plasma*

Component (units)	Quantity†
Glucose (mg/dl)	535 ± 78
Sodium (mEq/L)	172 ± 7
Potassium (mEq/L)	3.5 ± 0.2
Chloride (mEq/L)	73 ± 4
Bicarbonate (mEq/L)	15 ± 3
Calcium (mg/dl)	7.56 ± 0.4
Protein (g/dl)	5.5 ± 0.4
Albumin (% of total protein)	60 ± 6

*Analysis of 35 FFP units, 89% containing CPD preservative.
†Values expressed as mean ± SD.
Data from Ewalenko P, Deloof T, and Peeters J: Composition of fresh frozen plasma, *Crit Care Med* 14:145, 1986.

able in these situations, the albumin solution may be superior because it is more purified and contains a greater percentage of albumin ($\geq$93%). Because the cost of the two preparations is roughly equivalent, PPF offers no particular advantage over 5% albumin during acute perioperative fluid management.

Minor adverse reactions to PPF are similar in nature to those associated with albumin, but significant anaphylactoid reactions may also occur.[210,580] Rapid intravenous infusion of PPF (e.g., rates exceeding 10 ml/min)[67] or intraarterial administration during cardiopulmonary bypass[13] can produce hypotension. This problem apparently results from Hageman-factor fragments contained within the PPF solution. These fragments stimulate excessive in vivo bradykinin activation that ultimately produces hypotension.[13] PPF preparations are presently screened for high titers of these fragments; nevertheless, manufacturers now list cardiopulmonary bypass as a contraindication to the use of PPF.

Fresh Frozen Plasma

Fresh frozen plasma (FFP) is yet another natural colloid preparation. This plasma product is actually the fluid portion of a unit of whole blood that has been centrifuged, separated, and frozen within 6 hours of collection.[91] Thus each unit of FFP is derived from a single human blood donor. The usual volume of a unit of FFP is approximately 180 to 250 ml,[91,192] with the size of the component bag and the type of preservative (e.g., acid citrate dextrose or citrate phosphate dextrose) determined by the specific manufacturer. FFP contains minerals, lipids, carbohydrates, immunoglobulins, albumin, and both the labile and stable components of the coagulation, fibrinolytic, and complement systems (Table 46-31). The relative composition of a typical unit is as follows: 91% water, 7% protein, and 2% carbohydrates and lipids.[264] All of the plasma proteins remain intact and are functional when infused. The COP of FFP is essentially the same as that for normal human plasma. The risk of a hemolytic reaction—the result of infused antibody combining with the recipient's RBCs—due to FFP is extremely small. Nevertheless, blood banks normally provide ABO-compatible FFP.

Over the past 25 years, the use of FFP has paralleled the gradual acceptance of blood component therapy. Until recently, FFP was routinely used as an intravascular volume expander.[359,679] However, the risk of viral disease transmission (e.g., hepatitis B and C, cytomegalovirus, mononucleosis, and acquired immunodeficiency syndrome) has become an overwhelming concern. This risk theoretically increases in proportion to the number of donors used to generate the volume of administered FFP. In addition, the hyperosmolar, hyperglycemic, and hypernatremic nature of FFP has the potential for creating concentration and composition disturbances when infused in large amounts. Thus the routine use of FFP as a colloidal component of perioperative fluid therapy is no longer an acceptable practice; because safer alternative agents exist, there is no justification for using FFP as an intravascular volume expander. The administration of FFP should be limited to conditions or situations requiring the replacement of deficient coagulation proteins.[220]

Dextran

Dextrans are synthetic colloids that are composed of linear polysaccharide molecules. For clinical purposes, dextrans are designated by their average molecular weights (see Table 46-30), despite the fact that these solutions are actually polydisperse colloids containing both large and small molecules. Dextran 40, with an average molecular weight of 40,000 d (range 10,000 to 90,000 d), is available in a 500-ml bottle or bag as either 10% dextran 40 in 0.9% sodium chloride (77 mEq of sodium, pH 3.5 to 7) or 10% dextran 40 in 5% dextrose (pH 3 to 7). Dextran 70 has an average molecular weight of 70,000 d (range 20,000 to 200,000 d), and the 500-ml container of 6% dextran 70 in physiologic salt solution provides 77 mEq of sodium ion (pH 3 to 7). In vitro, the COP of dextran 40 is equivalent to that of a 17% albumin solution (i.e., approximately 70 mm Hg).[195] For dextran 70, the reported COP ranges from 40 to 60 mm Hg.[110,564] Despite exerting a higher oncotic pressure, the lower molecular weight dextran solution is more rapidly cleared by the kidney.[24] The threshold for the renal excretion of dextran is a molecular weight of roughly 50,000 d,[25] and particles less than 15,000 d are rapidly filtered and not resorbed. Within 24 hours after infusion, approximately 70% of dextran 40 and 50% of dextran 70 is excreted unchanged in the urine. Severe renal dysfunction prolongs the intravascular half-life and causes an accumulation of the smaller dextran molecules. On the other hand, if the creatinine clearance remains greater than 30 ml/min, both the elimination half-life and urinary recovery of dextran appear unchanged from normal. Dextran particles greater than 50,000 d are phagocytized by the reticuloendothelial system, degraded to glucose, and metabolized to carbon dioxide and water over several days.[485,727] A small portion of these larger molecules are excreted into the gastrointestinal tract and eliminated in the feces.[3]

The dextran solutions provide reliable PV expansion resulting from a colloidal osmotic effect (i.e., a fluid translocation from the interstitial to the intravascular compartment). Their effectiveness has been demonstrated during states of hypovolemia[147,393] and endotoxemia.[385,467,468] In most instances the dextran preparations produce a subacute expansion of PV that is approximately equal to the volume of solution infused. Acutely, dextran 40 will produce a greater increment in PV as compared with dextran 70; however, intravascular volume expansion is generally more prolonged with dextran 70. Each gram of dextran may retain as much as 25 ml of water within the intravascular compartment, at least for a short period.[195]

It has been demonstrated that dextran 40 can improve microcirculatory blood flow during hemorrhagic shock.[318] This effect may not be solely the result of volume expansion, hemodilution, and enhanced cardiac output.[128,404,617] It has been postulated that low molecular weight dextrans can favorably alter RBC rheology.[33,170,617] Dextran 40 may be absorbed by erythrocytes and prevent, diminish, or reverse RBC aggregation; decrease RBC rigidity; and ultimately reduce blood viscosity. However, there is no conclusive evidence that these rheologic improvements are due to the colloid molecules rather than the crystalloid diluent of dextran 40.[129,576] Nevertheless, the use of this solution may offer some advantage (when compared with other intravenous fluids) in treating certain types of shock or impending shock that are associated with RBC sludging and tissue hypoxia.

Although the dextrans are effective PV expanders, there are certain drawbacks to their use. Dextran 40 may interfere with the cross-matching of blood if a proteolytic enzyme technique is employed. Dextran 70 can induce RBC aggregation and rouleaux formation that may also impede cross-matching. Both solutions can produce a factitious hyperglycemia, and the lower molecular weight dextran solution can increase serum AST (SGOT) and ALT (SGPT) levels. Dextran 40 can produce a highly viscous urine (i.e., a specific gravity of up to 1.088) due to the renal excretion of particles weighing less than 50,000 d.[394] This viscous urine may actually obstruct the renal tubules and cause acute renal failure, especially in situations of impaired renal perfusion or function or severe dehydration and oliguria.[118] Anaphylactoid reactions ranging from mild cutaneous eruptions to shock[88,455] may occur in up to 5% of patients receiving dextran.[725] However, the overall incidence of severe reactions is considerably less than 1%.[411] In addition, the dextrans interfere with coagulation and thus have the potential for increasing perioperative blood loss.[232] Dextran infusions impair platelet adhesiveness, reduce factor VIII levels, and promote fibrinolysis. To minimize the clinical impact of these hemostatic changes, the dose of dextran should be limited to 1.5 g/kg/day.[169]

Hydroxyethyl Starches
Hetastarch

The hydroxyethyl starch (HES) compounds are a group of polydisperse synthetic colloids that structurally resemble glycogen (i.e., highly-branched glucose polymers). Hetastarch is a high molecular weight HES, with an average molecular weight of 450,000 d with 80% of the polymers falling in the range of 30,000 d to 2,400,000 d. However, for polydisperse colloids, the number-average molecular weight provides a better representation of the number of particles of a given size as opposed to the weight-average molecular weight, which is greatly influenced by the larger molecules in the particular solution.[110]* The frequently quoted number-average molecular weight for hetastarch is 69,000 d. This HES is available as 6% hetastarch in 0.9% sodium chloride and is supplied in 500-ml bottles or plastic bags. The COP of this solution is approximately 30 mm Hg, and each gram of hetastarch has a water-binding capacity of 20 ml. In patients with hypovolemia, hetastarch appears to produce a significantly greater increase in plasma COP when compared with an equal volume of 5% albumin.[304] In addition, this increased plasma COP lasts at least 2 days after an initial 1-L bolus. Numerous studies performed under a variety of conditions have demonstrated hetastarch to be an effective PV expander that may increase circulatory volume for as long as 24 to 36 hours after an initial infusion. In certain situations as much as 40% of the maximum PV expansion may persist for 24 hours.[452]

The disappearance of hetastarch from the body is a complicated process due to the heterogeneous nature of this HES compound.[562,791] Hetastarch is a complex mixture containing molecules of different size, shape, and structure that are present in various amounts. This mosaic of different molecular fractions governs the duration of both intravascular and total body elimination. Hetastarch excretion is primarily a function of the kidneys. Particles weighing less than 50,000 d are rapidly filtered and deposited in the urine with 40% to 50% of an administered dose eliminated within 48 hours.[791] Larger molecules are degraded enzymatically by α-amylases in the plasma and throughout the body. This is a dynamic and continuous process in which hetastarch molecules are excreted, large molecules are fractionated, and new— but smaller—molecules are formed. It may take as long as 48 days to eliminate 90% of the hetastarch within the body. Most of the enzymatically-produced smaller molecules are excreted by the kidneys, with less than 1% excreted in the bile[355] and less than 1% metabolized and exhaled as carbon dioxide.

There has been a minimum of toxicity associated with the use of hetastarch. Basal serum amylase concentrations may double after an infusion due to a stable hetastarch-amylase complex that retards amylase excretion.[374] These elevated amylase levels may persist for 3 to 5 days but are not indicative of pancreatic dysfunction.[375] The incidence of anaphylactoid reactions is less than one tenth of 1%.[580] The effect on hemostasis appears to be dose related. Large volumes of hetastarch in experimental studies have produced low levels of procoagulants and both quantitative and qualitative platelet abnormalities. However, multiple clinical trials have failed to demonstrate a significant coagulation disturbance associated with the use of hetastarch.[39,316,602,607,709] To prevent coagulopathies, it is often asserted that the dose of hetastarch should be kept below 20 ml/kg/day, but much larger doses have been given to patients without any untoward effects.[367,567,629] Thus there is an abundance of clinical data that fail to implicate hetastarch as a cause of significant bleeding complications. In addition, hetastarch has a negligible effect on the typing and cross-matching of blood.[707]

Pentastarch

Pentastarch is a so-called low molecular weight HES that has recently become available in this country. Its average molecular weight is 260,000 d (number-average molecular weight equal to 63,000 d), with 80% of the polymers falling between 10,000 to 1,000,000 d. Pentastarch is supplied in 500-ml bottles containing 10% pentastarch in 0.9% sodium chloride. Because of its lower average molecular weight and greater concentration, the water-binding capacity and COP of pentastarch are greater than the values for

---

* The average molecular weight usually reported for colloid solutions (e.g., 70,000 d for 6% dextran 70) is actually the weight-average molecular weight, which is defined as the sum of the number of molecules at each molecular weight multiplied by their mass and divided by the total weight of the molecules. The number-average molecular weight is simply the numeric average of the individual molecular weights.[562]

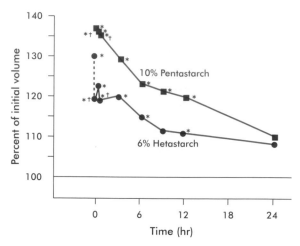

Fig. 46-25. Mean time course of plasma volume expansion in 10 normal subjects after infusion of 6% hetastarch (500 ml) and 10% pentastarch (500 ml). *, significant difference from baseline. +, significant difference between treatments. (From Quon CY: Clinical pharmacokinetics and pharmacodynamics of colloidal plasma volume expanders, *J Cardiothorac Anesth* 2(1) 2([suppl 1]):13, 1988.)

hetastarch by 10 ml/g and 10 mm Hg, respectively.[413] Thus it could be anticipated that pentastarch is a more potent volume expander than is hetastarch. In normal subjects the same dose of both agents reveals a greater expansion of PV with 10% pentastarch[562] (Fig. 46-25). The duration of effect for pentastarch (i.e., 8 to 12 hours) lies between that for 5% albumin and 6% hetastarch.[562]

Pentastarch molecules weighing less than 50,000 d undergo rapid renal excretion. As a result of the relatively small average molecular weight, the vascular half-life appears to be about 10 hours.[571] Total body elimination is also much faster than that occurring with the high molecular weight HES. Due to the structure and configuration of the pentastarch molecules, hydrolysis via α-amylase is rapid and results in an elimination half-life that is shorter than that for hetastarch. After a single 500-ml dose, 70% of the drug is eliminated in the urine within 24 hours and 80% within 1 week.[527] A small percentage of the drug undergoes a variable but overall slower elimination process.

The toxicity and side effects of pentastarch are very similar to those of hetastarch. After an infusion, there may be a transient elevation in the serum amylase concentration unrelated to pancreatic function. The incidence of anaphylactoid reactions appears to be extremely low. In terms of hemostasis, pentastarch may possibly have less impact on the coagulation and fibrinolytic systems than does hetastarch.[708] As much as 2 L of pentastarch have been administered after open-heart surgery with no apparent effect on the

monitored clinical and laboratory parameters of hemostasis.[415]

At present, pentastarch is approved for use only as an adjunct to leukapheresis.[527] However, clinical and laboratory trials are attempting to define its role as a PV expander in cases of sepsis,[571] hypovolemic shock,[759] cardiopulmonary bypass,[414] and postoperative fluid replacement.[415]

Crystalloid vs. Colloid Therapy

For the last several decades, relatively indiscriminate perioperative blood administration was a common practice. It was not until the risk of viral disease transmission became highly publicized that perioperative transfusion practices were substantially altered. In the absence of significant cardiovascular or cerebrovascular disease, the National Institutes of Health now discourages transfusion therapy if a patient's hemoglobin concentration is equal to or greater than 7 g/dl.[500] Thus asanguineous normovolemic hemodilution has become a clinical reality, but it remains controversial as to which type of intravenous fluid (i.e., crystalloid or colloid) will best achieve this goal.

Numerous clinical and laboratory investigations have been performed in an attempt to define the proper role of colloid solutions in the perioperative setting and in states of increased permeability and shock (e.g., cardiogenic, hypovolemic, distributive, and obstructive). Despite the use of many different fluid regimens, investigational end-points, and study goals, the accumulated data have failed to resolve the controversy surrounding the use of colloid preparations. Furthermore, no studies have attempted to address the effects of crystalloid vs. colloid replacement specifically in pediatric patients; all the reported clinical protocols to date have focused only on adults. For most of the conditions investigated, a clear-cut and reproducible advantage of one regimen (e.g., crystalloids) over the other (e.g., colloids) has not been conclusively demonstrated. Thus practicing at either end of the spectrum of colloid use (i.e., liberal use vs. no use) is inappropriate. Instead, a more selective approach is warranted, because there are instances in which colloids offer a definite benefit, a questionable benefit, and no benefit, when compared with crystalloid solutions. The prudent anesthesiologist will be cognizant of these situations and adjust perioperative fluid replacement accordingly.

Although asanguineous fluid replacement is often discussed in terms of crystalloids or colloids, this overly simplistic dichotomy is only applicable in a laboratory setting. In clinical practice the fluid options are actually crystalloids alone or crystalloids in combination with a colloid supplement. Maintenance water and electrolyte requirements must be fulfilled, and nonproteinaceous fluid losses (e.g., gastric drainage) must be replaced. Thus some volume of crystalloid solution will be continuously required. If a colloid supplement is deemed appropriate for the particular situation, then besides determining the volume and type of colloid to administer, one must also decide how much of which crystalloid should be given before, during, and after the colloid infusion. The provision of colloids therefore increases the complexity of fluid management, because the use of colloids is intricately intertwined with ongoing crystalloid therapy; inappropriate management of the crystalloid portion of fluid replacement may partially or completely offset the potential benefit of a colloid supplement. In most instances, body fluid deficits should be replaced with solutions that are similar in composition and/or function to the fluids that have been lost. Based on this rationale, colloids will most often be considered when there are significant losses of either plasma or blood.

Crystalloid solutions are generally the first line of therapy for maintenance and/or replacement of fluid deficits. There is no question that crystalloids—when given in appropriate quantities—can adequately replenish intravascular volume. However, depending on the fluid infused, the crystalloid requirement may be substantial; only 7% to 8% of water (i.e., 70 to 80 ml of 1000 ml D_5W), 20% of a balanced salt solution (i.e., 200 ml of 1000 ml lactated Ringer's), and 25% of physiologic saline (i.e., 250 ml of 1000 ml 0.9% sodium chloride) may be retained within the vascular compartment 1 hour after infusion. Pure crystalloid volume resuscitation therefore requires relatively large volumes of fluid and is frequently associated with tissue edema and reduced plasma COP. The duration of active fluid replacement is longer and the potential of recurrent hypovolemia is greater when colloids are omitted from the fluid regimen. Depending on the particular situation, these characteristics of crystalloid resuscitation may or may not have significant clinical importance.

When equal volumes of fluid are infused, colloid solutions are clearly more effective than are crystalloid solutions in restoring hemodynamic stability. Colloid resuscitation requires less volume, maintains or increases plasma COP, and provides a more prolonged period of homeostasis after the initial resuscitation. It is difficult to compare the extent and duration of PV expansion resulting from the various colloid preparations, because most of the reported studies differ significantly in terms of methodology (e.g., study group, baseline PV volume and COP, infusion rate of colloid, volume of infusate, method of PV quantification, and timing of PV measurements). It appears that most colloid preparations produce a PV increment between 50% and 150% of the administered volume.[502] It is usually acceptable to predict a 1-ml PV expansion for each 1 ml of administered colloid; one must realize, of course, this is only an approximation. However, a greater degree of volume expansion (milliliter for milliliter) can usually be anticipated with the use of the more hyperoncotic solutions (e.g., 25% albumin, 10% dextran 40, and 10% pentastarch). Thus colloids provide a definite advantage over crystalloids in situations of impending hypovolemic cardiovascular collapse, where it is essential that the repletion of intravascular volume be performed expediently. It is generally agreed that when volume resuscitation must be rapidly accomplished and intravenous access is a limiting factor, colloid supplementation is indicated.

There is considerably less agreement as to the role of colloid solutions in preventing pulmonary edema during volume resuscitation. Many of the studies evaluating this quandary suffer from the same limitations that have befallen the studies of colloidal PV expansion. In addition, some of the pulmonary edema studies use preselected volumes or predetermined filling pressures to guide fluid replacement, rather than physiologic end-points; in addition, some use mortality as a measure of outcome, although a lack of influence on survival may be an excessively stringent test for judging the difference between fluid regimens. Furthermore, the isolated use of certain physiologic parameters (e.g., shunt fraction,[647] alveolar-arterial oxygen gradient,[225] pulmonary venous oxygen content[87]) may fail to identify substantial increases in extravascular lung water.[225] Few of the reported studies have attempted to evaluate the effect of different fluid protocols in situations where an elevated pulmonary capillary pressure is superimposed on a moderately to severely ill subject (animal or human).[291,610] Unfortunately, these are but a few of the problems that must be confronted when attempting to interpret the crystalloid vs. colloid data. These shortcomings and inconsistencies in methodology no doubt contribute to the controversy surrounding the qualitative aspects of perioperative fluid replacement.

It is clear that plasma COP falls in the majority of patients during the recovery phase of shock and preshock states and after major surgery.[124,331,417,506,670] The dilution of albumin may be only one of several mechanisms responsible for this COP reduction.[160,331] Nevertheless, within the lung there is an increase in transcapillary fluid flux, but the diminished plasma COP by itself does not seem to produce pulmonary edema.[374,726,812] It appears that the enhanced interstitial fluid volume evokes a compensatory and protective increase in pulmonary lymph flow.[159,295,379] Thus, even though crystalloid resuscitation is associated with a greater increase in tissue fluid when compared with a colloid-based fluid resuscitation, this isolated occurrence may have little or no clinical significance.

Table 46-32 COP-PCWP gradient	
Condition	Gradient (mm Hg)
Normal	8-16
Pulmonary edema	< 4

More than 30 years ago it was originally demonstrated[284] and later confirmed[224] that left atrial pressure is a major determinant of lung water accumulation. These investigations revealed that extravascular water accumulation occurs at a significantly lower capillary pressure (i.e., left atrial pressure) in protein-depleted animals as compared with normal animals. Subsequent studies have underscored the importance of pulmonary capillary hydrostatic pressure as a key variable in the development of excess lung water.[719] This relationship between capillary pressure and lung water appears to be critically important during the resuscitation phase of hypovolemic or septic shock and also during states of increased capillary permeability (i.e., ARDS). Although an elevated capillary pressure seems to be the predominant factor, the propensity for developing pulmonary edema is also enhanced when less severe derangements of two or more predisposing factors (e.g., reduced plasma COP and elevated capillary pressure) coexist.

Clinically, the PCWP has been used as an estimate of pulmonary capillary hydrostatic pressure and the COP-PCWP gradient has been employed in an attempt to predict situations where pulmonary edema is likely to occur.[564] This gradient normally ranges from 8 to 16 mm Hg and reflects a tendency to retain fluid in the pulmonary vasculature (Table 46-32). A gradient of less than 4 mm Hg has been frequently associated with the development of pulmonary edema in a wide variety of conditions.* The proponents of colloid therapy assert that the proper use of colloidal supplements, in contrast with large quantities of crystalloid, will maintain the COP-PCWP gradient, diminish the risk of pulmonary edema,[566] and possibly enhance survival rates.[568,569]

However, the predictive reliability of the COP-PCWP gradient is not universally accepted.[121,228,453,752] There is some evidence that the PCWP is not an accurate predictor of the capillary hydrostatic pressure.[133] In addition, a high normal or even elevated PCWP may not exceed the critical capillary pressure, which is the highest pulmonary capillary pressure at which lung tissue can maintain a constant interstitial

volume without flooding the alveolar sacs with fluid. In intact dogs there appears to be a fairly good correlation between plasma COP and critical capillary pressure.[173] In critically ill individuals, however, it is possible that this relationship is altered in a patient-specific or condition-specific manner and influenced by the multiple determinants of effective lymphatic drainage, the dynamic interaction between interstitial volume and pressure, the functional state of the capillary membrane, or even the transpulmonary pressure changes resulting from mechanical ventilation. The problem in clinical practice is that although one or two of the Starling forces can be measured, the remaining forces and factors are either ignored or substituted with commonly accepted values that may or may not be pertinent for the particular physiologic state. A valid analysis of Starling forces in the lung requires measurement of the interstitial pressures,[283] as well as consideration of several additional factors: capillary permeability, the Staverman reflection coefficient, pulmonary lymph flow[807] and the influence of CVP,[172] interstitial space geometry and compliance,[283] and the distribution of fluid between solid and gel states within the interstitium.[121] In addition, the increment in volume resulting from either crystalloid or colloid infusions will increase capillary hydrostatic pressure such that vascular and cardiac compliance are also factors that will modulate the response to therapy.[110] It is conceivable that the COP-PCWP gradient may accurately predict the development of pulmonary edema only if there is no change, minimal change, or off-setting changes in these unmeasured factors and influences. Despite its limitations, the COP-PCWP gradient is widely used and is probably at least equal to (if not better than) any other objective clinical parameter for predicting the occurrence of increased extravascular lung water. Consequently, this gradient may be useful as an objective guideline for the administration of colloidal supplements.

In summary, it is clear that surgical patients undergoing fluid resuscitation of a substantial magnitude have the potential for developing perioperative pulmonary edema. However, the debate as to which type of fluid (crystalloid or colloid) will better minimize this risk has not been resolved. It appears that capillary pressure is the major factor determining the accumulation of extravascular lung water. There is some indication that colloid therapy may be beneficial in situations where an elevated pulmonary capillary pressure and a reduced plasma COP exist concurrently. The COP-PCWP gradient may be helpful in identifying patients at risk for the development of pulmonary edema who might benefit from colloidal supplementation in conjunction with measures to reduce the PCWP. On the other hand, colloids offer no apparent benefit in situations where

---

* References 158, 194, 482, 557, 558, 568-570, 760.

the plasma COP is reduced but the pulmonary capillary pressure remains within normal limits. As an isolated occurrence, a diminished plasma COP may produce peripheral edema but is not associated with pulmonary edema and impaired oxygenation unless the value is extremely low. Colloids, similar to most therapeutic agents, should not be considered innocuous, because there are side effects and certain toxicities occasionally associated with their use.[502] Thus the *routine* use of colloids—in most situations—cannot be justified, because there is little objective evidence for their superiority over crystalloids; in addition, there may be unacceptable financial and biologic costs associated with their use.[66] There is no question that the colloidal preparations are efficient PV expanders that can maintain or increase plasma COP. Nevertheless, colloid supplements should be selectively administered and only infused in those situations where they provide a definite or potential advantage when compared with crystalloid solutions.

TRANSFUSION THERAPY

Whether to augment the red cell mass in an anemic surgical patient is a perioperative dilemma frequently encountered in the practice of anesthesiology. Defining a threshold for initiating transfusion therapy and an end-point for cessation of that therapy is not always a simple task. In a critically ill, acutely anemic patient with hypotension, tachycardia, oliguria, lactic acidosis, and a large surgical blood loss, the need for blood replacement may be obvious. On the other hand, preoperative transfusion in an otherwise healthy patient with a chronic or subacute anemia may not necessarily be beneficial nor reduce the risks associated with the administration of anesthetics and surgery. In addition, a substantial number of surgical patients will have a clinical presentation that falls somewhere between these two extremes. Such patients may have a dual component anemia, where an acute operative blood loss is superimposed on a chronic anemia that is secondary to the surgical disease or an unrelated medical problem. Unfortunately, little scientific data exist on the indications for transfusion, the threshold for transfusion (i.e., the so-called minimally acceptable hemoglobin [Hb] or hematocrit [HCT] level), the end-point of transfusion (i.e., the optimal Hb or HCT level), or the benefit of transfusion therapy. The potential surgical and anesthetic risks may be totally unaffected or even enhanced by red blood cell (RBC) therapy. In certain situations the morbidity and mortality associated with the transfusion of blood may, in fact, exceed those for the surgical procedure.

The decision to infuse red blood cells should not be based on an isolated Hb or HCT value, but rather on the patient's physiologic status and a risk-benefit analysis of the proposed intervention. This will necessitate an understanding of (1) tissue-oxygen delivery and consumption, (2) the adaptive responses to anemia, and (3) the potential toxicities associated with RBC infusions. It is important not only to identify which patients will benefit from transfusion therapy, but also to determine the extent to which the red cell mass should be increased. Influential factors will include the duration (acute, subacute, or chronic) and degree of anemia, the patient's cardiopulmonary reserve, the planned surgical procedure, and the anticipated volume and rapidity of blood loss. In addition, the differences among various red cell preparations and the potential side effects or complications associated with each must be appreciated. The remainder of this chapter addresses each of these areas; however, the generalizations presented must be cautiously applied to an individual patient. All underlying medical and/or surgical problems should be given thoughtful consideration because such conditions may have a significant impact on the decision to initiate transfusion therapy.

Oxygen Supply and Demand Relationships

The transport of oxygen to the tissues is the single most important function in any aerobic organism. This transport, proceeding from the alveoli to the peripheral tissues, is dependent on convection, chemical reaction, and diffusion processes that occur along a route of decreasing oxygen tension (e.g., 100 mm Hg in the alveolus to approximately 1 mm Hg in the mitochondria). In spite of its complexity, this system ensures an adequate oxygen supply to even the most remotely situated cells. A significant impairment in oxygen delivery ($\dot{D}o_2$) can result in tissue hypoxia and ultimately death by anoxia. In general, there are four mechanisms by which tissue oxygenation may become compromised: (1) stagnant hypoxia—a lack of tissue perfusion, (2) hypoxic hypoxia—a failure of pulmonary gas exchange, (3) histotoxic hypoxia—a cessation of cellular respiration, and (4) anemic hypoxia—a failure in the oxygen-carrying capacity of blood. The following discussion addresses this latter mechanism.

When a gas that contains oxygen interfaces with plasma, the plasma oxygen concentration rises to a constant value. This quantity of dissolved oxygen is determined by the atmospheric pressure, the proportion of oxygen in the gas, and the solubility coefficient of oxygen for plasma (Henry's law):

$$\text{Dissolved O}_2 = C \times Po_2/P_{ATM}$$

where C is the solubility coefficient for oxygen in the plasma component of blood and is equal to 0.023 ml oxygen per milliliter of blood at 38° C, P_{ATM} is the atmospheric pressure, and Po_2 is the partial pressure of oxygen in the plasma. Rewriting this equation to express dissolved oxygen in milliliters of oxygen at STP per 100 ml of blood results in the following:

$$\text{Dissolved } O_2 = 100 \times$$
$$0.023/(760 - 47) \times P_{O_2} = 0.0031 \times P_{O_2}$$

It is apparent that at normal atmospheric pressure, and regardless of how elevated the oxygen tension may be, the amount of dissolved oxygen contained within blood is extremely small (Fig. 46-26). This quantity of oxygen will in no way by itself meet the body's metabolic requirements. However, the dissolved oxygen becomes an increasingly important component of the blood's oxygen-carrying capacity in severe anemia. Under normal circumstances the hemoproteins contained within RBCs significantly augment this oxygen-carrying capacity.

The RBC is highly specialized for carrying reversibly-bound oxygen from the lungs to the peripheral tissues. Of its intracellular protein, 95% is Hb, which provides the means for this direct binding and subsequent oxygen transport. The mature red blood cell is incapable of synthesizing new protein,[54,282] and herein lies the clinical significance of a reduced RBC mass; there is no mechanism by which a RBC can increase its absolute content of Hb. Therefore, once the intracellular Hb is fully saturated, the factor that limits the oxygen-carrying capacity (or oxygen content) of blood is the quantity of RBCs.

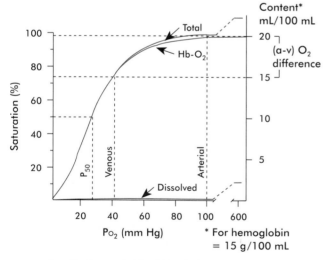

Fig. 46-26. Oxyhemoglobin dissociation curve relates hemoglobin saturation and the oxygen content of arterial blood to the arterial oxygen tension (P_{O_2}). Under normal conditions, the quantity of oxygen bound to hemoglobin (Hb-O$_2$) is the prime determinant of the arterial oxygen content. Raising the P_{O_2} to 600 mm Hg (by breathing 100% oxygen) increases the quantity of oxygen dissolved in the plasma and, hence, the total oxygen content. The arteriovenous (a-v) oxygen difference reflects the gradient in content between arterial and mixed venous blood.

The total concentration of oxygen in blood is the sum of oxygen dissolved in plasma and that bound to Hb. The oxygen bound to Hb can be determined with the aid of the following information: (1) 4 M of oxygen can bind to 1 M of Hb, (2) each mole of oxygen equals 22,400 ml of oxygen, and (3) the molecular weight of hemoglobin is 64,458.[611] Hence

$$1 \text{ g Hb} = (4 \times 22,400)/64,458 = 1.39 \text{ ml } O_2$$

In the literature, this result varies from 1.34 to 1.39, depending on the value used for the molecular weight of Hb, (i.e., 64,500 to 66,800 d)[12] and because it is often assumed that the theoretic maximum for the binding of oxygen to Hb is seldom achieved under normal circumstances.[12,246] The total oxygen content of blood (Ca$_{O_2}$) will depend on the degree to which a Hb molecule is saturated with oxygen (Sa$_{O_2}$) and the total amount of Hb contained in the blood. This content can be expressed as follows:

$$Ca_{O_2} = (1.39 \times Hb \times Sa_{O_2}) + .0031 \times Pa_{O_2}$$

From this equation, it is clear that the Sa$_{O_2}$ level and especially the Hb level are the major determinants of the oxygen-carrying capacity of blood. The oxygen content of blood in a patient with an Hb concentration of 14 g/dl, a Pa$_{O_2}$ level of 100 mm Hg, and an Sa$_{O_2}$ level of 100% would be slightly greater than 20 ml of O$_2$/dl of blood (i.e., 20 vol %). If the Hb level is reduced to 7 g/dl, the oxygen content will fall to 10 vol %. If the Pa$_{O_2}$ level is then increased to 500 mm Hg, the oxygen content will rise to only 11 vol %.

Despite the importance of the Ca$_{O_2}$ level, it is only one of two major determinants of tissue oxygen delivery. The other pivotal component is cardiac output (Q$_T$):

$$\dot{D}_{O_2} = Q_T \times Ca_{O_2}$$

In an average-sized healthy adult, D$_{O_2}$ will be approximately 1000 ml/min (5 L/min × 200 ml/L). However, the importance of $\dot{D}_{O_2}$ (especially in the presence of anemia) revolves around its relationship to oxygen consumption ($\dot{V}_{O_2}$) and its ability to provide a wealth of oxygen to all metabolically active tissues. Total body $\dot{V}_{O_2}$ can be calculated by means of the Fick equation:

$$\dot{V}_{O_2} = Q \times (Ca_{O_2} - C\bar{v}_{O_2})$$

where blood drawn from the main pulmonary artery is used to calculate the mixed venous oxygen content (C$\bar{v}_{O_2}$) by using the partial pressure and oxygen saturation of this venous blood (normally, the P$\bar{v}_{O_2}$ level is about 40 mm Hg and the S$\bar{v}_{O_2}$ level is roughly 75%). This arteriovenous oxygen content difference (normally 5 vol %) reflects the extent to which total oxygen availability matches total body metabolism or oxygen requirements. In no way does it represent the state of oxygen balance for a specific organ or tissue bed. A decrease in the Pvo_2 level indicates either a reduction in total oxygen supply or an increase in overall tissue oxygen demand.[208] Under normal circumstances the $\dot{V}o_2$ level is only 250 ml/min so that there is a moderate excess of oxygen delivery, and consequently, the risk of tissue hypoxia is minimized. This relationship between oxygen consumption and delivery is termed the oxygen-extraction ratio ($\dot{V}o_2/\dot{D}o_2$), which under basal conditions is approximately 24% to 28%.

Under normal circumstances the body's metabolic rate determines the amount of oxygen consumed. If, however, the delivery of oxygen to the tissues becomes drastically reduced, then cellular respiration will be compromised and the $\dot{V}o_2$ level will fall. This relationship, which has been demonstrated in both animal experiments[100,101,102] and human studies, is schematically depicted in Fig. 46-27. As oxygen delivery diminishes in the $\dot{D}o_2$-independent region of the curve, compensatory mechanisms are called on that ultimately increase the oxygen-extraction ratio. The overall $\dot{V}o_2$ level is therefore unaltered by variations in oxygen delivery. Unfortunately, the ability of tissue beds to increase their oxygen extraction is limited, and when further reductions in oxygen availability occur, a point is reached where cellular metabolism is compromised and the $\dot{V}o_2$ level decreases. This point, where the $\dot{V}o_2$ level becomes supply dependent, is described as the critical oxygen delivery ($\dot{D}o_{2\ crit}$)[100] and represents an oxygen delivery of approximately 8 to 10 ml/min/kg in patients undergoing coronary artery bypass surgery[633] but may range as high as 20 ml/min/kg in certain types of critically ill patients.*

---

* References 143, 303, 367, 469, 734, 735.

When the value for tissue oxygen availability lies within the $\dot{D}o_2$-dependent region of the curve, evidence of tissue hypoxia usually develops (e.g., lactate production, metabolic acidosis, lowered Pvo_2 level, reduced Svo_2 level, and a narrowed arteriovenous oxygen content difference).

Physiology of Anemia

From the preceding discussion, it should be evident that a major concern (at least from a hematologic standpoint) in an anemic surgical patient is the maintenance of an adequate blood oxygen content and tissue oxygen delivery. With acute or chronic reductions in the circulating red cell mass, a number of homeostatic compensatory mechanisms are normally used to achieve this goal.

One critically important adaptation to chronic anemia is an alteration in the oxygen affinity of Hb. Changes in oxygen affinity produce shifts in the oxyhemoglobin dissociation curve and are reflected by the P_{50} level (the partial pressure of oxygen at an Hb saturation of 50%). The normal P_{50} level is approximately 26 mm Hg, but this value increases in the presence of anemia. In other words, anemia results in a rightward shift of the oxyhemoglobin dissociation curve (i.e., a subnormal affinity of Hb for oxygen), which is due to a compensatory increase in concentration of erythrocytic 2,3-diphosphoglyceric acid (2,3-DPG).[208,732] The extent of elevation for both P_{50} and 2,3-DPG concentrations appears to parallel the severity of the anemia (Fig. 46-28). The enhanced P_{50} level will facilitate tissue oxygenation if oxygen availability is compromised by the anemia. It is possible that the 2,3-DPG–mediated alterations in the P_{50} concentration may compensate for as much as

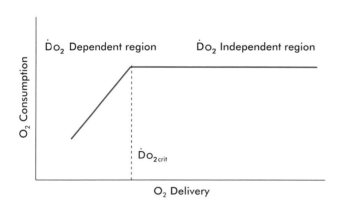

Fig. 46-27. Idealized representation of the relationship between oxygen delivery ($\dot{D}o_2$) and oxygen uptake ($\dot{V}o_2$). $\dot{D}o_2{}^{crit}$ represents the critical value for oxygen delivery (see text for details). (From Gutierrez G: Peripheral delivery and utilization of oxygen. In Dantzker DR, ed: *Cardiopulmonary critical care,* Orlando, 1986, Grune & Stratton.)

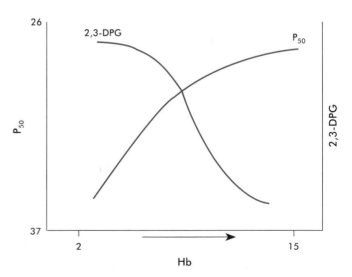

Fig. 46-28. Changes in 2,3-DPG and P_{50} with anemia. (Modified from Finch CA, Lenfant C: Oxygen transport in man, *New N Engl J Med* 286:407, 1972.)

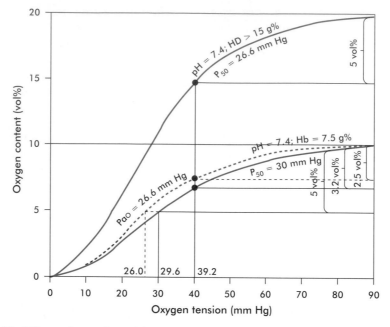

Fig. 46-29. Effects of anemia and increased P_{50} on the oxyhemoglobin dissociation curve. Normal oxyhemoglobin dissociation curve is shown at the top, with the curves in anemia displayed below. The dashed line represents the unshifted curve (normal P_{50}) and the solid line represents the curve in a compensated anemia (increased P_{50}). If the mixed venous (i.e., end-capillary) oxygen tension remains at 39.2 mm Hg, the shifted curve in anemia permits an increased oxygen extraction from 2.5 to 3.2 volume percent. If the normal 5 volume percent of oxygen were extracted, the resulting mixed venous oxygen tension would be 29.6 mm Hg as opposed to 26 mm Hg with the unshifted curve. (From Torrance J, Jacobs P, Restrepo A et al: Intraerythrocytic adaptation to anemia, *New N Engl J Med* 283:165, 1970.)

50% of the expected oxygen deficit in chronic anemia[12,732] (Fig. 46-29). Alveolar oxygen tensions are high enough so that the elevated P_{50} level does not significantly affect oxygen uptake by erythrocytes in the pulmonary capillaries. There is some evidence that a rightward shift of the oxyhemoglobin dissociation curve may occur within several hours of the onset of anemic hypoxia.[40]

The microcirculation is able to fine-tune tissue oxygenation through local regulatory mechanisms (e.g., capillary recruitment, capillary transit time, and erythrocyte flow).[681] Input from the autonomic nervous system, endogenous vasoactive substances, and pH level regulates the tone of arteriolar sphincters.[280] In the presence of anemia, vasodilatation occurs within metabolically active tissue beds, increasing blood flow and hence oxygen delivery. After an acute blood loss, arteriolar constriction occurs in areas that are relatively oxygen insensitive (e.g., skin, gastrointestinal tract), whereas a decrease in vascular resistance is observed in oxygen-sensitive organs (e.g., heart, brain).* The exact mechanism responsible for this dilatory effect is unknown, but it may resemble that seen in hypoxic hypoxia where lowered oxygen tensions result in dilatation of arterioles and capillary beds. The quantity of open capillaries in a tissue bed is determined by precapillary sphincters.[178] The distance that oxygen must diffuse to reach the most remote cells is determined by the number of capillaries that actually contain erythrocytes and the relative volume of interstitial fluid. In a healthy person at rest, the majority of capillaries merely contain plasma and only a small percentage contain red blood cells.[222] Hypoxia results in local tissue adenosine release, which in turn dilates the precapillary sphincters, providing an increased density of capillaries, which contain RBCs.[146,326,365,480] It is conceivable that a similar mechanism sustains oxygen delivery to vital structures during anemia.

Among the physiologic adaptations occurring with anemia, the changes in viscosity are extremely critical. Viscosity is the friction between adjacent layers of fluid as they move relative to one another.[724] This relative movement or shear rate depends on the diameter of the vessel and the rate of flow. Thus the sluggish blood flow associated with vessels of extremely small caliber accounts for the majority of resistance within the circulatory system.[281] Both the concentration and deformability of RBCs are key determinants of blood viscosity. A logarithmic rela-

---

* References 18, 196, 208, 247, 288, 301, 317, 348, 349, 447, 489, 746.

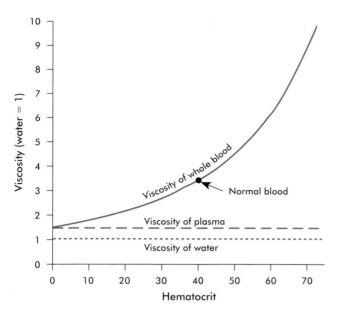

Fig. 46-30. Effect of hematocrit on viscosity. (From Guyton AC: Overview of the circulation and medical physics of pressure, flow, and resistence. In *Textbook of medical physiology,* ed 8, Philadelphia, 1991, WB Saunders.)

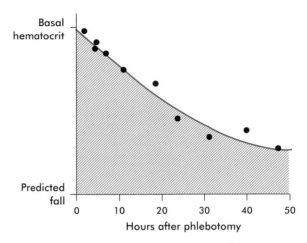

Fig. 46-31. Fall in hematocrit after an acute blood loss. Complete endogenous expansion of the blood volume and the lowest hematocrit value may not be appreciated for up to 72 hours. (From Adamson J, Hillman RS: Blood volume and plasma protein replacement following acute blood loss in normal man, *JAMA* 205:609, 1968.)

tionship exists between viscosity and the HCT concentration, such that as the HCT concentration progressively drops from 40%, the blood viscosity rapidly declines and eventually approaches that of plasma alone (only 1.5 times greater than water)[282] (Fig. 46-30). In turn, this diminished viscosity improves blood flow through minute vessels and may (depending on the Hb concentration, P_{50} level, and cardiac output) maintain a near-normal tissue $\dot{D}o_2$.

In the majority of instances where there is a chronic reduction in the circulating red cell mass, the total intravascular volume remains normal, or nearly normal, due to a compensatory expansion of the PV.[12,269,332] A loss of blood causes mobilization of interstitial protein and fluid that ultimately normalizes the circulating volume. After an acute hemorrhage, endogenous PV expansion (i.e., blood volume normalization) requires 20 to 60 hours to complete; during this period the HCT level* gradually falls[5,180,410]) (Fig. 46-31). Perioperatively, this restoration of the circulating blood volume can be accomplished within minutes to hours through the administration of crystalloids and/or colloids. If the intravascular volume is appropriately corrected, the hematocrit concentra-

tion will accurately reflect the preceding blood loss. In either case (i.e., endogenous or exogenous PV expansion), the combination of a diminished RBC mass and a normal blood volume is primarily responsible for the previously described reduction in viscosity.

The presence of acute or chronic anemia may substantially alter cardiac performance. Cardiac output is usually elevated in the presence of anemia.[77,588,628] With an acute and severe isovolemic anemia, cardiac output is enhanced by an increase in heart rate.[746] In mild chronic anemia the increased cardiac output is also the result of a tachycardia with no change in stroke volume.[259,269] When the hemoglobin concentration is chronically less than or equal to 7 g/dl, the heart rate is usually normal and the cardiac output is elevated as a consequence of an increased stroke volume.[77,593,594] If the hemoglobin concentration slowly decreases from 7 to 4 g/dl, an almost linear increase in cardiac output occurs[746] (Fig. 46-32), with the left ventricular end-diastolic pressure remaining normal and volume increasing.[269,588] Lowered blood viscosity[578] and reduced net systemic vascular tone[215] produce an augmentation of ventricular preload[258,275] and a reduction in ventricular afterload,[451,561,575] which favor the maintenance of the elevated stroke volume and hyperkinetic state associated with anemia.[259,269]

The heart has a higher rate of oxygen extraction than any other vital organ and normally uses 65% to 70% of the oxygen available in the coronary circulation.[598] Despite the increase in the P_{50} level, if myocardial oxygen demand increases during anemia (e.g., exercise, perioperative stress), oxygen extraction may quickly reach a maximum unless oxygen delivery is enhanced. There is evidence that suggests coronary

---

* The total number or volume of RBCs in the circulation is termed the red cell mass. The total quantity of blood (i.e., RBCs and plasma) in the circulation is the blood volume. The ratio of these two entities is a measure of concentration known as the body HCT (as opposed to the capillary HCT), which is closely reflected by the venous blood HCT concentration, Hb concentration, or the RBC count. If a HCT value is 45%, it implies that 45% of the blood volume is RBCs and the remainder is plasma.

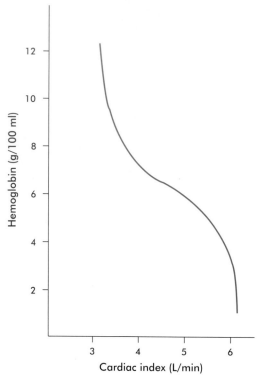

Fig. 46-32. Relationship between anemia and cardiac output. (Modified from Varat MA, Adolph RJ, and Fowler NO: The cardiovascular effects of anemia, *Am Heart J* 83:415, 1972.)

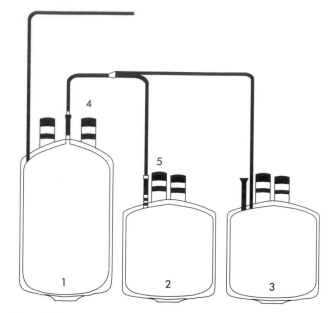

Fig. 46-33. Closed blood collection system for the preparation of AS-1 Prbcs: (1) primary collection bag with CPD preservative preservation solution *(1)*, satellite bag with Adsol preservative *(2)*, empty satellite bag for plasma *(3)*, and in-line cannulas *(4 and 5)*.

blood flow increases during anemia; acute anemia lowers coronary vascular resistance, whereas chronic anemia induces the formation of intercoronary collaterals.[181,811] However, these adaptations may not be possible in the presence of significant coronary atherosclerosis where the heart may be the first organ to develop anemic hypoxia. Healthy patients tolerate anemia because, percentage-wise, coronary blood flow increases more than does cardiac output.[2]

The gradual development of anemia may lead to cardiac hypertrophy, but an otherwise normal heart can tolerate moderately severe anemia (i.e., Hb concentration of 7 to 9 g/dl) for many years without demonstrating an impairment in function. If CHF or angina pectoris develops in patients with this degree of anemia, it usually signifies the presence of underlying heart disease. Chronic anemia alone does not often cause CHF, unless the Hb concentration falls below 4 g/dl.[588] However, in acute anemia, left ventricular function apparently can become compromised with less dramatic reductions in the level of Hb (e.g., less than 6 g/dl).[113]

Erythrocyte Preparations

The administration of blood and blood products is an important part of the practice of anesthesiology, because approximately 50% to 70% of all RBC

transfusions are given in the perioperative period.[531,560] The proper use of whole blood and/or its derivatives allows the performance of certain surgical procedures that would not otherwise be possible. In addition, there are situations in which transfusion therapy probably has a significant impact on perioperative morbidity and mortality, although no data support this contention. Transfusion of a specific portion of whole blood (i.e., component therapy) has become practical with the advent of "closed" collection systems composed of plastic blood containers. A typical system consists of a primary collection bag, integral tubing, in-line cannulas, and transfer or satellite bags (Fig. 46-33). This system can be kept sterile while differential speed centrifugation techniques allow separation of the various blood fractions. The individual components can be stored and then used when indicated by the clinical circumstances. The primary advantage of component therapy is that several patients may benefit from a single blood donation. Approximately 12 million units of whole blood are collected annually in the United States, and over 85% of these are fractionated into components.[697] Thus the use of component therapy has become a routine practice necessitating all anesthesic providers to be familiar with the characteristics and the potential side effects of the available preparations.

Preservative Solutions

Several different solutions can be added to either whole blood or packed RBCs to allow storage of these

Table 46-33   Biochemical changes of blood in various preservative solutions

Parameter	WB CPD		WB CPDA-1		PC CPDA-1		PC AS-3	PC AS-1
Storage time (Days)	0	21	0	35	0	35	42	49
pH level (at 37° C)	7.2	6.8	7.6	7.0	7.6	6.7	6.5	6.6
Plasma Hb level (mg/dL)	1.7	19	8.2	46	7.8	658*	†	‡
Plasma K^+ level (mEq/L)	3.9	21	4.2	27	5.1	79*	N/A	6.5
2,3-DPG level (% of initial)	100	44	100	< 10	100	< 10	< 10	< 5
ATP level (% of initial)	100	86	100	56	100	45	58	64
Viable RBCs (% of initial)	100	80	100	79	100	71	83	76

WB, whole blood; *PC*, packed red blood cells.
*Total PV approximately 70 ml.
†0.8% hemolysis.
‡0.5% hemolysis.
Modified from blood and blood components: preparation, storage and shipment. In Walker RH, ed:
Technical manual, ed 10, Arlington, Va, 1990, American Association of Blood Banks.

products. A variety of substances have been used to maintain the viability and function of stored erythrocytes. In general the preservative solutions contain additives that prevent coagulation, support glycolysis, and maintain adenosine triphosphate (ATP) generation. The particular preservative determines the blood product's storage or shelf life, which is defined by the requirement for 70% viability of the transfused RBCs at 24 hours after infusion. Transfused RBCs that circulate beyond 24 hours have a normal survival curve, whereas all nonviable RBCs are quickly removed from circulation.[739] The viability of stored RBCs correlates with ATP levels, which—regardless of the preservative—gradually fall over the shelf life of the product. ATP within erythrocytes is required for maintaining intracellular sodium and potassium concentrations, Hb function, glucose metabolism, and cell membrane deformability and integrity.[697] Reduced red cell ATP concentrations are associated with a loss of membrane lipid, increased cellular rigidity and osmotic fragility, and a spherical RBC configuration.[293]

Blood collected in a citrate-phosphate-dextrose (CPD) solution has an approved shelf life of 21 days. The citrate binds calcium and prevents clotting, the dextrose is an RBC energy source that maintains metabolism and ATP production, and the phosphate serves as a buffer.[540,560] When a larger quantity of dextrose and a small amount of adenine are added to the CPD solution, the shelf life of whole blood and packed RBCs is extended to 35 days.[477] Adenine increases the adenosine diphosphate level, which drives the glycolytic pathways toward ATP production—hence the greater survivability of RBCs preserved in CPD adenine-1 (CPDA-1). The shelf life

of packed RBCs can be extended to 42 days by adding a second preservative solution to one of the satellite bags.[740] Additive solution formula one (AS-1 or Adsol) contains sterile water, 900 mg of sodium chloride, 750 mg of mannitol, and both adenine and dextrose in quantities greater than those contained in the CPDA-1 solution.[310,680] The mannitol stabilizes the erythrocyte cell membrane,[310] which is important because much of the storage-induced lesion is due to loss of membrane surface area and flexibility.[781,782] This membrane damage appears to correlate with declining RBC and ATP concentrations. Nutricel or AS-3 preservative contains an even larger amount of adenine compared with the CPDA-1 and AS-1 solutions.[661] In addition, the composition of the anticoagulant and buffer in AS-3 are slightly different than those contained in other preservative solutions.

Regardless of which preservative or combination of preservatives are used, the RBC levels of 2,3-DPG rapidly and progressively decrease during storage.[476,477] Less than 10% of the normal quantity of 2,3-DPG is present after 2 weeks of RBC storage[55] (Table 46-33). The fall in the pH level during blood storage enhances the activity of 2,3-DPG phosphatase, which is responsible for the breakdown of 2,3-DPG within RBCs.[148] The reduced 2,3-DPG levels correlate with a lower than normal P_{50} level and an increased affinity of Hb for oxygen.[272,681] It is conceivable that tissue oxygen availability may remain limited despite the increment in RBC mass after a transfusion of 2,3-DPG depleted blood.[683,763] The importance of adequate red cell 2,3-DPG in transfused blood has been demonstrated in animal studies.[130,273,471,743,786] Human investigations, on the other hand, have not consistently demonstrated a relationship between physiologic performance and 2,3-DPG levels.* It is possible that only certain types of patients (e.g., those with a fixed cardiac output and moderate to severe perioperative stress) are at risk for impaired tissue oxygenation after the infusion of stored blood. At present, the clinical significance of transfusing 2,3-DPG depleted blood remains unclear. In otherwise healthy patients, it may require 24 to 48 hours to restore near-normal 2,3-DPG concentrations within the circulating transfused RBCs.[741] In critically ill patients, however, the time needed to achieve this restoration may be considerably extended.[742] During storage the levels of 2,3-DPG decrease at a slightly greater rate in AS-1 and AS-3 RBCs, compared with erythrocytes maintained in CPD or CPDA-1 solutions. Nevertheless, red cell ATP is better maintained in the preservatives with a higher adenine content, which permits a more rapid regeneration of 2,3-DPG after transfusion.

The metabolism of glucose by RBCs produces lactic acid, pyruvic acid, and carbon dioxide. No matter which preservative is used, these substances accumulate during RBC storage and generate a progressive pH decrement. The ensuing acidosis impairs the function of various enzyme systems, which—in turn—reduces cellular viability. To slow the rate of RBC metabolism and impede the accumulation of both volatile and fixed acids, blood is normally stored at 4° C (range, 1° C to 6° C). This cold storage results in greater posttransfusion RBC survival.[336]

Whole Blood

A unit of whole blood (WB) generally contains 450 ml ($\pm 10\%$) of blood and about 60 ml of preservative. The end product consists of RBCs, plasma, and nonviable granulocytes and platelets. The HCT concentration of WB is usually in the range of 35% to 45% but will vary in accordance with the donor's Hb concentration. Consequently, there may be significant variation in the total quantity of Hb contained within different units of WB, depending on the volume of the unit and the donor's HCT concentration.[792] The fluid portion of a WB unit may vary in size from roughly 180 to 300 ml. This fluid is predominately plasma but also includes a small amount of preservative. WB is stored in either CPD or CPDA-1, and thus the shelf life is either 21 or 35 days, respectively. The additive solutions (i.e., AS-1 and AS-3) are not used for preserving WB.[69]

Because of the widespread acceptance of component therapy, the use of WB has greatly diminished over the past 2 decades. Except for trauma centers,

most hospital blood banks stock only a minimal supply of WB. In fact, many hospitals do not routinely store WB because of its infrequent use and the immediate availability of acceptable therapeutic options.

The use of WB is essentially limited to situations in which there is an acute, severe, and combined deficit of both oxygen-carrying capacity (i.e., RBC mass) and PV. Thus stored WB is useful for treating hemorrhagic shock where it may simplify and expedite fluid resuscitation. In the past, when the possibility of a massive transfusion existed, "fresh" WB was frequently requested. WB stored for 72 hours contains only a relatively small quantity of viable platelets (i.e., at most, 20% of the original platelet mass).[368] However, as much as 45% of the stored platelets may remain viable for up to 24 hours. The use of "fresh" WB (i.e., less than 24 hours of storage) may keep the recipient's platelet count above 90,000/mm³ until the total transfusion exceeds 1.5 blood volumes.[458] However, with the advent of component therapy, the availability of WB has been dramatically reduced. It is therefore unrealistic to expect the procurement of "fresh" WB in large quantities. If the infusion of WB is deemed necessary, platelet concentrates should be provided as indicated by the patient's clinical condition and laboratory data (e.g., quantitative and qualitative platelet assessments).

WB is contraindicated for the treatment of chronic anemias, because the intravascular fluid volume is almost always normal in these conditions and the risk of fluid overload is excessive. The use of WB as a pure volume expander is also an unacceptable practice, because safer alternative agents are readily available. Furthermore, the labile clotting factors (i.e., V and VIII) progressively diminish in concentration during storage. Therefore WB is seldom used to replace deficient procoagulants, because FFP, cryoprecipitate, or specific factor concentrates are generally more effective.

Packed Red Blood Cells

Packed red blood cells (PRBCs), also referred to as packed cells or red cell concentrates, are separated from the plasma portion of WB within 6 hours of collection by either centrifugation or sedimentation. The plasma is then transferred to a satellite collection bag, with the red cell component remaining in the primary collection bag that contains CPDA-1 as a preservative. Enough plasma is removed to raise the HCT concentration of the PRBCs as high as 70% to 80%. If the erythrocytes are to be stored in AS-1, the primary collection bag will contain CPD preservatives. After the plasma is expressed, the red cell concentrate will be transferred to a satellite bag containing the AS-1 solution (see Fig. 46-33). The HCT concentration of AS-1 PRBCs ranges from 50%

---

to 60%. The volume of a unit of PRBCs (250 to 350 ml) is dependent on the donor's Hb concentration and the preservative solution; the AS-1 red cell product contains 50 to 60 ml more preservative volume than PRBCs collected in CPDA-1.

The use of CPDA-1 PRBCs requires that at least 100 ml of physiologic saline be added per unit to improve flow and minimize hemolysis.[104] The reconstitution of PRBCs with 5% dextrose in 0.45% sodium chloride, 5% dextrose in 0.9% sodium chloride, and Normosol-R (pH 7.4) will not cause hemolysis,[459] but the exposure of RBCs to dextrose may cause clumping. The use of lactated Ringer's solution will cause clotting due to the presence of calcium[600] and hypotonic solutions (e.g., 5% dextrose in water, 5% dextrose in 0.2% sodium chloride, PPF) will produce an osmotic hemolysis.[79,150] This pre-infusion dilution is unnecessary with AS-1 packed cells, because the viscosity is about half of that measured in the CPDA-1 product,[310] and the infusion flow rate for AS-1 erythrocytes is essentially equivalent to the flow rate for WB.[539]

All PRBC preparations contain some amount of plasma—usually between 40 and 100 ml. Therefore hemolytic reactions, IgA-mediated anaphylactic reactions, or leukocyte antigen–mediated allergic reactions may occur with the infusion of red cell concentrates. In addition, there are no data to support the contention that the smaller volume of transfused plasma (compared with WB) is associated with a reduced risk of posttransfusion hepatitis.[115] One further similarity between PRBCs and WB is that there are few or no viable platelets or granulocytes remaining in the product after 24 to 48 hours of storage irrespective of the particular preservative solution.

The transfusion of PRBCs is indicated for the relatively rapid correction of a clinically significant impairment in oxygen-carrying capacity. A unit of packed cells contains the same RBC mass as the originally donated unit of WB. Red cell concentrates are generally used to replace blood losses that are less than 30% to 50% of the total blood volume. These preparations are especially useful when RBC supplementation is required in patients who are prone to develop fluid overload (e.g., individuals with significant renal or myocardial dysfunction).

Miscellaneous Red Cell Preparations

Leukocytes and platelets contained within units of blood can produce both allergic and febrile, nonhemolytic transfusion reactions. These reactions are more likely to occur in multiparous women and multiply transfused patients, because these individuals frequently develop antibodies to leukocyte and/or platelet antigens.[729] In many cases, leukoagglutinins in the recipient cause immune damage to donor white cells (regardless of their viability), which may be associated with complement activation.[69] Symptoms are usually mild and include chills, fever, headache, malaise, nausea, and vomiting, but on occasion bronchospasm, hypotension, and even ARDS may develop.[109,176] Patients with severe or repeated reactions often do better when transfused with leukocyte-poor RBCs,[532] because the clinical reaction appears dependant on the number of white cells administered.[69] Leukocyte-poor RBCs are produced from red cell concentrates that have undergone a method of leukocyte removal (e.g., filtration, sedimentation, centrifugation, or washing).[69] The newer filtration techniques are highly efficient and remove more than 99% of the leukocytes.[449] Centrifugation of stored blood and removal of the buffy coat is the least efficient process for eliminating white cells but, until recently,[662] was the only method that maintained a closed system and allowed prolonged storage of the final product. The leukocyte-poor RBC preparation must retain at least 80% of the RBCs from the original blood product.

The white cell content of washed RBCs is similar to that of leukocyte-poor PRBCs, but in addition, the majority of plasma (greater than 99%) is eliminated. The washing process removes most of the plasma proteins, microaggregates, platelets, and leukocytes.[69,251] The washed RBC preparation eliminates many of the potential disadvantages of the plasma fraction contained in WB and PRBCs and probably decreases the degree of immunization against non–red cell antigens. The use of washed RBCs reduces the incidence of febrile, urticarial, and certain types of anaphylactic reactions. Washed RBCs may be beneficial in IgA-deficient patients who can have anaphylactic reactions when transfused with blood or blood components containing IgA. The washing process causes a loss of some red cells but does not affect the survival of those cells which are eventually transfused. Washed RBCs are prepared in an open system (i.e., the collection system's hermetic seal is broken; see Fig. 46-32) and therefore must be administered within 6 hours if stored at 20° to 24° C or 24 hours if stored at 1° to 6° C.

Frozen or deglycerolized RBCs retain the characteristics of the cells at the time of freezing. Thus freezing is the ideal form of storage for rare types of blood and for the long-term preservation of blood intended for autologous transfusion. The standards of the American Association of Blood Banks permit storage for up to 7 years, although RBCs properly frozen for as long as 21 years have demonstrated no evidence of deterioration. Glycerol is the most commonly used cryoprotective agent, because it offers both extracellular and intracellular protective effects by removing water from red cells and limiting red cell dehydration, respectively.[443,449] Depending on the concentration of glycerol, the rapidity of freezing, and the method of storage, the glycerolized RBCs are maintained at approximately $-80°$ C or $-150°$ C. Before transfusion, frozen RBCs must be thawed and washed to prevent glycerol-induced, in vivo hemolysis. The repetitive washing process (i.e., deglycerolization) minimizes the risk of antigenic immune reactions because of the near total removal of plasma, leukocytes, platelets, and microaggregate debris. The deglycerolized RBCs are concentrated by centrifugation to a HCT concentration of 90% and resuspended in physiologic saline at a HCT concentration of 70%.[443] The final product contains 80% of the originally donated red cell mass,[715] which must be infused within 24 hours of deglycerolization.

The in vivo survival and oxygen-carrying capacity of frozen RBCs are a function of the duration of erythrocyte storage between the time of donation and that of freezing.[335] Because most frozen RBCs are processed shortly after collection or have undergone rejuvenation,[744] the erythrocyte 2,3-DPG and ATP levels are normal and the ability of Hb to transport and release oxygen is similar to that observed with fresh WB.

The major disadvantage of frozen RBCs is the considerable increase in cost per unit of blood. In addition, the glycerolization, freezing, and deglycerolization processes do not totally remove the risk of viral disease transmission.[302] Furthermore, viable lymphocytes have been demonstrated after deglycerolization.[386] Thus, in the setting of severe immune compromise, the use of frozen RBCs does not eliminate the risk of a graft-vs.-host reaction.[69]

Indications for Transfusion

Historically, blood transfusions have been used to maintain a perioperative Hb concentration of 10 g/dl or a HCT concentration of 30%.[246,378,698,808] Presumably, the belief was that these minimal values ensured adequate oxygen availability to all vital structures, especially the heart, where the arteriovenous oxygen content difference within the coronary circulation of a resting adult is 12 vol %.[461] However, this rather limited viewpoint overlooks the many physiologic adjustments occurring with an acute stress (i.e., surgery, trauma, and so on) that serve to maintain adequate tissue $\dot{D}o_2$ in spite of a diminished oxygen content and increased $\dot{V}o_2$ level. Thus it seems that this rather arbitrary guideline for transfusion therapy was based more on tradition and personal bias than on scientific data. In patients undergoing surgery and the administration of an anesthetic, all attempts to define either a minimally acceptable or optimal level of Hb have failed to identify a single value or range of values

that clearly minimize perioperative morbidity and mortality rates.[12,111] Both past[263,572] and recent[695] studies have failed to demonstrate that the presence of anemia (independent of cause and coexisting conditions) confers an increased risk of complications during or after surgery. Patients with chronic renal failure have routinely undergone surgery and the administration of an anesthetic uneventfully with Hb levels of 5 to 8 g/dl.[486,604,745] Patients refusing transfusion because of religious beliefs have survived perioperative isovolemic hemodilution with HCT levels as low as 6% to 7%.[112,407,501,687] In addition, studies in healthy animals have revealed that the lower limit of anemia compatible with life appears to be a HCT concentration of approximately 6% to 8%,[619] and in situations where an acute hemorrhage (simulating an intraoperative blood loss) is superimposed on an isovolemic anemia, prehemorrhage HCT concentrations as low as 23% does not enhance mortality.[426] Thus there is evidence that suggests that surgical and anesthetic procedures can be safely performed on normovolemic patients with HCT (or Hb) levels considerably less than the traditional minimal requirement.

As indicated in the previous section, the heart is the vital organ most at risk for anemic hypoxia when the RBC mass is diminished. The limit of cardiac compensation in healthy but anemic primates appears to correlate with a HCT concentration of 10%.[774,775] In dogs, coronary blood flow progressively increases as the HCT concentration undergoes isovolemic reduction to a level of 10%.[343] Exercise-induced stress in animals with HCT concentrations of 18% appears to neither alter the distribution of myocardial blood flow nor induce ischemia.[2] Cardiac work and myocardial oxygen consumption remain stable as the HCT concentration is reduced to levels of 10% to 20%.[235,343,472] Therefore isovolemic reductions in the HCT concentration are associated with increases in the myocardial oxygen extraction ratio until a critical point is reached. Animal studies indicate that this critical level corresponds to a HCT concentration in the range of 10% to 20%.[343,774] In addition, the myocardial oxygen requirement is not related to stroke volume (the major determinant of cardiac output in severe anemia) but rather is related to heart rate and the ventricular pressure generated during systole.[472,596]

The available data suggest that normal cardiac function persists over a wide range of Hb or HCT levels, so long as isovolemic conditions are maintained. The implication is that patients who are free of heart disease and have an adequate circulating fluid volume may effectively compensate for HCT reductions as low as 20%. However, patients with fixed coronary stenoses or myocardial dysfunction may require a higher level of HCT to prevent ischemia.[236,587] In otherwise healthy but anemic dogs (i.e., HCT concentration of 20%), coronary flow reserve is significantly compromised after a transient arterial occlusion,[235] and HCT concentrations of 15% may cause a redistribution of coronary blood flow that results in subendocardial ischemia.[82] Although there is a paucity of experimental data, it seems logical that patients with significant heart disease have a diminished cardiac reserve, greater myocardial vulnerability, and an enhanced perioperative risk when compared with healthy patients with a similar degree of anemia. Thus it is not unreasonable to assume that such patients would benefit from a somewhat greater HCT concentration in the perioperative period.

At the other end of the perioperative Hb/HCT spectrum, studies in canine[139,319,578] and human[142,392,712] subjects indicate that optimal oxygen transport may occur with a HCT concentration between 30% and 40%. However, systemic oxygen transport values may not accurately reflect oxygenation in specific tissue beds, because changes in regional blood flow and oxygen extraction, viscosity, and P_{50} level are all influential but difficult to assess in a clinical setting.

It is clear that there are no objective and definitive criteria, based on scientific data, that can be used to guide transfusion therapy. Adults, children, and infants are usually administered RBCs in an effort to maintain a level of Hb or HCT that has been deemed most desirable for the patient's clinical status. However, this clinical approach is rather imprecise, and consequently, more physiologic measures of tissue oxygenation have been suggested.[256,334] It has been demonstrated that the traditionally monitored variables of heart rate, mean arterial pressure, and CVP may not adequately predict effective and successful resuscitation in hypovolemic patients; these variables are, at best, a crude reflection of cellular injury.[643,645,646,649,650] The monitoring of perfusion-related variables may be more efficacious for directing therapeutic interventions in certain types of hypovolemic patients (e.g., surgical patients with multiple trauma, burns, septic or hemorrhagic shock). The perfusion-related variables include cardiac output, arterial lactate concentrations, arterial base excess, mixed venous pH and Po_2 levels, arteriovenous oxygen content difference, $\dot{V}o_2$ level, $\dot{D}o_2$, and whole body oxygen debt. Although the interaction of the variables is complex,[722] sequential patterns of $\dot{D}o_2$, $\dot{V}o_2$ level, and oxygen debt may be critically important because these variables appear to most consistently predict clinical outcome and most accurately reflect the status of tissue perfusion and oxygenation.[643] Moreover, changes in these key variables that result from therapy (e.g., blood transfusion) provide an immediate and objective measure of the efficacy of

the particular intervention (see Fig. 46-33). Recent studies continue to demonstrate the utility of monitoring various combinations of these indices of tissue perfusion in both animal models[179,301] and patients.[116,168,644]

It is not uncommon for a critically ill, anemic, surgical patient to have a peripheral oxygen deficit, with both oxygen extraction and use unable to match the metabolic requirement. This problem is often evidenced by a diminished $\dot{V}o_2$ level, increased oxygen debt, and lactic acidosis. The abnormally low $\dot{V}o_2$ level is frequently flow dependent and will increase as $\dot{D}o_2$ is augmented.[694] By producing an increase in arterial oxygen content, transfusion therapy should theoretically be the most effective means of maximizing $\dot{D}o_2$ and thus improving the $\dot{V}o_2$ level.[93,272,681] In this subgroup of surgical patients, the combined use of Hb or HCT levels, filling pressures (i.e., CVP, PAOP), and perfusion-related variables should provide an objective indication of the need for transfusion therapy.

Pulmonary artery catheterization has conventionally been used as a diagnostic tool for evaluating myocardial performance in relation to left ventricular preload. The role of this monitoring modality has now expanded to include the following: (1) identification of deficient peripheral tissue perfusion, (2) evaluation of the efficacy of different therapeutic maneuvers to improve tissue perfusion, and (3) titration of an appropriate therapy to achieve optimal physiologic goals.[641] The provision of blood might best be directed by the use of perfusion-related variables,[105,265,363] but the placement of a pulmonary artery catheter in all patients who might require a blood transfusion is both impractical and unwarranted. Even when critically ill patients undergo invasive monitoring, there is evidence that suggests that perfusion-related variables are rarely used when deciding whether a transfusion is indicated.[737]

For many years, blood was considered innocuous, inexpensive, and readily available. This viewpoint certainly influenced past transfusion practices, but now—because of the overwhelming fear of transfusion-transmitted disease—there is a much more conservative attitude toward the use of blood and blood products. Physicians, hospitals, and regulatory agencies are scrutinizing the indications for transfusion. It is difficult to devise generic guidelines for the administration of blood, because of the diversity of patients and clinical situations. Young healthy patients may easily compensate for an acute or chronic anemia of substantial magnitude, but elderly patients may develop serious complications at a similar level of Hb or HCT. Irrespective of the ease of measurement, sole reliance on Hb and HCT values as a method of directing transfusion practices ignores the complex interaction between $\dot{D}o_2$ and the $\dot{V}o_2$ level. Nevertheless, because blood is often administered inappropriately and this therapy is frequently initiated as the result of a specific Hb or HCT level, the Food and Drug Administration has issued stringent guidelines for the use of RBC preparations.[738] This FDA bulletin states that adequate oxygen-carrying capacity can be achieved with a Hb concentration of 7 g/dl (and occasionally lower), as long as the patient's intravascular volume is sufficient to allow adequate tissue perfusion. It is implied that the transfusion trigger point should generally be 7 g/dl; however, certain conditions (e.g., coronary atherosclerotic heart disease) may warrant a greater Hb concentration.

On the other hand, a National Institutes of Health Consensus Conference does not support the use of a single criterion (e.g., a Hb concentration of less than 10 g/dl) as an indication for transfusion.[831] This NIH statement, however, does point out that otherwise healthy patients with a Hb concentration equal to—or greater than—10 g/dl rarely require perioperative transfusion, whereas patients with an acute blood loss resulting in a Hb concentration of less than 7 g/dl will frequently require RBC supplementation. In addition, it is noted that some patients with chronic anemia (e.g., those with chronic renal failure) may tolerate Hb values of less than 7 g/dl. The ASA essentially conforms with the NIH statement and notes that many patients can safely undergo surgery and the administration of an anesthesic with Hb levels of 7 g/dl or less as long as cardiac output, normovolemia, and an appropriate inspired oxygen concentration are maintained.[560]

It should be apparent that there is no single Hb or HCT value that will guarantee a safe level of tissue oxygenation in all surgical patients and that no single measure can replace good clinical judgement as the basis for decisions about perioperative transfusion. The transfusion of RBCs should be limited to situations where there is a need to maintain or enhance the oxygen-carrying capacity of blood.[560] Volume deficits associated with an adequate blood oxygen content should be replaced with crystalloid solutions using colloidal supplementation when indicated. The importance of an adequate asanguineous fluid resuscitation cannot be overemphasized, because RBC transfusions in euvolemic patients with moderate to severe anemia may not improve tissue oxygen metabolism.[168]

The decision to transfuse blood should be guided by a careful clinical assessment and aided by laboratory data (e.g., Hb or HCT values) in addition to filling pressures and perfusion-related variables (when indicated by the patient's condition). Furthermore, additional factors must be considered, including the duration of the anemia, the extent of the surgical procedure, the anticipated blood loss, and the presence of coexisting conditions such as myocardial ischemia, pulmonary dysfunction, or cerebrovascular disease. One must remember that there is no evidence that mild to moderate anemia, in and of itself, contributes to perioperative morbidity. Before the administration of blood, the benefit of improved tissue oxygenation must always be weighed against the risk of both long-term and short-term adverse consequences.

The transfusion of homologous blood carries a well-documented risk of both immune changes and infection. Hepatitis viruses are the most frequently transmitted infectious agents, with an incidence of approximately 1:100 to 1:300 per unit.[738,831] The risk of human immunodeficiency virus transmission has been variously estimated at 1:40,000 to 1:1,000,000.[11,74,757,831] The incidence of mild leukocyte-induced or platelet-induced immune reactions has been estimated at 1:100, whereas hemolytic transfusion reactions occur at a frequency of 1:6000.[729,831] The severity of this latter reaction is generally proportional to the amount of incompatible blood transfused, the type of incompatibility, and the length of time between transfusion and the initiation of treatment.[560]

Alternatives to Homologous Blood Transfusion

One alternative to homologous blood transfusion is the use of autologous blood. The predonation of blood for elective surgical procedures offers several advantages to the patient and the community. Unless the specimen is mishandled, alloimmunization and disease transmission are avoided, and thus autologous blood is usually the safest RBC preparation for any given patient. In addition, the homologous blood supply may not be reduced (depending on the patient's transfusion requirement) and may even be enhanced if the patient does not require perioperative transfusion, because the autologous preparation can enter the general blood pool if both the donor and his/her blood meet all the usual criteria. Although the indications for transfusion may become less stringent when autologous blood is available, the mere presence of this blood is not a mandate for transfusion.[697]

The requirements for autologous donation are less restrictive than those for general blood collection.[99,429] There are no upper and lower age limits; therefore cooperative children may be suitable candidates.[696] The frequency of donation can be no greater than once every 3 days, and blood is generally not collected if either the Hb or HCT concentration falls below 11 g/dl or 34%, respectively.[99] Phlebotomy cannot be performed within 72 hours of the scheduled surgical date, so as to allow restoration of the PV.

Autologous blood may also be salvaged intraoperatively and infused during or after the surgical procedure.[519] The semicontinuous flow, cell-washing centrifuge has reached a stage of development that makes it practical and cost effective to salvage as little as 2 to 3 units of PRBCs.[547] The widespread use of these autotransfusion devices without significant complications has been reported for patients undergoing cardiac, vascular, orthopedic, and liver transplantation procedures. Theoretic contraindications include surgery in the area of malignant tumors and surgery in a possibly contaminated field.[72] The salvaged RBCs undergo a washing cycle (with physiologic saline) to remove fat, bone chips, and/or other particulate matter. A significant amount of platelets and plasma may also be removed such that the patient's coagulation profile must be carefully monitored if large quantities of salvaged blood are reinfused.[518] Standard 170-μm filters should be used to remove microaggregates during the reinfusion process. Without refrigeration the salvaged blood should generally be infused within 4 hours of collection, and when processed and stored at 4° C, this blood is usable for 24 hours.

Acute normovolemic hemodilution can be an important component of a perioperative blood conservation program. The process involves the removal of WB immediately before or just after the induction of anesthesia and simultaneous replacement of the blood volume with an appropriate amount of asanguineous fluid.[346,431] Acute normovolemic hemodilution decreases homologous blood requirements, provides a source of fresh WB for transfusion at the end of surgery, and improves tissue perfusion through beneficial rheological alterations associated with the hemodilution. The blood withdrawn from the patient should be collected in a standard blood bag containing an anticoagulant. The amount of blood to be withdrawn (V) depends on the patient's (adult or child) estimated blood volume (EBV), the initial HCT level (HCT_i), the lowest desired intraoperative HCT level (HCT_D), and the average of these two levels (HCT_{AV}):[267]

$$V = EBV \times \frac{(HCT_i - HCT_D)}{HCT_{AV}}$$

This technique offers the advantage of minimizing the intraoperative reduction in RBC mass, because hemodilution decreases the HCT level of the blood lost during surgery. In addition, this technique is applicable to many surgical procedures and is associated with minimal hemodynamic alterations as long as the patient remains normovolemic.[431,696]

A potential alternative to the transfusion of homologous blood is the use of acellular oxygen-carrying compounds. The perflurocarbon (FC) preparations are derived from hydrocarbons, with fluorine substituted for hydrogen. Pure FCs are synthetic oils that are not miscible with plasma. Consequently, they must be prepared as an emulsion to prevent the formation of gaseous emboli. The FCs are potential oxygen carriers because of their relatively high oxygen solubility as compared with blood or plasma;[334,353] the pure compounds have a solubility coefficient which is 10 to 20 times greater than that of plasma. Unfortunately, when these agents are emulsified, their final concentration (in the infusible product) is substantially reduced, as is the maximal achievable oxygen content.[61] FCs carry oxygen in a physically dissolved form and not chemically combined to Hb. Thus the oxygen content is linearly related to the oxygen tension and the quantity of FC present in the solution (i.e., the flurocrit level). When administered to a patient, the total oxygen content can be considered the sum of three distinct oxygen carriers[255]:

$$[O_2] \text{ total} = [O_2] \text{ RBC} + [O_2] \text{ plasma} + [O_2] \text{ FC}$$

Cellular viability is dependent on total oxygen availability and not the mode of oxygen transport.[258] At an extremely high PO_2 level (i.e., FIO_2 level of 1.0), even plasma can become a significant carrier of oxygen; thus the need for FCs remains unclear.[255]

Fluosol-DA is the commercial FC product most readily available in the United States; however, none of the FC solutions have been licensed for clinical use. In addition to the FC, this 20% preparation contains a nonionic detergent, yolk phospholipids, hetastarch, and a variety of salts.[257] Fluosol-DA offers some value as an oxygen carrier, but there are several drawbacks to its use: (1) a high FIO_2 level is required, (2) the maximal amount that can be administered to a patient (40 ml/kg) limits the flurocrit level to about 5%, (3) when both the flurocrit and FIO_2 levels are maximized, the FC oxygen content in patients may be far less than the 5 vol % achievable in the laboratory, and (4) the Hb concentration must be considerably reduced before there is a "significant" contribution to the total arterial oxygen content.[257] Thus at present the FCs appear to be an inadequate RBC substitute, because they are unnecessary in moderate anemia and ineffective in severe anemia.[623]

Another acellular oxygen-carrying compound undergoing development is stroma-free hemoglobin (SFH). The unmodified Hb solution is prepared by washing and lysing outdated, stored human RBCs. A series of filtration steps removes the RBC membrane debris (i.e., stromata) from the Hb molecules, resulting in a solution of SFH.[61] Because red cell antigens are membrane bound, SFH is universally compatible and can be administered without regard for the recipient's blood type.[165] In addition, SFH is less viscous than blood, contains no microaggregates, can undergo long-term storage, and displays a normal oxygen-carrying capacity. SFH is produced with a Hb concentration of 7 g/dl so as to make the solution isooncotic.[255] One major problem with this agent is the loss of 2,3-DPG that occurs after rupture of the RBC membrane. This loss results in a reduced P_{50} level (12 to 14 mm Hg) as reflected in the oxygen content curve for SFH (Figs. 46-34 and 46-35). However, the addition of pyridoxal-phosphate to the SFH solution results in a preparation with a P_{50} concentration of approximately 20 to 22 mm Hg.[166] Furthermore, if this pyridoxylated SFH is polymerized, the Hb concentration can be increased to 15 g/dl while maintaining the COP of a 7 g/dl solution. Thus this pyridoxylated and polymerized SFH has a higher Hb concentration, a greater P_{50} level, a longer half-life, and an equivalent COP, as compared with the unmodified SFH. The pyridoxylated, polymerized SFH has proven to be an effective oxygen carrier in animals.[622] Also, in both animal studies and a limited clinical trial,[623] there have been no adverse hemostatic, hemodynamic, or nephrogenic effects. Although it has not yet been licensed by the FDA or approved for clinical use, the pyridoxylated, polymerized SFH appears to be the most promising of the acellular oxygen-carrying products. However, further studies will be necessary to determine its most appropriate clinical application(s).

Assessing the Adequacy of Fluid Replacement

It should be evident that there are a multitude of intravenous fluids and supplements available for use during the perioperative period. It should also be apparent that various combinations of these fluids and supplements may be required, depending on the clinical situation. Nevertheless, the uniform objective for administering these agents is to maintain vital organ perfusion and thus function. Unfortunately, there are no practical methods for the rapid and repetitive assessment of perioperative organ perfusion.[642] In addition, most methods for assessing organ function are either indirect (e.g., urine output) or influenced by so many variables that it is often difficult to interpret the significance of the acquired information (e.g., PA catheter data). Therefore, by default, perioperative organ perfusion and function are usually assessed by the use of relatively crude estimates, measures, and/or derivatives of cardiovascular function. Most of these relatively imprecise reflections of vital organ integrity are significantly influenced by anesthetic techniques and occasionally altered by the ambient operating room conditions.

Because perioperative fluid deficits are frequent in occurrence, a great deal of concern is directed toward the volume status of the intravascular compartment. Because of the administration of anesthetic agents, subjective information (as provided by the patient) is usually unavailable or unreliable. Therefore the assessment of volume status is predominantly based on the interpretation of various objective data. The patient's heart rate and systemic arterial blood pressure are the two parameters most often used to evaluate the intravascular volume. Ideally, proper fluid management would maintain these variables within their basal ranges, with hypovolemia producing a sinus tachycardia, a lowered mean arterial pressure, and a narrowed pulse pressure. Hypovolemia may also produce delayed capillary refilling (easily noted on the thenar eminence) and cool, dry, and pale skin. However, sympathetic stimulation and temperature changes unrelated to volume loss may also elicit these findings. Occasionally, invasive monitoring modalities are used to facilitate perioperative management. Mean central venous and pulmonary artery occlusion

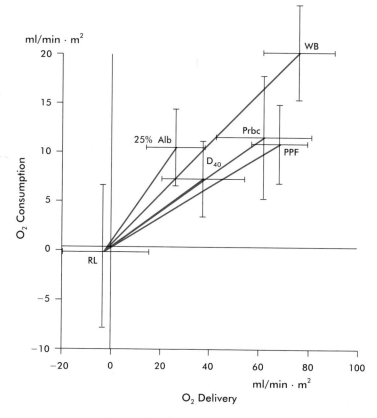

Fig. 46-34. Changes in $\dot{D}O_2$ plotted against their corresponding coresponding changes in $\dot{V}O_2$ after various fluid infusions (n = 400) in postoperative patients (n = 211). The increases in both $\dot{D}O_2$ and $\dot{V}O_2$ are significant following the infusion of 500 ml (1 U) whole blood *(WB)*, 100 ml 25% albumin *(Alb)*, 500 ml (2 U) packed red blood cells *(Prbc)*, 500 ml plasma protein fraction *(PPF)*, and 500 ml 10% dextran-40 *(D₄₀)*. The change in $\dot{D}O_2$ and $\dot{V}O_2$ following the infusion of 1000 ml lactated Ringer's solution *(RL)* is not significant. (From Shoemaker WC, Appel PL, and Kram HB: Oxygen-transport measurements to evaluate tissue perfusion and titrate therapy: dobutamine and dopamine effects, *Crit Care Med* 19:672, 1991.)

pressures reflecting adequate volume replacement are generally specific to the patient and situation; there are numerous factors that may determine the mean filling pressures that correlate with a normal (actual or functional) intravascular volume. In a patient who has no complications, however, a mean end-expiratory CVP and/or PAOP in the high-normal range may be an acceptable reflection of adequate volume replacement. A much less invasive estimate of intravascular volume can be obtained by altering the patient's position. When the patient is in the lithotomy position, a lack of change in the heart rate and blood pressure on placing him/her in the supine position often indicates adequate volume replenishment. In addition, at the end of a surgical procedure, the operating room table can be placed in a mild head-up (i.e., reverse Trendelenburg) position in an attempt to elicit a change in heart rate and blood pressure. Orthostasis of this nature may reflect a previously unrecognized volume deficit, but—on the other hand—a positive response must be cautiously interpreted; anesthetic agents or techniques may impair peripheral sympathetic tone, transiently enlarge the intravascular compartment, and evoke signs or symptoms of hypovolemia that may dissipate when sympathetic tone normalizes. In addition, urinary output is often used to gauge the adequacy of volume replacement. It is generally perceived that urine that appears dilute and is produced at a rate of greater than, or equal to, 0.5 ml/kg/hr reflects normovolemia or hypervolemia. Again, this may or may not be the case, because the quantity of quality of urine can be affected by anesthetic techniques and agents, perioperative medications, intrinsic renal disease, and a number of neurohumoral influences. Therefore determining the adequacy of volume replacement is not a simple task and should not be based on one or two objective parameters. Instead, the assessment of multiple parameters must be integrated to obtain a reasonably accurate estimate of volume status.

Assessing the adequacy of red blood cell replacement is intricately linked to the overall assessment of volume replenishment. Many of the problems inherent to the accurate assessment of asanguineous fluid replacement also apply to red cell transfusions. However, there are certain laboratory measurements that may help in the assessment of the effectiveness of red cell supplementation. An Hb concentration will accurately reflect the red cell mass so long as the ECF volume has been normalized and stabilized. The oxygen transport parameters (e.g., arteriovenous oxygen content difference) may also provide an estimate of the effectiveness of red cell replacement similar to an arterial lactate concentration and pH level.

In addition to these standard perfusion related variables recent evidence suggests that arteriovenous differences in carbon dioxide tension and pH level may be effective adjuncts for gauging the adequacy of volume resuscitation after hemorrhagic shock.[177]

Serial measurements of these parameters are generally more meaningful than is an isolated value, but are nonetheless limited in their usefulness because so many factors can have an impact on these measured or calculated values. Continuous mixed venous oximetry suffers from the same limitations but may be helpful when combined with other measures of tissue oxygen supply and demand.

Concentration abnormalities are water disturbances that are associated with changes in the serum sodium concentration. The patient's volume status and total body sodium content may not necessarily be reflected by the measured serum sodium concentration. On the other hand, a pure water loss or gain with a normal total body sodium content is generally associated with changes in the serum sodium and chloride concentrations, which are directly proportional in nature. Therefore, during an assessment of the effectiveness of various therapeutic interventions, the patient's volume status must be accurately defined and the laboratory data (e.g., both serum and urine electrolytes and osmolality concentrations, fractional excretion of sodium) should be interpreted in the context of the volume status.

Electrolyte disturbances or abnormalities of composition are generally identified and defined by the serum concentration of the particular ion. As previously discussed, the serum concentration of certain electrolytes may not necessarily reflect the total body ionic stores. However, there is no clinical method or means for assessing these body stores. Therefore, despite their shortcomings, the serum concentrations are commonly used to evaluate the effectiveness of

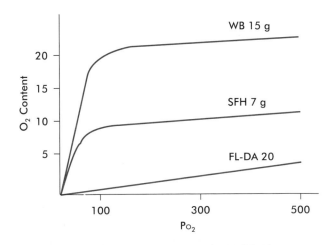

Fig. 46-35. Oxygen content curves for 15 g/dl of hemoglobin in whole blood *(WB)*, 7 g/dl of hemoglobin in a stroma-free hemoglobin solution *(SFH)*, and 20% flurosol-DA *(FL-DA 20)*. (From Gould SA, Moss GS, Rosen AL et al: Red cell substitutes. In Civetta JM, Taylor RW, and Kirby RR, eds: *Critical care,* Philadelphia, 1989, JB Lippincott.)

therapy. Depending on the severity of the disturbance, these electrolyte concentrations may be used in conjunction with ECG monitoring and repeated physical examinations (e.g., quality of deep tendon reflexes, muscle tone, muscle strength, and so on) to assess patient improvement.

It should be clear that assessing the adequacy of parenteral fluid therapy is, on occasion, a more difficult task than defining the initial perturbation. Volume depletion is probably the single most common perioperative disturbance; however, accurately defining the ECF volume status during or after the planned fluid resuscitation can be extremely difficult. The anesthesiologist must become the consummate clinician: he/she must evaluate multiple parameters, account for the effects of anesthetic agents and techniques, assimilate a wealth of objective data, and finally, determine the actual or functional state of the fluid compartments. Furthermore, this process must be repeated frequently and the therapeutic interventions adjusted in accordance with the derived conclusions. The ability to accurately assess the adequacy (or inadequacy) of perioperative fluid replacement is a clinical skill that must be honed through constant repetition.

SUMMARY

This chapter reviews the physiologic basis of parenteral fluid therapy, as well as the relevant aspects of patient management. A variety of crystalloids, colloids, electrolytes, and red cell preparations are currently available. To consistently provide high-quality anesthetic care, the practicing anesthesiologist must be familiar with this wealth of therapeutic options. The indications for the use of certain agents is clear-cut and well defined. For other agents, a theoretic benefit may exist but their clinical use is controversial and experimental. The cornerstone of fluid management is a careful, accurate, and ongoing assessment of the patient's status in terms of volume, concentration, and composition. This assessment should then be used to appropriately modify the initial plan for fluid management. However, it is extremely important that the anesthesiologist not limit his/her focus solely on the intraoperative phase of fluid replacement. Parenteral fluid therapy immediately before and after surgery is also crucial to patient outcome and should be incorporated into an appropriate *perioperative* fluid plan.

Certain facets of fluid therapy are applicable to all surgical patients. As a generalization, free water is necessary to replace both insensible losses and the water consumption resulting from energy metabolism. The administration of water is essential to prevent concentration abnormalities and intracellular dehydration. Electrolytes are needed to avoid pH, osmolality, and membrane depolarization disturbances. Protein may be required to prevent a decrease in COP and the development of interstitial edema. An infusion of red blood cells may be necessary to sustain an adequate level of tissue oxygen delivery. Isotonic solutions are indicated for replacing pure volume deficits, which are the most frequent cause of hypovolemia. In practice, a balanced salt solution containing both free water and electrolytes is often the predominant perioperative fluid administered. This solution can then be supplemented with red blood cells, colloid solutions, and/or additional electrolytes, as needed. The provision of these fluids and supplements should be based on the specific needs of each individual patient; the formulas and equations associated with fluid management are merely guidelines that often require considerable adjustment and "fine-tuning" in clinical situations.

REFERENCES

1. Aasheim GM: Hyponatremia during transurethral surgery. *Can Anaesth Soc J* 20:274, 1973.
2. Abendschein DR, Fewell JE, Carlson CJ et al: Myocardial blood flow during acute isovolemic anemia and treadmill exercise in dogs, *J Appl Physiol* 53:203, 1982.
3. Aberg B, Bloom EL, and Hansson E: Gastrointestinal excretion of dextran ^{14}C, *Acta Physiol Scand* 52:188, 1961.
4. Abouna B, Veazey PR, and Terry DM: IV infusion of hydrochloric acid for therapy of severe metabolic alkalosis, *Surgery* 75:194, 1974.
5. Adamson J, Hillman RS: Blood volume and plasma protein replacement following acute blood loss in normal man, *JAMA* 205:609, 1968.

6. Adrogue HJ, Madios NE: Changes in plasma potassium concentrations during acid-base disturbances, *Am J Med* 71:456, 1981.
7. Agus ZS, Goldberg M: Role of antidiuretic hormone in the abnormal water diuresis of anterior hypopituitarism in man, *J Clin Invest* 50:1478, 1971.
8. Agus ZS, Goldfarb S: Clinical disorders of calcium and phosphate, *Med Clin North Am* 65:385, 1981.
9. Al-Dahhan J, Haycock GB, Chantler C et al: Sodium homeostasis in term and preterm neonates: renal aspects, *Arch Dis Child* 58:335, 1983.
10. Al-Dahhan J, Haycock GB, Nichol B et al: Sodium homeostasis in term and preterm neonates: effect of salt supplementation, *Arch Dis Child* 59:945, 1984.

11. Aledort LM: Risks associated with homologous blood transfusion, *J Cardiothor Anesth* 2(suppl 1):2, 1988.
12. Allen JB, Allen FB: The minimum acceptable level of hemoglobin, *Int Anesthesiol Clin* 20(4):1, 1982.
13. Alving BM, Hohima Y, Pisano JJ et al: Hypotension associated with prekallikrein activator (Hageman-factor fragments) in plasma protein fraction, *N Engl J Med* 299:66, 1978.
14. Andreoli TE: Disorders of fluid volume, electrolytes, and acid-base balance. In Wyngaarden JB, Smith LH, eds: *Cecil textbook of medicine*, ed 18, Philadelphia, 1988, WB Saunders.
15. Androgue HF, Madias NE: Changes in plasma potassium concentration during

acute acid-base disturbances, *Am J Med* 71:456, 1981.

16. Arieff AI: Hyponatremia, convulsions, respiratory arrest and permanent brain damage after elective surgery in healthy women, *N Engl J Med* 314:1529, 1986.

17. Arieff AI: Treatment of symptomatic hyponatremia: neither haste nor waste, *Crit Care Med* 19:748, 1991 (editorial).

18. Arieff AI, Carroll HJ: Nonketotic hyperosmolar coma with hyperglycemia: clinical features, pathophysiology, renal function, acid-base balance, plasma-cerebrospinal fluid equilibria, and the effects of therapy in 37 cases, *Medicine* 51:73, 1972.

19. Arieff AI, Guisado R: Effects on the central nervous system of hypernatremic and hyponatremic states, *Kidney Int* 10:104, 1975.

20. Arieff AI, Guisado R: Effects on the CNS of hypernatremic and hyponatremic states, *Kidney Int* 10:104, 1976.

21. Arieff AI, Leach W, Park W et al: Systemic effects of $NaHCO_3$ in experimental lactic acidosis in dogs, *Am J Physiol* 242(F):586, 1982.

22. Arieff AI, Leach F, and Massry SG: Neurologic manifestations and morbidity of hyponatremia: correlation with brain water and electrolytes, *Medicine* 55:121, 1976.

23. Arroyo V, Bosch J, Gaya-Beltran D et al: Plasma renin activity and urinary sodium excretion as prognostic indicators in nonazotemic cirrhosis with ascites, *Ann Intern Med* 94:198, 1981.

24. Arturson G, Granath K, Thoren L et al: The renal excretion of low molecular weight dextran, *Acta Chir Scand* 127:543, 1964.

25. Arturson G, Wallenius G: The renal clearance of dextran of different molecular sizes in normal humans, *Scand J Clin Lab Invest* 16:81, 1964.

26. Assal J, Aoki TT, Manzano FM et al: Metabolic effects of sodium bicarbonate in management of diabetic ketoacidosis, *Diabetes* 23:405, 1974.

27. Auler JOC, Pereira MHC, Gomide Amaral RV et al: Hemodynamic effects of hypertonic sodium chloride during surgical treatment of aortic aneurysms, *Surgery* 101:594, 1987.

28. Aviram A, Pfau A, Czaczkes JW et al: Hyperosmolality with hyponatremia, caused by inappropriate administration of mannitol, *Am J Med* 42:648, 1967.

29. Ayus JC, Krothapalli RK, and Arieff AI: Changing concepts in treatment of severe symptomatic hyponatremia, *Am J Med* 78:897, 1985.

30. Ayus JC, Krothapalli RK, and Arieff AI: Treatment of symptomatic hyponatremia and its relation to brain damage. A prospective study, *N Engl J Med* 317:1190, 1987.

31. Ayus JC, Olivero JJ, and Frommer JP: Rapid correction of severe hyponatremia with intravenous hypertonic saline solution, *Am J Med* 72:43, 1982.

32. Badola RP, Chatterji S, Pandey K et al: Effects of calcium on neuromuscular block by suxamethonium in dogs, *Br J Anaesth* 43:1027, 1971.

33. Baker RJ, St Ville JM, Suzuki F et al: Evaluation of red cell equilibration in hemorrhagic shock, *Arch Surg* 90:538, 1965.

34. Bali IM, Dundee JW, and Doggart JR: The source of increased potassium following succinylcholine, *Anesth Analg* 54:680, 1975.

35. Bartter FC, Schwartz WB: The syndrome of inappropriate secretion of antidiuretic hormone, *Am J Med* 42:790, 1967.

36. Bastl CP, Sebastian A: Adrenal hormones. In Maxwell MH, Kleeman CR, and Narins RG, eds: *Clinical disorders of fluid and electrolyte metabolism,* ed 4, New York, 1987, McGraw-Hill.

37. Beck LH: Edema states and the use of diuretics, *Med Clin North Am* 65:291, 1981.

38. Behnke AR: Physiological studies pertaining to deep sea diving and aviation, especially in relation to the fat content and composition of the body, *Harvey Lect* 37:198, 1941-1942.

39. Belcher T, Lennox SC: Avoidance of blood transfusion in coronary artery surgery. A trial of hydroxyethyl starch, *Ann Thorac Surg* 36:365, 1985.

40. Bellingham AJ: The red cell in adaption to anaemic hypoxia, *Clin Haematol* 3:577, 1974.

41. Bellingham AJ, Delter JC, and Lanfant C: Regulatory mechanisms of hemoglobin oxygen affinity in acidosis and alkalosis, *J Clin Invest* 50:700, 1971.

42. Benabe JE, Martinez-Maldonado M et al: Hypercalcemic nephropathy, *Arch Int Med* 138:177, 1978.

43. Benabe JE, Martinez-Maldonado M: Disorders of calcium metabolism. In Maxwell MH, Kleeman CR, and Narins RG eds: *Clinical disorders of fluid and electrolyte metabolism,* ed 4, New York, 1987, McGraw-Hill.

44. Benumof JL: Special physiology of the lateral decubitus position, the open chest, and one-lung ventilation. In *Anesthesia for thoracic surgery,* Philadelphia, 1987, WB Saunders.

45. Benumof JL: The respiratory physiology and respiratory function during anesthesia. In Miller RD, ed: *Anesthesia,* ed 3, New York, 1990, Churchill-Livingstone.

46. Benumof JL, Mathers JM, and Wahrenbrock EA: Cyclic hypoxic pulmonary vasoconstriction induced by concomitant carbon dioxide changes, *J Appl Physiol* 41:466, 1976.

47. Berger JJ: Transurethral resection of the prostate, *Cumul Rev Clin Anesth* 1:162, 1981.

48. Bergstrom J: Muscle electrolytes in man, *Scand J Clin Lab Invest* 14(suppl):68, 1962.

49. Bergstrom WH, Wallace WM: Bone as the sodium and potassium reservoir, *J Clin Invest* 33:867, 1954.

50. Berl T, Anderson RJ, McDonald KM et al: Clinical disorders of water metabolism, *Kidney Int* 10:117, 1976.

51. Berl T, Schrier RW: Water metabolism in the hypoosmolar syndromes. In Brenner BM, Stein JH, eds: *Sodium and water homeostasis,* New York, 1978, Churchill-Livingstone.

52. Berry A: Respiratory support and renal function, *Anesthesiology* 55:655, 1981.

53. Berson SA, Yalow RS, Schreiber SS et al: Tracer experiments with ^{131}I-labeled human serum albumin: distribution and degradation studies, *J Clin Invest* 32:746, 1953.

54. Beutler E: Energy metabolism and maintenance of erythrocytes. In Williams WJ, Beutler E, Erslev AL et al, eds: *Hematology,* ed 4, New York, 1990, McGraw-Hill.

55. Beutler E, Meul A, and Wood LA: Depletion and regeneration of 2,3-diphosphoglyceric acid in stored red blood cells, *Transfusion* 9:109, 1969.

56. Bia MJ, DeFronzo RA: Extrarenal potassium homeostasis, *Am J Physiol* 240(F):257, 1981.

57. Bidani A: Electrolyte and acid-base disorders, *Med Clin North Am* 70:1013, 1986.

58. Biebisch G: Functional organization of proximal and distal tubular electrolyte transport, *Nephron* 6:260, 1969.

59. Bilbrey GL, Herbin L, Carter NW et al: Skeletal muscle resting membrane potential and potassium deficiency, *J Clin Invest* 52:3011, 1973.

60. Binstock ML, Mundy GR: Effect of calcitonin and glucocorticoids in combination on the hypercalcemia of malignancy, *Ann Intern Med* 93:269, 1980.

61. Biro GP: Current status of erythrocyte substitutes, *Can Med Assoc J* 129:237, 1983.

62. Biro GP, Blais P: Perfluorocarbon blood substitutes, *CRC Crit Rev Oncol/Hematol* 6:311, 1987.

63. Bishop RL, Weisfeldt ML: Sodium bicarbonate administration during cardiac arrest. Effect on arterial pH, PCO_2, and osmolality, *JAMA* 235:506, 1976.

64. Black RM: Disorders of serum sodium and serum potassium. In Rippe JM, Irwin RS, Alpert JS et al, eds: *Intensive care medicine,* Boston, 1985, Little, Brown.

65. Black RM: Metabolic acid-base disturbances. In Rippe JM, Irwin RS, Alpert JS et al, eds: *Intensive care medicine,* Boston, 1985, Little, Brown.

66. Blackburn GL, Driscoll DF: Time to abandon routine albumin supplementation, *Crit Care Med* 20:157, 1992 (editorial).

67. Bland JHL, Laver MB, and Lowenstein E: Vasodilator effect of commercial 5% plasma protein fraction solutions, *JAMA* 224:1721, 1973.

68. Blevins LS, Wand GS: Diabetes insipidus, *Crit Care Med* 20:69, 1992.

69. Blood and blood components: preparation, storage and shipment. In Walker RH, ed: *Technical manual,* ed 10, Arlington, 1990, American Association of Blood Banks.

70. Blood transfusion practice. In Walker RH, ed: *Technical manual,* ed 10, Arlington, 1990, American Association of Blood Banks.

71. Boton R, Gaviria M, and Batlle DC: Prevalence, pathogenesis and treatment of renal dysfunction associated with chronic lithium therapy, *Am J Kidney Dis* 10:329, 1987.

72. Boudreaux P, Bornside GH, and Cohn I: Emergency autotransfusion: partial cleansing of bacteria-laden blood by cell washing, *J Trauma* 23:31, 1983.

73. Boutros AZ, Ruess R, Olson L et al: Comparison of hemodynamic, pulmonary and renal effects of use of three types of fluids after major surgical procedures on the abdominal aorta, *Crit Care Med* 7:9, 1979.

74. Bove JR: Transfusion-associated hepatitis and AIDS: what is the risk? *N Engl J Med* 317:242, 1987.

75. Brackett NC, Cohen JJ, and Schwartz WB: Carbon dioxide titration curve of normal man. Effect of increasing degrees of acute hypercapnia on acid-base equilibrium, *N Engl J Med* 272:6, 1965.

76. Brackett NC, Wingo CF, Muren O et al: Acid-base response to chronic hypercapnia in man, *N Engl J Med* 280:124, 1969.

77. Brannon ES: The cardiac output in patients with chronic anemia as measured by the technique of right atrial catheterization, *J Clin Invest* 24:332, 1945.

78. Brantigan JW, Ziegler EC, Hynes KM et al: Tissue gases during hypovolemic shock, *J Appl Physiol* 37:117, 1974.

79. Braunwald E: The physical examination. In *Heart disease,* ed 4, Philadelphia, 1992, WB Saunders.

80. Braunwald E, Grossman W: Clinical aspects of heart failure. In *Heart disease,* ed 4, Philadelphia, 1992, WB Saunders.

81. Brautbar N, Massry SG: Disorders of magnesium metabolism. In Maxwell MH, Kleeman CR, and Narins RG, eds: *Clinical disorders of fluid and electrolyte metabolism,* ed 4, New York, 1987, McGraw-Hill.

82. Brazier J, Cooper N, Maloney JV et al: The adequacy of myocardial oxygen delivery in acute normovolemic anemia, *Surgery* 75:508, 1974.

83. Bready LL, Hoff BH, Boyd RC et al: Acute hyponatremia associated with transurethral surgery, *Anesthesiol Rev* 12:37, 1985.

84. Breslow MJ: Neuroendocrine responses to surgery. In Breslow MJ, Miller CF, and Rogers MC, eds: *Perioperative management,* St Louis, 1990, Mosby–Year Book.

85. Bricker NS: Sodium homeostasis in chronic renal disease, *Kidney Int* 21:886, 1982.

86. Brigham KL: Mechanisms of lung injury, *Clin Chest Med* 3:9, 1982.

87. Brigham KL, Kariman K, Harris TR et al: Correlation of oxygenation with vascular permeability-surface area but not with lung water in humans with acute respiratory failure and pulmonary edema, *J Clin Invest* 72:339, 1983.

88. Brisman R, Parks LC, and Haller JA: Anaphylactoid reactions associated with the clinical use of dextran 70, *JAMA* 204:824, 1968.

89. Brown MJ, Brown DL, and Murphy MB: Hypokalemia from β_2 receptor stimulation by circulating epinephrine, *N Engl J Med* 309:1414, 1983.

90. Brown RH, Rossini AA, Callaway CW et al: Caveat on fluid replacement in hyperglycemic, hyperosmolar, nonketotic coma, *Diabetes Care* 1:305, 1978.

91. Brozovic B, Brozovic M: Transfusion of plasma components and products. In *Manual of clinical blood transfusion,* London, 1986, Churchill-Livingstone.

92. Buckalew VM: Hyponatremia: pathogenesis and management, *Hosp Pract* 21:49, 1986.

93. Buran MJ: Oxygen consumption: In Snyder JV, ed: *Oxygen transport in the critically ill,* Chicago, 1987, Yearbook Medical Publishers.

94. Burch GE, Giles TD: The importance of magnesium deficiency in cardiovascular disease, *Am Heart J* 94:649, 1977.

95. Burnell JM, Teubuer EJ, and Simpson DP: Metabolic alkalosis accompanying potassium deprivation, *Am J Physiol* 227:329, 1974.

96. Burnell JM, Villamil MF, Uyeno BT et al: The effects in humans of extracellular pH change on the relationship between serum potassium concentration and intracellular potassium, *J Clin Invest* 35:935, 1956.

97. Buschle DF, Saklad M: A compatible solution for administration with blood, *Anesthesiology* 14:53, 1953.

98. Bushinsky DA, Coe FL, Katzenberg C et al: Arterial P_{CO_2} and chronic metabolic acidosis, *Kidney Int* 22:311, 1982.

99. Cable RG: Implementation of a predonation system, *Int Anesth Clin* 20:59, 1982.

100. Cain SM: Oxygen delivery and uptake in dogs during anemic and hypoxic hypoxia, *J Appl Physiol* 42:228, 1977.

101. Cain SM, Chapler CK: O_2 extraction by hind limb versus whole dog during anemic hypoxia, *J Appl Physiol* 45:966, 1978.

102. Cain SM, Chapler CK: Oxygen extraction by canine hind limb during hypoxic hypoxia, *J Appl Physiol* 46:1023, 1979.

103. Caldwell FT, Bowser BH: Critical evaluation of hypertonic solutions to resuscitate severely burned children. A prospective study, *Ann Surg* 189:546, 1979.

104. Calkins JM, Vaughan RW, Cork RC et al: Effects of dilution, pressure, and apparatus on hemolysis and flow rate in transfusion of packed erythrocytes, *Anesth Analg* 61:776, 1982.

105. Cane RD: Hemoglobin: how much is enough? *Crit Care Med* 18:1046, 1990.

106. Cannon PJ, Heinemann HO, Alpert MS et al: "Contraction" alkalosis after diuresis of edematous patients with ethacrynic acid, *Ann Intern Med* 62:979, 1965.

107. Cardenas-Rivero N, Chernow B, Stoiko MA et al: Hypocalcemia in critically ill children, *J Pediatr* 114:946, 1989.

108. Cardiovascular pharmacology I. In *Textbook of advanced cardiac life support,* Dallas, 1987, American Heart Association.

109. Carilli AD, Ramananurty MU, and Chang YS: Non-cardiogenic pulmonary edema following blood transfusion, *Chest* 74:310, 1978.

110. Carlson RW, Rattan S, and Haupt MT: Fluid resuscitation in conditions of increased permeability, *Anesthesiology Rev* 279(3):14, 1990.

111. Carpenter RL, Cullen BF: Hematologic and immune function. In Brown DL, ed: *Risk and outcome in anesthesia,* Philadelphia, 1988, JB Lippincott.

112. Carson JL, Spence RK, Poses RM, et al: Severity of anaemia and operative mortality and morbidity, *Lancet* 1:727, 1988.

113. Case RB, Berglung E, and Sarnoff SJ: Ventricular function. VII. Changes in coronary resistance and ventricular function resulting from acutely induced anemia and the effect thereon on coronary stenosis, *Am J Med* 18:397, 1955.

114. Chamberlain MJ: Emergency treatment of hyperkalemia, *Lancet* 1:464, 1964.

115. Chaplin H: Packed red blood cells, *N Engl J Med* 281:364, 1969.

116. Chappell TR, Rubin LT, Markham RV et al: Independence of oxygen consumption and systemic oxygen transport in patients with either stable pulmonary hypertension of refractory left ventricular failure, *Am Rev Respir Dis* 128:30, 1983.

117. Chernow B, Zaloga G, and McFadden E: Hypocalcemia in critically ill patients, *Crit Care Med* 10:848, 1982.

118. Chinitz JL, Kim KE, Onesti G et al: Pathophysiology and prevention of dextran-40 induced anuria, *J Lab Clin Med* 77:76, 1981.

119. Cholst IN, Steinberg SF, Tropper PL et al: The influence of hypermagnesemia on serum calcium and parathyroid hormone levels in human subjects, *N Engl J Med* 310:1221, 1984.

120. Ciabattoni G, Cinotti GA, Pierucci A et al: Effects of Sulindac and ibuprofen in patients with chronic glomerular disease. Evidence for the dependence of renal function on prostacyclin, *N Engl J Med* 310:279, 1984.

121. Civetta JM: A new look at the Starling equation, *Crit Care Med* 7:84, 1979.

122. Clark DD, Chang BS, Garella SG et al: Secondary hypocapnia fails to protect "whole-body" intracellular pH during chronic "HCL" acidosis in the dog, *Kidney Int* 23:336, 1983.

123. Clive DM, Stoff JS: Renal syndromes associated with non-steroidal anti-inflammatory drugs, *N Engl J Med* 310:563, 1984.

124. Cloutier CT, Lowery BD, and Carey LC: The effect of hemodilution resuscitation on serum protein levels in humans in hemorrhagic shock, *J Trauma* 9:514, 1969.

125. Cogan MC, Arieff AI: Sodium-wasting, acidosis and hyperkalemia induced by methicillin interstitial nephritis: evidence for selective distal tubular dysfunction, *Am J Med* 64:500, 1978.

126. Cohen EN: Patients with altered sensitivity, *Clin Anesth* 2:76, 1966.

127. Cohen L, Kitzes R: Magnesium sulfate and digitalis-toxic arrhythmias, *JAMA* 249:2808, 1983.

128. Cohn JN, Luria MH, Daddario RC et al: Studies in clinical shock and hypotension. V. Hemodynamic effects of dextran, *Circulation* 35:316, 1967.

129. Collens GM, Leedbrook J: The rheologic properties of low molecular weight dextrans: fact or fancy? *Am Heart J* 72:41, 1966.

130. Collins JA, Stechenberg L: The effects of the concentration and function of hemoglobin on the survival of rats after hemorrhage, *Surgery* 85:412, 1979.

131. Comroe JH: Transport and elimination of carbon dioxide. In *Physiology of respiration,* ed 2, Chicago, 1974, Year Book Medical Publishers.

132. Connor TB, Rosen BL, Blaustein MP et al: Hypocalcemia precipitating congestive heart failure, *N Engl J Med* 307:869, 1982.

133. Cope DK, Allison RC, Parmentier JC et al: Using pulmonary artery pressure profile after occlusion, *Crit Care Med* 14:16, 1986.

134. Cote' CJ, Lambertus JD, Daniels AL et al: Calcium chloride versus calcium gluconate: comparison of ionization and cardiovascular effects in children and dogs, *Anesthesiology* 66:465, 1987.

135. Cox M: Potassium homeostasis, *Med Clin North Am* 65:363, 1981.

136. Cox M, Guzzo M, Morrison G et al: Demeclocycline and therapy of hyponatremia, *Ann Intern Med* 86:113, 1977.

137. Cronin RE, Knochel JP: Magnesium deficiency, *Adv Intern Med* 28:509, 1983.

138. Cross JS, Gruber DP, Burchard KW et al: Hypertonic saline fluid therapy following surgery: a prospective study, *J Trauma* 29:817, 1989.

139. Crowell JW, Ford RG, and Lewis VM: Oxygen transport and hemorrhagic shock as a function of the hematocrit ratio, *Am J Physiol* 196:1033, 1959.

140. Cryer PE, Weiss S: Reduced plasma norepinephrine response to standing in autonomic dysfunction, *Arch Neurol* 33: 275, 1976.

141. Cuthbertson DP: Parenteral fluid therapy in relation to the metabolic response to injury, *Surg Gynec Obstet* 110:105, 1960.

142. Czer LSC, Shoemaker WC: Optimal hematocrit value in critically ill postoperative patients, *Surg Gynecol Obstet* 147:363, 1978.

143. Danek SJ, Lynch JP, Weg JG et al: The dependence of oxygen uptake on delivery in the adult respiratory distress syndrome, *Am Rev Respir Dis* 122:387, 1980.

144. Darrow DC, Yannet H: Changes in the distribution of body water accompanying increase and decrease in extracellular electrolytes, *J Clin Invest* 14:266, 1935.

145. Davenport: What happens in blood? In *The ABCs of acid-base chemistry,* ed 6, Chicago, 1974, The University of Chicago Press.

146. Davidson D, Stalcup SA: Systemic circulatory adjustments to acute hypoxia and reoxygenation in unanesthetized sheep, *J Clin Invest* 73:317, 1984.

147. Davidson IJA, Willms CD, Sandor ZF et al: Ringer's lactate with or without 3% dextran-60 as volume expanders during abdominal aortic surgery, *Crit Care Med* 19:36, 1991.

148. Dawson RB, Kocholaty WF, and Gray JL: Hemoglobin function and 2,3-DPG levels in blood stored at 4° C in ACD and CPD: pH effect, *Transfusion* 10:299, 1970.

149. Decaux G, Waterlox Y, Genene F et al: Treatment of the syndrome of inappropriate secretion of antidiuretic hormone by furosemide, *N Engl J Med* 304:329, 1981.

150. De Cesare WR, Bove JR, and Ebaugh FG: The mechanism of the effect of iso- and hyperosmolar dextrose-saline solution on in vivo survival of human erythrocytes, *Transfusion* 4:237, 1964.

151. DeCosse JJ, Randal HT, Habif DV et al: The mechanism of hyponatremia and hypotonicity after surgical trauma, *Surgery* 40:27, 1956.

152. De Felippe J, Timoner J, Velasco IT et al: Treatment of refractory hypovolemic shock by sodium 7.5% chloride injections, *Lancet* 2:1002, 1980.

153. DeFronzo RA: Intravenous potassium chloride therapy, *JAMA* 245:2446, 1981.

154. DeFronzo RA: Hyperkalemic states. In Maxwell MH, Kleeman CR, Narins RG, eds: *Clinical disorders of fluid and electrolyte metabolism,* ed 4, New York, 1987, McGraw-Hill.

155. DeFronzo RA, Goldberg M, and Agus ZS: Normal diluting capacity in hyponatremic patients: reset osmostat or a variant of SIADH, *Ann Intern Med* 84:538, 1976.

156. DeGowin RL: The thorax and cardiovascular system: the blood vessels. In *Bedside diagnostic examination,* ed 5, New York, 1987, MacMillan Publishing.

157. del Castillo J, Engback L: The nature of the neuromuscular block produced by magnesium, *J Physiol (Lond)* 124:370, 1954.

158. DeLuz P, Shubin H, Weil MH et al: Pulmonary edema related to changes in colloid osmotic pressure in patients after acute myocardial infarction, *Circulation* 51:350, 1975.

159. Demling RH, Harms B, Kramer G et al: Acute versus sustained hypoproteinemia and post-traumatic pulmonary edema, *Surgery* 92:79, 1982.

160. Denis R, Smith RW, Grabow D et al: Relocation of nonalbumin proteins after albumin resuscitation, *J Surg Res* 43:413, 1987.

161. Dennis RC, Hectman HB, Berger RL et al: Transfusion of 2,3-DPG–enriched red blood cells to improve cardiac function, *Ann Thorac Surg* 26:17, 1978.

162. Desai TK, Carlson RW, Thill-Baharozian M et al: A direct relationship between ionized calcium and arterial pressure among patients in an intensive care unit, *Crit Care Med* 16:578, 1988.

163. Desmond J: Complications of transurethral prostatic surgery, *Can Anaesth Soc J* 17:25, 1970.

164. Deutsch S: Pre- and post-operative fluid balance. In *Clinical fluid and electrolyte management,* Washington, 1976, Veterans Administration.

165. DeVenuto F: Hemoglobin solutions as oxygen delivering resuscitation fluids, *Crit Care Med* 10:238, 1982.

166. DeVenuto F: Modified hemoglobin solution as a resuscitation fluid, *Vox Sang* 44:129, 1983.

167. DeVore JS, Asran R: Magnesium sul-

168. Dietrich KA, Conrad SA, Hebert CA et al: Cardiovascular and metabolic response to red blood cell transfusion in critically ill volume-resuscitated nonsurgical patients, *Crit Care Med* 18:940, 1990.

169. Dodge C, Glass D: Crystalloid and colloid therapy, *Semin Anesth* 1:293, 1982.

170. Dormandy JA: Influence of blood viscosity on blood flow and the effect of low molecular weight dextrans, *Br Med J* 4:716, 1971.

171. Downey RS, Monafo WW: Metabolic response to injury in critical illness. In Civetta JM, Taylor RW, and Kirby RR, eds: *Critical care,* Philadelphia, 1988, JB Lippincott.

172. Drake R, Laine G: Pulmonary microvascular permeability to fluid and macromolecules, *J Appl Physiol* 64:487, 1988.

173. Drake R, Smith J, and Gabel J: Estimation of the filtration coefficient in intact dog lungs, *Am J Physiol* 238:H430, 1980.

174. D'Silva JL: The action of adrenaline on serum potassium, *J Physiol (Lond)* 82: 393, 1934.

175. D'Silva JL: The action of adrenaline on serum potassium, *J Physiol (Lond)* 86: 219, 1936.

176. Dubois M, Lotze MT, and Diamond WJ: Pulmonary shunting during leukoagglutinin-induced non-cardiac edema, *JAMA* 244:2186, 1980.

177. Ducey JP, Lamiell JM, and Gueller GE: Arterial-venous carbon dioxide tension difference during hemorrhage and resuscitation, *Crit Care Med* 20:518, 1992.

178. Duling BR: Local control of microvascular function: role in tissue oxygen supply, *Ann Rev Physiol* 42:373, 1980.

179. Dunham CM, Siegel JH, Weireter L et al: Oxygen debt and metabolic acidemia as quantitative predictors of mortality and the severity of the ischemic insult in hemorrhagic shock, *Crit Care Med* 19:231, 1991.

180. Ebert RV, Stead EA, and Gibson JG: Response of normal subjects to acute blood loss, *Arch Intern Med* 68:578, 1941.

181. Eckstein RW: Development of interarterial coronary anastomoses by chronic anemia. Disappearance following correction of anemia, *Circ Res* 3:309, 1955.

182. Edelman FS, Olney JM, James AH et al: Body composition: studies in the human being by the dilution principle, *Science* 115:447, 1952.

183. Edelman IS, Leibman J: The anatomy of body water and electrolytes, *Am J Med* 27:256, 1959.

184. Edelman IS, Leibman J, O'Meara MP et al: Interrelationships between serum sodium concentration, serum osmolarity and total exchangeable sodium, total exchangeable potassium and total body water, *J Clin Invest* 37:1236, 1958.

185. Edes TE, Ettayapuram V, and Sunderrajan: Heparin induced hyperkalemia, *Arch Intern Med* 145:1070, 1985.

186. Edwards R, Winnie AP, and Ramamurthy S: Acute hypocapneic hypokalemia:

an iatrogenic anesthetic complication. *Anesth Analg* 56:786, 1977.

187. Elliott JP: Magnesium sulfate as a tocolytic agent, *Am J Obstet Gynecol* 147: 277, 1983.

188. Ellman H, Dembin H, and Seriff N: The rarity of shortening of the QT interval in patients with hypercalcemia, *Crit Care Med* 10:320, 1982.

189. Emmett M, Norris RG: Clinical use of the anion gap, *Medicine* 56:38, 1977.

190. Engle WD: Development of fetal and neonatal renal function, *Semin Perinatol* 10:113, 1986.

191. Ettinger PO, Regan TJ, and Oldewartel HA: Hyperkalemia, cardiac conduction, and electrocardiogram: a review, *Am Heart J* 88:360, 1974.

192. Ewalenko P, Thierry D, and Peeters J: Composition of fresh frozen plasma, *Crit Care Med* 14:145, 1986.

193. Falk JL, Rackow EC, Fein IA et al: The effect of hetastarch, albumin and saline resuscitation on coagulation in shock patients, *Crit Care Med* 11:219, 1983.

194. Falk J, Rackow EC, Fein I et al: Colloid osmotic-pulmonary wedge pressure gradient and pulmonary edema during fluid resuscitation in patients with septic shock, *Chest* 86:287, 1984.

195. Falk JL, Rackow EC, and Weil MH: Colloid and crystalloid fluid resuscitation. In Shoemaker WC, Ayres S, Grenvick A et al, eds: *Textbook of critical care,* ed 2, Philadelphia, 1989, WB Saunders.

196. Fan F, Chen RYZ, Schuessler GB et al: Effect of hematocrit variations on regional hemodynamics in oxygen transport in the dog, *Am J Physiol* 238:H545, 1980.

197. Fanestil DD: Compartmentalization of body water. In Maxwell MH, Kleeman CR, Narins RG, eds: *Clinical disorders of fluid and electrolyte metabolism,* ed 4, New York, 1987, McGraw-Hill.

198. Feig PU: Hypernatremia and hypertonic syndromes, *Med Clin North Am* 65:271, 1981.

199. Feig PU, McCurdy DK: The hypertonic state, *N Engl J Med* 297:1444, 1977.

200. Feldberg W, Sherwood SL: Effects of calcium and potassium injected into the cerebral ventricles of the cat, *J Physiol (Lond)* 139:408, 1957.

201. Feldman SA: Effect of changes in electrolytes, hydration and pH upon the reactions to muscle relaxants, *Br J Anaesth* 35:546, 1963.

202. Feldman SA: The significance of acid-base balance. In Scurr C, Feldman S, eds: *Scientific foundations of anaesthesia,* Chicago, 1974, Year Book Medical Publishers.

203. Felig P: Diabetic ketoacidosis, *N Engl J Med* 290:1360, 1974.

204. Fencl V, Miller TB, and Pappenheimer JR: Studies on the respiratory responses to disturbances of acid-base balance, *Am J Physiol* 210:459, 1956.

205. Fichman MP, Vorher H, Kleeman CR et al: Diuretic-induced hyponatremia, *Ann Intern Med* 75:853, 1971.

206. Fillman EM, Hanson OL, and Gilbert LO: Radioisotopic study of effects of irrigating fluid in transurethral prostatectomy, *JAMA* 171:1488, 1959.

207. Finberg L: Hypernatremic (hypertonic) dehydration in infants, *N Engl J Med* 289:196, 1973.

208. Finch CA, Lenfant C: Oxygen transport in man, *N Engl J Med* 286:407, 1972.

209. Finch CA, Sawyer CG, and Flynn JM: Clinical syndrome of potassium intoxication, *Am J Med* 1:337, 1946.

210. Finlayson JS: Albumin substitutes, *Semin Thromb Hemostas* 6:85, 1980.

211. Fisken RA, Heath DA, and Somers S: Hypercalcemia in hospital patients, *Lancet* 1:202, 1981.

212. Flink EB: Therapy of magnesium deficiency, *Ann NY Acad Sci* 162:901, 1969.

213. Folkow B: Nervous control of the blood vessels, *Physiol Rev* 35:629, 1955.

214. Foster DW, McGarry JD: The metabolic derangements and treatment of diabetic ketoacidosis, *N Engl J Med* 309:159, 1983.

215. Fowler NO, Holmes JC: Blood viscosity and cardiac output in acute experimental anemia, *J Appl Physiol* 39:453, 1975.

216. Fraley DS, Adler S: Correction of hyperkalemia by bicarbonate despite constant blood pH, *Kidney Int* 12:354, 1977.

217. Fraley DS, Adler S, Bruns FJ et al: Stimulation of lactate production by administration of bicarbonate in a patient with a solid neoplasm and lactic acidosis, *N Engl J Med* 303:1100, 1980.

218. Franks DP, Cockett AT: Local hyponatremia of the urinary bladder during transurethral surgery, *Anesthesiology* 22: 15, 1961.

219. Fraser CL, Arieff AI: Fatal central diabetes mellitus and insipidus resulting from untreated hyponatremia: a new syndrome, *Ann Intern Med* 112:113, 1990.

220. Fresh-frozen plasma. Indications and risks (consensus conference), *JAMA* 253: 551, 1985.

221. Fried TA, Stein JH: Glomerular dynamics, *Arch Intern Med* 143:787, 1983.

222. Friedman WF: Congenital heart disease in infancy and childhood. In Braunwald E, ed: *Heart disease,* ed 3, Philadelphia, 1988, WB Saunders.

223. Fulop M: Hypercapnia in metabolic alkalosis, *NY State J Med* 76:19, 1976.

224. Gaar KA, Taylor AE, Owens LJ et al: Effect of capillary pressure in plasma protein on development of pulmonary edema, *Am J Physiol* 213:79, 1967.

225. Gabel JC, Drake RE, and Arens JF: Oxygenation as an indicator of lung fluid accumulation, *Anesthesiology* 51:S156, 1979.

226. Gabow PA: Disorders associated with an altered anion gap, *Kidney Int* 27:472, 1985.

227. Gabow PA, Kaehay WD, Fernessey PV et al: Diagnostic importance of an increased serum anion gap, *N Engl J Med* 303:854, 1980.

228. Gallagher TJ, Banner MJ, and Barnes PA: Large volume crystalloid resuscitation does not increase extravascular lung water, *Anesth Analg* 64:323, 1985.

229. Gambling DR, Birmingham CL, and Jenkins LC: Magnesium and the anaesthetist, *Can J Anaesth* 35:644, 1988.

230. Garella S, Chang BS, and Kahn SI: Dilutional acidosis and contraction al-

kalosis. Review of a concept, *Kidney Int* 8:279, 1975.

231. Garella S, Dana CL, and Chazan JA: Severity of metabolic acidosis as a determinant of bicarbonate requirements, *N Engl J Med* 289:121, 1973.

232. Garzon AA, Cheng C, Lerner B et al: Hydroxyethyl starch and bleeding, *J Trauma* 7:757, 1967.

233. Gault MH, Dixon ME, Doyle M et al: Hypernatremia, azotemia, and dehydration due to high-protein tube feeding, *Ann Intern Med* 68:778, 1968.

234. Geers AB, Koomans HA, Ross JC et al: Functional relationships in the nephrotic syndrome, *Kidney Int* 26:324, 1984.

235. Geha AS: Coronary and cardiovascular dynamics in oxygen availability during acute normovolemic anemia, *Surgery* 80: 47, 1976.

236. Geha AS, Baue A: Graded coronary stenosis and coronary flow during acute normovolemic anemia, *World J Surg* 2:645, 1978.

237. Geha DG: Blood gas monitoring. In Blitt CD, ed: *Monitoring in anesthesia and critical care medicine,* New York, 1985, Churchill-Livingstone.

238. Gennari EJ: Serum osmolality, *N Engl J Med* 310:102, 1984.

239. Gennari FJ: Respiratory acidosis and alkalosis. In Maxwell MH, Kleeman CR, and Narins RG, eds: *Clinical disorders of fluid and electrolyte metabolism,* ed 4, New York, 1987, McGraw-Hill.

240. Gennari FJ, Cohen JJ: Role of the kidney in potassium homeostasis: lessons from acid-base disturbances, *Kidney Int* 8:1, 1975.

241. Gennari FJ, Kassirer JP: Osmotic diuresis, *N Engl J Med* 291:714, 1974.

242. Gerst PH, Fleming WH, and Malm JR: Increased susceptibility of the heart to ventricular fibrillation during metabolic acidosis, *Circ Res* 19:63, 1966.

243. Ghoneim MM, Long JP: The interaction between magnesium and other neuromuscular blocking agents, *Anesthesiology* 32:23, 1970.

244. Giesecke AH, Egbert LD: Perioperative fluid therapy-crystalloids. In Miller RD, ed: *Anesthesia,* ed 2, New York, 1986, Churchill-Livingstone.

245. Giesecke AH, Walmsley AJ: Fluid replacement. In Israel JS, DeKornfeld TJ, eds: *Recovery room care,* ed 2, Chicago, 1987, Year Book Medical Publishers.

246. Gillies IDS: Anaemia in anaesthesia, *Br J Anaesth* 46:589, 1974.

247. Gilmour DG, Aitkenhead AR, Hothersall AP et al: The effect of hypovolemia on colonic blood flow in the dog, *Br J Surg* 67:82, 1980.

248. Glynn IM: Sodium and potassium movements in human red cells, *J Physiol* 134:278, 1956.

249. Goldberg M: Hyponatremia, *Med Clin North Am* 65:251, 1981.

250. Goldfarb S, Cox M, Singer I et al: Acute hyperkalemia induced by hyperglycemia: hormonal mechanisms, *Ann Intern Med* 84:426, 1976.

251. Goldfinger D, Lowe C: Prevention of adverse reactions to blood transfusion by the administration of saline-washed red blood cells, *Transfusion* 21:277, 1981.

252. Goldstein G: Serum potassium levels and anesthesia, *Curr Rev Clin Anesthesiol* 1:170, 1981.

253. Goodwin C, Dorethy J, Lam V et al: Randomized trial of efficacy of crystalloid and colloid resuscitation on hemodynamic response and lung water following thermal injury, *Ann Surg* 197:520, 1983.

254. Goodwin WE, Cason JF, and Scott WW: Hemoglobinemia and lower nephron nephrosis following transurethral prostatic surgery: use of a new nonhemolytic irrigating solution, 3% mannitol, as preventive, *J Urol* 65:1075, 1951.

255. Gould SA, Moss GS, Rosen AL et al: Red cell substitutes. In Civetta JM, Taylor RW, and Kirby RR, eds: *Critical Care*, Philadelphia, 1988, JB Lippincott.

256. Gould SA, Rice CL, and Moss GS: The physiologic basis of the use of blood and blood products, *Surg Annu* 16:13, 1984.

257. Gould SA, Rosen AL, and Sehgal LR: Fluosol-DA as a red cell substitute in acute anemia, *N Engl J Med* 314:1653, 1986.

258. Gould SA, Rosen AL, Sehgal LR et al: Red cell substitutes. Hemoglobin solution or fluorocarbon? *J Trauma* 22:736, 1982.

259. Graettinger JS, Parsons RL, and Campbell JA: A correlation of clinical and hemodynamic studies in patients with mild and severe anemia with and without congestive failure, *Ann Intern Med* 58:617, 1963.

260. Graf H, Leach W, and Arieff AI: Evidence for a detrimental effect of bicarbonate therapy in hypoxic lactic acidosis, *Science* 227:754, 1985.

261. Graham IFM: Preoperative starvation and plasma glucose concentrations in children undergoing outpatient anaesthesia, *Br J Anaesth* 51:161, 1979.

262. Graham LA, Caesar JJ, and Burger ASV: Gastrointestinal absorption and excretion of magnesium(28) in man, *Metabolism* 9:646, 1960.

263. Graves CL, Allen RM: Anesthesia in the presence of severe anemia, *Rocky Mt Med J* 67:35, 1974.

264. Gravlee GP, Hopkins MB: Blood plasma products. In Ellison N, Jobes DR, eds: *Effective hemostasis in cardiac surgery*, Philadelphia, 1988, WB Saunders.

265. Greenburg AG: To transfuse or not to transfuse—that is the question! *Crit Care Med* 18:1045, 1990.

266. Gronert GA, They RA: Pathophysiology of hyperkalemia induced by succinylcholine, *Anesthesiology* 43:89, 1975.

267. Gross JB: Estimating allowable blood loss: correction for dilution, *Anesthesiology* 58:277, 1983.

268. Gross JB, Imai M, and Kokko JP: A functional comparison of the cortical collecting tubule and the distal convoluted tubule, *J Clin Invest* 55:1284, 1975.

269. Grossman W, Braunwald E: High cardiac output states. In Braunwald E, ed: *Heart disease*, ed 3, Philadelphia, 1988, WB Saunders.

270. Gullick HD, Raisz LG: Changes in the renal concentrating ability associated with major surgical procedures, *N Engl J Med* 262:1309, 1960.

271. Gump FE, Kinney JM: Measurement of water balance: a guide to surgical care, *Surgery* 64:154, 1968.

272. Gutierrez G: Peripheral delivery and utilization of oxygen. In Dantzker DR, ed: *Cardiopulmonary critical care*, Orlando, 1986, Grune & Stratton.

273. Guy JT, Bromberg PA, Metz EN et al: Oxygen delivery following transfusion of stored blood. I. Normal rats, *J Appl Physiol* 37:60, 1974.

274. Guyton AC: Interstitial fluid pressure: II. Pressure-volume curves of interstitial space, *Circ Res* 16:452, 1965.

275. Guyton AC: The relationship of cardiac output to arterial pressure control, *Circulation* 64:1079, 1981.

276. Guyton AC: The systemic circulation. In *Textbook of medical physiology*, Philadelphia, 1986, WB Saunders.

277. Guyton AC: The body fluid compartments: extracellular and intracellular fluids; interstitial fluid and edema. In *Textbook of medical physiology*, ed 8, Philadelphia, 1991, WB Saunders.

278. Guyton AC: Energetics and metabolic rate. In *Textbook of medical physiology*, ed 8, Philadelphia, 1991, WB Saunders.

279. Guyton AC: Membrane potentials and action potentials. In *Textbook of medical physiology*, ed 8, Philadelphia, 1991, WB Saunders.

280. Guyton AC: Nervous regulation of the circulation and rapid control of arterial pressure. In *Textbook of medical physiology*, ed 8, Philadelphia, 1991, WB Saunders.

281. Guyton AC: Overview of the circulation, and medical physics of pressure, flow, and resistance. In *Textbook of medical physiology*, ed 8, Philadelphia, 1991, WB Saunders.

282. Guyton AC: Red blood cells, anemia and polycythemia. In *Textbook of medical physiology*, ed 8, Philadelphia, 1991, WB Saunders.

283. Guyton AC, Granger HJ, and Taylor AE: Interstitial fluid pressure, *Physiol Rev* 51:527, 1971.

284. Guyton AC, Lindsey AW: Effect of elevated left atrial pressure and decreased plasma protein concentration on the development of pulmonary edema, *Circ Res* 7:649, 1959.

285. Guyton AC, Richardson TQ: Effect of hematocrit on venous return, *Circ Res* 9:157, 1961.

286. Guyton AC, Taylor AE, and Granger HJ: Capillary exchange and normal fluid convection in the interstitial spaces. In *Circulatory physiology II: dynamics and control of the body fluids*, Philadelphia, 1975, WB Saunders.

287. Hagen GA, Frawley TF: Hyponatremia due to sulfonylurea compounds, *J Clin Endocrinol Metab* 31:570, 1970.

288. Haglund U, Jodal M, and Lundgren O: The small bowel in arterial hypotension and shock. In Shephend AP, Granger DN, eds: *Physiology of the intestinal circulation*, New York, 1984, Raven Press.

289. Halperin ML, Hammeke M, Josse RG et al: Metabolic acidosis in the alcoholic: a pathophysiologic approach, *Metabolism* 32:308, 1983.

290. Halter JB, Pflug AE, and Porte D: Mechanism of plasma catecholamine increases during surgical stress in man, *J Clin Endocrinol Metab* 45:936, 1977.

291. Hankeln K, Radel C, Beez M et al: Comparison of hydroxyethyl starch and lactated Ringer's solution on hemodynamics and oxygen transport of critically ill patients in prospective crossover studies, *Crit Care Med* 17:133, 1989.

292. Hantman D, Rossier B, Zohlman R et al: Rapid correction of hyponatremia in the syndrome of inappropriate secretion of antidiuretic hormone: an alternative treatment to hypertonic saline, *Ann Intern Med* 78:870, 1973.

293. Haradin RI, Weed RI, and Reed CF: Changes in physical properties of stored erythrocytes: relationship to survival in vivo, *Transfusion* 9:229, 1969.

294. Hariprasad MK, Eisinger RP, Nadler IM et al: Hyponatremia in psychogenic polydipsia, *Arch Intern Med* 140:1639, 1980.

295. Harms BA, Kramer GC, Bodai BI et al: Effect of hypoproteinemia on pulmonary and soft tissue edema formation, *Crit Care Med* 9:503, 1981.

296. Harper HA: Appendix: general and physical chemistry. In *Review of physiological chemistry*, ed 14, Los Altos, Calif, 1973, Lange Medical Publications.

297. Harper HA: The chemistry of respiration. In *Review of physiological chemistry*, ed 14, Los Altos, Calif, 1973, Lange Medical Publications.

298. Harper HA: The kidney and the urine. In *Review of physiological chemistry*, ed 14, Los Altos, Calif, 1973, Lange Medical Publications.

299. Harrington JT, Ismer JM, and Kassirer JP: Our national obsession with potassium, *Am J Med* 73:155, 1982.

300. Hart GR, Anderson RJ, Crumpler CP et al: Epidemic classical heat stroke: clinical characteristics and course of 28 patients, *Medicine* 61:189, 1982.

301. Hartmann M, Montgomery A, Jönsson K et al: Tissue oxygenation in hemorrhagic shock measured as transcutaneous oxygen tension, subcutaneous oxygen tension, and gastrointestinal intramucosal pH in pigs, *Crit Care Med* 19:205, 1991.

302. Haugen RK: Hepatitis after the transfusion of frozen red cells and washed red cells, *N Engl J Med* 301:393, 1979.

303. Haupt MT, Gilbert EM, and Carlson RW: Fluid loading increases oxygen delivery and consumption in septic patients with lactic acidosis, *Am Rev Respir Dis* 131:912, 1985.

304. Haupt MT, Rackow EC: Colloid osmotic pressure and fluid resuscitation with hetastarch, albumin and saline solutions, *Crit Care Med* 10:159, 1982.

305. Hauswirth O: Ionic mechanisms in heart muscle in relation to the genesis and the pharmacological control of cardiac arrhythmias, *Pharmacol Rev* 30:5, 1979.

306. Hayes MA: Current concepts: water and electrolyte therapy after operation, *N Engl J Med* 278:1054, 1968.

307. Hayes MA, Goldenberg IS: Renal effects of anesthesia and operation medi-

ated by endocrines, *Anesthesiology* 24: 487, 1963.

308. Hays RM: Dynamics of body water and electrolytes. In Maxwell MH, Kleeman CR, eds: *Clinical disorders of fluid and electrolyte metabolism,* ed 2, New York, 1972, McGraw-Hill.

309. Heath DA: The emergency management of disorders of calcium and magnesium, *Clin Endocrinol Metab* 9:487, 1980.

310. Heaton A, Miripol J, Aster R et al: Use of Adsol preservative solution for prolonged storage of low viscosity AS-1 red blood cells, *Br J Haematol* 57:467, 1984.

311. Hemmer M, Viguerat CE, Suter PM et al: Urinary antidiuretic hormone excretion during mechanical ventilation and weaning in man, *Anesthesiology* 52: 395, 1980.

312. Henry W: Experiments on the quality of gases absorbed by water at different temperatures and under different pressures, *Philos Trans R Soc* 93:29, 1803.

313. Herndon R, Meroney W, and Pearson C: The electrocardiographic effects of alteration in concentration of plasma chemicals, *Am Heart J* 50:188, 1955.

314. Heyl JT, Gibson JC, and Janeway CA: Studies on plasma proteins, *J Clin Invest* 22:763, 1943.

315. Hickam JB, Pryor WW: Cardiac output in postural hypotension, *J Clin Invest* 30:410, 1951.

316. Hicks GL, Jensen LA, Norsen LH et al: Platelet inhibitors and hydroxyethyl starch: safe and cost-effective interventions in coronary artery surgery, *Ann Thorac Surg* 39:422, 1985.

317. Hillman RS: Acute blood loss anemia. In Williams WJ, Beutler E, Erslev AJ et al, eds: *Hematology,* ed 3, New York, 1983, McGraw-Hill.

318. Hinshaw JR, Pories WJ, Harris PD et al: Effect of the molecular size of dextran on liver and kidney oxygen tension, *Surg Forum* 11:360, 1960.

319. Hint H: The pharmacology of dextran and the physiological background for the clinical use of Rheomacrodex and Macrodex, *Acta Anaes Belgica* 2:119, 1968.

320. Hirsch IA, Tomlinson DL, Slogoff S et al: The overstated risk of preoperative hypokalemia, *Anesth Analg* 67:131, 1988.

321. Holcroft JW, Vassar MJ, Turner JE et al: 3% NaCl and 7.5% NaCl/dextran 70 in the resuscitation of severely injured patients, *Ann Surg* 206, 1987.

322. Holliday MA, Kalayci MN, and Harrah J: Factors that limit brain volume changes in response to acute and sustained hypernatremia and hyponatremia, *J Clin Invest* 47:1916, 1968.

323. Holliday MA, Segar WE: Maintenance need for water in parenteral fluid therapy, *Pediatrics* 19:823, 1957.

324. Hollifield JW: Potassium and magnesium abnormalities: diuretics and arrhythmias in hypertension, *Am J Med* 77:28, 1984.

325. Hollinshead WH: The interphase of diabetes insipidus, *Mayo Clin Proc* 39:92, 1964.

326. Honig CR, Frierson JL: Role of adenosine in exercise vasodilatation in dog gracilis muscle, *Am J Physiol* 238:H708, 1980.

327. Hood VL, Danforth E, Horton ES et al: Impact of hydrogen ion on fasting ketogenesis: feedback regulation of acid production, *Am J Physiol* 11:F238, 1982.

328. Hornbein TF: Acid-base balance. In Miller RD, ed: *Anesthesia,* ed 2, New York, 1986, Churchill-Livingstone.

329. Horsey PJ: Applied physiology of the body fluids. In Scurr C, Feldman S, eds: *Scientific foundations of anaesthesia,* Chicago, 1974, W Heinemann.

330. Howland J: The fundamental requirements of an infant's nutrition, *Am J Dis Child* 2:49: 1911.

331. Hoye RC, Bennett SH, Geelhoed GW et al: Fluid volume and albumin kinetics occurring with major surgery, *JAMA* 222:1255, 1972.

332. Huber H, Lewis SM, and Szur L: The influence of anemia, polycythemia and splenomegaly on the relationship between venous hematocrit and red-cell volume, *Br J Haematol* 10:567, 1964.

333. Huckabee WE: Abnormal resting lactate: I. The significance of hyperlactatemia in hospitalized patients, *Am J Med* 30:833, 1961.

334. Huestis DW, Bove JR, and Case J: Red blood cell transfusion. In *Practical blood transfusion,* Boston, 1988, Little, Brown & Company.

335. Huggins C: Preparation and usefulness of frozen blood, *Ann Rev Med* 36:499, 1985.

336. Hughes-Jones NC: Storage of red cells at temperatures between +10° C and −20° C, *Br J Haematol* 4:249, 1958.

337. Humes HD, Narins RG, and Brenner BM: Disorders of water balance, *Hosp Pract* 3:133, 1979.

338. Hurlbert BJ, Edelman JD, and David K: Serum potassium levels during and after terbutaline, *Anesth Analg* 60:723, 1981.

339. International forum on oxygen carrying blood substitutes, *Vox Sang* 42:97, 1982.

340. Iseri LT, Freid J, and Barnes AR: Magnesium deficiency and cardiac disorders, *Am J Med* 58:837, 1975.

341. Israel S, Haworth JC, Dunn HG et al: Lactic acidosis in childhood, *Adv Pediatr* 22:267, 1975.

342. Jain U, Kalathiveetil J, Shah K et al: Severe transurethral resection of the prostate syndrome. Case report, *Anesthes Rev* 27:52, 1990.

343. Jan K, Chien S: Effect of hematocrit variations on coronary hemodynamics and oxygen utilization, *Am J Physiol* 233:H106, 1977.

344. James MFM: Clinical use of magnesium infusions in anesthesia, *Anesth Analg* 74:129, 1992.

345. Järnberg P, De Villota DE, Eklund J et al: Effects of positive and expiratory pressure on renal function, *Acta Anaesthesiol Scand* 22:508, 1978.

346. Jobes DR, Gallagher J: Acute normovolemic hemodilution, *Int Anesth Clin* 20:77, 1982.

347. Johnston SD, Lucas CB, Gerrick SJ et al: Altered coagulation after albumin supplements for treatment of oligemic shock, *Arch Surg* 114:379, 1979.

348. Jones MD, Traystman RJ, Simmons MA et al: Effects of changes in arterial O₂

content on cerebral blood flow in the lamb, *Am J Physiol* 240:H209, 1981.

349. Jönsson K, Jensen JA, Goodson WH et al: Assessment of perfusion in postoperative patients using tissue oxygen measurements, *Br J Surg* 74:263, 1987.

350. Jung A: Comparison of two parenteral diphosphonates in hypercalcemia of malignancy, *Am J Med* 72:221, 1982.

351. Kaehny WD: Pathogenesis and management of metabolic acidosis and alkalosis. In Schrier RW, ed: *Renal and electrolyte disorders,* Boston, 1976, Little, Brown.

352. Kafiluddi R, Kennedy RH, and Seifen E: Effects of buffer magnesium on positive inotropic agents in guinea pig cardiac muscle, *Eur J Pharmacol* 165:181, 1989.

353. Kahn RA, Allen RW, and Baldassare J: Alternate sources and substitutes for therapeutic blood components, *Blood* 66:1, 1985.

354. Kaissirer JP, London AM, Goldman DM et al: Pathogenesis of metabolis alkalosis in hyperaldosteronism, *Am J Med* 49:306, 1970.

355. Kalhorn TF, Yacobi A, and Sum CY: Biliary excretion of hydroxyethyl starch in man, *Biomed Mass Spectrom* 11:164, 1984.

356. Kapoor W: Hypotension and syncope. In Braunwald E, ed: *Heart disease,* ed 4, Philadelphia, 1992, WB Saunders.

357. Kaufman BS, Rackow EC, and Falk JL: A relationship between oxygen delivery and consumption during fluid resuscitation of hypovolemic and septic shock, *Chest* 85:336, 1984.

358. Kaye R: Diabetic ketoacidosis—the bicarbonate controversy (editorial), *J Peds* 87:156, 1975.

359. Keats AS: Cardiovascular anesthesia: perceptions and perspectives, *Anesthesiology* 60:467, 1984.

360. Keller U, Berter W: Prevention of hypophosphatemia by phosphate infusion during treatment of DKA and hyperosmolar coma, *Diabetes* 29:87, 1980.

361. Kharasch ED, Bowdle TA: Hypokalemia before induction of anesthesia and prevention by β₂ adrenoceptor antagonism, *Anesth Analg* 72:216, 1991.

362. Khilnani P: Electrolyte abnormalities in critically ill children, *Crit Care Med* 20:241, 1992.

363. Kickler TS: When should red cell transfusions be given? *J Intens Care Med* 5:197, 1990 (editorial).

364. Kien ND, Kramer GC, and White DA: Acute hypotension caused by rapid hypertonic saline infusion in anesthetized dogs, *Anesth Analg* 73:597, 1991.

365. Kille JM, Klabunde RE: Adenosine as a mediator of post contraction hyperthermia in dog gracilis muscle, *Am J Physiol* 246:H274, 1984.

366. Kingston ME, Al-Siba'i MB, and Skooge WC: Clinical manifestations of hypomagnesemia, *Crit Care Med* 14:950, 1986.

367. Kirklin JK, Lell WA, and Kouchoukos NT: Hydroxyethyl starch versus albumin for colloid infusion following cardiopulmonary bypass in patients undergoing myocardial revascularization, *Ann Thorac Surg* 37:40, 1984.

368. Kissmeyer-Nelson F, Gidergaard J: Platelets in blood stored in untreated

and siliconed glass bottles and plastic bags, *J Clin Pathol* 14:626, 1961.

369. Kleeman CR: CNS manifestations of disordered salt and water balance, *Hosp Pract* May:59, 1979.

370. Knepper MA, Rector FC: Urinary concentration and dilution. In Brenner BM, Rector FC, eds: *The kidney,* ed 4, Philadelphia, 1991, WB Saunders.

371. Koch SM, Taylor RW: Chloride ion in intensive care medicine, *Crit Care Med* 20:227, 1992.

372. Knochel JP, Reed G: Disorders of heat regulation. In Maxwell MH, Kleeman CR, Narins RG, eds: *Clinical disorders of fluid and electrolyte metabolism,* ed 4, New York, 1986, McGraw-Hill.

373. Knockel JP, Schlein FM: The mechanism of rhabdomyolysis in potassium depletion, *J Clin Invest* 51:1750, 1972.

374. Köhler H, Kirch W, and Horstmann HJ: Formation of high molecular aggregates between serum amylase and colloidal plasma substitutes, *Anaesthetist* 26:623, 1977.

375. Köhler H, Kirch W, and Horstmann HJ: Hydroxyethyl start-induced macroamylasemia, *Int J Clin Pharmacol* 15:428, 1977.

376. Kokko J: Chronic renal failure. In Wyngaarden JB, Smith LH, eds: *Textbook of medicine,* ed 18, Philadelphia, 1988, WB Saunders.

377. Kopriva CJ, Ratliff JL, Fletcher JR et al: Biochemical and hematological changes associated with massive transfusion of ACD-stored blood in severely injured combat casualties, *Ann Surg* 176:585, 1972.

378. Kowalyshyn TJ, Prager D, and Young J: A review of the present status of preoperative hemoglobin requirements, *Anesth Analg* 51:75, 1972.

379. Kramer GC, Harms BA, Gunther RA et al: The effects of hypoproteinemia on blood-to-lymph fluid transport in sheep lung, *Circ Res* 49:1173, 1981.

380. Krasner BS: Cardiac effects of magnesium with special reference to anesthesia: a review, *Can Anaesth Soc J* 26:181, 1979.

381. Krasner B, Girdwood R, and Smith H: The effect of slow releasing oral magnesium chloride on the QTc interval of the electrocardiogram during open heart surgery, *Can Anaesth Soc J* 28:329, 1981.

382. Kreimeier U, Frey L, Dentz J et al: Hypertonic saline dextran resuscitation during the initial phase of acute endotoxemia: effect on regional blood flow, *Crit Care Med* 19:801, 1991.

383. Kreisberg RA: Lactate homeostasis and lactic acidosis, *Ann Intern Med* 92:227, 1980.

384. Krejs GJ, Fordtran JS: Diarrhea. In Sleisenger MH, Fordtran JS, eds: *Gastrointestinal disease,* ed 3, Philadelphia, 1983, WB Saunders.

385. Kristensen J, Modig J: Ringer's acetate and dextran-70 with or without hypertonic saline in endotoxin induced shock in pigs, *Crit Care Med* 18:1261, 1990.

386. Kurtz SR, Van Deinse WH, and Valeri CR. The immunocompetence of residual lymphocytes at various stages of red cell cryopreservation with 40% W/V

387. Kurtzman N, Sabatini S: Metabolic alkalosis. In Maxwell MH, Kleeman CR, and Narins RG, eds: *Clinical disorders of fluid and electrolyte metabolism,* ed 4, New York, 1987, McGraw-Hill.

388. Kusano K, Braun-Werness JL, Vick DJ et al: Chlorpropamide action on renal concentration mechanisms in rats with hypothalamic diabetes insipidus, *J Clin Invest* 72:1298, 1983.

389. Kuschinsky W, Wahl M: Local, chemical and neurogenic regulation of cerebral vascular resistence, *Physiol Rev* 58:656, 1978.

390. Kwon NJ, Stolte AL, and Farina JP: Hypokalemia in rats produces resistance to dysrhythmias under halothane anesthesia, *J Cardiothorac Anesth* 3:532, 1989.

391. Ladenson JH, Lewis JW, and Boyd JC: Failure of total serum calcium corrected for protein, albumin, and pH to correctly assess free calcium status, *J Clin Endocrinol Metab* 46:986, 1978.

392. Laks H, O'Connor NJ, Pilon RN et al: Acute normovolemic hemodilution: effects of hemodynamics, oxygen transport and lung water in anesthetized man, *Surg Forum* 24:201, 1973.

393. Lamke LO, Liljedahl SO: Plasma volume expansion after infusion of 5%, 20% and 25% albumin solutions in patients, *Resuscitation* 5:85, 1976.

394. Langsjoen PH: Observations in the excretion of low molecular weight dextran, *Angiology* 16:148, 1965.

395. Laragh JH: The effect of potassium chloride on hyponatremia, *J Clin Invest* 33:807, 1954.

396. Laureno R, Karp BI: Pontine and extrapontine myelinolysis following rapid correction of hyponatremia, *Lancet* i:1439, 1988.

397. Layon AJ, Kirby RP: Fluids and electrolytes in the critically ill. In Civetta JM, Taylor RW, and Kirby RR, eds: *Critical care,* Philadelphia, 1988, JB Lippincott.

398. Layon J, Duncan D, Gallaghar TJ et al: Hypertonic saline as a resuscitation solution in hemorrhagic shock: effect on extravascular lung water in cardiopulmonary function, *Anesth Analg* 66:154, 1987.

399. Leaf A: Neurogenic diabetes insipidus, *Kidney Int* 15:572, 1979.

400. Lee C, Zaloga GP: Magnesium metabolism, *Semin Resp Med* 7:75, 1985.

401. Lehninger AL: Enzymes: mechanism, structure and regulation. In *Biochemistry,* New York, 1970, Worth Publishers.

402. Lehninger AL: Water. In *Biochemistry,* New York, 1970, Worth Publishers.

403. Lemann J, Adams ND, and Gray RW: Urinary calcium excretion in human beings, *N Engl J Med* 301:535, 1979.

404. Lepley D, Weisfeldt M, Close AS et al: Effect of low molecular weight dextran in hemorrhagic shock, *Surgery* 54:93, 1963.

405. Levinsky NG: Management of emergencies: VI. Hyperkalemia, *N Engl J Med* 274:1076, 1966.

406. Levy M, Allotey JB: Temporal relationships between urinary salt retention and

altered systemic hemodynamics in dogs with experimental cirrhosis, *J Lab Clin Med* 92:560, 1978.

407. Lichtenstein A, Eckhart WF, Swanson KJ et al: Unplanned intraoperative and postoperative hemodilution: oxygen transport and consumption during severe anemia, *Anesthesiology* 69:119, 1988.

408. Limas SL, Berl T, Robertson GL et al: Role of vasopressin in the impaired water secretion of glucocorticoid deficiency, *Kidney Int* 18:58, 1980.

409. Lipner HI, Ruzamy F, Dasgupta M et al: The behavior of carbenicillin as a nonreabsorbable anion, *J Lab Clin Med* 8:279, 1975.

410. Lister J, McNeill IF, Marshall VC et al: Transcapillary refilling after hemorrhage in normal man: basal rates and volumes; effect of norepinephrine, *Ann Surg* 158:698, 1963.

411. Ljungström KG, Renck H, Strandberg K et al: Adverse reactions to dextran in Sweden 1970-1979, *Acta Chir Scand* 149:253, 1983.

412. Loeb JN: The hyperosmolar state, *N Engl J Med* 290:1184, 1974.

413. London MJ: Perioperative fluid management, *Anesthesiology Rev* 27(3):44, 1990.

414. London MJ, Franks ME, Merrick SH et al: Pentastarch (low-molecular-weight hydroxyethyl starch): efficacy and clinical safety as a cardiopulmonary bypass priming solution, *Anesthesiology* 69: A208, 1988.

415. London MJ, Ho JS, Triedman JK et al: A randomized clinical trial of 10% pentastarch (low molecular weight hydroxyethyl starch) versus 5% albumin for plasma volume expansion after cardiac operations, *J Thorac Cardiovasc Surg* 97:785, 1989.

416. Lopes OU, Velasco IT, Guertzenstein PG et al: Hypertonic NaCl restores mean circulatory filling pressure in severely hypovolemic dogs, *Hypertension* 8:I195, 1986.

417. Lucas CE, Benishek DJ, and Ledgerwood AM: Reduced oncotic pressure after shock, *Arch Surg* 117:675, 1982.

418. Lucas CE, Ledgerwood AM: The fluid problem in the critically ill, *Surg Clin North Am* 63:439, 1983.

419. Lucas EC, Weaver D, Higgins RF et al: Effects of albumin vs. nonalbumin resuscitation on plasma volume and renal excretory function, *J Trauma* 18:564, 1978.

420. Maddox DA, Brenner BM: Glomerular ultrafiltration. In Brenner BM, Rector FC, eds: *The kidney,* ed 4, Philadelphia, 1991, WB Saunders.

421. Madias NE: Lactic acidosis, *Kidney Int* 29:752, 1986.

422. Madias NE, Schwartz WB, and Cohen JJ: The maladaptive renal response to secondary hypocapnia during chronic "HCL" acidosis in the dog, *J Clin Invest* 60:1393, 1977.

423. Madsen PO, Madsen RE: Clinical and experimental evaluation of different irrigating fluids for transurethral surgery, *Invest Urol* 3:122, 1965.

424. Maffley RH: The body fluids: volume,

composition, and physical chemistry. In Brenner BM, Rector FC, eds: *The kidney,* Philadelphia, 1976, WB Saunders.

425. Maffly LH, Leaf A: Intracellular osmolarity of mammalian tissues, *J Clin Invest* 37:916, 1958.

426. Malmberg PO, Woodson RD: Effect of anemia on oxygen transport in hemorrhagic shock, *J Appl Physiol* 47:882, 1979.

427. Maluf NSR, Boren JS, and Brandes GE: Absorption of irrigating solution and associated changes upon urethral electroresection the prostate, *J Urol* 75:824, 1956.

428. Mani M, Keh E, Kartha RK et al: Transurethral prostatic surgery revisited: a case in point, *Anesthesiol Rev* 3:15, 1976.

429. Mann M, Sacks HJ, and Goldfinger D: Safety of autologous blood donation prior to elective surgery for a variety of potentially "high-risk" patients, *Transfusion* 22:229, 1983.

430. Manthey AA: The effect of calcium on the desensitization of membrane receptors at the neuromuscular junction, *J Gen Physiol* 49:963, 1966.

431. Martin E, Hansen E, and Peter K: Acute limited normovolemic hemodilution: a method for avoiding homologous transfusion, *World J Surg* 11:53, 1987.

432. Marx GF, Orkin LR: Complications associated with transurethral surgery, *Anesthesiology* 23:802, 1962.

433. Maslowski AH, Ikram H, Nicholls MG et al: Haemodynamic, hormonal, and electrolyte responses to captopril in resistent heart failure, *Lancet* 1:71, 1981.

434. Mathieu D, Neviere R, Billard V et al: Effects of bicarbonate therapy on hemodynamics and tissue oxygenation in patients with lactic acidosis: a prospective, controlled clinical study, *Crit Care Med* 19:1352, 1991.

435. Mattar JA: Hypertonic and hyperoncotic solutions in patients, *Crit Care Med* 17:297, 1989 (editorial).

436. Mattar JA, Weil MH, and Shubin H: A study of the hyperosmolal state in critically ill patients, *Crit Care Med* 1:293, 1973.

437. Mattar JA, Yeil MH, Shubin H et al: Cardiac arrest in the critically ill. II. Hyperosmolal states following cardiac arrest, *Am J Med* 56:162, 1974.

438. Matthews CME: Effects of plasmapheresis on albumin pools in rabbits, *J Clin Invest* 40:603, 1961.

439. Mazzoni MC, Arfors BK, and Intaglietta M: Dynamic fluid redistribution in hyperosmotic resuscitation of hypovolemic hemorrhage, *Am J Physiol* 139:H629, 1988.

440. McCammon RL, Stoelting RK: Exaggerated increase in serum potassium following succinylcholine in dogs with beta blockade, *Anesthesiology* 61:723, 1984.

441. McConn R, Derrick JB: The respiratory function of blood: transfusion and blood storage, *Anesthesiology* 36:119, 1972.

442. McCurdy DK: Hyperosmolar hyperglycemic nonketotic diabetic coma, *Med Clin North Am* 54:683, 1970.

443. McDonald D, Kaplan JA: Blood and volume expanders. In Kaplan JA, ed: *Cardiac anesthesia,* vol 2, New York, 1983, Grune & Stratton.

444. McDonald KM, Anderson R, Miller PD et al: Hormonal control of renal water excretion, *Kidney Int* 10:38, 1976.

445. McGovern B: Hypokalemia and cardiac arrhythmias, *Anesthesiology* 63:127, 1985 (editorial).

446. Medalle R, Webb R, and Waterhouse C: Lactic acidosis and associated hypoglycemia, *Arch Intern Med* 128:273, 1971.

447. Mellander S: Contribution of small vessel tone to the regulation of blood volume and formation of oedema, *Proc R Soc Med* 61:55, 1968.

448. Menitove SM, Goldring RM: Combined ventilator and bicarbonate strategy in the management of status asthmaticus, *Am J Med* 74:893, 1983.

449. Meryman HT: Cryopreservation of blood and marrow cells: basic biological and biophysical considerations. In Petz LD, Swisher SN, eds: *Clinical practice of blood transfusion,* New York, 1981, Churchill-Livingstone.

450. Meryman HT, Hornblower M: The preparation of red cells depleted of leukocytes, *Transfusion* 26:101, 1986.

451. Messmer K, Sunder-Plassmann L: Hemodilution, *Progr Surg* 13:208, 1974.

452. Metcalf W, Papadopoulous A, Tufaro R et al: A clinical physiologic study of hydroxyethyl starch, *Surg Gynecol Obstet* 131:255, 1970.

453. Metildi LA, Shackford SR, Virgilio RW et al: Crystalloid versus colloid in fluid resuscitation of patients with severe pulmonary insufficiency, *Surg Gynecol Obstet* 158:207, 1984.

454. Meyer BJ, Meyer A, and Guyton A: Interstitial fluid pressure, *Clin Res* 22:263, 1968.

455. Michelson E: Anaphylactic reaction to dextrans, *N Engl J Med* 278:552, 1968.

456. Miller CE, Remenchik AP: Problems involved in accurately measuring the potassium content of the human body, *Ann NY Acad Sci* 110:175, 1963.

457. Miller M, Kalkos T, Moses AM et al: Recognition of partial defects in antidiuretic hormone secretion, *Ann Intern Med* 73:721, 1970.

458. Miller RD: The match transfusion. Intraoperative coagulation defects, *Annual refresher course lectures,* Washington, DC, 1974, America Society of Anesthesiologists Annual Meeting.

459. Miller RD: Transfusion therapy. In *Anesthesia,* ed 3, New York, 1990, Churchill-Livingstone.

460. Miller TA, Duke JH: Fluid and electrolyte management. In Dudrick SJ, ed: *Manual of preoperative and postoperative care,* ed 3, Philadelphia, 1983, WB Saunders.

461. Milnor WR: Regional circulations. In Mountcastle VB, ed: *Medical physiology,* St Louis, 1974, CV Mosby.

462. Mitchell JH, Sildenthal K, and Johnson RL: The effects of acid-base disturbances on cardiovascular and pulmonary function, *Kidney Int* 1:375, 1972.

463. Mitchell JH, Wildenthal K, and Johnson RL: The effect of acid-base disturbances on cardiovascular and pulmonary function, *Kidney Int* 1:375, 1973.

464. Mitchell RA, Singer MM: Respiration and cerebral spinal fluid pH in metabolic acidosis and alkalosis, *J Appl Physiol* 20:905, 1965.

465. Mithoefer JC, Porter WF, and Karetzky MS: Indications for the use of sodium bicarbonate in the treatment of intractable asthma, *Respiration* 25:201, 1968.

466. Mizock BA, Falk JL: Lactic acidosis in critical illness, *Crit Care Med* 20:80, 1992.

467. Modig J: Effectiveness of dextran-70 versus Ringer's acetate in traumatic shock in adult respiratory distress syndrome, *Crit Care Med* 14:454, 1986.

468. Modig J: Comparison of effects of dextran-70 and Ringer's acetate on pulmonary function, hemodynamics and survival in experimental septic shock, *Crit Care Med* 16:266, 1988.

469. Mohsenifar Z, Goldbach P, Tashkin DP et al: Relationship between O_2 delivery and O_2 consumption in the adult respiratory distress syndrome, *Chest* 84:267, 1983.

470. Molloy DW, Dhingra S, Solven F et al: Hypomagnesemia and respiratory muscle power, *Am Rev Respir Dis* 129:497, 1984.

471. Mondzelewski JP, Guy JT, Bromberg PA et al: Oxygen delivery following transfusion of stored blood. II. Acidotic rats, *J Appl Physiol* 37:64, 1974.

472. Monroe RG: Myocardial oxygen consumption during ventricular contractions and relaxation, *Circ Res* 14:294, 1964.

473. Moore FD: Determination of total body water and solids with isotopes, *Science* 104:157, 1946.

474. Moore FD: Common patterns of water and electrolyte change in injury, surgery and disease, *N Engl J Med* 258:277, 1958.

475. Moore FD, McMurrey JD, Parker HV et al: Body composition: total body water and electrolytes: intravascular and extravascular phase volumes, *Metabolism* 5:447, 1959.

476. Moore GL, Ledford ME, and Merydith A: The biochemical effects on CPDA-2-drawn red blood cells of delayed refrigeration prior to component preparation, *Transfusion* 22:485, 1982.

477. Moore GL, Peck CC, Sohmer PR et al: Some properties of blood stored in CPDA-1 solution, *Transfusion* 21:135, 1981.

478. Moran WH, Mittenberger FW, Shuayb WA et al: Relationship of antidiuretic hormone secretion to surgical stress, *Surgery* 56:99, 1964.

479. Mordes JP, Tranquada RE, and Rossini AA: Lactic acidosis. In Rippe JM, Irwin RS, and Alpert JS et al, eds: *Intensive care medicine,* Boston, 1985, Little, Brown.

480. Morff RJ, Granger HJ: Contribution of adenosine to arteriolar autoregulation in striated muscle, *Am J Physiol* 244:H567, 1983.

481. Morgan DB, Young RM: Acute transient hypokalemia: new interpretation of a common event, *Lancet* 2:751, 1982.

482. Morissette M, Weil MH, and Shubin H: Reduction in colloid osmotic pressure associated with fatal progression of car-

diopulmonary failure, *Crit Care Med* 3:115, 1975.

483. Moses AM, Notman DD: Diabetes insipidus and the syndrome of inappropriate anti-diuretic hormone secretion (SIADH), *Adv Intern Med* 27:73, 1982.

484. Moss GS, Lower RJ, Jilek J et al: Colloid or crystalloid in the resuscitation of hemorrhagic shock: a controlled clinical trial, *Surgery* 89:434, 1981.

485. Mowry RW, Millican RD: A histochemical study of the distribution and fate of dextran in tissues of the mouse, *Am J Pathol* 29:523, 1953.

486. Muller MC: Anesthesia for the patient with renal dysfunction, *Int Anaesthesiol Clin* 22:169, 1984.

487. Muller-Plathe O, Lindemann K: Ionized calcium versus total calcium, *Scand J Clin Lab Invest* 43(165):71, 1983.

488. Mundy GR, Raisz LG, Cooper RH et al: Evidence for the secretion of an osteoclast stimulating factor in myeloma, *N Engl J Med* 291:1041, 1974.

489. Murray JF: Venous oxygenation and circulatory responses to oxygen inhalation in acute anemia, *Am J Physiol* 207:228, 1964.

490. Nakayama S, Sibley L, Gunther RA et al: Small volume resuscitation with hypertonic saline (2400 mOsm/L) during hemorrhagic shock, *Circ Shock* 13:149, 1984.

491. Nanji AA: Drug-induced electrolyte disorders, *Drug Intell Clin Pharm* 17:175, 1983.

492. Nanninga LB: Calculation of free magnesium, calcium and potassium in muscle, *Biochem Biophys Acta* 54:338, 1961.

493. Narins RG: Acid-base disorders: definitions and introductory concepts. In Maxwell MH, Kleeman CR, and Narins RG, eds: *Clinical disorders of fluid and electrolyte metabolism*, ed 4, New York, 1987, McGraw-Hill.

494. Narins RG, Emmett M: Simple and mixed acid-base disorders: a practical approach, *Medicine* 59:161, 1980.

495. Narins RG, Gardner LB: Simple acid-base disorders, *Med Clin North Am* 65(2):321, 1981.

496. Narins RG, Goldberg M: Renal tubular acidosis: pathophysiology, diagnosis and treatment. Normal acid-base physiology. In Dolling HF, ed: *DM*, Chicago, 1977, Year Book Medical Publishers.

497. Narins RG, Jones ER, and Dornfeld LP: Alkali therapy of the organic acidoses: a critical assessment of the data and the case for judicious use of sodium bicarbonate. In Narins RG, ed: *Controversies in nephrology and hypertension*, New York, 1984, Churchill-Livingstone.

498. Narins RG, Jones ER, Stom MC et al: Diagnostic strategies in disorders of fluid, electrolyte and acid-base homeostasis, *Am J Med* 72:496, 1982.

499. Narins RG, Krishna GG, Bressler L et al: The metabolic acidoses. In Maxwell MH, Kleeman CR, and Narins RG, eds: *Clinical disorders of fluid and electrolyte metabolism*, ed 4, New York, 1987, McGraw-Hill.

500. National Blood Resource Education Program: Transfusion alert: indications for the use of red blood cells, platelets

and fresh frozen plasma, NIH publication 89-2974a, May, 1989.

501. Nearman HS, Eckhauser ML: Postoperative management of a severely anemic Jehovah's witness, *Crit Care Med* 2:142, 1983.

502. Nearman HS, Herman ML: Toxic effects of colloids in the intensive care unit, *Crit Care Med* 7:713, 1991.

503. Nerlich M, Gunther R, and Durling RH: Resuscitation from hemorrhagic shock with hypertonic saline or lactated Ringer's (effect on the pulmonary and systemic microcirculation), *Circ Shock* 10:179, 1983.

504. Ng ML, Levy MN, and Zieske HA: Effects of changes of pH and carbon dioxide tension on left ventricular performances, *Am J Physiol* 213:115, 1967.

505. Nicolas G, Kahn T, Sanchez A et al: Glucose-induced hyperkalemia in diabetic subjects, *Arch Intern Med* 141:49, 1981.

506. Nielsen O: Sequential changes in circulating total protein and albumin masses after abdominal vascular surgery, *Ann Surg* 202:231, 1985.

507. Nunn JF: Carbon dioxide. In *Applied respiratory physiology*, ed 3, London, 1987, Butterworths.

508. Nunn JF: Control of breathing. In *Applied respiratory physiology*, ed 3, London, 1987, Butterworths.

509. Nunn JF: Diffusion and alveolar/capillary permeability. In *Applied respiratory physiology*, ed 3, London, 1987, Butterworths.

510. Nunn JF: Distribution of pulmonary ventilation and perfusion. In *Applied respiratory physiology*, ed 3, London, 1987, Butterworths.

511. Oester A, Madsen PO: Determination of absorption of irrigating fluid during transurethral resection of the prostate by means of radioisotopes, *J Urol* 102:714, 1969.

512. Oh MS, Carroll HJ: Electrolyte and acid-base disorders. In Chernow B, ed: *The pharmacologic approach to the critically ill patient*, ed 2, Baltimore, 1988, Williams & Wilkins.

513. Oh MS, Carroll HJ: Disorders of sodium metabolism: hypernatremia and hyponatremia, *Crit Care Med* 20:94, 1992.

514. O'Kelley R, Magee F, and McKenna TJ: Routine heparin therapy inhibits adrenal aldosterone production, *J Clin Endocrinol Metab* 56:108, 1983.

515. Opie LH: Effect of extracellular pH on function and metabolism of isolated perfused rat heart, *Am J Physiol* 209:1075, 1965.

516. Orlinger CE, Eustace JC, Wunsch CD et al: Natural history of lactic acidosis after grand mal seizures, *N Engl J Med* 297:796, 1977.

517. Orloff MJ, Hutchin P: Fluid and electrolyte response to trauma and surgery. In Maxwell MH, Kleeman CR, eds: *Clinical disorders of fluid and electrolyte metabolism*, ed 2, New York, 1972, McGraw-Hill.

518. Orr MD: Autotransfusion: intraoperative scavenging, *Int Anesth Clin* 20:97, 1982.

519. Orr MD: Autologous transfusion: a via-

ble alternative, *J Cardiothorac Anesth* 2(1):7, 1988.

520. Oster JR, Epstein M: Acid-base aspects of ketoacidosis, *Am J Nephrol* 4:137, 1984.

521. Owen OE, Reichard GA: Human forearm metabolism during progressive starvation, *J Clin Invest* 50:1536, 1971.

522. Pace N, Kline L, Schachman HK et al: Studies on body composition. IV. Use of radioactive hydrogen for measurement in vivo of total body water, *J Biol Chem* 168:459, 1947.

523. Pace N, Rathbun EN: Studies of body composition. III. The body water and chemically combined nitrogen content in relation to fat content, *J Biol Chem* 158:685, 1945.

524. Paddle BM, Haugaard N: Role of magnesium in effects of epinephrine on heart contraction and metabolism, *Am J Physiol* 221:1178, 1971.

525. Parkinson CA, Belton SJ, and Pratt JH: The effect of captopril treatment on potassium-induced stimulation of aldosterone production in vitro, *Endocrinology* 114:1567, 1984.

526. Pastan SO, Braunwald E. Renal disorders and heart disease. In Braunwald E, ed: *Heart disease*, ed 4, Philadelphia, 1992, WB Saunders.

527. Pentaspan: Package insert, Wilmington, Delaware, 1989, DuPont Pharmaceuticals.

528. Percival RC, Yates AJP, Gray RES et al: Role of glucocorticoids in the management of malignant hypercalcemia, *Br Med J* 289:287, 1984.

529. Peretz DI, Scott HM, Duff J et al: The significance of lacticacidemia in the shock syndrome, *Ann NY Acad Sci* 119:1133, 1965.

530. Perez-Ayuso RM, Arroyo V, Camps J et al: Evidence that renal prostaglandins are involved in renal water metabolism in cirrhosis, *Kidney Int* 26:72, 1984.

531. *Perioperative red cell transfusion*, National Institutes of Health Consensus Development Conference Statement, 7(4), 1988.

532. Perkins HA, Payne R, Ferguson J et al: Nonhemolytic febrile transfusion reactions: quantitative effects of blood components with emphasis on isoantigenic incompatibility of leukocytes, *Vox Sang* 11:578, 1966.

533. Perlia CP, Gubisch NJ, Wolter J et al: Mithramycin treatment of hypercalcemia, *Cancer* 25:389, 1970.

534. Pettinger WA: Anesthetics and the renin-angiotensin-aldosterone axis, *Anesthesiology* 48:393, 1978 (editorial).

535. Petty C: Miscellaneous blood measurements. In Blitt CD, ed: *Monitoring in anesthesia and critical care medicine*, New York, 1985, Churchill-Livingstone.

536. Pick A: Arrhythmias and potassium in man, *Am Heart J* 72:295, 1966.

537. Pierce NF, Fedson DS, Brigham KL et al: The ventilatory response to acute base deficit in humans. Time course during development and correction of metabolic acidosis, *Ann Intern Med* 72:633, 1970.

538. Pildes RS: Neonatal hyperglycemia, *J Pediatr* 109:905, 1986.

539. Pineda AA, Rippeteau ND, Clare DE et al: Infusion flow rates of whole blood and AS-1-preserved erythrocytes: a comparison, *Mayo Clin Proc* 62:199, 1987.

540. Pisciotto PT, Snyder EL: Use and administration of blood and components. In Chernow B, ed: *The pharmacologic approach to the critically ill patient,* ed 2, Baltimore, 1988, Williams & Wilkins.

541. Pitts RF: The role of ammonia production and excretion in regulation of acid-base balance, *N Engl J Med* 284:32, 1971.

542. Pitts RF: Renal regulation of acid-base balance. In *Physiology of the kidney and body fluids,* ed 3, Chicago, 1974, Year Book Medical Publishers.

543. Pitts RF: Volume and composition of the body fluids. In *Physiology of the kidney and body fluids,* ed 3, Chicago, 1974, Year Book Medical Publishers.

544. Pizov R, Ya'ari Y, and Perel A: Systolic pressure variation is greater during hemorrhage than during sodium nitroprusside-induced hypotension in ventilated dogs, *Anesth Analg* 67:170, 1988.

545. Polak A, Haynic GD, Hays RM et al: Effects of chronic hypercapnia on electrolyte and acid-base equilibrium. I. Adaptation, *J Clin Invest* 40:1223, 1961.

546. Pollock AD, Arieff AI: Abnormalities of cell volume regulation and their functional consequence, *Am J Physiol* 239:F195, 1980.

547. Popovsky MA, Devine PA, and Taswell HF: Intraoperative autologous transfusion, *Mayo Clin Proc* 60:125, 1985.

548. Posner JB, Plum F: Spinal fluid pH and neurologic symptoms in systemic acidosis, *N Engl J Med* 277:605, 1967.

549. Price HL, Linde HW, Jones RE et al: Sympathoadrenal responses to general anesthesia in man and the relation to hemodynamics, *Anesthesiology* 20:563, 1959.

550. Prien T, Backhaus N, Pelster F et al: Effect of intraoperative fluid administration and colloid osmotic pressure on the formation of intestinal edema during gastrointestinal surgery, *J Clin Anesth* 2:317, 1990.

551. Pritchard JA: Management of preeclampsia and eclampsia, *Kidney Int* 18:259, 1980.

552. Prough DS, Johnson JC, Poole GV et al: Effects on intracranial pressure of resuscitation from hemorrhagic shock with hypertonic saline versus lactated Ringer's solution, *Crit Care Med* 13:407, 1985.

553. Prough DS, Johnson JC, Stump DA et al: Effects of hypertonic saline versus lactated Ringer's solution on cerebral oxygen transport during resuscitation from hemorrhagic shock, *J Neurosurg* 64:627, 1986.

554. Prough DS, Whitley JM, Olympio MA et al: Hypertonic/hyperoncotic fluid resuscitation after hemorrhagic shock in dogs, *Anesth Analg* 73:738, 1991.

555. Prough DS, Whitley JM, Taylor CL et al: Regional cerebral blood flow following resuscitation from hemorrhagic shock with hypertonic saline: influence of a subdural mass, *Anesthesiology* 75:319, 1991.

556. Prough DS, Whitley JM, Taylor CL et al: Regional cerebral blood flow following resuscitation from hemorrhagic shock with hypertonic saline, *Anesthesiology* 75:319, 1991.

557. Puri VK, Freund U, Carlson RW et al: Colloid osmotic and pulmonary wedge pressure in acute respiratory failure following acute hemorrhage, *Surg Gynecol Obstet* 147:537, 1978.

558. Puri VK, Weil MH, Michaels S et al: Pulmonary edema associated with reduction in plasma oncotic pressure, *Surg Gynecol Obstet* 151:344, 1980.

559. Quamme GA, Dirks KJ: Magnesium metabolism. In Maxwell MH, Kleeman CR, and Narins RG, eds: *Clinical disorders of fluid and electrolyte metabolism,* ed 4, New York, 1987, McGraw-Hill.

560. *Questions and answers about transfusion practices,* Committee on Blood and Blood Products, Park Ridge, Ill, 1987, The American Society of Anesthesiologists.

561. Quinones MA, Gaasch WH, and Alexander JK: Influence of acute changes in preload, afterload, contractile state and heart rate on ejection and isovolumic indices of myocardial contractility in man, *Circulation* 53:293, 1976.

562. Quon CK: Clinical pharmacokinetics and pharmacodynamics of colloidal plasma volume expanders, *J Cardiothorac Anesth* 2(1):13, 1988.

563. Rackow EC: Clinical significance of colloid oncotic pressure, *Anesthesiology Rev* 27(3):6, 1990.

564. Rackow EC: Fluid resuscitation in circulatory shock, *Anesthesiology Rev* 27(3):3, 1990.

565. Rackow EC, Falk JL, Fein IA et al: Comparison of albumin, hetastarch and saline solutions for resuscitation of patients with shock, *Crit Care Med* 10:230, 1982.

566. Rackow EC, Falk JL, Fein IA et al: Fluid resuscitation in shock: a comparison of cardiorespiratory effects of albumin, hetastarch and saline solutions in patients with hypovolemic and septic shock, *Crit Care Med* 11:839, 1983.

567. Rackow EC, Falk JL, and Weil MH: Coagulation profile during albumin and hetastarch fluid resuscitation in patients with septic shock, *Clin Pharmacol Ther* 39(2):220, 1986.

568. Rackow EC, Fein IA, and Leppo J: Colloid osmotic pressure as a prognostic indicator of pulmonary edema and mortality in the critically ill, *Chest* 72:709, 1977.

569. Rackow EC, Fein IA, and Siegel J: The relationships of colloid osmotic-pulmonary artery wedge pressure gradient to pulmonary edema and mortality in critically ill patients, *Chest* 82:433, 1982.

570. Rackow EC, Hormaechea E, Becker H et al: Colloid osmotic pressure, pulmonary artery wedge pressure and the time course for clearance of cardiogenic pulmonary edema, *Circulation* 58(II):109, 1978.

571. Rackow EC, Mecher C, Astiz ME et al: Effects of pentastarch and albumin infusion of cardiorespiratory function and coagulation in patients with severe sep-

sis and systemic hypoperfusion, *Crit Care Med* 17:394, 1989.

572. Rawstron RE: Anaemia and surgery: a retrospective analysis, *Aust NZ J Surg* 39:425, 1970.

573. Reeves WB, Andreoli TE: The posterior pituitary and water metabolism. In Wilson JD, Foster DW, eds: *Williams textbook of endocrinology,* ed 8, Philadelphia, 1992, WB Saunders.

574. Reichek N, Wilson J, Sutton MS et al: Noninvasive determination of left ventricular end systolic stress: validation of the method and initial application, *Circulation* 65:99, 1982.

575. Reineck HJ, Stein JH: Sodium metabolism. In Maxwell MH, Kleeman CR, and Narins RG, eds: *Clinical disorders of fluid and electrolyte metabolism,* ed 4, New York, 1987, McGraw-Hill.

576. Replogle RL, Kundler H, and Gross RE: Studies on the hemodynamic importance of blood viscosity, *J Thorac Cardiovasc Surg* 50:638, 1965.

577. Resuscitation of infants and children. In *Textbook of advanced cardiac life support,* Dallas, 1987, American Heart Association.

578. Richardson TQ, Guyton AC: Effects of polycythemia and anemia on cardiac output and other circulatory factors, *Am J Physiol* 197:1167, 1959.

579. Riley RL, Cournand A: "Ideal" alveolar air and the analysis of ventilation-perfusion relationships in the lungs, *J Appl Physiol* 1:825, 1949.

580. Ring J, Messmer K: Incidence and severity of anaphylactoid reactions to colloid volume substitutes, *Lancet* 1:466, 1977.

581. Risberg B, Webb WR, Osburn K et al: Pulmonary microvascular leakage after microembolization and hemodilution, *Surgery* 92:409, 1982.

582. Robertson GL, Aycinana P, and Zerbe RL: Neurogenic disorders of osmoregulation, *Am J Med* 72:339, 1982.

583. Robertson GL: Abnormalities of thirst regulation, *Kidney Int* 25:460, 1984.

584. Robson AM: Parenteral fluid therapy. In Behrman RE, Vaughan VC, eds: *Nelson textbook of pediatrics,* ed 13, Philadelphia, 1987, WB Saunders.

585. Rocha E, Silva M, Negraes JA et al: Hypertonic resuscitation from severe hemorrhagic shock: patterns of regional circulation, *Circ Shock* 19:165, 1986.

586. Rosa RM, Silva P, Young JB et al: Adrenergic modulation of extrarenal potassium disposal, *N Engl J Med* 302:431, 1980.

587. Rosberg B, Wulff K: Hemodynamics following normovolemic hemodilution in elderly patients, *Acta Anaesth Scand* 25:402, 1981.

588. Rosenthal DS, Braunwald E: Hematological-oncological disorders in heart disease. In Braunwald E, ed: *Heart disease,* ed 3, Philadelphia, 1988, WB Saunders.

589. Ross EJ, Christie SBM: Hypernatremia, *Medicine* 48:441, 1969.

590. Rossi NF, Schrier RW: Hyponatremic states. In Maxwell MH, Kleeman CR, Narins RG, eds: *Clinical disorders of fluid*

and electrolyte metabolism, ed 4, New York, 1987, McGraw-Hill.

591. Rothschild MA, Oratz M, and Schreiber SS: Albumin metabolism, *Gastroenterology* 64:324, 1973.

592. Rothschild MA: Labeled albumin: some recent contributions to current concepts concerning regulation of protein metabolism, *Mt Sinai J Med* 40:474, 1973.

593. Roy SB et al: Hemodynamic effects of chronic severe anemia, *Circulation* 28:346, 1963.

594. Roy SB et al: Determinants and distribution of high cardiac output in chronic severe anemia, *Indian Heart J* 18:325, 1966.

595. Rude RK, Singer FR: Magnesium deficiency and excess, *Annu Rev Med* 32:245, 1981.

596. Rushmer RF: Atherosclerosis: occlusive disease of coronary and peripheral arteries. In *Cardiovascular dynamics,* ed 4, Philadelphia, 1976, WB Saunders.

597. Rushmer RF: Effects of posture. In *Cardiovascular dynamics,* ed 4, Philadelphia, 1976, WB Saunders.

598. Rushmer RF: Peripheral vascular control. In *Cardiovascular dynamics,* ed 4, Philadelphia, 1976, WB Saunders.

599. Rushmer RF: The systemic arterial pressure. In *Cardiovascular dynamics,* ed 4, Philadelphia, 1976, WB Saunders.

600. Ryden SE, Oberman HA: Compatibility of common intravenous solutions with CPD blood, *Transfusion* 15:250, 1975.

601. Ryzen E, Martodam RR, Troxell M et al: Intravenous etidronate in the management of malignant hypercalcemia, *Arch Intern Med* 145:449, 1985.

602. Sade RM, Stroud MR, Crawford FA et al: A prospective randomized study of hydroxyethyl starch, albumin, and lactated Ringer's solution as priming fluid for cardiopulmonary bypass, *J Thorac Cardiovasc Surg* 89:713, 1985.

603. Salem MR, Bennett EJ, Schweiss JF et al: Cardiac arrest related to anesthesia: contributing factors in infants and children, *JAMA* 223: 238, 1975.

604. Samuel JR, Powell D: Renal transplantation. Anaesthetic experience of 100 cases, *Anaesthesia* 25:165, 1970.

605. Sarnaik AP, Meert K, Hackbarth R et al: Management of hyponatremic seizures in children with hypertonic saline. A safe and effective strategy, *Crit Care Med* 19:758, 1991.

606. Sato M, Pawlik G, and Heiss WD: Comparative studies of regional CNS blood flow autoregulation and responses to CO_2 in the cat, *Stroke* 15:91, 1984.

607. Saunders CR, Carlisle L, and Bick RL: Hydroxyethyl starch versus albumin in cardiopulmonary bypass prime solutions, *Ann Thorac Surg* 36:532, 1985.

608. Saxton CR, Seldin DW: Clinical interpretation of laboratory values. In Kokko JP, Tannen RL, eds: *Fluids and electrolytes,* Philadelphia, 1986, WB Saunders.

609. Scatchard G, Batchelder AC, and Brown A: Chemical, clinical and immunological studies on the products of human plasma fractionation. VI. The osmotic pressure of plasma and of serum albumin, *J Clin Invest* 23:458, 1944.

610. Schaeffer RC, Barnhart MI, and Carlson RW: Pulmonary fibrin deposition and increased microvascular permeability to protein following fibrin microembolism in dogs: a structure-function relationship, *Microvasc Res* 33:327, 1987.

611. Scherrer M, Bachofen H: The oxygen-combining capacity of hemoglobin, *Anesthesiology* 36:190, 1972.

612. Schertel ER, Valentine AK, Rademakers AM et al: Influence of 7% NaCl on the mechanical properties of the systemic circulation in the hypervolemic dog, *Circ Shock* 31:203, 1990.

613. Schiffer MA, Pakter J, and Clahr J: Mortality associated with hypertonic saline abortion, *Obstet Gynecol* 42:759, 1973.

614. Schneider AB, Sherwood LM: Calcium homeostasis and the pathogenesis and management of hypercalcemic disorders, *Metabolism* 23:975, 1974.

615. Schrier RW, Conger JD: Acute renal failure: pathogenesis, diagnosis, and management. In Schrier RW, ed: *Renal and electrolyte disorders,* Boston, 1976, Little, Brown.

616. Schulte TL, Hammer HJ, and Reynolds LR: Clinical use of Cytal in urology, *J Urol* 71:656, 1954.

617. Schumer W: Physiochemical and metabolic effects of low molecular weight dextran in oligemic shock, *J Trauma* 199:297, 1967.

618. Schwartz AB: Potassium-related cardiac arrhythmias and their treatment, *Angiology* 29:194, 1978.

619. Schwartz S, Frantz RA, and Shoemaker WC: Sequential hemodynamic and oxygen transport responses in hypovolemia, anemia and hypoxia, *Am J Physiol* 241: H864, 1981.

620. Schwartz WB, von Ypersele de Strihou C et al: Role of anions in metabolic alkalosis and potassium deficiency, *N Engl J Med* 279:630, 1968.

621. Scott R, Deane RF, and Callander R: Diseases of the prostate. In *Urology illustrated,* ed 2, New York, 1982, Churchill-Livingstone.

622. Sehgal LR, Gould SA, Rosen AL et al: Polymerized pyridoxylated hemoglobin: a red cell substitute with normal O_2 capacity, *Surgery* 95:433, 1984.

623. Sehgal LR, Rosen AL, Gould SA et al: Artificial blood, *Anesthesiology Rev* 27(3):38, 1990.

624. Seyberth HW, Segre GV, Morgan JL et al: Prostaglandins as mediators of hypercalcemia associated with certain types of cancer, *N Engl J Med* 293:1278, 1975.

625. Shackford SR: Hypertonic saline and dextran for intraoperative fluid therapy: more or less, *Crit Care Med* 20:160, 1992 (editorial).

626. Shackford SR, Fortlage DA, Peters RM et al: Serum osmolar and electrolyte changes associated with large infusions of hypertonic sodium lactate for intravascular volume expansion of patients undergoing aortic reconstruction, *Surg Gynecol Obstet* 164:127, 1987.

627. Shackford SR, Sise MJ, Fridlund PH et al: Hypertonic sodium lactate versus lactated Ringer's solution for intrave-nous fluid therapy in operations on the abdominal aorta, *Surgery* 94:41, 1983.

628. Sharpey-Schafer EP: Cardiac output in severe anemia, *Clin Sci* 5:125, 1944.

629. Shatney CH, Krishnapradad D, Militello PR et al: Efficacy of hetastarch and the resuscitation of patients with multisystem trauma and shock, *Arch Surg* 118: 804, 1983.

630. Shear L, Brandman LS: Hypoxemia and hypercapnia caused by respiratory compensation for metabolic alkalosis, *Am Rev Respir Dis* 107:836, 1973.

631. Sheldon GF: Diphosphoglycerate in massive transfusion and erythropoiesis, *Crit Care Med* 7:407, 1979.

632. Sherwood LM: The multiple causes of hypercalcemia in malignant disease, *N Engl J Med* 303:1412, 1980.

633. Shibutani K, Komatsu T, Kubal K et al: Critical level of oxygen delivery in anesthetized man, *Crit Care Med* 11:640, 1983.

634. Shimazaki S, Toshiharu Y, Tanaka N et al: Body fluid changes during hypertonic lactated saline solution therapy for burn shock, *J Trauma* 17:38, 1977.

635. Shires GT: Postoperative, posttraumatic management of fluids, *Bull NY Acad Med* 55:248, 1979.

636. Shires GT, Canizaro PC: Fluid, electrolyte and nutritional management of the surgical patient. In Schwartz SI, ed: *Principles of surgery,* ed 2, New York, 1974, McGraw-Hill.

637. Shires GT, Peitzman A, Albert S et al: Response of extravascular lung water to intraoperative fluids, *Ann Surg* 197:515, 1983.

638. Shires GT, Shires III GT: Routine perioperative fluid and electrolyte management. In Maxwell MH, Kleeman CR, and Narins RG, eds: *Clinical disorders of fluid and electrolyte metabolism,* ed 4, New York, 1987, McGraw-Hill.

639. Shires T, Williams J, and Brown F: Acute change in extracellular fluids associated with major surgical procedures, *Ann Surg* 154:803, 1961.

640. Shoemaker WC: Fluids and electrolytes in the acutely ill adult. In Schoemaker WC, Ayres S, Grenvik A et al, eds: *Textbook of critical care,* ed 2, Philadelphia, 1989, WB Saunders.

641. Shoemaker WC: Use and abuse of the Swan-Ganz catheter: are patients getting their money's worth? *Crit Care Med* 18:1294, 1990.

642. Shoemaker WC: Tissue perfusion in oxygenation: a primary problem in acute circulatory failure and shock states, *Crit Care Med* 19:595, 1991.

643. Shoemaker WC, Appel PL, Bland R et al: Clinical trial of an algorithm for outcome prediction in acute circulatory failure, *Crit Care Med* 10:390, 1982.

644. Shoemaker WC, Appel PL, and Kram HB: Measurement of tissue perfusion by oxygen transport patterns in experimental shock and high risk surgical patients, *Intensive Care Med* 16:S135, 1990.

645. Shoemaker WC, Boyd DR, Kim SF et al: Sequential oxygen transport and acid-base changes after trauma to the unanesthetized patient, *Surg Gynecol Obstet* 144:909, 1977.

646. Shoemaker WC, Czer LSC: Evaluation of the biologic importance of various hemodynamic and oxygen transport variables: which variables should be monitored in postoperative shock? *Crit Care Med* 7:424, 1979.

647. Sibbald WJ, Warshawski FJ, Short AK et al: Clinical studies of measuring extravascular lung water by the thermal dye technique in critically ill patients, *Chest* 5:725, 1983.

648. Sieber FE, Smith DS, Traystman RJ et al: Glucose: a reevaluation of its intraoperative use, *Anesthesiology* 67:72, 1987.

649. Siegel JH, Farrel EF, Goldwyn RM et al: The surgical implications of physiologic patterns in myocardial infarction shock, *Surgery* 72:126, 1972.

650. Siegel JH, Rivkind AI, Dalal SA et al: Early physiologic predictors of injury severity and death in blunt multiple trauma, *Arch Surg* 125:498, 1990.

651. Siesjö BK: Cerebral circulation and metabolism, *J Neurosurg* 60:883, 1984.

652. Sigaard-Andersen O: The pH, log P_{CO_2} blood acid-base nomogram revised, *Scand J Clin Lab Invest* 14:598, 1962.

653. Sigaard-Andersen O: Acid-base balance, *Scand J Clin Lab Invest* 15(70), 1963.

654. Sigaard-Andersen O, Engel K, Jorgensen K et al: A micro-method for determination of pH, carbon dioxide tension, base excess and standard bicarbonate in capillary blood, *Scand J Clin Lab Invest* 12:172, 1960.

655. Siggard-Anderson O, Thode J, and Fogh-Anderson N: What is "ionized calcium"? *Scand J Clin Lab Invest* 43(165):11, 1983.

656. Siker D: Pediatric fluids and electrolytes. In Gregory GA, ed: *Pediatric anesthesia,* ed 2, New York, 1989, Churchill-Livingstone.

657. Silva P, Brown RS, and Epstein FH: Adaptation to potassium, *Kidney Int* 11:466, 1977.

658. Silva P, Spokes K: Sympathetic system in potassium homeostasis, *Am J Physiol* 241:F151, 1981.

659. Silva P, Spokes K, and Epstein FH: Catecholamines in potassium homeostasis, *Kidney Int* 12:544, 1977.

660. Simmons MA, Adcock EW, Bard H et al: Hypernatremia and intracranial hemorrhage in neonates, *N Engl J Med* 291:6, 1974.

661. Simon TL, Marcus CS, Myhre BA et al: Effects of AS-3 nutrient additive solution on 42-49 day storage of red cells, *Transfusion* 27:178, 1987.

662. Simon T, Nelson EJ: Study of a new system for white cell removal from red blood cell concentrates by filtration prior to storage (abstract), *Transfusion* 27:530, 1987.

663. Singer FR, Neer RM, Murray TM et al: Mithramycin treatment of intractable hypercalcemia due to parathyroid carcinoma, *N Engl J Med* 283:634, 1970.

664. Singer FR, Sharp CF, and Rude RK: Pathogenesis of hypercalcemia in malignancy, *Mineral Electrolyte Metab* 2:161, 1978.

665. Singer I: Differential diagnosis of polyuria and diabetes insipidus, *Med Clin North Am* 65:303, 1981.

666. Singer I, Forrest JN: Drug-induced states of nephrogenic diabetes insipidus, *Kidney Int* 10:82, 1976.

667. Singh YN, Harvey AL, and Marshall IG: Antibiotic-induced paralysis of the mouse phrenic nerve-hemidiaphragm preparation, and reversability by calcium and neostigmine, *Anesthesiology* 48:418, 1978.

668. Skelton H: The storage of water by various tissues of the body, *Arch Int Med* 40:140, 1927.

669. Skillman JJ, Awwad HK, and Moore FD: Plasma protein kinetics of the early transcapillary refill after hemorrhage in man, *Surg Gynecol Obstet* 125:983, 1967.

670. Skillman JJ, Restall S, and Salzman EW: Randomized trial of albumin vs. electrolyte solutions during abdominal aortic operations, *Surgery* 78:291, 1975.

671. Skou JC: Enzymatic basis for active transport of Na^+ and K^+ across cell membranes, *Physiol Rev* 45:596, 1965.

672. Skowsky WR, Nikuchi I: The role of vasopressin in the impaired water excretion of myxedema, *Am J Med* 64:613, 1978.

673. Sladen RN: Effect of anesthesia and surgery on renal function, *Crit Care Clin* 3(2):373, 1987.

674. Slater JDH: The hormonal control of body sodium, *Postgrad Med J* 40:479, 1964.

675. Smith AL, Wollman H: Cerebral blood flow and metabolism: effects of anesthetic drugs and techniques, *Anesthesiology* 36:378, 1972.

676. Smith HJ, Antoonisen NR: Results of cardiac resuscitation in 254 patients, *Lancet* 1:1027, 1965.

677. Smith TW, Braunwald E, and Kelly RA: The management of heart failure. In Braunwald E, ed: *Heart disease,* Philadelphia, 1992, WB Saunders.

678. Smithline N, Gardner D: Gaps—anionic and osmolal, *JAMA* 236:1594, 1976.

679. Snyder AJ, Gottschall JL, and Menitove JE: Why is fresh-frozen plasma transfused? *Transfusion* 26:107, 1986.

680. Snyder EL, Hezzey A, Joyner R et al: Stability of red cell antigens during prolonged storage in citrate-phosphate-dextrose and a new preservative solution, *Transfusion* 23:165, 1983.

681. Snyder JV: Oxygen transport: the model and reality. In *Oxygen transport in the critically ill,* Chicago, 1987, Year Book Medical Publishers.

682. Sobel BE: Cardiac and noncardiac forms of acute circulatory collapse (shock). In Braunwald E, ed: *Heart disease,* Philadelphia, 1980, WB Saunders.

683. Sohmer PR, Dawson RB: The significance of 2,3-DPG in red blood cell transfusions, *Crit Rev Clin Lab Sci* 11:107, 1979.

684. Sokoll MD, Gergis SD: Antibiotics and neuromuscular function, *Anesthesiology* 55:148, 1981.

685. Solomon RJ, Katz JD: Disturbances of potassium homeostasis. In Stoelting RK, ed: *Advances in anesthesia,* vol 3, Chicago, 1986, Year Book Medical Publishers.

686. Sorensen SC: Theoretical considerations on the potential hazards of hyperventilation during anesthesia, *Acta Anaesthesiol Scand* 67:106, 1978.

687. Spence RK, Carson JA, Poses R et al: Elective surgery without transfusion: influence of preoperative hemoglobin level and blood loss on mortality, *Am J Surg* 159:320, 1990.

688. Sprung CL, Isikoff S, Hauser M et al: Comparison of measured and calculated colloid osmotic pressure of serum and pulmonary edema fluid in patients with pulmonary edema, *Crit Care Med* 8:613, 1980.

689. Sprung J, Cheng EY, Gamulin S et al: Effects of acute hypothermia and β-adrenergic receptor blockade on serum potassium concentration in rats, *Crit Care Med* 19:1545, 1991.

690. Stamy TA: The pathogenesis and implications of the electrolyte imbalance in ureterosigmoidostomy, *Surg Gynecol Obstet* 103:736, 1959.

691. Starling EH: On the absorption of fluids from the connective tissue spaces, *J Physiol (Lond)* 9:312, 1896.

692. Staub NC: Pulmonary edema, *Physiol Rev* 54:687, 1971.

693. Steele JM, Berger EY, Dunning MF et al: Total body water in man, *Am J Physiol* 162:313, 1950.

694. Steffes CP, Bender JS, and Levison MA: Blood transfusion and oxygen consumption in surgical sepsis, *Crit Care Med* 19:512, 1991.

695. Stehling L: Perioperative morbidity in anemic patients (abstract), *Transfusion* 29:37S, 1989.

696. Stehling L: The surgical patient: transfusion management. In Wilson SM, Levitt JS, and Strauss RG, eds: *Improving transfusion practice for pediatric patients,* Arlington, 1991, American Association of Blood Banks.

697. Stehling LC: Recent advances in transfusion therapy, *Adv Anesthesiol* 4:213, 1987.

698. Stehling L, Ellison N, Gotta A et al: A survey of transfusion practices among anesthesiologists, *Vox Sang* 62:60, 1987.

699. Sterns RH: Severe hyponatremia: the case for conservative management, *Crit Care Med* 20:534, 1992.

700. Sterns RH, Cox M, Feig PU et al: Internal potassium balance in the control of plasma potassium concentration, *Medicine* 60:339, 1981.

701. Sterns RH, Riggs JE, and Schochet SS: Osmotic demyelination syndrome following correction of hyponatremia, *N Engl J Med* 314:1535, 1986.

702. Sterns RH, Thomass DJ, and Herndon RM: Brain dehydration and neurologic deterioration after rapid correction of hyponatremia, *Kidney Int* 35:69, 1989.

703. Stewart AF: Therapy of malignancy-associated hypercalcemia: 1983, *Am J Med* 74:475, 1983.

704. Stewart AF, Horst R, Deftos LJ et al: Biochemical evaluation of patients with cancer—associated hypercalcemia, *N Engl J Med* 303:1377, 1980.

705. Stock JL: Disorders of calcium and

magnesium metabolism. In Rippe JM, Irwin RS, Alpert JS et al, eds: *Intensive care medicine,* Boston, 1985, Little, Brown.

706. Strauch BS, Ball MF: Hemodialysis in the treatment of severe hypercalcemia, *JAMA* 235:1347, 1976.

707. Strauss RG: Review of the effects of hydroxyethyl starch on the blood coagulation system, *Transfusion* 21:299, 1981.

708. Strauss RG, Stansfield C, Henriksen RA et al: Pentastarch may cause fewer effects on coagulation than hetastarch, *Transfusion* 28:257, 1988.

709. Strauss RG, Stump DC, Henriksen RA et al: Effects of hydroxyethyl starch on fibrinogen, fibrin clot formation and fibrinolysis, *Transfusion* 25:230, 1985.

710. Struthers AD, Whitesmith T, and Reid JL: Prior thiazide diuretic treatment increases adrenaline-induced hypokalemia, *Lancet* 1:1358, 1983.

711. Sulway MJ, Malins JM: Acetone in DKA, *Lancet* 2:736, 1970.

712. Sunder-Plasmann L, Klovenkorn WP, Holper K et al: The physiologic significance of acutely induced hemodilution: effects on hemodynamics, oxygen transport and lung water in anesthetized man, *Surg Forum* 24:201, 1973.

713. Surawicz B: Relationship between electrocardiogram and electrolytes, *Am Heart J* 73:814, 1967.

714. Sutton RAL, Dirks JH: Disturbances of calcium and magnesium metabolism. In Brenner BM, Rector FC, eds: *The kidney,* ed 4, Philadelphia, 1991, WB Saunders.

715. Szymanski IO, Carrington EJ: Evaluation of a large-scale frozen blood program, *Transfusion* 17:431, 1977.

716. Tannen RL: Disorders of potassium balance. In Brenner BM, Rector FC, eds: *The kidney,* ed 4, Philadelphia, 1991, WB Saunders.

717. Tarail R, Buchwald KW, Holland JF et al: Misleading reductions of serum sodium and chloride associated with hyperproteinemia in patients with multiple myeloma, *Proc Soc Exp Biol Med* 110:145, 1962.

718. Taylor AE: Capillary fluid filtration: Starling forces and lymph flow, *Circ Res* 49:557, 1981.

719. Taylor AE, Parker JC, Allison RC et al: Capillary exchange of fluid and protein. In Shoemaker WC, Ayres S, Grenvik A et al, eds: *Textbook of critical care,* ed 2, Philadelphia, 1989, WB Saunders.

720. Taylor G, Larson CP, and Restwich R: Unexpected cardiac arrest during anesthesia and surgery, an environmental study, *JAMA* 236:2758, 1976.

721. Taylor RO, Maxson ES, Carter FH et al: Volumetric, gravimetric and radioisotopic determination of fluid transfer in transurethral prostatectomy, *J Urol* 79: 490, 1958.

722. Tenney SM, Mithoefer JC: The relationship of mixed venous oxygenation to oxygen transport, *Am Rev Respir Dis* 125:474, 1982.

723. Textor SC, Bravo EL, Fouad F et al: Hyperkalemia in azotemic patients during angiotensin-converting enzyme inhibition and adosterone reduction with captopril, *Am J Med* 83:719, 1982.

724. Thomas DJ: Whole blood viscosity and cerebral blood flow, *Stroke* 13:285, 1982 (editorial).

725. Thompson WL: Rational use of albumin and plasma substitutes, *Johns Hop Med J* 5:220, 1975.

726. Thompson WL, Bacek LA, Powell SH et al: Albumin versus hydroxyethyl starch in hypoalbuminemic patients, *Clin Res* 78:718A, 1980.

727. Thompson WL, Britton JJ, and Walton RP: Persistence of starch derivatives and dextran when infused after hemorrhage, *J Pharmacol Exper Ther* 136:125, 1962.

728. Thoren L: Magnesium deficiency in gastrointestinal fluid loss, *Acta Chir Scand* 306:5, 1963.

729. Thulstrup H: The influence of leukocyte and thrombocyte incompatibility on non-hemolytic transfusion reactions, *Vox Sang* 21:233, 1971.

730. Thys DM, Kaplan JA: Cardiovascular physiology. In Miller RD, ed: *Anesthesia,* ed 3, New York, 1990, Churchill-Livingstone.

731. Tonnesen AS: Chrystalloids and cholloids. In Miller RD, ed: *Anesthesia,* ed 3, New York, 1990, Churchill-Livingstone.

732. Torrance J, Jacobs P, Restrepo A et al: Intraerythrocytic adaptation to anemia, *N Engl J Med* 283:165, 1970.

733. Traverso WL, Bellamy RF, Hollenbach SJ et al: Hypertonic sodium chloride solutions: effect on hemodynamics and survival after hemorrhagic shock in swine, *J Trauma* 27:32, 1987.

734. Tuchschmidt J, Fried J, Swinney R et al: Early hemodynamic correlates of survival in patients with septic shock, *Crit Care Med* 17:719, 1989.

735. Tuchschmidt J, Oblitas D, and Fried JC: Oxygen consumption in sepsis and septic shock, *Crit Care Med* 19:664, 1991.

736. Ukai M, Moran WH, and Zimmermann B: The role of visceral afferent pathways in vasopressin secretion and urinary excretory patterns during surgical stress, *Ann Surg* 168:16, 1968.

737. Ulstad DR, Godfrey PM, Robbins R et al: Red cell transfusion in a critical care unit, *J Intensive Care Med* 5:205, 1990.

738. Use of blood components, *FDA Drug Bulletin* 19(2):1, 1989.

739. Valeri CR: Viability and function of preserved RBCs, *N Engl J Med* 284:81, 1971.

740. Valeri CR: Measurement of viable Adsol-preserved human red cells, *N Engl J Med* 312:377, 1985.

741. Valeri CR, Collins FB: Physiologic effects of 2,3-DPG-depleted red cells with high affinity for oxygen, *J Appl Physiol* 31:823, 1971.

742. Valeri CR, Hirsch NM: Restoration of in vivo erythrocyte adenosine triphosphate 2,3-diphosphoglycerate, potassium ion and sodium ion concentrations following the transfusion of acid-citrate-dextrose-stored human red blood cells, *J Lab Clin Med* 73:722, 1969.

743. Valeri CR, Yarnoz M, Vecchione JJ et al: Improved oxygen delivery to the myocardium during hypothermia by transfusion with 2,3-DPG-enriched red blood cells, *Ann Thorac Surg* 30:527, 1980.

744. Valeri CR, Zaroulis CG, Vecchione JJ et al: Therapeutic effectiveness and safety of out-dated human red blood cells rejuvenated to restore oxygen transport function to normal, frozen, for 3 to 4 years at $-80°$ C, washed, and stored at $4°$ C for 24 hours prior to rapid infusion, *Transfusion* 20:159, 1980.

745. Vandam LD, Harrison H, Murray JA et al: Anesthetic aspects of renal homotransplantation in man, *Anesthesiology* 23:783, 1962.

746. Varat MA, Adolph RJ, and Fowler NO: Cardiovascular effects of anemia, *Am Heart J* 83:415, 1972.

747. Vaughan RS: Potassium in the perioperative period, *Br J Anaesth* 67:194, 1991.

748. Vaughan RS, Lunn JN: Potassium and the anaesthetist: a review, *Anaesthesia* 28:118, 1973.

749. Velasco IT, Pontieri V, Rocha E Silva M et al: Hyperosmotic NaCl and severe hemorrhagic shock, *Am J Physiol* 239: H664, 1980.

750. Venkataraman PS, Tsang RC, Steichen JJ et al: Early neonatal hypocalcemia in extremely preterm infants, *AJDC* 140: 1004, 1986.

751. Vincent HH, Boomsma F, Man in't Veld AJ et al: Effects of selective and nonselective beta agonists on plasma potassium and norepinephrine, *J Cardiovasc Pharmacol* 6:107, 1984.

752. Virgilio RW, Rice CL, Smith DE et al: Crystalloid versus colloid resuscitation: is one better? *Surgery* 85:129, 1979.

753. Vitez TS, Soper LE, and Soper PG: Chronic hypokalemia does not increase anesthetic dysrhythmias, *Anesth Analg* 61:221, 1982.

754. Vitez TS, Soper LE, Wong KC et al: Chronic hypokalemia and intraoperative dysrhythmias, *Anesthesiology* 63:130, 1985.

755. Walser M: Magnesium metabolism, *Rev Physiol Biochem Exp Pharm* 59:185, 1967.

756. Walter RH, Morgan FM, Songkhla YN et al: Water and electrolyte studies in cholera, *J Clin Invest* 38:1879, 1959.

757. Ward JW, Holmberg SD, Allen JR et al: Transmission of human immunodeficiency virus (HIV) by blood transfusions screened as negative for HIV antibody, *N Engl J Med* 318:473, 1988.

758. Warner GF, Sweet NJ, and Dobson EL: Sodium space and body sodium content, exchangeable with sodium-24 in normal individuals and in patients with ascites, *Circ Res* 1:486, 1953.

759. Waxman K, Holmes R, Tominaga G et al: Hemodynamic and oxygen transport effects of pentastarch in burn resuscitation, *Ann Surg* 209:341, 1989.

760. Weil MH, Henning RJ, Morissette M et al: Relationship between colloid osmotic pressure and pulmonary artery wedge pressure in patients with acute respiratory failure, *Am J Med* 64:643, 1978.

761. Weil MH, Michaels S, Puri VK et al: The stat laboratory. Facilitating blood gas and biochemical measurements for the

critically ill and injured, *Am J Clin Pathol* 76:34, 1981.

762. Weil MH, von Planta M, and Rackow EC: Acute circulatory failure (shock). In Braunwald E, ed: *Heart disease,* ed 4, Philadelphia, 1992, WB Saunders.

763. Weisel RD, Dennis RC, Manny J et al: Adverse effects of transfusion therapy during abdominal aortic aneurysectomy, *Surgery* 83:682, 1978.

764. Weissman P, Stienkman L, and Gregerian RI: Chlorpropamide hyponatremia. Drug induced inappropriate ADH activity, *N Engl J Med* 28:65, 1971.

765. West JB: Gas exchange. In *Pulmonary pathophysiology — the essentials,* Baltimore, 1982, Williams & Wilkins.

766. Whalley PJ, Pritchard JA: Oxytocin and water intoxication, *JAMA* 186:601, 1963.

767. Whang R, Flink EB, Dyckner T et al: Magnesium depletion as a cause of refractory potassium repletion, *Arch Intern Med* 145:1686, 1985.

768. Wharton RS, Mazze RI: Fluid and electrolyte problems. In Orkin FK, Cooperman LH, eds: *Complications in anesthesiology,* Philadelphia, 1983, JB Lippincott.

769. White RD, Goldsmith RS, Rodriquez R et al: Plasma tonic calcium levels following injection of chlorine, gluconate and gluceptate salts of calcium, *J Thorac Cardiovasc Surg* 71:609, 1976.

770. Widdowson EM, McCance RA, and Spray CM: The chemical composition of the human body, *Clin Sci* 10:113, 1951.

771. Widmer B, Gerhardt RE, Harrington JT et al: Serum electrolyte and acid-base composition: the influence of graded degrees of chronic renal failure, *Arch Intern Med* 139:1099, 1979.

772. Wiederhielm CA: Dynamics of transcapillary fluid exchange, *J Gen Physiol* (II): 29s, 1952.

773. Wilcox CS: Diuretics. In Brenner BM, Rector FC, eds: *The kidney,* ed 4, Philadelphia, 1991, WB Saunders.

774. Wilkerson DK, Rosen AL, Gould SA et al: Oxygen extraction ratio: a valid indicator of myocardial metabolism in anemia, *J Surg Res* 42:629, 1987.

775. Wilkerson DK, Rosen AL, Lakshman R et al: Limits of cardiac compensation in anemic baboons, *Surgery* 103:665, 1988.

776. Williamson JR, Safer B, Rich T et al: Effects of acidosis on myocardial contractility and metabolism, *Acta Med Scand* 587:95, 1975.

777. Wilson HK, Kener SP, Lea AS et al: Phosphate therapy in DKA, *Arch Intern Med* 142:517, 1982.

778. Wilson RF, Gibson D, and Percivel AK: Severe alkalosis in critically ill surgical patients, *Arch Surg* 105:197, 1972.

779. Winkler AW, Smith PK: The apparent volume of distribution of potassium injected intravenously, *J Biol Chem* 124: 589, 1938.

780. Wittmers LE, Bartlett M, and Johnson JA: Estimation of capillary permeability coefficient of inulin in various tissues of the rabbit, *Microvasc Res* 11:67, 1976.

781. Wolfe L: The red cell membrane and the storage lesion, *Clin Haematol* 14:259, 1985.

782. Wolfe LC: The membrane and the lesions of storage in preserved red cells, *Transfusion* 25:185, 1985.

783. Wong KC: Hypokalemia and dysrhythmias, *J Cardiothorac Anaesth* 3:529, 1989 (editorial).

784. Wong KC, Wen-Shin L: Anesthesia for urologic surgery. In Stoelting RK, ed: *Advances in anesthesia,* vol. III, Chicago, 1986, Year Book Medical Publishers.

785. Wong O, Metcalfe-Gibson A: The electrolyte content of faeces, *Proc R Soc Med* 58:1007, 1965.

786. Woodson RD, Wranne B, and Detter JC: Effect of increased blood oxygen affinity on work performance of rats, *J Clin Invest* 52:277, 1973.

787. Woolf PD: Hormonal responses to trauma, *Crit Care Med* 20:216, 1992.

788. Worthley LI, Thomas PD: Treatment of hyponatremic seizures with intravenous 29.2% saline, *Br Med J* 292:168, 1986.

789. Wright FS: Potassium transport by successive segments of the mammalian nephron, *Fed Proc* 40:2398, 1981.

790. Wright FS, Giebisch G: Renal potassium transport: contributions of individual nephron segments and populations, *Am J Physiol* 235:F515, 1978.

791. Yacobi A, Stoll RG, Sum CY et al: The pharmacokinetics of hydroxyethyl starch in normal subjects, *J Clin Pharmacol* 22:206, 1982.

792. Yeston NS, Niehoff JM, and Dennis RC: Transfusion therapy. In Civetta JM, Taylor RW, and Kirby RR, eds: *Critical care,* Philadelphia, 1988, JB Lippincott.

793. Younes RN, Aun F, Accioly CQ et al: Hypertonic solutions in the treatment of hypovolemic shock: a prospective, randomized study in patients admitted to the emergency room, *Surgery* 111:380, 1992.

794. Zaloga GP: Hyperosmolar states. In Civetta JM, Taylor RW, and Kirby RR, eds: *Critical care,* Philadelphia, 1988, JB Lippincott.

795. Zaloga GP: Calcium disorders, *Problems Crit Care* 4:382, 1990.

796. Zaloga GP: Hypocalcemic crisis, *Crit Care Clin* 7:191, 1991.

797. Zaloga GP: Hypocalcemia in critically ill patients, *Crit Care Med* 20:251, 1992.

798. Zaloga GP, Chernow B: Calcium metabolism, *Clin Crit Care Med* 5:169, 1985.

799. Zaloga GP, Chernow B: Hypocalcemia in critical illness, *JAMA* 256:1924, 1986.

800. Zaloga GP, Chernow B: Divalent ions: calcium, magnesium, and phosphorous. In Chernow B, ed: *The pharmacologic approach to the critically ill patient,* ed 2, Baltimore, 1988, Williams & Wilkins.

801. Zaloga GP, Chernow B, Cook D et al: Assessment of calcium homeostasis in the critically ill patient. The diagnostic pitfalls of the McLean Hastings Nomogram, *Ann Surg* 202:587, 1985.

802. Zaloga G, Eisenach JC: Magnesium, anesthesia, and hemodynamic control, *Anesthesiology* 74:1, 1991 (editorial).

803. Zaloga GP, Malcolm DS, Holaday J et al: Verapamil reverses calcium cardiotoxicity, *Ann Emerg Med* 16:637, 1987.

804. Zaloga GP, Roberts JE: Magnesium disorders, *Problems Crit Care* 4:425, 1990.

805. Zaloga GP, Wilkens R, Tourville J et al: A simple method for determining physiologically active calcium and magnesium concentrations in critically ill patients, *Crit Care Med* 15:813, 1987.

806. Zaloga GP, Willey SC, and Chernow B: Free fatty acids alter calcium binding. A cause for misinterpretation of serum calcium values and hypocalcemia in critical illness, *J Clin Endocrinol Metab* 64:1010, 1987.

807. Zarins CK, Rice CL, Smith DE et al: Role of lymphatics in preventing hypooncotic pulmonary edema, *Surg Forum* 27:257, 1976.

808. Zauder HL: Preoperative hemoglobin requirements, *Anesthesiol Clin North Am* 8:471, 1990.

809. Zerbe RL, Robertson GL: A comparison of plasma vasopressin measurements with a standard indirect test in the differential diagnosis of polyuria, *N Engl J Med* 305:1539, 1981.

810. Zerbe RL, Robertson GL: Osmotic and nonosmotic regulation of thirst and vasopressin secretion. In Maxwell MH, Kleeman CR, and Narins RG, eds: *Clinical disorders of fluid and electrolyte metabolism,* ed 4, New York, 1987, McGraw-Hill.

811. Zoll F, Wessler S, and Schlesinger MJ: Interarterial anastomoses in the human heart with particular reference to anemia and relative cardiac anoxia, *Circulation* 4:794, 1951.

812. Zrains CK, Rice CL, Peters RM et al: Lymph and pulmonary response to isobaric reduction in plasma oncotic pressure in baboons, *Circ Res* 43:925, 1978.

CHAPTER 47

Anesthesia Delivery System

JAMES B. EISENKRAFT

The anesthesia delivery system is the anesthesiologist's constant companion in the operating room. Whether a patient is to receive general anesthesia, regional anesthesia, or monitored anesthesia care, the delivery system must be checked and ready for use. **An understanding of the structure and function of the anesthesia delivery system is essential to the safe practice of anesthesia.**

The components of a contemporary basic anesthesia delivery system are depicted in Fig. 47-1. These

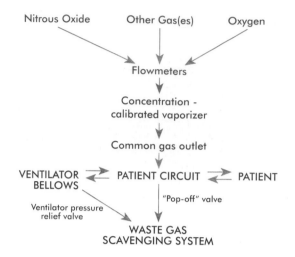

Nitrous Oxide   Other Gas(es)   Oxygen

Flowmeters

Concentration - calibrated vaporizer

Common gas outlet

VENTILATOR BELLOWS ⇄ PATIENT CIRCUIT ⇄ PATIENT

"Pop-off" valve

Ventilator pressure relief valve

WASTE GAS SCAVENGING SYSTEM

Fig. 47-1. Schematic of generic anesthesia delivery system.

include the anesthesia machine itself, which receives the gases oxygen (O_2), nitrous oxide (N_2O), and perhaps a third and fourth gas (e.g., helium [He], air, carbon dioxide [CO_2]) delivered under pressure. A controlled gas mixture in terms of concentration of O_2 and other gas(es), as well as total gas flow rates, is delivered to a concentration-calibrated vaporizer, where a measured amount of a potent inhaled agent may be added. The resulting fresh gas mixture of known composition and metered production rate leaves the anesthesia machine at the common gas outlet and flows to the patient circuit. The patient circuit represents a mini-environment with which the patient makes respiratory exchange and with whose contained gas tensions the patient's blood and brain equilibrate to produce the desired depth of anesthesia, as well as controlled tensions of CO_2, O_2, and other gases. Connected to the circuit may be an anesthesia ventilator bellows whereby the patient may be mechanically ventilated. Excess gases are vented from the anesthesia circuit via either the adjustable pressure-limiting (APL or "pop-off") valve or the ventilator pressure relief valve. The vented gases enter the waste gas scavenging system and are removed from the operating room, usually through the hospital suction.

The anesthesia delivery system has evolved considerably over the past several years. **The current voluntary consensus standard describing the features of a contemporary machine is that published by the American Society for Testing and Materials (ASTM) and designated F1161-88.**[4] This document, approved in July 1988 and published in March 1989, is entitled *Standard Specification for Minimum Performance and Safety Requirements for Components and Systems of Anesthesia Gas Machines*. It specifies the minimum performance and safety requirements to be used in the design of anesthesia gas machines for human use

to enhance safety of the patient and operator.[4] This standard supersedes the Z79.8-1979 anesthesia machine standard published in 1979 by the American National Standards Institute.[3] The F1161-88 is a consensus standard adopted voluntarily by the machine manufacturers. Certain accrediting and licensing bodies, however, may choose to adopt such standards in whole or in part and make them *requirements* for machines used in that locality. A summary of the important new aspects addressed in the F1161-88 standard is provided later in this chapter.

Presently, in the United States, the two largest manufacturers of anesthesia delivery systems (machines, ventilators, vaporizers, scavenging systems) are North American Dräger (Telford, Pa) and Ohmeda (a division of BOC Health Care, Madison, Wis). This chapter reviews the features of a basic anesthesia delivery system, referring to the Dräger and Ohmeda products where appropriate. **The approach is to trace the flow of gases and vapors from their storage sources, through the various components of the delivery system, and to understand the function of each. In this way the reader can more readily appreciate the rationale for the various checkout procedures and will have a framework from which to diagnose problems arising with the equipment.** A systematic approach to problems with the delivery system is presented elsewhere.[26] It is emphasized at the outset that **the machine manufacturer's operator's and service manuals represent the most comprehensive source of reference for any individual model of machine, and the reader is strongly encouraged to review the manual(s) relevant to his/her equipment. In the event of a severe machine malfunction, an alternate means for delivering O_2 or air to the patient should be kept immediately available. Thus a self-inflating (e.g., Ambu) bag and a full tank of O_2 should be available in each anesthetizing location.**

BASIC ANESTHESIA MACHINE

The flow arrangements of a basic two-gas anesthesia machine are shown in Fig. 47-2. The machine receives each of the two basic gases, O_2 and N_2O, from two supply sources: a tank or cylinder source and a pipeline source.

Oxygen

Oxygen has a molecular weight of 32 and a boiling point of $-183°$ C at a pressure of 760 mm Hg (14.7 PSIG*). Boiling point (the temperature at which O_2

---

* PSIG, Pounds/square inch gauge pressure. Gauges record pressure above or below existing atmospheric pressure.[52] Absolute pressure is designated PSIA. Thus atmospheric pressure = 760 mm Hg = 14.7 PSIA = 0 PSIG.

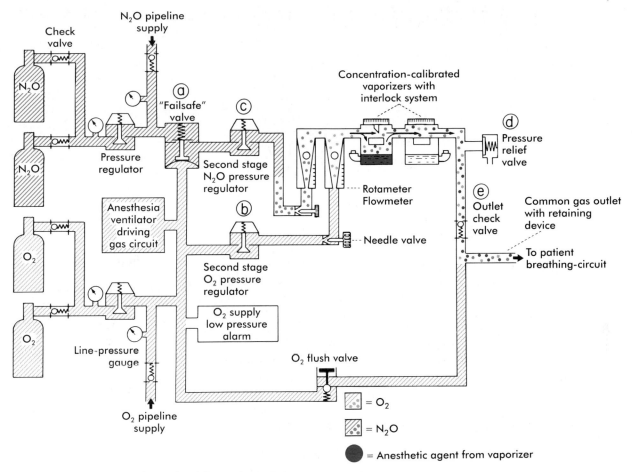

Fig. 47-2. Schematic of flow arrangements of contemporary anesthesia machine. "Failsafe" valve *a* in Ohmeda machines is termed a pressure sensor shutoff valve. In North American Dräger machines it is the O_2 failure protection device. Second-stage O_2 pressure regulator *b* is used in Ohmeda (but not North American Dräger Narkomed) machines. Second-stage N_2O pressure regulator *c* is used in Ohmeda Modulus machines having the Link 25 Proportion Limiting System; not used in North American Dräger machines. Pressure relief valve *d* is used in Ohmeda Modulus machines; not used in North American Dräger machines. Outlet check valve *e* is used in Ohmeda machines except Modulus II Plus and Modulus CD models; not used in North American Dräger machines. (Modified from *"Check-out": a guide for preoperative inspection of an anesthesia machine,* Park Ridge, Ill, 1987, The American Society of Anesthesiologists.)

changes from the liquid to the gas phase) is related to ambient pressure such that as pressure increases, so does the boiling point of O_2. However, a certain *critical temperature* is reached above which, no matter how much pressure is applied, the liquid O_2 boils to a gas. **The critical temperature for O_2 is $-118.8°$ C, and the *critical pressure*, which must be applied at this temperature to keep O_2 liquid, is 737 PSIA.**[57] **Because room temperature is 20° C and therefore well above critical temperature, O_2 can exist only as a gas at room temperature.** This has certain implications in understanding the contents of an O_2 tank.

Oxygen tanks form a backup supply in case of pipeline failure. Machines are usually equipped with one or two E cylinders, which hang on spe-

cific O_2 yokes. **The pin-index safety system ensures that the correct medical gas tank is hung in the correct yoke.** The system consists of two pins in the yoke, which fit into two holes in the tank valve. The two pins are in a unique configuration for O_2 and should never be removed from the hanger yoke. **Specific pin configurations exist for each of the medical gases supplied in small cylinders to prevent erroneous misconnections of gas supplies.** A tank should therefore never be force-fitted to a yoke.

Oxygen tanks are filled at the factory to a pressure of approximately 1900 PSIG at room temperature.[20] **When full, they contain a fixed number of gas molecules (fixed mass of gas) that obey Boyle's law,**

(i.e., Pressure × Volume = Constant), provided that temperature does not change. A full E cylinder of O_2 at a pressure of 1900 PSIG will evolve 660 L of gaseous O_2 at atmospheric pressure (14.7 PSIA, or 760 mm Hg). The internal volume (V_1) of an E cylinder is therefore approximately 5 L because, by Boyle's law, $P_1 \times V_1 = P_2 \times V_2$. Thus $1900 \times V_1 = 14.7 \times 660$. If the O_2 tank pressure reads 1000 PSIG, the tank is 1000/1900, or 52% full, and will generate only $660 \times 52\%$, or 340 L of O_2. If such a tank were being used at an O_2 flow rate of 6 L/min, it would empty in just under 1 hour (actually 340/6 = 57 minutes). It is important to understand these principles when O_2 cylinders are in use to supply the machine or to transport a ventilated patient. **If the anesthesia machine is equipped with two E cylinders of O_2, only one should be open and in use at any one time so that both tanks are not emptied simultaneously.**

In the hanger yoke for O_2 (and other medical gases) is a check valve to prevent leakage of gas out through the yoke if no cylinder is hanging in place and the machine is being supplied by the pipeline or from a second O_2 tank (see Fig. 47-2). If two O_2 tanks are hanging, **the check valve in the yoke prevents transfilling of gas from one tank to the other.** However, these check valves may leak, so if a hanger yoke does not have a tank hanging in it, a yoke plug should be inserted to prevent leakage of gas in the event of an incompetent check valve.

In many medical facilities the O_2 pipeline is supplied from a bulk liquid source that is more economical for the institution, depending on volume of O_2 use. Liquid O_2 is stored at temperatures of -150 to $-175°$ C under pressure in a storage vessel that resembles a large vacuum (Dewar) flask.[54] When gaseous O_2 is drawn from the top of the storage vessel, liquid O_2 boils to replace it. The boiling (change of phase) helps to keep the remaining liquid O_2 cold. The gas evolved is very cold; therefore it is passed through a heating coil and then through a **pressure regulator that maintains the pipeline pressure at 50 to 55 PSIG.** Alarms and safety devices, including relief valves and shut-off valves, ensure the safe functioning of the bulk O_2 storage and pipeline systems. **Pipeline O_2 is available in the operating rooms through manufacturer-specific outlets or gas-specific "quick couplers."**[20]

In the operating room, although the wall connectors are noninterchangeable among medical gases, so that an N_2O hose cannot be connected to an O_2 outlet, these connectors are also manufacturer specific (e.g., Schraeder, Ohmeda, Chemetron). **At the machine end of the pipeline hose is a connector that is gas specific by a national standard. The diameter-index safety system (DISS) specifies that the machine end of the medical gas connectors be of different diameter.**

The diameter- and pin-index safety systems ensure that the correct medical gas enters the correct part of the anesthesia machine.[14,19]

While O_2 from the pipeline supply enters the machine at a pressure of approximately 50 PSIG, O_2 from a full tank supply enters the yoke at pressures of 1900 PSIG. **The O_2 tank source is therefore regulated** (O_2 passes through a regulator valve) **and enters the machine at a nominal pressure of 45 PSIG (see Fig. 47-2).** Pressure regulators reduce a variable high input pressure (in this case 1900 PSIG) to a constant low output pressure (in this case 45 PSIG) for the gas whose pressure is being regulated. The tank supply serves as a backup in case the pipeline fails, and, once it has been checked, **the tank supply should be turned off if the pipeline source is being used.** If the O_2 tank(s) remains turned on while the machine is being supplied from the pipeline, O_2 is drawn preferentially from the pipeline (50 to 55 PSIG) because the regulator that controls flow from the O_2 tanks only permits flow when the pressure in the machine falls below about 45 PSIG (see Fig. 47-2). However, the pipeline pressure may at times fluctuate to below 45 PSIG, in which case O_2 would be drawn from an open tank. Thus, if the machine is being supplied from the O_2 pipeline, the O_2 tanks on the machine should be turned off to prevent the tank O_2 supply being drawn down and the backup tank supply being accidently depleted.

It is important to appreciate that as long as pipeline supply pressure (50 to 55 PSIG) exceeds pressure downstream of the first-stage O_2 regulator, the O_2 tank source will not supply the machine. If one wants to use the tank O_2 to supply the machine, the O_2 pipeline connector should first be disconnected from the wall. Thus, **if one suspects that a hypoxic gas is being delivered through the O_2 pipeline system at 50 to 55 PSIG (e.g., because of pipeline crossover or misfilling of the bulk O_2 supply tank), the machine pipeline connection must be disconnected from the wall outlet to permit the tank O_2 supply to be used.**

Having entered the machine at a pressure of 45 to 55 PSIG (from tank or pipeline), O_2 may flow or pressurize in several directions (see Fig. 47-2):

- **When the O_2 flush valve is opened, O_2 flows to the common gas outlet of the machine at a steady rate of 35 to 75 L/min.**[4] The O_2 flush bypasses the vaporizers, and the pressure in the patient circuit can potentially be high (up to 55 PSIG) when the flush is operated. Caution is therefore necessary when using the O_2 flush so as to prevent barotrauma.
- Oxygen pressurizes an O_2 supply failure alarm system such that if the O_2 supply pressure falls (usually below 30 PSIG), an alarm sounds. In the Ohmeda Modulus I, II, and Excel machines a

pressurized canister is used. This emits an audible alarm for at least 7 seconds when the pressure falls below threshold. In Dräger Narkomed and Ohmeda Modulus II Plus and Modulus CD machines, a pressure-operated electrical switch ensures a continuous audible alarm whenever the O_2 supply pressure falls below the threshold setting.[42,47]

- Oxygen provides the power source for a pneumatically driven anesthesia ventilator.

- Oxygen pressurizes and holds open a pressure-sensor shut-off valve that reduces or interrupts the supply of N_2O and other gases (e.g., CO_2, He, air) to their flowmeters if the O_2 supply pressure falls below the threshold setting. This, in relation to N_2O supply control, is the so-called "fail-safe" system designed to prevent the unintentional delivery of a hypoxic mixture to the flow control valves. The fail-safe system differs between Ohmeda and Dräger machines.

   In Ohmeda machines, when the O_2 supply pressure falls below 20 PSIG, the N_2O and other gas flowmeters are no longer supplied with gas. The pressure-sensor shut-off valve used by Ohmeda is an "all-or-nothing" or threshold arrangement that is open at O_2 pressures greater than 20 PSIG and closed at lower pressures.[42]

   The fail-safe valve in Dräger Narkomed machines is called an *oxygen failure protection device* (OFPD), and one exists for each gas supplied to the machine. As the O_2 supply pressure falls, OFPDs proportionately reduce the supply pressure of the other gases to their flowmeters. The supply of N_2O and other gases is interrupted completely when the O_2 supply pressure falls below 12 ± 4 PSIG.[47]

- Oxygen flows to the O_2 flow control valves and flowmeters (rotameters). Gas supply to the O_2 flowmeters differs between Ohmeda and Dräger machines.

   In contemporary Ohmeda machines the O_2 supply pressure to the flowmeter is regulated to 14 PSIG by a second-stage regulator.[42] This regulator (see Fig. 47-2) ensures a constant supply pressure to the Ohmeda O_2 flowmeter. Thus, if the O_2 supply pressure to the machine decreases below 45 to 50 PSIG, as long as it exceeds 14 PSIG, the flow set on the O_2 flowmeter is maintained. Without this regulator, if the O_2 supply pressure were to fall, the O_2 flow would decrease at the flowmeter, and if another gas (e.g., N_2O) were also being used, a hypoxic gas mixture could result at the flowmeter level.

   Dräger Narkomed anesthesia machine design does not require a second-stage O_2 pressure regulator valve (see Fig. 47-2). Dräger Narko-

med machines have an OFPD that interfaces the supply pressure of O_2 with that of N_2O and any other gas supplied to the machine.[47] A decrease in O_2 supply pressure causes a proportionate decrease in the supply pressure of each of the other gases to their flowmeters. As the O_2 supply pressure and flow decrease, all other gas flows are decreased in proportion to prevent creation of a hypoxic gas mixture at the flowmeter level (see also previous point about fail-safe valves).

The use (Ohmeda) or nonuse (Dräger) of a second-stage O_2 regulator affects the total gas flow emerging from the common gas outlet of the machine if the O_2 supply pressure were to fall. In an Ohmeda machine, as long as the O_2 supply pressure exceeds 20 PSIG, all set gas flows are maintained. In a Dräger machine, if the O_2 supply pressure falls from normal (45 to 55 PSIG), all gas flows decrease in proportion. A decrease in total gas flow from the machine common gas outlet may cause rebreathing, depending on the anesthetic circuit in use; a Mapleson (rebreathing) system is affected more than a circle system with CO_2 absorption.

Nitrous Oxide

As with O_2, N_2O may be supplied to the machine from the pipeline system at 50 to 55 PSIG or from a backup E cylinder supply on the machine. **N_2O has a molecular weight of 44 and a boiling point of $-88°$ C at 760 mm Hg (14.7 PSIA) pressure.[52] Because it has a critical temperature of 36.5° C (critical pressure, 1054 PSIG), N_2O can exist as a liquid at room temperature (20° C). E cylinders of N_2O are factory-filled to 90% to 95% capacity with liquid N_2O.[20] Above the liquid in the tank is N_2O vapor. Because the liquid agent is in equilibrium with its vapor or gas phase, the pressure exerted by the gaseous N_2O is its saturated vapor pressure (SVP) at the ambient temperature. At 20° C the SVP of N_2O is 750 PSIG.[52]**

A full E tank of N_2O generates approximately 1600 L of gas at 1 atmosphere pressure at sea level (14.7 PSIA). As long as some liquid N_2O is present in the tank and the ambient temperature remains at 20° C, the pressure in the N_2O tank will remain at 750 PSIG, which is the SVP of N_2O at 20° C.

Unlike with O_2, the content of a N_2O tank cannot be determined by reference to the N_2O tank pressure gauge. However, the content can be estimated by weighing the tank and subtracting the weight of the empty tank (tare weight) to determine what *weight* of N_2O remains. By Avogadro's volume, 44 g of N_2O occupy 22.4 L at standard temperature and pressure (STP, 760 mm Hg pressure; 273.15° K [0° C]). Once all the liquid N_2O has been used and the tank contains only gas, Boyle's law may be applied. In this situation, where the tank pressure is 750 PSIG (from gas only) and the internal volume of the E cylinder is approximately 5 L (see previous O_2 section), the volume of N_2O that will be evolved at a pressure of 760 mm Hg (14.7 PSIA) can be calculated. Thus $P_1V_1 = P_2V_2$; $750 \times 5 = 14.7 \times V_2$, or $V_2 = 255$ L. At this point the N_2O tank is 255/1600, or 16% full. An E tank of N_2O with a pressure of 400 PSIG would evolve $(400/750) \times 255$ L, or 136 L of N_2O.

Nitrous oxide from the tank supply enters the yoke at pressures up to 750 PSIG (at 20° C) and then passes through a regulator that reduces this pressure to 40 to 45 PSIG (see Fig. 47-2). The pin-index safety system is designed to ensure that only a N_2O tank may hang in a N_2O hanger yoke. As with O_2, a check valve in each yoke prevents the back leakage of N_2O if no tank is hung in the yoke.

The N_2O pipeline is supplied from banks of large N_2O tanks, usually H cylinders, each of which evolves 16,000 L of gas at atmospheric pressure.[20] **The pressure in the N_2O pipeline is regulated to 50 to 55 PSIG to supply the outlets in the operating room.** Having entered the anesthesia machine, N_2O must flow past the fail-safe valve to reach its flow control valve and rotameter.

In Ohmeda Modulus anesthesia machines that have the Link-25 Proportion Limiting System (see later discussion), a second-stage N_2O regulator further reduces gas pressure so that N_2O is supplied to its flowmeter at a nominal pressure of 26 PSIG (see Fig. 47-2). The actual downstream pressure of this regulator is adjusted at the factory or by a field service representative to ensure correct functioning of the proportioning system.

Fig. 47-3. O_2 flowmeter and flow control valve. (Modified from Bowie E, Huffman LM: *The anesthesia machine: essentials for understanding,* Madison, Wis, 1985, Ohmeda, BOC Health Care.)

Flowmeters

The proportions of O_2, N_2O, and other medical gases controlled by the anesthesia machine, as well as total gas flows delivered to the patient circuit, are adjusted by means of flow control valves and flowmeters (rotameters).[47] There may be one or two rotameters (Fig. 47-3) in series for each gas.[4] If two are present for any gas, the first permits accurate measurement of low flows (usually up to 1 L/min) and the other of flows up to 10 to 12 L/min. Thus, although more than one flow tube may exist for a gas, **only one flow control knob exists for each gas emerging at the machine common gas outlet.**[4] In North America the O_2 **flowmeter is positioned on the right side of the rotameter bank, downstream from the other flowmeters and closest to the common gas outlet.** In the event of a leak in one of the other flowmeter tubes, this

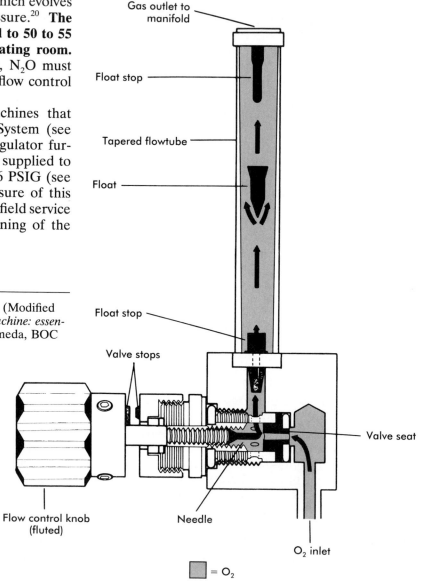

Gas outlet to manifold

Float stop

Tapered flowtube

Float

Float stop

Valve stops

Flow control knob (fluted)

Needle

Valve seat

O_2 inlet

$\blacksquare = O_2$

position is the one least likely to result in a hypoxic mixture.[21]

Rotameters are examples of constant-pressure, variable-orifice flowmeters. Their operation is based on the Thorpe tube principle.[20] Each rotameter consists of a tapered glass tube that has a small cross-sectional diameter at the bottom, is wide at the top, and contains a ball or bobbin. The area between the outside of the bobbin and the inside of the glass tube represents the variable orifice. A certain pressure difference across the bobbin is required to "float" the bobbin. As the orifice widens, greater and greater flows are required to create the same pressure difference across the bobbin, which floats higher in the tapered glass tube.

At low flow rates, gas flow is essentially laminar and Poiseuille's law applies.[67] Thus:

$$\text{Flow} = (\pi p r^4 / 8 v l) \propto p \propto v^{-1}$$

where p is the pressure drop across the bobbin, r is the radius of the tube, v is the viscosity of the gas, and l is the length of the bobbin or float.

When the orifice is larger and flows are greater, turbulence occurs,[52] in which case:

$$\text{Flow} \propto \sqrt{p}, \propto r^2 \propto \frac{1}{\text{Length}} \propto \frac{1}{\sqrt{\text{Density}}}$$

Rotameters are precision instruments. Flow tubes are manufactured for specific gases, calibrated with a unique float, and for use within a certain range of temperature and pressure. **Flowmeters are not interchangeable among gases.** If a gas is passed through a rotameter for which it has not been calibrated, the flows shown would likely be incorrect. Theoretic exceptions to this would be that at *low* flows, flow rates of gases with *similar viscosities* would be read identically (e.g., O_2 and He, 202 and 194 micropoise, respectively, and at *high flows,* gases of *similar density* (e.g., N_2O and CO_2, both with molecular weights of 44) would be read identically. Again, it is emphasized that flowmeters are *not* interchangeable among medical gases and for the Ohmeda machines they are now manufactured so that they cannot be interchanged.[42]

The gas flow to the rotameter tube is controlled by a touch-coded and color-coded knob linked to a needle valve (see Fig. 47-3). In the United States **the O_2 control knob is color-coded green (as is everything related to O_2), is fluted, and is larger in diameter than the other gas flow control knobs.**[9] **The N_2O control knob is smaller, color-coded blue, and not fluted.**

Anesthesia machine manufacturers offer as an option an O_2 flow that cannot be discontinued completely because either (1) a stop is provided to ensure a minimum O_2 flow of 200 to 300 ml/minute past the needle valve (Ohmeda, see Fig. 47-3)[9] or (2)

a gas flow resistor, which permits a similar flow of 200 to 300 ml/min to bypass a totally closed O_2 flow control needle valve, is provided (Dräger Narkomed).[47] In Dräger Narkomed machines the minimum O_2 flow feature functions in the "$O_2 + N_2O$" mode but not in the "ALL GASES" mode.[47]

Oxygen Ratio Monitoring and Proportioning Systems

A major consideration in the design of contemporary anesthesia machines is the prevention of the delivery of a hypoxic gas mixture. The fail-safe system described previously only serves to interrupt (Ohmeda) or proportionately reduce and ultimately interrupt (Dräger OFPD) the supplies of N_2O and other gases (e.g., air, He) to their flowmeters if the O_2 supply pressure to the machine is reduced. It does not prevent the delivery of a hypoxic mixture to the common gas outlet, and the term "fail-safe" is therefore somewhat of a misnomer.

In contemporary machines, O_2 and N_2O flow controls are physically interlinked either mechanically (Ohmeda) or mechanically and pneumatically (Dräger), so that a fresh gas mixture containing at least 25% O_2 is created at the level of the flowmeters when only N_2O and O_2 are being used.[42,47]

Ohmeda anesthesia machines use the Link-25 Proportion Limiting Control System to ensure an adequate percentage of O_2 in the gas mixture created.[42,43] In this system a gear with 14 teeth is integral with the N_2O flow control spindle, whereas a gear with 29 teeth "floats" on a threaded O_2 flow control valve spindle (Fig. 47-4). The two gears are connected together by a precision stainless steel link chain. For every 2.07 revolutions of the N_2O flow control spindle, an O_2 flow control, set to the lowest O_2 flow, rotates once because of the 14:29 ratio of gear teeth. Because the gear on the O_2 flow control spindle is thread-mounted so that it can rotate on the control valve spindle (rather than being integral with the spindle), O_2 flow can be increased independently of N_2O. However, regardless of the O_2 flow set, if the flow of N_2O is increased sufficiently, the gear on the O_2 spindle will engage with the O_2 flow control knob, causing it to rotate and thereby causing O_2 flow to increase.[42,43] If N_2O flow is now reduced, the O_2 flow remains high unless it is deliberately reduced by the user. The 75% N_2O:25% O_2 proportioning is completed because (1) the N_2O flow control valve is supplied from a second-stage gas regulator, which reduces N_2O pressure to a nominal 26 PSIG (adjusted as previously described) before it reaches the flow control valve, whereas the O_2 flow control valve is supplied at a pressure of 14 PSIG from a second-stage O_2 regulator (see Figs. 47-2 and 47-4). The Link-25 system permits the N_2O and O_2 flow control valves to

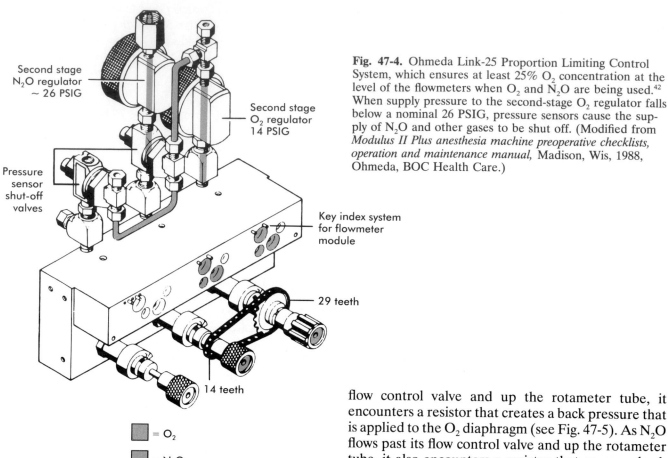

Second stage
N₂O regulator
~ 26 PSIG

Second stage
O₂ regulator
14 PSIG

Pressure
sensor
shut-off
valves

Key index system
for flowmeter
module

29 teeth

14 teeth

■ = O₂

■ = N₂O

Fig. 47-4. Ohmeda Link-25 Proportion Limiting Control System, which ensures at least 25% O_2 concentration at the level of the flowmeters when O_2 and N_2O are being used.[42] When supply pressure to the second-stage O_2 regulator falls below a nominal 26 PSIG, pressure sensors cause the supply of N_2O and other gases to be shut off. (Modified from *Modulus II Plus anesthesia machine preoperative checklists, operation and maintenance manual,* Madison, Wis, 1988, Ohmeda, BOC Health Care.)

be set independently of one another. However, whenever a N_2O concentration of more than 75% would be accidently set, the O_2 flow is automatically increased to maintain at least 25% O_2 in the resulting mixture. **This system thus increases the minimum flow of O_2 according to the N_2O flow set.**[42,43]

The Link-25 system interconnects only the N_2O and O_2 flow control valves. If the anesthesia machine has flow controls for other gases, (e.g., He, air) (see Fig. 47-4), a gas mixture containing less than 25% O_2 could potentially be set at the flowmeters.

In Dräger Narkomed machines the *oxygen ratio monitor controller (ORMC)* (Fig. 47-5) serves to limit the N_2O *flow according to the O_2 flow* and create a mixture of at least 25% O_2 at the flowmeter level when these two gases are being used.[47] At O_2 flow rates of less than 1 L/minute, even higher concentrations of O_2 are delivered. In addition, an alarm is activated when the ORMC is functioning to prevent a hypoxic mixture when the Narkomed machine is used in the "O_2 + N_2O" mode, but not in the "ALL GASES" mode (i.e., when air, helium, etc., might be switched into the system).[47]

The ORMC works as follows. As O_2 flows past its

flow control valve and up the rotameter tube, it encounters a resistor that creates a back pressure that is applied to the O_2 diaphragm (see Fig. 47-5). As N_2O flows past its flow control valve and up the rotameter tube, it also encounters a resistor that causes a back pressure on the N_2O diaphragm. The two diaphragms are linked by a connecting shaft, the ultimate position of which depends on the relative back pressures, and therefore flows, of N_2O and O_2. The left-hand end of the connecting shaft controls the orifice of a slave valve, which in turn controls the supply pressure of N_2O to its flow control valve. When the O_2 flow is high, the shaft moves to the left and opens the slave control valve (Fig. 47-5, *lower*). Conversely, if the N_2O flow is increased excessively, the shaft moves to the right, closing the slave valve orifice and limiting the supply pressure and thereby the flow of N_2O to its flow control valve. When the ORMC is acting to prevent a hypoxic mixture, the leaf spring contacts (see Fig. 47-5) are closed, annunciating an alarm. This alarm is disabled if the machine is in the "ALL GASES" mode.[47]

The Dräger ORMC differs from the Ohmeda Link-25 Proportion Limiting Control System in several ways. First, the ORMC does not require second-stage O_2 and N_2O regulators. Second, **the ORMC serves to limit the N_2O flow according to the O_2 flow, whereas the Link-25 system increases the O_2 flow as the N_2O flow is increased.** As with the Link-25 system, **the ORMC functions only between N_2O and O_2,** and there is no interlinking of O_2 with other gases (e.g., air, He) that might also be deliverable by the machine.

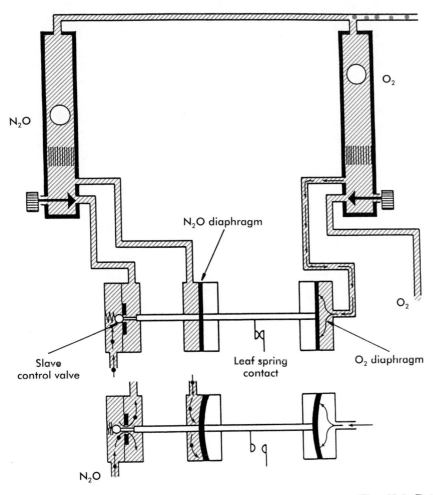

= O$_2$

= N$_2$O

Fig. 47-5. Dräger Oxygen Ratio Monitor Controller (ORMC). See text for details of operation. (From *Narkomed 3 anesthesia system technical service manual,* Telford, Pa, 1988, North American Dräger.)

Thus, while a third or fourth gas is in use, the proportioning systems afford no protection against a hypoxic mixture. Prevention of delivery of a hypoxic gas mixture when a third or fourth gas is supplied to the machine may be achieved by supplying that gas in a tank premixed with O$_2$ (e.g., 75% He/25% O$_2$).

Although elegant in design, both the ORMC and the Link-25 systems are subject to mechanical and pneumatic failure and should be tested according to the manufacturer's instructions during the preuse machine checkout.[43,46] Furthermore, if the systems are functioning correctly, they only ensure adequacy of greater than 25% O$_2$ at the flowmeter level. An O$_2$ leak downstream from the flowmeters could result in a hypoxic mixture emerging from the machine's common gas outlet. **An oxygen analyzer in the patient circuit is therefore essential if a potentially hypoxic mixture is to be detected and thereby prevented.** The controlled flows of O$_2$, N$_2$O, and other gases are mixed

in the manifold at the top of the flowmeter bank, and they flow to a concentration-calibrated anesthesia vaporizer (see Fig. 47-2).

ANESTHESIA VAPORIZERS

A vapor is the gas phase of an agent that is normally a liquid at room temperature and atmospheric pressure. Vaporizers facilitate the change of a liquid anesthetic into its vapor phase and add a controlled amount of this vapor to the flow of gases passing to the patient circuit.

Vapor, Evaporation, and Vapor Pressure

Consider halothane in a closed container at atmospheric pressure (760 mm Hg) and room temperature (20° C), Although most is in liquid form, some halothane molecules escape from the surface of the liquid to enter the space above as a vapor. Under steady conditions of temperature, an equilibrium is established between the molecules in the vapor phase and those in the liquid phase. The vapor phase molecules are in constant motion, striking the walls of the container to exert a vapor pressure. If the temperature is increased, more molecules enter the vapor phase (evaporate), resulting in an increase in vapor pressure. When the gas phase above the liquid contains all the halothane vapor that it can hold at that temperature, it is said to be saturated. The pressure from the halothane is its *saturated vapor pressure* (SVP) at that temperature.

The vapor pressure exerted by the vapor phase of a potent volatile agent depends only on the volatile agent and the ambient temperature (Fig. 47-6). The temperature at which vapor pressure becomes equal to atmospheric pressure and at which all the liquid agent changes to the vapor phase is termed the liquid's *boiling point*. The most volatile agents are those with the highest SVPs for any given temperature, and they therefore also have the lowest boiling points (e.g., desflurane and diethyl ether boil at 23.5° C and 35° C, respectively, at an ambient pressure of 760 mm Hg). Boiling point decreases with decreasing ambient pressure, such as occurs at high altitude.

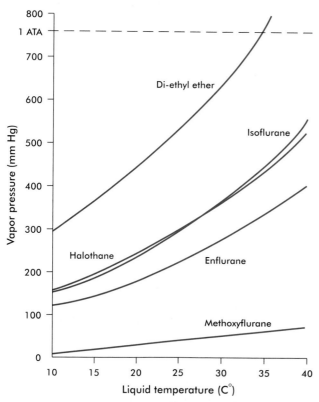

Fig. 47-6. Vapor pressure curves for the potent inhaled anesthetics. (From Eisenkraft JB: Vaporizers and vaporization of volatile anesthetics. In Eisenkraft JB, ed: *Progress in anesthesiology,* vol 2, San Antonio, Tx, 1988, Dannemiller Memorial Educational Foundation.)

Units of Vapor Concentration

Anesthetic vapor presence may be quantified either (1) as an absolute pressure, expressed in millimeters of mercury, or (2) in volumes percent of 1 atmosphere (i.e., volumes of vapor per 100 volumes of total gas).

By applying Dalton's Law, volumes percent is similar to the agent's fractional partial pressure:

$$\text{Vols \%} = \frac{\text{Partial pressure of agent}}{\text{Total ambient pressure}} \times 100$$

Dalton's Law of Partial Pressures

Dalton's law states that in a mixture of gases (or vapors) the pressure exerted by each gas is the same as that it would exert if it alone occupied the container.[52] Each gas (or vapor) exerts its pressure independently of the pressure of the other gases present. For example, in a container of dry air at atmospheric pressure (760 mm Hg), if O_2 represented 21% of all gases present, the pressure exerted by the O_2 (its partial pressure) would be 21% × 760, or 159.6 mm Hg.

Consider now air, which is fully saturated with water vapor at 37° C (normal body temperature). Vapor pressure depends on temperature. The SVP for water at 37° C is 47 mm Hg. O_2 now represents 21% of what remains (i.e., 713, or 760 − 47), having a partial pressure of 21% × 713, or 149.3 mm Hg.

Volumes percent expresses the relative ratio of gas molecules in a mixture, whereas partial pressure represents an absolute value. Anesthetic uptake and potency are directly related to partial pressure and only indirectly to volumes percent. This distinction will become more apparent when hyperbaric and hypobaric situations are considered later.

Minimum Alveolar Concentration

The minimum alveolar concentration of a potent inhaled anesthetic agent that produces immobility in 50% of patients undergoing a surgical incision (MAC) is used to indicate anesthetic potency or depth. MAC is typically expressed as volumes percent of alveolar (end-tidal) gas at 1 atmosphere pressure at sea level (760 mm Hg). Table 47-1 shows how MAC in familiar volumes percent can be expressed as a partial pressure in millimeters of mercury (mm Hg).[23] The reader is encouraged to think of MAC in terms of partial pressure (MAP or MAPP) rather than volumes percent because it is the partial pressure (tension) of the anesthetic in the brain that is responsible for the depth of anesthesia.[28,29] The term $P_{MAC\ 1}$ (Table 47-1) is used to express the partial pressure of a potent inhaled agent at a concentration of 1 MAC. Thus 1 MAC halothane is equivalent to a $P_{MAC\ 1}$ of 5.7 mm Hg.

Table 47-1   Expression of minimum alveolar concentration of anesthetic agent (MAC) as partial pressure at concentration of 1 MAC (P_{MAC1}) assuming ambient pressure of 760 mm Hg

Anesthetic agent	MAC (vol%)		P_{MAC1} (mm Hg)
Halothane	0.75 × 760	=	5.7
Enflurane	1.68 × 760	=	12.8
Isoflurane	1.15 × 760	=	8.7
Methoxyflurane	0.16 × 760	=	1.2
Desflurane*	6.0 × 760	=	45.6
	7.25 × 760	=	55.1
Sevoflurane†	1.7 × 760	=	12.9

*MAC of desflurane is age dependent: 18 to 35 years = 7.25%; 31 to 65 years = 6.0%.[56]
†Data from Katoh T, Ikeda K: The minimum alveolar concentration (MAC) of sevoflurane in humans, *Anesthesiology* 66:301, 1987.
From Eisenkraft JB: Anesthesia vaporizers. In Ehrenwerth J, Eisenkraft JB, eds: *Anesthesia equipment: principles and applications*, St Louis, 1992, Mosby–Year Book.

Latent Heat of Vaporization

Energy is needed to transfer molecules from the liquid to the vapor phase. This energy is called the *latent heat of vaporization* and is defined as the amount of heat (calories) required to convert unit mass (grams) of the liquid into vapor.[52] The latent heats of vaporization of volatile anesthetics at room temperature are halothane, 35 cal/g; enflurane and isoflurane, 41 cal/g; and methoxyflurane, 58 cal/g.[20]

The heat of vaporization is inversely related to ambient temperature so that the lower the temperature, the more heat required. Heat required to vaporize anesthetic agents is drawn from the remaining liquid and the surroundings. As vapor is generated, the temperatures of the vaporizer and liquid fall. This causes the vapor pressure to fall and would result in decreased vaporizer output if no compensatory mechanism were provided.

Specific Heat

Specific heat is the quantity of heat (calories) required to raise the temperature of unit mass (grams) of a substance by one degree of temperature (1° C).[52] Heat must be supplied to the liquid anesthetic in the vaporizer to maintain its temperature while heat is being lost in the process of evaporation.

Specific heat is also important to vaporizer construction material. Thus materials with high specific heat change temperature more gradually than those with low specific heats for the same amount of heat lost through vaporization. *Thermal capacity* is defined as the product of specific heat and mass and repre-

sents the amount of heat stored in the vaporizer body.[52]

Also of importance is the construction material's ability to conduct heat from the environment through to the contained liquid anesthetic. This is called *thermal conductivity,* defined in terms of how quickly heat is transmitted through a substance. **The ideal material for vaporizer construction would have a high specific heat and high thermal conductivity.** In this respect, copper comes close to the ideal, thus the Copper Kettle vaporizer. More recently, bronze and stainless steel have been used in vaporizer construction.[20]

Regulating Vaporizer Output: Measured Flow vs. Variable Bypass

The saturated vapor pressures of the three potent inhaled agents halothane, enflurane, and isoflurane at room temperature are 243, 175, and 241 mm Hg, respectively, and far in excess of those required clinically (Fig. 47-6 and Table 47-2). **The vaporizer therefore first creates a saturated vapor that must then be diluted by the bypass gas flow to result in clinically useful concentrations.** If this were not done, a lethal concentration of agent could be delivered to the anesthesia circuit.

Contemporary anesthesia vaporizers are concentration-calibrated and of the variable bypass design.[4] In a variable bypass vaporizer (e.g., Ohmeda Tec series, Dräger Vapor 19.1) the total fresh gas flow from the anesthesia machine flowmeters passes to the vaporizer. The vaporizer splits the incoming gas flow into a smaller flow, which enters the vaporizing chamber to emerge with the agent at saturated vapor concentration, and a larger bypass flow that, when mixed with the vaporizing chamber output, results in the desired or "dialed-in" concentration (Fig. 47-7).

In the now rarely used measured flow (non-concentration-calibrated) vaporizers, such as Copper Kettle (Foregger/Puritan-Bennett) or Verni-Trol (Ohmeda), a measured O_2 flow is set on a separate flowmeter to pass to the vaporizer, from which vapor at its SVP emerges. This is then diluted by an additional measured flow of gases from other (main) flowmeters on the anesthesia machine (Fig. 47-8). In this type of arrangement, several calculations are necessary to determine the anesthetic vapor concentration in the emerging gas mixture.

With either type of vaporizing arrangement, an efficient system must exist to create a saturated vapor concentration in the vaporizing chamber. This is achieved by having a large surface area for evaporation. In flow-over vaporizers (e.g., Dräger Vapor 19.1 series, Ohmeda Tec series) the area is increased by the use of wicks and baffles.[20] In bubble-through vaporizers (e.g., Copper Kettle, Verni-Trol), O_2 is

Table 47-2 Physical properties of potent volatile agents

Parameter	Halothane	Enflurane	Isoflurane	Methoxyflurane	Sevoflurane	Desflurane
Structure	$CHBrClCF_3$	$CHFClCF_2OCHF_2$	$CF_2HOCHClCF_3$	$CHCl_2CF_2OCH_3$	$CH_2FOCH(CF_3)_2$	$CF_2HOCFHCF_3$
Molecular weight	197.4	184.5	184.5	165.0	200	168
Boiling point at 760 mm Hg (° C)	50.2	56.5	48.5	104.7	58.5	23.5
SVP at 20° C (mm Hg)	243	175	238	20.3	160	664
Saturated vapor concentration at 20° C and 1 atmosphere absolute (vol%)	32	23	31	2.7	21	87
MAC at 1 atmosphere absolute (vol%)	0.75	1.68	1.15	0.16	1.7	6.0-7.25*
P_{MACl} (mm Hg)	5.7	12.8	8.7	1.22	12.9	46-55*
Specific gravity of liquid at 20° C	1.86	1.52	1.50	1.41	1.51	1.45
Vapor (ml) per liquid (g) at 20° C	123	130	130	145	120	143
Vapor (ml) per liquid (ml) at 20° C	226	196	195	204	182	207

*Age related; see Table 47-1.

SVP, Saturated vapor pressure; *MAC*, minimum alveolar concentration; P_{MACl}, partial pressure at concentration of 1 MAC.

From Eisenkraft JB: Anesthesia vaporizers. In Ehrenwerth J, Eisenkraft JB, eds: *Anesthesia equipment: principles and applications*, St Louis, 1992, Mosby–Year Book.

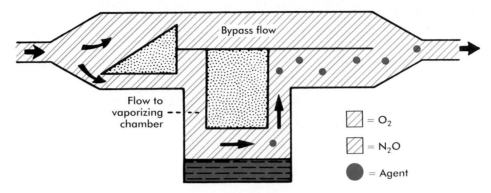

Fig. 47-7. Variable bypass vaporizer principle. These are concentration-calibrated and are of the flow-over design (*see text*). (From Eisenkraft JB: Vaporizers and vaporization of volatile anesthetics. In Eisenkraft JB, ed: *Progress in anesthesiology,* vol 2, San Antonio, Tx, 1988, Dannemiller Memorial Educational Foundation.)

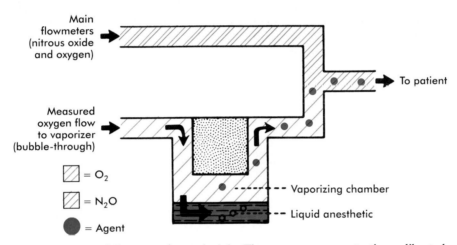

Fig. 47-8. Measured flow vaporizer principle. These are nonconcentration-calibrated and of the bubble-through design (*see text*). (From Eisenkraft JB: Vaporizers and vaporization of volatile anesthetics. In Eisenkraft JB, ed: *Progress in anesthesiology,* vol 2, San Antonio, Tx, 1988, Dannemiller Memorial Educational Foundation.)

bubbled through the liquid agent. The tiny bubbles, created by passage of O_2 through a sintered bronze disk in the Copper Kettle, represent large areas of liquid-gas interface over which evaporation of agent can quickly occur.

Calculation of vaporizer output

Assume that room temperature is kept constant at 20° C. The saturated vapor pressures of the three most frequently used potent inhaled agents are halothane, 243 mm Hg; enflurane, 175 mm Hg; and isoflurane, 238 mm Hg (see Table 47-2). If ambient pressure is 760 mm Hg, these SVPs represent 243/760 = 32% halothane; 175/760 = 23% enflurane; and 239/760 = 31% isoflurane, in terms of volumes percent of agent at 1 atmosphere (760 mm Hg).

A fundamental concept to the understanding of vaporizer function is that, under steady-state condi- tions, if a certain volume of carrier gas flows into a vaporizing chamber over a certain time, that same volume of carrier gas will exit the chamber over the same period. In the vaporizing chamber, however, anesthetic vapor at its SVP constitutes a mandatory fractional volume of the atmosphere (e.g., 32% in a halothane vaporizer at 20° C and 760 mm Hg ambient pressure). Therefore the volume of carrier gas constitutes the difference between 100% of the atmosphere in the vaporizing chamber and that from the anesthetic vapor.

With halothane at 20° C the carrier gas at any time represents 68% of the atmosphere in the vaporizing chamber. Thus, if 100 ml of carrier gas enters a vaporizing chamber containing halothane, the carrier gas represents 68% (100% − 32%) of the atmosphere, and the remaining 32% is halothane vapor. By simple proportions, the latter can be calculated to be

47 ml of halothane vapor (100/68 × 32). To recap, if 100 ml of carrier gas enters the vaporizing chamber per minute, the same 100 ml of carrier gas emerges, together with 47 ml of halothane vapor/min.

By applying Dalton's law, another way of expressing this is:

$$\frac{\text{SVP agent (mm Hg)}}{\text{Total pressure (mm Hg)}} = \frac{\text{Agent vapor (x ml)}}{\text{Carrier gas (y ml)} + \text{Agent vapor (x ml)}}$$

For halothane in the previous example, y = 100 ml/min. Therefore:

$$\frac{243}{760} = \frac{x}{(100 + x)}$$

from which x can be calculated to be 47 ml. Conversely, if x is known, the carrier gas flow (y) can be calculated. Thus a larger total volume of gas leaves the vaporizing chamber than enters it, the additional volume being anesthetic vapor at its saturated vapor concentration.

Measured flow vaporizers

Although it is not mentioned in the most recent machine standard,[4] it is valuable to first review the function of a measured flow vaporizer (e.g., Copper Kettle). This arrangement is used in the Ohmeda 885A field machine currently used by the U.S. military.

Suppose 1% (vol/vol) halothane is required at a total fresh gas flow rate to the patient circuit of 5 L/min (Fig. 47-9). This requires 50 ml halothane vapor to be evolved per minute by the vaporizer (1% × 5000 ml). In the vaporizing chamber, halothane represents 32% of the atmosphere, assuming temperature is kept constant at 20° C and therefore saturated vapor pressure is maintained at 243 mm Hg. Now if 50 ml of halothane vapor represents 32%, the carrier gas (O₂) must represent the other 68%, or 106 ml (50/32 × 68). Alternatively:

$$\frac{243}{760} = \frac{50}{y + 50}, \text{where } y = \text{carrier gas (O}_2\text{) flow} = 106 \text{ ml}$$

Thus, if 106 ml/min of O₂ flows through a measured flow vaporizer, 156 ml/min of gas emerge, of which 50 ml is halothane vapor and 106 ml O₂ is supplied to the vaporizer. This vaporizer output of 156 ml/min must be diluted by an additional fresh gas flow of 5000 − 156 = 4844 ml/min, to create a precise 1% halothane mixture (since 50 ml of halothane diluted in a total volume of 5000 ml = 1% by volume).

In clinical practice, however, the anesthesiologist would likely set flows of 100 ml/min to the measured flow vaporizer and 5 L/min of fresh gas on the main flowmeters, which results in a little less than 1% halothane (actually 47/5147 = 0.91%). Multiples of

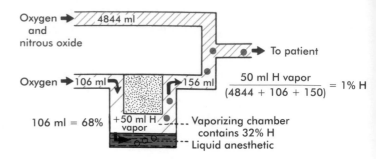

Fig. 47-9. Preparation of 1% (vol/vol) halothane by measured flow vaporizer. (From Eisenkraft JB: Vaporizers and vaporization of volatile anesthetics. In Eisenkraft JB, ed: *Progress in anesthesiology,* vol 2, San Antonio, Tx, 1988, Dannemiller Memorial Educational Foundation.)

either of these numbers are used to create other concentrations of halothane from a measured flow vaporizing system. Thus a 100 ml/min O₂ flow to the vaporizer and 2500 ml/min on the main flowmeters would give approximately 2% halothane (actually 1.78%). It is important to realize that if there is O₂ flow only to the vaporizer and no bypass gas flow is set on the main flowmeters, potentially lethal concentrations (approaching 32%) of halothane would be delivered to the anesthesia circuit, although at low flow rates.

Since halothane and isoflurane have similar vapor pressures at 20° C (see Table 47-2), the flows described for halothane are essentially the same as those to be set for isoflurane when similar concentrations of isoflurane are to be produced from a measured flow vaporizing system.

With enflurane (Fig. 47-10) the vaporizing chamber contains 23% enflurane vapor (175/760 = 23%). The O₂ flow therefore represents the other 77% of the atmosphere in the vaporizer. If 1% enflurane is required at a 3 L/min flow, 30 ml/min of enflurane vapor is needed. If 30 ml represents 23% of the atmosphere in the vaporizer, the carrier gas must represent 100 ml/min (30/23 × 77). Alternatively, using the formula given previously:

$$\frac{175}{760} = \frac{30}{30 + y}, \text{where } y = \text{O}_2 \text{ flow to vaporizer} = 100 \text{ ml/min}$$

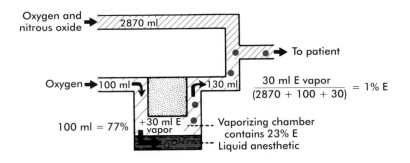

In practice mainflow is set to 3 L/min
Vaporizer flow is set to 100 ml/min
E output is 0.96% (i.e., 30 ml E vapor
diluted in [3000 + 100 + 30] ml)

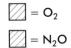 = O$_2$

= N$_2$O

= Enflurane

Fig. 47-10. Preparation of 1% (vol/vol) enflurane by measured flow (e.g., Copper Kettle) vaporizer. (From Eisenkraft JB: Vaporizers and vaporization of volatile anesthetics. In Eisenkraft JB, ed: *Progress in anesthesiology,* vol 2, San Antonio, Tx, 1988, Dannemiller Memorial Educational Foundation.)

Thus, if 100 ml/min of O$_2$ are bubbled through liquid enflurane contained in a measured flow vaporizer, 130 ml/min of gas emerge, including 30 ml/min of enflurane vapor. This must be diluted in a fresh gas flow of 3000 − 130 = 2870 ml/min to achieve 1%. In practice a bypass gas flow of 3000 ml would be set on the main flowmeters to give a resulting enflurane concentration of a little less than 1% (actually 30/3130 = 0.96%) (see Fig. 47-10).

Variable bypass

In the foregoing examples it was necessary to calculate both the O$_2$ flow to the measured flow vaporizer and the total bypass gas flow needed to produce the desired output concentrations of vapor. This is inconvenient and may give rise to errors, but one must understand the principles underlying the calculations involved because such vaporizing systems may still be in use (e.g., Ohmeda 885A field machine).

In the concentration-calibrated variable bypass design, the vaporizer splits the total flow of gas arriving from the machine flowmeters between a variable bypass and the vaporizer chamber containing the anesthetic agent (see Fig. 47-7). The ratio of these flows, the *splitting ratio,* depends on the anesthetic agent, the temperature, and the dialed-in vapor concentration set to be delivered to the patient circuit. Fig. 47-11 shows the schematic of a contemporary concentration-calibrated Dräger Vapor 19.1 vaporizer. Anesthetic output concentration is increased by

turning the concentration dial *(3),* which raises the control cone *(6),* allowing more saturated anesthetic vapor to leave the vaporizing chamber.

Review of the previous section for accurately delivering 1% halothane reveals that a 4950 ml/minute of incoming total gas flow must be split so that 106 ml enters the vaporizing chamber and 4844 ml enters the bypass (see Fig. 47-9). This results in a splitting ratio of 4844/106, or 46:1 (at a temperature of 20° C). **A variable bypass vaporizer (e.g., Dräger Vapor 19.1), when set to deliver 1% halothane, is therefore, in effect, set to a splitting ratio of 46:1.**

Consider an Enfluratec (concentration-calibrated variable bypass) vaporizer set to deliver 2% enflurane. What splitting ratio for incoming gases does this vaporizer achieve? If 100 ml/min of carrier gas enters the vaporizing chamber, 30 ml/min of enflurane vapor emerges and must be diluted in 1500 ml/min of total gas flow to produce a 2% concentration. Thus, if 1470 ml/min of carrier gas enters the vaporizer from the flowmeters and is split so that 1370 ml/min enters the bypass while 100 ml/min enters the vaporizing chamber, when the gas flows emerge, 2% enflurane will result. The splitting ratio is 1370/100, or 13.7:1.

The splitting ratios for variable bypass vaporizers used at 20° C are shown in Table 47-3. The reader is encouraged to calculate these ratios for himself/herself and to apply them to different total fresh gas flows arriving from the main flowmeters to the inlet of a concentration-calibrated variable bypass vaporizer.

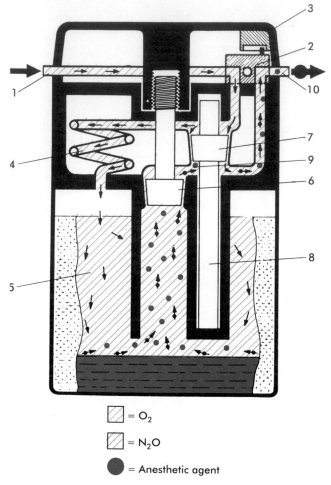

$\square$ = O₂

$\square$ = N₂O

● = Anesthetic agent

Fig. 47-11. Schematic of Dräger Vapor 19.1 vaporizer. When concentration knob *(3)* is in 0 (zero) position, on/off switch *(2)* is closed. Gas mixture enters vaporizer at fresh gas inlet *(1)* and leaves through fresh gas outlet *(10)* without entering vaporizer's interior. When concentration knob *(3)* is turned to any volume (%) concentration above 0.2 vol%, on/off switch *(2)* automatically opens and allows fresh gas to enter vaporizer's interior. Gas is immediately divided and follows two different routes. One part of fresh gas moves through thermostatically controlled bypass *(7)*, which compensates for temperature changes and maintains correct volume percent concentration vapor output as selected with concentration knob *(3)*. Other part of fresh gas moves through pressure compensator *(4)*, which prevents pressure changes that occur upstream or downstream from vaporizer to be transmitted into vaporizer and thus affect volume percent vapor output. From pressure compensator, gas continues into vaporizing chamber *(5)*. This chamber contains liquid anesthetic agent, which is absorbed and evaporated by special wick assembly. As fresh gas moves through vaporizing chamber, it is fully saturated with anesthetic vapor. Saturated gas leaves the chamber through control cone *(6)*. Cone is adjustable with concentration knob *(3)*. Saturated vapor and fresh gas that did not pass through vaporizing chamber are combined and leave through fresh gas outlet *(10)*. Combination of the bypass opening *(7)* and control cone opening *(6)* determines volume percent vapor output. Expansion element *(8)* reduces vaporizing chamber gas flow as temperature increases. (From *Narkomed 3 anesthesia system technical service manual,* Telford, Pa, 1988, North American Dräger.)

Table 47-3 Gas flow splitting ratios at 20° C*				
Halothane	**Enflurane**	**Isoflurane**	**Methoxyflurane**	**Sevoflurane**
1% 46 : 1	29 : 1	44 : 1	1.7 : 1	25 : 1
2% 22 : 1	14 : 1	21 : 1	0.36 : 1	12 : 1
3% 14 : 1	9 : 1	14 : 1	†	7 : 1

*Ratios are not given for desflurane, since the vaporizer for this agent will use a different design from that used for the above agents. See discussion at end of Key Points
†Maximum possible is 2.7% at 20° C (see Table 47-2).
From Eisenkraft JB: Anesthesia vaporizers. In Ehrenwerth J, Eisenkraft JB, eds: *Anesthesia equipment: principles and applications,* St Louis, 1992, Mosby–Year Book.

Concentration-calibrated vaporizers are agent specific and should only be used with the agent for which the unit is designed and calibrated. To produce a 1% vapor concentration, a halothane vaporizer makes a flow split of 46:1, whereas an enflurane vaporizer makes a flow split of 29.7:1 (Table 47-3). If an empty enflurane vaporizer set to deliver 1% were filled with halothane, the halothane vapor emerging would exceed 1% (actually 46/29.7 = 1.6%). An understanding of splitting ratios enables fairly accurate prediction of the concentration output of an agent-specific variable bypass vaporizer that has been erroneously filled with an agent for which it was not designed (see later discussion).

Efficiency and Temperature Compensation

Agent-specific concentration-calibrated vaporizers are located in the fresh gas line between the rotameters on the anesthesia machine and the machine common gas outlet (see Fig. 47-2). The vaporizers must be efficient and produce steady concentrations of agent over a fairly wide range of incoming gas flows. However, as the agent is vaporized and the temperature falls, SVP falls and vaporizing chamber output tends to decrease. With a measured flow vaporizer (e.g., Copper Kettle) or an uncompensated variable bypass vaporizer, this results in delivery of less anesthetic vapor to the patient circuit. For this reason, **all vaporizing systems must be temperature compensated.** This compensation may be manually or automatically achieved.

Measured flow vaporizers (e.g., Copper Kettle, Verni-Trol) incorporate a thermometer that measures the temperature of the liquid agent in the vaporizing chamber. A lower temperature translates to a lower SVP in this chamber, and reference to the vapor pressure curves (see Fig. 47-6) enables a resetting of vaporizer flows, bypass gas flows, or both to ensure correct output at the prevailing temperature. Such an arrangement can be tedious but does ensure the most accurate and rapid temperature compensation. The original Dräger Vapor vaporizer (as distinct from the modern Vapor 19.1 models fitted to contemporary Dräger Narkomed machines) is a variable bypass vaporizer in which temperature compensation is achieved manually by reference to a thermometer and grid of lines on the control dial whereby the desired output concentration is matched to liquid agent temperature. Turning the control dial changes the size of an orifice in the bypass flow in this unit.

Most contemporary variable bypass vaporizers (e.g., Ohmeda Tec series, Dräger Vapor 19.1) have automatic temperature compensation achieved by a temperature-sensitive valve in the bypass gas flow. When temperature rises, the valve in the bypass opens wider to create a higher splitting ratio. More gas flows through the bypass, and less gas enters the vaporizing chamber. A smaller volume of a higher concentration of vapor emerges from the vaporizing chamber. When mixed with an increased bypass gas flow, this volume maintains the vaporizer output reasonably constant when temperature changes are gradual and not extreme.

The design of the temperature-sensitive valve varies among the different types of vaporizer. In the vaporizing chamber, some vaporizers (e.g., Ohio) use a gas-filled bellows linked to a valve in the bypass gas flow.[9] As temperature increases, the bellows expands, causing the valve to open wider. Other vaporizers (e.g., Ohmeda Tec series) use a bimetallic strip. The principle of this is that a flap valve situated in the bypass flow is composed of two different metals that have different coefficients of expansion (change in length per unit length per unit change in temperature). As temperature rises, one surface of the flap expands more than the other, causing the flap to move in such a way that the valve orifice opens wider. The principle of differential expansion of metals is applied similarly in the Dräger Vapor 19.1 vaporizers, in which an expansion element reduces vaporizing chamber gas flow as temperature increases (see Fig. 47-11, component *8*).

The vapor pressures of the potent volatile anesthetics vary nonlinearly as a function of temperature (see Fig. 47-6). The automatic temperature compensation mechanisms described are linear in terms of expansion coefficients of materials. When these affect the size of the orifice that they control, however, the compensation mechanisms also become nonlinear. The situation is complex, depending on the geometry of the valves and the nature of the gas flow through them. The result is that the vapor output concentration at any given vaporizer setting remains constant only within a certain range of temperatures. For example, the Dräger Vapor 19.1 vaporizers are specified as accurate to ±15% of the concentration set when used within the temperature range of +15° C to +35° C at normal atmospheric pressure.[46, 47] At temperatures outside this range, the resulting concentration increases beyond the upper tolerance limit despite continuing compensation. The boiling point of the volatile agent must never be reached in the current variable bypass vaporizers designed for halothane, enflurane, isoflurane, methoxyflurane, and sevoflurane, since otherwise the vapor output concentration would be totally uncontrolled and lethal.

In some previous vaporizers (e.g., Fluotec Mark II) the temperature compensation valve was in the vaporizing chamber itself. The thymol preservatives added to halothane could cause sticking of this valve, so that in subsequent models and other modern vaporizers the temperature-compensating valve is situated in the bypass gas flow.[20]

Incorrect Filling of Vaporizers

Modern vaporizers are agent-specific. If an empty vaporizer designed for one agent is filled with an agent for which it was not designed, the vaporizer output may be erroneous. Since at room temperature the vaporizing characteristics of halothane and isoflurane are almost identical, this problem currently only applies to interchanging halothane or isoflurane with enflurane.

An even more dangerous situation would result if a vaporizer designed for methoxyflurane (SVP of 20.3 mm Hg at 20° C) were filled with halothane, enflurane, or isoflurane (see Table 47-2). Since methoxyflurane is seldom used now, this is, fortunately, now an unlikely occurrence. A methoxyflurane vaporizer filled with halothane and set to deliver 1% methoxyflurane (although 6 MAC, see Table 47-2) would deliver 14.8% (20 MAC) halothane. Set to 1 MAC (0.16%) methoxyflurane, the vaporizer makes a flow split of 16:1, similar to that of a halothane or iso-flurane variable bypass vaporizer set to deliver 2.7%.

The outputs of erroneously filled vaporizers are shown in Table 47-4. Erroneous filling affects the output concentration and consequently the MAC (MAP, MAPP) or potency output of the vaporizer.[11] Thus an enflurane vaporizer set to 2% (1.19 MAC) but filled with halothane will deliver 3.21% (4.01 MAC) halothane, that is, 3.3 times the anticipated anesthetic potency output.[11] Erroneous filling of vaporizers may be prevented by careful attention to the specific agent and the vaporizer when filling is performed. Agent-specific keyed filling mechanisms are available as options on modern vaporizers. Liquid anesthetic agents are commercially available packaged in bottles that have an agent-specific collar. An agent-specific filling device has one end that fits the collar on the agent bottle, and the other end fits only the vaporizer designed for that agent. These filling

Table 47-4   Output in percent and minimum alveolar concentration (MAC) in O₂ of erroneously filled vaporizers at 22° C

Vaporizers	Liquid	Setting (%)	Output (%)	Output MAC
Halothane	Halothane	1.0	1.00	1.25
	Enflurane	1.0	0.62	0.37
	Isoflurane	1.0	0.96	0.84
Enflurane	Enflurane	2.0	2.00	1.19
	Isoflurane	2.0	3.09	2.69
	Halothane	2.0	3.21	4.01
Isoflurane	Isoflurane	1.5	1.50	1.30
	Halothane	1.5	1.56	1.95
	Enflurane	1.5	0.97	0.57

From Bruce DL, Linde HW: Vaporization of mixed anesthetic liquids, *Anesthesiology* 60:342, 1984.

Halothane, enflurane, and isoflurane, when mixed, do not react chemically but do influence the extent of each other's ease of vaporization. Halothane facilitates the vaporization of both enflurane and isoflurane and in the process is itself more likely to vaporize.[36] The clinical consequences depend on the potencies of each of the mixed agents as well as the delivered vapor concentrations. If a halothane vaporizer 25% full is refilled to 100% with isoflurane and set to deliver 1%, the halothane output is 0.41% (0.51 MAC) and the isoflurane output 0.9% (0.78 MAC) (Table 47-5).[11] In this case the output potency of 1.29 MAC is not far from the 1.25 MAC (1% halothane) expected.

On the other hand, an enflurane vaporizer 25% full and set to deliver 2% (1.19 MAC) enflurane, which is filled to 100% with halothane, has an output of 2.43% (3.03 MAC) halothane and 0.96% (0.57 MAC) enflurane (Table 47-5).[11] This represents a total MAC of 3.6, or more than twice that intended. In any event, it is important that erroneous filling of vaporizers be avoided, and that if suspected, the vaporizer should be emptied, serviced, flushed, and refilled with the correct agent. Contemporary vaporizers are available with agent-specific filling devices that are designed to prevent erroneous filling, as well as to reduce operating room contamination.

Filling of Vaporizers

Vaporizers should only be filled as directed in their accompanying instructions. Overfilling or tilting of a vaporizer (free-standing or by tilting the whole anesthesia machine) may result in liquid agent entering parts of the anesthesia delivery system (e.g., vaporizer bypass flow) designed for gases only and might give rise to lethal concentrations of the agent. If a vaporizer has been tilted and there is concern that liquid agent has leaked into the gas delivery system, with no patient connected to the system, the vaporizer should be flushed with a high flow rate of O₂ (10 L/min) from the flowmeter (not the O₂ flush, which

though well intentioned, to date have not gained much popularity in use. The F1161-88 standard states that the filling mechanism *should* be fitted with a permanently attached standard, agent-specific keyed filling device to prevent accidental filling with the wrong agent.[4] **Agent-specific filling devices will assume greater importance with the introduction of desflurane into clinical use, an agent with an SVP of 664 mm Hg at 20° C** (see later discussion and Table 47-2).

Vaporization of Mixed Anesthetic Liquids

Perhaps a more likely scenario is that an agent-specific vaporizer that is partially filled with correct agent is topped off with an incorrect agent.[11] The situation here is more complex, it is less easily predicted in terms of vaporizer output, and large errors in delivered vapor administration can occur.

Table 47-5   Vaporizer output after incorrectly refilling from 25% full to 100% full

Vaporizer	Setting (%)	Refill liquid	Halothane %	Halothane MAC	Enflurane %	Enflurane MAC	Isoflurane %	Isoflurane MAC	Total MAC
Halothane	1.0	Enflurane	0.33	0.41	0.64	0.38	—	—	0.79
	1.0	Isoflurane	0.41	0.51	—	—	0.90	0.78	1.29
Enflurane	2.0	Halothane	2.43	3.03	0.96	0.57	—	—	3.60
Isoflurane	1.5	Halothane	1.28	1.60	—	—	0.57	0.50	2.10

From Bruce DL, Linde HW: Vaporization of mixed anesthetic liquids, *Anesthesiology* 60:342, 1984.

bypasses the vaporizer) and with the vaporizer concentration dial set to the maximum concentration setting.[69a]

Table 47-2 shows that **1 ml of liquid volatile agent produces approximately 200 ml of vapor at 20° C.** Thus, if small volumes of liquid agent enter the gas delivery system, it is easy to see how the lethal concentrations could arise. For example, if 1 ml of liquid halothane entered the common gas tubing, it would require 20 L of fresh gas to dilute the resulting vapor to a 1% concentration (1.3 MAC).

Effect of Carrier Gas on Vaporizer Output

The carrier gas used to vaporize the volatile agent in the vaporizing chamber may also affect vaporizer output. Thus, when the carrier gas flow through a variable bypass Ohio enflurane vaporizer was changed from N_2/O_2 to N_2O/O_2, the vaporizer output concentration decreased for about 15 minutes and then returned to normal.[59] Once the output was stable with a carrier gas of N_2O/O_2, changing back to N_2/O_2 resulted in an increase in vaporizer output for about 15 minutes (Fig. 47-12).

The explanation of this observed effect is the solubility of N_2O in the liquid volatile agents. Thus, when N_2O/O_2 begins to enter the vaporizing chamber, some N_2O gas dissolves in the liquid agent, and the vaporizing chamber output decreases until the liquid has become saturated with N_2O. Conversely, when N_2O is withdrawn as the carrier gas, the N_2O gas

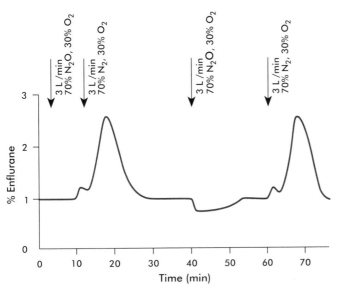

Fig. 47-12. Effect of carrier gas composition on output of Ohio enflurane variable bypass vaporizer (*see text for details*). (From Scheller M, Drummond JC: Solubility of N_2O in volatile anesthetics contributes to vaporizer aberrancy when changing carrier gases, *Anesth Analg* 65:88, 1986.)

dissolved in the liquid anesthetic comes out of solution and represents, in effect, additional gas flow to the vaporizing chamber. The solubility of N_2O in the liquid anesthetics is approximately 4.5 ml/ml of liquid anesthetic. Thus 100 ml of halothane liquid, when fully saturated, can dissolve approximately 450 ml of N_2O. Such a volume of N_2O, being added to the vaporizing chamber flow over a brief period when N_2O has been discontinued, causes the observed increase in vaporizer output concentration. This effect is not seen with measured flow vaporizers, since in this type of arrangement (e.g., Copper Kettle, Verni-Trol) the carrier gas is always O_2.[59]

Changes in Barometric Pressure

Although vaporizers are usually used at ambient pressures of around 760 mm Hg (1 atmosphere at sea level), they may be used under hypobaric conditions (e.g., at increased altitude) or under hyperbaric conditions (e.g., in a hyperbaric chamber).[33]

Hypobaric conditions

Few reports discuss the use of vaporizers under hypobaric conditions. The theoretic considerations applying to such use therefore are discussed here. Consider a variable bypass vaporizer set to deliver 1% halothane (1.3 MAC at 760 mm Hg atmospheric pressure) that is being used at an ambient pressure of 500 mm Hg (equivalent to altitude of 10,000 feet above sea level) and at a temperature of 20° C (Fig. 47-13). In the vaporizing chamber, halothane has an SVP of 243 mm Hg (temperature of 20° C), but this now represents 243/500 = 48.6 vol%. The vaporizer, set to deliver 1% under normal conditions, creates a splitting ratio of 46:1 (see Table 47-3) between bypass and vaporizing chamber flows.

If the total gas flow to the vaporizer is 4700 ml/min (Fig. 47-13), 100 ml/min of carrier gas enters the vaporizing chamber. This represents 51.4% of the volume there because halothane represents the other 48.6 vol% (100 − 51.4). Emerging from the chamber is 100 ml/min of carrier gas plus [(100/51.4) × 48.6] = 94.6 ml/min of halothane vapor. When the vaporizing chamber and bypass flows merge, the 94.6 ml/min of halothane vapor are diluted in a total volume of 4794.6 ml/min (4600 + 100 + 94.6 ml), giving a halothane concentration of 1.97 vol%, or approximately 2%. This would appear to be double the dialed-in concentration in terms of volumes percent.

Now consider partial pressures. If halothane represents 1.97% of the gas mixture by volume, its partial pressure in the emerging mixture is 1.97 × 500, or 9.85 mm Hg. In terms of anesthetic potency, this represents 9.85/5.7, or 1.73 MAC, since the $P_{MAC\,1}$ of halothane is 5.7 mm Hg (see Table 47-1).

Thus in theory, used at a pressure of 500 mm Hg,

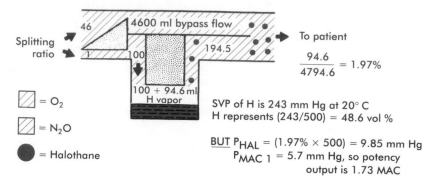

Fig. 47-13. Use of variable bypass halothane vaporizer under hypobaric conditions. Vaporizer is set to 1% (vol/vol) and is being used at ambient pressure of 500 mm Hg. (From Eisenkraft JB: Vaporizers and vaporization of volatile anesthetics, In Eisenkraft JB, ed: *Progress in anesthesiology,* vol 2, San Antonio, Tx, 1988, Dannemiller Memorial Educational Foundation.)

the variable bypass halothane vaporizer set to 1% (vol/vol) would deliver twice the set concentration in terms of volumes percent but only 1.73/1.33 MAC, or 1.3 times, the anesthetic potency. The same situation would result if a measured flow system were being used with the flows set as for 1% halothane at an ambient pressure of 760 mm Hg.

Hyperbaric conditions

Consider a variable bypass isoflurane vaporizer set to deliver 2% (1.74 MAC at 760 mm Hg atmospheric pressure) isoflurane vapor and being used at 20° C under conditions of 3 atmospheres pressure (3 × 760 = 2280 mm Hg), as may exist in a hyperbaric chamber (Fig. 47-14).

In the vaporizing chamber, the SVP of isoflurane is 238 mm Hg (see Table 47-2), and the isoflurane concentration is 10.4 vol% (238/2280). A variable bypass isoflurane vaporizer set to deliver 2% creates a splitting ratio of 21:1 for the fresh gas flow (see Table 47-3). If the total gas flow to the vaporizer is 2200 ml/min, 100 ml of carrier gas enters the vaporizing chamber per minute (see Fig. 47-14). This 100 ml represents 89.6% (100 − 10.4) of the total gas there; the remainder is isoflurane vapor. The amount of isoflurane vapor evolved is [(100/89.6) × 10.4] = 11.6 ml/minute. This volume, diluted in 2100 + 100 + 11.64 gives 11.6/2211.6, or 0.52% isoflurane vapor by volume. This is 0.26 (0.52/2.0) times what was set on the concentration dial in terms of volumes percent.

What about potency? The partial pressure of isoflurane in the emerging gas mixture is 11.9 mm Hg (0.52% × 2280). Dividing by the $P_{MAC\,1}$ for isoflurane of 8.7 mm Hg (see Table 47-1) gives a potency output of 1.37 MAC (11.9/8.7). Thus the isoflurane vaporizer, set to deliver 1.74 MAC under conditions of 1 atmosphere (760 mm Hg) pressure, delivers 1.37 MAC at 3 atmospheres, or about 0.80 times the anesthetic potency expected.

These examples show that, although changing ambient pressure has a great effect on vaporizer

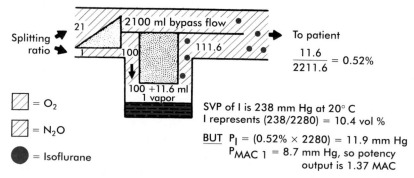

Fig. 47-14. Use of variable bypass isoflurane vaporizer under hyperbaric conditions. Vaporizer is set to 2% (vol/vol) and is being used at ambient pressure of 2280 mm Hg (3 atmospheres). (From Eisenkraft JB: Vaporizers and vaporization of volatile anesthetics. In Eisenkraft JB, ed: *Progress in anesthesiology,* vol 2, San Antonio, Tx, 1988, Dannemiller Memorial Educational Foundation.)

output in terms of volumes percent, the anesthetic potency (MAC) output is changed less drastically. In the examples discussed, it was assumed that the set splitting ratios (see Table 47-3) would be maintained constant as ambient pressure changed. In reality, however, changes in gas density occur with changes in ambient pressure and may affect the splitting ratios slightly. **From a practical point of view the anesthetic potency output expected for any given vaporizer setting is relatively unchanged, even though vapor concentration (vol/vol) may be altered considerably.**[33] **Again, it is emphasized that vaporizer output concentration expressed in volumes percent is of limited value unless converted to MAC units using the concept of pressures as described in the foregoing examples.**[23,33]

Arrangement of Vaporizers

Older anesthesia machines had up to three variable bypass vaporizers arranged in series such that fresh gas from the flowmeters passed through each vaporizer (although all through the bypass flow) to reach the common gas outlet of the anesthesia machine. Without an interlock system, which permits only one vaporizer to be in use at any time, one could have all three vaporizers turned on simultaneously. Apart from potentially overdosing the patient, the agent from the upstream vaporizer could contaminate the agent(s) in the vaporizer(s) downstream. During subsequent use the output of the downstream vaporizer would be contaminated. The resulting concentrations in the emerging gas and vapor mixture would be indeterminant and might even be lethal.[23]

With modern arrangements, only one vaporizer can be on at any time. The F1161-88 standard requires that to prevent cross-contamination of the contents of one vaporizer with agent from another, a system must be provided that isolates the vaporizers from each other and prevents gas from passing through the vaporizing chamber of one vaporizer and then through that of another.[4] This specification is met by use of an interlock system. Contemporary Dräger and Ohmeda anesthesia machines incorporate manufacturer-specific interlock systems.[43,47]

Calibration and Checking of Vaporizer Outputs

Vaporizers should be regularly serviced according to manufacturer's recommendations and their outputs checked to ensure that a malfunction does not exist. Thus the vaporizer dial is set to deliver a certain concentration. The actual output concentration is measured by an anesthetic agent analyzer sampling gas via a connector placed at the common gas outlet of the anesthesia machine.

Currently available practical vapor analysis methods include mass spectrometry, multiwavelength infrared spectroscopy, laser-Raman scattering, oscillating lipophilic-coated piezo-electric quartz crystal, and refractometry. The first three methods enable multiple agents to be identified and quantified in the presence of one another. Refractometry, single wavelength infrared agent analysis, and piezo-electric crystal technology are reliable if only one agent is present and has been qualitatively identified to the analyzer. The reader is referred elsewhere for a more detailed discussion of these technologies.[25a]

Preparation of Standard Vapor Concentrations

Although the physical methods for analysis mentioned in the previous section may be used to check vaporizer output, the agent analyzers themselves require calibration. For this a standard vapor concentration must be prepared.

Consider the preparation of a standard mixture of halothane in O_2. Avogadro's volume states that 1 molecule of a gas or vapor occupies 22.4 L at STP (760 mm Hg pressure, 0° C/273° K). Thus 197.4 g of halothane vapor occupies 22.4 L at STP, and 1 g occupies 22.4/197.4 L.

According to Charles' law (volume of a fixed mass of gas is proportional to absolute temperature if pressure remains constant), 1 g halothane occupies $22.4/197.4 \times 293/273 = 0.12$ L at 20° C (293° K). One milliliter of liquid halothane weighs 1.86 g (specific gravity of halothane is 1.86, see Table 47-2); therefore 1 ml of liquid halothane generates $22.4/197.4 \times 293/273 \times 1.86$, or 0.226 L of vapor. Thus 1 ml of liquid halothane produces 226 ml of vapor at 20° C.

Using this type of calculation, a predetermined volume of liquid agent can be accurately measured using a micropipette, then transferred to and vaporized in a chamber of known volume to produce a calibration standard gas mixture.

Desflurane

Desflurane (Suprane, Anaquest, Liberty Corner, NJ) is a new potent inhaled volatile anesthetic currently undergoing clinical investigation in the United States. The physical properties are shown in Box 47-1. With an SVP of 664 mm Hg at 20° C (Fig. 47-15) and a boiling point of 23.5° C, this agent is extremely volatile, which presents certain problems regarding vaporization and production of controlled concentration of vapor. At least four possible methods exist for controlling the vapor output concentration.[23]

Heated, pressurized vaporizer. This technique is employed in the Ohio DM (Direct Metering) 5000 machine, which has a heated, pressurized vaporizer. The agent is heated to 23.5° to 24° C, at which its vapor pressure is 770 mm Hg, and the machine upstream of the common gas outlet is pressurized to 1550 mm Hg by an altitude compensator (back pressure regulator).

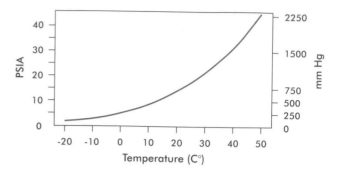

Fig. 47-15. Vapor pressure curve for desflurane. (Data courtesy Anaquest, Liberty Corner, NJ.)

In the vaporizer the desflurane vapor therefore represents 770/1550, or approximately 50% of the atmosphere by volume. A measured flow type of arrangement (see Fig. 47-8) is then used to dilute the 50% desflurane to clinically useful concentrations. The DM 5000 has been used in the United States for clinical trials of desflurane only. For the investigations an agent analyzer is also used to continuously monitor the anesthetic concentration in the patient circuit and to protect against possible overdosing.

Heating liquid to form vapor under pressure. Desflurane could be heated to greater than 24° C to form a gas under pressure, which is then metered into the main gas flow using a separate flow control system. A potential disadvantage of this arrangement is condensation of liquid agent in parts of the delivery system intended for gas only so that the desflurane vapor delivery system would have to be heated throughout to prevent this from occurring. This technology is available now in the Ohmeda Tec 6 vaporizer* (see footnote at end of Key Points for discussion).

Liquid injection. Desflurane liquid in pulsed, metered doses could be vaporized into known fresh gas flows to produce clinically useful concentrations. This system is analogous to fuel injection systems used in automobile engines and has been used in certain anesthesia delivery systems (Engström ELSA, Boston Anesthesia Machine).[1,17]

Cooled variable bypass vaporizer. If cooled to 5° C, desflurane has an SVP of about 250 mm Hg (Fig. 47-15) and could thus potentially be administered using a conventional variable bypass (Tec-type) vaporizer. Cooling a variable bypass vaporizer presents many technical problems and is energy inefficient.

If and when desflurane becomes generally available for clinical use, the vaporizing system will differ from those described for the presently available potent inhaled agents and will likely use one of the method-

ologies just described, all of which require a source of energy (electricity). General requirements of the desflurane vaporizer are that it will deliver accurate concentrations over a wide range of gas flows and that it should be easily retrofitted to contemporary anesthesia machines, replacing one of the existing machine-mounted and interlocked vaporizers.

COMMON GAS OUTLET AND OUTLET CHECK VALVES

The fresh gas mixture produced by the settings of the flowmeters for O_2, N_2O, and other gases, and vapor from one concentration-calibrated vaporizer exit the machine via the common gas outlet. Situated between the vaporizer and the common gas outlet, Ohmeda Modulus I and Modulus II machines have (1) an outlet check valve and (2) a pressure relief valve that opens at a pressure of 120 to 150 mm Hg (2.3 to 2.9 PSIG) (see Fig. 47-2). The pressure relief valve, as its name suggests, prevents the buildup of excessive pressures upstream of the outlet check valve. These components are located upstream from where the O_2 flush flow would join to pass to the common gas outlet. The Ohmeda Excel machine has an outlet check valve and a pressure relief valve (opening pressure threshold, 5 PSIG) that is located *downstream* of the outlet check valve.

The purpose of the outlet check valve, where present (Ohmeda Modulus I, Modulus II, and Excel but not Modulus II Plus or Modulus CD machines), is to prevent reverse gas flow, which could cause gas to go back into the vaporizer if the latter did not have its own outlet check valve or specialized design. This "pumping" effect, if not prevented, could cause increased vaporizer output concentrations.[23]

Dräger Narkomed machines are designed so as not to require an outlet check valve. Any pumping effect is eliminated by special design of the Vapor 19.1 vaporizer (see Fig. 47-11, component *4*). The Ohmeda Modulus II Plus and Modulus CD machines are equipped with Ohmeda Tec 4 or Tec 5 vaporizers, which incorporate a baffle system and specially designed manifold to prevent the pumping effect, making an outlet check valve unnecessary on these machines. Nevertheless, the Ohmeda Modulus II Plus and Modulus CD machines *do* have a pressure relief valve (see Fig. 47-2). Dräger Narkomed machines do not require a separate pressure relief valve.[47] In these machines, pressure relief opening (threshold approximately 18 PSIG), if required, takes place through the specially designed Vapor 19.1 vaporizers. The presence or absence of an outlet check valve and pressure relief valve is important for testing the low-pressure system of the anesthesia machine for leaks.[23a]

Some anesthesiologists have configured a jet ventilation system to be used in an emergency and to ventilate via a cricothyroid needle puncture. Such systems are connected to the machine's common gas outlet using a 15-mm connector, and ventilation is achieved by intermittent depression of the O_2 flush button. High-pressure tubing is used to conduct the O_2 from the common gas outlet to the cricothyroid cannula. One must realize that the driving pressure, and, therefore, efficacy, of such a system depends on whether the machine has an outlet check valve and the type and threshold opening pressure of any pressure relief valve. Thus in a Dräger Narkomed machine with Vapor 19.1 vaporizers, the driving pressure of the system at the common gas outlet would be approximately 18 PSIG. With an Ohmeda Modulus I or II, it would be 55 PSIG. With an Ohmeda Modulus II Plus or Modulus CD, the driving pressure would be much less (approximately 3 PSIG). Machine manufacturers do not advocate the use of such systems connected to the common gas outlet.[23a]

The F1161-88 standard requires that when the common gas outlet is connected to the breathing system by a fresh gas supply hose (the usual arrangement in most operating rooms), the common gas outlet should be provided with a manufacturer-specific retaining device.[4] It may have a 15 mm female fitting or a 15/22 mm coaxial fitting. Machines should have only one common gas outlet. The retaining device's purpose is to help prevent disconnection or misconnections between the machine common gas outlet and the patient circuit, which could result in patient injury. Dräger Narkomed machines have a bar-type retaining device, whereas Ohmeda machines use a spring-loaded bayonet-fitting retaining device.

ANESTHESIA MACHINE CHECKOUT

The anesthesia delivery system should be checked each day before administering anesthesia to the first patient and whenever any change has been made to the system. Such changes include replacing the ventilator bellows or anesthesia circuit and moving **the anesthesia machine, even within the operating room. Moving the machine may cause kinking or compression of tubing, which in turn may produce interference with gas delivery, ventilator function, or waste gas scavenging. Thus, in addition to a complete checkout at the start of each day, a shortened checkout of the delivery system should precede each administration of an anesthetic.**

In August 1986 the Food and Drug Administration (FDA) published its *Anesthesia Apparatus Checkout Recommendations,* which are shown in Box 47-2.[30] This checkout applies as a general guideline only, and the FDA encourages users to modify this checkout "to accommodate differences in equipment design and variations in local clinical practice. **Users should refer to the operator's manual for special procedures or precautions**" (bold added). In this respect the user must understand the basic arrangement and functions of the anesthesia machine components to apply the correct checkout procedure. This becomes apparent in the following sections.

Testing for Leaks in Anesthesia Machine and Breathing System

Item *16* in the FDA checkout describes how to check for leaks (Box 47-2).[30] This checkout evaluates the components of the delivery system that are downstream of the flowmeters. It should detect *gross* leaks that may result from cracked rotameter tubes, leaking gaskets and vaporizers, and leaks in the anesthesia circuit. In this generic test the adjustable pressure-limiting (APL, or "pop-off") valve is closed and the patient circuit is occluded at the patient end (Box 47-2, item *16a*). The system is then filled via the O_2 flush until the reservoir bag is just full, but negligible pressure exists in the system. Oxygen flow is set to 5 L/min (Box 47-2, item *16b*). Oxygen flow is then slowly decreased until pressure no longer rises above about 20 cm H_2O (Fig. 47-16). This set flow is said to approximate the total gas leak rate, which should be no greater than a few hundred ml/min (Box 47-2, item *16c*). The reservoir bag should then be squeezed to a pressure of about 50 cm H_2O to verify that the system is gas tight (Box 47-2, item *16d*). If a large enough leak is present, the circuit pressure may fall to zero (Fig. 47-17).

The advantages of this test routine are that it can be performed quickly and that it checks the patient circuit as well as the low-pressure parts of the machine in those models without an outlet check valve. Disadvantages of this routine are that it is relatively insensitive to small leaks and that, in those machines with an outlet check valve (e.g., Ohmeda Modulus I, Modulus II, and Excel models), only the patient circuit downstream of the outlet check valve would be tested for leaks.

The generic checkout is insensitive because it is

BOX 47-2
FDA ANESTHESIA APPARATUS CHECKOUT RECOMMENDATIONS—1986

This checkout or a reasonable equivalent should be conducted before administering anesthesia. This is a guideline that users are encouraged to modify to accommodate differences in equipment design and variations in local clinical practice. Such local modifications should have appropriate peer review. Users should refer to the operator's manual for special procedures or precautions.

*1. Inspect anesthesia machine for:
  a. Machine identification number.
  b. Valid inspection sticker.
  c. Undamaged flowmeters, vaporizers, gauges, supply hoses.
  d. Complete, undamaged breathing system with adequate CO_2 absorbent.
  e. Correct mounting of cylinders in yokes.
  f. Presence of cylinder wrench.

*2. Inspect and turn on:
  a. Electrical equipment requiring warm-up (ECG/pressure monitor, O_2 monitor, etc.).

*3. Connect waste gas scavenging system:
  a. Adjust vacuum as required.

*4. Check that:
  a. Flow-control valves are off.
  b. Vaporizers are off.
  c. Vaporizers are filled (not overfilled).
  d. Filler caps are sealed tightly.
  e. CO_2 absorber bypass (if any) is off.

*5. Check O_2 cylinder supplies:
  a. Disconnect pipeline supply (if connected) and return cylinder and pipeline pressure gauges to zero with O_2 flush valve.
  b. Open O_2 cylinder; check pressure; close cylinder and observe gauge for evidence of high-pressure leak.
  c. With the O_2 flush valve, flush to empty piping.
  d. Repeat b and c for second O_2 cylinder, if present.
  e. Replace any cylinder less than about 600 PSIG. At least one should be nearly full.
  f. Open less full cylinder.

*6. Turn on master switch (if present).

*7. Check N_2O and other gas cylinder supplies. Use same procedure as described in 5a and 5b, but open and *close* flow control valve to empty piping.
  NOTE: N_2O pressure below 745 PSIG indicates that the cylinder is less than ¼ full.

*8. Test flowmeters:
  a. Check that float is at bottom of tube with flow control valves closed (or at minimal O_2 flow if so equipped).
  b. Adjust flow of all gases through their full range and check for erratic movements of floats.

*9. Test ratio protection/warning system (if present). Attempt to create hypoxic O_2/N_2O mixture, and verify correct change in gas flows and/or alarm.

*10. Test O_2 pressure failure system:
  a. Set O_2 and other gas flows to midrange.
  b. Close O_2 cylinder and flush to release O_2 pressure.
  c. Verify that all flows fall to zero; open O_2 cylinder.
  d. Close all other cylinders and bleed piping pressures.
  e. Close O_2 cylinder and bleed piping pressure.
  f. *Close flow control valves.*

*11. Test central pipeline gas supplies:
  a. Inspect supply hoses (should not be cracked or worn).
  b. Connect supply hoses, verifying correct color coding.
  c. Adjust all flows to at least mid-range.
  d. Verify that supply pressures hold (45-55 PSIG).
  e. Shut off flow control valves.

*12. Add any accessory equipment to the breathing system. Add PEEP valve, humidifier, etc., if they might be used (if necessary remove after step 18 until needed).

13. Calibrate O_2 monitor:
  *a. Calibrate O_2 monitor to read 21% in room air.
  *b. Test low alarm.
  c. Occlude breathing system at patient end; fill and empty system several times with 100% O_2.
  d. Check that monitor reading is nearly 100%.

14. Sniff inspiratory gas.
  There should be no odor.

*15. Check unidirectional valves:
  a. Inhale and exhale through a surgical mask into the breathing system (each limb individually, if possible).
  b. Verify unidirectional flow in each limb.
  c. Reconnect tubing firmly.

†16. Test for leaks in machine and breathing system:
  a. Close APL (pop-off) valve and occlude system at patient end.
  b. Fill system via O_2 flush until bag just full, but negligible pressure in system. Set O_2 flow to 5 L/min.
  c. Slowly decrease O_2 flow until pressure *no longer rises* above about 20 cm H_2O. This

---

*If an anesthetist uses the same machine in successive cases, these steps need not be repeated or may be abbreviated after the initial checkout.
†A vaporizer leak can only be detected if vaporizer is turned on during this test. Even then, a relatively small but clinically significant leak may still be obscured.
Developed by the FDA, August 1986.

***BOX 47-2—*cont'd**
FDA ANESTHESIA APPARATUS CHECKOUT RECOMMENDATIONS—1986

---

approximates total leak rate, which should be no greater than a few hundred ml/min (less for closed-circuit techniques).

CAUTION: Check valves in some machines make it imperative to measure flow in step c when pressure *just stops rising.*

d. Squeeze bag to pressure of about 50 cm H_2O, and verify that system is tight.

17. Check exhaust valve and scavenger system:
    a. Open APL valve and observe release of pressure.
    b. Occlude breathing system at patient end and verify that negligible positive or negative pressure appears with either zero or 5 L/min flow and exhaust relief valve (if present) opens with flush flow.

18. Test ventilator:
    a. If switching valve is present, test function in both bag and ventilator mode.

b. Close APL valve if necessary and occlude system at patient end.
c. Test for leaks and pressure relief by appropriate cycling (exact procedure will vary with type of ventilator).
d. Attach reservoir bag at mask fitting, fill system, and cycle ventilator. Ensure filling/emptying of bag.

19. Check for appropriate level of patient suction.
20. Check, connect, and calibrate other electronic monitors.
21. Check final position of all controls.
22. Turn on and set other appropriate alarms for equipment to be used.
    (Perform next two steps as soon as practical.)
23. Set O_2 monitor alarm limits.
24. Set airway pressure and/or volume monitor alarm limits (if adjustable).

---

volume dependent. Thus in this test a large volume of gas (i.e., that contained in the circuit tubing, absorber, and reservoir bag) is compressed, and a change in reading on the pressure gauge is sought. The term *compliance* expresses the relationship between volume and pressure and is defined as change in volume per unit change in pressure. Because of the large volume of gas compressed and the high compliance of the distensible reservoir bag, relatively large changes in volume (i.e., leaks) may exist with minimal changes in pressure. The anesthetist performing the check is seeking a pressure drop as an indicator of gas leakage, but large leaks may go undetected by this test. Such leaks may be unimportant while high fresh gas flows are used but become more significant if gas flow rates are reduced subsequently during the maintenance of anesthesia.

The second limitation of the FDA generic checkout is related to the presence or absence of an outlet check valve, which, if present, separates the low-pressure part of the machine from the common gas outlet and circuit components downstream (see Fig. 47-2). Application of the generic leak check in this situation may fail to detect leaks in components downstream of the outlet check valve (Fig. 47-18). Furthermore, in the past, certain anesthesia delivery systems *configured by the user* placed a free-standing vaporizer in series between the common gas outlet of the machine and the fresh gas inlet of the patient circuit. Some of these free-standing vaporizers incorporated their own outlet check valve to prevent a

pumping effect on the vaporizer. If such an arrangement is being used, the generic leak check will test only as far proximally as the location of this check valve in the vaporizer's outlet.

The use of in-series free-standing vaporizers is not described in the F1161-88 standard and should be avoided. Further, because free-standing vaporizers were placed downstream of the machine's common gas outlet, use of the O_2 flush would deliver a "bolus" of potent inhaled agent to the patient circuit. This assumes that the tubing connections were not disrupted by the high pressures associated with use of the O_2 flush. A disconnect between the machine's common gas outlet and the free-standing vaporizer could also cause a low-concentration O_2 mixture to develop in the patient circuit during controlled ventilation (if a hanging bellows ventilator is being used),[13] thus the current requirement for a retaining device.[4] In addition, any vaporizer exclusion system (interlock) would be compromised with a free-standing arrangement. **Again, it is emphasized that the use of free-standing vaporizers downstream of the common gas outlet is not recommended and may be hazardous.**

The limitations of the FDA generic leak check demand that specialized leak checks of the low-pressure system must be used and that the machine operator's manual should be consulted for details. Those tests described for the Dräger Narkomed and Ohmeda machines are briefly reviewed to illustrate the differences in system design, function, and checkout.

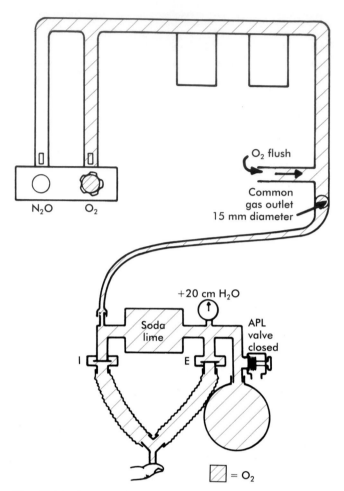

Fig. 47-16. Generic leak test in machine without outlet check valve (Box 47-2, item *16*). In this case, pressure of 20 cm of water is held with no gas flow, indicating both patient circuit and low-pressure parts of machine are gas tight. (From Eisenkraft JB: Anesthesia delivery system. Part II. In Eisenkraft JB, ed: *Progress in anesthesiology,* vol 3, San Antonio, Tx, 1989, Dannemiller Memorial Educational Foundation.)

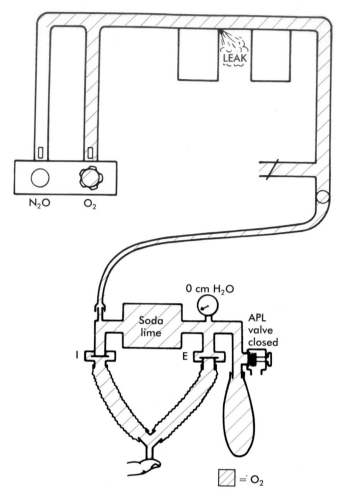

Fig. 47-17. In absence of outlet check valve, leak at vaporizer mount results in failure of system to hold pressure, which in this case falls to zero. Such a leak would not be detectable by this test if outlet check valve (see Fig. 46-18) were present. (From Eisenkraft JB: Anesthesia delivery system. Part II. In Eisenkraft JB, ed: *Progress in anesthesiology,* vol 3, San Antonio, Tx, 1989, Dannemiller Memorial Educational Foundation.)

Dräger Narkomed Machines: No Outlet Check Valve

North American Dräger recommends the following test procedure for checking the anesthesia breathing system and fresh gas delivery system.[45,46] In this test, all gas flow control (flowmeter) valves are closed, and the machine system's main power switch is turned to standby or off. In this way, no gas should flow to the flowmeters or from the common gas outlet. All vaporizer concentration dials are set to zero concentration. The inspiratory and expiratory valves are interconnected using a 22 mm–diameter circuit hose (Fig. 47-19). The shortest possible length of hose should be used to minimize contained gas volume. The "manual/automatic" selector valve is set to the manual (bag) position. The APL ("pop-off") valve is

closed (turned fully clockwise). The reservoir bag is removed, and the "test terminal" is attached to the bag mount. A sphygmomanometer squeeze bulb is connected to the hose barb on the test terminal.

The total volume of the circuit components has now been drastically reduced by removing the circle system tubing (a circle with each limb 152 cm [5 feet] in length has a volume of about 1200 ml) and the reservoir bag (3 L). The sphygmomanometer bulb is then squeezed by hand until the pressure shown on the breathing system pressure gauge indicates a pressure higher than 50 cm H_2O. The gauge is then observed for a pressure drop. The manufacturer specifies that 30 seconds or longer is required for a pressure decrease from 50 to 30 cm H_2O.[45,46] Because the volume of gas being compressed in this test is

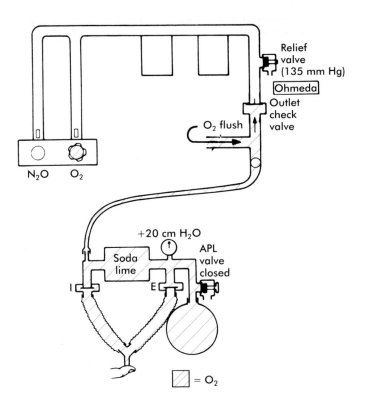

Fig. 47-18. Applications of generic checkout to system with outlet check valve (see Box 47-2, item *16*). In this case, application of positive back pressure of 20 cm H_2O causes check valve to close so that only components downstream (i.e., the circuit) are being tested for leaks. (From Eisenkraft JB: Anesthesia delivery system. Part II. In Eisenkraft JB, ed: *Progress in anesthesiology,* vol 3, San Antonio, Tx, 1989, Dannemiller Memorial Educational Foundation.)

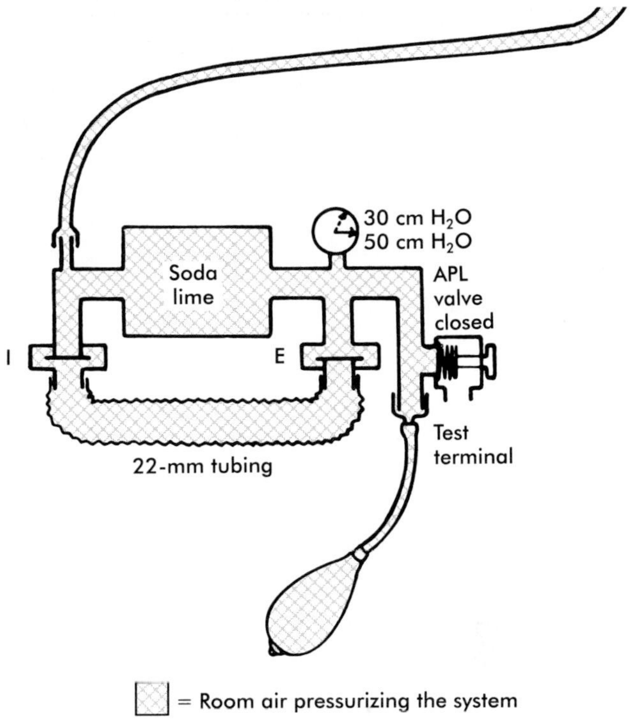

Fig. 47-19. North American Dräger Narkomed positive-pressure leak check. Thirty seconds or longer should be required for a pressure decrease from 50 to 30 cm H_2O. (From Eisenkraft JB: Anesthesia delivery system. Part II. In Eisenkraft JB, ed: *Progress in anesthesiology,* vol 3, San Antonio, Tx, 1989, Dannemiller Memorial Educational Foundation.)

minimal, small gas leaks result in decreased pressure, which is observable on the circuit pressure gauge.

The *positive-pressure leak check* should be repeated sequentially with each vaporizer turned on and set at any concentration above 0.4%. This will check for leaks in individual vaporizers (e.g., filler caps, selector switches, vaporizer mounts).[45,46]

The test specifications given in this section apply to an anesthesia breathing system without accessories (e.g., volumeter, sidestream gas analyzer, other adapters).[45,46] Test limits are exceeded when accessory items are included in the test. (The supplier of the accessory items should be contacted for leak specifications.)

Leaks in the patient circuit components can be distinguished from leaks in the low-pressure part of the Dräger Narkomed machine (no outlet check valve) as follows. If a leak has been identified using the combined circuit/machine positive-pressure leak check just described, the sphygmomanometer bulb can be connected to the machine's common gas outlet using a 15 mm connector and to a pressure gauge using a three-way stopcock. With this arrangement

only the machine (as opposed to machine and circuit in the previous test) is pressurized to 50 cm H_2O. A decrease in pressure then indicates a leak within the machine upstream of the common gas outlet. This test is possible because no outlet check valve is present in Dräger Narkomed machines.

Leaks in the patient circuit can be detected by systematically examining each component and connection in the circuit. If necessary, soap solution can be applied over joints suspected of leaking, with bubbles indicating the leakage site(s).

Ohmeda Machines: Outlet Check Valve Present

In certain Ohmeda machines an outlet check valve complicates positive-pressure testing of the machine's low-pressure system (see Fig. 47-18). Application of positive-pressure downstream from the valve causes it to close, and only components downstream of this valve (i.e., beyond the common gas outlet) would be checked for leaks. Positive-pressure ventilation and opening of the O_2 flush valve cause the check valve to close. For this reason, Ohmeda describes a *negative-pressure leak test* using a special suction bulb device

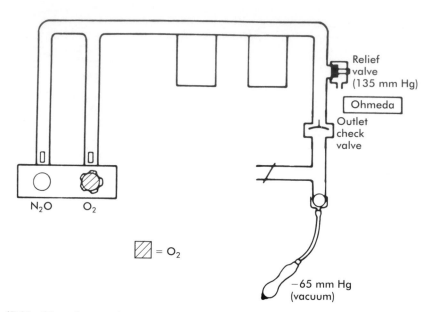

Fig. 47-20. Ohmeda negative-pressure leak check. See text for details. (From Eisenkraft JB: Anesthesia delivery system. Part II. In Eisenkraft JB, ed: *Progress in anesthesiology,* vol 3, San Antonio, Tx, 1989, Dannemiller Memorial Educational Foundation.)

that is supplied with each machine to which this test applies (Fig. 47-20).[42-44]

First, the adequacy of *the leak-testing device should be checked* by sealing the bulb's inlet connector and squeezing the bulb until it is collapsed. The bulb is then released and the time taken to reinflate observed. If reinflation occurs in less than 60 seconds, the device should be replaced.[42-44] The device is checked periodically (at times of machine servicing) to ensure that the vacuum produced by the evacuated bulb is at least -65 mm Hg (Fig. 47-20).

The device is then used to check the machine as follows.[42-44] First, the anesthesia machine system's master switch and all vaporizers are turned off so that no gases should be flowing in the machine's low-pressure parts. Each gas supply is then opened by turning on the cylinder valves or by connecting the pipeline supply. The flow control valves (rotameters) are turned fully open. The negative-pressure leak-testing bulb is attached to the machine's common gas outlet via a 15 mm connector. The hand bulb is repeatedly squeezed and released until it remains collapsed. If the bulb reinflates within 30 seconds or less (Fig. 47-21), a leak of as little as 30 ml/minute is present. The test procedure is repeated with each vaporizer on in turn to seek for leaks in individual vaporizers. If the source is not obviously correctable, the machine should be withdrawn from service.

When the leak tests are completed, the negative-pressure bulb is removed from the common gas outlet, and residual vapors are flushed out of the machine by turning on O_2 flow at 1 L/minute for 1 minute with all vaporizers off. Use of the O_2 flush control following

this check would not flush vapors out of the machine because the O_2 flush flow enters the system downstream from the vaporizers and from the outlet check valve. Because the leak check described is conducted with all the flow control valves open, components up to and including the machine's main on/off control switch are also tested for leaks.

The negative-pressure leak check described for Ohmeda machines results in the outlet check valve being held open by the -65 mm Hg vacuum (see Figs. 47-20 and 47-21) and air or gas being sucked into the system through any leaks. If such leaks were present while the machine was in service, anesthesia gases would escape from the system through such leaks.

Considering the basic internal arrangement of the Ohmeda Modulus I, Modulus II, and Excel machines, all of which have an outlet check valve, one might suggest that an internal machine leak could be detected by occluding the common gas outlet (by thumb or by clamping the fresh gas delivery tubing, as shown in Fig. 47-22). One then turns the machine on and observes the O_2 flow rate, which is possible at the rotameter, assuming that the O_2 flow rate would indicate the leakage rate (compare with FDA checkout procedure). The procedure described, however, would *not* necessarily indicate the true leakage rate because Ohmeda Modulus I and Modulus II machines also have a pressure relief valve (PRV) located between the vaporizers and the outlet check valve (see Figs. 47-20 to 47-22). This PRV opens at a pressure of 135 ± 15 mm Hg (approximately 2.3 to 2.9 PSIG) to release gas and prevent pressure buildup proximal to the outlet check valve. Ohmeda Excel machines have

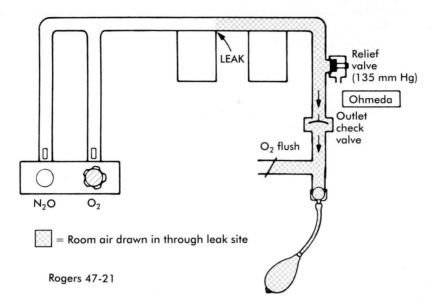

Rogers 47-21

Fig. 47-21. Ohmeda negative-pressure leak check. With a leak into machine, evacuated bulb reinflates. See text for details. (From Eisenkraft JB: Anesthesia delivery system. Part II. In Eisenkraft JB, ed: *Progress in anesthesiology,* vol 3, San Antonio, Tx, 1989, Danne-miller Memorial Educational Foundation.)

a PRV located downstream from the outlet check valve, between this valve and the common gas outlet. This PRV has an opening pressure of 5 PSIG. A PRV therefore limits the use of the procedure just described to testing for machine leaks only at pressures *below* the PRV's opening pressure. **Only the negative-pressure test described by Ohmeda in their operator's manual for that particular model should therefore be used.**

If, following testing, the anesthesia machine is found to have a leak, it should be withdrawn from use until an authorized agent has repaired the leak, rechecked the system, and certified that it is able to be put back into clinical service.

Ohmeda Modulus II Plus and Modulus CD Machines: No Outlet Check Valve

Although the most recently introduced Ohmeda models (Modulus II Plus, Modulus CD) *do not* have an outlet check valve (see Fig. 47-2), Ohmeda recommends the *negative* leak-testing procedure previously described to check for leaks in these models.[43] The negative-pressure leak check device could, in principle, be used to check for leaks in a Dräger Narkomed machine, but North American Dräger has not to date provided specifications for the application of such a leak-checking device on their products.

The 1986 FDA checklist is currently being revised. Results of a recent study[40a] suggested that the checklist did not improve the ability of the anesthesiologist to detect faults in an anesthesia machine. It was concluded that "rewriting of the FDA checklist

may be required to improve its utility as a clinical tool."[40a] Therefore, a revised version is being developed.[38] A draft of the proposed FDA Anesthesia Apparatus Checkout Recommendations, 1992, is shown in Box 47-3. It must be appreciated that this is only a draft version to be updated, if necessary, when the final version is published late in 1992.

The proposed checklist is simpler than its 1986 predecessor. It begins with checking to ensure that emergency ventilation equipment is available and functioning. A backup supply of O_2 and a self-inflating (Ambu-type) bag should be kept continuously available in the event that the delivery system fails. Note also the recommendation for use of a suction bulb to check the low pressure system of all machines.

ANESTHESIA CIRCUITS

The anesthesia circuit represents a minienvironment with which the patient makes respiratory exchange. The fresh gas flow from the anesthesia machine delivers known volumes and concentrations of O_2, N_2O, and potent inhaled anesthetic to the circuit, and gases are vented from the circuit to the scavenging system. In some arrangements, high fresh gas flows are used, in which case the patient's inspired gas concentrations approximate those in the fresh gas supply. Other circuits, such as the adult circle system, use lower fresh gas flows and rely on an absorption system for CO_2. In the circle system using low gas flows, the composition of the inspired gas may be quite different from that of the fresh gas inflow.

BOX 47-3
DRAFT OF FDA ANESTHESIA APPARATUS CHECKOUT RECOMMENDATIONS—1992

This checkout or a reasonable equivalent should be conducted before administering anesthesia. These recommendations are only valid for an anesthesia system that conforms to current and relevant standards and includes an ascending bellows ventilator and at least the following monitors: capnograph, pulse oximeter, oxygen analyzer, respiratory volume monitor (spirometer), and breathing system pressure monitor with high and low pressure alarms. This is a guideline that users are encouraged to modify to accommodate differences in equipment design and variations in local clinical practice. Such local modifications should have appropriate peer review. Users should refer to the operator's manual for special procedures or precautions.

Emergency Ventilation Equipment

*1. Verify backup ventilation equipment is available and functioning.

High Pressure System

*2. Check oxygen cylinder supply:
   a. Open O_2 cylinder and verify at least half full (about 1000 PSIG).
   b. Close cylinder.
*3. Check central pipeline supplies:
   a. Check that hoses are connected and pipeline gauges read 45 to 55 PSIG.

Low Pressure System

*4. Check initial status of low pressure system:
   a. Close flow control valves and turn vaporizers off.
   b. Check fill level and tighten vaporizers' filler caps.
   c. Remove O_2 monitor sensor from circuit.
*5. Perform leak check of machine low pressure system:
   a. Verify that the machine master switch and flow control valves are OFF.
   b. Attach "suction bulb" to common (fresh) gas outlet.
   c. Squeeze bulb repeatedly until fully collapsed.
   d. Verify bulb stays *fully* collapsed for at least 10 seconds.
   e. Open one vaporizer at a time and repeat "c" and "d" as above.
   f. Remove suction bulb and reconnect fresh gas hose.
*6. Turn on machine master switch and all other necessary electrical equipment
*7. Test flowmeters:
   a. Adjust flow of all gases through their full range, checking for smooth operation of floats and undamaged flowtubes.
   b. Attempt to create a hypoxic O_2/N_2O mixture and verify correct changes in flow and/or alarm.

Breathing System

*8. Calibrate O_2 monitor:
   a. Calibrate to read 21% in room air.
   b. Reinstall sensor in circuit and flush breathing system with O_2.
   c. Verify that monitor now reads greater than 90%.
9. Check initial status of breathing system:
   a. Set selector switch in "bag" mode.
   b. Check that breathing circuit is complete, undamaged, and unobstructed.
   c. Verify that CO_2 absorbent is adequate.
   d. Install breathing circuit accessory equipment to be used during the case.
10. Perform leak check of the breathing system:
   a. Set all gas flows to zero (or minimum).
   b. Close APL valve and occlude Y-piece.
   c. Pressurize breathing system to 30 cm H_2O with O_2 flush.
   d. Ensure that pressure remains at 30 cm H_2O for at least 10 seconds.

Scavenging System

11. Check APL valve and scavenging system:
   a. Pressurize breathing system to 50 cm H_2O and ensure its integrity.
   b. Open APL valve and ensure that pressure decreases.
   c. Ensure proper scavenging connections and waste gas vacuum.
   d. Fully open APL valve and occlude Y-piece.
   e. Ensure absorber pressure gauge reads zero when:
      (1) Minimum O_2 is flowing.
      (2) O_2 flush is activated.

Manual and Automatic Ventilation Systems

12. Test ventilation systems and unidirectional valves:
   a. Place a second breathing bag on Y-piece.
   b. Set appropriate ventilator parameters for next patient.

---

*If an anesthetist uses the same machine in successive cases, these steps need not be repeated or may be abbreviated after the initial checkout.
FDA draft ver2.9, 4/2/92. Final version to be published late in 1992. For further information on the checklist please contact Jay Crowley or Robert Cangelosi at Food and Drug Administration; Center for Devices and Radiological Health; HFZ-240, room 228; 1901 Chapman Avenue; Rockville, MD 20857. Phone: (301) 443-2436. FAX: (301) 443-8810.

BOX 47-3—*cont'd*
DRAFT OF FDA ANESTHESIA APPARATUS CHECKOUT RECOMMENDATIONS—1992

c. Set O_2 flow to 250 ml/min, other gas flows to zero.
d. Switch to automatic ventilation ("ventilator") mode.
e. Turn ventilator ON and fill bellows and breathing bag with O_2 flush.
f. Verify that during inspiration bellows delivers correct tidal volume and that during expiration bellows fills completely.
g. Check that volume monitor is consistent with ventilator parameters.
h. *Check for proper action of unidirectional valves.*
i. Exercise breathing circuit accessories to ensure proper function.
j. Turn ventilator OFF and switch to manual ventilation ("Bag/APL") mode.
k. Ventilate manually and assure inflation and deflation of artifical lungs and appropriate feel of system resistance and compliance.
l. Remove second breathing bag from Y-piece.

Monitors
13. Check, calibrate, and/or set alarm limits of all monitors:
   a. Capnometer.
   b. Oxygen analyzer.
   c. Pulse oximeter.
   d. Respiratory volume monitor (spirometer).
   e. Pressure monitor with high and low airway pressure alarms.

Final Position
14. Check final status of machine:
   a. Vaporizers off.
   b. APL valve open.
   c. Selector switch to "Bag."
   d. All flowmeters to zero (or minimum).
   e. Patient suction level adequate.
   f. Breathing system ready to use.

All anesthetic circuits are composed of corrugated 22-mm–diameter tubing, a reservoir bag, and connecting piece or elbow to the patient's airway. They may or may not also include a valve or valves. How these items are arranged gives the resulting circuit its functional characteristics.[39] Breathing systems are generally classified as rebreathing, having no CO_2 absorption system (i.e., Mapleson classification circuits A to F), or nonrebreathing, having a CO_2 absorber (e.g., circle system).

Rebreathing Systems

The circuits assigned letters according to Mapleson's classification[40] are illustrated in Fig. 47-23. In circuits *A, B,* and *C* the APL ("pop-off") valve is located near to the patient, whereas *D, E,* and *F* are T-piece arrangements with gas leaving the circuit a distance from the patient. Since there is no CO_2 absorber in any of these systems, the potential exists for the patient to inhale alveolar gas that has been previously exhaled and contains CO_2. The extent of rebreathing depends on the circuit anatomy, the patient's minute ventilation, pattern of ventilation, fresh gas flow rate, and whether ventilation is spontaneous or controlled.[40,66]

Mapleson A: Magill attachment

The Magill attachment is illustrated in Fig. 47-23 (circuit *A*). Fresh gas from the anesthesia machine enters at the end of the system farthest from the patient and closest to the reservoir bag and leaves via a spring-loaded adjustable pop-off valve located close to the patient. The system functions very differently during spontaneous vs. controlled ventilation. During spontaneous ventilation, as the patient begins to exhale, dead space gas enters the tubing and passes toward the reservoir bag. Meanwhile, fresh gas entering the system from the machine is stored in the reservoir bag. As exhalation continues, pressure rises in the system, and the pop-off valve opens to preferentially vent alveolar gas. If the fresh gas flow rate is high, dead space gas stored in the tubing may also be vented via the pop-off valve. During the next spontaneous inspiration the patient breathes in any dead space gas stored in the tubing, followed by fresh gas from the anesthesia machine and that stored in the reservoir bag. Mapleson[40] calculated and others[34] have confirmed that during spontaneous ventilation, a fresh gas flow rate equivalent to alveolar ventilation (i.e., about 70% of minute ventilation) will prevent rebreathing. However, as the fresh gas flow rate approaches alveolar ventilation, the system's vulnerability to producing rebreathing, as a result of an uneven ventilatory pattern, is increased.

When used during controlled ventilation, the Magill attachment becomes very inefficient in terms of fresh gas requirements. During controlled inspiration, when the bag is squeezed, the pop-off valve

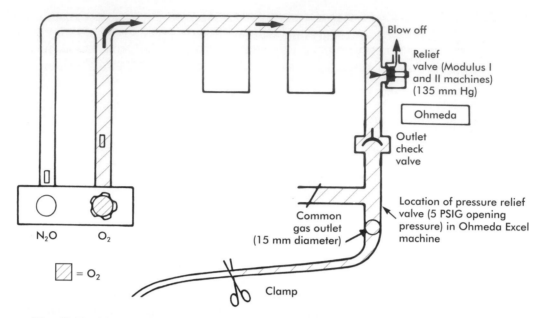

Fig. 47-22. Ohmeda system. Effect of occluding common gas outlet and turning on the O_2 flowmeter. Flow shown does not necessarily indicate leakage rate but may be showing rate of gas flow (blowoff) through pressure relief valve (PRV). See text for details. (From Eisenkraft JB: Anesthesia delivery system. Part II. In Eisenkraft JB, ed: *Progress in anesthesiology,* vol 3, San Antonio, Tx, 1989, Dannemiller Memorial Educational Foundation.)

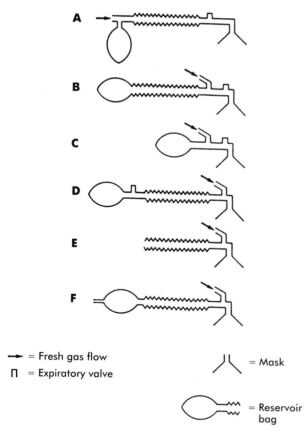

Fig. 47-23. Mapleson classification of rebreathing systems (see text for details on **A** to **F**). Mapleson A circuit is also known as Magill attachment. (From Conway CM: Anaesthetic breathing systems, *Br J Anaesth* 57:649, 1985.)

opens, causing release of fresh gas.[66] Alveolar gas that had become previously exhaled is not vented efficiently and is rebreathed. With controlled ventilation the most efficient removal of CO_2 occurs with a short inspiratory:expiratory (I:E) ratio, a large tidal volume, and a high fresh gas flow.[15,40] Fresh gas flow rates of three times the estimated minute ventilation have therefore been recommended during controlled ventilation with the Magill attachment.[69] Such high flows are wasteful of anesthetic gases and pose additional problems for waste gas scavenging.

Enthusiasm for the Magill attachment has resulted in potential modifications to address these problems. Thus, during controlled ventilation, the fresh gas requirement could be reduced by keeping the pop-off valve closed during inspiration. This is achieved in the Enclosed Magill System or the Miller modification (Fig. 47-24),[41] a system somewhat analogous to that used in contemporary double-circuit anesthesia ventilators (see later discussion). This modified system is reported to be as efficient during controlled ventilation as the Magill attachment is during spontaneous ventilation.[12,41]

As noted, because the pop-off valve in the Magill attachment is close to the patient, waste gas scavenging is a potential problem. This is addressed in the coaxial Mapleson A or Lack Breathing System (Fig. 47-25), which is functionally similar to the Mapleson A.[37]

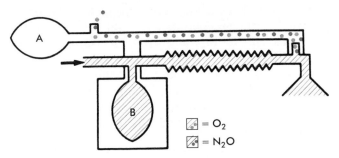

Fig. 47-24. Enclosed Magill System. Squeezing reservoir bag *(A)* causes pop-off valve to be held closed and results in compression of enclosed reservoir bag *(B)*. (From Miller DM, Miller JC: Enclosed afferent reservoir breathing systems, *Br J Anaesth* 60:469, 1988.)

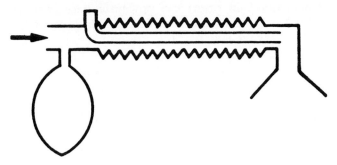

Fig. 47-25. Coaxial Mapleson A or Lack breathing system.

Mapleson B and C systems

In these systems (see Fig. 47-23, *B* and *C*) the site of fresh gas inflow and the pop-off valve are near the patient, whereas the circuit tubing and reservoir bag form a cul-de-sac in which a mixture of dead space, alveolar, and fresh gas may collect. The Mapleson C system, with a shorter length of tubing between patient and bag, is also known as the Waters to-and-fro system without absorber. These systems function similarly during both spontaneous and controlled ventilation. **Mapleson calculated that rebreathing is prevented with fresh gas flows of at least twice the minute ventilation.**[40,66] In contemporary anesthesia practice the B and C systems are rarely used.

Mapleson D systems

The Mapleson D system (see Fig. 47-23, *D*) **is basically a T piece with a long expiratory limb, the end of which has a reservoir bag and a pop-off valve. During spontaneous ventilation it is less efficient than the A system but more efficient than the B or C.**[40,66] On spontaneous exhalation, dead space, alveolar, and fresh gas enter the tubing, and as pressure increases, some of this gas mixture is vented. During the next spontaneous inspiration the patient inhales fresh gas from the anesthesia machine mixed with gas from the tubing, the composition of which depends on fresh gas flow, tidal volume, and duration of the patient's expiratory pause. If the latter is long, the tubing is flushed with fresh gas, which is then available to be inhaled on the next inspiration. If the pause is short, flushing is less and rebreathing of CO_2 becomes more likely. Large tidal volumes result in more alveolar gas entering the tubing, which also predisposes to rebreathing. **Mapleson**[40] **calculated that a fresh gas flow of at least two times the minute ventilation was required to prevent rebreathing.** This has been confirmed by others.[15,66]

When used during controlled ventilation, gas is distributed similarly in the circuit. Thus manual compression of the reservoir bag ensures that alveolar and dead space gas is released via the pop-off valve during inspiration and that fresh gas enters the patient's airway. During exhalation, dead space gas and fresh gas tend to enter the reservoir bag first before the pop-off valve opens to vent the remaining (mainly alveolar) gas. As with spontaneous ventilation, a fresh gas flow of two to three times the minute ventilation prevents rebreathing.[15,66]

The Mapleson D circuit originally described is rarely used now in the United States. However, a coaxial modification, the Bain circuit, is frequently used in pediatric anesthesia practice.

Bain circuit: coaxial Mapleson D

This system, introduced by Bain and Spoerel in 1972,[7] is shown in Fig. 47-26. Fresh gas from the anesthesia machine enters the inner (smaller-bore) tubing and is delivered to the patient end. Exhaled gas is carried via the outer tubing to the reservoir bag and pop-off valve. Both reusable and disposable versions are available. The outer tubing is now made from transparent material so that the inner tubing can be inspected for kinking or disconnection. Clearly, if disconnection occurred at the machine end, the whole system would become apparatus dead space and result in excessive rebreathing.

The Bain system may be used for spontaneous or assisted ventilation, or the reservoir bag may be

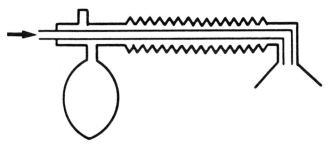

Fig. 47-26. Bain circuit: coaxial Mapleson D.

removed and an anesthesia ventilator hose attached to the bag mount for mechanical ventilation. Several studies have evaluated the fresh gas flow (FGF) requirements of the Bain system. Although some have found that during spontaneous ventilation, an FGF of 100 ml · kg^{-1} · min^{-1} produces normocarbia at the cost of increased minute ventilation,[7] another study reported that an FGF of 2.5 to 3 times the minute ventilation prevents rebreathing during spontaneous ventilation.[16] The slightly higher FGF requirement of the Bain circuit compared with the basic Mapleson D may be caused by turbulence at the patient end of the coaxial system, in turn causing failure to store fresh gas in the outer corrugated tubing.[39] During controlled ventilation the Bain circuit behaves more as a Mapleson D, and a FGF flow of 70 ml · kg^{-1} · min^{-1} results in normocarbia, provided minute ventilation is adequate (120 ml · kg^{-1} · min^{-1}). This applies in patients weighing more than 40 kg.[8]

A ventilation nomogram has been produced for the Bain circuit during controlled ventilation (Fig. 47-27).[63] This shows that the alveolar CO_2 tension (P$A CO_2$) can be estimated from a combination of FGF and minute ventilation ($\dot{V}_E$). **At high FGF, P$A CO_2$ becomes independent of FGF and dependent on ($\dot{V}_E$). At high ($\dot{V}_E$), P$A CO_2$ is independent of ($\dot{V}_E$) and becomes dependent on FGF.** The Bain circuit can thus be used to provide controlled rebreathing with hyperventilation, resulting in normal P$A CO_2$. Such predictive nomograms, while useful guides, will become of less importance as monitoring of end-tidal CO_2 by capnometry becomes widespread. The pop-off valve in the Bain circuit is located close to the machine; therefore scavenging from the Bain circuit is not a problem.

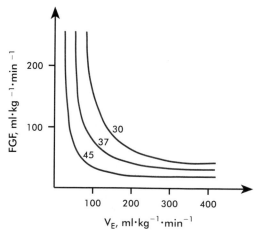

Fig. 47-27. Nomogram for predicting P$A CO_2$ from given combination of fresh gas flow (FGF) and minute ventilation ($\dot{V}_E$) for Bain system. Three isopleths indicate P$A CO_2$ of 30, 37, and 45 mm Hg. (From Seeley HF, Barnes PK, and Conway CM: Controlled ventilation with the Mapleson D system, *Br J Anaesth* 49:107, 1977.)

A preuse check of the Bain circuit is essential to ensure that the inner gas delivery tube has not become disconnected. If this occurred, it could lead to rebreathing. Two checkout methods have been described. In one[53] the patient end of the whole system is occluded, the pop-off valve is closed, and the system is filled with O_2 until the reservoir bag is distended. The patient end is then unoccluded, and O_2 is flushed into the circuit via the inner tube. The high O_2 flow produces a Venturi effect at the patient end of the circuit. The low pressure created at the end of the outer tubing causes O_2 to be drawn along the outer tubing from the bag, causing the reservoir bag to deflate. If a disconnection or a leak occurs in the inner tubing, flushing the circuit with O_2 would allow the high pressure to be transmitted from the inner to the outer tubing, and the reservoir bag would remain inflated or distend further.[53]

A second checkout method[62] of the Bain circuit is to set 50 ml/min of flow on one of the flowmeters and then occlude the distal (patient) end of the inner tube using the plunger of a small syringe. If the inner tube is intact, this should cause the gas flow to cease and the flowmeter bobbin to fall. The second test is preferred because if the inner tube has been omitted, the first test may give no indication that anything is wrong.[20]

Mapleson E and F systems

The Mapleson E and F systems are valveless, T-piece arrangements (see Fig. 47-23, *E* and *F*). The E system is modified from Ayre's original T-piece by the addition of corrugated tubing to the expiratory limb, which thereby becomes a reservoir of fresh gas during inspiration. During inspiration the patient breathes fresh gas from the machine and gas stored in the expiratory limb. The latter should have a capacity greater than the patient's expected tidal volume to prevent entrainment of room air during inspiration. During exhalation, exhaled gas enters the expiratory limb; during the expiratory pause, this limb is flushed with fresh gas, which is then available for the next inspiration.

The E system may be used for either spontaneous or controlled ventilation, the latter being achieved by intermittent occlusion of the expiratory limb by a "mechanical thumb" type of ventilator. **With the E system, rebreathing is avoided if a fresh gas flow of three times the minute ventilation is used.**[66]

The Mapleson F circuit is Jackson-Rees' modification of the Ayre's T-piece (Mapleson E) system (see Fig. 47-23, *E* and *F*).[32] In this system a reservoir bag and a means for venting waste gases are added to the end of the expiratory limb tubing. The venting piece is usually a valve with an adjustable orifice that is connected to a waste gas scavenging system.

The F system functions similarly to the Mapleson E, except that during exhalation a mixture of exhaled and fresh gas collects in the bag. On the next inspiration the patient inhales fresh gas from the machine and that stored in the expiratory limb. Addition of the reservoir bag to the E system provides a means to qualitatively monitor ventilation during spontaneous breathing, as well as a means to control ventilation by manually squeezing the reservoir bag. **Prevention of rebreathing is achieved using fresh gas flows of two to three times the minute ventilation.**[66]

The Ayre's T-piece and Jackson-Rees' systems have been popular for pediatric anesthesia because they are simple to assemble, are inexpensive, and, being valveless, offer low resistance to breathing. A disadvantage of all T-piece systems, however, is that because relatively high fresh gas flows are needed, they are less desirable for use in adults. They also cause greater loss of moisture from the airway if dry gases are used.[15,39,66]

Circle System

The circle system was introduced by Sword in 1926. In this system the components form a circle into which fresh gas can enter and from which excess gas can leave. Although several possible configurations are possible, the arrangement of the components of a contemporary circle system is shown in Fig. 47-28. Fresh gas enters just upstream from the inspiratory undirectional valve and during inspiration passes down the circle's inspiratory limb to the Y-piece connector. During expiration, gas passes along the expiratory limb to the expiratory undirectional valve. Just beyond the expiratory valve are the APL (pop-off) valve and a reservoir bag. Gas then passes through a canister containing a CO₂ absorbent (e.g., soda lime) and emerges to rejoin fresh gas entering the circuit from the anesthesia machine just upstream from the inspiratory valve.

In the system described, rebreathing of CO_2 is prevented by the absorption of CO_2 from exhaled gas before it is reinspired. At high fresh gas flows, however, CO_2 absorption becomes unnecessary, and some older circle systems even permitted bypass of the absorber canister. **At lower fresh gas flows, CO_2 absorption is necessary.** Eger[22] has suggested three basic rules for minimizing CO_2 rebreathing in a circle system:

- **A unidirectional valve must be present between the reservoir bag and the patient on both inspiratory and expiratory sides.**
- **Fresh gas must not enter the system between the expiratory unidirectional valve and the patient.**
- **The overflow valve must not be placed between the patient and the inspiratory unidirectional valve.**

Unidirectional gas flow occurs only in that part of the circle between the unidirectional valves and the patient. In the part of the circuit between the fresh gas inlet and the APL valve, gas flow is bidirectional (Fig. 47-28). Incompetence of either unidirectional valve permits bidirectional gas flow in the corrugated patient tubing, leading to rebreathing of previously exhaled CO_2.

The circle system is currently the most popular anesthesia system in use in the United States. It has the advantages of permitting low fresh gas flows, reduction of operating room pollution, and conservation of heat and humidity. Disadvantages of the circle system include a somewhat complex design with multiple components that could malfunction or be arranged incorrectly. It is also difficult predicting inspired gas composition within the circle, particularly if low fresh gas flows are being used.[39] The latter may cease to be a problem, however, as monitoring of anesthetic and respiratory gas concentrations becomes more common.

Absorption of carbon dioxide. The CO_2 absorber is the central component in a circle system. Contemporary canisters are large with a minimal gas space equal to the largest expected patient tidal volume. This design permits low gas flow rates, long dwell times,

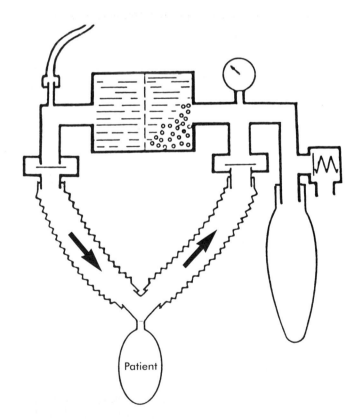

Fig. 47-28. Contemporary anesthesia circle system arrangement. (From Schreiber P: *Safety guidelines for anesthesia systems,* Telford, Pa, 1985, North American Dräger.)

and thereby more complete removal ("scrubbing") of CO_2. Canisters usually have two chambers so that one half of the absorbent (that in the upstream chamber) can be completely exhausted before removal. The chambers are then reversed so that the previously downstream chamber now becomes upstream.[65]

The two CO_2 absorbents most often used are soda lime and baralyme. Soda lime consists of 4% NaOH, 1% KOH, 14% to 19% H_2O, and the remainder $Ca(OH)_2$.[20] In addition, small amounts of silica or kieselguhr are added for hardening because this reduces the formation of dust. The absorptive efficacy of soda lime is inversely related to its hardness. The reaction of CO_2 with soda lime is as follows[65]:

(1) $CO_2 + H_2O \leftrightarrows H_2CO_3$
(2) $2H_2CO_3 + 2Na^+ + 2OH^- + 2K + 2OH^- \rightarrow$
$2Na^+ + CO_3^{2-} + 2K^+ + CO_3^{2-} + 4H_2O + Heat$
(3) $Ca(OH)_2 + H_2O \rightleftharpoons Ca^{2+} + 2OH^- + H_2O$
(4) $2Ca^{2+} + 4OH^- + 2Na^+ + CO_3^{2-} + 2K^+ + CO_3^{2-}$
$\rightleftharpoons 2CaCO_3 + 2Na^+ + 2OH^- + 2K^+ + 2OH^-$

Considerable heat is liberated during the course of this reaction. The preservation of heat and moisture within the system is considered to be a desirable feature.

Baralyme is a mixture of 20% $Ba(OH)_2$ and 80% $Ca(OH)_2$, with $Ba(OH)_2$ the more active ingredient.[20] Baralyme may also contain some KOH as an indicator. The reaction with CO_2 is as follows:

(1) $9CO_2 + 9H_2O \leftrightarrows H_2CO_3$
(2) $Ba(OH)_2, 8H_2O + CO_2 \leftrightarrows BaCO_3 + 9H_2O + Heat$
(3) $9H_2CO_3 + 9Ca(OH)_2 \leftrightarrows CaCO_3 + 18H_2O + Heat$
(4) $2KOH + H_2CO_3 \rightarrow K_2CO_3 + 2H_2O$
(5) $Ca(OH)_2 + K_2CO_3 \rightarrow CaCO_3 + 2KOH$

The water required for the reaction is supplied by the eight molecules of water in barium hydroxide octahydrate.

Absorptive surface area and gas flow through soda lime are a function of granule size. The smaller the size, the larger is the area for absorption but the greater is the resistance to gas flow. Conversely, large granules decrease absorption surface area, offer less resistance to flow, and may encourage channeling of gases through the soda lime, thereby decreasing CO_2 absorption. The most frequently used size of soda lime granule is therefore 4 to 8 mesh (i.e., ¼-inch to ⅛-inch diameter).[65] In theory, 100 g of CO_2 absorbent (soda lime) could absorb 26 L of CO_2. In practice the amount of CO_2 actually absorbed is less because of channeling of gas through the absorber.[20]

Indicators are added to the absorbent granules to show when they are becoming exhausted. These indicators are pH sensitive and are colorless when soda lime is fresh but become colored when pH decreases. The most frequently used indicator is ethyl violet, which changes from colorless to purple as absorption proceeds. It was chosen because the color change is conspicuous under even poor lighting conditions.[65]

A recent report indicates that even ethyl violet may be deactivated by fluorescent lighting and possibly temporally deactivated after a container is opened, even with storage in the dark.[6] Such deactivation increases the hazard of using CO_2 absorption, but such a hazard would be offset by continuous intraoperative capnography. The authors[6] recommend that the problem be minimized by using ultraviolet filters and incorporating additional ethyl violet in Sodasorb.

When using CO_2 absorption, the absorbent must be compatible with the anesthetic gases in use. In this regard, trichloroethylene may react with soda lime to produce dichloroacetylene, phosgene, and carbon monoxide, which are potentially neurotoxic gases. Trichloroethylene has not been used in the United States but was often used in the United Kingdom. Sevoflurane, a new potent inhaled anesthetic, is degraded by both soda lime and Baralyme.[68] Exposure of other fluorinated anesthetics (e.g., enflurane) to CO_2 absorbent may also produce carbon monoxide.[44a,44b]

ANESTHESIA VENTILATORS

Contemporary anesthesia ventilators, such as the Dräger AV-E and the Ohmeda 7000 and 7810 models, are examples of "bag-in-a-bottle" respirators. The basic principle is that the reservoir bag of an anesthesia circle system is replaced by a bellows in a bellows housing, and the APL (pop-off) valve is replaced by a ventilator pressure relief valve (PRV) (Fig. 47-29). Inspiration occurs when compressed gas enters the bellows housing. The bellows is compressed, and the PRV is held closed (Fig. 47-30). Gas contained within the bellows, as well as fresh gas entering the patient circuit from the anesthesia machine, are forced into the patient's lungs. At end-inspiration the bellows housing is no longer pressurized, the bellows refills (by gravity in the case of a hanging bellows, as in Fig. 47-29 and 47-30), and the PRV is able to open, venting excess patient circuit gas to the waste gas scavenging system.

Anesthesia ventilators are also described as double-circuit ventilators, one circuit being the driving gas circuit and the other the patient circuit. The interface between these two circuits is the ventilator bellows itself. Although both the Dräger AV-E and the Ohmeda 7000 and 7810 model ventilators are of the double-circuit design, their mechanisms of action differ in certain details, so a brief description of each is provided.

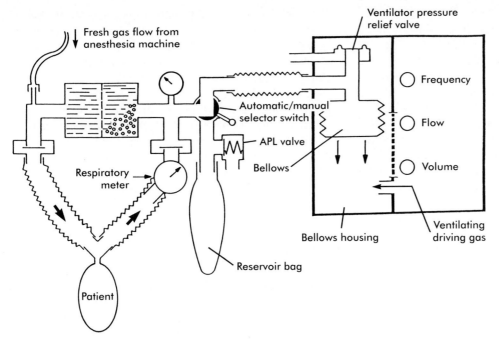

Fig. 47-29. Schematic of typical "bag-in-a-bottle" anesthesia ventilator. Reservoir bag and APL valve are switched out of circuit and replaced by ventilator bellows (bag) in bellows housing (bottle). (From Schreiber P: *Safety guidelines for anesthesia systems,* Telford, Pa, 1985, North American Dräger.)

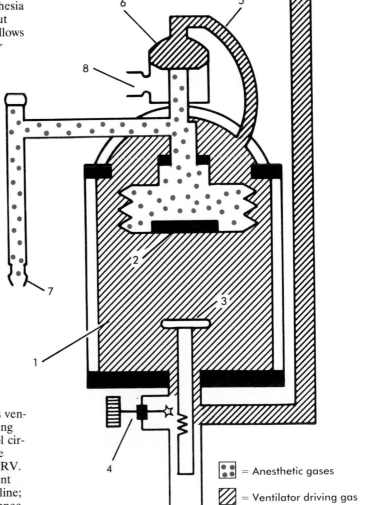

Fig. 47-30. Schematic of Dräger AV-E hanging bellows ventilator during inspiration. Hatched area represents driving gas under pressure, which comes from ventilator control circuits, enters bellows housing to compress and empty the bellows, and pressurizes and thereby closes ventilator PRV. *1,* Bellows housing; *2,* bellows; *3,* tidal volume adjustment plate; *4,* tidal volume control knob; *5,* relief valve pilot line; *6,* ventilator PRV; *7,* connector to patient circuit; *8,* connector to waste gas scavenging system. (From Eisenkraft JB: Potential for barotrauma or hypoventilation with the Dräger AV-E ventilator, *J Clin Anesth* 1:452, 1989.)

Ohmeda 7000

This ventilator is shown in Fig. 47-31. The Ohmeda 7000 consists of two basic units: a bellows housing and assembly and a control unit. The former may be separate from, or be mounted on, the control unit, as in Fig. 47-31. The driving gas circuit is considered first (Fig. 47-32).[48]

The driving gas supply of this ventilator, O_2 at a nominal pressure of 50 PSIG, passes to a pressure regulator whose output is set to 38 PSIG at 24 L/min of flow. From here the pressure-regulated O_2 flow passes to a block containing five solenoid flow control valves connected in parallel. These flow control valves are electronically opened during the inspiratory phase to direct O_2 flow through tuned orifices, which are calibrated for flows of 2, 4, 8, 16, and 32 L/min. The possible range for flow selection is 4 to 60 L/min in 2 L/minute increments. By controlling the duration of opening of each of the five solenoid valves, the control module determines the O_2 volume that passes into the collection chamber. This metered O_2 volume then enters the bellows housing, where it exerts pressure on the bellows and displaces an equal volume of anesthesia gas mixture from the bellows into the patient circuit. This displaced volume is the tidal volume.

The Ohmeda 7000 ventilator uses a standing bellows. According to the settings on the ventilator panel (tidal volume [V_T] equals set minute volume [MV] divided by set respiratory rate [RR], or $V_T = MV/RR$), the bellows empties until the predetermined tidal volume has been delivered. The bellows therefore does not empty completely unless a tidal volume of 1600 ml or greater is selected (Fig. 47-31). During inspiration the exhaust valve in the collection chamber (Fig. 47-32) is closed so that the driving gas does not escape. A ventilator PRV (pop-off valve) located in the base of the bellows is held closed by the driving gas pressure during inspiration so that gas passes from within the bellows to the patient circuit (Fig. 47-33).

Exhalation begins when the driving gas exhaust valve located in the control module opens, permitting driving gas to be vented from the bellows housing. This occurs because this gas is displaced by the bellows refilling with anesthesia gases from the patient's lungs and the fresh gas flow from the anesthesia machine. During exhalation, for the bellows to refill with anesthesia gases, a slight positive pressure must be maintained in the circuit. If the circuit were kept at atmospheric pressure during exhalation, circuit gas would preferentially flow out to

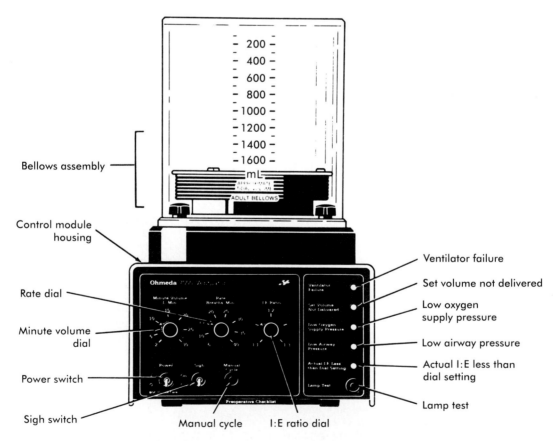

Fig. 47-31. Ohmeda 7000 Electronic Anesthesia ventilator. (Courtesy Ohmeda, BOC Health Care, Madison, Wis.)

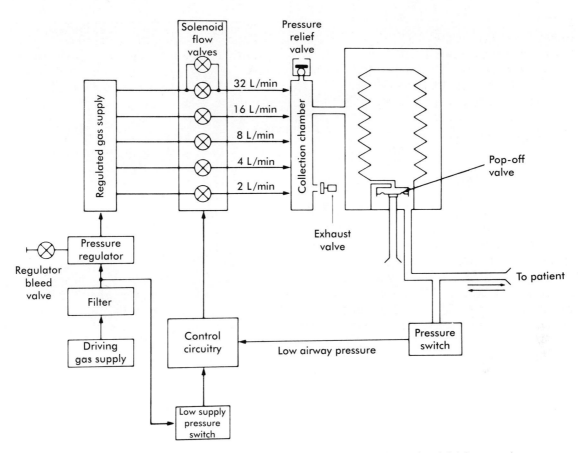

Fig. 47-32. Ohmeda 7000 Electronic Anesthesia ventilator. Schematic of driving gas circuit. (Courtesy Ohmeda, BOC Health Care, Madison, Wis.)

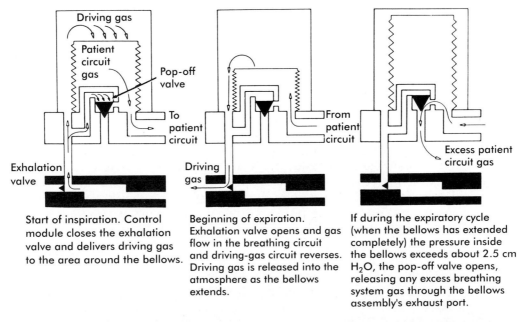

Start of inspiration. Control module closes the exhalation valve and delivers driving gas to the area around the bellows.

Beginning of expiration. Exhalation valve opens and gas flow in the breathing circuit and driving-gas circuit reverses. Driving gas is released into the atmosphere as the bellows extends.

If during the expiratory cycle (when the bellows has extended completely) the pressure inside the bellows exceeds about 2.5 cm H_2O, the pop-off valve opens, releasing any excess breathing system gas through the bellows assembly's exhaust port.

Fig. 47-33. Ohmeda 7000 and 7810 ventilators. Schematic of function of pop-off valve in bellows during inspiration and expiration (*see text for details*). (Courtesy Ohmeda, BOC Health Care, Madison, Wis.)

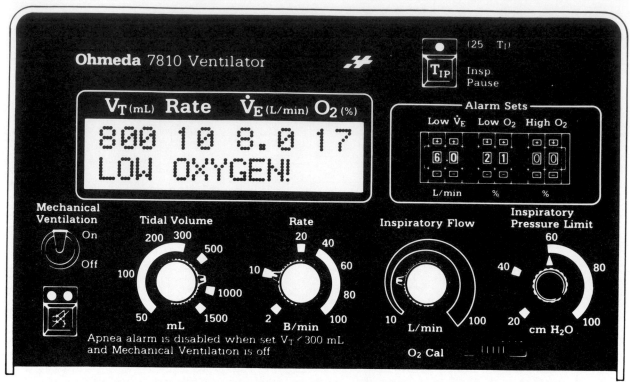

Fig. 47-34. Ohmeda 7810 Electronic Anesthesia ventilator. Schematic of control panel (*see text for details*). (Courtesy Ohmeda, BOC Health Care, Madison, Wis.)

the scavenging system, and the bellows would not reexpand. The ventilator PRV is therefore also a positive end-expiratory pressure (PEEP) valve exerting a pressure of about 2.5 cm H_2O on the gas contained within the patient circuit. At end-expiration, when the bellows has reached its limit of expansion and the circuit pressure has risen to greater than 2.5 cm H_2O, the ventilator PRV opens, and excess gas from the patient circuit is vented to the waste gas scavenging system.

The PRV in the driving gas collection chamber (see Fig. 47-32) represents a safety feature such that if the pressure in the driving gas circuit becomes too high (greater than 65 cm H_2O), the valve opens to relieve the excess pressure. This prevents such excessive pressure from being applied to the patient's airway.[48] The Ohmeda 7000 ventilator is electronically controlled and time cycled. Operator controls (see Fig. 47-31) are for minute volume, respiratory rate (thus $V_T = MV/RR$), and I:E ratio.[48]

Ohmeda 7810

The Ohmeda 7810 ventilator (Fig. 47-34) is very similar to the model 7000 but differs in certain features.[49] Driving gas is O_2 at 50 PSIG nominal pressure (Fig. 47-35). The O_2 passes to a primary regulator whose output is controlled to 26 PSIG. From here the O_2 passes to a pneumatic manifold,

where its flow into the bellows housing is controlled by a flow control valve. This sophisticated valve varies the opening of a flow orifice according to the current supplied to the valve's coil, thereby controlling O_2 flow. A combination of the current supplied to the coil and the time for which it is applied (valve opening size and time) is determined by the microprocessor and based on the operator control settings.

The pneumatic manifold in the model 7810 therefore replaces the five solenoid valves and tuned orifices of the model 7000 (see Fig. 47-32). The operator controls also differ in that the model 7810 the limits of tidal volume, rate, inspiratory flow, and inspiratory pressure (maximum, 100 cm H_2O) may be set directly (see Fig. 47-34). The I:E ratio, however, is not set directly but is calculated by the unit and displayed. The control unit also contains an O_2 analyzer and displays the O_2 concentration sensed in the patient circuit. It also incorporates pressure and volume alarms. In other respects, the 7810 ventilator functions are similar to the model 7000.[48,49]

Dräger AV-E

The Dräger AV-E ventilator is also a double-circuit, pneumatically powered design.[45-47] It consists of a control unit mounted above the flowmeters and vaporizers on a Dräger Narkomed machine and a bellows assembly (Fig. 47-36). A schematic of this

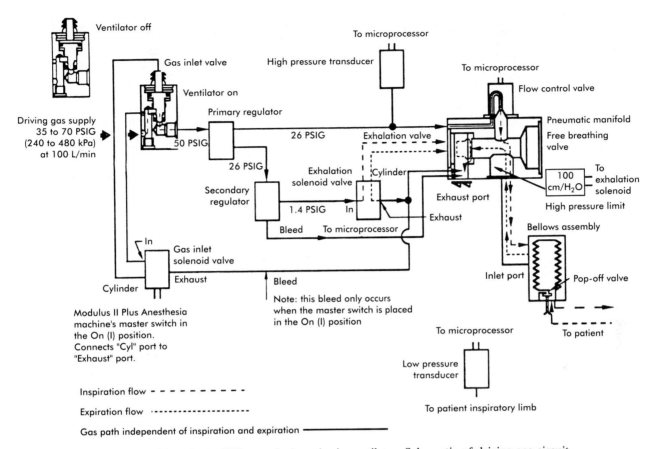

Fig. 47-35. Ohmeda 7810 Electronic Anesthesia ventilator. Schematic of driving gas circuit (*see text for details*). (Courtesy Ohmeda, BOC Health Care, Madison, Wis.)

ventilator is shown in Fig. 47-37. The following numbers in parentheses refer to Figs. 47-37 and 47-38. The driving gas circuit is described first.[51]

The ventilator is powered by O_2 at a driving pressure of 50 PSIG *(2)*. When the ventilator on/off switch *(3)* is turned on, O_2 pressure is supplied to a 1 PSIG switch *(4)*, which is activated and energizes the electronic circuit. The respiratory rate *(7)* and I:E ratio *(6)* controls (see *inset*, Fig. 47-36) are set as desired. Inspiration (Fig. 47-37) occurs when the solenoid valve *(9)* receives an electrical signal from the control unit *(5)*. This signal remains throughout inspiration and activates the solenoid valve *(9)* to allow O_2 at 50 PSIG to pass through it to activate the control valve *(10)*. Opening the control valve allows O_2 that has passed through the adjustable flow regulator *(11)* to pass through the control valve *(10)* to the venturi *(13)*. The inspiratory flow rate is adjusted by the flow regulator *(11)* (see flow control knob, Fig. 47-36), and the flow rate is monitored on a flow indicator gauge *(12)*. This indicator is really a pressure gauge, measuring pressure downstream from the flow regulator. The display on the gauge shows flow in three zones: high, medium, and low (see Fig. 47-36). During inspiration, back pressure from the

venturi *(13)* is conducted to a pilot actuator *(15)*, which is held closed. As the O_2 flows from the venturi *(13)*, room air is entrained through the muffler and entrainment port *(14)*.

The mixture of O_2 and entrained air is directed into the bellows chamber *(16)*. As pressure rises in the bellows chamber, the bellows is compressed. Anesthetic gases within the bellows are forced into the patient circuit via the breathing connector *(22)*. At the same time, driving gas pressure from the bellows housing *(16)* is transmitted via the relief valve pilot line *(20)* to hold the ventilator PRV *(21)* closed as long as the bellows housing is under pressure (i.e., throughout inspiration). In this ventilator the bellows is emptied completely with each inspiratory cycle. Thus tidal volume is determined by the extent to which the bellows is allowed to expand during exhalation, which in turn is adjusted by the tidal volume control knob *(19)* and bellows plate *(18)*. During the inspiratory pause the O_2 continues to flow from the venturi *(13)*. However, since the bellows is now fully compressed, no further air is entrained, and pressure is maintained in the bellows housing by the pressure of the O_2 jet from the venturi. Meanwhile, the chamber *(16)* contains

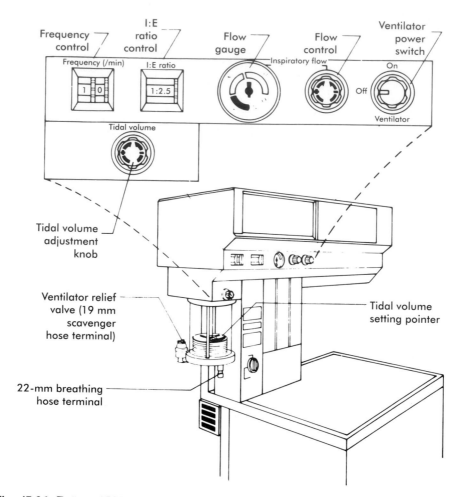

Fig. 47-36. Dräger AV-E anesthesia ventilator. Note standing bellows arrangement in diagram. Figs. 47-29 and 47-30 show a hanging bellows version. (Courtesy North American Dräger, Telford, Pa.)

(16) contains a mixture of air and O$_2$ with an average O$_2$ concentration of 33%.

Expiration (Fig. 47-38) begins when the electrical signal from the control unit *(5)* to the solenoid valve *(9)* stops. The solenoid valve is deactivated and closes, interrupting the supply of 50 PSIG O$_2$ to the control valve *(10)*, which therefore also closes. The preset O$_2$ flow from the flow regulator *(11)* is interrupted by the control valve *(10)*, causing a pressure drop at the venturi *(13)*, and no back pressure is supplied to pilot actuator *(15)*. The latter opens to allow gas from the bellows chamber *(16)* to be vented through the pilot actuator *(15)* and the entrainment port *(14)* of the venturi *(13)*. This exhausted driving gas leaves the ventilator through a muffler. A clean, dry muffler is essential for normal function of this ventilator. As the pressure falls in the bellows chamber *(16)*, the bellows *(17)* begins to refill. As long as any pressure remains in the bellows chamber *(16)*, the ventilator relief valve *(2)* is also pressurized and held closed.

Figs. 47-39 and 47-40 are schematics of the standing bellows version of the Dräger AV-E during inspiration and expiration, respectively. As with the standing bellows arrangement in the Ohmeda ventilators (7800, 7810), the Dräger AV-E ventilator relief valve applies about 2.5 cm H$_2$O PEEP to the gas in the patient circuit. Once the standing bellows has reached its preset limit of expansion (the next tidal volume) and circuit pressure exceeds 2.5 cm H$_2$O, the PEEP valve opens, permitting excess circuit gas to enter the waste gas scavenging system (Fig. 47-40).

In the Dräger AV-E the ventilator PRV is controlled via an external relief valve pilot line (see Figs. 47-37 and 47-38, item *20*), which is essentially a short length of plastic tubing. Kinking this tubing can cause ventilator malfunction. Occlusion during inspiration, when the valve is being held closed, causes it to remain closed thereafter, and excess gas cannot leave the anesthesia circuit. Consequently, pressure in the circuit rises and, if not relieved, could result in barotrauma.[25] A circuit continuing pressure or high pressure alarm should alert the clinician to such a situation. If the tubing is occluded during exhalation when the valve is not held closed, during the next

Fig. 47-37. North American Dräger AV-E ventilator. Schematic of ventilator function during *inspiration*. See text for details of operation. *1*, Electric power supply (117 volts AC); *2*, gas supply of O_2 (50 PSIG); *3*, ventilator on/off switch; *4*, electrical supply on/off switch (1 PSIG pressure switch); *5*, AV-E printed circuit; *6*, I:E ratio control; *7*, frequency control; *8*, solenoid pilot pressure line; *9*, solenoid valve; *10*, control valve; *11*, flow regulator; *12*, flow indicator gauge; *13*, venturi; *14*, Venturi entrainment port; *15*, pilot actuator; *16*, bellows chamber; *17*, bellows; *18*, tidal volume adjustment plate; *19*, tidal volume control; *20*, relief valve pilot line; *21*, ventilator relief valve; *22*, patient breathing system connector; *23*, waste gas scavenging system connector. (Courtesy North American Dräger, Telford, Pa.)

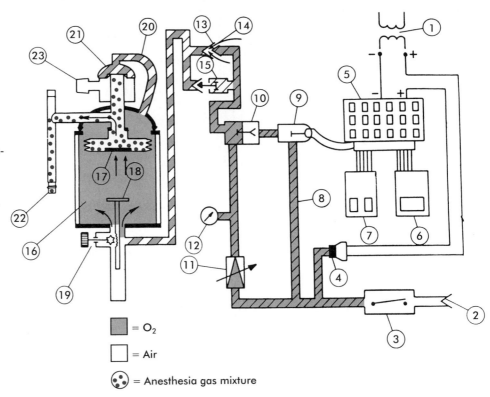

Fig. 47-38. Dräger AV-E ventilator. Schematic of ventilator function during *expiration*. See Fig. 47-37 for numbers and text for details. (Courtesy North American Dräger, Telford, Pa.)

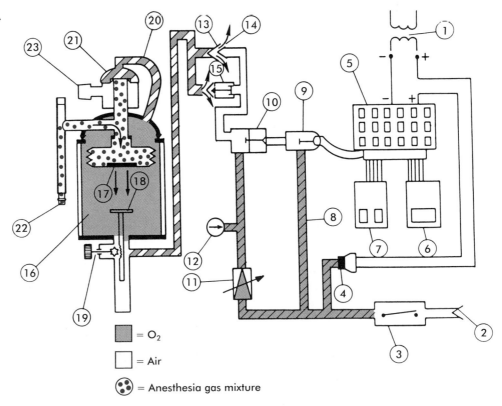

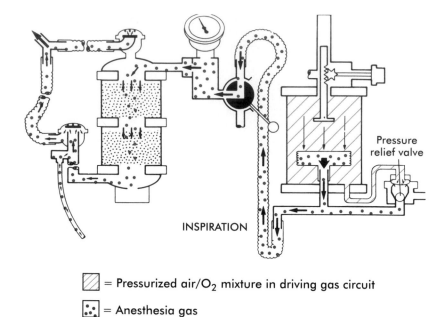

INSPIRATION

⬚ = Pressurized air/O$_2$ mixture in driving gas circuit

⬚ = Anesthesia gas

Fig. 47-39. North American Dräger AV-E standing bellows design showing events during *inspiration.* (Courtesy North American Dräger, Telford, Pa.)

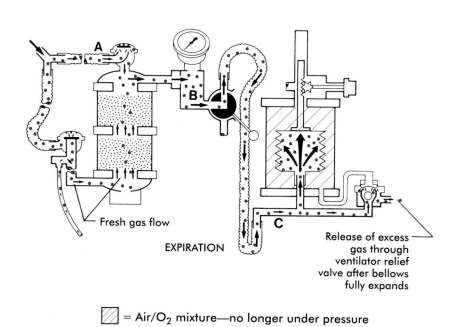

Fresh gas flow

EXPIRATION

Release of excess gas through ventilator relief valve after bellows fully expands

⬚ = Air/O$_2$ mixture—no longer under pressure

⬚ = Anesthesia gas

Fig. 47-40. North American Dräger AV-E standing bellows design showing events during *expiration. A, B,* and *C* represent possible positions for PEEP valve placement *(see text for details).* (Courtesy North American Dräger, Telford, Pa.)

inspiratory cycle, pressure cannot be transmitted through to the valve to hold it closed. Then patient circuit gas can leak out to the scavenging system rather than enter the patient circuit. This might result in hypoventilation of the patient. Incompetence of the PRV itself may also result in patient hypoventilation.[64] Again, contemporary circuit pressure volume or ventilation (CO_2) alarms should alert one to these situations.

Differences Among Ventilator Designs
Standing vs. hanging bellows ventilators

Contemporary anesthesia ventilators are of the standing bellows design; that is, they rise (fill) during exhalation and descend (empty) during inspiration. With a disconnection, in which circuit pressure becomes equal to atmospheric pressure, the bellows cannot refill during exhalation.

In the hanging bellows design (see Figs. 47-29 and 47-30), the bellows fills by gravity during exhalation so that the ventilator PRV does not require a PEEP design. With a circuit disconnection, room air is entrained into the patient circuit via the leak and the bellows refills, emptying through the leak on the next inspiration. For this reason the standing bellows design is preferred, although it is not required by the new standard describing specifications for anesthesia ventilators.[5] The standard states that if the ventilator incorporates a weighted descending bellows, the manufacturer shall specify the maximum negative pressure created (1) when the fresh gas flow to the circuit is shut off and (2) when the patient connecting port of the delivery system is obstructed just after a tidal volume is described and the ventilator shut off.

Dräger vs. Ohmeda: driving gas

The gas entering the bellows housing in an Ohmeda ventilator is 100% O_2 (see Figs. 47-32 and 47-35), whereas in the Dräger AV-E the gas is an air/O_2 mixture (see Fig. 47-37). With a leak (hole) in the bellows, driving gas enters the patient circuit and dilutes the gases there. This could cause O_2 enrichment with an Ohmeda ventilator but a decrease in the fraction of inspired O_2 with a Dräger AV-E if an FIO_2 >0.4 were set at the flowmeters.

In the Dräger ventilator the tidal volume is determined by setting the expansion limit of the bellows during expiration, since the bellows is emptied completely during inspiration. The bellows (see Figs. 47-39 and 47-40) is graduated from 0 ml below to 2000 ml at the top of the housing. In the Ohmeda design the bellows is graduated from 0 ml at the top to 1600 ml at the bottom of the bellows housing, since the tidal volume is displaced from the bellows by a metered volume of compressed O_2 (see Fig. 47-31). The Dräger AV-E ventilator uses a venturi and an

air/O_2 mixture to compress the bellows. This economizes on the use of compressed O_2. In the Ohmeda ventilator, O_2 consumption as the driving gas is a little greater than the set minute ventilation.[55]

In the Ohmeda ventilator the circuit PRV is flush-mounted inside the bellows (see Fig. 47-33). The design does not use a relief valve pilot line and is therefore not vulnerable to the effects of this line kinking (see Fig. 47-37, item 20).[25]

Ohmeda ventilators incorporate a PRV in the driving gas circuit (see Figs. 47-32 and 47-35). This may be preset to 65 cm H_2O (as in the 7000 model) or be adjustable (see Fig. 47-34, 7810 model, "Inspiratory Pressure Limit"). Most original Dräger AV-E ventilators do not have a PRV in the driving gas circuit. Such a valve (Dräger Pressure Limit Control), with variable relief pressure settings, is now available and may be retrofitted to standing bellows versions of these ventilators, thereby providing a pressure limit.[26]

Because the Dräger AV-E ventilator venturi requires entrainment of air (see Figs. 47-37 and 47-38), a clean muffler is essential. If the muffler becomes blocked for any reason, air is no longer entrained and inspiration cannot be completed. If blockage occurs during exhalation, gas cannot leave the ventilator bellows housing, and the bellows remain collapsed.[58]

Tidal Volume

During inspiration the anesthesia ventilator circuit PRV is held closed so that gas contained in the bellows enters the patient circuit rather than the scavenging system (see Fig. 47-39). Meanwhile, fresh gas continues to enter the patient circuit from the anesthesia machine throughout the ventilatory cycle, according to the rotameter settings on the machine.

When setting tidal volume (V_T) on a ventilator bellows to achieve a certain patient V_T, one must consider the fresh gas flow (FGF) rate from the anesthesia machine to the patient circuit.[31,60] Consider an anesthesia ventilator set to a frequency of 10 breaths/min, an I:E ratio of 1:2, and an FGF of 6 L/min (or 100 ml/sec) to the anesthesia circle. Each breath lasts 6 seconds (60 sec/10 breaths), with inspiration lasting 2 seconds and expiration 4 seconds (I:E, 1:2). During inspiration the ventilator PRV is closed so that both gas from the emptying bellows and FGF from the machine enter the patient circuit (see Fig. 47-39). Since FGF is 100 ml/sec, and each inspiration lasts 2 seconds, the V_T set on the ventilator bellows is potentially augmented by 200 ml. Changing the FGF, respiratory rate, or I:E ratio may therefore have a profound effect on circuit V_T, alveolar ventilation, and arterial CO_2 tension ($PaCO_2$).[31,60] Effect on $PaCO_2$ is illustrated in Fig. 47-41.

The additional minute ventilation to the circuit

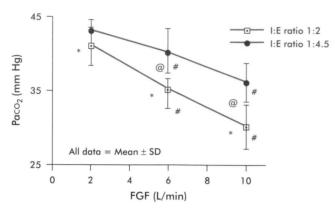

Fig. 47-41. Effect of fresh gas flow (FGF) and inspiratory:expiratory (I:E) ratio on arterial CO_2 tension (PaCO$_2$) in patients ventilated with anesthesia ventilator set to constant tidal volume (V$_T$). Increasing FGF or I:E ratio causes an increase in delivered V$_T$, increase in alveolar ventilation, and decrease in PaCO$_2$. (From Scheller MS, Jones BL, and Benumof JL: The influence of fresh gas flow and I:E ratio on tidal volume and arterial PCO$_2$ in mechanically ventilated surgical patients, *J Cardiothorac Anesth* 3:564, 1989.)

when using an anesthesia ventilator is approximated by the formula:

$$\text{Additional ventilation} = [I/(I + E)] \times FGF$$

This is divided by the respiratory rate to determine the augmentation of each ventilator bellows V$_T$.

In terms of V$_T$ actually delivered to the patient, this formula provides an approximation only. The actual augmentation of V$_T$ also depends on the patient's total thoracic compliance compared with that of the anesthesia circuit components. If the patient's total thoracic compliance is low, additional fresh gas inflow from the machine may be accommodated mainly by compression in the circuit. **Thus patient minute volume (MV) is given by:**

Set MV + [FGF × (I/I + E)] − [Gas volume compressed in circuit at peak inspiratory pressure × RR]

RR is the respiratory rate in breaths/min. **The compressed gas volume term can be calculated as the product of circuit compliance and peak inspiratory pressure.** Thus volume compressed in the circuit equals compliance of circuit (ml/cm H$_2$O) times peak inspiratory pressure. These considerations do not apply to intensive care unit ventilators, which are designed to be minute volume dividers and whose V$_T$ is not affected by FGF, I:E ratio, or rate.

Positive End-Expiratory Pressure

The deliberate application of PEEP to the patient's airway is not uncommon during anesthesia. PEEP may be applied by adding a free-standing PEEP valve between the circle system's expiratory limb and

the expiratory valve (e.g., Boehringer PEEP valve, Boehringer Laboratories, Wynnewood, Pa). Free-standing PEEP valves function well, but they may be used erroneously and may totally occlude the circuit if incorrectly placed in the circle's inspiratory limb.[26, 61]

The machine manufacturers, North American Dräger and Ohmeda, provide PEEP valves in their contemporary anesthesia delivery systems as an option. These purpose-designed valves are convenient and should also avoid the risk of erroneous valve placement. **However, one must consider the effects of possible placement positions of a PEEP valve in the anesthesia circuit.**

At end-exhalation the pressure in an anesthesia circuit during positive-pressure ventilation using a standing bellows ventilator is +2.5 cm H$_2$O because of the PEEP effect of the ventilator PRV (see Fig. 47-40). If a 10 cm H$_2$O PEEP valve is now added by the expiratory unidirectional valve (see Fig. 47-40, position *A*), that part of the circuit between the inspiratory and PEEP valves is at +10 cm H$_2$O compared with pressure beyond the valve. That part of the circuit between the PEEP valve and the ventilator is at +2.5 cm H$_2$O. On the next inspiration, gas from the compressed bellows enters the circuit and must compress that gas in the patient circuit that is at +2.5 cm H$_2$O by an additional +10 cm H$_2$O before any entering gas will flow past the inspiratory unidirectional valve to enter the circle's inspiratory limb. The volume of gas that leaves the ventilator bellows and is compressed in that part of the circuit that was at +2.5 cm H$_2$O represents wasted bellows V$_T$ since it is not available to ventilate the patient. If the PEEP valve is placed close to the ventilator bellows (see Fig. 47-40, position *C*), at end-exhalation most of the gas in the patient circuit is now at +10 cm PEEP. Thus a much smaller volume of gas leaving the bellows during inspiration must be compressed in the circuit before the patient begins to receive a V$_T$. Thus, once a V$_T$ has been set on an anesthesia ventilator bellows, addition of PEEP to the basic patient circuit may decrease delivered V$_T$, depending on the position of the PEEP valve in the patient circuit. In Fig. 47-40, bellows V$_T$ loss would be greatest with position *A* and least with position *C;* position *B* is intermediate.[27] Decreases in V$_T$ may be reflected in spirometer readings or in other monitors of patient ventilation (e.g., PaCO$_2$; end-tidal CO$_2$).

Advantages of placing the PEEP valve near to the expiratory unidirectional valve (see Fig. 47-40, position *A* or *B*), however, are that in these positions PEEP may be applied during spontaneous as well as during mechanical ventilation. The decrease in patient V$_T$ on application of PEEP at position *A* in Fig. 47-40 (such as would be obtained with insertion of a free-standing PEEP valve) is greatest at low bellows V_T settings.[27] It is also more significant with the Ohmeda design of ventilator (7000, 7810) than with the Dräger AV-E.[51] This is because the Dräger AV-E bellows empties completely during each inspiration, whereas the Ohmeda bellows empties only the set V_T into the circuit. Since an Ohmeda bellows has a capacity of 1600 ml (see Fig. 47-31), the compression volume in the circuit at end-inspiration is $1600 - V_T$ greater than in the Dräger AV-E ventilator system.

WASTE GAS SCAVENGING SYSTEMS

Trace concentrations of anesthetic (waste) gases have neither been fully incriminated nor fully exonerated as a health hazard to operating room personnel. However, all the concerned agencies, such as the National Institute for Occupational Safety and Health (NIOSH), the American Hospital Association (AHA), the Joint Commission on Accreditation of Healthcare Organizations (JCAHO), and the American Society of Anesthesiologists (ASA), encourage reduction of exposure to waste gases, including waste gas scavenging and monitoring of measures to reduce exposure.[24]

NIOSH has recommended environmental limits for the upper boundary of exposure as follows[18]:

Occupational exposure to halogenated anesthetic agents shall be controlled so that no worker is exposed at concentrations greater than 2 parts per million (ppm) of any halogenated anesthetic agent.... When such agents are used in combination with nitrous oxide, levels of the halogenated agent well below 2 ppm are achievable. In most situations, control of nitrous oxide to a time-weighted average (TWA) concentration of 25 ppm during the anesthetic administration period will result in levels of approximately 0.5 ppm of the halogenated agent.... Occupational exposure to nitrous oxide, when used as the sole anesthetic agent, shall be controlled so that no worker is exposed at TWA concentrations greater than 25 ppm during anesthetic administration. Available data indicate that with current control technology, exposure levels of 50 ppm and less for nitrous oxide are attainable in dental offices.

These recommended exposure limits were based on two reports. Whitcher et al. showed that these levels were readily attainable in the operating room when certain precautionary measures were taken.[71] Bruce and Bach found no decrement in the psycho-motor capacities of volunteers exposed for 4 hours at these levels.[10] Guidelines for waste gas scavenging are discussed and set out in an ASA publication[70] and in a standards document.[2]

Waste gases may leave the anesthesia circuit via the APL valve or via the ventilator PRV. In either case, tubing of 19-mm internal diameter is used, as distinct from the 22-mm internal diameter with anesthesia

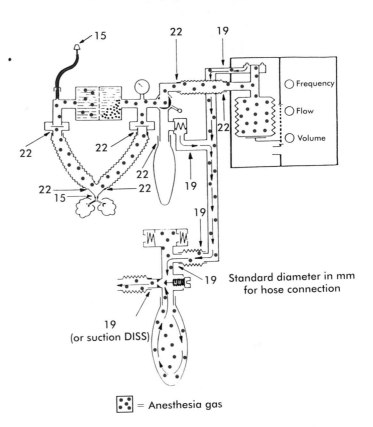

Fig. 47-42. Schematic of anesthesia circuit and scavenging system tubing showing diameters for hose connections. (From Schreiber P: *Safety guidelines for anesthesia systems,* Telford, Pa, 1985, North American Dräger.)

circuit and ventilator tubing, and the 15-mm internal diameter common gas outlet and endotracheal tube connector sizes (Fig. 47-42). The scavenging system *interfaces* the gas flow out of the patient circuit with the hospital suction system.[6a] Scavenging systems may be *open* or *closed*. Closed systems use spring-loaded valves to ensure that excessively high or low pressures are not applied to the patient circuit (see Fig. 47-42).[6a,45] Thus, if not connected to negative pressure (suction), excess pressure in the closed interface caused by gas entering it from the circuit is vented via the positive-pressure ("pop-off") relief valve, which opens at about $+5$ cm H_2O. If excessive suction might be applied to the circuit, one (Ohmeda interface) or two (Dräger closed interface, Fig. 47-43) negative-pressure relief ("pop-in") valves (-0.25 to -1.80 cm H_2O, depending on the system) would open to preferentially draw in room air. This would minimize the potential for application of negative pressure to the patient circuit.[6a, 26, 45]

Open-reservoir scavenging interfaces are valveless (Fig. 47-44) and use continually open relief ports to provide pressure relief.[50] Waste gas from the circuit is directed to the bottom of the canister, and the hospital suction system aspirates gas from the bottom

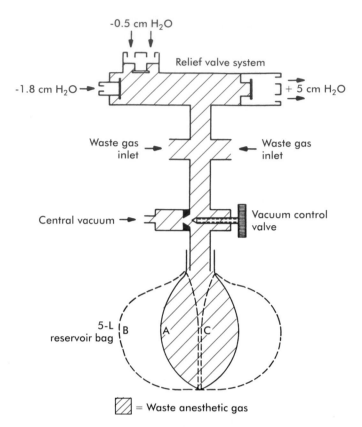

Fig. 47-43. North American Dräger Closed Scavenger Interface. (Schreiber P: *Safety guidelines for anesthesia systems,* Telford, Pa, 1985, North American Dräger.)

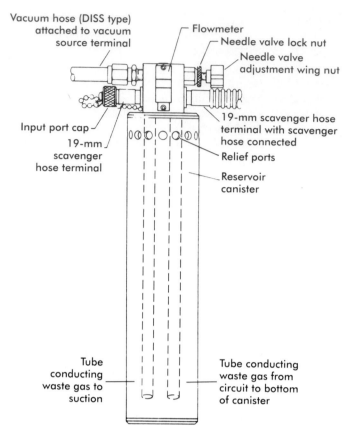

Fig. 47-44. North American Dräger Open-Reservoir Scavenging System. This interface uses continually open relief ports to provide positive and negative pressure relief (compare with valves in Fig. 47-43). An adjustable needle valve regulates waste gas exhaust flow, which is indicated on uncalibrated flowmeter. Flowmeter reading halfway between two white lines corresponds to suction flow rate of about 25 L/min. (Courtesy North American Dräger, Telford, Pa.)

of the canister. In this type of interface, the reservoir canister contains the excess waste gas and thereby accommodates a range of waste gas flow rates from the patient circuit. Since this type of interface depends on open relief ports for pressure relief, care must be taken to ensure that these ports remain unoccluded at all times. Items *17a* and *17b* of the FDA checklist (1986) describe, in principle, how the scavenging system should be checked out (see Box 47-2).

ANESTHESIA MACHINE STANDARD: ASTM F1161-88

The American Society for Testing and Materials (ASTM) document F1161-88 (published March 1989) represents a voluntary consensus among manufacturers, users, and other interested parties as to the *Standard Specification for Minimum Performance and Safety Requirements for Components and Systems of Anesthesia Gas Machines.*[4] It describes the performance characteristics of a contemporary anesthesia gas machine. F1161-88 supersedes the previous American National Standards Institute (ANSI) Z79.8-1979 standard. Important new considerations

in the F1161-88 standard are briefly discussed here. Numbers in parentheses indicate subsections in the original ASTM F1161-88 document.

Flow Control (Section 9.1)

Only one flow adjustment control for each gas delivered to the common gas outlet should be provided. Thus banks of flowmeters in parallel with separate high and low flow controls for the same gas are potentially hazardous. Some new anesthesia machines include a separate flow control and nipple for O_2 (for monitored anesthesia care). This does not violate the standard, since in this case the O_2 is not being delivered to the common gas outlet.

Concentration-Calibrated Vaporizers (12.1)

All vaporizers located within the fresh gas circuit should be concentration-calibrated. Control of the vapor concentration should be provided by means of calibrated knobs or dials (12.1.1). Measured flow vaporizers (e.g., Copper Kettle, Verni-Trol) are not mentioned and therefore probably no longer should be considered contemporary.

Common Gas Outlet (13.1.1)

When the common gas outlet is connected to the breathing system by a fresh gas supply hose, the common gas outlet should be provided with a retaining device. The outlet should have a manufacturer-specific fitting.

Alarms (16)

Alarm characteristics of monitors should be categorized as high, medium, or low priority. The alarms should be distinguishable audibly and visually, and the operator response should be immediate (high priority), prompt (medium priority), or an awareness (low priority). Contemporary machines should therefore incorporate an integrated and prioritized alarm system.

Oxygen Supply Precautions (17)

The machine should be designed so that whenever the O_2 supply pressure is reduced from normal (manufacturer specified) and until flow ceases, the set O_2 *concentration* should not decrease at the common gas outlet. The anesthesia circuit O_2 concentration should be measured, and the analyzer should sound a high-priority alarm when the concentration falls below the preset threshold. The machine should be designed so that the O_2 analyzer is enabled and

functioning anytime the machine is capable of delivering an anesthetic mixture.

Ventilatory Monitoring (18)

The anesthesia machine should have breathing pressure monitoring as well as either exhaled volume or ventilatory CO_2 monitoring.

The alarms associated with these monitors should be enabled and functioning automatically whenever the machine is in use.

The reader is referred to the original ASTM F1161-88 document for further information and the rationale for the stated requirements.[4]

SUMMARY

A basic understanding of the anesthesia delivery system and its components is important to the provision of safe patient care. The reader is encouraged to trace the flow of gases and vapors from their sources of storage, through his/her own particular delivery system, to waste gas scavenging. One should also consider the structure and function of each component in the gas pathway. In this way, malfunctions can be more readily identified and often more easily corrected by the user.[26] The reader is also strongly encouraged to review the operator's manual accompanying his/her anesthesia delivery system and in particular to *understand* the rationale behind the specific checkout procedures described.

KEY POINTS

- A basic understanding of the anesthesia delivery system and its components is important to the provision of safe patient care.

- The current voluntary consensus standard describing the features of a contemporary anesthesia machine is the ASTM F1161-88, published in 1989.

- A full oxygen tank (E cylinder) has a pressure of approximately 1900 PSIG and evolves 660 L of gaseous O_2 at atmospheric pressure (14.7 PSIA, 760 mm Hg). By applying Boyle's law, the pressure gauge can indicate fullness of the O_2 tank.

- Tank O_2 supply is regulated to enter the machine at 40 to 45 PSIG. Pipeline O_2 is regulated to 50 to 55 PSIG.

- The pin-index and diameter-index safety systems ensure that the correct medical gas enters the correct part of the machine.

- The "fail-safe" valve (pressure sensor shutoff valve, O_2 failure protection device) only ensures that if the

O_2 supply *pressure* is adequate, nitrous oxide (N_2O) and other gases may flow to their flow control valves. This valve does not ensure O_2 *flow*.

- N_2O can exist as a liquid at room temperature.

- N_2O E cylinders have a pressure of 750 PSIG (the saturated vapor pressure of N_2O at 20° C) as long as some liquid N_2O remains.

- Only one flow control knob should exist for each gas emerging at the common gas outlet.

- The O_2 flowmeter should be located downstream of all other gas flowmeters, i.e., it should be the one closest to the common gas outlet.

- On recent anesthesia machines the O_2 and N_2O flow controls are interlinked so that a gas mixture containing 25% or greater is created at the flowmeters when N_2O and O_2 are in use. Use of a third or fourth gas may "defeat" this feature.

- *An O_2 analyzer in the patient circuit is essential to detect a hypoxic mixture. It should be automatically* *enabled and the alarm set whenever the machine is capable of delivering an anesthetic gas mixture.*

■ Anesthesia vaporizers create a saturated vapor concentration of the anesthetic and then dilute it to clinically useful concentrations.

■ The ideal vaporizer construction material has high specific heat and thermal conductivity.

■ Modern vaporizers are variable bypass, concentration calibrated, and temperature compensated.

■ The volume of gas leaving a vaporizer is greater than that entering it by the addition of anesthetic vapor.

■ The output of a variable bypass, concentration-calibrated, agent-specific vaporizer is determined by the splitting ratio created by the dial setting. This determines what flow bypasses the vaporizing chamber (bypass flow) and what flow enters the vaporizing chamber to evolve the agent at its saturated vapor concentration.

■ Vaporizers are agent-specific. Erroneous filling should be avoided, and the use of agent-specific filling devices is encouraged.

■ Desflurane has a vapor pressure of 664 mm Hg at 20° C and boils at 23.5° C. *It cannot be used in current designs of variable bypass, concentration-calibrated vaporizers.* The most likely design will heat the liquid agent to form vapor under pressure. A concentration-dial rotary valve arrangement will then add controlled quantities of this vapor to the fresh gas flow. The vaporizing system for this agent will require energy (electricity) (See Tec 6 below).*

■ The anesthesia machine should be checked each day before anesthetizing the first patient and whenever any change has been made to the system. A shortened checkout should precede each administration of anesthesia. The checkout procedure should follow the directions given in the machine's operation and maintenance manual.

■ Presently, a positive-pressure check for leaks is recommended for Dräger Narkomed machines and a negative-pressure check for Ohmeda machines.

■ Use of free-standing vaporizers downstream from the common gas outlet may be hazardous and should be avoided.

■ Anesthesia circuits are classified as rebreathing (no CO_2 absorption) or nonrebreathing (have CO_2 absorber, e.g., circle system).

■ In all circuits, the higher the fresh gas flow, the

closer will inspired gas composition approach that of fresh gas.

■ Anesthesia ventilators are of "bag-in-a-bottle" or "double-circuit" design. The bellows is the interface between the patient circuit and the driving gas circuit.

■ Ohmeda ventilators (7000, 7800 series) are driven by 100% O_2, whereas the Dräger AV-E is driven by an air/O_2 mixture in the bellows housing.

■ Standing bellows ventilators are considered the preferred design. The bellows descend on inspiration and ascend on expiration. This design requires that the ventilator relief valve incorporate a positive end-expiratory pressure (PEEP) mechanism.

■ Having set the ventilator rate (f) and tidal volume (V_T) controls, one must appreciate that patient V_T is determined also by fresh gas flow (FGF), inspiratory:expiratory (I:E) ratio, circuit compliance, and peak inspiratory pressure:

$$\text{Patient } V_T = \left[(\text{Bellows } V_T) + \left(\frac{\text{FGF} \times \text{I}}{(\text{I} + \text{E}) \times \text{f}}\right)\right] -$$
$$[\text{Circuit compliance} \times \text{peak inspiratory pressure}]$$

■ Free-standing PEEP valves may be hazardous if added to the circuit incorrectly. PEEP valves are safer when designed as part of the circuit. Addition of PEEP to a circle decreases the V_T; the decrease depends on the position of the PEEP valve in the circle. The ideal position is as close to the ventilator bellows as possible.

■ Waste anesthesia gases should be scavenged.

■ NIOSH recommends that exposure of operating room workers to halogenated agents should be kept below 2 parts/million (ppm). N_2O levels should be controlled so that no worker is exposed at time-weighted average concentrations greater than 25 ppm. The latter guide should result in levels of approximately 0.5 ppm of the halogenated agents.

■ The ASTM F1161-88 standard calls for an integrated and prioritized alarm system, breathing pressure monitoring, and exhaled volume or ventilatory CO_2 monitoring.

■ In the event of a severe machine or gas delivery system malfunction, an alternative means for delivering O_2 (or room air) should be immediately available. Thus a self-inflating bag and full tank of O_2 should be available in each anesthetizing location.

---

*In anticipation of desflurane's approval by the FDA, Ohmeda has developed the *Tec 6 vaporizer.* This is a concentration-calibrated vaporizer designed to make the clinical administration of desflurane no different from that of the other commonly used potent inhaled agents in Tec-type vaporizers. The vaporizer is similar in appearance to the Tec 5 and can be mounted on a Selectatec manifold. In the Tec 6, liquid desflurane is heated to 39° C to produce vapor at a pressure of 1500 mm Hg (2 atmospheres absolute). This vapor is then metered into the main gas flow via a rotary valve controlled by the vaporizer concentration dial. The pressure of the vapor entering the rotary valve is continuously and automatically adjusted (by a pressure regulating valve that is in turn controlled by the output from a differential pressure transducer) to be equal to the pressure generated by the fresh gas inflow to a fixed restrictor. Unlike other concentration-calibrated vaporizers, such as the Tec 5 and Dräger Vapor 19.1, which are of the variable bypass design, in the Tec 6 no fresh gas enters the vaporizing chamber. The vaporizer is electrically powered, incorporating several heating elements as well as a sophisticated electronic control and alarm system. The 510 (k) application to the FDA for this vaporizer is currently under review. See reference 23.

KEY REFERENCES

American Society for Testing and Materials: *Standard specification for minimum performance and safety requirements for components and systems of anesthesia gas machines, F1161-88,* Philadelphia, 1989, The Society.

Bowie E, Huffman LM: *The anesthesia machine: essentials for understanding,* Madison, Wis, 1985, Ohmeda, BOC Health Care.

Conway CM: Anesthetic breathing systems, *Br J Anaesth* 57:649, 1985.

Dorsch JA, Dorsch SE: *Understanding anesthesia equipment,* ed 2, Baltimore, 1984, Williams & Wilkins.

Ehrenwerth J, Eisenkraft JB, eds: *Anesthesia equipment: principles and applications,* St Louis, 1992, Mosby–Year Book.

Eisenkraft JB, Sommer RM: Hazards of the anesthesia delivery system. In Ehrenwerth J, Eisenkraft JB,

eds: *Anesthesia equipment: principles and applications,* St Louis, 1992, Mosby–Year Book.

Food and Drug Administration: *Anesthesia apparatus checkout recommendations,* Rockville, Md, 1986, FDA. Revised update to be published late in 1992.

Parbrook GD, Davis PD, and Parbrook EO: *Basic physics and measurement in anesthesia,* ed 2, Norwalk, Conn, 1986, Appleton-Century-Crofts.

Schreiber P: *Safety guidelines for anesthesia systems,* Telford, Pa, 1985, North American Dräger.

Sykes MK: Rebreathing circuits, a review, *Br J Anaesth* 40:666, 1960.

Waste anesthetic gases in operative room air: a suggested program to reduce personnel exposure, Park Ridge, Ill, 1980, The American Society of Anesthesiologists.

REFERENCES

1. Alexander JP, Watters CH, Dodds WJC et al: The Engström Elsa anaesthetic machine: an electronic system for anaesthesia, *Anaesthesia* 45:746, 1990.

2. American National Standard for Anesthetic Equipment: *Scavenging systems for excess anesthetic gases,* ANSI Z79.11-1982, New York, 1982, American National Standards Institute.

3. American National Standards Institute: *Minimum performance and safety requirements for components and systems of continuous flow anesthesia machines for human use,* ANSI Z79.8-1979, New York, 1979, The Institute.

4. American Society for Testing and Materials: *Standard specification for minimum performance and safety requirements for components and systems of anesthesia gas machines, F1161-88,* Philadelphia, 1989, The Society.

5. American Society for Testing and Materials: *Standard specification for ventilators intended for use during anesthesia,* F1101-90, Philadelphia, 1990, The Society.

6. Andrews JJ, Johnston RV, Bee DE et al: Photodeactivation of ethyl violet: a potential hazard of Sodasorb, *Anesthesiology* 72:59, 1990.

6a. Azar I, Eisenkraft JB: Waste gas scavenging. In Ehrenwerth J, Eisenkraft JB, eds: *Anesthesia equipment: principles and applications,* St Louis, 1992, Mosby–Year Book.

7. Bain JA, Spoerel WE: A streamlined anaesthetic system, *Can Anaesth Soc J* 19:426, 1972.

8. Bain JA, Spoerel WE: Flow requirements for a modified Mapleson D system during controlled ventilation, *Can Anaesth Soc J* 20:629, 1973.

9. Bowie E, Huffman LM: *The anesthesia machine: essentials for understanding,* Madison, Wis, 1985, Ohmeda, BOC Health Care.

10. Bruce DL, Bach MJ: Effects of trace anaesthetic gases on behavioural performance of volunteers, *Br J Anaesth* 48:871, 1976.

11. Bruce DL, Linde HW: Vaporization of mixed anaesthetic liquids, *Anesthesiology* 60:342, 1984.

12. Bruce WE, Soni NC: Preliminary evaluation of the enclosed Magill breathing system, *Br J Anaesth* 62:144, 1989.

13. Capan L, Ramanathan S, Chalon J et al: A possible hazard with use of the Ohio Ethrane vaporizer, *Anesth Analg* 59:65, 1980.

14. *Compressed gas cylinder valve outlet and inlet connections,* pamphlet V-1, New York, 1977, Compressed Gas Association.

15. Conway CM: Anaesthetic breathing systems, *Br J Anaesth* 57:649, 1985.

16. Conway CM, Seeley HF, and Barnes PK: Spontaneous ventilation with the Bain anaesthetic system, *Br J Anaesth* 49:1245, 1977.

17. Cooper JB, Newbower RS, Moore JW et al: A new anesthesia delivery system, *Anesthesiology* 49:310, 1978.

18. *Criteria for a recommended standard — occupational exposure to waste anesthetic gases and vapors,* pub no 77-140, Cincinnati, 1977, US Department of Health, Education and Welfare, Public Health Service, Center for Disease Control, National Institute for Occupational Safety and Health.

19. *Diameter-index safety system,* New York, 1978, Compressed Gas Association.

20. Dorsch JA, Dorsch SE: *Understanding anesthesia equipment,* ed 2, Baltimore, 1984, Williams & Wilkins.

21. Eger EI II, Hylton RR, Irwin RH et al: Anesthetic flow meter sequence — a cause for hypoxia, *Anesthesiology* 24:396, 1963.

22. Eger EI II: Anesthetic systems: construction and function. In *Anesthetic uptake and action,* Baltimore, 1974, Williams & Wilkins.

23. Eisenkraft JB: Anesthesia vaporizers. In Ehrenwerth J, Eisenkraft JB, eds: *Anesthesia equipment: principles and applications,* St Louis, 1992, Mosby–Year Book.

23a. Eisenkraft JB: The anesthesia machine. In Ehrenwerth J, Eisenkraft JB, eds: *Anesthesia equipment: principles and applications,* St Louis, 1992, Mosby–Year Book.

24. Eisenkraft JB: Operating room pollution. In Eisenkraft JB, ed: *Progress in anesthesiology,* vol 1, San Antonio, 1987, Dannemiller Memorial Educational Foundation.

25. Eisenkraft JB: Potential for barotrauma or hypoventilation with the Dräger AV-E ventilator, *J Clin Anesth* 1:452, 1989.

25a. Eisenkraft JB, Raemer DB: Monitoring respiratory and anesthetic gases. In Ehrenwerth J, Eisenkraft JB, eds: *Anesthesia equipment: principles and applications,* St Louis, 1992, Mosby–Year Book.

26. Eisenkraft JB, Sommer RM: Hazards of the anesthesia delivery system. In Ehrenwerth J, Eisenkraft JB, eds: *Anesthesia equipment: principles and applications,* St Louis, 1992, Mosby–Year Book.

27. Elliott WR, Harris AE, and Philip JH: Positive end-expiratory pressure: implications for tidal volume changes in anesthesia machine ventilation, *J Clin Monit* 5:100, 1989.

28. Fink BR: How much anesthetic? *Anesthesiology* 34:403, 1971.

29. Fink BR: MAPP versus MAC, *Anesth Analg* 64:646, 1985.

30. Food and Drug Administration: *Anesthesia apparatus checkout recommendations,* Rockville, Md, 1986, FDA.

31. Gravenstein N, Banner MJ, and McLaughlin G: Tidal volume changes due to the interaction of anesthesia machine and anesthesia ventilator, *J Clin Monit* 3:187, 1987.

32. Jackson-Rees G: Anaesthesia in the newborn, *Br Med J* 2:1419, 1950.

33. James MFM, White JF: Anesthetic considerations at moderate altitude, *Anesth Analg* 63:1097, 1984.

34. Kain ML, Nunn JF: Fresh gas economics of the Magill circuit, *Anesthesiology* 29:964, 1968.

35. Katoh T, Ikeda K: The minimum alveolar concentration of sevoflurane in humans, *Anesthesiology* 66:301, 1987.

36. Korman B, Ritchie IM: Chemistry of halothane-enflurane mixtures applied to anesthesia, *Anesthesiology* 63:152, 1985.

37. Lack JA: Theatre pollution control, *Anaesthesia* 31:259, 1976.

38. Lees DE: FDA preanesthesia checklist being evaluated, revised, *Anesth Patient Safety Found Newslet* 6:25, 1991.

39. Magee PT: Anesthetic breathing systems. In Eisenkraft JB, ed: *Progress in anesthesiology,* vol 4, San Antonio, Tx, 1990, Dannemiller Memorial Educational Foundation.

40. Mapleson WW: The elimination of rebreathing in various semi-closed anaesthetic systems, *Br J Anaesth* 26:323, 1954.

40a. March MG, Crowley JJ: An evaluation of anesthesiologists' present checkout methods and the validity of the FDA checklist, *Anesthesiology* 75:724, 1991.

41. Miller DM, Miller JC: Enclosed afferent reservoir breathing systems, *Br J Anaesth* 60:469, 1988.

42. *Modulus II anesthesia system operation and maintenance manual,* Madison, Wis, 1987, Ohmeda, BOC Health Care.

43. *Modulus II Plus anesthesia machine preoperative checklists, operation and maintenance manual,* Madison, Wis, 1988, Ohmeda, BOC Health Care.

44. *Modulus II system service manual,* Madison, Wis, 1985, Ohmeda, BOC Health Care.

44a. Moon RE, Ingram C, Brunner EA et al: Spontaneous generation of carbon monoxide within anesthesia circuits, *Anesthesiology* 75(3A): 873, 1991 (abstract).

44b. Moon RE, Meyer EF, Scott D et al: Intraoperative carbon monoxide toxicity, *Anesthesiology* 73(3A): 1089, 1990 (abstract).

45. *Narkomed 2A anesthesia machine technical service manual, operating principles,* Telford, Pa, 1985, 1989, North American Dräger.

46. *Narkomed 3 anesthesia system operator's instruction manual,* Telford, Pa, 1986, North American Dräger.

47. *Narkomed 3 anesthesia system technical service manual,* Telford, Pa, 1988, North American Dräger.

48. *Ohmeda 7000 electronic anesthesia ventilator service manual,* Madison, Wis, 1985, Ohmeda, BOC Health Care.

49. *Ohmeda 7810 Electronic Anesthesia ventilator service manual,* Madison, Wis, 1989, BOC Health Care.

50. *Open reservoir scavenger operators instruction manual,* Telford, Pa, 1986, North American Dräger.

51. Pan PH, van der Aa JJ: Anesthesia ventilator performance, delivered tidal volume, and PEEP, *Anesthesiology* 73 (3A):A420, 1990 (abstract).

52. Parbrook GD, Davis PD, and Parbrook EO: *Basic physics and measurement in anesthesia,* ed 2, Norwalk, Conn, 1986, Appleton-Century-Crofts.

53. Pethick SL: Correspondence, *Can Anaesth Soc J* 22:115, 1975.

54. Petty C: *The anesthesia machine,* New York, 1987, Churchill Livingstone.

55. Raessler KL, Kretzman WE, and Gravenstein N: Oxygen consumption by anesthesia ventilators, *Anesthesiology* 69(3A): A271, 1988 (abstract).

56. Rampil IJ, Lockhart SH, Eger EI II et al: The electroencephalographic effects of desflurane in humans, *Anesthesiology* 74: 429, 1991.

57. Rau JL, Rau MY: *Fundamental respiratory therapy equipment,* Sarasota, Fla, 1977, Glenn Educational Medical Series.

58. Roth S, Tweedie E, and Sommer RM: Excessive airway pressure due to a malfunctioning anesthesia ventilator, *Anesthesiology* 65:532, 1986.

59. Scheller MS, Drummond JC: Solubility of N_2O in volatile anesthetics contributes to vaporizer aberrancy when changing carrier gases, *Anesth Analg* 65:88, 1986.

60. Scheller MS, Jones BL, and Benumof JL: The influence of fresh gas flow and I:E ratio on tidal volume and arterial PCO_2 in mechanically ventilated surgical patients, *J Cardiothorac Anesth* 3:564, 1989.

61. Schreiber P: *Safety guidelines for anesthesia systems,* Telford, Pa, 1985, North American Dräger.

62. Seed RF: A test for coaxial circuits, *Anaesthesia* 32:676, 1977.

63. Seeley HF, Barnes PK, and Conway CM: Controlled ventilation with the Mapleson D system, *Br J Anaesth* 49:107, 1977.

64. Sommer RM, Bhalla GS, Jackson JM et al: Hypoventilation caused by ventilator valve rupture, *Anesth Analg* 67:999, 1988.

65. *The Sodasorb manual of carbon dioxide absorption,* New York, 1962, Dewey and Almy Chemical Division, WR Grace.

66. Sykes MK: Rebreathing circuits, a review, *Br J Anaesth* 40:666, 1960.

67. Sykes MK, Vickers MD, and Hull CJ: *Principles of measurement for anesthetists,* Philadelphia, 1981, FA Davis.

68. Tanifuji Y, Takagi MS, Kobayashi K et al: The interaction between sevoflurane and soda lime or baralime, *Anesth Analg* 68:S285, 1989 (abstract).

69. Tyler CKG, Barnes PK, and Rafferty MP: Controlled ventilation with a Mapleson A (Magill) breathing system: reassessment using a lung model, *Br J Anaesth* 62:462, 1989.

69a. *Vapor 19.1 Vaporizer operating manual,* Lubeck, Germany, 1986, Drägerwerk AG.

70. *Waste anesthetic gases in operating room air: a suggested program to reduce personnel exposure,* Park Ridge, Ill, 1980, The American Society of Anesthesiologists.

71. Whitcher C, Piziali R, Sher R: *Development and evaluation of methods for the elimination of waste anesthetic gases and vapors in hospitals,* no (NIOSH) 75-137, Cincinnati, 1975, US Department of Health, Education and Welfare, Public Health Service, Center for Disease Control, National Institute for Occupational Safety and Health.

CHAPTER 48

Endotracheal Intubation

JAMES T. ROBERTS
SUSAN VASSALLO

APPROACHES TO INTUBATION

Endotracheal intubation is perhaps the single most useful airway-securing maneuver used by anesthesiologists. When it is performed properly it is life preserving. On the other hand, when it is performed improperly, it may well be life threatening. *In general there are four approaches to endotracheal intubation: (1) tactile blind, (2) nontactile blind, (3) indirect, and (4) direct.*

Tactile blind intubation was first described by Kite in the eighteenth century when he used a rigid endotracheal tube to facilitate resuscitation of near-drowning victims.[16] Two fingers are inserted to locate the epiglottis and the endotracheal tube is passed between them.

With nontactile blind endotracheal intubation an endotracheal tube is guided through the nasal passages to enter the larynx and trachea. A popular version of this approach uses a light wand, either nasally or orally, to guide the endotracheal tube.[1] The light position may be seen through the skin of the anterior neck if the room is darkened and thus directed into the trachea. The endotracheal tube is then advanced over the wand into the trachea.

Indirect laryngoscopy views the laryngeal opening through some optical device such as a flexible fiberoptic laryngoscope (Fig. 48-1), which is inserted either orally or nasally.[14] A rigid fiberoptic device such as the Bullard laryngoscope, or a mirrored rigid laryngoscope such as the Siker blade, is designed only for oral use.[13] The flexible fiberscope is designed to conform to the patient's anatomy whereas the rigid scopes force the patient's anatomy to conform to the instrument.

Direct laryngoscopy (Fig. 48-2) is the most widely used form of laryngoscopy for endotracheal intubation. Although a wide variety of laryngoscope blades are available, all have the unfortunate property of forcing the patient's anatomy to comform to the laryngoscope blade, which limits the use of the instruments in patients with abnormal anatomy.

Macewen, in 1878, was the first to report intubation for anesthesia.[8] Dr. Chevalier Jackson placed laryngoscopy on a firm footing with the development of the

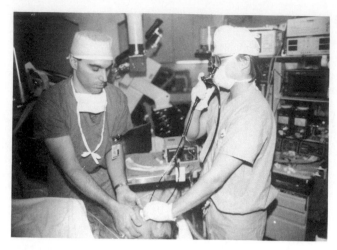

Fig. 48-1. Indirect laryngoscopy using the Olympus LF-1 flexible fiberoptic laryngoscope. The fiberbundle molds itself to the patient's pharyngeal anatomy rather than forcing the patient's anatomy to mold to a rigid steel or plastic blade, as is the case with most other laryngoscopes.

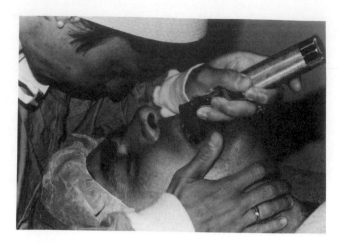

Fig. 48-2. Example of direct laryngoscopy using a no. 3 MacIntosh laryngoscope. (From Roberts JT: *Fundamentals of tracheal intubation,* New York, 1983, Grune & Stratton.)

Jackson laryngoscope to facilitate placement of endotracheal tubes. Highlights of endotracheal tube development are summarized in Box 48-1.

JUSTIFICATION FOR INTUBATION

Currently, justification for endotracheal intubation may be classified under five headings: inadequate oxygenation, inadequate ventilation, failure of the protective mechanisms of the larynx, trauma to the airway, and diagnostic or therapeutic measures.

Inadequate oxygenation of a patient may be determined subjectively when the patient develops a dusky appearance, or objectively by drawing an arterial blood gas sample or finding a low oximeter oxygen saturation reading.[11] Deficient tissue oxygenation may arise from inadequate delivery of oxygen to the alveoli from secondary to pneumothorax, atelectasis, multiple trauma, flail chest, postoperative splinting, intraoperative splinting, chronic obstructive pulmonary disease (COPD), restrictive lung disease, adult respiratory distress syndrome (ARDS), or restrictive lung disease. Poor transfer of oxygen across the alveoli may be the result of pulmonary edema, pneumonia, or pulmonary fibrosis. Pulmonary shunting may result from pulmonary emboli, fat emboli, or may be congenital in origin. Abnormal binding of oxygen to hemoglobin may be the result of carbon monoxide poisoning or abnormal hemoglobin species. Hypermetabolic states such as thyroid storm, hyperthermia, or malignant hyperthermia increase the demand for oxygen delivery to the cells. Endotracheal intubation helps ensure maximal oxygen delivery through the upper airway.

Inadequate ventilation may arise from malfunction of respiratory drive, failure of the ventilatory muscles, airway obstruction or intrinsic lung disease, and a failure of the bellows mechanism.[4] Respiratory drive is commonly affected by narcotics, volatile anesthetic agents, anoxia, brain trauma, and stroke. Loss of ventilatory power may be secondary to weakened intercostal muscles, paralyzed diaphragm, insecticide poisoning, Guillain-Barré syndrome, myasthenia gravis, or phrenic nerve injury. Airway obstruction may result from bilateral recurrent laryngeal nerve injury resulting in closure at the vocal cords or stenosis from direct tracheal injury.

Folding of the epiglottis over the laryngeal inlet protects the larynx and trachea during ingestion of food. Failure of this protective mechanism, which may result from drug overdose, a burn of the airway, stroke, or coma, often necessitates endotracheal intubation.[6] Endotracheal intubation also provides easy access to the airway for tracheal lavage or fiberoptic bronchoscopy.

FUNCTIONAL ANATOMY OF THE AIRWAY

Infants are obligatory nose breathers and they have a greater ratio of physiologic dead space to tidal volume than do adults. Although infants have no teeth, their tongues are relatively larger, they have larger adenoids, and the lower border of the larynx (the cricoid) is positioned more cephalad at the lower border of the C4 vertebra. In the infant the epiglottis is relatively larger, stiffer and positioned at an angle of 45 degrees to the trachea, whereas in the adult the epiglottis is relatively shorter, flatter, and parallel to the axis of the

BOX 48-1
HIGHLIGHTS OF ENDOTRACHEAL TUBE DEVELOPMENT

1543	Vesalius	Kept pig alive by intubation and ventilation
1667	Hooke	Ventilated a dissected dog
1705	Kite	Invented device for resuscitating drowning victims
1765	Home	Suggested tracheostomy
1796	Herholdt and Rafn	Blind intubation for drowning
1814	Desault	Nasotracheal intubation
1826	Bretonean	Silver cannula for intubation
1878	Macewen	First intubation for anesthesia
1880	O'Dwyer	Laryngeal stent for croup
1890	Hailes	Tube needed introducer but no extractor
1893	Eisenmenger	First cuffed oral tracheal tube
1897	Fisher	Introducer allowed immediate ventilation through the tube
1905	Kuhn	Laryngeal stent extended outside the mouth; suggested placing cuff on tube
1909	Jackson	Placed bronchoscopy on firm ground
1912	Feroud	Feroud tube needed introducer and extractor
1943	Grun and Knight	Used thin cuff to allow placement of tube through the nose
1970	Guess	Implant testing

trachea. The infant's vocal cords are approximately one half cartilaginous; in the adult there is a greater proportion that is ligamentous. The anterior edge of the thyroid cartilage lies almost vertically in the infant, whereas it tilts anteriorly in the adult. In the infant the cricoid ring is smaller than the rima glottis and the cricoid plate is slanted posteriorly. In the adult the cricoid plate slants vertically and enlarges with growth, which leaves the rima glottis the narrowest part of the upper airway. In the infant the vocal process is inclined inferiorly and medially, causing a concave surface to the vocal cord. In the adult the vocal cord surface is flat. Squamous epithelium covers the upper part of the epiglottis, the upper latereal walls of the vestibule, and the vocal cords. Ciliated columnar epithelium lines the ventricles, the inferior vestibule, and the larynx below the rima glottidis. The structure of the infant trachea compared to the adult is presented in Fig. 48-3. It is evident that edema will have a much greater effect on the infant trachea because of its much smaller cross-sectional area compared to the adult trachea. Also note the different shape of the adult trachea. The lunate configuration has a greater propensity to collapse of the posterior wall.

Nasal intubation is limited in the adult by the size of the external nares and the relative size of the nasal turbinates. Although both the inferior and middle turbinates obstruct passage of an endotracheal tube, it is the inferior turbinate that has a greater effect on limiting the size of the endotracheal tube used.

The position of the base of the tongue, the size of the tongue relative to the oral cavity, and the position of the upper teeth all may adversely affect the ease with which a laryngoscope blade can be inserted. A quick guide to the effect of these structures on the ease of laryngoscopy is the Mallampatti test, which is discussed later.

The larynx is composed of thyroid, cricoid, epiglottis, and arytenoid cartilages, and the hyoid bone, which are positioned as in Fig. 48-4. The relative motion of the parts of the larynx is governed by the intrinsic muscles of the larynx. Two nerves (superior and inferior laryngeal) innervate all of the intrinsic muscles (Table 48-1). The superior laryngeal nerves innervate the bilateral cricothyroideous muscles. All

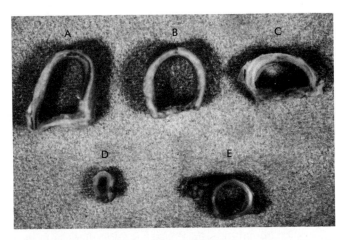

Fig. 48-3. Examples of cross sections of adult (*A* to *C*) and infant (*D* and *E*) tracheas. Note the wide variety of adult shapes. (From Roberts JT: *Fundamentals of tracheal intubation,* New York, 1983, Grune & Stratton.)

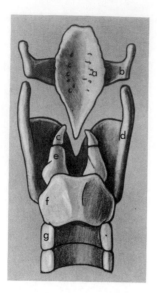

Fig. 48-4. Illustration of cartilages of the larynx. (From Roberts JT: *Fundamentals of tracheal intubation,* New York, 1983, Grune & Stratton.)

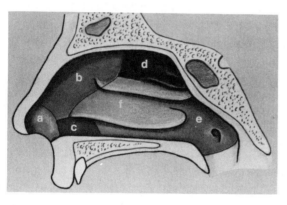

Fig. 48-5. Sensory distribution of the lateral nasal wall. (From Roberts JT: *Fundamentals of tracheal intubation,* New York, 1983, Grune & Stratton.)

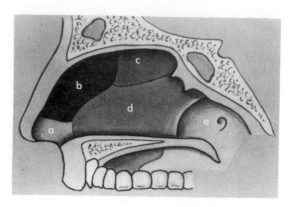

Fig. 48-6. Sensory distribution of the nasal septum. (From Roberts JT: *Fundamentals of tracheal intubation,* New York, 1983, Grune & Stratton.)

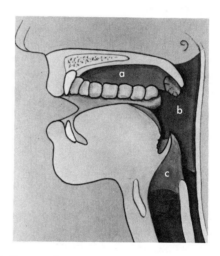

Fig. 48-7. Sensory innervation of the pharynx. (From Roberts JT: *Fundamentals of tracheal intubation,* New York, 1983, Grune & Stratton.)

Table 48-1   Intrinsic muscles of the larynx

Muscle	Function
Posterior cricoarytenoid glottis	Abducts vocal cords, closing
Lateral cricoarytenoid glottis	Adducts arytenoids, closing
Transverse arytenoid glottis	Adducts arytenoids, closing
Oblique arytenoid	Closes glottis
Aryepiglottic	Closes glottis
Vocalis	Relaxes tension of vocal folds
Thyroarytenoid	Relaxes tension of vocal folds
Cricothyroid	Increases tension of vocal folds

Table 48-2   Extrinsic muscles of the larynx

Muscle	Function
Sternohyoid	Changes position of thyroid cartilage and hyoid bone relative to each other and to the sternum
Sternothyroid	Modifies folding of thyrohyoid and aryepiglottic folds
Thyrohyoid	Same as above
Thyroepiglottic	Mucosal inversion or aryepiglottic fold
Stylopharyngeus cartilage	Indirectly assists folding of thyroid
Inferior pharyngeal constrictor	Assists swallowing
Thyropharyngeal	Assists swallowing
Cricothyroid	Tenses vocal folds

other intrinsic muscles of the larynx are innervated by the inferior (recurrent) laryngeal nerves. **The superior laryngeal nerves are singularly important because they innervate the only tensor of the vocal cords.** Blocking these nerves is easy and greatly facilitates an awake intubation (discussed later). The extrinsic muscles of the larynx are listed in Table 48-2.

Sensory innervation of the nasal passages is illustrated in Figs. 48-5 and 48-6. Use of a spray or a large cotton swab containing lidocaine and phenylephrine is recommended to anesthetize the nasal passages topically. Sensory innervation to the pharynx is supplied by the glossopharyngeal and palatine nerves (Fig. 48-7). **The base of the tongue, epiglottis, vallecula, and piriform recess down to the vocal cords may be anesthetized by blocking the superior laryngeal nerves either percutaneously or intraorally** (Fig. 48-8). The sensory fibers to the trachea should be anesthetized with a local anesthetic, either percutaneously or by the use of an intraoral spray. The trachea should not be anesthetized by blocking the inferior (recurrent) laryngeal nerves.

Stimulation of the autonomic nerves of the airway may be initiated by six types of receptors that reside in the respiratory tract. They respond to chemical, mechanical, and thermal stimuli such as pressure of a laryngoscope, aspiration of stomach contents, inhalation of volatile gases, inflation or deflation of the lungs, and thermal injury. Depending on the area of the respiratory tract stimulated, salivation, coughing, gagging and vomiting, laryngospasm, bronchospasm, inflation, deflation, or aspiration reflexes may be initiated.

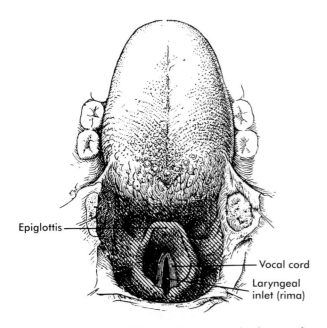

Fig. 48-8. Sensory distribution of the superior laryngeal nerve.

PREDICTING EASE OF INTUBATION

Potentially difficult intubations may be predicted by the several tests. The Mallampati test involves visual assessment of the oral cavity.[9] Laryngeal tilt measured with a bubble inclinometer is significant when the tilt is greater than 40 degrees from the horizontal.[15] A receding mandible, enlarged teeth, and a high arched palate are also indications that an intubation will be difficult to perform.

TRACHEAL INTUBATION IN THE AWAKE PATIENT

Endotracheal intubation on an awake patient poses problems that are either not encountered or encountered to a lesser degree in an anesthetized-paralyzed patient. These problems include failure to open the mouth adequately, patient anxiety, hypertension from laryngoscopy, reactive closure of the vocal cords, vomiting and gagging, or bronchospasm upon insertion of the endotracheal tube. To counter these problems, an awake intubation requires patient sedation combined with adequate topical anesthesia of the airway.[12]

A valuable technique for awake intubation begins with intravenous sedation using a combination of fentanyl and droperidol titrated to produce the desired sedative effect. During this initial sedation in the supine position, the operator applies 4% lidocaine ointment on an oral airway that is partially placed in the patient's mouth; adequate time is allowed for the ointment to melt (as a result of the patient's body temperature) and to coat the posterior pharynx (glossopharyngeal distribution).

The superior laryngeal nerves are then blocked bilaterally to anesthetize the base of the tongue, vallecula, epiglottis, and piriform recesses down to the vocal cords. The superior horns of the thyroid cartilage are palpated and the larynx is slightly displaced laterally toward the side of injection. The needle of the syringe with local anesthetic is advanced against the superior horn, then moved anteriorly until the needle slides off the superior horn. As the needle slides off the horn, it is advanced approximately 1 cm deeper. If no air is aspirated, 1 or 2 ml of 1% lidocaine is injected while the needle is withdrawn. This is repeated on the contralateral side.

This leaves only the trachea to be anesthetized. An atomizer with a long nozzle may be introduced gradually into the trachea transorally after good topical anesthesia is obtained. However, we prefer the percutaneous approach where the needle is inserted through the first tracheal ring, after which air is aspirated to ensure placement of the needle tip within the tracheal lumen; then the local anesthetic is

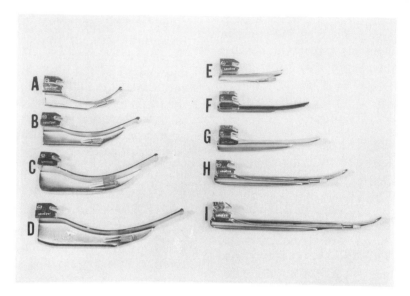

Fig. 48-9. The common MacIntosh (*A* to *D*)and Miller (*E* to I) laryngoscope blades.

injected. Injection produces coughing so the syringe must be held firmly to prevent movement of the needle tip. Thereafter, the laryngoscopy and intubation should not be rushed, and adequate time should be allowed for proper sedation and full topical anesthesia to be achieved.

ANESTHETIZING A PATIENT FOR TRACHEAL INTUBATION

Both general anesthesia and skeletal muscle relaxation are routinely used to facilitate endotracheal intubation. Thiopental sodium induces general anesthesia more rapidly than the newer intravenous agent propofol. Appropriate use of these agents is discussed elsewhere in the text (see Chapter 53).

Muscle relaxation may be achieved using either a depolarizing or nondepolarizing agent. Fine control of laryngeal muscles is achieved by a low ratio of muscle fibers to nerve endings, that is, 1:1. This low ratio allows a much lesser dose of muscle relaxant to be effective. **The goal of using a muscle relaxant is not only to relax the laryngeal muscles but also to relax the masseters.** The larger skeletal muscles have a much higher muscle fiber to nerve ending ratio, that is, 13:1. Thus, whereas a 20-mg dose of succinylcholine will relax laryngeal muscle, a much larger dose is required to relax the masseters to permit easier insertion of the laryngoscope blade.

OROTRACHEAL INTUBATION

Indications for orotracheal intubation have been discussed in the preceding section. Selection of an instrument and a specific technique for oral intuba-

tion depends on one's experience. The MacIntosh (curved) and Miller (straight) blades are the most widely used laryngoscopes (Fig. 48-9). The MacIntosh blade is designed to be placed anterior to the epiglottis and to lift it by pushing against the hyoepiglottic ligament. The Miller blade, on the other hand, is designed to be placed posterior to the epiglottis; lifting this blade then offers a more direct view of the laryngeal opening.

A recent addition to rigid blade instruments is the Bullard laryngoscope. The Bullard scope is shaped more like a retractor than the usual laryngoscope; as such it fits the patient's anatomy better. It is designed

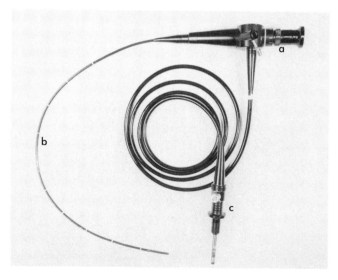

Fig. 48-10. The common parts of a flexible fiberoptic laryngoscope. *A,* Body; *B,* coherent light bundle; *C,* noncoherent bundle to the light source.

for the patient with a difficult anatomy, but as of the writing of this chapter, a Medline search revealed no research that critically evaluated the adult Bullard laryngoscope. The cost of this instrument is a considerable disadvantage.

The cost of a flexible fiberoptic laryngoscope approximates the cost of the Bullard laryngoscope. The flexible fiberscope, however, easily molds itself to the patient's anatomy, and it can be used for nasal intubations also. The flexible fiberoptic laryngoscope is now widely used. Fig. 48-10 illustrates a flexible fiberoptic laryngoscope. Detailed instructions have recently been published on its use.[13]

NASOTRACHEAL INTUBATION

Indications for nasotracheal intubation include failure of orotracheal intubation, inability to open the mouth because of arthritis or mandibular fracture, or intended dental work or facial surgery. Prolonged intubation in an ICU setting is more comfortable with nasal intubation.

Nasotracheal intubation may be facilitated by direct oral laryngoscopy, by blind intubation with or without a light wand, or by indirect laryngoscopy using a fiberoptic laryngoscope. When nasotracheal intubation is assisted by direct oral laryngoscopy with a no. 3 MacIntosh laryngoscope, the tip of the endotracheal tube is first inserted into the posterior pharynx. Once the tip of the endotracheal tube is seen in the posterior pharynx, it is advanced through the laryngeal opening directly, or with the aid of a Magill forceps (Fig. 48-11). It is important not to grasp and rupture the cuff of the endotracheal tube when forceps are used.

A nasal endotracheal tube may be blindly guided to the laryngeal entrance by listening to the patient's breath sounds at the adapter end of the endotracheal tube, and advancing the endotracheal tube when the

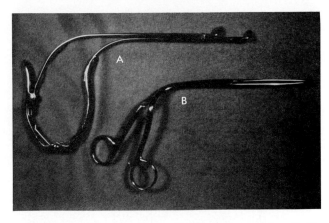

Fig. 48-11. Aillon *(A)* and Magill *(B)* forceps used to facilitate guiding an endotracheal tube placed through the nose toward the laryngeal opening. (From Roberts JT: *Fundamentals of tracheal intubation,* New York, 1983, Grune & Stratton.)

breath sounds are clearly heard. Maneuvers to position the larynx properly with regard to the endotracheal tube tip include (1) flexing or extending the patient's atlanto-occipital joint (Fig. 48-12); (2) slowly rotating, advancing, or withdrawing the endotracheal tube; (3) tilting the patient's head laterally toward the side of the nares into which the tube was placed (Fig. 48-13); or (4) manually displacing the patient's larynx to one or the other side, depending on where the tip of the tube lies (Fig. 48-14).

A light wand may be helpful when performing blind intubation (Fig. 48-15). The room lights should be dimmed to help in seeing the position of the light wand tip through the skin of the patient's neck.

It is preferable to perform nasotracheal intubation under indirect vision using a fiberoptic laryngoscope. The technique of fiberoptic laryngoscopy should emulate the following algorithm: the nasal passages should be sprayed with phenylephrine to prevent

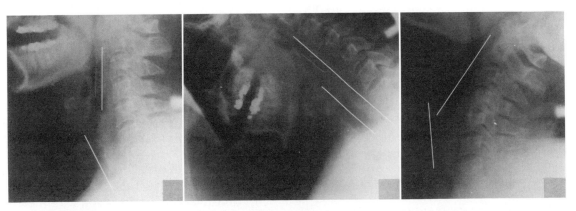

Fig. 48-12. Example of flexion and extension of the atlanto-occipital joint. (From Roberts JT: *Fundamentals of tracheal intubation,* New York, 1983, Grune & Stratton.)

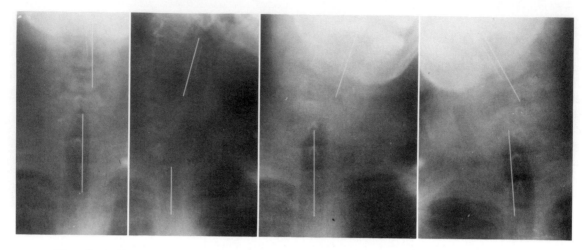

Fig. 48-13. Tilting the head sideways (toward the side of nasal insertion) may help guide the endotracheal tube during a blind nasal intubation. (From Roberts JT: *Fundamentals of tracheal intubation,* New York, 1983, Grune & Stratton.)

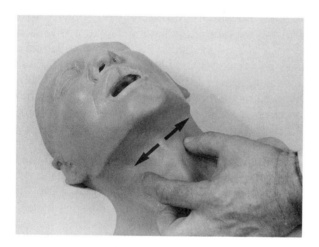

Fig. 48-14. Larynx may also be displaced laterally to guide the larynx toward the tip of the endotracheal tube.

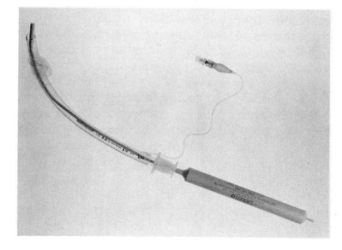

Fig. 48-15. Photograph of a light wand inserted through the lumen of an endotracheal tube.

hemorrhage as the endotracheal tube advances. An endotracheal tube 0.5 mm smaller than that used for oral intubation should be selected. The plastic adapter should be removed from the endotracheal tube. The endotracheal tube should be slid over the lubricated fiberbundle and the proximal end of the tube should be forced gently up onto the wider base of the fiberscope (Fig. 48-16). This keeps the endotracheal tube from falling off the fiberbundle during intubation. The visual path should be clear and the light source illuminated. The fiberscope should be looked through immediately as its tip enters the external nares. Oxygen should be attached to the side port of the fiberscope at +/− 7 L flow; blowing oxygen down the fiberscope channel should be controlled with the index finger. If there is a possibility of

being in the patient's esophagus, oxygen should not be insufflated.

The vocal cords should be observed and the fiberoptic scope should be advanced through the glottic opening. Once it is in the trachea near the carina, the endotracheal tube should be advanced over the fiberscope, which is now acting as a stylet. If the endotracheal tube hangs up on the right arytenoid this following procedure should be attempted: the endotracheal tube should be withdrawn by 1 cm, then the tube should be rotated 90 degrees counterclockwise before the tube is readvanced. The tube should now move easily past the obstructing arytenoid.

After the tube is in position with the endotracheal tube tip above the carina, the fiberscope should be withdrawn, and the plastic adapter reinserted and

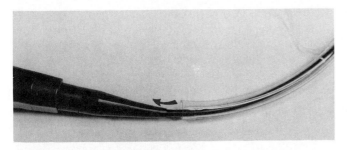

Fig. 48-16. With the adapter removed, the endotracheal tube is seated on the tapered portion of the flexible fiberoptic laryngoscope. This prevents the endotracheal tube from sliding along the fiberbundle and interfering with advancement of the fiberbundle.

connected to the anesthesia machine. Carbon dioxide should be checked for when the patient exhales. The cuff should be inflated and the tube should be positioned gently to permit adequate ventilation of both lungs (verified by auscultation). The fiberscope should be cleaned and sterilized to ready it for its next use. It should be stored in a sterile plastic bag to indicate sterility for the next user.

WHEN AN INTUBATION ATTEMPT FAILS

What happens when an intubation attempt fails? Hypoxia may or may not rapidly ensue, depending on whether the airway is partially or totally obstructed. Aerobic metabolism is impaired when the Pao_2 within the cellular mitochondria reaches a critical value. Neurons cease to function and the patient loses consciousness with a further decrease in blood oxygen content. Maintainance of oxygenation depends on volume of stored oxygen, and the rate of use of these stores. The primary storage site is the lungs (3500 ml). The blood itself carries only approximately 19.5 ml oxygen/100 ml blood. The rate of utilization of these oxygen stores depends on pH, the concentration of hemoglobin, the type of hemoglobin, body temperature, 2,3-DPG, and the circulating carbon monoxide concentration.

With failure of intubation, diminished ventilation may result in hypercapnia. Elevated CO_2 levels have both direct and indirect effects. Direct effects involve a decrease in the myocardial contractility, slowing of the heart rate, induction of hypotension with ganglionic blockade, and increased myocardial perfusion but decreased skeletal muscle perfusion. Other effects of elevated CO_2 include cerebral vasodilation, release of epinephrine and norepinephrine, and depressed activity of acetylcholine.

Indirect effects of an elevated CO_2 concentration, which depend on an intact autonomic nervous system, are what are usually clinically associated with hyper-

---

BOX 48-2
INSTRUMENTS TO HAVE
READILY AVAILABLE

MacIntosh laryngoscope blades (with batteries and bulbs)
Miller laryngoscope blades
Flexible fiberoptic laryngoscope (sterile)
Light source for flexible fiberscope
Variety of oral airways (Ovassapian, Williams, Patil, Olympus)
Appropriate anesthesia machine
Additional oxygen source and tubing
Ambu-bag
Selection of endotracheal tubes
Syringes and needles
Patil mask to permit ventilation during intubation
Suction catheters and tubing
Spray bottles for local anesthetics
Cotton-tipped applicators
Pulse oximeter
Capnograph

BOX 48-3
DRUGS TO HAVE READILY AVAILABLE

Midazolam	Atracurium
Diazepam	Vecuronium
Lorazepam	Atropine
Fentanyl	Glycopyrolate
Morphine	Sodium thiopental
Droperidol	Propofol
Succinylcholine	Lidocaine

---

capnia. These include an increased cardiac output, tachycardia, increased blood pressure, and increased myocardial oxygen consumption.

Drug metabolism may be altered during hypercapnia by the effects of changes in pH on drug binding and distribution. The patient may exhibit signs of agitation and restlessness. A partially closed glottis may hinder attempts at subsequent intubation when the glottis is displaced inferiorly by marked inspiratory efforts.

Instruments and drugs that should be readily available during attempted endotracheal intubation are listed in Boxes 48-2 and 48-3. **The initial response to a failed intubation attempt should be to ventilate the patient by mask. The subsequent course of action depends on whether there is an obstructed airway.**

Techniques for managing failed endotracheal intubation include (1) using a flexible fiberoptic technique, (2) inserting a Brain airway, (3) proceeding with a retrograde intubation, (4) using a blind technique (with or without a light wand), or (5) possibly resorting to another rigid laryngoscope like the Bullard laryngoscope. The prudent anesthesiologist should always have available a simple device for percutaneous transtracheal oxygenation such as illustrated in Fig. 48-17 and should be prepared to perform an emergency cricothyrotomy or tracheostomy.

In our experience, the preferred approach is to use a flexible fiberoptic laryngoscope via the oral route. Box 48-2 lists the minimal items required for this technique. Proper positioning of the patient is critical to the success of oral flexible fiberoptic intubation. As illustrated in Fig. 48-18, the patient's head should not rest on a blanket as indicated for direct laryngoscopy but should be flat against the operating room table mattress. Combined atlanto-occipital and cervical extension should be used unless cervical injury is

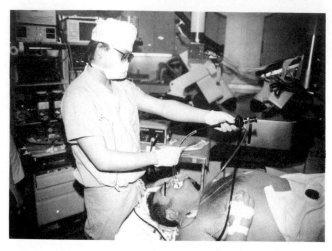

Fig. 48-18. Proper positioning of the patient for flexible fiberscopy. No pillows should be used and the patient's head is placed flat on table with atlanto-occipital extension to lift the epiglottis from the posterior pharyngeal wall. Table is dropped to aid in keeping the fiberscope extended.

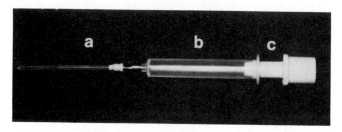

Fig. 48-17. Simple three-part (*a* to *c*) device for transtracheal oxygenation. (From Roberts JT: *Fundamentals of tracheal intubation,* New York, 1983, Grune & Stratton.)

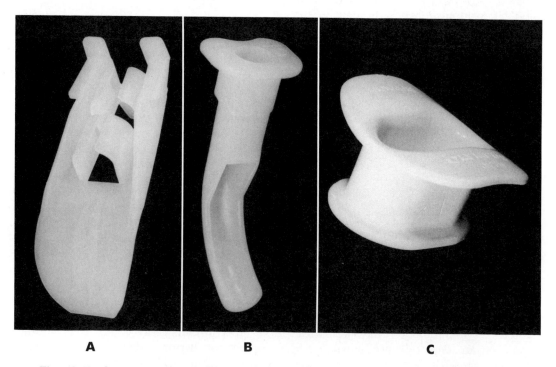

A   B   C

Fig. 48-19. Ovassapian (**A**), Williams (**B**), and Olympus (**C**) bite blocks commonly used to protect (and guide) the fiberscope during oral flexible fiberoscopy. (From Roberts JT, guest editor: Fiberoptics in anesthesia, *Anesth Clin North Am*, Philadelphia, 1991, WB Saunders.)

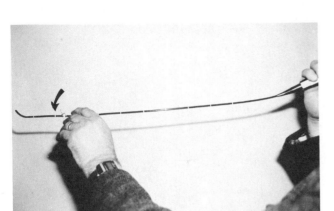

Fig. 48-20. The distal end of the fiberbundle is held at the second white band (10-cm mark) indicated by the arrow.

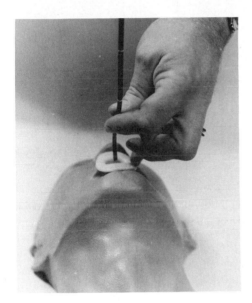

Fig. 48-21. Fiberscope should be inserted in the midline.

suspected. The operating room table should be lowered to allow the laryngoscopist to keep the flexible fiberscope extended and straight.

A bite block is essential to prevent injury to the fiberscope from the patient's teeth. Several common bite blocks are illustrated in Fig. 48-19. The fiberscope bundle should be grasped approximately 8 to 10 cm from the tip (Fig. 48-20) and inserted exactly in the midline of the tongue only to a depth of 8 to 10 cm (Fig. 48-21). Thereafter the scope is guided toward the laryngeal opening under direct vision through the fiberoptic eyepiece.

Four maneuvers of the fiberscope are all that are necessary to direct the scope properly. The first manipulation is to bend the tip of the scope in a vertical plane by adjusting the lever with the thumb, as shown in Fig. 48-22. Second, the instrument may be rotated along its long axis (Fig. 48-23). The handle of the scope, *not* the fiberbundle, should be rotated. Rotating the fiberbundle may cause disorientation. Rotating the scope without bending the tip does not change the image seen through the eyepiece. Once the desired path is centered in the view seen through the eyepiece, the scope should be *slowly* advanced. The channel of the fiberscope may also be used to facilitate passage into the trachea.

The sequence of views that can be seen as the scope advances toward the trachea are tongue, uvula, epiglottis with atlanto-occipital flexion, epiglottis with atlanto-occipital extension, vocal cords, trachea, carina, right mainstem bronchus, and left mainstem bronchus.

Another method of establishing an airway is to use the laryngeal mask airway. Fig. 48-24 illustrates the airway before insertion; Fig. 48-25 shows the position of the airway during anesthesia for MRI. Its advan-

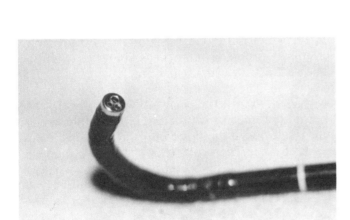

Fig. 48-22. Tip of the fiberscope bends in a vertical plane.

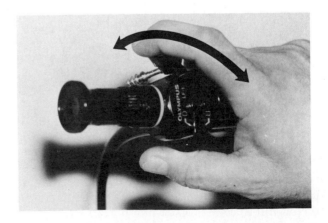

Fig. 48-23. The fiberscope should be rotated *at the handle,* rather than at the distal fiberbundle.

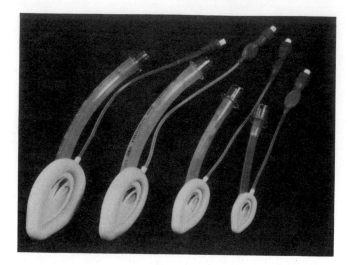

Fig. 48-24. Various sizes of the laryngeal mask airway. (Courtesy NG Goudsouzian, MD.)

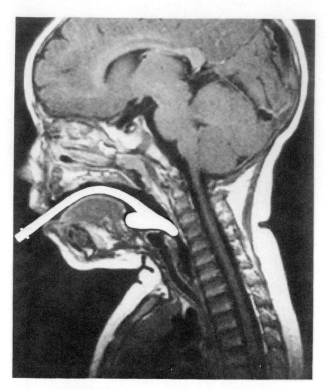

Fig. 48-25. MRI of the laryngeal mask airway *(shown in white)* in proper position. (Courtesy NG Goudsouzian, MD.)

tages include simplicity of use and the ability to connect the airway to a ventilator. Its disadvantages are its relatively high cost (although it may be resterilized), and the fact that it does not protect the airway against aspiration of stomach contents. Also, when laryngospasm is present, a laryngeal mask airway may aggravate the situation. Succinylcholine may or may not be indicated in the situation of a failed intubation attempt. Its use should be limited to situations in which the operator is confident that failure resulted from inadequate muscle relaxation, because the combination of muscle relaxation, apnea, and inability to intubate can be lethal.

Retrograde intubation is an alternate approach for dealing with a difficult airway. In this technique, a wire is passed percutaneously through the cricothyroid membrane, through the pharynx, and out of the mouth. An endotracheal tube or flexible fiberscope is then guided through the larynx over the wire, after which the wire is withdrawn and the endotracheal tube is advanced into the trachea.[10]

A blind nasal or oral intubation may be attempted also. A light wand may be useful but may require darkening the room, which may not be the best choice for observing the patient in a critical situation.

A rigid laryngoscope may be used for repeat attempts to intubate the trachea. The Bullard laryngoscope has been touted as a device for difficult intubations. Although the curvature of the blade more closely approaches the normal oral airway, and its fiberoptic channel allows viewing the tip of the blade, its use requires considerable experience. Its main disadvantages are that it forces the patient's anatomy to conform to a steel blade and that its use is limited to oral intubations only.

EXTUBATION OF THE TRACHEA

Success at intubation introduces an entirely new problem: that of successful and uncomplicated extubation. Criteria for extubation include indications of adequate ventilation, a negative inspiratory force of at least 20 cm H_2O, a vital capacity of at least 15 ml/kg body weight, or a forced expiratory volume during the first second of greater than 10 ml/kg body weight. Occasionally, a negative methylene blue test for aspiration may be helpful. A sustained head lift of greater than 5 seconds indicates adequate neuromuscular function. Satisfactory oxygenation may be assessed by arterial blood gases or by pulse oximetry.

Several problems may necessitate changing an endotracheal tube. A cuff may break or a large air leak may occur. The endotracheal tube may be partially obstructed. An oral tube may need to be replaced with another oral tube or with a nasal tube. When a nasal tube is selected, it should be inserted through the nose and a direct laryngoscopy should be performed with both tubes in sight in the pharynx. The original (oral) tube should be removed and the second tube should be advanced through the larynx. Another method involves inserting a long catheter (either a ureteral catheter or, preferably, a plastic catheter with a lumen for oxygen insufflation that is specifically designed for this purpose) through the existing endotracheal tube. The tube over the stylet should be removed and the new endotracheal tube should be passed over the stylet, which guides it into the trachea. A flexible fiberoptic scope may also be used by placing the new endotracheal tube over the fiberbundle, then inserting the fiberbundle into the pharynx until the laryngeal entrance is viewed. The malfunctioning tube is then withdrawn under direct vision and the flexible fiberbundle is advanced into the trachea as described previously.

RECOGNITION, PREVENTION, AND TREATMENT OF COMPLICATIONS

Significant complications may be associated with endotracheal intubation. These include esophageal intubation, laryngospasm, vomiting, gastroesophageal reflux and aspiration, undesirable physiologic reflexes, lacerations, hemorrhage, broken teeth, inadvertent extubation, changes in endotracheal tube position, endotracheal tube obstruction, bronchospasm, and disconnection from a ventilator.

Esophageal Intubation

Until recently esophageal intubation was almost entirely detected by auscultation of the chest and epigastrium. Today, good practice dictates the use of a capnometer to detect expired carbon dioxide, followed by auscultation of the chest and epigastrium. Esophageal intubation may be prevented by ensuring that the endotracheal tube is actually seen passing through the vocal cords. The problem with esophageal intubation lies not in the act itself but in not recognizing its presence and correcting it immediately.

Laryngospasm

Three muscle groups are associated with laryngospasm: the cricothyroids, the thyroarytenoids, and the lateral cricoarytenoids. Wyllie suggested in 1866 that laryngospasm of the true vocal cords prevents inspiration but not expiration of air. Spasm of the false cords, on the other hand, prevents both inspiration and expiration. Laryngospasm may be prevented by deep anesthesia before intubation, the use of a muscle relaxant before laryngoscopy, or prior blocking of the superior laryngeal nerves with a local anesthetic. Treatment of laryngospasm may involve applying positive pressure to the airway by mask, or the administration of intravenous succinylcholine.

Vomiting

Vomiting may occur following gagging during laryngoscopy. Cricoid pressure (the Sellick maneuver) has been shown to prevent expulsion of stomach contents into the pharynx. Insisting on NPO status before elective anesthesia should be required, but this alone cannot guarantee against aspiration of gastric contents. Intravenous administration of 300 mg of cimetidine and 0.125 mg of droperidol should be given to those patients deemed to be at increased risk for vomiting during anesthesia or endotracheal intubation.

Gastroesophageal Reflux and Aspiration

Aspiration may be prevented by cricoid pressure during intubation. The use of antibiotics to treat secondary bacterial infection is accepted but the use of steroids to treat chemical pneumonitis remains controversial.

Undesirable Physiologic Reflexes

Hypertension and tachycardia commonly accompany laryngoscopy and intubation.[5] These are preventable with adequate depth of anesthesia before laryngoscopy, or by a variety of adjuvant drugs that blunt hypertension and tachycardia (e.g., clonidine, esmolol). Usually the sympathetic response to laryngoscopy is less than the response to intubation, but both contribute, especially when laryngoscopy is prolonged.

Lacerations

Lacerations of the lips and oral mucosa are usually minor but quite common. Lubrication of the laryngoscope blade may help to minimize the intraoral problems; careful technique during insertion of the blade into the mouth will minimize the occurrence of lip lacerations.

Hemorrhage

Varying degrees of hemorrhage are associated with passing an endotracheal tube through a narrow nasal passage. Phenylephrine 0.25% spray helps to shrink the nasal mucosa and prevent bleeding.

Broken teeth

Broken teeth are one of the most common injuries resulting from laryngoscopy.[7] Using a force vector directed 2 feet above the umbilicus on the laryngoscope helps to relieve pressure on and damage to the upper teeth; occasionally a dental guard similar to that used by athletes may be used, although it may make visualization of the larynx more difficult because it decreases the distance between the upper and lower teeth.

Inadvertent Extubation

Surprise extubation can usually be prevented by proper sedation, good taping of the endotracheal tube, and adequate anesthesia or muscle relaxation.

Changes in Endotracheal Tube Position

The recommended positioning of an endotracheal tube when viewing a roentgenogram is as follows: the distance between the tip of the tube and the carina should be approximately 3 cm with the head flexed, 5 cm with the head neutral, and 7 cm with the head extended. Extreme positions can result in possible cuff pressure against the vocal cords if the patient's head position is extended, or possible right mainstem bronchus intubation if the head is flexed.[3]

Obstruction of the Endotracheal Tube

This is usually identified by the inability to pass a flexible suction catheter through the lumen of the endotracheal tube. A variety of objects may obstruct an endotracheal tube. These include solidified secretions, a foreign body in the lumen, flattening of the tip of the tube against the wall of the trachea, a soluble lubricant that dries and hardens, or as a result of the patient biting and obstructing the lumen of the endotracheal tube if an airway is not in place. Obstruction is usually rectified by replacing or modifying the tube in position.

Bronchospasm

Bronchial constriction may result from stimulation of tracheal sensory receptors near the carina. When bronchospasm occurs, it is important to verify endotracheal tube position before initiating drug therapy. Only then should drug therapy, with intravenous aminophylline or beta agonists, or with atomized bronchodilators, be initiated.

Disconnection from a Ventilator

All ventilators should now be equipped with fail-safe alarm systems to warn immediately of ventilator disconnections, which can be rapidly fatal. These, together with continuous monitoring of breath sounds, should prevent the lethal consequences of disconnection. None are foolproof, however, and constant vigilance is essential to prevent this devastating event.

SUMMARY

The safety of endotracheal intubation has increased significantly since 1880, when it was first performed by Sir William Macewen. Today its safety in skilled hands far outweighs its disadvantages.

Currently anesthesiologists have new technology at their disposal so that even patients with a "difficult airway" may often be managed safely by endotracheal (oral or nasal) intubation with a flexible fiberoptic laryngoscope.

KEY POINTS

- There are four approaches to endotracheal intubation: tactile blind, nontactile blind, indirect, and direct.

- There are five reasons for endotracheal intubation: inadequate oxygenation, inadequate ventilation, failure of the protective mechanisms of the larynx, trauma to the airway, and diagnostic or therapeutic measures.

- The base of the tongue, epiglottis, vallecula, and piriform recess down to the vocal cords may be anesthetized by blocking the superior laryngeal nerves either percutaneously or intraorally.

- Potentially difficult intubations may be predicted by the Mallampati test, which involves visual assessment of the oral cavity, or by the laryngeal tilt test, which uses a bubble inclinometer to document a tilt greater than 40 degrees from the horizontal. A receding mandible, enlarged teeth, a high arched palate are also indications of an impending difficult intubation.

- Both general anesthesia and skeletal muscle relaxation are routinely used to facilitate endotracheal intubation. A muscle relaxant is used to relax not only the laryngeal muscles but also the masseters.

- The initial response to a failed intubation attempt should be to ventilate the patient by mask. The subsequent course of action depends on whether there is an obstructed airway.

- Techniques for managing failed endotracheal intubation include (1) using a flexible fiberoptic technique, (2) inserting a laryngeal mask airway, (3) proceeding with a retrograde intubation, (4) using a blind technique (with or without a light wand), or (5) possibly resorting to another rigid laryngoscope such as the Bullard laryngoscope.

- Significant complications associated with endotracheal intubation include esophageal intubation, laryngospasm, vomiting, gastroesophageal reflux and aspiration, undesirable physiologic reflexes, lacerations, hemorrhage, broken teeth, inadvertent extubation, changes in endotracheal tube position, endotracheal tube obstruction, bronchospasm, and disconnection from a ventilator.

- The safety of endotracheal intubation has increased significantly since 1880, when it was first performed by Sir William Macewen. Today, its safety in skilled hands far outweighs its disadvantages.

KEY REFERENCES

Fink B, Demarest R: *Laryngeal biomechanics,* Cambridge, Mass, 1978, Harvard University Press.

Reed AP, Han DG: Preparation of the patient for awake fiberoptic intubation, *Anesth Clin North Am,* Philadelphia, 1991, WB Saunders.

Roberts JT: *Fundamentals of tracheal intubation,* New York, 1983, Grune & Stratton.

Roberts JT: Preparing to use the flexible fiberoptic laryngoscope, *J Clin Anesthesiol* 3:Jan/Feb, 1991.

Roberts JT, Ali HH, and Shorten GD: Using the bubble inclinometer to measure laryngeal tilt and predict difficulty of laryngoscopy, *J Clin Anesthesiol* (in press).

REFERENCES

1. Ainsworth QP, Howells TH: Transilluminated tracheal intubation, *Br J Anaesth* 62(5):494.
2. Blanc VF, Tremblay NAG: The complications of tracheal intubation: a new classification with a review of the literature, *Anesth Analg* 53:202, 1974.
3. Conrardy PA, Goodman LR, Lainge F et al: Alteration of endotracheal tube position: flexion and extension of the neck, *Crit Care Med* 4:8, 1976.
4. Cote CJ, Liu LM, Szyfelbein SK et al: Intraoperative events diagnosed by expired carbon dioxide monitoring in children, *Can Anaesth Soc J* 33(3;pt 1):315, 1986.
5. Derbyshire DR, Chmielewski A, Fell D et al: Plasma catecholamine responses to tracheal intubation, *Br J Anaesth* 55:855, 1983.

6. Fink B, Demarest R: *Laryngeal biomechanics,* Cambridge, Mass, 1978, Harvard University Press.
7. Lind GL, Spiegel EH, and Munson ES: Treatment of traumatic tooth avulsion, *Anesth Analg* 61:469, 1974.
8. Macewen W: Clinical observations on the introduction of tracheal tubes by the mouth instead of performing tracheostomy or laryngotomy, *Br Med J* 2:163, 1880.
9. Mallampati SR et al: *Can Anaesth Soc J* 32:429, 1985.
10. Powell WF, Ozdil T: A translaryngeal guide for tracheal intubation, *Anesth Analg* 46:231, 1967.
11. Redden RL, Biery KA, and Campbell RL: Arterial oxygen desaturation during awake endotracheal intubation, *Anesth Prog* 37(4):201, 1990.

12. Reed AP, Han DG: Preparation of the patient for awake fiberoptic intubation, *Anesth Clin North Am*, Philadelphia, 1991, WB Saunders.
13. Roberts JT: *Fundamentals of tracheal intubation,* New York, 1983, Grune & Stratton.
14. Roberts JT: Preparing to use the flexible fiberoptic laryngoscope, *J Clin Anesth* 3:Jan/Feb, 1991.
15. Roberts JT, Ali HH, and Shorten GD: Using the bubble inclinometer to measure laryngeal tilt and predict difficulty of laryngoscopy, *J Clin Anesth* (in press).
16. Sykes WS: *Essays on the first hundred years of anaesthesia,* Huntington, New York, 1972, Robert E Krieger.

CHAPTER 49

Mechanism of Action of General Anesthetic Agents

JAMES K. ALIFIMOFF
KEITH W. MILLER

The question of how general anesthetics render both insensibility to pain and unconsciousness has remained a pharmacologic enigma since the first public demonstration of general anesthesia almost 150 years ago. The solution to this mystery has been complicated by several factors. First, the central nervous system (CNS) is extremely complex, and we possess only a rudimentary understanding of its physiology. Furthermore, physiologists have made extremely slow progress in unraveling the mechanisms responsible for maintaining consciousness. Finally, there is no physiologic definition of the general anesthetic state, that is, there is no set of physiologic changes that can be equated consistently with anesthesia in patients.

Thus, experimentally, the resolution of the question of how general anesthetics act has been fraught with great difficulty. When considering the overall problem of how general anesthetics exert their effects, the question can be addressed on three levels. First, where in the CNS do these drugs act? Second, where is their cellular site of action? That is, do general anesthetics act presynaptically or postsynaptically or along the nerve axon itself? Finally, what is their molecular mechanism of action? The focus of this chapter is to examine each of these questions.

CENTRAL NERVOUS SYSTEM SITE OF ACTION

The site of action in the central nervous system (CNS) for general anesthetics is difficult to determine because neurophysiologists have no consensus of opinion regarding the region or regions of the brain responsible for the maintenance of consciousness. One theory ascribes consciousness to a discrete area of the CNS,[98] whereas another states that consciousness is a function of the integration of many brain areas working together.[58] Thus general anesthetics may induce loss of consciousness either through inhibition of a discrete region or through global depression of CNS excitability.

Early neurophysiologists thought that the cerebral cortex was the brain area responsible for the control of consciousness.[105] However, it was soon discovered that large regions of the cortex could be ablated without loss of consciousness. In contrast, tumors of the brainstem frequently resulted in coma. This led to the consideration that some brainstem structure was responsible for modulating consciousness. The specific region that has received the most attention as the site of consciousness and thus the site of action of general anesthetics is the brainstem reticular activating system. Interest in the reticular activating system derives from early observations made by Morruzzi and Magoun that stimulation of this brain region in anesthetized animals resulted in signs of both electroencephalographic (EEG) and behavioral arousal. Further experiments showed that anesthetics blocked brainstem activity before blocking main sensory pathways and that this differential blockade did not require an intact cerebral cortex.[34] From these experiments the idea developed that general anesthetics acted by blocking the consciousness-maintaining activity of the brainstem reticular activating system on the cortex.

However, if this hypothesis were correct, the brainstem reticular activating system should be vital to the maintenance of consciousness in the unanesthetized state. Studies have shown, however, that gross lesions in the reticular activating system abolish the EEG response to stimulation but animals still remain behaviorally awake.[26] Thus the reticular activating system cannot be the site of action of general anesthetics. Although early experiments showed reversible inhibition of brainstem reticular activating system activity by general anesthetics,[3,111] other experiments demonstrated variable effects in that anesthetics either increased, decreased, or did not alter brainstem reticular activating system activity.[19,22,89,126]

Where else in the CNS might general anesthetics act? General anesthetics have been shown to inhibit CNS excitatory transmission and to prolong inhibitory effects in parts of the CNS other than the brainstem reticular activating system. For example, halothane inhibits excitatory transmission in the cerebral cortex,[4,101] the olfactory cortex,[104] and the hippocampus.[109] Halothane also prolongs inhibitory postsynaptic effects in the olfactory cortex.[92,117] **However, although much data exist on anesthetic effects in various brain regions, no set is sufficiently complete or consistent to allow one to conclude that anesthetics exert their actions through one specific effect in one CNS region.** Thus the approach has been to attempt to study the effect of general anesthetics on a cellular rather than a global level.

CELLULAR SITE OF ACTION

Neurophysiologists agree that general anesthetics disrupt the transmission of neuronal impulses in the CNS. Since the early work of Sowton and Sherrington[123] and that of Larabee and Posternak,[63] **it has been known that general anesthetics block synaptic transmission at concentrations much lower than those required to block axonal conductance.** For this reason, the synapse has become the focus of studies on general anesthetics' cellular site of action. Since anesthetics may be viewed as having effects at either excitatory or inhibitory synapses, one would expect depressant actions on excitatory postsynaptic potentials (EPSPs) and/or enhancement of inhibitory postsynaptic potentials (IPSPs).

Effect of Anesthetics on Excitatory Postsynaptic Potentials

Studies in both the peripheral nervous system[63,123] and the CNS have shown that EPSPs are sensitive to the action of general anesthetics.* Work with preparations from the olfactory cortex[103,104,108] has demonstrated inhibition of EPSPs without any change in axonal conductance of neural impulses by small axons and with no change in latency of the synaptic potential. However, conflicting results have been obtained in hippocampal preparations. Some investigators have shown significant EPSP inhibition at low concentrations of anesthetics,[9,109] whereas others have only been able to do so at supra clinical concentrations.[37,69,87] This variable depression of EPSPs at clinical concentrations of anesthetics suggests that either depression of EPSPs does not play a significant role as a unitary mechanism of general anesthetic action (see following discussion) or that this particular brain region (i.e., hippocampus) is not relevant to anesthetic action.

Effect of Anesthetics on Inhibitory Postsynaptic Potentials

It is now well established that gamma-aminobutyric acid (GABA) is the principal inhibitory neurotransmitter in the CNS.[59,60,73] One possible mechanism of anesthetic action is through enhancement of inhibitory synapses rather than through inhibition of excitatory synapses. Barbiturates greatly enhance GABAergic IPSPs,[68,92] as manifested by prolongation of GABA-evoked channel opening, which results in longer inhibitory postsynaptic currents and IPSPs.[6,38] Similar effects have been found with steroid anesthetics.[71]

Unfortunately, when considering the volatile anesthetics, confusing results again begin to surface.

---

* References 62,92,103,104,108,109,136.

Although some investigators have reported prolongation of inhibitory postsynaptic currents in the olfactory cortex[117] and of IPSPs in the hippocampus,[38,88] others have actually observed a *reduction* of IPSPs with both halothane and isoflurane.[37,87,125,135] One possible explanation is that halothane-mediated depression of IPSPs is not caused directly by but rather through depression of excitatory synapses acting on GABAergic inhibitory cells.[61] Thus to clarify this dichotomy of effect, more information is needed on the effects of inhalational agents on monosynaptic IPSPs in the absence of excitatory transmission.[61]

Although anesthetics' effects on synaptic transmission are not entirely unequivocal, ample evidence exists to conclude that certain anesthetics do block synaptic transmission in certain neural pathways. However, exactly where along the pathway of synaptic transmission do anesthetics work? Synaptic transmission is a process that can be conveniently divided into four separate events:

- Axonal conductance of an impulse along the afferent axon
- Release of neurotransmitter into the synaptic cleft
- Binding of the neurotransmitter to specific receptors in the postjunctional membrane
- Conductance changes leading to propagation of the action potential

Axonal conduction has already been established as not being relevant to discussions of the mechanisms of anesthetic action, since inhibition occurs only at supraclinical concentrations of anesthetics long after the inhibition of synaptic transmission. The other possible sites of action of anesthetic agents on synaptic transmission are considered in more detail.

Action of anesthetics on neurotransmitter release

A presynaptic site of action could account for depression of EPSPs as well as for augmentation of IPSPs. Evidence suggests that several anesthetics inhibit neurotransmitter release in peripheral nerves,[132] sympathetic ganglia,[72] and the CNS. Barbiturates inhibit the release of L-aspartate and L-glutamate (excitatory neurotransmitters) while enhancing the release of GABA (inhibitory neurotransmitters) in the olfactory cortex[16] as well as other CNS areas.[53,86,99] In contrast, some anesthetics have no effect on either GABA or aspartate release from presynaptic nerve terminals.[53]

Although most evidence suggests that anesthetics inhibit excitatory and enhance inhibitory neurotransmitter release, this provides no molecular mechanism. It is unlikely that alterations in neurotransmitter release are secondary to alterations in CNS concentrations of neurotransmitters, since these have been shown to either be elevated[18] or remain constant[99] on exposure to anesthetics. Physiologic evidence also supports anesthetics not interfering with either the synthesis or the storage of neurotransmitters in presynaptic terminals.[103,104,106,109,122] Thus alterations in neurotransmitter release apparently must be caused by the direct actions of anesthetics on the neurosecretory process itself. The mechanism of this remains unknown.[106]

Action of anesthetics on postsynaptic receptors

Although there is strong evidence that anesthetics modulate neurotransmitter release, there is equally compelling evidence that they affect postsynaptic receptors. Barbiturates reduce the sensitivity of neurons in the cerebral cortex,[17] cunate nucleus,[39] and olfactory cortex[108] to ionophoretically applied L-glutamate. Interestingly, halothane does not alter the excitatory effects of ionophoretically applied L-glutamate,[39,108] suggesting that in this case halothane may inhibit neurotransmitter release from presynaptic terminals. With inhibitory neurotransmitters, pentobarbital increases the effects of GABA at the frog neuromuscular junction[93] as well as in mouse spinal neurons.[102] This potentiation of GABA's effect results from an increase in the channel's open time[7] rather than from an increase in the GABA receptor's affinity or from decreased uptake.[47,86]

Various anesthetics have also been shown to interact with isolated postsynaptic nicotine acetylcholine receptors. Single-channel studies with inhalational agents[13] and butanol[70] show brief interruptions of open-channel currents without changes in conductance, whereas inhalational, barbiturate, and alcohol anesthetics also inhibit nicotinic channels.[81] In addition, the barbiturates are allosteric modulators at both GABA[94] and acetylcholine receptors.[79] However, the binding of barbiturates to either the GABA[127] or the acetylcholine receptor[21] does not correlate with anesthetic potency.

Summary

On a cellular level, the most likely site of action of general anesthetics is the synapse. Inhibition of synaptic conduction by general anesthetics occurs at lower concentrations than effects on the axonal conduction of neural impulses. Importantly, however, anesthetics have no effect on synaptic transmission that is *common* to all synapses and all anesthetics. For example, at excitatory synapses, some anesthetics inhibit neurotransmitter release, whereas others enhance it. Likewise, effects on postsynaptic receptors vary. A group of neurons may exist within the CNS that is essential to the maintenance of consciousness and on which all anesthetic agents have the same effect. However, at present no evidence suggests that such a population does exist.[106]

The implications of this for theories on general

anesthesia are profound. **Two theories of action of general anesthetics have arisen from the complexity of these observations. The** *unitary theory* **of general anesthesia, first promulgated by Claude Bernard,**[10] **holds that all general anesthetics exert their actions by a common mechanism. In contrast, the** *degenerate theory* **of anesthetic action postulates that different classes of anesthetics have different mechanisms of actions.**[105] One class of anesthetic might act at a binding site on a protein in one brain region, whereas another class might act at a different binding site in a separate brain region. For example, halothane might inhibit glutamatergic EPSPs in the hippocampus, whereas the barbiturates might enhance GABAergic IPSPs in the thalamus. Alternatively, different classes of anesthetics might act at multiple sites on the same receptor system.

Faced with these major gaps in our understanding, two primary strategies have evolved in an attempt to elucidate the molecular basis of anesthetic action. The first approach is *pharmacologic,* **which obtains information by studying the relative potencies of anesthetics in animals. The second approach is** *mechanistic,* **in which the effects of general anesthetics on well-defined molecular models are studied to determine molecular mechanisms.** These mechanisms may be unique to the model being studied or may occur more generally. In this latter case the mechanism might then be generalized to those that cause anesthesia at some as yet unknown CNS site.

PHARMACOLOGY OF GENERAL ANESTHESIA

Since the site of action of anesthetics remains unknown, all theories of general anesthesia are based on observations of anesthetics' effects in animals. Reliable potency data in whole animals are of unequivocal importance to the testing of hypotheses concerning these drugs' mechanism of action. An anesthetic's potency is measured by determining the response of an animal to a well-defined stimulus. Two end points have commonly been used: (1) an animal's ability to right itself after it has been turned over (righting reflex) and (2) an animal's ability to respond with a purposeful movement when subjected to a painful stimulus, usually a tail clamp.

The loss of righting reflex as a definition of general anesthesia has been used with small animals, mainly mice[110] and tadpoles, which equilibrate rapidly with anesthetics and which allow large numbers to be tested. Quantal concentration-response relationships are obtained,[131] and anesthetic potency is defined as the concentration at which half the animals have lost their righting reflex (EC_{50}). The tail clamp has been employed with larger animals so that their physiologic

state may be more easily monitored. With larger mammals, however, equilibration with anesthetic agents is slow and alveolar concentrations must be determined. Eger et al. have called the concentration at which half the animals do not respond purposefully the *minimum alveolar concentration* (MAC) and have used this as the measure of potency.[74,115] Unfortunately, a drawback to the use of MAC measurement as an index of potency is that it is limited to volatile agents.

The use of tadpoles in anesthetic concentration-response determination has many advantages.[1,2,95,96] First, it circumvents the limitation of MAC to volatile agents. Second, it avoids ambiguities caused by the complex pharmacokinetics of intravenous agents. The amount of anesthetic is present in such excess in the aqueous medium during concentration-response experiments that factors relating to protein binding, differential metabolism, or even the production of active metabolites are negated. Other advantages are that the drug concentration to which the tadpole is exposed can easily be controlled and that drugs equilibrate rapidly and gain access to the CNS. Finally and most importantly, after equilibration, the drug concentration in the aqueous medium is equal to the drug concentration in the aqueous phase surrounding its site of action in the CNS. Thus one can reliably determine the aqueous concentration of an anesthetic at its site of action, even though the location of this site is unknown.

Observations of the effects of general anesthetics on animals and the careful determination of anesthetic potency as described have resulted in several pharmacologic characteristics, or "probes," of general anesthesia. These include:

- Lack of specificity
- The cutoff in anesthetic potency
- Lack of stereoselectivity
- Pressure reversal

These pharmacologic criteria are important because critical tests can be applied to purported models of the anesthetic target site. Any acceptable theory of molecular mechanism of action of general anesthetics must be able to account for this pharmacology. Each of these characteristics is considered in detail.

Lack of Specificity

General anesthesia is caused by a remarkable number of structurally diverse molecules, from the simple inert gas xenon to such complex molecules as althesin and α-chloralose (Fig. 49-1), suggesting that no single, structurally specific receptor mediates general anesthesia. At the beginning of the twentieth century, Meyer[75] and Overton,[95,96] working independently, made the remarkable observation that the potencies of a broad array of general anesthetics correlated well

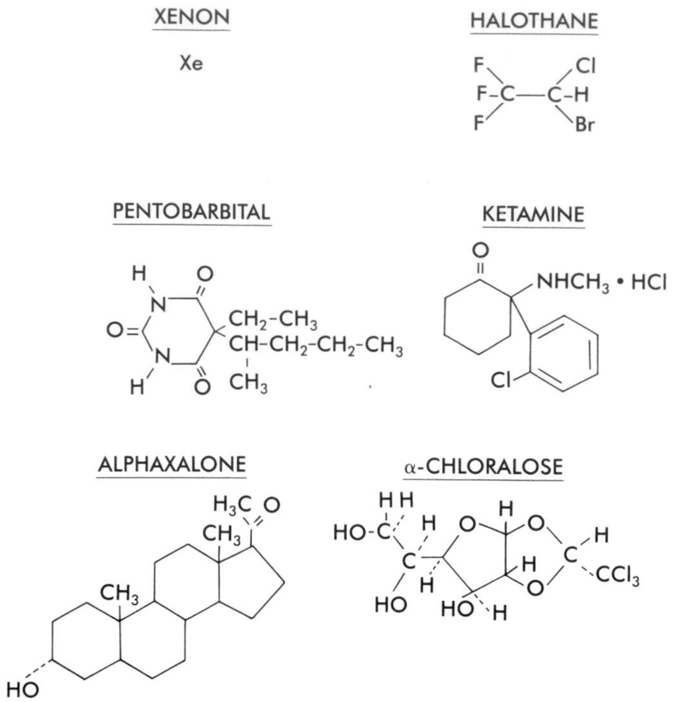

Fig. 49-1. Structures of some representative general anesthetics. (From Janoff AS, Miller KW: A critical assessment of the lipid theories of general anaesthetic action. In Chapman D, ed: *Biological membranes*, vol 4, London, 1982, Academic Press.)

Table 49-1 Anesthetic potency and thermodynamic activity of some representative anesthetics that both obey and disobey Ferguson's rule

Anesthetic	EC_{50}*	Activity $\times 10^2$
Obey Ferguson's rule		
Butanol	12 mM	1.3
Hexanol	0.7 mM	1.2
Octanol	0.06 mM	1.3
Halothane	0.23 mM	1.2
Disobey Ferguson's rule		
Decanol	0.013 mM	4.1
Dodecanol	0.005 mM	25
Methane (CF_4)	11 atm	0.23
Ethane (C_2F_6)	18 atm	0.44

*Median effective concentration.

with their solubilities in a simple organic solvent, olive oil. **This correlation of anesthetic potency with lipid solubility has become known as the *Meyer-Overton rule* and provides a remarkably accurate means of predicting anesthetic potency.** However, a much more powerful and informative, although less precise, correlation is that of anesthetic potency with ideal solubility. In 1939 Ferguson[27] proposed that general anesthetic potency correlated with the thermodynamic activity (equivalent to ideal solubility) of the anesthetic. Thus, whatever concentration of an anesthetic is required to produce a given level of anesthesia, the thermodynamic activity would be the same. For the volatile anesthetics, *Ferguson's rule* can be written as follows:

$$a_{50} = P_{50}/P_o$$

where P_{50} is the partial pressure of an anesthetic at a median effective concentration (EC_{50}), P_o is the anesthetic's vapor pressure at the physiologic temperature, and a_{50} is the thermodynamic activity.[78] For nonvolatile anesthetics:

$$a_{50} \sim EC_{50}/C_{Sat}$$

where C_{Sat} is the concentration of anesthetic in a saturated aqueous solution.

An important feature to note is that Ferguson's rule is a correlation between anesthetic potency and vapor pressure. It is distinguished from the Meyer-Overton rule in that vapor pressure is a property of the anesthetic molecule itself and contains no information on how that anesthetic interacts with other substances. On the other hand, a molecule's anesthetic potency must depend on the strength of interaction between the anesthetic and its site of action. Therefore anesthetics that obey Ferguson's rule provide little information on the site of action of general anesthetics, and one must look to deviant anesthetics to provide meaningful information on interactions between anesthetics and their site of action. On the other hand, a site where Ferguson's rule is disobeyed by usually obedient anesthetics is not related to the anesthetic site but may be related to some more specific pharmacologic action.

When testing theories of anesthetic action, it is important to divide anesthetics in two groups. The first group is drugs with potencies predicted by Ferguson's rule; they provide a necessary but not a sufficient test of a model. They can reject it but not support it. The other group is anesthetics that disobey Ferguson's rule and consequently provide a much more critical test of a model (Table 49-1). Models that can successfully account for the potencies of anesthetics that disobey Ferguson's rule have a much higher probability of being correct than those that do not.

Fig. 49-2 provides an example. The left-hand panel is a test of Ferguson's rule for several gaseous and volatile anesthetics. Most of the drugs fall on the line, with the notable exception of three gaseous anesthetics with potencies more than an order of magnitude less than predicted (P_{50} higher). These agents are the

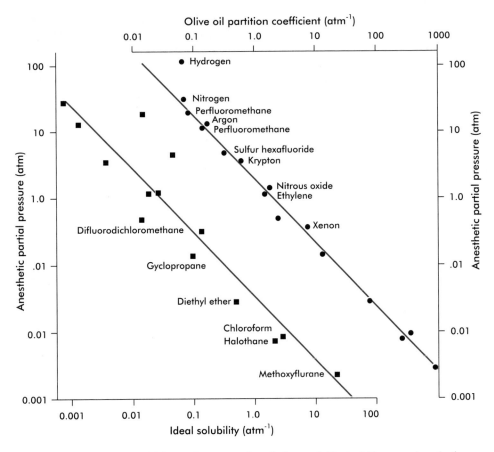

Fig. 49-2. Ferguson's and Meyer-Overton rules. *Left panel,* Test of Ferguson's rule (correlation of anesthetic potency with ideal solubility) portrayed graphically. *Right panel,* Test of Meyer-Overton rule. (From Miller KW: The nature of the site of general anesthesia, *Int Rev Neurobiol* 27:1, 1985.)

fully fluorinated hydrocarbon derivatives of methane (CF_4) and ethane (C_2F_6) as well as sulfur hexafluoride (SF_6). In contrast, the potencies of these anesthetics are accounted for by the Meyer-Overton rule. Thus these drugs' ability to disobey Ferguson's rule provides a rigorous test of models of the anesthetic target site. A model that can account for the behavior of anesthetics that disobey Ferguson's rule is much more powerful than one that can only account for molecules fulfilling the correlation. Interestingly only a few anesthetics have been found that disobey Ferguson's rule (Table 49-1).

Cutoff Effect

Many homologous series of chemical compounds are anesthetics. This is fortuitous because it allows one to study structure-activity relationships for general anesthetics. An example of one such homologous series of general anesthetics is the primary alcohols. Starting with methanol ($C_N = 1$), the first member of the series, anesthetic potency increases logarithmically with the number of carbon atoms in the alcohol's hydrocarbon chain (C_N) until a point is reached where

anesthetic potency suddenly and unexpectedly disappears. Dodecanol ($C_N = 12$) is the most potent anesthetic in the series, but potency disappears completely at tridecanol ($C_N = 13$) (Table 49-2).

This "cutoff" effect of anesthetic potency was first observed by Ferguson,[27] but we have since shown the effect to occur in other homologous series of anesthetics (e.g., alkanes, fluorocarbons, secondary alkanols). Interestingly, the cutoff is not simply a function of the length of the anesthetic molecule's hydrocarbon chain. Introducing a double bond into a primary alkanol converts it into a alkenol and extends the position of cutoff from tridecanol ($C_N = 13$) to hexadecanol ($C_N = 16$). Also, altering the position of the hydroxyl group from the first carbon atom to a secondary position extends the position of the cutoff effect by one carbon atom, such as from 1-tridecanol ($C_N = 13$) to 2-tetradecanol ($C_N = 14$) (Pacquette A, Alifimoff JK, Miller KW, unpublished observations). The n-alkanes demonstrate a cutoff between decane and dodecane,[36,91] whereas the fully fluorinated alkanes cut off at a very short chain length, octafluoropropane (C_3F_8).[82]

Stereoselectivity

Another pharmacologic criterion of general anesthesia is the lack of stereoselective effects. For example, both d-halothane and l-halothane inhibit synaptic transmission and disorder spin-labeled bilayers nonstereoselectively.[56] Unfortunately the tremendous cost of synthesizing d- and l-halothane has prevented the in vivo determination of their anesthetic poten-

cies. Bulter and Dickson[14] were the first to demonstrate that optical isomers of an alcohol anesthetic, 2-butanol, were not stereoselective. Not until recently, however, did investigators show that the more potent isomers of the homologous series were also nonselective.[1] This is significant because, when stereoselectivity does occur, it is often present in the most potent members of a series. Although some intravenous agents may demonstrate modest stereoselectvity, it is difficult to preclude differential metabolism as a reason for this.[113]

Table 49-2 Anesthetic potencies of primary alcohols (alkanols) illustrating cutoff

Alcohol	EC_{50}*
Methanol	590 ± 41 mM
Ethanol	190 ± 16 mM
Propanol	73 ± 2.4 mM
Butanol	10.8 ± 0.77 mM
Pentanol	2.9 ± 0.11 mM
Hexanol	570 ± 37 µM
Heptanol	230 ± 11 µM
Octanol	57 ± 2.5 µM
Nonanol	37 ± 2.4 µM
Decanol	12.6 ± 0.48 µM
Undecanol	8.1 ± 0.81 µM
Dodecanol	4.7 ± 0.33 µM
Tridecanol	Not anesthetic
Tetradecanol	Not anesthetic

*Median effective concentration.
From Alifimoff JK, Firestone LL, and Miller KW: Anesthetic potencies of primary alkanols: implications for the molecular dimensions of the anaesthetic site, *Br J Pharmacol* 96:9, 1989.

Pressure Reversal

The final pharmcologic characteristic of general anesthesia is that it is reversed by high pressure. This phenomenon was first discovered in 1950 in tadpoles by Johnson and Flagler[50] and has since been observed in various other species.[66] Fig. 49-3 shows a typical concentration-response relationship for phenobarbital in mice. As the total pressure is raised with the nonanesthetic gas helium, from 2 to 50 to 100 atm, the EC_{50} for the concentration-response relationship shifts progressively to the right; that is, pressure antagonizes the effect of the anesthetic on the righting reflex.[84]

When considering the phenomenon of pressure reversal of general anesthesia, two questions arise:

- Is pressure per se or helium responsible for the reversal of anesthesia?
- Is pressure reversal a specific effect occurring at the general anesthetic's site of action, or is pressure reversal simply a generalized CNS excitaton counteracting a global depression?

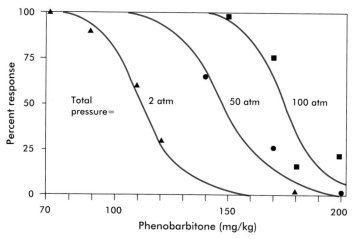

Fig. 49-3. Pressure reversal of general anesthesia in mice. Groups of 14 mice were injected with phenobarbital intraperitoneally and exposed to high pressures of helium in presence of 1 atmosphere of oxygen. Dose of phenobarbital is given on x axis, and percentage of animals with intact righting reflex is given on y axis. (From Miller KW, Wilson MW: The pressure reversal of a variety of anesthetic agents in mice, *Anesthesiology* 48:104, 1978.)

Fig. 49-4 may answer this first question. EC_{50}s for ethyl carbamate were determined in a pressure bomb at 1 atm and at several different pressures up to 110 atm. The EC_{50} doubled over this range. Then a space was allowed to remain in the bomb, and it was pressurized with a gas that dissolved in the remaining solution. The anesthetic gases argon and nitrogen decreased the EC_{50} for ethyl carbamate. When helium was used, the EC_{50} decreased relative to control at the same hydrostatic pressure. Thus helium contributes an anesthetic effect of its own.[20] If helium could be dissolved without raising the pressure, it would be an anesthetic. However, its *net* effect is close to that of pressure.

The second question on the mechanistic significance of pressure reversal is not as straightforward. Many investigators have boldly assumed that pressure reversal is a specific action at the site of anesthetic action rather than a global phenomenon. They have concluded that those sites demonstrating pressure reversal are more probably sites for general anesthetic action than sites where pressure reversal is not observed. For example, pressure has been shown to reverse the motor and sensory effects of ethyl carbamate on the CNS.[3] Likewise, anesthetic block of axonal conduction shares some features of pressure reversal in vivo.[55] However, at several sites, most notably the nicotinic acetylcholine receptor, pressure reversal does not occur.[54] Thus, although one can explain pressure reversal data by the assumption that anesthetics and pressure act at the same site, one must also consider the alternative.[120]

Pressure reversal in vivo has been demonstrated with all anesthetics studied to date, although the degree of pressure reversal may vary with the agent.[85] In contrast, pressure does not reverse anesthetic effects in invertebrates when glycine is not a neurotransmitter.[129] Fig. 49-5 illustrates the effects of hydrostatic pressure on both tadpoles and freshwater shrimp. In contrast to the tadpole, hydrostatic pressure rather than antagonizing ethanol's effects actually enhances them in the shrimp. These data suggest

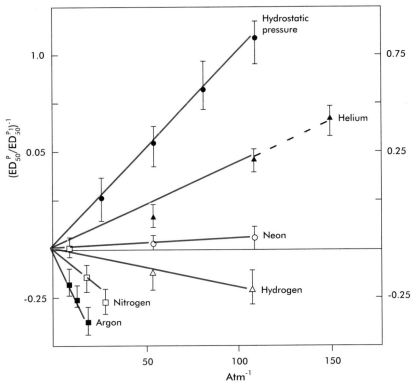

Fig. 49-4. Median effective concentration (EC_{50}) of ethyl carbamate (urethane) is altered by raising pressure on tadpoles swimming in a bomb. Change is expressed by ratio of EC_{50} at 1 atm to that determined at pressure minus 1. For example, EC_{50} of ethyl carbamate at 110 atm of hydrostatic pressure is twice that at 1 atm. Hydrostatic and helium pressure reduce potency of ethyl carbamate (pressure reversal). Neon does not change EC_{50} whereas the anesthetic gases hydrogen, nitrogen, and argon decrease EC_{50}. Atmosphere minus 1 equals absolute pressure in atmospheres minus 1. Ambient pressure is thus represented as zero. (From Dodson BA, Furmaniuk ZW, and Miller KW: The physiological effects of hydrostatic pressure are not equivalent to those of helium pressure on *Rana pipiens, J Physiol [Lond]* 362:233, 1985.)

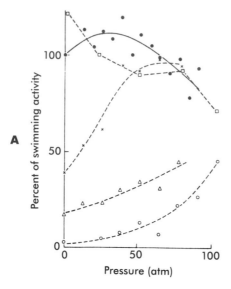
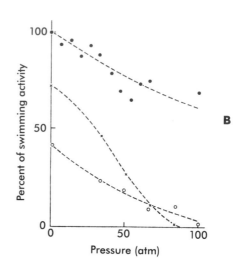

Fig. 49-5. Lack of pressure reversal in shrimp. **A,** Swimming activity of tadpoles as atmospheric pressure is increased from ambient to 100 atm in absence of ethanol *(black circles)* and at different concentrations of ethanol. At all concentrations, pressure antagonizes anesthetic effect. **B,** Swimming activity of shrimp in absence of ethanol *(black circles)* and at two other concentrations. In contrast to tadpole, pressure enhances ethanol's effect in shrimp. (From Smith EB, Bowser-Riley F, and Daniels S: New observations on the mechanism of pressure-anesthetic interactions. In Roth SH, Miller KW eds: *Molecular and cellular mechanisms of anesthetics,* New York, 1986, Plenum Medical.)

that pressure's effect may be mediated through a specific pathway.

■ ■ ■

In summary the pharmacologic probes of the site of action of general anesthetics—lack of specificity, cutoff, lack of stereoselectivity, and pressure reversal—have all arisen from observations of the effects of general anesthetics on small animals. Their importance to the overall question of the mechanism of action of general anesthetics is pivotal in that any model system that purports to realistically serve as an experimental model or any theory of anesthetic action must be able to account for this pharmacology. If, for example, a model of the anesthetic site shows a cutoff in potency for the primary alcohol anesthetics but does not show a lack of stereoselectivity for the secondary alcohol anesthetics, its relevance must be considered dubious.

MOLECULAR SITE OF ACTION

There are three predominant schools of thought as to where, on a molecular level, general anesthetics might exert their effects. One group of investigators has interpreted the Meyer-Overton rule to support the hypothesis that the primary site of action of anesthetics is the lipid bilayer.[46] **Through primary actions on these lipid structures, anesthetics render adjacent neurotransmitter receptor proteins inexcitable. Other**

investigators have used this same correlation to support the hypothesis that anesthetics act directly on neurotransmitter receptor proteins themselves.[29] **Finally, a third theory holds that anesthetics act not at a protein site or at a lipid site, but rather at a mixed site at the lipid-protein interface**[34,44,65] **(Fig. 49-6).**

Lipid Theories of Anesthetic Action
Lipid solubility hypothesis

In 1906 Hans Meyer[75] stated the *lipid solubility hypothesis* of anesthetic action, summarizing it as follows: "the narcotizing substance enters into a loose physico chemical combination with the vitally important lipoids of the cell, perhaps with the lethicin, and in doing so changes their nomal relationship to the other cell constituents. . . ." This rather remarkable conclusion pointed to the cell membrane as the direct target of anesthetics years before Davson and Danielli proposed the first important hypothesis of the structure of biologic membranes.

In its simplest form the lipid solubility theory of anesthetic action correlates anesthetic potency with an anesthetic's solubility in a simple organic solvent, olive oil. However, this theory is most relevant when the lipid site of action is taken to be a cholesterol-containing bilayer rather than an organic solvent. The lipid solubility theory predicts that anesthetics should cause equal degrees of anesthesia when they attain equal concentrations in the cell membrane of excit-

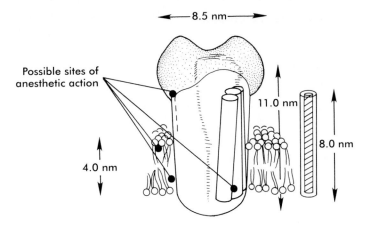

Fig. 49-6. Possible sites of anesthetic action. (Modified from Kistler J, Stroud RM, Klymkowsky MW et al: Structure and function of an acetylcholine receptor, *Biophys J* 37:371, 1982.)

able tissue. The lipid solubility theory can be expressed in more rigorous terms as:

$$C_{50} = \lambda \cdot EC_{50}$$

where C_{50} is the anesthetic's concentration in lipid, λ is the anesthetic's lipid solubility or the membrane-buffer partition coefficient, and the EC_{50} is the anesthetic's concentration in the aqueous phase that anesthetizes half a population of animals.

A critical feature of the lipid solubility hypothesis is that it predicts that anesthesia occurs when an anesthetic's concentration reaches a value of 25 to 50 mmol/L in the lipid bilayer. Unfortunately the hypothesis fails several of the critical pharmacologic tests examined earlier. First, it cannot account for the cutoff effect. At one time, solubility in lipid bilayers was thought to account for the cutoff in potency of the primary alcohol anesthetics in that drugs up to the point of cutoff were able to acheive a concentration within the lipid bilayer of 35 to 50 mmol/L. However, nonanesthetic alcohols (e.g., tetradecanol, hexadecanol) were unable to achieve this minimum critical concentration within the bilayer. Thus they were unable to induce anesthesia because their lipid solubilities or partition coefficiencts (λ) decreased for some unknown reason.[46] More recent work, however, suggests that the nonanesthetic alcohols are able to attain sufficient membrane concentrations but still are unable to cause anesthesia.[32] Furthermore, the lipid solubility theory is unable to account for pressure reversal. If lipid solubility were to account for pressure reversal, the anesthetic molecules would have to be squeezed out of the model solvent (or lipid bilayer) as the pressure increases. However, any such "squeezing" is too small in magnitude to explain pressure reversal.[83] Thus this hypothesis must be either cast aside or modified to account for the pharmacology of general anesthetics.

General lipid perturbation hypothesis

An important question unanswered by the lipid solubility hypothesis is how the anesthetic, once in the lipid bilayer, disrupts the function of integral membrane proteins. A modification of the lipid solubility hypothesis attempts to explain this. The *lipid perturbation hypothesis* suggests that once inside the lipid bilayer, anesthetics are able somehow to perturb its structure so as to render inexcitable neurotransmitter receptor proteins. Possible mechanisms of this perturbation are discussed later, but a generalized statement of the lipid perturbation hypothesis can be written as follows:

$$E_{50} = C_{50} \cdot T_P$$

where E_{50} represents some functional change in the excitable membrane that leads to half a population of animals being anesthetized, P_L is a perturbation of the lipid bilayer produced by a unit concentration of anesthetic in the bilayer, and T_P describes the transmission of that lipid perturbation to the membrane protein's function.[45]

The theory assumes that the transmission of the lipid perturbation to the membrane protein is constant and ascribes various meanings to P_L, as discussed following. Also, since the anesthetic's concentration in the bilayer (C_{50}) is usually a constant, P_L will be constant; that is, the size of the perturbation will be proportional to the amount of anesthetic in the membrane. However, notable exceptions to these generalizations exist. C_{50} will deviate from a constant, whereas P_L deviates in the opposite direction to keep E_{50} constant, such as would have to occur to account for pressure reversal. Another exception is when the lipid composition differs from that at the site of anesthesia. If P_L has a small value, it would explain why proteins in some membranes are less affected by anesthetics. The value of T_P should also be independent of the anesthetic but dependent on the protein to explain why some proteins are more sensitive to anesthetics than others.

One question has aroused the most interest about the lipid perturbation theory: what is the nature of the perturbation?

Nature of the Lipid Perturbation
Membrane expansion theories

A simple lipid perturbation that accounts for pressure reversal and also suggests a mechanism by which the function of ion channel proteins is inhibited is membrane expansion. This is expressed as the *critical volume hypothesis,* **which states that anesthesia occurs when a hydrophobic phase expands beyond a critical amount.** Pressure simply compresses this phase, reversing anesthesia. If the hydrophobic phase is taken to be a lipid bilayer, then membrane expansion may not only account for pressure reversal of anesthesia but may also suggest simple physical mechanisms that inhibit transmembrane ion channels. For example, a change in membrane thickness would change the potential gradient across a neuronal membrane, thus affecting voltage gating of a channel. Investigators have explored such a model for the actions of general anesthetics on sodium channels.[24]

Substantial evidence shows that membranes do expand when exposed to anesthetics. The surface area of membrane lipids, spread as an air-water interface, is increased at clinical concentrations of anesthetics and also decreases on exposure to nonanesthetic gases.[8] Alkane anesthetics cause membrane expansion in black lipid films[42] as well as in squid axon membranes.[43] Likewise, erythrocyte membranes expand on exposure to anesthetics.[11,112,118] Measurement of the volume expansion of various lipid bilayers exposed to anesthetics shows that at physiologic concentrations, expansion ranges from 0.2% to 0.6%, close to the degree of expansion predicted by the critical volume hypothesis necessary to account for pressure reversal of anesthesia. Interestingly, work on red cells shows that their area expands much more than their volume, probably because the bilayer becomes thinner as its area increases.[57]

Lipid phase transition

Another simple lipid perturbation that may be responsible for anesthesia is related to lipid phase transitions. The lipids that form biologic membranes are not heterogeneous but rather are distributed randomly either within a single leaflet of the bilayer or across it.[124] A homogeneous mixture of lipids can separate into two phases of different composition. This phase separation may be induced by various factors, such as the presence of proteins, pH, ionic strength, temperature, or calcium concentration.

One mechanism by which lateral phase transitions might affect excitable membrane proteins[130] is as follows. The lipid surrounding an excitable protein exists in two phases: a solid, high-density gel phase and a liquid, low-density crystalline phase. The opening of the ion channel requires a lateral expansion of the protein as it undergoes a conformational change. This lateral expansion compresses the surrounding liquids, coverting some of the expanded liquid crystalline phase to the compressed gel phase (Fig. 49-7). When anesthetic molecules partition into the lipid membrane surrounding the protein, they cause the bilayer to undergo a phase transition so that more lipid exists in the expanded liquid crystalline phase. The membrane protein is now unable to undergo the conformation changes that allow ion channels to open.

Unfortunately, little convincing data support lipid phase transition as being the critical membrane peturbation that renders excitable membrane proteins inexcitable. The lipid phase transition theory fails several critical pharmacologic tests of the anesthetic target site. Such phase transitions are reversed by only a few tens of atmospheres of pressure.[52,90] In addition, the *cis* and *trans* isomers of the Δ^9-hexadecanols, which have equal anesthetic potencies, result in opposite changes in solid/fluid phase equilibria.[100]

Membrane disordering

Another lipid perturbation that may be of mechanistic importance to general anesthesia evolved from spectroscopic studies. These showed that when general anesthetics dissolve in the lipid bilayer, they cause the closely packed, parallel array of lipid molecules to take up a more disordered arrangement. This increase in fluidity in turn perturbs the functioning of neurotransmitter proteins within the lipid bilayer, leading to inexcitability. Experiments have shown that such changes in the bilayer's lipid fluidity can affect protein function. A 6% change in order parameter has been shown to cause a ten fold change in Na^+/K^+-stimulated adenosine triphosphatase (ATPase) activity.[116]

Studies using spin-labeled lipids have shown that such diverse anesthetics as ketamine, steroid anesthetics,[64] and α-chloralose disorder cholesterol-containing lipid bilayers,[97] whereas nonanesthetic steroids do not.[64] Interestingly only lipid bilayers that contain cholesterol in approximately equal molar ratios to phospholipid are disordered by anesthetics in proportion to their in vivo potencies. Lipid bilayers that do not contain cholesterol are disordered by volatile anesthetics but ordered by barbiturates, alphaxalone, and ketamine.[45]

The lipid perturbation hypothesis can account for several pharmacologic criteria of general anesthesia.

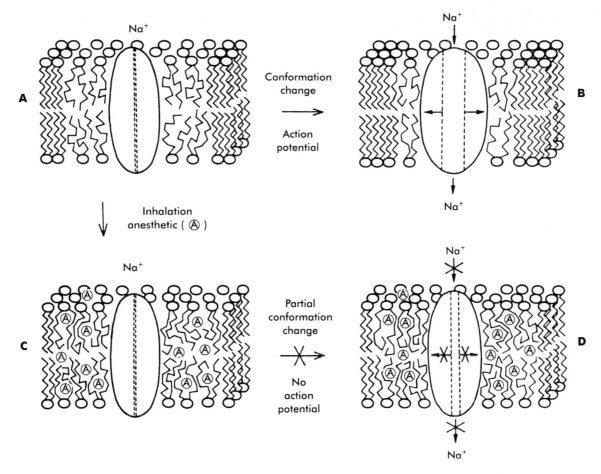

Fig. 49-7. Lateral phase separation theory of general anesthesia. **A,** Phospholipid bilayer containing sodium channel in closed conformation. **B,** Channel has undergone hypothetical conformational change, which is accomplished by packing high-volume disordered lipid into low-volume arrays. **C,** Anesthetic molecules have melted regions of ordered lipid. **D,** Protein is now unable to expand or change conformation. Excitation cannot occur. (From Trudell JR: A unitary theory of anesthesia based on lateral phase separations in nerve membranes, *Anesthesiology* 46:5, 1977.)

First, it is able to correctly predict the position of the in vivo cutoff in anesthetic potency of the primary alcohols. Fig. 49-8 shows that the ability of these alcohols to disorder lipids in *Torpedo* postsynaptic membranes cuts off at the same point as does general anesthesia in the tadpole.[80] Furthermore, optical isomers of the secondary alcohol general anesthetics disorder these same membranes nonstereoselectively.[28] Finally, the limited data available on pressure show that lipid disordering accounts for pressure reversal. Both ion permeability and order parameters change in opposite directions by anesthetics and by pressure.[15,51]

Critical Evaluation of Lipid Theories of Anesthetic Action

The solubility of an anesthetic in a lipid bilayer is able to account for the potencies of a vast array of anesthetics spanning a range of potencies of approx-imately 10,000-fold, and it provides a very satisfactory explanation of Meyer's and Overton's original observations. However, it does not account for either pressure reversal or cutoff. Modifying the theory to encompass lipid perturbations enables it to account for pressure reversal,[15] the cutoff in potency of the primary alcohol anesthetics,[80] and lack of stereoselectivity.[28]**

However, the lipid perturbation theory has not been able to explain how anesthetics might lead to selective perturbation of membranes and how these changes are then translated into functional inhibition of protein function. The structural perturbations that anesthetics induce in the lipid bilayer are about 1%. Without an explanation of how these changes are translated into inhibition of protein function, it is difficult to understand how such small changes can have such dramatic functional consequences.

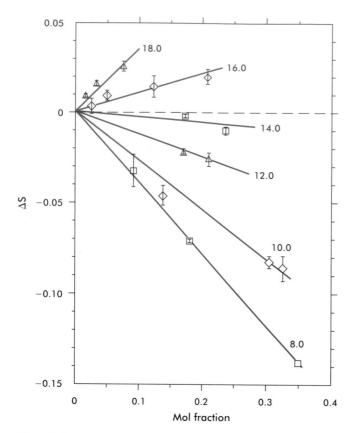

Fig. 49-8. Change in spectroscopic lipid order parameter (ΔS) as function of the mol fraction of alkanol in membranes from the marine ray, *Torpedo*. The anesthetic alcohols otanol, decanol, and dodecanol disorder lipid bilayer, whereas the nonanesthetic alcohol tetradecanol results in no change in order parameter. The nonanesthetic alcohols hexadecanol and octadecanol actually order membranes. (From Miller KW, Firestone LL, Alifimoff JK et al: Nonanesthetic alcohols dissolve in synaptic membranes without perturbing their lipids, *Proc Natl Acad Sci* 86:1084, 1989.)

Protein Theories of Anesthetic Action

Just as some investigators have interpreted Meyer's and Overton's original observations on anesthetic potency and lipid solubility to mean that the primary site of anesthetic action is the lipid bilayer, others have interpreted this to mean that anesthetics act directly on proteins. **General anesthetics have long been known to interact directly with proteins.** This is not surprising, since half the amino acids in proteins have hydrophobic side chains. **Two types of anesthetic-protein interactions can be distinguished, specific and nonspecific.** In specific interactions only a narrow range of anesthetics participate at a given site. In nonspecific interactions a wide range of anesthetics participate, and this type appears to mimic general anesthesia.

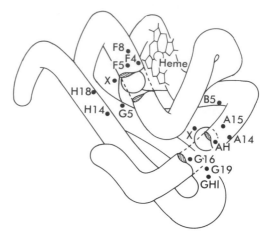

Fig. 49-9. Binding of xenon to myoglobin. (From Settle W: Function of the myoglobin molecule as influenced by anesthetic molecules. In Featherstone RM, ed: *Guide to molecular pharmacology-toxicology,* Part II, New York, 1973, Marcel Dekker.)

Specific anesthetic-protein interactions

The best example of a specific anesthetic-protein interaction is xenon with the globular protein myoglobin. Myoglobin is a relatively small protein consisting of a single polypeptide chain and heme group. It has been crystallized and its three-dimensional structure determined by x-ray diffraction.[119,128] The molecule is extremely compact, and the interior consists almost entirely of nonpolar hydrophobic amino acid residues, with the heme group located in a crevice. A few anesthetics have been shown to bind directly to the myoglobin molecule. At a partial pressure of 2.5 atm, xenon binds at an interior site near the heme, as illustrated in Fig. 49-9. Difluorodichloromethane, which is slightly larger than xenon, also binds in the same pocket but must push apart some adjacent amino acid side chains. Anesthetics larger than difluorodichloromethane do not bind because of spatial limitations, whereas other anesthetics such as ethane, which are small enough to fit into the binding site, do not bind because their intermolecular forces are too weak. Finally, some anesthetics, such as krypton and nitrous oxide, are simply too small.

A more interesting interaction between an anesthetic and a protein is halothane with muscle adenylate kinase because of the fact that halothane is a triggering agent for malignant hyperthermia. Halothane competitively inhibits the production of adenosine diphosphate, (ADP) by adenylate kinase.[114] X-ray diffraction studies have shown that halothane binds deep within the protein's interior in a hydrophobic pocket in much the same way as xenon does to myoglobin. **Unfortunately the interaction**

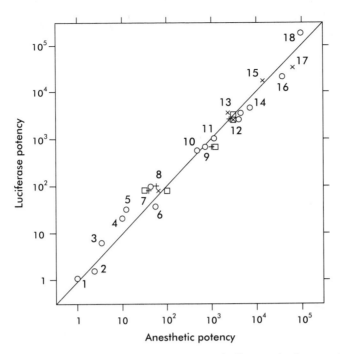

Fig. 49-10. Inhibition of firefly luciferase by diverse volatile anesthetics correlates with their in vivo anesthetic potency. *1,* Methanol; *2,* ethanol; *3,* acetone; *4,* propanol; *5,* butanone; *6,* paraldehyde; *7,* diethyl ether; *8,* butanol; *9,* benzyl alcohol; *10,* chloroform; *11,* hexanol; *12,* halothane; *13,* methoxyflurane; *14,* octanol; *15,* pentane; *16,* nonanol; *17,* hexane; *18,* decanol. (From Franks NP, Lieb WR: Do general anesthetics act by competitive binding to specific receptors? *Nature* 310:599, 1984.)

occurs only supraclinical concentrations of halothane, so its relevance to either malignant hyperthermia or anesthesia is questionable. Although many other examples of this type of specific anesthetic-protein interaction exist,[12,77,78] their relevance to the molecular mechanism(s) of anesthetic action is highly doubtful.

Nonspecific anesthetic-protein interactions

An interesting observation on the effects of anesthetics is that they cause luminescent bacteria[41,49,133] to cease to glow. In bacteria, anesthetics inhibit luminescence by directly competing with an alkyl aldehyde co-factor for a site on the enzyme.[76] Work on firefly luciferase also shows competitive inhibition but with a different cofactor, *D*-luciferin, in the light-emitting reaction.[30]

Experiments on a purified, lipid-free preparation of firefly luciferase have shown that a variety of anesthetics are able to inhibit this enzyme's light-emitting activity. In addition, the in vivo anesthetic potencies of these drugs correlate quite well with their potencies as enzymatic inhibitors of the luciferase reaction, and the potencies span six orders of magnitude[30] (Fig. 49-10). More importantly, however, the inhibition of firefly luciferase occurs with clinical concentrations of anesthetics. Franks and Lieb[30] have interpreted these data to mean that general anesthetics act by competing with endogenous ligands for specific receptors in the CNS.

How well does the luciferase model account for the pharmacology of general anesthetics? Firefly luciferase demonstrates a cutoff in anesthetic potency for both the alcohol and the *n*-alkane anesthetics.[31] However, the cutoff for the primary alcohols occurs between hexadecanol ($C_N = 16$) and heptadecanol ($C_N = 17$) and possibly even higher.[80] One can contrast this with the in vivo cutoff for anesthetic potency that occurs after dodecanol ($C_N = 12$).[1] The luciferase model also predicts incorrectly that hexanol and heptanol should have equal anesthetic potency in vivo (see Table 49-2). Also, the ability of steroids to inhibit luciferase correlates poorly with their anesthetic potency.[5]

The effect of optical isomers of anesthetic alcohols on luciferases has not been examined, although the co-factor in the reaction, *D*-luciferin, is optically active. Thus stereoselective anesthetic effects could occur. Finally, the inhibition of bacterial luciferase by anesthetics is reversed by pressure.[48] This observation prompted the first experiments with pressure reversal in animals. However, the bacterial enzyme is much less sensitive to pressure reversal than whole animals because the effects of some anesthetics (e.g., sodium barbital) are not reversed. In contrast, firefly luciferase does not demonstrate reversal of anesthetic inhibition by pressure.[33]

Fluorine-19 nuclear magnetic resonance (NMR) studies in animals may be more relevant to protein theories of general anesthetic action. NMR methods have enabled direct observation of fluorinated anesthetics in vivo.[134] NMR studies in rats have shown that halothane's anesthetic effect correlated with an apparent saturable binding site in the brain.[25] More recent studies[23] contradict this claim and have led to a critical assessment of the application of NMR to this problem.[67]

Critical Evaluation of Protein Theories of Anesthetic Action

Although anesthetics have been shown to interact with different proteins, most of these interactions (e.g., xexon with myoglobin) occur only at concentrations higher than those used clinically. In contrast, the inhibition of firefly luciferase is the only anesthetic protein interaction that comes close to obeying the Meyer-Overton rule. Luciferase demonstrates a cutoff for the primary alcohol anesthetics and n-alkanes. Unfortunately the cutoff does not agree with the in vivo cutoff. Similarly the luciferase model does not demonstrate pressure reversal. Despite these difficulties, the advantage of luciferase as a model of the anesthetic target site is that it provides a possible mechanism whereby anesthetics might render receptors inoperable; this may be competitive inhibition of neurotransmitter or, more likely, neuromodulator binding by anesthetics. One must remember that the demonstration of a binding site on a protein such as luciferase does not constitute proof that such sites actually exist in the CNS. However, among the many neurotransmitter receptor proteins in the CNS, more relevant examples may be found. Whether or not protein theories of anesthetic action survive as plausible will be determined by their ability to account for the pharmacology of general anesthetics.

Lipid-Protein Interaction Theories of General Anesthetic Action

Both the lipid theories and the protein theories of anesthetic action have certain limitations. A third possible site of action for general anesthetics is at the lipid-protein interface (see Fig. 49-6).[24,44,65,129] The lipids in direct association with transmembrane receptor proteins are known as the *boundary lipid.* These lipids are in dynamic equilibrium with the lipid molecules in the bulk bilayer. Theoretic studies

suggest that the surface of the protein molecules within the bilayer is rough[40] and that the boundary lipid molecules wrap themselves around these rough spots. Conceivably, anesthetics might displace critical lipid molecules necessary for the functional integrity of transmembrane proteins and might produce inexcitability. Unfortunately, progress in this area has been painfully slow because of technical difficulties, and the pharmacology of general anesthesia has not been extensively examined in any of the available model systems.

Recent studies on the nicotinic acetylcholine receptor, a chemically gated transmembrane cation channel (see Fig. 49-6), show that general anesthetics decrease the affinity of the lipid for the lipid-protein interface. Anesthetics do so selectively, with some lipids affected more than others, suggesting some degree of specificity of action. The few anesthetics examined all exerted this effect, but much remains to be done before firm conclusions may be drawn.[34] In particular, interpretation in a way that relates these data to lipid perturbations' ability to affect protein function (T_p in previous equation) is still rudimentary.

CONCLUSION

The mechanism of action of general anesthesia remains a pharmacologic enigma. **Just as there is no consensus of opinion among neurophysiologists as to what region of the CNS is responsible for consciousness, there is no consensus among pharmacologists as to where in the CNS anesthetics act.** There is, however, clear evidence that on a cellular level, anesthetics act at the synapse, but the mechanisms of synaptic inhibition remains unclear, owing largely to the tremendous complexity of the CNS and its interdependence. This has resulted in the opinion of some pharmacologists that a unitary mechanism of action is unlikely, but this remains to be validated.

Although no physiologic definition of the general anesthetic state is available, a well-characterized pharmacologic one does exist. Unfortunately a specific antagonist for general anesthesia is lacking, and this blunts the power of the pharmacologic approach. Therefore much more work must be done to provide additional pharmacologic probes that can be applied to well-defined models. To proceed critically, one must proceed slowly and systematically.

The lipid theories of anesthetic action have withstood a wider battery of pharmacologic tests than any protein model evaluated. Most proteins have failed to provide a successful model of the anesthetic site. The luciferases may have more relevant application, but even this is questionable. Other proteins in the CNS may provide better models, but it will be difficult to separate direct from indirect effects for any membrane-bound protein. On the other hand, the lipid theories will remain unproved until a direct mechanism can be established regarding how membrane perturbation leads to inhibition of protein function.

KEY POINTS

■ How general anesthetics render both insensibility to pain and unconsciousness remains an enigma. While data on the anesthetic effects in various regions of the brain are abundant, no set is sufficiently complete or consistent to support anesthetic actions occurring through one specific effect in one region of the CNS. The most likely site of action of general anesthetics, on a cellular level, is the synapse.

■ General anesthetics block synaptic transmission at concentrations much lower than required to block axonal conductance.

■ The two theories of action of general anesthetics are the *unitary theory*, which holds that all general anesthetics exert their actions by a common mechanism, and the *degenerate theory*, which postulates that different classes of anesthetics have different mechanisms of action.

■ Two primary strategies are used to elucidate the molecular basis of anesthetic action: (1) the *pharmacologic approach* studies the relative potencies of anesthetics in animals and (2) the *mechanistic approach* studies the effects of general anesthetics on well-defined molecular models.

■ Because general anesthesia can be produced by several structurally diverse molecules from the simple inert gas xenon to such complex molecules as althesin and α-chloralose, we must assume that no single, structural specific receptor serves as mediator.

■ The correlation of anesthetic potency with lipid solubility is expressed in the Meyer-Overton rule; it provides an accurate means of predicting anesthetic potency.

■ Three schools of thought exist as to where, on a molecular level, general anesthetics might exert their effects: (1) primarily on the lipid bilayer, (2) directly on neurotransmitter receptor proteins, or (3) at a mixed site at the lipid-protein interface.

■ Membrane expansion is a simple lipid perturbation that accounts for pressure reversal and suggests how ion channel protein function is inhibited. This is expressed as the critical volume hypothesis, which states that anesthesia occurs when a hydrophobic phase expands beyond a critical amount.

■ The solubility of an anesthetic in a lipid bilayer accounts for the varying potencies of anesthetics and provides an explanation of Meyer's and Overton's original data. However, it does not account for either pressure reversal or cut-off. Modifiying the theory to encompass liquid perturbations accounts for pressure reversal, the cut-off in potency of the primary alcohol anesthetics, and lack of stereoselectivity but not how anesthetics might lead to selective perturbation of membranes and how these changes are then translated into inhibition of protein function.

■ General anesthetics interact directly with proteins in two ways: specific (e.g., xenon with the globular protein myoglobin or halothane with muscle adenylate kinase) and nonspecific. Most interactions occur only at concentrations higher than those used clinically.

KEY REFERENCES

Brett RJ, Dilger JP, and Yland KF: Isoflurane causes "flickering" of the acetylcholine receptor channel: observations using the patch clamp, *Anesthesiology* 69:161,1988.

Franks NP, Lieb WR: Where do general anesthetics act? *Nature* 274:339, 1978.

Kendig JJ, Trudell JR, and Cohen EN: Halothane stereoisomers: lack of sterospecificity in two model systems, *Anesthesiology* 39:518, 1973.

Lever MJ, Miller KW, Paton WDM et al: Pressure reversal of anesthesia, *Nature (Lond)* 231:368, 1971.

Miller KW: The nature of the site of general anesthesia, *Int Rev Neurobiol* 27:1, 1985.

REFERENCES

1. Alifimoff JK, Firestone LL, and Miller KW: Anesthetic potencies of secondary alcohol enantiomers, *Anesthesiology* 66: 55, 1987.
2. Alifimoff JK, Firestone LL, and Miller KW: Anesthetic potencies of primary alkanols: implications for the molecular dimensions of the anaesthetic site, *Br J Pharmacol* 96:9, 1989.
3. Angel A: Effect of anaesthetics on nervous pathways. In Gray TC, Nunn JF, and Utting JE eds: *General anaesthesia* London, 1980, Butterworths.
4. Angel A, Gratton DA: The effect of anaesthetic agents on cerebral cortical responses in the rat, *Br J Pharmacol* 76:541, 1982.
5. Banks P, Peace CB: Enzyme inhibition by steroid anaesthetics derived from progesterone, *Br J Anaesth* 57:512, 1985.
6. Barker JL, McBurney RN: Phenobarbitone modulation of post-synaptic GABA receptor function on cultured mammalian neurons, *Proc R Soc Lond (Biol)* 206:318, 1979.
7. Barker SL, Ransom BR: Pentobarbitone pharmacology of mammalian central neurons grown in tissue culture, *J Physiol (Lond)* 280:355, 1980.
8. Bennett DB, Papahadjopoulos D, and Bangham AD: The effect of raised pressure of inert gases on phospholipid membranes, *Life Sci* 6:2527, 1967.
9. Berg-Johnsen J, Langmoen: Isoflurane hyperpolarizes neurons in rat and human cerebral cortex, *Acta Physiol Scand* 130:679, 1987.
10. Bernard C: *Lecons sur les anesthetiques et sur l'asphyxie,* Paris, 1875, Bailliers.
11. Bull MH, Brailsford JD, and Bull BS: Erythrocyte membrane expansion due to volatile anesthetics, the l-alkanols, and benzyl alcohol, *Anesthesiology* 57:399, 1982.
12. Braswell LM, Kitz RJ: The effects *in vitro* of volatile anesthetics on the activity of cholinesterases, *J Neurochem* 29: 665, 1977.
13. Brett RJ, Dilger JP, and Yland KF: Isoflurane causes "flickering" of the acetylcholine receptor channel: observations using the patch clamp, *Anesthesiology* 69:161, 1988.
14. Butler TC, Dickson HL: The anesthetic potency of optical antipodes. I. The secondary butyl alcohols, *J Pharmacol Exp Ther* 69:225, 1940.
15. Chin JH, Trudell JR, and Cohen EN: The compression-ordering and solubility-disordering effects of high pressure gases on phospholipid bilayers, *Life Sci* 18:489, 1976.
16. Collins GGS: Release of endogenous amino acid neurotransmitter candidates from rat olfactory cortex slices: possible regulatory mechanisms and the effects of pentobarbitone, *Brain Res* 190:517, 1980.
17. Crawford JM, Curtis DR: Pharmacological studies on feline Betz cells, *J Physiol (Lond)* 186:121, 1966.
18. Crossland J, Merrick AJ: The effect of anaesthesia of acetylcholine content of brain, *J Physiol (Lond)* 125:56, 1954.
19. Darbinjan TM. Golovchinsky VB, and Plehotkina SI: The effects of anesthetics on reticular and cortical activity, *Anesthesiology* 34:219, 1971.
20. Dodson BA, Furmaniuk ZW, and Miller KW: The physiological effects of hydrostatic pressure are not equivalent to those of helium pressure on *Rana pipiens, J Physiol (Lond)* 362:233, 1985.
21. Dodson BA, Uhr RR, and Muller KW: Relative potencies for barbiturate binding to acetylcholine receptor, *Br J Pharmacol* 101:710, 1990.
22. Dubois MY, Sato S, Chassy J et al: Effects of enflurane on brainstem auditory evoked responses in humans, *Anesth Analg* 61:898, 1982.
23. Eger, Litt:
24. Elliot JR, Haydon DA: The actions of neutral anaesthetics on ion conductances of nerve membranes, *Biochim Biophys Acta* 988:257, 1989.
25. Evers AS, Berkowitz BA, and d'Avignon DA: Correlation between the anaesthetic effect of halothane and saturable binding in the brain, *Nature* 328:157, 1987.
26. Feldman SM, Waller HJ: Dissociation of electrocortical actvation and behavioral arousal, *Nature (Lond)* 196:1320, 1962.
27. Ferguson J: The use of chemical potentials as indices of toxicity, *Proc R Soc (Biol)* 127:387, 1939.
28. Firestone LL, Alifimoff JK, and Miller KW: Anesthetic and lipid disordering potencies of secondary alcohol stereoisomers, *Anesthesiology* 67(3A):A380, 1987.
29. Franks NP, Lieb WR: Where do general anesthetics act? *Nature* 274:339, 1978.
30. Franks NP, Lieb WR: Do general anesthetics act by competitive binding to specific receptors? *Nature* 310:599, 1984.
31. Franks NP, Lieb WR: Mapping of general anesthetic target sites provides a molecular basis for cut-off effects, *Nature* 316:349, 1985.
32. Franks NP, Lieb WR: Partitioning of long-chain alcohols into lipid bilayers; implications for mechanisms of general anesthesia, *Proc Natl Acad Sci* 83:5116, 1986.
33. Franks NP, Lieb WR: Personal communication.
34. Fraser DM, Louro SRW, Laszlo HI et al: A study of the effect of general anesthetics on lipid-protein interactions in acetylcholine receptor enriched membranes from *Torpedo nobiliana* using nitroxide spin-labels, *Biochemistry* 29: 2664, 1990.
35. French JD, Verzeano M, and Magoun HW: A neural basis of the anesthetic state, *Arch Neurol Psychiatry* 69:519, 1953.
36. Fuhner H: Die narkotische wirkung des benzins und seiner bestandteile (pentan, hexan, heptan, octan) *Biochem Zeit* 115: 235, 1935.
37. Fujiwara N, Higashi H, Fujita S et al: Mechanisms of halothane action on synaptic transmission in motoneurons of the newborn rat spinal cord *in vitro, J Physiol* 412:155, 1988.
38. Gage PW, Robertson B: Prolongation of inhibitory postsynaptic currents of pentobarbitone, halothane and ketamine in CA1 pyramidal cells in rat hippocampus, *Br J Pharmacol* 85:675, 1985.
39. Galindo A: Effects of procaine, pentobarbital and halothane on synaptic transmission in the central nervous system, *J Pharmacol Exp Ther* 169:185, 1969.
40. Guy HR: A structural model of the acetylcholine receptor channel based on partition energy and helix packing calculations, *Biophys J* 45:249, 1984.
41. Halsey MJ, Smith EB: Effects of anaesthetics on luminous bacteria, *Nature* 227:1363, 1970.
42. Haydon DA, Hendry BM, Levinson SR et al: The molecular mechanisms of anaesthesia, *Nature* 268:356, 1977.
43. Haydon DA, Requena J, and Urban BW: Some effect of aliphatic hydrocarbons on the electrical capacity and ionic currents of the squid giant axon membrane, *J Physiol (Lond)* 309:229, 1980.
44. Heidmann T, Oswald RE, and Changeux J-P: Multiple sites of action for noncompetitive blockers on acetylcholine receptor rich membrane fragments from *Torpedo marmorata, Biochemistry* 22:3112, 1983.
45. Janoff AS, Miller KW: A critical assessment of the lipid theories of general anaesthetic action. In Chapman D, ed: *Biological membranes,* vol 4, London, 1982, Academic Press.
46. Janoff AS, Pringle MJ, and Miller KW: Correlation of general anesthetic potency with solubility in membranes, *Biochim Acta* 649:125, 1981.
47. Jessell TM, Richards CD: Barbiturate potentiation of hippocampal p.s.p.s. is not mediated by blockade of GABA uptake, *J Physiol (Lond)* 269:42P, 1977.
48. Johnson FH, Brown DES, and Marsland DA: Pressure reversal of the action of certain narcotics, *J Cel Comp Physiol* 20:269:1942.
49. Johnson FH, Eyring H, and Polissar MJ: *The kinetic basis of molecular biology,* New York, 1954, Wiley.
50. Johnson FH, Flagler EA: Hydrostatic pressure reversal of narcosis in tadpoles, *Science* 112:91, 1951.
51. Johnson SM, Miller KW, and Bangham AD: The opposing effects of pressure and general anaesthetics on the cation permeability of liposomes of varying lipid composition, *Biochim Biophys Acta* 307:42, 1973.
52. Kamaya H, Ueda I, Moore PS et al: Antagonism between high pressure and anesthetics in the thermal phase transi-

tion of dipalmitoyl phosphatidycholine bilayer, *Biochim Biphys Acta* 550:131, 1979.

53. Kendall TJG, Minchin MCW: The effects of anaesthetics on the uptake and release of amino acid neurotransmitters in thalamic slices, *Br J Pharmacol* 75:219, 1982.

54. Kendig JJ: Anesthetics and pressure in nerve cells. In Fink BR, ed: *Molecular mechanisms of anesthesia,* vol 2, *progress in anesthesiology,* New York, 1982, Raven Press.

55. Kendig JJ, Grossman Y: Homogeneous and branching axons: differing responses to anesthetics and pressure. In Roth SH, Miller KW eds: *Molecular and cellular mechanisms of anesthetics,* New York, 1986, Plenum Medical.

56. Kendig JJ, Trudell JR, and Cohen EN: Halothane stereoisomers: lack of stereospecificity in two model systems, *Anesthesiology* 39:518, 1973.

57. Kita Y, Miller KW: The partial molar volumes of some n-alkanols in erythrocyte ghosts and lipid bilayers, *Biochemistry* 21:2840, 1982.

58. Koffka K: Principals of Gestalt psychology, New York, 1935, Harcourt Brace.

59. Krnjevic K: transmitters in the cerebral cortex. In *Proceedings of the XXII International Congress on Physiology and Science,* Tokyo, 1965, International Congress Series no 87, New York, 1965, Excerpta Medica Foundation.

60. Krnjevic K: Chemical nature of synaptic transmission in vertebrates, *Physiol Rev* 54:418, 1974.

61. Krnjevic K: Cellular mechanisms of anaesthesia, *Ann NY Acad Sci,* 1991 (in press).

62. Kullman DM, Martin RL, and Redman SJ: Reduction by general anesthetics of group I_a excitatory postsynaptic potentials and currents in the spinal cord, *J Physiol (Lond)* 412:277, 1989.

63. Larrabee MG, Posternak JM: Selective action of anesthetics on synapses and axons in mammalian sympathetic ganglia, *J Neurophysiol* 15:91, 1952.

64. Lawrence DK, Gill EW: Structurally specific effects of some steroid anesthetics on spin-labeled liposomes, *Mol Pharmacol* 11:280, 1975.

65. Lee AG: Model for the action of local anaesthetics, *Nature* 262:545, 1976.

66. Lever MJ, Miller KW, Paton WDM et al: Pressure reversal of anesthesia, *Nature (Lond)* 231:368, 1971.

67. Litt, 1990.

68. MacDonald RL, Barker JL: Enhancement of GABA-mediated postsynaptic inhibition in cultured mammalian spinal cord neurons: a common mode of anticonvulsant action, *Brain Res* 167:323, 1979.

69. MacIver MB, Roth SH: Inhalation anaesthetics exhibit pathway specific and differential actions in hippocampal synaptic responses *in vitro, Br J Anaesth* 60:680, 1988.

70. MacLarnon JG, Pennefather P, and Quastel DMJ: Mechanism of nicotinic channel blockade by anesthetics. In

Roth SH, and Miller KW eds: *Molecular and cellular mechanisms of anesthetics,* New York, 1986, Plenum Medical.

71. Majewska MD, Harrison NJ, Schwartz RD et al: Steroid hormone metabolites are barbiturate-like modulators of the GABA receptor, *Science* 232:1004, 1986.

72. Matthews EK, Quilliam JP: Effects of central depressant drugs upon acetylcholine release, *Br J Pharmacol Chemother* 22:415, 1970.

73. McGeer PL, Eccles JC, and McGeer EG: *Molecular neurobiology of the mammalian brain,* New York, 1987, Plenum Press.

74. Merkel G, Eger EI II: A comparative study of halothane and halopropane anesthesia, including method for determining equipotency, *Anesthesiology* 24: 346, 1963.

75. Meyer HH: The theory of narcosis, *Harvey Lect* 99:11, 1906.

76. Middleton AJ, Smith EB: General anaesthetics and bacterial luminescence. II. The effect of diethyl ether on the *in vitro* light emission of *Vibrio fischeri, Proc R Soc Lond (Biol)* 193:173, 1976.

77. Miller JC, Miller KW: Approaches to mechanisms of action of general anesthetics. In *MTP international review of sciences: physiological and pharmacological series,* Baltimore, 1975, Butterworths/University Park Press.

78. Miller KW: The nature of the site of general anesthesia, *Int Rev Neurobiol* 27:1, 1985.

79. Miller KW, Braswell LM, Firestone LL et al: General anesthetics act both specifically and nonspecifically on acetylcholine receptors. In Roth SH, Miller KW, eds: *Molecular and cellular mechanisms of anesthetics,* New York, 1986, Plenum Medical.

80. Miller KW, Firestone LL, Alifimoff JK et al: Non-anesthetic alcohols dissolve in synaptic membranes without perturbing their lipids, *Proc Natl Acad Sci* 86:1084, 1989.

81. Miller KW, Firestone LL, and Forman SA: General anesthetic and specific effects of ethanol on acetylcholine receptors, *Ann NY Acad Sci* 492:71, 1987.

82. Miller KW, Paton WDM, Smith EB et al: Physiochemical approaches to the mode of action of general anesthetics, *Anesthesiology* 36:339, 1972.

83. Miller KW, Paton WDM, Smith RA et al: The pressure reversal of anesthesia and the critical volume hypothesis, *Mol Pharmacol* 9:131, 1973.

84. Miller KW, Wilson MW: The pressure reversal of a variety of anesthetic agents in mice, *Anesthesiology* 48:104, 1978.

85. Miller KW, Wilson MW and Smith, RA: Pressure resolves two sites of action of inert gases, *Mol Pharmacol* 14:950, 1978.

86. Minchin MCW: The effect of anaesthetics on the uptake and release of γ-aminobutyrate and D-aspartate in rat brain slices, *Br J Pharmacol* 73:681, 1981.

87. Miu P, Puil E: Isoflurane-induced impairment of synaptic transmission in hippocampal neurons, *Exp Brain Res* 75:354, 1989.

88. Mody I, MacIver MB, adn Tanelian DL: Calcium mediates the halothane induced prolongation of spontaneous inhibitory post-synaptic currents (SIPSCs) in hippocampal neurons, *Soc Neurosci Abstr* 16, 1990.

89. Mori K, Winters WD: Neural background of sleep and anesthesia, *Int Anesthesiol Clin* 13:67, 1975.

90. Mountcastle DB, Biltonen RL, and Halsey MJ: Effect of anesthetics and pressure on the thermotropic behavior of multilamellar dipalmitoylphosphatidylcholine liposomes, *Proc Natl Acad Sci* 75:4906, 1978.

91. Mullins LJ: In Lajtha A, ed: *Handbook of neurochemistry* , vol 6, New York, 1971, Plenum Press.

92. Nicoll RA: The effects of anesthetics on synaptic excitation and inhibition in the olfactory bulb, *J Physiol (Lond)* 233:803, 1972.

93. Nicoll RA: Pentobarbital: action on frog motoneurons, *Brain Res* 96:119, 1975.

94. Olsen RW: Drug interactions at the GABA receptor–ionophore complex, *Annu Rev Pharmacol Toxicol* 22:245, 1982.

95. Overton CE: *Studien uber die Narkose,* Jena, 1901, Fisher.

96. Overton CE: *Studies of narcosis,* Lipnick NL, ed, London, 1991, Chapman and Hall.

97. Pang KYY, Miller KW: Cholesterol modulates the effect of membrane perturbers in phospholipid vesicles and biomembranes, *Biochem Biophys Acta* 511:1, 1978.

98. Penfield W, Rasmussen T: *The cerebral cortex of man,* New York, 1950, MacMillan.

99. Potashner SJ, Lake N, Langlois EA et al: Pentobarbital: differential effects on amino acid transmitter release. In Fink BR, ed: *Molecular mechanisms of anesthesia,* vol 2, *Progress in anesthesiology,* New York, 1980, Raven Press.

100. Pringle MJ, Brown KB, and Miller KW: Can the lipid theories of anesthesia account for the cutoff in anesthetic potency in homologous series of alcohols? *Mol Pharmacol* 19:49, 1981.

101. Rabe LS, Moreno L, Rigor BM et al: Effects of halothane on evoked field potentials recorded from cortical and subcortical nuclei, *Neuropharmacology* 19:813, 1980.

102. Ransom BR, Barker JL: Pentobarbital selectively enhances GABA mediated postsynaptic inhibition in tissue cultured mouse spinal meurons, *Brain Res* 144: 530, 1976.

103. Richards CD: On the mechanism of barbiturate anesthesia, *J Physiol (Lond)* 227:749, 1972.

104. Richards CD: On the mechanism of halothane anesthesia, *J Physiol (Lond)* 233:439, 1973.

105. Richards CD: In search of the mechanisms of anesthesia, *Trends Neurosci* 3:9, 1980.

106. Richards CD: Actions of general anesthetics on synaptic transmission in the CNS, *Br J Anaesth* 55:201, 1983.

107. Richards CD, Hesketh TR: Implications for theories of anesthesia of antagonism between anesthetic and non-anesthetic steroids, *Nature (Lond)* 256:179, 1975.

108. Richards CD, Russell WJ, and Smaje JC: The action of ether and methoxyflurane on synaptic transmission in isolated preparation of the mammalian cortex, *J Physiol (Lond)* 248:121, 1975.

109. Richards CD, White AE: The actions of volatile anesthetics on synaptic transmission in the dentate gyrus, *J Physiol (Lond)* 252:241, 1975.

110. Robbins BH: Preliminary studies of the anesthetic activity of fluorinated hydrocarbons, *J Pharmacol Exp Ther* 86:197, 1946.

111. Rosner BS, Clark DL: Neurophysiologic effects of general anesthetics. II. Sequential regional actions in the brain, *Anesthesiology* 39:59, 1973.

112. Roth SH: Physical mechanisms of anesthesia, *Annu Rev Pharmacol Toxicol* 19:159, 1979.

113. Ryder S, Way WL, and Trevor AJ: Comparative pharmacology of optical isomers of ketamine in mice, *Eur J Pharmacol* 49:15, 1978.

114. Sachsenheimer W, Pai EF, Schultz GE et al: Halothane binds in the adenine-specific niche of crystalline adenylate kinase, *FEBS Lett* 79:310, 1977.

115. Saidman LJ, Eger E II: Effect of nitrous oxide and of narcotic premedication on the alveolar concentration of halothane required for anesthesia, *Anesthesiology* 25:302, 1964.

116. Sinesky M, Pinkerton F, Sutherland E et al: Rate limitation of the $(Na^+ + K^+)$-stimulated adenosine-triphosphatase by membrane acyl chain ordering, *Proc Natl Acad Sci* 76:4893, 1979.

117. Scholfield CN: Potentiation of inhibition by general anaesthetics in neurones of the olfactory cortex *in vitro, Pflugers Arch* 383:249, 1980.

118. Seeman P: Membrane actions of anesthetics and tranquilizers, *Pharmacol Rev* 24:583, 1972.

119. Settle W: Function of the myoglobin molecule as influenced by anesthetic molecules. In Featherstone RM, ed: *Guide to molecular pharmacology-toxicology,* Part II, New York, 1973, Marcel Dekker.

120. Smith EB, Bowser-Riley F, and Daniels S: New observations on the mechanism of pressure-anesthetic interactions. In Roth SH, Miller KW eds: *Molecular and cellular mechanisms of anesthetics,* New York, 1986, Plenum Medical.

121. Somjen GG: Effects of ether and thiopental on spinal presynaptic terminals, *J Pharmacol Exp Ther* 140:396, 1963.

122. Somjen GG, Gill M: The mechanism of the blockade of synaptic transmission in the mammalian spinal cord by diethyl ether and by thiopental, *J Pharmacol Exp Ther* 140:19, 1963.

123. Sowton SCM, Sherrington CS: On the relative effects of chloroform upon the heart and other muscular organs, *Br Med J* 2:181, 1905.

124. Storch J, Kleinfield AM: The lipid structure of biological membranes, *Trends Biol Sci* 10:418, 1985.

125. Takenoshita M, Takahashi T: Mechanisms of halothane action on synaptic transmission in motoneurons of the newborn rat spinal cord *in vitro, Brain Res* 402:303, 1987.

126. Thornton C, Heneghan CPH, James MFM et al: Effects of halothane or enflurane with controlled ventilation on auditory evoked potentials, *Br J Anaesth* 56:315, 1984.

127. Ticku MK, Rastogi SK: Barbiturate-sensitive sites in the benzodiazepine-GABA receptor–ionophore complex. In Roth SH, Miller KW eds: *Molecular and cellular mechanisms of anesthtics,* New York, 1986, Plenum Medical.

128. Tilton RF Jr, Kuntz ID Jr, and Petsko GA: Cavities in proteins: structure of a metmyoglobin-xenon complex solved to 1.9 Å, *Biochemistry* 23:2849, 1984.

129. Trudell JR: A unitary theory of anesthesia based on lateral phase separations in nerve membranes, *Anesthesiology* 46:5, 1977.

130. Trudell JR, Hubbell WL, and Cohen EN: The effect of two inhalational anesthetics on the order of spin-labeled phospholipid vesicles, *Biochim Biophys Acta* 291:321, 1973.

131. Waud DR: On biological assays involving quantal responses, *J Pharmacol Exp Ther* 183:577, 1972.

132. Weakley JN: Effect of barbiturates on 'quantal' synaptic transmission in spinal motorneurons, *J Physiol (Lond)* 204:63, 1969.

133. White DC, Dundas CR: Effect of anaesthetics on emission of light by luminous bacteria, *Nature* 226:456, 1970.

134. Wyrwicz AM, Pszenny MH, Tillman PC et al: Noninvasive observations of fluorinated anesthetics in rabbit brain by fluorine-19 nuclear magnetic resonance, *Science* 222:428, 1983.

135. Yosjimura M, Higashi H, Fujita S et al: Selective depression of hippocampal inhibitory post-synaptic potentials and spontaneous firing by volatile anesthetics, *Brain Res* 340:363, 1985.

136. Zorychta E, Capek R: Depression of spinal monosynaptic transmission of diethyl ether: quantal analysis of unitary synaptic potentials, *J Pharmacol Exp Ther* 207:825, 1978.

CHAPTER 50

Pharmacology of Inhalational Anesthetics

DAVID E. LONGNECKER
FRANCIS L. MILLER

The anesthetic state of unconsciousness and absence of all sensations may be achieved using a variety of drugs administered by different routes, but, in practice, general anesthesia is produced by the inhalation of anesthetic gases. The administration of drugs by inhalation may seem awkward and complicated to other physicians but is familiar to all anesthesiologists. The inhalational route is immediately accessible: the anesthesiologist is always aware of respiration and can control airway functions in order to ensure adequate delivery of oxygen (O_2) and removal of carbon dioxide (CO_2) and is, thus, in a good position to control the delivery or removal of inhaled drugs.

Inhalational anesthetics are used today because the gases may be administered and excreted via the lungs and the depth of anesthesia can be readily altered by this mechanism. These gases produce characteristic changes in respiration and circulation, which may be used as indications of dose requirements; however, these requirements may vary depending on the surgical stimulus, associated medications, and the patient's physical condition. Measurement of anesthetic gas partial pressures in respiratory gases by mass spectrometry enhances further the precision, safety, and individual dosage of the inhalational anesthetics to an extent not achievable with injectable agents. However, intelligent and safe use of inhalational agents requires an understanding of the physical and pharmacologic properties of these agents and of the physiologic responses of the patient to drugs and surgical stimuli.

Historically, intravenous techniques were not available until late in the nineteenth century. The recreational inhalation of gases and vapors led to the discovery and popularization of anesthetics for surgery, first of diethyl ether by William Morton in 1846 and then of nitrous oxide (N_2O) by Gardner Quincy Colton in 1863.[59] The early anesthetics, N_2O, ether, and chloroform, were sufficient to fill needs for the next century. However, the undesirable properties of earlier anesthetics led to the development of new inhalational agents that displaced ether and the other once-popular anesthetics. Diethyl ether and cyclopropane were flammable, chloroform produced unexplained cardiac arrest, trichlorethylene formed the toxic gases phosgene and carbon monoxide in the presence of soda lime, and methoxyflurane caused renal tubular damage because its rapid metabolism released fluoride ions. These varied and subtle problems were recognized only after periods of clinical use; therefore, newer agents have been subject to much more intense initial scrutiny than were their predecessors.

The purpose of this chapter is to discuss the chemical, physical, biophysical, and pharmacologic properties of the inhalational general anesthetic agents. The agents that are in current use, N_2O, isoflurane (Forane), enflurane (Ethrane), and halothane (Fluothane) are listed in Table 50-1 for comparison. The table also includes the properties of two new anesthetics undergoing laboratory and clinical testing, sevoflurane and desflurane. The discussion primarily concerns the four agents in current use, but the scientific basis for the use of these anesthetics applies to all of the anesthetic agents of the past and the future.

Table 50-1 General properties of inhalational anesthetics

Property	N_2O	Isoflurane	Enflurane	Halothane	Desflurane	Sevoflurane
Molecular weight	44	184.5	184.5	197.4	168	218
Boiling point (°C)	−88.5	48.5	56.5	50.2	23.5	58.5
Specific gravity (25° C)	1.53*	1.5	1.52	1.86	1.45	1.50
Vapor pressure (20° C) (mm Hg)	38,770 (gas)	238	172	243	664	160
MAC (in O_2) (%)	105	1.28	1.58	0.75	4.6-6	1.71
MAC (in 70% N_2O) (%)	–	0.56	0.57	0.29		0.66
AD_{95}	–	1.68	1.88	0.90		2.07
MAC-awake (multiple)	0.6-0.8			0.52	0.53	
MAC as partial pressure (mm Hg)	800	9.7	12.0	5.7	34.9-45.6	13.0
Partition coefficients (37° C)						
Blood-gas	0.47	1.4	1.8	2.3	0.42	0.59
Brain-blood	1.1	2.6	1.4	2.9	1.3	1.7
Muscle-blood	1.2	4.0	1.7	3.5	2.0	3.1
Fat-blood	2.3	45	36	60	27	48
Rubber-gas	1.2	62	74	120	20	30
Flammability (in 70% N_2O/30% O_2) (%)		7	5.8	4.8	17	10
Stability						
Alkali	Stable	Stable	Stable	Some instability	Stable	Very unstable
Ultraviolet	Stable	Stable	Stable	Unstable		
Metal	Stable	Stable	Stable	Corrodes	Stable	Stable
Preservative	None	None	None	Thymol	None	None
Recovered as metabolites (%)	0.0	0.2	2.4	20		

*Specific gravity for N_2O is for the gas relative to air but for other anesthetics is for the liquid relative to water.
MAC, Minimum alveolar concentration; AD_{95}, anesthetic depth or the dose that prevents movement in 95% of subjects in response to standard surgical incision.

CHEMICAL PROPERTIES

The chemical structures necessary for anesthetic effects are widely different, suggesting that no one specific receptor or site for activity exists. The structure-function relationship is discussed in Chapter 49.

The chemical structure determines the stability of the molecule and its resistance to degradation by physical variables, such as heat, light, and materials it will contact in use, as well as its resistance to metabolic breakdown in the body and thus its potential for toxicity. The chemical structures of the inhaled anesthetics are diagrammed in Fig. 50-1. The agents are discussed separately.

Nitrous Oxide

N_2O is a simple linear compound that is highly stable and undergoes no degradation on exposure to the normal physical conditions in which it is used clinically, and it is not metabolized in the body. It is the only inorganic compound currently in use for anesthesia, although other inorganic substances also have anesthetic effects, notably nitrogen and certain noble gases at sufficient pressures. N_2O supports combustion almost as well as O_2, so that substituting N_2O for O_2 during electrocautery or laser surgery of the airway is not helpful in preventing ignition injuries.

The purity of N_2O is a major concern, and contaminants include other oxides of nitrogen (nitric oxide, nitrogen dioxide) that can cause damage because of production of free radicals in aqueous solution.[2] Strict manufacturing safeguards are necessary. Theoretically, N_2O can generate hydroxyl free radicals in the presence of gamma radiation in aqueous solution ($N_2O + e^- \rightarrow OH^. + OH^- + N_2$), but this is not a practical issue because of the small amount of N_2O in tissue at anesthetic partial pressures.[113] Waste N_2O from medical uses is only a small part of the total contribution from human activities to atmospheric N_2O; solar ultraviolet light interacts with N_2O and atomic O_2 to produce nitric oxide, which contributes to destruction of ozone.[68] Photodissociation of chlorine-containing anesthetics may also contribute to the burden of long-lived atmospheric ozone destructive compounds, but the fluoride-containing anesthetics may not since the active fluoride species are several orders of magnitude less effective at destroying ozone than the chlorides.

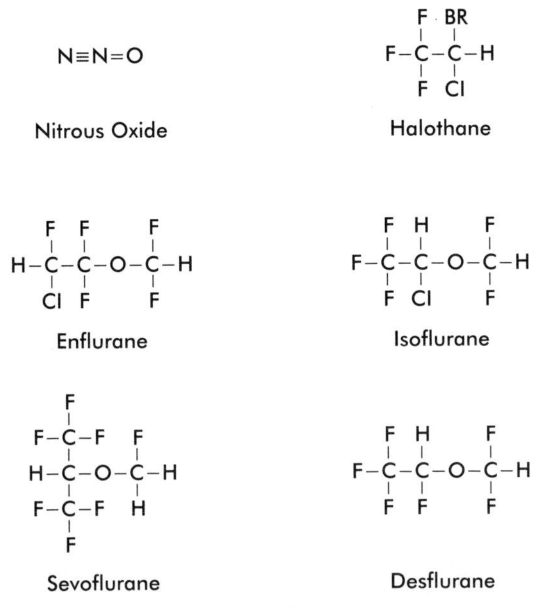

Halothane

Halothane is an alkane, a halogen-substituted ethane derivative that was introduced to clinical use in 1956. This molecule was an extraordinary improvement on the earlier ethers and alkanes with or without halogen substitutions and rapidly replaced other general anesthetic drugs. Chemical stability is greatly improved over the explosive gases, ether and cyclopropane; halothane is flammable but only at concentrations much greater than those used clinically (but that may be achieved within anesthetic machine piping). Halothane is also somewhat unstable in the presence of physical factors typically associated with anesthesia (see Table 50-1). Prolonged exposure corrodes metal and degrades some plastic parts of the anesthetic circuit. Halothane oxidizes spontaneously and is broken down by ultraviolet light so that 0.01% thymol is added to liquid halothane as a stabilizer. Isoflurane, enflurane, and desflurane are not so affected and do not require a stabilizer. Halothane is also adsorbed and broken down by contact with dry soda lime.[38] The effect is sufficient to slow induction; as the soda lime is humidified by use, halothane may be released, increasing inspired concentration.[39]

Two problems with halothane led to the introduction of enflurane and isoflurane after a systematic evaluation of the structure-activity characteristics of several anesthetic molecules. These were sensitization of the myocardium to dysrhythmias with use of the drug and the metabolism or biotransformation of halothane, which was thought to contribute to hepatotoxicity. These will be discussed in a following section.

Enflurane and Isoflurane

Alkanes induce cardiac toxicity because of sensitization of the myocardium to catecholamines. The introduction of the ether link in enflurane and

Fig. 50-1. Chemical structure of inhaled anesthetics. Note that isoflurane and enflurane are structural isomers.

isoflurane greatly reduced this tendency. The substitution of fluorine for chlorine and bromine increased stability while decreasing potency and solubility. Thus, in enflurane and isoflurane, undesirable characteristics have been greatly reduced or eliminated by the removal of bromide and the introduction of the ether link. Enflurane and isoflurane are isomers differing only in their structure; they have the same chemical formulas and thus the same molecular weight. However, their physical and pharmacologic properties differ in important ways.

Sevoflurane and Desflurane

The investigational anesthetics, sevoflurane and desflurane, carry these themes further. Thus the low solubility of both agents is desirable but at the expense of decreased potency; the potency of sevoflurane is increased by a bulky propyl side chain.

Substitution of fluoride for the chloride in isoflurane further enhances stability. Thus desflurane is currently the most stable of all the ether derivatives. Plasma fluoride is not increased measurably. Desflurane is also the least soluble of the currently available halogenated anesthetics.

PHYSICAL PROPERTIES

The physical properties of the inhalational agents, such as boiling point, vapor pressure, specific gravity, and molecular weight, determine the design requirements for precision vaporizers and affect other quantitative and economic concerns.

The boiling point of N_2O is $-88.5°$ C (see Table 50-1); therefore, it is a gas at room temperature. However, when compressed to 50 atmospheres (atm) (or 745 PSIG), N_2O is a liquid at room temperature and is supplied in cylindric steel tanks for clinical use. As the N_2O is used, the liquid vaporizes and the pressure remains nearly constant, until the tank is almost empty. The latent heat of vaporization cools the tank outlet valves and pressure gauges. This equipment is therefore designed to encourage diffusion of heat from the atmosphere to the sites of cooling to prevent malfunction.[84] Rapid emptying, which cools the remaining liquid, can severely reduce the pressure of an even almost full tank. The tank's weight rather than the pressure of its contents is the only reliable guide to how much of the liquid remains, although this measurement is impractical when the tank is in use. The temperature transition point felt on the outside of a vertical tank in use may allow gross estimates of filling. When flows of 6 L/min or more are used, the liquid may cool below the freezing point of water and frost may appear on the tank's outside surface below the liquid level; at $0°$ C the tank pressure will be 30 atm, (or about 450 PSIG).[54]

Desflurane poses a similar challenge to practical use. Because the boiling point is near room temperature, evaporative cooling quickly decreases vapor pressure and, therefore, the delivered partial pressure if a conventional apparatus is used.

Isoflurane, enflurane, and halothane are colorless liquids at room temperature. The saturated vapor pressure of isoflurane (see Table 50-1) at $20°$ C is 238 mm Hg. Therefore, if a flow of gas is directed through a chamber with wicks or baffles, arranged so as to allow saturation of the gas flow with isoflurane, the emerging gas and vapor mixture will have a partial pressure of 238 mm Hg of isoflurane, whereas the original inflowing gas will make up the remaining partial pressure to the total atmostpheric pressure (normally about 760 mm Hg at sea level). The concentration of isoflurane in the saturated gas mixture is therefore about 31% (i.e., 100 × [238/760]), a concentration that would be rapidly fatal if inhaled. A modern vaporizer for isoflurane is heavily constructed of metal to act as a source of the latent heat of vaporization as a small flow of gas is continuously saturated with anesthetic vapor.[20] In the earliest version of these vaporizers (e.g., Copper Kettle, Vernitrol) the desired concentration in the inspired gas mixture was achieved by adjusting a second (diluent) gas flow to mix with the saturated isoflurane gas flow, with manual adjustments for changes of saturated vapor pressure with temperature. These vaporizers were neither temperature nor flow compensated, and considerable possibilities for error occurred when these "measured flow" type of vaporizers were used. These vaporizers have been almost entirely replaced by "variable bypass" vaporizers (e.g., Dräger Vapor or Tec series) in which the desired concentration is achieved by simply turning a graduated dial (Fig. 50-2). The separation of gas flows to generate the correct output concentration, at the prevailing temperature and total gas flow, is incorporated in the engineering design of the vaporizer, which is thus automatically temperature and flow compensated (see Chapter 47 for a more complete description of apparatus).

Inhaled anesthetics may be quantified by partial pressure, with units of mm Hg, and by percent of the total gas volume. It is common practice to refer to anesthetic gas concentration in percentage units (e.g., the inspired concentration of isoflurane is 2%). However, as is emphasized in later sections of this chapter, the partial pressure of the anesthetic is a more fundamental measure. For example, at sea level with a normal barometric pressure of 760 mm Hg, a 2% concentration of isoflurane will contain a partial pressure of 15 mm Hg (0.02 × 760). However, in an operating room 6000 feet above sea level (e.g., just above that of Denver), the normal barometric pres-

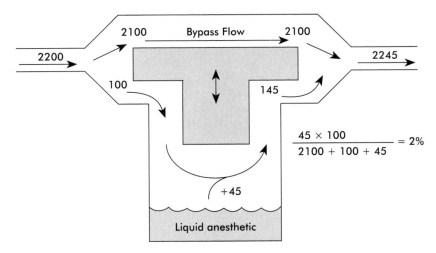

Fig. 50-2. Gas flows in variable bypass vaporizer for preparation of 2% isoflurane gas mixture. Splitting ratio for gas flows is 21:1 assuming constant temperature of 20° C. The gas flows in milliliters per minute are indicated by numbers in figures. (Diagram after style of Eisenkraft JB: Vaporizers and vaporization, *Prog Anesthesiol* 2 [24], 1989.)

sure is 609 mm Hg, and 2% isoflurane contains a partial pressure of only 12 mm Hg. For a variable bypass vaporizer set to 2% isoflurane, the constants are the saturated vapor pressure of isoflurane (238 mm Hg) and the gas dilution ratio of the vaporizer (21:1 for the ratio of diluent gas to gas flow entering the anesthetic chamber of an isoflurane vaporizer set to 2%), both of which are independent of barometric pressure. If the barometric pressure is 609 mm Hg, however, calculation of the actual volumes of gas leaving the vaporizer shows that the final concentration of the isoflurane will be 2.8% instead of the 2% set on the dial, and the partial pressure will be closer to 17 mm Hg instead of the 15 mm Hg obtained at sea level.

The saturated vapor pressure for enflurane is 172 mm Hg, and its saturated concentration is about 23%. The variable bypass vaporizer for this agent, therefore, has a slightly different dilution ratio but otherwise uses the same principles. Because the vapor pressure of halothane (243 mm Hg) is nearly that of isoflurane, the same partial pressure can be achieved with either agent in the same vaporizer. However, the safe partial pressures of these agents are different, and overdosage may occur with a vaporizer containing halothane that is thought to contain isoflurane. For this reason and for convenience and economy in the use of the agents, each of the volatile inhalational anesthetics is administered via a different vaporizer, labelled for use only with that agent.

More than one vaporizer is usually installed on a modern anesthesia apparatus, thus introducing the possibility of contamination of a vaporizer by anesthetic vapor of another type. Vaporizers are therefore interlocked to prevent simultaneous use. Some va-

porizers also include agent-specific filling devices to prevent contamination by the addition of the wrong agent to the vaporizer. The consequences of this type of error include both overdose and underdose, depending on the type of agent and type of vaporizer.

In the case of the isoflurane vaporizer accidentally misfilled with halothane, at sea level the bypass ratio is still 21:1 for a 2% setting. The vapor pressure for halothane is 243 mm Hg, and the delivered concentration is not greatly different from the dialed concentration, 2.1%; however, the effect of this dose of halothane will be much greater than the effect of what is thought to be 2% isoflurane.

A vaporizer used with halothane must be cleaned frequently because the stabilizing agent, thymol, necessary to prevent halothane breakdown, accumulates with time and forms a gummy deposit in the vaporizer that impairs its efficiency and is difficult to remove. The other volatile agents do not contain a stabilizing agent.

BIOPHYSICAL PROPERTIES

At induction with an inhaled anesthetic, the patient does not lose consciousness immediately, and consciousness does not return immediately when the anesthetic is discontinued. The explanation for this is found in the biophysical property of solubility in blood and body tissues, which determines uptake, distribution, and elimination characteristics. The pharmacokinetics of this process were first described by Kety in 1950.[58] The biophysical property of solubility also correlates with potency, which is discussed in the section on mechanism of anesthesia.

The aim in administering an inhalational anes-

thetic is to achieve a brain partial pressure sufficient to obtain the desired effect. Because the brain is a very well-perfused organ, the partial pressure of anesthetic in the arterial blood and that in the brain approach equilibrium quite rapidly. The exchange of anesthetic across the alveolar membranes is generally very efficient, so the arterial partial pressure of anesthetic is close to that in the alveolar gas, and the partial pressure of anesthetic in the brain will follow closely the alveolar partial pressure of that anesthetic. The problem in practice is to consider the factors determining the alveolar partial pressure.

The anesthesiologist must understand the principles of anesthetic gas uptake and distribution in order to understand and predict the effect of various physiologic and pathologic conditions on the rate of induction, rate of emergence, and depth of anesthesia for the particular agent in use. The anesthesiologist controls only the output of anesthetic gas by varying fresh gas flows and the dial setting on a vaporizer to cause changes in the partial pressure of anesthetic in the brain, but the relationship between the vaporizer setting and the effect on the brain is somewhat vague and may be confusing unless the pharmacokinetic principles are understood.

Many pharmacokinetic factors affect the distribution of a drug administered as an inhaled gas. The effect of the anesthetic is in the brain; thus the effective concentration of an anesthetic gas is related to the partial pressure of the gas in brain tissue. The anesthetic molecules must move from the anesthetic liquid in the vaporizer to the dissolved anesthetic in the brain. Within this path, several partial pressure gradients may exist that will influence the rate of delivery of anesthetic. It is useful to divide the path for uptake into three components: (1) delivery to the airways, (2) uptake into pulmonary capillary blood, and (3) uptake into tissue.

The difference in partial pressure between a gas phase (alveolar gas) and a liquid phase (blood) determines the movement of the anesthetic molecules between the phases. Because more anesthetic is in the gas phase initially, the net direction of movement is from the alveolar gas to the blood. As anesthetic accumulates in the blood, molecules begin to diffuse back from the blood into the alveolar gas as well. Eventually the rate of diffusion in both directions is equal, and the net exchange of anesthetic molecules is zero. This is the definition of equilibrium; in practice, however, this state is never achieved because the blood is also giving up molecules of anesthetic to other phases (tissues).

The partial pressure may be the best measure of concentration for describing diffusion and for expressing dosage and potency, but the solubilities as expressed by partition coefficients characteristic of

the individual anesthetic agents are independent of the partial pressure and are critically important in determining the uptake and distribution properties of each agent. The desire for inhalational anesthetics with low partition coefficients has driven the search for new agents beyond isoflurane and enflurane.

Partition Coefficients

The most basic and important concept is that the concentration of agent in gas or solution can be expressed as a partial pressure. Anesthetic gases conform very nearly to the ideal gas laws, so that fractional concentration:

$$C_{gas} = \frac{P_{gas}}{P_{total}} = \frac{V_{gas}}{V_{total}}$$

The second most important concept is stated by Henry's law: the amount of gas dissolved in a liquid is proportional to the partial pressure of the gas (this is certainly the case for the agents in current use, but not all gases conform because of the presence of saturable binding sites on hemoglobin or other molecules). More completely, the concentration of dissolved gas in a liquid is determined by the partial pressure, the solubility of the gas in that liquid, and the temperature. Solubility is usually expressed as the Ostwald solubility coefficient measured at a standard temperature, usually 37° C:

$$Ò = \frac{V_{gas\ dissolved}}{V_{liquid}}$$

Solubility is also expressed as a partition coefficient (λ), or the ratio of the solubilities for two media, such as in *blood-brain partition coefficient*, which describes the ratio of solubility of an agent for blood to that for brain. The solubility of anesthetics in the blood and tissues determines how much drug uptake is required to increase partial pressures to anesthetic levels in the brain and thus how long induction and emergence require.

A partition coefficient describes the ratio of concentrations at equilibrium of anesthetic in two different phases. For example, in a volume of blood in equilibrium with 2% enflurane at 37° C and an atmospheric pressure of 760 mm Hg, the concentration of enflurane in the gas phase is 2 ml of enflurane vapor/dl of gas (or 2 vol %) and the partial pressure of enflurane is $(760 - 47) \times 0.02 = 14.2$ mm Hg. The partial pressure in the liquid phase must also be 14.2 mm Hg. However, the volume of anesthetic vapor contained in the blood can be measured independently, and it is found to be 3.6 ml of enflurane/dl of blood or (3.6 vol %). At the same partial pressure the blood may contain 3.6 vol % enflurane, whereas the gas phase contains 2 vol %; this is expressed as the blood-gas partition coefficient ($3.6/2 = 1.8$). Blood-tissue coefficients may be measured and expressed in a similar manner (see Table 50-1).

Several points are critical to the practical use of inhalational anesthetics and all other gases and vapors. First, the net direction of exchange of gas molecules between any two phases is always directed from the phase with greater partial pressure to that with lesser. Second, the partial pressure in a nongas phase is always defined ultimately with reference to a gas phase. Third, the actual quantity or volume of anesthetic vapor that is contained in the nongas phase depends on the partial pressure and its solubility in that particular tissue.

Returning to the enflurane example, if the blood equilibrated with gas containing enflurane at 14.2 mm Hg is exposed to brain, muscle, and fat tissue until they also are in equilibrium (in practice this will never be achieved), then the entire system demonstrates no further net exchange between the phases, and the partial pressure throughout is 14.2 mm Hg. Measurement of the concentrations of enflurane in the different tissues shows that the brain, muscle, and fat, respectively, contain 1.4, 1.7, and 36 times greater volumes of enflurane vapor than does the same quantity of blood; these are the values of the brain-blood, muscle-blood, and fat-blood partition coefficients in Table 50-1. Compared with the gas phase, the blood, brain, muscle, and fat therefore contain 1.8, 2.5, 3.1, and 65 times more anesthetic in terms of volume of enflurane/volume of tissue, although the partial pressure of enflurane is the same (14.2 mm Hg) throughout. Before equilibrium (Fig. 50-3) enflurane moves from gas to blood, then to brain, muscle, and fat in the direction of least partial pressure, even though the concentrations in the brain, muscle, and fat soon exceed those in blood and gas.

The blood-gas partition coefficient is affected by a number of factors besides temperature; cellular and serum constituents are also known to affect solubility. Hematocrit increases enflurane solubility but decreases isoflurane solubility; the difference for isoflurane between plasma and red blood cells is as much as 20%. Other serum constituents are also important, particularly at low hematocrits. For aqueous solutions, increasing osmolarity of nonprotein constituents will decrease the isoflurane blood-gas partition coefficient slightly,[64] whereas lipids and protein, notably albumin, may increase the coefficient. Thus the blood-gas partition coefficients for all of the halogenated agents increase postprandially.[81]

Although the blood-gas partition coefficient for N_2O is the least among the inhalational agents, it is still 31 times greater than that of nitrogen. Any body cavities that contain gaseous nitrogen and are not open to the atmosphere will exchange nitrogen for N_2O in proportion to the partial pressure difference

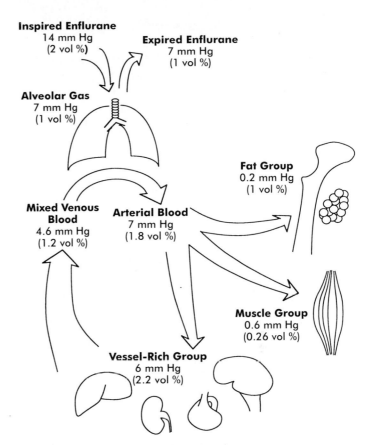

Fig. 50-3. Distribution of partial pressures (mm Hg) and concentration (vol %) for enflurane in body tissues calculated for 10 minutes after beginning ventilation with 2% enflurane in inspired gas. Figure illustrates that at this time alveolar gas concentration and partial pressure are about half that of inspired gas. Anesthetic flow is in direction of decreasing partial pressure, and this is indicated quantitatively by size and direction of arrows. The partial pressures show that the vessel-rich group of tissues is close to equilibrium with blood and the muscle and fat group are still far from equilibrium. Note that the concentration (vol %) of enflurane in tissues depends on partition coefficients and that anesthetic uptake continues into vessel-rich and fat groups, even though concentration (vol %) in fat group is already greater than that of blood.

between the gas and the blood phases. However, for an equal change in partial pressure, approximately a 30 times greater volume of N_2O will replace the nitrogen removed per unit of time, and therefore the body cavity will be greatly expanded. At equilibrium, when 80% N_2O is used, the maximum size increase of a gas bubble in blood would be fourfold larger than the initial size (Fig. 50-4).[26]

This phenomenon explains at least in part the distortion of hearing observed before loss of consciousness as N_2O enters the middle ear. The ear is a closed noncompliant space, and large pressures may be generated but are normally vented by patent ducts.

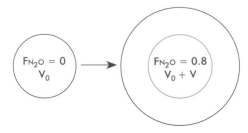

Fig. 50-4. Volume increase of air bubble in blood equilibrated with N_2O. Starting volume V_0 increases to $V_0 + V_{N_2O}$ at equilibrium (before nitrogen diffuses out). Fractional concentration of N_2O at equilibrium with blood is same in alveolar gas and inside bubble. Therefore:

$$F_{N_2O} = \frac{V_{N_2O}}{V_{N_2O} + V_0}$$

or, rearranging:

$$V_0 = \frac{V_{N_2O}(1 - F_{N_2O})}{F_{N_2O}}$$

The size change is:

$$\frac{V_{new}}{V_0} = \frac{V_0 + V_{N_2O}}{V_0}$$

Substituting V_0 from the second expression:

$$\frac{V_{new}}{V_0} = \frac{1}{1 - F_{N_2O}}$$

Thus, if 80% N_2O is being used ($F_{N_2O} = 0.8$), bubble volume increases fourfold.

Of greater significance, however, is the potential for complications to develop in patients with gas-filled cavities related to pathologic (e.g., bowel obstruction or rupture, pneumothorax, pneumopericardium) or therapeutic events (e.g., tympanic membrane closure, air injected for encephalography, sulfur hexafluoride for intraocular procedures). Air emboli will also expand rapidly and cause hemodynamic changes or death at three to four times smaller volumes than if N_2O was not used. The use of N_2O is contraindicated in such circumstances; other volatile agents will exchange in the same way, but the volume of the agents is too small to be of significance.

Uptake, Distribution, and Elimination

When the anesthetic vaporizer dial is set to the required percentage, the fresh gas flow will almost immediately contain the anesthetic vapor at the selected partial pressure, but the inspired gas partial pressure will take some time to approach this value. There are three reasons for this delay. First, the circuit itself contains a volume of gas that must be replaced by the fresh gas. The kinetics of transfer of fresh gas to a well-mixed circuit are described by a simple first-order rate equation for concentration:

$$C = C_0 (1 - e^{-T/\tau})$$

where τ is a time constant and C_0 the inspired concentration. In this case, since all the drug is in the gas phase, the concentration may also be expressed as partial pressure. The time constant for such a system can be calculated by dividing the gas volume of the circuit by the fresh gas inflow rate. If, as in Fig. 50-5, a circle system is used with a total gas volume of 8 L (reservoir bag = 3 L; CO_2 absorber = 3 L; anesthetic hose, connections, and valves = 2 L) and a fresh gas flow of 4 L/min, then the time constant is 2 minutes (8/4). The change of anesthetic concentration in the system is exponential, and at 1, 2, and 3 time constants the anesthetic will be 63%, 86.5%, and 95%, respectively, of the fresh gas flow value. Thus, with a dial setting of 2% enflurane, the concentration in the circle system will be about 1.26%, 1.73%, and 1.9% at 2, 4, and 6 minutes, respectively. The time constant can be reduced by increasing the gas flow rate, reducing the circuit volume by emptying the reservoir bag, or by "overpressure" with an initial concentration of anesthetic greater than that finally desired. At very high flows, the circuit gas does not mix with fresh gas but is exhausted through the "pop-off," so that the time constant is very small.

The "wash-in" of circuit gas to the patient's functional residual capacity (FRC) must also be included in the calculations. The result is not only an increased delay before alveolar gas achieves the inspired concentration, but also a delay in the circuit gas equilibration with fresh gas by the transport of agent to the lung volume. If mixing were similar to the circuit, the additional volume could be included in the calculation of the time constant for the circuit. In fact, the exchange of the lung volume with inspired gas is determined by respiratory rate and tidal volume, and the increase in concentration after several inspirations is determined by the initial inspired concentration and by the ratio between FRC and minute ventilation ($\dot{V}_A$) (Fig. 50-6). For practical purposes, the error between the extremes of four breaths/min and higher respiratory rates is minimal at one time constant (FRC/$\dot{V}_A$). The delay in achieving alveolar concentrations may thus be shortened by increasing $\dot{V}_A$. Lung gas concentrations during breath holding or coughing or when the airway is not secure will not rapidly approach inspired concentration.

A second factor that delays the rate of increase of the anesthetic concentration in the circuit is the high solubility of the anesthetic in some rubber and plastic materials. The rubber-gas solubility shown in Table 50-1 is sufficient to reduce initially the anesthetic concentration when inspiratory gas is in contact with hoses made of rubber. In addition, the CO_2 absorbent is known to adsorb anesthetic agents and to cause breakdown. This is generally most apparent at induction or during high fresh gas flow rates, when the absorber is dry. For isoflurane or

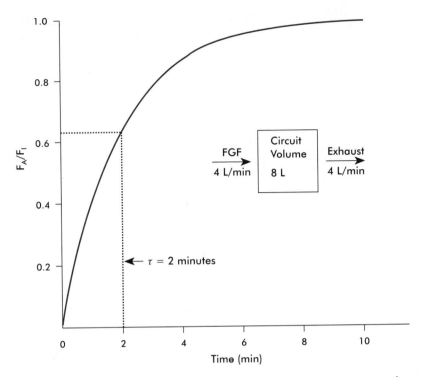

Fig. 50-5. Circuit gas concentration as fresh gas is added: one-compartment pharmacokinetic model. Circuit volume is 8 L, fresh gas flow *(FGF)* is 4 L/min, and mixing is complete. Excess gas is exhausted. Circuit concentration of anesthetic reaches 63% of fresh gas concentration at one time constant, or 2 minutes.

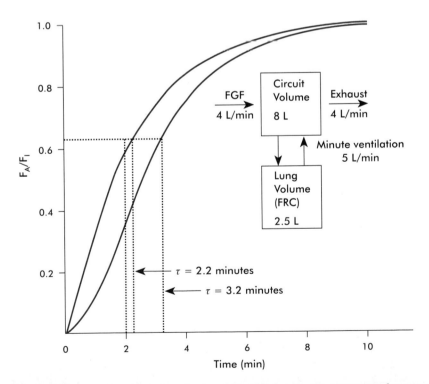

Fig. 50-6. Circuit gas concentration as fresh gas is added: two-compartment pharmacokinetic model. Lung with a functional residual capacity *(FRC)* of 2.5 L is ventilated at 5 L/min. Circuit gas concentration is slightly delayed compared with the first-order model, whereas lung concentration is further delayed by approximately one lung time constant $(FRC/\dot{V}_A)$, or 1 minute.

desflurane an additional 75 to 140 ml would be required to replace the adsorbed gas in a conventional apparatus.[66] For sevoflurane breakdown is significant and may be as high as 0.66 ml/min at 22° C at 2% concentration. Breakdown is accelerated at low flows because the absorber temperature is increased by the exothermic reaction between CO_2 and the absorbent.[109]

The third and most important factor in a circle system is the uptake of anesthetic by the patient. The anesthetic partial pressure in the expired limb of the circuit is less than in the inspired limb, and therefore the rate of rise of the circuit partial pressure toward the fresh gas partial pressure is slower and more complex than accounted for by a single exponential time constant.

The alveolar fractional concentration of anesthetic (FA_x) is determined by the balance of delivery (by ventilation, $\dot{V}_A$) of an inspired fractional concentration (FI_x) of anesthetic and the uptake by the blood ($\dot{V}_x$):

$$\frac{FA_x}{FI_x} = 1 - \frac{\dot{V}_x}{(FI_x \cdot \dot{V}_A)}$$

At induction, uptake is maximal, $\dot{V}_x$ is equal to delivered anesthetic ($\dot{V}_A \cdot FI_x$), so that FA/FI = 0. With long exposure time, uptake is minimal, and FA/FI approaches 1.

Uptake by the blood ($\dot{V}_x$) is determined by the blood:gas partition coefficient (λ), cardiac output ($\dot{Q}$), and the difference of anesthetic partial pressure between alveolar gas and mixed venous blood ($PA_x - P\bar{v}_x$), according to the Fick equation:

$$\dot{V}_x = \lambda \cdot \dot{Q} \cdot \left(\frac{PA_x - P\bar{v}_x}{P_B}\right)$$

where P_B is the barometric pressure.

The equations combine to the complete expression:

$$\frac{FA_x}{FI_x} = 1 - \lambda \left(\frac{1}{FI_x}\right) \left(\frac{\dot{Q}}{\dot{V}_A}\right) \left(\frac{PA_x - P\bar{v}_x}{P_B}\right)$$

This equation summarizes all the relationships discussed earlier that determine the curves of Fig. 50-7. **The approach of the alveolar and thus the brain partial pressure to that of the inspired gas is delayed by high solubility, increased cardiac output, or a large difference between the alveolar and the mixed venous partial pressures and is accelerated by increasing the inspired partial pressure of anesthetic or by increasing the alveolar ventilation.**

Initially, during induction, venous concentration is zero, and uptake will be maximal and proportional to solubility and cardiac output. If the substitution of $P\bar{v}_x = 0$ is made in the equation for uptake, one may derive a simpler relationship:

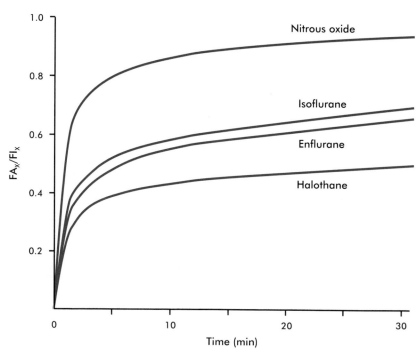

Fig. 50-7. Increase of alveolar fractional concentration *(FAₓ)* toward that of inspired concentration *(FIₓ)* with time is compared for different agents. Note more rapid rise for the less-soluble anesthetics. (Modified from Eger EI II: *Isoflurane [Forane],* ed 2, Madison, Wis, 1981, BOC Inc.)

$$\frac{FA_x}{FI_x} = \frac{1}{\left(1 + \dfrac{\dot{Q} \cdot \lambda}{\dot{V}_A}\right)}$$

The significance of this form of the uptake equation is that, for a given cardiac output and ventilation, FA/FI is determined solely by the agent's solubility. Thus, for halothane, with ($\lambda = 2.47$) and cardiac output equal to minute ventilation, the maximum alveolar concentration reached would be less than 29% of the inspired; thus, to achieve a minimum anesthetic concentration of 0.8% halothane, an inspired concentration of almost 2.8% would be required. For isoflurane, ($\lambda = 1.3$), alveolar gas would be 43% of inspired, and an inspired concentration of 2.5% would be required for anesthetic effect. For a less soluble gas, such as nitrous oxide ($\lambda = 0.47$), the alveolar concentration would be 68% of inspired; unfortunately, the inspired concentration cannot be increased to the desired 161%. FA/FI may also be increased by increasing the minute ventilation.

As the highly perfused tissues (brain, heart, liver, kidney) take up anesthetic, the venous blood partial pressure increases, uptake from the alveoli decreases, and alveolar partial pressure increases. Less-well-perfused tissues (muscle, skin) take up anesthetic more slowly, and the venous blood leaving these tissues is lower in partial pressure than for the well-perfused tissues. Finally, poorly perfused tissues

(bone, cartilage, fat) take up small quantities but do not greatly affect the initial rise in blood partial pressures (Fig. 50-8). The equations of tissue uptake are similar to the uptake from alveoli:

$$\dot{V}_{tissue} = \lambda_{tissue} \cdot \dot{Q}_{tissue} \cdot \left(\frac{Pa_x - P\bar{v}_{x_{tissue}}}{P_B}\right)$$

where the tissue solubilities and perfusions are estimated. For each tissue, the total anesthetic content may be determined assuming a uniformly perfused compartment and follows the equation for first-order kinetics of drug distribution. The mixed venous partial pressure is determined by summing the products of tissue perfusion and $Pv_{x_{tissue}}$.

Thus body composition will have an effect on the duration of induction, on the dose of anesthetic required to maintain anesthesia, and on the duration of the elimination phase during emergence, mainly by determining the partial pressure of anesthetic in mixed venous blood. Multicompartmental pharmacokinetic models thus describe the most important factors in the induction, maintenance, and elimination of the anesthetic drugs.

A major complicating factor is that one effect of anesthetics is to change both cardiac output and the distribution of perfusion to tissues, as well as ventilation, so that the uptake and elimination of tracer quantities will be different from the kinetics of

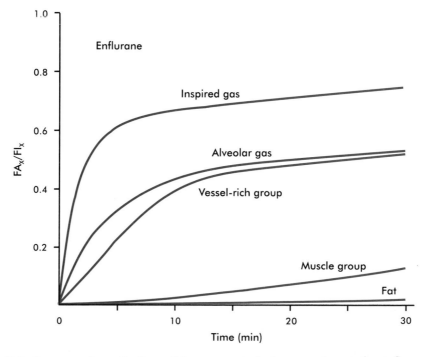

Fig. 50-8. Increase of anesthetic partial pressures in body compartments for enflurane. Vessel-rich group (which includes brain) lags behind alveolar concentration until about 10 minutes of administration. Muscle group lags substantially more, not reaching 10% of fresh gas concentration until 30 minutes.

clinically useful quantities of anesthetic. Thus the most accurate model of uptake and distribution would include physiologic parameters that depend on tissue concentrations.

Pathologic alterations in ventilation and circulation also affect uptake and elimination. The classification of pulmonary disorders into dead space and right-to-left shunt illustrates the problem. In the case of dead space, ventilation is "wasted," and no uptake from the affected alveoli occurs; thus during uptake, the measured alveolar partial pressure is greater than expected and arterial less than expected; the difference is larger for more-soluble anesthetics, and uptake is delayed. If arterial CO_2 partial pressure ($Paco_2$) is maintained by increasing total ventilation, however, no effect of dead space on uptake occurs, merely on the observed difference between arterial and end-tidal partial pressures. In the case of right-to-left shunt, the effect on uptake depends on anesthetic solubility; for poorly soluble anesthetics, uptake is delayed; for the more-soluble anesthetics, uptake is only slightly delayed.[108] In the nonhomogeneous lung with a broad ventilation/perfusion ($\dot{V}/\dot{Q}$) distribution, the effect is complex, but for the most part, uptake is delayed, and the difference between end-tidal and arterial concentrations is increased.

Left-to-right shunts are unlikely to affect uptake: total effective body perfusion does not change for small shunts (except for some congenital heart defects or maturing arteriovenous [AV] malformations). Although total cardiac output is increased, the mixed venous blood perfusing the lung cannot take up anesthetic any faster than determined by alveolar concentration. However, this type of shunt may reduce the effect of right-to-left shunt, since in this case the blood shunted from left to right is less saturated and can take up additional anesthetic.

At the end of an anesthetic, the inspired concentration is reduced to zero, but the patient does not awaken. The same principles are in effect as during induction, except that the rate of decrease of the anesthetic depends on the tissue saturation by anesthetic, which is more complete with longer duration of administration. If complete saturation (after infinitely long administration) and equilibration have occurred, the rate of decrease in alveolar concentration is equal to the rate of rise of anesthetic on induction. In reality, however, alveolar concentration (and arterial concentration) initially decreases rapidly to mixed venous levels (at a rate determined by the FRC/$\dot{V}_A$ ratio). Thereafter, the rate of decrease is determined by the same equation that determines uptake:

$$\frac{F\bar{v}_X - FA_X}{F\bar{v}_X} = \frac{1}{\left(1 + \dfrac{\dot{Q} \cdot \lambda}{\dot{V}_A}\right)}$$

Thus, after the initial rapid washout of the circuit and FRC, alveolar concentrations will be 71% of mixed-venous halothane concentration; 57% for isoflurane, and 32% for N_2O.

With time, tissue concentrations decrease, and mixed-venous concentration also decreases, at a rate determined by the relative perfusions, solubilities, and sizes of the tissue compartments, as well as by the difference between arterial and tissue partial pressures (which is determined by tissue saturation). Thus the washout of anesthetic depends greatly on the duration of administration as well as solubility.

The rate of induction may be increased by the use of overpressure; during elimination, the alveolar-to-expired concentration gradient is fixed by the mixed-venous partial pressure. Thus, awakening must be anticipated by discontinuation of inspired gas before the end of the procedure. Other mechanisms that may hasten elimination include increasing minute ventilation. For very soluble agents (e.g., ether, methoxyflurane), this will greatly decrease alveolar partial pressure but have no great effect on the washout from tissues. For poorly soluble agents (e.g., nitrous oxide), alveolar concentration will not decrease greatly. For agents of intermediate solubility (e.g., isoflurane), the effect is most pronounced for both alveolar concentration and tissue washout. The increase in ventilation, however, must not be so great that the decrease in $Paco_2$ causes cerebral vasoconstriction and slows brain washout.

An increase in cardiac output will delay the decrease in alveolar partial pressure but hasten tissue washout, again more for agents with intermediate solubilities. Both an increase in cardiac output and ventilation (common during recovery from painful procedures) do not initially change the rate of decrease of alveolar partial pressure. However, tissue washout is increased, and brain concentration will decrease rapidly.

Concentration-Related Effects

Two phenomena that substantially modify the pharmacokinetics of uptake are the concentration effect and the second gas effect. At low concentrations the alveolar gas concentration of the inspired agent is reduced in proportion to uptake.

When a high concentration of gas is administered, large volumes of gas are removed by alveolar uptake. Although N_2O is relatively insoluble, the use of high concentrations (typically 70% with the balance in O_2) means that large volumes of gas will be exchanged. Measured uptake in humans is 30 L, with almost complete arterial saturation within 20 minutes (Fig. 50-9).[96] Two phenomena may then occur. The first is an increase in inspired volume caused by continued negative inspiratory pressure at the end of inspiration,

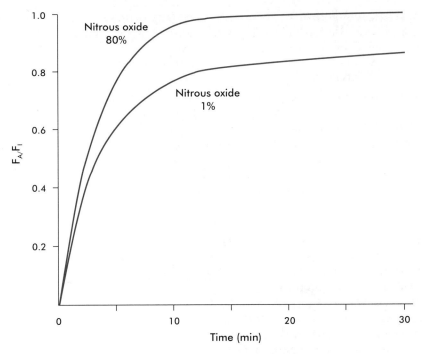

Fig. 50-9. Enhancement of alveolar concentration of N_2O by the concentration effect. At 80% inspired N_2O, uptake of large volumes of alveolar gas accelerate increase in alveolar gas to nearly that of inspired at 10 minutes; for 1% N_2O, FA/FI is less than 0.8 at 10 minutes and increases slowly thereafter.

as gas is taken up. The increased minute ventilation decreases the alveolar washin time constant (FRC/ $\dot{V}_A$).

The second effect is concentration of the anesthetic caused by the replacement of the absorbed gas with inspired gas enriched with respect to the absorbed gas. The result is that alveolar gas is reduced only slightly in concentration by uptake. At the extreme, when the administered gas concentration is 100% (safely achieved only with O_2), no change in concentration will occur. The result of both these phenomena is a marked increase in the rate that alveolar gas concentration approaches the inspired concentration.

The rapid uptake of large volumes of a gas such as N_2O may accelerate the rate of increase (wash-in) of alveolar concentration of a second gas administered along with N_2O. Replacement of the absorbed volume of N_2O will also replace the absorbed second gas, thus accelerating the rate of increase of the concentration of that gas.[30] However, complete replacement of volume may not occur in anesthetized patients; the FRC may be decreased as a result. This will increase the concentration of the remaining gases.[107] The relative contributions of the two phenomena are determined by the rate of uptake of the second gas. For very soluble gases, the residual gas in the lung will be almost depleted by uptake; thus there will be insignificant concentrating effect from lung volume

loss; thus enhancement of inspired ventilation is more important. For insoluble gases, the reverse is true.

The second gas effect also has implications for O_2 exchange. If a breath of 80% N_2O/20% O_2 is given and then held, the N_2O uptake is very rapid in comparison to O_2, so the alveolar O_2 tension (PAo_2) will actually rise during breath holding, in proportion to the decrease in lung volume.[46] In practice, however, Pao_2 may actually decrease, as the alveoli may collapse from the loss of FRC. This phenomenon is thought to occur during 100% O_2 breathing but occurs more rapidly when high concentrations of N_2O are inspired.

The reverse phenomenon, an increase in lung volume and expired minute ventilation during elimination of N_2O, also has implications for O_2 and CO_2 exchange. At the end of a period of equilibration with N_2O, a breath of room air is inspired (21% O_2/79% nitrogen). The mixed-venous blood continues to deliver N_2O to the alveoli, and excretion is proportional to cardiac output and N_2O tension. Thus the inspired O_2 and nitrogen are both diluted by the N_2O, and arterial concentrations of O_2 and CO_2 may be reduced. This phenomenon has been called *diffusion anoxia* and is maximal during the early phase of N_2O excretion, usually by 2 to 3 minutes after air breathing begins.[31] The effect is diminished by ensuring adequate and continued ventilation, but administration of 100% O_2 for several minutes, until the greatest volume of N_2O has been excreted, ensures adequate oxygenation. The effect of the diluted alveolar CO_2 may be to further depress ventilation.

Clinical Application of Pharmacokinetics

Uptake and elimination kinetics play an essential part in the administration of all inhalational agents. The precise formulations of the uptake equations are not as important as is the realization that the fresh gas, circuit, and inspired and end-tibal (or alveolar) partial pressures of the anesthetic differ systematically and that their relationship changes with time during induction and maintenance and is reversed during elimination. Thus, in practice, the delay in achieving the desired alveolar partial pressures must be anticipated by administering or discontinuing the anesthetic gases before a change in brain partial pressures is needed, as well as by manipulating fresh gas flows and circuit characteristics. The use of gas-measuring devices (e.g., mass spectrometer) to follow the end-expiratory partial pressures of the inhaled anesthetics are particularly helpful in understanding these phenomena.

The rate of uptake at the start of an anesthetic is so large that it is usual to increase the partial pressure of a volatile anesthetic in the inspired gas as rapidly as the patient will tolerate to a value several times the desired alveolar partial pressure. This technique of overpressure during the first few minutes thus compensates for the early rapid uptake and hastens the approach to the slower rising phase of the curves shown in Fig. 50-7.

It is important to realize that neither cardiac output nor total ventilation are constant during induction or maintenance. A surgical stimulus early in an anesthetic will increase cardiac output. This abruptly increases blood uptake and decreases alveolar and thus arterial and brain partial pressures. The patient will then react strongly unless the stimulus has been anticipated by the alert anesthesiologist by increasing either ventilation or inspired anesthetic partial pressure. Later, when mixed-venous partial pressures are increased, the effect of a change in cardiac output is less abrupt; a stimulus merely increases uptake slightly. The arousal then increases ventilation and thus delivery of anesthetic. An increase in inspired gas partial pressure at this point decreases ventilation and thus anesthetic delivery, so blood partial pressures change by only a small amount. This self-regulating behavior is the major advantage of spontaneous ventilation during the maintenance of anesthesia.

Later in the course of anesthesia, if the same inspired gas partial pressure is maintained, the alveolar and total body content of anesthetic will continue to increase, particularly in the muscle and fat

groups of tissues. This results in delayed awakening and increased metabolism as these tissues release their anesthetic back into the blood during postoperative recovery. The inspired partial pressure must be reduced with time according to the principles discussed here to maintain an appropriate brain partial pressure during the course of the anesthetic. The determination of that partial pressure is discussed in the next section.

Near the end of surgery the inspired anesthetic partial pressure is reduced to zero, and recovery from anesthesia commences. The elimination of the anesthetic follows the same principles discussed for uptake, but the elimination curves are not a mirror image of the uptake curves for two reasons. First, it is not possible to reduce the inspired partial pressure to less than zero, and therefore no comparable maneuver exists during recovery to that of overpressure during induction, whereby the elimination of anesthetic can be accelerated. Second, when the inspired anesthetic is discontinued, the first compartments from which the anesthetic is cleared are those of the vessel-rich tissues that are in equilibrium with the arterial blood. In contrast, the partition coefficient of fat is so great that at this time the tissue partial pressure of the anesthetic is still less than that of the arterial blood. These tissues continue to take up anesthetic from the blood even after the inspired anesthetic has been discontinued. This effect hastens the initial decrease and therefore awakening from anesthesia but also may delay the complete elimination of the drug for days.

GENERAL PHARMACOLOGIC PROPERTIES

The central nervous system (CNS) is the primary target organ for the inhalational anesthetics. The safety of these agents is related to the ratio of the dose of anesthetic required to produce anesthesia (loss of consciousness) to the dose required to produce effects on other systems, primarily the cardiovascular and respiratory systems.

Theory and Concepts of Anesthesia

The biophysical mechanisms of anesthesia are not well established (see Chapter 49), but a complete theory of anesthetic action requires knowledge of the neurophysiologic basis of consciousness and the action of anesthetics on neuronal functioning. Woodbridge[118] conceived that anesthesia included four components: hypnosis or amnesia, analgesia or absence of painful perceptions, absence of muscle movement, and absence of reflex responses to noxious stimuli. Not all components are required for every procedure for every patient, and some of these components may be provided by specific drugs.

However, the inhalational anesthetics are unique in their ability to provide all four of these components from a single drug.

Estimating Anesthetic Requirements

Historically, much attention was paid to physical signs that correlated with depth of anesthesia. Particularly with diethyl ether, a combination of respiratory, circulatory, pupillary, and reflex response signs allowed a reasonable prediction of when a patient was sufficiently anesthetized for surgery. The concept of estimating the anesthetic dosage ("depth") was introduced by Snow,[103] who divided ether anesthesia into stages, and Guedel,[42] who introduced the refinement of "planes" of anesthesia.

First stage is the time between first administration to the unanesthetized individual until the loss of consciousness; this stage may have enough associated analgesia that some surgical stimuli are painless, but the patient is conscious and may respond to a surgical stimulus. With the *second stage* the patient loses awareness and recall. Delirium and excitement occur, in which behavior is uncontrolled, often violent, with coughing and vomiting, hypertension and tachycardia, ending with the transition to the next stage if administration continues. The anesthesiologist's goal is to bring the patient through this stage as quickly as possible; in practice, a rapid induction with an IV agent is preferred instead of inhalational agent alone. The *third stage* is surgical anesthesia, with restored regular spontaneous respiration and normal vital signs. The eyelid reflex is suppressed, and spontaneous movement stops. The eyes may move and pupils are small. The third stage can be divided into "planes"; all the stages and planes are distinguished by certain outward signs, such as pupil size, patterns of respiration, and response to stimulation. In plane 1, respiration is full, both thoracic and diaphragm muscles act in synchrony; eyes may move, and pupils remain small. In plane 2, respiration begins to diminish; the eyes are in fixed midline position, and pupils begin to dilate; lacrimation may occur on entering this plane but decreases progressively. In plane 3, diaphragmatic movement continues but thoracic muscle contractions are diminished and delayed. The pupils continue to dilate. In plane 4, thoracic paralysis is complete, and diaphragmatic motion diminishes. *Fourth stage* is the deepest state, with cessation of spontaneous respiration, medullary cardiac reflexes, and possible death.

Although the modern description of anesthesia retains some of the language of Snow, many signs were specific to ether and have little use in gauging depth when modern agents are used. For example, when halothane, isoflurane, or enflurane are used, pupils are constricted and unresponsive to light over

the clinically useful range of doses. The rapidity of transitions with modern agents prevents the use of clinical signs as complete monitors of depth. The use of premedications and narcotics often interferes with pupillary signs, and muscle relaxants may abolish limb or respiratory movements so that circulatory and reflex responses are all that remain.

However, changes in respiration and circulation are still useful to judge the depth of anesthetic. Circulatory responses depend on individual anesthetic properties as well as the patient's physiologic state, and therefore the depth of anesthesia is primarily judged by experience and the individual response to surgical stimulation. It is appropriate for the depth of anesthesia to vary about a level that just abolishes the motor and autonomic response to surgery. In general an anesthetic administration that demonstrates no circulatory response to surgery (i.e., no changes in blood pressure or pulse rate) has probably used more anesthetic than is necessary. On the other hand, movement in response to incision is poorly received by the surgical team and may be dangerous to the patient, such as during neurosurgery or ophthalmic procedures. Not only is it necessary to progressively reduce the inspired partial pressure with time, as discussed in the preceding section, but it is also appropriate to change the anesthetic depth to match the surgical stimulation. Often the initial skin preparation and surgical incision and final skin closure are stronger stimuli than the procedure itself, and the depth should be adjusted to anticipate the periods of maximal and minimal stimulation.

Minimum Alveolar Concentration

The matching of anesthetic administration to the requirements of the patient, surgeon, and surgical procedure has been greatly assisted by the measure of potency represented by the MAC, introduced by Eger et al.[27] **MAC is the minimum alveolar concentration (in percent of atmospheric pressure) of anesthetic that prevents movement in 50% of subjects in response to a standard surgical incision.** Experimentally, MAC is established for each agent by maintaining a particular alveolar partial pressure for about 15 minutes to achieve near equilibrium with brain tissue and then instituting a painful stimulus (skin incision in humans) and recording whether or not movement occurs in response to the stimulus. The percent of the subjects moving is then plotted against the alveolar or end-tidal anesthetic concentration, and the 50% response rate is interpolated. The major advantage of the MAC concept is the relative constancy of the measure within a species. **In practice, a wide range of concentrations of anesthetic may actually be used, but MAC as a measure of dosage allows predictable**

administration and direct estimation of depth of anesthesia from measured gas concentrations in expired gas.

The values for MAC for each of the inhalational agents are listed in Table 50-1. When administered with O_2, the order of increasing potency is N_2O, desflurane, sevoflurane, enflurane, isoflurane, and halothane; the values vary from 105% with N_2O to 0.75% with halothane. By convention, the values are provided in terms of percent concentration of alveolar gas, but the relevant units are really partial pressure, and this should be considered whenever anesthesia is to be conducted under hyperbaric or hypobaric conditions.

Certain defined factors alter MAC. The MAC for halothane increases from 0.8% at birth to 1.08% at 6 months to 1 year of age, progressively decreasing until a slight increase at puberty, and steady decreasing thereafter (Fig. 50-10, *A*). With increasing age the MAC requirement is reduced by 40% by age 80.[37] The change with age is slightly less for enflurane, isoflurane, sevoflurane, and desflurane.[111]

Body temperature decreases MAC for halothane as much as 50% for each 10° C decrease (or about 5% for each degree; Fig. 50-10, *B*).[25] In pregnancy, MAC requirement is decreased by as much as 40%, a factor useful in reducing neonatal depression after cesarean section.[87] CNS stimulants and depressants such as amphetamines or alcohol moderately increase or decrease requirements. Other factors, such as gender, general health, obesity, duration of anesthesia, or hematocrit, do not affect MAC. The intensity of stimulus does not appear to change MAC once it is above a certain level.

The range of interindividual variability is small; within a species the standard deviation is 10% to 20%. In species other than humans, MAC may be quite different. For instance, in the dog the MAC for N_2O is 190% and in the mouse 225%, which are quite different from human values. For isoflurane the MAC in dogs is 1.39%, which is more similar to the human value.[57]

Extremes of physiology may affect MAC, probably because the CNS does not function properly under those conditions. Hypercarbia (Pco_2 greater than 100), hypoxia (Po_2 less than 40), CNS acidosis (cerebrospinal fluid [CSF] pH less than 7.0) and hypotension (blood pressure less than half normal) decrease MAC. In rats a circadian rhythm is known to affect the MAC for halothane by about 5% to 10%; whether this is true for humans is unknown. Tolerance is thought to occur to sedatives such as alcohol; tolerance may also exist to N_2O, but for the human CNS, no change appears to occur in MAC during prolonged anesthesia. However, the effect of these agents on other organ systems may change over time.

Genetic factors may affect MAC; certain breeds of mice may be less sensitive to N_2O.

Emergence occurs at a constant and predictable fraction of MAC, or "MAC-awake." For halothane, this is 59% of MAC, and for isoflurane, 29% of MAC, when slow washout is performed.[35] This explains some of the variability in time to recovery for the anesthetics. Despite the greater solubility of halothane, the recovery time of 9 minutes compares favorably with isoflurane at 15 minutes, the unexpected difference resulting from the smaller difference between MAC and MAC-awake for halothane. MAC-awake is not greatly affected by prior naracotic medication.[41]

MAC is analogous to any other effective dose for 50% of group (ED_{50}) value computed from a pharmacologic dose-response curve; what is unusual is the particular stimulus and the particular response. Once MAC was defined for the inhalational anesthetics, the influence of many factors that were known or hypothesized to influence anesthesia from empiric observations could be confirmed and tested. The effects of age, body temperature, pregnancy, drugs, and disease (Fig. 50-10) are important examples. Further, the potency of different inhalational agents and of combinations of anesthetics can be compared using the MAC concept. In general, a half MAC of each of two inhalational agents is equivalent to one MAC of either; not only does this observation have clinical use, but it also suggests that the fundamental mechanism by which these agents induce anesthesia is the same.

The MAC for N_2O is 105%. The alveolar partial pressure of N_2O alone must exceed the normal atmospheric pressure and is achievable only under hyperbaric conditions. However, the additivity of the anesthetic properties of the inhalational agents is used by employing a 70% mixture of N_2O in O_2 while adding a volatile agent to achieve the desired anesthetic effect. So common is this technique that Table 50-1 includes the MAC values for the volatile agents in the presence of 70% N_2O, which are appropriately reduced. Among the advantages of this combination are the reduced quantity of either agent that is required, the rapidity with which the N_2O partial pressure can be changed, and the reduced cardiovascular depression observed compared with use of a volatile agent alone.

The addition of other drugs to the inhalational anesthetic may have the effect of reducing MAC requirements. When adding inhaled anesthetics, the substitution is proportional, and total MAC is the sum of the individual MAC values (Fig. 50-10, *C*). Sedatives such as barbiturates and benzodiazepines contribute a real but limited MAC equivalent (Fig. 50-10, *D*).[89] Narcotics may contribute substantially to the MAC requirement,[44] but a "ceiling effect" pre-

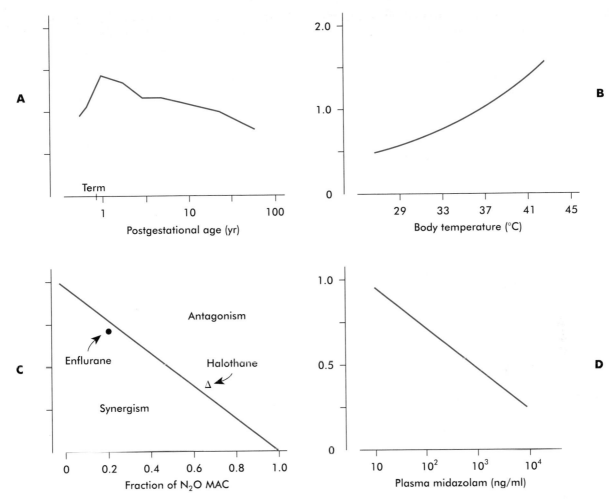

Fig. 50-10. Influence of age, body temperature, N_2O, and midazolam on minimum alveolar concentration (MAC). **A,** Change in relative MAC is shown as a function of age in years on a logarithmic scale. Soon after birth, MAC value is similar to that of young adults but increases to 1.4 times that value at 1 year. Thereafter MAC declines with age. **B,** Normal MAC value at 37° C is increased or decreased as a direct function of body temperature. **C,** Additive effect of halothane or enflurane MAC with MAC for N_2O is illustrated. **D,** Influence of increasing doses of midazolam, a common premedicant and anesthetic adjuvant agent, in MAC for enflurane. In *B* and *D* data are for dogs. (**A,** Data modified from Le Dez KM, Lerman J: The minimum alveolar concentration [MAC] of isoflurane in preterm neonates, *Anesthesiology* 67:301, 1987. **B,** Data from Steffey EP, Eger EI: Hyperthermia and halothane MAC in the dog, *Anesthesiology* 41:392, 1974. **C,** Modified from Torri G, Damia G, and Fabiani ML: Effect of nitrous oxide on the anesthetic requirement of enflurane, *Br J Anaesth* 46:468, 1974. **D,** Data from Hall RZ, Schwieger IM, and Hug CC: The anesthetic efficacy of midazolam in the enflurane-anesthetized dog, *Anesthesiology* 68:862, 1988.)

vents narcotics from being complete anesthetics.[82] Muscle relaxants are generally ineffective at replacing the inhaled agents; however, by preventing movement at marginal partial pressures of the inhaled anesthetic, they can be used to limit the dose requirement while improving surgical conditions. The MAC requirement may also decrease because of inhibition of muscle afferent stimulation. Acute amphetamine ingestion increases MAC in a dose-related fashion; chronic use decreases MAC, suggesting a role for

central catecholamines in modifying anesthetic effects.[53]

Because MAC is defined in terms of the most frequently used index of anesthetic depth (AD), response to a surgical incision, it is immediately useful as a guide to practical administration. It is not satisfactory to have 50% of patients moving during surgery, and usually 1.5 to 2.5 times the MAC is required to maintain anesthesia solely with an inhalational agent. Much higher partial pressures are required to suppress cardiovascular responses to the incision. Another measure of dose is the AD_{95} (AD_{50} corresponds to MAC), which may correspond better to the "clinical" dose of anesthetic. These are 0.90, 1.68, and 1.88% for halothane, isoflurane, and enflurane, respectively.[18]

MAC is not, however, a complete measure of anesthetic effect. MAC is a single point on a curved dose-response relationship, which also has parameters of slope, baseline, and maximal effect. It is also not a realistic dose because a 50% response rate is unacceptable in patients undergoing surgery. MAC is defined only for movement after a standard incision stimulus. An anesthetized patient typically responds to a stimulus by coughing, straining, or breathing deeply. A good anesthesiologist anticipates the response by increasing dose before the stimulus occurs. An increase in depth of respiration and in heart rate and blood pressure are normal with the incision and are used to estimate anesthetic depth. These secondary responses are usually suppressed at some multiple of MAC that is predictable for each agent. A measure of the dose required to suppress hemodynamic responses is "MAC-bar," or the anesthetic dose sufficient to block adrenergic response (norepinephrine blood concentration) to incision in half of patients.[92] This is 1.45 MAC for halothane, 1.60 MAC for enflurane, and 1.66 MAC for desflurane. MAC-bar may be reduced to a value less than MAC by the addition of other drugs, especially narcotics.[44]

MAC is usually stated in percent of atmospheric pressure. The partial pressure of the gas is the important variable. Thus, at high altitudes, a mixture containing 70% N_2O is not as potent as at sea level, nor is the 30% O_2 that makes up the remainder of the gas sufficient to ensure safety.

Finally, MAC is defined for an estimate of alveolar partial pressure of agent when the effective partial pressure is in the brain. Normally, alveolar gas is in equilibrium with arterial blood, which is nearly in equilibrium with well-perfused tissues. Disorders of the circulation or lung that alter gas exchange may also cause a discrepancy between alveolar and arterial anesthetic partial pressures.

Other monitors for anesthetic dose may be useful, such as the electroencephalogram (EEG). As the depth of anesthesia is increased with the inhalational agents, the electrical activity of the cerebral cortex slows with progressive replacement of fast low-voltage activity by slow waves of greater amplitude, and at very high doses of anesthetic, electrical silence occurs. Because of the complexity and detail of the EEG, several more concise indices of EEG activity have been developed.[65] These indices correlate well with anesthetic partial pressures in controlled experiments, but in clinical circumstances the interpretation

is often obscured by hypoxemia, cerebral ischemia, artifacts, and the effects of other drugs.[28] The EEG is therefore a useful indicator of change but cannot yet be used alone as a reliable index of anesthetic depth. Furthermore, the inhalational agents may interfere with the interpretation of the EEG during evoked potential monitoring.

Thus no single monitor of depth is sufficient, so the anesthesiologist must use judgment in interpreting all these indicators. Gas concentration monitors are helpful, but do not prevent relative overdose or underdose in certain populations. The correct dose is difficult to define but is determined by the balance between good surgical conditions and adverse pharmacologic effects. The correct dose is also constantly changing as the level of surgical stimulation changes during the course of a procedure.

Awareness During General Anesthesia

Published descriptions of the first demonstrations of anesthesia include accounts by the patient of awareness of the procedure or of apparent verbal responses by the patient without subsequent recall. As the specialty matured, the incidence of recall diminished, but later the practice of using paralytic agents prevented the assessment of dose by observation of movement. The problem of recall has become a primary concern for the practice of anesthesia; even with modern practice, the incidence of recall has not vanished. A recent retrospective analysis of the risk factors for awareness recommended that patients not be heavily dosed with relaxants and that the anesthesiologist pay close attention to physiologic signs of response to incision (e.g., sweating) to avoid recall.[43] However, biophysical and pharmacokinetic factors may contribute to the incidence of unanticipated awareness and may be understood from the principles presented in this chapter. For example, the incidence of recall was more frequent at high altitude; this is predictable if the administration of anesthetic is guided by percentage concentration rather than partial pressure. The onset of anesthesia with the inhalational agent is delayed by uptake, and therefore induction of anesthesia with IV agents of short duration may not allow enough uptake of inhalational agent to reach anesthetic concentration in the brain. Finally, the partial pressure of anesthetic in the alveolus is generally less than that delivered to the circuit; the difference may be exaggerated by gas exchange abnormalities or by increased uptake in certain patients.

PHARMACOLOGIC PROPERTIES

The inhaled anesthetics have pharmacologic properties that are primarily unique for the individual

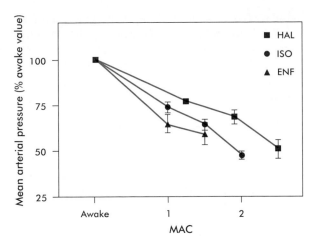

Fig. 50-11. Effects of halothane, isoflurane, or enflurane anesthesia on arterial blood pressure in humans. (Modified from data in Eger EI II: Isoflurane: a review, *Anesthesiology* 55:559, 1981.)

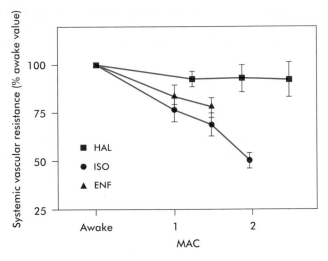

Fig. 50-12. Effects of halothane, isoflurane, or enflurane anesthesia on systemic vascular resistance in humans. (Modified from data in Calverley RK, Smith NT, Prys-Roberts C et al: Cardiovascular effects of enflurane anesthesia during controlled ventilation in man, *Anesth Analg* 57:619, 1978; Eger EI II, Smith NT, Stoelting RK et al: Cardiovascular effects of halothane in man, *Anesthesiology* 32:396, 1970; and Sonntag H, Donath U, Hillebrand W et al: Left ventricular function in conscious man and during halothane anesthesia, *Anesthesiology* 48:320, 1978.)

agents. However, at least some features are common among the potent halogenated hydrocarbons—halothane, enflurane, and isoflurane. Each is a respiratory depressant, as evidenced by depression of the ventilatory response to CO_2 (see Fig. 50-15), and each causes dose-dependent hypotension (Fig. 50-11). However, even among these structurally similar compounds, differences in the effect on organs, tissues, and physiologic functions exist. Further, the effects of these anesthetics are modified considerably by N_2O, an adjuvant frequently used to supplement the potent vapors. The adjuvant's purpose is to decrease the undesirable effects of those vapors on various physiologic functions. The use of N_2O in this way is so common that it seems appropriate to begin with a description of this adjuvant before describing the individual agents whose use N_2O frequently modifies.

Nitrous Oxide

N_2O is the first of the inhalational anesthetics, having been in use for more than 100 years. It is still probably the most often employed anesthetic primarily because of its adjuvant function. However, N_2O is rarely used as the sole anesthetic in modern anesthesia practice because it lacks the potency required to produce adequate anesthesia for most patients. As noted earlier, the MAC for N_2O is 105%, implying that it would need to be administered under hyperbaric conditions to produce adequate anesthesia. Rather, N_2O is usually administered as the inhalational component of "balanced" anesthesia (a misnomer that describes the combination of inhaled N_2O plus IV supplementation with narcotics, barbiturates, or propofol, often with the simultaneous administration of skeletal muscle relaxants.) Even in balanced anesthesia, the lack of N_2O potency occasionally

results in recall of intraoperative events, especially in those patients in whom muscle relaxants are used to produce skeletal muscle relaxation during the surgical procedure.

As noted, **the major use of N_2O is as a supplement to other inhalational or IV anesthetics. This use is based on the observations that (1) the contributions of each inhaled anesthetic in the breathing mixture are additive, and (2) the side effects of the potent vapors are dose dependent. Thus the goal is to administer a combination of inhaled anesthetics that will produce complete anesthesia while avoiding the arterial hypoxemia that might accompany "pure" N_2O anesthesia or the cardiovascular, pulmonary, and metabolic effects (among others) of anesthesia with the potent vapor only.** A common practice is to administer 70% N_2O in O_2, combined with a reduced concentration of the potent vapor. The increased inspired O_2 concentration ($FIO_2 = 0.3$) provides a margin of safety against arterial hypoxia, whereas the N_2O contributes approximately two thirds of the anesthetic requirement, allowing the potent vapor to be reduced to one third of that which would be required in the absence of N_2O.

Induction

N_2O is also often used to speed the induction of anesthesia produced by inhalational anesthetics. Because of its physical properties, both a second gas effect and a concentration effect (see previous section) enhance the uptake of the accompanying potent vapor. These physical properties of N_2O speed the induction of anesthesia during the initial few minutes of inhalation anesthesia and facilitate the smooth transition from awake to the anesthetized state.

Circulatory actions

N_2O tends to activate the sympathetic nervous system, an effect that is evident when it is administered in combination with other potent vapors or with IV narcotics. N_2O-halothane anesthesia, compared with halothane only, results in small but measurable increases in cardiac output and arterial blood pressure.[51] Similar but less marked effects are seen when N_2O is added to enflurane or isoflurane anesthesia.

N_2O also alters the hemodynamic response to narcotic anesthesia. Compared with IV morphine only, the addition of N_2O causes increased systemic vascular resistance (SVR) and decreased cardiac output in humans, although arterial pressure remains essentially unchanged.[117]

Each of these responses likely results from the actions of N_2O on the sympathetic nervous system. In cats, N_2O increased the neuronal firing rates in preganglionic sympathetic nerves,[34] an effect consistent with the increase in circulating norepinephrine seen with N_2O inhalation in humans.[102] Vasoconstriction also occurs in the renal and splanchnic vasculature of animals when N_2O is added to halothane anesthesia.[97] Together, these data imply that N_2O activates the sympathetic nervous system by a yet undefined mechanism, and the combination of sympathetic activation from N_2O combined with the decreased requirement for potent vapors, which are associated with greater cardiovascular depression, results in considerably less hypotension than might be expected in patients under anesthesia produced with equipotent concentrations of the potent vapors only.

Respiratory actions

Compared with the potent vapors, the actions of N_2O on respiration are relatively minor. N_2O reduces the ventilatory drive to hypoxia[119] but has little effect on the response to CO_2 except when N_2O is added to the potent vapors, when it contributes to additional respiratory depression.[51]

Actions on brain and central nervous system

The actions of N_2O on the cerebral vasculature remain somewhat controversial. In animals the addition of N_2O to a background of halothane anesthesia causes a decrease in cerebrovascular resistance and a consequent increase in cerebral blood flow.[97] Similar but less consistent effects have been observed in humans, leading some to be cautious about the use of

this anesthetic in patients with decreased intracerebral compliance (e.g., from tumor or hematoma).[47,90] However, the cerebrovascular response to CO_2 remains intact during N_2O administration, and autoregulation of cerebral blood flow is maintained in the presence of nitrous oxide as well.[116]

Actions on other organs

N_2O has little effect on hepatic or gastrointestinal (GI) function or on the function of most other organs, including muscles. N_2O does not produce skeletal muscle relaxation itself, and it does not potentiate the actions of the muscle relaxants significantly.

Biotransformation

N_2O appears to be eliminated almost entirely by pulmonary ventilation, although small but measurable amounts diffuse out through the skin as well. Little evidence suggests that significant amounts are biotransformed during or after typical exposures for clinical anesthesia.

Emergence

Just as the physical properties of N_2O (relative insolubility) result in rapid uptake of the drug during induction of anesthesia, the reverse (rapid elimination from the lungs) occurs when N_2O is discontinued. If N_2O is suddenly discontinued and the patient is allowed to breath room air immediately, the movement of large volumes of N_2O from the blood into the alveoli can result in transient hypoxemia, termed *diffusional anoxia.*[31] Diffusional anoxia or hypoxemia can be avoided by the administration of supplemental O_2 during the initial minutes after N_2O breathing has ceased.

Complications

N_2O is approximately 30 times more soluble in blood than nitrogen, and N_2O readily exchanges with the nitrogen that may be present in gas-containing structures in the body (see section on partition coefficients). If sufficient space exists, the gas-containing cavity will expand considerably in the presence of N_2O. The expansion of a pneumothorax or of the gas contained in obstructed bowel during N_2O breathing are typical examples of this physical phenomenon. When insufficient space exists for expansion because of the volume of N_2O, the pressure in the closed cavity may greatly increase. This can occur in the cranial vault after pneumoencephalography or when pneumocephalus is present after trauma or surgery.

Bone marrow depression occurs during the prolonged administration of N_2O to animals,[62] and anemia may result. N_2O inhibits the actions of methionine synthetase, an enzyme involved in vitamin

B_{12} metabolism, leading to impaired bone marrow function.[17] Although theoretic concerns have been expressed about the actions of N_2O on the hemopoietic system, little evidence suggests that this is a problem during the limited exposure typical of most procedures, and considerable practical experience indicates that the concern is unfounded under all but the most unusual circumstances.[24]

The effects of long-term repeated exposure to N_2O, as might occur among operating room personnel, are of greater concern. A neuropathy that resembles that of vitamin B_{12} deficiency has been reported in dentists who use N_2O regularly in their practice[63]; this effect is presumed to result from the combination of N_2O's actions on methionine synthetase and the chronic exposure to unusually high N_2O concentrations as the physician works in the oral cavity, near the source of atmospheric pollution with N_2O, which is often administered by a small nasal mask.

Halothane

Although halothane (1,1,1-trifluoro-2-bromo-2-chloroethane) is today used less frequently in the United States than it was previously, its pharmacologic properties are important because it was the first in a series of short-chain halogenated alkanes or ethers that are the backbone of modern anesthesia practice.

Halothane had profound effects on the practice of anesthesia and surgery after it was introduced into clinical practice in 1956. Unlike cyclopropane or diethyl ether, halothane was not flammable in clinical concentrations, thus allowing the use of electrocautery for the surgeon and the introduction of extensive electronic monitoring for the anesthesiologist. Unlike ether, halothane produced rapid induction and emergence from anesthesia and permitted rapid changes in anesthetic depth with ease. However, its potency and marked dose-dependent circulatory depression, especially compared with diethyl ether, required increased precision for safe administration and increased vigilance to prevent respiratory and circulatory collapse. Although it is now used less frequently in adults, halothane remains popular for anesthesia in pediatric patients.

Induction

Halothane's potency and lack of airway irritation result in rapid, smooth induction of anesthesia by inhalation only, especially when it is administered in combination with 60% to 70% N_2O to speed induction further. In children, this combination is often continued for maintenance of anesthesia, whereas in adult patients it is common to replace halothane with one of the newer halogenated hydrocarbons after inhalation induction of anesthesia.

Circulatory actions

The most prominent circulatory effect of halothane is dose-dependent arterial hypotension (see Fig. 50-11). Although halothane dilates cutaneous arteries and veins and thus leaves a visual impression that implies significant vasodilation, the overall effect on SVR is relatively minor even at deep levels of halothane anesthesia (Fig. 50-12); in essence, the decrease in blood pressure results from an associated decrease in cardiac output[23] **(Fig. 50-13).** Unlike N_2O, halothane anesthesia does not stimulate the sympathetic nervous system, and the cardiodepressant effects remain

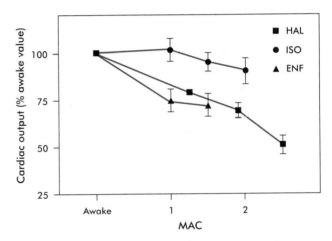

Fig. 50-13. Effects of halothane, isoflurane, or enflurane anesthesia on cardiac output in humans. (Modified from data in Eger EI II: Isoflurane: a review, *Anesthesiology* 55:559, 1981.)

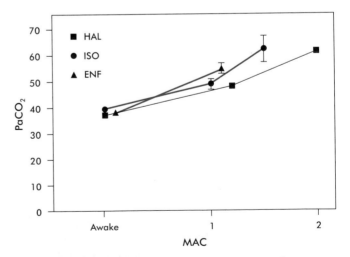

Fig. 50-14. Effects of halothane, isoflurane, or enflurane anesthesia on arterial carbon dioxide tension in humans. (Modified from data in Eger EI II: Isoflurane: a review, *Anesthesiology* 55:559, 1981.)

relatively unopposed. Rather remarkable hypotension can result in the absence of surgical stimulation. Surgical stimulation activates sympathoadrenal responses (both adrenal medullary and cortical) during halothane anesthesia and blunts the magnitude of the hypotension, at least during light or moderate levels of anesthesia.

An associated decrease in coronary blood flow accompanies halothane anesthesia, but anaerobic metabolism does not occur.[80,104] The decrease in coronary blood flow appears to be a response to the decreased O_2 requirement of the myocardium as myocardial work is decreased (both systemic flow and arterial pressure are reduced), not a cause for the decline in cardiac output.

Halothane's negative inotropic actions appear to result from alterations in intracellular calcium mechanisms that affect the contractile function of actomyosin, not from the drug's direct actions on contractile proteins or muscle per se. Decreased influx through the calcium slow channel,[71] increased binding by plasma membranes,[94] and decreased uptake of calcium by the sarcoplasmic reticulum[52] all act to inhibit intracellular calcium flux, leading to decreased cardiac output.

Cardiac rate and rhythm may be altered by halothane anesthesia as well. The usual effect is a slight decrease in cardiac rate, resulting from multiple sites of action on both pacemaker cells and the His-Purkinje system[1], and from apparent increases in vagal activity. Slow nodal rhythms with unsynchronized atrial contraction are not unusual during halothane anesthesia. These effects are usually reversible by pharmacologic blockade of vagal activity by atropine. Increasing the heart rate by this mechanism is a relatively common method to counter the hypotension associated with halothane anesthesia in patients not receiving beta-adrenergic blocking drugs for associated medical conditions, such as coronary artery disease.

Tachydysrhythmias may occur during halothane anesthesia, especially with an associated increase in circulating catecholamines. **Ventricular ectopy during halothane anesthesia resulting from beta-adrenergic stimulation occurs when exogenous epinephrine is administered in doses that would have no effect on cardiac rhythm in awake patients.**[56] The guidelines for the safe administration of epinephrine during halothane anesthesia require that no more than 100 μg in 10 minutes or 300 μg/hour be administered in adults. Children tolerate much greater doses of epinephrine during halothane anesthesia, although the mechanisms for this difference are not defined.[55]

Organ blood flows are altered considerably by halothane anesthesia.[98] Although effects can be observed in almost every organ, the principal responses occur in the cerebral, coronary (discussed earlier), cutaneous, renal, and hepatic circulations.

Cerebral vasodilation occurs in response to halothane, resulting in increases in cerebral blood flow despite the decrease in cardiac output.[101] The cerebral vasculature remains responsive to CO_2, and thus cerebral vasodilation can be at least partly prevented by hyperventilation before and during halothane anesthesia. Nevertheless, **the potential increase in intracranial pressure (ICP) that accompanies dilatation of the cerebral vasculature limits the use of the drug in patients with space-occupying lesions of the intracranial cavity, such as tumors or hematoma.**

Halothane causes marked dose-dependent vasodilation of the cutaneous vasculature, leading to decreased vascular resistance (arteriolar dilatation) and increased vascular capacitance (venular dilatation) in the skin circulation.[69,98] The increase in skin blood flow is so significant that venous blood samples from cutaneous veins accurately reflect arterial pH and Pco_2 during halothane anesthesia.[115] The same effect is seen during isoflurane or enflurane anesthesia.

Halothane anesthesia causes a significant (30% to 40%) decrease in renal blood flow, an effect that results from decreased perfusion pressure rather than increased renal vascular resistance.[77] An associated decrease occurs in urine volume and glomerular filtration, both of which are promptly reversible when halothane is discontinued.

Halothane has important actions on the splanchnic circulation, leading to decreased total hepatic blood flow.[98] **Portal venous flow is decreased in response to decreased blood flow in the GI viscera, and this is accompanied by hepatic arterial vasoconstriction as well. In contrast to other potent halogenated anesthetics, halothane abolishes the normal reciprocal relationship between portal venous and hepatic arterial flows, leading to the possibility for tissue ischemia and cellular hypoxia in the liver.**[98] Whether these alterations in hepatic circulation contribute to any of the hepatic complications associated with halothane remains unknown, but experimental evidence suggests that arterial hypoxemia (and thus tissue hypoxia) contributes to the development of hepatic dysfunction after halothane administration to animals.[78]

Respiratory actions

Alveolar hypoventilation and arterial hypercarbia occur in a dose-dependent manner when halothane anesthesia is administered with spontaneous respiration (Fig. 50-14). Halothane also causes an increased gradient for O_2 between the alveoli and the blood (A-a gradient), indicating that O_2 transfer is impaired. Although the effect on respiratory drive is less prominent during surgical stimulation, ventilation is usually assisted or controlled during anesthesia, and the O_2 concentration in the inspired gas is usually increased to at least 30% to counter the actions of halothane on respiratory drive and O_2 exchange.

The respiratory depression associated with halothane is characterized by rapid shallow respirations, leading to arterial hypercarbia as the tidal volume tends to decrease toward the dead space volume. In awake humans, this effect would be countered by the increased ventilatory drive associated with acute hypercarbia, but this response is blunted in a dose-dependent manner by halothane.[60] The ventilatory response to hypoxemia is abolished by halothane anesthesia as well.[60] Halothane impairs the central neural control of respiration, but the dominant effect appears to be related to alterations in the ventilatory response to CO_2.[88] Together, it is evident that many of the control mechanisms that regulate ventilatory drive are no longer active during halothane anesthesia. The effect of deep halothane anesthesia can be devastating during spontaneous ventilation since the combination of progressive hypoventilation and impaired O_2 transfer, combined with blunted (or absent) responses to CO_2 and O_2, can lead to hypoxemia and profound hypercarbia.

Actions on brain and central nervous system

Halothane anesthesia, compared with the awake state, produces slowing and increased amplitude of the EEG, although these effects are countered to some extent by surgical stimulation, which tends to partially restore the faster components, especially during light levels of anesthesia.[5] Cerebral metabolism decreases in a dose-dependent manner in response to halothane, and a relative excess of perfusion exists to meet the brain's metabolic demands during anesthesia with this drug.[101]

Actions on other organs

Halothane does not depress the skeletal muscle (twitch) response to electrical stimulation of motor nerves. However, it potentiates the actions of non-depolarizing relaxants, such as pancuronium or *d*-tubocurarine, moderately. However, this effect is more pronounced with enflurane or isoflurane. Uterine smooth muscle relaxation occurs in response to clinical doses of halothane, an effect that can be either beneficial or detrimental depending on the circumstances. Uterine relaxation can assist the operator when version of the fetus is required during delivery, but uterine relaxation also can contribute to inadequate uterine tone and resultant hemorrhage after delivery.

Biotransformation

The major route of elimination of halothane is through the lungs, but a significant amount (10% to 20%) is biotransformed in the liver; small amounts diffuse out through the skin as well. Hepatic biotransformation occurs through the cytochrome P_{450} system, resulting in the release of bromide and chloride ions and the formation of fluorine-containing compounds, mostly trifluoroacetic acid.[95] Many believe that the hepatic complications (see later discussion) associated with halothane result from its considerable biotransformation.

Emergence

Awakening after halothane anesthesia is generally quite prompt, although patients often remain groggy for several hours. This may result from the combined residual effect of the anesthetic plus the actions of barbiturates, narcotics, and benzodiazepines often administered as part of modern anesthetic care. Although bromine is released during biotransformation, it appears not to contribute significantly to delayed emergence or prolonged lethargy in most patients who receive moderate doses (and durations) of halothane anesthesia.[112]

Nausea and vomiting may occur in the early postanesthesia interval, but these are greatly reduced with halothane compared with the earlier inhalation anesthetics, such as dimethyl ether. Although a common (and unfortunate) tendency exists to attribute postoperative nausea and vomiting to the anesthetic, it is apparent that these events are often not caused by the anesthetic per se. The incidence of postoperative nausea and vomiting depends on a variety of factors, including gender, surgical site, associated use of N_2O, and administration of narcotics perioperatively.

Complications

Reversible events comprise the most frequent complications associated with halothane. These include hypotension, respiratory depression, alterations in cardiac rhythm, and sensitivity of the myocardium to catecholamines. A much more dramatic and serious complication involves hepatic dysfunction after halothane administration.

Data from the National Halothane Study[8] indicate that a rare but real incidence of severe hepatic dysfunction, even hepatic necrosis, is associated with halothane anesthesia. A typical response involves anorexia, lethargy, low-grade fever, eosinophilia, and biochemical evidence (bilirubin and hepatic enzyme abnormalities) of hepatic dysfunction. Often, other factors, such as previous drug therapy or blood transfusion, confound the diagnosis. A metabolite capable of activating an immune response may be present.[106] Although the incidence is low (approximately 1 in 10,000 halothane anesthetics in adults, but much less frequently in children), the death rate is reported to be approximately 50% with the severe syndrome. The threat of hepatic dysfunction is perhaps the major factor that has led to the decreasing use of halothane for anesthesia in adults. **The severe response occurs more often after repeated exposures to halothane and is frequently associated with obesity or episodes of intraoperative hypotension. The precise etiology remains uncertain but is presumed to be related to the metabolic products of the biotransformation of halothane, leading to immunologically mediated hepatic necrosis, which is perhaps enhanced by cellular hypoxia from decreased hepatic perfusion.**

Isoflurane

Isoflurane (1-chloro-2,2,2-trifluoroethyl difluoromethyl ether) is a potent and relatively insoluble halocarbon anesthetic that is often used for inhalation anesthesia in the United States. It is an isomer of enflurane but it has many unique pharmacologic properties. As with enflurane, isoflurane is not flammable and is stable in anesthetic vaporizers and anesthetic delivery circuits. It has gained great popularity for a variety of reasons, including the virtual absence of serious hepatic toxicity, minimal biotransformation, and ease of administration.

Induction

The combination of relatively low solubility and considerable potency results in rapid induction by inhalation of isoflurane. Although it does not stimulate tracheobronchial secretions or activate airway reflexes, some patients complain that isoflurane produces a "burning" sensation in the airway if high concentrations are administered rapidly. Many anesthesiologists prefer to induce anesthesia with halothane and then switch promptly to the inhalation of isoflurane for maintenance of anesthesia if an inhalation induction is planned. As with the other inhalational agents, IV induction with an ultrashort-acting barbiturate obviates any of these issues, and both patients and practitioners usually prefer this approach because it provides a rapid, smooth onset of anesthesia.

Circulatory actions

Progressive dose-related hypotension accompanies isoflurane anesthesia; the magnitude of the effect is similar to that seen during halothane anesthesia[23]

(see Fig. 50-11), although the hemodynamic mechanisms responsible for the hypotension are unique to this drug.

In contrast with halothane or enflurane, isoflurane anesthesia is characterized by well-maintained cardiac output, even during moderately deep anesthesia[23] (see Fig. 50-13). Although decreased contractile force is observed in the isolated heart exposed to isoflurane, this effect is not prominent in intact humans or animals.

Isoflurane produces dose-dependent decreases in systemic vascular resistance, and this peripheral circulatory effect is almost entirely responsible for the hypotension that occurs during light-to-moderate levels of isoflurane anesthesia.

Coronary arteries dilate during isoflurane anesthesia, and coronary blood flow is usually greater with this drug than with other potent anesthetics.[98] This would suggest initially that isoflurane has salutary effects on the coronary circulation, although the interpretation of these hemodynamic effects is clouded somewhat by other factors. First, the increased coronary blood flow may be a response to the increased myocardial work associated with the greater cardiac output that occurs with this drug compared with the other potent vapors. Second, theoretic concerns exist that the coronary vasodilation that accompanies isoflurane could result in a coronary "steal" phenomenon, similar to that observed with the vasodilator, sodium nitroprusside, in patients with coronary vascular architecture that facilitates coronary "steal." It is estimated that approximately 25% of patients with significant coronary artery disease have areas of myocardium that depend on blood flow through collateral vessels for

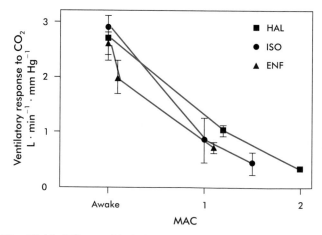

Fig. 50-15. Effects of halothane, isoflurane, or enflurane anesthesia on the ventilatory response to carbon dioxide challenge in humans. (Modified from data in Eger EI II: Isoflurane: a review, *Anesthesiology* 55:559, 1981.)

blood supply.[6] Preferential dilatation of normal vessels could divert ("steal") blood away from these collaterals, leading to ischemia in the collateral-dependent region. The possibility of this phenomenon has been demonstrated in animals,[7] and myocardial ischemia during isoflurane anesthesia (which resolved when halothane was substituted to continue anesthesia) has been reported in isolated cases.[40] However, vast experience exists in patients with ischemic heart disease who receive isoflurane anesthesia for myocardial revascularization procedures; the clinical experience and the investigative evidence[99] suggest that isoflurane is as safe as other anesthetics under these circumstances. (However, these patients almost routinely receive beta-adrenergic blockers that prevent the tachycardia typically observed during isoflurane anesthesia in patients not receiving these medications, so the results in cardiac surgical patients do not translate easily to the general population.)

Tachycardia frequently occurs during isoflurane anesthesia.[105] It appears to be more common in younger patients and may be quite pronounced (heart rate greater than 100) when isoflurane is accompanied by other drugs, such as pancuronium, that also increase heart rate. Abnormalities of cardiac rhythm infrequently occur with isoflurane, and exogenous epinephrine is well tolerated during anesthesia with this drug.

Cerebral blood flow increases and the cerebral vasculature dilates in response to isoflurane. Most available evidence suggests that the extent of these effects is less with isoflurane than with halothane,[29] although some recent studies suggest that the effects may be quite similar.[98]

Cutaneous blood flow is increased considerably with isoflurane, as it is with halothane or enflurane.[98,105] This appears to be a common response to anesthesia with each of the potent vapors, although details of the mechanism for this response have not been determined.

Renal blood flow is decreased by isoflurane, primarily because of decreased perfusion pressure rather than changes in regional vascular resistance.[75]

Total hepatic blood flow is decreased by isoflurane, but the extent of this response is less than that with halothane or enflurane anesthesia.[98] **Hepatic O_2 transport, hepatic oxygenation, and hepatic arterial compensation for decreased portal venous flow (reciprocity of hepatic blood flow) all appear to be better maintained during isoflurane than during enflurane or halothane anesthesia.**[13,36,98]

Respiratory actions

As with the other potent vapors, isoflurane impairs both ventilatory drive and O_2 transport from the alveoli to the arterial blood, leading, in particular, to hypercarbia during anesthesia (see Fig. 50-14). The ventilatory responses to both hypoxemia and hypercarbia are depressed by isoflurane, perhaps to a greater extent than seen with the other potent vapors.[49] Isoflurane causes bronchodilatation and inhibits bronchoconstriction, a common effect among the potent vapors.[48]

Alterations in pulmonary mechanics (decreased pulmonary compliance and decreased FRC), combined with impairment of hypoxic pulmonary vasoconstriction,[19] contribute to the alterations in gas exchange seen with isoflurane and with the other potent vapors as well.[73]

Actions on brain and central nervous system

Cerebral metabolism is decreased considerably during isoflurane anesthesia, and this effect is evident at a relatively lighter level of isoflurane compared with halothane or enflurane anesthesia. The EEG shows progressive development of slow waves that culminate in electrical silence without evidence of the seizure activity seen with enflurane. Isoflurane alone causes increases in ICP, but this effect is blunted or eliminated when isoflurane is combined with hypocarbia.[79] In animals, isoflurane provides some protection from ischemia or hypoxemia,[85] and the combination of these effects has led to a preference for isoflurane anesthesia for neurosurgical anesthesia.

Actions on other organs

Isoflurane causes skeletal muscle relaxation and enhances the actions of the nondepolarizing skeletal muscle relaxant drugs. Uterine muscle is relaxed by isoflurane, an effect similar to that observed with halothane or enflurane.

Urine flow is decreased in response to the decreases in renal blood flow and glomerular filtration rate that occur during isoflurane anesthesia. As with the other potent vapors, these effects are dissipated rapidly after the drug is discontinued.

Hepatic function is not impaired significantly by isoflurane, and hepatic failure or necrosis is not attributed to this anesthetic. Isoflurane is relatively unique in this regard, and it is presumed that the absence of hepatic sequelae can be attributed to support of liver blood flow (and O_2 transport), to decreased metabolism of the drug (see following discussion), or to a combination of these factors.

Biotransformation

Only small quantities (approximately 0.2%) of isoflurane are metabolized; the extent of biotransformation is approximately 1/100th that of halothane and 1/10th that of enflurane.[50] The quantities of these metabolites, including fluoride and trifluoroacetic acid, are insufficient to cause significant cell injury or toxicity.

Emergence

Emergence from anesthesia is prompt after isoflurane is discontinued. The incidence of nausea and vomiting is similar to that seen with other agents and probably reflects associated factors more than the drug's inherent qualities.

Complications

The most common concerns associated with isoflurane involve the cardiovascular system and represent the spectrum of its pharmacologic properties rather than any specific toxicity. Hypotension, similar to that seen with the other potent vapors, is especially evident in the absence of significant surgical stimulation. Tachycardia and the remote possibility of coronary blood flow "steal" cause some concern in patients who have coronary artery disease. However, the relative absence of hepatic complications is a significant advantage of the drug. Overall, isoflurane is remarkable for its lack of significant complications, and this probably accounts for its popularity among inhalation anesthetics.

Enflurane

Enflurane (1,1,2-trifluoro-2-chloroethyl difluoromethyl ether) is a halogenated hydrocarbon anesthetic that is approximately one-half as potent as halothane. It achieved several years of popularity as an alternative to halothane, although its use has declined considerably since the introduction of isoflurane. Enflurane's principal advantages over halothane appear to be a reduced incidence of hepatic dysfunction and relative freedom from cardiac dysrhythmias when used in combination with epinephrine.

Induction

Although induction with enflurane is prompt, most clinicians believe that inhalation induction of anesthesia is more easily accomplished and more rapid with halothane. Induction is generally supplemented with IV ultrashort-acting barbiturates to provide prompt loss of consciousness, but continued administration of inhaled enflurane usually results in a smooth, quiet transition to surgical levels of anesthesia.

Circulatory actions

Light-to-moderate levels of anesthesia with enflurane result in a progressive decrease in blood pressure that is similar to that seen with halothane anesthesia[23] (see Fig. 50-11). **However, attempts to achieve deep levels of enflurane anesthesia are often accompanied by profound hypotension,**[10] **indicating that the margin between adequate anesthesia and unacceptable hypotension is quite narrow for this drug. The decrease** **in blood pressure results from balanced effects on both the heart and the peripheral circulation, as evidenced by decreases in both cardiac output and SVR.** As with halothane and isoflurane, enflurane does not increase circulating catecholamines or stimulate the sympathetic nervous system.

Myocardial depression, as evidenced by decreases in contractility, occurs in both the isolated heart and in intact humans. Myocardial O_2 consumption decreases as myocardial work is diminished because of decreases in both cardiac output and arterial pressure, but enflurane does not appear to result in myocardial ischemia or increased anaerobic metabolism in the heart.

Cerebral blood flow is increased and cerebral vascular resistance decreased by enflurane anesthesia.[101] Although the magnitude of the increase in cerebral blood flow appears to be somewhat less than that observed during halothane anesthesia, the effect is still considerable, leading to a 50% to 75% increase in flow during clinical levels of anesthesia.

As with halothane, marked increases occur in cutaneous flow associated with decreased cutaneous vascular resistance. Renal blood flow is decreased by approximately 25% and is accompanied by a similar decrease in glomerular filtration.[4]

Total hepatic blood flow, especially portal venous flow, is decreased by enflurane, but the normal reciprocal relationship between portal flow and hepatic arterial flow is preserved.[98] Increased heart rate frequently occurs during enflurane anesthesia, and the occasional slow nodal rhythm that occurs during halothane anesthesia is rarely seen with enflurane. The heart is not sensitized to the administration of exogenous catecholamines, and dysrhythmias are infrequent during enflurane anesthesia.

Respiratory actions

Enflurane causes mild bronchodilation and inhibits bronchoconstriction, as do both halothane and isoflurane. **It produces dose-dependent respiratory depression and hypercarbia,**[23] manifested primarily by decreased tidal volume but with less tachypnea than seen with halothane or isoflurane. **Ventilatory drive is blunted severely; the responses to both O_2 and CO_2 are impaired to a greater extent by enflurane than by halothane.**[49] Respiratory depression, although profound, is countered to some extent by surgical stimulation, and assisted or controlled ventilation is used during most procedures. As with halothane, the pulmonary O_2 exchange is impaired by enflurane anesthesia, and the alveolar-arterial (A-a) gradient for O_2 is increased. Consequently, enflurane is usually administered in a breathing mixture that contains at least 30% O_2.

Actions on brain and central nervous system

Tonic-clonic muscle activity, associated with EEG evidence of seizure activity, may occur with deeper levels of enflurane,[12] especially if hypocarbia is also present. The EEG pattern is one of increased frequency and amplitude, followed by burst suppression and spike complexes that are typical of seizure activity. Intermittent tonic-clonic jerking movements may be present in the facial and limb muscles if skeletal muscle relaxants have not been administered. These responses are infrequent and inconsistent, and it is not clear why they occur in occasional patients but not in others. Curiously, it appears that enflurane does not increase the incidence or severity of seizures when administered to epileptic patients, but many clinicians avoid its use in this population.

Enflurane causes dose-dependent decreases in cerebral metabolism and cerebral metabolic O_2 consumption.[101] The combination of increased brain blood flow and reduced brain metabolism implies a relative excess of perfusion to the brain during enflurane anesthesia. The increase in cerebral blood flow is not beneficial during neurosurgical procedures since the decrease in cerebrovascular resistance results in an increase in vascular volume that leads to increased total brain volume and increased ICP, especially in those with intracranial space-occupying lesions. Systemic hypoxia usually dilates the cerebral vasculature and increases brain blood flow, presumably as a compensatory mechanism to maintain O_2 transport to the brain, but this response is reversed by enflurane, leading to increased cerebrovascular resistance and decreased flow during hypoxia. This effect could lead potentially to brain cellular hypoxia.[21]

Actions on other organs

Dose-related skeletal muscle relaxation occurs during enflurane anesthesia.[93] This effect appears to result from alterations at a postjunctional site in the neuromuscular junction and perhaps from actions in the CNS as well. The actions of nondepolarizing skeletal muscle relaxants are enhanced considerably in the presence of enflurane, and the doses of these drugs can be reduced almost 50% during enflurane anesthesia.

Both glomerular filtration and urine flow are decreased in association with the reduction in renal blood flow that accompanies enflurane. As with halothane, these effects disappear rapidly when anesthesia is discontinued. Fluoride, which may produce renal effects, is a product of enflurane metabolism (see complications section).[95]

Major alterations in hepatic function can occur after enflurane anesthesia although they are quite rare. Hepatic necrosis after repeated administration has been reported, and it is perhaps wise to avoid multiple administrations over short intervals in the same patient if other anesthetics can be substituted.

Biotransformation

The extent of metabolism of enflurane is less than that for halothane, principally because the fluorine and chlorine (without bromine) are not easily cleaved from this stable ether molecule. Most (80% to 90%) of the inhaled enflurane is eliminated in expired air, and a small fraction diffuses out through the skin. The remainder (2% to 3%) is metabolized by the hepatic cytochrome P_{450} enzyme system.[11] Metabolic products include fluoride and difluoromethoxydifluoroacetic acid.[95] Nephrotoxicity caused by fluoride is a concern only when the dose (either depth or duration of anesthesia) in MAC hours exceeds that of most clinical conditions, although many avoid the use of enflurane if renal function is severely compromised.

Emergence

As would be expected from its physical and pharmacologic properties (solubility and potency), emergence from enflurane anesthesia is generally prompt, and no tendency exists for laryngospasm or unusual excitement. Shivering may occur but is no more common with this drug than with other potent inhalation anesthetics.

Complications

Major complications unique to enflurane occur infrequently. Reasons for its declining popularity may involve the narrow margin between adequate anesthesia and unacceptable hypotension more than any specific toxicity of the drug. Seizure activity (discussed previously) is rare, self-limited, and without apparent sequelae. Hepatic dysfunction is also rare. **Biotransformation of enflurane may lead to the release of free fluoride, especially when anesthesia is prolonged[74,95] or when renal dysfunction is present. However, the usual levels of fluoride required to produce nephrotoxicity (40 to 50 μmol) are rarely exceeded except during dramatically prolonged enflurane anesthesia.**

OTHER POTENT INHALATIONAL ANESTHETICS

Three other potent vapors deserve mention, although they are not currently in frequent use in anesthesia practice. Methoxyflurane was used often and still is used occasionally, especially for obstetric analgesia and anesthesia. Desflurane and sevoflurane are newer halogenated ethers that are in active clinical trials in the United States at this time. Other agents, such as diethyl ether, divinyl ether, ethylene, fluroxene, and cyclopropane, were used frequently at one time but have been replaced almost entirely by the modern potent vapors. These older drugs were often associated with problems that included flammability, unpleasant induction and emergence, nausea and vomiting, or ventricular dysrhythmias (e.g., cyclopropane).

Methoxyflurane

This halogenated ether (1,1-difluoro-2,2-dichloroethyl methyl ether) is remarkable for two characteristics: its remarkable potency (MAC of 0.16%) and solubility in blood and fat (blood-gas partition coefficient of 12.0). Despite its potency, the extreme solubility results in slow induction and emergence, making it difficult to provide prompt emergence and recovery from anesthesia. Dose-related hypotension occurs, but cardiac dysrhythmias occur infrequently.

The major concern with methoxyflurane involves biotransformation of the drug to toxic metabolites. Methoxyflurane is metabolized to a greater extent than any other potent vapor,[95] and the products of this biotransformation in the liver include difluoromethoxyacetic acid, dichloroacetic acid, oxalic acid, and free fluoride; the latter two are nephrotoxic. When administered in clinical concentrations for only 2 hours, metabolism of methoxyflurane can produce plasma fluoride concentrations that exceed 40 μM, and renal tubular damage occurs. The clinical syndrome is characterized by large volumes of dilute urine, by inability to concentrate urine even in response to challenge with antidiuretic hormone (ADH), and by hypernatremia and azotemia.[15,16,76] Recovery of renal function is extremely slow, and significant mortality is associated with the syndrome.

Although some advocate the use of methoxyflurane for brief procedures or for analgesia during labor (it is a potent analgetic in subanesthetic concentrations), little reason appears to exist to use this drug in either circumstance; the pharmacokinetics are inappropriate for brief procedures, and there are now better ways to provide analgesia during labor (e.g., epidural analgesia).

Desflurane

Desflurane (1-fluoro-2,2,2-trifluoroethyl difluoromethyl ether) is a new halocarbon inhalation anesthetic that is notable for its insolubility in blood (leading to very rapid changes in blood levels of the drug) and for its lack of biotransformation in the body. Its principal advantage appears to be rapid patient emergence from anesthesia.[100,120] Its principal disadvantages involve difficulty handling the drug because of its physical properties (it boils at essentially room temperature and thus requires specially constructed

vaporizers, see Chapter 47) and airway irritation during inhalation induction.

Induction of anesthesia by inhalation of desflurane would be expected to be rapid because of its insolubility in blood.[122] However, this theoretic advantage is countered considerably by airway irritation, which leads to coughing, breath holding, and laryngospasm during induction.[123] It is unlikely that this agent will be used frequently for inhalation induction of anesthesia. These problems are not evident when inhalation is preceded by a sleep dose of an IV induction agent (e.g., thiopental or propofol), a practice that is much more common than inhalation induction except in children, in whom inhalation induction with halothane is probably preferred.

The circulatory actions of desflurane are generally similar to those of isoflurane.[9,86,114] Arterial hypotension results from actions on the peripheral circulation (decreased SVR) rather than from decreased systemic blood flow. Cardiac output may be even better maintained with desflurane than with isoflurane. Cerebrovascular effects of desflurane also are similar to those of isoflurane;[70] decreased cerebrovascular resistance and increased cerebral blood flow occur although the responsiveness to CO_2 remains intact. The coronary vascular effects of desflurane have been examined in animal models (dogs) with coronary stenoses, and there is no evidence of coronary blood flow "steal" under these conditions.[45]

Based on current (incomplete) knowledge, it appears that the respiratory effects of desflurane are similar to those of isoflurane;[67] tachypnea, decreased tidal volume, and resultant hypercarbia all occur with spontaneous ventilation.

Desflurane causes progressive suppression of EEG activity without evidence of epileptiform activity; therefore, its pharmacologic actions resemble those of isoflurane.[91]

The biotransformation of desflurane is minuscule, even compared with that of isoflurane. Serum fluoride concentrations and urinary excretion of fluoride are unchanged during and after desflurane anesthesia.[110] Although slight increases in serum trifluoroacetic acid occur, the levels (0.17 μmol/L) are approximately one-tenth those seen with isoflurane anesthesia. Although clinical experience is inadequate to allow firm conclusions, hepatic or renal complications caused by biotransformation of this drug apparently would be rare based on present evidence.

Rapid emergence from anesthesia may be the major advantage of desflurane since evidence indicates that awakening and recovery of cognitive function is remarkably prompt after brief procedures.[32] This may be a valuable property in busy operating suites where rapid turnover of patients is required and in surgical outpatients who would especially benefit from rapid recovery of mental facilities.

Sevoflurane

Sevoflurane (1,1,1,3,3,3-hexafluoro-2-propyl fluoromethyl ether) is currently in use for clinical anesthesia in Japan and in clinical trials in the United States. As with desflurane, it is notable for its lack of solubility in blood[72] and tissues,[121] leading to rapid induction and emergence from anesthesia. The cardiovascular effects (decreased SVR and arterial pressure) of this drug are generally similar to those of isoflurane.[3,14]

Sevoflurane depresses respiration and hypercarbia results, but the extent of this effect appears to be less than that seen with halothane. Tidal volume and the durations of inspiration and expiration are greater with sevoflurane compared with isoflurane, suggesting that sevoflurane has different actions on the central neural control of respiration.[61] However, the net result for clinical practice is similar to that of other potent vapors; all are potent respiratory depressants.

The biotransformation of sevoflurane is significant, leading to increases in plasma fluoride that could produce renal toxicity after longer procedures. The increase in plasma fluoride usually correlates with the duration of exposure, but it exceeded the threshold for renal toxicity (50 μmol/L) in 10% of surgical patients in a recent study.[33] Although creatinine and blood urea nitrogen did not change overall, these results suggest that sevoflurane administration may be limited to short procedures only, if it is released by the U.S. Food and Drug Administration after completion of clinical trials.

SELECTION OF INHALATIONAL AGENTS

The selection of a particular anesthetic technique and of the appropriate anesthetic drugs is based on a rational analysis of the patient's condition and the planned surgery.

The ideal anesthetic is stable in the long term under normal physical conditions (temperature, humidity, light, alkali) found in the anesthesia apparatus; nonflammable in air, O_2, or N_2O; and easily handled in liquid or gas form. It must be potent, allowing use with enriched O_2, and poorly soluble in blood and tissue, allowing rapid induction and emergence. It should be nonirritating to the airway, nontoxic in anesthetic or trace partial pressures even during long exposure, and nonmetabolizable. It should have minimal and predictable cardiovascular and respiratory effects and no adverse interactions with other drugs. It should be easily produced and inexpensive.

How close to this ideal can we approach? The relative merits and disadvantages of each anesthetic prevent absolute assignment of the "best" anesthetic agent. From the present discussion it should also be

---

Table 50-2   Clinical qualities of inhalational anesthetics

Anesthetic	Strengths	Weaknesses
Nitrous oxide	Analgesia Rapid uptake and elimination Little cardiac or respiratory depression	Sympathetic stimulation Expansion of closed air spaces Requires high concentration Interferes with vitamin B_{12} metabolism
Halothane	Inexpensive Effective in low concentrations Little airway instability Uterine relaxation	Chemically less stable Slow uptake and elimination Biodegradable Hepatic necrosis Cardiac depression and dysrhythmias
Enflurane	Good muscle relaxatoin Stable cardiac rate and rhythm	Pungent odor Seizure activity on EEG
Isoflurane	Good muscle relaxation Stable cardiac rate and rhythm Decreased CSF pressure	Pungent odor Expensive Strong vasodilator
Desflurane	Rapid uptake and elimination Stable molecule	Pungent odor Low boiling point Strong vasodilator Expensive
Sevoflurane	Rapid uptake and elimination	Biodegradable Strong vasodilator Expensive

apparent that various differences make one agent preferable to another in a particular set of circumstances. These relative indications and contraindications are summarized in Table 50-2.

The new agents, desflurane and sevoflurane, may approach the ideal in some ways and depart in others. Both agents have very low gas-blood and blood-tissue partition coefficients that allow rapid induction and emergence. Desflurane is difficult to handle and will require new vaporizers and may possibly be limited to closed-circuit administration because of cost; sevoflurane resembles isoflurane in physical properties. Desflurane is almost inert under normal conditions

and has less metabolic breakdown than isoflurane; sevoflurane is very unstable in alkali and is metabolizable to products, including fluoride. Both anesthetics cause cardiovascular and respiratory depression, which is dose related and similar to that for isoflurane. Thus the search for the "ideal" agent continues, but evidence shows major progress toward this goal, especially during the past 20 years.

The inhalational anesthetic agents have the advantages of ease of administration, ability to regulate and monitor dosages, rapid reversibility, and relative inertness in the body. Few other drugs can match this record of safety and usefulness.

KEY POINTS

- The aim in administering an inhalational anesthetic is to achieve a brain partial pressure sufficient to obtain the desired effect. Because the brain is a very well-perfused organ, the partial pressure of anesthetic in the arterial blood and that in the brain approach equilibrium quite rapidly. The exchange of anesthetic across the alveolar membranes is generally very efficient so that the arterial partial pressure of anesthetic is close to that in the alveolar gas and the partial pressure of anesthetic in the brain will follow closely the alveolar partial pressure of that anesthetic. The problem in practice is to consider the factors determining the alveolar partial pressure.

- The difference in partial pressure between a gas phase (alveolar gas) and a liquid phase (blood) determines the movement of the anesthetic molecules between the phases.

- Solubility is also expressed as a partition coefficient (γ) or the ratio of the solubilities for two media, such as in *blood-brain partition coefficient*, which describes the ratio of solubility of an agent for blood to that for brain. The solubility of anesthetics in the blood and tissues determines how much drug uptake is required to increase partial pressure to anesthetic levels in the brain, and thus how long induction and emergence require.

- When the anesthetic vaporizer dial is set to the required percentage, the fresh gas flow will almost immediately contain the anesthetic vapor at the selected partial pressure but the inspired gas partial pressure will take some time to approach this value. Delay results because (1) the circuit itself contains a volume of gas that must be replaced by the fresh gas, (2) the anesthetic is highly soluble in some rubber and plastic materials, and (3) the anesthetic is taken up by the patient.

- The approach of the alveolar partial pressure to that of the inspired gas is delayed by (1) high solubility, (2) increased cardiac output, or (3) a large difference between the alveolar and the mixed venous partial pressures. It is accelerated by (1) increasing the inspired partial pressure of anesthetic or (2) increasing the alveolar ventilation.

- Uptake and elimination kinetics play an essential part in the administration of all inhalational agents. The precise formulations of the uptake equations are not as important as is the realization that the fresh gas, circuit, and inspired and end-tidal (or alveolar) partial pressures of the anesthetic differ in a systematic manner. Their relationship (1) changes with time during induction and maintenance and is (2) reversed during elimination. In practice, the delay in achieving the desired alveolar partial pressure must be anticipated by administering or discontinuing the anesthetic gases before a change in brain partial pressure is needed and by manipulating fresh gas flows and circuit characteristics.

- MAC is the minimum alveolar concentration (in percent of atmospheric pressure) of anesthetic that prevents movement in 50% of subjects in response to a standard surgical incision. MAC is analogous to any other ED_{50} value computed from a pharmacologic dose-response curve; what is unusual is the particular stimulus and the particular response.

- Nitrous oxide is used primarily to supplement other inhalational or intravenous anesthetics. Its use is based on the observations that (1) the contributions of each inhaled anesthetic in the breathing mixture are additive and (2) the side effects of the potent vapors are dose dependent. Thus a combination of inhaled anesthetics that will produce complete anesthesia is administered. This method avoids both the arterial hypoxemia that might accompany "pure" nitrous oxide anesthesia and the cardiovascular, pulmonary, and metabolic effects (among others) of anesthesia with the potent vapor only.

- Nitrous oxide is approximately 30 times more soluble in blood than is nitrogen, and it readily exchanges with the nitrogen that may be present in the gas-containing structures of the body. If there is sufficient space, a gas-containing cavity will expand considerably in the presence of nitrous oxide (i.e., bowel or thoracic cavity); if there is no room to expand, then the pressure in that cavity will increase markedly (i.e., intracranial pressure).

- Nitrous oxide inhibits the actions of methionine synthetase, an enzyme involved in vitamin B_{12} metabolism, leading to impaired bone marrow function, but this is usually not significant in routine clinical practice.

- The most prominent circulatory effect of halothane is dose-dependent arterial hypotension. Although halothane dilates cutaneous arteries and veins and thus leaves a visual impression that implies significant vasodilation, the overall effect on systemic vascular resistance is relatively minor even at deep levels of halothane anesthesia. Essentially, the decrease in blood pressure results from an associated decrease in cardiac output.

- Ventricular ectopy during halothane anesthesia, resulting from beta-adrenergic stimulation, occurs when exogenous epinephrine is administered in doses that would have no effect on cardiac rhythm in awake patients.

- The potential increase in intracranial pressure that accompanies dilatation of the cerebral vasculature limits the use of halothane in patients with space-occupying lesions of the intracranial cavity, such as tumors or hematoma.

- Halothane has important actions on the splanchnic circulation, leading to decreased total hepatic blood flow. Portal venous flow is decreased in response to decreased blood flow in the gastrointestinal viscera, and this is accompanied by hepatic arterial vasoconstriction also. Unlike other potent halogenated anesthetics, halothane abolishes the normal reciprocal relationship between portal venous and hepatic arterial flows, leading to the possibility for tissue ischemia and/or cellular hypoxia in the liver.

- Alveolar hypoventilation and arterial hypercarbia occur in a dose-dependent manner when halothane anesthesia is administered with spontaneouos respiration.

- The major route of elimination of halothane is through the lungs, but a significant amount (10% to 20%) is biotransformed in the liver; small amounts diffuse out through the skin also.

- There is a rare but real incidence of severe hepatic dysfunction, even hepatic necrosis, associated with halothane anesthesia. The severe response is more common after repeated exposures to halothane and is often associated with obesity or episodes of intraoperative hypotension. The precise etiology remains uncertain, but it is presumed to be related to the metabolic products of the biotransformation of halothane leading to immunologically mediated hepatic necrosis and is perhaps enhanced by cellular hypoxia resulting from decreased hepatic perfusion.

- Isoflurane anesthesia is accompanied by progressive dose-related dependent hypotension; the magnitude of the effect is similar to that seen during halothane anesthesia.

- In contrast to halothane or enflurane, isoflurane anesthesia is characterized by well maintained cardiac output, even during moderately deep anesthesia.

- Isoflurane produces dose-dependent decreases in systemic vascular resistance, and this peripheral circulatory effect is almost entirely responsible for the hypotension that occurs during light-to-moderate levels of isoflurane anesthesia.

- Hepatic oxygen transport, hepatic oxygenation, and hepatic arterial compensation for decreased portal venous flow (reciprocity of hepatic blood flow) all appear to be better maintained during isoflurane than during enflurane or halothane anesthesia.

- As with the other potent vapors, isoflurane impairs both ventilatory drive and the transport of oxygen from the alveoli to the arterial blood, leading especially to hypercarbia during anesthesia.

- Only small quantities of isoflurane are metabolized; the extent of biotransformation is approximately 1/100th that of halothane and 1/10th that of enflurane.

- Light-to-moderate levels of anesthesia result in a progressive decrease in blood pressure with enflurane anesthesia that is similar to that seen with halothane or isoflurane. However, deep levels of enflurane anesthesia are often accompanied by profound hypotension, indicating that the margin between adequate anesthesia and unacceptable hypotension is quite narrow for this drug. The decrease in blood pressure results from decreases in both cardiac output and systemic vascular resistance.

- Enflurane produces dose-dependent respiratory depression and hypercarbia. Ventilatory drive is blunted severely; the responses to both oxygen and carbon dioxide are impaired to a greater extent by enflurane than by halothane.

■ Biotransformation of enflurane may lead to the release of free fluoride, especially when anesthesia is prolonged or when renal dysfunction is present. However, the usual levels of fluoride required to produce nephrotoxicity are rarely exceeded except during dramatically prolonged enflurane anesthesia.

KEY REFERENCES

Calverley RK, Smith NT, Prys-Roberts C et al: Cardiovascular effects of enflurane anesthesia during controlled ventilation in man, *Anesth Analg* 57:619, 1978.

Eger EI II: Isoflurane: a review, *Anesthesiology* 55:559, 1981.

Eger EI II, Saidman LJ, and Brandsteter B: Minimum alveolar anesthetic concentration: a standard of anesthetic potency, *Anesthesiology* 26:756, 1965.

Eger EI II, Smith NT, Stoelting RK et al: Cardiovascular effects of halothane in man, *Anesthesiology* 32:396, 1970.

Gelman S: General anesthesia and hepatic circulation, *Can J Physiol Pharmacol* 65:1762, 1987.

Hornbein TF, Martin WE, Bonica JJ et al: Nitrous oxide effects on the circulatory and ventilatory responses to halothane, *Anesthesiology* 31:250, 1969.

Knill RL, Gelb AW: Ventilatory responses to hypoxia and hypercapnia during halothane sedation and anesthesia in man, *Anesthesiology* 49:244, 1978.

Smith AL, Wollman H: Cerebral blood flow and metabolism: effects of anesthetic drugs and techniques, *Anesthesiology* 36:378, 1972.

Stevens WC, Cromell TH, Halsey MJ et al: The cardiovascular effects of a new inhalation anesthetic, Forane, in human volunteers at constant arterial carbon dioxide tension, *Anesthesiology* 35:8, 1971.

Stoelting RK, Longnecker DE: Effect of right-to-left shunt on rate of rise in arterial anesthetic concentration, *Anesthesiology* 36:352, 1972.

REFERENCES

1. Atlee JL, Alexander SC: Halothane effects on conductivity of the AV node and His-Purkinje system in the dog, *Anesth Analg* 56:378, 1977.
2. Austin AT: The chemistry of the higher oxides of nitrogen as related to the manufacture, storage and administration of nitrous oxide, *Br J Anaesth* 39:345, 1967.
3. Bernard JM, Wouters PF, Doursout MJ et al: Effects of sevoflurane and isoflurane on cardiac and coronary dynamics in chronically instrumented dogs, *Anesthesiology* 72:659, 1990.
4. Bevan DR: *Renal function in anesthesia and surgery*, New York, 1979, Grune & Stratton.
5. Bimar J, Bellville JW: Arousal reaction during anesthesia in man, *Anesthesiology* 47:449, 1977.
6. Buffington CW, Davis KB, Gillispie S et al: The prevalence of steal-prone coronary anatomy in patients with coronary artery disease: an analysis of the coronary artery surgery study registry, *Anesthesiology* 69:721, 727, 1988.
7. Buffington CW, Romson JL, Levine A et al: Isoflurane induces coronary steal in a canine model of chronic coronary occlusion, *Anesthesiology* 66:280, 1987.
8. Bunker JP, Forrest WH Jr, Mosteller F et al: *The National Halothane Study: a study of the possible association between halothane anesthesia and postoperative hepatic necrosis*, Bethesda, Md, 1969, National Institutes of Health.
9. Cahalan MK, Weiskopf RB, Eger EI II et al: Hemodynamic effects of desflurane/nitrous oxide anesthesia in volunteers, *Anesth Analg* 73:157, 1991.
10. Calverley RK, Smith NT, Prys-Roberts C et al: Cardiovascular effects of enflurane anesthesia during controlled ventilation in man, *Anesth Analg* 57:619, 1978.
11. Carpenter RL, Eger EI II, Johnson BH et al: The extent of metabolism of inhaled anesthetics in humans, *Anesthesiology* 65:201, 1986.
12. Clark DL, Rosner BD: Neurophysiologic effects of general anesthetics. I. The electroencephalogram and sensory evoked responses in man, *Anesthesiology* 38:564, 1973.
13. Conzen PF, Hobbhahn J, Goetz AE et al: Splanchnic oxygen consumption and hepatic surface oxygen tensions during isoflurane anesthesia, *Anesthesiology* 69:643, 1988.
14. Conzen PF, Vollmar B, Habazettl H et al: Systemic and regional hemodynamics of isoflurane and sevoflurane in rats, *Anesth Analg* 74:79, 1992.
15. Cousins MJ, Mazze RI: Methoxyflurane nephrotoxicity: a study of dose-response in man, *JAMA* 225:1611, 1973.
16. Crandell WB, Pappas SG, and Macdonald A: Nephrotoxicity associated with methoxyflurane anesthesia, *Anesthesiology* 27:591, 1966.
17. Deacon R, Lumb M, Perry J et al: Selective inactivation of vitamin B_{12} in rats by nitrous oxide, *Lancet* 2:1023, 1978.
18. de Jong RH, Eger EI II: AD_{50} and AD_{95} values of common inhalational anesthetics in man, *Anesthesiology* 42:384, 1975.
19. Domino KB, Borowec L, Alexander CM, et al: Influence of isoflurane on hypoxic pulmonary vasoconstriction in dogs, *Anesthesiology* 64:423, 1986.
20. Dorsch JA, Dorsch SE: *Understanding anesthesia equipment*, ed 2, Baltimore, 1984, Williams & Wilkins.
21. Durieux ME, Sperry RJ, and Longnecker DE: Effects of hypoxemia on regional blood flow during anesthesia with halothane, enflurane, and isoflurane, *Anesthesiology* 76:402, 1992.
22. Eger EI II: *Anesthetic uptake and action*, Baltimore, 1974, Williams & Wilkins.
23. Eger EI II: Isoflurane: a review, *Anesthesiology* 55:559, 1981.
24. Eger EI II: *Nitrous oxide/N_2O*, New York, 1985, Elsevier.
25. Eger EI II, Johnson BH: MAC of I-653 in rats, including a test of the effect of body temperature and anesthetic duration, *Anesth Analg* 66:974, 1987.
26. Eger EI II, Saidman LJ: Hazards of

nitrous oxide anesthesia in bowel obstruction and pneumothorax, *Anesthesiology* 26:61, 1965.

27. Eger EI II, Saidman LJ, and Brandsteter B: Minimum alveolar anesthetic concentration: a standard of anesthetic potency, *Anesthesiology* 26:756, 1965.

27a. Eger EI II, Smith NT, Stoelting RK et al: Cardiovascular effects of halothane in man, *Anesthesiology* 32:396, 1976.

28. Eger EI II, Stevens WC, Cromwell TH: The electroencephalogram in man anesthetized with Forane, *Anesthesiology* 35:504, 1971.

29. Eintrei C, Leszniewski W, and Carlsson C: Local application of ^{133}xenon for measurement of regional cerebral blood flow (rCBF) during halothane, enflurane, and isoflurane anesthesia in humans, *Anesthesiology* 63:391, 1985.

30. Epstein RM, Rackow H, Salanitre E et al: Influence of the concentration effect on the uptake of anesthetic mixtures, *Anesthesiology* 25:364, 1964.

31. Fink BR: Diffusion anoxia, *Anesthesiology* 16:511, 1955.

32. Fletcher JE, Sebel PS, Murphy MR et al: Psychomotor performance after desflurane anesthesia: a comparison with isoflurane, *Anesth Analg* 73:260, 1991.

33. Frink EJ Jr, Ghantous H, Malan TP et al: Plasma inorganic fluoride with sevoflurane anesthesia: correlation with indices of hepatic and renal function, *Anesth Analg* 74:231, 1992.

34. Fukunaga AF, Epstein RM: Sympathetic excitation during nitrous oxide–halothane anesthesia in the cat, *Anesthesiology* 39:231, 1973.

35. Gaumann DM, Mustaki J-P, and Tassonyi E: MAC-awake of isoflurane, enflurane and halothane evaluated by slow and fast alveolar washout, *Br J Anaesth* 68:81, 1992.

36. Gelman S: General anesthesia and hepatic circulation, *Can J Physiol Pharmacol* 65:1762, 1987.

37. Gregory GA, Eger EI II, and Munson ES: The relationship between age and halothane requirement in man, *Anesthesiology* 30:488, 1969.

38. Grodin WK, Epstein MAF, Epstein RA: Soda lime adsorption of isoflurane and enflurane, *Anesthesiology* 62:60, 1985.

39. Grodin WK, Epstein RA: Halothane adsorption complicating the use of soda-lime to humidify anesthetic gases, *Br J Anaesth* 54:555, 1982.

40. Gross JB: Myocardial ischemia during isoflurane anesthesia: the effect of substituting halothane, *Anesthesiology* 70:1012, 1989.

41. Gross JB, Alexander CM: Awakening concentrations of isoflurane are not affected by analgesic doses of morphine, *Anesth Analg* 67:27, 1988.

42. Guedel AE: *Inhalation anesthesia,* ed 2, New York, 1951, Macmillan.

43. Guerra F: Awareness and recall, *Int Anesthesiol Clin* 24:75, 1986.

44. Hall RI, Murphy MR, Hug CC Jr: The enflurane sparing effect of sufentanil in dogs, *Anesthesiology* 67:518, 1987.

45. Hartman JC, Pagel PS, Kampine JP et al: Influence of desflurane on regional distribution of coronary blood flow in a chronically instrumented canine model of multivessel coronary artery obstruction, *Anesth Analg* 1991 72:289, 1991.

46. Heller ML, Watson TR Jr: The role of preliminary oxygenation prior to induction with high nitrous oxide mixtures: polarographic PaO$_2$ study, *Anesthesiology* 23:219, 1962.

47. Henriksen HT, Joergensen PB: The effect of nitrous oxide on intracranial pressure in patients with intracranial disorders, *Br J Anaesth* 45:486, 1973.

48. Hirshman CA, Edelstein G, Peetz S et al: Mechanism of action of inhalational anesthesia on airways, *Anesthesiology* 56:107, 1982.

49. Hirshman GG, McCullough RE, Cohen PJ et al: Depression of hypoxic ventilatory response by halothane, enflurane and isoflurane in dogs, *Br J Anaesth* 49:957, 1977.

50. Holaday DA, Fiseroua-Bergerova V, Latto IP et al: Resistance of isoflurane to biotransformation in man, *Anesthesiology* 43:325, 1975.

51. Hornbein TF, Martin WE, Bonica JJ et al: Nitrous oxide effects on the circulatory and ventilatory responses to halothane, *Anesthesiology* 31:250, 1969.

52. Housmans PR, Murat I: Comparative effects of halothane, enflurane and isoflurane at equipotent anesthetic concentrations on isolated ventricular myocardia of the ferret, *Anesthesiology* 69:451, 1988.

53. Johnston RR, Way WL, and Miller RD: Alteration of anesthetic requirement by amphetamine, *Anesthesiology* 36:357, 1972.

54. Jones PL: Some observations on nitrous oxide cylinders during emptying, *Br J Anaesth* 46:534, 1974.

55. Karl HW, Swedlow DB, Lee KW et al: Epinephrine-halothane interactions in children, *Anesthesiology* 58:142, 1983.

56. Katz RL, Matteo RS, and Papper EM: The injection of epinephrine during general anesthesia. II. Halothane, *Anesthesiology* 23:597, 1962.

57. Kazama T, Ikeda K: Comparison of MAC and the rate of rise of alveolar concentration of sevoflurane with halothane and isoflurane in the dog, *Anesthesiology* 68:435, 1988.

58. Kety SS: The physiologial and physical factors governing the uptake of anesthetic gases by the body, *Anesthesiology* 11:517, 1950.

59. Keys TE: *The history of surgical anesthesia,* New York, 1978, Robert Krieger.

60. Knill RL, Gelb AW: Ventilatory responses to hypoxia and hypercapnia during halothane sedation and anesthesia in man, *Anesthesiology* 49:244, 1978.

61. Kochi T, Izumi Y, Isono S et al: Breathing pattern and occlusion pressure waveform in humans anesthetized with halothane or sevoflurane, *Anesth Analg* 73:327, 1991.

62. Lassen HCA, Henriksen E, Neukirch F et al: Treatment of tetanus: severe bone-marrow depression after prolonged nitrous-oxide anesthesia, *Lancet* 1:527, 1956.

63. Layzer RB: Myeloneuropathy after prolonged exposure to nitrous oxide, *Lancet* 2:1227, 1978.

64. Lerman J, Willis MM, Gregory GA, and Eger EI II: Osmolarity determines the solubility of anesthetics in aqueous solutions at 37° C, *Anesthesiology* 59:554, 1983.

65. Levy WJ, Shapiro HM, Maruchak G et al: Automated EEG processing for intraoperative monitoring: a comparison of techniques, *Anesthesiology* 53:223, 1980.

66. Liu J, Laster MJ, Eger EI II et al: Absorption and degradation of sevoflurane and isoflurane in a conventional anesthetic circuit, *Anesth Analg* 72:785, 1991.

67. Lockhart SH, Rampil IJ, Yasuda N et al: Depression of ventilation by desflurane in humans, *Anesthesiology* 74:484, 1991.

68. Logan M, Farmer JG: Anaesthesia and the ozone layer, *Br J Anaesth* 63:645, 1989.

69. Longnecker DE, Harris PD: Dilatation of small arteries and veins in the bat during halothane anesthesia, *Anesthesiology* 37:423, 1972.

70. Lutz LJ, Milde JH, and Milde LN: The cerebral functional, metabolic, and hemodynamic effects of desflurane in dogs, *Anesthesiology* 73:125, 1990.

71. Lynch C: Differential depression of myocardial contractility by halothane and isoflurane *in vitro, Anesthesiology* 64:620, 1986.

72. Malviya S, Lerman J: The blood/gas solubilities of sevoflurane, isoflurane, halothane, and serum constituent concentrations in neonates and adults, *Anesthesiology* 72:793, 1990.

73. Marshall BE: Hypoxic pulmonary vasoconstriction, *Acta Anaesth Scand* 34(suppl 94):37, 1990.

74. Mazze RI, Calverley RK, and Smith NT: Inorganic fluoride nephrotoxicity: prolonged enflurane and halothane anesthesia in volunteers, *Anesthesiology* 46:265, 1977.

75. Mazze RI, Cousins MJ, and Burr GA: Renal effects and metabolism of isoflurane in man, *Anesthesiology* 40:536, 1974.

76. Mazze RI, Rosen M, and Mushin WM: Methoxyflurane as an obstetric analgesic: a comparison with trichloroethylene, *Br Med J* 2:1554, 1966.

77. Mazze RI, Schwartz FD, Slocum HC et al: Renal function during anesthesia and surgery. I. The effects of halothane anesthesia, *Anesthesiology* 24:279, 1963.

78. McLain GE, Sipes G, and Brown BR: An animal model of halothane hepatotoxicity: roles of enzyme induction and hypoxia, *Anesthesiology* 51:321, 1979.

79. McPherson RW, Brian JE, and Traystman RJ: Cerebrovascular responsiveness to carbon dioxide in dogs with 1.4% and 2.87% isoflurane, *Anesthesiology* 70:843, 1989.

80. Merin RG, Kumazawa T, and Luka NL: Myocardial function and metabolism in

the conscious dog and during halothane anesthesia, *Anesthesiology* 44:402, 1976.

81. Munson ES, Eger EI II, Tham MK, and Embro WJ: Increase in anesthetic uptake, excretion, and blood solubility in man after eating, *Anesth Analg* 57:224, 1978.

82. Murphy MR, Hug CC Jr: The anesthetic potency of fentanyl in terms of its reduction of enflurane MAC, *Anesthesiology* 57:485, 1982.

83. Murphy MR, Hug CC Jr: The enflurane sparing effect of morphine, butorphanol and nalbuphine, *Anesthesiology* 57:489, 1982.

84. Mushin WW, Jones PL: *Physics for the anaesthetist,* ed 4, Boston, 1987, Blackwell.

85. Newberg LA, Michenfelder JD: Cerebral protection by isoflurane during hypoxemia or ischemia, *Anesthesiology* 59:29, 1983.

86. Pagel PS, Kampine JP, Schmeling WT et al: Comparison of the systemic and coronary hemodynamic actions of desflurane, isoflurane, halothane, and enflurane in the chronically instrumented dog, *Anesthesiology* 74:539, 1991.

87. Palahniuk RJ, Shnider SM, Eger EI II: Pregnancy decreases the requirement for inhaled anesthetic agents, *Anesthesiology* 41:82, 1974.

88. Pavlin EG, Hornbein TR: Anesthesia and the control of ventilation. In Cherniak NS, Widdicombe JG, eds: *The respiratory system,* vol 2, part 1, Bethesda, Md, 1986, American Physiological Society.

89. Perisho JA, Buechel DR, and Miller RD: The effect of diazepam (Valium) on minimum alveolar anaesthetic requirement in man, *Can Anaesth Soc J* 18:536, 1971.

90. Phirman JR, Shapiro HM: Modification of nitrous oxide–induced intracranial hypertension by prior induction of anesthesia, *Anesthesiology* 46:150, 1977.

91. Rampil IJ, Lockhart SH, Eger EI II et al: The electroencephalographic effects of desflurane in humans, *Anesthesiology* 74:434, 1991.

92. Roizen MF, Horrigan RW, and Frazer BM: Anesthetic doses blocking adrenergic (stress) and cardiovascular responses to incision-MAC BAR, *Anesthesiology* 54:390, 1981.

93. Rupp SM, McChristian JW, and Miller RD: Neuromuscular effects of atracurium during halothane, nitrous oxide and enflurane, nitrous oxide anesthesia on humans, *Anesthesiology* 63:16, 1985.

94. Rusy BF, Komai H: Anesthetic depression of myocardial contractility: a review of possible mechanisms, *Anesthesiology* 67:745, 1987.

95. Sakai T, Takaori M: Biodegradiation of halothane, enflurane, and methoxyflurane, *Br J Anaesth* 50:785, 1978.

96. Severinghaus JW: The rate of uptake of nitrous oxide in man, *J Clin Invest* 33:1183, 1954.

97. Seyde WC, Ellis JE, and Longnecker DE: The addition of nitrous oxide to halothane decreases renal and splanchnic flow and increases cerebral blood flow in rats, *Br J Anaesth* 58:63, 1986.

98. Seyde WC, Longnecker DE: Anesthetic influences on regional hemodynamics in normal and hemorrhaged rats, *Anesthesiology* 61:686, 1984.

99. Slogoff S, Keats AS: Randomized trial of primary anesthetic agents on outcome of coronary artery bypass operations, *Anesthesiology* 70:179, 1989.

100. Smiley RM, Ornstein E, Matteo RS et al: Desflurane and isoflurane in surgical patients: comparison of emergence time, *Anesthesiology* 74:425, 1991.

101. Smith AL, Wollman H: Cerebral blood flow and metabolism: effects of anesthetic drugs and techniques, *Anesthesiology* 36:378, 1972.

102. Smith NT, Eger EI II, Stoelting RK et al: The cardiovascular and sympathomimetic responses to the addition of nitrous oxide to halothane in man, *Anesthesiology* 32:410, 1970.

103. Snow J: *On the inhalation of the vapor of ether in surgical operations,* London, 1847, John Churchill.

104. Sonntag H, Donath U, Hillebrand W et al: Left ventricular function in conscious man and during halothane anesthesia, *Anesthesiology* 48:320, 1978.

105. Stevens WC, Cromell TH, Halsey MJ et al: The cardiovascular effects of a new inhalation anesthetic, Forane, in human volunteers at constant arterial carbon dioxide tension, *Anesthesiology* 35:8, 1971.

106. Stock JGL, Strunin L: Unexplained hepatitis following halothane, *Anesthesiology* 63:424, 1985.

107. Stoelting RK, Eger EI II: An additional explanation for the second gas effect: a concentrating effect, *Anesthesiology* 30:273, 1969.

108. Stoelting RK, Longnecker DE: Effect of right-to-left shunt on rate of rise in arterial anesthetic concentration, *Anesthesiology* 36:352, 1972.

109. Strum DP, Johnson BH, Eger EI II: Stability of sevoflurane in soda lime, *Anesthesiology* 67:779, 1987.

110. Sutton TS, Koblin DD, Gruenke LD et al: Fluoride metabolites after prolonged exposure of volunteers and pa-

tients to desflurane, *Anesth Analg* 73:180, 1991.

111. Taylor RH, Lerman J: Minimum alveolar concentration of desflurane and hemodynamic responses in neonates, infants, and children, *Anesthesiology* 75:975, 1991.

112. Tinker JH, Gandolfi AJ, and Van Dyke RA: Elevation of plasma bromide levels in patients following halothane anesthesia: time correlation with total halothane dosage, *Anesthesiology* 44:194, 1976.

113. Webster NR, Nunn JF: Molecular structure of free radicals and their importance in biological reactions, *Br J Anaesth* 60:98, 1988.

114. Weiskopf RB, Cahalan MK, Ionescu P et al: Cardiovascular actions of desflurane with and without nitrous oxide during spontaneous ventilation in humans, *Anesth Analg* 73:165, 1991.

115. Williamson DC, Munson ES: Correlation of peripheral venous and arterial blood gas values during general anesthesia, *Anesth Analg* 61:950, 1982.

116. Wollman H, Alexander SC, Cohen PJ et al: Cerebral circulation during general anesthesia and hyperventilation in man: thiopental induction to nitrous oxide and *d*-tubocurarine, *Anesthesiology* 26:329, 1965.

117. Wong KD, Martin WE, Hornbein TF et al: The cardiovascular effects of morphine sulfate with oxygen and with nitrous oxide in man, *Anesthesiology* 38:542, 1973.

118. Woodbridge PD: Changing concepts concerning depth of anesthesia, *Anesthesiology* 18:536, 1957.

119. Yacoub O, Doell D, Kryger MH et al: Depression of hypoxic ventilatory response by nitrous oxide, *Anesthesiology* 45:385, 1976.

120. Yasuda N, Lockhart SH, Eger EI II et al: Kinetics of desflurane, isoflurane, and halothane in humans, *Anesthesiology* 74:489, 1991.

121. Yasuda N, Targ AG, and Eger EI II: Solubility of I-653, sevoflurane, isoflurane, and halothane in human tissues, *Anesth Analg* 69:370, 1989.

122. Yasuda N, Targ AG, Eger EI II et al: Pharmacokinetics of desflurane, sevoflurane, isoflurane, and halothane in pigs, *Anesth Analg* 71:340, 1990.

123. Zwass MS, Fisher DM, Welborn LG et al: Induction and maintenance characteristics of anesthesia with desflurane and nitrous oxide in infants and children, *Anesthesiology* 76:373, 1992.

CHAPTER 51

Pharmacology of Intravenous Sedative Agents

BEVERLY K. PHILIP

Intravenous (IV) sedatives are widely used in the clinical practice of anesthesia, from premedication to intraoperative supplementation to postoperative sedation. By far the most commonly used IV sedatives are the benzodiazepines. Many benzodiazepines have been synthesized and marketed; those compounds available for IV administration and used in anesthesia in the United States include diazepam (Valium), midazolam (Versed), and lorazepam (Ativan). An IV benzodiazepine antagonist, flumazenil, is also available. Oral formulations of diazepam, as well as other benzodiazepines, can be used for preoperative sedation. Droperidol, alone and in neuroleptic combina-

tions (as Innovar), is also sometimes used for premedication and intraoperative sedation.

BENZODIAZEPINES

Physiochemical Properties

The benzodiazepines structurally consist of a benzene ring fused to a diazepine ring (Fig. 51-1).[76] All clinically used 1,4-benzodiazcpine compounds also have an aryl or cyclohexenyl group at the 5 position; this is the structural unit needed to retain central nervous system (CNS) sedative properties.[30] Substitutions at other positions enable the development of many compounds with minor modifications in clinical activity. Diazepam and lorazepam are structurally similar, whereas midazolam is structurally different, with an imidazole ring at the 1,2 position.

Mechanisms of Action

An understanding of the pharmacology of the benzodiazepine sedatives begins with the neurotransmitter concept. Neurotransmitters carry signals from one cell to another and may have either excitatory or inhibitory effects on signal transmissions.[64] Gamma-aminobutyric acid (GABA) is the most important inhibitory neurotransmitter in the brain.[35,64] GABA is synthesized and stored in presynaptic axon terminals and is released into the synapse by calcium ions at the time of a nerve action potential. GABA is then available to act on nonspecific receptors located on the postsynaptic membrane of target neurons. Activation of the GABA receptor is associated with the opening of chloride channels in the postsynaptic membrane. The influx of chloride ions results in hyperpolarization of the cell membrane and the

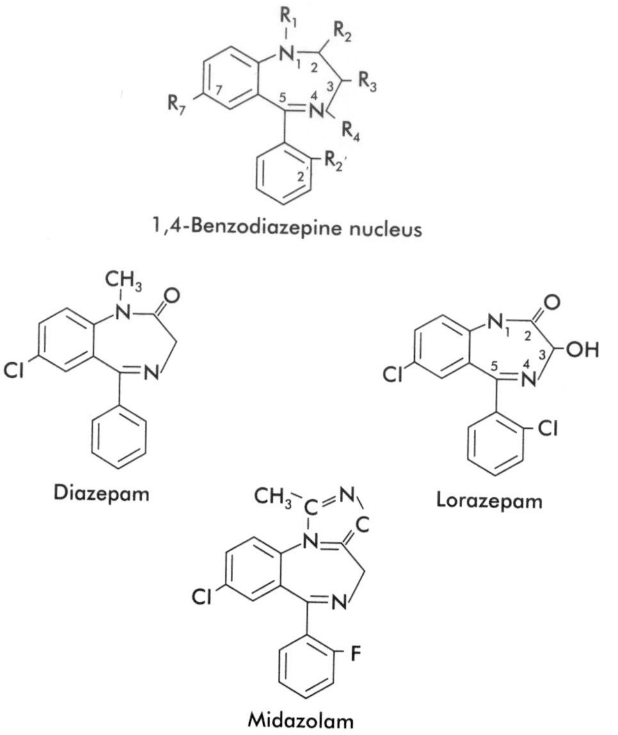

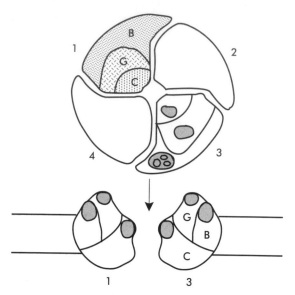

1,4-Benzodiazepine nucleus

Diazepam

Lorazepam

Midazolam

Fig. 51-1. Structure of benzodiazepines. (From Wood M: *Intravenous anesthetic agents.* In Wood M, Wood AJJ: *Drugs and anesthesia,* Baltimore, 1990, Williams & Wilkins.)

Fig. 51-2. Hypothetic diagram of gamma-aminobutyric acid (GABA)–benzodiazepine receptor–chloride channel complex. Complex is seen from extracellular site *(top)* on section through cell membrane. Complex is shown to be composed of four monomers. The monomers contain three major anatomic and functional domains: chloride channel part *(C),* GABA receptor *(G),* and benzodiazepine receptor *(B).* Each domain carries ligand-binding site (shown on monomer 3): on benzodiazepine receptor sites for agonists, inverse agonists, and antagonists. (Modified from Haefely W: *The biologic basis of benzodiazepine actions.* In Smith DE, Wesson DR, eds: *The benzodiazepines—current standards for medical practice,* Lancaster, England, 1985, MTP Press.)

inhibitory effect of GABA. Neurons with GABA are primarily interneurons and represent either feed-forward or feedback inhibition systems.[35]

Highly specific receptors for benzodiazepines have been identified. Electrophysiologic and biochemical experiments indicate that these receptors are located in close association with GABA receptors in the nervous system.

Structurally, benzodiazepine receptors are part of a tetrameric α_2/β_2 supramolecular complex consisting of the GABA receptor, the chloride channel, and the benzodiazepine receptor (Fig. 51-2).[35] The benzodiazepine receptor may be on the alpha subunits. **Activation of the benzodiazepine receptor induces conformational changes in the GABA receptor, enhancing binding of GABA to its receptor and thereby increasing chloride ion flow. Physiologically, benzodiazepines potentiate the action of GABA, causing a shift to the left in the GABA dose–chloride conductance response curve. Benzodiazepine receptors are distributed unevenly in the brain, with the highest number in the cerebral cortex, the limbic system, and the cerebellar cortex.**

Glycine is thought to be the major inhibitory neurotransmitter in the brainstem and spinal cord.[64] Benzodiazepines have affinity for glycine receptors, and it has been suggested that benzodiazepines may

have additional glycine-mimetic activity through that mechanism.

The mechanisms of actions of benzodiazepines on the neurotransmitter system can be correlated with their pharmacologic effects (Fig. 51-3). The anticonvulsant property of benzodiazepines may be mediated by their GABA-facilitating effect. Seizure activity can be induced by interference with GABA transmission, and benzodiazepines can prevent these seizures. **Sedative properties of benzodiazepines may be mediated through GABA neurotransmission, possibly in the cortex. Glycine mediates inhibition of motor neurons in the spinal cord; the muscle-relaxant properties of benzodiazepines may therefore be related to their glycine-mimetic activity. Benzodiazepine interaction with the inhibitory transmitter glycine may also result in the antianxiety effect of benzodiazepines, via inhibition of afferent conduction to higher anxiety centers at the level of the brainstem. Neurochemical mechanisms have not been postulated for the production of amnesia by benzodiazepines.**

Three distinct classes of active agents, or ligands, have been identified at the benzodiazepine receptor. Agonist ligands potentiate GABA efficacy and in-

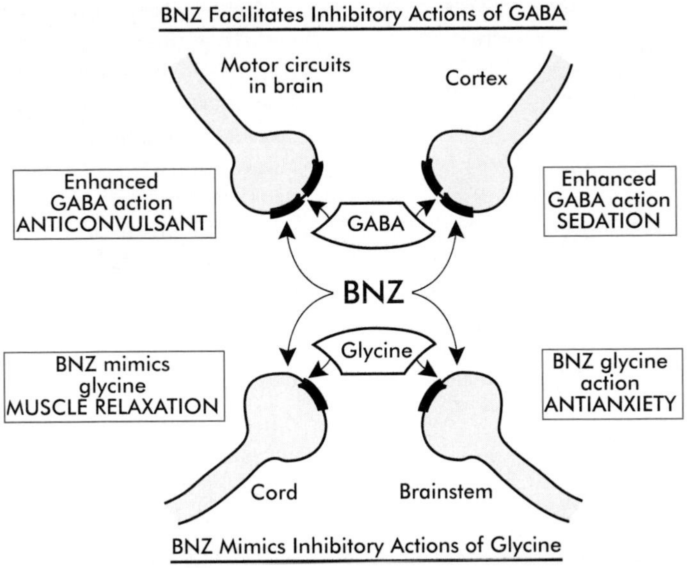

BNZ Facilitates Inhibitory Actions of GABA

Motor circuits in brain · Cortex

Enhanced GABA action ANTICONVULSANT · GABA · Enhanced GABA action SEDATION

BNZ

BNZ mimics glycine MUSCLE RELAXATION · Glycine · BNZ glycine action ANTIANXIETY

Cord · Brainstem

BNZ Mimics Inhibitory Actions of Glycine

Fig. 51-3. Summary of possible mechanisms for pharmacologic properties of benzodiazepine drugs *(BNZ)*. *GABA,* Gamma-aminobutyric acid. (From Richter JJ: Current theories about the mechanisms of benzodiazepines and neuroleptic drugs, *Anesthesiology* 54:66, 1981.)

clude the classic therapeutic benzodiazepine drugs. Inverse agonist ligands decrease GABA efficacy. These ligands have, in general, anxiogenic proconvulsant properties and are represented by compounds such as the beta-carbolines. Benzodiazepine-receptor antagonists are able to block the effect of both agonists and inverse agonists without activity of their own. An endogenous ligand at the benzodiazepine receptor has not yet been identified, but evidence suggests that it has GABA-inhibitory (inverse agonist) activity.[49]

AGONISTS
Diazepam
Pharmacology

Diazepam is the classic benzodiazepine used for sedation in anesthesia. It is insoluble in water and highly lipid soluble. After IV administration, the drug undergoes rapid entry into cerebrospinal fluid, followed by redistribution from blood primarily into fatty tissues. Redistribution has been shown to occur relatively rapidly (10 to 15 minutes) and is primarily responsible for the disappearance of acute clinical effect.[70] Pharmacokinetic parameters for diazepam and the other therapeutic benzodiazepines are compared in Table 51-1.

Diazepam has a large volume of distribution and low hepatic clearance, resulting in an elimination half-life of 20 to 40 hours in adult patients and even longer in the elderly.[48] Diazepam is highly bound to plasma albumin (approximately 98%). Factors that

alter protein binding and tissue distribution can lead to altered diazepam elimination. Marked prolongation of diazepam elimination is seen in patients with hepatic cirrhosis and increased age, and a shortened half-life occurs in patients with renal failure.

Diazepam undergoes hepatic metabolism initially via oxidative processes to form desmethyldiazepam, methyloxazepam, and oxazepam (Fig. 51-4). These metabolites are pharmacologically active, and each has a long elimination half-life. Plasma levels of the primary metabolite desmethyldiazepam increase over 48 hours, with an elimination half-life of 51 to 120 hours. Diazepam metabolites are then secondarily biotransformed by conjugation with glucuronic acid. Oxidative metabolism can be impaired by old age, decreased hepatic function, and the presence of metabolic inhibitor drugs such as cimetidine; conju-

Table 51-1 Comparative pharmacokinetics of the therapeutic benzodiazepines

Drug	Distribution half-life (min)	Elimination half-life (hr)	Clearance (ml/min/kg)	Volume of distribution (L/kg)
Diazepam	10-15	20-40	0.25-0.50	1.0-1.5
Midazolam	7-10	2.0-2.5	4.0-8.0	1.1-1.8
Lorazepam	3-10	10-20	0.75-1.0	0.8-1.3

Modified from Swerdlow BN, Holley FO: Intravenous anesthetic agents: pharmacokinetic-pharmacodynamic relationships, *Clin Pharmacokinet* 12:79, 1987.

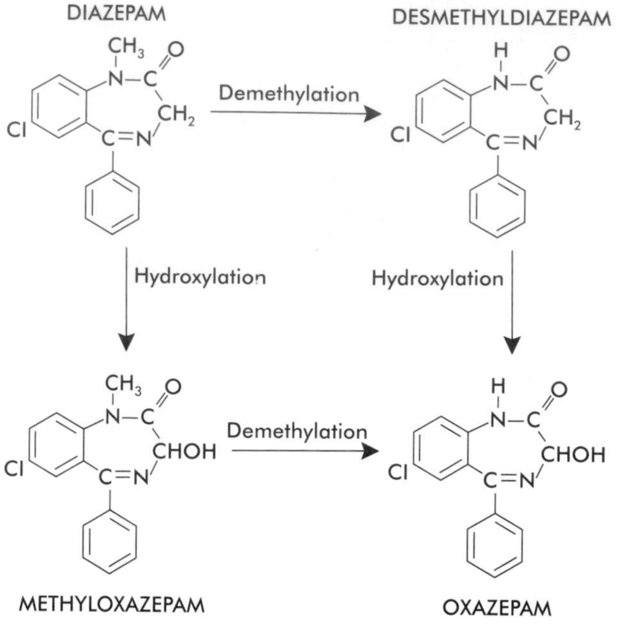

DIAZEPAM   DESMETHYLDIAZEPAM

Fig. 51-4. Hepatic metabolism of diazepam. (From Mandelli M, Tognoni G, and Garrattini S: Clinical pharmacokinetics of diazepam, *Clin Pharmacokinet* 3:72, 1978.)

gative processes are not affected by these factors. The glucuronides formed are pharmacologically inactive and are excreted in the urine.

Diazepam is well absorbed orally, with peak effects at 30 to 60 minutes. Absorption is delayed by the coadministration of food or aluminum-containing antacids. The oral formulation is dependable and preferable for preoperative medication. The alternative intramuscular route is painful, and absorption is erratic.

The major drawbacks of diazepam administered intravenously are local pain and phlebitis. Because diazepam is insoluble in water, it is formulated in organic solvents, including propylene glycol and ethyl alcohol (Valium). The incidence of venous sequelae after diazepam is greater when injected into smaller veins and increases with time: 23% after 2 to 3 days and 39% after 7 to 10 days.[36] Also, a faster rate of injection is associated with a higher incidence of immediate pain. Flushing the vein with saline may reduce thrombophlebitis.

Organ effects

Diazepam and all benzodiazepines have potent anticonvulsant properties. In the treatment of epilepsy, diazepam acts to prevent propagation and generalization of seizure activity. Diazepam is particularly useful as a supplement to local and regional anesthesia because it increases the seizure threshold for local anesthetic drugs. This should not, however, be construed as reason to exceed the permissible dose of local anesthetic.[60]

Respiratory function is variably affected by low, sedative doses of IV diazepam 0.1 mg/kg[6] and is depressed by moderate, soporific doses of the drug. Diazepam 0.4 mg/kg depresses the ventilatory response to carbon dioxide, increases the dead space/tidal volume ratio, and increases arterial carbon dioxide tension (Pa_{CO_2}). These effects are present within 1 minute and last 25 to 30 minutes[34] (Fig. 51-5). Depression of ventilation is intensified with the coadministration of narcotics.

Cardiovascular effects of diazepam are minimal. Doses of 0.5 mg/kg given to normal subjects produce a slight reduction in systolic blood pressure and no significant change in heart rate, pulmonary artery pressure, cardiac output, or systemic vascular resistance.[50] The concomitant administration of 50% nitrous oxide with diazepam produces minimal additional change; a slight reduction in cardiac output compared with values in the awake patient is associated with a decrease in systemic resistance.

Diazepam decreases muscle tone. This effect is mediated through the spinal internuncial neurons and involves GABAergic presynaptic inhibition. The neuromuscular junction is not involved.[15] Diazepam's effect on the cerebellar cortex may also contribute to muscle relaxation and incoordination.

High lipid solubility permits rapid transfer of diazepam across the placenta and into the fetus. Diazepam administration has been linked to increased birth defects, and it should be avoided in the first trimester of pregnancy. Diazepam administered to the parturient also has adverse effects on the newborn, including hypotonia and impairment of temperature regulation.[12]

Clinical use

Diazepam is able to produce amnesia, which can be a useful component of sedation. Oral diazepam has minimal amnestic effect: after 60 minutes, 5% lack of recall with 10 mg and 15% lack of recall with 20 mg.[45] IV doses of 5 mg and 10 mg of diazepam are required to produce a lack of recall lasting approximately 30 minutes in 50% and 90% of patients, respectively.[18] A more rapid rate of diazepam injection generates amnesia more frequently. However, these doses are excessive for sedation of the ambulatory patient. Retrograde amnesia after administration of IV diazepam has been variably reported.

Diazepam is not useful for anesthetic sleep induction because of slow variable onset as well as prolonged awakening and recovery. Diazepam is widely used to produce preoperative and intraoperative sedation for a broad range of diagnostic and therapeutic procedures with the patient under local and regional anesthesia. Sedation peaks rapidly, but total clinical effects may be prolonged. Ataxia and

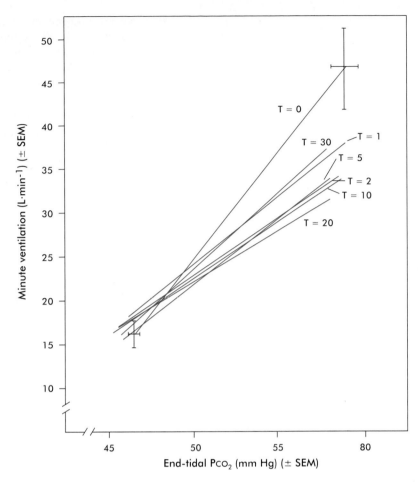

Fig. 51-5. Two-point carbon dioxide response curves before (*time = 0 minutes*) and after IV diazepam (0.4 mg/kg). (From Gross JB, Smith L, and Smith TC: Time course of ventilatory response to carbon dioxide after intravenous diazepam–nitrous oxide in patients with coronary artery disease, *Anesthesiology* 57:18, 1982.)

dizziness sufficient to delay discharge are present in 8% and 16% of subjects, respectively, 1 hour after administration of 10 mg of IV diazepam.[7] After 20 mg, ataxia and dizziness are present in 40% and 30% of subjects, respectively. Furthermore, after a period of early recovery, drowsiness and an increase in plasma concentration of diazepam have been reported at 6 to 8 hours, probably from enterohepatic recirculation as well as desmethyldiazepam effect (Fig. 51-6). **To avoid oversedation, diazepam should be used in 2.5 mg increments at 2- to 3-minute intervals. Individual dose response is widely variable, and dosage must be reduced in the elderly.**[48] **Diazepam should not be considered a sedative drug with short duration of action. Patients should be cautioned that they may feel tired for a day or more after its administration.**

Midazolam
Pharmacology
Midazolam has a chemical structure that is different from other therapeutic benzodiazepines.[40] At pH less

than 4 the diazepine ring structure is open (Fig. 51-7); this confers solubility in aqueous media. Midazolam can therefore be formulated without irritating solvents, and venous irritation or thrombosis is rare. At a pH greater than 4 the diazepine ring closes, with a half-life of about 10 minutes. The closed ring form is lipophilic at physiologic pH. This permits easy passage across the blood-brain barrier and therefore rapid onset of drug effect after IV administration.

After an IV dose, midazolam undergoes rapid redistribution with a 7- to 10-minute half-life (see Table 51-1). **The volume of distribution at steady state is similar to that of other IV benzodiazepines. Hepatic clearance, however, is much faster, approximately 50% of hepatic blood flow and 10 times that of diazepam. The net result is a significantly shorter elimination half-life of 2 to 2½ hours.** After an oral dose, uptake is rapid, with maximal plasma concentrations at ½ to 1 hour (Fig. 51-8). Bioavailability after oral administration is 30% to 50% and is related to extensive first-pass hepatic metabolism.

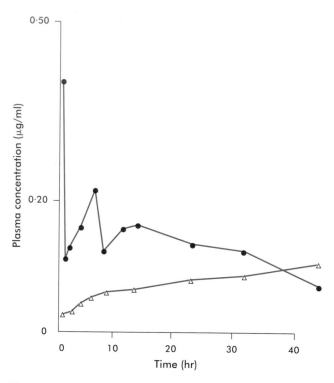

Fig. 51-6. Plasma concentrations of diazepam (●) and des-methyldiazepam (△) after IV administration of diazepam (20 mg). (From Baird ES, Hailey DM: Delayed recovery from a sedative: correlation of the plasma levels of diazepam with clinical effects after oral and intravenous administration, *Br J Anaesth* 144:803, 1972.)

Midazolam undergoes oxidative metabolism in the liver to 1- and 4-hydroxymidazolam (Fig. 51-9). The 1-OH form predominates in humans. This metabolite has intrinsic activity (in animal tests) of approximately one-tenth the potency of the parent compound. The elimination half-life of 1-OH midazolam is about 1 hour, and its effect should be included in assessing clinical response to midazolam.[13] The hydroxylated metabolites of midazolam are further conjugated to inactive glucuronides and excreted in the urine. Midazolam is highly protein bound (approximately 96%), primarily to albumin.

The duration of midazolam's clinical effect depends primarily on the rate of redistribution from

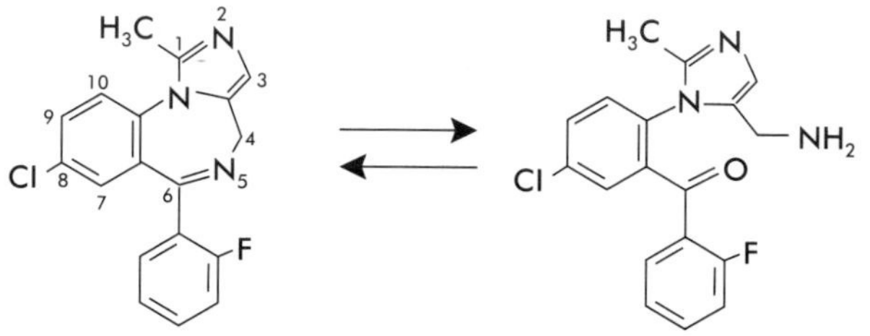

Fig. 51-7. The pH-dependent, ring–opening phenomenon characteristic of midazolam. (From Kanto JH: Midazolam: the first water-soluble benzodiazepine, *Pharmacotherapy* 5:138, 1985.)

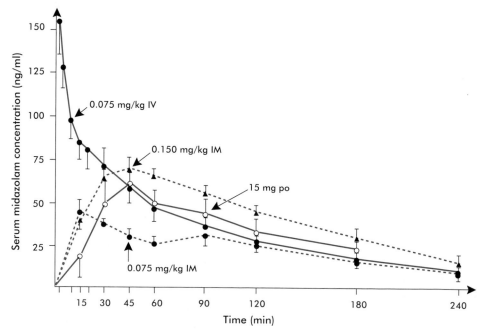

Fig. 51-8. Serum concentrations of midazolam after single doses of midazolam by oral *(po)*, intramuscular *(IM),* and intravenous *(IV)* routes. (From Kanto JH: Midazolam: the first water-soluble benzodiazepine, *Pharmacotherapy* 5:138, 1985.)

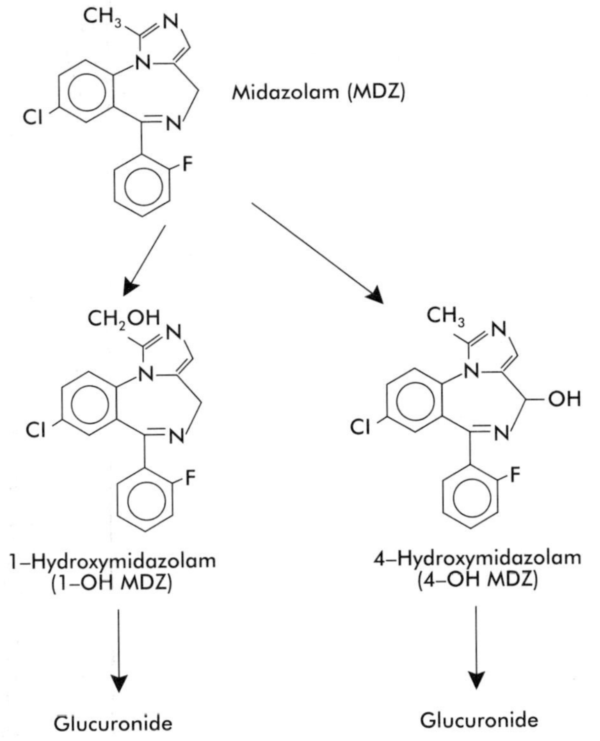

Fig. 51-9. Biotransformation of midazolam. (From Kanto JH: Midazolam: the first water-soluble benzodiazepine, *Pharmacotherapy* 5:138, 1985.)

active sites in the central compartment (specifically brain) to inactive peripheral sites. A larger volume of distribution occurs with larger adipose tissue mass, and the size of single doses of midazolam may need to be increased in morbidly obese patients in proportion to their total weight.[32] Other factors associated with increased tissue distribution include female gender, pregnancy, age, and renal insufficiency.

The elimination half-life of midazolam is prolonged when peripheral distribution is increased. Elimination of midazolam is also extended when hepatic microsomal metabolism is impaired; this occurs in patients with hepatic cirrhosis and in the elderly, particularly males.[26,63] Drug elimination becomes the significant factor in termination of midazolam's effect during prolonged oral administration and during continuous infusions. Therefore infusion rates in elderly men should be reduced by approximately 50%. Midazolam's effect is enhanced with pretreatment by the H_2-receptor antagonists cimetidine and ranitidine; higher peak midazolam plasma levels are produced through a reduction in midazolam hepatic clearance.

Organ effects

Intracranial pressure is stable even with anesthetic induction doses of midazolam. However, 0.25 mg/kg **doses do not prevent the increase in intracranial pressure associated with laryngoscopy and intubation (Fig. 51-10).[29] Midazolam also reduces cerebral metabolic rate and cerebral blood flow in a dose-related fashion while maintaining a relatively normal metabolism/flow ratio. These data suggest that midazolam may be helpful for hypoxic brain protection.[63]**

Midazolam causes a reduction in ventilatory response to carbon dioxide. The level of depression after midazolam 0.15 mg/kg is similar to that seen after diazepam 0.3 mg/kg in healthy patients.[23] Patients with chronic obstructive pulmonary disease demonstrate midazolam-induced respiratory depression that peaks more slowly and returns to baseline later. Hypoxic ventilatory responses are depressed as well after sedative doses of midazolam 0.1 mg/kg.[1] Midazolam also can produce dose-related apnea. Both apnea and hypoxemia secondary to hypoventilation occur more frequently with the coadministration of opioids. Healthy volunteers given midazolam 0.05 mg/kg alone experience no apnea (15 seconds without spontaneous ventilation) or hypoxemia (pulse saturation less than 90% for 10 seconds). When midazolam is given with fentanyl 2 μg/kg, apnea occurs in 50% of the volunteers and hypoxemia in 92% (Table 51-2).[5]

Hemodynamic changes are observed after induction doses of midazolam. In healthy patients given 0.15 mg/kg, systolic and diastolic blood pressures are reduced by 5% and 10%, respectively, and heart rate is increased by 18%. In patients with ischemic heart disease given 0.2 to 0.3 mg/kg, the cardiac index and left-sided and right-sided heart filling pressures are maintained, but systemic vascular resistance may decrease by 15% to 33%.[63] **Hemodynamic changes produced by midazolam are similar to those produced by induction doses of thiopental 3 mg/kg but somewhat greater than diazepam 0.25 to 0.50 mg/kg (Fig. 51-11).**

Clinical use

Midazolam is an effective amnestic. Anterograde amnesia after 5 mg of IV midazolam is greatest 2 to 5 minutes after injection and lasts 20 to 40 minutes.[20] Complete amnesia for picture card recall develops in 67% of patients and partial amnesia in 93%. Amnesia, however, is not ensured even after a substantial 5 mg IV bolus; 33% of the patients did not develop complete amnesia.[20] Brief amnesia has been reported after only 2 mg and was not associated with patient drowsiness.[58] It should be emphasized that some patients become distressed when they cannot recall perioperative events. The potential for amnesia should be discussed with patients in advance, and all perioperative instructions should be given both verbally and in writing.

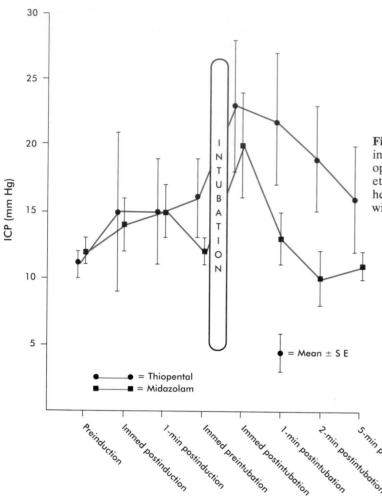

Fig. 51-10. Intracranial pressure *(ICP)* during induction and intubation with midazolam (0.25 mg/kg) compared with thiopental (4 mg/kg). (From Giffin J, Cottrell J, Shwiry B, et al: Intracranial pressure, mean arterial pressure and heart rate following midazolam or thiopental in humans with brain tumors, *Anesthesiology* 60:491, 1984.)

Midazolam can be used to temporarily obtund consciousness during the placement of local or regional blocks. This effect can be achieved using doses of 0.15 to 0.40 mg/kg. Midazolam dosage should be reduced in the elderly, who appear to have increased CNS sensitivity for midazolam.[33] Signs of adequate induction are both loss of lash reflex and

loss of response to verbal command; the former alone is unreliable. Speed of induction is variable, somewhat slower than seen with the barbiturates[52] and similar to that seen with diazepam.[25] Awakening after induction with midazolam (0.20 mg/kg) can be achieved after a 20-minute ambulatory anesthetic.[11] The level of postoperative sedation after 30 minutes of recovery was lower than with thiopental (4 mg/kg), but a difference was no longer present after 60 minutes. Speed of recovery is enhanced with the benzodiazepine antagonist flumazenil (see later discussion).[61]

Premedication[16] or coadministration[73] of an opioid decreases the induction dose of midazolam. This effect is synergistic and is seen even with subanalgetic doses of opioid (Fig. 51-12).[41] The increased ease of induction that occurs when benzodiazepines and opioids are given together is of particular concern if the anesthetic plan is local or regional anesthesia with sedation. The change from conscious to "unconscious" sedation carries increased risk of loss of protective reflexes and loss of airway patency. For this use, particular attention should be given to administer

Table 51-2 Occurrence of apnea and hypoxemia when midazolam (0.05 mg/kg) and fentanyl (2 μg/kg) are given alone or together		
Drugs	**Apnea**	**Hypoxemia**
Midazolam	0/12	0/12
Fentanyl	0/12	6/12
Midazolam plus fentanyl	6/12*	11/12*

*p < 0.05, compared with drugs alone.
From Bailey PL, Pace NL, Ashburn MA et al: Frequent hypoxemia and apnea after sedation with midazolam and fentanyl, *Anesthesiology* 73:826, 1990.

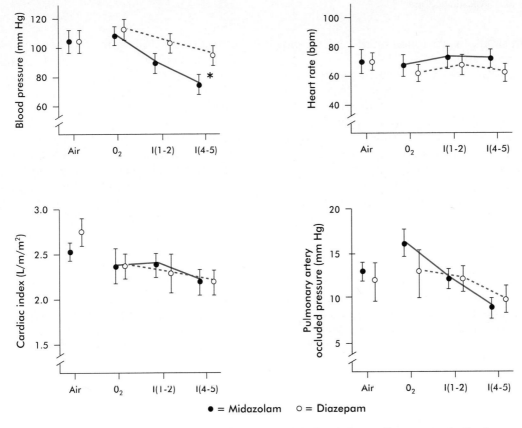

Fig. 51-11. Hemodynamic variables in patients with ischemic heart disease anesthetized with midazolam (0.2 mg/kg IV) and diazepam (0.5 mg/kg IV). Determinations were made with patients breathing room air, breathing 100% oxygen, 1 to 2 minutes after intubation *(I [1-2]),* and 4 to 5 minutes after induction *(I [4-5]).* * $p < 0.05$, midazolam vs. diazepam. (From Reves JG, Fragen RF, Vinik HR, and Greenblatt DJ: Midazolam: pharmacology and uses, *Anesthesiology* 62:310, 1985.)

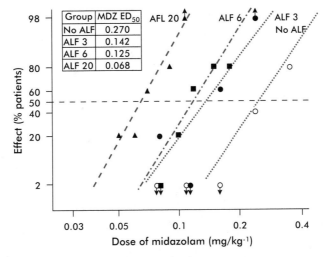

Fig. 51-12. Effect of alfentanil *(ALF)* on the midazolam *(MDZ)* dose-response curves for induction of anesthesia. *No ALF* (O), midazolam dose-response curve without addition of alfentanil (saline only). *ALF 3* (●), *ALF 6* (■), and *ALF 20* (▲), midazolam dose-response curves with addition of alfentanil in doses 3, 6, and 20 µg/kg, respectively. Each symbol represents effect in a subgroup of five patients at indicated dosage. *Inset* represents midazolam ED_{50} (effective dose for 50% of group) values for the four dose-response curves. (Modified from Kissin I, Vinik HR, Castillo R, and Bradley EL: Alfentanil potentiates midazolam-induced unconsciousness at subanalgesic doses, *Anesth Analg* 71:65, 1990.)

drug doses in small, titrated increments and to allow time to observe possible effects.[57]

Midazolam is used for preoperative sedation. The oral formulation is effective at 15 mg doses for the adult,[40] but it is not available in the United States. For children, midazolam 0.5 mg/kg has been given in apple juice. This dose allows improved parental separation and smoother anesthetic induction for 15 to 40 minutes after midazolam administration.[75] The intramuscular route is popular. Midazolam 5 mg given intramuscularly to adults has provided preoperative sedation, less anxiety, and impaired recall.[69] Recovery was not prolonged. However, this dose-time combination might be more applicable to routine inpatient rather than outpatient premedication. The IV route for presurgical sedation is often used. **Midazolam 5 mg IV generates sedation and anxiolysis within 1 to 2 minutes. Motor performance recovers in 34 minutes, and subjects are awake and walking unaided within 73 minutes.**[19]

Large doses of midazolam, however, result in prolonged drowsiness. Also, administration of inappropriately large doses of midazolam can result in excessive adverse effects, particularly respiratory depression. Cardiorespiratory arrests have been reported, particularly in the elderly during endoscopic procedures. Midazolam should be given in small 1 to 2 mg increments, and individual patient response varies considerably. Similar dose increments can be used to establish sedation during local and regional anesthesia.

Plasma levels of midazolam and clinical endpoints have been correlated (Fig. 51-13). A midazolam con-

centration of 300 ng/ml has been found to provide adequate hypnosis during total IV anesthesia for surgical procedures.[56] At midazolam concentration of 150 to 200 ng/ml, patients are arousable and become able to respond verbally; at concentrations of 150 to 100 ng/ml, patients appear drowsy. Amnesia is present at concentrations above 100 ng/ml, and sedation persists until concentrations decline below 75 ng/ml.[55]

Plasma levels of midazolam can be used to demonstrate the enhanced sedation that occurs when opioids and midazolam are given together.[55] Patients are more sedated at similar plasma midazolam concentrations when alfentanil is also being administered, with a leftward shift in the midazolam plasma concentration–effect curve (Fig. 51-14).

Midazolam has been compared with diazepam for supplementation of ambulatory regional anesthesia. Patients undergoing spinal, epidural, or brachial plexus blocks have received moderate doses of a benzodiazepine, either midazolam 0.10 mg/kg or diazepam 0.18 mg/kg.[14] The degree of intraoperative sedation is similar after either sedative using these doses. However, when residual sedation is evaluated after 2 hours of recovery, 80% of the patients who receive midazolam are awake. After the same period of recovery from diazepam, only 65% of patients are awake. Amnestic effectiveness under these conditions can also be compared. Fifty percent of patients who receive 0.10 mg/kg of midazolam remember nothing of their surgery, but only 18% of patients who receive 0.18 mg/kg of diazepam are completely amnestic. **Midazolam, rather than diazepam, allows more rapid recovery and provides more effective amnesia when**

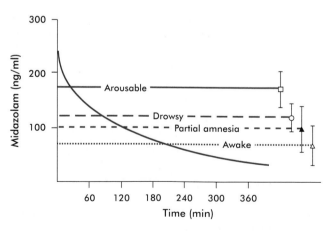

Fig. 51-13. Concentration-time profile of midazolam showing mean (±SD) concentrations associated with various pharmacodynamic endpoints. (From Persson MP, Nilsson A, and Hartvig P: Relations of sedation and amnesia to plasma concentrations of midazolam in surgical patients, *Clin Pharmacol Ther* 43:324, 1988.)

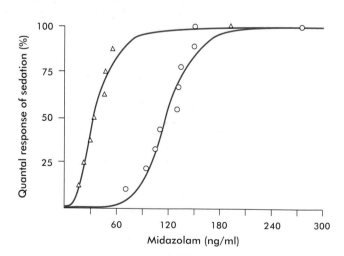

Fig. 51-14. Concentration-response curve during patient recovery for steps from arousable to drowsy. ○, After midazolam sedation with epidural block. △, After midazolam plus alfentanil for total IV anesthesia. (Modified from Persson MP, Nilsson A, and Hartvig P: Relation of sedation and amnesia to plasma concentrations of midazolam in surgical patients, *Clin Pharmacol Ther* 43:324, 1988.)

used for sedation during local anesthesia for ambulatory dental[4] and endoscopic[68] procedures as well.

Midazolam can be administered by infusion to provide a stable level of sedation during surgery. If midazolam is to be used by continuous infusion, care must be taken to provide only that amount needed to produce the desired level of effect. One must also terminate the infusion at an appropriate time to avoid excessive sedation after the procedure and prolonged recovery times. When giving midazolam by infusion to supplement local or regional anesthesia, a satisfactory level of sedation should be achieved first by incremental titration of a loading dose, using boluses or rapid infusion. Loading doses of 0.01 to 0.07 mg/kg have been used. A maintenance infusion rate of 0.04 to 0.10 mg/kg/hour, sufficient to continue the desired level of sedation, may then be given.[59] Wide individual variability exists. Both loading and maintenance doses are reduced in the elderly.

Midazolam has additional usefulness for sedation in adult and pediatric intensive care units. Infusion rates of approximately 0.04 mg/kg/hour (range, 0.01 to 0.20 mg/kg/hour)[44] have been used with opioids for postsurgical care or alone for sedation during mechanical ventilation. Loading doses are scaled to achieve the desired effect: 0.03 to 0.06 mg/kg for "cooperative and tranquil patients" to 0.2 mg/kg for "asleep" patients. After a mean 18 hours of sedation, recovery to time of extubation is about 3¼ hours.

Lorazepam
Pharmacology

Lorazepam is approximately 5 to 10 times more potent than diazepam. After IV administration, lorazepam shows a rapid distribution half-life of 3 to 10 minutes.[31] Compared with diazepam, lorazepam is only moderately lipid soluble and moderately highly (approximately 90%) protein bound. The steady-state volume of distribution is slightly smaller and hepatic clearance slightly faster, resulting in an intermediate-duration elimination half-life of 10 to 20 hours[70] (see Table 51-1). Lorazepam is metabolized primarily in the liver to pharmacologically inactive glucuronides, which are excreted in the urine. Lorazepam distribution is not significantly affected by increasing age or renal or liver disease. Elimination half-life may be prolonged in patients with hepatic cirrhosis because of nonmetabolic factors, including changes in lorazepam protein binding and tissue distribution.

Lorazepam is relatively insoluble in water, and the parenteral formulation of lorazepam includes solvents such as polyethylene glycol. However, lorazepam is associated with less pain on injection or venous thrombosis than diazepam.[36] Unlike diazepam, intramuscular absorption of lorazepam is reliably effective.

Clinical duration of action with lorazepam is not explained solely by the pharmacokinetic half-lives given previously. A delay in the onset of effect occurs after lorazepam administration, and peak clinical effect lags behind peak serum concentration.[70] This has been observed after both oral and IV routes of administration. The delay may be caused by lorazepam's relatively lower lipid solubility, compared with diazepam, and therefore slower entry into the CNS. Also, duration of clinical effect may be longer than with diazepam despite lorazepam's shorter elimination half-life. This may result from tighter lorazepam binding to the CNS receptor site, with slower redistribution to peripheral tissues.

The effects of lorazepam on cardiovascular and respiratory systems resemble those of diazepam.

Clinical use

Doses of 2 and 4 mg of lorazepam have been compared for their amnestic and sedative effects. Oral administration of lorazepam at either dose results in sedation, which appears within 30 minutes and increases for 2 hours. The sedative effect persisted for the 4 hours studied.[45] Intramuscular lorazepam has similar time course of sedative effect. After IV administration of 2 or 4 mg of lorazepam, sedation appeared within 5 minutes and lasted for the 4 to 6 hours of the study.[53] This would suggest that a dose of 2 mg of lorazepam suffices for preoperative sedation.

The amnestic effect of lorazepam, however, is dose dependent. Anterograde amnesia after oral lorazepam 2 mg peaks at 30% lack of recall at 2 hours and declines to 15% at 4 hours. After 4 mg of oral lorazepam, lack of recall is approximately 70% at 2 and 3 hours and declines to only 40% at 4 hours.[45] After IV administration of 2 mg of lorazepam, amnesia develops in 50% of patients at 30 minutes and lasts ½ hour. After 4 mg of IV lorazepam, amnesia develops in 70% of patients at 15 minutes, and the effect persists over 4 hours.[53] Increased and prolonged amnesia may be achieved with a 4-mg dose.

The sedative and amnestic actions of IV lorazepam have been compared with diazepam.[17] **Two mg of lorazepam provides sedation of equivalent efficacy to 10 mg of diazepam. Four mg of lorazepam produces amnesia that begins more slowly and lasts longer than after 10 to 20 mg of diazepam (Fig. 51-15). Lorazepam is also more effective than diazepam in suppressing sequelae produced by ketamine, probably because of lorazepam's greater amnestic properties.**

The long duration of sedation and amnesia after lorazepam, by any route of administration, suggests that it should not be used when rapid awakening of patients after surgery is desired.

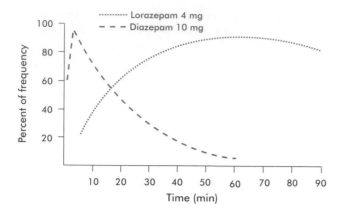

Fig. 51-15. Percentage frequency of patients' loss of ability to recall objects shown at various intervals following IV administration of lorazepam (4 mg) and diazepam (10 mg). (From Dundee JW, McGowan WAW, Lilburn JK et al: Comparison of the actions of diazepam and lorazepam, *Br J Anaesth* 51:439, 1979.)

NONSPECIFIC BENZODIAZEPINE ANTAGONISTS

The sedative, psychomotor, and amnestic effects of clinically used benzodiazepines can persist after a procedure is completed. A variety of drugs have been tried, some empirically, to terminate the benzodiazepine effect.

Aminophylline

Aminophylline is a methylxanthine that has analeptic and cardiorespiratory stimulant properties. These properties are probably mediated through blocking the receptors of the inhibitory CNS neurotransmitter adenosine. Aminophylline is not active at the central benzodiazepine receptor. Low doses of aminophylline, 1 to 2 mg/kg, have been used to reverse the sedative, respiratory depressant, and psychomotor effects of benzodiazepines with moderate but inconsistent efficacy.[27] Caffeine is also effective by a similar mechanism.

Physostigmine

Physostigmine is an anticholinesterase that can cross the blood-brain barrier. Physostigmine combines with the enzyme acetylcholinesterase to form a carbamyl-ester compound. This reversible inactivation of acetylcholinesterase allows increased cholinergic neurotransmission. Physostigmine may therefore act as an analeptic agent through accumulation of acetylcholine at muscarinic cholinergic receptors in the ascending reticular activating system.[71] Physostigmine does not affect the benzodiazepine receptor directly or the GABA neurotransmitter system. **Physostigmine, 1 to 2 mg in the adult, has been used for reversing sedation caused by benzodiazepines, but often with inconsis-**

Table 51-3   Pharmacokinetic data for flumazenil

Distribution half-life (min)	Elimination half-life (hr)	Clearance (L/min)	Volume of distribution (L/kg)
≤5	0.7-1.3	0.5-1.3	0.6-1.6

Data from Amrein R, Hetzel W, Bonetti EP et al: Clinical pharmacology of Dormicum (midazolam) and Anexate (flumazenil), *Resuscitation* 16:55, 1988; and Klotz U, Kanto J: Pharmacokinetics and clinical use of flumazenil (RO 15-1788), *Clin Pharmacokinet* 14:1, 1988.

tent or limited efficacy. Cholinergic side effects include vomiting (hyperperistalsis), bradycardia, and increased salivation and perspiration.

Naloxone

Naloxone, the mu receptor opioid antagonist, is not effective against pure benzodiazepine-induced sedation or respiratory depression, except perhaps at pharmacologic doses (15 mg).[39]

SPECIFIC ANTAGONIST: FLUMAZENIL
Pharmacology

While screening imidazobenzodiazepine derivatives for clinical efficacy, researchers identified a group of compounds with a high affinity for the benzodiazepine receptor but with no CNS effects. These compounds were then found to have specific antagonist activity.[37] Flumazenil (Mazicon) is the antagonist that has undergone the most extensive testing and clinical use.

Flumazenil is a mildly lipophilic, weak base that can be prepared in aqueous solutions using a dilution of 0.1 mg/ml.[2] Average pharmacokinetic data can be found in Table 51-3. **After IV injection, onset of flumazenil's effect is rapid. Peak levels occur in plasma within 5 minutes and in the cerebral cortex and cerebellum within 5 to 8 minutes (Fig. 51-16).[54] A lower protein binding of approximately 50%, compared with 96% for the agonist benzodiazepine midazolam, contributes to the rapidity of onset. Rapid distribution coupled with a high liver extraction rate (60%) produce a relatively short duration of action. Flumazenil is metabolized in the liver predominantly to a free carboxylic acid derivative and then immediately to the glucuronide (Fig. 51-17); both compounds are inactive. From 90% to 95% of the metabolized drug is excreted in the urine and 5% to 10% in feces; less than 0.1% of the parent drug is excreted in the urine. Oral flumazenil has low bioavailability (16%) because of the extensive hepatic clearance. The pharmacokinetic profile of flumazenil is not significantly altered**

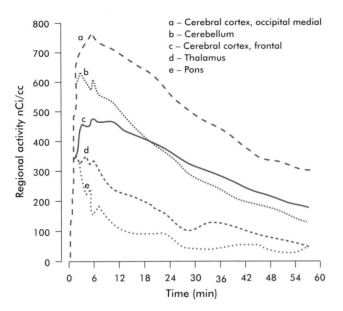

a – Cerebral cortex, occipital medial
b – Cerebellum
c – Cerebral cortex, frontal
d – Thalamus
e – Pons

Fig. 51-16. Radioactivity in brain regions of a healthy man after IV injection of carbon-11-labelled (^{11}C) RO 15-1788 (flumazenil); *nCi,* nanocuries. (From Persson A, Ehrin E, Eriksson L et al: Imaging of ^{11}C-labelled Ro-1788 binding to benzodiazepine receptors in the human brain by positron emission tomography, *J Psychiatr Res* 19:609, 1985.)

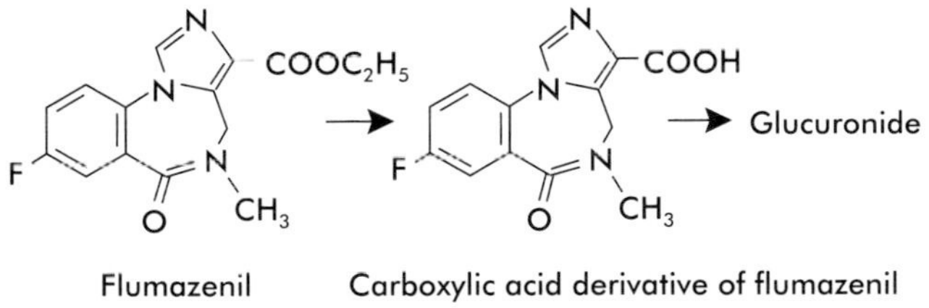

Flumazenil   Carboxylic acid derivative of flumazenil

Fig. 51-17. Flumazenil and its metabolism. (From Amrein R, Hetzel W, Bonetti EP et al: Clinical pharmacology of Dormicum [midazolam] and Anexate [flumazenil], *Resuscitation* 16:S5, 1988.)

by the coadministration of another therapeutic benzodiazepine,[43] and vice versa.

Flumazenil has clear competitive antagonist activity, whether given before, simultaneously with, or after a therapeutic benzodiazepine.[42] Antagonist activity has been shown for all benzodiazepine effects modulated through the CNS benzodiazepine receptor, including sedative, amnestic, muscle relaxant, and anticonvulsant effects. Flumazenil can antagonize all the therapeutic benzodiazepines tested and the few other drugs that are active at the CNS benzodiazepine receptors. Flumazenil has no antagonist effect on substances that do not act at the central benzodiazepine receptor (e.g., barbiturates, opiates, alcohol).[2] Antagonist activity has been demonstrated both with research subjects given benzodiazepine and flumaze-

nil and with patients given benzodiazepine for diagnostic and therapeutic procedures. Symptoms consistent with benzodiazepine withdrawal have been reported in benzodiazepine-dependent individuals.

In addition to its predominantly antagonist properties, flumazenil may have weak, generalized central arousal or anxiogenic (inverse agonist-like) activity. This effect is variable and depends on the basal condition and measurement performed.[42] Flumazenil also does have weak anticonvulsant (agonist-like) activity. Flumazenil is directly able to reverse hepatic coma, a transient effect that occurs via modulation of the GABA neurotransmitter system.

Flumazenil and the therapeutic benzodiazepines demonstrate reciprocal dose-dependent action. The therapeutic benzodiazepines produce clinical effects in a dose-related spectrum; for example, low doses of midazolam cause anxiolysis, and high doses are needed for hypnosis. Reversal of benzodiazepine effects occurs in a sequence opposite to the order of their appearance[2] (Table 51-4). Also, the dose of antagonist needed is reciprocal to the dose of therapeutic benzodiazepine. For example, high doses of flumazenil are needed to reverse anxiolysis. This allows the clinician some differential selectivity in reversing excess benzodiazepine effect, such as hypnosis to sedation while retaining anxiolysis.

Organ Effects

Flumazenil has little intrinsic toxicity. Single doses of up to 600 mg orally or 100 mg intravenously have been well tolerated.[42] Flumazenil reversal has been shown to have no effect on hemodynamic parameters when assessed in patients undergoing cardiac catheterization.[28] Patients were sedated with diazepam (mean, 11.4 ± 4.4 mg) and then awakened after the procedure with flumazenil (0.24 ± 0.1 mg), with no change

Table 51-4   Reciprocal dose-dependent effects of benzodiazepines (e.g., midazolam) and flumazenil

Midazolam	Effects	Flumazenil
Low dose	Anxiolysis	High dose
↓	Anticonvulsion	↑
	Slight sedation	
	Reduced attention	
	Amnesia	
	Intense sedation	
	Muscle relaxation	
High dose	Hypnosis	Low dose

Modified from Amrein R, Hetzel W, Bonetti EP et al: Clinical pharmacology of Dormicum (midazolam) and Anexate (flumenazil), *Resuscitation* 16:S5, 1988.

in heart rate, mean systemic arterial pressure, mean pulmonary artery pressure, left ventricular end-diastolic pressure, cardiac index, or pulmonary or systemic vascular resistances. Hemodynamic changes are not observed in postoperative cardiac or neurologic patients even in the presence of flumazenil-induced anxiety.

Flumazenil (0.1 mg/kg) injected alone produces no changes in cerebral blood flow in healthy subjects.[24] This dose also normalizes midazolam-induced decreases in cerebral blood flow as well as electroencephalographic (EEG) changes. Increases in cerebral blood flow and intracranial pressure to transiently above-normal values have been reported in heavily sedated animals given flumazenil[22] and in human patients after severe head injury with unstable intracranial pressure treated with midazolam. This suggests caution in the use of flumazenil for patients with decreased intracranial compliance.

Clinical Use

Flumazenil has been used to reverse residual benzodiazepine sedation in patients during local and regional anesthesia, using doses of 0.2 to 0.4 mg.[66] Subjective awakening occurs in 1 minute.[67] Amnesia is retained for events during benzodiazepine sedation and before antagonist administration, but flumazenil inhibits benzodiazepine anterograde amnesia for 5 to 60 minutes after its administration.[65] In general, the duration of flumazenil's action depends on the activity and dose of the previously administered benzodiazepine, the dose of flumazenil, and the time elapsed between administration of the agonist and the antagonist.[71]

Flumazenil may be used to reverse residual sedation after general anesthesia induced with a benzodiazepine. After the completion of midazolam-induced laparoscopy, patients have received increments of flumazenil to a mean total of 0.83 ± 0.04 mg (range, 0.6 to 1.0 mg).[61] They show significant subjective and objective improvement in sedation and in psychomotor coordination (Fig. 51-18). By 2 hours after surgery, the scores of the flumazenil-treated group are no longer different from the placebo-treated group, and both groups continue to recover. In studies involving longer-acting benzodiazepines, resedation has been reported. Caution must be observed to avoid premature discharge of ambulatory surgery patients during the time that flumazenil is effective.

Flumazenil also has potential use in the treatment of accidental or intentional benzodiazepine overdose in the emergency room or intensive care unit (ICU).[3] Flumazenil is consistently effective in reversing unconsciousness caused only by benzodiazepines with minimal side effects, using doses of 0.2 to 1.0 mg. The use of flumazenil for reversal in a mixed-drug

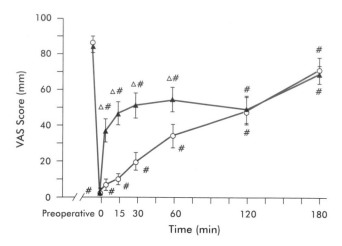

Fig. 51-18. Visual analog sedation scales (0, most sedated — 100, most alert) after midazolam-induced ambulatory laparoscopy. Flumazenil (▲) vs. placebo (○). △, p < 0.05, vs. placebo-treated group. #, p < 0.05, vs. preoperative control (within group). (From Philip BK, Simpson TH, Hauch MA et al: Flumazenil reverses sedation after midazolam-induced general anesthesia in ambulatory surgery patients, *Anesth Analg* 71:370, 1990.)

overdose, however, may result in increased side effects and may reveal the toxic effects of the other compounds ingested. Flumazenil is effective in interrupting or terminating benzodiazepine-induced ICU sedation, assessing level of consciousness, or facilitating weaning from mechanical ventilation. The most common side effect in ICU patients is agitation (6.5%). One must remember the short duration of flumazenil's activity and the potential need for repeat dosage or administration by infusion.[8]

The most common minor side effect reported after flumazenil administration in anesthesia is nausea and/or vomiting (10.8%).[3] **Nausea occurs more often when flumazenil is given to patients after general anesthesia for surgery than after conscious sedation or ICU use, which suggests a contribution from other anesthetic agents or the surgical procedure itself.**[10] **Interestingly, the overall incidence of vomiting alone after general anesthesia is not different with flumazenil than with placebo.**[3] Transient minor effects include tears, tremors, dizziness, and anxiety (each less than 1%). To minimize side effects, flumazenil should be given in incremental doses of 0.1 mg after an initial 0.2 mg, titrated to the desired level of arousal.

DROPERIDOL
Pharmacology

Droperidol has been used for many years as a sedative for surgical and diagnostic procedures. **Droperidol is a butyrophenone derivative, chemically related to**

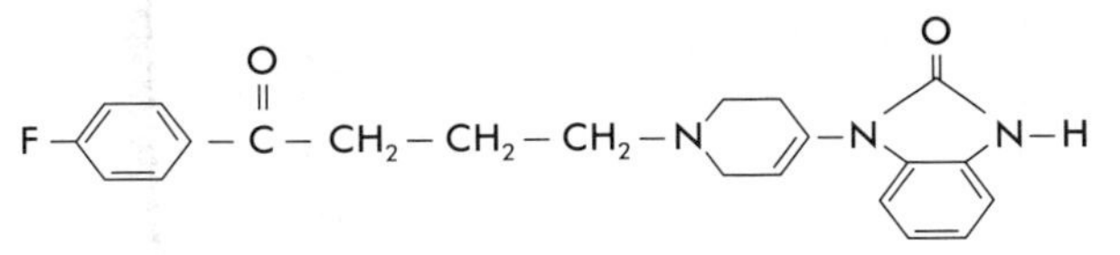

Fig. 51-19. Structure of droperidol.

haloperidol (Fig. 51-19).[38] **Butyrophenones act as dopamine antagonists in the central and peripheral nervous systems. Butyrophenones are thought to occupy postsynaptic GABA receptors and thereby block dopaminergic synapses.**

Studies in humans reveal a rapid distribution half-life of 10 to 14 minutes and elimination half-life of 103 to 134 minutes.[21] Droperidol is extensively metabolized in the liver, with less than 1% excreted in the urine as intact drug. Droperidol's metabolite is found in both urine and feces, suggesting biliary excretion as well. Significant levels of droperidol metabolite are seen for 8 to 12 hours following drug administration. The peak clinical effects after droperidol last 2 to 3 hours, but a significant clinical effect is detectable for at least 10 hours. This suggests clinical activity for the metabolite, possibly coupled with high CNS receptor affinity and retention of the drug.

Organ Effects

Organ effects of droperidol are generally minimal. Large doses of droperidol, 0.3 mg/kg, do not significantly affect respiration when assessed by carbon dioxide rebreathing techniques, although wide individual variation of response occurs.[62] Hypoxic ventilatory drive is stimulated by droperidol, via its dopamine receptor–blocking activity on the carotid body.[74] **Cardiovascular effects reflect mild alpha-adrenergic blocking activity, resulting in reduced systemic vascular resistance with an increase in venous capacitance.[72] Vasodilatation and decreased blood pressure are seen. Clinically significant hypotension may develop in patients with hypovolemia.**

Clinical Use

Droperidol produces a sense of detachment, lack of responsiveness, and apparent tranquility. It has therefore been used as a preoperative and intraoperative sedative in doses of 2.5 to 5 mg intravenously or 5 to 10 mg intramuscularly. **Droperidol is more often used with an opioid, producing neuroleptanalgesia. The combination of droperidol (2.5 mg/ml) and fentanyl (0.05 mg/ml) is sold as Innovar.**

Early enthusiastic use of droperidol alone and as Innovar generated many reports of complications, including prolonged and excessive sedation, extrapyramidal symptoms, and apprehension and anxiety despite apparent drowsiness. Great disparity exists between the observer's assessment of "sedation" and the patient's assessment of drug effect.[46] Patients sometimes became anxious, agitated, and confused to the extent that they canceled previously desired elective surgery. The incidence of refusal was 4.7% in a series of 121 military patients for plastic surgery[9] and 0.7% in a series of 1438 private patients scheduled for sterilization or plastic surgery procedures.[47]

In addition, the dose of the butyrophenone component of Innovar is too large and the effect too long lasting relative to the short-acting analgetic component. Its use for sedation during longer procedures requires supplementation with additional fentanyl, and respiratory depression can occur. Innovar may be used for sedation during longer diagnostic and surgical procedures, including endoscopies, burn dressings, and radiologic studies. However, Innovar is in general not recommended for ambulatory surgical procedures when rapid recovery with minimal side effects is desired.[57]

Droperidol is a potent antiemetic. Lower doses of 0.005 to 0.017 mg/kg (0.625 to 1.25 mg in adults) have been shown to be significantly effective in reducing postoperative vomiting in adults and children after general or regional anesthesia for inpatient or outpatient surgery. Droperidol is effective as an antiemetic given prophylactically or postoperatively to treat symptoms. Excessive sedation rarely occurs at these doses. However, extrapyramidal reactions, as well as anxiety and restlessness that persist after discharge, have been reported in ambulatory surgery patients receiving prophylactic, low doses of droperidol (0.6 to 1.2 mg) for antiemetic therapy.[51]

KEY POINTS

- Benzodiazepine receptors are located in close association with gamma-aminobutyric acid (GABA) receptors in the nervous system. Activation of GABA receptors increases chloride ion flow. Benzodiazepine receptors are distributed unevenly, with the greatest number in the cerebral cortex, limbic system, and the cerebellar cortex. Benzodiazepines potentiate the action of GABA, causing a

- shift to the left in the GABA dose–chloride conductance response curve and producing sedation.

- Benzodiazepines may have glycine-mimetic activity, possibly producing their muscle relaxant and antianxiety properties through this mechanism.

- Diazepam has a large volume of distribution and low hepatic clearance, resulting in an elimination half-life of 20 to 40 hours in adult patients and even longer in the elderly. It is highly bound to plasma albumin. Prolongation of diazepam elimination occurs with hepatic cirrhosis or increased age, whereas shortened half-life occurs with renal failure.

- Intravenous diazepam causes local pain and phlebitis. Respiratory function is depressed by moderate, soporific doses. Diazepam depresses the ventilatory response to CO_2, increases the dead space/tidal volume ratio, and increases $Paco_2$. Depression of ventilation is intensified when narcotics are coadministered.

- Diazepam is rapidly transferred across the placenta and into the fetus and has been linked to increased birth defects; therefore it should be avoided in the first trimester of pregnancy. Diazepam administered to the parturient also has adverse effects on the newly born infant, including hypotonia and impaired temperature regulation.

- Midazolam reduces cerebral metabolic rate and cerebral blood flow equivalently and may provide protection for the brain against hypoxia. Midazolam also causes a reduction in ventilatory response to CO_2 similar to that seen with diazepam. Patients with chronic obstructive pulmonary disease respond and recover more slowly from midazolam's respiratory depressant effects. Apnea and hypoxemia secondary to hypoventilation occur more frequently when midazolam is coadministered with opioids.

- Large doses of midazolam result in prolonged drowsiness and in respiratory depression, especially evident in the elderly during endoscopic procedures.

- Lorazepam is approximately 5 to 10 times as potent as diazepam and, after IV administration, shows a rapid distribution half-life (3 to 10 minutes). Its elimination half-life is 10 to 20 hours. Clinical onset of effect, however, is delayed and clinical duration is prolonged. Lorazepam is metabolized primarily in the liver, and its distribution is not significantly affected by increasing age, renal disease, or liver disease. Elimination half-life may be prolonged in the presence of hepatic cirrhosis.

- Lorazepam provides sedation, amnesia, and suppression of emergence sequelae produced by ketamine. The long duration of sedation and amnesia after lorazepam, by any route of administration, suggests that it should not be used when rapid awakening after surgery is desired.

- Physostigmine can be used to reverse sedation due to benzodiazepines but often has inconsistent or limited efficacy. Cholinergic side effects include vomiting (hyperperistalsis), bradycardia, increased salivation, and perspiration.

- The action of flumazenil, a specific benzodiazepine antagonist, is rapid after IV injection. Rapid distribution coupled with a high liver extraction rate produces a relatively short duration of action. The most common minor side effect reported after flumazenil administration in anesthesia is nausea and/or vomiting.

- Droperidol is a butyrophenone derivative, chemically related to haloperidol. Butyrophenones act as dopamine antagonists in the central and peripheral nervous systems. They occupy postsynaptic GABA receptors and thereby block dopaminergic synapses.

- Droperidol is metabolized in the liver. Significant levels of droperidol metabolite are seen for 8 to 12 hours following drug administration; the peak clinical effects after droperidol last 2 to 3 hours, but significant clinical effect is detectable for at least 10 hours.

- Cardiovascular effects of droperidol include mild alpha-adrenergic blocking activity, resulting in vasodilation and decreased blood pressure. Droperidol is also a potent antiemetic. Anxiety, agitation, and extrapyramidal symptoms are side effects seen.

KEY REFERENCES

Greenblatt DJ: Benzodiazepines, *N Engl J Med* 291:1011, 1974.

Klotz U, Kanto J: Pharmacokinetics and clinical use of flumazenil (RO 15-1788), *Clin Pharmacokinet* 14:1, 1988.

Martin IL: The benzodiazepines and their receptors: 25 years of progress, *Neuropharmacology* 26:957, 1987.

Philip BK, Simpson TH, Hauch MA et al: Flumazenil reverses sedation after midazolam-induced general anesthesia in ambulatory surgery patients, *Anesth Analg* 71:370, 1990.

Reves JG, Fragen RF, Vinik HR et al: Midazolam: pharmacology and uses, *Anesthesiology* 62:310, 1985.

Shafer A, White PF, Urquhart ML et al: Outpatient premedication: use of midazolam and opioid analgesics, *Anesthesiology* 71:495, 1989.

Kreienbuhl G: Der Einfluss der Pramedikation auf die subjektiven postanaesthetischen Beschwerden bei ambulanten (Tagesklinik-) Patienten, *Anaesthesist* 29:421, 1980.

REFERENCES

1. Alexander CM, Gross JB: Sedative doses of midazolam depress hypoxic ventilatory responses in humans, *Anesth Analg* 67: 377, 1988.
2. Amrein R, Hetzel W, Bonetti EP et al: Clinical pharmacology of Dormicum (midazolam) and Anexate (flumazenil), *Resuscitation* 16:S5, 1988.
3. Amrein R, Leishman B, Bentzinger C et al: Flumazenil in benzodiazepine antagonism, *Med Toxicol* 2:411, 1987.
4. Aun C, Flynn PJ, Richards J et al: A comparison of midazolam and diazepam for intravenous sedation in dentistry, *Anaesthesia* 39:589, 1984.
5. Bailey PL, Place NL, Ashburn MA et al: Frequent hypoxemia and apnea after sedation with midazolam and fentanyl, *Anesthesiology* 73:826, 1990.
6. Baird PL, Andriano KP, Goldman M et al: Variability of the respiratory response to diazepam, *Anesthesiology* 64: 460, 1986.
7. Baird ES, Hailey DM: Delayed recovery from a sedative: correlation of the plasma levels of diazepam with clinical effects after oral and intravenous administration, *Br J Anaesth* 144:803, 1972.
8. Bodenham A, Brownlie G, Dixon JS et al: Reversal of sedation by prolonged infusion of flumazenil (Anexate, RO 15-1788), *Anaesthesia* 43:376, 1988.
9. Briggs RM, Ogg MJ: Patients' refusal of surgery after Innovar premedication, *Plast Reconstr Surg* 51:158, 1973.
10. Brogden RN, Goa KL: Flumazenil, *Drugs* 35:448, 1988.
10a. Chiolero et al: *Intensive Care Med* 14:196, 1988.
11. Crawford ME, Carl P, Andersen RS et al: Comparison between midazolam and thiopentone-based balanced anaesthesia for day-case surgery, *Br J Anaesth* 56:165, 1984.
12. Cree JE, Meyer J, and Hailey DM: Diazepam in labour: its metabolism and effect on the clinical condition and ther-

mogenesis of the newborn, *Br Med J* 4:251, 1973.
13. Crevoisier C, Ziegler WH, Eckert M et al: Relationship between plasma concentration and effect of midazolam after oral and intravenous administration, *Br J Clin Pharmacol* 16:51S, 1983.
14. Dixon J, Power SJ, Grundy EM et al: Sedation for local anaesthesia: comparison of intravenous midazolam and diazepam, *Anaesthesia* 39:372, 1984.
15. Dretchen K, Ghoneim MM, and Long JP: The interaction of diazepam with myoneural blocking agents, *Anesthesiology* 34: 463, 1971.
16. Dundee JW, Halliday NJ, McMurray TJ et al: Pretreatment with opioids, *Anaesthesia* 41:159, 1986.
17. Dundee JW, McGowan WAW, Lilburn JK et al: Comparison of the actions of diazepam and lorazepam, *Br J Anaesth* 51:439, 1979.
18. Dundee JW, Pandit SK: Anterograde amnestic effects of pethidine, hyoscine and diazepam in adults, *Br J Pharmacol* 44:140, 1972.
19. Dundee JW, Samuel IO, Toner W et al: Midazolam: a water-soluble benzodiazepine, *Anaesthesia* 35:454, 1980.
20. Dundee JW, Wilson DB: Amnesic action of midazolam, *Anaesthesia* 35:459, 1980.
21. Fischler M, Bonnet F, Trang H et al: The pharmacokinetics of droperidol in anesthetized patients, *Anesthesiology* 64:486, 1986.
22. Fleischer JE, Milde JH, Moyer TP et al: Cerebral effects of high-dose midazolam and subsequent reversal with Ro 15-1788 in dogs, *Anesthesiology* 68:234, 1988.
23. Forster A, Gardaz JP, Suter PM et al: Respiratory depression by midazolam and diazepam, *Anesthesiology* 53:494, 1980.
24. Forster A, Juge O, Louis M et al: Effects of a specific benzodiazepine antagonist (RO 15-1788) on cerebral blood flow, *Anesth Analg* 66:309, 1987.
25. Fragen RJ, Caldwell NJ: Awakening

characteristics following anesthesia induction with midazolam for short surgical procedures, *Arzneim Forsch Drug Res* 31:2261, 1981.
26. Garzone PD, Kroboth PD: Pharmacokinetics of the newer benzodiazepines, *Clin Pharmacokinet* 16:337, 1989.
27. Geller E, Halpern P, Weinbrun A et al: Reversal agents in anaesthesia, *Acta Anaesthesiol Scand* 32:S28, 1988.
28. Geller E, Niv D, Nevo Y et al: Early clinical experience in reversing benzodiazepine sedation with flumazenil after short procedures, *Resuscitation* 16:S49, 1988.
29. Giffin J, Cottrell J, Shwiry B et al: Intracranial pressure, mean arterial pressure and heart rate following midazolam or thiopental in humans with brain tumors, *Anesthesiology* 60:491, 1984.
30. Greenblatt DJ: Benzodiazepines, *N Engl J Med* 291:1011, 1239, 1974.
31. Greenblatt DJ: Clinical pharmacokinetics of oxazepam and lorazepam, *Clin Pharmacokinet* 6:89, 1981.
32. Greenblatt DJ, Sellers EM, and Shader RI: Drug disposition in old age, *N Engl J Med* 306:1081, 1982.
33. Greenblatt DJ, Abernathy DR, Lockniskar A et al: Effect of age, gender and obesity on midazolam kinetics, *Anesthesiology* 61:27, 1984.
34. Gross JB, Smith L, and Smith TC: Time course of ventilatory response to carbon dioxide after intravenous diazepam, *Anesthesiology* 57:18, 1982.
35. Haefely W: The biologic basis of benzodiazepine actions. In Smith DE, Wesson DR, eds: *The benzodiazepines — current standards for medical practice,* Lancaster, England, 1985, MTP Press.
36. Hegarty JE, Dundee JW: Sequelae after the intravenous injection of three benzodiazepines — diazepam, lorazepam and flunitrazepam, *Br Med J* 2:1384, 1977.
37. Hunkeler W, Möhler H, Pieri L et al: Selective antagonists of benzodiazepines, *Nature* 290:514, 1981.

38. Janssen PAJ, Niemegeers CJE, Schellekens KHL et al: The pharmacology of dehydrobenzperidol, *Arzneim Forsch* 13:205, 1963.

39. Jordan C, Lehane JR, and Jones JG: Respiratory depression following diazepam: reversal with high-dose naloxone, *Anesthesiology* 53:293, 1980.

40. Kanto JH: Midazolam: the first water-soluble benzodiazepine, *Pharmacotherapy* 5:138, 1985.

41. Kissin I, Vinik HR, Castillo R et al: Alfentanil potentiates midazolam-induced unconsciousness at subanalgesic doses, *Anesth Analg* 71:65, 1990.

42. Klotz U, Kanto J: Pharmacokinetics and clinical use of flumazenil (RO 15-1788), *Clin Pharmacokinet* 14:1, 1988.

43. Klotz U, Ziegler G, Ludwig L et al: Pharmacodynamic interaction between midazolam and a specific benzodiazepine antagonist in humans, *J Clin Pharmacol* 25:400, 1985.

44. Kong KL, Willatts SM, and Prys-Roberts C: Isoflurane compared with midazolam for sedation in the intensive care unit, *Br Med J* 298:1277, 1989.

45. Kothary SP, Brown ACD, Pandit UA et al: Time course of antirecall effect of diazepam and lorazepam following oral administration, *Anesthesiology* 55:641, 1981.

46. Kreienbuhl G: Der Einfluss der Pramedikation auf die subjektiven postanaesthetischen Beschwerden bei ambulanten (Tagesklinik-) Patienten, *Anaesthesist* 29:421, 1980.

47. Lee CM, Yeakel AE: Patient refusal of surgery following Innovar premedication, *Anesth Analg* 54:224, 1975.

48. Mandelli M, Tognoni G, and Garrattini S: Clinical pharmacokinetics of diazepam, *Clin Pharmacokinet* 3:72, 1978.

49. Martin IL: The benzodiazepines and their receptors: 25 years of progress, *Neuropharmacology* 26:957, 1987.

50. McCammon RL, Hilgenberg JC, and Stoelting RK: Hemodynamic effects of diazepam and diazepam–nitrous oxide in patients with coronary artery disease, *Anesth Analg* 59:438, 1980.

51. Melnick B, Sawyer R, Karambelkar D et al: Delayed side effects of droperidol after ambulatory general anesthesia, *Anesth Analg* 69:748, 1989.

52. Pakkanen A, Kanto J: Midazolam compared with thiopentone as an induction agent, *Acta Anaesthesiol Scand* 26:143, 1982.

53. Pandit SK, Heisterkamp DV, and Cohen PJ: Further studies of the anti-recall effect of lorazepam: a dose-time-effect relationship, *Anesthesiology* 45:495, 1976.

54. Persson A, Ehrin E, Eriksson L et al: Imaging of ^{11}C-labelled Ro 15-1788 binding to benzodiazepine receptors in the human brain by positron emission tomography, *J Psychiatr Res* 19:609, 1985.

55. Persson MP, Nilsson A, and Hartvig P: Relation of sedation and amnesia to plasma concentrations of midazolam in surgical patients, *Clin Pharmacol Ther* 43:324, 1988.

56. Persson P, Nilsson A, Hartvig P et al: Pharmacokinetics of midazolam in total I.V. anaesthesia, *Br J Anaesth* 59:548, 1987.

57. Philip BK: Ambulatory anesthesia, *Semin Surg Oncol* 6:177, 1990.

58. Philip BK: Hazards of amnesia after midazolam in ambulatory surgical patients, *Anesth Analg* 66:97, 1987.

59. Philip BK: Infusion in regional blocks. In Vinik HR, ed: *Midazolam infusion for anesthesia and intensive care,* Princeton, 1989, Exerpta Medica.

60. Philip BK: Supplemental medication for ambulatory procedures under regional anesthesia, *Anesth Analg* 64:1117, 1985.

61. Philip BK, Simpson TH, Hauch MA et al: Flumazenil reverses sedation after midazolam-induced general anesthesia in ambulatory surgery patients, *Anesth Analg* 71:370, 1990.

62. Prokocimer P, Delavault E, Rey F et al: Effects of droperidol on respiratory drive in humans, *Anesthesiology* 59:113, 1983.

63. Reves JG, Fragen RF, Vinik HR et al: Midazolam: pharmacology and uses, *Anesthesiology* 62:310, 1985.

64. Richter JJ: Current theories about the mechanisms of benzodiazepines and neuroleptic drugs, *Anesthesiology* 54:66, 1981.

65. Ricou B, Forster A, Brückner A et al: Clinical evaluation of a specific benzodiazepine antagonist, *Br J Anaesth* 58:1005, 1986.

66. Riishede L, Krogh B, Nielsen JL et al: Reversal of flunitrazepam sedation with flumazenil, *Acta Anaesthesiol Scand* 32:433, 1988.

67. Rodrigo MRC, Rosenquist JB: The effect of Ro 15-1788 (Anexate) on conscious sedation produced with midazolam, *Anaesth Intensive Care* 15:185, 1987.

68. Sainpy D, Boileau S, and Vicari F: Etude comparative du midazolam et du diazepam intraveineux comme agents de sedation en endoscopie digestive, *Ann Fr Anesth Reanim* 3:177, 1984.

69. Shafer A, White PF, Urquhart ML et al: Outpatient premedication: use of midazolam and opioid analgesics, *Anesthesiology* 71:495, 1989.

70. Swerdlow BN, Holley FO: Intravenous anesthetic agents: pharmacokinetic-pharmacodynamic relationships, *Clin Pharmacokinet* 12:79, 1987.

71. Vatashsky E, Beilin B, Razin M et al: Mechanism of antagonism by physostigmine of acute flunitrazepam intoxication, *Anesthesiology* 64:248, 1986.

72. Videcoq M, Desmonts JM, Marty J et al: Effect of droperidol on peripheral vasculature: use of cardiopulmonary bypass as a study model, *Acta Anaesthesiol Scand* 31:370, 1987.

73. Vinik HR, Bradley EL, and Kissin I: Midazolam-alfentanil synergism for anesthetic induction in patients, *Anesth Analg* 69:213, 1989.

74. Ward D: Stimulation of hypoxic ventilatory drive by droperidol, *Anesth Analg* 63:106, 1984.

75. Weldon BC, Watcha M, and White PF: Oral midazolam premedication: optimal timing and effect of atropine, *Anesthesiology* 73:A1243, 1990.

76. Wood M: Intravenous anesthetic agents. In Wood M, Wood AJJ: *Drugs and anesthesia,* Baltimore, 1990, Williams & Wilkins.

CHAPTER 52

Mechanisms of Opioid Analgetic Actions

DANIEL B. CARR

ANDRZEJ W. LIPKOWSKI

Background: What is an Opioid?
Endogenous Opioid Peptides and Synthetic Analogs
Opioid Receptors
Transducing Opioid Signals: "Second Messengers"
Proto-Oncogenes: "Third Messengers"
Opioid Analgesia
How Opioids Act: Summary

Twenty years ago, opioid research was a quiet field sparsely populated by pharmacologists, toxicologists, medicinal chemists, and addiction researchers. Since then, studies of the diverse physiology of the endogenous opioid system and its biochemical basis have flourished, often revealing new results just as the field appeared well understood. Novel opioids continue to appear for use in pain relief (often through "new" routes, e.g., epidural sufentanil) and now occupy a key place in cardiovascular anesthesiology.* Other innovative applications of opioids will undoubtedly continue to emerge, possibly employing their recently recognized immunomodulatory† and antiarrhythmic[42,64,220] actions.

This chapter describes how opioids produce their clinically valuable effects. Such effects include analgesia but also encompass other diverse actions, even in the unconscious anesthetized patient, whose perception is absent.[32,158,159,208] For example, opioids may decrease such undesirable perioperative occurrences as tachycardia,[27,47,82,217,267] systemic or pulmonary hypertension,[159,208] negative nitrogen balance, and ventricular fibrillation.[42,64,220] Because the basis for the biologic effects of any opioid, whether "natural" or newly engineered, is a particular molecular shape, this shape is described at the outset along with relevant nomenclature. To interconnect opioid drugs' diverse actions, this chapter then describes how, where, and when their endogenous opioid counterparts are secreted within the body. Next, some changes produced within cells when opioids bind to their receptors on the cell membrane are discussed. This section also highlights opioid receptors, since they form the basis for optimizing treatment with currently available opioids (e.g., by drug coadministration) or for engineering new opioid compounds.[9,83,120,206,291]

The final portion of this chapter, how opioids influence cell networks for pain transmission, follows closely the earlier, more basic discussion. It is organized according to the sequence of events, each modified by opioids, that ensues after a painful stimulus, such as a surgical incision or tissue trauma. Throughout, we acknowledge the controversy that exists regarding aspects of opioid action that appeared to be firm "facts" as recently as 5 years ago.

BACKGROUND: WHAT IS AN OPIOID?

Terms that apply to morphinelike compounds have evolved rapidly in the past decade, and unfortunate inconsistencies still exist in their usage. At present, the word "narcotic" is avoided because it has pejorative legal and regulatory meanings that apply not only to morphine but also to unrelated classes of controlled substances such as barbiturates. **Traditionally, *opiates* are morphinelike alkaloids derived from**

---

* References 5, 13, 28, 77, 87, 106, 209, 243.
† References 17, 61, 92, 93, 168, 179, 180, 192, 232, 233, 235, 238, 239, 253.

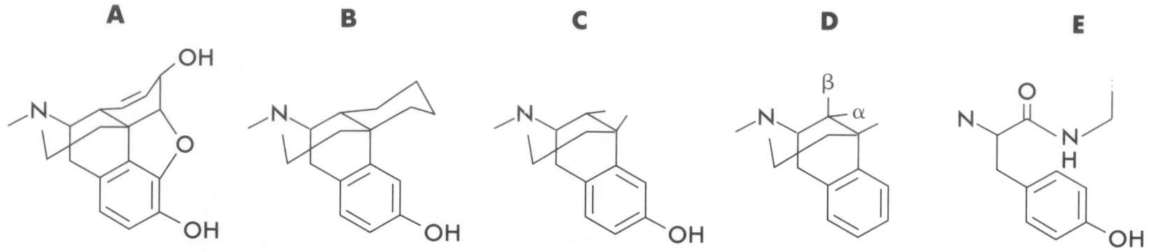

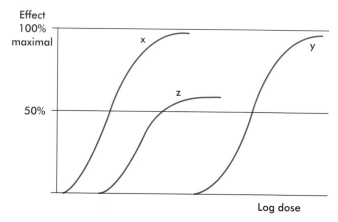

Fig. 52-1. Structural motif common to all morphinelike opioids. Progressive removal of ring structures converts five-ring alkaloid morphine (**A**), to four-ring morphinan (**B**), to three-ring benzomorphan (**C**), to two-ring phenylpiperidine (**D**), to tyramine moiety typical of endogenous opioid peptides (**E**). (From Carr DB: Opioids, *Int Anesthesiol Clin* 26:273, 1988.)

poppy seeds,[119] **although a few recent reports point to their presence in mammals as well, possibly from intestinal flora.**[68,268] **Besides morphine, opiates include codeine and thebaine, five- or six-ring alkaloids of the phenanthrene class.** Reducing the number of rings to four yields *morphinans;* to three, *benzomorphans;* and to two, *phenylpiperidines.*[121,254] Endogenous opioid peptides begin with the amino acid tyrosine, which has a single ring. As shown in Fig. 52-1, **all morphinelike compounds share this tyrosine-like portion of their structure.**[113] Any of these agents can produce morphinelike analgesia, constipation, and tolerance (or withdrawal if abruptly stopped). The term *opioid* encompasses this entire group of substances, without restriction as to origin or specific structure.

By far the best characterized endogenous opioids are peptides. At times the word "endorphins" has been used to refer to all endogenous opioid peptides, a practice to be discouraged because it invites confusion between families of molecules (e.g., pro-ACTH/endorphin) and the entire superfamily.

Although the tyrosine moiety is crucial for any compound's ability to produce morphinelike effects, other regions of opioid molecules may be responsible for biologic actions distinct from those produced by morphine.[251] **Opioid peptides that lack an amino terminus tyrosine (called *des-Tyr* derivatives) are devoid of morphinelike activity but produce effects in the central nervous system (CNS), such as enhancement of memory, and in the periphery, such as binding to complement.**[65] **Such actions are termed** *nonopioid* **and are not blocked by the opioid antagonist naloxone.** They evidently result from binding of regions distinct from the morphinelike amino terminus to receptors distinct from the conventional opioid types. Naloxone itself has biologic effects outside of opioid systems.[221] Further, subtypes of opioid receptors (see later section) appear to be "blind" to opioid peptides but retain high affinity for opioid alkaloids.[74] Studies of the nonopioid properties of many opioids are attracting growing interest. Unless otherwise

Fig. 52-2. Distinctions between potency and partial agonism. Drug *x* is more potent than drug *y*, but both can evoke a full biologic effect and thus are termed *agonists* (or *full agonists*). Drug *z* can evoke a half-maximal effect at a dosage between those required for drugs *x* or *y* to evoke the same effect; therefore drug *z* is less potent than *x* and more potent than *y*. However, the maximal possible effect evoked by drug *z* is below that evoked by drugs *x* or *y*, and so drug *z* is termed a *partial agonist*. (Redrawn from Gilman AG, Goodman LS, Rall TW et al, eds: *The pharmacological basis of therapeutics,* ed 7, New York, 1985, Macmillan.)

stated, however, the remainder of this chapter concerns only the morphinelike, naloxone-reversible *opioid* effects of such compounds.

Concerning such actions, a few remaining terms deserve clarification because they are widely misunderstood. **Drugs such as morphine or fentanyl produce dose-dependent biologic responses in vivo and are termed** *agonists* **or** *full agonists.* **In contrast, other opioids such as buprenorphine evoke a submaximal plateau response, even as their dosage is increased indefinitely, and thus are called** *partial agonists.* **The phenomenon of partial agonism is distinct from the concept of potency; in the normal clinical dosage range, a 0.3 mg dose of buprenorphine produces analgesia equivalent to a 10 mg dose of morphine (Fig. 52-2). Finally, other opioids, such as butorphanol, are agonists at one type of opioid receptor and antago-**

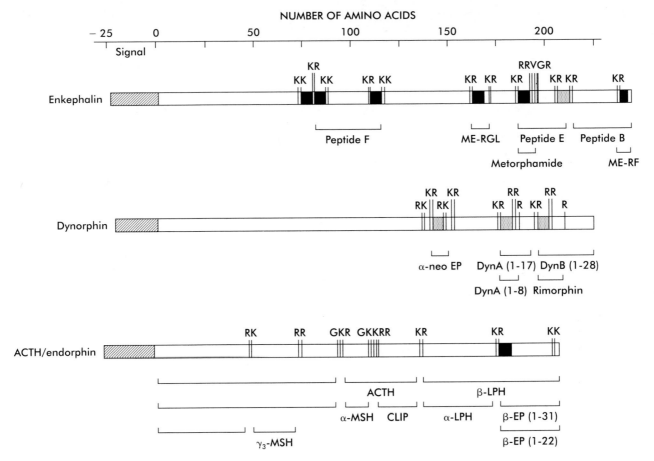

Fig. 52-3. Three opioid precursor families have been identified according to precursor from which members of each family are derived. Principal biologically active fragments are indicated. *F,* phenylalanine; *G,* glycine; *K,* lysine; *L,* leucine; *R,* arginine; *V,* valine. (From Carr DB, Lipkowski AW, and Silbert BS: Biochemistry of the opioid peptides. In Estafanous FG, ed: *Opioids in anesthesia II,* Boston, 1990, Butterworth-Heinemann.)

nists at a second type. Thus they have received the seemingly illogical designation *mixed agonist-antagonist,* or simply *agonist-antagonist.*[36]

ENDOGENOUS OPIOID PEPTIDES AND SYNTHETIC ANALOGS

Opioid drugs can produce their effects because they mimic the actions of endogenous opioid peptides on their receptors.[83] **Three families of such peptides exist, with each family derived from a common precursor molecule (Fig. 52-3): pre-proopiomelancortin (POMC), preproenkephalin, and preprodynorphin (preproenkephalin B).**[58,212] The expression of each precursor is controlled separately, as is the expression of a single precursor in different regions. The POMC precursor was characterized in detail using recombinant DNA (deoxyribonucleic acid) methods. POMC is the common precursor of beta-endorphin and adrenocorticotropic hormone (ACTH), melanocyte-stimulating hormone (MSH), and related compounds.[73]

The different anatomic distributions of met-enkephalin and POMC, as well as the absence of leu-enkephalin from the amino acid sequence of POMC, motivated a successful search for a separate precursor for the enkephalins. The first enkephalin precursor to be characterized was proenkephalin A, containing six copies of met-enkephalin and one copy of leu-enkephalin. Recognition in hypothalamic extracts of still other distinct peptides, alpha-neo-endorphin and dynorphin, initiated a search for a third precursor. This search ended in 1982 with the elucidation of the complementary DNA (cDNA) sequence encoding the third precursor, named pre-prodynorphin (preproenkephalin B), which contains three copies of leu-enkephalin and also gives rise to dynorphin, alpha-neo-endorphin, and rimorphin (dynorphin B). Similarities between the structures of each family lead to the view that the three precursors in aggregate form a superfamily.

Before the initial discovery of endogenous opioid peptides in the mid-1970s, considerable knowledge had already amassed concerning the biosynthesis of

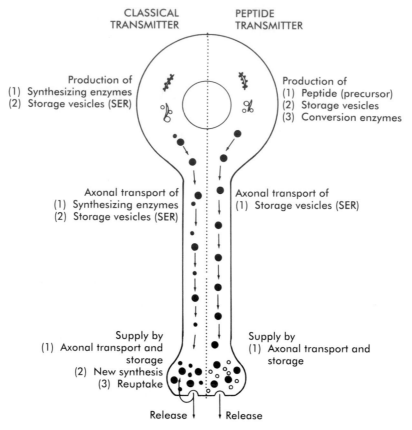

Fig. 52-4. Contrasting modes of synthesis and secretion of peptides and "classical" (i.e., small monoamine) neurotransmitters. Omitted for simplicity are differences in quality of postsynaptic potentials evoked by either type of compound during neurotransmission. (Redrawn from Hökfelt T: Peptidergic neurones, *Nature* 284:515, 1980.)

peptides and relationships between peptide structure and biologic activity.* However, the study of peptides is comparatively young and has benefitted in recent years from concurrent technologic advances for peptides' characterization, synthesis, and genetic study.[18,128,194] Such research has disclosed substantial roles for nonopioid peptides, such as calcitonin and calcitonin gene-related peptide, substance P and other tachykinins, corticotropin-releasing factor (CRF), and somatostatin, in nociceptive and neuroendocrine regulation.[45] Conciseness, however, rules out any attempt to survey here the extensive, expanding field of nonopioid analgetic peptides.[282]

Peptides have a chemical structure more complex than that of "classic" monoamine neurotransmitters. Differences in biosynthesis, axonal transport, secretion, regulation, and modes of action further distinguish these two classes of compounds (Fig. 52-4). Classic neurotransmitters are low-molecular-weight monoamines such as adrenaline, acetylcholine, serotonin, and gamma-aminobutyric acid (GABA), each

of which is the product of a sequence of enzymatic modifications of a single amino acid precursor. **Neuropeptides often are co-released along with classic transmitters from the same neurons, in keeping with earlier findings that biogenic amines and peptide hormones are present within the same endocrine cells.[111,164]**

A peptide's structure is determined by its primary sequence of amino acids. Within an aqueous milieu, this primary sequence folds or coils itself to form secondary helices or sharp turns (Fig. 52-5).[251] This conformation may assume an amphiphilic form when the peptide resides at the interface between the lipid cell membrane and the aqueous extracellular environment (Fig. 52-6).[127,142] **The unique steric forms assumed by side groups on amino acids underlie the characteristic biologic actions of related peptides.[251] Schwyzer[229] is credited with the insight that certain segments of a peptide molecule constitute an "address" for recognition and binding by a family of target receptor(s). Other "message" portions fine-tune the receptor selectivity of the resultant peptides and give rise to distinct profiles of physiologic action within the cell (Fig. 52-7).**

* References 35, 38, 41, 122, 195, 196.

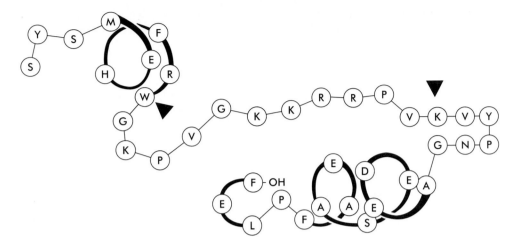

Fig. 52-5. Primary sequence of amino acids within peptide gives rise to peptide's conformation. Side groups *(not shown)* on each amino acid interact with each other and surrounding solution to create helices, sharp turns, or random coils. In this classic example from Schwyzer, particular sequences within adrenocorticotropic hormone (ACTH) molecule (e.g., positions 4 to 10) are "messages" by virtue of their characteristic structure. (Redrawn from Schwyzer R: ACTH: a short introductory review, *Ann NY Acad Sci* 297:3, 1977.)

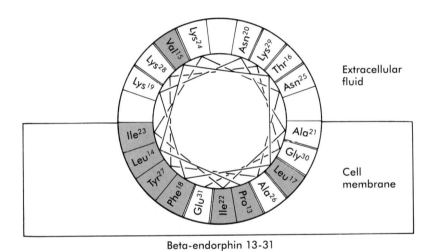

Beta-endorphin 13-31

Fig. 52-6. Helical conformation of peptide presents polar amino acids to exterior of cell membrane and nonpolar, lipophilic amino acids to membrane itself. In this amphiphilic, alpha-helical conformation—viewed here along axis of helix generated by residues 13 through 31 of beta-endorphin—peptide coil resides, detergent-like, at interface between membrane and exterior. (Redrawn from Kaiser ET, Kézdy FJ: Amphiphilic secondary structure: design of peptide hormones, *Science* 223:249, 1984.)

Changing a letter within a written word, or switching one word for another within a sentence, may make a text more forceful or alter its impact. Similarly, new peptide analogs that contain addresses and messages modified from those of their natural counterparts may offer therapeutically attractive potency, selectivity, and stability profiles. Many ingenious strategies have been employed to synthesize thousands of "designer peptides" in the past 20 years (Table 52-1).

A common strategy is substitution of an unnatural D-isomer of an amino acid in place of the native L-isomer at one or more positions, thereby rendering the compound resistant to enzymatic degradation. Such modification is quite limited as to the position where it may occur without interfering with the active conformation. A new peptide analog may be rendered resistant to enzymatic degradation with minimal change in its spatial structure. This is done by reversing the primary amino acid sequence and

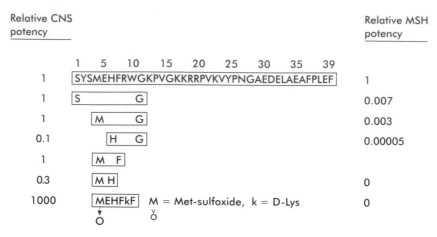

Fig. 52-7. Schwyzer's summary of evidence that truncated forms of a peptide that contain message for one biologic activity may retain this activity and lose other activities. In this case, relative potencies of ACTH, truncated sequences, and truncated analog sequence are compared in assays to determine potency on central nervous system *(CNS)* for acquisition and retention of learned behavior vs. activity on skin darkening (melanocyte-stimulating hormone, *MSH*). (Redrawn from Schwyzer R: ACTH: a short introductory review, *Ann NY Acad Sci* 297:3, 1977.)

Table 52-1 Strategies for design of new peptides

Design	Advantages
Truncated "message" sequences	More potent
Substitute D amino for L amino acids	More stable
Retro-inverso forms	More stable
Cyclized forms	More stable, more selective
Hybrids (e.g., alkaloid message, peptide address)	More stable, more selective
Bivalent forms	More selective

linking successive amino acids with a D peptide bond instead of the natural L form, producing a so-called retroenantiomeric analog. Cyclic analogs are made by joining two amino acid residues that normally are apart when the peptide is in its native conformation. They may demonstrate higher selectivity and biologic activity by concentrating in nonpolar regions such as brain.[181] Cyclic analogs also resist enzymatic degradation because they have no exposed "end" to serve as a substrate for enzyme action..

Such strategies for prolonging peptide half-life have been complemented by other approaches aimed at altering the receptor binding affinities of the resulting analogs.[29,188] Administering only the message and omitting irrelevant portions of the sequence can greatly enhance potency[229] (see Fig. 52-7). Cou-

pling an opiate alkaloid message to a peptide address[153] or linking pairs of enkephalin analogs by methylene bridges of variable chain length[152,234] can yield remarkably selective compounds. Such unconventional structures suggest the neologism "peptoids!"

In contrast to these chemical tours de force, the many opioid, phenylpiperidine, or tyramine derivatives differ from one another essentially at their side groups only. Substitutions of these groups affect not only receptor affinities but also other properties, such as protein binding, pK, lipophilicity, and potency. Possibilities for modification of "classic" monoamine neurotransmitters are also limited to introducing a few side groups onto a single amino acid substrate, such as tyrosine or histidine.

As with all natural peptides, endogenous opioids are derived from larger precursors that undergo proteolytic processing to yield biologically active daughter molecules[18] (Fig. 52-8).

Since the discovery of the pentapeptide (i.e., five amino acid length) enkephalins in 1975, many larger opioid peptides have been isolated. These share with the enkephalins an *N*-terminus tetrapeptide fragment, Tyr-Gly-Gly-Phe-.[266] The metabolism of endogenous opioid peptides or their synthetic analogs is quite different from morphine and related (i.e., alkaloid) analgetics. Because biologic peptides are generated from precursors, the concentration of a particular endogenous opioid peptide reflects two opposed processes, formation and degradation.[228] Both processes represent important regulatory steps in opioid peptide action, since distinct mechanisms exist whereby the inactive precursor is converted to

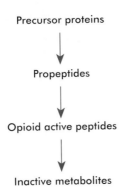

Precursor proteins

↓

Propeptides

↓

Opioid active peptides

↓

Inactive metabolites

Fig. 52-8. Proteolytic processing of precursor protein. Large precursors are enzymatically processed within cells to liberate propeptides that are secreted extracellularly or further processed intracellularly. Enzymatic cleavage of propeptides generates peptides with opioid bioactivity; these peptides are further processed to yield metabolites that lack opioid bioactivity. Although labelled *inactive* here, end metabolites often possess biologic activities that are nonopioid in nature. (From Carr DB, Lipkowski AW, and Silbert BS: Biochemistry of the opioid peptides. In Estafanous FG, ed: *Opioids in anesthesia II*, Boston, 1990, Butterworth-Heinemann.)

the physiologically active peptide and then further metabolized to inactive fragments and amino acids.[287]

OPIOID RECEPTORS

The concept that cellular receptors mediate drug action was originated by Langley in the nineteenth century. By the 1950s, sophisticated studies of opioid stereochemistry were being conducted on the assumption that such relationships derived from opioid drugs fitting into receptors. **In the 1960s Martin inferred the existence of at least two types of opioid receptors, based on observations of the biphasic effect that certain opioids such as nalorphine had on morphine analgesia in patients.**[90,114,167] Observations revealed that low doses of nalorphine diminished morphine analgesia but that analgesia reemerged at high doses of nalorphine. This led Martin to deduce that nalorphine acted as an antagonist to morphine at a shared receptor target but was active as an analgetic at a second receptor insensitive to morphine.

Later, Martin observed distinct clinical syndromes in addicts given or withdrawing from various opioids, which led him to enlarge the initial concept of receptor dualism. Using a canine model, he compared analgetic, autonomic, and behavioral responses to single opioid drug doses in dogs habituated to morphine or cyclazocine (another opioid). Martin identified three clusters of responses to three prototypic drugs: morphine, ketocyclazocine, and *N*-allyl normetazocine (also termed SKF-10,047) (Table 52-2). Based on this clustering, **Martin postulated that morphine acts on a hypothetic *mu* receptor to produce**

miosis, bradycardia, analgesia, and indifference to the environment. Ketocyclazocine, as with morphine, constricts pupils and reduces the flexor reflex. Unlike morphine, however, it produces sedation rather than indifference, has little effect on the skin twitch reflex, and does not reduce symptoms of morphine withdrawal. Thus ketocyclazocine's effects are identified with actions on a second receptor, named *kappa*. Distinct from both these drugs is N-allyl normetazocine (SKF-10,047), which causes sympathetic and behavioral arousal through a third receptor, *sigma*. Drug actions mediated by any of the three drugs are reversible by naloxone, although progressively higher doses of naloxone are required to antagonize kappa and sigma effects compared with mu.[165]

Martin's classification, employing in vivo animal studies to refine clinical observations, has undergone refinement, but its essence is still valid. It has been supported by other in vivo approaches (besides cross-tolerance assays) that differentiate between prototype opioid agonists.[50,57,109,189,222] These approaches include observations of effects on motor and exploratory behavior of rats in a Y maze.[57] Other training studies require the subject to gauge similarities between known and test opioid drugs to receive a reward[50] or avoid an averse stimulus.[189,222] Still other whole-animal approaches to distinguishing the opioid receptor type important for a given effect (e.g., analgesia) involve titration of antagonist doses required to neutralize an agonist's effects. A difference in the concentration of antagonist required to reverse the actions of two agonists provides quantitative evidence that these agonists produce their effects via different opioid receptors.[149,166,223] Related to this technique is the observation that a drug's opioid receptor selectivity may be inferred from its relative efficacy against experimental pain of different origins (e.g., thermal vs. pressure stimuli) (Fig. 52-9).[258,260]

For all the merit of whole-animal approaches, one must always be cautious interpreting such results, since many factors influence absorption, distribution, biotransformation, and excretion of drugs and thus their concentration at receptors.[30,37,65,139,149] Whole-animal preparations may not distinguish between simultaneous drug actions through different mechanisms at distinct sites. This is important because opioids are known to produce analgetic effects at peripheral, spinal, and supraspinal sites by diverse mechanisms (see following discussion).* Even when all variables are controlled as much as possible (e.g., during intrathecal administration of receptor-selective opioids), one cannot predict an individual animal's analgetic responses with certainty.

---

* References 2, 4, 70, 76, 78, 94, 125, 137, 175, 177, 231, 262, 276.

Table 52-2   Prototypic opioid receptors

	Morphine	Ketocyclazocine	N-allyl normetazocine (SKF-10,047)
Flexor reflex	Marked depression A = B	Marked depression	Modest depression C ≠ A, B
Skin twitch reflex	Marked depression	Modest depression B ≠ A	No depression C ≠ A, B
Pupils	Constriction A = B	Constriction	Dilatation C ≠ A, B
Body temperature	Depression	Slight depression	Slight elevation C ≠ A
Respiratory rate	Increased (panting)	No effect B ≠ A	Increased C ≠ B
Sedation	Yes A = B	Yes	No C ≠ A, B
Canine delirium	No A = B	No	Yes C ≠ A, B
Pulse rate	Decreased	No effect B ≠ A	Increased C ≠ A, B
Abstinence			
Morphine-dependent dogs	Suppressed; did not precipitate	Neither suppressed nor precipitated B ≠ A	Precipitated C ≠ A, B
Cyclazocine-dependent dogs	Suppressed A = B	Suppressed; did not precipitate B ≠ A	?
Receptor	Mu (μ)	Kappa (κ)	Sigma (σ)

A, Morphine; B, Ketocyclazocine; C, N-allyl normetazocine.
From Martin WR: Multiple opioid receptors: a little about their history and some implications related to evolution, *Life Sci* 28:1547, 1981.

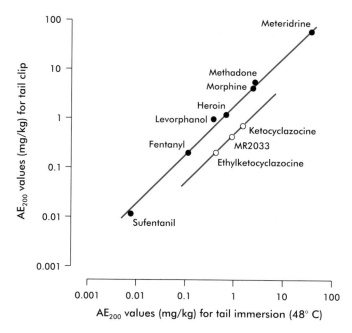

Fig. 52-9. Opioid potencies depend on type of experimental pain used to assess their analgetic effects. If potencies based on pressure ("tail clip") vs. thermal ("immersion") nociceptive testing are compared, opioids cluster along regression lines according to whether they are mu or kappa agonists. Mu agonists (*closed circles*) have greater potency on thermal testing, and kappa agonists (*open circles*) are more potent in a pressure model. *AE200*, Dose of drug needed to produce analgetic effect 200% above control levels. (Redrawn from Upton N, Sewell RDE, Spencer PSJ: Differentiation of potent mu- and kappa-opiate agonists using heat and pressure antinociceptive profiles and combined potency analysis, *Eur J Pharmacol* 78:421, 1982.)

To overcome the inherent imprecision in studies of opioid receptors' relative contribution to a biologic effect in vivo, many sophisticated methods have been devised. Unfortunately, as these methods have become more and more distant from the bedside or whole animal, the meaning of the term *opioid receptor* has been undermined or at least altered irreversibly from Martin's idea of operationally defined substrates for distinct in vivo syndromes produced by different opioids. Further confusion has arisen even in description of in vivo analyses. In certain contexts the word "receptor" refers only to the binding or recognition component of a macromolecular complex, whereas at other times it connotes an entity with the dual functions of ligand binding and physiologic response.

In vitro methods that rely on whole-organ responses, such as opioids' ability to inhibit electrically induced contraction of smooth muscle from guinea pig ileum or mouse vas deferens,[191] are closest to the in vivo bioassays.[149] The smooth muscle bioassay is of historic importance because it was used by Kosterlitz and colleagues to identify and characterize the enkephalins in fractions tracked through progressive purification steps from pig brain. **The same group also deduced the existence of a fourth opioid receptor type (termed *delta* for "deferens") based on observations of different potency rankings of a test panel of drugs when applied to mouse vas deferens vs. guinea pig ileum.[157] The three opioid receptor types most relevant to analgesia are mu, delta, and kappa.** Examples of some highly receptor-selective

Table 52-3 Some receptor-selective opioid agonists

Type of receptor	Example
Mu	Tyr-dAla-Gly-N-methyl-Phe-Gly-ol (DAMGO)
	Tyr-Pro-Phe-Pro-NH$_2$ (PL 017)
Delta	Tyr-dAla-Gly-Phe-dLeu (DADLE)
	Cyclic Tyr-d-Pen-Gly-Phe-d-Pen (DPDPE)
Kappa	U-50,488H (NOTE: not a peptide)

opioid agonists available for investigational use are presented in Table 52-3.

Less closely linked to a biologic effect are the many studies that examine one or another aspect of ligand binding to tissues or purified cell membranes. These studies infer the presence of a new "receptor" type or subtype based, for example, on curve-fitting formulas applied to measurements of radiolabelled tracer binding to the membranes or tissue under study.* Although hundreds of studies have taken such abstract approaches, they have sometimes generated confusing results by equating receptor binding with biologic effect.[134] Martin,[166] Li et al.,[151] and other investigators have called attention to the lack of correlation between in vitro measures of opioid drug binding to receptors and pharmacologic effects in vivo, such as analgetic potency. Such discrepancies between in vivo and in vitro testing, not unique to opioids,[207] presumably reflect intermediate signalling steps known to separate the receptor binding of many compounds from their biologic sequelae.[154]

For these reasons, it is probably not appropriate to speak of any binding site as a receptor unless its occupancy produces a physiologic response consistent with that receptor's known function in vivo. Before applying this criterion, preliminary requirements exist for identifying a biologically relevant binding site. First, unlabelled ligand should, as its concentration is increased, displace progressively greater amounts of labeled ligand, consistent with reversible ligand binding to a finite number of sites (saturability). Next, structurally unrelated ligands should be ineffective in displacing the labelled ligand (specificity). In particular, the biologically inactive d isomer of an opioid should not bind to a putative opioid receptor, but the l form should bind (stereospecificity). Even though certain opioid receptors have relatively low affinity for naloxone, displaceability of ligand by

naloxone is often another criterion for an opioid binding site.[46] These criteria for stereospecific, saturable binding sites were met in the initial descriptions of "the" opioid receptor.[193,252,237]

Taking the current view that it is valid to deem a binding site a "receptor" only if its exposure to an opioid produces an appropriate physiologic response, then progress on the molecular characterization of opioid receptors has been frustratingly slow. By comparison, much more is known about the structure of other cell surface receptors, many of which have been purified and their genes cloned. Loh and Smith[155] have cited three reasons for slow progress to date on molecular characterization (i.e., gene cloning) of opioid receptors. First, harvesting of opioid receptors in soluble form is technically difficult and usually results in a loss of stereospecific ligand binding. Second, no biochemical marker exists at the membrane level to serve as a surrogate for a macroscopic biologic response, such as analgesia or smooth muscle paresis. Third, opioid receptors are heterogeneous, and ligands used for binding studies are not perfectly selective; thus membrane receptor isolates are rarely pure. Despite these difficulties, several groups have progressed toward cloning the opioid receptors, and their results to date have been startling and perplexing.* (Parallel progress has also been made in identifying and characterizing, on a molecular basis, the binding sites for nonopioid derivatives of the opioid peptides.[205])

Loh et al.[155] have reported initial work on isolating the cDNA sequence for a delta opioid binding site. They found no homology between the amino acid sequence of this protein and any of the known sequences in data banks. Molecular characterization of the mu opioid receptor reviewed by Loh and Smith[155] began with the purification of a 58-kilodalton binding protein derived from cow brain. In contrast to other opioid binding proteins purified by others, the Loh group's protein required reconstitution with acidic lipids to bind opioids. Such a lipid requirement reflects the mode of cellular action of opioid-receptor complexes and is present for other hormone-receptor complexes as well.[105] Peptide fragments of this purified protein were isolated and corresponding oligonucleotide probes prepared, then used to clone and sequence its DNA. Comparison of the binding site's protein sequence to a computerized database revealed a high degree of homology to vertebrate proteins involved in cell adhesion or cell recognition.[225] Such proteins include neural cell adhesion molecule (N-CAM), carcinoembryonic antigen (CEA), and myelin-associated glycoprotein. A weaker homology, probably still indicative of a common evolutionary relationship, is present between this protein and receptors for interleukin-6 (IL-6) and platelet-derived growth factor (PDGF). Overall, these homologous molecules are considered to belong to an immunoglobulin superfamily of proteins, in which the conserved structural motif is of disulfide-bonded, folded regions. Loh and Smith[155] have termed this opioid binding site *opioid-binding cell-adhesion molecule* (OBCAM).

The identification of OBCAM as a protein within the immunoglobulin superfamily is both satisfying and puzzling. The satisfaction reflects a potentially strong connection with recent findings of multiple immunologic effects[160] of opioids (see later discussion). The puzzling part is that the quasi-immunoglobulin structure of OBCAM is unexpected; at least a decade of evidence has accumulated showing that opioid receptors are coupled to the adenylate cyclase second-messenger system. This coupling takes place via guanine neucleotide binding-regulatory proteins *(G proteins),* as described in the next section. Many hormones and neurotransmitters act through well-characterized receptors (many now cloned) that activate G proteins. It now appears that receptors coupled to G proteins have seven hydrophobic domains that function as transmembrane spanning segments. This number is consistent with the "six to eight" active membrane sites in a recent opioid receptor model proposed by Martin to account for opioid structure-activity relationships.[166] However, OBCAM's predicted structure is devoid of the transmembrane or intracellular regions considered mandatory for G protein–coupled receptors.

At present, OBCAM's structure appears most to resemble that of other receptors known to terminate within the cell membrane that effect cellular responses by causing membrane phospholipid breakdown. Other recognition and adhesion molecules within the immunoglobulin superfamily (N-CAM, CEA, etc.) are also linked to membrane phospholipids. Thus, for the opioid receptors, one must still await the knowledge spurt that has followed molecular characterization of other receptors, such as the adrenergic. For the adrenergic receptor, specific functions have been assigned to individual transmembrane domains through functional analyses of permutations of sets of synthetic receptor subunit hybrids ("chimeras").[135]

TRANSDUCING OPIOID SIGNALS: "SECOND MESSENGERS"

Viewing the opioid itself as a "first messenger" whose arrival at the cell membrane produces an activated opioid + receptor complex, subsequent events within a cell are "second messengers" within internal cellular signal pathways. Such internal biochemical signals are few in number but generate the entire repertoire of cellular responses to the environment: contraction, depolarization, secretion, adhesion, or growth (or inhibition of these processes).[54,72,119,126]

Several signal methods, two of which are uniquely important for opioid action, arose early in evolution and have been conserved from single-celled organisms to humans. The first employs cyclic adenosine monophosphate (cAMP),[44] and the second relies on membrane phospholipid breakdown and calcium ion fluxes.[45,226] In both mechanisms, signal molecules rapidly diffuse within a cell and produce their effects by changing the structure of cellular proteins, either directly by binding to such proteins or indirectly by activating an enzyme (*phosphorylase)* that attaches a phosphate group to them.

Either path may be activated when a drug, hormone, opioid, or any other external signal (e.g., a growth factor) binds to its receptor, thereby changing that receptor's conformation.[26,49] **This conformational change is transmitted across the cell membrane through one of seven transmembrane receptor domains and interacts with a G protein.**[81,182] **G proteins inhibit (G_i) or stimulate (G_s) adenylate cyclase**[91] **and perform other functions (G_o) not directly related to the regulation of cAMP. For example, G_o and the several known forms of G_i couple receptors for various hormones and neurotransmitters to potassium and calcium channels, and G_s activates certain calcium channels.**

The availability of recombinant DNA technology and the discovery that specific bacterial toxins inactivate isolated steps within G protein signalling pathways have permitted detailed, ongoing elucidation of this system. G proteins consist of three subunits, alpha, beta, and gamma, designated in order of decreasing molecular weight. Guanosine diphosphate (GDP) or triphosphate (GTP) are the inactivating and activating ligands, respectively, for G proteins. The activated ligand-receptor complex catalyzes the dissociation of GDP from the alpha subunit of the G protein trimer, which then binds GTP, at which point the alpha subunit dissociates. The alpha subunit interacts with and regulates one or more intracellular effectors, such as ion channels (Fig. 52-10). A membrane receptor that interacts with G_i is termed R_i, and one that interacts with G_s is termed R_s.

Dynorphin and other peptides involved in nociception (e.g., bradykinin, substance P) at times may bypass the step of receptor binding and may interact with G proteins by "docking" their amphiphilic portion in the cell membrane. However, an impressive body of evidence has established that many or most important opioid effects result from opioid recep-

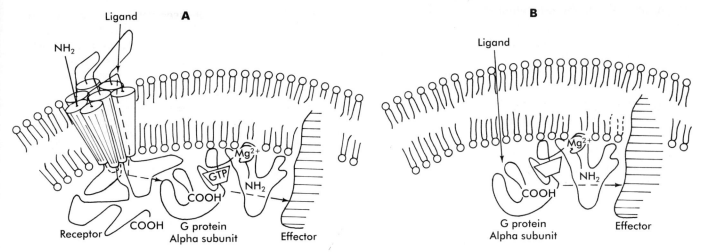

Fig. 52-10. A, A ligand typically activates an intracellular G protein by binding to extracellular surface of a receptor, causing intracellular changes in conformation to one of seven transmembrane domains. **B,** This receptor step may be bypassed if ligand can enter membrane by means of an amphiphilic interaction (see Fig. 52-6). (Redrawn from Mousli M, Bueb JL, Bronner C et al: G protein activation: a receptor-independent mode of action for catonic amphiphilic neuropeptides and venom peptides, *TIPS* 11:358, 1990.)

tor–G_i **protein interactions.** Thus, beginning in the mid-1970s, Klee and Nirenberg[133] and Koski[136] showed inhibitory effects of opioids on basal and prostaglandin E_1–stimulated cAMP generation in cultured neuroblastoma-glioma cells. Acute opioid exposure lowered cAMP production in this cell line (that has delta receptors only). cAMP production returned to normal with continued exposure, only to exceed normal levels on acute opioid withdrawal, suggesting a mechanism for opioid tolerance and dependence.[136]

More recent data suggest that an opioid agonist's potency influences the rate at which it induces tolerance in vivo.[89,247] Early results on G protein coupling of opioid receptors have been confirmed in brain membrane preparations and extended to encompass mu and kappa opioid receptors as well as delta.[59] A strong experimental argument for the dependence of opioid analgesia on G_i derives from observations that pertussis toxin (a selective deactivator of G_i) inhibits (1) the antinociceptive effect of morphine, (2) the depressant electrophysiologic effects of opioids on cultured dorsal horn networks, and (3) the antinociceptive effects of intrathecally administered mu, delta, and kappa opioid agonists.[123,199]

The coupling of opioid receptors to ion channels is a complementary mechanism for opioid action that does not exclude G_i protein activation. Indeed, G proteins are capable of activating ion channels (e.g., for calcium) directly without the involvement of adenylate cyclase.[67] Intracellular calcium has a leading role as an ionic second messenger for a broad range of ligands, including opioids.[21,43,210,269] Levels of

intracellular calcium regulate essential cellular processes (e.g., neurotransmitter release, action potential generation) and bind to calmodulin, thereby activating this widely distributed regulatory protein. Opioids inhibit transmembrane calcium currents as well as certain actions of the activated calcium-calmodulin complex.[211]

Calcium channel blockers given in vivo potentiate opioid analgesia produced by drugs[110] or environmental stress[129] and suppress the morphine withdrawal syndrome.[19,202] **Kappa opioid agonists may accomplish their effects by directly binding to calcium channels[86,162] (or a subtype thereof).[97] In contrast, agonists of the mu or delta type have a primary effect of increasing potassium conductance, thereby shortening the duration of the action potential and only secondarily decreasing calcium conductance.[185,186] The potassium channel coupled to the mu receptor appears identical to that coupled to the delta receptor, as well as to potassium channels coupled to certain other neurotransmitter receptors (e.g., acetylcholine, norepinephrine, dopamine, adenosine, somatostatin).[187]**

We should note that this overview is general and that new exceptions and anomalies are constantly being reported.[45] For example, the selective kappa agonist U-50,488H has been reported to interact with sodium channels in guinea pig hippocampal neurons. Also, activation of mu receptors has been found to inhibit transient high- and low-threshold calcium currents in rat dorsal root ganglion.

The preceding evidence indicates that intracellular processes triggered by opioids culminate in inhibition of neurotransmitter release and slowing of neuronal

firing rate. Where excitatory neural effects of opioids have been observed (e.g., in the hippocampus), these have previously been attributed to "disinhibition" (i.e., inhibition of interneurons that are themselves inhibitory). However, recent studies of sensory neuron action potentials in cell cultures indicate that selective opioid agonists can have a direct excitatory effect on such neurons. These excitatory effects are prevented by naloxone and are evident at low (nanomolar) concentrations, in contrast to the inhibitory effects that predominate at higher (micromolar) concentrations. Crain and Shen[60] have found that the excitatory effects of low doses of morphine are prevented by cholera toxin A, a selective deactivator of G_s. At higher doses, the G_i-mediated opioid inhibitory effects outlined previously outweigh opioid G_s-dependent effects. **Opioids, having biphasic excitatory or inhibitory actions on the same cell may explain otherwise perplexing observations. These include morphine hyperalgesia in occasional patients, itch in many patients given spinal opioids,[6] or naloxone-reversible hyperalgesia after low doses of morphine in some animal models of pain.[277]** Other explanations for the complex effects of naloxone relate to the system of diffuse, noxious inhibitory controls described later.

Changes in intracellular cAMP, cGMP, calcium, or calmodulin activate protein kinases, diverse enzymes that phosphorylate substrates ranging from hormone receptors to ion channels to G proteins.[54,119,138,270] **Protein kinases are thus cellular effectors, regulated by second messengers and influenced by opioids along with other drugs and hormones.[48,49,126,270] Many biologic molecules, excitable membrane proteins in particular, have their functions altered and thereby regulated by protein kinase–dependent phosphorylation.** Protein kinase C, a multifunctional protein kinase, is found throughout all tissues but is enriched in brain synaptic membranes. Its activation follows hormone-receptor (or drug-receptor) binding through a second messenger step involving membrane phospholipid breakdown.[14,183]

This brief survey can only hint at the wealth of information on intracellular signalling accumulated through the efforts of laboratories over many decades. None of the second messenger mechanisms listed is unique to opioid actions, and much detail has been omitted.

PROTO-ONCOGENES: "THIRD MESSENGERS"

The time frame for second messenger action is brief, but all who treat or study pain recognize that pain may persist long after a brief noxious stimulus. For example, chronic "phantom" pain is normal after limb amputation. **In the past few years the gene *c-fos* (originally identified within tumors) has been implicated as a "third messenger" that mediates such long-term activation of pain transmission neurons throughout the CNS.*** To help one understand why studies of *c-fos* (and its protein product Fos) have spurred such interest, this section briefly reviews what is meant by "oncogenes," describes their recently recognized functions in normal (i.e., nonmalignant) tissue, and summarizes some emerging results of studies of *c-fos* and related genes in the context of pain. This outline cannot do justice to the explosion in knowledge about the roles of growth factors and oncogenes in the normal or damaged nervous system. However, it illustrates the interdisciplinary cross-fertilization that is a hallmark of present-day pain research.

Oncogenes **are portions of DNA that, when expressed within normal cells, "transform" such cells into neoplastic forms whose growth and division are no longer restrained by normal controls.**[3,102,265] Oncogenes were first discovered within carcinogenic viruses and act by mimicking or amplifying one or more steps within the normal sequence by which growth factors or hormones induce the division or growth of normal cells.[63] As reviewed earlier, these steps include (1) binding of hormones or growth factors to their receptors, (2) activation of G proteins or protein kinases, (3) phosphorylation of cellular proteins, and (4) binding and activation of specific regions of the genome within the cell nucleus. Close homology, in some cases identity, exists between the DNA sequences of viral oncogenes and certain DNA sequences within normal cells.[100] The latter are therefore termed *proto-oncogenes* or *cellular oncogenes* (*c-oncs*) and mediate many aspects of growth or mitosis in normal, nonmalignant cells, such as in response to growth factors.

C-fos, a proto-oncogene within normal cells, derives its name from a homologous viral oncogene (*"v-fos"*) that induces osteosarcomas in mice. Within the nucleus of an activated cell, this gene's protein product, Fos, dimerizes with another nuclear protein, Jun (the product of the *c-jun* proto-oncogene).[62] This dimer in turn binds to a nuclear regulatory site, AP-1, that functions in the transcription of adjacent target genes for cellular products, such as the enkephalin precursor and other neuropeptides (Fig. 52-11). Fos-Jun dimerization begins within minutes of intracellular signalling by diverse second messengers, such as ion fluxes, AMP, or diacylglycerol, or after transsynaptic activation by neurotransmitters.[51] Curran and Franza[62] have compared the association of Fos,

---

* References 25, 79, 102, 115, 174, 200.

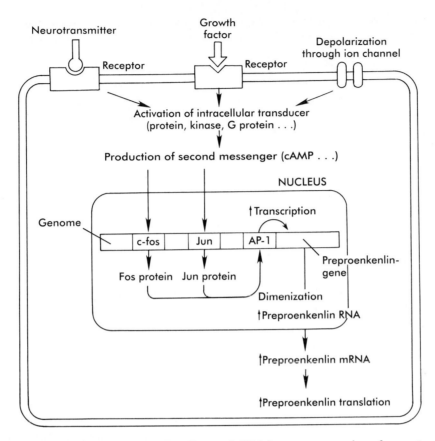

Fig. 52-11. Interactions between Fos, Jun, and AP-1 increase expression of many target genes, including preproenkephalin precursor in spinal cord neurons (see Fig. 52-12). In this example, neuronal activation follows cell surface stimulation (caused by receptor binding of a neurotransmitter or growth factor) or depolarization (caused by or independent of neurotransmitter action). Intracellular second messengers such as cyclic adenosine monophosphate (cAMP) stimulate expression of the proto-oncogenes *c-fos* and *c-jun*. The corresponding protein products Fos and Jun form a heterodimer that binds to AP-1, a distinct regulatory site activating transcription of (in this case) the preproenkephalin gene.

Jun, and AP-1 binding sites in the nucleus to ligand-receptor interactions at the cell membrane. They described this nuclear process as a "third messenger." That is, "a primordial signalling system adapted for use by selected target genes in different cell types."[62]

Hunt, Pini, and Evan,[115] following suggestions that nuclear protein products such as Fos might participate in persistent neural changes that follow transient stimuli,[95] found that noxious heat or chemical stimuli induced *c-fos* in dorsal horn neurons. Sagar, Sharp, and Curran[219] described the appearance of Fos in nuclei within polysynaptic pain transmission pathways after electrical stimulation of rat sensorimotor cortex. They deemed this type of investigation "metabolic mapping at the cellular level."

Correlative studies of *c-fos* responses together with neuropeptide levels, with or without opioid analgesia, have great relevance to opioid physiology. Draisci and Iadarola[69] measured messenger ribonucleic acid (mRNA) for *c-fos* in spinal cord dorsal horn neurons

during peripheral inflammation in rat paw, along with mRNA levels for dynorphin and enkephalin precursors. Immediate large rises in *c-fos* mRNA coincided with modest increases in enkephalin precursor mRNA, followed in several hours by marked, prolonged rises in dynorphin mRNA that persisted for at least a day (Fig. 52-12).[213] Basbaum and Fields[8] and colleagues[197] others have used *c-fos* to investigate the lamina-specific actions of morphine on inhibiting cellular excitation. They have also found dose-dependent decreases in the number of Fos-containing neurons in rat spinal cord with systemic morphine administration (Fig. 52-13).

Studies of the involvement of proto-ocogenes in analgesia, still at an early stage and far from consolidated, indicate that opioids may prevent activation of pain transmission neurons by inhibiting the early expression of *c-fos* and the resulting cascade of physiologic sequelae that ensue after a painful stimulus.[197,255] This hypothesis confirms related observations that expression of the proenkephalin gene, a

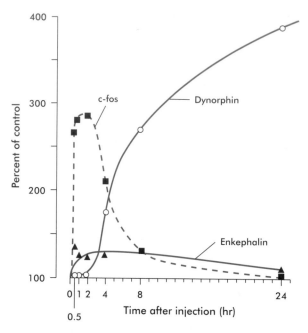

Fig. 52-12. Hindpaw inflammation produced by injection of carrageenan rapidly stimulates *c-fos*, enkephalin, and dynorphin gene expression in rat dorsal lumbar spinal cord. Shown on the ordinate is messenger RNA content expressed as percentage of control values. (From Draisci G, Iadarola MJ: Temporal analysis of increases in *c-fos*, pre-prodynorphin and preproenkephalin mRNAs in rat spinal cord, *Mol Brain Res* 6:31, 1989.)

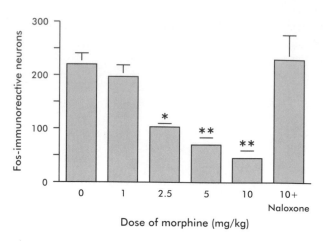

Fig. 52-13. Pretreatment with systemic morphine reduces number of rat spinal cord neurons containing detectable amounts of Fos protein following noxious stimulus (hindpaw formalin injection) delivered 20 minutes after drug treatment. (From Presley RW, Ménétrey D, Levine JD et al: Systemic morphine suppresses noxious stimulus-evoked Fos protein–like immunoreactivity in the rat spinal cord, *J Neurosci* 10:323, 1990.)

physiologic target for Fos and Jun,[184,242] is reduced by systemic morphine administration.[259] On the other hand, one must be cautious before concluding that oncogene studies are the Rosetta stone of pain research. *C-fos* activation is not specific for pain pathways; it also occurs in the retina after light exposure,[218] the hippocampus after seizure, or even outside the nervous system. Also, many other processes and participants besides *Fos, Jun,* and AP-1 influence neuropeptide gene expression.[52,200]

OPIOID ANALGESIA

Pain is the subjective counterpart of first, second, and third cellular messengers and intercellular signals that occur concurrently throughout the neuraxis, usually in response to tissue damage. No molecular structure or weight, DNA sequence, binding constant, or chromatographic profile exists for pain, but no physiologic process has been analyzed in greater detail.*

Pain is a highly dynamic process. Wall, Woolf, and others[53,264,274,277] **have found that (1) the arrival of C fiber afferent impulses sets off prolonged, widespread** increases of spinal cord neuronal excitability (**Fig. 52-14**); (2) **once the hyperexcitable state is established, it is necessary to use very high doses of narcotics to suppress it; but (3) "if small narcotic doses are given before the barrage arrives, the triggered central hyperexcitability never occurs." This work provides, in the words of Wall,**[263] **"A rationale for preoperative treatment in which small manipulations may prevent the cord ever reaching a hyperexcitable state in which the cord later responds excessively to inputs which would not be painful if the cord were not primed."**

The cellular anatomy of opioids' beneficial effects on pain transmission pathways is in keeping with their generally inhibitory effects on single cells: **opioid action typically reduces neurotransmission across excitatory synapses.**[1,8,101] A prototype of the integration of opioid physiology and neuroanatomy is in the spinal cord's dorsal horn, where enkephalin neurons presynaptically inhibit the release of substance P from nociceptive afferent C fibers (**Fig. 52-15**).[16,71,108,236,288]

Inhibition of excitatory synaptic transmission is termed *neuromodulation*. **Opioids are neuromodulators not only of substance P transmission in the dorsal horn, but also of dopamine in basal ganglia and of adrenergic transmission in innervated myocardium,**[28,141,203,267] **to cite just two examples of this prototypic opioid mechanism.**[85,198] Tens of thousands of research reports, reviews, and monographs on all aspects of opioid analgesia overwhelm any attempt to convey more than a glimpse of this complex process. Even if one gives less attention to chronic pain

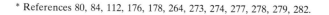

* References 80, 84, 112, 176, 178, 264, 273, 274, 277, 278, 279, 282.

mechanisms and focuses on acute pain because of its daily importance to anesthesiologists' practice, one can only highlight selected research findings.[31,56,66,240]

The varied means by which opioids produce analgesia in vivo may be categorized according to actions directly at the site of trauma (i.e, outside the CNS), within the spinal cord, or at supraspinal sites.

Controversy has existed concerning the effectiveness of peripherally administered opioids. Recently a consensus has emerged that negative conclusions[24,230,286] reflect observations in uninjured tissue, whereas analgesia results from injections into inflamed tissue. Opioid receptors have been identified in peripheral nerves (both somatic and sympathetic),* as well as on white blood cells† and vascular smooth muscle.[124,283] Opioids given directly into the site of peripheral inflammation inhibit the release of substance P,[22,147,148,280,284] as well as the generation of bradykinin,[104,116,117] and block prostaglandin-induced hyperalgesia.[75,76,124,204] Hargreaves et al.[103] have found (in a rat model of carrageenan-induced foot pad inflammation) that analgesia from a peripherally administered kappa opioid agonist occurs at doses inadequate to produce systemic analgesia. This analgesia is stereospecific and dose related and accompanied by a decrease in edema.[7,23,125,216] Parallel findings been reported as well by Stein and Herz[244,245,246] and others[215] for peripheral actions of mu-, kappa-, and delta-selective opioids. Many additional studies point to a role for endogenous opioids, along with other neuropeptides, in modulating white cell functions (Box 52-1).[99,131]

Use of spinal opioid effects clinically (a curiosity when introduced in 1978[257]) is today a valuable part of daily anesthesia practice to control postoperative and cancer pain.[31,55,275] Neuroanatomic substrates for and neurophysiologic effects of spinal opioid effects are presented in virtually every text[273,274] and monograph[289] on pain. The dorsal horn receives primary

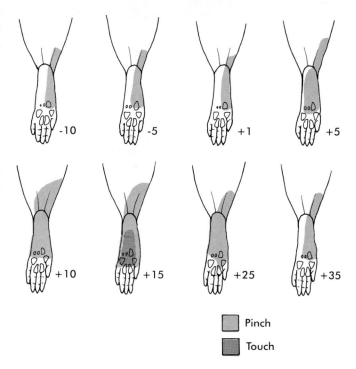

Fig. 52-14. Expansion of pinch receptive field of dorsal horn neuron after brief nociceptive stimulus. Note that 15 minutes after stimulus, neuron responds to touch, a lower-intensity stimulus. (From Cook AJ, Woolf CJ, Wall PD et al: Dynamic receptive field plasticity in rat spinal cord dorsal horn following C-primary afferent input, *Nature* 325:151, 1987.)

---

* References 12, 20, 70, 78, 94, 125, 137, 140, 170, 198, 241, 262, 285.
† References 17, 92, 156, 168, 179, 192, 214, 232, 233, 235, 238, 239, 253.

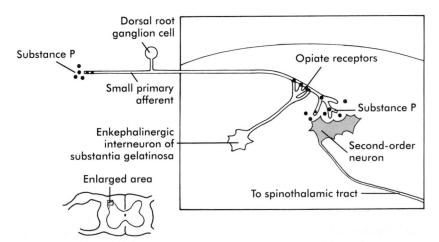

Fig. 52-15. Enkephalin interneuron inhibits substance P release from C fiber primary afferent in spinal cord's dorsal horn. (Redrawn from Bishop B: Pain: its physiology and rationale for management. Part II. Analgesic systems of the CNS, *Phys Ther* 60:21, 1980.)

BOX 52-1
ACTIONS OF OPIOIDS ON WHITE
BLOOD CELLS

Stimulate polymorphonuclear cell chemotaxis
Increase macrophage superoxide production
Activate mast cell serotonin release
Decrease lymphocyte antibody production
Increase natural killer cell activity

From Sibinga NES, Goldstein A: Opioid peptides and opioid receptors in cells of the immune system, *Annu Rev Immunol* 6:219, 1988.

---

afferent axons from neurons whose cell bodies are in the dorsal root ganglia. Sharp, well-localized "first" pain after tissue injury results from afferent impulses arriving via myelinated A delta fibers. Dull, achy, poorly localized, prolonged "second" pain arrives later over nonmyelinated C fibers. A delta and C fibers terminate mainly in the superficial layers of the dorsal horn (*substantia gelatinosa*) and in the deeper areas (*nucleus proprius*) corresponding to layers IV and V in the traditional (Rexed) classification.

Spinal neurons responding only to pain, and thus termed *nociceptive specific* or *high threshold,* are densest in the superficial area. Cells responding to less intense as well as painful stimuli are more abundant in the deeper layers and have variously been termed *wide dynamic range, convergent,* or *polymodal.*

As outlined previously and in Figs. 52-14 and 52-15, **spinally or systemically administered opioids reduce neurotransmitter (e.g., substance P) release from synapses of primary afferents**[16] **and also prevent enlargement of cutaneous receptive fields evoked by A delta and C fiber impulses. However, these opioids have little effect on spinal responses evoked by A beta afferents.** Opioids inhibit spinal neuron responses to C fiber stimulation more than to a delta fiber stimulation.[15] **Opioids prevent the summation of excitatory postsynaptic potentials (EPSPs) that otherwise follow prolonged C fiber input, thereby inhibiting dorsal horn neuronal excitation in response to painful input (Fig. 52-16).**

The action of opioids to prevent EPSP summation occurs at low doses of morphine and corresponds to the prevention of flexor reflex conditioning in vivo by C fiber afferent stimuli.[53,277] **Once C fiber facilitation of flexor withdrawal is established, 10-fold higher doses of morphine are required to reverse it compared with the doses to prevent this process from occurring.** Opioid inhibition of dorsal horn EPSPs may contribute to clinically valuable effects. These include recruiting additional dermatomes of sensory *anesthe-*

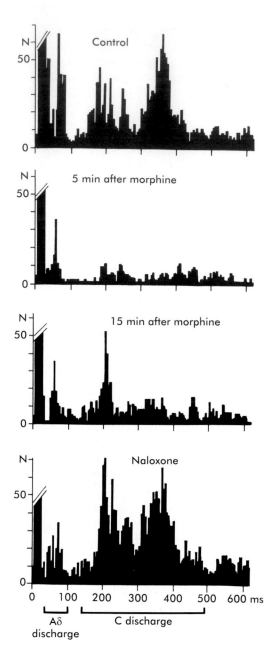

Fig. 52-16. Systemic morphine administration abolishes summation of postsynaptic potentials in spinal cord dorsal horn produced by electrical stimulation of a peripheral nerve. Note more complete suppression of C fiber responses compared with A delta fiber responses. (From LeBars D, Guilbaud G, Jurna I et al: Differential effects of morphine on responses of dorsal horn lamina V type cells elicited by A and C fibre stimulation in the spinal cat, *Brain Res* 115:518, 1976.)

sia by systemic morphine during epidural infusion of local anesthetic[161] or delaying the onset of postoperative pain through opioid premedication combined with intraoperative local anesthetic nerve blocks.[172,263]

In the 1950s Beecher[10] and others considered that opioids might inhibit spinal cord nociceptive processing through descending pathways of supraspinal

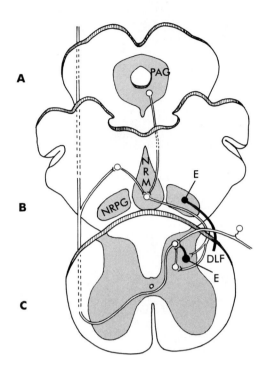

Fig. 52-17. Model for opioid-mediated descending analgesia originally proposed by Basbaum and Fields in the late 1970s. Opioid receptors stimulate neurons originating in periaqueductal gray *(PAG)* of midbrain **(A)**, as well as in nucleus raphe magnus *(NRM)* of medulla **(B)**. Descending enkephalinergic neurons originate from NRM and NRPG and travel to spinal cord segments *(C)* via dorsolateral funiculi *(DLF)*. Spinal enkephalin *(E)* interneurons within each segment also inhibit afferent nociceptive transmission. (From Basbaum A, Fields H: Endogenous pain control systems: brainstem spinal pathways and endorphin circuitry, *Annu Rev Neurosci* 7:309, 1984.)

origin.[118] Basbaum and Fields[8] in the mid-1970s proposed a model of descending opioid-mediated analgesia to consolidate then-current findings on opioids' sites of action. In this model (Fig. 52-17), opioids reinforce inhibition through pathways that originate in sites such as the periaqueductal gray of the midbrain. These pathways continue caudally via dorsolateral tracts to spinal segments, where they inhibit pain transmission in the dorsal horn.

Descending opioid analgetic pathways, normally quiescent, become active to yield "stress-induced" analgesia during environmental challenge,[132,256] **"stimulation-produced" analgesia on central electrical stimulation, or opioid analgesia after drug administration.**[1,10,101,250] These descending analgetic effects depend on mu opioid receptor mechanisms. Kappa receptors appear less active in this descending analgetic pathway, since spinal transection does not reduce kappa opioid agonists' analgetic effect at the level of the distal cord.[175,177,201] Some stressors, such as cold ambient temperature, produce analgesia through nonopioid peptide or monoamine mechanisms. An-

algesia from a single type of stress, such as foot shock, may have opioid or nonopioid features (e.g., naloxone reversibility) according to its frequency and escapability.

Although there is no question that analgesia resulting from stress, central electrical stimulation, or systemic opioid administration depends on activation of supraspinal pathways, detailed understanding of these phenomena has evolved considerably in the past decade. Portions of the classic Basbaum-Fields model survive, such as neurochemical mediation by monoamine systems and anatomic mediation through the dorsolateral funiculi. Other features of that model have been replaced, essentially, by their opposites. Specifically, **the concept that descending, opioid-sensitive pathways act directly to inhibit nociceptive transmission at the spinal level has been superseded by a construct in which pain perception depends on a contrast between "background" somesthetic neuronal activity and nociceptive signals.**[143-146] Analgesia results when the contrasting activity between these two pools is reduced either by increasing background somesthetic input or by decreasing the primary nociceptive signal (Fig. 52-18).

In this model, advanced by LeBars et al.,[143-146] nociceptive excitatory signals arising at the spinal level induce *diffuse noxious inhibitory controls* (DNIC) of supraspinal origin. Neurophysiologic studies have established that DNIC reduce spontaneous nonnociceptive activity in convergent neurons at many spinal segments, including those where the pain signals arise. DNIC also augment pain perception by exaggerating the contrast between the primary nociceptive signal and background neural activity. The DNIC response corresponds well with other amplifying processes triggered by painful stimuli described earlier.

Direct electrophysiologic studies have shown that morphine given intracerebrally or at low systemic doses blocks DNIC so that somesthetic background activity is restored, lessening pain perception. Morphine given systemically at high doses or intrathecally acts to depress nociceptive transmission directly at the spinal level, further reducing the contrast between background neural activity and primary nociceptive signal and thereby increasing analgesia. Briefly, **in the DNIC schema the supraspinal action of morphine *decreases* descending inhibitory activity on non-nociceptive wide dynamic range neurons at many levels. In the classic Basbaum-Fields model, however, morphine acts supraspinally to *increase* descending inhibition on segmental pain transmission neurons.**

The current model, although more complex than the initial Basbaum-Fields one, appears better suited to explain various observations, such as the complex effects of naloxone.[11,98,221] The DNIC model also has

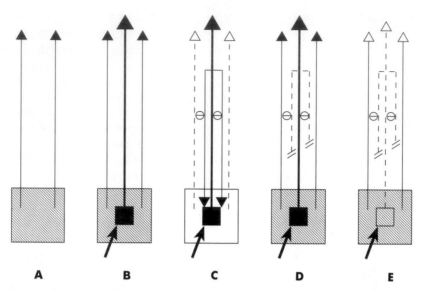

Fig. 52-18. Model advanced by LeBars and colleagues to explain range of stimulation- and drug-induced opioid analgetic and hyperanalgetic effects. **A,** Background somesthetic activity of wide dynamic range (WDR) neurons. Activation of nociceptive-specific neurons *(dark central square)* along with WDR neurons by noxious stimulus **(B)** evokes excitatory input to brain that triggers diffuse noxious inhibitory controls (DNIC), shown as paired descending arrows in **C. D,** Low doses of systemic morphine, or intraventricular morphine, suppress DNIC and thereby restore somesthetic background activity. **E,** Higher doses of systemic morphine, or intrathecal morphine, inhibit segmental nociceptive processing, resulting in more intense analgesia than at lower doses. (Modified from references 143-146.)

been supported by ongoing studies that employ electrophysiologic measures in humans (e.g., the R III reflex) to quantitate inhibitory opioid effects on spinal reflexes in vivo.[271,272] Because multiple descending analgesia systems involving diverse mechanisms most likely exist, future models probably will integrate ever-growing knowledge of these mechanisms. For example, Randich and Maixner recently observed that vagectomy abolishes analgesia from systemic morphine adminstration. This observation suggests that vagal afferent impulses may be an important, previously overlooked mechanism for opioid-induced supraspinal activation.[203a] **Rostral supraspinal sites such as the hippocampus, basal ganglia, hypothalamus, and cortex are also rich in opioids and their receptors. These sites are presumptive targets for opioid effects on cognitive, emotional, and neuroendocrine dimensions of clinical pain.**[150,163,169,248]

HOW OPIOIDS ACT: SUMMARY

The preceding survey has described some basic aspects of opioid actions. These aspects include (1) structural requirements for a molecule to mimic the actions of morphine, (2) properties of receptors that recognize such molecules, (3) changes within single cells that follow opioid + receptor binding, and (4) opioid effects on groups of cells (inside and outside the CNS) that result in analgesia. Of these four topics, descriptions of the latter three prepared 5 years ago would not be hopelessly dated.

It is now clear that **opioids given after tissue injury alter (and in typical clinical doses, uniformly inhibit) synergistic processes that, if untreated, amplify and prolong the initial brief nociceptive stimulus (Table 52-4).** These same benefits can be obtained with lower doses of opioids if given before the onset of pain, in keeping with anesthesiologists' longstanding practical wisdom that lower doses of opioids are needed to "stay ahead of pain" rather than to "catch up to it."

In the periphery, processes evoked by tissue injury and suppressed by opioids include the release of algetic mediators that sensitize nociceptors and trigger inflammation. Systemic immune responses are also altered by opioids, in part through "nonopioid" mechanisms. In the spinal cord, opioids impede synaptic transmission, block amplification of the pain signal, and diminish expression of proto-oncogenes and opioid peptide precursors. Supraspinally, opioids reduce descending DNIC and thereby lessen the contrast between pain signals and background somesthetic "noise." Further rostrally, opioids alter hormonal, cognitive, and emotional responses to pain.[248]

Besides analgesia, opioids have other important effects on autonomic and neuroendocrine events that

Table 52-4 Opioid analgesia: sites and processes

Site	Processes
At site of tissue injury and inflammation	Decrease peptide mediator (bradykinin, substance P) release Reduce prostaglandin-induced hyperalgesia Reduce edema Influence white cell processes (?) Directly act on opioid receptors in peripheral nerve
At spinal segment	Decrease substance P-mediated neurotransmission from C (± A delta) fiber to second-order neuron Block summation of excitatory postsynaptic potentials in second-order neuron Prevent expansion of receptive fields and reduction of excitatory thresholds of second-order neurons Prevent neuronal gene expression (c-fos, opioid precursor molecules)
Supraspinally	Augment endogenous, descending, opioid-sensitive suppression of spinal pain signal transmission ([?] reduce DNIC or augment descending inhibition) Alter (mostly reduce) neuroendocrine and autonomic "stress" responses by acting on brainstem-limbic and hypothalamic opioid receptors Alter cognitive and emotional processing of painful input by acting on limbic and cortical opioid receptors

are initiated by tissue injury and augmented by persistent nociception. These include beneficial cardiovascular (e.g., antifibrillatory)[42] actions and a reduction in systemic "stress" hormone secretion.[30,41] In certain frail patient populations, presumably because of these beneficial effects, opioid administration may reduce postoperative morbidity or mortality. Since these other opioid effects are outside the scope of this chapter's focus on analgesia, they have been omitted; the reader should consult other discussions in this textbook or the literature for more information. Further significant topics relevant to opioids, such as the means to measure their concentrations or assess their potency, or problems involved in selecting an opioid analgesic according to the precise nature of the painful stimulus, are similarly covered elsewhere.[36,224,249]

In our view the aim of acute pain treatment in physiologic terms is to dissociate the event of tissue injury (over which anesthesiologists normally have no control) from the collection of undesirable nociceptive, autonomic, and neuroendocrine responses that customarily ensue.[261] Because of their unrivaled multiplicity of sites and mechanisms of action, opioids are uniquely valuable means for achieving this goal.[173]

ACKNOWLEDGEMENTS

We are grateful for the unswerving support of Dr. Richard J. Kitz for studies on pain under the auspices of the Department of Anesthesia at the Massachusetts General Hospital. Drs. Kenneth Hargreaves, Daniel LeBars, Edward McCleskey, and Walter Zieglgänsberger generously provided pre- and reprints but did not have the opportunity to review and correct drafts of this chapter. Dr. Chawki Haddad brought to the authors' attention the 1978 account of therapeutic use of intraspinal opioids. Miss Evelyn Hall provided expert secretarial assistance during preparation of this manuscript.

KEY POINTS

- "Opioids" are morphinelike alkaloids derived from poppy seeds; they may also be present in mammals, possibly originating in intestinal flora. Codeine and thebaine, five- or six-ring alkaloids of the phenanthrene class, are also "opioids."

- A portion of the structure of all morphinelike compounds resembles the amino acid, tyrosine. The tyrosine portion of opioids is essential for morphinelike action. Other regions of opioid molecules may produce biologic effects different from those produced by morphine.

- Morphine and fentanyl produce dose-dependent biologic responses and are termed "agonists" or "full agonists." Other opioids, such as buprenorphine, evoke a submaximal plateau response despite indefinite increases in dosage; these are called "partial agonists." Opioids such as butorphanol are agonists at one type of opioid receptor and antagonists at a second type and are called "mixed agonist-antagonists."

- Since the discovery of enkephalins in 1975, numerous opioid peptides have been isolated that share with the enkephalins an N-terminus tetrapeptide fragment, Tyr-Gly-Gly-Phe-.

- In the 1960s Martin inferred the existence of at least two types of opioid receptors. He postulated that morphine acts upon a hypothetic "mu" receptor to produce miosis, bradycardia, analgesia, and indifference to the environment. In contrast, ketocyclazocine constricts pupils and reduces the flexor reflex but produces sedation rather than indifference, has little effect on the skin twitch reflex, and does not alter symptoms of morphine withdrawal. Hence Martin postulated that the effects of ketocyclazocine are identified with actions on a second receptor, the "kappa" receptor. A third receptor, the "sigma" receptor, theoretically accounts for the sympathetic and behavioral arousal caused by N-allyl normetazocine ("SKF-10,047").

- The opioid may be considered a "first messenger" whose arrival at the cell membrane produces an activated opioid + receptor complex. Subsequent intracellular events are "second messengers" and follow internal cell signalling pathways.

- Second messengers that arose early in evolution and are retained in man are important for opioid action. One employs cyclic adenosine monophosphate (cAMP) and another uses membrane phospholipid breakdown and calcium ion fluxes. In both mechanisms, signal molecules rapidly diffuse within a cell and act by changing the structure of cellular proteins. Either path may be activated when an opioid binds to its receptor. Binding changes that receptor's conformation and this conformational change is transmitted across the cell membrane to interact with a G protein. G proteins inhibit (G_i) or stimulate (G_s) adenylyl cyclase. Many important opioid effects result from opioid receptor-G_i interactions.

- Intracellular calcium is an important ionic second messenger for many ligands, including opioids. Opioids inhibit transmembrane calcium currents as well as certain actions of the activated calcium-calmodulin complex.

- Second messenger action is brief, but pain may persist long after the initial noxious stimulus. Long-term activation of pain transmission neurons throughout the central nervous system is mediated by a "third messenger," the *c-fos* proto-oncogene. Oncogenes are portions of DNA that transform normal cells into neoplastic forms whose growth and division are no longer restrained by normal controls. Studies of proto-oncogenes in analgesia indicate that opioids may prevent activation of pain transmission neurons by inhibiting the early expression of *c-fos* and the physiologic effects of painful stimulus.

- Pain is the subjective counterpart of first, second, and third cellular messengers and intercellular signals that occur concurrently throughout the neuraxis, usually in response to tissue damage.

- Opioid release typically reduces neurotransmission across excitatory synapses, and the beneficial effects of opioids to reduce or prevent signal amplification in pain transmission networks reflects their inhibitory effects at the cellular level.

- Inhibition of excitatory synaptic transmission is termed "neuromodulation": opioids are neuromodulators of substance P transmission in the dorsal horn, of dopamine in basal ganglia, and of adrenergic transmission in innervated myocardium.

- Spinal or systemically administered opioids reduce neurotransmitter release from synapses of primary afferents. They also prevent enlargement of cutaneous receptive fields evoked by A-delta and C-fiber impulses. They have little effect on spinal responses evoked by A-beta afferents.

- Opioids prevent the summation of excitatory postsynaptic potentials that otherwise follow prolonged C-fiber input, thereby inhibiting dorsal horn neuronal excitation in response to painful input.

- Pain perception depends on a contrast between "background" somesthetic neuronal activity and nociceptive signals. Analgesia results when the contrasting activity between these two pools is reduced. Contrast may be reduced either by increasing background somesthetic input or by decreasing the primary nociceptive signal. Morphine given intracerebrally or at low systemic doses restores somesthetic background activity, thereby lessening pain perception. Morphine given systemically at high doses or intrathecally depresses nociceptive transmission at the spinal level, further reducing contrast.

- Opioids given after tissue injury uniformly inhibit synergistic processes that, if untreated, amplify and prolong the initial brief nociceptive stimulus. Lower doses of opioids given before the onset of pain have the same effect as higher doses given afterwards.

- In the spinal cord, opioids impede synaptic transmission, block amplification of the pain signal, and diminish expression of proto-oncogenes and opioid peptide precursors. Supraspinally, opioids lessen the contrast between pain signals and background somesthetic "noise."

- The aim of acute pain treatment is to dissociate the event of tissue injury from the undesirable nociceptive, autonomic, and neuroendocrine responses that customarily ensue. Because of their unrivaled multiplicity of sites and mechanisms of action, opioids are a uniquely valuable means for achieving this goal.

KEY REFERENCES

Cousins MJ, Cherry DA, and Gourlay GK: Acute and chronic pain: use of spinal opioids. In Cousins MJ, Bridenbaugh PO, eds: *Neural blockade in clinical anesthesia and management of pain,* ed 2, Philadelphia, 1988, JB Lippincott.

Draisci G, Iadarola MJ: Temporal analysis of increases in c-fos, preprodynorphin and preproenkephalin mRNAs in rat spinal cord, *Mol Brain Res* 6:31, 1989.

Janssen PAJ: Stereochemical anatomy of morphinomimetics. In Loh HH, Ross DH, eds: *Neurochemical mechanisms of opiates and enkephalins,* New York, 1979, Raven Press.

Joris J, Dubner R, and Hargreaves KM: Opioid analgesia at peripheral sites: a target for opioids released during stress and inflammation? *Anesth Analg* 66:1277, 1987.

Randich A, Maixner W: Interactions between cardiovascular and pain regulatory mechanisms, *Neurosci Biobehav Rev* 8:343, 1984.

Sibinga NES, Goldstein A: Opioid peptides and opioid receptors in cells of the immune system, *Ann Rev Immunol* 6:219, 1988.

Upton N, Sewell RDE, and Spencer PSJ: Differentiation of potent mu- and kappa-opiate agonists using heat and pressure antinociceptive profiles and combined potency analysis, *Eur J Pharmacol* 78:421, 1982.

Wall PD: The prevention of postoperative pain, *Pain* 33:289, 1988.

Willer JC, Le Bars D, and De Broucker T: Diffuse noxious inhibitory controls in man: involvement of an opioidergic link, *Eur J Pharmacol* 182:347, 1990.

Yaksh TL: Neurologic mechanisms of pain. In Cousins MJ, Bridenbaugh PO, eds: *Neural blockade in clinical anesthesia and management of pain,* ed 2, Philadelphia, 1988, JB Lippincott.

REFERENCES

1. Advokat C: The role of descending inhibition in morphine-induced analgesia, *Trends Pharmacol Sci* 9:330, 1988.
2. Aghajanian G: Tolerance of locus coeruleus neurons to morphine and suppression of withdrawal responses to morphine, *Nature* 276:186, 1979.
3. Alberts B et al, eds: *Molecular biology of the cell,* ed 2, New York, 1989, Garland.
4. Atweh SF, Kuhar MJ: Distribution and physiological significance of opioid receptors in the brain, *Br Med Bull* 39:47, 1983.
5. Bailey PL, Stanley TH: Pharmacology of intravenous narcotic anesthetics. In Miller RD, ed: *Anesthesia,* ed 2, New York, 1986, Churchill-Livingstone.
6. Ballantyne JC, Loach AB, and Carr DB: Itching after epidural and spinal opiates, *Pain* 33:149, 1988.
7. Bartho L, Szolcsanyi J: Opiate agonists inhibit neurogenic plasma extravasation in the rat, *Eur J Pharmacol* 73:101, 1981.
8. Basbaum A, Fields H: Endogenous pain control systems: brainstem spinal pathways and endorphin circuitry, *Annu Rev Neurosci* 7:309, 1984.
9. Beckett AH, Casy AF: Synthetic analgesics: stereochemical considerations, *J Pharm Pharmacol* 6:986, 1954.
10. Beecher HK: The measurement of pain, *Pharmacol Rev* 9:59, 1957.
11. Bell JA: Naloxone-induced facilitation of C-fiber reflexes is induced by chronic morphine, *Eur J Pharmacol* 168:101, 1989.
12. Bentley G, Newton S, and Star J: Evidence for an action of morphine and the enkephalins on sensory nerve endings of the mouse peritoneum, *Br J Pharmacol* 73:325, 1981.
13. Bernton EW, Long JB, and Holaday JW: Opioids and neuropeptides: mechanisms in circulatory shock, *Fed Proc* 44:290, 1985.
14. Berridge MJ: Inositol triphosphate and diacylglycerol as second messengers, *Biochem J* 220:345, 1984.
15. Bing Z, Villaneuva L, and LeBars D: Effects of systemic morphine upon Aδ- and C-fibre evoked activities of subnucleus reticularis dorsalis neurones in the rat medulla, *Eur J Pharmacol* 164:85, 1989.
16. Bishop B: Pain: its physiology and rationale for management. II. Analgesic systems of the CNS, *Phys Ther* 60:21, 1980.
17. Blalock JE, Smith EM: A complete regulatory loop between the immune and neuroendocrine systems, *Fed Proc* 44:108, 1985.
18. Bloom FE: Neurotransmitters: past, present, and future directions, *FASEB J* 2:32, 1988.
19. Bongianni F, Carla V, Moroni F et al: Calcium channel inhibitors suppress the morphine-withdrawal syndrome in rats, *Br J Pharmacol* 88:561, 1986.
20. Bosnjak Z, Seagard JL, Roerig DL et al: The effects of morphine on sympathetic transmission in the stellate ganglion of the cat, *Can J Physiol Pharmacol* 64:940, 1986.
21. Bradford HF, Crowder JM, and White EJ: Inhibitory actions of opioid compounds on calcium fluxes and neuro-transmitter release from mammalian cerebral cortical slices, *Br J Pharmacol* 88:87, 1986.
22. Brodin E, Gazelius B, Panopoulos P et al: Morphine inhibits substance P release from peripheral sensory nerve endings, *Acta Physiol Scand* 117:567, 1983.
23. Brown J, Kissel J, and Lish P: Studies on the acute inflammatory response. I. Involvement of the central nervous system in certain models of inflammation, *J Pharmacol Exp Ther* 160:231, 1968.
24. Bullingham R, O'Sullivan G, McQuay H et al: Perineural injection of morphine fails to relieve postoperative pain in humans, *Anesth Analg* 62:164, 1983.
25. Bullitt E: Induction of c-fos-like protein within the lumbar spinal cord and thalamus of the rat following peripheral stimulation, *Brain Res* 493:391, 1989.
26. Cabot MC, McKeehan WL, eds: *Mechanisms of signal transduction by hormones and growth factors,* New York, 1987, Alan R Liss.
27. Caffrey JL, Wooldridge CB, and Gaugl JF: The interaction of endogenous opiates with autonomic circulatory control in the dog, *Circ Shock* 17:233, 1985.
28. Caffrey JL, Wooldridge CB, and Gaugl JF: Naloxone enhances myocardial responses to isoproterenol in dog isolated heart-lung, *Am J Physiol* 250:H749, 1986.
29. Calimlim JF, Wardell WM, Sriwatanakul K et al: Analgesic efficacy of parenteral metkephamid acetate in treatment of postoperative pain, *Lancet* 1:1374, 1982.

30. Carr DB: Caveats in the measurement and interpretation of chemical mediators of pain and analgesia. In Max MB, Portenoy RK, and Laska E, eds: *The design of analgesic clinical trials,* New York, 1991, Raven Press.

31. Carr DB: Pain. In Firestone LL, Lebowitz P, and Cook C, eds: *Clinical anesthesia procedures of the Massachusetts General Hospital,* ed 3, Boston, 1988, Little Brown.

32. Carr DB, Athanasiadis CG, Skourtis CT et al: Quantitative relationships between plasma beta-endorphin immunoactivity and hemodynamic performance in preoperative cardiac surgical patients, *Anesth Analg* 68:77, 1989.

33. Carr DB, Ballantyne JC: Endorphins and analgesia, *Compr Ther* 13:7, 1987.

34. Carr DB, Bergland R, Hamilton A et al: Endotoxin-stimulated opioid peptide secretion: two pools and feedback control in vivo, *Science* 217:845, 1982.

35. Carr DB, Carr JM: Role of brain opiates in pain relief. In Stoll BA, Parbhoo S, eds: *Bone metastasis: monitoring and treatment,* New York, 1983, Raven Press.

36. Carr DB, Fisher JE: Opiate receptors, endogenous ligands, and anesthesia: a synopsis. In Estafanous FG, ed: *Opioids in anesthesia,* Boston, 1984, Butterworths.

37. Carr DB, Jones KJ, Bergland RM et al: Causal links between plasma and CSF endorphin levels in stress: vector-ARMA analysis, *Peptides* 6 (suppl 1):5, 1985.

38. Carr DB, Lipkowski AW: Neuropeptides and pain, *Agressologie* 31:173, 1990.

39. Carr DB, Lipkowski AW, and Silbert BS: Biochemistry of the opioid peptides. In Estafanous FG, ed: *Opioids in anesthesia. II,* Boston, 1990, Butterworth-Heinemann.

40. Carr DB, Murphy MT: Operation, anesthesia, and the endorphin system. *Int Anesthesiol Clin* 26:199, 1988.

41. Carr DB, Rosenblatt M: Endorphins in the normal and abnormal pituitary. In Black P et al, eds: *Secretory tumors of the pituitary gland,* New York, 1984, Raven Press.

42. Carr DB, Saini V, and Verrier RL: Opioids and cardiovascular function: neuromodulation of ventricular ectopy. In Kulbertus HE, Franck G, eds: *Neurocardiology,* New York, 1988, Futura.

43. Chapman DB, Way EL: Modification of endorphin/enkephalin analgesia and stress-induced analgesia by divalent cations, a cation chelator and an inophore, *Br J Pharmacol* 75:389, 1982.

44. Christie MJ, Williams JT, and North RA: Cellular mechanisms of opioid tolerance: studies in single brain neurons, *Mol Pharmacol* 32:633, 1987.

45. Chrubasik J: Spinal analgesia by neuropeptides, *Schmerz-Pain-Douleur* 3:103, 1987.

46. Civelli O, Machida C, Bunzow J et al: The next frontier in the molecular biology of the opioid system: the opioid receptors, *Mol Neurobiol* 1:373, 1987.

47. Clo C, Muscari C, Tantini B et al: Reduced mechanical activity of perfused rat heart following morphine or en-kephalin peptides administration, *Life Sci* 37:1327, 1985.

48. Clouet DH, O'Callaghan JP: Role of protein kinases in opiate actions in brain. In Loh HH, Ross DH, eds: *Neurochemical mechanisms of opiates and endorphins,* New York, 1979, Raven Press.

49. Cohen P, Houslay MD, eds: *Molecular mechanisms of transmembrane signalling,* New York, 1985, Elsevier.

50. Colpaert FC, Lal H, Niemegeers CJ et al: Investigations on drug produced and subjectively experienced discriminative stimuli. I. The fentanyl cue, a tool to investigate subjectively experienced narcotic drug actions, *Life Sci* 16:705, 1975.

51. Comb M, Hyman SE, and Goodman HM: Mechanisms of trans-synaptic regulation of gene expression, *Trends Neurosci* 10:473, 1987.

52. Comb M, Mermod N, Hyman SE et al: Proteins bound at adjacent DNA elements act synergistically to regulate human proenkephalin cAMP inducible transcription, *EMBO J* 7:3793, 1988.

53. Cook AJ, Woolf CJ, Wall PD et al: Dynamic receptive field plasticity in rat spinal cord dorsal horn following C-primary afferent input, *Nature* 325:151, 1987.

54. Cooper JR, Bloom FE, and Roth RH: *The biochemical basis of neuropharmacology,* ed 5, New York, 1986, Oxford University Press.

55. Cousins MJ, Cherry DA, and Gourlay GK: Acute and chronic pain: use of spinal opioids. In Cousins MJ, Bridenbaugh PO, eds: *Neural blockade in clinical anesthesia and management of pain,* ed 2, Philadelphia, 1988, JB Lippincott.

56. Cousins MJ, Phillips GD, eds: *Acute pain management,* New York, 1986, Churchill-Livingstone.

57. Cowan A: Simple *in vivo* tests that differentiate prototype angonists at opiate receptors, *Life Sci* 28:1559, 1981.

58. Cox BM: Endogenous opioid peptides: a guide to structures and terminology, *Life Sci* 31:1645, 1982.

59. Cox BM: Molecular and cellular mechanisms in opioid tolerance. In Basbaum AI, Bessom J-M, eds: *Towards a new pharmacotherapy of pain,* New York, 1991, John Wiley & Sons.

60. Crain SM, Shen K-F: Opioids can evoke direct receptor-mediated excitatory effects on sensory neurons, *Trends Pharmacol Sci* 11:77, 1990.

61. Crone LA, Conley JM, Clark KM et al: Recurrent herpes simplex virus labialis and the use of epidural morphine in obstetric patients, *Anesth Analg* 67:318, 1988.

62. Curran T, Franza BR: Fos and Jun: the AP-1 connection, *Cell* 55:395, 1988.

63. Darnell J, Lodish H, and Baltimore D: *Molecular cell biology,* ed 2, New York, 1990, Scientific American.

64. Da Silva RA, Verrier RL, and Lown B: Protective effect of the vagotonic action of morphine sulphate on ventricular vulnerability, *Cardiovasc Res* 12:167, 1978.

65. DeWied D: Pituitary neuropeptides and behavior. In Hokfelt T, Luft R, eds: *Central regulation of the nervous system,* New York, 1978, Plenum.

66. Dodson ME, ed: *The management of postoperative pain,* vol 8, *Current topics in anaesthesia,* Baltimore, 1985, Edward Arnold.

67. Dolphin AC: Nucleotide binding proteins in signal transduction and disease, *Trends Neurosci* 10:53, 1987.

68. Donnerer J, Oka K, Brossi A et al: Presence and formation of codeine and morphine in the rat, *Proc Natl Acad Sci USA* 83:4566, 1986.

69. Draisci G, Iadarola MJ: Temporal analysis of increases in c-fos, preprodynorphin and preproenkephalin mRNAs in rat spinal cord, *Mol Brain Res* 6:31, 1989.

70. Dubner R, Gebhart GF, and Bond MR, eds: *Proceedings of the Fifth World Congress on Pain,* New York, 1988, Elsevier.

71. Duggan AW: Electrophysiology of opioid peptides and sensory systems, *Br Med Bull* 39:65, 1983.

72. Duggan AW, North RA: Electrophysiology of opioids, *Pharmacol Rev* 35:219, 1984.

73. Eipper BA, Mains RE: Structure and biosynthesis of proadrenocorticotropin/endorphin and related peptides, *Endocr Rev* 1:1, 1980.

74. Evans CJ, von Zastrow M: A state of the delta opioid receptor that is 'blind' to opioid peptides yet retains high affinity for the opiate alkaloids. In van Ree JM et al, eds: *New leads in opioid research,* Amsterdam, 1990, Excerpta Medica.

75. Ferreira SH, Nakamura M: Prostaglandin hyperalgesia: the peripheral analgesic activity of morphine, enkephalins and opioid antagonists, *Prostaglandins* 18:191, 1979.

76. Ferreira S, Nakamura M: Prostaglandin hyperalgesia. II. The peripheral analgesic activity of morphine, enkephalins and opioid antagonists, *Prostaglandins* 23:53, 1979.

77. Feuerstein G: The opioid system and central cardiovascular control: analysis of controversies, *Peptides* 6(suppl 2):51, 1985.

78. Fields H, Emson PC, Leigh BK et al: Multiple opiate receptor sites on primary afferent fibers, *Nature* 284:351, 1980.

79. Fitzgerald M: C-fos and the changing face of pain, *Trends Pharmacol Sci* 13:439, 1990.

80. Foley KM, Inturrisi CE, eds: Opioid analgesics in the management of clinical pain. In Bonica JJ ed: *Advances in pain research and therapy,* New York, 1986, Raven Press.

81. Frances B, Puget H, Moisand C et al: Apparent precoupling of κ- but not μ-opioid receptors with a G protein in the absence of agonist, *Eur J Pharmacol* 189:1, 1990.

82. Franz DN, Hare BD, and McCloskey KL: Spinal sympathetic neurons: possible sites of opiate-withdrawal suppression by clonidine, *Science* 215:1643, 1982.

83. Freidinger RM: Non-peptide ligands for peptide receptors, *Trends Pharmacol Sci* 10:270, 1989.

84. Freye E: *Opioid agonists, antagonists and mixed narcotic analgesics: theoretical background and considerations for practical use,* Berlin, 1987, Springer Verlag.

85. Gaddis R, Dixon W: Modulation of peripheral adrenergic neurotransmission by met-enkephalin, *J Pharmacol Exp Ther* 221:282, 1982.

86. Gandhi VC, Ross DH: The effect of kappa agonist U50-488H on [³H] nimodipine receptor binding in rat brain regions, *Eur J Pharmacol* 150:51, 1988.

87. Gann DS, Ward DG, and Carlson DE: Neural control of ACTH: a homeostatic reflex, *Recent Prog Horm Res* 34:357, 1978.

88. Garzon J, Schulz R, and Herz A: Evidence for the epsilon-type of opioid receptor in the rat vas deferens, *Mol Pharmacol* 28:1, 1985.

89. Gebhart GF: Some mechanistic insights into opioid tolerance, *Anesthesiology* 73:1065, 1990.

90. Gilbert PE, Martin WR: The effects of morphine- and nalorphine-like drugs in the nondependent, morphine-dependent and cyclazocine-dependent spinal dog, *J Pharmacol Exp Ther* 198:66, 1976.

91. Gilman AG: G proteins and regulation of adenylyl cyclase, *JAMA* 262:1819, 1989.

92. Gilman SC, Schwartz JM, Milner RJ et al: Beta-endorphin enhances lymphocyte proliferative responses, *Proc Natl Acad Sci USA* 79:4226, 1982.

93. Gilmore W, Weiner LP: The opioid specificity of beta-endorphin enhancement of murine lymphocyte proliferation, *Immunopharmacology* 17:19, 1989.

94. Gissen AJ, Gugino LD, Datta S et al: Effects of fentanyl and sufentanil on peripheral mammalian nerves, *Anesth Analg* 66:1272, 1987.

95. Goelet P, Castellucci VF, Schacher S et al: The long and short of long-term memory: a molecular framework, *Nature* 322:419, 1986.

96. Goldstein A: Binding selectivity profiles for ligands of multiple receptor types: focus on opioid receptors, *Trends Pharmacol Sci* 8:456, 1987.

97. Gross RA, Macdonald RL: Dynorphin A selectively reduces a large transient (N-type) calcium current of mouse dorsal root ganglion neurons in cell culture, *Proc Natl Acad Sci USA* 84:5469, 1987.

98. Hamilton AJ, Black PM, and Carr DB: Contrasting actions of naloxone in experimental spinal cord trauma and cerebral ischemia: a review, *Neurosurgery* 17:845, 1985.

99. Hamilton AJ, Carr DB, LaRovere JM et al: Endotoxic shock elicits greater endorphin secretion than hemorrhage, *Circ Shock* 19:47, 1986.

100. Hanahan D: Transgenic mice as probes into complex systems, *Science* 246:1265, 1989.

101. Hanaoka K, Ohtani M, Toyooka H et al: The relative contribution of direct and supraspinal descending effects upon spinal mechanisms of morphine analgesia, *J Pharmacol Exp Ther* 207:476, 1978.

102. Hanley MR: Proto-oncogenes in the nervous system, *Neuron* 1:175, 1988.

103. Hargreaves KM, Dubner R, and Joris J: Peripheral action of opiates in the blockade of carrageenan-induced inflammation. In Dubner R, Gebhart GF, and Bond MR, eds: *Pain research and clinical management,* vol 3, Amsterdam, 1988, Elsevier.

104. Hargreaves KM, Wells L, and Solodkin A: Opiates inhibit release of immunoreactive bradykinin from inflamed tissue, as evaluated by peripheral microdialysis probes, *Abstr Soc Neurosci* 15:148, 1989.

105. Hasegawa J-I, Loh HH, and Lee NM: Lipid requirement for μ opioid receptor binding, *J Neurochem* 49:1007, 1987.

106. Hassen AH, Feuerstein G, Pfeiffer A et al: Delta versus mu receptors: cardiovascular and respiratory effects of opiate agonists microinjected into nucleus tractus solitarius of cats, *Regul Pept* 4:299, 1982.

107. Hayes A, Kelly A: Profile of activity of K receptor agonists in the rabbit vas deferens, *Eur J Pharmacol* 110:317, 1985.

108. Henderson G: Electrophysiological analysis of opioid action in the central nervous system, *Br Med Bull* 39:59, 1983.

109. Herling S, Woods JH: Discriminative stimulus effects of narcotics: evidence for multiple receptor-mediated actions, *Life Sci* 28:1571, 1981.

110. Hoffmeister F, Tettenborn D: Calcium agonists and antagonists of the dihydropyridine type: antinociceptive effects, interference with opiate-mu-receptor agonists and neuropharmacological actions in rodents, *Psychopharmacology* 90:299, 1986.

111. Hökfelt T, Johansson O, Ljungdahl A et al: Peptidergic neurones, *Nature* 284:515, 1980.

112. Hollt V, Sanchez-Blazquez P, and Garzon J: Multiple opioid ligands and receptors in the control of nociception, *Philos Trans Soc Lond (Biol)* 308:299, 1985.

113. Horn AS, Rogers JR: Structural and conformational relationships between the enkephalins and the opiates, *Nature* 260:795, 1976.

114. Houde RW, Wallenstein SL: Clinical studies of morphine-nalorphine combinations, *Fed Proc* 15:440, 1956.

115. Hunt SP, Pini A, Evan G: Induction of c-fos-like protein in spinal cord neurons following sensory stimulation, *Nature* 328:632, 1987.

116. Inoki R, Hayashi T, Kudo T et al: Effects of morphine and acetylsalicylic acid on kinin forming enzyme in rat paw, *Arch Int Pharmacodyn* 228:126, 1977.

117. Inoki R, Toyoda T, and Yamamoto I: Elaboration of a bradykinin-like substance in dog canine pulp and its inhibition by narcotic and non-narcotic analgesics, *Arch Pharmacol* 279:387, 1973.

118. Irwin S et al: The effects of morphine, methadone and meperidine on some reflex responses of spinal animals to nociceptive stimulation, *J Pharmacol Exp Ther* 101:132, 1951.

119. Jaffe JH, Martin WR: Opioid analgesics and antagonists. In Gilman AG, Goodman LS, Rall TW et al, eds: *The pharmacological basis of therapeutics,* ed 7, New York, 1985, MacMillan.

120. Janssen PAJ: The development of new synthetic narcotics. In Estafanous FG, ed: *Opioids in anesthesia,* Boston, 1984, Butterworth.

121. Janssen PAJ: Stereochemical anatomy of morphinomimetics. In Loh HH, Ross DH, eds: *Neurochemical mechanisms of opiates and enkephalins,* New York, 1979, Raven Press.

122. Janssen PAJ, Van der Eycken CAM: The chemical anatomy of potent morphine-like analgesics. In Burger A, ed: *Drugs affecting the central nervous system,* vol 2, New York, 1968, Marcel Dekker.

123. Johnson SM et al: Pertussis toxin reduces the inhibitory action of morphine and ADP-ribosylates G proteins in guinea pig myenteric neurons. In van Ree JM et al, eds: *New leads in opioid research,* Amsterdam, 1990, Excerpta Medica.

124. Joris J, Costello A, Dubner R et al: Opiates suppress carrageenan-induced edema and hyperthermia at doses that inhibit hyperalgesia, *Pain* 43:95, 1990.

125. Joris J, Dubner R, and Hargreaves KM: Opioid analgesia at peripheral sites: a target for opioids released during stress and inflammation? *Anesth Analg* 66:1277, 1987.

126. Kaczmarek LK, Levitan IB, eds: *Neuromodulation,* New York, 1987, Oxford University Press.

127. Kaiser ET, Kézdy FJ: Amphiphilic secondary structure: design of peptide hormones, *Science* 223:249, 1984.

128. Kandel ER, ed: *Molecular neurobiology in neurology and psychiatry,* New York, 1987, Raven Press.

129. Kavaliers M: Stimulatory influences of calcium channel antagonists on stress induced opioid analgesia and locomotor activity, *Brain Res* 408:403, 1987.

130. Kavanaugh MP, Tester BC, Scherz MW et al: Identification of the binding subunit of the sigma-type opiate receptor by photoaffinity labeling with 1-(4-azido-2-methyl [6-³H] phenyl)-3-(2-methyl [4,6-H³] phenyl) guanidine, *Proc Natl Acad Sci USA* 85:2844, 1988.

131. Kayser V, Guildbaud G: The analgesic effects of morphine, but not those of the enkephalinase inhibitor thiorphan, are enhanced in arthritic rats, *Brain Res* 267:131, 1983.

132. Kelly DD, ed: *Stress-induced analgesia,* New York, 1986, New York Academy of Sciences.

133. Klee WA, Nirenberg M: A neuroblastoma-glioma hybrid cell line with morphine receptors, *Proc Natl Acad Sci USA* 71:3474, 1974.

134. Klotz IM: Numbers of receptor sites from Scatchard graphs: facts and fantasies, *Science* 217:1247, 1982.

135. Kobilka BK, Kobilka TS, Daniel K et al: Chimeric alpha₂-, beta₂-adrenergic receptors: delineation of domains involved in effector coupling and ligand binding specificity, *Science* 240:1310, 1988.

136. Koski G, Klee W: Opiates inhibit adenylate cyclase by stimulating cyclic GTP hydrolysis, *Proc Natl Acad Sci USA* 78:4185, 1981.

137. Kosterlitz HW, Wallis DI: The action of morphine-like drugs on impulse transmission in mammalian nerve fibers, *Br J Pharmacol* 22:499, 1964.

138. Krebs EG: Role of the cyclic AMP-dependent protein kinase in signal transduction, *JAMA* 262:1815, 1989.

139. Labella FS, Pinsky C, and Havlicek V: Morphine derivatives with diminished opiate receptor potency show enhanced central excitatory activity, *Brain Res* 174:263, 1979.

140. Laduron P: Axonal transport of opiate receptors in the capsaicin sensitive neurones, *Brain Res* 294:157, 1984.

141. Laurent S, Marsh JD, and Smith TW: Enkephalins increase cyclic adenosine monophosphate content, calcium uptake, and contractile state in cultured chick embryo heart cells, *J Clin Invest* 77:1436, 1986.

142. Lear JD, Wasserman ZR, and DeGrado WF: Synthetic amphiphilic peptide models for protein ion channels, *Science* 240:1177, 1988.

143. LeBars D, Dickenson AH, and Besson JM: Opiate analgesia and descending control systems. In Bonica JJ, ed: *Advances in pain research and therapy,* vol 5, New York, 1983, Raven Press.

144. LeBars D, Guilbaud G, Jurna I et al: Differential effects of morphine on responses of dorsal horn lamina V type cells elicited by A and C fibre stimulation in the spinal cat, *Brain Res* 115:518, 1976.

145. LeBars D, Villaneuva L: Electrophysiological evidence for the activation of descending inhibitory controls by nociceptive afferent pathways. In Fields HL, Besson J-M, eds: *Progress in brain research,* Amsterdam, 1988, Elsevier Science.

146. LeBars D et al: Aspects of sensory processing through convergent neurons. In Yaksh TL, ed: *Spinal afferent processing,* New York, 1986, Plenum.

147. Lembeck F, Donnerer J: Opioid control of the function of primary afferent substance P fibres, *Eur J Pharmacol* 114:241, 1985.

148. Lembeck F, Donnerer J, and Bartho L: Inhibition of neurogenic vasodilation and plasma extravasation by substance P antagonists, somatostatin and (D-Met2, Pro5) enkephalinamide, *Eur J Pharmacol* 85:171, 1982.

149. Leslie FM: Methods used for the study of opioid receptors, *Pharmacol Rev* 39:197, 1987.

150. Lewis ME, Mishkin M, Bragin E et al: Opiate receptor gradients in monkey cerebral cortex: correspondence with sensory processing hierarchies, *Science* 211:1166, 1981.

151. Li CH, Tseng LF, Ferrara P et al: Beta-endorphin: dissociation of receptor binding activity from analgesic potency, *Proc Natl Acad Sci USA* 77:2303, 1980.

152. Lipkowski AW, Konecka AM, and Sadowski B: Double-enkephalins—synthesis, activity on guinea pig ileum and analgesic effect, *Peptides* 3:697, 1982.

153. Lipkowski AW, Tam SW, and Portoghese PS: Peptides as receptor selectivity modulators of opiate pharmacophores, *J Med Chem* 29:1222, 1986.

154. Loeb JN, Strickland S: Hormone binding and coupled response relationships in systems dependent on the generation of secondary mediators, *Mol Endocrinol* 1:75, 1987.

155. Loh HH, Smith AP: Molecular characterization of opioid receptors, *Annu Rev Pharmacol Toxicol* 39:123, 1990.

156. Lopker A, Abood LG, Hoss W et al: Stereoselective muscarinic acetylcholine and opiate receptors in human phagocytic leukocytes, *Biochem Pharmacol* 29:1361, 1980.

157. Lord JAH, Waterfield AA, Hughes J et al: Endogenous opioid peptides: multiple agonists and receptors, *Nature* 267:495, 1977.

158. Lowenstein E: Narcotics in anesthesia: past, present, and future. In Estafanous FG, ed: *Opioids in anesthesia,* Boston, 1984, Butterworths.

159. Lowenstein E, Hallowell P, Levine FH et al: Cardiovascular response to large doses of intravenous morphine in man, *N Engl J Med* 281:1389, 1969.

160. Lumpkin MD: The regulation of ACTH secretion by IL-1, *Science* 238:452, 1986.

161. Lund C, Mogensen T, Hjortso NC et al: Systemic morphine enhances spread of sensory analgesia during postoperative bupivicaine infusion, *Lancet* 1:1156, 1985.

162. Macdonald RL, Werz MA: Dynorphin A decreases voltage-dependent calcium conductance of mouse dorsal root ganglion neurones, *J Physiol* 377:237, 1986.

163. Mansour A, Khachaturian H, Lewis ME et al: Anatomy of CNS opioid receptors, *Trends Neurosci* 11:308, 1988.

164. Martin WR: Multiple opioid receptors: a little about their history and some implications related to evolution, *Life Sci* 28:1547, 1981.

165. Martin WR: Opioid antagonists, *Pharmacol Rev* 19:463, 1967.

166. Martin WR: Pharmacology of opioids, *Pharmacol Rev* 35:283, 1984.

167. Martin WR, Eades CG, Thompson JA et al: The effects of morphine- and nalorphine-like drugs in the nondependent and morphine-dependent chronic spinal dog, *J Pharmacol Exp Ther* 197:517, 1976.

168. Mathews PM, Froelich CJ, Sibbitt WL Jr et al: Enhancement of natural cytotoxicity by beta-endorphin, *J Immunol* 130:1658, 1983.

169. Maurer R: Multiplicity of opiate receptors in different species, *Neurosci Lett* 30:303, 1982.

170. Mays KS, Lipman JJ, Schnapp M: Local analgesia without anesthesia using peripheral perineural morphine injections, *Anesth Analg* 66:417, 1987.

171. McKnight AT, Corbett AD, Marcoli M et al: Hamster vas deferens contains delta-opioid receptors, *Neuropeptides* 5:97, 1984.

172. McQuay HJ, Carroll D, and Moore RA: Postoperative orthopaedic pain—the effect of opiate premedication and local anesthetic blocks, *Pain* 33:291, 1988.

173. Melzack R: The tragedy of needless pain: a call for social action. In Dubner R, Gebhart GF, and Bond MR, eds: *Proceedings of the Fifth World Congress on Pain,* New York, 1988, Elsevier.

174. Menétrey D, Gannon A, Levine JD et al: Expression of c-fos protein in interneurons and projection neurons of the rat spinal cord in response to noxious somatic, articular, and visceral stimulation, *J Comp Neurol* 285:177, 1989.

175. Millan MJ: K-Opioid receptors and analgesia, *Trends Pharmacol Sci* 11:70, 1990.

176. Millan MJ: Multiple opioid systems and pain, *Pain* 27:303, 1986.

177. Millan MJ, Czlonkowski A, Lipkowski A et al: Kappa-opioid receptor-mediated antinociception in the rat. II. Supraspinal in addition to spinal sites of action, *J Pharmacol Exp Ther* 251:342, 1989.

178. Millan MJ, Morris BJ, Colpaert FC et al: A model of chronic pain in the rat: response of multiple opioid systems to adjuvant-induced arthritis, *J Neurosci* 6:899, 1986.

179. Miller GC, Murgo AJ, and Potnikoff NP: Enkephalins—enhancement of active T-cell rosettes from lymphoma patients, *Clin Immunol Immunopathol* 26:446, 1983.

180. Morley JE, Benton D, and Solomon GF: The role of stress and opioids as regulators of the immune response. In McCubbin JA, Kaufman PG, and Nemeroff CB, eds: *Stress, neuropeptides, and systemic disease,* San Diego, 1991, Academic Press.

181. Mosberg HI, Hurst R, Hruby VJ et al: Conformationally constrained cyclic enkephalin analogs with pronounced delta opioid receptor agonist selectivity, *Life Sci* 32:2565, 1983.

182. Mousli M, Bueb JL, Bronner C et al: G protein activation: a receptor-independent mode of action for catonic amphiphilic neuropeptides and venom peptides, *Trends Pharmacol Sci* 11:358, 1990.

183. Nishizuka Y: The role of protein kinase C in cell surface signal transduction and tumour promotion, *Nature* 398:693, 1984.

184. Noguchi K, Morita Y, Kiyama H et al: Preproenkephalin gene expression in the rat spinal cord after noxious stimuli, *Mol Brain Res* 5:227, 1989.

185. North RA: Opioid receptor types and membrane ion channels, *Trends Neurosci* 9:114, 1986.

186. North RA, Williams JT: Opiate activation of potassium conductance inhibits calcium action potentials in rat locus coeruleus neurones, *Br J Pharmacol* 80:225, 1983.

187. North RA, Williams JT, Surprenant A et al: Mu and delta receptors belong to a family of receptors that are coupled to potassium channels, *Proc Natl Acad Sci USA* 84:5487, 1987.

188. Onofrio BM, Yaksh TL: Intrathecal delta-receptor ligand produces analgesia in man, *Lancet* 1:1386, 1983.

189. Overton DA, Bhatta SK: Investigation of narcotics and antitussives using drug discrimination techniques, *J Pharmacol Exp Ther* 211:401, 1979.

190. Pasternak GW: Multiple morphine and enkephalin receptors and the relief of pain, *JAMA* 259:1362, 1988.

191. Paton WDM: The action of morphine and related substances on contraction and on acetylcholine output of coaxially stimulated guinea pig ileum, *Br J Pharmacol Chemother* 12:119, 1957.

192. Payan DG, McGillis JP, Renold FK et al: Neuropeptide modulation of leukocyte function, *Ann NY Acad Sci* 496: 182, 1987.

193. Pert CV, Snyder SH: Opiate receptor: demonstration in nervous tissue, *Science* 179:1011, 1973.

194. Pollak JM, ed: *Regulatory peptides,* Cambridge, Mass, 1989, Birkhauser.

195. Portoghese PS: A new concept on the mode of interaction of narcotic analgesics with receptors, *J Med Chem* 8:609, 1965.

196. Protoghese PS: Relationships between stereostructure and pharmacological activities, *Annu Rev Pharmacol* 10:51, 1970.

197. Presley RW, Menétrey D, Levine JD et al: Systemic morphine suppresses noxious stimulus–evoked Fos protein–like immunoreactivity in the rat spinal cord, *J Neurosci* 10:323, 1990.

198. Prosdocimi M, Finesso M, and Gorio A: Enkephalin modulation of neural transmission in the cat stellate ganglion: pharmacological actions of exogenous opiates, *J Auton Nerv Syst* 17:217, 1986.

199. Przewlocki R, Costa T, Lang J et al: Pertussis toxin abolishes the antinociception mediated by opioid receptors in rat spinal cord, *Eur J Pharmacol* 144:91, 1987.

200. Przewlocki R, Haarman I, Nikolarakis K et al: Prodynorphin gene expression in spinal cord is enhanced after traumatic injury in the rat, *Brain Res* 464:37, 1988.

201. Przwelocki R, Stala L, Greczek M et al: Analgesic effects of mu-, delta- and kappa-opiate agonists and, in particular, dynorphin at the spinal level, *Life Sci* 33(suppl 1):649, 1983.

202. Ramkumar V, El-Fakahany EE: Prolonged morphine treatment increases rat brain dihydropyridine binding sites, *Eur J Pharmacol* 146:73, 1988.

203. Randich A, Maixner W: Interactions between cardiovascular and pain regulatory mechanisms, *Neurosci Biobehav Rev* 8:343, 1984.

203a. Randich A, Thurston CL, Ludwig P S et al: Antinociception and cardiovascular responses produced by intravenons morphine: the role of vagal, afferents, *Brain Res* 543:256, 1991.

204. Rios L, Jacobs J: Local inhibition of inflammatory pain by naloxone and its N-methyl quaternary analog, *Eur J Pharmacol* 96:277, 1983.

205. Ronken E, Tonnaer JADM, and Wiegant VM: Molecular identification of 60 kDa binding site for non-opioid gamma-type endorphins in rat brain membranes. In van Ree JM et al, eds: *New leads in opioid research,* Amsterdam, 1990, Excerpta Medica.

206. Roques BP: What are the relevant features of the distribution, selective binding, and metabolism of opioid peptides and how can these be applied to drug design? In Basbaum AI, Bessom J-M, eds: *Towards a new pharmacology of pain,* New York, 1991, John Wiley & Sons.

207. Rosenblatt M: Peptide hormone antagonists that are effective in vivo: lessons from parathyroid hormone, *N Engl J Med* 315:1004, 1986.

208. Rosow CE: Cardiovascular effects of narcotics. In Covino BG, Fozzard HA, Rehder K et al, eds: *Effects of anesthesia,* Bethesda, Md, 1985, American Physiological Society.

209. Rosow CE, Moss J, Philbin DM et al: Histamine release during morphine and fentanyl anesthesia, *Anesthesiology* 56: 93, 1982.

210. Ross DH, Cardenas HL: Nerve cell calcium as a messenger for opiate and endorphin actions. In Loh HH, Ross DH, eds: *Neurochemical mechanisms of opiates and endorphins,* New York, 1979, Raven Press.

211. Ross DH, Cardenas HL: Opiates inhibit calmodulin activation of a high-affinity Ca^{2+}-stimulated Mg^{2+}-dependent ATPase in synaptic membranes, *Neurochem Res* 12:41, 1987.

212. Rossier J: Opioid peptides have found their roots, *Nature* 298:221, 1982.

213. Ruda MA, Iadarola MJ, Cohen LV et al: *In situ* hybridization histochemistry and immunocytochemistry reveal an increase in spinal dynorphin biosynthesis in a rat model of peripheral inflammation and hyperalgesia, *Proc Natl Acad Sci USA* 85:622, 1988.

214. Ruff MR, Wahl SM, Mergenhagen S et al: Opiate receptor-mediated chemotaxis of human monocytes, *Neuropeptides* 5:363, 1985.

215. Russell N, Schaible H-G, and Schmidt R: Opiates inhibit the discharges of fine afferent units from inflamed knee joint of the cat, *Neurosci Lett* 76:196, 1987.

216. Russell N et al: Peripheral opioid effects upon neurogenic plasma extravasation and inflammation, *Br J Pharmacol* 86: 788P, 1985.

217. Ruth JA, Eiden LE: Leucine-enkephalin modulation of catecholamine positive chronotropy in rat atria is receptor-specific and calcium-dependent, *Neuropeptides* 4:101, 1984.

218. Sagar SM, Sharp FR: Light induces a Fos-like nuclear antigen in retinal neurons, *Mol Brain Res* 7:17, 1990.

219. Sagar SM, Sharp FR, Curran T: Expression of *c-fos* protein in brain: metabolic mapping at the cellular level, *Science* 240:1328, 1988.

220. Saini V, Carr DB, Hagestad EL et al: Antifibrillatory mechanism of the narcotic agonist fentanyl, *Am Heart J* 115: 598, 1988.

221. Sawynok J, Pinsky C, and LaBella FS: On the specificity of naloxone as an opiate antagonist, *Life Sci* 25:1621, 1979.

222. Schaefer GJ, Holtzman SG: Discriminative effects of morphine in the squirrel monkey, *J Pharmacol Exp Ther* 201:67, 1977.

223. Schild HO: pA₂ and competitive drug antagonism, *Br J Pharmacol* 4:277, 1949.

224. Schmauss C, Yaksh TL: *In vivo* studies on spinal opiate receptor systems mediating antinociception. II. Pharmacological profiles suggesting a differential association of mu, delta, and kappa receptors with visceral chemical and cutaneous stimuli in the rat, *J Pharmacol Exp Ther* 228:1, 1984.

225. Schofield PR, McFarland KC, Hayflick JS et al: Molecular characterization of a new immunoglobulin superfamily protein with potential roles in opioid binding and cell contact, *EMBO J* 8:489, 1989.

226. Schroeder JE, Fischbach PS, Zheng D et al: Activation of mu opioid receptors inhibits transient high and low threshold Ca^{++} currents, but spares a sustained current, *Neuron* 6:13, 1990.

227. Schulz R, Wuster M, and Herz A: Pharmacological characterization of the epsilon-opiate receptor, *J Pharmacol Exp Ther* 216:604, 1981.

228. Schwartz J-C et al: Physiological roles of "enkephalinase" (enkephalin dipeptidyl carboxypeptidase) and a bestatin sensitive aminopeptidase in the inactivation of enkephalins. In Ehrenpreis S, Sicuteri F, eds: *Degradation of endogenous opioids: its relevance in human pathology and disease,* New York, 1983, Raven.

229. Schwyzer R: ACTH: a short introductory review, *Ann NY Acad Sci* 297:3, 1977.

230. Senami M, Aoki M, Kitahata LM et al: Lack of opiate effects on cat C polymodal nociceptive fibers, *Pain* 17:81, 1986.

231. Seybold VS, Elde RP: Receptor autoradiography in the thoracic spinal cord: correlation of neurotransmitter binding sites with sympathoadrenal neurons, *J Neurosci* 4:2533, 1984.

232. Sharp BM, Keane WF, Suh HJ et al: Opioid peptides rapidly stimulate superoxide production by human polymorphonuclear leukocytes and macrophages, *Endocrinology* 117:793, 1985.

233. Shavit Y, Lewis JW, Terman GW et al: Opioid peptides mediate the suppressive effect of stress on natural killer cytotoxicity, *Science* 223:188, 1984.

234. Shimohigashi Y, Costa T, Chen HC et al: Dimeric tetrapeptide enkephalins display extraordinary selectivity for the delta opiate receptor, *Nature* 297:333, 1982.

235. Sibinga NES, Goldstein A: Opioid peptides and opioid receptors in cells of the immune system, *Annu Rev Immunol* 6:219, 1988.

236. Siggins GR, Gruol DL: Mechanisms of transmitter action in the vertebrate nervous system. In Mountcastle VB, Bloom FE, and Geiger SR, eds: *Handbook of physiology,* section 1, vol 4, Bethesda, Md, 1986, American Physiological Society.

237. Simon EJ, Hiller JM, and Edelman I: Stereospecific binding of the potent narcotic analgesic [3H] etorphine to rat-brain homogenate, *Proc Natl Acad Sci USA* 70:1947, 1973.

238. Simpkins CO, Dickey CA, and Fink MP: Human neutrophil migration is en-

hanced by beta-endorphin, *Life Sci* 34: 2251, 1984.

239. Smith EM, Blalock JE: Human lymphocyte production of corticotropin and endorphin-like substances: association with leukocyte interferon, *Proc Natl Acad Sci USA* 78:7530, 1981.

240. Smith G, Covino BG: *Acute pain,* Boston, 1985, Butterworths.

241. Smith T, Buchan P: Peripheral opioid receptors located on the rat saphenous nerve, *Neuropeptides* 5:217, 1984.

242. Sonnenberg JL, Rauscher FJ III, Morgan JI et al: Regulation of proenkephalin by *fos* and *jun, Science* 246:1622, 1989.

243. Stanley TH, Gray NH, Stanford W et al: Effects of high-dose morphine on fluid and blood requirements in open-heart operation, *Anesthesiology* 38:536, 1973.

244. Stein C, Millan MJ, Yassouridis A et al: Antinociceptive effects of mu and kappa agonists in inflammation are enhanced by a peripheral opioid receptor-specific mechanism, *Eur J Pharmacol* 155:255, 1988.

245. Stein C, Millan MJ, Shippenberg TS et al: Peripheral effects of fentanyl upon nociception in inflamed tissue of the rat, *Neurosci Lett* 84:225, 1988.

246. Stein C, Millan MJ, Shippenberg TS et al: Peripheral opioid receptors mediating antinociception in inflammation: evidence for involvement of mu, delta and kappa receptors, *J Pharmacol Exp Ther* 248:1269, 1988.

247. Stevens CW, Yaksh TL: Magnitude of opioid dependence after continuous intrathecal infusion of μ- and δ-selective opioids in the rat, *Eur J Pharmacol* 166:467, 1989.

248. Swanson LW, Sawchenko PE: Hypothalamic integration: organization of the paraventricular and supraoptic nuclei, *Annu Rev Neurosci* 6:269, 1983.

249. Szyfelbein SK, Osgood PF, and Carr DB: The assessment of pain and plasma beta-endorphin immunoactivity in burned children, *Pain* 22:173, 1985.

250. Takagi H et al: The effect of analgesics on the spinal reflex activity of the cat, *Jpn J Pharmacol* 4:176, 1955.

251. Taylor JW, Kaiser ET: The structural characterization of beta-endorphin and related peptide hormones and neurotransmitters, *Pharmacol Rev* 38:291, 1986.

252. Terenius L: Characteristics of the "receptor" for narcotic analgesics in synaptic plasma membrane fraction from rat brain, *Acta Pharmacol Toxicol* 33:377, 1973.

253. Teschemacher H, Schweigerer L: Opioid peptides: do they have immunological significance? *Trends Pharmacol Sci* 6:368, 1985.

254. Thorpe DH: Opiate structure and activity—a guide to understanding the opiate receptor, *Anesth Analg* 63:143, 1984.

255. Tölle TR, Castro-Lopes JM, Coimbra A et al: Opiates modify induction of c-fos proto-oncogene in the spinal cord of the rat following noxious stimulation, *Neurosci Lett* 111:46, 1990.

256. Tricklebank MD, Curzon G, eds: *Stress-induced analgesia,* New York, 1984, Wiley.

257. Tricoire M: *La morphine intrarachidienne dans le traitement de la douleur chez les cancereux,* doctoral thesis, Toulouse, France, 1978, Universite Paul Sabatier.

258. Tyers MB: A classification of opiate receptors that mediate antinociception in animals, *Br J Pharmacol* 69:503, 1980.

259. Uhl GR, Ryan JP, and Schwartz JP: Morphine alters preproenkephalin gene expression, *Brain Res* 459:391, 1988.

260. Upton N, Sewell RDE, and Spencer PSJ: Differentiation of potent mu- and kappa-opiate agonists using heat and pressure antinociceptive profiles and combined potency analysis, *Eur J Pharmacol* 78:421, 1982.

261. Usdin E, Kvetnansky R, and Axelrod J, eds: *Stress: the role of catecholamines and other neurotransmitters,* New York, 1984, Gordon and Breach.

262. Van der Kooy D: Hyperalgesic functions of peripheral opiate receptors. In Kelly DD, ed: *Stress-induced analgesia,* New York, 1986, New York Academy of Sciences.

263. Wall PD: The prevention of postoperative pain, *Pain* 33:289, 1988.

264. Wall PD, Melzack R, eds: *Textbook of pain,* ed 2, New York, 1988, Churchill-Livingstone.

265. Watson JD et al: *Molecular biology of the gene,* ed 4, Reading, Mass, 1987, Benjamin/Cummings.

266. Way EL: Review and overview of four decades of opiate research. In Loh HH, Ross DH, eds: *Neurochemical mechanisms of opiates and enkephalins,* New York, 1979, Raven Press.

267. Weinstock M, Schorer-Apelbaum D, and Rosin AJ: Endogenous opiates mediate cardiac sympathetic inhibition in response to a pressor stimulus in rabbits, *J Hypertens* 2:639, 1984.

268. Weitz CJ, Lowney LI, Faull KF et al: Morphine and codeine from mammalian brain, *Proc Natl Acad Sci USA* 83:9784, 1986.

269. Werz MA, MacDonald RL: Opioid peptides with differential affinity for mu and delta receptors decrease sensory neuron calcium-dependent action potentials, *J Pharmacol Exp Ther* 227:394, 1983.

270. West RE, Miller RJ: Opiates, second messengers and cell response, *Br Med Bull* 39:53, 1983.

271. Willer JC, De Broucker R, and Le Bars D: Encoding of nociceptive thermal stimuli by diffuse noxious inhibitory controls in humans, *J Neurophysiol* 62:1028, 1989.

272. Willer JC, Le Bars D, and De Broucker T: Diffuse noxious inhibitory controls in man: involvement of an opioidergic link, *Eur J Pharmacol* 182:347, 1990.

273. Willis WD Jr: Control of nociceptive transmission in the spinal cord. In Autrum H, Ottoson D, Perl ER et al, eds: *Progress in sensory physiology,* vol 3, New York, 1982, Springer-Verlag.

274. Willis WD Jr: *The pain system: the neural basis of nociceptive transmission in the mammalian nervous system,* New York, 1985, Karger.

275. Wood MM, Cousins MJ: Iatrogenic neurotoxicity in cancer patients, *Pain* 39:1, 1989.

276. Wood PL, Rackham A, and Richard J: Spinal analgesia: comparison of the mu agonist morphine and the kappa agonist ethylketazocine, *Life Sci* 28:2119, 1981.

277. Woolf CJ, Wall PD: Morphine-sensitive and morphine-insensitive actions of C-fibre input on the rat spinal cord, *Neurosci Lett* 64:221, 1986.

278. Yaksh T: Opioid receptor systems and the endorphins: a review of their spinal organization, *J Neurosurg* 67:157, 1987.

279. Yaksh TL: Neurologic mechanisms of pain. In Cousins MJ, Bridenbaugh PO, eds: *Neural blockade in clinical anesthesia and management of pain,* ed 2, Philadelphia, 1988, JB Lippincott.

280. Yaksh TL: Substance P release from knee joint afferent terminals: modulation by opioids, *Brain Res* 458:319, 1988.

281. Yaksh TL, Durant PA, Gaumann DM et al: The use of receptor-selective agents as analgesics in the spinal cord: trends and possibilities, *J Pain Symptom Management* 2:129, 1987.

282. Yaksh TL, Rudy TA: Narcotic analgesics: CNS sites and mechanisms of action as revealed by intracerebral injection techniques, *Pain* 4:299, 1978.

283. Yamamoto Y, Hotta K, and Matsuda T: Effect of met-enkephalin on the spontaneous activity of the smooth muscle of the rat portal vein, *Life Sci* 34:993, 1984.

284. Yonehara N, Iami Y, and Inoki R: Effects of opioids on the heat stimulus–evoked substance P release and thermal edema in the rat hind paw, *Eur J Pharmacol* 151:381, 1988.

285. Young WS et al: Opioid receptors undergo axonal flow, *Science* 210:76, 1980.

286. Yuge O, Matsumoto M, Kitahata LM et al: Direct opioid application to peripheral nerves does not alter compound action potentials, *Anesth Analg* 64:667, 1985.

287. Zakarian S, Smyth DG: Beta-endorphin is processed differently in specific regions of rat pituitary and brain, *Nature* 296:250, 1982.

288. Zieglgänsberger W: Central control of nociception. In Mountcastle VB, Bloom FE, and Geiger SR, eds: *Handbook of physiology,* Baltimore, 1986, Williams & Wilkins.

289. Zieglgänsberger W: Opioid actions on mammalian spinal neurons, *Int Rev Neurobiol* 25:243, 1984.

290. Zukin RS, Eghbali M, Olive D et al: Characterization and visualization of rat and guinea pig brain kappa opioid receptors: evidence for kappa₁ and kappa₂ opioid receptors, *Proc Natl Acad Sci USA* 85:4061, 1988.

291. Zukin RS et al: Group report: what is the molecular basis of opioid antinociception and how does this information point to new drug design? In Basbaum AI, Besson J-M, eds: *Towards a new pharmacology of pain,* New York, 1991, John Wiley & Sons.

CHAPTER 53

Pharmacology of Intravenous Anesthetic Agents

JAN VAN HEMELRIJCK
JERRY M. GONZALES
PAUL F. WHITE

Many different drugs are currently available for intravenous induction of anesthesia; however, the "ideal" intravenous anesthetic has not yet been developed. The physical and pharmacologic properties an ideal intravenous anesthetic agent should possess are listed in Box 53-1.

BOX 53-1
THE "IDEAL" INTRAVENOUS ANESTHETIC AGENT

Stable in aqueous solution
No pain on injection, venoirritation, or tissue damage from accidental perivenous administration
Very low potential to release histamine or precipitate hypersensitivity reactions
Rapidly metabolized to pharmacologically inactive substances, with minimal accumulation when administered by repeated bolus doses or continuous infusion
Rapid and smooth onset of action, without excitatory phenomena such as muscle movements, hypertonus, or hiccoughing
Produces a steep dose-response relationship so that changes in the rate of administration result in rapid changes in the depth of anesthesia when administered by continuous infusion
Rapid and smooth return of consciousness, even after prolonged administration for maintenance of anesthesia or sedation
Produces a decrease in cerebral metabolism proportional to the decrease in cerebral blood flow and does not raise intracranial pressure
Minimal cardiovascular and respiratory depressant effects with no adverse effects on other organ systems
Allows rapid recovery without postoperative side effects, such as nausea and vomiting, psychomimetic symptoms, dizziness, headache, or prolonged sedation ("hangover")

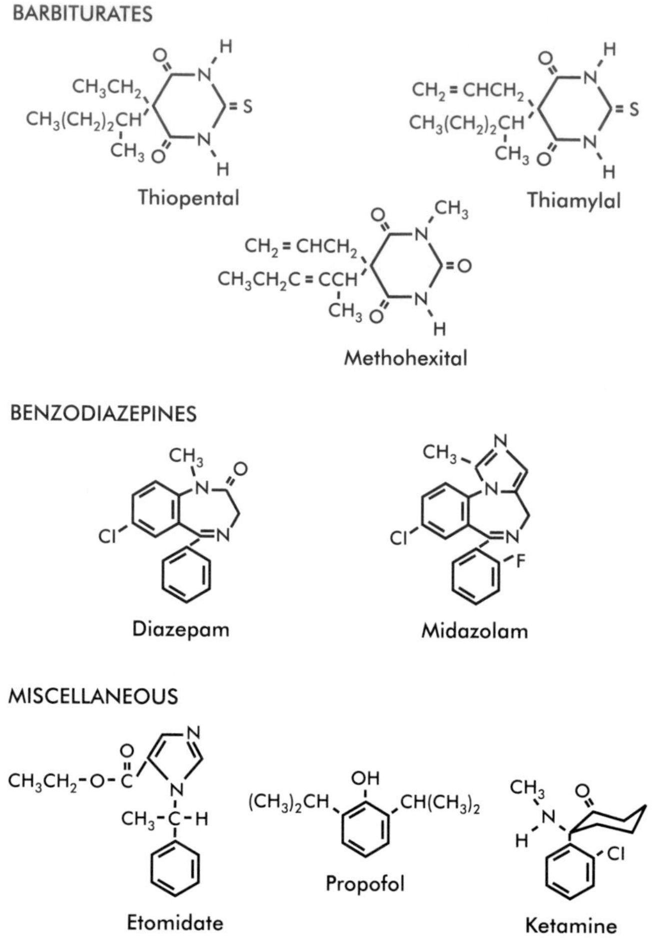

BARBITURATES

Thiopental

Thiamylal

Methohexital

BENZODIAZEPINES

Diazepam

Midazolam

MISCELLANEOUS

Etomidate

Propofol

Ketamine

Fig. 53-1. Chemical structures of the currently available intravenous anesthetics. (From Fragen RJ, Avran MJ: Comparative pharmacology of drugs used for the induction of anesthesia. In Miller RK, Kirby RR, Ostheimer GW et al, eds: *Year book of anesthesia.* Chicago, 1986, Year Book Medical Publishers.)

Since its introduction into clinical practice in 1934, thiopental has become the "gold standard" of intravenous anesthetic agents to which all newer agents must be compared (Fig. 53-1). Despite its proved usefulness, safety, and widespread acceptance, thiopental is far from being the ideal intravenous anesthetic. Many newer drugs have been introduced into clinical practice over the last few decades. Some have proved to be extremely valuable in specific clinical situations. These newer compounds combine some of the characteristics of the ideal intravenous anesthetic but fail in aspects where other drugs succeed. None of these agents combine *all* of the desired properties of an ideal anesthetic. For some of these drugs, major disadvantages have lead to restricted indications (e.g., ketamine, etomidate) or to their withdrawal from clinical use (e.g., Althesin, propanidid). The aim of this chapter is to compare the pharmacologic charac-

teristics of the intravenous anesthetics that are currently available for clinical use. Since the desired pharmacologic properties are not equally important in every clinical situation, this comparative evaluation was structured to enable the anesthesiologist to make the choice that best fits the needs of the individual patient. In addition to the discussion about currently available drugs, interesting aspects of "historical drugs" will also be mentioned.

CHEMISTRY
Barbiturates

The commonly used barbiturates are thiopental, methohexital, and, to a lesser extent, thiamylal (Table 53-1). Thiopental and thiamylal are thiobarbiturates, while methohexital is an oxybarbiturate. All three are water-soluble molecules available as sodium salts and must be dissolved in isotonic sodium chloride (0.9%) or water. Typically, solutions of 2.5% thiopental, 1% to 2% methohexital, and 2% thiamylal are used. Their chemical stability in aqueous solution is limited. Solutions of thiobarbiturates are stable for a maximum of 2 weeks if refrigerated. Solutions of methohexital in water are stable for up to 6 weeks. When barbiturates are added to Ringer's lactate or to an acidic solution containing other water-soluble drugs, precipitation will occur and may even occlude the intravenous catheter. **The typical solution of thiopental (2.5%) is highly alkaline (pH >10) and can be irritating to the tissues if injected extravenously. Solutions of 2.5% thiopental do not cause pain on injection and venoirritation is rare. However, even a 1% methohexital solution causes some discomfort when injected into small veins.** Nevertheless, unlike thiopental, it can be safely administered to induce anesthesia by intramuscular injection.[201] Intraarterial injection of barbiturates can be a serious complication as crystals can form in the arterioles and capillaries, causing intense vasoconstriction, thrombosis, and tissue necrosis.[46]

Benzodiazepines

The three benzodiazepines of interest to anesthesiologists are diazepam, lorazepam, and midazolam. Diazepam and lorazepam are insoluble in water, and their formulation contains propylene glycol, a tissue irritant that causes pain on injection and venous irritation.[99] As expected, absorption after intramuscular administration is highly unpredictable. Diazepam is also available in an emulsion formulation (Diazemuls), which rarely causes pain or thrombophlebitis but is associated with a slightly lower bioavailability.[57,145] Diazepam cannot be mixed with solutions of other drugs. **Midazolam is a newer benzodiazepine, which is available in a water-soluble**

Table 53-1   Physiochemical properties of IV anesthetic agents

Drug group	Drug name (generic)	Available solutions (pH and/or pKa)	Venous irritation
Barbiturates			
Thiobarbiturates	Thiopental	(pKa 7.5)	+ + +
	Thiamylal	Sodium salts, to be diluted in water or saline (pH > 10); precipitation in Ringer's lactate or acid solutions	Less with more diluted solutions
Oxybarbiturates	Methohexital	(pKa 7.9)	
Benzodiazepines	Diazepam	0.5% in 40% propylene glycol and 10% alcohol; 0.5% emulsion formulation	+ + + + / −
	Lorazepam	0.4% in propylene glycol	+
	Midazolam	0.5% buffered aqueous solution (pH 3.5); compatible with saline, D_5W, Ringer's lactate, formulations of acidic salts	−
Imidazoles	Etomidate	Water soluble at acidic pH, lipophilic at physiologic pH (pKa 4.24); 0.2% solution in 30% propylene glycol (ph 5); 10% solution in ethanol (not available in the United States)	+ + +
Substituted phenols Alkylphcnols	Propofol	1% solution in an aqueous emulsion containing 10% soya bean oil, 2.25% glycerol, and 1.2% egg phosphatide (pKa 11)	+ +
Eugenols	Propanidid*	Cremophor EL, water insoluble	
Arylcyclohexylamines	Ketamine	1 or 5% aqueous solution (pH 3.3-5.5; pKa 7.5)	−
Steroids	Alphaxalone/ alphadolone*	Cremophor EL, water insoluble, 0.9% alphaxalone, 0.3% alphadolone	

*Not available for patient use in most countries.

formulation (Versed). **Midazolam's parenteral solution (pH 3.5) causes minimal local irritation after intravenous or intramuscular injection. At physiologic pH, an intramolecular rearrangement occurs that changes the physicochemical properties of midazolam such that it becomes more lipid soluble**[185] (Fig. 53-2). Midazolam can be mixed with saline, Ringer's lactate solution, and solutions of acidic salts of other drugs.

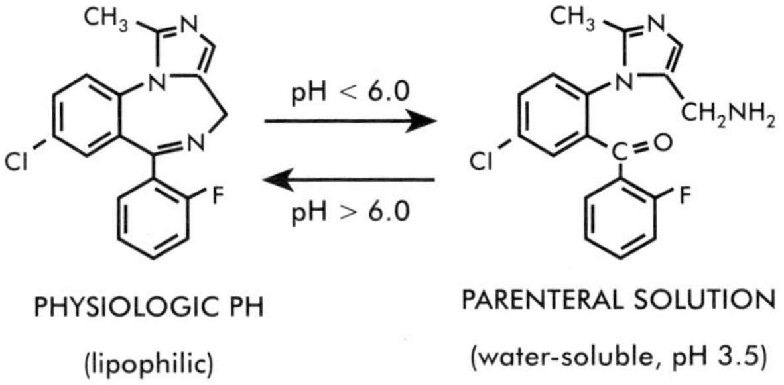

Etomidate

Etomidate is a novel carboxylated imidazole-containing anesthetic compound that is structurally unrelated to any other anesthetic. Only the D-isomer of etomidate possesses anesthetic activity. Like midazolam (which also contains an imidazole nucleus), etomidate is water soluble at an acidic pH and lipophilic at a physiologic pH. The aqueous solution of etomidate is unstable. **The most commonly available formulation of etomidate (Amidate) is the 0.2%**

Fig. 53-2. Effect of pH on the chemical structure of midazolam. (From White PF: Pharamacologic and clinical aspects of preoperative medication, *Anesth Analg* 65:963, 1986.)

solution in 35% propylene glycol. Propylene glycol, a solubilizing agent, is responsible for the high incidence of pain on injection[227] and occasional veno-irritation. This formulation should not be diluted or mixed with other drugs. A 12.5% formulation in ethanol is available in some countries for administration by continuous intravenous infusions (in saline or dextrose in water).

Propofol

Propofol, a 2,6-diisopropylphenol compound, is virtually insoluble in aqueous solution. Following initial introduction of propofol in a chromophore EL formulation, the drug was withdrawn from clinical testing because of the high incidence of anaphylactic reactions to the chromophore solvent. Subsequently, 1% propofol has been reintroduced in an egg lecithin emulsion formulation, which consists of 10% soya bean oil, 2.25% glycerol, and 1.2% egg phosphatide. Pain on injection into small veins occurs in a high proportion of patients,[15,16] but injection into large veins or prior administration of lidocaine or an opioid analgetic ameliorates the pain. It is not recommended that the emulsion be mixed with other drugs or intravenous fluids; however it can be safely administered into isotonic dextrose or saline. Propanidid is a eugenol derivative with a substituted phenol structure that is structurally related to propofol. It was also available in a chromophore EL formulation, but it has been withdrawn from clinical use for the same reason that the original propofol formulation was.

Ketamine

Ketamine (pKa 7.5) is an arylcyclohexylamine that is structurally related to phencyclidine (PCP). The drug is highly water-soluble and is available in a 1%, 5%, and 10% aqueous solutions that are moderately acidic (pH 3.5 to 5.5). As with other water-soluble drugs, it cannot be mixed with diazepam or barbiturates. Ketamine does not cause pain on injection or tissue irritation. The molecule contains a chiral center producing two optical isomers. The S(+) isomer would appear to offer some clinical advantages over the racemic mixture [or the R(−) isomer] because it is a more effective anesthetic and analgetic drug with a more rapid recovery and lower incidence of emergence delirium.[220]

Althesin

Althesin was the only intravenous steroid anesthetic to be made available for clinical use. Althesin was a mixture of two water-insoluble steroids (alphaxalone and alphadolone), with alphaxalone being the most pharmacologically active of the two steroid compounds. Alphadolone is half as potent as alphaxalone and was included to enhance the solubility of the

formulation. Althesin was available in the chromophore EL formulation; however, it too was withdrawn from clinical use because of the occurrence of severe anaphylactic reactions.

PHARMACODYNAMICS
Central Nervous System (CNS) Effects

Several theories have been proposed to explain the mechanism of action of sedative hypnotics on the central nervous system. The concept of a common "nonspecific" mechanism of action of all general anesthetics has largely been abandoned. **Intravenous anesthetics act to enhance inhibitory or inhibit excitatory neurotransmission (see Fig. 53-3). Several intravenous hypnotics exert their effect by enhancing the function of the inhibitory gamma-aminobutyric acid (GABA) neurotransmitter system.*** When the $GABA_A$-receptor is activated, transmembrane chloride conductance increases, resulting in hyperpolarization of the postsynaptic cell membrane and functional inhibition of the postsynapic neuron. Sedative-hypnotic drugs can interact with different components of the $GABA_A$-receptor complex. Benzodiazepines bind to specific receptor sites that are part of a larger complex that includes a GABA binding site. The configuration of the receptor complex increases the efficiency of the coupling between the GABA-occupied receptor and the chloride ion-channel.[36,126] The interaction of barbiturates with another component of the $GABA_A$-receptor complex appears to decrease the rate of dissociation of GABA from its receptor.[84,94] Etomidate and propofol may also enhance GABA neurotransmission.[34,35,223] The interaction of different hypnotics with the GABA-receptor may involve different receptor populations. **Ketamine causes a functional dissociation between the thalamocortical and limbic systems. Ketamine interacts with brain acetylcholine and spinal opiate receptors and blocks the open channel of the NMDA receptor.**[116,127,202]

Effects on cerebral metabolism, blood flow, and intracranial pressure

The influence of sedative-hypnotics on cerebral metabolism, cerebral hemodynamics, and intracranial pressure is of particular importance for neuroanesthesia (Table 53-2). In patients with reduced cerebral compliance a small increase in cerebral blood volume can cause a life-threatening increase in intracranial pressure. **Most sedative-hypnotic drugs cause a proportional reduction in cerebral metabolism and cerebral blood flow, resulting in a decrease in**

---

* References 36, 84, 94, 126, 146, 147, 223.

EXTRACELLULAR

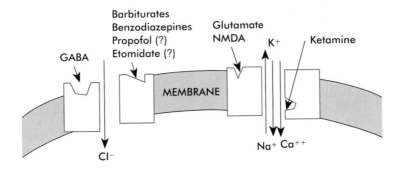

INTRACELLULAR

Fig. 53-3. This model depicts the postsynaptic site of action of GABA and glutamate within the central nervous system. GABA decreases the excitability of neurons by its action at the GABA$_A$ receptor complex. When GABA occupies the binding site of this complex, it allows inward flux of chloride ion resulting in hyperpolarizing of the cell and therefore the subsequent resistance of the neuron to stimulation by excitatory transmitters. Barbiturates, benzodiazepines, and probably propofol and etomidate decrease neuronal excitability by enhancing the effect of GABA at this complex, facilitating this inhibitory effect in the postsynaptic cell. Glutamate (or its analog NMDA) is excitatory. When glutamate occupies the binding site on the NMDA subtype of glutamate receptor, the channel opens and allows Na$^+$, K$^+$, and Ca^{++} to either enter or leave the cell, as shown in the figure. Flux of these ions leads to depolarization of the postsynaptic neuron and initiation of an action potential and activation of other pathways. Ketamine blocks this open channel and prevents further ion flux, thus inhibiting the excitatory response to glutamate. This model does not attempt to represent any structural information pertaining to subunits or binding sites.

intracranial pressure. It has been suggested that barbiturates also possess "neuroprotective" properties secondary to a decrease in oxygen demand (as a result of a decrease in cellular metabolism).[133] Alternative explanations that have been suggested for the cerebroprotective effects of barbiturates and benzodiazines include a reverse steal ("Robin Hood effect") of cerebral blood flow, free-radical scavenging, and excitatory amino-acid receptor blockade.

Barbiturates produce a proportional decrease in cerebral metabolism and blood flow, thereby lowering intracranial pressure.[98] Cerebral perfusion improves if thiopental reduces intracranial pressure to a greater degree than systemic arterial pressure.[154,179] Because of these properties, thiopental is used to improve brain relaxation during neurosurgery and to improve cerebral perfusion pressure after brain injury. Although barbiturate therapy can be used to control intracranial pressure after brain injury, the results of outcome studies are no better than with other aggressive forms of cerebral antihypertensive therapy.[51,169,206] Based on evidence from experimental studies[76,189,193] and a large randomized prospective multi-institutional study,[2] it has been suggested that barbiturates have no place in the therapy following resuscitation of a cardiac arrest patient. In contrast,

Table 53-2   Central nervous system effects of IV anesthetic agents*

Drug name	CMRO$_2$	CBF	CPP	ICP
Thiopental	− −	− −	−/0/+	− −
Methohexital	− −	− −	−/0/+	− −
Etomidate	− −	− −	0/+	− −
Propofol	− −	− −	−/− −	−
Benzodiazepines	−	−/0	0	−
Ketamine	+	+ +	−/0/+	+

*− − = marked decrease, − = mild decrease, 0 = no change, + = mild increase, + + = marked increase

barbiturates are frequently used for cerebroprotection during incomplete ischemia (e.g., carotid endarterectomy, temporary occlusion of cerebral arteries, profound hypotension, cardiopulmonary bypass). Several animal studies indicate that barbiturates improve the brain's tolerance of incomplete ischemia.[131,132,184] These results are supported by one study involving patients undergoing normothermic cardiopulmonary bypass. This study showed that patients treated with high-dose barbiturates had a lower incidence of neuropsychiatric disorders after bypass surgery than the control patients.[143]

Like the barbiturates, etomidate lowers cerebral metabolism, cerebral blood flow, and intracranial pressure.[137,162] The hemodynamic stability associated with etomidate may help to maintain adequate cerebral perfusion pressure. Etomidate can be successfully used for both induction and maintenance of anesthesia for neurosurgery.[174] However, etomidate's inhibition of adrenocortical synthetic function may limit its clinical usefulness for long-term treatment of elevated intracranial pressure. In animals, smaller doses of etomidate have been reported to exert a cerebroprotective effect in the case of incomplete ischemia.[10] However, higher doses of etomidate caused a spiking EEG pattern with an increase in cerebral metabolism.[67]

Propofol decreases cerebral metabolism and blood flow, as well as intracranial pressure.[158,190,196,199] However, when larger doses are administered, the marked lowering of systemic arterial pressure can significantly decrease cerebral perfusion pressure.[198] Cerebrovascular autoregulation in response to changes in systemic arterial pressure is not affected by the drug.[61,199] Preliminary evidence for a possible neuroprotective effect has recently been reported.[209]

Benzodiazepines also decrease both cerebral metabolism and blood flow. It has been suggested that high doses of benzodiazepines might reduce cerebral metabolism to levels approaching those seen with the barbiturates.[142] However, a study in dogs demonstrated a "ceiling" effect with respect to the decrease in cerebral metabolism produced by increasing doses of midazolam (with a maximum reduction of 25% to 40%). In contrast to the barbiturates, midazolam was unable to produce a burst suppressive pattern or isoelectricity on the EEG.[62] Presumably, this "ceiling" effect is due to the fact that maximal metabolic suppression is reached when the benzodiazepine receptors are fully saturated. A 40% to 50% decrease in cerebral metabolic rate for oxygen with midazolam resulted in an improvement in neurologic outcome and survival after incomplete ischemia in rats,[10] while an in vitro study of rat hypocampal slices suggests neuroprotective effects that are not mediated by the GABAergic system.[1]

Ketamine is generally considered to be contraindicated for neuroanesthesia and for all patients with increased intracranial pressure or decreased cerebral compliance because it increases cerebral metabolism, cerebral blood flow, and intracranial pressure. In normal dogs, the ketamine-induced increase in intracranial pressure was prevented by hyperventilation and diazepam pretreatment.[6] However, it is not determined if these techniques are effective in attenuating ketamine's cerebrovascular effects in patients with abnormal brain compliance. Ketamine blocks the ion channel of the N-methyl-D-aspartate (NMDA) receptor and may therefore possess some inherent protective effect against brain ischemia. However, results of animal experiments are contradictory.[3,31,124] These differing findings may be explained by the fact that the final outcome in the whole animal will be determined by many factors that are influenced by ketamine, including metabolic changes, alterations of cerebral blood flow regulation, and effects on other neurotransmitter systems.

With the exception of ketamine, all sedative-hypnotics lower intraocular pressure (IOP). In fact, the changes in IOP generally reflect the effects of the intravenous agent on systemic arterial pressure. However, none of the available sedative-hypnotic drugs protects against the transient elevation in intraocular pressure that occurs following administration of succinylcholine, laryngoscopy, and intubation.

Effects on EEG

Most intravenous hypnotics have similar encephalographic effects (Fig. 53-4). A transient activation of high frequency activity (e.g., 15 to 30 Hz waves) is seen at low brain concentrations of an anesthetic agent. This is followed by an increase in slower wave forms with higher amplitude and finally by a burst suppression pattern at high brain concentrations. Most sedative-hypnotics have been reported to cause occasional seizure activity.[135,136] Interestingly, the same drugs also possess anticonvulsant properties. When considering the possible epileptogenic properties of drugs, it is important to differentiate between true epileptic activity and myoclonic phenomena. True epileptic activity refers to a sudden alteration in central nervous system activity resulting from a high voltage electrical discharge at either cortical or subcortical sites and spreading to the thalamic and brainstem centers. Myoclonus can have an epileptic or nonepileptic origin depending on the electroencephalographic (EEG) findings.[125]

Barbiturates cause predictable dose-dependent EEG changes and possess potent anticonvulsant activity. Continuous infusions of thiopental have been used to control refractory status epilepticus in intubated and ventilated patients.[17,226] However, low doses of thiopental may induce brief periods of spike wave activity in epileptic patients. Methohexital has well-established epileptogenic effects in patients with psychomotor epilepsy.[165] In fact, low dose methohexital is frequently used to activate cortical EEG seizure discharges in patients with temporal lobe epilepsy.[150] In epileptic patients, the frequency of epileptiform EEG activity during induction of anesthesia with methohexital is significantly less than that which

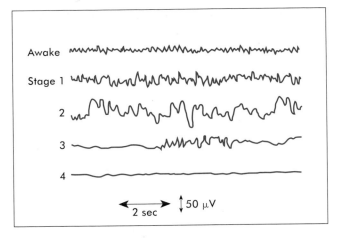

Fig. 53-4. Changes in EEG pattern with increasing concentrations of thiopental. Loss of consciousness (hypnosis) occurs early during stage 1. (From Hudson RJ et al.: A model for studying depth of anesthesia and tolerance to thiopental, *Anesthesiology* 59:3301, 1983).

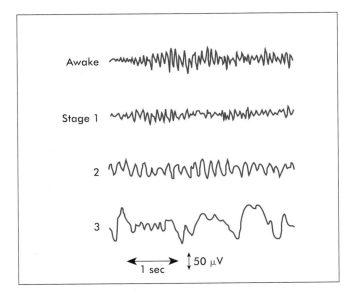

Fig. 53-5. Progressive changes in the EEG produced by ketamine. Stages 1 to 3 are achieved with racemic ketamine and its S(+) isomer. With R(−) ketamine, stage 2 was the maximal EEG depression produced. (From Schüttler J, Stanski DR, White PF et al: Pharmacodynamic modeling of the EEG effect of ketamine and its enantiomers in man, *J Pharmacokinet Biopharm* 15:241, 1987.)

occurs during their normal periods of sleep, indicating that even methohexital has some anticonvulsant activity.[148] Methohexital frequently causes muscle tremors and other signs of excitatory activity (e.g., hiccoughing). Premedication with benzodiazepines, more rapid administration, and the use of higher doses will decrease the occurrence of these side effects.[222]

Etomidate produces an EEG pattern similar to that produced by thiopental, except there is no increased beta activity at lower doses. Etomidate produces a significant increase of the amplitude of somatosensory evoked potentials, while only minimally increasing their latency.[107,130,183] Etomidate has also been used to facilitate the interpretation of somatosensory evoked potentials when the signal quality is poor. **Involuntary myoclonic movements are common during induction of anesthesia with etomidate, but this may be reduced by premedication with diazepine or fentanyl plus atropine.**[22] Current evidence suggests that an alteration in the balance of inhibitory and excitatory influences in the thalamocortical tract is responsible for this myoclonic-like activity. It is unclear whether this epileptic or nonepileptic activity is cortical or subcortical in origin.[135,136] The frequency of myoclonic activity can be attenuated by prior administration of opioid analgesics.[22] Etomidate can induce convulsion-like EEG potentials in epileptic patients without the appearance of myoclonic or convulsion-like motor activity.[148] Etomidate also possesses anticonvulsant properties and has been used to terminate status epilepticus.[85]

Propofol produces cortical EEG changes that are similar to those seen with thiopental.[190,225] Induction of anesthesia with propofol is occasionally accompanied by excitatory motor activity. Whether these movements represent true seizure activity or merely nonepileptic myoclonia is unclear.[135,136] Propofol also possesses profound anticonvulsant properties and has been successfully used to terminate therapy-resistant status epilepticus.[224]

Benzodiazepines cause an increase in the amplitude of the beta wave activity with a reduction in alpha activity and a transient increase in the amplitude of the delta and theta frequency waves.[59,153] Benzodiazepines are potent anticonvulsants[135,136] and are frequently used to treat status epilepticus.

Cortical EEG recordings following a ketamine induction are characterized by the appearance of fast beta activity (30 to 40 Hz), followed by moderate-voltage theta activity mixed with high-voltage delta waves recurring at 3- to 4-second intervals.[170] At higher doses, ketamine produces a unique burst suppression EEG pattern (Fig. 53-5). Myoclonic and seizure-like activity are not uncommon in normal (nonepileptic) patients. However, EEG evidence for a cortical epileptic origin is lacking.[135,136] In contrast, ketamine can activate epileptogenic foci in patients with known seizure disorders.[11,58] In patients without CNS disease, ketamine also appears to possess anticonvulsant activity.[60]

Respiratory System Effects

All intravenous anesthetics have significant effects on the respiratory system. The respiratory depression produced by intravenous anesthetics are compared for normal patients and those with chronic obstructive pulmonary disease in Table 53-3. Although induction agents may directly stimulate coughing and airway irritation or increase airway sensitivity, most airway problems are caused by manipulation of the airway during light levels of anesthesia rather than being caused by a direct drug effect. **Ketamine has a prominent bronchodilatory effect,**[181] **while others do not significantly alter bronchial smooth muscle tone.** In the presence of active bronchospasm, ketamine should be considered for intravenous induction.

In contrast to the other agents, protective airway reflexes are more likely to be preserved with ketamine. However, it must be emphasized that one should not assume that the use of ketamine obviates the need for tracheal intubation in the patient with a full stomach, since tracheal soiling and aspiration have been reported.[24,151]

Table 53-3 Respiratory depressant effects of IV anesthetic agents in healthy patients (normals) and those with chronic obstructive pulmonary disease (COPD)*

Drug name	Normals	COPD
Barbiturates	+ +	+ + +
Propofol	+ +	+ + (?)
Etomidate	+	+
Benzodiazepines	+	+ + +
Ketamine	0/+	0/+

*0 = none, + = minimal, + + = moderate, + + + = marked depression.

Most intravenous induction agents produce dose-dependent respiratory depression characterized by a decrease in tidal volume and minute ventilation, as well as a transient rightward shift in the CO_2 response curve. Ketamine is the exception among intravenous anesthetics; it causes little, if any, respiratory depression in clinically relevant doses. Following rapid injection of large bolus doses of each agent except ketamine, transient apnea occurs and lasts 30 to 90 seconds. Etomidate is associated with less respiratory depression than the barbiturate compounds or propofol.[28,70] An antisialagogue is recommended with ketamine to prevent excessive salivation. **The respiratory depression associated with the use of benzodiazepines is enhanced in patients with chronic respiratory disease,**[77] **and synergetic depression occurs when opioid analgesics are coadministered with benzodiazepines (e.g., midazolam-fentanyl combination).**

Cardiovascular System Effects

Many different factors contribute to the hemodynamic changes associated with the induction of anesthesia. The patient's preexisting cardiovascular disease, fluid status, resting sympathetic nervous system tone, the residual effects of chronically administered drugs, preinduction agents, and the speed of injection of induction agent all influence the cardiovascular response to the induction of anesthesia. In addition, cardiovascular changes can be attributed directly to the pharmacologic action of the anesthetic and analgetic drugs (Table 53-4). Anesthetic agents can depress the central and peripheral autonomic nervous system, blunt the compensatory baroreceptor reflex mechanisms, directly depress the myocardium, and decrease preload and afterload. Profound hemodynamic effects are usually seen at induction when a high drug concentration is achieved in the central compartment or in the presence of hypovolemia. Additionally, the cardiocirculatory effects of intrave-

Table 53-4 Cardiovascular effects of IV anesthetic agents*

Drug name	Mean arterial pressure (MAP)	Heart rate (HR)	Cardiac output (CO)	Contractility (dp/dt)	Systemic vascular resistance (SVR)	Venous dilatation (CVP)
Thiopental	−	+	−	−	−/+	+ +
Methohexital	−	+ +	−	−	−/+	+
Etomidate	0	0	0	0	0	0
Propofol	− −	−	−	−	− −	+ +
Ketamine	+ +	+ +	+	+/−†	+/−†	0
Diazepam	0/−	−/+	0	0	−/0	+
Midazolam	0/−	−/+	0/−	0	−/0	+

*+ = increase, 0 = no change, − = decrease.
†Change is dependent on sympathetic reserve.

nous anesthetics may be accentuated in the elderly or in the presence of preexisting cardiovascular disease.

Thiopental decreases cardiac output, systemic arterial pressure, and peripheral vascular resistance.[26] **Decreased cardiac output is due to a decrease in venous return caused by peripheral pooling and direct myocardial depression.** The effects of methohexital are similar to thiopental; however, an equipotent dose of methohexital produces somewhat less hypotension because the ability to increase the heart rate in response to decreased blood pressure is better preserved.[129]

Etomidate produces little, if any, cardiovascular depression in healthy patients. Even in the presence of cardiovascular disease, etomidate has minimally depresses the cardiovascular system.* Etomidate may have advantages for poor-risk patients and in those situations where preservation of a normal systemic arterial pressure is crucial.

Propofol's cardiovascular depressant effects are more profound than those of thiopental.[56,78] **Both direct myocardial depression**[32,138] **and decreased systemic vascular resistance**[149] **have been implicated as important factors in producing hypotension following large bolus doses of propofol.** Propofol alters the baroreflex mechanism, resulting in a smaller increase in heart rate for a given decrease in arterial pressure.[39] Age also affects the cardiocirculatory response to propofol and caution is mandatory when propofol is administered to the elderly.[49]

In contrast, ketamine stimulates the cardiovascular system, because of stimulation of the sympathetic nervous system, primarily by direct stimulation of CNS structures but also by peripheral stimulation.[219] This explains the increase in arterial pressure and heart rate usually seen on induction of anesthesia with

---

* References 37, 71, 82, 92, 103, 171, 191.

ketamine. However, ketamine directly depresses the myocardium, and this becomes apparent in the seriously ill patient with depleted catecholamine reserves. In animals the drug has been shown to possess some antidysrhythmic activity. Ketamine may compromise the balance between myocardial oxygen supply and demand in patients with coronary artery disease.[63,192] Since ketamine also increases pulmonary artery pressure, it may be contraindicated in adult patients with poor right ventricular reserve.[95] Interestingly, in children this effect seems to be attenuated, and induction of anesthesia with ketamine is safe.[83]

Benzodiazepines produce relatively small changes in cardiocirculatory performance. However, both midazolam and diazepam produce decreases in systemic vascular resistance and blood pressure,[4,166] which may be masked when intubation quickly follows the administration of these agents. The failing heart may benefit from a moderate decrease in preload and afterload produced by benzodiazepines, but the effect on blood pressure may be more marked in hypovolemic patients.[139,168]

Miscellaneous Effects

Intravenous anesthetics have varying effects on hepatic, renal, and endocrine function (Table 53-5). For example, all intravenous anesthetic agents except ketamine increase antidiuretic hormone secretion. Increases in this stress hormone can result in a reduction of urine output.[46,181] Glucose tolerance appears to be decreased during anesthesia. However, the observed hyperglycemia may simply reflect the hormonal response to surgical stress. Liver function is not affected by standard doses of intravenous anesthetics.[13,47,100] Changes in liver and renal blood flow are secondary to changes in cardiac output.

Etomidate produces a high incidence of postoperative nausea and emesis, especially when used in combination with opioid analgetics for short outpa-

---

Table 53-5 Miscellaneous effects of IV anesthetic agents*

Drug name	Liver function tests	Renal blood flow	Adrenocortical function	Safety in porphyria
Barbiturates	Low dose: no effect; high dose and prolonged infusions: increased liver enzymes	−	0	No
Etomidate	0	0	Blocks cortico-steroid synthesis	No
Ketamine	0	+	0	Yes
Propofol	0	− −	0	Unknown
Diazepam	0	0/−	0	Maybe
Midazolam	0	0/−	0	Maybe

*0 = no effect, − = mild decrease, − − = moderate decrease, + = mild increase.

tient procedures. In contrast, propofol may have antiemetic properties, since the incidence of emetic sequelae after outpatient anesthesia with propofol appears to be extremely low.[128] When propofol is used as part of a "balanced" (propofol-alfentanil-N₂O) technique, the incidence of nausea and vomiting appers to be significantly lower than with alfentanil-N₂O alone.

The increased mortality in critically ill patients sedated with an etomidate infusion[112] has been attributed to its effect on cortisol synthesis.* Etomidate inhibits the activity of the 17 α-hydroxylase and 11 β-hydroxylase enzymes necessary for the synthesis of cortisol, aldosterone, 17-hydroxyprogesterone, and corticosterone. Even after an induction dose of etomidate, adrenal suppression persists for 5 to 8 hours.[204] However, the clinical importance of short-term blockade of cortical synthesis is not known.

In general, the intravenous sedative-hypnotic drugs do not have analgetic properties. Thiopental is antianalgetic (i.e., it appears to lower the pain threshold). In contrast, ketamine produces profound somatic analgesia. Although ketamine's ability to bind to spinal opiate receptors may contribute to its analgetic effects, analgesia is primarily caused by a dissociation of electrical activity between the thalamic and limbic systems (which are responsible for the interpretation of pain signals). This dissociation may be caused by ketamines ability to block the channel of the NMDA receptor.

Barbiturates may precipitate episodes of acute intermittent porphyria (AIP), and their use in patients who are predisposed to AIP is absolutely contraindicated. Etomidate, especially when used by infusion,[80] and benzodiazepines are relatively contraindicated since they are potentially porphyrogenic. Ketamine can be regarded as safe, while the safety of propofol is unknown.

HYPERSENSITIVITY (ALLERGIC) REACTIONS

Allergic reactions to intravenous anesthetics or their solubilizing agents can be severe and even life-threatening. The intravenous route of administration bypasses the normal "protective barriers" against entrance of foreign molecules. All the induction agents except etomidate have been shown to cause some histamine release.[43] However, the incidence of severe anaphylactic reactions is low with the currently available induction agents. The high frequency of allergic reactions to the "older" chromophore EL-containing formulations (1 in 1000 administrations)

that led to their early withdrawal possibly resulted from direct action on mast cells, classic complement activation, complement activation through the alternative pathway, antigen-antibody (IgE) reactions, and anaphylactoid reactions of the "mixed type."

Following thiopental administration, the plasma level of histamine increases to about 350% of normal and decreases to normal values after approximately 10 minutes.[114] A transient urticarial rash can be associated with the use of barbiturates. Severe anaphylactic reactions, however, are extremely uncommon.[55,211] The incidence of allergic reactions to the new egg lecithin emulsion formulation of propofol, ketamine, and benzodiazepines appears to be very low. Etomidate does not increase plasma histamine levels and, although anaphylactic reaction to etomidate has been reported,[186] it is probably the intravenous anesthetic least likely to induce a hyperactivity reaction.[208]

PHARMACOKINETICS

An understanding of basic pharmacokinetic principles is essential to understanding the pharmacologic actions of intravenous anesthetics. A knowledge of the pharmacokinetic properties of intravenous anesthetics will allow the anesthesiologist to develop optimal dosing strategies (Table 53-6).

Lipid Solubility

A high degree of lipid solubility will facilitate diffusion across cellular membranes including the blood brain barrier. Only the non-ionized form of molecules is sufficiently lipid soluble to readily cross membranes. The ratio of the non-ionized-to-ionized fraction depends on the pKa of the drug and the pH of the body fluids. The rapid onset of the central nervous system effect of the intravenous anesthetics can be explained by their high lipid solubility and the high proportion of the cardiac output perfusing the brain (20%). Both etomidate and midazolam undergo an intramolecular rearrangement at physiologic pH, resulting in closed ring structures with enhanced lipid solubility.

Protein Binding

Most intranveous anesthetics reversibly bind to plasma and tissue proteins. The number of binding sites is usually saturable; however, for most of these drugs only a small fraction of the available binding sites are occupied at clinically relevant drug concentrations. Nevertheless, the very high plasma concentrations that are achieved immediately after an intravenous bolus injection can result in saturation of the protein-binding sites. Only the unbound drug can diffuse across membranes and exert pharmacologic activity. Therefore the diffusion rate is more limited

---

* References 64, 66, 155, 156, 173, 205.

Table 53-6   Pharmacokinetic profiles for IV anesthetic agents

Drug name	Distribution half-life (min)	Elimination half-life (hr)	Clearance (ml/min)	Volume of distribution (L)	Protein binding (%)
Thiopental	2-4	10-12	120-180	100-200	85
Methohexital	5-6	2-5	700-900	60-80	85
Diazepam	10-15	20-40	15-35	60-100	98
Lorazepam	3-10	10-20	50-70	50-90	98
Midazolam	7-15	2-4	300-550	70-130	94
Etomidate	2-4	2-5	800-1400	200-400	75
Propofol	2-4	1-3	1400-2800	200-500	98
Ketamine	11-17	2-3	1250-1400	200-250	12
Alphaxalone-alphadolone	NA	0.5-1	1200-1800	60-100	NA
Propanidid	3	0.16	NA	NA	NA

NA = not available.

for drugs with a high degree of protein binding. When several agents competing for the same binding sites are administered, or when the protein concentration in the blood is decreased by disease (e.g., hepatic failure), a higher fraction of the unbound drug may be available and its central pharmacologic effect will be enhanced. This is particularly true for drugs with a high degree of protein binding. Only unbound drug is available for uptake and metabolism in the liver. Extensively protein-bound drugs have a limited rate of hepatic metabolism as a result of a decreased hepatic extraction ratio (i.e., the fraction of the hepatic blood flow cleared of drug).

Redistribution and Elimination

The primary mechanism for terminating the central effect of intravenous anesthetics administered for induction of anesthesia is their redistribution from the central, highly perfused compartment (e.g., blood, brain) to the larger and less-well perfused "peripheral" compartments. Even for drugs with a high hepatic extraction ratio, the hepatic elimination does not usually play a major role in terminating the drug's central effects.[89] The redistribution half-life ($t_{1/2}\alpha$) is the time to redistribute one half of the central distribution volume of a drug to a larger peripheral or total distribution volume of the drug. The size of the peripheral compartment for a drug is a function of its volume of distribution at steady state (Vd_{ss}).

Most intravenous anesthetic agents are eliminated via hepatic metabolism followed by renal excretion of their more water-soluble metabolites. Some metabolites have pharmacologic activity and can be responsible for prolonged drug effects (e.g., desmethyldiazepam, norketamine). There is considerable pharamacokinetic variability in the clearance rates for commonly used intravenous anesthetic drugs. Al-

though a high degree of protein binding usually results in a low hepatic extraction ratio, certain drugs have a high hepatic extraction ratio and elimination clearance despite extensive protein binding (e.g., propofol), indicating that protein binding is not always a rate limiting factor. For most drugs, the hepatic enzyme systems are not saturated at clinically relevant drug concentrations, and the rate of drug elimination will be an exponential function of the drug's concentration (i.e., first order kinetics). However, when high steady-state plasma concentrations are achieved with high doses or prolonged infusions (e.g., thiopental > 40 µg/ml), the enzymes can become fully saturated and the elimination rate becomes independent of the drug concentration as the elimination system is operating at maximal capacity (i.e., zero-order kinetics). Propofol's elimination clearance rate (ml/kg/min) exceeds hepatic blood flow, suggesting that an extrahepatic route of elimination contributes to its clearance (e.g., lungs).

The elimination half-life ($t_{1/2}\beta$) is the time required to clear half of the distribution volume of circulating drugs. The $t_{1/2}\beta$ thus depends on the volume to be cleared (the distribution volume) and the efficiency of the metabolic clearance system. The wide variation in elimination half-life values for the intravenous anesthetics is a reflection of the large differences in their clearance values, because their volumes of distribution are similar (see Table 53-6). Drugs with a short elimination half-life are more suited for administration by continuous infusion. When a drug infusion is administered without a loading dose, 3 to 5 times that $t_{1/2}\beta$ is required to reach a steady-state plasma concentration. The steady-state plasma concentration depends only on the rate of administration and the clearance rate of the drug. When an infusion is discontinued, the rate at which the plasma concentration decreases depends largely on the terminal elimination half-life value. For drugs with short elimination half-lives (e.g., propofol, etomidate, ketamine, methohexital, and midazolam), the plasma concentration decreases at a rate that allows for an acceptably rapid recovery. Drugs with longer elimination half-life values (e.g., thiopental and diazepam) are usually administered by continuous intravenous infusion for conditions requiring long-term treatment (e.g., elevated intracranial pressure, prolonged sedation, or anticonvulsive treatment). Titration of the drug to achieve the desired clinical effect is necessary in this situation to avoid drug accumulation and the resultant prolonged drug action after the infusion is discontinued.[187]

Factors Affecting Pharmacokinetics and Metabolism

Aging, preexisting diseases, operative site, physiologic factors, drug interactions, and coadministration of volatile anesthetics can all influence the pharmacokinetics of intravenous drugs by altering their disposition, degree of protein binding, and efficiency of hepatic and renal elimination processes.[29,30,44]

Older patients require significantly lower doses of intravenous anesthetic agents, because of both increased sensitivity and alterations in pharmacokinetic variables.* **With increasing age, the volume of distribution of lipophilic drugs increases because of a decrease in lean body mass and total body water and a proportional increase in total body fat.**[18,96] **The increased distribution volume together with a decreased hepatic clearance leads to a prolongation of the elimination half-time.** Prolongation of the elimination half-time produces higher steady-state plasma concentrations at any given infusion rate. A decrease of the volume of the central compartment had been reported for thiopental and etomidate, resulting in higher initial drug concentrations in the central compartment, and it was alleged to explain the decreased anesthetic requirement in the elderly.[5,87] More recently, it has been suggested that slowed redistribution from the vessel-rich tissues to lean muscle is responsible for the age-related decrease in the induction dose requirement.[9]

The hepatic clearance of drugs with a high (e.g., etomidate, propofol, ketamine) or intermediate (e.g., methohexital, midazolam) extraction ratio depends largely on hepatic blood flow, as most of the drug is removed from the blood as it flows through the liver (i.e., perfusion-limited clearance) (Table 53-7). The elimination rate of drugs with low hepatic extraction ratios (thiopental, diazepam, lorazepam) depends on

---

* References 30, 48, 49, 86, 87, 96, 104, 121, 172.

Table 53-7 Relative hepatic extraction ratio equation for IV anesthetics

Low	Intermediate	High
Diazepam: 0.01-0.025	Midazolam: 0.2	Etomidate: 0.7
Thiopental: 0.1-0.2	Methohexital: 0.5-0.6	Ketamine: 0.8
		Propofol: >1

the enzymatic activity of the liver and is independent of hepatic blood flow (capacity-limited clearance). Hepatic clearance decreases during upper abdominal surgery and, as a result, higher blood levels of drugs with a high hepatic extraction ratio are achieved at any given infusion rate.[7,178] With aging, a decreased cardiac output and a redistribution of blood flow can partly explain the lower clearance rate for drugs with perfusion limited clearance. Coadministration of volatile anesthetics, which decrease liver blood flow, has no influence on the elimination of thiopental,[69] but it decreases the clearance of etomidate,[197] ketamine,[141] methohexital,[188] and presumably, propofol. Other factors that decrease hepatic blood flow include hypocapnia,[90] congestive heart failure, volume depletion, circulatory collapse, beta-adrenergic blockade, norepinephrine administration, and general anesthesia.

Hepatic disease can influence the pharmacokinetics of drugs in several different ways. The protein content of plasma may be altered, thereby changing the degree of protein binding; hepatic blood flow may be increased or decreased and hepatic shunting may occur. Also, in hepatic failure the enzymatic activity of the liver can be depressed. Therefore the influence of hepatic disease on pharmacokinetics and dynamics is difficult to predict in the individual patient. Renal disease can also alter the concentration of plasma and tissue proteins, as well as the degree of protein binding, thereby producing changes in free drug concentrations and in the rate of clearance by the liver.[19]

Thiopental is metabolized in the liver mainly to hydroxythiopental and the carboxylic acid derivative. These metabolites are more water-soluble and have little hypnotic activity. When high doses of thiopental are administered, a desulfuration reaction may occur with the production of pentobarbital, which does depress the central nervous system. Hepatic and renal disease decrease the plasma protein binding of thiopental, increasing the free fraction of the drug[20,68] and resulting in enhanced sensitivity to thiopental.[45] Methohexital is metabolized in the liver to inactive hydroxy derivatives. The clearance of methohexital, which has a moderate hepatic extraction ratio, depends more heavily on liver blood blow than thiopental.

Diazepam is metabolized to active metabolites (e.g., desmethyldiazepam, 3-hydroxydiazepam) that can prolong its sedative effect.[75,157] These metabolites undergo secondary conjugation to form inactive water-soluble glucuronide conjugates. Drugs that inhibit the oxidative metabolism of diazepam include the H_2-receptor blocking drug cimetidine.[105] Severe liver disease reduces the protein binding of diazepam, thereby increasing the free fraction of drug. An increased Vd_{ss} and decreased hepatic metabolic function, though, result in delayed clearance.[106] Chronic renal disease decreases protein binding, and the increased free drug fraction result in enhanced hepatic metabolism and a shorter elimination half-time.[97,144] In elderly patients, the elimination rate of diazepam decreases because of changes in tissue distribution and protein binding.[74,106]

Lorazepam is directly conjugated to glucuronic acid to form pharmacologically inactive metabolites.[52] Age and renal disease have little influence on the kinetics of lorazepam; however, severe hepatic disease decreases its clearance rate.[111] Midazolam undergoes extensive oxidation by hepatic enzymes to form hydroxylated metabolites that are excreted in the urine.[81] The primary metabolite (1-hydroxymethylmidazolam), however, has some central nervous system depressant activity. The clearance rate of midazolam is five times that of lorazepam and ten times greater than diazepam.[152] Although changes in liver blood flow can markedly affect the clearance of midazolam, age has little influence on midazolam's elimination half-life.[8]

Etomidate is metabolized extensively in the liver and by plasma ester hydrolysis, forming inactive water-soluble metabolites. A significant decrease in plasma protein binding has been reported in the presence of uremia and hepatic cirrhosis.[14,21,195] Severe hepatic disease causes a prolongation of the elimination half-life secondary to an increased volume of distribution.[21,195]

Propofol is rapidly and extensively metabolized to inactive, water-soluble sulphate and glucuronic acid conjugates that are eliminated by the kidney.[33,182,215] In addition to the liver's ability to metabolize propofol, extrahepatic clearance mechanisms may also be involved in the drug's rapid elimination (e.g., pulmonary circulation). Changes in liver blood flow would be expected to produced marked alterations in propofol's clearance rate as a result of its high hepatic extraction ratio. However, no changes in propofol's pharmacokinetics have been reported to date in the presence of hepatic or renal disease.

Ketamine is extensively metabolized by hepatic microsomal cytochrome P-450 enzymes. Its primary metabolite, norketamine, is one third to one fifth as potent as ketamine. The metabolites of norketamine are excreted by the kidney as water-soluble hydroxylated and glucoronidated conjugates. Although ketamine has a high hepatic clearance rate, its large distribution volume results in a moderately long elimination half-time. The high hepatic extraction ratio would suggest that alterations in hepatic blood flow could significantly influence ketamine's clearance rate.

CLINICAL USES OF INTRAVENOUS ANESTHETICS
Induction of Anesthesia

The induction and recovery characteristics of the available intravenous anesthetic agents are summarized in Tables 53-8 and 53-9. The suggested induction doses are for healthy ASA physical status I and II patients undergoing elective operations. **Because of pharmacokinetic (e.g., altered clearance and distribution volumes) and pharmacodynamic differences (e.g., altered sensitivity), the induction dose should be adjusted to the needs of the individual patient.** Advanced age, preexisting disease states (e.g., hypothyroidism, hypovolemia), premedication and co-administration of adjuvant drugs (e.g., opioid analgetics, alpha$_2$-adrenergic agonists) will decrease the dose of the induction agent required to produce unconsciousness. Whenever there is concern regarding a possible abnormal response, assessing the effect of 10% to 20% of the usual induction dose (i.e., "test dose") may identify those patients for whom a dosage adjustment is necessary. Before administering more drug, adequate time should be allowed for the drug to exert its effect, especially for induction agents with a slow onset time (e.g., midazolam) or in the presence of a slow circulation time (e.g., congestive heart failure).

Barbiturates have a rapid onset of effect, usually within one arm-to-brain circulation time. Thiamylal is only slightly more potent than thiopental, while methohexital is two to three times more potent. The duration of unconsciousness after a single bolus of the barbiturates is short because these drugs are rapidly redistributed from vessel-rich organs to lean muscle and fat. The clearance rate for methohexital is three to four times higher than for thiopental and thiamylal, resulting in an elimination half-time of 3 to 5 hours for methohexital compared to 10 to 12 hours for thiopental.[89] Full recovery from the central nervous system effects of methohexital may, therefore, be significantly more rapid than for thiopental, especially when repeated doses or continuous infusions are

Table 53-8   Induction characteristics of IV anesthetic agents

Drug name	Induction dose (mg/kg)	Onset (sec)	Duration (min)	Excitatory activity*	Pain on injection*
Thiopental	3-6	<30	5-10	+	+
Thiamylal	3-6	<30	5-10	+	+
Methohexital	1-3	<30	5-10	+ +	+ +
Diazepam	0.3-0.6	45-60	15-30	0	+ + +
Lorazepam	0.03-0.06	60-120	60-120	0	+ +
Midazolam	0.2-0.4	30-60	15-30	0	0
Etomidate	0.2-0.3	15-45	3-12	+ + +	+ + +
Propofol	1.5-3	15-45	5-10	+	+ +
Ketamine	1-2	45-60	10-20	+	0

*0 = none, + = minimal, + + = moderate, + + + = severe.

Table 53-9   Recovery characteristics of IV anesthetic agents

Drug name	Emergence	Frequency of emetic sequelae
Barbiturates	Moderate-to-severe hangover	Low-to-moderate
Etomidate	Mild hangover	Very high
Ketamine	Hallucinations and emergence delirium	Moderate-to-high
Propofol	Minimal hangover, possible euphoria	Antiemetic effect (?)
Diazepam	Prolonged sedation and hangover	Minimal
Midazolam	Sedation, residual amnesia, rebound insomnia	Minimal

administered.[23,109,110] Nevertheless, recovery of fine motor skills will still require 6 to 8 hours after an induction dose of methohexital.[72,109]

There is wide variation in the dose-response relationship for the benzodiazepines,[25,160] especially in unpremedicated, healthy, elective surgery patients. **Diazepam and lorazepam have slower onset times, and the effect produced is somewhat unpredictable. As a result of these characteristics, benzodiazepines are not ideal for routine induction of general anesthesia.[12,161,200] Midazolam has a slightly more rapid onset and may be a useful alternative induction agent for special indications (e.g., situations where nitrous oxide is contraindicated, total intravenous anesthesia).[214] Return of consciousness takes substantially longer with benzodiazepines than with other sedative-**hypnotic drugs. The slow hepatic clearance of diazepam and lorazepam is responsible for their prolonged postanesthetic effects (e.g., sedation, fatigue). In addition, there is a marked temporal lag between the peak concentration in the plasma and the clinical effect of lorazepam.[73] Due to its more extensive hepatic metabolism, midazolam's elimination half-time is significantly shorter. However, recovery of cognitive function is slower after sedation with midazolam compared to methohexital, etomidate,[194] or propofol.[140] Despite the shorter elimination half-time of midazolam, objective measures of recovery have failed to demonstrate a more rapid return to baseline function compared with diazepam.[108]

Etomidate is characterized by a rapid onset and recovery, which compares favorably with the barbiturates. The duration of central nervous system depression after a single induction bolus of etomidate is dose dependent, with return of consciousness occurring after 3 to 12 minutes. Recovery of cognitive and psychomotor function is intermediate between thiopental[88] and methohexital.[134]

Intravenous administration of propofol results in a rapid loss of consciousness comparable to the barbiturates.[163,164] Recovery from propofol's sedative-hypnotic effects is also rapid.[101,210] The duration of its central effects increases in a dose-dependent fashion.[102] In contrast to the barbiturates, there appears to be less residual postoperative sedation, fatigue ("hangover"), and cognitive and psychomotor impairment with propofol.[117]

Ketamine also has a rapid onset of action on the central nervous system following intravenous administration. With the usual induction dose (1 to 2 mg/kg IV), consciousness returns after 10 to 15 minutes. However, full recovery from ketamine's central effects is much slower. After a delay of 2 to 8 minutes, intramuscular ketamine (4 to 8 mg/kg) produces anesthesia for a period of 20 to 40 minutes.

The induction dose is higher in children under 6 months of age and also increases with repeated administration as a result of the development of tolerance.

Propanidid had a rapid onset and a particularly short duration of sedative-hypnotic action that was followed by a fast and complete recovery.[42] Althesin had an onset of action comparable to that of the barbiturates and was characterized by an extremely short elimination half-time and a rapid return of consciousness, although full recovery of psychomotor function was occasionally prolonged.[38,109]

Maintenance of Anesthesia

Volatile anesthetics are still the most popular agents for maintenance of anesthesia because they reliably produce unconsciousness, control autonomic nervous system activity, and relax skeletal muscle. Volatile anesthetics are also easily delivered, their concentration titrated, and they are reliably eliminated. As intravenous drugs with rapid onset and short recovery times and easy-to-use infusion systems have become available, their use may compare favorably with the use of volatile anesthetics.

The traditional administration of intravenous drugs by intermittent bolus doses results in a "depth" of anesthesia (and analgesia) that oscillates above and below the desired level. Due to rapid distribution and redistribution of the drug, the high peak blood concentration after each bolus is followed by a rapid decrease, producing fluctuating drug levels in the blood and brain. The magnitude of the drug level fluctuation depends on the size of the bolus dose and the frequency of administration. Wide variations in plasma concentration can result in hemodynamic and respiratory instability due to rapid changes in the depth of anesthesia. By more closely titrating the drug administration to the desired clinical effect, it is possible to minimize the "peak and valley" pattern in blood concentration. By providing a narrower band of blood (and brain) concentrations, it might be possible to improve anesthetic conditions and hemodynamic stability, as well as decrease side effects and recovery times with intravenous anesthetics.[213] Administration of intravenous anesthetics by a variable-rate infusion is a logical extension of the incremental bolus method of drug titration, as a continuous infusion is equivalent to the sequential administration of infinitely small bolus doses.

To more rapidly achieve a therapeutic blood concentration, it is necessary to administer a loading dose. To maintain the desired drug concentration, a maintenance infusion will be necessary.[203] Although a drug can be titrated to produce and maintain the desired clinical effect, a knowledge of basic pharmacokinetic principles is helpful in more accurately

Table 53-10   Plasma concentrations (Cp) and pharmacokinetic variables used to calculate loading dose (LD) and initial maintenance infusion rate (MIR)

Drug name	Cp (μg/ml)	Vc (L/kg)	Vd$_{ss}$ (L/kg)	Clearance (ml/kg/min)
Thiopental	5-20	0.4	2.5	3
Methohexital	1-4	0.3	2	11
Midazolam	0.05-1	0.4	1.5	7
Etomidate	0.1-0.5	0.3	4	17
Propofol	1-10	0.3	2	30
Ketamine	0.5-2.5	0.5	3	18

predicting the intravenous dosage requirements. The loading dose (LD) and initial maintenance infusion rate (MIR) can be calculated from previously determined population pharmacokinetic variables (Table 53-10):

$$LD = Cp \ (\mu g/ml) \times Vd_{ss} \ (ml/kg)$$
$$MIR = Cp \ (\mu g/ml) \times Cl \ (ml/kg/min)$$

where Cp = plasma drug concentration; Vd_{ss} = distribution volume; and Cl = drug clearance.

The loading dose can be administered as a bolus or as a rapid loading infusion. The latter method produces less fluctuation in the plasma drug concentration and fewer side effects. The required plasma concentration depends on the desired pharmacologic effect (e.g., hypnosis, sedation, muscle relaxation), the concomitant use of other drugs (with additive, potentiating, or antagonistic pharmacologic actions), the type of operation (e.g., superficial, intraabdominal, intracranial),[7,178] and the individual patient's sensitivity to the drug (e.g., age, drug history, preexisting diseases). Obviously, preexisting diseases (e.g., cirrhosis, congestive heart failure, renal failure) can markedly alter the pharmacokinetic variables. In general, children have higher clearance rates. Distribution volumes also tend to be greater in the elderly because of an age-related decline in muscle mass and a greater proportion of body fat. The use of the central (initial) distribution volume (Vc) in place of the distribution volume (Vd$_{ss}$) in the loading dose equation may underestimate the required LD, whereas use of the larger steady state (total) distribution volume Vd$_{ss}$ value will result in drug levels that transiently exceed those that are desired (Fig. 53-6). If a smaller LD is administered, a higher initial MIR will be required. The initial MIR must replace the amount of drug that is removed from the brain by both redistribution and elimination processes. As the

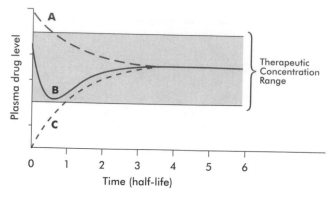

Fig. 53-6. Simulated drug level curves when a constant infusion is administered following a "full" loading dose equal to [Cp] × Vd_{ss} *(A)*; a smaller loading dose equal to [Cp] × Vc *(B)*; or in the absence of a loading dose *(C)*. (From White PF: Clinical uses of intravenous anesthetic and analgesic infusions, *Anesth Analg* 68:161, 1989).

redistribution phase assumes less importance, the MIR will decrease because it is then solely dependent on the drug's elimination and the desired plasma concentration.

Although computer programs are available that allow prediction of concentration time profiles for intravenous anesthetics and analgesics, their clinical usefulness is unclear given the marked pharmacokinetic and pharmacodynamic variability that exists among surgical patients.[122,123,177,178] If a continuous infusion is to be used in an optimal manner to suppress responses to surgical stimulation, the drug's maintenance infusion rate should be varied according to the individual patient responses. Using a MIR great enough to suppress responses to the most intense surgical stimuli will lead to excessive drug accumulation, postoperative side effects, and delayed recovery. Gradual signs of inadequate or excessive anesthesia can be treated by making 25% to 50% changes in the MIR. Abrupt increases in autonomic activity can be treated by giving a small bolus dose (10% to 25% of the initial loading dose) and then increasing the MIR if the surgical stimulus is sustained.[216] Alternatively, vasodilators, beta-adrenergic antagonists, and α_2-adrenergic agonists can be used to blunt the hemodynamic responses to more stressful surgical stimulation, thereby decreasing the analgetic and anesthetic requirements.[175] There is no simple clinical sign to use in determining the optimal maintenance infusion rate during intravenous anesthesia. Most anesthesiologists rely on somatic and autonomic signs for assessing depth of anesthesia, titrating intravenous drugs in the same manner as the volatile anesthetics. The most sensitive clinical signs of depth of anesthesia appear to be changes in muscle tone and ventilatory pattern. However, if the patient has been given muscle

relaxants, the anesthesiologist must rely on signs of autonomic hyperactivity (e.g., tachycardia, hypertension, lacrimation, diaphoresis). Changes in peripheral vascular resistance may be a more reliable indicator of depth of anesthesia than the commonly used hemodynamic signs because blood pressure also depends on the ability of the heart to maintain cardiac output in the face of an increased afterload. The heart rate response to surgical stimulation may be more useful than the blood pressure response in determining the need for additional intravenous anesthetic drugs. However, in the presence of drugs with marked effects on heart rate (e.g., beta-adrenergic antagonists, opioid analgetics), the signs of autonomic hyperactivity may be partially masked, diminishing their usefulness as guides for anesthetic delivery. Thus blood pressure and heart rate responses to surgical stimulation appear to be a less useful guide with intravenous techniques than with volatile anesthetics.[217] Unfortunately, autonomic activity can be effectively blunted during intravenous anesthesia without assuring unconsciousness. A simple, noninvasive monitor of the depth of anesthesia, with a consistent dose-response relationship for commonly used anesthetic drugs that would reliably predict a patient's response to surgical stimulation, would be extremely valuable for use with intravenous anesthetic techniques. Electromyographic (EMG) activity of the frontalis muscles increases significantly in patients who move in response to a specific surgical stimuli,[27] however, EMG changes occur late, and interpretation can be obscured by muscle relaxant drugs. The electroencephalographic (EEG) changes depend largely on the anesthetics used, although a common pattern can be recognized with increasing depression of central nervous system function. Univariate descriptors of EEG activity appear to be of limited clinical use.[113] In a recent study, no correlation could be found between spectral edge frequency and hemodynamic response to surgical stimuli during propofol–nitrous oxide anesthesia.[217] Although lower esophageal contractility (LEC) monitoring was reported to correlate with autonomic responses during surgery in adults anesthetized with volatile anesthetics,[53,54,115] it was less useful in children.[207] When evaluated during "balanced" anesthesia, LEC monitoring was of limited usefulness in assessing depth of anesthesia.[176]

The newer, shorter-acting sedative-hypnotics are better suited for continuous administration techniques than the more traditional agents because they can be more accurately titrated to meet the unique and changing needs of the individual patient (Box 53-2). Since none of the currently available intravenous drugs can provide for a complete anesthetic state without producing undesirable side effects and prolonged recovery times, it is necessary to administer a combination of intravenous agents that provide for hypnosis, amnesia, analgesia, blunting of autonomic responses, and muscle relaxation. Sedative-hypnotics (e.g., methohexital, midazolam, propofol, etomidate, ketamine), opioid analgetics (e.g., fentanyl, alfentanil, sufentanil), and muscle relaxants (e.g., vecuronium, atracurium, mivacurium) can be successfully administered using continuous infusion techniques as alternatives to volatile agents and/or nitrous oxide.*

Sedation

Sedation is frequently desirable during local or regional anesthesia to produce amnesia and enhance patient comfort during the operation. Although intermittent bolus injections of sedative-hypnotic drugs (e.g., diazepam, 2.5 to 5 mg; midazolam, 1.25 to 2.5 mg; thiopental 25 to 75 mg) are commonly administered, the effect is often short-lasting because of rapid redistribution and/or elimination. Continuous infusion techniques are more suitable to achieve and maintain a stable level of sedation.

Infusions of subhypnotic doses of barbiturates (thiopental, 1 to 5 mg/min; methohexital, 0.5 to 2.5 mg/min) have been used for sedation. Prolonged infusion of methohexital is associated with a more rapid recovery than thiopental because the clearance rate of methohexital is three to four times higher, resulting in a shorter elimination half-life (3 to 5 vs. 10 to 12 hours). Thus when thiopental is used for long-term sedation (e.g., for sedation of ventilator-dependent patients in the ICU), recovery can be prolonged.

Benzodiazepines remain the most widely used drugs for sedation and relief of acute situational anxiety during the perioperative period. Midazolam has a steeper dose-response curve than diazepam[221]; therefore careful titration is necessary to avoid oversedation. Midazolam infusion (0.05 to 5 μg/kg/min) can be used for sedation in ICU patients. Use of a midazolam infusion has been shown to control agitation and decrease requirements without producing cardiovascular or respiratory instability.[180,221] However, marked variability exists in individual patient dose-effect relationships. In addition, tolerance may develop to the CNS effects of midazolam with prolonged infusion. The sedative-amnestic and recovery characteristics of methohexital, etomidate, and midazolam when infused during regional anesthesia have been compared.[194] Although midazolam provided more effective intraoperative sedation and amnesia, recovery of psychomotor function was slower with midazolam than with either methohexital or etomidate. Etomidate has been used to provide effective sedation

---

* References 40, 41, 65, 91, 167, 178.

> **BOX 53-2**
> **USES OF CONTINUOUS INFUSIONS OF SEDATIVE, HYPNOTIC, AND ANALGETIC DRUGS**
>
> I. Adjunctive (supplemental) agents during surgery
>   A. Sedative-hypnotic infusions
>   1. Local or regional anesthesia
>   2. Outpatient (ambulatory) surgery
>   3. Neurosurgery
>   B. Opioid analgetic infusions
>   1. General and orthopedic surgery
>   2. Scoliosis fusion surgery
>   3. Cardiac surgery
>   C. Ketamine infusions
>   1. One-lung anesthesia
>   2. Cardiac tamponade
>   3. Supplement local or regional anesthesia
> II. Total intravenous anesthetic techniques
>   A. Sedative-hypnotic/opioid/muscle relaxant
>   B. Benzodiazepine/ketamine/muscle relaxant
> III. Postoperative sedation and/or analgesia
>   A. Opioid analgetic infusions
>   B. Sedative-hypnotic infusions
>   C. Ketamine infusions

for ICU patients[50]; however, because of the drugs effect on adrenocortical synthetic function, this technique is no longer used.

Propofol sedation may offer advantages over the other sedative-hypnotics because of its short duration of effect, rapid recovery, and minimal side effects.[118-120] A carefully titrated subhypnotic dose of propofol (0.5 to 1 mg/kg followed by 3 to 4.5 mg/kg/h) produces excellent sedation with minimal cardiorespiratory depression and a short recovery period.[218] Compared to midazolam, propofol sedation may allow for more rapid weaning of critically ill patients from artificial ventilation.[79,119] Recent investigation would suggest that tolerance to the CNS effects of propofol may also develop with prolonged administration.

Low-dose ketamine infusions (5 to 25 μg/kg/min) can be used for sedation during local or regional anesthetic procedures, as well as in the ICU setting. Midazolam, 0.07 to 0.15 mg/kg infused over 3 to 5 minutes, followed by ketamine, 0.25 to 0.5 mg/kg intravenous over 1 to 3 min, produced excellent sedation, amnesia, and analgesia without significant cardiorespiratory depression during the injection of local anesthetic solutions for cosmetic (facial) surgery.[221] Ketamine also significantly decreases the opioid analgetic requirement when used for sedation in ICU patients.[93]

SUMMARY

It is obvious that many of the goals desirable in an ideal intravenous anesthetic have not been achieved with the currently available drugs. Nevertheless, each of these sedative-hypnotic drugs possesses characteristics that may be useful in specific clinical situations.

Thiopental remains the most widely used intravenous anesthetic even though it is unstable in solution, produces significant cardiocirculatory and respiratory depression, and is associated with a high incidence of postoperative drowsiness and sedation. Thiamylal appears to be almost identical to thiopental both pharmacokinetically and pharmacodynamically. Although recovery from anesthesia with methohexital appears to be faster than with thiopental, methohexital produces more pain on injection and excitatory side effects (e.g., myoclonus, hiccoughing).

Etomidate has minimal cardiovascular and respiratory depressant effects and is therefore extremely useful in high-risk patients. Etomidate has not been associated with histamine release and is associated with an extremely low incidence of hypersensitivity reactions. Unfortunately, pain on injection, excitatory phenomena, adrenocortical suppression, and a high incidence of postoperative nausea and vomiting limit the use of etomidate to special situations in which it offers significant advantages over other available intravenous anesthetics.

Propofol is the drug of choice in situations where a rapid and smooth recovery is required, as for outpatient anesthesia. Recovery from propofol anesthesia is characterized by the absence of a "hangover effect" and a low incidence of nausea and vomiting. The cardiovascular depressant effects produced by propofol appear to be more pronounced than those of thiopental. Elderly and hypovolemic patients are particularly sensitive to propofol's cardiovascular effects.

Ketamine produces somatic analgesia, bronchodilation, and sympathetic nervous system stimulation. Induction of anesthesia is possible with intramuscular administration of ketamine, which may be useful when intravenous access is difficult to establish. Ketamine may be indicated in the presence of hypovolemic shock, bronchospastic disease, right-to-left intracardiac shunts, and cardiac tamponade. Unfortunately, the adverse cerebrodynamic effects of ketamine and its psychomimetic effects during emergence are serious drawbacks to the more widespread use of the drug.

When administered alone, benzodiazepines have variable effectiveness as induction agents. In the usual doses, however, benzodiazepines are associated with minimal cardiorespiratory depression. Benzodiazepines also produce reliable amnesia and therefore, they are valuable adjunctive agents (e.g., acute sedation before induction of anesthesia, in the absence of nitrous oxide). Midazolam has important clinical advantages over diazepam (e.g., less pain and venous irritation, and a shorter elimination half-life without active metabolites).

The shorter elimination times of methohexital, midazolam, and propofol make these drugs extremely useful for administration by continuous infusion for maintenance of anesthesia or sedation. While the search for the ideal intravenous anesthetic agent continues, the challenge for the anesthesiologist is to choose the sedative-hypnotic that most closely matches the needs of the specific clinical situation.

KEY POINTS

- Intravenous anesthetics depress the level of consciousness by enhancing the function of GABA inhibitory synapses or inhibiting NMDA excitatory synapses. Except for ketamine, the intravenous drugs decrease cerebral metabolism, O_2 consumption, and cerebral blood flow.

- Except for ketamine and etomidate, the intravenous drugs depress the cardiovascular and respiratory systems. Smaller doses of the induction agent should be used in the elderly or debilitated.

- Because of high lipid solubility and a high proportion of cardiac output perfusing the brain, the intravenous drugs have a rapid onset and offset of effect. Termination of initial peak effect of intravenous drugs is due to redistribution from the central compartment and is not due to metabolism or elimination. Smaller doses of the induction agent should be used in the elderly or debilitated.

- Barbiturates are hyperanalgetic at low doses. The induction dose of thiopental is 3 to 6 mg/kg. Thiopental is the standard to which all intravenous anesthetics are compared.

- The induction dose of thiamylal is 3 to 6 mg/kg. Thiamylal is nearly identical to thiopental in clinical use.

- The induction dose of methohexital is 1 to 3 mg/kg. Patients recover quicker after methohexital than after thiopental. The injection of methohexital may cause mild pain.

- Benzodiazepines cause less cardiovascular and respiratory depression than barbiturates. Benzodiazepines may produce greater respiratory depression in patients with COPD and may exaggerate the respiratory effects of narcotics. Benzodiazepines are slower to act and last longer than other classes of intravenous anesthetic drugs. Benzodiazepines are useful for conscious sedation and anxiolysis.

- The induction dose of diazepam is 0.3 to 0.6 mg/kg. Diazepam contains 35% propylene glycol preparation, which is venoirritating and causes pain on injection.

- The induction dose of lorazepam is 0.03 to 0.06 mg/kg. Lorazepam contains 35% propylene glycol preparation.

- The induction dose of midazolam is 0.2 to 0.4 mg/kg. Midazolam is water soluble in acidic solution but undergoes intramolecular recombination at physiologic pH to become more lipid soluble. Midazolam has a more rapid onset and offset of effect than diazepam or lorazepam.

- The induction dose of etomidate is 0.2 to 0.3 mg/kg. The most common formulation of etomidate is 35% propylene glycol preparation.

- Etomidate has minimal effects on cardiovascular system but depresses corticosteroid synthesis. There is a high incidence of postoperative nausea and vomiting with etomidate. Etomidate may cause involuntary myoclonic movements on induction. There is no histamine release and extremely low incidence of hypersensitivity reactions with etomidate.

- The induction dose of propofol is 1.5 to 3.0 mg/kg. The preparation of propofol in 10% soya bean oil, 2.25% glycerol, and 1.2% egg phosphatide causes pain on injection.

- Propofol causes greater cardiovascular depression than thiopental. Propofol produces the quickest recovery after induction. Propofol may cause euphoria and an antiemetic effect.

- The induction dose of ketamine is 1 to 2 mg/kg. Ketamine produces a profound somatic analgesia.

- Ketamine increases cerebral O_2 consumption, cerebral blood flow, and intracranial pressure. Ketamine stimulates the sympathetic nervous system centrally and peripherally leading to bronchodilation and possibly increased heart rate, blood pressure, and cardiac output. Ketamine produces a dissociative state and may cause hallucinations and emergence delirium.

- Ketamine is not venoirritating and may be used as an IM induction agent (4 to 8 mg/kg). Ketamine is safe in acute intermittant porphyria.

KEY REFERENCES

Haefely WE: Benzodiazepines, *Int Anesthesiol Clinics* 26:262, 1988.

Kates RA, Stack RS, Hill RF et al: General anesthesia for patients undergoing percutaneous transluminal coronary angioplasty during acute myocardial infarction, *Anesth Analg* 65:815, 1986.

Olsen RW: Barbiturates, *Int Anesthesiol Clin* 26:254, 1988.

Renou AM, Verenhiet J, Macrez P et al: Cerebral blood flow and metabolism during etomidate anaesthesia in man, *Br J Anaesth* 50:1047, 1978.

Reves JG, Fragen RJ, Vinik HR et al: Midazolam: pharamacology and uses, *Anesthesiology* 62:310, 1985.

Sebel PS, Lowdon JD: Propofol: a new intravenous anesthetic, *Anesthesiology* 71:260, 1989.

Wagner RL, White PF: Etomidate inhibits adrenocortical function in surgical patients, *Anesthesiology* 61:647, 1984.

White PF: Clinical uses of intravenous anesthetic and analgesic infusions, *Anesth Analg* 68:161, 1989.

White PF, Way WL, and Trevor AJ: Ketamine — its pharmacology and therapeutic uses, *Anesthesiology* 56:119, 1982.

REFERENCES

1. Abramowicz AE et al: The effect of midazolam and gabaergic inhibition on anoxic damage in the rat hippocampal slice, *Anesth Rev* 15:84, 1988.
2. Abramson NS: Randomized clinical study of thiopental loading in comatose survivors of cardiac arrest, *N Engl J Med* 314:397, 1986.
3. Albin MS et al: Ketamine hydrochloride fails to protect against acute global hypoxia, *Anesth Rev* 15:80, 1988.
4. Al-Khudairi D et al: Hemodynamic effects of midazolam and thiopentone during induction of anaesthesia for coronary artery surgery, *Br J Anaesth* 54:831, 1982.
5. Arden JR, Holley FO, and Stanski DR: The effect of increasing age on etomi-

date pharmacokinetics, *Anesthesiology* 61:A421, 1984.

6. Artru A, Katz RA: Cerebral blood volume and CSF pressure following administration of ketamine in dogs: modification by pre- and post-treatment with hypocapnia or diazepam, *J Neurosurg Anesth* 1:8, 1989.

7. Ausems ME, Hug CC Jr, Stanski DR et al: Plasma concentrations of alfentanil required to supplement nitrous oxide anesthesia for general surgery, *Anesthesiology* 64:362, 1986.

8. Avram MJ, Fragen RJ, and Caldwell NJ: Midazolam kinetics in women of two age groups, *Clin Pharmacol Ther* 34:505, 1983.

9. Avram MJ, Krejcie TC, and Henthorn TK: The relationship of age to the pharmacokinetics of early drug distribution. The concurrent disposition of thiopental and indocyanine green, *Anesthesiology* 72:403, 1990.

10. Baughman VL et al: Cerebral metabolic depression and brain protection produced by midazolam and etomidate in the rat, *J Neurosurg Anaesth* 1:22, 1989.

11. Bennett DR, Madsen JA, Jordan WS et al: Ketamine anesthesia in brain-damaged epileptics: electroencephalographic and clinical observations, *Neurology* 23:449, 1973.

12. Berggren L, Eriksson I: Midazolam for induction of anesthesia in outpatients, a comparison with thiopentone, *Acta Anaesth Scand* 25:492, 1981.

13. Blunnie WP, Zacharias M, Dundee JW et al: Liver enzyme studies with continuous intravenous anaesthesia, *Anaesthesia* 36:152, 1981.

14. Bonnardot JP et al: Pharmacokinetics of etomidate: comparison in normal and hepatic patients. *Anaesthesia*, Volume of summaries, Abstract 23, Sixth European Congress of Anesthesiology, London, 1982.

15. Briggs LP, White M: The effects of premedication on anaesthesia with propofol (Diprivan), *Postgrad Med J* 61(3):35, 1985.

16. Briggs LP, Clarke RS, Dundee JW et al: Use of diisopropylphenol as main agent for short procedures, *Br J Anaesth* 53:1197, 1981.

17. Brown AS, Horton JM: Status epilepticus treated by intravenous infusions of thiopentone sodium, *Br Med J* 1:27, 1967.

18. Bruce A, Andersson M, Arvidsson B et al: Body composition: prediction of normal body potassium, body water and body fat in adults on the basis of body height, body weight and age, *Scand J Clin Lab Invest* 40:461, 1980.

19. Burch PF, Stanski DR: Decreased protein binding and thipental kinetics, *Clin Pharmacol Ther* 32:212, 1982.

20. Burch PG, Stanski DR: Pharmacokinetics of thiopental in renal failure, *Anesthesiology* 55:A176, 1981.

21. Carlos R, Calvo R, and Brill S: Plasma protein binding of etomidate in patients with renal failure or hepatic cirrhosis, *Clin Pharmacokin* 4:144, 1979.

22. Carlos R, Innerarity S: Effect of pre-

medication on etomidate anaesthesia, *Br J Anaesth* 51:1159, 1979.

23. Carson IW, Graham J, and Dundee JW: Clinical studies of induction agents. XLIII. Recovery from althesin—a comparative study with thiopental and methohexitone, *Br J Anaesth* 47:358, 1975.

24. Carson IW, Moore J, Balmer JR et al: Laryngeal competence with ketamine and other drugs, *Anesthesiology* 38:128, 1973.

25. Cartwright PD, Pingel SM: Midazolam and diazepam in ketamine anaesthesia, *Anaesthesia* 39:439, 1984.

26. Chamberlain JH, Sede RGFL, and Chung DCW: Effect of thiopentone on myocardial function, *Br J Anaesth* 49:865, 1977.

27. Chang T, Dworsky WA, and White PF: Continuous electromyography for monitoring depth of anesthesia, *Anesth Analg* 53:315, 1980.

28. Choi SD, Spaulding BC, Gross JB et al: Comparison of the ventilatory effects of etomidate and methohexital, *Anesthesiology* 62:442, 1985.

29. Christensen JH, Anderson F: Individual variation in response to thiopental, *Acta Anaesth Scand* 22:303, 1978.

30. Christensen JH, Andreasen F, and Jansen JA: Pharmacokinetics and pharmacodynamics of thiopentone: a comparison between young and elderly patients, *Anaesthesia* 31:398, 1982.

31. Church J, Zeman S, and Lodge D: The neuroprotective action of ketamine and MK-801 after transient cerebral ischemia in rats. *Anesthesiology* 69:702, 1988.

32. Claeys MA, Gepts E, and Camu F: Hemodynamic changes during anaesthesia induced and maintained with propofol, *Br J Anaesth* 60:3, 1988.

33. Cockshot ID: Propofol (Diprivan) pharmacokinetics and metabolism, an overview, *Postgrad Med J* 61:45, 1985.

34. Collins GGS: Effects of the anaesthetic 2,6-diisoprophylphenol on synaptic transmission in the rat olfactory cortex slice, *Br J Pharmacol* 95:939, 1988.

35. Concas A, Santoro G, Mascia MP et al: The general anaesthetic propofol enhances the function of γ-aminobutyric acid-coupled chloride channel in the rat cerebral cortex, *N Neurochem* 55:2135, 1990.

36. Costa E: The role of gamma-butyric acid in the action of 1,4-benzodiazepines, *Trends Pharmacol Sci* 1:41, 1979.

37. Craido A et al: Induction of anesthesia with etomidate: hemodynamic study of 36 patients, *Br J Anaesth* 52:803, 1980.

38. Craig J, Cooper GM, and Sear JW: Recovery from day-care anesthesia: comparison between methohexitone, althesin and etomidate, *Br J Anaesth* 54:447, 1982.

39. Cullen PM, Turtle M, Prys-Roberts C et al: Effects of propofol anesthesia on baroreflex activity in humans, *Anesth Analg* 66:1115, 1987.

40. de Grood PMRM, Harbers JB, van Egmond J et al: Anaesthesia for laparosocpy: a comparison of five techniques including propofol, etomidate,

thiopentone and isoflurane. *Anaesthesia* 42:815, 1987.

41. de Grood PMRM, Mitsukuri S, van Egmond J et al: Comparison of etomidate and propofol for anesthesia in microlaryngeal surgery, *Anaesthesia* 42:366, 1987.

42. Doenicke A, Kugler J, Kalmar L et al: Klinisch experimentelle untersuchungen mit propanidid, *Anaesthesist* 22:255, 1973.

43. Doenicke A, Lorenz W, Beigl R et al: Histamine release after intravenous application of short-acting hypnotics, *Br J Anaesth* 45:1097, 1973.

44. Dundee JW: The influence of body weight, sex and age on the dosage of thiopentone, *Br J Anaesth* 26:164, 1954.

45. Dundee JW, Richards RK: Effect of azotemia upon the action of intravenous barbiturate anesthesia, *Anesthesiology* 15:333, 1954.

46. Dundee JW, Wyant GM: *Intravenous anaesthesia,* ed 2, Edinburgh and London, 1985, Churchill-Livingstone.

47. Dundee JW, Fee JP, Moore J et al: Changes in serum enzyme levels following ketamine infusions, *Anaesthesia* 35:12, 1980.

48. Dundee JW, Hassard TH, McGowan WA et al: The induction dose of thiopentone: a method of the study and preliminary illustrative results. *Anaesthesia* 37:1176, 1982.

49. Dundee JW, Robinson FP, McCollum JS et al: Sensitivity to propofol in the elderly, *Anaesthesia* 41:482, 1986.

50. Edbrooke DL, Newby DM, Mather SJ et al: Safer sedation for ventilated patients—a new application for etomidate, *Anaesthesia* 37:765, 1982.

51. Eisenberg HM, Frankowski RF, Contant CF et al: High dose barbiturate control of elevated intracranial pressure in patients with severe head injury, *J Neurosurg* 69:15, 1988.

52. Elliot HW: Metabolism of lorazepam, *Br J Anaesth* 48:1017, 1976.

53. Evans JM, Bithell JF, and Vlachnikolis IG: Relationship between lower esophageal contractility, clinical signs and halothane concentration during general anesthesia and surgery in man, *Br J Anaesth* 59:1346, 1987.

54. Evans JM, Davies WL, and Wise CC: Lower esophageal contractility: a new monitor of anesthesia, *Lancet* 1:1151, 1984.

55. Evans JM, Keogh JAM: Adverse reactions to intravenous anesthetic induction agents, *Br J Med* 2:235, 1977.

56. Fahy LT, Van Mourik GA, and Utting JE: A comparison of the induction characteristics of thiopentone and propofol (2,6-diisopropyl phenol), *Anaesthesia* 40:939, 1985.

57. Fee JPH, Collier PS, and Dundee JW: Bioavailability of three formulations of intravenous diazepam, *Acta Anaesthesiol Scand* 30:337, 1986.

58. Ferrer-Allado T, Brechner VL, Dymond A et al: Ketamine-induced electroconvulsive phenomena in the human limbic and thalmic regions, *Anesthesiology* 38:333, 1973.

59. Fink M, Weinfeld RE, Schwartz MA et al: Blood levels and electroencephalographic effects of diazepam and bromazepam, *Clin Pharmacol Ther* 20:184, 1976.

60. Fisher M: Use of ketamine hydrochloride in the treatment of convulsions, *Anaesth Intens Care* 2:266, 1974.

61. Fitch W et al: Responsiveness of the cerebral circulation to acute alterations in mean arterial pressure during the administration of propofol, *J Neurosurg Anesth* 1:375, 1989.

62. Fleischer JE, Milde JH, Moyer TP et al: Cerebral effects of high-dose midazolam and subsequent reversal with RO 15-1788 in dogs, *Anesthesiology* 68:234, 1988.

63. Folts JD, Afonso S, Rowe GG et al: Systemic and coronary hemodynamic effects of ketamine in intact anaesthetized and unanaesthetized dogs, *Br J Anaesth* 47:686, 1975.

64. Fragen RJ, Shanks CA, and Molpeni A: Etomidate, *Lancet* 2:265, 1983.

65. Fragen RJ, Avram MJ, Henthorn TK, et al: A pharmacokinetically designed etomidate infusion regimen for hypnosis, *Anesth Analg* 62:654, 1983.

66. Fragen RJ, Shanks CA, Molteni A et al: Effects of etomidate on hormonal response to surgical stress, *Anesthesiology* 61:652, 1984.

67. Gancher S, Laxer KD, and Kreiger W: Activation of epileptogenic foci by etomidate, *Anesthesiology* 61:616, 1984.

68. Ghoneim MM, Pandya HB: Plasma protein binding of thiopental in patients with impaired renal or hepatic function, *Anesthesiology* 42:545, 1975.

69. Ghonein NM, Van Hamme MJ: Pharmacokinetics of thiopentone: effects of enflurane and nitrous oxide anaesthesia and surgery, *Br J Anaesth* 50:1237, 1978.

70. Giese JL, Stanley TH: Etomidate: a new intravenous anesthetic induction agent, *Pharmacotherapy* 3:251, 1983.

71. Gooding JM, Weng JT, Smith RA et al: Cardiovascular and pulmonary response following etomidate induction of anesthesia in patients with demonstrated cardiac disease, *Anesth Analg* 50:40, 1979.

72. Green R, Long HA, Elliott CJ et al: A method of studying recovery after anesthesia—a critical measurement of recovery following methohexital and thiopental using a complex performance task, *Anaesthesia* 18:189, 1963.

73. Greenblatt DJ, Shader RI, Franke K et al: Pharmacokinetics and bioavailability of intravenous, intramuscular and oral lorazepam in humans, *J Pharmaco Sci* 68:57, 1978.

74. Greenblatt DJ, Allen MD, Harmatz JS et al: Diazepam disposition determinants, *Clin Pharmacol Ther* 27:301, 1980.

75. Greenblatt DJ, Laughren TP, Allen MD et al: Plasma diazepam and desmethyldiazepam concentrations during long term diazepam therapy, *Br J Clin Pharmacol* 11:35, 1981.

76. Grisvold SE et al: Thiopental treatment after global brain ischemia in pigtailed monkeys, *Anesthesiology* 60:88, 1984.

77. Gross JB, Smith TC: Ventilation after midazolam and thiopental in subjects with COPD, *Anesthesiology* 55:A384, 1981.

78. Grounds RM, Twigley AJ, Carli F et al: The haemodynamic effects of intravenous induction, comparison of the effects of thiopentone and propofol, *Anaesthesia* 40:735, 1985.

79. Grounds RM, Lalor JM, Lumley J et al: Propofol infusion for sedation in the intensive care unit: preliminary report, *Br Med J* 296:397, 1987.

80. Harrison PG, Moore MR, and Meissner TM: Porphyrogenicity of etomidate and ketamine as continuous infusions: screening in the DDC-primed rat model, *Br J Anaesth* 57:420, 1985.

81. Heizman P, Eckert M, and Ziegler WH: Pharmacokinetics and bioavailability of midazolam in man, *Br J Clin Pharmacol* 16:43S, 1983.

82. Hempelmann G, Hempelmann W, Piepenbrock S et al: Blood gas analysis and hemodynamic studies on heart surgery patients using etomidate, *Anaesthesist* 23:423, 1974.

83. Hickey PR, Hansen DD, Cramolini GM et al: Pulmonary and systemic hemodynamic responses to ketamine in infants with normal and elevated pulmonary vascular resistance, *Anesthesiology* 62:287, 1985.

84. Ho IK, Harris RA: Mechanism of action of barbiturates, *Am Rev Pharmacol Toxical* 121:83, 1981.

85. Hoffmann P, Schokkenhoff B: Etomidate as an anticonvulsant agent, *Anaesthesist* 33:142, 1984.

86. Homer TD, Stanski DR: The effect of increasing age on thiopental requirement, *Anesthesiology* 59:A530, 1983.

87. Homer TD, Stanski DR: The effect of age on thiopental disposition, *Anesthesiology* 62:714, 1985.

88. Horrigan RW, Moyers JR, Johnson BH et al: Etomidate vs thiopental with and without fentanyl, a comparative study of awakening in man, *Anesthesiology* 52:362, 1980.

89. Hudson RJ, Stanski DR, and Burch PG: Pharmacokinetics of methohexital and thiopental in surgical patients, *Anesthesiology* 59:215, 1983.

90. Hughes RL, Mathie R, Fitch W et al: Liver blood flow and oxygen consumption during hypocapnia and IPPV in the greyhound, *J Applied Physiol* 47:290, 1979.

91. Idvall J, Ahlgren I, Aronsen KR et al: Ketamine infusions—pharmacokinetics and clinical effects, *Br J Anaesth* 51:1167, 1979.

92. Janssen PAJ, Niemegeers CJE, and Marsbrook RPH: Etomidate, a potent non-barbiturate hypnotic. Intravenous etomidate in mice, rats, guinea-pigs, rabbits and dogs, *Arch-Int Pharmacodyn Ther* 214:92, 1975.

93. Joachimsson PO, Hedstrand U, and Eklund A: Low dose ketamine infusion for analgesia during postoperative ventilator treatment, *Acta Anaesth Scand* 30:697, 1986.

94. Johnston GAR, Willow M: GABA and barbiturate receptors, *Trends Pharmacol Sci* 3:328, 1982.

95. Johnstone M: The cardiovascular effects of ketamine in man, *Anaesthesia* 31:873, 1976.

96. Jung D, Mayersohn M, Perrier D et al: Thiopental disposition as a function of age in female patients undergoing surgery, *Anesthesiology* 56:263, 1982.

97. Kangas L, Kanto J, Forsström J et al: Protein binding of diazepam and N-demethyldiazepam in patients with poor renal function, *Clin Nephrology* 4:114, 1976.

98. Kassel NF, Hitchon PW, and Yesh MK: High dose barbiturate therapy. The effect of sodium thiopental on cerebral blood flow, oxygen metabolism and electrical activity, *J Cerebr Blood Flow Metab* 1:411, 1984.

99. Kawar P, Dundee JW: Frequency of pain on injection and venous sequelae following the i.v. administration of certain anaesthetics and sedatives, *Br J Anaesth* 54:935, 1982.

100. Kawar P, Briggs LP, Bahar M et al: Liver enzyme studies with disoprofol (ICI 35868) and midazolam, *Anaesthesia* 37:305, 1982.

101. Kay B, Rolly G: ICI 35868, a new intravenous induction agent, *Acta Anaesth Belg* 28:303, 1977.

102. Kay B, Stephenson DF: Dose-response relationship for disoprofol (IC I35 868; Diprivan), *Anaesthesia* 36:863, 1981.

103. Kettler D, Sonntag H, Donath U et al: Hemodynamik, Myokardmechanik, Sauerstoffbedarf und Sauerstoffversorgung des menschlichen Herzens unter Narkoseeinleitung mit Etomidate, *Anaesthesist* 23:116, 1974.

104. Kirkpatrick T, Cockshott ID, Douglas EJ et al: Pharmacokinetics of propofol (Diprivan) in elderly patients, *Br J Anaesth* 60:146-150, 1988.

105. Kloz U, Reimann I: Delayed clearance of diazepam due to cimetidine, *N Engl J Med* 302:1012, 1980.

106. Klotz U, Avant GR, Hoyumpa A et al: Effects of age and liver disease on disposition and elimination of diazepam in adult man, *J Clin Invest* 55:347, 1975.

107. Koht A, Schutz W, Schmidt G et al: Effects of etomidate, midazolam, and thiopental on median nerve somatosensory evoked potentials and the additive effects of fentanyl and nitrous oxide, *Anesth Analg* 67:435, 1988.

108. Korttila K, Tarkkanen J: Comparison of diazepam and midazolam for sedation during local anaesthesia for bronchoscopy, *Br J Anaesth* 57:581, 1985.

109. Korttila K, Linnoila M, Ertama P et al: Recovery and simulated driving after intravenous anesthesia with thiopental, methohexital or alphadione, *Anesthesiology* 43:291, 1975.

110. Korttila K, Ghoneim MM, Jacobs L et al: Evaluation of instrumented force platform as a test to measure residual effects of anesthetics. *Anesthesiology* 55:625, 1981.

111. Kraus JW, Desmond PV, Marshall JP et al: Effects of aging and liver disease

on disposition of lorazepam, *Clin Pharmacol Ther* 24:411, 1978.

112. Ledingham IM, Watt I: Influence of sedation on mortality in criticlly ill multiple trauma patients, *Lancet* 1:1270, 1983.

113. Levy WJ: Intraoperative EEG patterns: implications for EEG monitoring, *Anesthesiology* 60:430, 1984.

114. Lorenz W, Doenicke A, Meyer R et al: Histamine release in man by propanidid and thipentone: pharmacological effects and clinical consequences, *Br J Anaesth* 44:355, 1972.

115. Maccioli GA, Kuni DR, Silvay G et al: Response of lower esophageal contractility to changing concentrations of halothane or isoflurane: a multicentre study, *J Clin Monitoring* 4:247, 1988.

116. MacDonald JF, Miljkovic Z, and Pennefather P: Use-dependent block of excitatory amino acid currents in cultured neurons by ketamine, *J Neurophysiol* 58:251, 1987.

117. MacKenzie N, Grant IS: Comparison of the new emulsion formulation of propofol with methohexitone and thiopentone for induction of anaesthesia in day cases, *Br J Anaesth* 57:725, 1985.

118. MacKenzie N, Grant IS: Comparison of propofol with methohexitone in the provision of anesthesia for surgery under regional blockade, *Br J Anaesth* 57:1167, 1985.

119. MacKenzie N, Grant IS: Propofol for intravenous sedation, *Anaesthesia* 42:3, 1987.

120. MacKenzie N, Grant IS: Propofol infusion for sedation in the intensive care unit, *Br Med J* 294:774, 1987.

121. Macklon AF, Barton M, James O et al: The effects of age on the pharmacokinetics of diazepam, *Clin Sci* 59:479, 1980.

122. Maitre PO, Ausems ME, Vozeh S et al: Evaluating the accuracy of using poplation pharmacokinetic data to predict plasma concentrations of alfentanil, *Anesthesiology* 68:59, 1988.

123. Maitre PO, Vozeh S, Heykants J et al: Population pharmacokinetics of alfentanil: the average dose-plasma concentration relationships and interindividual variability in patients, *Anesthesiology* 66:3, 1987.

124. Marco FW, Goodrich JE, and Dominick MA: Ketamine prevents ischemic neuronal injury, *Brain Res* 452:329, 1988.

125. Marsden CD, Hallett M, and Fahn S: The nosology and pathophysiology of myoclonus. In Marsden CD, Fahn S, eds: *Movement disorders,* London, 1982, Butterworths.

126. Martin IL: The benzodiazepine receptor: functional complexity, *Trends Pharmacol Sci* 5:343, 1984.

127. Mayer ML, Westbrook GL, and Vyklicky L: Sites of antagonist action on N-methyl-D-aspartatic acid receptors studied using fluctuation analysis and a rapid perfusion technique, *J Neurophysiol* 60:645, 1988.

128. McCollum JSC, Milligan KR, and Dundee JW: The antiemetic action of propofol, *Anaesthesia* 43:239, 1988.

129. McMillan JC et al: The effect of methohexitone on myocardial blood flow and oxygen consumption in the dog, *Br J Anaesth* 46:729, 1974.

130. McPherson RW, Levitt R: Effect of time and dose on scalp recorded somatosensory evoked potential wave augmentation by etomidate, *J Neurosurg Anesth* 1:16, 1989.

131. Michenfelder JD, Milde JH: Influence on anesthetics on metabolic, functional and pathological responses to regional cerebral ischemia, *Stroke* 6:405, 1975.

132. Michenfelder JD, Milde JH, and Sundt TM Jr: Cerebral protection by barbiturate anesthesia, *Arch Neurol* 33:345, 1976.

133. Michenfelder JD, Theye RA: Cerebral protection by thiopental during hypoxia, *Anesthesiology* 39:510, 1973.

134. Miller BM, Hendry JGB, and Lees NW: Etomidate and methohexital, a comparative clinical study in outpatient anesthesia, *Anaesthesia* 33:450, 1978.

135. Modica PA, Tempelhoff R, and White PF: Pro- and anticonvulsant effects of anesthetics. Part I, *Anesth Analg* 70:303, 1990.

136. Modica PA, Tempelhoff R, and White PF: Pro- and anticonvulsant effects of anesthetics. Part II, *Anesth Analg* 70:433, 1990.

137. Moss E, Powell D, Gibson RM et al: Effect of etomidate on intracranial pressure and cerebral perfusion pressure, *Br J Anaesth* 51:347, 1979.

138. Mulier JP, Wouters PF, Van Aken H et al: Cardiodynamic effects of propofol in comparison to thiopental: assessment with a transesophageal echocardiographic approach, *Anesthesiology* 71: A29, 1989.

139. Muller, Schleussner E, Stoyanov M et al: Haemodynamische Wirkungen und charakteristika der Narkoseeinleitung mit Midazolam, *Drug Res* 31:2227, 1981.

140. Negus JB, White PF: Use of sedative infusions during local and regional anesthesia. A comparison of midazolam and propofol, *Anesthesiology* 69:A711, 1988.

141. Nimmo WS, Clements JA: Ketamine. In Prys-Roberts C, Hug CC Jr, eds: *Pharmacokinetics of anaesthesia,* Boston, 1984, Blackwell Scientific Publications.

142. Nugent M, Artru AA, and Michenfelder JD: Cerebral metabolic, vascular and protective effects of midazolam maleate, *Anesthesiology* 56:172, 1982.

143. Nussmeier NA, Arlund C, and Slogoff S: Neuropsychiatric complications after cardiopulmonary bypass: cerebral protection by a barbiturate, *Anesthesiolgoy* 64:171, 1986.

144. Ochs HR et al: Diazepam kinetics in chronic renal failure, *Clin Pharmacol Ther* 29:270, 1981.

145. Olesen AS, Huttel MS: Local reactions to i.v. diazepam in three different formulations, *Br J Anaest* 52:609, 1980.

146. Olsen RW: Drug interactions at the GABA receptor-ionophore complex, *Ann Rev Pharmacol Toxical* 22:245, 1982.

147. Olsen RW, Wong EH, Stauber GB et al: Biochemical pharmacology of the gamma-aminobutyric acid receptor/ionophore protein, *Fed Proc* 43:2773, 1984.

148. Opitz A, Marschall M, Degen R et al: General anesthesia in patients with epilepsy and status epilepticus. In Delgado-Escueta AV, Wastedain CG, Treiman DM et al, eds: *Status epilepticus: mechanisms of brain damage and treatment,* New York, 1983, Raven Press.

149. Patrick MR, Blair IJ, Feneck PO et al: A comparison of the hemodynamic effects of propofol (Diprivan) and thiopentone in patients with coronary artery disease, *Postgrad Med J* 61:23, 1985.

150. Paul R, Harris R: A comparison of methohexitone and thiopentone in electrocortiography, *J Neurol Neusurg Psychiat* 33:100, 1970.

151. Penrose BH: Aspiration pneumonitis following ketamine induction for a general anesthetic, *Anesth Analg Curr Res* 51:41, 1976.

152. Persson P, Nilsson A, Hartrig P et al: Pharmacokinetics of midazolam in total intravenous anesthesia, *Br J Anaesth* 59:548, 1987.

153. Pichlmayr I, Lips U, and Kunkel H: Premedication. In Pichlmayr I, Lips U, and Kunkel H, eds: *The electroencephalogram in anaesthesia,* Berlin, 1984, Springer-Verlag.

154. Pierce EC Jr, Lambertsen CJ, Deutsch S et al: Cerebral circulation and metabolism during thiopental anesthesia and hyperventilation in man, *J Clin Invest* 41:1664, 1962.

155. Preziosi V: Etomidate, sedative and neuroendocrine changes, *Lancet* 2:276, 1983.

156. Preziosi V, Vacca M: Etomidate and the corticotrophic axis, *Arch Int Pharmacodyn Ther* 256:308, 1982.

157. Randall LO, Scheckel CL, and Banziger RF: Pharmacology of the metabolites of chlordiazepoxide and diazepam, *Curr Ther Res* 7:590, 1965.

158. Ravussin P, Guinard JP, Ralley F et al: Effect of propofol on cerebrospinal fluid pressure and cerebral perfusion pressure in patients undergoing craniotomy, *Anaesthesia* 43:37, 1988.

159. Rees DI, Howell ML: Ketamine-atracurium by continuous infusion as the sole anesthetic for pulmonary surgery, *Anesth Analg* 65:860, 1986.

160. Reeves JG et al: Midazolam: pharmacology and uses, *Anesthesiology* 62:310, 1985.

161. Reiton JA, Porter W, and Braunstein M: Comparison of psychomotor skills and amnesia after induction of anesthesia with midazolam or thiopental, *Anesth Analg* 65:933, 1986.

162. Renou AM, Verenhiet J, and Macrez P et al: Cerebral blood flow and metabolism during etomidate anaesthesia in man, *Br J Anaesth* 50:1047, 1978.

163. Rogers KM, Dewar KM, McCubbin TD et al: Preliminary experience with ICI 35868 as an IV induction agent: comparison with althesin, *Br J Anaesth* 52:807, 1980.

164. Rutter DV, Morgan M, Lumley J et al: ICI 35868 (Diprivan): a new intravenous induction agent, *Anaesthesia* 35:1188, 1980.

165. Ryder W: Methohexitone and epilepsy, *Br Dent J* 126:343, 1969.

166. Samuelson PN et al: Midazolam versus diazepam: different effects on systemic vascular resistance, *Drug Res* 31:2268, 1980.

167. Scheepstra GL, Booij LH, Rutten CL et al: Propofol for induction and maintenance of anesthesia: comparison between younger and older patients, *Br J Anaesth* 62:54, 1989.

168. Schulte-Sasse U, Hess W, and Tarnow J: Haemodynamic responses to induction of anaesthesia using midazolam in cardiac surgical patients, *Br J Anaesth* 54:1053, 1982.

169. Schwartz ML et al: A prospective randomized comparison of pentobarbital and mannitol, *Can J Neurol Sci* 11:434, 1984.

170. Schwartz MS, Virden S, and Scott DF: Effects of ketamine on the electroencephalogram, *Anaesthesia* 29:135, 1974.

171. Scorgie B: Etomidate infusion: its use in anesthesia for general surgery, *Anaesthesia* 38:63, 1983.

172. Sear JW, Cooper GM, and Kumar V: The effect of age on recovery: a comparison of the kinetics of thiopentone and althesin, *Anaesthesia* 38:1151, 1983.

173. Sear JW, Allen MC, Gales M et al: Suppression by etomidate of normal cortisone response to anesthesia and surgery, *Lancet* 2:1028, 1983.

174. Sear JW, Walters FJ, Wilkins DG et al: Etomidate by infusion for neuroanesthesia. Kinetic and dynamic interactions with nitrous oxide, *Anaesthesia* 39:12, 1984.

175. Segal IS et al: Perioperative use of transdermal clonidine as an adjunctive agent, *Anesth Anagl* 68:S250, 1989.

176. Sessler DI, Stoen R, Olofsson CI et al: Lower esophageal contractility predicts movement during skin incision in patients anesthetized with halothane, but not with nitrous oxide and alfentanil, *Anesthesiology* 70:42, 1989.

177. Shafer A, Sung M-L, and White PF: Pharmacokinetics and pharmacodynamics of alfentanil infusions during general anesthesia, *Anesth Analg* 65:1021, 1986.

178. Shafer A, Doze VA, Shafer SL et al: Pharmacokinetics and pharmacodynamics of propofol infusions during general anesthesia, *Anesthesiology* 69:348, 1988.

179. Shapiro HM: Intracranial hypertension: therapeutic and anesthetic considerations, *Anesthesiology* 43:445, 1975.

180. Shapiro HM, Westphal LM, White PF et al: Midazolam infusion for sedation in the intensive care unit—effect on adrenal function, *Anesthesiology* 66:396, 1986.

181. Silvay G: Ketamine, *Mt Sinai J Med* 50:300, 1983.

182. Simons et al: Blood concentration, metabolism and elimination after subanesthetic intravenous dose of 14C-propofol ("Diprivan") to male volunteers, *Postgrad Med J* 61:64, 1985.

183. Sloan TB, Ronai AK, Toleikis JR et al: Improvement of intraoperative somatosensory evoked potentials by etomidate, *Anesth Analg* 67:582, 1988.

184. Smith AL, Hoff JT, Nielsen SL et al: Barbiturate protection in acute focal cerebral ischemia, *Stroke* 5:76, 1974.

185. Smith MT, Eadie MJ, and Brophy TO: The pharmacokinetics of midazolam in man, *Eur J Clin Pharm* 19:271, 1981.

186. Sold MJ, Rothhammer A: Lebensbedrohliche anaphylaktoide Reaktion nach Etomidat, *Anaesthesist* 34:208, 1985.

187. Stanski DR, Mihm FG, Rosenthal MH et al: Pharmacokinetics of high-dose thiopental used in cerebral resuscitation, *Anesthesiology* 53:169, 1980.

188. Stanski DR: Pharmacokinetics of barbiturates, In Prys-Roberts C, Hug CC Jr, eds: *Pharmokinetics in anaesthesia*, Boston, 1984, Blackwell Scientific Publications.

189. Steen PA, Milde JH, and Michenfelder JD: No barbiturate protection in a dog model of complete cerebral ischemia, *Ann Neurol* 5:343, 1979.

190. Stephan H et al: Einfluss von Disoprivan auf die Durchblutung und den Sauerstoffverbrauch des Gehirns und die CO2 Reaktivitaet des Himgefaesses beim Menschen, *Anaesthesist* 36:60, 1987.

191. Tarnow J, Hess W, and Kline W: Etomidate, althesin and thiopentone as induction agents for coronary artery surgery, *Can Anaesth Soc J* 27:338, 1980.

192. Tarnow J, Hess W, Schmidt D et al: Narkoseeinleitung bei Patienten mit koroaner Herzkrankheit: Flunitrazepam, Diazepam, Ketamin, Fentanyl, *Anaesthesist* 28:9, 1979.

193. Todd MM, Chadwick HS, Shapiro HM et al: The neurologic effects of thiopental therapy following experimental cardiac arrest in cats, *Anesthesiology* 57:76, 1982.

194. Urquhart ML, White PF: Comparison of sedative infusions during regional anesthesia. Methohexital, etomidate and midazolam, *Anesth Analg* 68:249, 1988.

195. Van Beem HBH et al: Pharmacokinetics of etomidate in patients with liver cirrhosis. *Anesthesia*, Volume of summaries, Abstract 426, Sixth European Congress of Anaesthesiology, London, 1982.

196. Vandesteene A, Trempont V, Engelman E et al: Effect of propofol on cerebral blood flow and metabolism in man, *Anaesthesia* 43:37, 1988.

197. Van Hamme MJ, Ghoneim MM, and Ambre JJ: Pharmacokinetics of etomidate, a new intravenous anesthetic, *Anesthesiology* 49:274, 1978.

198. Van Hemelrijck J et al: The effects of propofol on ICP and cerebral perfusion pressure in patients with brain tumors, *Anesthesiol Rev* 15:67, 1988.

199. Van Hemelrijck J, Fitch W, Mattheussen M et al: Effect of propofol on the cerebral circulation and autoregulation in the baboon, *Anesth Analg* 71:49, 1990.

200. Varner PD, Ebert JP, McKay RD et al: Methohexital sedation for children undergoing CT-scan, *Anesth Analg* 64:643, 1985.

201. Verma R, Ramasubramanian R, and Sachar RM: Anesthesia for termination of pregnancy, midazolam compared with methohexital, *Anesth Analg* 64:792, 1985.

202. Vincent JP, Cavey D, Kamenka JM et al: Interaction of phencyclinidines with the muscarinic and opiate receptors in the central nervous system, *Brain Res* 152:176, 1978.

203. Wagner JG: A safe method for rapidly achieving plasma concentration plateaus, *Clin Pharmacol Ther* 16:691, 1974.

204. Wagner RL, White PF: Etomidate inhibits adrenocortical function in surgical patients, *Anesthesiology* 61:647, 1984.

205. Wagner RL, White PF, Kan PB et al: Inhibition of adrenal steroidogenesis by the anesthetic etomidate, *N Engl J Med* 310:1415, 1984.

206. Ward JD, Becker DP, Miller JD et al: Failure of prophylactic barbiturate coma in the treatment of severe head trauma, *J Neurosurg* 62:383, 1985.

207. Watcha NE, White PF: Failure of lower esophageal contractility to predict patient movement in children anesthetized with halothane and nitrous oxide, *Anesthesiology* 71:664, 1989.

208. Watkins J: Etomidate: an "immunologically safe" anesthetic agent? *Anaesthesia* 40:1015, 1985.

209. Wear D, Goodchild CS, and Graham DL: Propofol: effect on indices of cerebral ischemia, *J Neurosurg Anesth* 1:284, 1989.

210. Weightman WM, Zacharias M: Comparison of propofol and thiopentone anaesthesia (with special reference to recovery characteristics), *Anaesth Intens Care* 15:389, 1987.

211. Westacott P, Ramachandran PR, and Jancelewicz A: Anaphylactic reaction to thiopentone: a case report, *Can Anaesth Soc J* 31:434, 1984.

212. Westphal LM, Cheng EY, White PF et al: Use of midazolam for sedation following cardiac surgery, *Anesthesiology* 67:257, 1987.

213. White PF: Use of continuous infusion versus intermittent bolus administration of fentanyl or ketamine during outpatient anesthesia, *Anesthesiology* 59:294, 1983.

214. White PF: The role of midazolam in outpatient anethesia, *Anesth Rev* 12:55, 1985.

215. White PF: Propofol, pharmacokinetics and pharmacodynamics, *Sem Anesth* 7:4, 1988.

216. White PF: Clinical uses of intravenous anesthetic and analgesic infusions, *Anesth Analg* 68:161, 1989.

217. White PF, Boyle WA: Relationship between hemodyamic and electroencephalographic changes during general anesthesia, *Anesth Analg* 68:177, 1989.

218. White PF, Negus JB: Sedative infusions during local or regional anesthesia—a comparison of propofol and midazolam, *J Clin Anesth* 3:32, 1991.

219. White PF, Way WL, and Trevor AJ: Ketamine—its pharmacology and therapeutic uses, *Anesthesiology* 56:119, 1982.

220. White PF, Ham J, Way WL et al: Pharmacology of ketamine isomers in surgical patients, *Anesthesiology* 52:231, 1980.

221. White PF, Vasconez LO, Mathes SA et al: Comparison of midazolam and diazepam for sedation during plastic surgery, *J Plast Reconstruc Surg* 81:703, 1988.

222. Whitman JG: Intravenous induction agents, *Clin Anesthesiol* 2:515, 1984.

223. Willow MA: Comparison of the actions of pentobarbitone and etomidate on [3H] GABA binding to crude synaptosomal rat brain membranes, *Brain Res* 220:427, 1981.

224. Wood PR, Brown GPR, and Pugh S: Propofol infusion for the treatment of status epilepticus, *Lancet* 1:480, 1988.

225. Yate PM, Maynard DE, Major E et al: Anesthesia with ICI 35868 monitored by the cerebral function analysing monitor (CFAM), *Eur J Anesthesiol* 3:159, 1986.

226. Young GB et al: Anesthetic barbiturates in refractory status epilepticus, *Can J Neurol Sci* 7:291, 1980.

227. Zacharias M, Clarke RS, Dundee JW et al: An evaluation of three preparations of etomidate, *Br J Anaesth* 50:925, 1978.

CHAPTER 54

Pharmacology of Opioid Analgetic Agents

CARL ROSOW

Chemistry
Opioid Agonists
  Pharmacodynamics
  Pharmacokinetics
  Intraoperative use of opioid agonists
Opioid Antagonists
  Naloxone
  Naltrexone
  Nalmefene
Opioid Agonist-Antagonists
  General properties
  Analgesia
  Sedation
  Respiratory depression
  Smooth muscle effects
  Cardiovascular effects
  Antagonist effects
  Tolerance and abuse liability

Opioid analgetics are used in nearly every facet of modern anesthesia practice. They are used as premedicants or sedatives (Chapter 51), intravenous anesthetics (Chapter 53), postoperative analgetics (Chapter 65), and intraspinal analgetics (Chapter 64). Unfortunately, they are also abused by patients (Chapter 30) and physicians (Chapter 102).

In Chapter 53, we saw that the opioids may be divided into three groups based upon their pharmacodynamic activity: *pure agonists* (morphine, fentanyl, etc.), *pure antagonists* (naloxone, naltrexone), and *mixed agonist-antagonists* (nalbuphine, butorphanol, etc.). Opioids may also be grouped on the basis of

their chemical groups or their postulated interactions with opioid receptor subtypes (mu, kappa, delta, sigma, episilon, etc.). In this chapter the clinical pharmacology of opioids will be reviewed according to their pharmacodynamic classification.

CHEMISTRY

Opium is a complex mixture of alkaloids obtained from the seed pods of *Papaver somniferum*, the opium poppy. The two naturally occurring *opiate* analgetics are the phenanthrene alkaloids, morphine and codeine. **The term *opioid* applies to any natural or synthetic compound that has morphinelike properties. All the clinically available opioids are structurally related to morphine.** The chemical structure of morphine is shown in Fig. 54-1, *A*. It is a five-ring system with several distinctive features: there are two hydroxyl groups (one phenolic and one alcoholic), a quaternary carbon atom at position 13, and a piperidine ring with a methyl group on the nitrogen. Morphine is optically active, and only the levorotatory form is analgetically active. Codeine is morphine that has been O-methylated at position 3.

When the methyl substituent on the piperidine nitrogen is replaced by a bulkier chemical group (e.g., allyl, cyclopropyl, cyclobutyl), the compound usually takes on antagonist properties. For example, the N-allyl derivatives of morphine and oxymorphone are the antagonists, nalorphine and naloxone respectively.

The first semisynthetic opioids (heroin, hydromorphone) were made by simple substitution, but the morphine molecule may be modified extensively without loss of agonist activity. Meperidine, a totally

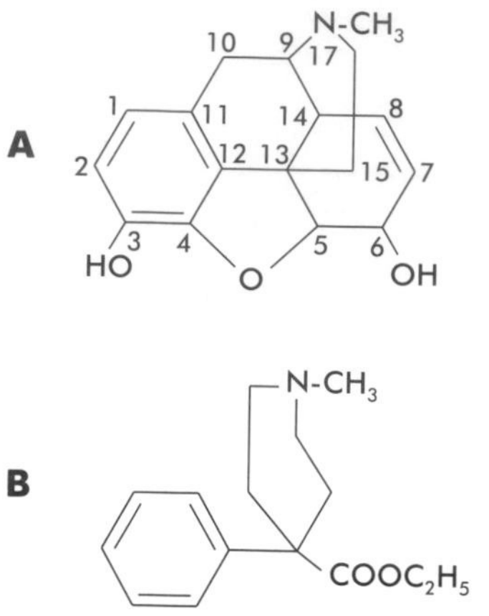

Fig. 54-1. Structural formulas of morphine (**A**) and meperidine (**B**).

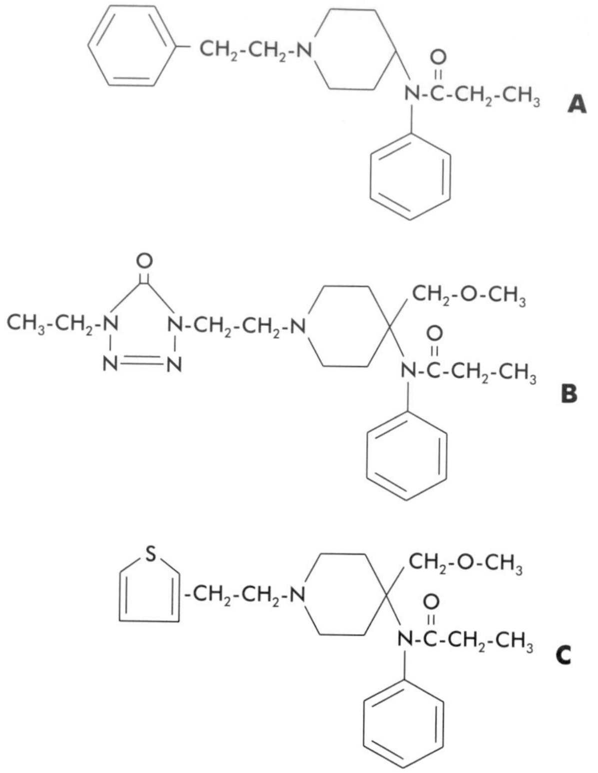

Fig. 54-2. Structural formulas of fentanyl (**A**), alfentanil (**B**), and sufentanil (**C**).

synthetic phenylpiperidine (Fig. 54-1, *B*), retains only the piperidine ring and fragments of the morphine structure. Fentanyl, sufentanil, and alfentanil are 4-anilinopiperidines that are structurally related to meperidine (Fig. 54-2).

OPIOID AGONISTS

Pharmacodynamics

General properties

The most widely used opioid analgetics are the pure agonists, and all of these are relatively selective for mu opioid receptors. Unlike the volatile anesthetics, opioid agonists produce a group of highly specific depressant and stimulant effects by acting at discrete sites within the central nervous system. For example, morphine stimulates the vagal nuclei in the medulla while depressing respiratory centers only a few millimeters away. The acute and chronic effects of opioids are listed in Box 54-1.

Given their common mechanism of action, it is easy to see why morphine, meperidine, fentanyl, and the fentanyl congeners have very similar pharmacodynamic effects. The few qualitative differences between them (e.g., histamine release) usually do not involve specific opioid receptor mechanisms. However, the various opioids differ greatly in their physicochemical properties as well as in speed of onset and duration of action, so the clinical selection of an opioid is frequently based on pharmacokinetic considerations.

CNS effects

Analgesia and mood effects. The opioids produce selective relief of pain at doses that do not produce sleep or impair sensation. As has been discussed previously in this text, **opioid analgetic effects prob-**

ably result from actions at several different levels of the neuraxis.[42] **The processing of pain information is inhibited by a direct spinal effect at the dorsal horn; the rostrad transmission of pain signals is decreased by activation of descending inhibitory pathways in the brainstem**[1]**; finally, the emotional response to pain is altered by opioid actions on the limbic cortex. There is recent evidence that opioids may also act at receptors located peripherally on sensory neurons.**[161]

Opioids affect both the perception of pain and the response to pain, but it is difficult to make the distinction in most clinical circumstances. Patients given morphine will typically report that pain is still present, but the intensity is decreased and it no longer bothers them as much. The relief of pain and anxiety will often result in sleep, but sometimes mood elevation or frank euphoria may occur. The euphoriant effect or sense of well-being produced by opioid agonists is thought to be one of the most important reasons for their abuse.[77]

Sufficient doses of opioids will relieve almost any pain, although some types of pain are typically more responsive than others. Prolonged, burning pain, for example, is more effectively blunted than the brief, sharp pain of an incision. Neuropathic pain (e.g., pain of nerve root compression) can be very resistant to opioid treatment.[8] **Intraoperatively the opioids can**

BOX 54-1
ACUTE AND CHRONIC EFFECTS OF OPIOIDS

Acute

Analgesia	Miosis
Respiratory depression	Nausea and vomiting
Sedation	Skeletal muscle rigidity
Euphoria	Smooth muscle spasm
Vasodilation	Constipation
Bradycardia	Urinary retention
Cough suppression	Biliary spasm

Chronic

Tolerance
Physical
  dependence

Table 54-1   Dose, time to peak effect, and duration of analgesia for intravenous opioid agonists and agonist-antagonists*

Opioid	Dose† (mg)	Peak (min)	Duration‡ (hr)
Morphine	10	20-30	3-4
Meperidine	80	5-7	2-3
Hydromorphone	1.5	15-30	2-3
Oxymorphone	1.0	15-30	3-4
Methadone	10	15-30	3-4
Fentanyl	0.1	3-5	.5-1
Sufentanil	0.01	3-5	.5-1
Alfentanil	0.75	1.5-2	.2-.3
Pentazocine	60	15-30	2-3
Butorphanol	2	15-30	2-3
Nalbuphine	10	15-30	3-4
Buprenorphine	0.3	<30	5-6
Dezocine	10	15-30	3-4

*Data for fentanyl derivatives are derived from intraoperative studies, the remainder are from postoperative pain studies.
†Approximately equianalgetic doses (see text).
‡Average duration of first, single dose.

produce sufficient analgesia to reduce or abolish autonomic and somatic responses to surgical stimuli. In this circumstance they are almost always combined with other central nervous system depressants (see discussion on intraoperative use).

Table 54-1 lists some commonly used opioid agonists along with their recommended doses and durations of action. The relative potencies of most older opioids have been determined in postoperative pain models, but similar data for the fentanyl series are not available. The doses in the table are for comparison only, and the actual doses given during administration of anesthesia will vary greatly depending on the application. "Equianalgetic" doses can be very difficult to determine when opioids with very different analgetic time-effect curves are being compared (Fig. 54-3). Fentanyl is often stated to have 80 to 100 times the potency of morphine, a figure that takes into account both the intensity and duration of effect (i.e., the area under the curve is measured). If one considered only the peak intensity of effect, fentanyl might appear to be 200 times as potent as morphine. Because the anesthesiologist typically looks for peak analgetic and toxic effects following an intravenous bolus, the latter number may be more useful.

Sedation-hypnosis. In usual analgetic doses, morphine-like drugs may produce drowsiness, feelings of heaviness, and difficulty concentrating. Unlike benzodiazephines, opioids do not usually produce amnesia in subhypnotic doses. At higher doses sedation becomes more pronounced, and, eventually, hypnosis may occur. It is important to remember that doses of opioids that are sufficient to produce apnea and profound analgesia do not always produce sleep in healthy individuals.[12,155] The use of opioids alone to produce both hypnosis and analgesia has resulted in numerous cases of intraoperative awareness. Sleep is much more likely to occur in elderly or debilitated patients or in those given small doses of benzodiazepines. High doses of morphine, fentanyl, or its congeners produce a cortical EEG pattern that is superficially similar to deep sleep.[150] The average frequency decreases, and large-amplitude delta waves predominate.

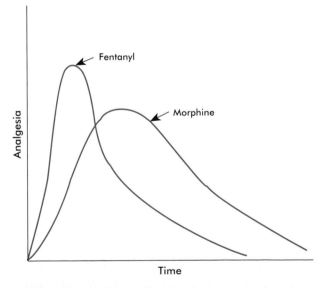

Fig. 54-3. Idealized time-effect curves for fentanyl and morphine. Estimated potency of fentanyl is higher if only peak analgesia is considered and duration ignored (see text).

CNS toxicity. **Dysphoria and agitation occur infrequently after analgetic doses of most opioids, although their incidence is higher with meperidine and codeine. True seizures can be produced by meperidine because its major metabolite, normeperidine, is a potent convulsant. This is most likely to occur after large doses, or if the patient has renal failure and cannot excrete the metabolite**[163] (see discussion of pharmacokinetics).

In laboratory animals, extremely high doses of morphine or fentanyl will produce seizure activity, but this does not occur at the concentrations achieved in clinical practice.[114] Opioid-induced hypertonus of skeletal muscle (see discussion of muscle rigidity) can sometimes lead to myoclonic movements that have been mistaken for seizures.

Administration of opioids can raise cerebrospinal fluid pressure if ventilation is not controlled and Pa_{CO_2} is allowed to rise. Opioid premedication should generally be avoided when elevated intracranial pressure (ICP) is suspected; ICP may rise further, and the opioid effects may mask changing neurologic signs. These drugs are very useful, however, during induction of anesthesia in neurosurgical patients. When ventilation is controlled, fentanyl and sufentanil have little effect on cerebral metabolic rate and blood flow and therefore do not increase ICP.[15,107,154]

Respiratory depression. **Opioids produce a dose-related depression of the ventilatory response to CO_2 by a direct effect on respiratory centers in the medulla.**[79] **Morphine has also been shown to blunt the response to hypoxia.**[174] In awake subjects given an analgetic dose of morphine the intercept of the CO_2 response curve is shifted to the right, and (depending upon the measurement technique) there may also be a decrease in slope (Fig. 54-4). Both the rate and the rhythm of breathing are affected: as the dose of opioid is increased, respiratory rate will slow, but the effect of this may be partially offset by an increase in tidal volume. **It is important to remember that a decrease in respiratory rate is not a very sensitive indicator of opioid effect. A patient's drive to breathe may be abnormal despite an apparently normal respiratory rate and state of consciousness. Sleep depresses the response to CO_2 and potentiates the respiratory depression caused by opioids.**[45]

At usual analgetic doses the opioids rarely cause clinically significant respiratory depression unless there is preexisting pathology (such as hypothyroidism or pulmonary or CNS disease) or previous drug administration (alcohol, general anesthetics, or benzodiazepines).

Very large doses of opioids will eventually result in inadequate ventilation. Breathing may become irregular or even take on a Cheyne-Stokes pattern. There may be complete inattention to breathing; otherwise

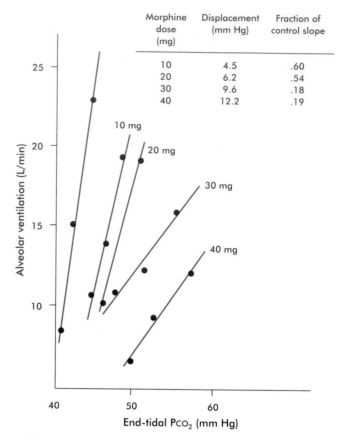

Morphine dose (mg)	Displacement (mm Hg)	Fraction of control slope
10	4.5	.60
20	6.2	.54
30	9.6	.18
40	12.2	.19

Fig. 54-4. CO_2 response curves from one subject who received four doses of morphine 10 mg intravenously at 40-minute intervals. (From Keats AS: The effect of drugs on respiration in man, *Ann Rev Pharmacol Toxicol* 25:41, 1985.)

responsive patients may hypoventilate to the point of cyanosis unless they are reminded to breathe. Respiratory depression is, of course, the major toxicity of opioids and nearly always the cause of death from overdose.

Equianalgetic doses of all opioids produce equivalent amounts of respiratory depression. There is no convincing evidence that any analgetic is more or less dangerous than morphine in this regard. Despite experimental evidence that analgesia and respiratory depression may be mediated by different receptor subtypes (mu_1 and mu_2, respectively), no highly selective agonist or antagonist has been developed for clinical use.[128]

Both analgesia and respiratory depression are reduced by administration of an opioid antagonist or by the development of tolerance. This has two important clinical implications:

- **Tolerant individuals who require large amounts of opioid for relief of pain are not at proportionately increased risk of respiratory depression.**
- **Respiratory depression is difficult to reverse without reversing some analgesia (see discussion of naloxone).**

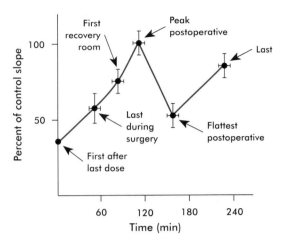

Fig. 54-5. Recurrent ventilatory depression expressed as slope of CO_2 response curve (percentage of awake control) vs. time. First data point obtained after last intraoperative dose of fentanyl. Response recovered, then subsequently declined when patients were no longer stimulated (see text). (From Becker LD et al: Biphasic respiratory depression after fentanyl-droperidol or fentanyl alone used to supplement nitrous oxide anesthesia, *Anesthesiology* 44:291, 1976.)

A number of case reports have described "recurrent" or "delayed" ventilatory depression after administration of anesthetics with fentanyl or alfentanil.[16,74] Becker et al. showed that CO_2 sensitivity could recover after fentanyl-N_2O anesthesia, only to decline once again over the next hour (Fig. 54-5). It is likely that these events are actually caused by varying levels of stimulation: opioid-induced respiratory depression is antagonized by pain and movement during emergence and transfer to the recovery area; it may reappear if the patient goes back to sleep.

Cough suppression. **Opioids suppress cough by depressing cough centers in the medulla. This effect apparently involves different receptor mechanisms than those mediating analgesia or respiratory depression.** Cough is effectively suppressed by dextro-isomers of opioids (e.g., dextromethorphan), compounds that have no analgetic activity. The molecular modification that selectively increases antitussive potency is replacement of the 3-hydroxyl group on morphine with a bulkier group. Thus, cough suppression is greatest with heroin (R = CH_3COO), strong with codeine (R = CH_3O), and very weak with meperidine (R = H).[126]

Pupillary constriction. **Opioids stimulate the Edinger-Westphal nucleus of the oculomotor nerve to produce miosis.**[91] **The pinpoint pupil is a pathognomonic sign of opioid overdose (until hypoxia supervenes).** Miosis is rapidly reversed with naloxone, and it may be overcome with sufficient doses of atropine or ganglionic blockers. Miosis occurs after relatively small doses of most opioids, so it is not very useful as

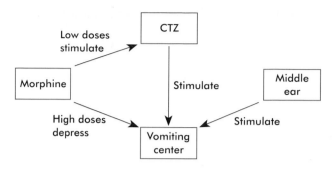

Fig. 54-6. Mechanisms of opioid-induced nausea and vomiting (see text for details). (From Rosow CE: Newer synthetic opioid analgesics. In Smith G, Covino BG, eds: *Acute pain,* London, 1985, Butterworths.)

an indicator of the intensity of opioid effect. Absence of miosis suggests absence of opioid effect, however.

Nausea and vomiting. **Opioids produce complex effects on vomiting centers in the medulla (Fig. 54-6). There is direct stimulation of the chemoreceptor trigger zone (CTZ) in the area postrema on the floor of the fourth ventricle. This, in turn, activates the vomiting center proper, which is a deeper structure.**[17] The emetic effects are markedly potentiated by stimulation of the vestibular apparatus, so ambulatory patients are much more likely to vomit than those lying quietly. Postoperatively, patients frequently become nauseated when they have to move from stretcher to bed. Wang has shown that high doses of opioids can actually have antiemetic effects by depressing the vomiting center proper.[170] It is not clear at which dose a given opioid becomes antiemetic.

The emetic effects involve a complex interaction of dopaminergic, cholinergic, and serotonergic mechanisms. Antiemetic drugs have been developed that interact with each of these neurotransmitter systems: butyrophenones (droperidol), benzamides (metoclopramide), and phenothiazines (prochlorperazine) are dopamine antagonists; scopolamine and various antihistamines are cholinergic antagonists; and ondansetron inhibits nausea by blocking a subset of serotonin receptors.

Muscle rigidity. The opioids have no significant effects on nerve conduction, at the neuromuscular junction or at the skeletal muscle membrane.[49] In animals they produce minimal depression of monosynaptic and polysynaptic spinal reflexes, but the clinical relevance of this is not known.[106] **A much more important effect is the generalized hypertonus of skeletal muscle, which can be produced by large intravenous doses of most opioid agonists. Although morphine can produce rigidity, the problem is most commonly associated with fentanyl, alfentanil, and sufentanil.**

Opioid-induced rigidity was originally thought to

be restricted to the abdominal and thoracic musculature, but it is now known that muscles of the neck and extremities are involved as well.[18] The incidence and severity of the problem are greatest when large amounts of opioids are infused rapidly, but rigidity can occur with doses of only 1 to 2 μg/kg of fentanyl. This effect is usually seen at induction of anesthesia, just before, or at loss of consciousness. When very large amounts of opioid have been administered (e.g., for cardiac surgery), rigidity may occur upon emergence.[110] Rigidity is more likely to occur in older patients and when nitrous oxide is administered along with the opioid.[147]

In its most severe form, "lead pipe" muscle rigidity can totally prevent mechanical ventilation. The difficulty is caused, in part, by loss of chest wall compliance as well as constriction of laryngeal and pharyngeal muscles. Some have suggested that supraglottic obstruction is the more important problem.[6,147] Substantial amounts of positive pressure are sometimes needed for effective ventilation, and this can lead to decreased venous return, gastric insufflation, and so forth. Fortunately, rigidity is effectively treated (or prevented) by administering relatively small doses of muscle relaxants.

Opioids are believed to produce rigidity by actions at mu receptors in the striatum. Opioids increase the rate of striatal dopamine biosynthesis and inhibit the release of the inhibitory neurotransmitter gamma-amino butyric acid (GABA).[32] The benzodiazepines facilitate GABA neurotransmission, but they are not uniformly effective in preventing rigidity. In the rat, microinjection of opioid antagonists at certain raphe nuclei will selectively block rigidity.[175]

Cardiovascular effects

At normal analgetic doses opioids produce minimal cardiovascular effects. Bradycardia and peripheral vasodilation are seen at higher doses and when opioids are combined with other anesthetic drugs.

Opioids produce bradycardia by a specific stimulant effect on the central nuclei of the vagus nerves. In animals, microinjection of naloxone at these sites will antagonize the bradycardia, but not the analgesia, produced by intravenous fentanyl.[89] The bradycardic effect is most likely to occur when large doses of opioids are administered rapidly. It may be prevented or reversed by atropine, pancuronium, and other vagolytic drugs.[137] Opioid-induced bradycardia may be more frequent when a relaxant such as vecuronium is used because it lacks vagal blocking effects.[54] Meperidine, which is weakly atropinic, does not usually cause bradycardia.

The opioid-induced increase in vagal tone leads to a prolongation of AV conduction. There is also evidence of a direct depressant effect on the SA node.[166]

Morphine and fentanyl decrease central sympathetic tone, and this has been demonstrated to raise the threshold for ventricular fibrillation in the dog.[145]

Opioids produce peripheral vasodilation by depressing vasomotor centers in the medulla. Analgetic doses frequently cause orthostatic hypotension, and higher doses may significantly reduce venous return. There appear to be opioid actions on both resistance and capacitance vessels.[62] Zelis has shown that an analgetic dose of morphine increases blood flow through forearm skeletal muscle without altering systemic pressure.[178] This effect is thought to represent a centrally mediated lysis of sympathetic tone. Lowenstein et al. demonstrated that morphine's effect on skeletal muscle vascular resistance is neurally mediated and markedly increased under conditions of high sympathetic activity.[95] This is consistent with clinical observations: opioids are more apt to cause hypotension in patients with conditions that elevate the baseline level of sympathetic tone (e.g., hypovolemia, coronary artery disease, congestive failure).

There have been several studies suggesting a direct effect of opioids on vascular smooth muscle, but this is not universally accepted.[44,62] In the case of morphine, some vasodilation is caused by the release of histamine (discussed later).

Venodilation is also produced, and this may lead to significant pooling of blood, especially in the splanchnic vasculature. There is evidence in the dog that morphine causes blood to be sequestered in hepatic sinusoids, but it is not known if this is an important effect in man.[56,90] In both humans and animals opioid-induced venodilation seems to occur later and last longer than the effect on arterioles.[62,68]

At clinically relevant concentrations the opioids do not produce significant myocardial depression. The combination of slow heart rate, peripheral vasodilation, and minimal direct myocardial effects makes opioid-based anesthesia particularly useful for patients with cardiac ischemia or failure. When hypotension does occur, it frequently responds to simple measures like elevation of the legs and administration of intravenous fluids.

Histamine release

True allergic responses to opioids are very rare, although IgE-mediated anaphylaxis to meperidine has been reported.[92] Many opioids, but not all, produce a nonimmunologic release of histamine from tissue mast cells. This is most often seen as local itching, redness, or hives near the site of intravenous injection. Sometimes a patient will experience generalized flushing. When sufficient histamine is liberated, it may cause decreases in systemic vascular resistance, hypotension, and tachycardia.[142] The cardiovascular effects (but not the histamine release)

may be prevented by pretreatment with H₁ and H₂ antagonists like chlorpheniramine and cimetidine.[130]

This is a nonspecific effect that depends upon competitive displacement of the amine by opioid molecules. Because the more potent opioids present lower concentrations to tissue mast cells, they are less likely to cause release. **Morphine and meperidine release histamine (especially when large doses are administered for cardiac anesthesia), but the potent opioids fentanyl, sufentanil, and alfentanil do not**[43,143,155] **(Fig. 54-7).** Chemical structure also influences this process,

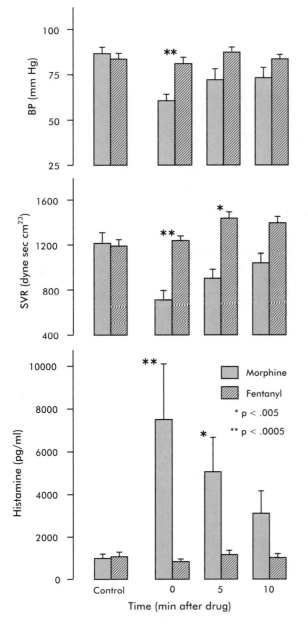

Fig. 54-7. Plasma histamine increases while mean arterial pressure *(BP)* and systemic vascular resistance *(SVR)* decrease in cardiac surgical patients given morphine 1 mg/ kg, IV. These effects do not occur after fentanyl 50 μg/kg, IV. (Rosow CE et al: Histamine release during morphine and fentanyl anesthesia, *Anesthesiology* 56:93, 1982.)

because even equimolar concentrations of fentanyl and morphine do not cause equivalent histamine release.[64]

Opioids should be used with great care on patients with asthma even though histamine release is not likely to be the primary cause of bronchospasm. These drugs may exacerbate preexisting bronchospasm by depressing cough and respiratory drive, and by drying airway secretions.

Frequently patients given opioids will complain of itching and warmth over the neck and face, especially over the malar area. Epidural administration of opioids can produce very troublesome generalized itching.[13] This effect is thought to be a dysesthesia produced at the brainstem level. It is not reliably treated with antihistamines, and it can be produced by opioids like fentanyl, which do not release histamine.

Smooth muscle effects

Intestine and stomach. Chronic administration of opioids frequently necessitates the administration of laxatives and stool softeners to treat constipation. This effect may also be used therapeutically in the treatment of diarrheal syndromes. **Opioids produce spasm of smooth muscle all along the GI tract. The mechanism involves both CNS effects and peripheral actions on opioid receptors in the bowel.**[162] **Both the small and large bowel become hypertonic, but rhythmic propulsive activity is diminished.** The delay in intestinal transit time and spasm of the anal sphincter are the causes of opioid-induced constipation.

The increase in resting tone is especially pronounced in patients with ulcerative colitis, and opioids may predispose the patient to the development of toxic megacolon. Meperidine and some of the agonist-antagonist opioids appear to cause less constipation.[156] Treatment of diarrhea is usually accomplished with opioids like diphenoxylate and loperamide. These compounds are poorly absorbed, so therapeutic doses do not usually produce central effects.

It is important to remember that opioids delay gastric emptying, and this may slow the absorption of oral medications, which are administered concomitantly. Food may not pass into the proximal jejunum for many hours, so surgical patients given opioids may remain at risk for aspiration despite nominal NPO status.

Biliary system. Opioids cause contraction of smooth muscle along the biliary tree and spasm of the sphincter of Oddi. In some individuals this can precipitate biliary colic. Intraoperatively, the same effect has been reported to cause false-positive cholangiograms and even to prevent instrumentation of the common duct.[28] The biliary effects may be completely antagonized by naloxone and partially reversed by glucagon, nitroglycerin, or atropine.[7,135]

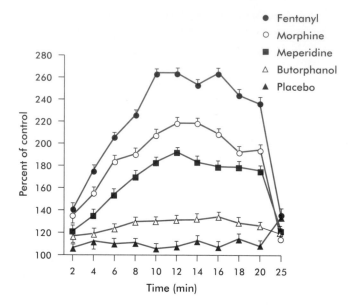

Fig. 54-8. Percentage change in common bile duct pressure vs. time following equianalgetic doses of several opioids. Patients were undergoing cholecystectomy with basal enflurane anesthesia. After 20 minutes, the effect was reversed by naloxone. (From Radnay PA et al: Common bile duct pressure changes after fentanyl, morphine, meperidine, butorphanol and naloxone, *Anesth Analg* 63:441, 1984.)

The biliary effects of meperidine appear to be smaller than those of morphine or fentanyl, but are still significant[135] (Fig. 54-8). The agonist-antagonist opioids have much smaller smooth muscle effects (see the following discussion).

Urinary tract. Opioids increase the contractions of the ureter although they relieve the pain caused by ureteral stones. They also increase the tone of the detrusor muscle of the bladder and the urinary sphincter by both central and peripheral mechanisms.[35] This may cause a sense of urinary urgency but an inability to void. Sufficient opioid may also make a patient inattentive to the stimulus of bladder distension. Urinary retention occurs much more commonly in men, and it is an especially frequent side effect when opioids are administered into the lumbar epidural space.

Hormonal effects

Morphine inhibits the release of gonadotropin-releasing hormone and corticotropin-releasing factor by acting on the hypothalamus.[167] The concentrations of testosterone and cortisol in plasma are decreased because the secretion of pituitary trophic hormones is inhibited.[29] Opioids also increase plasma levels of certain hormones such as growth hormone and prolactin. Over the short term, most of these hormonal changes are probably not clinically significant. Perhaps more importantly, surgery and pain can produce large increases in many hormones (the

so-called "stress" response), and opioids are able to blunt or abolish these responses (see discussion on intraoperative use).

Effects on pregnancy and the neonate

Opioids have no specific teratogenic effects, but chronic opioid use by the mother may lead to "addiction" in utero (actually physical dependence). Neonatal withdrawal may occur shortly following delivery, and, in some instances, may be life threatening.

Parenteral opioids are commonly used to treat labor pain. Because they cross the placenta readily, they may cause respiratory depression in the neonate. Morphine has been shown to produce more depression in the neonate than meperidine.[173] The newborn infant has an incompletely developed blood-brain barrier, so a dose of morphine that is appropriate for the mother may produce excessive effects in the baby. Meperidine is more lipophilic, and its effects in mother and infant are more comparable. Meperidine takes time to accumulate in the fetus, so the neonate may actually be less affected if the opioid is given very close to the time of delivery.[112,153] Naloxone may be required to reverse the effects of meperidine given repeatedly during a long labor.

Meperidine is preferred in obstetric applications for other reasons. Morphine is thought to depress uterine contractions and antagonize the effects of oxytocics. Meperidine may actually increase uterine contracility, and it does not seem to impair the progression of normal labor.[14]

Tolerance

There appear to be two types of tolerance to opioid action. When a large dose is administered by bolus or rapid infusion, *acute tolerance* or *tachyphylaxis* may occur. Acute tolerance to various opioid effects has been demonstrated in animals, but it is not clear whether this phenomenon occurs in clinical practice.[9] Bovill et al. have suggested that acute tolerance may occur to the hypnotic effect of large doses of alfentanil.[21] Tolerance can sometimes occur very rapidly when opioid infusions are used for sedation in intensive care settings.

The more common problem of *chronic tolerance* occurs when opioids are administered over longer periods of time. The first indication of tolerance is frequently a decrease in the duration of analgesia after each dose, but eventually the intensity of effect declines as well. Tolerance may be overcome, in most cases, by an increase in the dose of the opioid. Occasionally, a patient will present with profound tolerance, and huge doses may be required to produce an adequate effect.[140] Regional blocks and nonopioid methods of pain relief may be better choices in this circumstance.

When tolerance to an opioid occurs, there is simultaneous development of *cross-tolerance* to all other opioid agonists. In general, tolerance develops most rapidly to the effects we have described as depressant (analgesia, respiratory depression, euphoria), but much less tolerance occurs to some of the stimulant effects like constipation or pupillary constriction. For example, a heroin addict who is placed on chronic methadone treatment becomes tolerant to the euphoriant effect but frequently continues to have miosis and constipation. Similarly, constipation is a common problem for the terminal cancer patient who requires large doses of morphine for relief of pain.

Physical dependence

After sufficient doses have been administered, all opioids induce a state of physical dependence. Abruptly stopping the drug or administering an antagonist then causes a stereotypic withdrawal syndrome. The symptoms of withdrawal can be rapidly terminated with small doses of intravenous morphine. This topic is discussed in more detail in Chapter 102.

Some authorities believe that medically induced physical dependence is common, and clinically imperceptible dependence may actually be present after only a few injections of a potent opioid. In most cases withdrawal may occur without the patient or physician being aware of it. Physical dependence is not the same thing as *psychologic dependence* or *addiction,* which includes the dimension of compulsive drug-seeking behavior. The data of Porter and Jick suggest that addiction resulting from appropriate medical treatment is a very unusual event.[133] Irrational fear of causing patients to become addicted has been cited as a frequent cause for the inadequate treatment of acute pain.[99]

When a patient with known physical dependence is to be detoxified, he/she is commonly switched to methadone, and the dose is reduced slowly. This produces a mild though protracted withdrawal syndrome. However, when a person addicted to heroin or methadone presents emergently for medical treatment, he/she is generally not an appropriate candidate for detoxification (see Chapter 102).

Pharmacokinetics

As discussed previously, the onset or duration of effect is most often the basis for selection of a particular opioid. The clinically available opioid agonists vary greatly in their physicochemical properties and therefore in their absorption and distribution throughout the body. Important physicochemical properties of several opioids are listed in Table 54-2, and pharmacokinetic parameters for the same drugs are listed in Table 54-3. It should be noted that there is tremendous variability in the published values for

Table 54-2 Physicochemical properties of some opioid agonists

Drug	pKa	Percent of ionized drug (pH 7.4)	Partition coefficient*
Morphine	7.9/9.4	76	1.4
Meperidine	8.5	95	38.8
Fentanyl	8.4	91	860
Sufentanil	8.0	80	1778
Alfentanil	6.5	11	130

*The n-octanol/water partition coefficient (corrected for the percentage of drug unionized at pH 7.4) is a measure of liquid solubility.

most of these pharmacokinetic parameters. Some of this variability reflects true differences between patient populations, whereas some is the result of sampling times and other technical aspects of measurement.

Morphine

Morphine is the least lipophilic of the opioids listed, and this has two important implications for its pharmacokinetics: morphine penetrates biologic membranes more slowly than lipophilic opioids, and it is less likely to accumulate in lipid membranes or fatty tissues. The plasma pharmacokinetics of morphine are similar to those of a fat soluble drug. It is rapidly absorbed after intramuscular, subcutaneous, or oral administration.[25] After an intravenous bolus, plasma concentrations decline rapidly as the drug is distributed into well-perfused tissues. Only about 25% to 35% is bound to plasma proteins, primarily albumin.[125] The steady-state volume of distribution is very large, and it is probably made up of nonfatty tissues.

Morphine is eliminated primarily by hepatic biotransformation with about 5% to 15% excreted unchanged in the urine. The rate of hepatic clearance is very high, and this accounts for the relatively short elimination half-life. The hepatic extraction of morphine is approximately 0.7; that is, 70% is cleared in one pass through the liver. Morphine is therefore subject to flow-dependent elimination, and factors that decrease hepatic blood flow will prolong its elimination. High hepatic clearance also means that morphine is subject to a large first-pass effect, and larger doses are required when the drug is given orally.

Over 90% of a dose of morphine is metabolized and excreted within 24 hours. The primary route of metabolism is conjugation in the liver to produce morphine 3-glucuronide and morphine 6-glucuronide. A small amount of morphine is N-demethylated to form normorphine.[111] These polar metabolites are

Table 54-3 Pharmacokinetic properties of some opioid agonists

Drug	T1/2α (min)	T1/2β (hr)	Vdss (L/kg)	Clearance (ml/kg/min)	Protein binding (%)
Morphine	1.7 (19.8)	3-4	3.2-4.7	12.4-15.2	30
Meperidine	7-11	3-4	2.8-4.2	10.1-16.4	64
Fentanyl	1.8 (13.2)	4-7	3.2-4.2	11.2-13.3	84
Sufentanil	17.7	2.5	1.7	13.0	92
Alfentanil	11.6	1-1.6	0.86	6.4	92

then excreted in the urine and bile.[25] Morphine 6-glucuronide, which may constitute 15% of total morphine metabolites, has been shown to possess greater analgetic activity than the parent molecule.[129] The presence of a potent active metabolite may contribute to morphine's long duration of action.

The plasma pharmacokinetics of morphine do *not* parallel its clinical effects. In spite of morphine's rapid distribution and elimination, the onset and offset of analgesia are rather slow. Morphine enters the central nervous system with difficulty, and peak analgetic effects may not occur for 15 to 30 minutes after intravenous injection. Hug demonstrated in dogs that peak respiratory depression did not occur for 30 to 60 minutes following an intravenous bolus of

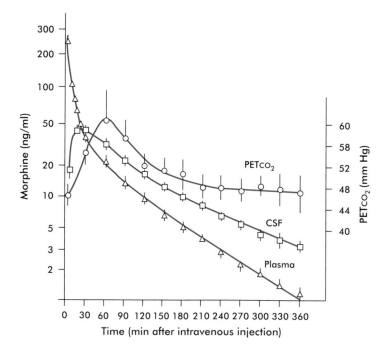

Fig. 54-9. Concentration of morphine in plasma and CSF and end-tidal CO2 (PETCO2) vs. time in six dogs given 0.3 mg/kg and allowed to breathe spontaneously (see text for details). (Hug CC Jr, Murphy MR: Fentanyl disposition in cerebrospinal fluid and plasma and its relationship to ventilatory depression in the dog, *Anesthesiology* 50:342, 1979.)

morphine[72] (Fig. 54-9). During the recovery period, Hug showed that concentrations of cerebrospinal fluid declined more slowly than those in plasma, and the decline in ventilatory depression was slower still.

Herz has shown that only a small fraction of a dose of morphine injected into animals enters the brain. At the time of peak effect, the concentration of morphine in the brain is much less than that in the blood.[65] Redistribution of morphine from brain to blood is delayed because plasma concentrations must drop substantially before the concentration gradient favors movement of drug out of the CNS.

Meperidine

This substituted phenylpiperidine is significantly more lipid soluble than morphine although its plasma pharmacokinetics are similar. The onset of analgetic effect is faster than morphine, and the duration is shorter (2 to 3 hours). Meperidine is rapidly distributed into a large apparent volume of distribution, and it has a very high rate of clearance by hepatic biotransformation.[102,168] The high hepatic extraction means that meperidine undergoes significant (48% to 56%) first-pass metabolism. The elimination half-life has been estimated as 3 to 7 hours—which is similar to or longer than that of morphine. Meperidine is more highly protein bound than morphine (65%-80%), and it is bound mainly to alpha-1-acid glycoprotein.

Meperidine is rapidly N-demethylated to form normeperidine; the other major metabolites are meperidinic acid and normeperidinic acid. Less than 7% of a dose is excreted unchanged in the urine. The metabolism of meperidine plays a significant role in its pharmacodynamics. In the mouse, normeperidine is an analgetic with about half the potency of meperidine; unfortunately, in both mouse and man it is a potent convulsant.[108] This toxic metabolite has an elimination half-life of 8 to 12 hours, so significant amounts may accumulate. Seizures have occurred in patients with renal failure (who could not excrete normeperidine) and in cancer patients who received high doses of meperidine over long periods of time.[163]

A large amount of data has been obtained on the correlation between meperidine plasma concentration and its pharmacodynamic effects. For meperidine the relationship between plasma level and analgesia is both predictable and useful. Austin et al. titrated meperidine to analgetic effect in postsurgical patients. For each individual, the change from no pain relief to excellent pain relief occurred over a very narrow range of plasma concentrations, and this level was fairly consistent over a 2-day period.[11] In contrast, there was a large variability (40%) in meperidine requirement between individuals. These data are remarkably similar to those describing the relationship of alfentanil concentration to intraoperative analgetic response[10] (see section on intraoperative analgesia). The data on meperidine have been used to demonstrate that our traditional dosage regimens for relief of acute pain often result in inadequate or excessive plasma concentrations.

Fentanyl

This potent synthetic opioid is extremely fat soluble, which accounts for its rapid onset and relatively short duration. After intravenous administration fentanyl is rapidly distributed to the brain, heart, and other highly perfused tissues (the "central compartment").[71] Unlike morphine, fentanyl crosses the blood-brain barrier easily, and its peak effect occurs in only 3 to 5 minutes. Within a short time, the drug is then distributed extensively throughout the body (steady-state volume of distribution is more than 4 L/kg), so plasma levels drop precipitously. Herz has shown in rabbits that only 3 to 5 minutes after an intravenously administered dose of fentanyl the level of drug in brain is over 10 times that in plasma.[65] This large concentration gradient then favors redistribution of fentanyl away from the central nervous system, and thus terminates the effect (the similarity to thiopental should be apparent).[71]

When redistribution is mostly completed, the elimination phase begins, and plasma levels fall much more slowly. Fentanyl is biotransformed in the liver to inactive metabolites, primarily norfentanyl and several hydroxylation products.[52] Only 6% to 8% is excreted unchanged in the urine. The hepatic clearance of fentanyl is very high (12 to 13 ml/kg/min), and more than 60% is cleared in one pass. The large distribution volume, however, means that most of the drug remains extravascular and unavailable for biotransformation. The long elimination half-life of fentanyl (3 to 4 hours) is a function of the slow rate at which it reenters the central compartment.[105]

Fentanyl concentration in the plasma correlates well with CSF concentration and pharmacodynamic effect. Fentanyl plasma pharmacokinetics therefore predict some of its more important pharmacodynamic properties:

- **When low doses (1 to 3 μg/kg) are administered, redistribution (half-life 13 minutes) terminates the effect, and the drug appears short-acting[118] (Fig. 54-10). A dose of 100 to 200 μg of fentanyl generally lasts less than 1 hour.**
- When much larger doses are given (e.g., >20 μg/kg), redistribution is not sufficient to bring plasma concentrations to subtherapeutic levels. Termination of effect depends instead on the much slower elimination process, and the drug appears long-acting[118] (see Fig. 54-10). The distribution and elimination half-lives do not change with dosage (fentanyl obeys first-order kinetics throughout the clinical dose range).[117]
- **The long elimination half-life means that repeated intravenous boluses of fentanyl are very likely to produce cumulative effects.**
- **The high hepatic extraction ratio (0.6) means the clearance of fentanyl is limited by hepatic blood flow. Factors that lower hepatic blood flow (e.g., intraabdominal surgery, cardiopulmonary bypass) can decrease elimination of fentanyl.**
- **Because fentanyl undergoes substantial first-pass metabolism, the oral route is inefficient. The drug is well absorbed when given transdermally,**

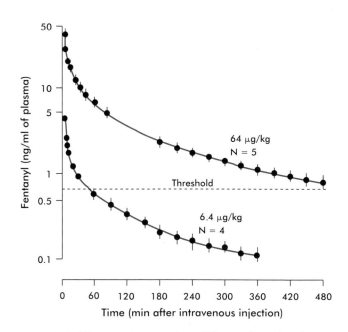

Fig. 54-10. Plasma concentration of fentanyl vs. time in dogs given either 6.4 or 64 μg/kg intravenously. Threshold represents the concentration above which depression of ventilation occurs (see text for details). Effects of the lower dose are terminated by redistribution; those of the higher dose are terminated by elimination. (From Murphy MR, Olson WA, and Hug CC Jr: Pharmacokinetics of ³H-fentanyl in the dog anesthetized with enflurane, *Anesthesiology* 50:13, 1979.)

intranasally, or via the oral mucosa.[53,121] These routes bypass the portal circulation and result in high blood levels.

Sufentanil

This thienyl derivative of fentanyl is more potent and even more fat soluble. In most respects its pharmacokinetics resemble those of fentanyl[23] (see Table 54-3). The drug is rapidly and extensively distributed, and the effects of small doses are terminated by redistribution. The elimination half-life of sufentanil is shorter than that of fentanyl, because its volume of distribution is slightly smaller, and the hepatic clearance is greater (extraction ratio = 0.7). Sufentanil is metabolized by N-dealkylation and O-demethylation.

Sufentanil has had extensive use in cardiac surgery, where it is given in very large doses (8-30 μg/kg).[138] At these doses, opioid effects are terminated by elimination rather than redistribution. Profound analgesia and respiratory depression last for many hours, although extubation is usually possible earlier than with comparable doses of fentanyl.[146] The kinetics are dramatically affected by cardiopulmonary bypass: plasma levels drop with hemodilution, but the huge amounts sequestered in lung and muscle cause a secondary increase when the bypass is discontinued.[124] Large amounts of sufentanil can also be bound to oxygenators and tubing in the bypass circuit.

The fat solubility of sufentanil allows it to be absorbed rapidly through intact skin and mucous membranes.[61] When it is given epidurally, it produces a block that is rapid in onset, and fairly short in duration.[82]

Alfentanil

Alfentanil is a slightly less potent congener of fentanyl, and has an extremely rapid onset and short duration of effect.[160] Peak analgetic and respiratory depressant effects occur in less than 2 minutes, and the duration of the effects of small doses (10 μg/kg) may last only 15 minutes. There has been intense interest in this drug, because its short duration seems particularly suitable for perioperative use in outpatients. The pharmacokinetics of alfentanil are unusually well studied; some of the more important pharmacokinetic parameters are listed in Table 54-3.

The pharmacokinetic behavior of fentanyl and alfentanil is qualitatively similar. A single bolus of alfentanil undergoes rapid redistribution and then slower elimination. Termination of alfentanil effects after small doses still depends upon redistribution, and the effects of larger doses (100-200 μg/kg) may be prolonged. Alfentanil is less lipophilic than fentanyl, and it has much less tendency to bind nonspecifically in muscle and fat. This is reflected in smaller initial and steady-state volumes of distribution.[24]

Alfentanil is rapidly metabolized by N-dealkylation and O-demethylation, and very little of the drug is excreted unchanged in the urine.[24,63] The relatively small steady-state volume of distribution is less than one quarter that of fentanyl. This means that considerably more alfentanil remains in the blood stream and is thus available for hepatic metabolism. In spite of the fact that the liver clears alfentanil more slowly than fentanyl, the total body clearance is faster and the elimination half-life is shorter.[160]

The elimination half-life of alfentanil is about 80 to 100 minutes in most healthy patients. This is substantially shorter than fentanyl, so alfentanil is much less likely to produce cumulative effects after repeated doses. Rapid elimination also makes this opioid particularly suitable for administration by continuous infusion.[10,152]

Like fentanyl and sufentanil, alfentanil is sufficiently fat soluble to enter the CNS with ease. Its onset is markedly faster, which is apparently the result of several factors:

- The central compartment for alfentanil is smaller, so the initial plasma level (before distribution) is higher. A larger concentration gradient, therefore, drives alfentanil from blood to CSF.
- Alfentanil has a pKa of 6.5, which means that it exists in predominantly unionized form at body pH. Fentanyl, by contrast, has a pKa of 8.4 and is 90% ionized. Not only does more alfentanil remain in the central compartment, but more of it exists in a diffusible (uncharged) form.
- Compared to fentanyl, alfentanil probably undergoes much less nonspecific binding in brain tissue. It is 22 times less soluble than fentanyl in rat brain.[20] Theoretically, this leaves a larger concentration of drug available for specific receptor binding, and occupancy of these sites may occur more rapidly.

Faster receptor occupancy is somewhat conjectural, but the time for equilibration between brain and plasma is unequivocally more rapid with alfentanil than fentanyl.[69] Scott et al. investigated volunteers given a brief infusion of either fentanyl or alfentanil at a sufficient rate to produce slowing of the electroencephalogram (EEG)[148] (Fig. 54-11). Both opioids produced a decrease in the average EEG frequency as the plasma level increased; when the infusions were terminated, the EEG reverted to normal fast frequencies. In the fentanyl group, there was a delay of 2 to 3 minutes before measurable slowing occurred, and these effects persisted for 20 to 30 minutes after the infusion was discontinued. In the alfentanil group, the onset and offset of effect were much more closely correlated to the rise and fall in plasma levels. It is a reasonable (but unproven) assumption that other brain effects, like

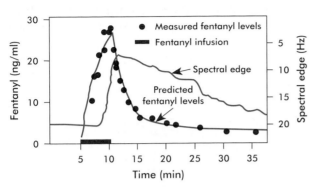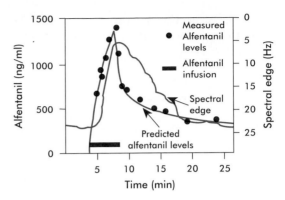

Fig. 54-11. Plasma concentration of fentanyl or alfentanil vs. time with simultaneous measurement of EEG spectral edge. Volunteers were given 150 μg/min fentanyl or 1500 μg/min alfentanil. Increasing opioid effect is depicted as a decrease in average EEG frequency and spectral edge. Changes in spectral edge follow plasma concentrations more closely for alfentanil (see text for details). (From Scott JC, Ponganis KV, and Stanski DR: EEG quantitation of narcotic effect: the comparative pharmacodynamics of fentanyl and alfentanil, *Anesthesiology* 62:234, 1985.

analgesia and respiratory depression, will also track plasma levels very closely.

Intraoperative Use of Opioid Agonists

Although opium extracts were used hundreds of years ago in "soporific sponges," the modern concept of an opioid-based general anesthetic did not evolve until quite recently. Gray and Rees defined general anesthesia as a "triad" consisting of narcosis (i.e., hypnosis), analgesia, and muscle relaxation.[55] The opioids by themselves do not produce muscle relaxation, and even high doses may sometimes fail to produce sleep. In the days before muscle relaxants, endotracheal tubes, and controlled ventilation, high doses of morphine were tried alone as total anesthetics and found to be both dangerous and only marginally effective.

Balanced anesthesia

In 1942, Griffiths introduced curare, which made it possible for muscle relaxation to be achieved during relatively light levels of anesthesia.[57] **The first attempts at "balanced" anesthesia used curare together with thiopental and nitrous oxide, but these techniques usually failed to block autonomic responses to surgical stimuli. In 1947, Neff et al. introduced a more satisfactory anesthetic that included small doses of meperidine in combination with thiopental, curare, and nitrous oxide.[120] Although the individual components have changed over the years, this technique is the basis for modern balanced anesthesia.**

In the 1950s the major tranquilizers (phenothiazines and butyrophenones) were introduced into clinical practice. DeCastro and Mundeleer described a technique called *neuroleptanalgesia* in which a butyrophenone (e.g., droperidol) was combined with fentanyl.[33] This combination does not necessarily cause sleep or amnesia, but it produces analgesia, apparent indifference to stimuli, immobility, and autonomic stability. When nitrous oxide is added to produce sleep, the technique is called *neuroleptanesthesia*. This form of balanced anesthesia is still somewhat popular in Europe and the United States.

Intraoperative analgesia

Analgesia is sometimes difficult to assess or even to define in a patient who is not awake. In general, we consider intraoperative analgesia to be a reduction in autonomic and somatic responses to noxious surgical stimuli. The cardiovascular responses to incision, laryngoscopy, and other painful events are blunted much more effectively by opioids than by most other intravenous agents[100] (Fig. 54-12).

Analgesia may also be measured by the decreasing requirement for other anesthetic agents. **The administration of opioids potentiates the hypnotic effects of barbiturates and benzodiazepines (and probably propofol)[17,81] (Fig. 54-13). By reducing the amount of hypnotic administered, an opioid can sometimes produce more rapid emergence. The opioids also produce a dramatic, dose-related decrease in the need for volatile anesthetics, and they are frequently used for this specific purpose. The minimum alveolar** concentration (MAC) of enflurane, for example, is decreased as the plasma concentration of fentanyl is increased[115] (Fig. 54-14). For pure opioid agonists, this effect seems to reach a plateau when the MAC has been reduced by about 70%. The mixed agonist-antagonists produce lower maximal effects.[116]

The amount of opioid analgetic required varies tremendously from patient to patient. Shafer et al.

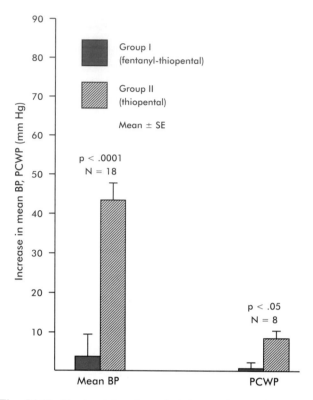

Fig. 54-12. Fentanyl 8 μg/kg, administered intravenously, prevents the increase in mean systemic and wedge pressure following laryngoscopy and intubation. All patients were given thiopental and pancuronium. (From Martin DE et al: Low-dose fentanyl blunts circulatory responses to tracheal intubation, *Anesth Analg* 61:680, 1982.)

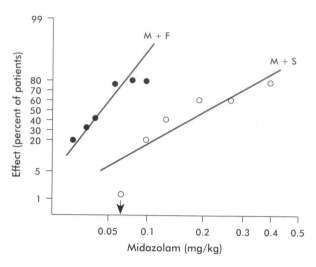

Fig. 54-13. Percentage of patients asleep vs. dose of midazolam on a log-probit plot. Curve is shifted to the left in the presence of fentanyl 1.9 μg/kg (M + F) compared to midazolam plus saline (M + S). (From Ben-Schlomo I: Midazolam acts synergistically with fentanyl for induction of anesthesia, *Br J Anaesth* 64:45, 1990.)

found a great deal of individual variability in both alfentanil pharmacokinetics and in the response to a given level of drug in plasma.[152] Administration of alfentanil at a fixed infusion rate resulted in inadequate anesthesia in some patients and postoperative respiratory depression in others. The population pharmacokinetics of alfentanil have recently been reviewed by Maitre et al.[97]

The requirement for opioid also depends upon the nature of the surgical stimulus. Ausems and Hug demonstrated this in patients receiving nitrous oxide and a continuous infusion of alfentanil.[10] The infusions were titrated to clinical response, and plasma concentrations were measured simultaneously. The Cp50 (the plasma concentration necessary to prevent a response in 50% of patients) was calculated for each stimulus. The study showed, for example, that the Cp50 for tracheal intubation was 475 ng/ml of alfentanil, but skin closure required only 150 ng/ml (Fig. 54-15). These investigators also found twofold to threefold differences in opioid sensitivity between individuals, but for each patient, the change between adequate and inadequate analgesia occurred over a very small range of plasma concentrations. The

challenge for the anesthesiologist is to find the clinical endpoint that establishes this narrow range for the individual patient.

How does one titrate an opioid intraoperatively? Decreasing respiratory rate or depth is usually a reliable sign of increasing opioid effect if the case permits spontaneous ventilation. More commonly, the rise in blood pressure and other autonomic responses to a "painful" stimulus are gauged. Unfortunately, autonomic responses are nonspecific and may be produced by many conditions that do not involve pain. Unlike the volatile anesthetics, the opioids do not produce graded cardiovascular depression as depth increases. Normal blood pressure does not necessarily mean that the anesthetic level is appropriate, because large overdoses of most opioids are well tolerated as long as ventilation is supported. Thus far other physiologic endpoints such as processed EEG, EMG, cortical-evoked potentials, lower esophageal contractility, and so forth have not been found to be reliable monitors of anesthetic depth.

The dose of opioid will also need to be modified according to the patient's age and physical condition. Opioid pharmacodynamics are altered in patients who are elderly,[149] hypovolemic, or debilitated, in those with significant CNS disease, and in those who have received other CNS depressants. Opioid pharmacokinetics are altered at the extremes of age and in a variety of disease states. The clearance of morphine, meperidine, fentanyl, and alfentanil is probably decreased in the elderly and the neonate. Pharmacokinetic differences due to age are frequently less than

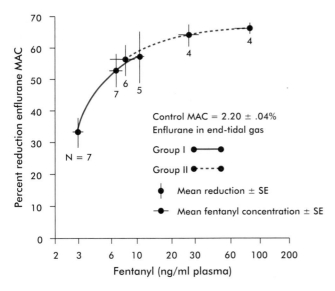

Fig. 54-14. Percentage decrease in MAC for enflurane vs. plasma concentration of fentanyl in the dog. Maximal effect is about 70% decrease in MAC for other opioid agonists as well (see text for details). (From Murphy MR, Hug CC Jr: The anesthetic potency of fentanyl in terms of its reduction of enflurane MAC, *Anesthesiology* 57.485, 1982.)

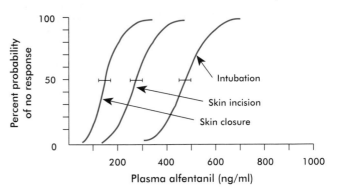

Fig. 54-15. Percentage probability of no response to various stimuli vs. plasma concentration of alfentanil. Patients received 66% nitrous oxide and muscle relaxants. During balanced anesthesia, much lower concentrations of alfentanil are required for skin incision and closure than for intubation. (From Ausems ME et al: Plasma concentrations of alfentanil required to supplement nitrous oxide anesthesia for general surgery, *Anesthesiology* 65:362, 1986.)

those attributable to the variability between individuals. Hepatic dysfunction must usually be severe before it produces a substantial change in opioid pharmacokinetics. The clearances of morphine,[83,103] sufentanil,[27] and alfentanil[39] are reduced in cirrhosis, but those of fentanyl[59] are not greatly affected. Interestingly, renal failure can cause an increase in the effect of morphine,[2,26] and there have been several cases of respiratory depression reported in such patients. The mechanism may be delayed renal excretion of morphine's active metabolite.

High-dose opioid anesthesia

Some aspects of high-dose opioid anesthesia will be discussed in more depth in Chapter 72. In 1969 Lowenstein et al. showed that high doses of morphine (>1 mg/kg) with controlled ventilation, 100% oxygen, and a muscle relaxant could be used to produce profound analgesia and sleep.[94] Hemodynamics were not changed appreciably in patients without heart disease; in patients with aortic valvular disease, hemodynamics actually improved because preload and afterload were reduced. Within a few years, morphine was being widely used as a sole anesthetic agent in cardiac surgery. At that time, the coronary bypass graft was a new procedure, and many morphine anesthetics were given to relatively healthy patients with angina. The drawbacks of the technique rapidly became apparent[93]:

■ Rapid administration of morphine could pro-

duce hypotension caused by histamine release and neurally mediated vasodilation (see discussion of cardiovascular effects).

■ Sleep was not reliably produced, and cases of intraoperative awareness occurred.

■ The addition of nitrous oxide produced myocardial depression and increases in pulmonary vascular resistance.[86]

■ Respiratory depression lasted for many hours, and prolonged mechanical ventilation was required.

■ In spite of the large analgetic dose, hypertension frequently occurred during surgical manipulations.

A 1973 study showed that increasing the dose of morphine to nearly 10 mg/kg did not create a satisfactory anesthetic.[158] This huge dose of morphine produced profound venodilation, unacceptable hypotension, and increased fluid requirements. Patients became edematous, and peripheral perfusion was sufficiently compromised to produce metabolic acidosis. These untoward effects were probably partly the result of splanchnic pooling and partly the result of histamine release.

In an effort to create an opioid anesthetic with fewer side effects, Stanley evaluated high doses of fentanyl in a variety of cardiac surgical populations.[96,157] Doses as high as 50 to 100 μg/kg were found to produce relatively modest decreases in systemic pressure and total peripheral resistance. As noted earlier, even huge doses of fentanyl did not release histamine.[142] These differences have turned out to be clinically significant, and during the last 10 years the use of fentanyl has virtually replaced that of morphine for this indication. Sufentanil was introduced more recently and, in doses of 8 to 30 μg/kg, it seems to share all of fentanyl's hemodynamic advantages as an opioid anesthetic.[138]

Why give such huge doses of these opioids? If no other anesthetic agents are administered, very large doses are *required* to produce sleep.[12,155] Profound analgesia has several advantages in this patient population: induction is usually smooth and well tolerated, even by patients with limited myocardial reserve; most hemodynamic responses to surgery are suppressed. This type of anesthesia can also block the release of many "stress" hormones (catecholamines, insulin, growth hormone, ADH, cortisol, renin, etc.) during major surgery.[22,85,151] The long duration of the opioid effect also allows for a smooth transition to mechanical ventilation in the immediate postoperative period.

The limitations of high-dose fentanyl and sufentanil are qualitatively similar to those of morphine anesthesia: intraoperative awareness is less common, but still a possibility. Recall has been reported after fentanyl doses as high as 90 μg/kg.[113] Prolonged ventilatory depression still occurs, and addition of nitrous oxide can still produce myocardial depression. Even very high plasma concentrations of fentanyl or sufentanil will not block all hemodynamic and hor-

monal responses to surgery[131] (Fig. 54-16). Certain reflex cardiovascular responses seem particularly resistant; for example, the reflex hypertension and tachycardia that is elicited by manipulation of the heart and great vessels. The stress hormonal responses that occur during cardiopulmonary bypass are not completely eliminated by opioids.[22,151]

In clinical practice, "pure" opioid anesthesia (without adjuvant anesthetic drugs) is rarely performed. Most patients receive premedication and a variety of inhalation or intravenous agents to control hemodynamics during surgery. Even a small dose of hypnotic or a volatile anesthetic can have marked cardiovascular effects when it is given in this setting. High-dose fentanyl, for example, produces a dramatic fall in peripheral resistance when the patient has been premedicated with intravenous diazepam.[165]

The paradox of opioid anesthesia is that it is used both for suppression and preservation of autonomic function. Opioids suppress autonomic responses to pain, but they are used to anesthetize critically ill patients because they preserve many essential hemodynamic reflexes. Unlike the volatile anesthetics, morphine does not block arteriolar constriction in response to sympathetic nerve stimulation or circulating catecholamines.[172] Unlike the volatile anesthetics, a fentanyl-diazepam combination does not block high- or low-pressure baroreceptor responses.[37]

Perhaps the most interesting perspective on high-dose opioid anesthesia came from a study by Wynands et al. who compared high-dose fentanyl anesthesia in patients with good or poor left ventricular function.[177] In spite of the fact that comparable plasma concentrations of fentanyl were maintained in the two groups, hypertensive episodes occurred almost exclusively in patients with good left ventricular function. Rather than being a sign of inadequate fentanyl, the occurrence of hypertension was a predictor for adequate myocardium. These patients tolerate—and require—supplemental intravenously administered or inhaled anesthetic agents.

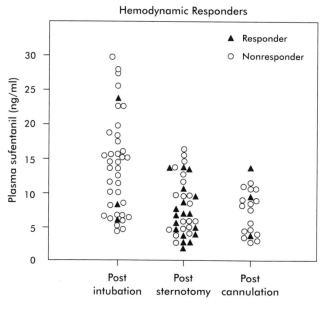

Fig. 54-16. Presence or absence of hemodynamic response vs. plasma concentration of sufentanil at three times during cardiac surgery. Patients undergoing coronary revascularization received only sufentanil, 100% oxygen, and muscle relaxant. Response was defined as increase in blood pressure of 15% or more over control value while awake. Given alone, even extremely high concentrations of sufentanil did not block all responses. (From Philbin DM et al: Fentanyl and sufentanil anesthesia revisited: how much is enough? *Anesthesiology* 73:5, 1990.)

OPIOID ANTAGONISTS
Naloxone

The only pure antagonist currently available for parenteral use is naloxone (Fig. 54-17, *A*), the N-allyl derivative of oxymorphone. Naloxone acts as a competitive antagonist at all opioid receptors, but it has greatest affinity for mu receptors. Small doses of naloxone reliably reverse or prevent the effects of pure opioid agonists and most mixed agonist-antagonists. The block is reversible and competitive, so it can be overcome by additional agonist. Naloxone probably has no effect on nonnarcotic anesthetics, although this remains somewhat controversial.[36,40,41]

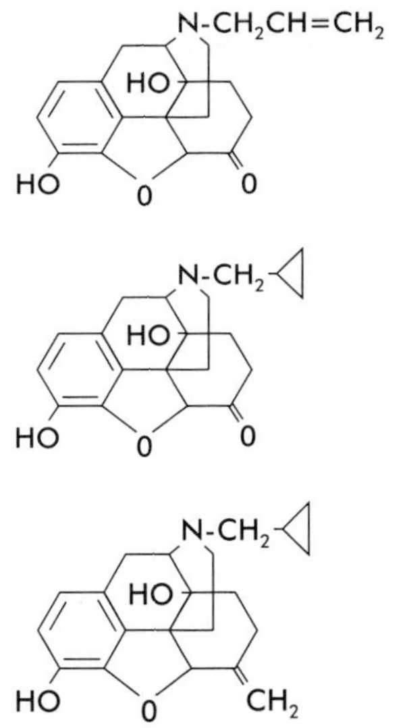

Fig. 54-17. Structural formulas of naloxone (**A**), naltrexone (**B**), and nalmefene (**C**).

Given alone, naloxone is nearly devoid of clinically demonstrable effects. In man, large doses (4 mg/kg) cause a mild increase in heart rate and systolic blood pressure,[31] as well as slowing of EEG alpha-wave activity.[169] Animal studies have also shown that naloxone can reduce food intake, alter sleep patterns, and improve spatial learning. In some disease states such as septic shock, large doses can have a pressor effect. This may be the result of antagonism of elevated endogenous opioid peptides.[19]

Naloxone is rapidly distributed and easily crosses the blood-brain barrier. Plasma and brain levels fall precipitously because of rapid redistribution.[122] The drug is rapidly cleared by hepatic biotransformation, mainly to the 3-glucuronide.[111] The clearance is very high (approximately 30 ml/kg/min), which suggests that extrahepatic elimination may be occurring. The terminal elimination half-life is 1 to 2 hours. **The onset of antagonist effect is extremely rapid, but because of rapid redistribution and elimination, the duration of action is quite brief. An IV dose of 0.4 mg will usually antagonize morphine for less than 1 hour; increasing the dose does not increase the duration appreciably.**[38]

Mild overnarcotization is a common problem in the postoperative setting. Small doses of naloxone (0.04 mg/kg in an adult, repeated every 3 minutes) can be given intravenously, usually with dramatic improvement. In many cases there is partial reversal of analgesia as well, but this can be minimized by careful dosing. Patients who receive naloxone need continued observation, and possibly repeated doses. Postoperative respiratory compromise is frequently caused by a combination of factors, and therapy with naloxone does not eliminate the need to search for and treat conditions like residual paralysis, bronchospasm, and airway edema.

Naloxone is used to reverse opioids in several other clinical settings:

- In the delivery suite naloxone may be used in depressed neonates whose mothers received opioids during labor. Clark showed that 0.01 mg/kg via an umbilical catheter was usually sufficient.[30] Acidotic infants were slower to reverse and sometimes required a second dose.
- In the emergency ward, 0.4 to 0.8 mg of naloxone is usually administered in cases of suspected heroin overdose. Naloxone is also useful as an aid in the differential diagnosis of coma; if a patient fails to respond to naloxone, non-opioid causes should be considered.
- Patients who receive epidural or intrathecal opioids are frequently troubled by side effects like pruritus and urinary retention (see Chapter 65). An IV infusion of naloxone will prevent or reverse these side effects, but it may also produce an unacceptable reduction in analgesia.[58]

Opioid reversal can sometimes have important hemodynamic consequences. Increases in systemic pressure, heart rate, and plasma levels of catecholamines can occur. This may be because of the sudden onset of pain, but these effects have been reproduced experimentally in the absence of painful stimuli.[109] There have been several case reports of fulminant pulmonary edema, dysrhythmias, and even death in young, previously healthy individuals given naloxone.[5] In one case, the dose of naloxone was only 0.1 mg.[127] The etiology of this rare, catastrophic response is not known.

Naltrexone

This is the N-cyclopropylmethyl derivative of oxymorphone (Fig. 54-17, *B*). It is a relatively pure antagonist like naloxone. It is available only in an oral preparation. The main clinical use of naltrexone is in the treatment of previously detoxified heroin addicts. When high doses are given chronically, naltrexone will block the euphoriant effects of injected heroin and thus help to prevent relapse.

Naltrexone is rapidly absorbed and undergoes 95% first-pass metabolism to 6-beta-naltrexol. This is an active metabolite that probably accounts for most of naltrexone's activity.[50] The metabolite accumulates during chronic treatment; it has an elimination half-life of 12.9 hours, so significant antagonist effects may persist for 2 to 3 days after naltrexone is stopped.

In the event that a patient on naltrexone requires emergency surgery or treatment for acute pain, he or she should be managed (if possible) with regional anesthesia, nonsteroidal antiinflammatory analgetics, and other nonopioid methods. If opioids are necessary, naltrexone antagonism is competitive and may be overcome with high doses of morphine or fentanyl.

Nalmefene

Nalmefene is a potent, extremely long-lasting pure antagonist that is currently undergoing clinical trials. It is the 6-methylene derivative of naltrexone (Fig. 54-17, *C*). Gal and DiFazio have shown that 2 mg of nalmefene can block the effects of repeated fentanyl injections for more than 8 hours.[47] The long duration of nalmefene is probably because of its extensive distribution and long terminal half-life (9 hours).

Reversal with nalmefene can probably cause some of the undesirable autonomic activation seen with naloxone. A single dose of nalmefene should certainly prevent renarcotization in most cases, and infusions are unlikely to be necessary. Nalmefene should be titrated carefully, because it can potentially eliminate all opioid analgesia for a very long period of time.

OPIOID AGONIST-ANTAGONISTS
General Properties

The agonist-antagonist opioids are synthetic and semisynthetic analgetics that are structurally related to morphine (Fig. 54-18). They have been used primarily for moderate to severe acute pain, although the indications for their perioperative use have been broadened in recent years.[141] All these compounds produce some degree of competitive antagonism to morphine and the other pure agonists.

Nalorphine, the original agonist-antagonist, is no longer used clinically, but its pharmacologic properties illustrate the most important features of the class:

Agonist effects

Nalorphine was known to be a morphine antagonist in animals, but traditional laboratory screening did not predict any analgetic activity. Lasagna and Beecher tested nalorphine in postoperative pain and were surprised to discover that it was nearly equipotent with morphine.[87]

Antagonist effects

Houde and Wallenstein found that nalorphine could reverse morphine analgesia, but this was highly dependent on the ratio of morphine to nalorphine.[67] A relatively low dose of nalorphine might reverse morphine, but a higher dose could actually produce a net increase in effect (the agonist effects predominated).

Abuse liability

Nalorphine was extremely unlikely to be diverted or abused. When nalorphine was administered to subjects who were physically dependent upon morphine,

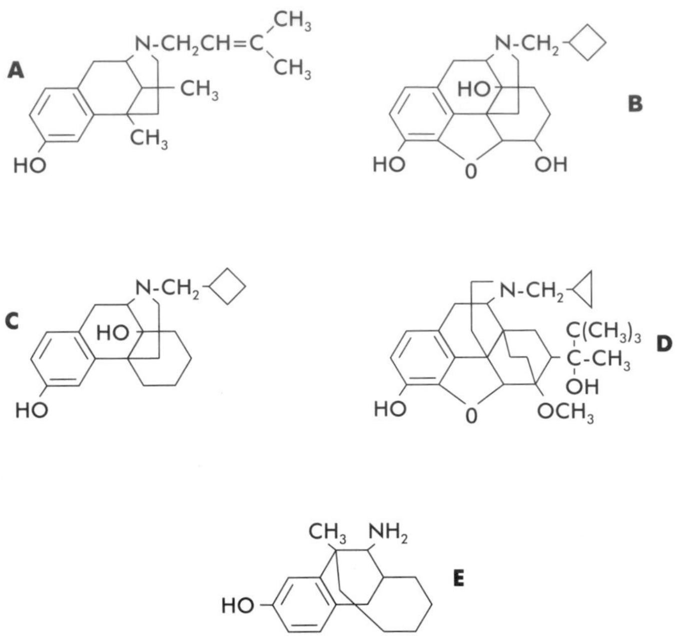

Fig. 54-18. Structural formulas of pentazocine (**A**), nalbuphine (**B**), butorphanol (**C**), buprenorphine (**D**), and dezocine (**E**).

it precipitated a violent withdrawal syndrome.[176] Former heroin addicts did not experience euphoria or perceive the drug as being similar to morphine.

Toxic effects

Nalorphine produced some typical opioid side effects like respiratory depression, sedation, miosis, and so forth. Unfortunately, analgetic doses could also produce severe psychotomimetic reactions.[87]

The distressing hallucinations and dysphoria made nalorphine clinically unacceptable as an analgetic, although it was used for many years as an antagonist. Nalorphine was an important milestone in opioid pharmacology because it demonstrated for the first time that addiction liability and potent analgesia might be separated. All the more modern agonist-antagonists have been products of an intense search for strong analgetics that are less likely to be abused.

The previous chapter has already introduced the concept of multiple opioid receptors and the theoretic basis for mixed agonist and antagonist activity. In this section some aspects of receptor theory will be discussed again in order to understand the clinical pharmacology of these drugs.

Nalorphine and all the other agonist-antagonists behave as *partial agonists;* these drugs tend to have shallower dose-response curves and produce lower maximal effects than fentanyl or morphine[136] (Fig. 54-19, *A*). Although this means there is a "ceiling" to the analgetic effects, the toxic effects are limited as

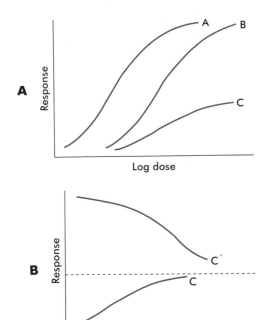

Table 54-4   Agonist vs. antagonist potency of opioid mixed agonist-antagonists

Drug	Analgetic potency (morphine = 1)	Morphine antagonist potency (nalorphine = 1)
Pentazocine	0.2	0.02
Nalbuphine	1	0.25
Butorphanol	5	— *
Buprenorphine	25	10
Dezocine	1	— †

*Weak antagonist; see text.
†Strong antagonist in animals.

Fig. 54-19. A, Idealized log dose response curves for two agonists (*A* and *B*) and a partial agonist (*C*) with an intrinsic activity of approximately 0.4. **B,** Idealized log dose response curve for the interaction of a partial agonist with a pure agonist. Curve *(C)*, the partial agonist alone; curve *(C')*, increasing doses of the partial agonist in the presence of a high concentration of pure agonist. The final level of response is 0.4 × maximum. (From Rance MJ: Multiple opiate receptors — their occurrence and significance, *Clin Anaesthesiol* 1:183, 1983.).

well.[80] **All the clinically available agonist-antagonists may be grouped according to the scheme proposed by Martin et al.[101,139]:**

- **Kappa partial agonists: Nalorphine, pentazocine, butorphanol, and nalbuphine are believed to produce their analgetic and sedative effects by interacting with kappa opioid receptors. Each of them has binding affinity but no efficacy at mu receptors, and therefore acts as a competitive antagonist to morphine. Naloxone acts as a competitive antagonist at both mu and kappa sites.**

- **Mu partial agonists: Buprenorphine and dezocine are believed to act selectively at mu receptors. Buprenorphine, for example, has been shown to have extremely high affinity but limited efficacy at mu receptors.[60] When given alone, its effects are similar to those of morphine. When given after morphine, it competes with the full agonist and causes a reduction in opioid effect[136] (Fig. 54-19, *B*).**

These drugs vary widely in their potencies, both as analgetics and antagonists (Table 54-4). Neither agonist vs. antagonist potency nor mu/kappa interac-

tion has proved to be a predictor of clinical utility or patient acceptance.

Analgesia

All the agonist-antagonists have been shown to be effective in a variety of acute and chronic pain states. They have been given intramuscularly, orally, sublingually, intranasally, intravenously by bolus or continuous infusion, and in patient-controlled analgesia systems. At the present time only pentazocine is commercially available in a nonparenteral preparation. The agents and their recommended doses are listed in Table 54-1. None of these drugs is currently approved for epidural or intrathecal use, although they have all been reported to be effective by this route.

All these opioids have been used as part of a balanced anesthetic technique, but their partial agonist properties are not an advantage in this setting. When given alone, even extremely large doses of nalbuphine or butorphanol will not produce a state of "anesthesia" like fentanyl or its derivatives.[159] Compared with morphine or fentanyl, the agonist-antagonists produce more limited decreases in the requirements for potent volatile anesthetics.[116] Dezocine is a partial agonist with somewhat more efficacy than the other agonist-antagonists.[98] In animals, dezocine has been shown to reduce enflurane MAC by up to 50%.[144]

Sedation

The kappa-type agonist-antagonists produce drowsiness and mood effects that are different from those of the pure agonists. Kappa agonists have been described as producing "apathetic sedation"; this may reflect the localization of kappa receptors in deeper layers of the cerebral cortex.[51] Patients given pentazocine, nalbuphine, or butorphanol may experience floating and dissociation, but usually do not experience mood elevation.[66] After analgetic doses these patients often appear extremely sedated, yet remain

capable of surprisingly lucid conversation. With pentazocine, patients are increasingly likely to experience "weird" feelings, dysphoria, or even hallucinations as the dose is raised. These unpleasant effects are relatively infrequent with butorphanol or nalbuphine. The subjective effects of buprenorphine and dezocine are similar to morphine throughout the dose range.

Most physicians are familiar with the pleasant mental detachment produced by morphine and use it as a sign that the drug is working. Because euphoria does not usually occur with the agonist-antagonists, there is a tendency to equate lack of mood elevation with lack of analgesia. Kaiko et al. has demonstrated that these effects are separable.[76] They assessed both analgetic and mood effects of meptazinol (an agonist-antagonist opioid available in the U.K.) and morphine. Both drugs improved pain scores, but only morphine produced a dose-related improvement in mood. The lack of mood effect is believed to be an important factor in the low abuse liability of these drugs.[77]

The sedative effects of some agonist-antagonists may be used to advantage. Butorphanol was evaluated as a premedicant in elective surgical patients, and it produced useful sedation in doses lower than those routinely used for analgesia.[34] Its effects on body perception, anxiety, and psychomotor testing were similar to those of midazolam. Unlike the benzodiazepine, it produced very little anterograde amnesia. In this patient population, there was no evidence of dysphoria or hallucinations.

Respiratory Depression

As stated previously, these opioids are all partial agonists, and their toxic effects are limited in intensity. Respiratory depression reaches a maximum after about 30 mg of nalbuphine[48] or 2 to 4 mg of butorphanol,[119] and even larger doses are well tolerated by most patients. Severe depression is still possible in sensitive individuals, those with concomitant CNS or pulmonary disease, and those receiving other depressant drugs. Respiratory depression may be reversed with naloxone but *not* with another agonist-antagonist.

A ceiling effect for respiration has also been demonstrated with the use of buprenorphine. This is important because buprenorphine has very high affinity for mu receptors and is not reliably antagonized by naloxone.[46,60,84] Even 16 mg of naloxone failed to reverse buprenorphine in one study. Dezocine is said to produce maximal respiratory depression after 30 mg, but a dose of 0.5 mg/kg produced apnea in one study subject (Rosow, 1992, unpublished observations).

Smooth Muscle Effects

Nalbuphine, butorphanol, and pentazocine do not cause significant elevation of intrabiliary pressure in animals or humans.[7,104,135] These agents may be particularly useful for patients who experience biliary colic after morphine. Buprenorphine is believed to cause biliary effects that are slightly more pronounced.[164] The agonist-antagonists appear to have small effects on smooth muscle in the intestine and bladder, and they cause less constipation and urinary retention than drugs that are similar to morphine.[156]

Cardiovascular Effects

The cardiovascular effects of buprenorphine and nalbuphine generally appear similar to those of morphine. Pentazocine produces unusual cardiovascular effects, both in normal individuals and in those with ischemic heart disease.[3] Unlike morphine, pentazocine may increase heart rate, systemic and pulmonary artery pressure, and LV end-diastolic pressure. These effects may be secondary to elevations in plasma catecholamines. Because these changes are likely to elevate myocardial oxygen consumption, pentazocine may be a poor choice for patients with ischemia or infarction.

Butorphanol (2 mg) can also increase pulmonary artery pressure, but heart rate and systemic pressure usually decrease slightly.[132] The rise in pulmonary artery pressure apparently does not increase as the dose is raised: in one study, doses of butorphanol greater than 25 mg were used safely during coronary artery bypass surgery.[4]

There have been few cardiovascular studies of the partial agonist dezocine, although it does not produce obvious hemodynamic changes in the doses recommended for analgesia.

Antagonist Effects

The approximate agonist and antagonist potencies of these drugs are listed in Table 54-4. **Nalbuphine and buprenorphine are strong antagonists, and they have been used clinically for this purpose.[88] The available evidence suggests that reversal with an agonist-antagonist is no safer or more reliable than reversal with naloxone.[73]**

Administration of an opioid antagonist to an opioid-dependent patient will precipitate withdrawal, and this has occurred after therapeutic doses of pentazocine, nalbuphine, and buprenorphine. Butorphanol is a very weak antagonist, and it produces only mild withdrawal in addicts who are maintained on 30 mg of methadone per day.[134] As stated previously, a low level of physical dependence may occur in patients who receive opioid agonists over long periods, and this subclinical state may be unmasked by administration of an antagonist. It seems prudent to avoid agonist-antagonists in patients who have had significant prior treatment with morphine, meperidine, oxycodone, and other such drugs.

In theory, administering an agonist-antagonist can create a problem if one subsequently gives a pure agonist (for example, nalbuphine premedication followed by fentanyl intraoperatively). In practice this does not seem to be a problem.

Tolerance and Abuse Liability

It is possible to give these drugs parenterally for long periods of time, but there are few clinical data on such use. Repeated injections of pentazocine have been reported to cause a fibrous myopathy in animals.[123]

At this writing, pentazocine is the only agonist-antagonist available for oral use (sublingual buprenorphine has been used for some time in the United Kingdom). Long-term studies on ex-heroin addicts showed that tolerance and physical dependence do occur after repeated administration of agonist-antagonist opioids. Withdrawal is usually brief and unlike that of morphine. Most importantly, withdrawal is not usually accompanied by drug-seeking behavior.

The agonist-antagonist opioids were developed primarily as less abusable substitutes for morphine-like drugs. There has been remarkably little abuse or diversion of the kappa agonists, and addicts tend to avoid them. Pentazocine tablets were abused parenterally for a few years, but the problem was solved by a reformulation in 1983. The World Health Organization Expert Committee on Drug Dependence has reviewed the abuse of agonist-antagonists and concluded that there is no basis for instituting narcotic controls.[75]

KEY POINTS

- The term "opioid" applies to any natural or synthetic compound that has morphinelike properties. All of the clinically available opioids are structurally related to morphine.

- The most widely used opioid analgetics are the pure agonists, and all of these are relatively selective for mu opioid receptors. Unlike the volatile anesthetics, opioid agonists produce a group of highly specific depressant and stimulant effects by acting at discrete sites within the central nervous system.

- Opioid analgetic effects probably result from actions at several different levels of the neuraxis. The processing of pain information is inhibited by a direct spinal effect at the dorsal horn. The rostrad transmission of pain signals is decreased by activation of descending inhibitory pathways in the brainstem; finally, the emotional response to pain is altered by opioid actions on the limbic cortex.

- Sufficient doses of opioids will relieve almost any pain, although some types of pain are typically more responsive than others. Prolonged, burning pain is more effectively blunted than the brief, sharp pain of an incision. Neuropathic pain can be very resistant to opioid treatment. Intraoperatively, the opioids can produce sufficient analgesia to reduce or abolish autonomic and somatic responses to surgical stimuli.

- In usual analgetic doses, morphinelike drugs may produce drowsiness, feelings of heaviness, and difficulty concentrating. Opioids do not usually produce amnesia in subhypnotic doses. With higher doses, sedation becomes more pronounced, and hypnosis may occur. Doses of opioids that are sufficient to produce apnea and profound analgesia do not always produce sleep in healthy individuals.

- Dysphoria and agitation occur infrequently after analgetic doses of most opioids although the incidence is higher with meperidine and codeine.

- True seizures can be produced by meperidine because its major metabolite, normeperidine, is a potent convulsant. Although rare, these are more likely to occur after large doses or in patients with renal failure who cannot excrete the metabolite.

- Opioids produce a dose-related depression of the ventilatory response to CO_2 by a direct effect on respiratory centers in the medulla. Morphine has been shown to blunt the response to hypoxia also.

- Equianalgetic doses of all opioids produce equivalent amounts of respiratory depression. There is no convincing evidence that any analgetic is more or less dangerous than morphine in this regard.

- Tolerant individuals who require large amounts of opioid for relief of pain are not at proportionately increased risk for respiratory depression.

- Respiratory depression is difficult to reverse (e.g., with naloxone) without reversing some analgesia.

- Opioids suppress cough by depressing cough centers in the medulla. This effect involves different receptor mechanisms than those mediating analgesia or respiratory depression.

- Opioids stimulate the Edinger-Westphal nucleus of

the oculomotor nerve to produce miosis. The pinpoint pupil is a pathognomonic sign of opioid overdose (until hypoxia supervenes).

- Opioids produce complex effects on vomiting mechanisms in the medulla. There is direct stimulation of the chemoreceptor trigger zone in the area postrema on the floor of the fourth ventricle. This, in turn, activates the vomiting center.

- Generalized hypertonus of skeletal muscle can be produced by large intravenous doses of most opioid agonists. Although morphine can produce rigidity, the problem is most commonly associated with fentanyl, alfentanil, and sufentanil.

- In its most severe form, "lead pipe" muscle rigidity can totally prevent mechanical ventilation. The difficulty is due to loss of chest wall compliance as well as constriction of laryngeal and pharyngeal muscles. Fortunately, rigidity is effectively treated (or prevented) by administering relatively small doses of muscle relaxants.

- In normal analgetic doses, opioids produce minimal cardiovascular effects. Bradycardia and peripheral vasodilation are seen with higher doses and when opioids are combined with other anesthetic drugs.

- True allergic responses to opioids are very rare. Many, but not all, opioids produce a nonimmunologic release of histamine from mast cells, most often seen as local itching, redness, or hives near the site of intravenous injection. Sometimes a patient will experience generalized flushing. When sufficient histamine is liberated, it may cause decreases in systemic vascular resistance, hypotension, and tachycardia.

- Opioids should be used with great care in persons with asthma to avoid the exacerbation of pre-existing bronchospasm by depressing cough and respiratory drive and drying airway secretions.

- Opioids produce spasm of smooth muscle all along the GI tract. Both small and large bowel become hypertonic, but rhythmic propulsive activity is diminished. The mechanism involves both CNS effects and peripheral actions on opioid receptors in the bowel.

- Opioids cause contraction of smooth muscle along the biliary tree and spasm of the sphincter of Oddi, sometimes precipitating biliary colic. Opioids increase the ureteral contractions although they relieve the pain of ureteral stones. They also increase the tone of the detrusor muscle of the bladder and urinary sphincter.

- Opioids have no specific teratogenic effects, but chronic opioid use by the mother may lead to "addiction" in utero (actual physical dependence). Neonatal withdrawal may occur shortly following

delivery, and, in some instances, may be life threatening.

- When tolerance to an opioid occurs, there is simultaneous development of *cross-tolerance* to all other opioid agonists.

- Morphine is the least lipophilic of the opioids, implying that morphine penetrates biologic membranes more slowly than lipophilic opioids and it less likely to accumulate in lipid membranes or fatty tissues.

- Morphine is eliminated primarily by hepatic biotransformation, with about 5% to 15% excreted unchanged in the urine. The rate of hepatic clearance is very high, accounting for the relatively short elimination half-life. About 70% is cleared in one pass through the liver, and morphine is therefore subject to flow-dependent elimination. Factors that decrease hepatic blood flow prolong its elimination. High hepatic clearance also means that morphine is subject to a large first-pass effect, and larger doses are required when the drug is given orally.

- The plasma pharmacokinetics of morphine do *not* parallel its clinical effects. Despite rapid distribution and elimination, the onset and offset of morphine analgesia are rather slow. Morphine enters the central nervous system with difficulty, and peak analgetic effects may not occur for 15 to 30 minutes after intravenous injection.

- The metabolism of meperidine plays a significant role in its pharmacodynamics. Less than 7% of a dose is excreted unchanged in the urine. Meperidine is rapidly N-demethylated to form normeperidine; the other major metabolites are meperidinic acid and normeperidinic acid. Normeperidine is a potent convulsant, and its elimination half-life is 8 to 12 hours, so significant amounts may accumulate. Seizures have occurred in patients with renal failure (who could not excrete normeperidine) and in cancer patients who received high doses of meperidine over long periods of time.

- Fentanyl is a potent synthetic opioid that is extremely fat-soluble, accounting for its rapid onset and relatively short duration. Unlike morphine, fentanyl crosses the blood-brain barrier easily, and peak effect occurs in only 3 to 5 minutes. Within a short time, the drug is extensively distributed throughout the body so plasma levels decrease precipitously. This large concentration gradient favors redistribution of fentanyl away from the central nervous system and thus terminates its effect. When low doses of fentanyl are administered, redistribution terminates the effect, and the drug appears short-acting.

- Fentanyl's long elimination half-life means that repeated IV boluses are very likely to produce cumulative effects. The high hepatic extraction ratio means that the clearance of fentanyl is limited by hepatic blood flow. Factors that lower hepatic blood flow can prolong the duration of fentanyl. Since fentanyl undergoes substantial first-pass metabolism, the oral route is inefficient. It is well absorbed when given transdermally, intranasally, or via the oral mucosa.

- Alfentanil is a slightly less potent congener of fentanyl with an extremely rapid onset and short duration of effect. Peak analgetic and respiratory depressant effects occur in less than 2 minutes, and the duration of small doses may last only 15 minutes.

- In 1947, a "balanced" anesthetic technique was developed which included small doses of meperidine in combination with thiopental, curare, and nitrous oxide. Although the individual components have changed over the years, this technique is the basis for modern balanced anesthesia.

- The administration of opioids potentiates the hypnotic effects of barbiturates and benzodiazepines. By reducing the amount of hypnotic administered, an opioid can sometimes produce more rapid emergence from anesthesia. The opioids also produce a dramatic, dose-related decrease in the requirement for volatile anesthetics, and they are frequently used for this specific purpose.

- The only pure opioid antagonist currently available for parenteral use is naloxone, the N-allyl derivative of oxymorphone. Naloxone acts as a competitive antagonist at all opioid receptors, but it has greatest affinity for mu receptors. Small doses of naloxone reliably reverse or prevent the effects of pure opioid agonists and most mixed agonist-antagonists. The onset of antagonist effect is extremely rapid, but, due to rapid redistribution and elimination, the duration of action is quite brief, and the effects of the opioid may recur.

- All of the clinically available agonist-antagonists may be grouped as either kappa partial agonists or mu partial agonists. The agonist-antagonist opioids are synthetic and semisynthetic analgetics structurally related to morphine. They are used primarily for moderate-to-severe acute pain. All of these compounds produce some degree of competitive antagonism to morphine and the other pure agonists.

- The kappa-type agonist-antagonists produce drowsiness and mood effects that are different from those of the pure agonists. This has been described as "apathetic sedation," and may reflect the localization of kappa receptors in deeper layers of the cerebral cortex. Patients given pentazocine, nalbuphine, or butorphanol may experience floating and dissociation but usually not mood elevation. After analgetic doses, these patients often appear extremely sedated yet remain capable of surprisingly lucid conversation. With pentazocine, patients are increasingly likely to experience bizarre feelings, dysphoria, or even hallucinations as the dose is raised. These unpleasant effects are relatively infrequent with butorphanol or nalbuphine. The subjective effects of buprenorphine and dezocine are morphine-like throughout the dose range.

KEY REFERENCES

Ausems ME et al: Plasma concentrations of alfentanil required to supplement nitrous oxide anesthesia for general surgery, *Anesthesiology* 65:362, 1986.

Austin KL, Stapleton JV, and Mather LE: Relationship between blood meperidine concentrations and analgesic response: a preliminary report, *Anesthesiology* 53:460, 1980.

Forrest WH, Bellville JW: The effect of sleep plus morphine on the respiratory response to carbon dioxide, *Anesthesiology* 25:137, 1964.

McClain DA, Hug CC Jr: Intravenous fentanyl kinetics, *Clin Pharmacol Ther* 28:106, 1980.

Murphy MR, Hug CC Jr: The anesthetic potency of fentanyl in terms of its reduction of enflurane MAC, *Anesthesiology* 57:485, 1982.

Philbin DM et al: Fentanyl and sufentanil anesthesia revisited: how much is enough? *Anesthesiology* 73:5, 1990.

Way WL, Costley EC, and Way EL: Respiratory sensitivity of the newborn infant to meperidine and morphine, *Clin Pharmacol Ther* 6:454, 1965.

REFERENCES

1. Advokat C: The role of descending inhibition in morphine-induced analgesia, *Trends Pharm Sci* 9:330, 1988.
2. Aitkenhead AR et al: Pharmacokinetics of single-dose intravenous morphine in normal volunteers and patients with end-stage renal failure, *Br J Anaesth* 58:813, 1984.
3. Alderman EL et al: Hemodynamic effects of morphine and pentazocine differ in cardiac patients, *N Engl J Med* 27:623, 1972.
4. Aldrete JA et al: Comparison of butorphanol and morphine as analgesics for coronary bypass surgery: a double-blind randomized study, *Anesth Analg* 62:78, 1983.
5. Andrée RA: Sudden death following naloxone administration, *Anesth Analg* 59:782, 1980.
6. Arandia HY, Patil VU: Glottic closure following large dose of fentanyl, *Anesthesiology* 66:574, 1987.
7. Arguelles JE et al: Intrabiliary pressure changes produced by narcotic drugs and inhalation anesthetics in guinea pigs, *Anesth Analg* 58:120, 1979.
8. Arner S, Meyerson BA: Lack of analgesic effects of opioids on neuropathic and idiopathic forms of pain, *Pain* 33:11, 1988.
9. Askitopoulou H et al: Acute tolerance to fentanyl during anesthesia in dogs, *Anesthesiology* 63:255, 1985.
10. Ausems ME et al: Plasma concentrations of alfentanil required to supplement nitrous oxide anesthesia for general surgery, *Anesthesiology* 65:362, 1986.
11. Austin KL, Stapleton JV, and Mather LE: Relationship between blood meperidine concentrations and analgesic response: a preliminary report, *Anesthesiology* 53:460, 1980.
12. Bailey PL et al: Anesthetic induction with fentanyl, *Anesth Analg* 64:48, 1985.
13. Ballantyne JC, Loach AB, and Carr DB: Itching after epidural and spinal opiates, *Pain* 33:149, 1988.
14. Ballar S, Toaff ME, and Toaff R: Effects of intravenous meperidine and meperidine with promethazine on uterine activity and fetal heart rate during labor, *Israel J Med Sci* 12:1141, 1976.
15. Baughman VL et al: Cerebral vascular and metabolic effects of fentanyl and midazolam in young and aged rats, *Anesthesiology* 67:314, 1987.
16. Becker LD et al: Biphasic respiratory depression after fentanyl-droperidol or fentanyl alone used to supplement nitrous oxide anesthesia, *Anesthesiology* 44:291, 1976.
17. Ben-Schlomo I: Midazolam acts synergistically with fentanyl for induction of anesthesia, *Br J Anaesth* 64:45, 1990.
18. Benthuysen JL et al: Physiology of alfentanil-induced rigidity, *Anesthesiology* 64:440, 1986.
19. Bernton EW, Long JB, and Holaday JW: Opioids and neuropeptides: mechanisms in circulatory shock, *Fed Proc* 44:290, 1985.
20. Björkman S et al: Comparative tissue concentration—profiles of fentanyl and alfentanil in man predicted from tissue-to-blood partition data obtained in rats, *Anesthesiology* 72:865, 1990.
21. Bovill JG et al: Influence of high-dose alfentanil anaesthesia on the EEG: correlation with plasma concentrations, *Br J Anaesth* 55:199S, 1983.
22. Bovill JG et al: The influence of sufentanil on endocrine and metabolic responses to cardiac anesthesia, *Anesth Analg* 62:391, 1983.
23. Bovill JG et al: The pharmacokinetics of sufentanil in surgical patients, *Anesthesiology* 61:502, 1984.
24. Bower S, Hull CJ: Comparative pharmacokinetics of fentanyl and alfentanil, *Br J Anaesth* 54:871, 1982.
25. Brunk SF, Delle M: Morphine metabolism in man, *Clin Pharmacol Ther* 16:51, 1974.
26. Chauvin M et al: Morphine pharmacokinetics in renal failure, *Anesthesiology* 66:327, 1987.
27. Chauvin M et al: Sufentanil pharmacokinetics in patients with cirrhosis, *Anesth Analg* 68:1, 1989.
28. Chessick KC, Black S, and Hoye SJ: Spasm and operative cholangiography, *Arch Surg* 110:53, 1975.
29. Cicero TJ et al: Function of the male sex organs in heroin and methadone users, *N Engl J Med* 292:882, 1975.
30. Clark RB, Beard AG, and Barclay DL: Naloxone in the newborn infant, *Anesth Rev* (Dec):9, 1975.
31. Cohen MR et al: Physiological effects of high dose naloxone administration to normal adults, *Life Sci* 30:2025, 1982.
32. Costall B, Fortune DH, and Naylor RJ: Involvement of mesolimbic and extrapyramidal nuclei in the motor depressant action of narcotic drugs, *J Pharm Pharmacol* 30:566, 1978.
33. De Castro J, Mundeleer R: Anesthesie sans barbituratiques: la neuroleptanalgesie, *Anesth Analg* (Paris) 16:1022, 1959.
34. Dershwitz M et al: Comparison of the sedative effects of butorphanol and midazolam, *Anesthesiology* 74:717, 1991.
35. Dray A, Metsch R: Opioids and central inhibition of urinary bladder motility, *Eur J Pharmacol* 98:155, 1984.
36. Duncalf D, Nagashima H, and Duncalf RM: Naloxone fails to antagonize thiopental anesthesia, *Anesth Analg* 59:558, 1978.
37. Ebert TJ et al: Fentanyl-diazepam anesthesia does not attenuate cardiopulmonary baroreflex-mediated vasoconstrictor responses to controlled hypovolemia in humans, *Anesth Analg* 67:548, 1988.
38. Evans JM et al: Degree and duration of reversal by naloxone of effects of morphine in conscious subjects, *Br Med J* 1:589, 1974.
39. Ferrier C: Alfentanil pharmacokinetics in patients with cirrhosis, *Anesthesiology* 62:480, 1985.
40. Finck AD, Ngai SH: Opiate receptor mediation of ketamine analgesia, *Anesthesiology* 56:291, 1982.
41. Finck AD, Ngai SH, and Berkowitz BA: Antagonism of general anesthesia by naloxone in the rat, *Anesthesiology* 46:241, 1977.
42. Fine PG, Hare BD: The pathways and mechanisms of pain and analgesia: a review and clinical perspective, *Hosp Formul* 20:972, 1985.
43. Flacke JW et al: Histamine release by four narcotics: a double-blind study in humans, *Anesth Analg* 66:723, 1987.
44. Flaim SF, Visman LA, and Zelis R: The effects of morphine on isolated cutaneous canine vascular smooth muscle, *Res Commun Chem Pathol Pharmacol* 16:191, 1977.
45. Forrest WH, Bellville JW: The effect of sleep plus morphine on the respiratory response to carbon dioxide, *Anesthesiology* 25:137, 1964.
46. Gal TJ: Naloxone reversal of buprenorphine induced respiratory depression, *Anesthesiology* 69:A818, 1988.
47. Gal TJ, DiFazio CA: Prolonged antagonism of opioid action with intravenous nalmefene, *Anesthesiology* 64:175, 1986.
48. Gal TJ, DiFazio CA, and Moscicki J: Analgesic and respiratory depressant activity of nalbuphine: a comparison with morphine, *Anesthesiology* 57:367, 1982.
49. Gissen AJ et al: Effects of fentanyl and sufentanil on peripheral mammalian nerves, *Anesth Analg* 66:1272, 1987.
50. Gonzales JP, Brogden RN: Naltrexone: a review of its pharmacodynamic and pharmacokinetic properties and therapeutic efficacy in the management of opioid dependence, *Drugs* 35:192, 1988.
51. Goodman RR, Snyder SH: Autoradiographic localization of kappa opiate receptors to deep layers of the cerebral cortex may explain unique sedative and analgesic effects, *Life Sci* 31:1291, 1982.
52. Goromaru T et al: Identification and quantitative determination of fentanyl metabolites in patients by gas chromatography–mass spectrometry, *Anesthesiology* 61:73, 1984.
53. Gourlay GK et al: The transdermal administration of fentanyl in the treatment of postoperative pain: pharmacokinetics and pharmacodynamic effects, *Pain* 37:193, 1989.
54. Gravlee GP et al: Rapid administration of a narcotic and neuromuscular blocker: a hemodynamic comparison of fentanyl, sufentanil, pancuronium and vecuronium, *Anesth Analg* 67:39, 1988.
55. Gray TC, Rees GJ: The role of apnoea in anaesthesia for major surgery, *Br Med J* 2:891, 1952.

56. Green JF, Jackman AP, and Krohm KA: Mechanism of morphine-induced shifts in blood volume between extracorporeal reservoir and the systemic circulation of the dog under conditions of constant blood flow and vena caval pressures, *Circ Res* 42:479, 1978.

57. Griffith HR, Johnson GE: The use of curare in general anesthesia, *Anesthesiology* 3:418, 1942.

58. Gueneron JP et al: Effect of naloxone infusion on analgesia and respiratory depression after epidural fentanyl, *Anesth Analg* 67:35, 1988.

59. Haberer JP et al: Fentanyl pharmacokinetics in anaesthetized patients with cirrhosis, *Br J Anaesth* 54:1267, 1982.

60. Heel RC et al: Buprenorphine: a review of its pharmacological properties and therapeutic efficacy, *Drugs* 17:81, 1979.

61. Henderson JM et al: Pre-induction of anesthesia in pediatric patients with nasally administered sufentanil, *Anesthesiology* 67:671, 1988.

62. Henney RP et al: The effects of morphine on the resistance and capacitance vessels of the peripheral circulation, *Am Heart J* 72:242, 1966.

63. Henthorn TK, Avram MJ, and Krejcie TC: Alfentanil clearance is independent of the polymorphic debrisoquin hydroxylase, *Anesthesiology* 71:635, 1989.

64. Hermens JM et al: Comparison of histamine release in human skin mast cells induced by morphine, fentanyl, and oxymorphone, *Anesthesiology* 62:124, 1985.

65. Herz A, Teschemacher JH: Activities and sites of antinociceptive action of morphine like analgesics. In Harper NJ, Simmonds AB, eds: *Advances in drug research*, New York, 1971, Academic Press.

66. Houde RW: Analgesic effectiveness of the narcotic agonist-antagonists, *Br J Clin Pharmacol* 7:297S, 1979.

67. Houde RW, Wallenstein SL: Clinical studies of morphine-nalorphine combination, *Fed Proc* 15:440, 1956.

68. Hsu HO, Hickey RF, and Forbes AR: Morphine decreases peripheral vascular resistance and increases capacitance in man, *Anesthesiology* 50:98, 1979.

69. Hug CC Jr: Lipid solubility, pharmacokinetics, and the EEG: are you better off today than you were four years ago? *Anesthesiology* 62:221, 1985.

70. Hug CC Jr, Murphy MR: Fentanyl disposition in cerebrospinal fluid and plasma and its relationship to ventilatory depression in the dog, *Anesthesiology* 50:342, 1979.

71. Hug CC Jr, Murphy MR: Tissue redistribution of fentanyl and termination of effect in rats, *Anesthesiology* 55:369, 1981.

72. Hug CC Jr et al: Pharmacokinetics of morphine injected intravenously into the anesthetized dog, *Anesthesiology* 54:38, 1981.

73. Jaffe RS et al: Nalbuphine antagonism of fentanyl-induced ventilatory depression: a randomized trial, *Anesthesiology* 68:254, 1988.

74. Jaffe RS, Coalson D: Recurrent respiratory depression after alfentanil administration, *Anesthesiology* 70:151, 1989.

75. Johanson CE, Yanagita T, eds: WHO symposium on drug dependence: benefit-risk ratio assessment of agonist-antagonist analgesics, *Drug Alcohol Dep* 20:289, 1987.

76. Kaiko RF et al: Intramuscular meptazinol and morphine in postoperative pain, *Clin Pharmacol Ther* 37:589, 1985.

77. Kalant H, Grupp LA: Drug abuse and drug dependence. In Kalant H, Roschlau WHE, eds: *Principles of medical pharmacology*, ed 5, Toronto, 1989, BC Decker.

78. Kaufman JJ, Semo NM, and Koski WS: Microelectrometric titration measurement of the pKas and partition and drug distribution coefficients of narcotics and narcotic antagonists and their pH and temperature dependence, *J Med Chem* 18:647, 1975.

79. Keats AS: The effect of drugs on respiration in man, *Ann Rev Pharmacol Toxicol* 25:41, 1985.

80. Keats AS, Telford J: Studies of analgesic drugs: respiratory effects of narcotic antagonists, *J Pharmacol Exp Ther* 151:126, 1966.

81. Kissin I et al: Alfentanil potentiates midazolam-induced unconsciousness in subanalgesic doses, *Anesth Analg* 71:65, 1990.

82. Klepper ID et al: Analgesic and respiratory effects of extradural sufentanil in volunteers and the influence of adrenaline as an adjuvant, *Br J Anaesth* 59:1147, 1987.

83. Klotz U et al: The effect of cirrhosis on the disposition and elimination of meperidine in man, *Clin Pharmacol Ther* 16:667, 1974.

84. Knape JT: Early respiratory depression resistant to naloxone following epidural buprenorphine, *Anesthesiology* 64:382, 1986.

85. Kono K et al: Renal function and stress response during halothane or fentanyl anesthesia, *Anesth Analg* 60:552, 1981.

86. Lappas DG et al: Left ventricular performance and pulmonary circulation following addition of nitrous oxide to morphine during coronary artery surgery, *Anesthesiology* 43:61, 1975.

87. Lasagna L, Beecher HK: The analgesic effectiveness of nalorphine and nalorphine-morphine combinations in man, *J Pharmacol Exp Ther* 112:356, 1954.

88. Latasch L, Probst S, and Dudziak R: Reversal by nalbuphine of respiratory depression caused by fentanyl, *Anesth Analg* 63:814, 1984.

89. Laubie M, Schmitt H, and Vincent M: Vagal bradycardia produced by microinjections of morphine-like drugs into the nucleus ambiguus in anesthetized dogs, *Eur J Pharmacol* 59:287, 1979.

90. Leaman DM et al: Effect of morphine on splanchnic blood flow, *Br Heart J* 40:569, 1978.

91. Lee HK, Wang SC: Mechanism of morphine-induced miosis in the dog, *J Pharmacol Exp Ther* 192:415, 1975.

92. Levy JH, Rockoff MA: Anaphylaxis to meperidine, *Anesth Analg* 61:301, 1982.

93. Lowenstein E: Morphine "anesthesia" —a perspective, *Anesthesiology* 35:563, 1971.

94. Lowenstein E et al: Cardiovascular response to large doses of intravenous morphine in man, *N Engl J Med* 28:1389, 1969.

95. Lowenstein E et al: Local and neurally mediated effects of morphine on skeletal muscle vascular resistance, *J Pharmacol Exp Ther* 180:359, 1972.

96. Lunn JK et al: High-dose fentanyl anesthesia for coronary artery surgery: plasma fentanyl concentration and influence of nitrous oxide on cardiovascular responses, *Anesth Analg* 58:390, 1979.

97. Maitre PO et al: Population pharmacokinetics of alfentanil: the average dose-plasma concentration relationship and interindividual variability in patients, *Anesthesiology* 66:3, 1987.

98. Malis JL, Rosenthale ME, and Gluckman MI: Animal pharmacology of Wy-16225, a new analgesic agent, *J Pharmacol Exp Ther* 194:488, 1975.

99. Marks RM, Sachar EJ: Undertreatment of medical inpatients with narcotic analgesia, *Ann Int Med* 78:173, 1973.

100. Martin DE et al: Low-dose fentanyl blunts circulatory responses to tracheal intubation, *Anesth Analg* 61:680, 1982.

101. Martin WR et al: The effects of morphine- and nalorphine-like drugs in the non-dependent and morphine-dependent chronic spinal dog, *J Pharmacol Exp Ther* 197:517, 1976.

102. Mather LE et al: Meperidine kinetics in man: intravenous injection in surgical patients and volunteers, *Clin Pharmacol Ther* 17:21, 1975.

103. Mazoit JX et al: Pharmacokinetics of unchanged morphine in normal and cirrhotic subjects, *Anesth Analg* 66:293, 1987.

104. McCammon RL, Stoelting RK, and Madura JA: Effects of butorphanol nalbuphine and fentanyl on intrabiliary tract dynamics, *Anesth Analg* 63:139, 1984.

105. McClain DA, Hug CC Jr: Intravenous fentanyl kinetics, *Clin Pharmacol Ther* 28:106, 1980.

106. McClane TK, Martin WR: Effects of morphine, nalorphine, cyclazocine and naloxone on the flexor reflex, *Int J Neuropharmacol* 6:89, 1967.

107. Milde LN, Milde JH, and Gallagher WJ: Cerebral effects of fentanyl in dogs, *Br J Anaesth* 63:710, 1989.

108. Miller JW, Anderson HH: The effect of N-demethylation on certain pharmacologic actions of morphine, codeine and meperidine in the mouse, *J Pharmacol Exp Ther* 112:191, 1954.

109. Mills CA et al: Cardiovascular effects of fentanyl reversal by naloxone at varying arterial carbon dioxide tensions in dogs, *Anesth Analg* 67:730, 1988.

110. Mirenda J, Tabatabai M, and Wong K: Delayed and prolonged rigidity greater than 24 hours following high-dose fentanyl anesthesia, *Anesthesiology* 69:624, 1988.

111. Misra AL: Metabolism of opiates. In Adler ML, Manara L, and Samanin R,

eds: *Factors affecting the action of narcotics,* New York, 1978, Raven Press.

112. Morrison JC et al: Metabolites of meperidine in the fetal and maternal serum, *Am J Obst Gynecol* 126:997, 1976.

113. Mummaneni N, Rao TLK, and Montoya A: Awareness and recall with high-dose fentanyl-oxygen anesthesia, *Anesth Analg* 59:948, 1980.

114. Murkin JM et al: Absence of seizures during induction of anesthesia with high-dose fentanyl, *Anesth Analg* 63:489, 1984.

115. Murphy MR, Hug CC Jr: The anesthetic potency of fentanyl in terms of its reduction of enflurane MAC, *Anesthesiology* 57:485, 1982.

116. Murphy MR, Hug CC Jr: The enflurane sparing effect of morphine, butorphanol and nalbuphine, *Anesthesiology* 57:489, 492, 1982.

117. Murphy MR, Hug CC Jr, and McClain DA: Dose-independent pharmacokinetics of fentanyl, *Anesthesiology* 59:537, 1983.

118. Murphy MR, Olson WA, and Hug CC Jr: Pharmacokinetics of ^{3}H-fentanyl in the dog anesthetized with enflurane, *Anesthesiology* 50:13, 1979.

119. Nagashima H et al: Respiratory and circulatory effects of intravenous butorphanol and morphine, *Clin Pharmacol Ther* 19:738, 1976.

120. Neff N, Mayer EC, and De La Luz Perales M: Nitrous oxide and oxygen anesthesia with curare relaxation, *Calif Med* 66:67, 69, 1947.

121. Nelson PS et al: Comparison of oral transmucosal fentanyl citrate and an oral solution of meperidine, diazepam, and atropine for premedication in children, *Anesthesiology* 70:616, 1989.

122. Ngai SH et al: Pharmacokinetics of naloxone in rats and man: basis for its potency and short duration of action, *Anesthesiology* 44:398, 1976.

123. Oh SJ: Experimental pentazocine-induced fibrous myopathy, *Alab J Med Sci* 14:64, 1977.

124. Okutani R et al: Effect of hypothermic hemodilutional cardiopulmonary bypass on plasma sufentanil and catecholamine concentrations in humans, *Anesth Analg* 67:667, 1988.

125. Olsen GD: Morphine binding to human plasma proteins, *Clin Pharmacol Ther* 17:31, 1975.

126. Parkhouse J, Pleuvry BJ, and Rees JMH, eds: *Analgesic drugs,* Oxford, 1979, Blackwell Scientific.

127. Partridge L, Ward CF: Pulmonary edema following low-dose naloxone administration, *Anesthesiology* 65:709, 1986.

128. Pasternak GW, Zhong AZ, and Tecott L: Developmental differences between high and low affinity opiate binding sites: their relationship to analgesia and respiratory depression, *Life Sci* 27:1185, 1980.

129. Paul D et al: Pharmacological characterization of morphine-6β-glucuronide, a very potent morphine metabolite, *J Pharmacol Exp Ther* 251:477, 1989.

130. Philbin DM et al: The use of H_1 and H_2 histamine antagonists with morphine anesthesia: a double-blind study, *Anesthesiology* 55:292, 1981.

131. Philbin DM et al: Fentanyl and sufentanil anesthesia revisited: how much is enough? *Anesthesiology* 73:5, 1990.

132. Popio KA et al: Hemodynamic and respiratory effects of morphine and butophanol, *Clin Pharmacol Ther* 23:281, 1978.

133. Porter J, Jick H: Addiction rare in patients treated with narcotics, *N Engl J Med* 302:123, 1980.

134. Preston KL, Bigelow GE, and Liebson IA: Butorphanol precipitated withdrawal in opioid dependent human volunteers, *J Pharmacol Exp Ther* 246:441, 1988.

135. Radnay PA et al: Common bile duct pressure changes after fentanyl, morphine, meperidine, butorphanol and naloxone, *Anesth Analg* 63:441, 1984.

136. Rance MJ: Multiple opiate receptors—their occurrence and significance, *Clin Anaesthesiol* 1:183, 1983.

137. Reitan JA et al: Central vagal control of fentanyl-induced bradycardia during halothane anesthesia, *Anesth Analg* 57:31, 1978.

138. Rosow CE: Sufentanil citrate: a new opioid analgesic for use in anesthesia, *Pharmacotherapy* 4:11, 1984.

139. Rosow CE: Newer synthetic opioid analgesics. In Smith G, Covino BG, eds: *Acute pain,* London, 1985, Butterworths.

140. Rosow CE: Acute and chronic tolerance: relevance for clinical practice. In *Problems of drug dependence,* Research Monograph 76, National Institutes on Drug Abuse, Washington DC, 1987, US Govt Printing Office.

141. Rosow CE: Agonist-antagonist opioids: theory and clinical practice, *Can J Anaesth* 36:3:S5, 1989.

142. Rosow CE et al: Histamine release during morphine and fentanyl anesthesia, *Anesthesiology* 56:93, 1982.

143. Rosow CE et al: Hemodynamics and histamine release during induction with sufentanil or fentanyl, *Anesthesiology* 60:489, 1984.

144. Rowlington JC, Moscicki JC, and DiFazio CA: Anesthetic potency of dezocine and its interaction with morphine in rats, *Anesth Analg* 62:899, 1983.

145. Saini V et al: Antifibrillatory action of the narcotic agonist fentanyl, *Am Heart J* 115:598, 1988.

146. Sanford TJ et al: A comparison of morphine, fentanyl and sufentanil anesthesia for cardiac surgery, *Anesth Analg* 65:259, 1986.

147. Scamman FL: Fentanyl-O_2-N_2O rigidity and pulmonary compliance, *Anesth Analg* 62:332, 1983.

148. Scott JC, Ponganis KV, and Stanski DR: EEG quantitation of narcotic effect: the comparative pharmacodynamics of fentanyl and alfentanil, *Anesthesiology* 62:234, 1985.

149. Scott JC, Stanski DR: Decreased fentanyl and alfentanil dose requirements with age. A simultaneous pharmacokinetic and pharmacodynamic evaluation, *J Pharmacol Exp Ther* 240:159, 1987.

150. Sebel PS et al: Effects of high-dose fentanyl anesthesia on the electroencephalogram, *Anesthesiology* 55:203, 1981.

151. Sebel PS et al: Hormonal responses to high-dose fentanyl anaesthesia, *Br J Anaesth* 53:941, 1981.

152. Shafer A, Sung ML, and White PF: Pharmacokinetics and pharmacodynamics of alfentanil infusions during general anesthesia, *Anesth Analg* 65:1021, 1986.

153. Shnider SM, Moya F: Effects of meperidine on the newborn infant, *Am J Obst Gynecol* 89:1009, 1964.

154. Shupak RC, Harp JR: Comparison between high-dose sufentanil-oxygen and high-dose fentanyl-oxygen for neuroanesthesia, *Br J Anaesth* 57:375, 1985.

155. Silbert BS et al: The effect of diazepam on induction of anesthesia with alfentanil, *Anesth Analg* 65:71, 1986.

156. Stanciu C, Bennet JR: Colonic response to pentazocine, *Br Med J* 1:312, 1974.

157. Stanley TH, Webster LR: Anesthetic requirements and cardiovascular effects of fentanyl-oxygen and fentanyl-diazepam-oxygen anesthesia in man, *Anesth Analg* 57:411, 1978.

158. Stanley TH et al: The effects of high dose morphine on fluid and blood requirements in open-heart operations, *Anesthesiology* 38:356, 1973.

159. Stanley TH et al: The cardiovascular effects of high-dose butorphanol-nitrous oxide anaesthesia before and during operation, *Can Anaesth Soc J* 30:337, 1983.

160. Stanski DR, Hug CC Jr: Alfentanil—a kinetically predictable narcotic analgesic, *Anesthesiology* 57:435, 1982.

161. Stein C et al: Analgesic effect of intraarticular morphine after arthroscopic knee surgery, *N Engl J Med* 325:1123, 1991.

162. Steward JJ, Weisbrodt NW, and Burks TF: Central and peripheral actions of morphine on intestinal transit, *J Pharmacol Exp Ther* 205:547, 1978.

163. Szeto HH: Accumulation of normeperidine, an active metabolite of meperidine in patients with renal failure or cancer, *Ann Int Med* 86:738, 1977.

164. Tigerstedt I et al: The effect of buprenorphine and oxycodone on the intracholedochal passage pressure, *Acta Anaesth Scand* 25:99, 1981.

165. Tomichek RC et al: Diazepam-fentanyl interaction—hemodynamic and hormonal effects in coronary artery surgery, *Anesth Analg* 62:881, 1983.

166. Urthaler F, Isobe JH, and James T: Direct and vagally mediated chronotropic effects of morphine studied by selective perfusion of the sinus node of awake dogs, *Chest* 68:222, 1975.

167. Van Ree JM et al: Effects of morphine on hypothalamic noradrenaline and on pituitary-adrenal activity in rats, *Neuroendocrinology* 22:305, 1976.

168. Verbeeck RK, Branch RA, and Wilkinson GR: Meperidine disposition in man: influence of urinary pH and route of

administration, *Clin Pharmacol Ther* 30: 619, 1981.

169. Volavaka J et al: Electroencephalographic and other effects of naloxone in normal men, *Life Sci* 25:1267, 1979.

170. Wang SC: Emetic and antiemetic drugs. In Root WS, Hoffman FG, eds: *Physiological pharmacology II (Part B)*, New York, 1963, Academic Press.

171. Wang SC, Glaviano VV: Locus of emetic action of morphine and hydergine in dogs, *J Pharmacol Exp Ther* 111:329, 1954.

172. Ward JW, McGrath RL, and Weil JV: Effects of morphine on the peripheral vascular response to sympathetic stimulation, *Am J Cardiol* 29:656, 1972.

173. Way WL, Costley EC, and Way EL: Respiratory sensitivity of the newborn infant to meperidine and morphine, *Clin Pharmacol Ther* 6:454, 1965.

174. Weil JV et al: Diminished ventilatory response to hypoxia and hypercapnia after morphine in normal man, *N Engl J Med* 292:1103, 1975.

175. Weinger MB et al: Brain sites mediating opiate-induced muscle rigidity in the rat: methylnaloxonium mapping study, *Brain Res* 544:181, 1991.

176. Wikler A, Fraser HF, and Isabell H: N-allylnormorphine: effect of single doses and precipitation of acute "abstinence syndromes" during addiction to morphine, methadone or heroin in man (postaddicts), *J Pharmacol Exp Ther* 109:8, 1953.

177. Wynands JE et al: Oxygen-fentanyl anesthesia in patients with poor left ventricular function: hemodynamics and plasma fentanyl concentrations, *Anesth Analg* 476, 1983.

178. Zelis R et al: The cardiovascular effects of morphine. The peripheral capacitance and resistance vessels in human subjects, *J Clin Invest* 54:1247, 1974.

CHAPTER 55

Intravenous Access and Delivery Principles

JAMES H. PHILIP

Intravenous (IV) administration of fluids and drugs is an important part of the routine care of patients, especially those undergoing anesthesia and surgery. The IV infusion is essential as a route of drug administration. In addition to facilitating induction, IV drugs are administered throughout the surgical procedure both as part of the anesthetic technique and as a way to meet surgical needs. Whenever fluid or blood is lost during surgery, replacement must be considered, sometimes with great immediacy and sometimes electively. Also, the patient's insensible losses over and above those from surgery must be replaced.

Every year in the United States, at least 20 million patients receive IV fluids.[13,43] Although clinicians generally regard IV fluid administration as safe and effective, IV site complications occur frequently,[44,45] These include phlebitis,[14] thrombosis, catheter obstruction, and fluid extravasation.[24,46,48] From the anesthesiologist's standpoint, the obvious result of these complications is inability to administer the intended drugs and fluids to the patient.

IV systems used in anesthesia range from the most simple to the most complex. Drugs can be administered from a syringe with needle into the flowing IV stream that is powered by gravity. At the other extreme, pumps or controllers can create the continuous infusion, and a syringe or other pumps can administer drugs. These drugs can be controlled manually by the clinician or by a computer, which determines the patient's drug needs based on a pharmacokinetic model with or without the assistance from the patient's physiologic variables.

This chapter summarizes alternative drug and fluid administration techniques and devices in the framework of a simple physical, physiologic model so that one can understand fluid flow in IV systems and patient veins.

HISTORY

Until the 1970s, IV infusion was performed with simple systems.[37] An elevated, fluid-filled bottle provided the energy while the clinician (nurse or physician) adjusted a roller clamp until the correct rate of drop formation was observed in the plastic drip chamber. As clinicians questioned the limitations of their tools, they discovered certain inadequacies in the conventional approach. In 1966 La Cour[22] and Ferechak et al.[7] in 1971 showed that the rate of drop formation is not an accurate measure of flow rate because of the influence of temperature, fluid composition, and diameter and shape of the drip chamber orifice. Flack and Whyte[8] showed that cold flow (creep) in the tubing underlying the roller clamp contributes to flow variation, and Ziser et al.[49] found this change to be greater than 15% over 45 minutes.

Venous physiology has been studied much more extensively than the technology of fluid infusion. Special focus has been placed on vein collapse. A review of that literature explains our current knowledge. In 1912 Starling (with Knowlton[19]) used a collapsible thin-walled rubber tube to produce constant back pressure (afterload) in his studies of heart failure. Although he claimed control of resistance with his device, he did produce constant pressure afterload with what we now call a *Starling resistor*.

Many years later, Holt[15] investigated venous collapse and the resulting decreased venous flow, attributing it to changing resistance. In 1954 Duomarco and Rimini[6] demonstrated the importance of energy and hydraulic gradients along veins. Rodbard and Saiki[40] found that "flow through widely patent elastic tubes followed the laws for flow through rigid pipes." They also noted that when air compressed a thin-walled venous model externally, wall flutter was seen and heard. Flutter ceased when external compressing pressure was raised.

Rodbard[39] showed that critically high flow velocities occur when veins collapse and explained the paradoxic increase in flow from vessel distension produced by adding downstream resistance. He showed later that constant flow in various body tissues can be produced by the same collapse phenomenon.[38]

In 1963 Permutt and Riley[26] explained that under conditions of tube collapse, flow is independent of the pressure drop from inlet to outlet. Rather, flow "depends on the difference between inlet pressure and critical closing pressure" (i.e., occlusion pressure or external pressure, P_{ext}). They used the term *vascular waterfall* to describe this phenomenon, applied by Starling in 1912.

In 1969 Holt[16] and Conrad[5] analyzed the physics of the collapse process observed in rubber tubes. Conrad's photos of a partly collapsed tube have been reprinted many times in texts and treatises that summarize the literature.[3,10,23] Later, Kresch and Noordergraaf[21] performed additional analyses of collapsible rubber tubes, whereas Katz et al.[18] found that "the significant variable is transmural pressure." Griffiths[11] noted that when collapse occurs, fluid flows at sonic velocity (i.e., the velocity of pressure waves in the tube). Brower and Noordergraaf[2] then showed

that "negative resistance" can explain the results of collapsed-tube studies. Further analysis by Shapiro[42] developed the one-dimensional theory of steady flow in thin-walled tubes partly collapsed by negative transmural pressure. Guyton[12] has written extensively on both vein and tissue pressures. The compliance of collapsible vessels has also been studied.[20]

The models just described explain the behavior of thin-walled rubber tubes subjected to external pressure that exceeds internal pressure. The incomplete collapse of rubber tubes makes the analysis complex. Ironically, in vivo and in vitro veins probably do not behave in this complex way; they collapse completely[9,18,25] (unpublished data, D. Joseph and the author). Inapplicable analysis has confused our understanding of the behavior of clinical IV systems.

SIMPLE IV SYSTEM

The simplest IV system consists of an elevated fluid-filled bag or bottle, a length of flexible tubing, a catheter cannulating the patient's vein, and the patient's venous system, which ultimately terminates at the heart, specifically the right atrium. An adjustable roller clamp compresses the tubing at one point, slowing fluid flow and allowing manual control by a clinician. The rate at which drops form is assessed visually, and the roller clamp is adjusted manually as needed. Depending on the type and brand of the tubing system, drop size is 1/10, 1/15 ml (macrodrop), or 1/60 ml (microdrop).

The flow rate through the IV system depends on several factors. The height of the IV bag less the pressure in the patient's vein determines the driving pressure for flow. The resistance of the catheter plus tubing system then determines flow:

$$F = \Delta P/R$$

where F is flow, ΔP is pressure difference, and R is resistance. In this analysis, F and ΔP are generally measured and R is computed.

The pressure difference depends on both fluid height in the bag or bottle and pressure in the patient's vein. The latter is more complex than is usually realized.

Veins possess two characteristics that slow fluid flow: resistance to fluid flow and opening pressure. Resistance is caused by the long, narrow nature of veins, which causes pressure loss along their length. Venous blood flow is usually assumed to be laminar, a subject discussed later in this chapter. Opening pressure for the vein depends on the forces exerted by tissues outside the vein along its course.

Before fluid is forced through the vein, venous pressure is essentially indeterminate. That is, the pressure measured may take on any value less than the obstructing or external pressure. Once fluid flows through the vein, pressure rises to the opening pressure. Then venous resistance affects fluid flow, and pressure rises as flow increases. These concepts and their application are developed further throughout this chapter.

PRESSURE-FLOW RELATIONSHIPS AND MODERN THEORY

To understand fluid flow in IV systems, one can use a conceptual model. The model describes the fluid flow behavior of any IV system and patient. Actual components of the system are depicted as combinations of one or more ideal components. The behavior of actual components can be predicted and measured using the model along with simple measurements.

The system is comprised of a selection of components from Table 55-1. Fig. 55-1 shows the theoretic pressure-flow relationship (PFR) for each component. The simplest configuration of actual components, a gravity flow administration system with rate manually controlled by a roller clamp, is shown in Fig.

55-2. Pressures at various locations, depicted as the heights of the vertical bars above the reference level, are shown under the condition that flow is 200 ml/hour.

The model's behavior can be viewed as follows. Pressure at the free-air surface at the top of the bag or bottle is zero (gauge), that is, atmospheric pressure. Lower in the tubing, the pressure head proximal to the roller clamp is determined by the height of the free-air surface above the roller clamp, combined with fluid density and gravity. Specifically, pressure equals height times fluid density times the acceleration of gravity. When the liquid is water and pressure is expressed in centimeters of water (cm H_2O), pressure is equal to the water height in centimeters. The density of most clinical solutions differs little from one (1.00).

Because an air-filled drip chamber intervenes between bag and roller clamp, the head height is diminished by the height of the air column. The diminution of pressure occurs because within the air-filled chamber, pressure is the same everywhere. No vertical pressure gradient exists in the air-filled chamber. The tubing is drawn vertically from the

Table 55-1   Ideal and actual IV system components*

Actual component	Ideal component	Symbol
Bag	Pressure source	P_{bag}
DS roller clamp	Variable resistor	R_{clamp}
Tubing	Low-resistance conduit	R_{tube}
Catheter	Resistor	R_{cath}
Normal peripheral vein	Resistor	R_{vein}
Extravascular tissue	Resistor	R_{tisuse}
Central vein	Conduit with no resistance	$R_{cv} = 0$
Heart	Pressure source	P_{cv} = central venous pressure
Obstruction	Starling resistor = Collapsible tube	P_{ext}
Inflated blood pressure cuff	Collapsible tube (CT)	P_{ext}, R_{vein}
Venous tourniquet	CT	P_{ext}, R_{vein}
Collapsible tube	CT	P_{ext}, R_{tube}
Problem IV site	CT	P_{ext}, R_{vein}
Catheter against vein wall	CT	P_{obs}, R_{vein}
Volumetric pump	Flow source	F_{pump}
Volumetric controller		
Variable resistor	Variable resistor	R_{cont}
Variable duty cycle	Variable pressure source	$P_{effective}$
Observation of drop rate	Flow measure	F_{drop}
Electronic pressure transducer	Pressure sensor	P
Water manometer	Pressure sensor	P

*Actual components behave similarly to theoretic components.

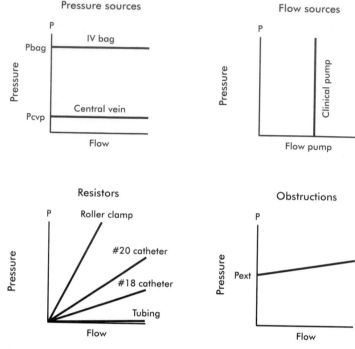

Fig. 55-1. Theoretic pressure-flow relationship (PFR) for various system components, including pressure sources, flow sources, resistors, and obstructions (i.e., collapsible tubes, Starling resistors). (From Philip JH: A model for the physics and physiology of fluid administration, *J Clin Monit* 5:123, 1989.)

bottle outlet and then horizontal until entering the patient's vein, which is at the same height as the heart (right atrium). This simplifies the physics to make the system more understandable.

In Fig. 55-2 the roller clamp has been adjusted to a resistance that provides a flow rate of 200 ml/hour. In clinical practice the clinician adjusting the clamp is unaware of actual resistance. He/she simply rotates the roller clamp until proper flow rate is judged by measuring the rate of drop formation observed in the drip chamber. Here, pressure just distal to the roller clamp is measured to be 16 cm H_2O with this particular combination of system components and patient. From the values for pressure difference across the clamp and the value for flow, roller clamp resistance can be computed.

Next, the origin of the pressure distal to the roller clamp must be considered. From the standpoint of the tubing system, the pressure at the catheter tip originates in the patient. The peripheral venous pressure measured in this situation can best be understood by realizing that the resistance of the vein cannot be zero. Thus the flow of blood back to the heart makes peripheral venous pressure slightly higher than central venous pressure (CVP), in the absence of fluid infusion and intervening obstruction. The pressure increment often is quite small (3 cm H_2O or less).[1,31,47] With partial venous obstruction (see later discussion) venous pressure may be significantly greater.

PRESSURE-FLOW RELATIONSHIP DATA

The PFR for the tubing-catheter-patient system can be measured in experimental situations and in clinical practice. This can be done with a volumetric pump and a pressure-monitoring device such as a pressure transducer or even a water column. One particular commercial IV infusion pump can facilitate this. The IVAC variable-pressure volumetric infusion pump, Model 560 (IVAC Corp., San Diego), produces constant flow and measures pressure during infusion and when the pump is stopped. In this pump, flow is created by a linear peristaltic mechanism that provides a flow pattern composed of successive 1 μl volumes. Just distal to the pumping mechanism, a pressure transducer presses against an in-line pressure-sensing disk contained in the IV tubing. The pressure-monitoring pump measures pressure with an accuracy of ± 2 mm Hg.[17,33,36] Pressure is measured in both the presence and the absence of flow.

Using the pump, the PFR has been measured for many tubing systems, catheters, other devices, and patients. Because of flow limitations in the pump (1000 ml/hour = 1 L/hour), effects of high flow on system nonlinearity cannot be studied with this device. High flow effects are presented in the section on nonlinearity. Resistance units (RU) are mm Hg/L/hour.

From experiments using the pump, the following facts have been determined.[30] An elevated IV bag behaves as a pressure source, with pressure equal to

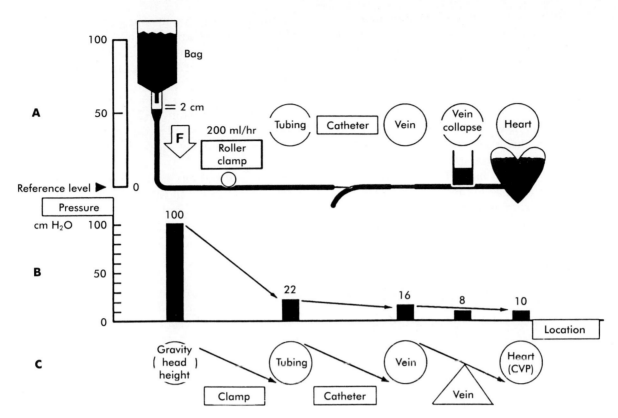

Fig. 55-2. Model for manually controlled IV administration system and patient. **A,** Pictorial schematic diagram of model's components. **B,** Pressures (cm H_2O) observed in various locations. **C,** Flow chart showing pressures (*circles*), resistances (*rectangles*), collapsible tubes (*triangles*), and pressure drops (*arrows*). In **A,** elevated fluid-filled bag acts as pressure source (P = 100 cm H_2O in **B**) equal to height of its free-air surface above reference level. Roller clamp is resistor, arbitrarily adjusted for F (flow) = 200 ml/hour in **A**. Catheter provides additive resistance in fluid path to patient. Vein acts as hydraulic resistor as well but can collapse if external pressure (8 cm H_2O in **B**) exceeds internal pressure (16 cm H_2O in **B**). Collapse does not occur here because internal pressure exceeds external pressure. Finally, heart acts as pressure source (sink) for venous return. (From Philip JH: A model for the physics and physiology of fluid administration, *J Clin Monit* 5:123, 1989.)

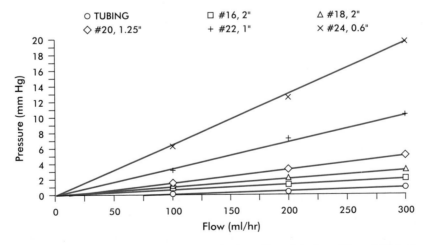

Fig. 55-3. PFR for five catheter sizes (16 × 2 inches, 18 × 2 inches, 20 × 1.25 inches, 20 × 1 inch, 24 × 1 inch). Pressures were measured at flows of 0, 100, 200, and 300 ml/hour, and resistance was computed as slope of least-squares regression line. Resistances are tabulated in Table 55-2. (From Philip JH: A model for the physics and physiology of fluid administration, *J Clin Monit* 5:123, 1989.)

the height of the free-air surface of the fluid above the reference level, less the height of the intervening air gap in the drip chamber.

IV tubing behaves as a low-resistance conduit relative to other system components:

$$R_{tubing} = 3 \pm 2 \text{ (SEM) RU}$$

A roller clamp behaves as a variable resistor. Once set, a roller clamp behaves the same ($\pm 5\%$) when connected to a flow source (IV pump) as with a pressure source (elevated bag). Typical roller clamp resistance during normal IV flow is 300 to 800 RU, depending on flow rate desired.

An IV catheter behaves as a resistor that offers more resistance than IV tubing. In the flow range of 0 to 300 ml/hour, the PFR is linear and resistance takes on a unique value for each catheter size.

The PFR for systems composed of an IV catheter (Fenwall QuickCath) plus a tubing system (Travenol 2C0001) is plotted in Fig. 55-3. Measured total resistances ($\pm$ SEM) for no. 16, no. 18, no. 20, no. 22, and no. 24 catheters are 6 ± 1, 10 ± 0, 17 ± 2, 34 ± 1, and 66 ± 3 RU, respectively. When measured tubing resistance (3 ± 2 RU, previous equation) was subtracted from each, respective mean catheter resistances were 3, 7, 14, 31, and 63 RU (Table 55-2).

A normal patient vein behaves as a resistor, with resistance similar to that of a 20-gauge IV catheter. The distribution of patient resistance for the veins of 46 surgical patients is shown in Fig. 55-4. The population statistics for normal vein resistance were $R_{vein} = 22 \pm 20$ (SD) RU (range, 0 to 91 RU; median, 22 RU)

In addition to resistance, veins showed a second parameter that limited flow. In some patients, this was caused by external compression between the IV site and the heart (see later section on obstructions). In other patients, this pressure was the CVP itself. For the 46 veins studied, opening pressure was $P_o = 15 \pm 8$ (SD) mm Hg (range, 2 to 35 mm Hg).

The central venous circulation offers essentially no resistance to fluid flow. All resistance encountered distal to the catheter tip is attributed to the peripheral venous system. However, the central venous system does provide a back pressure equal to CVP. This pressure must be considered when assessing fluid flow through the system.

Table 55-2	Catheter resistances*			
Gauge	Catheter plus tubing (R ± SEM)		Catheter alone (R ± SEM)	
16	6	1	3	2
18	10	0	7	2
20	17	2	14	3
22	34	1	31	2
24	66	3	63	4
None	3	2	0	2

*Resistance (R) in resistance units (RU) = 1 mm Hg/L/hour.

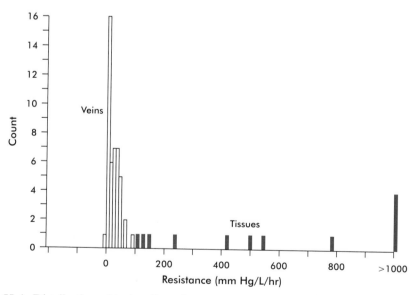

Fig. 55-4. Distribution of hydraulic resistance measured in 46 veins and 12 infiltrations. Veins, *open bars;* infiltrations, *closed bars.* (From Philip JH: A model for the physics and physiology of fluid administration, *J Clin Monit* 5:123, 1989.)

PATHOLOGIC SITUATIONS
Fluid Infusion into Tissues

The extravascular tissue near a vein behaves as a resistor that offers significantly more resistance than the vein. In the limited populations reported in the literature, tissue resistance is significantly greater than vein resistance. In addition, pressures measured at low flow are generally not elevated greatly above zero-flow pressures.

For tissues, resistance (R_{tissue}), estimated P_o, and initial pressure after infiltration (P_{init}) were R_{tissue} = 1125 ± 1376 (SD) RU, P_o = 44 ± 61 mm Hg, and P_{init} = 8 ± 8 mm Hg. Fig. 55-4 shows the distribution of tissue resistance superimposed on the distribution of vein resistance just described. R_{vein} and R_{tissue} were different significantly when tested with Student's t test (p < 0.001) and confirmed with Mann-Whitney U test (Z = −5.31). P_{init} for tissues was not significantly different from $P_{o,vein}$. Volunteers remarked that infiltration at a low infusion rate (and thus low pressure) was not painful.

Obstructions to Fluid Flow: Starling Resistors

Many clinical situations produce vein collapse, causing the vein to behave as a Starling resistor. An inflated blood pressure (BP) cuff behaves as a Starling resistor, with P_o close to the external pressure applied and little, if any, change in vein resistance. The PFR for a BP cuff on a typical patient is shown in Fig. 55-5. A venous tourniquet applied proximal to the IV site likewise behaves as a Starling resistor, raising P_o to 25 to 45 mm Hg and not affecting R significantly. Fig. 55-6 shows the PFR for a typical tourniquet-obstructed vein.

In vitro studies have shown that an elevated collapsible tube behaves as a Starling resistor, with P_o approximately equal to the elevation of the collapsed segment. Also, an externally compressed collapsible tube behaves as a Starling resistor, with P_o equal to external pressure.

Little information or data are available concerning IV sites that function erratically. It is known that a problem IV site can behave as a Starling resistor, with high obstructing pressure. In the one case reported,[30] an IV catheter was in place but was not running well ("problem IV"). Although the IV bag was 80 cm above the patient's heart and IV site, no fluid flow was detectable. A small fluid bolus injected via syringe into the IV tubing flowed easily, but spontaneous gravity-powered flow did not follow, even after catheter manipulation. When the IV bag was elevated 30 cm (12 inches), flow was observed to begin. After the IV site was determined to be functioning acceptably with bag elevated, the PFR was measured. Fig. 55-7 shows that resistance was 129 RU and P_o was 80 mm Hg equals 109 cm H_2O. Analyzing the clinical situation and experimental data suggests that opening pressure for the Starling resistor was higher than the initial bag height, resulting in no flow initially. Elevating the bag slightly raised infusion pressure and resulted in significant flow.

A catheter manipulated against a vein wall also can behave as a Starling resistor. In the one case reported,

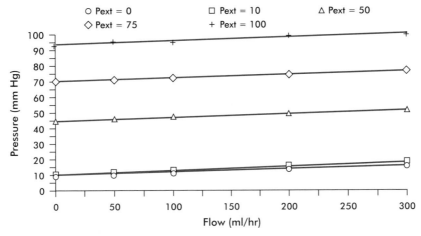

Fig. 55-5. PFR for typical patient vein obstructed by an external blood pressure cuff. Note that applying pressurized cuff raises opening pressure (P_o) to approximately cuff pressure. Resistance is relatively unaffected. *Pext,* external pressure = cuff pressure. (From Philip JH: A model for the physics and physiology of fluid administration, *J Clin Monit* 5:123, 1989.)

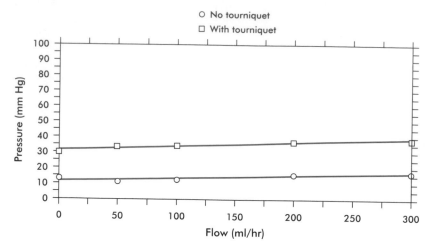

Fig. 55-6. PFR for typical patient vein obstructed by clinician-applied venous tourniquet. Note that applying tourniquet raises P_o from 12 to 32 mm Hg. Resistance is relatively unaffected. (From Philip JH: A model for the physics and physiology of fluid administration, *J Clin Monit* 5:123, 1989.)

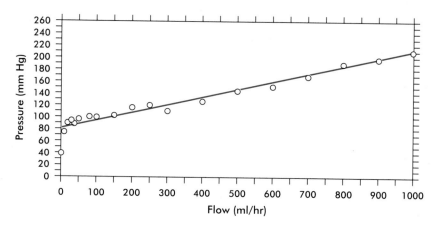

Fig. 55-7. PFR for "problem IV" site in patient. (From Philip JH: A model for the physics and physiology of fluid administration, *J Clin Monit* 5:123, 1989.)

"normal vein" resistance was $R_{vein} = 30 \pm 9$ (SD) RU and $P_o = 7 \pm 1$ mm Hg. When a "positional IV" was created by manipulating the catheter against the vein wall, $R_{vein\ against\ wall} = 27 \pm 0$ (SD) RU and $P_o = 36 \pm 0$ mm Hg.

SYSTEM NONLINEARITY

When IV flow rate is low (less than 3000 ml/hour for most catheters and systems), the PFR is linear. However, when flow is increased significantly, the PFR loses its linear shape. Nonlinearity greatly affects flow prediction during rapid fluid infusion, as is required during volume resuscitation.

In 1983 Philip and Philip[27] showed that the PFR for IV tubing systems and other fluid conduits is distinctly nonlinear and can be represented as:

$$P = (R_L \times F) + (R_T \times F^2)$$

Fig. 55-8 shows this. In the same study, by sequentially removing tubing sections, the authors showed that the R_L and R_T (multipliers of flow and flow squared) parameters are intrinsic properties of the tubing and do not result from flow perturbations at the entry or exit of the tubing system. They also showed that:

$$P = A \times F^n$$

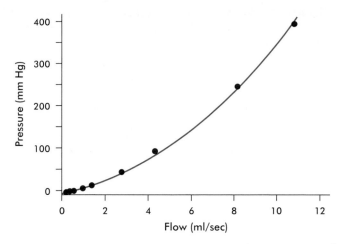

Fig. 55-8. PFR for IV infusion system. Fitted line is best least-squares estimated parabola to fit relationship $P = (R_L \times F) + (R_T \times F^2)$ (see text). (From Philip BK, Philip JH: Characterization of [nonlinear] flow in intravenous infusion systems, *IEEE Trans Biomed Eng* 30:702, 1983.)

does not fit the experimental data without systematic bias. Whether the observations represent concomitant laminar and turbulent flow in the same tubing section has not been established.

Finally, Philip and Philip[27] showed that stopcocks and check valves are almost exclusively F^2 devices, whereas 5 μ filters (MP-5, Travenol) are exclusively linear (F only) devices. Later, the same authors showed that an F^2 term is also required in analyzing the PFR for IV catheters.[28]

To understand the impact of interposing or removing devices to enhance fluid flow, the system's nonlinearity cannot be ignored. **The nonlinear PFR characteristics can be used to predict flow capability in IV infusion systems and assist clinical decisions on devices to be included or eliminated.**[29]

System nonlinearity can be ignored when flows are low enough. In 1988 Philip and Philip[35] tried to identify situations in which nonlinearity was not significant. To do so, they defined F_E as the flow at which pressure drop was twice the linear pressure drop. At flows less than 0.1 F_E, the system could be considered linear, and flow could easily be predicted from pressure by linear extrapolation. At flows above 1/10 F_E, the effects of nonlinearity must be considered. Later, the order of device removal or replacement was assessed using increased flow capability as a criterion.[29] The order was (1) fluid warmer removal, (2) 16-gauge to 14-gauge catheter change, (3) standard-bore to wide-bore tubing change, (4) 14-gauge to 12-gauge catheter change, (5) stopcock removal or change, (6) 12-gauge to 10-gauge catheter change, and finally (7) catheter elimination with the tubing directly connected to the patient's vein. Inter-

estingly, removal of the stopcock was not required until the infusion system was composed of only wide-bore tubing and a 12-gauge catheter.

CLINICAL FLUID INFUSION
Gravity Flow

During routine anesthesia and surgery, fluid requirements in adults range from approximately 100 ml/hour to 100 ml/minute and more. Before anesthesia, an IV catheter is inserted in a vein and fastened securely, usually with adhesive tape. The size of the IV catheter is chosen to allow for the patient's expected fluid requirement. However, one should always recognize that rapid blood loss can occur during almost any surgical procedure and that the anesthesiologist must be prepared for such an occurrence.

When selecting catheter size, one must consider known information about the resistance of catheters, IV systems, and patient veins. The resistance of each of these flow impediments adds to the others to form the total resistance to flow. Thus total resistance to fluid flow (R_{total}) is the sum of the resistance of IV tubing, catheter, intervening devices, and the patient's vein.

The 22 RU median value for vein resistance and Table 55-2 (catheter resistances) together offer insight into the choice of catheter size. For a typical vein with resistance $R_{vein} = 22$ RU, a 20-gauge catheter (R = 17 RU) approximately doubles resistance and halves flow. Changing from a 20-gauge to an 18-gauge catheter decreases total resistance from 39 RU to 32 RU, producing a resistance decrease of 18%, which causes a flow increase of 18%. Increasing catheter size from 18 gauge to 16 gauge decreases resistance and increases flow by 13%.

The typical (22 RU) vein cannulated with a 17 RU, 20-gauge catheter provides a total resistance of 39 RU. If the pressure bag or bottle is 110 cm above the patient's heart, infusion pressure equals 110 cm H_2O minus CVP (approximately 10 cm H_2O), yielding a 100 cm H_2O pressure head. Since 1 mm Hg = 1.34 cm H_2O and 1 cm H_2O = 76 mm Hg, pressure head = 76 mm Hg. Thus: F = P/R = 76 mm Hg/39 mm Hg/L/hour = 1.95 L/hour, or approximatley 2000 ml/hour. For a 10 drop/ml drip chamber: Drop rate = 10 drops/ml × 2000 ml/hour × 1 hour/ 3600 seconds = 5.6 drops/second. This usually forms a steady stream. If a clinical IV infusion seems to flow much more slowly than this, the impediment imposed by the patient's venous system probably is greater than the typical 22 RU used in this example. Most likely a very small vein has been cannulated or the cannulated vein is not functioning normally. In conclusion, when a small IV catheter (20 gauge) produces low flow of IV fluid, the major flow impediment is probably not the IV catheter but rather the patient's vein.

With gravity as the driving force for fluid flow through an IV system, a major limitation in flow arises from the limited pressure head available. The IV bag or bottle can typically be placed no higher than 1 m above the patient's heart. This height limits the hydrostatic pressure that can be applied by gravity alone. However, since the pressure that reaches the patient's vein is often much lower than that applied by the pressure source because of resistive losses in the catheter and other components, higher pressures are usually safe. This is especially true when a small catheter size has been selected and a large vein is cannulated. In this situation, positive pressure can be applied, as described in the next section.

High-Flow Resuscitation

Rapid fluid resuscitation is often required during anesthesia and surgery. Since both pressure and resistance limit flow, both should be optimized to accomplish rapid fluid flow. Resistance is lowered initially by removing restrictions imposed by roller clamps. Ideally, only one roller clamp is present between bag and patient to reduce the likelihood that a second control will be left unadjusted. Resistance can be further reduced by removing interposing devices that may contribute to total resistance. When nonlinearity is considered, the order of device removal or change is (1) remove the blood warmer, (2) change catheter from 16 to 14 gauge, (3) remove check valve, (4) change catheter from 14 to 12 gauge, (5) replace regular tubing with wide-bore tubing, (6) change catheter from 12 to 10 gauge, (7) remove

stopcocks, (8) remove the 10-gauge catheter, and (9) insert the sterile tubing end directly in the vein.[35]

As an alternative to reducing resistance, pressure can be increased to increase flow. Pressure can be increased in either of two ways. Some IV sets contain an integral manual pump that allows the clinician to produce liquid flow by volume displacement. This labor-intensive approach allows bolus administration at any time, completely under the anesthesiologist's control. Also, this technique allows fluids contained in glass bottles (e.g., 5% albumin) to be infused with assistance.

An alternative approach increases infusion pressure with a pressure infuser, a pneumatic device that encircles the fluid-filled IV bag. Many competing devices are available. The maximum pressure suggested by manufacturers is usually 300 mm Hg, although much higher pressures are possible (JH Philip, unpublished data, 1990). Several different models of pressure infusers are available.

With the original pressure-infuser design, the clinician uses a manual bulb-inflater pump similar to that used with a sphygmomanometer cuff. Once the infuser is filled with air under pressure, infuser pressure drops as fluid is infused and leaves the bag, which is encircled by the infuser. Often a snap clamp is applied to the tubing between the bag and inflation bulb because of the misconception that infuser pressure falls as a result of leaks in the inflation bulb. Although inflation bulbs do leak, the ever-present leaks are typically small and are only significant when fluid is infused extremely slowly, as with an Intraflo (Abbott/Sorenson Co.) or other continuous low-flow device designed to infuse 3 ml/hour.

To maintain constant driving pressure for infusion, the pressure infuser can be attached to a constant pressure source. Again, the maximum recommended pressure is 300 mm Hg. When the infuser is used in this way, a constant pressure head is applied to the IV system–patient combination. This has the advantage of flow continuing at its initial rate, since additional gas enters the infuser to maintain a constant volume in the infuser–IV bag combination.

Whenever fluid is infused under pressure, increased vigilance is required to avoid infusion of air into the venous system. Despite the danger of air infusion, IV fluid manufacturers add potentially dangerous volumes of air to IV bags. Volumes as large as 70 ml may be present.[32] Whenever fluid is administered under pressure, it is best to remove all air from the IV bag.

As the IV bag empties below 100 to 200 ml, most pressure infusers fail to apply their set pressure effectively to the bag, and infusion pressure drops. In an emergency situation, it might be best to discard the residual 100 ml of fluid and change bags rather than try to infuse the last drop. Some infuser designs may be more effective, but such information has not been published.

Several pressure infusers can be attached to a single pressure source to facilitate rapid changing of crystalloid- and blood-containing bags during emergencies. One such device[34] can provide 479 ml/min of lactated Ringer's solution or 318 ml/min of diluted packed RBC through standard IV tubing without a catheter. Several other devices have been described[4,41] or are commercially available.

MECHANICAL FLUID INFUSION SYSTEMS
IV Controllers

Many devices are available to adjust or control the flow of fluid infused. IV controllers use gravity as a pressure source and manipulate the fluid path to adjust flow. Flow is usually monitored by an electronic drop sensor that causes the instrument to vary its slowing of the infusion.

Variable-resistance flow controllers vary the resistance of the infusion system by constricting or otherwise increasing the resistance of the tubing system.

Variable-duty-cycle controllers interrupt the application of pressure to the fully open IV tubing system and thereby control effective pressure applied from the fluid bag or bottle. The maximal effective pressure is limited by the bag height and also by the maximal duty cycle allowed by the infusion device.

Some IV infusion controllers are capable of monitoring the IV site for deterioration. Devices that quantify either the resistance imposed or the duty cycle applied have the capacity to perform monitoring. Some instruments sound an alarm when flow is too low, considering the instrument's purposeful limitation of flow.

Controllers' accuracy is limited by the flow-monitoring system's accuracy. Since many instruments use drop counting, variations in drop size described earlier play an important limiting role.

IV Pumps

Fluid pumps use positive displacement to provide regulated fluid infusion. Positive displacement can be provided by peristaltic fingers, a reciprocating syringe, or other mechanisms.

Because pumps use positive displacement, they may be capable of overcoming high resistance or back pressure to fluid infusion. This property can be advantageous in some situations. However, in the patient with fluid extravasation, some danger clearly exists.

Many pumps are incapable of detecting problems downstream from the pump unless these problems produce a significant pressure rise. Such pressure rise could result from total obstruction of the catheter or tubing. Situations such as fluid extravasation usually produce only a small rise in pressure because of resistance to infusion. Most pumps fail to detect such conditions. Complications of extravascular injection clearly become more problematic when the patient is unable to complain, as during general anesthesia.

Other Fluids

When fluids other than dilute crystalloid solutions are infused, the PFR may differ from that expected. The difference may be in the slope of the PFR line or in the shape of this relationship. When viscosity varies, the linear slope is expected to change. Differences in density could influence the nonlinear component.

Solutions containing dextrose (JH Philip, unpublished data, 1985) provide increased effective viscosity, as manifested by increased resistance with increased dextrose concentration. The specific relationship is:

$$R_{D_cW} = R_{water} (1 + C^2/1000)$$

where C is the dextrose concentration expressed in percent (%) and D_cW represents dextrose with concentration $C\%$ in water. (Actual slope of the regression line is 1.09 ± 0.05, with 95% confidence interval $= 0.94 - 1.23$).

Applying this relationship, the resistance of $D_{50}W$ equals that of water $\times 1 + 50^2/1000 = 1 + 2500/1000 = 1 + 2.5 = 3.5$. Therefore, to achieve the same flow with $D_{50}W$ as with water, pressure must be increased by a factor of 3.5. Alternatively, at the same pressure head, flow diminishes to $1/3.5 = 0.28$ of the flow for dilute crystalloid.

From the resistance-concentration relationship, it can also be shown that relative viscosities of 1, 2, 3, and 4 are obtained with dextrose concentrations of 0%, 30%, 43%, and 52%. Similar analysis revealed that Intralipid has a relative viscocity of 1.36, equivalent to that of 17% dextrose in water. Osmolyte (for gastric infusion) has a relative viscosity of 6.57.

DRUG ADMINISTRATION

The IV route is used extensively for drug administration during anesthesia. Drugs can be administered with several different infusion profiles. The most common drug infusion regimens are bolus injection and constant infusion. Occasionally, careful pharmacokinetic control is used. The most common form uses an exponential decay in infusion rate to link bolus infusion to continuous infusion.

Delivery Devices

Many commercial devices are available for drug delivery, and several different technologies are available. Peristaltic pumps are usually reserved for nondrug fluid infusion because of the interface to an IV bag. However, many clinicians use a Buratrol or other device as a reservoir for the drug and then use a conventional fluid pump.

Syringe pumps appear better suited to drug infusion, since a small drug volume lends itself to containment in a syringe. Many competing devices are available.

Some drug infusion pumps are designed to facilitate drug administration on a milligrams/kilograms of weight basis. Others specifically facilitate use of individual drugs by using drug-specific labels. Still other drugs are capable of control by a computer that can infuse according to a prospective pharmacokinetic model or can vary drug infusion pharmacodynamically in response to monitored physiologic changes in the patient.

SUMMARY

IV therapy is an essential part of every anesthesia procedure. The IV infusion system connected to a patient can be analyzed according to simple physical and physiologic principles, and the resulting model can predict the IV infusion system behavior in many situations.

Devices are available to accommodate almost any need in fluid or drug administration. As new devices become available, the anesthesiologist must understand their operating principles and the physics that underlies them to recognize appropriate applications.

KEY POINTS

- The simplest IV system consists of an elevated, fluid-filled container, a length of flexible tubing, a catheter cannulating the patient's vein, and the patient's venous system.
- Flow through the IV system is determined by driving pressure and resistance of the catheter and tubing system.
- Driving pressure equals the height of the free-air surface of the fluid above the reference level, less the height of the intervening air gap in the drip chamber.
- IV tubing behaves as a low-resistance conduit relative to other system components: $R_{tubing} = 3 \pm 2$ (SEM) resistance units (RU). 1 RU = 1 mm Hg/L/hour.
- A roller clamp behaves as a variable resistor in that, once set, it behaves the same ($\pm 5\%$) when connected to a flow source (IV pump) as to a pressure source (elevated bag). Typical roller clamp resistance during normal IV flow is 300 to 800 RU, depending on flow rate desired.
- An IV catheter behaves as a resistor that offers more resistance than does IV tubing, so that in the flow range of 0 to 300 ml/hour, the pressure-flow relationship (PFR) is linear and resistance takes on a unique value for each catheter size.
- A normal patient vein behaves like a resistor with resistance similar to that of a 20-gauge IV catheter. The central venous circulation offers essentially no resistance to fluid flow.

- The extravascular tissue near a vein behaves as a resistor that offers significantly more resistance than does the vein.
- Many clinical situations produce vein collapse, causing the vein to behave as a Starling resistor.
- When IV flow rate is low, the pressure-flow relationship is linear. When flow is increased significantly, the pressure-flow relationship becomes nonlinear and this significantly affects flow prediction during rapid fluid infusion, as is required during volume resuscitation.
- Great care must always be taken to avoid infusion of air into the venous system whenever fluid is infused under pressure; this is especially so since IV fluid manufacturers add volumes of air as large as 70 ml to IV bags, which preferably should be removed before use.
- Numerous mechanical systems are available to adjust or control the flow of the fluid infused. Simple controllers use gravity as the pressure source and a variable resistor to adjust the rate of infusion. The accuracy of controllers is limited by the accuracy of the flow monitoring mechanism, which often consists of a drop counting system that is limited by the variations in the size (and fluid volume) of the drops. Further, the pressure source varies because of patient movement and changes in the height of the bed.
- Fluid pumps use positive displacement to provide regulated fluid infusion. Positive displacement is

provided by peristaltic compression, by a reciprocating syringe, or by other mechanisms. Such systems can infuse fluid despite variations in downstream resistance, an effect that can be beneficial (e.g., by eliminating changes in fluid administration due to patient movement) or detrimental (e.g., subcutaneous extravasation of fluid), depending on the conditions. Many pump systems incorporate a pressure monitor that can detect complete obstruction of the outflow system but may not detect subcutaneous extravasation.

- Several systems are available to facilitate intravenous drug administration. Many are now programmed to calculate the infusion rate, when data about patient weight, drug concentration, and desired dose (mg/kg) are provided. Although not foolproof, such devices should eliminate many of the risks of human error, especially in situations where the clinician has multiple tasks to perform simultaneously, as in complex anesthesia procedures.

KEY REFERENCES

Permutt S, Riley RL: Hemodynamics of collapsible vessels with tone: the vascular waterfall, *J Appl Physiol* 18:924, 1963.

Philip BK, Philip JH: Prediction of low capability in intravenous infusion systems: implications for fluid resuscitation, *J Clin Monit* 6:113, 1990.

Philip JH: A model for the physics and physiology of fluid administration, *J Clin Monit* 5:123, 1989.

Shapiro AH: Steady flow in collapsible tubes, *J Biomech Eng* 99:126, 1977.

REFERENCES

1. Allen P: A standardization of the Lewis method of venous pressure determination, *Can Med Assoc J* 59:560, 1948.
2. Brower RW, Noordergraaf A: Pressure-flow characteristics of collapsible tubes: a reconciliation of seemingly contradictory results, *Ann Biomed Eng* 1:333, 1973.
3. Caro CG, Pedley TJ, Schroter RC et al: *The mechanics of the circulation,* Oxford, 1978, Oxford University Press.
4. Chapman RB, Keep P: The Norfolk and Norwich infusion box, *Anaesthesia* 35:1211, 1980.
5. Conrad WA: Pressure-flow relationships in collapsible tubes, *IEEE Trans Biomed Instrum* 16:284, 1969.
6. Duomarco JL, Rimini R: Energy and hydraulic gradients along systemic veins, *Am J Physiol* 178:215, 1954.
7. Ferenchak P, Collins JJ, and Morgan AP: Drop size and rate in parenteral infusion, *Surgery* 70:674, 1971.
8. Flack FC, Whyte TD: Behaviour of standard gravity-fed administration sets used for intravenous infusion, *Br Med J* 3:439, 1974.
9. Franklin KJ: *A monograph on veins,* Springfield, Ill, 1937, Charles C Thomas.
10. Fung YC: *Biodynamics: circulation,* New York, 1984, Springer-Verlag.
11. Griffiths DJ: Steady fluid flow through veins and collapsible tubes, *Med Biol Eng* 9:597, 1971.
12. Guyton AC: *Textbook of medical physiology,* Philadelphia, 1976, WB Saunders.

13. Haug JN, Politser PE: *Socio-economic fact book for surgery,* Chicago, 1987, American College of Surgeons.
14. Hershey CO, Tomford JWT, McLaren CE et al: The natural history of intravenous catheter-associated phlebitis, *Arch Intern Med* 144:1373, 1984.
15. Holt JP: The collapse factor in the measurement of venous pressure, *Am J Physiol* 134:292, 1941.
16. Holt JP: Flow through collapsible tubes and through in situ veins, *IEEE Trans Biomed Instrum* 16:274, 1969.
17. Hutchinson PM, Yeoman PM, and Byrne AJ: Evaluation of the IVAC 560 volumetric pump, *Anaesthesia* 40:996, 1985.
18. Katz AI, Chen Y, and Moreno AH: Flow through a collapsible tube: experimental analysis and mathematical model, *Biophys J* 9:1261, 1969.
19. Knowlton FP, Starling EH: The influence of variations in temperature and blood-pressure on the performance of the isolated mammalian heart, *J Physiol (Lond)* 44:206, 1912.
20. Kresch E: Compliance of flexible tubes, *J Biomech* 12:825, 1979.
21. Kresch E, Noordergraaf A: A mathematical model for the pressure-flow relationship in a segment of vein, *IEEE Trans Biomed Instrum* 16:335, 1969.
22. La Cour D: Drop size in intravenous infusion, *Acta Anaesthesiol Scand* 24:35, 1966.

23. Leith DE: Physiological waterfalls, *Physiol Teacher (Am Physiol Soc)* 5:6, 1976.
24. MacCara ME: Extravasation: a hazard of intravenous therapy, *Drug Intell Clin Pharmacol* 17:713, 1983.
25. Moreno AH, Katz AI, Gold LD et al: Mechanics of distension of dog veins and other very thin-walled tubular structures, *Circ Res* 27:1069, 1970.
26. Permutt S, Riley RL: Hemodynamics of collapsible vessels with tone: the vascular waterfall, *J Appl Physiol* 18:924, 1963.
27. Philip BK, Philip JH: Characterization of [nonlinear] flow in intravenous infusion systems, *IEEE Trans Biomed Eng* 30:702, 1983.
28. Philip BK, Philip JH: Characterization of [nonlinear] flow in intravenous catheters, *IEEE Trans Biomed Eng* 33:529, 1986.
29. Philip BK, Philip JH: Prediction of flow capability in intravenous infusion systems: implications for fluid resuscitation, *J Clin Monit* 6:113, 1990.
30. Philip JH: A model for the physics and physiology of fluid administration, *J Clin Monit* 5:123, 1989.
31. Philip JH, Joseph DM: Peripheral venous pressure can be an accurate estimate of central venous pressure, *Anesthesiology* 61:A166, 1986 (abstract).
32. Philip JH, Philip BK: Avoiding air infusion with pressurized infusion systems: a new hazard, *Anesth Analg* 64:381, 1985.
33. Philip JH, Philip BK: Hydrostatic central venous pressure measurement by IVAC

560 infusion pump, *Med Instrum* 19:232, 1985.

34. Philip JH, Philip BK: Pressurized infusion system for fluid resuscitation, *Anesth Analg* 63:770, 1984.

35. Philip JH, Philip BK: Simplified [linear] approach to assessing intravenous flow characteristics in the therapeutic infusion range, *IEEE Trans Biomed Eng* 35:1093, 1988.

36. Philip JH, Philip BK, and Lehr JL: Accuracy of hydrostatic pressure measurement with a disposable dome transducer, *Med Instrum* 19:273, 1985.

37. Plumer AL, Cosentino F: *Principles and practice of intravenous therapy,* Chicago, 1987, Scott Foresman.

38. Rodbard S: Autoregulation in encapsulated, passive, soft-walled vessels, *Am Heart J* 46:648, 1963.

39. Rodbard S: Flow through collapsible tubes: augmented flow produced by resistance at the outlet, *Circulation* 11:290, 1955.

40. Rodbard S, Saiki H: Flow through collapsible tubes, *Am Heart J* 11:715, 1955.

41. Rosenblatt R, Dennis P, and Draper LD: A new method for massive fluid resuscitation in the trauma patient, *Anesth Analg* 62:613, 1983.

42. Shapiro AH: Steady flow in collapsible tubes, *J Biomech Eng* 99:126, 1977.

43. Simmons BP: Guidelines for prevention of intravascular infections, *Natl IV Ther Assoc* 5:41, 1982.

44. Turco SJ: Hazards associated with parenteral therapy, *Am J IV Ther Clin Nutr* 8:9, 1981.

45. Turnidge J: Hazards of peripheral intravenous lines, *Med J Aust* 141:37, 1984.

46. Upton J, Mulliken JB, and Murray JE: Major intravenous extravasation injuries, *Am J Surg* 137:497, 1979.

47. Warren JV, Stead EA: The effect of the accumulation of blood in the extremities on the venous pressure of normal subjects, *Am J Med Sci* 205:501, 1943.

48. Wetmore N: Extravasation—the dreaded complication, *Natl IV Ther Assoc* 8:47, 1985.

49. Ziser M, Feezor M, and Slolaut MW: Regulating intravenous flow: controller versus clamps, *Am J Hosp Pharm* 36:1090, 1979.

Index